Evidence-Based Cardiology
THIRD EDITION

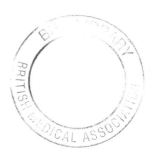

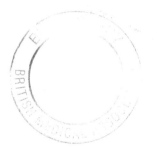

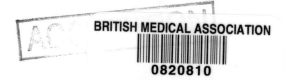

Evidence-Based Cardiology

THIRD EDITION

EDITED BY

Salim Yusuf

Heart and Stroke Foundation of Ontario Research Chair,
Professor of Medicine, McMaster University,
Director, Population Health Research Institute,
Vice President Research, Hamilton Health Sciences,
Hamilton, Ontario, Canada

John A Cairns

Professor of Medicine and Former Dean,
Faculty of Medicine, University of British Columbia,
Vancouver, BC, Canada

A John Camm

British Heart Foundation Professor of Clinical Cardiology,
Head of Cardiac and Vascular Sciences,
St George's University of London, London, UK

Ernest L Fallen

Professor Emeritus, McMaster University,
Faculty of Health Sciences, Hamilton, Ontario, Canada

Bernard J Gersh

Consultant in Cardiovascular Diseases and Internal Medicine, Mayo Clinic;
Professor of Medicine, Mayo Clinic College of Medicine, Rochester, MN, USA

⊛WILEY-BLACKWELL

A John Wiley & Sons, Ltd., Publication

This edition first published 2010 © 1998, 2003, 2010 by Blackwell Publishing Ltd

BMJ Books is an imprint of BMJ Publishing Group Limited, used under licence by Blackwell Publishing which was acquired by John Wiley & Sons in February 2007. Blackwell's publishing programme has been merged with Wiley's global Scientific, Technical and Medical business to form Wiley-Blackwell.

Registered office: John Wiley & Sons Ltd, The Atrium, Southern Gate, Chichester, West Sussex, PO19 8SQ, UK

Editorial offices: 9600 Garsington Road, Oxford, OX4 2DQ, UK

The Atrium, Southern Gate, Chichester, West Sussex, PO19 8SQ, UK

111 River Street, Hoboken, NJ 07030-5774, USA

For details of our global editorial offices, for customer services and for information about how to apply for permission to reuse the copyright material in this book please see our website at www.wiley.com/wiley-blackwell

The right of the author to be identified as the author of this work has been asserted in accordance with the Copyright, Designs and Patents Act 1988.

Library of Congress Cataloging-in-Publication Data

Evidence-Based Cardiology / edited by Salim Yusuf . . . [et al.]. – 3rd ed.
     p. ; cm.
   Includes bibliographical references and index.
   ISBN 978-1-4051-5925-8 (alk. paper)
1. Heart–Diseases–Handbooks, manuals, etc.   2. Evidence-based medicine–Handbooks, manuals, etc.
I. Yusuf, Salim, 1952–
   [DNLM: 1. Cardiovascular Diseases–therapy.   2. Cardiology–methods.   3. Evidence-Based Medicine–methods.
WG 166 E93 2010]
   RC669.15.S53 2010
   616.1'2–dc22

2009026216

ISBN: 978-1-4051-5925-8

A catalogue record for this book is available from the British Library.
Set in 9.5 on 12 pt Palatino by SNP Best-set Typesetter Ltd., Hong Kong

Printed and bound in Singapore by Fabulous Printers Pte Ltd

2   2010

Contents

Contents

The colour plate section can be found facing p. 940

List of contributors

Victor Aboyans MD, PhD
Hospital Physician, Department of Thoracic and Cardiovascular Surgery, and Angiology, Dupuytren University Hospital, Limoges, France

Sonia S. Anand MD, PhD, FRCPC
Professor of Medicine, McMaster University, Hamilton, Ontario, Canada

Jeffrey L. Anderson MD, FACC, FAHA, MACP
Professor of Internal Medicine, University of Utah School of Medicine; Associate Chief of Cardiology and Vice Chair for Research, Intermountain Medical Center, Salt Lake City, UT, USA

Craig Anderson MBBS, PhD, FRACP, FAFPHM
Director, Neurological and Mental Health Division, Professor of Stroke Medicine and Clinical Neuroscience, The George Institute for International Health, University of Sydney and the Royal Prince Alfred Hospital, Sydney, Australia

Paul W. Armstrong MD
Distinguished University Professor, University of Alberta, Edmonton, Alberta, Canada

Stephanie Atkinson PhD
Professor and Associate Chair (Research), Department of Pediatrics, Associate Member, Department of Biochemistry and Biomedical Science, McMaster University, Hamilton, Ontario, Canada

Colin Baigent BM, BCh, FFPH, FRCP
Professor of Epidemiology, University of Oxford, Clinical Trial Service Unit and Epidemiological Studies Unit (CTSU), Oxford, UK

Adrian Baranchuk MD
Kingston General Hospital, Queen's University, Kingston, Ontario, Canada

Conor D. Barrett MD
Instructor in Medicine, Harvard Medical School, Cardiac Arrhythmia Service, Massachusetts General Hospital Heart Center, Boston, MA, USA

Elisabeth Bédard MD
Adult Congenital Heart Centre and Centre for Pulmonary Hypertension, Royal Brompton Hospital, London, UK

David G. Benditt MD, FACC, FRCPC, FHRS
Professor of Medicine, Co-Director, Cardiac Arrhythmia Center, University of Minnesota Medical School, Minneapolis, MN, USA

William E. Boden MD, FACC
Professor of Medicine and Preventive Medicine, University at Buffalo, School of Medicine and Public Health; Clinical Chief, Division of Cardiovascular Medicine, University at Buffalo; Chief of Cardiology, Buffalo General and Millard Fillmore Hospitals, Buffalo, NY, USA

Barry A. Boilson MD, MRCPI
Fellow in Cardiac Transplantation Medicine, Mayo Clinic, Rochester, MN, USA

Robert H. Boone MD, FRCPC, MSc(Epi)
Clinical Assistant Professor, Interventional Cardiology, St. Paul's Hospital, Providence Health Care, University of British Columbia, Vancouver, BC, Canada

Morgan L. Brown MD
Research Fellow, Division of Cardiovascular Surgery, Mayo Clinic, Rochester, MN, USA

Brian H. Buck MD, MSc, FRCPC
Assistant Professor, Division of Neurology, Department of Medicine, University of Alberta, Edmonton, Alberta, Canada

Christopher E. Buller MD, FRCPC
Professor of Medicine, University of British Columbia; Head, Division of Cardiology, Vancouver General Hospital, Vancouver, BC, Canada

David J. Burkhardt MD
Texas Cardiac Arrhythmia Institute, St. David's Medical Center, Austin, TX, USA

John A. Cairns MD, FRCPC
Professor of Medicine and Former Dean, Faculty of Medicine, University of British Columbia, Vancouver, BC, Canada

A. John Camm MD
British Heart Foundation Professor of Clinical Cardiology, Head of Cardiac and Vascular Sciences, St George's University of London, London, UK

Blase A. Carabello MD
Professor of Medicine, Vice-Chairman, Department of Medicine, WA Tex and Deborah Moncrief Jr. Center, Baylor College of Medicine, Medical Care Line Executive, Veterans Affairs Medical Center, Houston, TX, USA

Matthew Chan FANZCA
Department of Anaesthesia and Intensive Care, The Chinese University of Hong Kong, Hong Kong Special Administrative Region, China

Chi Keong Ching MBBS, MRCP (UK)
Consultant Cardiologist and Electrophysiologist, Department of Cardiology, National Heart Centre Singapore, Mistri Wing, Singapore

Clara K. Chow MBBS, FRACP, PhD
Senior Research Fellow, Population Health Research Institute, McMaster University, Hamilton, Ontario, Canada

Victor Chu MD, FRCS(C)
McMaster University, Hamilton Health Sciences, Hamilton, Ontario, Canada

Michael Colquhoun BSc, FRCP, MRCGP
Honorary Lecturer, School of Medicine, Cardiff University, Cardiff, UK

Patrick J. Commerford MD
Cardiac Clinic, Department of Medicine, University of Cape Town, Groote Schuur Hospital, Cape Town, South Africa

Stuart J. Connolly MD, FRCPC
Director, Division of Cardiology, McMaster University, Hamilton, Ontario, Canada

Heidi M. Connolly MD
Professor of Medicine, Mayo Clinic, Rochester, MN, USA

Leslie T. Cooper Jr MD
Professor of Medicine, Mayo Clinic College of Medicine; Chief, Section of Vascular Medicine, Mayo Clinic, Rochester, MN, USA

Michael H. Criqui MD, MPH
Professor and Chief, Division of Preventive Medicine, Department of Family and Preventive Medicine, University of California, San Diego School of Medicine, La Jolla, CA, USA

Michael S. Cunnington BMedSci, MB BS (Hons), MRCP
British Cardiovascular Society/Swire Research Fellow, Institute of Human Genetics, Newcastle University, Newcastle-upon-Tyne, UK

Dawood Darbar MBChB, MD, FACC
Associate Professor of Medicine and Pharmacology, Director, Vanderbilt Arrhythmia Service, Vanderbilt University School of Medicine, Nashville, TN, USA

Tirone E. David MD
Professor of Surgery, University of Toronto, Head of Cardiovascular Surgery, Peter Munk Cardiac Centre, Toronto General Hospital, Toronto, Canada

Philip J. Devereaux MD, PhD, FRCP(C)
Departments of Clinical Epidemiology and Biostatistics and Medicine, McMaster University, Faculty of Health Sciences, Hamilton, Ontario, Canada

Luigi Di Biase MD
Electrophysiologist Research Fellow, Department Dean of Medicine, University of Texas Medical Branch at Austin, Texas Cardiac Arrhythmia Institute, St. David's Medical Center, Austin, TX, USA; Department of Cardiology, University of Foggia, Foggia, Italy

Kim A. Eagle MD, MACC
Albion Walter Hewlett Professor of Internal Medicine, Chief of Clinical Cardiology, Director, Cardiovascular Center, University of Michigan, Ann Arbor, MI, USA

John Eikelboom MBBS, MSc, FRACP, FRCPA, FRCPC
Associate Professor, Department of Medicine, McMaster University, Hamilton, Ontario, Canada

Claude S. Elayi MD
Assistant Professor of Medicine, Division of Cardiovascular Medicine, Gill Heart Institute, University of Kentucky, Lexington, KY, USA

Perry M. Elliott MBBS, MD, FRCP
Reader in Inherited Cardiac Disease, University College London, London, UK

Jonathan R. Emberson BA, MSc, PhD
Senior Statistician, University of Oxford, Clinical Trial Service Unit and Epidemiological Studies Unit (CTSU), Oxford, UK

R. Alan Failor MD
Clinical Professor of Medicine, Division of Metabolism, Endocrinology and Nutrition, University of Washington, Seattle, WA, USA

Ernest L. Fallen MD, FRCPC
Professor Emeritus, McMaster University Faculty of Health Sciences, Hamilton, Ontario, Canada

Shafie S. Fazel MD, PhD
Senior Resident, Division of Cardiac Surgery, Peter Munk Cardiac Center, Toronto General Hospital, University of Toronto, Toronto, Canada

Francisco Fernández-Avilés PhD, MD
Professor of Medicine, Head of the Department of Cardiology, Hospital General Universitario Gregorio Marañón, Complutense University, School of Medicine, Madrid, Spain

David Fitchett MD, FRCPC
Director, Cardiac ICU, St. Michael's Hospital Toronto, Associate Professor of Medicine, University of Toronto, Toronto, Ontario, Canada

Keith A. A. Fox BSc (Hons) MBChB, FRCP, FESC, FMedSci, FACC
FACC Professor of Cardiology, Centre for Cardiovascular Science, University of Edinburgh, Edinburgh, UK

Curt D. Furberg MD, PhD
Professor, Division of Public Health Sciences, Wake Forest University School of Medicine, Winston-Salem, NC, USA

Michael A. Gatzoulis MD, PhD, FACC, FESC
Professor of Cardiology, Congenital Heart Disease and Consultant Cardiologist, Adult Congenital Heart Centre and Centre for Pulmonary Hypertension, Royal Brompton Hospital, and the National Heart & Lung Institute, Imperial College, London, UK

Jacques Genest Jr MD, FRCPC
Professor, Faculty of Medicine, McGill University, Novartis Chair in Medicine at McGill University, Director, Division of Cardiology University Health Center/ Royal Victoria Hospital, Montreal, Quebec, Canada

Bernard J. Gersh MB, ChB, DPhil
Consultant in Cardiovascular Diseases and Internal Medicine, Mayo Clinic; Professor of Medicine, Mayo Clinic College of Medicine, Rochester, MN, USA

List of contributors

Hertzel C. Gerstein MD, MSc, FRCPC
Division of Endocrinology and Metabolism, Population Health Research Institute, Department of Medicine, McMaster University and Hamilton Health Sciences, Hamilton, Ontario, Canada

Raymond J. Gibbons MD
Arthur M. and Gladys D. Gray Professor of Medicine, Division of Cardiovascular Diseases, Mayo Clinic, Rochester, MN, USA

Michael M. Givertz MD
Cardiovascular Division, Brigham and Women's Hospital, Harvard Medical School, Boston, MA, USA

Paul J. Hauptman MD
Professor of Internal Medicine, Saint Louis University School of Medicine, St. Louis, MO, USA

Jeffrey S. Healey MD, MSc, FRCP(C)
Associate Professor of Medicine, McMaster University, Hamilton, Ontario, Canada

Mark A. Hlatky MD
Professor of Health Research and Policy & Professor of Medicine (Cardiovascular Medicine), Stanford University School of Medicine, Stanford, CA, USA

Rodney Horton MD
Texas Cardiac Arrhythmia Institute, St. David's Medical Center, Austin, TX, USA

Marjan Jahangiri FRCS
Professor of Cardiac Surgery, Department of Cardiothoracic Surgery, St. George's University of London, London, UK

Prabhat Jha MD, DPhil
Centre for Global Health Research, St. Michael's Hospital, University of Toronto, Toronto, Ontario, Canada

Michael Joy OBE, MD, FRCP, FACC, FESC, FRAeS
Professor of Clinical Cardiology, Postgraduate Medical School, Surrey University, Guildford, and, Cardiologist, Medical Department, UK Civil Aviation Authority, West Sussex, UK

Prince Kannankeril MD, MSCI
Assistant Professor, Vanderbilt, Department of Pediatrics, University Medical Centre, Nashville, TN, USA

Clive Kearon MB, MRCPI, FRCPC, PhD
Professor of Medicine, McMaster University, Hamilton, Ontario, Canada

Bernard D. Keavney MD
Professor of Cardiology, Institute of Human Genetics and Department of Cardiology, Newcastle University, Newcastle-upon-Tyne, UK

Rohit Khurana BMBCh, PhD, MRCP
Fellow, Interventional Cardiology, Vancouver General Hospital, Division of Cardiology, University of British Columbia, Vancouver, BC, Canada

Michael Klein MD
Clinical Professor of Medicine, Boston University, School of Medicine, Boston, MA, USA

Kornelia Kotseva MD, PhD, FESC
Senior Clinical Research Fellow, Consultant Cardiologist, Cardiovascular Medicine, National Heart and Lung Institute, Imperial College, London, UK

Stavros Kounas MD
The Heart Hospital, University College London, London, UK

Antonios Kourliouros MD
Department of Cardiothoracic Surgery, St George's University of London, London, UK

Sudhir Kushwaha MD
Associate Professor of Medicine, Mayo Clinic, Rochester, MN, USA

Malcolm Law FRCP, FMedSci
Professor of Epidemiology and Preventive Medicine, Centre for Environmental and Preventive Medicine, Queen Mary School of Medicine and Dentistry, Wolfson Institute of Preventive Medicine, London, UK

Lori-Ann Linkins MD, MSc, FRCPC
Associate Professor, McMaster University, Thromboembolism/Hematology, Hamilton, Ontario, Canada'

Fei Lu MD, PhD, FACC, FHRS
Associate Professor of Medicine, Director, Cardiac Electrophysiology Laboratories, Cardiac Arrhythmia Center, University of Minnesota Medical School, Minneapolis, MN, USA

Andrew J. Lucking BMedSci(Hons), MBChB(Hons), MRCP
Clinical Research Fellow, University of Edinburgh, Edinburgh, UK

Benedito Carlos Maciel MD
Full Professor of Medicine, Division of Cardiology, Department of Internal Medicine, Medical School of Ribeirão Preto, University of São Paulo, Ribeirão Preto, Brazil

Brendan P. Madden MD, MSc, FRCPI, FRCP
Professor of Cardiothoracic Medicine, St George's Hospital, London, UK

Sunil Mankad MD
Associate Professor of Medicine, Mayo Clinic College of Medicine, Director, Transesophageal Echocardiography, Co-Director, Education, Echocardiography, Mayo Clinic, Rochester, MN, USA

Johannes F. E. Mann MD
Professor of Medicine, Friedrich Alexander University of Erlangen, Head, Department of Nephrology and Hypertension, Schwabing General Hospital, Ludwig Maximilians University, Munich, Germany

Ali J. Marian MD
Professor of Molecular Medicine and Internal Medicine (Cardiology), Director, Center for Cardiovascular Genetics, Institute of Molecular Medicine, The University of Texas Health Science Center, Houston, TX, USA

J. Antonio Marin-Neto MD, PhD, FACC
Full Professor of Medicine and Director, Cardiology Division, Department of Internal Medicine, Medical School of Ribeirão Preto, University of São Paulo, Ribeirão Preto, Brazil

Barry J. Maron MD
Director, Hypertrophic Cardiomyopathy Center, Minneapolis Heart Institute Foundation, Minneapolis, MN, USA

Bongani M. Mayosi DPhil, FCP(SA)
Professor of Medicine, Groote Schuur
Hospital and University of Cape Town,

Gerald V. Naccarelli MD
Bernard Trabin Chair in Cardiology;
Professor of Medicine; Chief, Division of

Jeffrey L. Probstfield MD
Director, Clinical Trials Service Unit,
Professor of Medicine (Cardiology),
University of Washington School of
...A, USA

...ty MD, PhD
...and Epidemiology,
...lth Research Unit,
...ington, Seattle, WA, USA

...kee MD
...icine, McMaster
...milton Health Sciences,
...Canada

... Rahimtoola MB,
...C, DSc(Hon)
...fessor, University of
...ia, George C. Griffith
...ology, Professor of
...chool of Medicine at
...thern California, Los
...A

...r MD, PhD, FACC, FACP,
...r, Anis Rassi Hospital,

...Reddy MD
...ardiology, All India
...ical Sciences, New Delhi,

... Rihal MD
...sion of Cardiovascular
...Clinic Rochester; Professor
...yo Clinic College of
...ester, MN, USA

...erts MD, FRCPC, MACC
...CEO, Professor of Medicine
...uddy Canadian
...Genetics Centre, University
...t Institute, Ottawa, Ontario,

...cchiccioli MD
...Cardiovascular Research
...sity of Glasgow, Glasgow,

...Roden MD
...ledicine and Pharmacology,
...s Institute, Assistant
...r for Personalized Medicine,
...iversity School of Medicine,
...TN, USA

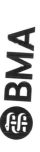

Annika Rosengren MD
Professor of Medicine, Department of
Medicine, Sahlgrenska University Hospital/
Ostra, Göteborg, Sweden

Scott Sakaguchi MD
Associate Professor of Medicine, Cardiac
Arrhythmia Center, University of
Minnesota Medical School, Minneapolis,
MN, USA

Zainab Samad MD
Fellow, Division of Cardiology, Department
of Internal Medicine, Duke University
Medical Center, Durham, NC, USA

Pedro L. Sánchez MD, PhD
Head of Section, Department of Cardiology,
Associate Professor; Hospital General
Universitario Gregorio Marañón, School of
Medicine, Complutense University, Madrid,
Spain

Irina Savelieva MD
Department of Cardiology, Division of
Cardiac and Vascular Science, St George's
University of London, London, UK

Ernesto L. Schiffrin MD, PhD,
FRSC, FRCPC, FACP
Physician-in-Chief and Chair, Department
of Medicine, Sir Mortimer B. Davis-Jewish
General Hospital, McGill University,
Montreal, Quebec, Canada

André Schmidt MD, PhD
Assistant Professor, Cardiology Division,
Medical School of Ribeirão Preto,
University of São Paulo, Ribeirão Preto,
Brazil

Jon-David R. Schwalm BSc, MD,
FRCPC
Chief Cardiology Resident, McMaster
University, Hamilton General Hospital Site,
Hamilton, Ontario, Canada

Arya M. Sharma MD, PhD, FRCPC
Professor of Medicine, Chair for Obesity
Management & Research, University of
Alberta, Edmonton, Alberta, Canada

Ashfaq Shuaib MD, FRCPC, FAHA
Professor of Medicine and Neurology;
Director, Stroke Program, University of
Alberta, Edmonton, Alberta, Canada

Marcus Vinicius Simões MD
Medical School of Ribeirão Preto,
University of São Paulo, Ribeirão Preto,
Brazil

Samuel C. Siu MD, SM
Gunton Professor and Chair of Cardiology,
Schulich School of Medicine and Dentistry,
University of Western Ontario, London,
Ontario, Canada

Elsayed Z. Soliman MD, MSc, MS
Associate Director, Epidemiological
Cardiology Research Center (EPICARE),
Assistant Professor, Department of
Epidemiology and Prevention, Wake Forest
University School of Medicine, Winston-
Salem, NC, USA

Ray W. Squires PhD
Professor of Medicine, Mayo Clinic College
of Medicine, Rochester, MN, USA

Garrick C. Stewart MD
Clinical Fellow, Division of Cardiovascular
Medicine, Brigham and Women's Hospital,
Harvard Medical School, Boston, MA, USA

Jack C.J. Sun MD, MSc
Division of Cardiac Surgery, McMaster
University, Hamilton, Ontario, Canada

Thoralf M. Sundt III MD
Consultant, Division of Cardiovascular
Surgery, Professor of Surgery, Mayo Clinic,
Rochester, MN, USA

Karl Swedberg MD, PhD
Head, Department of Emergency and
Cardiovascular Medicine, Professor of
Medicine, Sahlgrenska Academy,
University of Gothenburg, Sahlgrenska
University Hospital/ Östra, Göteborg,
Sweden

Faisal S. Syed MD
Department of Cardiology, University of
Newcastle-upon-Tyne, Newcastle, UK

Koon K. Teo MB, PhD, FRCPC, FRCPI
Professor of Medicine, Division of
Cardiology, Department of Medicine,
Population Health Research Institute,
McMaster University, Hamilton, Ontario,
Canada

Pierre Theroux CM, MD, FACC
Professor of Medicine, Montreal Heart
Institute, University of Montreal, Quebec,
Canada

Peter L. Thompson MD, FRACP,
FACP, FACC, MBA
Clinical Professor, Cardiologist and
Director of Research, Sir Charles Gairdner
Hospital, Clinical Professor of Medicine
and Population Health, University of
Western Australia, Perth, Australia

William D. Toff MD, FESC
Department of Cardiovascular Sciences,
University of Leicester, Leicester, UK

Thomas T. Tsai MD, MSc
Interventional Cardiology Fellow,
Cardiovascular Center, University of
Michigan Hospitals, Ann Arbor, MI, USA

Jack V. Tu MD, PhD
Institute for Clinical Evaluative Sciences,
University of Toronto & Schulich Heart
Centre, Sunnybrook Health Sciences Centre,
Toronto, Canada

Zoltan G. Turi MD
Professor of Medicine, Robert Wood
Johnson Medical School, Director,
Structural Heart Disease Program, Cooper
University Hospital, Camden, NJ, USA

Ameeth Vedre MD
Cardiovascular Center, University of
Michigan, Ann Arbor, MI, USA

Rachel M. Wald MD, FRCPC
Staff Cardiologist, University Health
Network and Hospital for Sick Children,
Assistant Professor, Department of
Pediatrics, University of Toronto, Toronto,
Canada

Albert L. Waldo MD
Department of Medicine, Case Western
Reserve, University School of Medicine,
Division of Cardiovascular Medicine,
University Hospitals Case Medical Center,
Cleveland, OH, USA

Andrew Wang MD
Associate Professor of Medicine; Director,
Cardiovascular Disease Fellowship
Program, Duke University Medical Center,
Durham, NC, USA

Deirdre Ward MRCPI
Director, Centre for Cardiovascular Risk in
Younger Persons, Institute of
Cardiovascular Science, Trinity College
Dublin, Dublin, Republic of Ireland

John G. Webb MD, FRCPC, FACC
McLeod Professor of Valvular Heart
Disease Intervention, Director,
Interventional Cardiology and Cardiac
Catheterization, St. Paul's Hospital,
Vancouver, BC, USA

William S. Weintraub MD
Christiana Care Health System, Center for
Heart & Vascular Health, Newark,
Delaware, USA

Robert C. Welsh MD, FRCPC
Associate Professor; Director, Cardiac
Catheterization and Interventional
Cardiology; University of Alberta &
Mazankowski Alberta Heart Institute,
Edmonton, Alberta, Canada

David A. Wood MSc, FRCP, FRCPE,
FFPHM, FESC
Garfield Weston Professor of
Cardiovascular Medicine at the National
Heart and Lung Institute, Imperial College
London, UK

David A. Wood MD FRCPC
Interventional Cardiology, Director,
Undergraduate Cardiovascular Medical
Education, Clinical Assistant Professor,
University of British Columbia, Vancouver,
BC, Canada

Salim Yusuf DPhil, FRCPC, FRSC
Heart and Stroke Foundation of Ontario
Research Chair, Professor of Medicine,
McMaster University; Director, Population
Health Research Institute, McMaster
University, Hamilton Health Sciences; Vice
President Research, Hamilton Health
Sciences, Hamilton, Ontario, Canada

Witold Zatonski MD, PhD
Director of the Cancer Epidemiology and
Prevention Division, The M. Sklodowska-
Curie Memorial Cancer Center and Institute
of Oncology, Warsaw, Poland

Preface to the third edition

'I had' said he 'come to an entirely erroneous conclusion which shows, my dear Watson, how dangerous it always is to reason from insufficient data'.

Sir Arthur Conan Doyle

Sherlock Holmes not only sought sufficient data, he scrutinized them with critical appraisal – two necessary prerequisites for an effective evidence based strategy. And so it is that clinical decision-making has come to rely more and more on best external evidence derived from well-executed large-scale clinical trials.

This is a big book. However, it can be used to best advantage in two ways: as a reference tome to gain in-depth understanding of a wide array of cardiovascular disorders, and as a source where clinicians can find and apply the best evidence to guide their management of specific cardiovascular conditions.

In 1964 over 50% of clinical research publications were devoted to clinical physiology experiments. There were no papers on clinical trials that year. The emphasis then was less on treatment and more on exploring mechanisms of disease. This changed in the 1980s so that by 2004 more than 20% of clinical research articles contained reports from large-scale clinical trials compared to only 3% that were laboratory based. This shift in emphasis from bench-to-bedside-to-community led to a startling paradox in which irrefutable evidence for the effectiveness of certain therapies not only assisted practising clinicians and their patients but begged the scientific question – "*How* and *why* does the therapeutic intervention work?" A clarion call for a community-to-bench paradigm.

In the preface to the second edition we stated, prophetically, that "Evidence-based medicine is a work in progress – a rapidly changing field – which cannot rest on its laurels, but must constantly be updated as newer and more effective treatments emerge". Although the very nature of book publication hardly competes with the instant gratification of "late breaking" trials presented at meetings or on-line, nevertheless the expert contributors of this compendium have successfully provided a clear and comprehensive overview of best evidence for the diagnosis and management of most cardiovascular disorders.

As with previous editions we continue to subscribe to the dictum that clinical decision-making ought to be an amalgam of best external evidence combined with clinical expertise and awareness of patients' needs and preferences. Although evidence-based guidelines are derived from clinical trial results, the reader should bear in mind that guidelines are disease (not patient) specific. In this context caution is urged whenever attempts are made to equate guidelines with standards of care. Not only are there multiple co-morbidities in over 60% of elderly patients but there are multiple co-medications as well. If one parses many of the studies outlined in this book one often finds that the effectiveness of a given therapy is proportional to disease severity and overall risk, whereas the harm of the intervention is often risk independent.

It is also recognized that clinical trials, irrespective of their strengths, need to be interpreted in the context of large registry databases that might reflect clinical practice on a wider scale. Trials have their strengths and limitations, as do registry studies, and both should be considered as complementary and not exclusive to each other.

This edition, like those before it, is comprised of four sections. Part I addresses some key concepts related to both evidence-based cardiology and critical appraisal. Part II is devoted to prevention and preventive strategies. Part III comprises several sections encompassing the management of specific cardiovascular disorders, and Part IV is a section on clinical applications describing how external evidence is used in individual case studies. There are several new features including major vascular complications in susceptible patients undergoing non-cardiac surgery; evidence-based cardiology as applied to employment fitness in specific occupations such as transportation and aviation; ablation therapy for atrial fibrillation; arrhythmias due to monogenic disorders; different forms of cardiomyopathy including Chagas' disease and adult congenital heart disease.

The editors are pleased to acknowledge the helpful guidance, advice and patience from Mary Banks, Helen Harvey and Simone Heaton of Wiley-Blackwell.

Salim Yusuf
John A Cairns
A John Camm
Ernest L Fallen
Bernard J Gersh

Classification of recommendations and levels of evidence

Classification of recommendations and levels of evidence used in *Evidence-Based Cardiology* are as follows:

Classification of recommendations

Class I: Evidence and/or general agreement that a given procedure or treatment is beneficial, useful and effective.

Class II: Conflicting evidence and/or a divergence of opinion about the usefulness/efficacy of a procedure or treatment.

Class IIa: Weight of evidence/opinion is in favor of usefulness/efficacy.

Class IIb: Usefulness/efficacy is less well established by evidence/opinion.

Class III: Evidence and/or general agreement that a given procedure or treatment is not useful/effective and in some cases may be harmful.

Levels of evidence

Level A: Well-conducted, large and reliable RCTs (one or more) or their overview with clear results.

Level B: RCTs (one or more) or their overview with significant limitations.

Level C:

1) High quality and persuasive cohort studies, case control studies or case series.

2) Lower quality evidence from non-randomized studies including opinions of experts.

These **classes of recommendations** are identical to those used by the ACC/AHA/ESC in their Guidelines documents, and the **levels of evidence** are very similar. Comprehensive approaches are used, which incorporate many different types of evidence (e.g. RCTs, non-RCTs, epidemiologic studies and laboratory data), and examine the architecture of the information for consistency, coherence and clarity. Classes of recommendation and levels of evidence appear in blue type either within the text (e.g. **Class I, Level A**) or within a table in the chapter. The system is applicable only to preventive or therapeutic interventions. It is not applicable to many other types of data such as descriptive, genetic or physiologic.

List of abbreviations

Abbreviations commonly used in this book

AADs	antiarrhythmic drugs
ABI	Ankle Brachial Index
ACC	American College of Cardiology
ACD	absolute claudication distance
ACE	angiotensin-converting enzyme
ACS	acute coronary syndrome
ADA	adenine deaminase
ADMA	asymmetric dimethylarginin
AF	atrial fibrillation
AHA	American Heart Association
AIS	acute ischemic stroke
ALI	Acute limb ischemia
AMI	acute myocardial infarction
AMR	antibody-mediated rejection; acute mitral regurgitation
AR	aortic regurgitation
ARB	angiotensin receptor blockers
ARF	acute rheumatic fever
ARR	absolute risk reduction
ARVC	arrhythmogenic right ventricular cardiomyopathy
ARVD	arrhythmogenic right ventricular dysplasia
AS	aortic stenosis
ASA	acetylsalicylic acid
ASD	atrial septal defect
ASMR	age-standardized mortality rates
ATP	adenosine triphosphate
AVA	aortic valve area
AVB	atrioventricular block
AVR	aortic valve replacement
AVSD	atrioventricular septal defect
AVV	atrioventricular valve
BAV	bicuspid aortic valve
BNP	brain natriuretic peptide
BUN	blood urea nitrogen
CABG	coronary artery bypass graft
CAD	coronary artery disease
CAV	cardiac allograft vasculopathy
CBF	cerebral/coronary blood flow
CCB	calcium channel blocker
CCC	Chagas' cardiomyopathy
CCMR	chronic compensated mitral regurgitation
CDMR	chronic decompensated mitral regurgitation
CETP	cholesteryl ester transfer protein
CHD	coronary heart disease
CHF	congestive heart failure
CK	creatine kinase
CKD	chronic kidney disease
CLI	critical limb ischemia
CMR	cardiac magnetic resonance
CMV	cytomegalovirus
COPD	chronic obstructive pulmonary disease
CPVT	catecholaminergic polymorphic ventricular tachycardia
Cr	Creatinine
CRP	C-reactive protein
CSS	carotid sinus syndrome
CTA	computed tomographic angiography
CTEPH	chronic thromboembolic pulmonary hypertension
CTI	cavotricuspid isthmus
CTPA	computed tomographic pulmonary angiography
CVD	cardiovascular disease
CVRF	cardiovascular risk factors
DAD	delayed afterdepolarizations
DALYs	disability-adjusted life-years
DCM	dilated cardiomyopathy
DBP	diastolic blood pressure
DSA	digital subtraction angiography
EAD	early afterdepolarizations
EBV	Epstein–Barr virus
ECMV	encephalomyocarditis virus
EF	ejection fraction
EKG	electrocardiogram
EMB	endomyocardial biopsy

EPS	electrophysiologic testing	NCD	non-communicable diseases
ESC	European Society of Cardiology	NNT	number needed to treat
ESR	erythrocyte sedimentation rate	NRT	nicotine replacement therapy
FISH	fluorescence *in situ* hybridization	NSAIDs	non-steroidal anti-inflammatory drugs
GAS	group A streptococcal	NSVT	non-sustained ventricular tachycardia
GFR	glomerular filtration rate	NVAF	non-valvular atrial fibrillation
GSD	glycogen storage disease	OAC	oral anticoagulants
HAART	highly active antiretroviral therapy	OLAT	organized left atrial tachyarrhythmia
HCM	hypertrophic cardiomyopathy	OR	odds ratio
HCt	haematocrit	PAD	peripheral arterial disease
HDL	high-density lipoprotein	PAH	pulmonary arterial hypertension
HFSA	Heart Failure Society of America	PAP	pulmonary artery pressures
HIC	high-income countries	PARs	population-attributable risks
HIT	heparin-induced thrombocytopenia	PAU	penetrating atherosclerotic ulcer
HIV	human immunodeficiency virus	PBAV	percutaneous balloon aortic valvuloplasty
HRQoL	health-related quality of life	PBMV	percutaneous balloon mitral valvuloplasty
IART	intra-atrial re-entrant tachycardia	PCA	percutaneous angioplasty
ICD	implantable cardioverter-defibrillator; initial claudication distance	PCI	percutaneous coronary intervention
		PDA	patent ductus arteriosus
ICH	intracerebral hemorrhage	PDGF	platelet-derived growth factor
IE	infective endocarditis	PFO	patent foramen ovale
IFG	impaired fasting glucose	POTS	postural orthostatic tachycardia syndrome
IGT	impaired glucose tolerance	PPA	plexogenic pulmonary arteriopathy
ILR	implantable loop recorder	PR	pulmonary regurgitation
IMH	intramural hematoma	PS	pulmonary stenosis
INR	international normalized ratio	PSVT	paroxysmal supraventricular tachycardia
ISHLT	International Society for Heart and Lung Transplantation	PTLD	post-transplant lymphoproliferative disorder
		PUFA	polyunsaturated fatty acids
IV	intravenous	PV	pulmonary valve
IVUS	intravascular ultrasound	PVAR	paravalvular aortic regurgitation
LCSD	left cardiac sympathetic denervation	PVE	prosthetic valve endocarditis
LDH	lactate dehydrogenase	PVI	pulmonary vein isolation
LDL	low-density lipoprotein	PVR	pulmonary vascular resistance
LMIC	low- and middle-income countries	PVS	pulmonary valve stenosis
LMWH	low molecular weight heparin	PVT	prosthetic valve thrombosis
LoB	line of block	QALYs	quality-adjusted life-years
LR	likelihood ratio	QoL	quality of life
LSCA	left subclavian artery	RAS	renin-angiotensin system
LSD	lysosomal storage disorders	RCT	randomized controlled/clinical trial
LV	left ventricle/ventricular	RF	radiofrequency
LVEF	left ventricular ejection fraction	RHD	rheumatic heart disease
LVH	left ventricular hypertrophy	RR	relative risk
LVOT	LV outflow tract	RRR	relative risk reduction
LVOTO	left ventricular outflow tract obstructions	RV	right ventricle/ventricular
LVSD	left ventricular systolic dysfunction	SAECG	signal-averaged ECG
MACE	major adverse cardiovascular events	SAH	subarachnoid hemorrhage
MCOT	mobile cardiac outpatient telemetry	SAM	systolic anterior motion
MDTD	maximum daily therapeutic dose	SAS	subvalvar aortic stenosis
METS	metabolic equivalents	SBP	systolic blood pressure
MI	myocardial infarction	SFA	saturated fatty acids
MS	mitral stenosis	SIDS	sudden infant death syndrome
MTT	Myocarditis Treatment Trial	SND	sinus node dysfunction
MUFA	monounsaturated fatty acids	SNPs	single nucleotide polymorphisms
MVR	mitral valve replacement	STEMI	ST segment elevated myocardial infarction

SUNDS	sudden unexplained nocturnal death syndrome	TSH	thyroid-stimulating hormone
SVAS	supravalvar aortic stenosis	TTE	transthoracic echocardiography
TAVR	transcatheter aortic valve replacement	TV	tricuspid valve
TCPC	total cavopulmonary connection	TWA	T-wave alternans
TE	thromboembolic	UFH	unfractionated heparin
TEE	transesophageal echocardiography	VF	ventricular fibrillation
TGA	transposition of the great arteries	VKAs	vitamin K antagonists
TIA	transient ischemic attack	VSD	ventricular septal defect
TLOC	transient loss of consciousness	VT	ventricular tachycardia
TOF	tetralogy of Fallot	VTE	venous thromboembolism
TR	tricuspid regurgitation	VUI	venous ultrasound imaging

General concepts and critical appraisal

Salim Yusuf, Editor

1

Evidence-based decision making: patient–physician interface

Philip J Devereaux,[1] Marc Pfeffer[2] and Salim Yusuf[1]

[1] Departments of Clinical Epidemiology and Biostatistics and Medicine, McMaster University, Hamilton, Ontario, Canada

[2] Brigham and Women's Hospital, Boston, MA, USA

Introduction

In 1836 Elisha Bartlett, the editor of the *American Journal of Medical Sciences*, heralded a study as "one of the most important medical works of the present century, marking the start of a new era in science."[1] What evoked such praise and suggested a paradigm shift was Dr Pierre Louis' systematic collection and numerical presentation of data on blood letting. Louis adopted a Baconian approach of collecting vast amounts of data on a large number of patients (by the standards of the early 1800s), which allowed him to systematically evaluate the efficacy of blood letting. Louis argued that large numbers of patients and enumeration were necessary to equalize differences between treatment groups since "by so doing, the errors (which are inevitable), being the same in two groups of patients subjected to different treatment, mutually compensate each other, and they may be disregarded without sensibly affecting the exactness of the results."[2] Louis subsequently went on to state: "a therapeutic agent cannot be employed with any discrimination or probability of success in a given case, unless its general efficacy, in analogous cases, has been previously ascertained" and thus, "without the aid of statistics nothing like real medicine is possible."[3]

The prevailing concept of illness, at the time, was that the sick were contaminated, whether by some toxin or contagion, or an excess of one humor or another. This understanding of illness contained within it the idea that these states were improved by opening a vein and letting the sickness run out. Louis' finding that blood letting hastened the death of the ill was a bombshell. George Washington had 2.4 liters of blood drained from him in the 15 hours prior to his death; he had been suffering from a fever, sore throat, and respiratory difficulties for 24 hours.[4] Some have suggested that Washington was murdered.[5–7]

While this is a relatively recent example, the plea for comparative evaluation is mentioned as early as the Old Testament. Throughout history there have been repeated exhortations to quantify medical or health problems and to compare outcomes in patient groups managed differently, with the goal of setting state policy or assisting individual physicians.

In this chapter we will consider what evidence-based medicine is and then discuss an approach to evidence-based decision making. We will use a clinical case to highlight the components of this approach which include: clinical state and circumstances, patient preferences and actions, research evidence, and clinical expertise. At the end of the chapter we will review the application of these components of evidence-based decision making as they apply to our patient and provide a decision aid that clinicians can use in such a case. This chapter is an overview of core concepts and other chapters in this book (e.g. clinical trials and meta-analysis) provide more in-depth coverage of specific topics.

What is evidence-based medicine?

Although the foundations for evidence-based medicine were laid over several centuries, an explicit philosophy with its attendant concepts, definitions, and models has been largely developed as a formal doctrine only during the last few decades. Evidence-based medicine is about solving clinical problems. Initially, the focus of evidence-based medicine was largely on finding the best objective quantifiable research evidence relevant to the particular problem, and applying that evidence in resolving the particular issue.[8] This early focus de-emphasized "intuition,

Evidence-Based Cardiology, 3rd edition. Edited by S. Yusuf, J.A. Cairns, A.J. Camm, E.L. Fallen, and B.J. Gersh. © 2010 Blackwell Publishing, ISBN: 978-1-4051-5925-8.

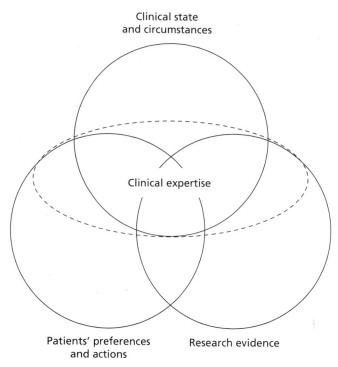

Figure 1.1 Current model of evidence-based clinical decision making.

Approach to evidence-based clinical decision making

Clinical scenario

A family physician refers a patient who has just moved cities to live with his daughter. The physician is requesting our input on the appropriateness of antithrombotic therapy. The patient is an 80-year-old male with a history of hypertension who 10 months ago, on routine exam, was diagnosed with atrial fibrillation. The patient suffered a major gastrointestinal bleed, requiring hospitalization, urgent endoscopy, and a transfusion 1 month prior to his diagnosis of atrial fibrillation. At the time of his bleed, the patient on endoscopy was diagnosed with a duodenal ulcer and *Helicobacter pylori*. The patient has been free of any gastrointestinal symptoms since his bleed 11 months ago and he received appropriate antibiotic and acid suppression therapy. Within 2 weeks of the patient's diagnosis of atrial fibrillation he underwent a transesophageal echocardiogram in his former city of residence and this demonstrated normal valvular and left ventricular function and a left atrium measurement of 6.5 cm without evidence of thrombus. An attempt at cardioversion was unsuccessful. The patient is very worried about having a stroke as his wife was left dependent on him for 2 years prior to her death, following a major stroke. The referring physician, who recently had a patient who suffered a serious gastrointestinal bleed while on warfarin, is very concerned about the risk of bleeding given this patient's age and history of gastrointestinal bleeding.

unsystematic clinical experience, and pathophysiologic rationale as sufficient grounds for clinical decision making" and stressed "the examination of evidence from clinical research."[9] Subsequent versions of evidence-based decision making have emphasized that research evidence alone is rarely sufficient to make a clinical decision.[10] Research evidence by itself seldom tells us what to do in individual situations, but rather it provides useful information that allows us to make more informed decisions. Clinicians must always view evidence in the context of the individual patient and then weigh the potential benefits versus the risks, costs, and inconveniences of each action. Ideally the patient's values and preferences affect these issues[10]

An initial description of evidence-based medicine from an editorial in 1996 provided the following definition: "Evidence-based medicine is the conscientious and judicious use of current best evidence from clinical care research in the management of individual patients."[10] The editorial also included the caveat that the definition of evidence-based medicine will evolve as new types of information emerge and therefore will be continuously refined. The concepts of evidence-based medicine have evolved considerably and the current model is outlined in Figure 1.1.[8] In the next section we use this model of evidence-based clinical decision making to help resolve a common clinical scenario.

Model for evidence-based clinical decisions

Figure 1.1 depicts a model for evidence-based clinical decisions,[8] which has more recently been redefined as "the integration of best research evidence with clinical expertise and patient values."[11] This model represents a desirable approach to how clinical decisions should be made. However, we acknowledge that, at present, many clinical decisions are not made this way. For instance, at present, clinicians' individual preferences (as distinct from clinical expertise) often play a large role in their actions, leading to large "practice variations" in managing similar cases. For example, when faced with critically ill patients with identical circumstances, different clinicians may, according to their preferences, institute aggressive life-prolonging interventions or withdraw life support.[12] Our model acknowledges that patients' preferences should be considered first and foremost, rather than clinicians' preferences, whenever it is possible and appropriate to do so (i.e. the patient wants to be involved in the decision making and they have the capacity to understand the outcomes and their consequences when explained by their physician). Although this model may look static, clinical decision making commonly requires an iterative approach whereby decisions are re-evaluated to ensure that they are still appropriate as evolving information comes to light. Integrating clinical state and circumstances, patient preferences and actions, and research evidence requires judgment and clinical expertise, thus constituting an overarching element. We will describe each of the components of the model, and the role of clinical expertise in integrating them.

Clinical state and circumstances

A patient's clinical state and circumstances often play a dominant role in clinical decisions. Clinical trials provide us with results reflective of the average patient within the treatment groups of the trial. Rarely is a patient in clinical practice the same as the average patient from a clinical trial. Individual patients have unique characteristics that typically put them at lower or higher risk of the outcome or treatment side effect than the average patient in the trial. As such, optimal clinical decisions should be individualized to the patient's clinical state. If a patient is at very high risk of a future vascular event but at low risk of any complication from a drug (e.g. a patient with a low-density lipoprotein value of 8.0 mmol/L post myocardial infarction and no contraindication to statin therapy), or conversely at low risk of the outcome and high risk of a treatment's complications (e.g. a 40-year-old man with atrial fibrillation without any associated stroke risk factors who has experienced a major gastrointestinal bleed 2 weeks ago), the clinical state of the patient may dominate the clinical decision-making process.

It is notable that the circles of clinical state and circumstances and research evidence overlap. Frequently research evidence can inform us about the influence of the clinical state and circumstances. Considering our patient, the pooled data from five randomized controlled trials (RCTs) evaluating the efficacy of warfarin in patients with non-valvular atrial fibrillation (NVAF) demonstrated an average annual stroke rate of 4.5% and major bleeding rate of 1% in patients not receiving antithrombotic therapy.[13] The investigators who combined the five RCTs used the control patient data to develop a clinical prediction tool to estimate the annual risk of stroke. Independent risk factors that predicted stroke in control patients were increasing age, a history of hypertension, diabetes, and prior stroke or transient ischemic attack (TIA).[13] These trials likely exclude patients with a history of bleeding 11 months prior to enrollment and as a result we would not want to rely upon these trials to estimate our patient's risk of severe bleeding; however, we believe, and research suggests,[14] that the estimate of stroke from the clinical prediction tool (which takes into account age) is relevant to our patient even though he is older than the average patient in the trials. Using this model, our patient's annual risk of stroke is predicted to be about 8%, which is higher than that of the average control patient in the five RCTs whose annual stroke rate was 4.5%.[13]

A clinical prediction tool has also been developed for predicting the risk of major bleeding (defined as the loss of 2 units of blood within 7 days or life-threatening bleeding) while taking warfarin therapy.[15] Independent risk factors that predict major bleeding in patients taking warfarin include age >65, history of stroke, history of gastrointestinal bleeding, recent myocardial infarction, anemia, renal failure, and diabetes (note that many of the factors that predict a higher risk of stroke also increase the risk of bleeding). Our patient's annual risk of major bleeding of 8% also differs from that of the average patient receiving warfarin in the five RCTs whose annual risk of major bleeding was 1.3%. We are unaware of any clinical prediction tool for predicting major bleeding while taking aspirin and the atrial fibrillation trials had inadequate power to estimate this risk. The results of the meta-analysis by the antithrombotic trialists' collaboration suggest that aspirin increases the risk of major bleeding from 1% to at least 1.3%.[16] This likely is an underestimation in our patient who is older than the average patient who participated in the atrial fibrillation trials, and in this setting of suboptimal information we estimate our patient's annual risk of major bleeding is approximately 2% with aspirin therapy.

The clinical circumstances we find ourselves in (e.g. our ability to administer and monitor a treatment) may be very different from that of an RCT. For example, the patient may not be able to obtain frequent tests of the intensity of anticoagulation. However, for a patient with the same clinical characteristics, we can frequently optimize clinical circumstances to decrease the risk of an outcome or treatment side effect. For example, we can decrease the risk of bleeding due to warfarin therapy by more intensive monitoring to ensure that the international normalized ratio (INR) is maintained in the range of 2–3. Thus, an "evidence-based" decision about anticoagulation for a patient with atrial fibrillation is not only determined by the demonstrated efficacy of anticoagulation and its potential adverse effects,[17] but will vary based on the patient's clinical state and according to individual clinical circumstances.

Patients' preferences and actions

Patients may have no views or, alternatively, unshakable views on their treatment options, depending on their condition, personal values and experiences, degree of aversion to risk, healthcare insurance and resources, family, willingness to take medicines, accurate or misleading information at hand, and so on.[8] Accordingly, individuals with very similar clinical states and circumstances may choose very different courses of action despite being presented with the same information about the benefits, risks, inconveniences, and costs of an intervention.

For our patient with NVAF, research evidence informs us about the differing preferences of patients and their physicians for antithrombotic therapy in atrial fibrillation when they weigh the competing risks of stroke and bleeding.[18] In this study,[18] participants (i.e. both physicians and patients) reviewed flipcharts describing in detail the acute and long-term consequences of a major and minor stroke and a major bleeding event. Participants were instructed that the likelihood of a minor or major stroke was equal. The participants then underwent a probability trade-off technique which determined the minimum number of strokes participants needed to be prevented before they felt antithrombotic therapy was justified (this value was determined for both warfarin and aspirin), given the associated increased risk of bleeding, costs and inconveniences. The same technique was also used to determine the maximum number of excess bleeds the participant considered acceptable with antithrombotic therapy (determined both for warfarin and aspirin), given the benefits in terms of stroke reduction with this therapy. This study demonstrates significant variability between physicians and patients in their weighing of the potential outcomes associated with atrial fibrillation and its treatment. Patients required less stroke reduction and were more tolerant of the risk of bleeding than physicians. For example, on average, patients were willing to accept the risk of 17 extra major bleeding events in 100 patients over a 2-year period if warfarin prevented eight strokes among these 100 patients. Physicians, however, were only willing to accept 10 major bleeding events for the same level of benefit. Furthermore, physicians varied significantly among themselves in how much bleeding risk they thought was acceptable for a given stroke reduction associated with an antithrombotic agent. Hence different physicians would make very different recommendations to the same patient with identical risks of bleeding and stroke. This underscores the importance of having patient values and preferences drive clinical decision making. It is the patient who is at risk of the outcome and hence, when willing and able, they should be the one to weigh the potential benefits versus the risks, costs, and inconveniences.

There is debate regarding the optimal way to elicit and incorporate patient preferences into clinical decision making. One method is to discuss the potential benefits and risks with a patient and then qualitatively incorporate your impression of the patient's preferences into the clinical decision. Alternatively, at least two quantitative approaches exist: decision analytic modeling and probability trade-off technique. In a decision analytic model, a standard gamble, time trade-off or visual analog scale technique is used to determine the utility (patient value/preference) for the various outcomes. This information is then fed into a decision tree that includes the probabilities of the outcomes for all clinical decisions being considered. Using the decision tree, calculations are undertaken to determine what course of action optimally fits the patient's prefer-

ences. Probability trade-off technique presents patients with the probabilities for the various interventions being considered and then asks them to make a decision based on this information. This allows a direct and quantitative incorporation of the patient's preferences. The only study we are aware of that has directly compared these two quantitative approaches demonstrated that over twice as many patients stated they would base their preferences on the results of the probability trade-off as opposed to the decision analysis.[19]

Regardless of what their preferences may be, patients' actions may differ from both their preferences and their clinicians' advice.[20] For example, a patient may prefer to lose weight, quit smoking and take their medications as prescribed, but their actions may fall short of achieving any of these objectives. Alternatively, they may follow the treatment as prescribed, even if they resent its imposition, adverse effects, and costs. Unfortunately, clinicians' estimates of their patients' adherence to prescribed treatments have no better than chance accuracy.[21] Thus, physicians' decisions for care will better meet the model's specifications if they are able to assess whether their patients will follow, or are following, the agreed-upon decision.[21]

We recognize that at present formal incorporation of patients' preferences is rarely done in clinical practice. This may be related to lack of training of physicians in these approaches, a reluctance to tread unfamiliar ground, and also in many circumstances the lack of accurate quantitative information on risk and benefits as well as clinical risk prediction tools. However, this is likely to change as clinical models can be derived from large databases and hand-held computers can be utilized to quantitate risks and benefits at the bedside.

Research evidence

We support a very broad definition of research evidence, namely "any empirical observation about the apparent relation between events."[22] In keeping with this definition research evidence includes everything from the unsystematic observation of a single physician to a systematic review of large RCTs. Not all evidence is created equal and hence there exists a hierarchy of evidence that varies depending on whether one is addressing a diagnostic, prognostic or therapeutic decision. We will focus on the hierarchy of evidence for therapeutic decisions (Box 1.1).

All evidence has value and clinicians should give appropriate consideration to the best evidence available in the hierarchy, even if it is not at the top of the hierarchy. Therefore, the unsystematic observations of colleagues should not be dismissed when no higher level evidence exists. Indeed, unsystematic observations can lead to many important insights and experienced clinicians usually develop a respect for the insights of their astute colleagues.

However, it is equally important to recognize that unsystematic observations commonly are limited by the small number of observations, variability in outcomes, lack of objectivity, and the difficulties in integrating (e.g. taking into account the natural history of a disorder, placebo effect, and a patient's desire to please) and drawing inferences from observations.[23] Clinicians should also realize that even for the highly cited animal studies demonstrating a beneficial treatment effect and published in a leading scientific journal, only a minority will be confirmed in human trials.[24]

All evidence has limitations. Although the majority of advances in medicine are initially uncovered through individual observations, physiologic studies, observational studies or randomized controlled trials evaluating surrogate endpoints, there have also been several extremely misleading findings that have, at times, resulted in harm. It is important to remember that contradictory results across studies on the hierarchy of evidence table are not isolated to one or two instances (Table 1.1).

Perhaps the most powerful example is the story of antiarrhythmic therapy. Despite encouraging evidence that encainide and flecainide could prevent premature ventricular beats after a myocardial infarction, a large RCT demonstrated a higher mortality rate with these drugs compared to placebo, such that these drugs resulted in an extra death for every 20 patients treated with encainide or flecainide.[39] It is estimated that more Americans were killed by these drugs than died in the Vietnam War.[40]

Ideally we would have evidence from all levels of the hierarchy and the evidence would be coherent across all levels. This would represent the most persuasive evidence.

BOX 1.1 Hierarchy of evidence for treatment decisions*

Coherence of evidence from multiple sources
Systematic review of several well-designed, large randomized controlled trials
Single large randomized controlled trial
Systematic review of several well-designed small randomized controlled trials
Single small randomized controlled trial
Systematic review of several well-designed observational studies
Single observational study
Physiologic studies
Unsystematic observation from a physician
Animal study

This hierarchy is not meant to represent a rigid structure. At times a single observation may be very powerful (e.g. defibrillation for ventricular fibrillation) or observational studies may provide unequivocal evidence (e.g. smoking cessation and decreased risk of lung cancer). However, in most cases where treatment effects are likely moderate, outcomes variable or the clinical course unpredictable, clinicians may find the hierarchy proposed useful.

Table 1.1 Some examples of contradictory results across studies at various positions in the hierarchy of evidence

Results from lower level evidence	Results from higher level evidence
Milrinone demonstrated improvement in left ventricular function during exercise.[25]	A large RCT[26] and meta-analysis of several RCTs[27] demonstrated a 28% relative increase in mortality with milrinone compared to placebo.
An observational study of extracranial to intracranial bypass surgery suggested a "dramatic improvement in the symptomatology of virtually all patients" undergoing the procedure.[28]	A large RCT demonstrated a 14% relative increase in the risk of fatal and non-fatal stroke in patients undergoing this procedure compared to medical management.[29]
A meta-analysis of 16 cohort studies and three cross-sectional angiographic studies (including studies of women with known coronary artery disease) demonstrated a relative risk of 0.5 (95% CI 0.44–0.57) for coronary artery disease among women taking estrogen.[30]	A moderate size secondary prevention RCT did not demonstrate any reduction in coronary heart disease events but did demonstrate an increase in thromboembolic events in patients receiving estrogen.[31] A primary prevention RCT (Women's Health Initiative) of 16,608 women demonstrated that hormone replacement therapy increases the risk of coronary artery disease (hazard ratio (HR) 1.29), stroke (HR 1.41), pulmonary emboli (HR 2.13), and breast cancer (HR 1.26).[32]
A secondary analysis of an RCT suggested that lower doses of ASA were associated with a higher risk of perioperative stroke and death in patients undergoing carotid endarterectomy.[33]	A large prospective RCT showed a higher risk of perioperative stroke, myocardial infarction, or death with high-dose ASA.[33]
A physiologic study demonstrated beta-blockers result in a decline in ejection fraction and increases in end-diastolic volume in patients with prior myocardial infarction.[34]	A meta-analysis of 18 RCTs[35] and three large trials (CIBIS-2,[36] MERIT-HF,[37] and COPERNICUS[38]) in patients with heart failure found a 32% relative risk reduction in death in patients receiving beta-blockers.

However, this rarely happens as even RCTs by chance may frequently demonstrate contradictory findings, especially when they are small. Therefore, physicians should always aim for the highest level of evidence for clinical decision making. Clinicians can still make strong inferences particularly when there is evidence from a systematic review of several well-designed large RCTs or simply a large single pragmatic RCT. The RCT is such a powerful tool because randomization is our only means to reduce bias in treatment comparisons by controling for unknown prognostic factors.[41] Therefore, RCTs have the potential to provide the most valid (i.e. likelihood that the trial results are unbiased) estimates of treatment effect.[42] Furthermore, large RCTs with broad eligibility criteria enhance the generalizability of their findings.

A common error in interpreting evidence relates to the confidence clinicians should have in a study based upon statistical significance despite its size and number of events. Consider two hypothetical RCTs that are both evaluating the effect of a new investigational drug versus placebo on patient mortality in patients at risk of a myocardial infarction. Both of these trials use identical methodology (e.g. blinding, complete patient follow-up, intention-to-treat principle). The first trial randomizes 100 patients to receive investigational drug A and 100 patients to receive placebo, and fewer patients assigned the investigational drug die (1 versus 9 patients, $P = 0.02$). The second trial randomizes 4000 patients to receive investigational drug B and 4000 patients to receive placebo, and fewer patients assigned the investigational drug die (200 versus 250 patients, $P = 0.02$). Given that both trials used the same methodology and achieved the same level of statistical significance, some would assume we should view both results with similar confidence. This, however, is not the case.

Although the P values in our hypothetical trials suggest that the results have the same probability of representing a true finding, we propose that there is a substantial difference in the fragility of the demonstrated P values. In the first trial if we were to add two events to the treatment group the P value would become 0.13 whereas adding two events to the treatment group in the second trial would have no meaningful impact on the P value which would remain 0.02. When one considers that there are at least nine independent risk factors associated with myocardial infarction,[43] the prevalence of these factors in patients suffering a myocardial infarction varies from 18% to 65%, and many of these risk factors have substantially larger associations with myocardial infarction (e.g. odds ratio 2.87 for current smoker versus never) than the moderate effects that are plausible in interventional trials, it is not difficult to understand how the effect seen in our first hypothetical trial could have easily occurred due to an imbalance in risk factors, whereas the size of our second trial substantially minimizes the likelihood of a meaningful imbalance in prognostic factors that could explain the result of our second trial.

The number of participants and events that represents the transition from a small trial to a large trial is a matter of debate and ongoing investigation. It is important to recognize that the number of both participants and events is relevant. Some have argued that cardiovascular trials with event rates of 10% require at a minimum several thousand participants and at least 350 events and ideally 650 events to provide convincing evidence of a moderate size treatment effect (i.e. a relative risk reduction of 20–30%).[44] Indeed, if the true effect of size is a 15% relative risk reduction, studies with over 1000 outcome events may be required. In the case of a more prevalent outcome or the rare case of a true large treatment effect, fewer participants and events are required. We encourage clinicians when assessing evidence to not simply assume that a P value <0.05 represents a true finding but to consider the sample size, number of events, and the fragility of the P value and to exercise caution when making clinical decisions based upon data from small trials. Research demonstrates that highly cited studies in leading medical journals are not uncommonly contradicted (16%) or demonstrated to have exaggerated treatment effects (16%) in subsequent studies, and the only identified factor explaining this outcome is that the initial trial had a small sample size.[45]

Another issue clinicians have to consider regarding research evidence is the applicability to their current patient. If a patient fulfills most of the eligibility criteria from a trial then most physicians would view the evidence as applicable to their patient, assuming the trial is high quality. If a patient does not fulfill most of the eligibility criteria, we recommend that physicians ask themselves if there is a strong biologic reason to believe their patient would respond quite differently to the intervention from the patients who participated in the trial. As stated above, it is likely that most of the atrial fibrillation trials excluded patients who had a history of gastrointestinal bleeding within 11 months of randomization. Given this, we think the results from the atrial fibrillation trials regarding bleeding risk are not applicable to our patient, and this is why we used a clinical model based upon a study that included patients with a prior history of gastrointestinal bleeding to estimate our patient's risk of severe bleeding with warfarin. However, we do not have a strong biologic rationale to suspect that the stroke benefit demonstrated in the trials is not applicable to our patient, and research suggests that despite his age we can expect a similar benefit.[14]

Considering our case of the patient with NVAF, the highest level of evidence comes from a systematic review of all the RCTs that have evaluated antithrombotic therapy in patients with atrial fibrillation.[17] This systematic review included six warfarin versus placebo RCTs that included a total of 2900 patients and 186 strokes, and six aspirin versus placebo RCTs that included a total of 3337 patients and 376 strokes, and demonstrated that warfarin reduced the relative risk of stroke (ischemic and hemorrhagic) by 62%, and aspirin by 22%.[17]

Considering the risk of bleeding associated with warfarin therapy, there is an RCT of 325 patients with 25 major bleeding events that demonstrates a 50% decrease in the risk of bleeding if a patient is willing to undergo education, training, and self-monitoring of prothrombin time.[46]

Clinical expertise

Evidence-based decision making requires clinical expertise to establish and balance the patient's clinical state and circumstances, preferences and actions, and the best research evidence. Before a therapeutic decision can be considered, clinical expertise is required to get the diagnosis and prognosis right. As shown above, clinical prediction tools can be extremely helpful in determining a patient's prognosis but they are unlikely to eliminate the need for sound clinical judgment acquired through clinical experience.

Sizing up the clinical circumstances has never been more challenging, as commonly there exist several potential interventions, some of which require technical expertise for their effective and safe delivery. Getting the evidence right requires the skill to identify, evaluate, and apply the evidence appropriately. Communicating with patients has always been considered important. This takes on greater importance, given that there is a growing desire on the part of patients to be involved in decisions relating to their health.[47] Expertise is required to provide patients with the information they need, to elicit their preferences and to incorporate their preferences into the decision.

Currently there is no consensus on how this information should be presented to patients and how their preferences should be incorporated. However, research suggests that information should not be presented to patients in relative terms (e.g. warfarin will decrease your risk of stroke by 62%) because patients assume their baseline risk is 100% even when they are instructed it is not.[48] A recent systematic review of RCTs compared decision aids (i.e. interventions designed to help people make specific choices among options by providing information on the options and outcomes relevant to the patient's health) to traditional ways of involving/informing patients in decision making and demonstrated that decision aids, compared with usual care, improved average knowledge scores of patients for the options and outcomes by 20% (95% CI 13–25), reduced decisional conflict scores (i.e. patients felt more certain, informed, and clear about values in their decision), and increased patient participation in decision making.[49] Where available, decision aids provide a potential means to facilitate information presentation, incorporation of preferences, and participation in the decision making process.

The varying roles of the components of evidence-based clinical decisions

Depending on the circumstances, any of the circles in the new model could dominate. Varying the size of the circles to reflect their actual contribution to the clinical decision could visually portray this concept. Sometimes the clinical state or circumstance dominates the clinical decision. For example, a patient who is at very high risk of an outcome and low risk of a complication may have their clinical state dominate the decision-making process. A patient living in a remote area may not have access to anticoagulation monitoring and this would likely dominate the decision-making process. Patients' preferences can be so strong that they act as the driving factor in the decision-making process. For example, some patients will not take blood products regardless of the clinical situation. Research evidence can be the main factor in decision making when the benefit of an intervention is moderate to large in size and the risk of treatment small, as with ACE inhibitors in coronary artery disease or heart failure, or cholesterol lowering with statins. Finally, clinical expertise can dominate especially when it is related to technical capabilities.

Approach to decision making

We advocate a shared decision-making process between the physician and patient with both as active partners.[47] There is evidence to support better health outcomes when shared decision making occurs.[50] Considering a therapeutic decision, the physician must incorporate the clinical state and circumstances into the relevant evidence to help inform the patient and then elicit the patient's values regarding the potential benefits, risks, costs, and inconveniences associated with the intervention. If a patient chooses not to take an effective therapy that the physician believes is in the patient's best interest then the physician's role is to ensure that the patient's choice represents a difference in values (e.g. monetary concerns) as opposed to a misunderstanding about the probable benefits, risks, inconveniences, and costs. Regardless of a patient's wishes (e.g. CABG surgery in the setting of extensive coronary artery disease without graftable distal vessels, non-therapeutic use of narcotics) no physician is required to provide an intervention that they feel is unethical, illegal or not in the patient's best interest. Although more patients want shared decision making, some may choose to take a passive role in the decision-making process.[47] For example, a patient may ask the physician "If it were you or your loved one what would you do?" This question permits the physician to present an evidence-based background, the uniqueness of the clinical state and circumstances, and the doctor's explicit values associated with their recommendation. If a physician does this they will provide the patient with a helpful understanding of their recommendation, and if a patient disagrees they can then express their perspective. Finally, after making a decision it is important to ensure that the patient understands that even the best evidence-based decision does not guarantee the patient that they will not suffer a negative outcome.

Application to our patient

For our patient the evidence would suggest an annual 8% risk of stroke and 1% risk of major bleeding without any antithrombotic therapy. With warfarin therapy we would expect the annual risk of stroke to decrease to 3% and the risk of major bleeding to increase to 8%. This risk of major

bleeding could potentially be reduced to 4% if the patient was willing to undergo self-monitoring of their prothrombin time and an education program as discussed above; however, it is important to acknowledge that our confidence in this intervention is not strong as the results are based upon one small trial with few events.[46] With aspirin therapy we would expect the annual risk of stroke to decrease to 6% and the risk of major bleeding to increase to 2%.

As discussed above, there is no consensus on how to present this information to our patient or incorporate his preferences. The patient expresses that he would like to participate in the decision-making process and you then share with him a decision aid for patients with atrial fibrillation that describes atrial fibrillation (Table 1.2), a major and minor stroke (Table 1.3), a severe bleed (Table 1.4), and

Table 1.2 Atrial fibrillation: the most common disorder of the heartbeat

Risk	Chances of developing atrial fibrillation increase with age and it occurs in approximately 10% of all people above the age of 75
Physical Symptoms	Irregular and usually rapid beating of the heart, sensed as a fluttering in the chest. Some patients feel no symptoms and are unaware that they have atrial fibrillation
Complications	Stroke • Atrial fibrillation increases the risk of a clot developing in the heart. This clot can be swept up towards the brain, causing a stroke • The chance of developing a stroke with atrial fibrillation increases with either age greater than 65 years, high blood pressure, diabetes, heart failure, or a history of strokes or "mini-strokes" • The risk of developing a stroke with atrial fibrillation varies, depending on how many of these risk factors you have
Treatment	• There are medications that thin the blood, which help to prevent clots and therefore stroke • Because the blood is thinned there is an increased risk of bleeding

Table 1.3 Strokes can be minor or major in severity. If you have a stroke as a result of atrial fibrillation, your chance of having a minor or major stroke are equal

	Minor stroke	Major stroke
Physical symptoms	You suddenly cannot move or feel one arm and one leg	You suddenly are unable to move one arm and one leg You cannot swallow
Mental symptoms	You are unable to fully understand what is being said to you You have difficulty expressing yourself	You are unable to understand what is being said You are unable to speak
Pain	You feel no physical pain	You feel no physical pain
Recovery	You are admitted to hospital Your weakness, numbness and problem with understanding improve, but you still feel weak or numb in one arm and one leg You are able to do almost all of the activities you did before the stroke You can function independently You leave the hospital after 1 week	You are admitted to hospital You cannot dress The nurses feed you You cannot walk After 1 month of physiotherapy you are able to wiggle your toes and lift your arm off the bed You remain this way for the rest of your life
Further risk	You have an increased risk of having more strokes	Another illness will probably cause your death

Table 1.4 Severe bleeding while taking warfarin or ASA: an example of a stomach bleed

Physical	You feel unwell for 2 days, then suddenly you vomit blood
Treatment	You are admitted to hospital
	You stop taking warfarin or ASA
	A doctor puts a tube down your throat to see where you are bleeding from
	You receive sedation to ease the discomfort of the test
	You do not need an operation
	You receive blood transfusions to replace the blood you lost
Recovery	You stay in hospital for 1 week
	You feel well at the end of your hospital stay
	You need to take pills for the next 6 months to prevent further bleeding
	After that you are back to normal

Bleeding from the stomach is the most common type of serious bleeding while taking warfarin or ASA; however, rarely other serious forms of bleeding can occur, such as bleeding within the head after a fall.

Warfarin or ASA can also cause minor bleeding, including bruising and nose bleeds.

Taking warfarin can mean costs and inconvenience to yourself and family. For example: need for blood tests; parking/transportation; cost of warfarin.

Taking ASA can mean costs to yourself.

For example: cost of ASA.

Without any blood thinning medication
Chance of stroke over next 2 years
is ____ out of 100
Chance of severe bleeding over next 2 years
is ____ out of 100

ASA
Chance of stroke over next 2 years
is ____ out of 100
Chance of severe bleeding over next 2 years
is ____ out of 100

Warfarin
Chance of stroke over next 2 years
is ____ out of 100
Chance of severe bleeding over next 2 years
is ____ out of 100

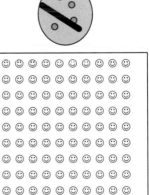 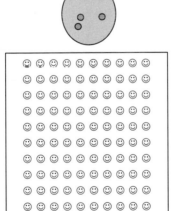 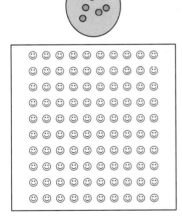

Figure 1.2 Patient decision aid.

a probability trade-off for no treatment, aspirin, and warfarin therapy (Fig. 1.2), which you individualize for him, filling in the specific numbers and coloring the faces relevant to his care. The description of major and minor stroke and a severe bleed are slight modifications of the descriptions developed and tested by Man-Son-Hing and colleagues.[51] After careful consideration of this information, our patient decides he wants to take warfarin therapy. He recognizes his increased risk of bleeding but places sub-

stantially more weight on avoiding a stroke than a severe bleed.

Once this evidence-based clinical decision is reached, our job is not over. The patient will need monitoring to ensure he is able to follow through on his clinical decision. One advantage of the decision aid provided (including his individualized probability trade-off) is that the patient can take the information home and does not have to rely on his memory to recall the facts discussed during your meeting.

Limitations of the evidence-based clinical decision model

This model does not consider the important roles that society, governments or healthcare organizations can play in decision making. We purposely restricted ourselves to decisions made by patients and their healthcare providers to allow a focused exploration of the issues involved in their immediate decision-making process. However, a healthcare organization may pre-empt these decisions. For example, not funding primary percutaneous transluminal coronary angioplasty in acute myocardial infarction can have an impact on health outcomes and will impose a clinical decision on all patients and physicians by eliminating this option. Alternatively, the system may fund preferentially, and at a higher level, a theoretically more attractive but more expensive and in reality no more effective therapy (e.g. dual-chamber pacemaker compared to single-chamber pacemaker for bradyarrhythmia) and this can distort the information presentation to patients, recommendations, and decisions made by physicians and healthcare providers. Physicians will have to factor in such issues when considering their patient's clinical circumstances.

Conclusion

The foundations for evidence-based medicine were established over the centuries but the specific philosophies, concepts, definitions, and models have essentially evolved over the past few decades. Evidence-based medicine is about solving clinical problems. Evidence-based decision making depends upon utilizing clinical expertise to integrate information about a patient's clinical setting and circumstances with the best research evidence while incorporating the patient's preferences and actions. Although there have been substantial advances throughout the last few decades, if evidence-based decision making is to achieve its full potential there is a need for further research to inform both the evidence base and the process of decision making. This chapter has provided an introduction to the concepts of evidence-based decision making, and subsequent chapters expand on the points we have discussed, describing different aspects of evaluating evidence and applying them.

References

1. Loius PCA. Researches on the effects of blood-letting in some inflammatory diseases, and on the influence of tartarised antimony and vesication in pneumonitis. *Am J Med Sci* 1836;**18**:102–11.

2. Loius PCA. Researches on the Effects of Bloodletting in Some Inflammatory Diseases and on the Influence of Tartarised Antimony and Vesication in Pneumonitis. Boston: Hilliard, Gray, 1836.

3. Louis PCA. Medical statistics. *Am J Med Sci* 1837;**21**:525–8.

4. Morens DM. Death of a president. *N Engl J Med* 1999; **341**(24):1845–9.

5. Lloyd JU. Who killed George Washington? *Eclectic Med J* 1923;**83**:353–6, 403–8, 453–6.

6. Marx R. A medical profile of George Washington. *American Heritage* 1955;**6**:43–47:106–7.

7. Pirrucello F. How the doctors killed George Washington. *Chicago Tribune Magazine*, 1977.

8. Haynes RB, Devereaux PJ, Guyatt GH. Clinical expertise in the era of evidence-based medicine and patient choice. *ACP J Club* 2002;**136**(2):A11–14.

9. Evidence-based medicine working group. Evidence-based medicine. A new approach to teaching the practice of medicine. *JAMA* 1992;**268**(17):2420–5.

10. Haynes RB, Sackett DL, Gray JM, Cook DJ, Guyatt GH. Transferring evidence from research into practice: 1. The role of clinical care research evidence in clinical decisions. *ACP J Club* 1996;**125**(3):A14–16.

11. Sackett DL, Straus S, Richardson SR, Rosenberg W, Haynes RB. Evidence-Based Medicine: How to Practice and Teach EBM, 2nd ed. London: Churchill Livingstone, 2000.

12. Cook DJ, Guyatt GH, Jaeschke R, Reeve J, Spanier A, King D *et al.* Determinants in Canadian health care workers of the decision to withdraw life support from the critically ill. Canadian Critical Care Trials Group. *JAMA* 1995;**273**(9):703–8.

13. Atrial fibrillation investigators. Risk factors for stroke and efficacy of antithrombotic therapy in atrial fibrillation. Analysis of pooled data from five randomized controlled trials. *Arch Intern Med* 1994;**154**(13):1449–57.

14. Evans A, Kalra L. Are the results of randomized controlled trials on anticoagulation in patients with atrial fibrillation generalizable to clinical practice? *Arch Intern Med* 2001;**161**(11):1443–7.

15. Beyth RJ, Quinn LM, Landefeld CS. Prospective evaluation of an index for predicting the risk of major bleeding in outpatients treated with warfarin. *Am J Med* 1998;**105**(2):91–9.

16. Antithrombotic Trialists' Collaboration. Collaborative meta-analysis of randomised trials of antiplatelet therapy for prevention of death, myocardial infarction, and stroke in high risk patients. *BMJ* 2002;**324**(7329):71–86.

17. Hart RG, Benavente O, McBride R, Pearce LA. Antithrombotic therapy to prevent stroke in patients with atrial fibrillation: a meta-analysis. *Ann Intern Med* 1999;**131**(7):492–501.

18. Devereaux PJ, Anderson DR, Gardner MJ, Putnam W, Flowerdew GJ, Brownell BF *et al.* Differences between perspectives of physicians and patients on anticoagulation in patients with atrial fibrillation: observational study. *BMJ* 2001;**323**(7323):1218–22.

19. Man-Son-Hing M, Laupacis A, O'Connor AM, Coyle D, Berquist R, McAlister F. Patient preference-based treatment thresholds and recommendations: a comparison of decision-analytic modeling with the probability-tradeoff technique. *Med Decis Making* 2000;**20**(4):394–403.

20. Haynes RB. Improving patient adherence: state of the art, with a special focus on medication taking for cardiovascular disor-

ders. In: Burke LE, Okene IS, eds. Patient Compliance in Health-care and Research. American Heart Association Monograph Series. Armonk, NY: Futura Publishing Co., 2001:3–21.

21. Stephenson BJ, Rowe BH, Haynes RB, Macharia WM, Leon G. The rational clinical examination. Is this patient taking the treatment as prescribed? *JAMA* 1993;**269**(21):2779–81.

22. Guyatt G, Haynes B, Jaeschke R *et al.* Introduction: the philosophy of evidence-based medicine. In: Guyatt G, Rennie DR, eds. Users' Guides to the MEDICAL LITERATURE. Chicago: AMA Press, 2002:3–12.

23. Nisbett R, Ross L. Human Inference. Englewood Cliffs, NJ: Prentice-Hall, 1980.

24. Hackam DG, Redelmeier DA. Translation of research evidence from animals to humans. *JAMA* 2006;**296**(14):1731–2.

25. Timmis AD, Smyth P, Jewitt DE. Milrinone in heart failure. Effects on exercise haemodynamics during short term treatment. *Br Heart J* 1985;**54**(1):42–7.

26. Packer M, Carver JR, Rodeheffer RJ, Ivanhoe RJ, DiBianco R, Zeldis SM *et al.* Effect of oral milrinone on mortality in severe chronic heart failure. The PROMISE Study Research Group. *N Engl J Med* 1991;**325**(21):1468–75.

27. Yusuf S, Teo KK. Inotropic agents increase mortality in patients with congestive heart failure. American Heart Association 63rd Scientific Sessions, November 12–15 1990, Dallas, Texas.

28. Popp AJ, Chater N. Extracranial to intracranial vascular anastomosis for occlusive cerebrovascular disease: experience in 110 patients. *Surgery* 1977;**82**(5):648–54.

29. EC/IC Bypass Study Group. Failure of extracranial-intracranial arterial bypass to reduce the risk of ischemic stroke. Results of an international randomized trial. *N Engl J Med* 1985;**313**(19):1191–200.

30. Stampfer MJ, Colditz GA. Estrogen replacement therapy and coronary heart disease: a quantitative assessment of the epidemiologic evidence. *Prev Med* 1991;**20**(1):47–63.

31. Hulley S, Grady D, Bush T, Furberg C, Herrington D, Riggs B *et al.* Randomized trial of estrogen plus progestin for secondary prevention of coronary heart disease in postmenopausal women. Heart and Estrogen/progestin Replacement Study (HERS) Research Group. *JAMA* 1998;**280**(7):605–13.

32. Rossouw JE, Anderson GL, Prentice RL, LaCroix AZ, Kooperberg C, Stefanick ML *et al.* Risks and benefits of estrogen plus progestin in healthy postmenopausal women: principal results from the Women's Health Initiative randomized controlled trial. *JAMA* 2002;**288**(3):321–33.

33. Taylor DW, Barnett HJ, Haynes RB, Ferguson GG, Sackett DL, Thorpe KE *et al.* Low-dose and high-dose acetylsalicylic acid for patients undergoing carotid endarterectomy: a randomised controlled trial. ASA and Carotid Endarterectomy (ACE) Trial Collaborators. *Lancet* 1999;**353**(9171):2179–84.

34. Coltart J, Alderman EL, Robison SC, Harrison DC. Effect of propranolol on left ventricular function, segmental wall motion, and diastolic pressure-volume relation in man. *Br Heart J* 1975;**37**(4):357–64.

35. Lechat P, Packer M, Chalon S, Cucherat M, Arab T, Boissel JP. Clinical effects of beta-adrenergic blockade in chronic heart failure: a meta-analysis of double-blind, placebo-controlled, randomized trials. *Circulation* 1998;**98**(12):1184–91.

36. CIBIS-II Investigators and Committees. The Cardiac Insufficiency Bisoprolol Study II (CIBIS-II): a randomised trial. *Lancet* 1999;**353**(9146):9–13.

37. The MERIT-HF Study Group. Effect of metoprolol CR/XL in chronic heart failure: Metoprolol CR/XL Randomised Intervention Trial in Congestive Heart Failure (MERIT-HF). *Lancet* 1999;**353**(9169):2001–7.

38. Packer M, Coats AJ, Fowler MB, Katus HA, Krum H, Mohacsi P *et al.* Effect of carvedilol on survival in severe chronic heart failure. *N Engl J Med* 2001;**344**(22):1651–8.

39. Echt DS, Liebson PR, Mitchell LB, Peters RW, Obias-Manno D, Barker AH *et al.* Mortality and morbidity in patients receiving encainide, flecainide, or placebo. The Cardiac Arrhythmia Suppression Trial. *N Engl J Med* 1991;**324**(12):781–8.

40. Moore TJ. Excess mortality estimates. In: Deadly Medicine: Why Tens of Thousands of Heart Patients Died in America's Worst Drug Disaster. New York: Simon & Schuster, 1995:281–9.

41. Kunz R, Oxman AD. The unpredictability paradox: review of empirical comparisons of randomised and non-randomised clinical trials. *BMJ* 1998;**317**(7167):1185–90.

42. Chalmers I. Unbiased, relevant, and reliable assessments in health care: important progress during the past century, but plenty of scope for doing better. *BMJ* 1998;**317**(7167): 1167–8.

43. Yusuf S, Hawken S, Ounpuu S, Dans T, Avezum A, Lanas F *et al.* Effect of potentially modifiable risk factors associated with myocardial infarction in 52 countries (the INTERHEART study): case-control study. *Lancet* 2004;**364**(9438):937–52.

44. Yusuf S, Collins R, Peto R. Why do we need some large, simple randomized trials? *Stat Med* 1984;**3**(4):409–22.

45. Ioannidis JP. Contradicted and initially stronger effects in highly cited clinical research. *JAMA* 2005;**294**(2):218–28.

46. Beyth RJ, Quinn L, Landefeld CS. A multicomponent intervention to prevent major bleeding complications in older patients receiving warfarin. A randomized, controlled trial. *Ann Intern Med* 2000;**133**(9):687–95.

47. Guyatt G, Montori V, Devereaux PJ, Schunemann H, Bhandari M. Patients at the center: in our practice, and in our use of language. *ACP J Club* 2004;**140**(1):A11–12.

48. Malenka DJ, Baron JA, Johansen S, Wahrenberger JW, Ross JM. The framing effect of relative and absolute risk. *J Gen Intern Med* 1993;**8**(10):543–8.

49. O'Connor AM, Rostom A, Fiset V, Tetroe J, Entwistle V, Llewellyn-Thomas H *et al.* Decision aids for patients facing health treatment or screening decisions: systematic review. *BMJ* 1999;**319**(7212):731–4.

50. Naik AD, Kallen MA, Walder A, Street RL Jr. Improving hypertension control in diabetes mellitus: the effects of collaborative and proactive health communication. *Circulation* 2008;**117**(11):1361–8.

51. Man-Son-Hing M, Laupacis A, O'Connor A, Wells G, Lemelin J, Wood W *et al.* Warfarin for atrial fibrillation. The patient's perspective. *Arch Intern Med* 1996;**156**(16):1841–8.

2 Obtaining incremental information from diagnostic tests

Raymond J Gibbons
Mayo Clinic, Rochester, MN, USA

Consider the following case history. A 75-year-old male presents with a history of exertional chest pain. The patient describes substernal chest pain that he perceives as a "pressure sensation" occurring when he walks too fast, uphill or in the cold. It is relieved by rest within a few minutes. On two recent occasions, he tried a friend's nitroglycerin tablets and obtained even more rapid relief of his symptoms. His symptoms have never occurred at rest. The patient has a history of diabetes mellitus, hypertension and hypercholesterolemia. He smokes one pack of cigarettes a day. Several male family members died of coronary artery disease before the age of 60. The patient underwent carotid artery surgery a year ago for treatment of transient ischemic attacks.

On the basis of his age, gender, chest pain description, and risk factors, this patient is highly likely to have significant obstructive coronary artery disease (CAD). The added, or incremental, value of any stress test for the diagnosis of the presence of disease in such a situation is very small. Out of 100 patients with this presentation, perhaps only one or two will not have obstructive CAD. The potential contribution of stress testing is therefore restricted to only these one or two patients.

This example demonstrates the importance of the concept of incremental value for diagnostic tests. In the current era of healthcare reform, it is no longer sufficient that a test simply provide "more information". The more appropriate current questions are:

- is it likely to influence clinical decision making?
- at what cost?
- will more informed decisions lead to better outcomes?

The demonstration of the incremental value of diagnostic tests requires rigorous methodology. The principles of the required methodology should be credited primarily to Dr George Diamond and his colleagues at Cedar Sinai Medical Center in Los Angeles.[1-3] First and foremost, such an analysis should reflect clinical decision making. Since clinical assessment is performed before any diagnostic tests, and usually at lower cost, parameters available from this assessment should be considered separately without any information from subsequent testing. The analysis should preferably focus on hard, demonstrable endpoints such as significant obstructive CAD, severe (three-vessel or left main) coronary artery disease, myocardial infarction or death. Although alternative endpoints, such as functional impairment, unstable angina, and the need for revascularization, are often included to increase statistical power, such endpoints have major limitations with respect to reversibility, subjectivity, and definite impact on patient outcome.

The analysis should create appropriate models that include all available important variables. An experienced clinician always takes the patient's age, gender, and history into account in making his or her clinical decision regarding patient management, even when testing results are available. These important clinical parameters must therefore be included in any final model that reflects the clinical decision-making process. The analysis must demonstrate that the additional information is statistically significant in an appropriate patient population. Analyses that demonstrate additional information in older, "sicker" inpatient populations should not be casually extrapolated to younger, "less sick" outpatients in whom testing is customarily performed. Finally, the test must provide information that is clinically significant and cost effective. In very large patient samples, differences that have little, if any, clinical significance for individual patient management may emerge as statistically significant. The potential impact on patient management in *some* patients must compare favorably with the incremental cost of the test in *all* the patients who must be tested.

This chapter will attempt to elucidate this methodology using the published data with respect to the diagnosis of significant obstructive CAD, non-invasive screening for

Evidence-Based Cardiology, 3rd edition. Edited by S. Yusuf, J.A. Cairns, A.J. Camm, E.L. Fallen, and B.J. Gersh. © 2010 Blackwell Publishing, ISBN: 978-1-4051-5925-8.

severe CAD, and patient outcome. All of these examples are drawn from the arena of ischemic heart disease, because this entity dominates clinical practice in cardiology, and the published literature is voluminous and extensive. However, the same principles apply to other disease entities, both cardiac and non-cardiac.

Clinical assessment

As outlined above, the initial step in any analysis designed to demonstrate incremental value is the consideration of all the information available prior to performance of the test. This will always include the results of the history and physical examination, and may sometimes include the results of other tests already performed. This section focuses on the information available from clinical assessment.

Diagnosis of coronary artery disease

As demonstrated by the earlier example, clinicians often encounter patients with chest pain and suspected CAD. The ability of clinical assessment to predict the likelihood of significant obstructive CAD has been demonstrated in numerous studies. The likelihood of significant disease based on clinical assessment is appropriately labeled the "pretest probability", in statistical terms.

Age, gender, and the patient's chest pain description are the most important clinical parameters for estimating the likelihood of CAD.[4] Older patients, men, and patients with chest pain that is typical, or classic, for angina pectoris are more likely to have coronary disease. Although multiple different systems have been used to classify chest pain, the simplest and easiest was proposed by Diamond.[5] He suggested a classification based on three elements – substernal location, precipitation by exertion, and relief by rest or nitroglycerin. If all three elements are present, the chest

pain is classified as "typical angina". If two elements are present, the chest pain is classified as "atypical angina". If only one or none is present, the chest pain is classified as "non-anginal chest pain".

Table 2.1 shows published estimates of pretest probability on the basis of age, gender, and chest pain description.[4] It is obvious that there is a very wide range of pretest probability, ranging from 1% for a 35-year-old woman with non-anginal chest pain to 94% for a 65-year-old man with typical angina. Note that a 50-year-old man with atypical angina has about a 50% probability of disease.

A more comprehensive attempt to consider all clinical characteristics, including risk factors for atherosclerosis, was published from the Duke University Medical Center databank.[6] In addition to the three parameters previously discussed, this analysis found that evidence for previous infarction, smoking, hyperlipidemia, ST and T wave changes on the resting electrocardiogram (ECG), and diabetes were all highly significant predictors of the presence of coronary artery disease. Figure 2.1 shows a published nomogram for men that incorporates all of these parameters. Careful inspection of this figure demonstrates that the impact of clinical parameters other than age, gender, and chest pain is variable. ECG and historical evidence of previous infarction have a major impact, diabetes and ECG ST-T changes have a modest impact, and lipids and smoking have a minimal impact. For example, a 50-year-old male with atypical angina has a 46% pretest probability of disease in the absence of smoking, hyperlipidemia or diabetes, a 48% pretest probability in the presence of both smoking and hyperlipidemia, and a 65% pretest probability if he has diabetes as well. In the presence of ECG Q-waves and a history of MI, his pretest probability exceeds 90%.

Recent evidence, particularly from the NHLBI-sponsored Women's Ischemic Syndrome Evaluation (WISE) Study,[7,8] has suggested that this traditional approach significantly underestimates the presence of obstructive CAD in women,

Table 2.1 Pretest probability of coronary artery disease

Age (years)	Pretest probability (%)							
	Asymptomatic		Non-anginal chest pain		Atypical angina		Typical angina	
	F	M	F	M	F	M	F	M
30–39	<1	2	1	5	4	22	26	70
40–49	1	6	3	14	13	46	55	87
50–59	4	9	8	22	32	59	79	92
60–69	8	11	19	28	54	67	91	94

From Diamond and Forrester.[4] Reprinted by permission of the *New England Journal of Medicine*, and Diamond GA.

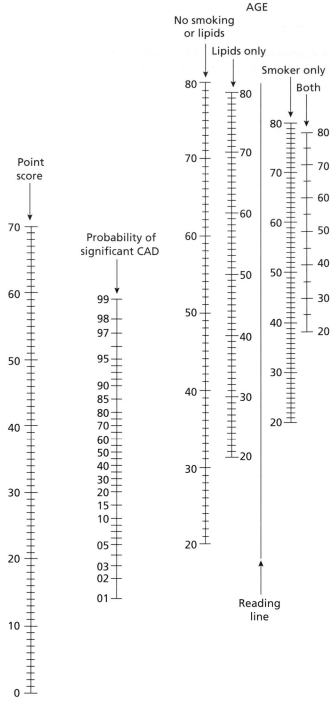

History – ECG
Point score

Angina – Typical – 26
Atypical – 10
Non-angina – 0

Previous MI
History only – 11
ECG Q waves – 12
Both – 30

ECG ST-T Changes – 6
Diabetes mellitus – 7

Directions for use

Step 1: Calculate the history ECG score and
locate point on left scale

Step 2: Using the appropriate age scale extrapolate
to the reading line for age (right scale)

Step 3: Place a ruler between the
point score and age (moved
to the reading line)

Step 4: Read off the probability of
significant CAD on the
center scale

Figure 2.1 Nomogram for predicting the probability of significant coronary artery disease (CAD) in men. ECG, electrocardiogram; MI, myocardial infarction. (After Pryor et al.[6]) Example: a 50-year-old, white male with atypical angina and diabetes mellitus, but no ECG ST changes, previous MI, smoking or hyperlipidemia. Point score on left scale = 10 + 7 = 17. Appropriate reading line on right labeled "no smoking or lipids". Connect age 50 on this reading line to point score of 17 with a straight edge. This intersects the middle line at 60, indicating that this is the percentage probability of significant CAD.

particularly younger women. Moreover, many women without obstructive disease continue to have symptoms and a poor quality of life.[9–11] Many of these have evidence of microvascular dysfunction.[12] There is a growing interest in the development of gender-specific tools for the assessment of ischemic heart disease in women, but the evidence is not yet robust enough to support the widespread use of a new approach.

Non-invasive screening for severe coronary artery disease

Not surprisingly, clinical parameters are also very important in estimating the likelihood of severe (three-vessel or left main) CAD.[13] The same parameters that are most important for predicting the presence of disease – age, gender, and chest pain description – remain important. In addition, diabetes mellitus and history or ECG evidence of myocardial infarction are also very important. The simplest approach to estimating the likelihood of severe disease was published by Hubbard *et al*.[14] They assigned one point each for: male gender; typical angina; history and ECG evidence of myocardial infarction; diabetes; and insulin use. Thus, the point score had a minimum value of 0 and a maximum value of 5. Figure 2.2 shows a nomogram for the probability of severe CAD based on age and this point score. It is quickly apparent that age is an extremely important parameter for predicting severe disease.

A more comprehensive analysis on a larger number of patients was published from the Duke University Medical Center databank.[15] In addition to the five parameters already mentioned, these workers found that the duration of chest pain symptoms, other risk factors (blood pressure, hyperlipidemia, and smoking), a carotid bruit, and chest pain frequency were also important determinants of the likelihood of severe CAD. However, the magnitude of their additional effect was modest.

Prediction of patient outcome

The ability of clinical assessment to predict patient outcome has been demonstrated in numerous previous studies. The largest and most important of these came from the Duke

University databank[16] and the Coronary Artery Surgical Study Registry.[17] Many of the same parameters that predict the presence of disease and the presence of severe disease are also associated with adverse patient outcome. Age, gender, chest pain description, and previous myocardial infarction all have independent value in predicting patient outcome. In addition, history and physical examination evidence for congestive heart failure, history and physical examination evidence of vascular disease, unstable chest pain characteristics, and other ECG findings, such as ST and T-wave changes, left bundle branch block, and intra-ventricular conduction delay, all have prognostic value. It is not generally appreciated how well clinical parameters perform in this regard. The Duke group reported that 37% of the patients undergoing stress testing at their institution had a predicted average annual mortality of 1% or less over the next three years, on the basis of clinical assessment.[17]

Several studies have shown that a normal resting ECG, and the absence of a history of prior infarction, predict a normal ejection fraction with 90% confidence,[18,19] and therefore a favorable prognosis.[20–22]

Approaches to the assessment of incremental value

Once the information available from clinical assessment (and other tests already performed) has been considered, there are a variety of conceptual and statistical approaches that can be employed to assess the incremental value of the test in question. This section will present examples of three such approaches.

Diagnosis of CAD

The application of multiple different stress tests for the diagnosis of coronary artery disease has been extensively studied. The most common approach used in this setting to demonstrate the incremental value of a new test employs Bayes' theorem.[23] This theorem indicates that the likelihood of disease following testing (post-test probability) can be calculated from the test characteristics (sensitivity and specificity) and the pretest probability. This calculated post-test probability is often plotted graphically as a function of pretest probability (Fig. 2.3).

In Figure 2.3, the pretest probability is shown on the *x*-axis and the post-test probability is shown on the *y*-axis. The dotted line represents the line of identity. The vertical distance from this line to the upper solid curve represents the increase in the probability of disease as a result of a positive test. In analogous fashion, the vertical distance from this dotted line to the lower solid curve represents the decrease in probability as a result of a negative test. The solid vertical lines describe three different clinical situations.

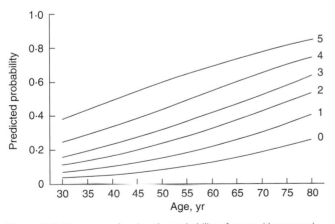

Figure 2.2 Nomogram showing the probability of severe (three-vessel or left main) coronary artery disease based on a five-point score. One point is awarded for each of the following variables – male gender, typical angina, history, and electrocardiographic evidence of MI, diabetes, and use of insulin. Each curve shows the probability of severe coronary disease as a function of age. (From Hubbard *et al*,[14] with permission.)

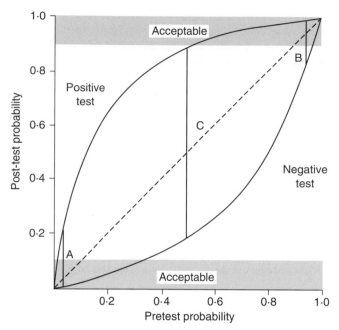

Figure 2.3 Relationship between pretest probability and post-test probability. The solid curves for positive and negative tests are plotted for a test with 80% sensitivity and a 90% specificity. Post-test probabilities that are acceptable for diagnosis (90% and 10%) are shown in the shaded zones. Line A represents a patient with a very low pretest probability; line B, a patient with a high pretest probability; line C, a patient with an intermediate probability. (Modified from Berman DS, Garcia EV, Maddahi J. Thallium-201 scintigraphy in the detection and evaluation of coronary artery disease. In: Berman DS, Mason DT, eds. *Clinical Nuclear Cardiology*. New York: Grune and Stratton, 1981, with permission.)

Line A represents a patient with a very low pretest probability, such as a 40-year-old woman with non-anginal pain. A negative test changes probability very little. A positive test increases probability somewhat, but the post-test probability remains well under 50%, and the test is most likely a "false positive".

Line B represents a patient with a high pretest probability of disease, such as a 65-year-old man with typical angina. A positive test will increase the probability only slightly. A negative test will decrease the probability of disease somewhat, but the post-test probability remains substantially greater than 50%, so that the test is most likely a "false negative".

The final situation (line C) represents a patient with an intermediate probability of disease, such as a 50-year-old male with atypical angina. A positive test in such a patient would increase the probability of disease substantially to near 90%. On the other hand, a negative test would decrease the probability of disease substantially to approximately 18%.

Thus, it is evident that the incremental value of diagnostic testing is greater in patients with an intermediate probability of disease, a principle that is broadly recognized.[23] However, it is also recognized that this kind of analysis has

a number of limitations. The single curves for positive and negative tests do not take into account the degree of test abnormality. The test results are therefore better displayed for a whole range of values for a parameter that helps distinguish normal from abnormal. The best known example of this would be the magnitude of ST segment depression on treadmill exercise testing.[24] In addition, multiple other parameters are reported during a treadmill exercise test, which help to distinguish severely abnormal tests from only mildly abnormal tests.[25] Ideally, all of these parameters would be incorporated into a single "score" and a series of curves would be plotted.

Next, construction of such curves relies on the premise that the sensitivity of tests will be identical for any population of patients with disease regardless of disease prevalence. This assumption is usually invalid. As demonstrated in the previous section, those parameters which help to identify the presence of disease also help to identify the presence of severe disease. In general, the sensitivity of most tests is greater in patients with more severe disease. It is therefore quickly evident that sensitivity would be expected to vary with the prevalence of disease. This point has been demonstrated by several investigators[26] and provides justification for the use of logistic regression analysis for diagnostic purposes.[27] Despite these limitations, Bayesian analysis serves as a useful framework for understanding the potential incremental value of diagnostic tests.

Post-test referral bias, also known as work-up bias or verification bias, occurs whenever the results of the test in question influence the subsequent performance of the "reference" test (sometimes referred to as the "gold standard"). This bias has been recognized for more than 20 years.[28] An early survey of the literature on exercise testing showed that only two of 33 studies avoided this bias.[29] The recognition of the importance of this phenomenon was emphasized in a landmark paper in 1983, which described the "declining specificity" of radionuclide angiography as a result of this bias.[30] Almost 20 years ago, a monograph from the Institute of Medicine emphasized this well-established concept.[31] The key question to ascertain whether postreferral bias is present is "did the results of the test being evaluated influence the decision to perform reference standard?".[32]

Although this bias potentially occurs for any diagnostic test, it is particularly important for non-invasive diagnostic tests for CAD. Patients with positive non-invasive tests are often referred to coronary angiography (the "reference" test). In contrast, patients with negative tests are often sent home without coronary angiography. The effects of this preferential referral to coronary angiography are to markedly decrease the observed specificity of the test in question and modestly increase its sensitivity.

The clearest solution to the problem of post-test referral bias is to avoid it completely by studying patients in whom the decision to proceed with the "reference" test is made before the performance of the diagnostic test in question.[31] For the diagnosis of CAD, this standard is incredibly difficult and rarely achieved. A more feasible alternative is the mathematical correction of sensitivity and specificity for post-test referral bias using one of two published formulae and information about all of the patients who were studied using the diagnostic test in question and did not proceed with coronary angiography.[33,34] There are a number of published studies demonstrating the effect of these corrections on the observed test performance for exercise electrocardiographic testing,[35] exercise echocardiography,[36] and exercise single photon computed tomography (SPECT) perfusion imaging.[37] Correction for referral bias markedly increases the specificity and modestly decreases the sensitivity of these tests. As a result, the predictive value of a positive test is improved, but the predictive value of a negative test decreases. It is generally difficult to confirm the validity of these corrections. However, a carefully designed prospective study of exercise echocardiography in women performed as part of the WISE study reported sensitivity and specificity values that were very close to those reported after correction for referral bias.[38]

Post-test referral bias has numerous important implications for the interpretation of the diagnostic literature.[38] Many of the reported sensitivity and specificity values are very likely to be erroneous.[38] Widespread misconceptions exist regarding gender differences in test performance. The post-test probability of CAD is higher for either a positive or negative test than that which would be calculated from Bayes' theorem using the reported values of sensitivity and specificity.[37]

Non-invasive screening for severe CAD

The incremental value of testing for the diagnosis of severe CAD has been studied using both Bayesian analysis and logistic regression analysis. When the latter analysis is conducted properly, all the previously discussed clinical parameters that are associated with severe coronary disease are incorporated into a model that is used to predict the probability of severe CAD. The output of such a model is a probability that ranges between 0 and 1. It is critically important that these candidate variables be "forced" into the model, even if they are statistically insignificant in the population under study. Most study populations are too small to have adequate power to detect the true significance of these variables, which has been demonstrated in very large subsets. For example, age should always be forced into such models, even if it does not appear to be significant in the particular population in question, because there is abundant evidence that it should always be considered (and indeed usually is by clinicians).

Using this approach, a second model should then be constructed which includes all the clinical parameters, as well as pertinent new parameters from the test in question. If these parameters have statistical significance independent of the clinical parameters, the test has incremental value. This approach is demonstrated in Table 2.2, which shows the improvement in the logistic regression model for severe CAD reported by Christian et al,[22] when the exercise test was added to clinical parameters, and when thallium imaging parameters were added to clinical and exercise parameters. Note that age and sex are both included in the clinical and exercise model (as well as the clinical, exercise and thallium-201 model). Magnitude of ST depression and (peak heart rate times peak systolic blood pressure) both added significantly to the clinical variables in the clinical and exercise model. An alternative approach is to construct the receiver operating characteristic (ROC) curves, which display sensitivity and specificity as a function of the predicted probability of severe disease (the output of a logistic regression model). The area under the ROC curve can then be compared between the model that incorporates clinical parameters and the model that incorporates clinical parameters and the new test parameters. Methods are available for determining the statistical significance of changes in the area under these two ROC curves.[39] An example of this approach is shown in Figure 2.4, taken from Christian et al.[22] The clinical significance of these differences in the models (assessed by either x^2 analysis or ROC curves) is discussed later.

Prediction of patient outcome

The demonstration of incremental prognostic value for diagnostic tests is obviously extremely important for clinical decision making. It requires strict adherence to the rigorous standards that were outlined previously. In general, very few of the published studies demonstrating prognostic value of diagnostic tests meet the strict criteria necessary to demonstrate *incremental* prognostic value for these tests. The statistical model most often used for this purpose is a linear proportional hazards, or Cox, model.[40] When strictly applied, all the previous information available to the clinician, from either clinical assessment or previous testing, should be incorporated into a linear proportional hazards model that predicts time to an event. Once again, parameters that have been clearly demonstrated in larger populations to be significant must be "forced" into such models to make sure that their contribution is not neglected. The events in question should preferably be hard endpoints such as death and myocardial infarction. As previously mentioned, unstable angina and the need for revascularization are alternative endpoints that are often included to enhance statistical power, but these have major limitations.

One of the earliest examples of a rigorously constructed analysis demonstrating incremental prognostic value of cardiac imaging was published by Pollock et al.[41] They tested the association between various combinations of

Table 2.2 Logistic regression multivariate analysis: prediction of three-vessel or left main (coronary artery) disease

Model	Direction	Odds ratio (95% CI)	P value
Clinical			
Diabetes mellitus	Present	2.0 (1.3–3.1)	0.001
Typical angina	Present	2.3 (1.4–3.9)	0.001
Sex	Male	3.2 (1.4–4.0)	0.007
Age[a]	Older	1.4 (1.1–1.9)	0.01
$x^2 = 31.3$			
Clinical and exercise			
Diabetes mellitus	Present	1.9 (1.2–3.0)	0.005
Typical angina	Present	1.9 (1.1–3.3)	0.02
Sex	Male	2.3 (0.9–5.3)	0.07
Age[a]	Older	1.2 (0.9–1.7)	0.16
Magnitude of ST depression	More	1.5 (1.3–1.8)	<0.001
Peak heart rate times peak systolic blood pressure[b]	Lower	0.9 (0.86–0.95)	<0.001
$x^2 = 65.0$			
Clinical, exercise, and thallium-201			
Diabetes mellitus	Present	1.9 (1.2–3.0)	0.004
Typical angina	Present	1.8 (1.1–3.2)	0.03
Sex	Male	2.2 (0.9–5.3)	0.07
Age[a]	Older	1.2 (0.9–1.7)	0.17
Peak heart rate times peak systolic blood pressure[b]	Lower	0.9 (0.86–0.95)	<0.001
Magnitude of ST depression	More	1.4 (1.2–1.7)	0.001
Global T1–201 score (delayed – after exercise)	Higher	1.1 (1.0–1.1)	0.02
$x^2 = 70.4$			

[a] Increments of 10 years (each 10-year increase in age increases the odds of severe disease 1.4-fold).
[b] Increments of 1000 units. From Christian *et al*,[22] with permission.

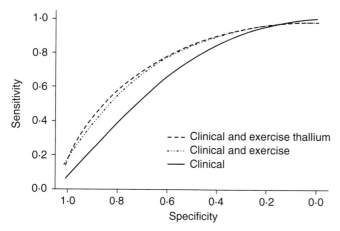

Figure 2.4 Receiver operator characteristic curves for three logistic curve regression multivariate models for the prediction of severe coronary disease. (From Chirstian *et al*[22] with permission).

variables and time to death or myocardial infarction, in a linear proportional hazards model using the x^2 statistic. Clinical and exercise variables were significantly better than clinical variables alone. Similarly, a model that added thallium redistribution to clinical and exercise variables was significantly better than the combination of clinical and exercise variables.

A subsequent rigorous analysis was reported by Christian *et al*[22] in patients with a normal resting electrocardiogram. Using a similar approach, these investigators reported that a model adding thallium variables to clinical and exercise variables did not add significantly to the model using clinical and exercise variables. In contrast, Kwok *et al*[42] performed a similar analysis on patients with non-specific ST-T abnormalities on their resting ECG. Exercise thallium variables added significantly to clinical and exercise variables in predicting patient outcome. The findings of Kwok *et al* may explain the positive findings reported by Pollock *et al*, as Pollock *et al* included many patients with abnormal resting ECGs in their study.

Pollock *et al*, Christian *et al*, and Kwok *et al* studied patients who were symptomatic with chest pain, and developed clinical models incorporating symptoms for their specific populations. In contrast, studies of asymptomatic populations should preferably use the Framingham risk score as a beginning clinical model, since it was developed and validated over decades in a population-based study.

Novel biomarkers such as high-sensitive C-reactive protein and brain natriuretic peptide identify asymptomatic individuals who are at increased risk for adverse outcomes such as death and myocardial infarction. However, when they were carefully assessed for their incremental value compared to the Framingham risk score, they added little (Fig. 2.5)[43] as measured by the concordance statistic.

In contrast, severe coronary calcification by computed tomographic (CT) scanning appears to add significantly to the Framingham risk score (Fig. 2.6), as reported by Greenland et al.[44] In particular, CT calcification may help identify patients with intermediate-risk Framingham scores who merit more intensive risk factor modification, although the ability of such an approach to improve patient outcomes has not yet been demonstrated.

Clinical significance and cost effectiveness

Even when statistically significant incremental value has been demonstrated for a diagnostic test using appropriate rigorous methodology, the clinical significance of the findings must be equally rigorously examined. The two fundamental issues that should be addressed are the actual impact of this incremental value on clinical decision making and, where possible, cost effectiveness. The available published data on diagnostic testing in coronary disease that will be presented here use only rudimentary concepts with respect to decision analysis. Formal cost analysis also requires understanding of a much greater body of published knowledge, which will not be presented here. The elementary examples presented here will only demonstrate the principle.

Diagnosis of CAD

The clinical significance of diagnostic testing can best be understood in terms of decision-making thresholds.[45] From the standpoint of diagnosis, a test will be useful primarily if it moves a significant number of patients from an "uncertain" pretest probability to an "acceptably certain" post-test probability. The exact criteria, or threshold, to be used in these classifications are clearly a matter of judgment; many investigators have chosen post-test probabilities of less than 10% and greater than 90% as criteria for definitive diagnosis.[36] Thus, non-invasive testing will be useful for diagnosis if it moves a reasonable number of patients into the shaded zone shown in Figure 2.3.

Although treadmill testing has clear incremental value for diagnosis, particularly in patients with intermediate pretest probability, as discussed earlier, its ability to move patients across such thresholds of probability appears to be very limited. Goldman et al[46] examined the ability of treadmill exercise variables to classify 329 patients with CAD. Their results are summarized in Table 2.3. The pretest model was very powerful, as it classified 84% of the patients correctly. Table 2.3 shows the number of additional patients classified correctly for given thresholds of probability. For example, if 10% was considered an acceptable threshold to "rule out" CAD, eight of 324 patients were moved across this threshold but only six were moved correctly. Similarly, for a 90% threshold to "rule in" CAD, 53 patients were moved across this threshold but only 33 were moved across

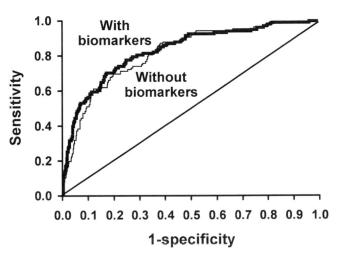

Figure 2.5 Receiver operator characteristic (ROC) curves showing sensitivity and specificity of Framingham risk score without novel biomarkers (dotted curve) and with addition of five novel biomarkers (solid curve) for five-year mortality. Although these curves were statistically different, the C (concordance) statistic increased only modestly from 0.80 to 0.82 with the addition of biomarkers. (From Wang et al,[43] with permission.)

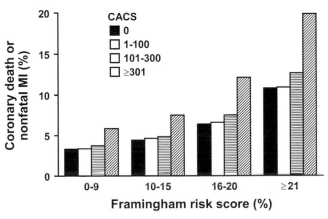

Figure 2.6 Rate of coronary death or non-fatal myocardial infarction (MI) over seven years in asymptomatic patients grouped by their coronary artery calcium score (CACS) and their Framingham risk score (expressed on the predicted rate of death or MI over 10 years). (From Greenland et al,[44] with permission.)

Table 2.3 Effect of treadmill exercise test results in moving patients across various diagnostic thresholds

Threshold probability	Patients moved across (n)	Correctly moved	Incorrectly moved	Net increase in diagnoses (correct/incorrect)
0.10	8	6	2	4
0.90	53	33	20	13
Either 0.10 or 0.90	61	39	22	17 (5%)

From Goldman et al,[46] by permission of the American Heart Association, Inc.

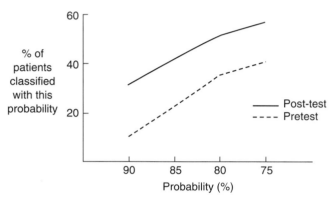

Figure 2.7 Percentage of patients classified with a given probability of coronary disease before and after exercise radionuclide angiography. The prospective study group of 76 patients excluded males of 40 years or older with typical angina. (From Gibbons et al,[47] with permission.)

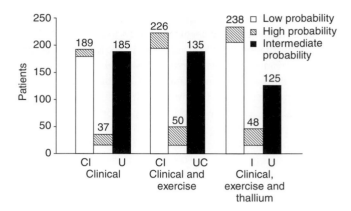

Figure 2.8 Correct (C), incorrect (I), and uncertain (U) classification of patients with three-vessel or left main coronary artery disease by the use of logistic regression multivariate models. Low, intermediate, and high probability defined using: clinical variables only; clinical and exercise variables; clinical, exercise, and thallium-201 variables. (From Christian et al,[22] with permission.)

correctly. As a result, the net total number of patients who were correctly moved into the diagnostic zone in Figure 2.3 was only 17, or 5% of the patient population. Thus, the clinical significance of the incremental value provided by the treadmill test appears to be very limited.

Similar rigorous analyses have been published for radionuclide angiography.[47] The results of one of these are displayed in Figure 2.7. The study group excluded men with typical angina over the age of 40 in order to eliminate most patients with a high pretest probability. Logistic regression models developed on a retrospective population were applied prospectively to a group of 76 patients. As demonstrated in Figure 2.7, eight (11%) of the 76 patients could be classified with 90% certainty on the basis of clinical variables alone. Following radionuclide angiography, 24 patients (32%) could be classified directly. Thus, the incremental value of exercise radionuclide angiography in moving patients across clinically meaningful decision thresholds appeared to be much greater than for the treadmill exercise test, as 21% of the patients were correctly classified by the radionuclide angiogram.

Similar findings have been reported for planar thallium imaging.[48,49] Unfortunately, no rigorous analyses are available for SPECT imaging using either thallium or sestamibi or both, primarily because post-test selection bias has greatly limited the feasibility of such studies in the current era.

Non-invasive screening for severe CAD

The same threshold approach has been applied to the non-invasive identification of severe CAD. Here the ability of tests to move patients across somewhat different thresholds of probability, as assessed by logistic regression models, has been tested. Christian et al[22] defined a low-probability group for severe CAD as <0.15, a high-risk group as >0.35, and an intermediate group as 0.15–0.35. These thresholds were chosen to correspond to earlier work from Duke University reporting on the utility of the early positive treadmill test.[50] Figure 2.8 shows the results that were obtained using this approach. Using clinical parameters alone, 189 patients (46% of the study group) were correctly classified as low or high probability. Thirty-seven patients (9%) were incorrectly classified as low or high probability. The remaining 185 patients (45% of the study group) had an intermediate probability, and were therefore in an uncertain category. The addition of exercise parameters correctly classified an additional 37 patients at the expense of 13 additional incorrect classifications, for a net of 24 additional correct classifications (6% of the study group). The addition of thallium parameters led to 12 additional correct classifications and two fewer incorrect classifications, for a net increase of 14 correct classifications (3% of the study group). These workers then used Medicare reimbursement figures to calculate the cost per additional correct classification. For exercise testing, the cost per additional correct patient classification was $1524. For thallium scintigraphy, the cost was $20 550 per additional correct classification.

Thus, this analysis demonstrated that the clinical impact was modest, and the cost was high, when thallium imaging was used in patients with a normal resting ECG to try to identify patients with severe CAD non-invasively. Although thallium scintigraphy clearly had statistically significant incremental value, it did not appear to be cost effective for this purpose.

Prediction of patient outcome

The issues of clinical significance and cost effectiveness are particularly pertinent to the application of diagnostic tests for the prediction of the patient outcome. These applications often involve relatively low-risk patient groups with few subsequent events. Tests applied to the entire population may identify a subset of patients who are at considerably increased risk compared to the remainder of the population.[51,52] These results will be highly statistically significant and generate very impressive P values and risk ratios. However, it must be recognized that the absolute rate of events often remains quite low in the patient subset at "increased" risk. Furthermore, the cost of this identification is often prohibitive when viewed on a per event or per patient basis.

This concept was nicely demonstrated in a study by Berman et al[53] on symptomatic patients with a low clinical likelihood of CAD studied by SPECT sestamibi. During 20 months of follow-up, only patients with an abnormal sestamibi study suffered death or myocardial infarction. This difference was statistically highly significant ($P = 0.007$). However, this increment in prognostic value was clearly not cost effective, as noted by the authors. Although the cost analysis by the authors was quite detailed, the cost ineffectiveness of this approach is readily apparent with very simple analysis. The 107 patients in the abnormal group suffered only three events during 20 months of follow-up. In order to identify the abnormal group, testing was required in 548 patients. Using a Medicare reimbursement figure of $700 per test,[22] more than $383 000 of testing would be required to identify the abnormal cohort. The cost of testing alone would therefore exceed $127 000 per possible event prevented. This simple analysis ignores the additional costs that would accrue from the subsequent cardiac catheterizations and coronary revascularizations that would be necessary in the high-risk group in order to attempt to prevent the three events. (There is obviously no certainty that the three events could actually be prevented by revascularization.)

Attempts to screen asymptomatic individuals to prevent subsequent CAD events are well intentioned but have similar limitations. "Targeting" individuals at "greater" risk will improve but not eliminate the problem. For example, Greenland et al demonstrated the incremental prognostic value of CT calcification in asymptomatic individuals with intermediate-risk Framingham scores.[44] However, they had to test 640 individuals to identify a subset of 118 with a calcium score of >300, who suffered 16 cardiac events (including an estimated 3 deaths) over seven years of follow-up. At $250 per CT scan, the cost of testing alone (without cardiac catheterization or revascularization) would exceed $10,000 per possible event prevented, and $50,000 per possible death prevented.

As a general principle, it should be recognized that non-invasive testing for the assessment of prognosis is far less cost effective in subsets of patients at intrinsically low risk.

Conclusion

Clinicians should recognize that an evidence-based approach to the evaluation of the incremental value of diagnostic tests is not simple or straightforward. Unfortunately, it is far easier for both clinicians and investigators to use simple, less rigorous, approaches that appear to demonstrate important incremental value for each new diagnostic test. Although convenient, such approaches lead to incorrect conclusions and generally overestimate the added value of each new testing modality. The examples presented in this chapter should provide a framework for thinking clinicians to more carefully evaluate new publications on new diagnostic tests. However difficult these analyses may be, and however disappointing the results, the escalating costs of healthcare demand an approach of rigorous methodology and thoughtful analysis to make certain that the *incremental* value of a diagnostic test is not only statistically significant, but clinically significant and cost effective.

References

1. Diamond G. Penny wise. *Am J Cardiol* 1988;**62**:806–8.
2. Bobbio M, Pollock BH, Cohen I, Diamond GA. Comparative accuracy of clinical tests for diagnosis and prognosis of coronary artery disease. *Am J Cardiol* 1988;**62**:896–900.
3. Ladenheim ML, Kotler TS, Pollock BH, Berman DS, Diamond GA. Incremental prognostic power of clinical history, exercise electrocardiography and myocardial perfusion scintigraphy in suspected coronary artery disease. *Am J Cardiol* 1987;**59**: 270–7.
4. Diamond GA, Forrester JS. Analysis of probability as an aid in the clinical diagnosis of coronary artery disease. *N Engl J Med* 1979;**300**:1350–8.
5. Diamond GA. Letter: a clinical relevant classification of chest discomfort. *J Am Coll Cardiol* 1983;**1**:574–5.

6. Pryor DB, Harrell FE Jr, Lee KL, Califf RM, Rosati RA. Estimating the likelihood of significant coronary artery disease. *Am J Med* 1983;**75**:771–80.

7. Shaw LJ, Bairey Merz CN, Pepine CJ *et al.* Insights from the NHLBI-Sponsored Women's Ischemia Syndrome Evaluation (WISE) Study: Part I: gender differences in traditional and novel risk factors, symptom evaluation, and gender-optimized diagnostic strategies. *J Am Coll Cardiol* 2006;**47**(3 suppl):S4–S20.

8. Bairey Merz CN, Shaw LJ, Reis SE *et al.* Insights from the NHLBI-Sponsored Women's Ischemia Syndrome Evaluation (WISE) Study: Part II: gender differences in presentation, diagnosis and outcome with regard to gender-based pathophysiology of atherosclerosis and macrovascular and microvascular coronary disease. *J Am Coll Cardiol* 2006:**47**(3 suppl):S21–9.

9. Johnson BD, Shaw LJ, Pepine CJ *et al.* Persistent chest pain predicts cardiovascular events in women without obstructive coronary artery disease: results from the NIH-NHLBI-sponsored Women's Ischaemia Syndrome Evaluation (WISE) study. *Eur Heart J* 2006;**27**(12):1387–9.

10. Marroquin OC, Kip KE, Mulukutla SR *et al.* Inflammation, endothelial cell activation, and coronary microvascular dysfunction in women with chest pain and no obstructive artery disease. *Am Heart J* 200;**1501**:109–15.

11. Shaw LJ, Merz CN, Pepine CJ *et al.* The economic burden of angina in women with suspected ischemic heart disease: results from the National Institutes of Health, National Heart, Lung, and Blood Institute sponsored Women's Ischemia Syndrome Evaluation. *Circulation* 2006;**114**(9):894–904.

12. Johnson BD, Shaw LJ, Pepine CJ *et al.* Women and cardiovascular heart disease: clinical implications from the Women's Ischemia Syndrome Evaluation (WISE) Study. Are we smarter? *J Am Coll Cardiol* 2006;**47**(3 suppl):S59–62.

13. Weiner DA, McCabe CH, Ryan TJ. Identification of patients with left main and three vessel coronary disease with clinical and exercise test variables. *Am J Cardiol* 1980;**46**:21–7.

14. Hubbard BL, Gibbons RJ, Lapeyre AC, Zinsmeister AR, Clements IP. Identification of severe coronary artery disease using simple clinical parameters. *Arch Intern Med* 1992;**152**: 309–12.

15. Pryor DB, Shaw L, Harrell FE Jr *et al.* Estimating the likelihood of severe coronary artery disease. *Am J Med* 1991;**90**:553–62.

16. Pryor DB, Shaw L, McCants CB *et al.* Value of the history and physical in identifying patients at increased risk for coronary artery disease. *Ann Intern Med* 1993;**118**:81–90.

17. Weiner DA, Ryan TJ, McCabe CH *et al.* The role of exercise testing in identifying patients with improved survival after coronary artery bypass surgery. *J Am Coll Cardiol* 1986;**8**:741–8.

18. O'Keefe JH Jr, Zinsmeister AR, Gibbons RJ. Value of electrocardiographic findings in predicting rest left ventricular function in patients with chest pain and suspected coronary artery disease. *Am J Med* 1989;**86**:658–62.

19. Rihal CS, Davis KB, Kennedy JW, Gersh BJ. The utility of clinical, electrocardiographic, and roentgenographic variables in the prediction of left ventricular function. *Am J Cardiol* 1995;**75**:220–3.

20. Connolly DC, Elveback LR, Oxman HA. Coronary heart disease in residents of Rochester, Minnesota. IV. Prognostic value of the resting electrocardiogram at the time of initial diagnosis of angina pectoris. *Mayo Clin Proc* 1984;**59**:247–50.

21. Gibbons RJ, Zinsmeister AR, Miller TD, Clements IP. Supine exercise electrocardiography compared with exercise radionuclide angiography in noninvasive identification of severe coronary artery disease. *Ann Intern Med* 1990;**112**:743–9.

22. Christian TF, Miller TD, Bailey KR, Gibbons RJ. Exercise tomographic thallium-201 imaging in patients with severe coronary artery disease and normal electrocardiogram. *Ann Intern Med* 1994;**121**:825–32.

23. Epstein SE. Implications of probability analysis on the strategy used for noninvasive detection of coronary artery disease. *Am J Cardiol* 1980;**46**:491–9.

24. Rifkin RD, Hood WB Jr. Bayesian analysis of electrocardiographic exercise stress testing. *N Engl J Med* 1977;**297**:681–6.

25. Cohn K, Kamm B, Feteih N, Brand R, Goldschlager N. Use of treadmill score to quantify ischemic response and predict extent of coronary disease. *Circulation* 1979;**59**:286–96.

26. Currie PJ, Kelly MJ, Harper RW *et al.* Incremental value of clinical assessment, supine exercise electrocardiography, and biplane exercise radionuclide ventriculography in the prediction of coronary artery disease in men with chest pain. *Am J Cardiol* 1983;**52**:927–35.

27. Morise AP, Detrano R, Bobbio M, Diamond GA. Development and validation of a logistic regression-derived algorithm for estimating the incremental probability of coronary artery disease before and after exercise testing. *J Am Coll Cardiol* 1992;**20**:1187–96.

28. Ransohoff DF, Feinstein AR. Problems of spectrum and bias in evaluating the efficacy of diagnostic tests. *N Engl J Med* 1978;**299**:926–30.

29. Philbrick JT, Horwitz RI, Feinstein AR. Methodologic problems of exercise testing for coronary artery disease: groups, analysis and bias. *Am J Cardiol* 1980;**46**:807–12.

30. Rozanski A, Diamond GA, Berman D, Forrester JS, Morris D, Swan HJC. The declining specificity of exercise radionuclide ventriculography. *N Engl J Med* 1983;**309**:518–22.

31. Council on Health Care Technology, Institute of Medicine. *Assessment of Diagnostic Technology in Health Care.* Washington, DC: National Academy Press, 1989.

32. Jaeschke R, Guyatt G, Sackett DL. Users' guides to the medical literature. *JAMA* 1994;**271**:389–91.

33. Diamond GA. An alternative factor affecting sensitivity and specificity of exercise electrocardiology (editorial). *Am J Cardiol* 1986;**57**:1175–80.

34. Begg CB, Greenes RA. Assessment of diagnostic tests when disease verification is subject to selection bias. *Biometrics* 1983;**39**:207–15.

35. Morise AP, Diamond GA. Comparison of the sensitivity and specificity of exercise electrocardiography in biased and unbiased populations of men and women. *Am Heart J* 1995;**130**:741–7.

36. Roger VL, Pellikka PA, Bell MR, Chow CWH, Bailey KR, Seward JB. Sex and test verification bias: impact on the diagnostic value of exercise echocardiology. *Circulation* 1997;**95**:405–10.

37. Miller TD, Hodge DO, Christian TF, Milavetz JJ, Bailey KR, Gibbons RJ. Effects on adjustment for referral bias on the sensitivity of specificity of single photon emission computed tomography for the diagnosis of coronary artery disease. *Am J Med* 2002;**112**:290–7.

38. Gibbons RJ, Chatterjee K, Daley J *et al.* ACC/AHA/ACP-ASIM guidelines for the management of patients with chronic

stable angina: a report of the American College of Cardiology/American Heart Association Task Force on Practice Guidelines (Committee on the Management of Patients With Chronic Stable Angina). *J Am Coll Cardiol* 1999;**33**:2092–7.

39. Wieand S, Gail M, James K, James B. A family of non-parametric statistics for comparing diagnostic tests with paired or unpaired data. *Biometrika* 1989;**76**:585–92.

40. Cox DR. Regression models and life tables. *J R Stat Soc B* 1972;**34**:197–220.

41. Pollock SG, Abbott RD, Boucher CA, Beller GA, Kaul S. Independent and incremental prognostic value of tests performed in hierarchical order to evaluate patients with suspected coronary artery disease. Validation of models based on these tests. *Circulation* 1992;**85**:237–48.

42. Kwok JM, Christian TF, Miller TD *et al.* Incremental prognostic value of exercise single-photon emission computed tomographic (SPECT) thallium 201 imaging in patients with ST-T abnormalities on their resting electrocardiograms. *Am Heart J* 2005; **149**(1):145–51.

43. Wang TJ, Gona P, Larson MG *et al.* Multiple biomarkers for the prediction of first major cardiovascular events and death. *N Engl Med* 2006;**355**:2631–9.

44. Greenland P, LaBree L, Azen SP *et al.* Coronary artery calcium score combined with framingham score for risk prediction in asymptomatic individuals. *JAMA* 2004;**291**(2):210–15.

45. Diamond GA, Forrester JS, Hirsch M *et al.* Application of conditional probability analysis to the clinical diagnosis of coronary artery disease. *J Clin Invest* 1980;**65**:1210–21.

46. Goldman L, Cook EF, Mitchell N *et al.* Incremental value of the exercise test for diagnosing the presence or absence of coronary artery disease. *Circulation* 1982;**66**:945–53.

47. Gibbons RJ, Lee KL, Pryor DB *et al.* The use of radionuclide angiography in the diagnosis of coronary artery disease: a logistic regression analysis. *Circulation* 1983;**68**:740–6.

48. Detrano R, Yiannikas J, Salcedo EE *et al.* Bayesian probability analysis: a prospective demonstration of its clinical utility in diagnosing coronary disease. *Circulation* 1984;**69**: 541–7.

49. Melin JA, Wijns W, Vanbutsele RJ *et al.* Alternative diagnostic strategies for coronary artery disease in women: demonstration of the usefulness and efficiency of probability analysis. *Circulation* 1985;**71**:535–42.

50. McNeer JF, Margolis JR, Lee KL *et al.* The role of the exercise test in the evaluation of patients for ischemic heart disease. *Circulation* 1978;**57**:64–70.

51. Rautaharju PM, Prineas RJ, Eifler WJ *et al.* Prognostic value of exercise electrocardiogram in men at high risk of future coronary heart disease: multiple risk factor intervention trial experience. *J Am Coll Cardiol* 1986;**8**:1–10.

52. Giagnoni E, Secchi MB, Wu SC *et al.* Prognostic value of exercise EKG testing in asymptomatic normotensive subjects: a prospective matched study. *N Engl J Med* 1983;**309**:1085–9.

53. Berman DS, Hachamovitch R, Hosen K *et al.* Incremental value of prognostic testing in patients with known or suspected ischemic heart disease: a basis for optimal utilization of exercise technetium-99 m sestamibi myocardial perfusion single-photon emission computed tomography. *J Am Coll Cardiol* 1995;**26**:639–47.

3 Clinical trials and meta-analysis

Jonathan R Emberson and Colin Baigent
Clinical Trial Service Unit, Oxford, UK

Introduction

Although large effects on survival arising from certain treatments may occasionally be obvious from simple observation (as, for example, when cardioversion for ventricular fibrillation avoids otherwise certain death), the vast majority of interventions have only moderate effects on major outcomes and hence are impossible to evaluate without careful study. Unfortunately, enthusiasm for the biologic foundations of a particular therapeutic approach often leads to exaggerated hopes for the effects of treatment on major clinical outcomes. These hopes may be based on dramatic laboratory measures of efficacy or on the types of surrogate outcome that are commonly studied before drugs go into Phase III or IV studies; for example, a drug may almost completely prevent experimental ischemia progressing to infarction or practically abolish experimental thrombosis. However, these large effects on surrogate endpoints very rarely translate into large effects on major clinical outcomes; the overwhelming message from over three decades of clinical trials in cardiology is that the net effects of most treatments are typically moderate in size. This chapter explains why large-scale randomized evidence, either in a single "mega-trial" or in a meta-analysis of similar trials, is generally an absolute requirement if such moderate effects on major outcomes are to be characterized reliably.

It is important to appreciate that progress in cardiologic practice, and in the prevention of cardiovascular disease, has been and remains dependent on the availability of large-scale randomized trials and of appropriately large-scale meta-analyses of such trials. In the management and prevention of acute myocardial infarction (MI), for example, these methods have helped to demonstrate that fibrinolytic

therapy,[1–4] aspirin,[2,4,5] blood pressure-lowering treatments,[6] and statins[7,8] all produce net benefits which, although individually moderate in size, have together produced a substantial improvement in the prognosis of acute MI. Similarly, the demonstration that angiotensin-converting enzyme (ACE) inhibitors and beta-blockers produce moderate reductions in the risk of death, cardiovascular disease and rates of hospitalization for worsening heart failure[9,10] has improved the outcome of patients with chronic heart failure.

Clinical trials: minimizing biases and random errors

Any clinical study whose main objective is to assess moderate treatment effects must ensure that any biases and any random errors that are inherent in its design are both substantially smaller than the effect to be measured.[11] Biases in the assessment of treatment can be produced by differences between randomized arms in factors other than the treatment under consideration. Observational (that is, nonrandomized) studies, in which the outcome is compared between individuals who received the treatment of interest and those who did not, can be subject to large biases.[12] Avoidance of biases can only be guaranteed by proper randomized allocation of treatment, blinded outcome assessment and appropriate statistical analysis, with no unduly data-dependent emphasis on specific subsets of the overall evidence (Box 3.1).[11,13]

Avoidance of moderate biases

Proper randomization to prevent foreknowledge of treatment allocation

The fundamental reason for random allocation of treatment in clinical trials is to maximize the likelihood that each type of patient will have been allocated in similar proportions to the different treatment strategies being investigated.[14] A key requirement is that treatment allocation should be con-

Evidence-Based Cardiology, 3rd edition. Edited by S. Yusuf, J.A. Cairns, A.J. Camm, E.L. Fallen, and B.J. Gersh. © 2010 Blackwell Publishing, ISBN: 978-1-4051-5925-8.

1. Negligible biases (that is, guaranteed avoidance of MODERATE biases)
   - Proper randomization (non-randomized methods cannot guarantee the avoidance of moderate biases)
   - BLINDING of treatment allocation, if feasible, and of outcome assessment
   - Analysis by ALLOCATED treatments (that is, an "intention-to-treat" analysis)
   - Chief emphasis on OVERALL results (with no unduly data-derived subgroup analyses)
   - Systematic META-ANALYSIS of all the relevant randomized trials (with no unduly data-dependent emphasis on the results from particular studies)
2. Small random errors (that is, guaranteed avoidance of MODERATE random errors)
   - LARGE NUMBERS OF EVENTS (with minimal data collection as detailed statistical analyses of masses of data on prognostic features generally add little to the effective size of a trial)
   - Systematic META-ANALYSIS of all the relevant randomized trials

cealed at the point of randomization since, if the next treatment allocation can be deduced by those entering patients, decisions about whether to enter a patient may be affected and, as a result, those allocated one treatment might differ systematically from those allocated another.[15] For example, in the Captopril Prevention Project (CAPPP) trial,[16] envelopes containing the antihypertensive treatment allocation could be opened before patients were irreversibly entered into the study. Highly significant differences in pre-entry blood pressure between the treatment groups, which were too large to have been due to chance, may well have been the result of this design weakness.[17] Proper randomization therefore requires that trial procedures are organized in a way that ensures that the decision to enter a patient is made irreversibly and without knowledge of the trial treatment to which a patient will be allocated. Once randomized, it is also generally desirable to "blind" both the patient and their doctor (whenever feasible) to the allocated treatment, for reasons discussed below.

Blinding of treatment allocation and of outcome assessment

While randomization should ensure a valid, i.e. unbiased, assessment of the effectiveness of a study drug, substantial bias can still be introduced if there is the potential for subjective judgment in the reporting, evaluation or data processing of clinical events (particularly when such judgments are made with knowledge, or suspected knowledge, of the treatment allocation) or if patients or their doctors are themselves aware of the treatment to which they have been randomized (since their subsequent healthcare and health behaviors may differ systematically from the comparison group in a way that influences clinical outcomes). Patients (and their doctors) should therefore be blinded to the randomized treatment wherever possible and, critically, study outcomes should be evaluated by people who are *unaware of the allocated treatment*.

Of course, some drugs may produce characteristic side effects which cannot effectively be hidden from a doctor or, indeed, from a well-informed patient. In some types of trials it may be impossible to blind a patient to the treatment received (e.g. surgical intervention trials). Moreover, even when blinding of patients and doctors is theoretically possible, in some circumstances it could act as a barrier to the practical feasibility of the study through the introduction of unnecessary complications and cost (for instance, in a trial where the doses of different study drugs need to be adjusted during the follow-up period). To overcome such problems, PROBE[18] (Prospective Randomized Open-label Blinded Endpoint) study designs are increasingly being employed (e.g. in the Anglo-Scandinavian Cardiac Outcomes Trial (ASCOT)[19] and the Incremental Decrease in Endpoints through Aggressive Lipid lowering (IDEAL) study[20]). The key feature of a PROBE design is that patients are aware of the study medication to which they have been randomized, as are their doctors. (It is important to note that, while patients and their doctors are unblinded to treatment allocation in a PROBE trial, it remains critically important that randomization procedures prevent foreknowledge of the next treatment to be allocated, and that outcome assessors are blinded to study allocation.) A potential for bias exists, however, if knowledge of a patient's study medication results in any differential reporting of study outcomes by study staff or differential use of concomitant drugs. This can be largely mitigated by the use of clearly defined and verifiable outcomes, blinded outcome adjudication and various means of evaluation of all or a random subset of patients to assess whether events have been missed, and whether any "missingness" is differential. The potential advantages of PROBE designs include their reduced cost and their similarity to standard clinical practice. However, it is important that these benefits are not achieved at the expense of moderate biases in estimates of treatment effects.

Intention-to-treat analyses

Even when studies have been properly randomized and blinded, moderate biases can still be introduced by inappropriate analysis or interpretation. This can happen, for example, if patients are excluded after randomization, particularly when the prognosis of the excluded patients in one treatment group differs from that in the other (such as might occur, for example, if non-compliant participants were excluded after randomization). This point is well illustrated by the Coronary Drug Project,[21] which compared clofibrate versus placebo among around 5000 patients with a history of coronary heart disease. In this study, patients who took at least 80% of their allocated clofibrate ("good compliers") had substantially lower five-year mortality than "poor compliers", who did not (15.0% vs 24.6% respectively; $P = 0.0001$). However, there was a similar difference in outcome between good and poor compliers in the placebo group (15.1% vs 28.3%; $P < 0.00001$), suggesting that good and poor compliers were prognostically different even after allowing for any benefits of actually taking clofibrate.[21] Under the null hypothesis of no treatment effect, the least biased assessment of the treatment effect is that which compares all those allocated to one treatment versus all those allocated to the other (that is, an "intention-to-treat" analysis), irrespective of what treatment they actually received.[22]

Because some degree of non-compliance with allocated treatments may be unavoidable in randomized trials, intention-to-treat analyses will tend to underestimate the effects produced by full compliance. However, "on treatment" (or "per protocol") analyses, which estimate treatment effects through analyses of compliant patients, are potentially biased; it is more appropriate to calculate an "adjustment" based on the level of compliance and then to apply this to the estimate of the treatment effect provided by the intention-to-treat comparison.[23] For example, in a meta-analysis of the randomized trials of prolonged use of antiplatelet therapy among patients with occlusive vascular disease, the average compliance one year after treatment allocation seemed to be around 80%.[24] Application of this estimate of compliance to the proportional reduction of about 30% in non-fatal MI and stroke estimated from intention-to-treat analyses of these trials suggests that full compliance with antiplatelet therapy might produce reductions in risk of about 35–40%.

Inappropriate use and interpretation of subgroup analyses

In the medical literature a particularly important source of bias is unduly data-dependent emphasis on selected trials or on particular subgroups of patients. Such emphasis is often entirely inadvertent, arising from a perfectly reasonable desire to understand the randomized trial results in terms of who to treat, which treatments to prefer or disease mechanisms. However, whatever its origins, selective emphasis on particular parts of the evidence can often lead to seriously misleading conclusions. This is because the identification of categories of patients for whom treatment is particularly effective (or ineffective) requires surprisingly large quantities of data. Even if the real sizes of the treatment effects do vary substantially among subgroups of patients, subgroup analyses are so statistically insensitive that they may well fail to demonstrate these differences. On the other hand, if the real proportional risk reductions are about the same for everybody, subgroup analyses can vary so widely just by the play of chance that the results in selected subgroups may be exaggerated. Indeed, it can be shown that if an overall treatment effect is conventionally statistically significant at the 5% level (i.e. $P = 0.05$), and patients are randomly split into two equal-sized groups, then there is a 1 in 3 chance that there will be a statistically significant treatment effect in one group and a non-significant effect in the other.[25] Thus, even when significant "interactions" are found, they may be a poor guide to the sizes (and even the directions) of any genuine differences, owing more to chance than to reality.

However, even if true differences in the effect of a treatment do exist between different groups of patients, then under certain circumstances, the overall treatment effect can still provide a better estimator of the effect in any given subgroup than the estimate actually derived from that subgroup (the mathematical theory of James-Stein estimators provides formal mathematical support for this).[26] The logical basis for placing emphasis on overall trial results is that, when there is definite and consistent evidence of benefit (and negligible hazard) in all categories of patients that have been studied extensively (such as for statins in the prevention of major vascular events)[8], then although the relative benefit in another (relatively unstudied) category might not be exactly the same, it is unlikely to be vastly different and, in particular, is extremely unlikely to be zero. Nonetheless, "exploratory" data-derived subgroup analyses are still widely reported in medical journals and at scientific meetings, with potential adverse consequences for medical care.

An example of how subgroup analyses have resulted in inappropriate management of patients is provided by the early trials of aspirin for the secondary prevention of stroke. Here, emphasis on the results in men led to a situation where, for almost 20 years, the US Food and Drug Administration approved the use of aspirin only for men; subsequent evidence shows this to have been a mistake, with aspirin reducing the risk of vascular events among high-risk people by about one quarter irrespective of sex.[24] A further example is provided by the large Italian GISSI-1 trial comparing streptokinase versus control after acute MI. The overall results favored streptokinase but subgroup analyses suggested that streptokinase was beneficial only in patients without prior MI. Fortunately, the GISSI investigators were circumspect about this finding[3] and their caution turned out to have been wise, as a subsequent overview of all the large fibrinolytic trials showed that the proportional benefits were similar, irrespective of a history of MI.[1] Many thousands of patients with a previous history of MI might well have been denied fibrinolytic therapy, however, if the apparent pattern of the results in the GISSI-1 subgroups had been believed.

Avoidance of moderate random errors

Trials may produce false-negative results

Whereas the avoidance of moderate biases requires careful attention to both the randomization process and the analysis and interpretation of the available trial evidence, the avoidance of moderate random errors requires large studies. When making inferences about the likely true effect of a drug based on observations in a clinical trial, there are two types of error that can be made. A type I error occurs if a trial reaches a false-positive result, i.e. when it appears that a beneficial treatment effect has been demonstrated but the drug is actually ineffective. The second, type II, error occurs when a trial achieves a false-negative result, i.e. when the estimated effect of a beneficial treatment fails to reach statistical significance. A critical part of the design of any clinical study is a decision about how small these type I (α) and type II (β) error rates need to be. Together with an estimate of the minimum size of the effect one wishes to detect, these error rates determine the number of events required in a trial. The smaller the desired type I and type II error rates for a trial, the more patients that trial will need to recruit to be able to demonstrate any true treatment effects. Conversely, for a fixed sample size, the "power" (which is the *a priori* probability, $1 - \beta$, of avoiding a false negative) of a trial to detect "meaningful" treatment effects reduces rapidly if the true magnitude of a treatment effect has been overestimated at the design stage. For example, as illustrated in Figure 3.1, in a trial of 10 000 participants in which one-fifth

of the control group has the primary endpoint, the power (at a type I error rate of 1%) to detect a true relative risk reduction of 20% would be excellent (>99%), but the power to detect a true reduction of 10% would be less than 1 in 2.

The power of a trial to identify a true treatment effect is greatly reduced if the true relative risk reduction is smaller than anticipated. However, it is also reduced if the study outcome occurs in a smaller than expected proportion of those randomized. Trials of major outcomes therefore need to accumulate large numbers of primary endpoints before the results can be guaranteed to be statistically (and hence medically) convincing. For example, the early trials of intravenous fibrinolytic therapy for acute myocardial infarction were individually too small to provide reliable evidence about any moderate effects of this treatment on mortality, although several did identify an increased risk of serious bleeding. As a result, fibrinolytic therapy was not used routinely until the GISSI-1[3] and ISIS-2[2] "mega-trials" provided such definite evidence of benefit that treatment patterns changed rapidly.[27] It is worth noting, however, that GISSI-1 and ISIS-2 each included more than 10 000 patients and 1000 deaths but had they only been one-tenth as large, the observed reduction in mortality would not have been conventionally significant and would therefore have had much less influence on medical practice.

When a clinical trial fails to demonstrate a statistically significant difference between two treatment groups, either there is not a true difference or, if there is, the trial was too small to detect it. In some circumstances, however, an appropriate objective may be the demonstration that two or more treatments are equally effective, in which case the statistical framework for the trial analysis is quite different from that required when the aim is to demonstrate treatment differences. The underlying model assumptions in such an "equivalence" study are essentially a reversal of those used in a conventional study design: the null hypothesis, rather than being one of no true difference between treatments, is that a small true difference Δ of size at least δ, say, exists between treatments (i.e. $|\Delta| \geq \delta$ where $\delta > 0$) and the aim is to accumulate evidence against this hypothesis. Hence, if the null hypothesis is rejected, the implication is that $|\Delta| < \delta$, i.e. the effects of each treatment differ by no more than the small amount δ. Similarly, in a non-inferiority trial, where the object is to demonstrate that a new drug is at least as good as an existing one, the null hypothesis would be expressed as $\Delta \leq -\delta$ (assuming that positive values of Δ are taken to mean that the new drug is better than the old one). Rejection of this hypothesis would imply that $\Delta > -\delta$; that is, the new drug has either similar or superior effects to the old one. Appropriate selection of the null hypothesis for a given clinical question plays a critical role not only in determining the sample size needed, but also in dictating how the results should be interpreted. Unfortunately, there are numerous examples

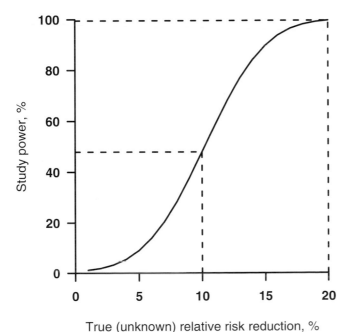

Figure 3.1 Power to detect different relative risk reductions in a trial of 10 000 patients (5000 active vs 5000 control), an outcome rate of 20% in the control group and a type I error rate of 0.01.

of trials that were designed to test for a difference between two drugs, but were subsequently interpreted under a different null hypothesis.

Effect of non-compliance on study power

Even in a situation where a trial is designed to have sufficient statistical power to address its primary hypothesis, study power can quickly be eroded through higher than expected levels of non-compliance. This is because the sample size needed to achieve a given power is inversely proportional to the *square* of the difference, between treatment groups, in the proportions taking study treatment or a non-study equivalent. For example, suppose a trial of 10 000 patients was originally designed so that it had 80% power, at a type I error rate of 5%, to address its primary hypothesis, but that the sample size calculations assumed full compliance among all trial participants. Then suppose that during the trial 20% of those allocated active treatment stop taking it ("drop outs") and 10% of those allocated control start taking the active treatment, or non-study equivalent, instead ("drop ins"). In these circumstances, the actual sample size that would have been needed to maintain study power is 20 000 patients (since $10\,000/[1 - 0.2 - 0.1]^2 \approx 20\,000$). It is therefore crucial that strenuous efforts are made to maintain compliance during a trial. In the Clopidogrel in Unstable angina to prevent Recurrent Events (CURE) trial,[28] for instance, many patients having a percutaneous coronary intervention were treated with open-label clopidogrel during the procedure and so discontinued allocated treatment; these patients were encouraged to restart afterwards in order to maximize the likelihood of the trial reaching a clear result for its primary outcome of cardiovascular death, non-fatal myocardial infarction or stroke.

Need for large-scale randomized trials

If the aim is to detect a moderate difference in a major clinical outcome then randomization is essential to avoid moderate biases and large numbers of events are required to avoid moderate random errors. The only study design that can be guaranteed to detect such differences, therefore, is a large-scale randomized trial. Trials of the effects of treatments on major outcomes can only be made large if they are kept as simple as possible. In particular, as many as possible of the main barriers to rapid recruitment need to be removed. An important way in which trial design can facilitate this is to limit the amount of information that is recorded. For example, data recorded at baseline can often be restricted to important clinical details, including at most only a few major prognostic factors and only a few variables that are thought likely to influence substantially the benefits or hazards of treatment. Similarly, the information recorded at follow-up need not be extensive and can be limited to those major outcomes that such studies have been designed to assess, and to approximate measures of compliance.

(Other outcomes that are of interest but which do not need to be studied on such a large scale may be best assessed in separate smaller studies or in subsets of these large studies when this is practicable.) Likewise, complicated eligibility criteria and inappropriately detailed consent procedures,[29] both of which consume time and resources unnecessarily, can prevent the recruitment of large numbers of patients. Furthermore, if trials are complex they are likely to involve a high cost per patient, which again tends to limit their size. Either way, complexity is rarely a virtue in trials designed to assess major outcomes, whereas simplicity can sometimes lead to the rapid randomization of very large numbers of patients, and to results that change clinical practice within very short periods of time.[2,27]

Large-scale randomized trials are costly, but their value for money can be greatly enhanced by randomizing patients twice or more to different types of treatments. Such "factorial designs" can assess more than one study hypothesis at little additional cost, and there are numerous examples illustrating the efficiency of this design for improving clinical care. For instance, in the MRC/BHF Heart Protection Study, 20 536 patients at high risk of vascular disease were randomized both to daily simvastatin or matching placebo and to antioxidant therapy or matching placebo (so that one-quarter of the patients received both simvastatin and antioxidant therapy, one quarter received simvastatin only, one quarter received antioxidant therapy only, and one-quarter received neither).[7,30] This "2 × 2" factorial design allowed the Heart Protection Study to assess the separate effects of simvastatin and antioxidant therapy on the risk of death from any cause (with each comparison involving about 10 000 patients allocated to active drug versus 10 000 allocated placebo). Factorial designs also provide the ideal setting for testing whether the size of the effect of one treatment depends on whether another is given (i.e. whether there are any "interactions" between treatments), though surprisingly large numbers of patients are needed for this purpose. A common concern over the use of factorial designs is the potential for adverse drug interactions, potentially affecting patient safety, compliance or study power. However, a review of factorial trials published between 2000 and 2002 found that treatment interactions were rare – in only two out of 31 tests for interaction (from 26 trials) were "significant" interactions detected.[31]

The "uncertainty principle"

For ethical reasons, randomization is appropriate if, and only if, both the doctor and the patient feel substantially uncertain as to which trial treatment is best. The "uncertainty principle" maximizes the potential for recruitment within this ethical constraint (see Box 3.2). In addition, if many hospitals are collaborating in a trial then wholehearted use of the uncertainty principle encourages clinically appropriate heterogeneity in the resulting trial

BOX 3.2 The uncertainty principle

A patient can be entered if, and only if, the responsible physician is substantially uncertain as to which of the trial treatments would be most appropriate for that particular patient. A patient should not be entered if the responsible physician or the patient is, for any medical or non-medical reason, reasonably certain that one of the treatments that might be allocated would be inappropriate for this particular individual (in comparison either with no treatment or with some other treatment that could be offered to the patient in or outside the trial).[32]

population which, in large trials, may add substantially to the practical value of the results. Among the early trials of fibrinolytic therapy, for example, most of the studies had restrictive entry criteria that precluded the randomization of elderly patients, and so those trials contributed nothing of direct relevance to the important clinical question of whether treatment was useful in older patients. Other trials that did not impose an upper age limit, however, did include some elderly patients and were therefore able to show that age alone is not a contraindication to fibrinolytic therapy.[1]

Thus, homogeneity of those randomized may be a serious defect in clinical trial design, whereas heterogeneity may be a scientific strength; after all, trials do need to be relevant to a very heterogeneous collection of future patients. Therefore, adoption of the "uncertainty principle" not only ensures ethicality and clinically useful heterogeneity, but is also easily understood and remembered by busy collaborating clinicians, thereby helping to encourage the randomization of large numbers of patients.

Interim analyses, stopping rules and the DMC

Trials can only be made large if they have proper oversight. Trial management committees, trial steering committees and data monitoring committees all have important roles to play in the successful running of a large trial. For instance, if sufficient evidence accumulates during a trial that one treatment is clearly better than the other, and that the results would be expected to have a substantial impact on clinical practice, the trial may need to be stopped or modified. Such oversight is typically the responsibility of the trial's Data Monitoring Committee (DMC; also sometimes called the Data and Safety Monitoring Board – DSMB), upon review of unblinded "interim" analyses. The DMC balances the welfare of the patients in the trial against the welfare of future patients, whose care may be affected by the results of the trial. If a trial is stopped early, the estimate of the treatment effect will be less precise and, as a consequence, might fail to have a major influence on future clinical practice. (On average, it will also be biased, overestimating the effect of treatment that would have been observed had the trial been allowed to run its course.[33])

Hence, a key question that the DMC should consider prior to recommending the termination of a trial is whether the current evidence is likely to lead to a material change in clinical practice. If the answer is no, then sufficient uncertainty probably remains for the trial to be allowed to continue. However, as the number of planned interim analyses increases, so does the overall type I error rate. If, for example, one employs the conventional $p < 0.05$ "threshold" value at which to reject the null hypothesis, the actual false-positive rate is 8% for two analyses (i.e. one interim analysis and one final analysis), almost 15% for five analyses and nearly 20% for 10 analyses.[34]

Various "stopping rules" have therefore been proposed to help maintain the overall type I error rate of a trial when multiple interim analyses are planned.[35] The O'Brien–Fleming rule, for instance, increases the stringency of the nominal significance level for rejecting the null hypothesis at each interim analysis, thereby offering an opportunity for early termination only when initial results are extreme, while essentially maintaining the type I error rate of the predetermined final analysis.[36] Similarly, an approach proposed by Haybittle[37], and later supported by Peto et al[22], recommends termination of a trial at an interim analysis only if the evidence against the null hypothesis is very strong (e.g. $P < 0.001$), so that the overall type I error rate after the final analysis (should the trial continue that far) is essentially unaffected.

Large-scale meta-analysis

Because meta-analyses are appearing in medical journals with increasing frequency it is useful to be able to judge the reliability of such reviews and, in particular, the extent to which confounding, biases or random errors could lead to misleading conclusions. (In randomized trials, "confounding" exists when a comparison of a treatment with a control group involves the routine co-administration in one group, but not the other, of another intervention that might affect the outcome.) To avoid any possibility of confounding, and to avoid any uncertainty about which trials to consider, meta-analyses should generally include only unconfounded properly randomized trials. The main problems that then remain are those of biases and random errors.

Small-scale meta-analyses may be unreliable

Two types of bias could affect the reliability of a meta-analysis: those that occur within individual trials and those that relate to the selection of trials. More empirical research into the numerous biases that can occur within randomized trials would be valuable. However, it is clear from existing studies that, for example, inadequate concealment of treatment allocation and inadequate blinding do quite often result in exaggerated estimates of treatment effect,[38,39] and that the inappropriate postrandomization exclusion of particular patients is common.[40] Including such trials in a meta-analysis would most likely manifest as an increase in heterogeneity of treatment effect between the studies (possibly in addition to a systematic bias). Such "methodological" defects can have unpredictable consequences for a particular trial, however, and no generalization about the size, or even direction, of the resultant bias is possible.

Publication bias

A particular problem in performing a meta-analysis involves the process of identifying all relevant trials. Unfortunately, the subset of trials that is eventually published (and hence which is conventionally available) is often a biased sample of the trials that have been done. Trials are more likely to be submitted for publication if their results are strikingly positive than if they are negative or null.[41–44] Such "publication bias" can, along with other sources of bias, produce surprisingly impressive-looking evidence of effectiveness for treatments that are actually useless.[45] The particular circumstances in which publication bias has contributed to producing misleading estimates of treatment are difficult to identify, and it is still more difficult to generalize about the exact size of any bias when it does occur. The problem with incomplete ascertainment is likely to be particularly acute within small meta-analyses that contain no more than a few hundred major outcomes and which consist mainly of small published trials. This is because results from trials with only a limited number of endpoints are subject to large random errors, and such trials are therefore particularly likely to generate implausibly large effect estimates. If publication bias then results in emphasis on the more promising of these small trial results, the remaining summary odds ratios are likely to be unreliable.[46]

One example where publication bias might have influenced interpretation of treatment effects is in the trials of magnesium among people who have had a myocardial infarction (Fig. 3.2). In the early 1990s there was considerable optimism that infusions of magnesium might limit the damage arising from blockage of the coronary artery. Eight small trials,[47–54] including a total of only about 1500 patients, had in aggregate found a statistically significant, but implausibly large, benefit (42/754 deaths among those allocated magnesium versus 86/740 among the controls, $2P < 0.001$), leading some to argue that magnesium should be widely used without the need for further randomized evidence. Nevertheless, two subsequent trials, one (LIMIT-2)[55] involving 2300 patients and the other (ISIS-4)[56] involving 58 000 patients, were set up to assess the possible effects of magnesium much more reliably. The first, published in 1992, yielded a moderately promising reduction in mortality risk of about one quarter.[55] However, a few years later, the much larger ISIS-4 trial yielded a completely unpromising result,[56] so that the overall evidence by that time (including four more small trials identified after LIMIT-2)[57–60] based on ~60 000 randomized patients was non-significantly adverse (Fig. 3.2). However, some cardiologists still remained hopeful that magnesium might prove to be effective among specific subgroups, such as older patients who could be treated within a few hours of reperfusion therapy or those not eligible for reperfusion therapy. Accordingly, the MAGIC trial subsequently randomized 6200 such patients to magnesium versus placebo but, in 2002, reported that there was no evidence of any benefit to such patients.[61]

The lesson to be learned here is that, unless the particular circumstances of a small-scale meta-analysis suggest that publication bias is unlikely, it may be best to treat such results as no more than "hypothesis generating". On the

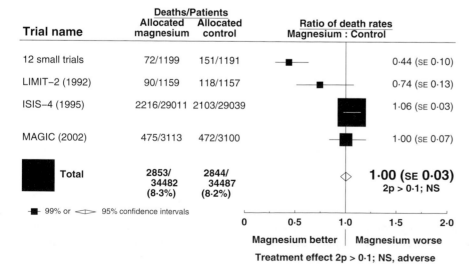

Figure 3.2 Magnesium in acute myocardial infarction: one-month mortality.

other hand, a thoroughly conducted meta-analysis that in aggregate contains sufficient numbers of major outcomes to constitute "large-scale" randomized evidence[1,8,24] is unlikely to be materially affected by publication bias and, provided there are no serious uncontrolled biases (see above) within the individual component trials, is likely to be fairly trustworthy – although, even then, inappropriate subgroup analyses may generate mistaken conclusions. A further lesson to be learned is that in the absence of large-scale randomized evidence, formal statistical tests for publication bias, for instance those based on detecting asymmetry in plots of trial effect size against associated standard errors, can be severely underpowered[62] and therefore misleadingly reassuring. For instance, based on the 12 small magnesium trials prior to LIMIT-2, ISIS-4 and MAGIC, Egger's test for funnel plot asymmetry[63] gives a P-value of 0.24 (i.e. no evidence of publication bias). Only when all the trials are considered together does the evidence for publication bias become clear ($P = 0.0001$).

"Fixed-effect" versus "random-effect" methods

Two general approaches exist for combining the results from different trials in a meta-analysis: "fixed-effect" and "random-effect" methods. In a fixed-effect method, a weighted average of the like-with-like comparisons within each trial is calculated (with bigger trials having proportionally more weight than smaller trials). Consequently, the resulting effect estimate is not directly influenced by any heterogeneity among the true effects of treatment in different trials. This terminology is, however, unsatisfactory, for it misleadingly suggests that any heterogeneity between the true effects of treatment in different trials is assumed to be zero, whereas no such unjustified assumptions are involved.[64] A better terminology for the fixed-effect method, therefore, might be "assumption free". Random-effect methods, on the other hand, estimate the heterogeneity in treatment effects across trials and incorporate this variability into the estimate of the overall result. However, this approach relies on the assumption that the different trial designs were randomly selected from some underlying set of possibilities (i.e. it assumes representativeness) which, in most cases, is extremely unlikely to be true. Indeed, in certain circumstances, such "assumed representativeness" methods can lead to small, potentially seriously biased studies gaining an inappropriately large statistical weight at the expense of larger, more reliable studies, which can lead to importantly wrong answers: applied to the 15 separate magnesium trials in Figure 3.2, a standard "random-effects" meta-analysis yields a summary odds ratio of 0.67 (95% CI 0.52–0.85; $2P < 0.001$), suggesting, quite incorrectly, that magnesium reduces mortality by about one-third.

Use of meta-regression to investigate heterogeneity

It is not uncommon for clinical trials of a particular drug to give rise to somewhat different estimates of treatment effect (indeed, one would expect them to give slightly different estimates because of sampling variation). However, if these differences are substantially larger than would be expected by chance alone (i.e. when there is statistically significant heterogeneity between the trial results), it may be possible to identify reasons for the differences.[65] In particular, "meta-regression" can be used to relate the primary results of each trial to underlying features of the trial population, in the same way that standard regression techniques relate observations made on individuals to potential "explanatory variables".[66] Say, for instance, that the effectiveness of a drug depends on the dose used, the duration of treatment, and the age of the patient, and that all of these factors differed, on average, between a series of reported trials. Essentially, meta-regression would allow one to look at the trial results "adjusted" for these differences, to see if the apparently disparate results can be explained by them, and to allow estimation of any residual heterogeneity.

For example, in the Cholesterol Treatment Trialists' collaboration of 14 randomized controlled trials of statin therapy, the relative reduction in the risk of vascular events in the different trials was found to be linearly related to the LDL cholesterol reduction achieved in the trials (i.e. the difference in mean follow-up LDL cholesterol levels observed between those patients allocated a statin and those allocated placebo).[8] As a consequence, substantial statistical heterogeneity ($\chi^2 = 37.4$ on 13 degrees of freedom, $P = 0.0004$) between the effects on major vascular events in each of the 14 trials was observed (since the trials in which a big lipid difference between the treatment groups was observed tended to find larger proportional reductions in major vascular events than the trials in which smaller lipid differences were observed). However, by standardizing the trial results to correspond to a common 1 mmol/L difference in LDL cholesterol between the two treatment groups, the between-trial statistical heterogeneity was greatly reduced ($\chi^2 = 10.1$, $P = 0.70$) and was no longer statistically significant.[8]

However, it is important to note that while meta-regression techniques can sometimes lead to an improved understanding of the reasons for apparent differences in trial results, they are susceptible to ecologic bias (also known as aggregation bias),[67] which is the bias that can be introduced through examination of associations at the "study" rather than at the "individual" level. Figure 3.3, for example, shows a hypothetic example in which, for each of four different studies A–D, the true relationship between a particular risk exposure and the incidence of disease is positive and linear. However, when average levels of the

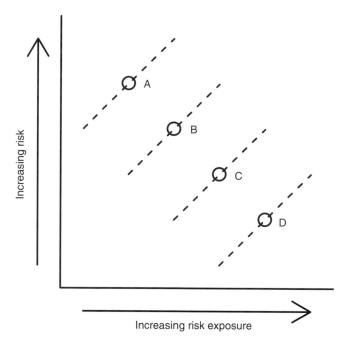

Figure 3.3 Hypothetical example of the potential effects of ecologic bias. The circles represent average risk exposure levels and average disease incidence rates observed in four hypothetical studies A–D. At the "study level" (i.e. drawing a line through the four circles) there is a clear inverse association between exposure to the risk factor and disease risk. However, this masks the fact that, within each study, the opposite is observed. The "ecological bias" (which, in this case, must have arisen because of large differences between the studies in at least one important risk factor) has, therefore, totally reversed the direction of the true risk–relationship.

risk exposure for each study are plotted against average disease incidence rates, the relationship is apparently inverse. The cause of this bias would typically be other differences between the studies that importantly modify individual risk (i.e. the bias could be due to confounding). It is therefore important that, when ecologic analyses are performed, estimates are standardized for potential confounders wherever possible. Nonetheless, such statistical adjustments might only be able to partially remove these effects. The only way to guarantee avoiding ecologic bias is to obtain information on individual participants.

Individual patient data meta-analyses

Meta-analyses based on individual patient data (IPD) rather than aggregate patient data (i.e. from summary information presented in publications) are generally thought of as the "gold standard" of meta-analysis.[68] While it may be more costly and time consuming to perform an IPD meta-analysis, it offers several clear advantages. Data can be checked centrally and the quality of the randomization and follow-up procedures assessed. Furthermore, it may be possible to use common definitions and outcomes

in all the studies, and analytical methods can be standardized. In particular, the availability of IPD permits the use of detailed "time-to-event" analyses for estimation of the effects of treatment on patient survival. The collection of detailed information in a really large meta-analysis that includes several thousand major outcomes, such as death[1] or cancer recurrence,[69,70] also makes it feasible to identify particular groups of individuals in whom the benefits or hazards of treatment are especially great. (Where it has been possible to establish co-operation between trialists before any of the trial results are known, having just a few prespecified subgroup hypotheses can provide some protection against unduly data-dependent emphasis on particular results in an IPD meta-analysis.[71]) In some conditions (such as breast cancer[69]) IPD meta-analyses can also be updated over time to take account of continued follow-up of patients beyond "in-trial" treatment periods, allowing for reliable estimation of long-term treatment effects many years after the individual trials have ended. Collaboration with trialists from across the world may also lead to a more global and balanced interpretation of the results.

Can observational studies substitute for large-scale randomized trials/ meta-analyses?

As the resources will never be sufficient to allow large, simple trials to address all the questions of clinical interest, there have been suggestions that observational studies might be able to provide reliable estimates of the effects of particular treatments. Non-randomized studies do not necessarily provide inaccurate estimates of the effects of treatments, but the point is that they cannot be *guaranteed* to produce reliable estimates because of biases that are inherent in their design. Even when treated and control groups appear similar in key prognostic factors, non-randomized studies can still give seriously misleading results, leading to over- or underestimations of treatment effects which can be large enough to lead studies to falsely conclude significant findings of benefit or harm.[72] It may well be difficult or impossible to avoid such biases or to adjust for their effects.[73] A review of different statistical methods for adjusting estimated treatment differences in non-randomized studies (e.g. using standardization, regression or propensity score methods) found that adequate correction was only possible when selection depended on a single factor (moreover, in some situations, adjusted results were *more* biased than unadjusted results).[72] When non-randomized studies suggest that certain treatments have surprisingly large effects, such findings are often refuted when those treatments are assessed in large randomized trials.[74] For example, the claims of hazards with digoxin in heart failure,[75] based on non-randomized evidence, were not confirmed by the very large randomized DIG (Digitalis Investigation Group) trial.[76] Even if non-randomized comparisons happen to get the right answer then nobody will really know that they have done so.

However, there are several scenarios in which a randomized controlled trial may be unnecessary, inappropriate, impossible or inadequate.[77] Rare adverse effects with extreme relative risks can often be recognized reliably by careful clinical observation or by other non-randomized methods, and such relative risks are sometime best quantified in case–control or cohort studies (as for the greatly increased risk of rhabdomyolysis from taking cerivastatin with the fibrate drug gemfibrizol).[78,79] Non-randomized observational studies are also unavoidable when there are substantial ethical or legal obstacles to performing a randomized controlled trial or when the outcome of interest is in the distant future (for example, the long-term consequences of oral contraceptives may not manifest for decades), making it difficult to perform a trial. However, when the primary aim is to assess moderate treatment effects (whether beneficial or adverse) on major outcomes within a reasonable time frame, non-randomized studies are of limited practical value.

Conclusion

Many interventions in cardiology practice produce only moderate effects on major outcomes such as death or serious disability. However, even a moderate effect of treatment, if demonstrated clearly enough for that treatment to be widely adopted, can prevent disabling events or death in substantial numbers of people. Moreover, if, as in the treatment of acute myocardial infarction, more than one moderately effective treatment can eventually be identified, the combination of two or three improvements individually moderate in outcome may collectively result in substantial health gains. In some instances sufficient information is already available from large-scale randomized trials – or, better still, from meta-analyses of those trials – to allow the balance of risk and benefit of particular treatments to be defined for particular patients. But many important questions have still not been answered reliably, and there remains a need for many more large "streamlined" mega-trials, and meta-analyses of such trials, to help resolve some of the outstanding clinical uncertainties in the management of cardiovascular disease.

References

1. Fibrinolytic Therapy Trialists' (FTT) Collaborative Group. Indications for fibrinolytic therapy in suspected acute myocardial infarction: collaborative overview of early mortality and major morbidity results from all randomised trials of more than 1000 patients. *Lancet* 1994;**343**:311–22.

2. ISIS-2 (Second International Study of Infarct Survival) Collaborative Group. Randomised trial of intravenous streptokinase, oral aspirin, both, or neither among 17,187 cases of suspected acute myocardial infarction: ISIS-2. *Lancet* 1988;**2**:349–60.

3. GISSI (Gruppo Italiano per lo Studio della Streptochinasi nell'Infarto Miocardico). Effectiveness of intravenous thrombolytic treatment in acute myocardial infarction. *Lancet* 1986;**1**:397–402.

4. Collins R, Peto R, Baigent C, Sleight P. Aspirin, heparin, and fibrinolytic therapy in suspected acute myocardial infarction. *N Engl J Med* 1997;**336**:847–60.

5. Antithrombotic Trialists' Collaboration. Collaborative meta-analysis of randomised trials of antiplatelet therapy for prevention of death, myocardial infarction, and stroke in high risk patients. *BMJ* 2002;**324**:71–86.

6. Blood Pressure Lowering Treatment Trialists' Collaboration. Effects of different blood-pressure-lowering regimens on major cardiovascular events: results of prospectively-designed overviews of randomised trials. *Lancet* 2003;**362**:1527–35.

7. Heart Protection Study Collaborative Group. MRC/BHF Heart Protection Study of cholesterol lowering with simvastatin in 20,536 high-risk individuals: a randomised placebo-controlled trial. *Lancet* 2002;**360**:7–22.

8. Cholesterol Treatment Trialists Collaboration. Efficacy and safety of cholesterol-lowering treatment: prospective meta-analysis of data from 90,056 participants in 14 randomised trials of statins. *Lancet* 2005;**366**:1267–78.

9. SOLVD Investigators. Effect of enalapril on survival in patients with reduced left ventricular ejection fractions and congestive heart failure. *N Engl J Med* 1991;**325**:293–302.

10. MERIT-HF. Effect of metoprolol CR/XL in chronic heart failure: Metoprolol CR/XL Randomised Intervention Trial in Congestive Heart Failure (MERIT-HF). *Lancet* 1999;**353**:2001–7.

11. Collins R, MacMahon S. Reliable assessment of the effects of treatment on mortality and major morbidity, I: clinical trials. *Lancet* 2001;**357**:373–80.

12. MacMahon S, Collins R. Reliable assessment of the effects of treatment on mortality and major morbidity, II: observational studies. *Lancet* 2001;**357**:455–62.

13. Collins R, Peto R, Gray R, Parish S. Large scale randomized evidence: trials and overviews. In: Weatherall D, Ledingham JGG, Warrell DA, eds. *Oxford Textbook of Medicine, Vol. 1*. Oxford: Oxford University Press, 1996.

14. Armitage P. The role of randomization in clinical trials. *Stat Med* 1982;**1**:345–52.

15. Kunz R, Oxman AD. The unpredictability paradox: review of empirical comparisons of randomised and non-randomised clinical trials. *BMJ* 1998;**317**:1185–90.

16. Hansson L, Lindholm LH, Niskanen L *et al.* Effect of angiotensin-converting-enzyme inhibition compared with conventional therapy on cardiovascular morbidity and mortality in hypertension: the Captopril Prevention Project (CAPPP) randomised trial. *Lancet* 1999;**353**:611–16.

17. Peto R. Failure of randomisation by "sealed" envelope. *Lancet* 1999;**354**:73.

18. Hansson L, Hedner T, Dahlof B. Prospective randomized open blinded end-point (PROBE) study. A novel design for

intervention trials. Prospective Randomized Open Blinded End-Point. *Blood Press* 1992;**1**:113–19.

19. Sever PS, Dahlof B, Poulter NR *et al*. Prevention of coronary and stroke events with atorvastatin in hypertensive patients who have average or lower-than-average cholesterol concentrations, in the Anglo-Scandinavian Cardiac Outcomes Trial – Lipid Lowering Arm (ASCOT-LLA): a multicentre randomised controlled trial. *Lancet* 2003;**361**:1149–58.

20. Pedersen TR, Faergeman O, Kastelein JJ *et al*. Design and baseline characteristics of the Incremental Decrease in End Points through Aggressive Lipid Lowering study. *Am J Cardiol* 2004;**94**:720–4.

21. Influence of adherence to treatment and response of cholesterol on mortality in the coronary drug project. *N Engl J Med* 1980;**303**:1038–41.

22. Peto R, Pike MC, Armitage P *et al*. Design and analysis of randomized clinical trials requiring prolonged observation of each patient. I. Introduction and design. *Br J Cancer* 1976;**34**:585–612.

23. Cuzick J, Edwards R, Segnan N. Adjusting for non-compliance and contamination in randomized clinical trials. *Stat Med* 1997;**16**:1017–29.

24. Antiplatelet Trialists' Collaboration. Collaborative overview of randomised trials of antiplatelet therapy I: Prevention of death, myocardial infarction, and stroke by prolonged antiplatelet therapy in various categories of patients. *BMJ* 1994;**308**:81–106.

25. Peto R. Statistical aspects of cancer trials, In: Halnan KE, ed. *Treatment of Cancer*. London: Chapman and Hall, 1982.

26. Efron BMC. Stein's paradox in statistics. *Sci Am* 1977; **236**:119–27.

27. Collins R, Julian D. British Heart Foundation surveys (1987 and 1989) of United Kingdom treatment policies for acute myocardial infarction. *Br Heart J* 1991;**66**:250–5.

28. Yusuf S, Zhao F, Mehta SR, Chrolavicius S, Tognoni G, Fox KK. Effects of clopidogrel in addition to aspirin in patients with acute coronary syndromes without ST-segment elevation. *N Engl J Med* 2001;**345**:494–502.

29. Doyal L. Informed consent in medical research. Journals should not publish research to which patients have not given fully informed consent – with three exceptions. *BMJ* 1997;**314**:1107–11.

30. Heart Protection Study Collaborative Group. MRC/BHF Heart Protection Study of antioxidant vitamin supplementation in 20,536 high-risk individuals: a randomised placebo-controlled trial. *Lancet* 2002;**360**:23–33.

31. McAlister FA, Straus SE, Sackett DL, Altman DG. Analysis and reporting of factorial trials: a systematic review. *JAMA* 2003;**289**:2545–53.

32. Collins R, Doll R, Peto R. Ethics of clinical trials. In: Williams CJ, ed. *Introducing New Treatments for Cancer: Practical, Ethical and Legal Problems*. Chichester: John Wiley, 1992.

33. Hughes MD, Pocock SJ. Stopping rules and estimation problems in clinical trials. *Stat Med* 1988;**7**:1231–42.

34. Armitage P, McPherson CK, Rowe BC. Repeated significance tests on accumulating data. *J R Stat Soc (Series A)* 1969;**132**: 235–44.

35. Demets DL. Practical aspects in data monitoring: a brief review. *Stat Med* 1987;**6**:753–60.

36. Fleming TR, Harrington DP, O'Brien PC. Designs for group sequential tests. *Control Clin Trials* 1984;**5**:348–61.

37. Haybittle JL. Repeated assessment of results in clinical trials of cancer treatment. *Br J Radiol* 1971;**44**:793–7.

38. Schulz KF, Chalmers I, Altman DG, Grimes DA, Dore CJ. The methodologic quality of randomization as assessed from reports of trials in specialist and general medical journals. *Online J Curr Clin Trials* 1995; Doc No 197.

39. Schulz KF, Chalmers I, Hayes RJ, Altman DG. Empirical evidence of bias. Dimensions of methodological quality associated with estimates of treatment effects in controlled trials. *JAMA* 1995;**273**:408–12.

40. Schulz KF, Grimes DA, Altman DG, Hayes RJ. Blinding and exclusions after allocation in randomised controlled trials: survey of published parallel group trials in obstetrics and gynaecology. *BMJ* 1996;**312**:742–4.

41. Dickersin K, Min YI. Publication bias: the problem that won't go away. *Ann NY Acad Sci* 1993;**703**:135–46; discussion 146–8.

42. Dickersin K, Min YI, Meinert CL. Factors influencing publication of research results. Follow-up of applications submitted to two institutional review boards. *JAMA* 1992;**267**:374–8.

43. Dickersin K, Chan S, Chalmers TC, Sacks HS, Smith H Jr. Publication bias and clinical trials. *Control Clin Trials* 1987;**8**:343–53.

44. Easterbrook PJ, Berlin JA, Gopalan R, Matthews DR. Publication bias in clinical research. *Lancet* 1991;**337**:867–72.

45. Counsell CE, Clarke MJ, Slattery J, Sandercock PA. The miracle of DICE therapy for acute stroke: fact or fictional product of subgroup analysis? *BMJ* 1994;**309**:1677–81.

46. Egger M, Smith GD. Misleading meta-analysis. *BMJ* 1995; **310**:752–4.

47. Morton BC, Nair RC, Smith FM, McKibbon TG, Poznanski WJ. Magnesium therapy in acute myocardial infarction – a double-blind study. *Magnesium* 1984;**3**:346–52.

48. Rasmussen HS, McNair P, Norregard P, Backer V, Lindeneg O, Balslev S. Intravenous magnesium in acute myocardial infarction. *Lancet* 1986;**1**:234–6.

49. Smith LF, Heagerty AM, Bing RF, Barnett DB. Intravenous infusion of magnesium sulphate after acute myocardial infarction: effects on arrhythmias and mortality. *Int J Cardiol* 1986;**12**:175–83.

50. Abraham AS, Rosenmann D, Kramer M *et al*. Magnesium in the prevention of lethal arrhythmias in acute myocardial infarction. *Arch Intern Med* 1987;**147**:753–5.

51. Feldstedt M, Boesgaard S, Bouchelouche P *et al*. Magnesium substitution in acute ischaemic heart syndromes. *Eur Heart J* 1991;**12**:1215–18.

52. Shechter M, Hod H, Marks N, Behar S, Kaplinsky E, Rabinowitz B. Beneficial effect of magnesium sulfate in acute myocardial infarction. *Am J Cardiol* 1990;**66**:271–4.

53. Ceremuzynski L, Jurgiel R, Kulakowski P, Gebalska J. Threatening arrhythmias in acute myocardial infarction are prevented by intravenous magnesium sulfate. *Am Heart J* 1989;**118**:1333–4.

54. Bertschat F. Antiarrhythmic effects of magnesium infusions in patients with acute myocardial infarction. *Magnesium Bull* 1989;**11**:155–8.

55. Woods KL, Fletcher S, Roffe C, Haider Y. Intravenous magnesium sulphate in suspected acute myocardial infarction: results of the second Leicester Intravenous Magnesium Intervention Trial (LIMIT-2). *Lancet* 1992;**339**:1553–8.

56. ISIS-4 (Fourth International Study of Infarct Survival) Collaborative Group. Randomised factorial trial assessing early oral captopril, oral mononitrate, and intravenous magnesium sulphate in 58,050 patients with suspected acute myocardial infarction. *Lancet* 1995;**345**:669–85.

57. Shechter M, Hod H, Chouraqui P, Kaplinsky E, Rabinowitz B. Magnesium therapy in acute myocardial infarction when patients are not candidates for thrombolytic therapy. *Am J Cardiol* 1995;**75**:321–3.

58. Thogersen A, Johnson O, Wester P. Effects of magnesium infusion on thrombolytic and non-thrombolytic treated patients with acute myocardial infarction. *Int J Cardiol* 1993;**39**:13–22.

59. Raghu C, Peddeswata P, Seshagiri D. Protective effect of intravenous magnesium in acute myocardial infarction following thrombolytic therapy. *Int J Cardiol* 1999;**71**:209–15.

60. Gyamlani G, Kulkarni A. Benefits of magnesium in acute myocardial infarction: timing is crucial. *Am Heart J* 2000;**139**:703.

61. Magnesium in Coronaries (MAGIC) Trial Investigators. Early administration of intravenous magnesium to high-risk patients with acute myocardial infarction in the Magnesium in Coronaries (MAGIC) Trial: a randomised controlled trial. *Lancet* 2002;**360**:1189–96.

62. Sterne JA, Gavaghan D, Egger M. Publication and related bias in meta-analysis: power of statistical tests and prevalence in the literature. *J Clin Epidemiol* 2000;**53**:1119–29.

63. Egger M, Davey Smith G, Schneider M, Minder C. Bias in meta-analysis detected by a simple, graphical test. *BMJ* 1997;**315**:629–34.

64. Yusuf S, Peto R, Lewis J, Collins R, Sleight P. Beta blockade during and after myocardial infarction: an overview of the randomized trials. *Progress Cardiovasc Dis* 1985;**27**:335–371.

65. Thompson SG. Why sources of heterogeneity in meta-analysis should be investigated. *BMJ* 1994;**309**:1351–5.

66. Thompson SG, Sharp SJ. Explaining heterogeneity in meta-analysis: a comparison of methods. *Stat Med* 1999;**18**: 2693–708.

67. Greenland S, Morgenstern H. Ecological bias, confounding, and effect modification. *Int J Epidemiol* 1989;**18**:269–74.

68. Chalmers I. The Cochrane Collaboration: preparing, maintaining, and disseminating systematic reviews of the effects of health care. *Ann NY Acad Sci* 1993;**703**:156–63; discussion 163–5.

69. Early Breast Cancer Trialists' Collaborative Group. Systemic treatment of early breast cancer by hormonal, cytotoxic, or immune therapy. 133 randomised trials involving 31,000 recurrences and 24,000 deaths among 75,000 women. *Lancet* 1992;**339**:71–85.

70. Early Breast Cancer Trialists' Collaborative Group. Systemic treatment of early breast cancer by hormonal, cytotoxic, or immune therapy. 133 randomised trials involving 31,000 recurrences and 24,000 deaths among 75,000 women. *Lancet* 1992;**339**:1–15.

71. Cholesterol Treatment Trialists' (CTT) Collaboration. Protocol for a prospective collaborative overview of all current and planned randomized trials of cholesterol treatment regimens. *Am J Cardiol* 1995;**75**:1130–4.

72. Deeks JJ, Dinnes J, D'Amico R *et al.* Evaluating non-randomised intervention studies. *Health Technol Assess* 2003;**7**:iii–x, 1–173.

73. Sheldon TA. Please bypass the PORT. *BMJ* 1994;**309**:142–3.

74. Peto R. Clinical trial methodology. *Biomedicine* 1978;**28**:24–36.

75. Yusuf S, Wittes J, Bailey K, Furberg C. Digitalis – a new controversy regarding an old drug. The pitfalls of inappropriate methods. *Circulation* 1986;**73**:14–18.

76. Digitalis Investigation Group. The effect of digoxin on mortality and morbidity in patients with heart failure. *N Engl J Med* 1997;**336**:525–33.

77. Black N. Why we need observational studies to evaluate the effectiveness of health care. *BMJ* 1996;**312**:1215–18.

78. Graham DJ, Staffa JA, Shatin D *et al.* Incidence of hospitalized rhabdomyolysis in patients treated with lipid-lowering drugs. *JAMA* 2004;**292**:2585–90.

79. Law M, Rudnicka AR. Statin safety: a systematic review. *Am J Cardiol* 2006;**97**:52C–60C.

4 Understanding concepts related to health economics

Mark A Hlatky
Stanford University School of Medicine, Stanford, CA, USA

Introduction

Economics is concerned with how to allocate scarce resources among alternative uses efficiently and effectively. It is a fundamental principle of economics that resources are limited relative to human wants, and that those resources have alternative uses.[1] Consequently, when people say that the cost of healthcare has grown too high, they mean that the quantity of resources flowing toward medical care has grown to the point where additional funds cannot be spent on other things that society values, such as education, public safety, environmental protection, public works, pensions for the retired or disabled, or assistance to the poor. The fact that most people put a very high value on health does not mean that they are willing to provide limitless resources to medical care. Indeed, the goal of improving health and longevity may also be served by non-medical expenditures on programs such as nutritional supplements, a safe and clean water supply, police and fire protection or safety improvements to roads.

The cost of medical care has been rising steadily for the past 40 years in all developed countries[2] but it has only been in the past decade that the level of expenditure has become so large as to cause alarm among policy makers, payers, and the general public (Table 4.1). The steady expansion of healthcare has now begun to meet substantial resistance in the large industrial countries, and new policies and payment mechanisms have been introduced to contain the rising cost of medical care. As a consequence, physicians must now consider cost as they design programs to prevent, diagnose, and treat disease. Cardiovascular diseases consume a large share of healthcare resources (Table 4.2), so cardiovascular specialists must be particularly knowledgeable about health economics.

Evidence-Based Cardiology, 3rd edition. Edited by S. Yusuf, J.A. Cairns, A.J. Camm, E.L. Fallen, and B.J. Gersh. © 2010 Blackwell Publishing, ISBN: 978-1-4051-5925-8.

This chapter will attempt to outline the major principles of health economics relevant to cardiovascular medicine. First, some general concepts of health economics will be presented. Second, methods to identify and compare the costs of cardiovascular interventions will be described. Finally, the principles of cost-effectiveness analysis will be discussed.

General concepts

Various societies have adopted different systems to pay for healthcare and these systems reflect societal values and the historical experience within each country. The United Kingdom has a national health service, Canada has national health insurance, France and Germany have public/private financing for healthcare, and the United States has a perplexing and evolving patchwork of public and private health insurance systems. These are very different systems for financing healthcare and yet each is faced with the same issues of how to allocate the limited resources available to best provide healthcare. Each country is also facing the same steady rise of healthcare costs, despite the wide differences in the ways they finance healthcare.

Provision of cardiovascular services requires resources in all societies, irrespective of the method of financing or delivering healthcare. Coronary bypass surgery, for example, is very resource intensive, requiring cardiac surgeons, a cardiac anesthesiologist or anesthetist, a perfusionist, several nurses, and considerable quantities of specialized supplies and equipment. Postoperative care also requires skilled nurses and physicians, with support from specialized supplies, equipment, and facilities. Each health professional involved in cardiac surgery spends the scarce resource of time to care for the patient – time that could be put to other valuable uses, such as care for other patients. The drugs used, the disposable supplies, the operating room equipment, even the hospital building, all cost money. All of these are true costs to the system, even if the coronary bypass operation is performed "for free" – that is, without

Table 4.1 US national healthcare expenditures, 2006

Category	US$ (billions)	Percentage
Hospital care	651.8	33
Physician services	447.0	22
Other professional services	215.7	11
Drugs, supplies	275.2	14
Nursing home care	126.1	6
Home healthcare	53.4	3
Public health	61.7	3
Administration	156.8	8
Total*	1987.7	100

* per capita, $6641
Source: Health Affairs 2007;26:w242–w253

Table 4.2 Resources devoted to cardiovascular care in the USA, 2005

Category	Cardiac n (×10³)	Percentage of total use
Deaths[a]	802	33%
Hospital admissions[b]	6159	18%
Myocardial infarction	683	
Heart failure	1079	
Cerebrovascular disease	985	
Operations and procedures[b]	6989	16%
Cardiac catheterization	1209	
Coronary bypass surgery	355	
Coronary angioplasty	1265	
Pacemaker related	384	
Physician office visits[c]	82	8%
Electrocardiograms	31	
Prescriptions[c]	335301	17%

*Sources: [a]NCHS Monthly Vital Statistics Report 2007;56(No. 5)
[b]NCHS Advance Data 2007 (No. 385)
[c]NCHS Advance Data 2007 (No. 387)Sources: [a]NCHS Monthly Vital Statistics Report 2007;56(No. 5)*

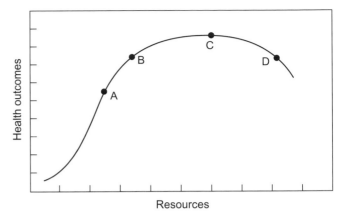

Figure 4.1 General relationship between increasing healthcare resources (horizontal axis) and health outcomes (vertical axis). At point A, outcomes are improving rapidly with increased resources and treatment is cost effective. At point B, outcomes are still improving with increased resources, but at a rate that is not cost effective. At point C, increased resources are no longer improving outcome (that is, "flat of the curve"), and at point D increased resources actually lead to worse outcomes, through iatrogenic complications and overtreatment.

an acute myocardial infarction, for example, survival would be improved as more resources are applied, such as pre-hospital transportation, electrocardiographic monitoring, access to defibrillation, and a competent team to deliver coronary care. Outcomes might be further improved by reperfusion therapy, but with a greater increment in survival from using a cheaper, basic approach (streptokinase, for example) relative to no therapy than from more expensive alternatives (such as tissue plasminogen activator or primary angioplasty). The extra benefit from adding even more aggressive care will be smaller still, and at some point the patient may be harmed by overly aggressive care. Helping physicians to define the optimal point on this curve (Fig. 4.1) is one of the goals of economic analysis.

Determination of costs

The cost of producing a particular healthcare service can be defined in a variety of ways. The cost of performing a coronary angiogram can be used as a specific example that will illustrate the various aspects of cost and how the cost might be measured.

Performing a coronary angiogram requires a variety of resources, including radiographic equipment, trained personnel (including an angiographer and technical assistants), and specialized supplies such as catheters, radiographic contrast, and sterile drapes. The equipment needed is very expensive to purchase and the healthcare facility where it is installed may require special modifications to insure proper radiation shielding and adequate electrical power. The capital cost for a coronary angiography laboratory will be

charge to the patient. The scene in the operating room, the postoperative recovery areas, and the hospital wards is much the same in the United Kingdom, Canada, France, Germany, and the United States despite the different ways in which these societies pay for medical care. The resources used in the care of patients and the increasing sophistication of that care drive healthcare costs up in each of these countries, irrespective of the way in which such care is paid for.

Another basic concept of economics is the so-called "law of diminishing returns". This concept is illustrated in Figure 4.1, in which the quantity of resources used in healthcare is plotted on the horizontal axis and the resulting health benefits on the vertical axis. In the case of the patient with

considerable, perhaps $2–3 million, depending on the type of equipment purchased. The laboratory will have a physical lifespan of perhaps 7–10 years, although technologic innovations may lead to replacement of the equipment before the end of its physical lifespan. The cost of building an angiography suite represents a large *fixed cost* for coronary angiography, a cost that is roughly the same whether the laboratory performs 200 or 2000 angiograms per year. The cost per case is lower in the high-volume laboratory, however, because the fixed equipment costs can be spread over more cases. Thus, if the equipment costs $2.5 million and has a useful life of 10 years, the prorated share of fixed costs for each patient in the low-volume laboratory performing 200 cases per year is:

$$\text{Fixed costs/case} = \frac{\$2\,500\,000}{(200\,\text{cases/yr})(10\,\text{years})} = \$1250/\text{case}$$

whereas in the high-volume laboratory (2000 cases per year) the prorated share of fixed costs per case would be:

$$\text{Fixed costs/case} = \frac{\$2\,500\,000}{(2000\,\text{cases/yr})(10\,\text{years})} = \$125/\text{case}$$

Procedures that have high fixed costs will be performed with greater economic efficiency in centers that have sufficient volume to spread those fixed costs over a larger number of individual patients. (There may be additional advantages to larger procedure volumes as well, since the technical proficiency is higher and clinical outcomes of many procedures are usually better when performed in higher volume clinical centers.[3–5]) Procedures with lower fixed costs will have a smaller effect of volume on costs.

In contrast to the fixed equipment costs, the cost of supplies consumed in performing coronary angiography varies directly with the volume of cases performed, and the supply cost per case will be fairly constant irrespective of the volume of cases performed (apart from the small effect of discounts available to large-volume purchasers). The cost of laboratory staff falls in between these two extremes, in that the hours worked in the catheterization laboratory by technical staff can be varied somewhat according to the volume of cases performed, but some staff effort is required regardless of patient volumes, such as supervisors.

Hospital overhead is also a real cost but one that is less directly linked to any one medical service or procedure. Hospitals must pay for admitting offices, the medical records department, central administration, the laundry service, the cafeteria, housekeeping and utilities, to name just a few areas. These costs cannot be tied easily to the coronary angiography procedure in the same way as the cost of the catheters or radiographic contrast. Most facilities assign a share of these costs to patient care services according to a formula such as the step-down method. Discussion of specific methods to allocate hospital overhead is beyond the scope of this chapter but can be found in several articles and books.[6,7]

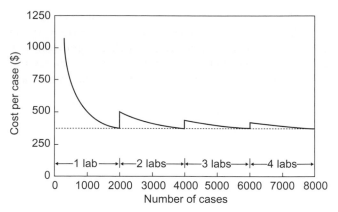

Figure 4.2 Cost per case for coronary angiography as a function of clinical volume. Assumes fixed costs per laboratory of $250000 per year, and marginal (that is, variable) costs of $250 per case. When volume reaches 2000 cases per year in a laboratory, the model assumes an additional laboratory will be built. The dotted line indicates the "long run average" cost per case of $375.

The overall effect of procedure volume on the cost per case is illustrated in Figure 4.2. In general, the cost per case declines as more cases are performed, up to the limit of the facility's capacity (for example, 2000 cases). If volume increases further, more facilities must be built, increasing the cost per case, as more fixed costs are spread over a few more patients. Figure 4.2 also illustrates the distinction between concepts of "marginal cost" and long run "average cost". The marginal cost is the added cost of doing one more case. In an already equipped and staffed coronary angiography laboratory, the marginal cost of performing one more procedure is just the cost of the disposable supplies consumed in the case: the catheters, radiographic contrast, and other sterile supplies. In the example of Figure 4.2, the marginal cost is $250 per case. The marginal cost is lower than the average cost per case ($375 per case), which also includes a prorated share of the salaries of the laboratory staff, depreciation of the laboratory equipment costs, and the facility's overhead costs.

It is important to distinguish "cost per case" from "total health system costs". The example above suggests that it is more economically efficient to perform 2000 procedures per year in one center (total cost $750000/year) than it is to perform 500 procedures per year in each of four centers (total cost $1500000/year). Of course, if the four centers each performed 2000 procedures per year instead of 500 procedures, the total cost to the health care system would be higher overall ($3000000/year) even though the cost per case would have been reduced (from $750/case to $375/case).

Estimation of costs

The cost of providing a specific service, such as coronary bypass surgery, can be established in several alternative ways. In principle, one valid way to measure cost would be to identify a competitive market for medical service, and note the charge (price) for coronary bypass surgery in that market. While competitive market pricing might work well for commodities such as consumer electronic devices or farm products, it is not well suited to medical care, where there are few competitive markets. An alternative method is to take note of the charges for a service and apply correction factors to estimate cost more accurately. A third method to estimate costs is to examine in detail the resources used to provide a service, and apply price weights to the resources used.[8]

Most health economic studies currently use this third method to measure the costs of care. The price weights are taken from standardized reimbursement schedules (for hospital or outpatient services) or average prices (for drugs and supplies) paid in the community. A consistent set of price weights should be used, taking all the prices from the US Medicare system, for instance, or all from the US private insurance market.

International perspectives

With the advent of large multicenter clinical trials that enroll patients from several countries, interest has developed in cost comparisons between countries for the same service. Cost estimation as part of large randomized trials will enhance clinical decision making, as the randomized design is the strongest way to compare all outcomes of therapeutic alternatives, including cost. Extension of cost comparisons across national borders introduces a number of technical and conceptual issues that deserve discussion.

Different countries measure cost in their respective national currencies, so that readers in another country need to convert between units (for example, UK pounds or euros to US dollars). These conversions can be done using currency exchange rates or the closely related purchasing power parity factors. The differences between countries in units of measurement are fairly simple to address.

A more thorny issue in international comparisons is differences in the relative prices of the resources used to provide a service and differences in resource profiles used to provide a service. Thus, if the cost of service *j* is defined as:

$$\text{Cost}_j = \sum (\text{Quantity})_{ij} \times (\text{Price})_{ij}$$

then cost may differ among countries due to differences in the quantity of resources used to provide a service, price differentials for the same resources, or both. A specific example will help illustrate these concepts (Table 4.3). Care of a patient with acute myocardial infarction given thrombolysis includes the cost of the drug, the cost of basic hospital care, and the cost of additional tests and treatments in the convalescent phase. Table 4.3 presents hypothetical

Table 4.3 Effect of differences in medical prices on costs of alternative treatments

	Country 1		Country 2	
	Tx A	Tx B	Tx A	Tx B
Drug ($)	2000	200	1500	150
Nursing hours	50	54	50	54
Nursing wages ($)	30	30	35	35
Total ($)	3500	1820	3250	2040
Cost savings ($)	1680		1210	
Cost ratio B/A	52%	63%		

Tx, treatment

Table 4.4 Effect of differences in resource utilization on costs of alternative treatments

	Country 1		Country 2	
	Tx A	Tx B	Tx A	Tx B
Drug/nursing ($)	3500	1820	3250	2040
Coronary angiography	40%	60%	10%	15%
Angio cost ($)	1000	1000	1000	1000
Total ($)	3900	2420	3350	2190
Cost savings ($)	1480		1160	
Cost ratio (B/A)	62%	65%		

Tx, treatment

costs of basic care in two countries, with monetary values expressed in dollar units for simplicity. The costs of drugs in Country 1 are higher than in Country 2, where drug prices are strictly regulated. The time spent by the hospital staff to care for the patient are quite similar in Country 1 and Country 2 (50 hours per patient for Treatment A and 54 for Treatment B, a difference due to lower complication rates with Treatment A). The average hourly compensation for hospital staff is, however, higher in Country 2, so that total personnel costs are higher as well. Thus, both cost savings and the relative costs of Treatment A and B are different in these two healthcare systems, due to different prices for the same resources used to care for a myocardial infarct patient.

There may also be differences in the level of resource use between countries, especially for discretionary procedures such as coronary angiography. Suppose that the use of Treatment A cuts the use of coronary angiography by one-third, partially offsetting the higher cost of the drug. If, however, the baseline rates of angiography are different between countries, the cost implications of reducing angiography by one-third in each country will be quite different (Table 4.4). A reduction by one-third in the high rate of angiography in Country 1 (from 60% to 40%) provides a $200 cost offset per patient, whereas a reduction by one-third in the low rate of angiography in Country 2 (from 20% to 15%) provides only a $50 cost offset per patient.

International comparisons of the cost of therapies can thus be affected by (a) differences in resource use patterns that reflect differences in practice style and the organization of medical care, and (b) differences between countries in the prices attached to specific resources, such as healthcare wages, drugs, and supplies. Data from cost studies can be most readily applied in different practice environments if the study provides information on both resource consumption patterns and price weights attached to the specific resources used, as well as a summary cost measure. This detail is needed for readers to understand the applicability of the cost findings to their own practice settings.

Cost-effectiveness analysis

The cost of providing a particular medical service can be measured, but determination of whether the service provides good value for the money spent is a more difficult judgment. Cost-effectiveness analysis is a method of weighing the cost of a service in light of the health effects it confers in an attempt to facilitate the ultimate value judgment about whether the service is "worth" the cost.

Cost-effectiveness analysis is one of several alternative analytic methods, each with its own strengths and limitations.[6] If two alternative therapies are either known to yield identical results or can be shown to be clinically equivalent, they can be compared on the basis of cost alone. This form of analysis, which is termed "cost-minimization analysis", is particularly appropriate for commodities such as drugs, supplies, and equipment that can be expected to yield equivalent results when applied clinically. In such situations, the relative costs of the alternatives become the predominant consideration.

Many alternative therapies are known to differ both in clinical outcomes and in cost. In this situation, both the difference in cost and the difference in effectiveness of the therapeutic alternatives must be measured and weighed against each other. When the effectiveness on intervention is measured in clinical terms (for example, lives saved, years of life added), the analysis is termed "cost effectiveness". If the clinical measures of effectiveness are translated into monetary units, the term "cost–benefit analysis" is applied. Cost–benefit analysis has been used to guide public policy in areas outside medicine, such as in the construction of transportation systems or whether to remove or reduce environmental exposures. Cost–benefit analysis measures the effects of programs in monetary terms, so that net cost (in dollars) can be compared with net benefits (in dollars). Since there is great reluctance on the part of

physicians and health policy makers to assign a dollar value to saving a life or improving a patient's function, cost-effectiveness analysis rather than cost–benefit analysis has been applied predominantly to medical problems.

Cost-effectiveness analysis was first applied to medical programs only 30 years ago[9,10] and has since been widely used.[11–13] The principles of cost-effectiveness analysis for medical programs have been examined in detail by a task force convened by the United States Public Health Service.[14–16] A group of experts attempted to establish consensus on a number of methodologic issues, with the goal of standardizing the technical aspects of cost-effectiveness analysis among studies, thereby enhancing their comparability. The principles articulated by this group are reasonable and should guide this important field in its next 20 years.

A basic principle of cost-effectiveness analysis is that the analysis should compare alternative programs and not look at any single program in isolation. Thus, a drug to treat life-threatening arrhythmias might be compared with placebo, or an implantable cardioverter defibrillator might be compared with a drug. In essence, cost-effectiveness analysis must always answer the question "cost effective compared with what?".

Another principle is that the costs included in cost-effectiveness analysis should be comprehensive. The cost of a specific therapy should include the cost of the intervention itself (for example, thrombolytic therapy for acute myocardial infarction) and the costs of any complications the therapy induced (for example, bleeding), less any cost savings due to reduction of complications (such as heart failure). The need for other concomitant therapy should also be included, which is particularly important when assessing the cost effectiveness of screening programs or diagnostic testing strategies. The length of follow-up should be sufficient to include all relevant costs and benefits – such as readmissions to the hospital due to treatment failures. Nonmonetary costs directly related to the medical intervention should also be included, such as the cost of home care by the patient's family, since omission of these costs would bias assessments toward programs that rely on unpaid work by family members or volunteers. Other costs not directly related to the intervention, however, such as the patient's lost wages or pension costs, are omitted by convention from the measured costs in a cost-effectiveness analysis.

Another important issue in cost-effectiveness analysis is the perspective taken by the analysis. There is general agreement that the analysis should include all relevant costs, regardless of who pays them. This principle is known as "taking the societal perspective" and it assures a complete accounting of costs in the analysis. A hospital, for instance, may not care about the out-of-pocket costs paid directly by the patient but these are real costs and should be considered in the analysis.

Medical costs may accrue over long periods of time, especially in preventive programs or the treatment of chronic disease. Time scales of more than a year or so bring up two related but distinct issues – inflation and discounting. The nominal value of any currency changes over time; a dollar in 1998 had more purchasing power than a dollar in 2008. Studies conducted over long time periods will need to correct for the changing value of currencies, typically by application of the Consumer Price Index (or the GDP deflator). Application of the Consumer Price Index removes the effect of inflation but does not address the separate issue of time preference for money. Even in a country free of inflation, citizens would prefer to receive $100 today than a promise they will be paid $100 in a year. One might have to promise to pay more money in a year, say $103, to compensate for the delay. The same is true in health programs: we would prefer to be paid today instead of in the future, and we would also prefer to pay our obligations in the future rather than today. Use of a discount rate provides a way to correct for the lower value of future costs relative to current costs. The technical experts' consensus is that future costs should be discounted at a rate equivalent to the interest paid on safe investments such as government bonds in an inflation-free environment, or about 3% per year. The effect of alternative discount rates between 0% and 5–10% per year should also be checked to document the sensitivity of the analysis to future costs.

In summary, a cost-effectiveness analysis should include all medical costs, including those of complications of therapy and adverse effects prevented. The study should be of sufficient duration to measure all relevant costs and benefits of the treatment. All costs and benefits should be included, regardless of who bears or receives them. In studies covering more than a year or so, corrections should be made for inflation, and 3% per year discount rate should be applied to follow-up costs.

Measuring effectiveness

The effectiveness of an intervention in practice can be measured in a variety of ways, with different outcome measures most appropriate for specific applications. Physiologic endpoints are often used in clinical trials, with the result of therapy assessed by a laboratory measure such as millimeters of mercury for blood pressure or episodes of non-sustained ventricular tachycardia on an electrocardiographic monitor. Laboratory measures are useful in judging the physiologic effects of therapy and its mechanism of action, but these surrogate markers may not predict the ultimate effect of therapy on mortality and morbidity, as vividly illustrated by the results of the Cardiac Arrhythmia Suppression Trial.[16] Physiologic endpoints are also tied closely to one specific disease, making comparisons against other benchmark therapies difficult. The patient and public are most concerned with the effect of therapy on survival and on their ability to function – that is, upon the length and quality of life. A common denominator measure of effectiveness is thus the life-years of expected survival or quality-adjusted life-years (QALYs). This measure is relevant to patients and to the public and can be applied to virtually any therapy.

Mortality is a common endpoint in clinical trials and leads directly to the measure of life-years of survival. The mean life expectancy of a cohort of patients is equal to the area under a standard survival curve. The difference in life expectancy between two therapies is therefore equal to the difference in the areas under their respective survival curves. Since many clinical studies do not follow patient cohorts long enough to observe complete survival times for all patients, some assumptions and modeling of long-term survival may be needed to estimate the full survival benefit of therapy for a cost-effectiveness analysis.[17]

Improvement in quality of life is often as important to patients as reducing mortality, and it is often the main goal of therapies, such as the relief of disabling angina or improvement in exercise tolerance. A quality of life measure can be translated into a scale that ranges from a low of 0.0 (the worst possible health state, usually taken as death) to 1.0 (perfect health). This quality of life measure is multiplied by the length of time a patient spends in the health state to yield a QALY. Thus:

$$QALY = \sum Q_i \times t_i$$

where QALY = the quality-adjusted life-years, Q_i = the quality factor for follow-up period "i" and t_i = the length of time spent in period "i". This equation shows that the effectiveness of a treatment, as measured in QALYs, can be improved by enhancing either the patient's quality of life (Q_i) or the patient's length of life (t_i), or both.

Calculation of cost effectiveness

After the costs of therapy and the medical effectiveness of therapy have been assessed, cost effectiveness (CE) can be calculated as:

$$CE \ ratio = \frac{Cost_2 - Cost_1}{QALY_2 - QALY_1}$$

where $Cost_1$ and $Cost_2$ represent the costs of program 1 and program 2, respectively, and $QALY_1$ and $QALY_2$ represent the effectiveness of programs 1 and 2, respectively.

There are several implications of using this formula. First, cost-effectiveness ratios that are positive (that is, >0) result if and only if one alternative has both higher cost and greater effectiveness – that is, $Cost_2 > Cost_1$ and $QALY_2 > QALY_1$ (or the reverse: $Cost_2 < Cost_1$ and

$QALY_2 < QALY_1$). Cost-effectiveness ratios of less than zero are not generally important for decision making, since they arise only when one alternative has both lower costs and greater clinical effectiveness than the other; for example, $Cost_2 > Cost_1$ and $QALY_2 < QALY_1$. In this case, program 1 is superior in all respects: it has better outcomes and lower cost than program 2 and thus is said to "dominate" the alternative. The decision of which program to recommend is therefore simple.

Most commonly, one of two therapeutic alternatives has higher costs and greater effectiveness, and use of the formula yields a cost-effectiveness ratio greater than zero. One treatment may have a cost-effectiveness ratio of $5000 per year of life saved and another might have a ratio of $75 000 per year of life saved. Since it is problematic to assign a dollar value to life, interpretation of these ratios is best made by consideration of benchmarks – other generally accepted therapies that serve as a rough gauge to an "acceptable" cost-effectiveness ratio. Renal dialysis is a form of therapy that most people would consider expensive, and yet dialysis is an intervention that the USA and most other industrialized countries provide as a life-saving therapy. The end-stage renal disease program in the USA costs about $50 000 a year per patient and if this therapy were withdrawn, the patient would die. Thus, renal dialysis has a cost-effectiveness ratio of $50 000 per year of life saved (or if one considers the reduced quality of life for a dialysis patient, perhaps $75 000 per quality-adjusted year of life saved). Therapies with cost-effectiveness ratios considerably more favorable than renal dialysis (that is, <$20 000) would be considered very cost effective, whereas therapies with cost effective ratios much higher (say >$125 000) would be considered too expensive.

Different societies may come to different conclusions about the level of cost effectiveness they consider good value. Wealthy countries with high per capita incomes are more willing to pay for expensive therapies than are poor countries. For instance, the percentage of gross domestic product and per capita health spending in Eastern Europe is much less than in Western Europe or North America, and these countries have not chosen to provide expensive services such as bypass surgery as readily or as frequently. The World Health Organization has suggested three times GDP per capita as a rough guide for the cost-effectiveness threshold.

A therapy that is cost effective is not necessarily affordable in the setting of limited resources. In particular, the aggregate effect of a new therapy on healthcare expenditures depends on both the number of patients treated and the incremental cost per patient. Expensive treatments for common diseases may raise costs by billions of dollars (e.g. coronary stents, implantable defibrillators). Decisions to adopt new technologies will consider the aggregate budgetary impact, not just the cost-effectiveness ratio.

Decisions about funding programs might be more equitable and rational when guided by the relative cost effectiveness of programs. When studies use similar methods to measure cost and effectiveness, cost-effectiveness ratios can be compared to rank the economic attractiveness of alternatives. Tables comparing various treatments, such as Table 4.5, have been termed "league tables" because of

Table 4.5 Cost effectiveness of selected cardiovascular therapies

Strategy	Patient group	Cost effectiveness[a]
Statin	Post-MI	Saves dollars and lives
	Men 45–54	
	Chol ≥250	
ACE inhibitor	CHF	Saves dollars and lives
	EF <35%	
Radiofrequency ablation	WPW, post cardiac arrest	Saves dollars and lives
Physician counseling	Smoking	$1300
Beta-blocker	Post-MI	$3600
	High-risk	
CABG	Left main CAD	$9200
	Severe angina	
Beta-blocker	Post-MI	$20 200
	Low-risk	
Statin	Primary prevention	$20 200
	Men 55–64	
	Chol >300	
	Three risk factors	
tPA vs SK	Acute MI	$32 800
ICD	Sustained VT	$35 000
CABG	Two-vessel CAD	$42 500
	Angina	
Statin	Primary prevention	$78 300
	Men 55–64	
	Chol >300	
	No other risk factors	
PCI	Mild angina (COURAGE)	$168 000[18]
CABG	Single-vessel CAD	$1 142 000
	Mild angina	
Statin	Primary prevention	$2 024 800
	35–44 year old women	
	Chol >300	
	No other risk factors	

[a] $ values, dollars per year of life added.
ACE, angiotensin- converting enzyme inhibitor; CABG, coronary artery bypass graft; CAD, coronary artery disease; CHF, congestive heart failure; Chol, Cholesterol; EF, ejection fraction; ICD, implantable cardioverter defibrillator; MI, myocardial infarction; tPA, tissue plasminogen activator; SK, streptokinase; VT, ventricular tachycardia; WPW, Wolff–Parkinson-White syndrome.
Source: adapted from Kupersmith et al.[10–12]

their similarity to the athletic league standings published in newspapers. Given the uncertainty inherent in measuring cost and effectiveness of medical interventions, and the methodologic variations among studies, only relatively large differences in cost-effectiveness ratios should be considered significant. Thus, a program with a cost-effectiveness ratio of $5000 per life year added is much better than one with a ratio of $30 000. Programs with ratios of $25 000 and $30 000 are so close that no firm conclusion about the relative values should be drawn.

A league table of cost-effectiveness ratios may help guide policy decisions about which therapies to provide within a health care system, but other factors also affect such decisions. The total budgetary impact of a therapy is the product of the number of treated patients and the net cost per patient. Two therapies with similar cost-effectiveness ratios may have quite different impacts on the health care budget, which policy-makers must consider as well. Furthermore, cost-effectiveness concerns economic efficiency, but policymakers also have to consider the distribution of resources and ensure fairness. They may decide to cover the only available therapy for a certain disease, even though it has a less favorable cost-effectiveness ratio than a second-line treatment for a different disease.

Patient selection and cost effectiveness

Drugs and procedures in medicine are applied to different patient groups for different clinical indications. The medical effectiveness of therapies varies considerably according to patient selection. Cholesterol-lowering therapy, for instance, will extend the life expectancy of a patient with multiple cardiac risk factors more than it will for a patient with the same cholesterol level and no other cardiac risk factors. Coronary bypass surgery provides greater life extension to a patient with left main coronary artery obstruction than it does to a patient with single vessel disease.[18] The cost-effectiveness ratio for these therapies will therefore vary among patient subgroups due to the impact of patient characteristics on the clinical effectiveness of therapy, which forms the denominator of the cost-effectiveness ratio. Similarly, the cost of a particular therapy may also vary according to patient characteristics, since the therapy itself may be more or less expensive according to different patient subgroups, or the likelihood of costly complications may be higher or lower in different groups of patients.

The clinical effectiveness of a therapy is generally the most important factor determining cost effectiveness. The reasons for this importance are (a) that clinical effectiveness of a therapy generally varies more among patients than does the cost of therapy, and (b) the value of the cost-effectiveness ratio is more sensitive to changes in the denominator (effectiveness) than to changes in the numera-

tor (cost). In the last analysis, a therapy must be clinically effective before it can be cost effective. Cost-effectiveness analysis relies more on the assessment of medical effectiveness than it does on determination of cost.

Diagnostic tests and cost effectiveness

Cost-effectiveness analysis has been applied primarily to assess specific therapies or therapeutic strategies, for which it is natural to measure effectiveness in terms of patient outcome. The principles of cost effectiveness can be extended to analyze screening tests and diagnostic strategies as well, but some additional factors must also be considered.

Therapies are expected to improve patient outcome *directly*, by intervening in the pathophysiology of disease processes. In contrast, a diagnostic test is expected to provide the physician with information about the patient, which in turn is expected to improve management and thereby *indirectly* improve patient outcome. The value of a test is therefore linked closely with patient selection for therapy, and the value of testing may well change as new therapies are developed or alternative tests become available.

The information provided by a test may be used in different decisions, and the test may be more or less useful in these different settings. An exercise electrocardiogram, for example, can be used as a diagnostic test for coronary disease, a prognostic test for patients with recent myocardial infarction, a monitoring test to assess the effect of anti-ischemic therapy or even as a way to establish target heart rates for an exercise training program. The efficacy and cost effectiveness of applying the exercise electrocardiogram will be different for these varied uses of the information provided by the test. The value of the test will depend on the indication for which it is used, much as the value of a beta-blocker will vary whether it is used to treat hypertension or as secondary prevention after a myocardial infarction.

The same test (for example, the exercise ECG) applied for the same purpose (such as diagnosis of coronary disease) will provide more information in some groups of patients than in others. As discussed elsewhere in this book, a diagnostic test provides more value if used when the pretest probability of disease is intermediate than when it is either very high or very low. The test has the most value when the result is likely to change the estimated probability of disease such that clinical management is changed. Tests that never change patient management cannot change patient outcome, which is the "bottom line" in assessing cost effectiveness.

Conclusion

Economic analysis is designed to assist decisions about the allocation of scarce resources. Physicians now must address the cost implications of clinical decisions, and be aware of the effects on scarce resources. Economic efficiency is but one of many goals, however, and issues of fairness and humaneness are also central to medical care and must be considered as well.

References

1. Fuchs VR. *Who Shall Live? Health, Economics and Social Choice.* New York: Basic Books, 1974.
2. OECD. *Health Data 2008: Statistics and Indicators for 30 Countries.* Paris: Organization for Economic Cooperation and Development, 2008.
3. Jollis JG, Peterson ED, DeLong ER *et al.* The relation between the volume of coronary angioplasty procedures at hospitals treating Medicare beneficiaries and short-term mortality. *N Engl J Med* 1994;**331**:1625–9.
4. Kimmel SE, Berlin JA, Laskey WK. The relationship between coronary angioplasty procedure volume and major complications. *JAMA* 1995;**274**:1137–42.
5. Hannan EL, Racz M, Ryan T, *et al.* Coronary angioplasty volume-outcome relationships for hospitals and cardiologists. *JAMA* 1997;**279**:892–8.
6. Drummond MF, O'Brien BJ, Stoddart GL, Torrance GW. *Methods for the Economic Evaluation of Healthcare Programmes*, 2nd edn. Oxford: Oxford University Press, 1997.
7. Finkler SA. The distinction between costs and charges. *Ann Intern Med* 1982;**96**:102–10.
8. Hlatky MA, Lipscomb J, Nelson C *et al.* Resource use and cost of initial coronary revascularization. Coronary angioplasty versus coronary bypass surgery. *Circulation* 1990;**82**(suppl IV):IV-208-IV-213.
9. Weinstein MC, Stason WB. Foundations of cost effectiveness analysis for health and medical practices. *N Engl J Med* 1977;**296**:716–21.
10. Detsky AS, Naglie IG. A clinician's guide to cost effectiveness analysis. *Ann Int Med* 1990;**113**:147–54.
11. Kupersmith J, Holmes-Rovner M, Hogan A, Rovner D, Gardiner J. Cost effectiveness analysis in heart disease, Part I: general principles. *Prog Cardiovasc Dis* 1994;**37**:161–84.
12. Kupersmith J, Holmes-Rovner M, Hogan A, Rovner D, Gardiner J. Cost effectiveness analysis in heart disease, Part II: preventive therapies. *Prog Cardiovasc Dis* 1995;**37**:243–71.
13. Kupersmith J, Holmes-Rovner M, Hogan A, Rovner D, Gardiner J. Cost effectiveness analysis in heart disease, Part III: ischemia, congestive heart failure, and arrhythmias. *Prog Cardiovasc Dis* 1995;**37**:307–46.
14. Russell LB, Gold MR, Siegel JE, Daniels N, Weinstein MC. The role of cost effectiveness analysis in health and medicine. Panel on Cost effectiveness in Health and Medicine. *JAMA* 1996;**276**:1172–7.
15. Weinstein MC, Siegel JE, Gold MR, Kamlet MS, Russell LB. Recommendations of the Panel on Cost effectiveness in Health and Medicine. *JAMA* 1996;**276**:1253–8.
16. Siegel JE, Weinstein MC, Russell LB, Gold MR. Recommendations for reporting cost effectiveness analyses. Panel on Cost effectiveness in Health and Medicine. *JAMA* 1996;**276**:1339–41.
17. Mark DB, Hlatky MA, Califf RM *et al.* Cost effectiveness of thrombolytic therapy with tissue plasminogen activator as compared with streptokinase for acute myocardial infarction. *N Engl J Med* 1995;**332**:1418–24.
18. Yusuf S, Zucker D, Peduzzi P *et al.* Effect of coronary artery bypass graft surgery on survival: overview of 10-year results from randomised trials by the Coronary Artery Bypass Graft Surgery Trialists Collaboration. *Lancet* 1994;**344**:563–70.
19. Weintraub WS, Boden WE, Zhang A *et al.* Cost effectiveness of percutaneous coronary intervention in optimally treated stable coronary patients. *Circ Cardiovasc Qual Outcomes* 2008;**1**:12–20.

5

Major vascular complications in patients undergoing non-cardiac surgery: magnitude of the problem, risk prediction, surveillance, and prevention

Philip J Devereaux,[1] Matthew Chan[2] and John Eikelboom[3]

[1] Departments of Clinical Epidemiology and Biostatistics and Medicine, McMaster University, Hamilton, Ontario, Canada
[2] Department of Anesthesia, The Chinese University of Hong Kong, Hong Kong, China
[3] Department of Medicine, McMaster University, Hamilton, Ontario, Canada

Magnitude of the problem

Throughout the last few decades, non-cardiac surgery has made substantial advances in treating diseases and improving patient quality of life, and as a result, the number of patients undergoing non-cardiac surgery is growing. A recent study used surgical data from 56 countries around the world to determine that globally there are over 230 million major surgical procedures undertaken annually.[1] The fact that cardiac and pediatric surgery only account for a minority of major surgical cases suggests that over 200 million adults undergo major non-cardiac surgery annually.

Non-cardiac surgery is associated with an increased risk of major vascular complications (i.e. vascular death, non-fatal myocardial infarction, non-fatal cardiac arrest, and non-fatal stroke). A recent review found only one study, by Lee and colleagues,[2] that evaluated the incidence of major perioperative vascular complications in a prospective cohort that fulfilled the following criteria: more than 300 patients, the patients were relatively unselected (i.e. not restricted to patients referred to internal medicine or to patients with or at high risk of coronary artery disease), not restricted to a specific type of surgery (e.g. orthopedics), and required patients to have at least one measurement of a cardiac biomarker or enzyme after surgery.[3] This study suggests that major perioperative vascular events occur in 1.4% (95% confidence interval (CI) 1.0–1.8%) of adults undergoing elective non-cardiac surgery. Conservative estimates suggest that at least half of the 200 million adults

undergoing non-cardiac surgery are in an at-risk age group.[4] These data together with the data from the Lee study suggests that worldwide, 1–1.8 million adults suffer a major perioperative vascular complication annually.

There is concern, however, that this is a substantial underestimation of the actual incidence. The recent Peri-Operative ISchemic Evaluation (POISE) trial included 8351 patients from 190 hospitals in 23 countries in a randomized controlled trial comparing the effects of a beta-blocker relative to placebo among patients undergoing non-cardiac surgery.[5] The incidence of major perioperative vascular complications in the POISE trial was more than three times higher than what was predicted by the Revised Cardiac Risk Index, which was developed from the study by Lee and colleagues. This suggests the possibility that the current incidence of major perioperative vascular complications is substantially higher than the estimate from the Lee study. Several limitations associated with the Lee study support this position. Lee *et al* did not include stroke as an outcome, and excluded patients undergoing emergency surgery.[2] Emergent cases represent about 10% of non-cardiac surgeries[6] and patients undergoing emergency surgery are at higher risk of major perioperative vascular events than patients undergoing elective surgery (odds ratio (OR) 2.6, 95% CI 1.2–5.6).[7] The data from Lee and colleagues are over 15 years old. Considering that patients with coronary artery disease are living longer and there has been a practice pattern shift towards advanced care for the elderly (including surgery), this suggests that older patients with high burdens of coronary artery disease are now surviving to develop other conditions that require an operation and these elderly patients are undergoing surgery.

These limitations support the finding in the POISE trial, and this suggests that the current worldwide incidence of adults suffering a major perioperative vascular

Evidence-Based Cardiology, 3rd edition. Edited by S. Yusuf, J.A. Cairns, A.J. Camm, E.L. Fallen, and B.J. Gersh. © 2010 Blackwell Publishing, ISBN: 978-1-4051-5925-8.

complication in the first 30 days after surgery is probably in the range of 3–5.4 million annually. This is in the range of the global incidence of new patients acquiring human immunodeficiency virus (HIV) annually,[8] and identifies major perioperative vascular complications as a similarly common and important public health problem.

Preoperative risk prediction

Need for preoperative risk prediction

Accurate estimation of perioperative vascular risk in patients undergoing non-cardiac surgery is important to guide perioperative management and to allow patients and physicians to make informed decisions about the appropriateness of surgery. The majority of non-cardiac surgeries are elective procedures. An accurate estimate of risk facilitates patient and physician decision making. For example, if an elderly female with multiple risk factors undergoing hip arthroplasty for osteo-arthritis was accurately informed that her risk of a major perioperative vascular event was 10–12%, she may decide to defer surgery for a year, living with suboptimal quality of life until after her granddaughter's wedding. Further, accurate perioperative cardiac risk prediction can inform management decisions (e.g. whether to delay or cancel surgery or type of anesthetic approach) and monitoring decisions (e.g. whether a patient should go to a telemetry unit after surgery).

Clinical risk prediction

Researchers have developed two types of clinical models – generic and Bayesian – to estimate perioperative cardiac risk in patients undergoing non-cardiac surgery. The generic risk models estimate a patient's risk of a perioperative cardiac event through determination of how many predictors of risk (e.g. history of coronary artery disease, diabetes, emergency surgery) an individual patient fulfills.

The Bayesian risk models modify the average cardiac event rate for a specific surgery or group of comparable surgeries (pretest probability) through use of a patient's individual index score (likelihood ratio), which is based upon how many predictors of risk (e.g. history of coronary artery disease, diabetes) an individual patient fulfills. The result provides an estimate of the patient's risk of a perioperative cardiac event (post-test probability).

Four clinical models developed to predict perioperative cardiac events fulfill the following criteria: assessed in >300 patients, validated at least within the original study, and not restricted to a specific type of non-cardiac surgery (e.g. vascular surgery).[2,7,9,10] Table 5.1 presents information on the studies that developed these clinical models and Table 5.2 presents their scoring systems. All studies had a small to moderate number of events and were underpowered to assess the independent effect of each variable given the number of variables assessed. These clinical models were designed to predict cardiac outcomes of varying importance, and no model included stroke. Table 5.3 presents the studies that have evaluated the predictors of stroke in patients undergoing non-cardiac surgery.[11–15] Although there are few studies and most observed few events, they do suggest overlap between the predictors of stroke and major cardiac events in patients undergoing non-cardiac surgery. The study with the most number of perioperative strokes (i.e. 61 strokes) suggests that perioperative stroke is a serious outcome (i.e. 18% died and 31% were care dependent at discharge).[15]

The Revised Cardiac Risk Index is the simplest of the models to use and is more predictive than the Original Cardiac Risk Index.[2,7] Of the two Bayesian models, the Veterans Affairs Model is simpler to use and the one study that compared these two models suggested the Veterans Affairs Model was as predictive as the Modified Cardiac Risk Index.[7] Although several studies have compared the predictive accuracy of the generic and Bayesian risk models,[2,7,9,16,17] only two have used pretest probabilities in the Bayesian models based upon contemporary data from the hospitals included in the studies.[7,9] The most recent of

Table 5.1 Studies that have developed clinical models to predict cardiac events in patients undergoing non-cardiac surgery

Study	Name of model	Type of model	N	Outcome	Number of events
Goldman[10]	Original Cardiac Risk Index	Generic	1001	Cardiac death, MI, pulmonary edema or ventricular tachycardia	58
Detsky[9]	Modified Cardiac Risk Index	Bayesian	455	Cardiac death, MI or pulmonary edema	30
Lee[2]	Revised Cardiac Risk Index	Generic	4315	Cardiac arrest, MI, pulmonary edema, complete heart block	92
Kumar[7]	Veterans Affairs Model	Bayesian	1121	Cardiac death, MI, pulmonary edema, cardiac arrest, unstable angina, new or worsening CHF without pulmonary edema	91

MI, myocardial infarction; CHF, congestive heart failure.

Table 5.2 Clinical models to predict cardiac events in patients undergoing non-cardiac surgery

Original Cardiac Risk Index[10]		Modified Cardiac Risk Index[9]				Revised Cardiac Risk Index[2]		Veterans Affairs Model[7]			
Computation of cardiac risk score		Pre-test probability		Index score		Computation of cardiac risk score		Pretest probability		Index score	
Variables	Pts	Surgery	Risk	Variables	Pts	Variables	Pts	Surgery	Risk	Variables	Pts
Age >70	5	Aortic	16%	MI within 6 mo	10	High-risk Sx	1	Aortic	32%	MI within 6 mo	25
MI within 6 mo	10	Carotid	15%	MI >6 mo	5	IHD	1	Carotid	10%	Emergency Sx	15
S₃ gallop or JVD	11	Peripheral vas	6%	CCSC angina 3	10	Prior CHF	1	Peripheral vasc	15%	MI >6 mo	10
Important VAS	3	Orthopedic	14%	CCSC angina 4	20	Prior CVA	1	Misc vasc Sx	10%	Prior CHF	10
Abn rhythm	7	Intrathoracic/	8%	U/A ≤3 mo	10	Insulin	1	Intra-abdominal/	13%	Abn rhythm	10
>5 PVCs/min	7	intraperitoneal	3%	APE <1 wk	10	therapy	1	Intrathoracic	3%		
Poor status	3	Head and neck	2%	APE ever	5	Cr >2 mg/dL	1	Interm-risk Sx	1%		
High-risk Sx	3	Minor		Critical VAS	20			Low-risk Sx			
Emergency Sx	4			Abn rhythm	5						
				>5 PVCs	5						
				poor status	5						
				Age >70	5						
				Emergency Sx	10						

Pts	Risk of event	A patient's post-test probability of an event is determined by using the total index score to modify the pretest probability using a likelihood ratio nomogram specific for this index				Pts	Risk of event	A patient's post-test probability of an event is determined by using the total index score to modify the pretest probability using a likelihood ratio nomogram specific for this index			
0–5	0.9%					0	0.5%				
6–12	7%					1	1.3%				
13–25	13%					2	4%				
≥26	78%					≥3	9%				

abn rhythm, rhythm other than sinus or premature atrial contractions on last preoperative electrocardiogram; APE, alveolar pulmonary edema; CCSC, Canadian Cardiovascular Society Class; CHF, congestive heart failure; Cr, creatinine; CVA, stroke or transient ischemic attack; IHD, ischemic heart disease; JVD, jugular vein distension; mo, months; poor status, $PO_2 < 60$, $PCO_2 > 50$ mmHg, K < 3.0, $HCO3 < 20$ meq/L, blood urea nitrogen >50, creatinine >3.0 mg/dL, abnormal serum glutamic oxalacetic transaminase, signs of chronic liver disease, or patient bedridden from non-cardiac causes; Pts, points; PVCs, premature ventricular contractions; U/A, unstable angina; vasc, vascular; VAS, valvular aortic stenosis; low-risk Sx, low-risk surgery (e.g. ophthalmology, maxillofacial, plastic, low-risk orthopedic, urologic, general surgery and non-thoracotomy thoracic procedures); Interm-risk Sx, intermediate risk surgery (e.g. neurosurgery, ENT surgery, major orthopedic surgery); high-risk Sx, high-risk surgery (e.g. intraperitoneal, intrathoracic, or aortic surgery); misc vasc Sx, miscellaneous vascular surgery (e.g. all lower extremity amputations, arteriovenous access procedures).

these two studies demonstrated superior prediction capabilities of the Bayesian risk models.[7]

Despite this finding, the current predictive accuracy of the Modified Cardiac Risk Index and the Veterans Affairs Model is uncertain because there is no high-quality study that has established contemporary complication rates for individual surgeries or groups of comparable surgeries, and it is unknown if contemporary complication rates at one institution are applicable to another institution. Further, it is unclear whether the Bayesian models would demonstrate superior prediction capabilities if the generic risk models included more specific surgeries or groups of comparable surgeries as risk factors, because it is likely that the type of surgery a patient undergoes influences the probability of a vascular complication.

The Vascular events In non-cardiac Surgery patIents cOhort evaluatioN (VISION) Study is a prospective cohort study of 40 000 patients undergoing non-cardiac surgery in several countries around the world (ClinicalTrials.gov, number NCT00512109). A primary objective of this study is to develop a current clinical risk estimation model for predicting major perioperative vascular complications. Until further studies like the VISION Study are complete, physicians need a practical clinical risk index. The Revised Cardiac Risk Index from the Lee study is the simplest to use in clinical practice, and several studies have validated the factors included in the index as independent predictors of major perioperative vascular complications.[18] The Revised Cardiac Risk Index consists of six equally weighted risk factors: high-risk surgery (intraperitoneal, intrathoracic

Table 5.3 Predictors of stroke in patients undergoing non-cardiac surgery

Study	Enrolment years	Design	Patient population	Events	Predictors of perioperative stroke
Larsen[11]	1981–1983	Single center prospective cohort study	2463 patients >40 years old who had elective or acute non-cardiac surgery; carotid surgery cases were excluded	3 TIAs and 6 strokes	Prior CVD, coronary artery disease, PVD, and hypertension predicted perioperative stroke and TIA in unadjusted analyses ($P < 0.001$, <0.001, <0.05, and <0.05, respectively)
Landercasper[12]	1981–1988	Single center retrospective cohort study	Patients who had general anesthesia were included, those who had cerebrovacular or neurosurgery were excluded; 173 of the 7690 patients had a prior history of stroke	5 strokes	Prior stroke predicted perioperative stroke in unadjusted analysis ($P < 0.001$)
Parikh[13]	NR	Single center case–control study	19 patients who suffered a perioperative stroke after general or vascular surgery and 19 controls matched for age and procedure operated on during the same time period; patients who had carotid endarterectomies were excluded	19 strokes	Prior hypertension, neurologic symptoms, abnormal cardiac rhythm predicted perioperative stroke in unadjusted analyses ($P = 0.02$, 0.02, and 0.04, respectively)
Rockman[14]	1988–1993	Singe center retrospective cohort study	Patients who had a carotid endarterectomy were included; those who had surgery for recurrent carotid stenosis and non-atherosclerotic disorders were excluded; 183 of the 606 patients had a prior history of stroke	13 strokes	Prior stroke predicted perioperative stroke in unadjusted analysis ($P = 0.01$)
Limberg[15]	1986–1996	Single center case–control study	61 patients who suffered an ischemic stroke after non-cardiac surgery and 122 randomly selected controls matched for age, sex, procedure, and year of surgery; patients who had heart, brain, vessel or neck surgery were excluded	61 strokes (ischemic)	AOR for prior CVD = 13 (95% CI 2.1–74); AOR for COPD = 9 (95% CI 2.5–31); AOR for PVD = 8 (95% CI 2.3–28); AOR for admission MAP = 1.04 (95% CI 1.01–1.07)

AOR, adjusted odds ratio; CVD, cerebrovascular disease; COPD, chronic obstructive pulmonary disease; PVD, peripheral vascular disease; MAP, mean arterial pressure; TIA, transient ischemic attack; NR, not reported; neurologic symptoms, optic migraine, transient ischemic attack, and stroke.

or suprainguinal vascular surgery), history of ischemic heart disease, history of congestive heart failure, history of cerebrovascular disease (i.e. stroke or transient ischemic attack), use of insulin therapy for diabetes, and a preoperative serum creatinine >175 μmol/L (>2.0 mg/dL). Table 5.4 presents data from the original study and demonstrates the percentage risk of patients suffering a major perioperative cardiac event (i.e. cardiac death, non-fatal myocardial infarction, and non-fatal cardiac arrest) and the corresponding 95% confidence intervals, based on the number of risk factors met. As stated above, the observed event rate in the recent large international POISE trial demonstrated an observed event rate that was three times higher than that predicted by the Revised Cardiac Risk Index. Therefore, physicians may want to double or triple the estimates from Table 5.4 until further data are available.

Non-invasive cardiac stress testing

Although clinical risk indices help to identify patients at risk of a major vascular complication, they underestimate risk in a substantial proportion of patients.[3,17] This likely occurs because for a prolonged period of time prior to undergoing surgery, many patients have limited mobility (e.g. patients with arthritis, peripheral vascular disease, cancer). Some of these patients have underlying cardiac disease but are not active enough to experience symptoms. Although it is likely that researchers will develop more accurate clinical risk indices, it is also likely that a substantial proportion of patients undergoing non-cardiac surgery (e.g. patients with limited mobility, diabetes) will require further evaluation beyond clinical symptoms to optimize their risk assessments.

To address this problem researchers have assessed the prognostic capabilities of non-invasive cardiac stress tests (e.g. stress echocardiography, nuclear scintigraphy imaging), prior to non-cardiac surgery.[3] A recent meta-analysis evaluating these two tests demonstrated that they have only moderate negative likelihood ratios (stress echocardiography 0.23 and stress perfusion imaging 0.44), and

Table 5.4 Perioperative cardiac risk estimation based upon predictors in the Revised Cardiac Risk Index

Number of risk factors	Percentage risk of patients suffering a major perioperative cardiac event	95% CI
0	0.4%	0.1–0.8%
1	1.0%	0.5–1.4%
2	2.4%	1.3–3.5%
>3	5.4%	2.8–7.9%

This table is reproduced with permission from Devereaux et al.[3]
Risk factors = high-risk surgery (intraperitoneal, intrathoracic or suprainguinal vascular surgery), history of ischemic heart disease (defined as a history of myocardial infarction, positive exercise test, current complaint of ischemic chest pain or nitrate use, or ECG with pathologic Q waves; patients with prior coronary bypass surgery or angioplasty were included only if they had such findings after their procedure), history of congestive heart failure (defined as a history of heart failure, pulmonary edema or paroxysmal nocturnal dyspnea; an S3 gallop or bilateral rales on physical examination, or a chest radiograph showing pulmonary vascular resistance), history of cerebrovascular disease (i.e. stroke or transient ischemic attack), use of insulin therapy for diabetes, and a preoperative serum creatinine >175 μmol/L (>2.0 mg/dL).
Major perioperative cardiac event = cardiac death, non-fatal myocardial infarction or non-fatal cardiac arrest; note that this table does not include postoperative cardiogenic pulmonary edema and complete heart block, which were included as outcomes in the Lee index.

more than a third of the patients who suffered a major perioperative cardiovascular event had a negative test result.[19] The studies that directly compared these tests suggested there was no difference between the two tests regarding their positive likelihood ratios. When either of these tests had a moderate-to-large defect it was associated with a positive likelihood ratio of 8; however, this test result was only present in a small proportion of patients (i.e. <15% of the patients undergoing one of these tests).

These data likely represent a best-case scenario for these tests because the results report the direct association between the non-invasive cardiac stress test and the risk of a major perioperative cardiovascular outcome. Because of the cost and time associated with these tests, the more relevant data are whether these non-invasive cardiac stress tests provide additional predictive value, beyond clinical variables, for the occurrence of major perioperative cardiovascular events. Most of the studies have not assessed whether these non-invasive cardiac stress tests provide independent prognostic information. The studies that have undertaken multivariable analysis are unreliable because they did not include all the known independent clinical variables or the analysis had too few events for the number of variables assessed.[20–24] The results and the limitations of these data leave considerable uncertainty as to the role of non-invasive cardiac stress testing prior to non-cardiac surgery.

Preoperative BNP and NT-proBNP measurement

Ventricular myocytes secrete brain natriuretic peptide (BNP), a prohormone, and its inactive cleavage product N-terminal fragment of the prohormone (NT-proBNP) into the blood in response to myocardial stretch and ischemia.[25,26] Plasma BNP and NT-proBNP are powerful predictors of death and major adverse cardiovascular events in patients with stable coronary artery disease, acute coronary syndromes, and congestive heart failure.[27–31] Table 5.5

Table 5.5 Adjusted association between pre-operative BNP/NT-proBNP level and perioperative cardiovascular event

Study and year of publication	Marker and threshold (pg/mL)	Outcome	No of events/no of patients in study	Adjusted OR (95% CI)
Dernellis 2006[32]	BNP (189)	Cardiac death, non-fatal MI, pulm. edema, VT	96/1590	34 (17–69)
Feringa 2006[33]	NT-proBNP (533)	Death, non-fatal MI	13/170	17 (3–106)
Cuthbertson 2007[34]	BNP (40)	Death, myocardial injury, arrhythmia†	12/204	7 (2–29)
Cuthbertson 2007[35]	BNP (170)	Cardiac death, myocardial injury	11/40	14 (2–98)
Cardinale 2007[36]	NT-proBNP (various*)	Atrial fibrillation	72/400	28 (13–59)
Yun 2008[37]	NT-proBNP (201)	Cardiac death, non-fatal MI, pulm. edema, non-fatal stroke	25/279	8 (2–27)

MI, myocardial infarction; pulm., pulmonary; VT, ventricular tachycardia; ACS, acute coronary syndrome.
* Authors employed six age- and sex-dependent thresholds;
† resulting in hemodynamic compromise or requiring intervention.

reports six studies that have evaluated the independent association between a preoperative BNP or NT-proBNP measurement and major perioperative cardiovascular events.[32–37] All studies suggest that an elevated preoperative BNP or NT-proBNP measurement is a strong independent predictor of a major perioperative cardiovascular event. Although there are limitations to these studies regarding the number of events, variations in the outcomes and thresholds evaluated, and the width of the confidence intervals, these results are encouraging. A large substudy (10 000 patients) of the VISION Study currently under way is evaluating the prognostic capabilities of preoperative NT-proBNP and will provide further insights into whether NT-proBNP, a relatively cheap and easily accessible test compared to the non-invasive cardiac stress tests, can enhance perioperative clinical risk predictions.

Perioperative myocardial infarctions

Considering the major perioperative vascular complications (i.e. vascular death, non-fatal myocardial infarction, non-fatal cardiac arrest, and non-fatal stroke) myocardial infarction is the most common event. For example, in the POISE trial 1.6% of patients suffered a vascular death, 0.7% suffered a stroke, 0.5% suffered a non-fatal cardiac arrest, and 5.0% suffered a myocardial infarction in the first 30 days.[5]

Pathophysiology of perioperative myocardial infarction

Rupture of atherosclerotic plaque with superimposed arterial thrombosis constitutes the underlying pathophysiology in the majority of *non-operative* myocardial infarctions.[38] Between 64% and 100% of patients with non-operative myocardial infarctions have coronary artery plaque fissuring[39,40] and 65–95% have an acute luminal thrombus.[40–44]

A commonly proposed mechanism of perioperative myocardial infarction relates to myocardial oxygen supply demand mismatch.[45] Fluid shifts, catecholamine surges, hypotension, anemia, pain, hypothermia, and hypoxia can occur during and after major non-cardiac surgery and transiently increase myocardial oxygen demand.[3] In coronary vessels with high-grade stenoses or occlusions, the supply response may be limited, resulting in supply/demand mismatch myocardial infarction. Consistent with this hypothesis, two small retrospective autopsy studies (<70 patients in total) that reported the coronary pathology of patients who suffered a fatal perioperative myocardial infarction revealed that two-thirds of patients had significant left main or three-vessel coronary artery disease.[46,47] Most of the patients did not exhibit plaque fissuring and only about one-third had an intracoronary thrombus. Although these

data require cautious interpretation because the timing of the autopsies relative to the myocardial infarctions may have allowed resolution of intracoronary thrombus, these data suggest that a substantial proportion of fatal perioperative myocardial infarctions may be secondary to an increase in oxygen demand in the setting of a fixed coronary artery stenosis.

Although POISE does not provide direct evidence regarding the pathophysiology of perioperative myocardial infarction, some of the findings challenge the theory that perioperative myocardial infarction result from an increase in oxygen demand in the setting of fixed coronary artery stenoses.[5] In POISE, perioperative beta-blockers prevented myocardial infarctions (beta-blockers 4.2% v placebo 5.7%; hazard ratio (HR) 0.73; 95% CI 0.60–0.89; $P = 0.0017$) but increased clinically significant hypotension (systolic blood pressure less than 90 mmHg that someone intervened upon; beta-blockers 15.0% vs placebo 9.7%; HR 1.55; 95% CI 1.38–1.74; $P < 0.0001$). Clinically significant hypotension had the largest population-attributable risk for perioperative death and perioperative stroke but appeared to have minimal impact on the risk of perioperative myocardial infarction. Because myocardial oxygen supply is critically dependent on maintaining coronary blood flow during diastole, hypotension of sufficient severity to cause stroke and death would be expected to further compromise coronary perfusion in patients with pre-existing fixed coronary artery stenosis, thereby increasing the risk of perioperative myocardial infarction with beta-blockers rather than reducing the risk. Therefore, the POISE results suggest the possibility that other mechanisms beyond increased oxygen demand in the setting of a fixed coronary artery stenosis are involved in the pathogenesis of perioperative myocardial infarction.

An additional or alternative mechanism of perioperative myocardial infarction is that the acute stress of surgery and mechanical tissue injury induce a hypercoagulable state that increases the risk of coronary thrombus formation at the sites of a fissured plaque or low coronary flow. This mechanism might also explain the reduction in perioperative myocardial infarction seen with beta-blockers in POISE because sympathetic hyperactivity promotes hypercoagulability by upregulating coagulation and platelets and downregulating fibrinolysis, and this effect can be suppressed by beta-blocker therapy.[48–51]

Consistent with the thrombosis hypothesis, a small study of 21 patients who suffered a perioperative myocardial infarction who had undergone a coronary angiography prior to vascular surgery revealed that the majority of non-fatal perioperative myocardial infarctions occurred in arteries without high-grade stenoses, suggesting that these events may result from acute coronary artery thrombosis superimposed on fissured coronary artery plaques.[52] Further, evidence to support this hypothesis comes from the Coronary Artery Revascularization Prophylaxis (CARP) trial[53] which randomized 510 patients undergoing elective vascular surgery, who had at least one coronary artery with a ≥70% stenosis that was suitable for revascularization, to receive coronary artery revascularization or no coronary artery revascularization before vascular surgery. This trial did not demonstrate a significant reduction in perioperative myocardial infarctions in the patients who first underwent coronary revascularization prior to their non-cardiac surgery. If hemodynamically significant stenoses are the major cause of perioperative myocardial infarctions, it is surprising that there was no reduction in the risk of a perioperative myocardial infarction despite coronary revascularization prior to non-cardiac surgery.

These limited and conflicting data regarding the pathophysiology of perioperative myocardial infarction highlight the need for large studies to provide insights. Such studies will inform the selection of appropriate preventive and management interventions to evaluate in subsequent large randomized controlled trials.

Diagnosing perioperative myocardial infarction

A recent review identified studies assessing patients undergoing non-cardiac surgery, that required patients to have at least one measurement of a cardiac biomarker or enzyme after surgery, and reported whether patients who suffered a perioperative myocardial infarction experienced cardiac symptoms.[54] This review identified three studies that included a total of 1309 patients, and 38 of these patients suffered a perioperative myocardial infarction.[55–57] Although the small sample size requires cautious interpretation, the findings were striking. Of the patients who suffered a perioperative myocardial infarction, only 14% experienced chest pain and only 53% had any potential sign or symptom that could have suggested a myocardial infarction.

These results are similar to the findings in the recent POISE trial, which also monitored cardiac biomarkers or enzymes in all patients for the first 3 days after surgery. Box 5.1 presents the definition used for myocardial infarction in the POISE trial, in which only 35% of the patients suffering a perioperative myocardial infarction had ischemic symptoms.[5] The fact that approximately 75% of these myocardial infarctions occurred within the first 48 hours after surgery helps to explain why so many patients may not have experienced ischemic symptoms (i.e. this is a period when the majority of patients receive high-dose analgesic medication to blunt surgical discomfort). These data suggest perioperative myocardial infarctions present differently from the majority of myocardial infarction in the emergency room and that perioperative myocardial infarctions are at high risk of going undetected if troponin measurements are not monitored for the first few days after surgery. The ongoing VISION Study will provide further

---

BOX 5.1 Diagnostic criteria for perioperative myocardial infarction in the POISE trial

The diagnosis of perioperative myocardial infarction required any one of the following

Criterion 1 A typical rise of troponin or a typical fall of an elevated troponin or a rapid rise and fall of CK-MB. Patients also had to have one of the following:
1. ischemic signs (e.g. chest, arm or jaw discomfort; shortness of breath)
2. development of pathologic Q waves in two contiguous leads on an ECG
3. ECG changes indicative of ischemia in at least two contiguous leads
4. coronary artery intervention (e.g. percutaneous coronary intervention)
5. new or presumed new cardiac wall motion abnormality on echocardiography or new or presumed new fixed defect on radionuclide imaging

Criterion 2 Pathologic findings of an acute myocardial infarction

ECG, electrocardiogram.

---

insights into this issue in a large unselected population of patients undergoing non-cardiac surgery who are having troponins monitored throughout the first 3 days after surgery.

Do perioperative myocardial infarctions matter and is surveillance justified?

A relevant question is whether a perioperative myocardial infarction alters prognosis to an extent that would justify routine monitoring for this event. In the POISE trial both asymptomatic and symptomatic perioperative myocardial infarctions were independent predictors of death at 30 days (OR 3.45; 95% CI 2.20–5.41 and OR 3.31; 95% CI 1.78–6.15, respectively). Smaller studies have also suggested that an elevation of a troponin measurement after surgery is an independent predictor of death in the first year after surgery.[58,59] These data suggest perioperative myocardial infarctions alter prognosis in an important way.

Another relevant question is whether detecting perioperative myocardial infarctions that would have otherwise gone unrecognized will allow physicians to improve patient outcomes. A present, there are no randomized controlled trials evaluating interventions among patients suffering a perioperative myocardial infarction. Therefore, it remains unproven that physicians detecting perioperative myocardial infarction can improve patient outcomes, but there is a strong rationale to suspect that the detection of perioperative myocardial infarctions will enhance patient outcomes.

Between 10% and 20% of patients suffering a perioperative myocardial infarction will die prior to hospital discharge,[57,60] and it is logical to assume that early detection of a myocardial infarction will afford physicians the greatest opportunity to prevent death, as is the case in the nonoperative setting. A number of strategies for managing detected perioperative myocardial infarctions are more likely to benefit than harm patients, including: (1) more frequent monitoring of vital signs to allow early detection and reversal of cardiovascular instability; (2) management in a telemetry monitored unit or cardiac care unit; (3) identifying and correcting potential contributing factors (e.g. hypoxia, anemia); (4) optimal intravascular volume management to minimize the risk of heart failure; and (5) a few therapies known to benefit patients suffering a non-operative myocardial infarction (e.g. acetyl-salicylic acid (ASA), angiotensin-converting enzyme (ACE) inhibitor).[61]

We believe that it is also reasonable to suspect that even patients who would survive to hospital discharge, despite having suffered an undetected perioperative myocardial infarction, can benefit from detection of their myocardial infarction. Approximately 10% of patients who suffer a perioperative myocardial infarction with or without signs or symptoms will suffer a major cardiac event within 1 year of hospital discharge after surgery.[57,62,63] Given that the majority of these patients have some degree of underlying coronary artery stenosis,[46,47,52] it would seem prudent to offer these patients long-term management with known beneficial secondary prophylaxis cardiac interventions (e.g. beta-blocker, HMG CoA reductase inhibitor (statin)), until definitive perioperative myocardial infarction randomized controlled trials are conducted.

Prevention of perioperative vascular complications

The plethora of triggers and activated mechanisms (e.g. pain, fasting, hypothermia, bleeding/anemia, platelet activation, hypercoagulability, inflammation, sympathetic activation)[3] that may result in a perioperative myocardial infarction suggests many potential prophylactic interventions. This multitude of triggers and mechanisms also suggests it is unrealistic to expect that any single intervention, which is likely to affect no more than a few triggers or mechanisms, will have a large effect. Realistic moderate-sized treatment effects can, however, have substantial impact in preventing major vascular complications among the 200 million adults globally who undergo non-cardiac surgery annually.

Beta-blockers

In the 1970s, physicians were encouraged to withhold beta-blockers prior to surgery out of concern that beta-blockers would inhibit compensatory cardiovascular responses when patients developed hypotension in the perioperative setting.[64] As research suggested that tachycardia was associated with increased myocardial oxygen demand and perioperative cardiovascular events this led to physicians (starting in the 1980s) to propose using perioperative beta-blockers as a means to prevent major perioperative cardiovascular complications.[65] Two small trials in the 1990s (total sample 312 patients) with methodologic limitations (unblinded, stopped early for unexpected large treatment effects, failure to follow intention-to-treat principle) suggested perioperative beta-blockers had a large treatment effect in preventing major cardiovascular events and death.[66,67] Based upon physiologic rationale and the results of these two trials, guideline committees recommended giving perioperative beta-blockers to patients undergoing non-cardiac surgery who were considered at risk for a major perioperative cardiovascular event.[68,69] In 2006 two moderate-sized trials (1417 patients in total), which did not suffer from the methodologic limitations of the early trials, reported no benefit with perioperative beta-blockers.[70,71] Despite these new data, guideline committees continued to recommend perioperative beta-blockers.[72]

Most recently, the POISE trial evaluated the effect of a perioperative beta-blocker versus placebo in 8351 patients recruited in 190 hospitals in 23 countries.[5] POISE included patients with or at risk of atherosclerotic disease who were undergoing non-cardiac surgery. The intervention was extended-release metoprolol succinate (metoprolol CR) or matching placebo. Patients had to have a systolic blood pressure (SBP) ≥100 mmHg and a heart rate ≥50 beats per minute (bpm) in order to receive the study drug. The dosing regimen in POISE was designed so that patients could get 200 mg of the study drug (i.e. metoprolol CR or matching placebo) during the first 24 hours.[73] Patients received 100 mg 2–4 hours prior to surgery and then another 100 mg 6 hours after surgery. Patients thereafter received 200 mg of the study drug daily for 30 days. If a patient's heart rate was below 45 bpm or their SBP < 100 mmHg, their study drug was withheld until their heart rate or SBP recovered and then they restarted the study drug at 100 mg orally once a day. Patients whose heart rate was 45–49 bpm and SBP >100 mmHg delayed taking the study drug for 12 hours until their hemodynamic measurements recovered.

In the POISE trial 99.8% of the patients completed the 30-day follow-up and all analyses were undertaken according to the intention-to-treat principle. Fewer patients in the metoprolol CR group (244, 5.8%) suffered the primary outcome (i.e. a composite of cardiovascular death, non-fatal myocardial infarction, and non-fatal cardiac arrest) compared to the placebo group (290, 6.9%) (HR for the metoprolol group, 0.84; 95% CI 0.70–0.99; P = 0.04).[5] This beneficial effect resulted from a reduction in myocardial infarction (176, 4.2%, in the metoprolol group compared to 239, 5.7%, in the placebo group; HR 0.73; 95% CI 0.60–0.89; P = 0.002). In contrast to this beneficial effect there was an excess of deaths in the metoprolol CR group (129, 3.1%) compared to the placebo group (97, 2.3%) (HR 1.33; 95% CI 1.03–1.74; P = 0.03). Further, there were more strokes in the metoprolol group (41, 1.0%) than in the placebo group (19, 0.5%) (HR 2.17; 95% CI 1.26–3.74; P = 0.005).

To many, the excess of deaths and strokes was a surprise finding. These findings are, however, supported by a recently published meta-analysis of high-quality perioperative beta-blocker randomized controlled trials by Bangalore and colleagues.[74] This meta-analysis, which included the POISE data, demonstrated a higher death rate among patients assigned a beta-blocker (160, 2.8%) compared to control (127, 2.3%) (OR 1.27; 95% CI 1.01–1.61; I^2 27%), and a higher risk of non-fatal strokes among patients assigned a beta-blocker (38, 0.7%) compared to control (17, 0.3%) (OR 2.16; 95% CI 1.27–3.68; I^2 0%).[74]

Further analyses in the POISE trial offer insights into whether and how metoprolol CR may have resulted in an excess of deaths and strokes. More patients assigned metoprolol CR (625, 15.0%) compared to placebo (404, 9.7%) experienced clinically significant hypotension (i.e. a SBP < 90 mmHg that someone had to do something about) (HR 1.55; 95% CI 1.38–1.74; P < 0.0001). *Post hoc* multivariable analyses were undertaken and population-attributable risks (PARs) were reported, which represent the proportion of all outcomes attributable to the relevant risk factor if causality were proven. Clinically significant hypotension had the largest PAR (37.3%) for death and the largest intraoperative/postoperative PAR (14.7%) for stroke. These findings suggest that an important pathway through which perioperative metoprolol CR caused death and stroke might be clinically significant hypotension.

The finding of excess deaths related to shock with perioperative beta-blockers is similar to the signal seen in the world's largest non-operative beta-blocker trial (i.e. the COMMIT trial), which randomized 45 852 patients to metoprolol CR or placebo in acute myocardial infarction.[75] In the COMMIT trial there was no impact on 30-day mortality but there was a statistically significant increase in death due to shock with beta-blocker therapy.[75] The main difference between POISE and COMMIT was that clinically significant hypotension was more common in the perioperative setting in POISE than in the acute myocardial infarction setting in COMMIT, and this may explain why the overall balance of total mortality went up in POISE and was neutral in COMMIT.[5,75]

Questions raised after POISE

Some authors have suggested that the beta-blocker dose used in POISE was too high.[76] Would a lower dose of a perioperative beta-blocker provide the benefits seen in POISE without the demonstrated risks? POISE used metoprolol CR (a long-acting beta-blocker) and targeted a dose that represents 50% of the maximum daily therapeutic dose (MDTD). Considering the two small positive beta-blocker trials – that have a total sample that is 4% of POISE's sample size – upon which the guidelines primarily based their recommendations, the first of these trials used atenolol (a long-acting beta-blocker) and targeted a dose that represents 50% of the MDTD.[66] The second used bisoprolol (a long-acting beta-blocker) starting at a dose that represents 25% of the MDTD and allowed titration to 50% of the MDTD.[67] The next largest perioperative beta-blocker trial after POISE is the DIPOM trial, which randomized 921 patients.[70] DIPOM used metoprolol CR and targeted a dose that represents 25% of the MDTD. The 30-day data from DIPOM demonstrated a trend towards excess deaths and strokes with metoprolol CR despite using half the POISE dose. Consistent with these findings are the results of the recent perioperative beta-blocker meta-analysis by Bangalore and colleagues that demonstrated a consistent finding of excess deaths and strokes with various perioperative beta-blockers and dosing regimens.[74] Although it is possible that a different perioperative beta-blocker dosing regimen may provide the benefits seen in POISE while avoiding the risks, the current evidence suggests this is unlikely.

Some authors have suggested that there is a benefit to starting a beta-blocker earlier than the initiating time used in POISE.[76] Considering that POISE demonstrated that a beta-blocker resulted in a beneficial effect when starting just a few hours prior to surgery (e.g. reduction in risk of myocardial infarction), the relevant question is whether starting a beta-blocker weeks prior to surgery would make the drug safe. Although this is possible, the POISE results offer insights that suggest it is not probable. In POISE 9.7% of the patients in the placebo group developed clinically significant hypotension. Therefore, a titrated beta-blocker dose that appears effective preoperatively is unlikely to inform what dose of a beta-blocker is safe after surgery when clinically significant hypotension is common. Another relevant question relates to the practicality of seeing patients preoperatively, initiating a beta-blocker, and seeing them a few more times before surgery to titrate their beta-blocker. Given that worldwide there are likely 100 million at risk adults undergoing noncardiac surgery annually and most preoperative clinics see patients very close to the time of surgery, the practicality of starting and titrating a beta-blocker before surgery is questionable.

Another relevant question is how physicians should manage patients undergoing non-cardiac surgery who are already taking a beta-blocker. POISE does not directly inform this question, because it excluded patients who were already taking a beta-blocker prior to surgery. Issues to consider include the following: the potential exacerbation of cardiac ischemia that may occur from stopping a beta-blocker acutely before a patient undergoes surgery; and the beta-blocker dose that is safe in the non-operative setting may still exacerbate clinically significant hypotension after surgery and result in the negative consequences demonstrated in POISE. Until a large, adequately powered trial is undertaken to directly inform this issue, physicians may want to consider halving the patient's beta-blocker dose around the time of surgery (i.e. starting on the morning of surgery and continuing for the first few days after surgery) and to only administer the beta-blocker if the patient's SBP is >115–120 mmHg. This suggestion tries to balance the concern about beta-blocker withdrawal ischemia and exacerbating clinically significant hypotension after surgery with a beta-blocker. This suggestion is not, however, informed from strong direct evidence, and therefore physicians will have to individualize the perioperative management of each patient who is on a beta-blocker until strong direct evidence becomes available.

Take-away message from POISE

POISE suggest that for every 1000 patients with a similar risk profile undergoing non-cardiac surgery, metoprolol CR would prevent 15 patients from suffering a myocardial infarction, three from undergoing cardiac revascularization, and seven from developing new clinically significant atrial fibrillation. POISE also suggests that metoprolol CR would result in an excess of eight deaths, five patients suffering a stroke, 53 experiencing clinically significant hypotension, and 42 experiencing clinically significant bradycardia. Patients who would place three times more value on avoiding a perioperative stroke (a majority of which resulted in death, incapacitation or a patient requiring help with everyday activities) compared to a perioperative myocardial infarction (a minority of which resulted in death or ischemic symptoms), or who are unwilling to accept a probable increase in mortality, would not want a perioperative beta-blocker.

POISE has another take-away message that goes beyond perioperative beta-blockers. Guidelines have recommended perioperative beta-blockers for over a decade. Even if only 10% of physicians acted on the guideline recommendations throughout the last decade (several studies suggest >30% of physicians prescribed a perioperative beta-blocker to the at-risk patients),[77–79] 100 million patients would have received a beta-blocker around the time of surgery. If the results of POISE are widely applicable, throughout the last decade 800 000 patients would have died prematurely and 500 000 patients would have suffered a stroke because they were given a beta-blocker around the time of surgery. This highlights the risk in assuming a perioperative beta-blocker regimen has benefit without substantial harm, and the importance and need for large randomized trials in the surgical setting.

Alpha-2 agonists

Like beta-blockers, alpha-2 agonists attenuate the stress response but through a different mechanism. Alpha-2 agonists act on central and presynaptic receptors to inhibit the release of norepinephrine, causing an overall reduction in central sympathetic outflow.[80,81] A meta-analysis of alpha-2 agonists included 12 non-cardiac surgery randomized controlled trials that assessed three alpha-2 agonists (clonidine, dexmedetomidine, mivazerol).[82] The authors of this systematic review reported separately the results for patients who had vascular surgery and patients who had non-vascular non-cardiac surgery. The meta-analysis demonstrated a statistically significant reduction in both deaths (39 events; relative risk (RR) 0.47; 95% CI 0.25–0.90) and myocardial infarction (110 events; RR 0.66; 95% CI 0.46–0.94) with alpha-2 agonist therapy among the patients who underwent vascular surgery. The investigators found no effect on mortality (31 events; RR 1.09; 95% CI 0.52–2.09) and myocardial infarction (62 events; RR 1.25; 95% CI 0.83–2.21) among the patients who underwent non-vascular non-cardiac surgery. The six trials that reported hypotension did not support an increase with administration of an alpha-2 agonist around the time of non-cardiac surgery (RR 1.03; 95% CI 0.89–1.21; P for heterogeneity 0.22).

Clonidine is the most widely available alpha-2 agonist, and it has a number of effects that make it attractive as a potential agent to prevent major cardiovascular complications around the time of non-cardiac surgery. Perioperative clonidine results in documented sympatholysis,[83,84] anesthetic/sedative/ anxiolytic/analgesic effects,[85–87] and anti-shivering effects[88] and is able to reduce tissue necrosis factor (TNF)-alpha and myocardial oxygen uptake.[89,90] A meta-analysis of two small randomized control trials (total sample size 358 patients) and another small randomized controlled trial (sample size 190 patients), published since the systematic review, have demonstrated that perioperative administration of clonidine reduces the incidence of myocardial ischemia in patients undergoing non-cardiac surgery without significantly affecting hemodynamic stability.[84,91] This is in contrast to a meta-analysis of trials of perioperative beta-blockers that demonstrated a clear increase in hypotension requiring treatment across 10 non-cardiac surgery trials (RR 1.27; 95% CI 1.04–1.56; I^2 6%).[92] Although these results are encouraging, they warrant a cautious interpretation. Confirmation of these results is required in a large, well-designed trial.

ASA

Immediately after non-cardiac surgery, patients experience a rise in circulating platelet release products.[93] Platelet surface catalyzing coagulation reactions facilitate thrombin generation and these events may promote thrombus formation and lead to arterial occlusion in the perioperative setting.[3] Acute withdrawal of chronic ASA results in a prothrombotic state (i.e. increased thromboxane A2 and decreased fibrinolysis).[94,95] Given these physiologic changes, ASA initiation or continuation for chronic users, which inhibits platelet aggregation, may prevent major perioperative vascular events.[96]

A systematic review of antiplatelet therapy versus placebo in patients undergoing infrainguinal bypass surgery identified 10 randomized controlled trials, of which six evaluated the effects of ASA.[97] There were 76 vascular events (i.e. vascular death, non-fatal myocardial infarction or non-fatal stroke) among the 893 patients randomized to antiplatelet therapy compared to 92 vascular events among the 872 patients randomized to placebo (OR 0.76; 95% CI 0.54–1.05).

In contrast to this encouraging evidence, the Pulmonary Embolism Prevention (PEP) trial suggested worse cardiac ischemic outcomes with ASA therapy in patients undergoing surgery for a hip fracture.[98] There were 105 cardiac ischemic events (i.e. death due to ischemic heart disease or non-fatal myocardial infarction) among the 6679 patients randomized to ASA compared to 79 cardiac ischemic events among the 6677 patients randomized to placebo (HR 1.33; 95% CI 1.00–1.78). More ASA patients (197) compared to placebo patients (1570 suffered a postoperative bleeding episode requiring a transfusion (relative risk increase (RRI) 24%; 95% CI 1–53%). In the PEP trial ASA therapy did, however, prevent pulmonary emboli (HR 0.43; 95% CI 0.18–0.60).

Given the clear evidence that ASA prevents cardiovascular events in the non-operative setting,[99] the conflicting randomized controlled trial evidence surrounding the impact of ASA on perioperative vascular events, and the likelihood of increased bleeding risk with perioperative ASA, there is a need for a large randomized controlled trial to determine the balance of benefits and risks of ASA in patients undergoing non-cardiac surgery. Until such a trial is completed, physicians will have to weigh the increased risk of bleeding against the potential but yet unproven vascular benefits.

Statins

Some authors have suggested the statins may prevent major perioperative vascular complications through plaque stabilization and improved endothelial function.[100] A recent meta-analysis of 10 non-cardiac surgery observational studies demonstrated a reduction in the composite outcome of death and acute coronary syndrome among patients receiving a perioperative statin (OR 0.70; 95% CI 0.53–0.91); however, this benefit was only seen among the retrospective studies (OR 0.65; 95% CI 0.50–0.84) and was not demonstrated in the pooled estimate from the three prospective cohort studies (OR 0.91; 95% CI 0.65–1.27).[101] A recent large retrospective cohort study raised a safety concern related to perioperative statin use when it demonstrated an increased adjusted risk of delirium after non-cardiac surgery associated with statin use (OR 1.33; 95% CI 1.16–1.53).[102] The authors suggest this increased risk of delirium with statin use may have occurred as a result of altered cerebral blood flow autoregulation.[102,103]

Three randomized controlled trials have evaluated the effects of a perioperative statin among patients undergoing non-cardiac surgery, but two of these studies are only published in abstract form as of January 2009. The one full-text published trial randomized 50 patients to receive atorvastatin and 50 patients to receive placebo who were undergoing vascular surgery.[104] Patients started taking the study drug at least 2 weeks prior to vascular surgery and continued for a period of 45 days. Four patients in the atorvastatin group and 13 in the placebo group suffered the primary outcome (a composite of cardiac death, non-fatal myocardial infarction, ischemic stroke, and unstable angina) at 6 months after surgery (relative risk reduction 69%; 95% CI 18–89%). One of the trials reported in abstract form was an unblinded trial that randomized 1066 patients to fluvastatin XL 80 mg daily or control therapy starting a median of 34 days prior to non-cardiac surgery.[105] There was no effect on the primary outcome (a composite of cardiac death and myocardial infarction) at 30 days after surgery, with 3.2% of fluvastatin patients and 4.9% of control patients experiencing the primary outcome (HR 0.65; 95% CI 0.35–1.10). There were, however, only 43 primary events in this trial. The second trial, only available in abstract form, randomized 253 patients to fluvastatin XL 80 mg daily and 247 patients to placebo, a median of 34 days prior to vascular surgery.[106] Fewer patients in the fluvastatin group (27 patients, 10.9%) experienced the primary outcome (myocardial ischemia) compared to the placebo group (47 patients, 18.9%) (OR 0.56; 95% CI 0.35–0.89). The abstract also reports that fewer fluvastatin patients suffered the secondary outcome (a composite of cardiac death and non-fatal myocardial infarction) (OR 0.48; 95% CI 0.24–0.95); however, there were only 37 secondary events.

A meta-analysis evaluating the effect of early statin therapy in almost 18000 patients suffering an acute coronary syndrome demonstrated no statistically significant effect on myocardial infarction until 24 months and no effect on cardiovascular death until 24 months.[107] These results contrast the quick and large effects suggested in the small perioperative trials.

Given the limited nature of the current perioperative statin efficacy data, the contrasting non-operative data, and the potential safety concern, it is difficult to outline a firm perioperative statin recommendation. Until a large trial with a lot of events is undertaken, physicians will have to weigh the limited available data when deciding whether to prescribe a perioeprative statin.

Neuraxial blockade

Uncontrolled pain after surgery leads to stimulation of the sympathetic system and activation of coagulation cascade, which leads to an increase in heart rate, arterial pressure, myocardial oxygen demand, and hypercoagulability.[3] Effective epidural blockade provides superior analgesia and may therefore reduce perioperative vascular events.[108] A meta-analysis of 141 trials involving 9559 patients demonstrated a decrease in the incidence of death (total of 247 deaths) after surgery with neuraxial blockade (epidural and spinal anesthesia) (OR 0.70; 95% CI 0.54–0.90), and neuraxial blockade also demonstrated a significant reduction in vascular events (venous thrombotic events, myocardial infarctions), bleeding requiring a transfusion, and pneumonia.[109] A subsequent meta-analysis of 11 trials that included 1173 patients evaluated the effects of postoperative epidural analgesia and demonstrated a trend towards a lower rate of perioperative myocardial infarction (total of 44 myocardial infarctions) with epidural analgesia (OR 0.56; 95% CI 0.30–1.03).[110]

Since the publication of these meta-analyses, two moderate-sized randomized controlled trials have been published. Despite better postoperative pain relief, the Multicenter Australian Study of Epidural Anesthesia (MASTER) trial found no effect of epidural anesthesia and analgesia on death (5.2% versus 4.3% in the treatment and control group, respectively) and cardiovascular events (25.7% versus 24.0% in the treatment and control group, respectively) among the 915 participants who underwent major abdominal surgery.[108] Similarly, the Veterans Affairs Co-operative Study (VACS, n = 1021) failed to observe a benefit with epidural anesthesia/analgesia (death occurred in 20 versus 17 patients and myocardial infarction in 44 versus 57 patients assigned to the treatment and control groups, respectively).[111] The lack of significant findings in these two trials may simply relate to their limited power. But these are the two largest trials and relatively free of biases.

Cardiac revascularization

The Coronary Artery Revascularization Prophylaxis (CARP) trial evaluated the management strategy of preoperative coronary artery revascularization prior to non-cardiac surgery.[53] Patients undergoing elective vascular surgery for an abdominal aortic aneurysm or severe claudication were recommended for coronary angiography. Patients were eligible if they had at least one coronary artery with a ≥70% stenosis that was suitable for revascularization; 33% of the patients who participated in the trial had three-vessel coronary artery disease. The trial excluded patients with unstable angina, left main coronary artery stenosis ≥50%, a left ventricular ejection fraction <20% or severe aortic stenosis.

It randomized 258 patients to receive coronary artery revascularization before vascular surgery and 252 patients to receive *no* coronary artery revascularization before vascular surgery, and patients were followed for a mean of 2.7 years. Among the patients assigned to coronary artery revascularization, 38% underwent CABG surgery, 55% underwent PCI, and 7% did not receive coronary revascularization. The primary outcome of total mortality during the long-term follow-up demonstrated 70 deaths in the revascularization group and 67 in the no revascularization group (RR 0.98; 95% CI 0.70–1.37).

A recent pilot trial randomized 101 patients undergoing major vascular surgery who demonstrated extensive cardiac ischemia on their preoperative cardiac stress test.[112] Coronary angiography in the patients assigned to coronary revascularization prior to non-cardiac surgery demonstrated three-vessel coronary disease in 67% of the patients. The primary outcome (a composite of death and myocardial infarction) at 30 days after the index surgical procedure occurred in 21 patients (43%) assigned to receive coronary revascularization prior to their vascular surgery and in 17 (33%) assigned to receive *no* coronary artery revascularization before their vascular surgery (HR 1.4; 95% CI 0.73–2.8).

Although these two trials do not exclude the possibility of a reduction in risk from preoperative coronary artery revascularization prior to non-cardiac surgery, they do not support any benefit from this invasive, time-consuming, and costly intervention.

Conclusion

Non-cardiac surgery is common, and annually several million patients will suffer a major vascular complication in the first 30 days after surgery. Clinical risk factors such as coronary artery disease and cerebrovascular disease can help to identify patients at risk of a major perioperative vascular complication. A preoperative NT-proBNP measurement may substantially enhance perioperative vascular risk prediction and troponin measurements for the first few days after surgery hold great promise as a surveillance strategy to allow physicians to avoid missing the majority of perioperative myocardial infarctions. The results of the POISE trial, which demonstrated that a perioperative beta-blocker prevented myocardial infarctions but at a cost of excess strokes and deaths, highlight why large perioperative trials are necessary. There is encouraging evidence that several interventions (e.g. clonidine) may prevent major perioperative vascular complications; however, there is an urgent need for large trials to evaluate these interventions. Current evidence does not support a management strategy of coronary artery revascularization prior to non-cardiac surgery.

References

1. Weiser T, Regenbogen S, Thompson K *et al.* An estimation of the global volume of surgery: a modelling strategy based on available data. *Lancet* 2008;**372**(9633):139–44.

2. Lee T, Marcantonio E, Mangione C *et al.* Derivation and prospective validation of a simple index for prediction of cardiac risk of major noncardiac surgery. *Circulation* 1999;**100**(10): 1043–9.

3. Devereaux P, Goldman L, Cook D, Gilbert K, Leslie K, Guyatt G. Perioperative cardiac events in patients undergoing noncardiac surgery: a review of the magnitude of the problem, the pathophysiology of the events and methods to estimate and communicate risk. *CMAJ* 2005;**173**(6):627–34.

4. Mangano D. Peri-operative cardiovascular morbidity: new developments. *Baillière's Clin Anaesthesiol* 1999;**13**(3): 335–48.

5. Devereaux P, Yang H, Yusuf S *et al.* Effects of extended-release metoprolol succinate in patients undergoing non-cardiac surgery (POISE trial): a randomised controlled trial. *Lancet* 2008;**371**(9627):1839–47.

6. Khuri S, Daley J, Henderson W *et al.* The National Veterans Administration Surgical Risk Study: risk adjustment for the comparative assessment of the quality of surgical care. *J Am Coll Surg* 1995;**180**(5):519–31.

7. Kumar R, Mckinney W, Raj G *et al.* Adverse cardiac events after surgery: assessing risk in a veteran population. *J Gen Intern Med* 2001;**16**(8):507–18.

8. The Global HIV/AIDS pandemic, 2006. *Morb Mortal Wkly Rep* 2006;**55**(31):841–4.

9. Detsky A, Abrams H, Mclaughlin J *et al.* Predicting cardiac complications in patients undergoing non-cardiac surgery. *J Gen Intern Med* 1986;**1**(4):211–19.

10. Goldman L, Caldera D, Nussbaum S *et al.* Multifactorial index of cardiac risk in noncardiac surgical procedures. *N Engl J Med* 1977;**297**(16):845–50.

11. Larsen S, Zaric D, Boysen G. Postoperative cerebrovascular accidents in general surgery. *Acta Anaesthesiol Scand* 1988;**32**(8): 698–701.

12. Landercasper J, Merz B, Cogbill T *et al.* Perioperative stroke risk in 173 consecutive patients with a past history of stroke. *Arch Surg* 1990;**125**(8):986–9.

13. Parikh S, Cohen J. Perioperative stroke after general surgical procedures. *NY State J Med* 1993;**93**(3):162–5.

14. Rockman C, Cappadona C, Riles T *et al.* Causes of the increased stroke rate after carotid endarterectomy in patients with previous strokes. *Ann Vasc Surg* 1997;**11**(1):28–34.

15. Limburg M, Wijdicks E, Li H. Ischemic stroke after surgical procedures: clinical features, neuroimaging, and risk factors. *Neurology* 1998;**50**(4):895–901.

16. Gilbert K, Larocque B, Patrick L. Prospective evaluation of cardiac risk indices for patients undergoing noncardiac surgery. *Ann Intern Med* 2000;**133**(5):356–9.

17. Chan A, Livingstone D, Tu J. The Goldman and Detsky Cardiac-Risk Indices: do they work in patients undergoing hip-fracture surgery? *Ann Rcpsc* 1999;**32**(6):337–41.

18. Devereaux PJ. Commentary on index identified patients at high risk of cardiac complications following non-urgent, non-cardiac surgical procedures. *Evidence-Based Cardiovasc Med* 2000;**4**:13.

19. Beattie W, Abdelnaem E, Wijeysundera D, Buckley D. A Meta-analytic comparison of preoperative stress echocardiography and nuclear scintigraphy imaging. *Anesth Analg* 2006;**102**(1): 8–16.

20. Vanzetto G, Machecourt J, Blendea D *et al.* Additive value of thallium single-photon emission computed tomography myocardial imaging for prediction of perioperative events in clinically selected high cardiac risk patients having abdominal aortic surgery. *Am J Cardiol* 1996;**77**(2):143–8.

21. Coley C, Field T, Abraham S, Boucher C, Eagle K. Usefulness of dipyridamole-thallium scanning for preoperative evaluation of cardiac risk for nonvascular surgery. *Am J Cardiol* 1992; **69**(16):1280–5.

22. Brown K, Rowen M. Extent of jeopardized viable myocardium determined by myocardial perfusion imaging best predicts perioperative cardiac events in patients undergoing noncardiac surgery. *J Am Coll Cardiol* 1993;**21**(2):325–30.

23. Boersma E, Poldermans D, Bax J *et al.* Predictors of cardiac events after major vascular surgery: role of clinical characteristics, dobutamine echocardiography, and beta-blocker therapy. *JAMA* 2001;**285**(14):1865–73.

24. Poldermans D, Arnese M, Fioretti P *et al.* Improved cardiac risk stratification in major vascular surgery with dobutamine-atropine stress echocardiography. *J Am Coll Cardiol* 1995;**26**(3): 648–53.

25. Levin E, Gardner D, Samson W. Natriuretic peptides. *N Engl J Med* 1998; **339**(5): 321–8.

26. Goetze J, Christoffersen C, Perko M *et al.* Increased cardiac BNP expression associated with myocardial ischemia. *FASEB J* 2003; **17**(9):1105–7.

27. Kragelund C, Gronning B, Kober L, Hildebrandt P, Steffensen R. N-Terminal Pro-B-type natriuretic peptide and long-term mortality in stable coronary heart disease. *N Engl J Med* 2005; **352**(7):666–75.

28. De Lemos J, Morrow D, Bentley J *et al.* The prognostic value Of B-type natriuretic peptide in patients with acute coronary syndromes. *N Engl J Med* 2001;**345**(14):1014–21.

29. Tsutamoto T, Wada A, Maeda K *et al.* Attenuation of compensation of endogenous cardiac natriuretic peptide system in chronic heart failure: prognostic role of plasma brain natriuretic peptide concentration in patients with chronic symptomatic left ventricular dysfunction. *Circulation* 1997; **96**(2):509–16.

30. Berger R, Huelsman M, Strecker K *et al.* B-type natriuretic peptide predicts sudden death in patients with chronic heart failure. *Circulation* 2002;**105**(20):2392–7.

31. Blankenberg S, Mcqueen M, Smieja M *et al.* Comparative impact of multiple biomarkers and N-terminal pro-brain natriuretic peptide in the context of conventional risk factors for the prediction of recurrent cardiovascular events in the Heart Outcomes Prevention Evaluation (HOPE) Study. *Circulation* 2006; **114**(3):201–8.

32. Dernellis J, Panaretou M. Assessment of cardiac risk before non-cardiac surgery: brain natriuretic peptide in 1590 patients. *Heart* 2006; **92**(11):1645–50.

33. Feringa H, Bax J, Elhendy A *et al.* Association of plasma N-terminal pro-B-type natriuretic peptide with postoperative cardiac events in patients undergoing surgery for abdominal aortic aneurysm or leg bypass. *Am J Cardiol* 2006;**98**(1): 111–15.

34. Cuthbertson B, Amiri A, Croal B *et al.* Utility of B-type natriuretic peptide in predicting perioperative cardiac events in patients undergoing major non-cardiac surgery. *Br J Anaesth* 2007;**99**(2):170–6.

35. Cuthbertson B, Card G, Croal B, Mcneilly J, Hillis G. The utility of B-type natriuretic peptide in predicting postoperative cardiac events and mortality in patients undergoing major emergency non-cardiac surgery. *Anaesthesia* 2007;**62**(9):875–81.

36. Cardinale D, Colombo A, Sandri M *et al.* Increased perioperative N-terminal pro-B-type natriuretic peptide levels predict atrial fibrillation after thoracic surgery for lung cancer. *Circulation* 2007;**115**(11):1339–44.

37. Yun K, Jeong M, Oh S *et al.* Preoperative plasma N-terminal pro-brain natriuretic peptide concentration and perioperative cardiovascular risk in elderly patients. *Circ J* 2008;**72**(2): 195–9.

38. Falk E, Shah P, Fuster V. Coronary plaque disruption. *Circulation* 1995;**92**(3):657–71.

39. Falk E. Plaque rupture with severe pre-existing stenosis precipitating coronary thrombosis. Characteristics of coronary atherosclerotic plaques underlying fatal occlusive thrombi. *Br Heart J* 1983;**50**(2):127–34.

40. Horie T, Sekiguchi M, Hirosawa K. Coronary thrombosis in pathogenesis of acute myocardial infarction. Histopathological study of coronary arteries in 108 necropsied cases using serial section. *Br Heart J* 1978;**40**(2):153–61.

41. Sinapius D. [Relationship between coronary-artery thrombosis and myocardial infarction]. *Dtsch Med Wochenschr* 1972;**97**(12): 443–8.

42. Chapman I. Relationships of recent coronary artery occlusion and acute myocardial infarction. *J Mt Sinai Hosp N Y* 1968;**35**(2): 149–54.

43. Spain D. Pathologic spectrum of myocardial infarction. In: Likoff W, Segal B, Insull W *et al*, eds. Atherosclerosis And Coronary Heart Disease. New York: Grune and Stratton, 1972;133–9.

44. Davies M, Woolf N, Robertson W. Pathology of acute myocardial infarction with particular reference to occlusive coronary thrombi. *Br Heart J* 1976;**38**:659–64.

45. Landesberg G. The pathophysiology of perioperative myocardial infarction: facts and perspectives. *J Cardiothorac Vasc Anesth* 2003;**17**(1):90–100.

46. Dawood M, Gutpa D, Southern J, Walia A, Atkinson J, Eagle K. Pathology of fatal perioperative myocardial infarction: implications regarding pathophysiology and prevention. *Int J Cardiol* 1996;**57**(1):37–44.

47. Cohen M, Aretz T. Histological analysis of coronary artery lesions in fatal postoperative myocardial infarction. *Cardiovasc Pathol* 1999;**8**(3):133–9.

48. Von Kanel R, Dimsdale J. Effects of sympathetic activation by adrenergic infusions on hemostasis in vivo. *Eur J Haematol* 2000; **65**(6):357–69.

49. Von Kanel R, Mills P, Ziegler M, Dimsdale J. Effect Of beta2-adrenergic receptor functioning and increased norepinephrine on the hypercoagulable state with mental stress. *Am Heart J* 2002;**144**(1):68–72.

50. Yun A, Lee P, Bazar K. Can thromboembolism be the result, rather than the inciting cause, of acute vascular events such as stroke, pulmonary embolism, mesenteric ischemia, and venous thrombosis? A maladaptation of the prehistoric trauma response. *Med Hypotheses* 2005;**64**(4):706–16.

51. Hjemdahl P, Larsson P, Wallen N. Effects of stress and beta-blockade on platelet function. *Circulation* 1991;**84**(6 suppl): Vi44–61.

52. Ellis S, Hertzer N, Young J, Brener S. Angiographic correlates of cardiac death and myocardial infarction complicating major nonthoracic vascular surgery. *Am J Cardiol* 1996;**77**(12): 1126–8.

53. Mcfalls E, Ward H, Moritz T *et al.* Coronary-artery revascularization before elective major vascular surgery. *N Engl J Med* 2004;**351**(27):2795–804.

54. Devereaux P, Goldman L, Yusuf S, Gilbert K, Leslie K, Guyatt G. Surveillance and prevention of major perioperative ischemic cardiac events in patients undergoing noncardiac surgery: a review. *CMAJ* 2005;**173**(7):779–88.

55. Mangano D, Browner W, Hollenberg M, London M, Tubau J, Tateo I. Association of perioperative myocardial ischemia with cardiac morbidity and mortality in men undergoing noncardiac surgery. The Study of Perioperative Ischemia Research Group. *N Engl J Med* 1990;**323**(26):1781–8.

56. Ashton C, Petersen N, Wray N *et al.* The incidence of perioperative myocardial infarction in men undergoing noncardiac surgery. *Ann Intern Med* 1993;**118**(7):504–10.

57. Badner N, Knill R, Brown J, Novick T, Gelb A. Myocardial infarction after noncardiac surgery. *Anesthesiology* 1998;**88**(3): 572–8.

58. Filipovic M, Jeger R, Probst C *et al.* Heart rate variability and cardiac troponin I are incremental and independent predictors of one-year all-cause mortality after major noncardiac surgery in patients at risk of coronary artery disease. *J Am Coll Cardiol* 2003;**42**(10):1767–76.

59. Oscarsson A, Eintrei C, Anskar S *et al.* Troponin T-values provide long-term prognosis in elderly patients undergoing non-cardiac surgery. *Acta Anaesthesiol Scand* 2004;**48**(9): 1071–9.

60. Shah K, Kleinman B, Rao T, Jacobs H, Mestan K, Schaafsma M. Angina and other risk factors in patients with cardiac diseases undergoing noncardiac operations. *Anesth Analg* 1990;**70**(3): 240–7.

61. Devereaux P, De Beer J, Villar J *et al.* Perioperative myocardial infarction: a silent killer. *CJGIM* 2006;**1**:9–13.

62. Mangano D, Browner W, Hollenberg M, Li J, Tateo I. Long-term cardiac prognosis following noncardiac surgery. The Study of Perioperative Ischemia Research Group. *JAMA* 1992;**268**(2): 233–9.

63. Lopez-Jimenez F, Goldman L, Sacks D et al. Prognostic value of cardiac troponin T after noncardiac surgery: 6-month follow-up data. *J Am Coll Cardiol* 1997;**29**(6):1241–5.

64. Sear J, Giles J, Howard-Alpe G, Foex P. Perioperative beta-blockade, 2008: what does Poise tell us, and was our earlier caution justified? *Br J Anaesth* 2008;**101**(2):135–8.

65. Stone J, Foex P, Sear J, Johnson L, Khambatta H, Triner L. Myocardial ischemia in untreated hypertensive patients: effect of a single small oral dose of a beta-adrenergic blocking agent. *Anesthesiology* 1988;**68**(4):495–500.

66. Mangano D, Layug E, Wallace A, Tateo I. Effect of atenolol on mortality and cardiovascular morbidity after noncardiac surgery. Multicenter Study of Perioperative Ischemia Research Group. *N Engl J Med* 1996;**335**(23):1713–20.

67. Poldermans D, Boersma E, Bax J et al. The effect of bisoprolol on perioperative mortality and myocardial infarction in high-risk patients undergoing vascular surgery. Dutch Echocardiographic Cardiac Risk Evaluation Applying Stress Echocardiography Study Group. *N Engl J Med* 1999;**341**(24):1789–94.

68. Palda V, Detsky A. Perioperative assessment and management of risk from coronary artery disease. *Ann Intern Med* 1997;**127**(4):313–28.

69. Eagle K, Berger P, Calkins H et al. ACC/AHA guideline update for perioperative cardiovascular evaluation for noncardiac surgery – executive summary. A report of the American College of Cardiology/American Heart Association Task Force on Practice Guidelines (Committee to Update the 1996 Guidelines on Perioperative Cardiovascular Evaluation for Noncardiac Surgery). *Circulation* 2002;**105**(10):1257–67.

70. Juul A, Wetterslev J, Gluud C et al. Effect of perioperative beta blockade in patients with diabetes undergoing major noncardiac surgery: randomised placebo controlled, blinded multicentre trial. *BMJ* 2006;**332**(7556):1482.

71. Yang H, Raymer K, Butler R, Parlow J, Roberts R. The effects of perioperative beta-blockade: results of the Metoprolol After Vascular Surgery (MAVS) study, a randomized controlled trial. *Am Heart J* 2006;**152**(5):983–90.

72. Fleisher L, Beckman J, Brown K et al. ACC/AHA 2007 Guidelines on Perioperative Cardiovascular Evaluation and Care for Noncardiac Surgery: Executive Summary. A report of the American College of Cardiology/American Heart Association Task Force on Practice Guidelines (Writing Committee to Revise the 2002 Guidelines on Perioperative Cardiovascular Evaluation for Noncardiac Surgery) Developed in Collaboration with the American Society of Echocardiography, American Society of Nuclear Cardiology, Heart Rhythm Society, Society of Cardiovascular Anesthesiologists, Society for Cardiovascular Angiography and Interventions, Society for Vascular Medicine and Biology, and Society for Vascular Surgery. *J Am Coll Cardiol* 2007;**50**(17):1707–32.

73. Devereaux PJ, Yang H, Guyatt G et al. Rationale, design, and organization of the Perioperative Ischemic Evaluation (Poise) trial: a randomized controlled trial of metoprolol versus placebo in patients undergoing noncardiac surgery. *Am Heart J* 2006;**152**(2):223–30.

74. Bangalore S, Wetterslev J, Pranesh S, Sawhney S, Gluud C, Messerli F. Perioperative beta blockers in patients having non-cardiac surgery: a meta-analysis. *Lancet* 2008;**372**(9654):1962–76.

75. Chen Z, Pan H, Chen Y et al. Early intravenous then oral metoprolol in 45,852 patients with acute myocardial infarction: randomised placebo-controlled trial. *Lancet* 2005;**366**(9497):1622–32.

76. Fleisher L, Poldermans D. Perioperative beta blockade: where do we go from here? *Lancet* 2008;**371**(9627):1813–14.

77. Lindenauer P, Fitzgerald J, Hoople N, Benjamin E. The potential preventability of postoperative myocardial infarction: underuse of perioperative beta-adrenergic blockade. *Arch Intern Med* 2004;**164**(7):762–6.

78. Schmidt M, Lindenauer P, Fitzgerald J, Benjamin E. Forecasting the impact of a clinical practice guideline for perioperative beta-blockers to reduce cardiovascular morbidity and mortality. *Arch Intern Med* 2002;**162**(1):63–9.

79. Taylor R, Pagliarello G. Prophylactic beta-blockade to prevent myocardial infarction perioperatively in high-risk patients who undergo general surgical procedures. *Can J Surg* 2003;**46**(3):216–22.

80. Muzi M, Goff D, Kampine J, Roerig D, Ebert T. Clonidine reduces sympathetic activity but maintains baroreflex responses in normotensive humans. *Anesthesiology* 1992;**77**(5):864–71.

81. Dorman T, Clarkson K, Rosenfeld B, Shanholtz C, Lipsett P, Breslow M. Effects of clonidine on prolonged postoperative sympathetic response. *Crit Care Med* 1997;**25**(7):1147–52.

82. Wijeysundera D, Naik J, Beattie W. Alpha-2 adrenergic agonists to prevent perioperative cardiovascular complications: a meta-analysis. *Am J Med* 2003;**114**(9):742–52.

83. Ellis J, Drijvers G, Pedlow S et al. Premedication with oral and transdermal clonidine provides safe and efficacious postoperative sympatholysis. *Anesth Analg* 1994;**79**(6):1133–40.

84. Wallace A, Galindez D, Salahieh A et al. Effect of clonidine on cardiovascular morbidity and mortality after noncardiac surgery. *Anesthesiology* 2004;**101**(2):284–93.

85. Hidalgo M, Auzani J, Rumpel L, Moreira N Jr, Cursino A, Caumo W. The clinical effect of small oral clonidine doses on perioperative outcomes in patients undergoing abdominal hysterectomy. *Anesth Analg* 2005;**100**(3):795–802.

86. Quintin L, Bouilloc X, Butin E et al. Clonidine for major vascular surgery in hypertensive patients: a double-blind, controlled, randomized study. *Anesth Analg* 1996;**83**(4):687–95.

87. Ghignone M, Calvillo O, Quintin L. Anesthesia and hypertension: the effect of clonidine on perioperative hemodynamics and isoflurane requirements. *Anesthesiology* 1987;**67**(1):3–10.

88. Kranke P, Eberhart L, Roewer N, Tramer M. Pharmacological treatment of postoperative shivering: a quantitative systematic review of randomized controlled trials. *Anesth Analg* 2002;**94**(2):453–60.

89. Nader N, Ignatowski T, Kurek C, Knight P, Spengler R. Clonidine suppresses plasma and cerebrospinal fluid concentrations of TNF-alpha during the perioperative period. *Anesth Analg* 2001;**93**(2):363–9.

90. Quintin L, Viale J, Annat G et al. Oxygen uptake after major abdominal surgery: effect of clonidine. *Anesthesiology* 1991;**74**(2):236–41.

91. Nishina K, Mikawa K, Uesugi T et al. Efficacy of clonidine for prevention of perioperative myocardial ischemia: a critical appraisal and meta-analysis of the literature. *Anesthesiology* 2002;**96**(2):323–9.

92. Devereaux PJ, Beattie W, Choi P *et al.* How strong is the evidence for the use of perioperative beta blockers in non-cardiac surgery? Systematic review and meta-analysis of randomised controlled trials. *BMJ* 2005;**331**(7512):313–21.

93. Naesh O, Friis J, Hindberg I, Winther K. Platelet function in surgical stress. *Thromb Haemost* 1985;**54**(4):849–52.

94. Beving H, Zhao C, Albage A, Ivert T. Abnormally high platelet activity after discontinuation of acetylsalicylic acid treatment. *Blood Coagul Fibrinolysis* 1996;**7**(1):80–4.

95. Fatah K, Beving H, Albage A, Ivert T, Blomback M. Acetylsalicylic acid may protect the patient by increasing fibrin gel porosity. Is withdrawing of treatment harmful to the patient? *Eur Heart J* 1996;**17**(9):1362–6.

96. Mcdaniel M, Pearce W, Yao J *et al.* Sequential changes in coagulation and platelet function following femorotibial bypass. *J Vasc Surg* 1984;**1**(2):261–8.

97. Robless P, Mikhailidis D, Stansby G. Systematic review of antiplatelet therapy for the prevention of myocardial infarction, stroke or vascular death in patients with peripheral vascular disease. *Br J Surg* 2001;**88**(6):787–800.

98. The PEP investigators. Prevention of pulmonary embolism and deep vein thrombosis with low dose aspirin: Pulmonary Embolism Prevention (PEP) trial. *Lancet* 2000;**355**(9212):1295–302.

99. Antithrombotic Trialists' Collaboration. Collaborative meta-analysis of randomised trials of antiplatelet therapy for prevention of death, myocardial infarction, and stroke in high risk patients. *BMJ* 2002;**324**(7329):71–86.

100. O'Neil-Callahan K, Katsimaglis G, Tepper M *et al.* Statins decrease perioperative cardiac complications in patients undergoing noncardiac vascular surgery: the Statins for Risk Reduction in Surgery (STARRS) study. *J Am Coll Cardiol* 2005;**45**(3):336–42.

101. Kapoor A, Kanji H, Buckingham J, Devereaux PJ, Mcalister F. Strength of evidence for perioperative use of statins to reduce cardiovascular risk: systematic review of controlled studies. *BMJ* 2006;**333**(7579):1149.

102. Redelmeier D, Thiruchelvam D, Daneman N. Delirium after elective surgery among elderly patients taking statins. *CMAJ* 2008;**179**(7):645–52.

103. Redelmeier D. New thinking on postoperative delirium. *CMAJ* 2007;**177**:424.

104. Durazzo A, Machado F, Ikeoka D *et al.* Reduction in cardiovascular events after vascular surgery with atorvastatin: a randomized trial. *J Vasc Surg* 2004;**39**(5):967–75; discussion 975–6.

105. Dunkelgrun M, Boersma E, Gemert Ak-V *et al.* Abstract 4536: bisoprolol and fluvastatin for the reduction of perioperative cardiac mortality and myocardial infarction in intermediate-risk patients undergoing non-cardiovascular surgery; a randomized controlled trial. *Circulation* 2008;**118**:S906–C907.

106. Poldermans D, Schouten O, Benner R *et al.* Abstract 2886: fluvastatin XI Use is associated with improved cardiac outcome after major vascular surgery. Results from a randomized placebo controlled trial: decrease III. *Circulation* 2008;**118**:S792.

107. Hulten E, Jackson J, Douglas K, George S, Villines T. The effect of early, intensive statin therapy on acute coronary syndrome: a meta-analysis of randomized controlled trials. *Arch Intern Med* 2006;**166**(17):1814–21.

108. Rigg J, Jamrozik K, Myles P *et al.* Epidural anaesthesia and analgesia and outcome of major surgery: a randomised trial. *Lancet* 2002;**359**(9314):1276–82.

109. Rodgers A, Walker N, Schug S *et al.* Reduction of postoperative mortality and morbidity with epidural or spinal anaesthesia: results from overview of randomised trials. *BMJ* 2000;**321**(7275): 1493.

110. Beattie W, Badner N, Choi P. Epidural analgesia reduces postoperative myocardial infarction: a meta-analysis. *Anesth Analg* 2001;**93**(4):853–8.

111. Park W, Thompson J, Lee K. Effect of epidural anesthesia and analgesia on perioperative outcome: a randomized, controlled Veterans Affairs Cooperative study. *Ann Surg* 2001;**234**(4): 560–9; discussion 569–71.

112. Poldermans D, Schouten O, Vidakovic R *et al.* A clinical randomized trial to evaluate the safety of a noninvasive approach in high-risk patients undergoing major vascular surgery: the Decrease-V pilot study. *J Am Coll Cardiol* 2007;**49**(17): 1763–9.

6

Implementing evidence-based medicine in cardiology

Brahmajee K Nallamothu,[1] Thomas T Tsai[1] and Jack V Tu[2]
[1] University of Michigan, Ann Arbor, MI, USA
[2] Schulich Heart Program, Sunnybrook Health Sciences Center, Toronto, Canada

Introduction

Remarkable advancements have been made over the last several decades in our understanding of the basic mechanisms and treatments related to cardiovascular diseases. This has led to dramatic improvements in public health. Between 1960 and 2000, for example, overall life expectancy for newborns in the United States increased by nearly seven years with approximately 70% of these gains in survival resulting specifically from lower rates of cardiovascular death.[1] For coronary artery disease (CAD) alone, age-adjusted mortality fell by more than 50% during the past two decades.[2] Similar patterns of improvements in survival have also been noted for patients with heart failure, despite an overall rising prevalence of this condition due to aging populations.[3,4]

Importantly, many of these benefits have been attributed to the discovery of evidence-based therapies in cardiology. Aspirin, beta-blockers, angiotensin-converting enzyme (ACE) inhibitors and statins can reduce the risk of death after acute myocardial infarction (AMI) by 20–35%.[5,6] The timely use of acute reperfusion therapy in ST elevation myocardial infarction lowers mortality by an additional 25%.[7] In heart failure, ACE inhibitors, angiotensin receptor blockers (ARB) and aldosterone blockers have all been linked to significant improvements in quality of life as well as lower rates of hospital admissions and mortality in patients with impaired left ventricular (LV) systolic function.[8] Similar advances have been noted in atrial fibrillation with anticoagulation therapy,[9] acute stroke management with fibrinolytic therapy,[10] and in the primary and secondary prevention of cardiovascular events using aspirin, statins and lifestyle modifications like smoking cessation counseling.[11]

Evidence-Based Cardiology, 3rd edition. Edited by S. Yusuf, J.A. Cairns, A.J. Camm, E.L. Fallen, and B.J. Gersh. © 2010 Blackwell Publishing, ISBN: 978-1-4051-5925-8.

Development of new therapies has been the traditional role of large national biomedical enterprises like the National Institutes of Health (NIH), as well as the pharmaceutical and device industries. Over the last several decades, this framework has been enormously successful in expanding the "evidence" behind much of what we know. However, it has clearly fallen short in its ability to guide these same scientific breakthroughs into routine clinical practice. Despite established data supporting their use, long-term adherence rates to evidence-based therapies such as aspirin, beta-blockers and statins in patients with CAD remain low in community-based practices across the United States, at between 45% and 70%.[12] For heart failure, long-term adherence rates for ACE inhibitors may be as low as 20%.[12] In fact, some estimates suggest that it takes on average 17 years for new therapies to be adopted into widespread clinical practice.[13] Simply increasing the use of existing evidence-based therapies in cardiology would have profound implications for the healthcare system and enhance the public health as much as new discoveries.

Practice gaps, knowledge translation and quality improvement science

The practice gaps between "what we know" and "what we do" have been well documented and widely recognized by policy makers and providers, although the reasons for them are less certain.[14] Moreover, these practice gaps are not limited to any single country or healthcare system but have been shown in a variety of regions and settings.[15] Strategies to address these challenges were introduced years ago but gained much more momentum during the 1990s, evolving from approaches that relied on the passive diffusion of knowledge to recent efforts to incorporate information technology and systems engineering into a transformation of the healthcare delivery system. Yet despite these advances, substantial practice gaps remain in medicine and these have been difficult to overcome. In its landmark report in 2001, the Institute of Medicine (IOM) referred to these practice gaps as the "quality chasm" and called for renewed efforts to develop better systematic approaches for bringing evidence to the bedside.[16]

Accordingly, this chapter focuses on strategies for improving the implementation of evidence-based cardiology based on research in knowledge translation. Knowledge translation has been described variably but a frequently cited definition is the one proposed by the Canadian Institutes of Health Research:

> "Knowledge translation is a dynamic and iterative process that includes synthesis, dissemination, exchange and ethically sound application of knowledge to improve the health of [populations], provide more effective health services and products and strengthen the health care system."[17]

Furthermore, the scientific investigation of specific methods to promote the use of research findings in clinical practice may be considered "quality improvement" science or research.[18] In different settings, similar concepts have been labeled as "knowledge transfer research" and "implementation science or research". In this chapter, we most frequently use the terms "knowledge translation" and "quality improvement science".

In the following sections, we discuss (1) the overall scope of the problem in practice gaps, (2) possible barriers identified in translating evidence to clinical practice, and (3) specific approaches that have been studied in quality improvement science to overcome these barriers. Many of the issues raised here are universal to medicine but we try to focus on examples in cardiology while still highlighting broader themes. We end the chapter by briefly discussing unique challenges faced in quality improvement science, including the growing tension between the immediate desire to improve quality and the rigor required for objectively studying its improvement.

Practice gaps: scope of the problem

Evidence-based medicine has been described as "the conscientious, explicit, and judicious use of current best evidence in making decisions about the care of individual patients".[19] The application of evidence-based medicine therefore is necessarily dependent upon the existence of a mature base of knowledge that can inform providers of what treatments are appropriate (and inappropriate) in specific clinical settings. Despite the fact that persistent voids continue to remain in some key clinical areas within cardiology, no specialized field of medicine is as well developed or evidence-based. This makes cardiology ideally suited in many ways for providers to optimize their use of evidence-based approaches. Yet even in areas of cardiology with a clear base of evidence, like acute myocardial infarction (AMI), heart failure, atrial fibrillation and hypertension, the practice gaps between "what we know" and "what we do" remain large and extend across the entire spectrum of care from inpatient to outpatient settings (Table 6.1).

Hospital setting

Practice gaps in the inpatient setting have been demonstrated for a number of disease processes in cardiology. For

Table 6.1 Recent examples of practice gaps in cardiovascular disease

Condition	Example
Coronary artery disease	*Beta-blocker use:* • Hospital data from 2004 indicate that mean performance at US hospitals for beta-blockers at admission remains at 85% (Jha *et al* 2005[86]) • Outpatient data from 1998 to 2000 indicate that 45% of patients with prior myocardial infarction remain on long-term beta-blockers (McGlynn *et al* 2003[12])
Heart failure	*ACE inhibitor use:* • Inpatient data from 2002 to 2003 found that median rates of compliance with ACE inhibitors in hospitalized patients with heart failure and left ventricular systolic dysfunction are suboptimal at 72% (Fonarow *et al* 2005[25]) • Outpatient data suggest that only 60–65% of Medicare patients with heart failure and left ventricular systolic dysfunction who are discharged on ACE inhibitors remain on these agents 90 days after their hospitalization (Butler *et al* 2004[87])
Atrial fibrillation	*Anticoagulation:* • Among 5333 inpatients and outpatients with atrial fibrillation enrolled in 35 countries in the Euro Heart Survey between 2003 and 2004, 67% of eligible patients and 49% of ineligible patients were prescribed oral anticoagulation therapy (Nieuwlaat *et al* 2005[29])
Hypertension	*Blood pressure management:* • NHANES data from 1999 to 2000 suggest that only 31% of patients with hypertension in the US had blood pressures under adequate control. Furthermore, 31% were not even aware of their disease (Wang and Wang 2004[88]) • REACH Registry data found 55% of patients with a history of atherothrombosis and hypertension to have elevated blood pressures noted at their clinic visit (Bhatt *et al* 2006[31])

example, acute reperfusion therapy with either fibrinolytic therapy or primary percutaneous coronary intervention (PCI) in ST elevation myocardial infarction reduces mortality and morbidity. While the use of acute reperfusion therapy has improved over recent years, recent data suggest that worldwide, as many as a third of eligible patients still do not receive it even at centers capable of delivering both treatments.[20] Furthermore, the overall effectiveness of acute reperfusion therapy is highly dependent upon its timely delivery, but both fibrinolytic therapy and primary PCI are often administered after long delays. Data from just a few years ago suggest that fewer than 50% of patients in the United States were treated with primary PCI within 90 minutes or fibrinolytic therapy within 30 minutes.[21] Similar practice gaps have been noted in other countries, including those in the developing world. In India, for example, evidence-based therapies like acute reperfusion therapy, beta-blockers, ACE inhibitors (or ARBs) and statins are used in between 50% and 60% of hospitalized patients with acute coronary syndromes.[22]

Others have documented wide regional variation in the appropriate use of cardiac catheterization and PCI after AMI (including data that suggest both under- and overutilization).[23,24] In a recent analysis of nearly 45000 patients, investigators noted that regions of the United States with a higher intensity of invasive procedure utilization performed cardiac catheterization at increased rates in both appropriate (i.e. for an ACC/AHA Class I indication) and inappropriate (i.e. for an ACC/AHA Class III indication) situations.[24] In addition, the use of invasive procedures was inversely correlated to the baseline risk of the patient assessed by their Global Registry of Acute Coronary Events (GRACE) risk score.

Similar patterns of practice gaps in the inpatient setting (including recent trends toward improvement) have also been demonstrated in heart failure and atrial fibrillation.[25,26] For example, the initial Euro Heart Surveys found rates of ACE inhibitor and beta-blocker use of 61.8% and 36.9%, respectively, among hospitalized patients with heart failure,[27] although these numbers have improved somewhat in more recent surveys.[28] Among inpatients and outpatients patients with atrial fibrillation enrolled at 182 hospitals in 35 countries in the Euro Heart Survey, roughly two-thirds of eligible patients were prescribed oral anticoagulation therapy.[29] Furthermore, oral anticoagulation therapy was not targeted at those patients who were the highest risk for stroke but instead depended upon nonclinical factors such as the availability of outpatient laboratory monitoring.[30]

Outpatient setting

In 2003, McGlynn *et al* published a landmark study demonstrating that just over 50% of patients received "recommended" care for a variety of healthcare conditions in the outpatient setting, using a complex survey design of 12 metropolitan areas of the United States between 1998 and 2000.[12] Recommended care in this study primarily focused on processes of care that were defined using the RAND-UCLA modified Delphi method to specific identify quality indicators through expert panels. Although rates of compliance with recommended care were generally higher for CAD (68%) and heart failure (64%) than other disease-specific conditions, critical practice gaps were still noted. For example, only 45% and 61% of patients with myocardial infarction received beta-blockers and aspirin, respectively, despite the absence of clear contraindications and strong evidence of long-term benefit with both. Rates of recommended care associated with atrial fibrillation were even less and dropped below 25%. Furthermore, the investigators noted broad differences in practice gaps based on the "mechanism" required for performing recommended care, regardless of the healthcare condition. Care that was related to direct encounters with providers or medications had the highest proportion of compliance at approximately 70%, whereas counseling or education was performed in fewer than 20% of cases (Table 6.2).

Similar findings were also noted in the international REACH registry, which enrolled nearly 68000 patients 45 years or older with evidence of atherosclerotic disease from 5473 physician practices across 44 countries.[31] Physician practices in this registry included a broad mix of clinical practices such as primary care providers and specialists; urban, rural and suburban environments; and office-based and hospital-based settings. Importantly, this study noted suboptimal adherence rates with statins (69%) and antiplatelet agents (79%) in these patients, as well as evidence for undertreatment of hypertension, with 50% of patients found to have elevated baseline blood pressures above 140/90 mmHg.

Disparities and the risk-treatment paradox

Key patterns have emerged from these studies with important clinical and policy implications. First, practice gaps that have been documented in clinical practice have consistently been largest among vulnerable populations, including the elderly, minority patients and women. These appear to be particularly evident for expensive and resource-intensive procedures, such as coronary revascularization and implantable cardioverter defibrillators (ICDs).[32–34] The extent to which these practice gaps are due to biological factors, reduced access to care, or systematic biases in the delivery of care to vulnerable populations is unclear. A similar association between practice gaps and socioeconomic status has also been recognized, including examples from developing countries. In the CREATE

Table 6.2 Adherence to outpatient quality indicators by mechanism in a random sample of US adults from 12 metropolitan areas (from McGlynn et al 2003[12])

Indicator area	No. of indicators	No. of participants eligible	Total no. of times indicator eligibility was met	Percentage of recommended care received (95% CI)*
Encounter or other intervention	30	2843	4,329	73.4 (71.5–75.3)
Medication	95	2964	8,389	68.6 (67.0–70.3)
Immunization	8	6700	9,748	65.7 (64.3–67.0)
Physical examination	67	6217	19,428	62.9 (61.8–64.0)
Laboratory testing or radiography	131	5352	18,605	61.7 (60.4–63.0)
Surgery	21	244	312	56.9 (51.3–62.5)
History	64	6711	36,032	43.4 (42.4–44.3)
Counseling or education	23	2838	3,806	18.3 (16.7–20.0)

*CI denotes confidence interval. All pairwise differences were statistically significant at $P < 0.001$ except those between medication and encounter or other intervention ($P = 0.02$), physical examination and immunization ($P = 0.001$), surgery and immunization ($P = 0.004$), and surgery and physical examination ($P = 0.05$). The difference between surgery and laboratory testing or radiography was not significant ($P = 0.39$).

registry, for example, 30-day mortality was significantly higher in poor hospitalized patients with acute coronary syndromes when compared with rich patients in 50 cities across India. Importantly, this mortality difference was largely explained by differences in rates of evidence-based therapy use. Studies such as the CREATE registry have provided invaluable insights by focusing on low- and middle-income countries where 80% of the global burden of cardiovascular disease exists. In general, there remains a paucity of data from these countries on practice gaps and additional work is urgently needed to improve our understanding of clinical practice patterns in these regions.

Second, there is evidence supporting a "risk-treatment" paradox for many evidence-based therapies. That is, those patients who may stand to benefit the most from a therapy paradoxically are the least likely to receive it. Among nearly 1500 patients in the EFFECT cohort with heart failure and LV systolic dysfunction, ACE inhibitor, ARB and beta-blocker use were inversely associated with the severity of the patient's condition and their predicted risk of death in the upcoming year.[35] After accounting for potential contraindications to therapy, low-risk patients were more likely to receive ACE inhibitors or ARBs (adjusted hazard ratio (HR), 1.6) and beta-blockers (adjusted HR, 1.8) than high-risk patients (both I < 0.001). Similarly, another population-based study from Ontario found statin use to be significantly lower among high-risk patients with established CAD or diabetes mellitus.[36] Interestingly, recent data suggest that much of the risk-treatment paradox may be explained by clinical factors not typically captured in administrative data, including functional limitations and depressive symptoms.[37]

Barriers to knowledge translation

A number of common barriers to implementing evidence-based medicine in clinical practice have been identified. We focus here primarily on barriers related to provider-level (e.g. physician and hospital) and system-level factors. While we recognize the importance of patient-level factors in the use of evidence-based therapies, it is beyond the scope of this discussion. One simple conceptual model for understanding these barriers suggests that incorporating new therapies into clinical practice proceeds from changes in *knowledge* to *attitudes* to *behavior* (Fig. 6.1).[38,39] This model mirrors other approaches that emphasized the progression from awareness to acceptance to adoption among providers,[40] but slightly differs by noting that each step is potentially independent of others in the process. For example, behavior can be changed through incentives at the organizational-level without necessarily improving knowledge or attitudes among providers.

Knowledge

Improving knowledge relies on providing new information to clinicians primarily through increasing their awareness of the published literature. The enormous size and complexity of contemporary biomedical research make this a particularly challenging barrier to implementing evidence-based medicine. For example, in 2006 the top 10 clinical cardiovascular journals alone published 4065 articles, averaging 78 articles per week. It is clearly impossible for busy providers in clinical practice today to stay on top of the latest developments even in a specialized field like cardiol-

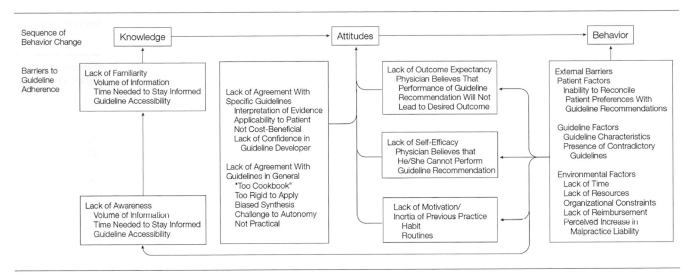

Figure 6.1 Barriers to use of guidelines and evidence-based medicine. (From Cabana et al,[38] with permission.)

ogy. An understanding of this barrier has led to the development of guidelines and evidence-based summaries to synthesize the published literature by professional organizations and other groups. In fact, it is one of the key motivations for writing this textbook.

Attitudes

Even when providers become familiar with the available evidence, recommendations may be incomplete or confusing. This can lead to barriers to changing the attitudes of providers (i.e. their acceptance of new evidence). For example, summary clinical guidelines and consensus statements from expert panels may be large, unmanageable or poorly developed.[41] Conflicting recommendations also can arise if different (and sometimes competitive) organizations produce separate guidelines for the same disease process. Finally, attitudes can limit acceptance when providers feel that recommendations inadequately reflect the nuances of clinical practice, making them less applicable to their patients or their healthcare system.

Behavior

Barriers to the adoption of behavior can still exist even when providers have moved beyond awareness and acceptance of evidence. Adoption of behaviors can be particularly challenging since it requires that changes occur in the actual performance of a task at the provider or organizational level. For providers, barriers to adoption can vary from factors as ordinary as the influence of habit and routine to more complex issues that reflect lack of time or resources.[42] Organizational-level factors that impact on behavior include reimbursement or payment structures for

providing care as well as the availability of or access to specialized services and medications.

Finally, it is important to recognize that patients can also indirectly influence the adoption of new recommendations by providers. A perceived lack of adherence to lifestyle recommendations by patients has been described as a frequent reason by providers for inconsistent recommendations about smoking cessation.[43] This also can be problematic in cases where patients often have set expectations for receiving a particular service. For example, providers may be reluctant not to pursue cardiac catheterization in an active individual with a low-risk stress test who believes it is necessary based on personal experiences (e.g. "My father had it done!").

Multiple barriers

It is rare for a single barrier to be responsible for the limited use of an evidence-based therapy. Instead multiple barriers often contribute to poor implementation, and barriers identified in one clinical environment may be less relevant for other areas or settings. For example, high out-of-pocket drug costs may be a pertinent barrier to statin use in patients with CAD, while limited availability of a high-quality program may be an important barrier for cardiac rehabilitation. In patients interested in smoking cessation, drug costs for nicotine replacement therapy and the availability of counseling programs could play important roles. Similarly, in urban areas barriers to timely access for primary PCI could be accomplished by redesigning emergency medical services to integrate new technologies like prehospital electrocardiography (ECG).[44] However, large geographic distances between hospitals with and without cardiac catheterization laboratories would limit the applicability of this approach in rural healthcare systems.[45]

Important socioeconomic factors can also affect patterns of adoption for evidence-based therapies, especially depending upon the structure of the healthcare delivery system into which these therapies are introduced. For example, an important reason why behavior modifications such as smoking cessation, nutritional counseling and cardiac rehabilitation may be difficult to implement is that most physicians are not traditionally trained in the skills required for these activities and reimbursement is disproportionately low for them. In contrast, physicians have a greater proclivity for performing diagnostic tests and therapeutic procedures since these are what they are often trained to do best and because their reimbursement is more aligned with these services. This has a potentially perverse effect on a healthcare system by encouraging overuse of expensive procedures (even when marginally effective) and underuse of useful simple diagnostic and therapeutic approaches (even when evidence-based and cost effective).[46]

An important limitation of existing literature in quality improvement science is that interventions are often developed without researchers first rigorously studying what local barriers may be contributing to insufficient knowledge translation. Furthermore, even when intervention-based studies report the presence of local barriers, descriptions frequently lack adequate detail. In a large review of studies examining barriers to guideline use among physicians, Cabana and colleagues found that just half of all intervention-based studies reported more than one category of barriers in their results.[38] Without a better appreciation of what barriers may have been present at baseline, it is impossible for readers to judge whether the findings associated with an intervention would be applicable in their own clinical practices.

Strategies for quality improvement

There have been a number of studies exploring different strategies for overcoming barriers to the implementation of evidence-based medicine in cardiology and improving quality. These strategies have evolved significantly over the years from simple educational interventions (i.e. one-time dissemination of educational materials) targeted at improving provider knowledge to complex and multifaceted approaches designed to leverage information and systems-based technologies (i.e. computerized order entry and reminders). On the "road map" for moving basic research into clinical practice, Dougherty and Conway have distinguished research in quality improvement science from other translational research and identified it as the third translational step (i.e. "T3") (Fig. 6.2).[47] While the first two translational steps focus primarily on moving evidence from basic science research to clinical efficacy (i.e. "T1") and clinical effectiveness (i.e. "T2"), T3 research should be focused on understanding how evidence-based medicine can be reliably delivered to broad populations of patients across different healthcare settings.

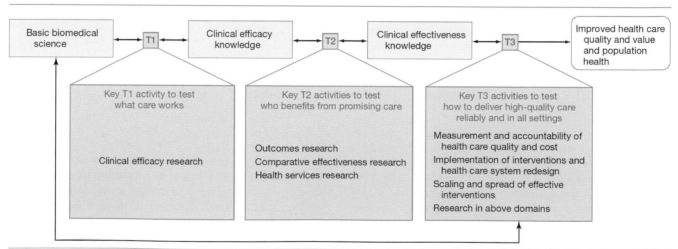

T indicates translation. T1, T2, and T3 represent the 3 major translational steps in the proposed framework to transform the health care system. The activities in each translational step test the discoveries of prior research activities in progressively broader settings to advance discoveries originating in basic science research through clinical research and eventually to widespread implementation through transformation of health care delivery. Double-headed arrows represent the essential need for feedback loops between and across the parts of the transformation framework.

Figure 6.2 The three translational steps on the roadmap from evidence into clinical practice. (From Dougherty and Conway,[47] with permission.)

Evolution of strategies

According to David Naylor, strategies aimed at knowledge translation have developed in four phases over the years, evolving as our understanding of barriers improved.[48] The first group of strategies initially relied exclusively on "passive diffusion" of evidence-based medicine into clinical practice (i.e. "Just publish it").[48] In this scenario, providers were largely responsible for accessing, reviewing and then incorporating new evidence by themselves. During this time period, proponents believed that the key to quality improvement was to educate providers to be efficient consumers of evidence-based medicine. Given the growing size and complexity of the medical literature, however, it soon became obvious that it was impossible for most providers to remain abreast of current developments, even within a narrow field, without help. This led to the second group of strategies aimed at developing guidelines and consensus statements to synthesize the literature for providers (i.e. an "active diffusion" of information exemplified by the documents that are now routinely produced by the American College of Cardiology (ACC) and American Heart Association (AHA)).[48]

However, simply producing guidelines does not always change clinical practice in a reliable manner. The third group of strategies, which arose from this understanding, represents what Naylor refers to as the "Era of Industrialization".[48] Strategies during this time reflected a growing interest in applying quality improvement tools from other industries to measuring, evaluating and then managing provider behavior. Rather than specific interventions, these strategies frequently emphasized incremental process-of-care improvements and were exemplified by the concepts of continuous quality improvement (CQI) and total quality management (TQM) adopted by the manufacturing industry during the 1980s.[49] Moving beyond a framework of CQI/TQM, the most recent group of strategies has focused on incorporating advances in information technology and systems engineering to completely redesign clinical pathways.[48] These strategies are exemplified by computerized ordering and reminder systems, as well as the development of clinical information tools to aid in informed decision making between patients and providers.

A general framework for categorizing strategies

One useful framework for categorizing strategies aimed at improving the implementation of evidence-based medicine is by the level of care within the healthcare system that the strategy is targeting. The Cochrane Collaboration's Effective Practice and Organization of Care (EPOC) group has used this type of framework to identify four categories of quality improvement interventions: *provider-level*, *organizational-level*, *financial-level*, and *regulatory-level* interventions.[50] Provider-level (i.e. professional) interventions include those aimed at continuing medical education, audit and data feedback. Organizational-level interventions are those aimed at the systems level that might include the incorporation of physician extenders or nursing in case management programs. Financial-level interventions are aimed at using economic incentives to influence clinical practice. Regulatory-level interventions include strategies such as public reporting of processes of care or outcomes, changes in medical liability or regionalization of specialized services. Specific examples from each of these categories that have been frequently discussed in the literature are presented in greater detail in Table 6.3.[51]

Education

Interventions aimed at improving provider awareness of guidelines or evidence-based recommendations are among the most studied in the published literature. Specific approaches include workshops or conferences targeted at large groups of providers, distribution of printed or electronic material to inform providers of new developments through mass media, and "academic detailing" that uses a trained individual to target and inform a particular provider (or group) about an explicit recommendation. Local opinion leaders are often utilized in these approaches. These types of interventions are frequently used in cardiology when guidelines have been updated or new therapies are discovered.

Reminder systems

Another common area of focus for interventions is the use of reminder systems that target providers. Paper-based or electronic reminder systems have been utilized to prompt providers to recognize patient-specific information during an encounter. When electronic, these reminder systems can also be supplemented with decision support tools to guide providers toward appropriate referrals or medication adjustments when indicated. These types of interventions have been used successfully during outpatient visits for notifying providers of cardiovascular risk assessment and helping with decisions about initiating statins.[52]

Audit and data feedback

The use of audit and feedback systems has been well studied at both the provider and organizational levels. This type of intervention frequently presents data to individual clinicians, groups of clinicians, a hospital or even a larger healthcare system. Data that are typically reported include summaries of the proportion of eligible patients within their practice or institution that receive a treatment or other

Table 6.3 Common examples of quality improvement interventions (from Shojania and Grimshaw 2005[18])

Strategy definition and examples	Effectiveness
Provider education – examples: • Conferences or printed educational materials detailing current recommendations for management of a particular condition • Educational outreach visits to providers' offices, usually targeting more specific aspects of care, such as appropriate medication choices for a target condition	• Generally ineffective if judged on the basis of improving patient outcomes • If judged in terms of increasing provider knowledge, can be effective
Provider reminder systems and decision support (systems for prompting health professionals to recall information relevant to a specific patient or clinical encounter; when accompanied by a recommendation such systems are classified as clinical decision support) – examples: • Sheet on front of chart alerting provider to date of the patient's most recent mammogram and its result • Computer-generated suggestion to intensify diabetes medications based on most recent HbA1c values	• Reminders often effective if well integrated with workflow • Decision support sometimes effective, but less so for the more complex situations in which it would be most desirable
Audit and feedback (summary of clinical performance for an individual provider or clinic, transmitted back to the provider) – example: • Reports to providers or provider groups summarizing percentages of their eligible patients who have achieved a target outcome (cholesterol below a certain value) or received a target process of care (counseling about smoking cessation), accompanied by recommended targets	• Small to modest (at best) benefits for various forms of audit and feedback (such as report cards, benchmarking) • Variations in format may explain some of the observed variations in effectiveness, in addition to providers' attitudes toward the accuracy or credibility of the reports
Patient education – examples: • Individual or group sessions with nurse educator for patients with diabetes • Medication education from a pharmacist for patients with heart failure	• Modest to large effects for some conditions and patient populations
Organizational change – example: • Changes in the structure or organization of the healthcare team or setting designed to improve processes or outcomes of care	• Mostly positive results for case management and disease management programs • Mixed results for total quality management and continuous quality improvement
Financial incentives, regulation, and policy – examples: • Financial bonuses for achieving target level of compliance with targeted processes of care • Change from fee-for-service to salaried or capitated reimbursement systems	• Some evidence for achieving target goals, but also for concerning decreases in access and conflicts of interest in physician–patient relationships

recommendation relative to national or local peer providers. The National Cardiovascular Data Registry (NCDR) sponsored by the American College of Cardiology provides this type of benchmarking information routinely to hospitals on established quality indicators. Regional examples of audit and data feedback have shown substantial quality improvements in PCI and coronary artery bypass grafting (CABG). For example, use of quarterly data feedback to clinicians and hospitals in a statewide PCI registry was associated with improved clinical outcomes and reduced practice variation in quality indicators related to vascular complications, contrast-related nephropathy and stroke.[53]

Disease and case management programs

These types of programs include any structured system designed for co-ordinating the diagnosis, treatment or ongoing management of a patient through a person or team in collaboration with the primary provider. Many of these programs have been studies in heart failure and have suggested benefits in reducing resource utilization and improving quality of life.[54] However, the heterogeneous nature of heart failure and case management programs often makes it difficult to tease out what (if any) aspects of these types of interventions are most responsible for their effectiveness and their potential generalizability to other clinical settings. This has led to tremendous challenges with implementing disease and case management programs in clinical practice.[55]

Financial and regulatory interventions

Financial interventions aim to improve the use of evidence-based medicine in clinical practice by modifying reimbursement systems for providers. The goal of these types of interventions is to reward behavior by providers and organizations that promotes quality and efficiency of care. Examples include changes from fee-for-service to capitated reimbursement systems as well as pay-for-performance programs. Pay-for-performance programs have drawn recent attention since these efforts attempt to tie evidence of improvement in quality indicators to increased reimbursement for services. Regulatory interventions include public reporting of outcomes and process-of-care measures. In some states like New York and California, public reporting has already been well established for several years for CABG.[56] This is also true in the United Kingdom where the Healthcare Commission now provides a national system with information on outcomes after CABG for hospitals and surgeons.[57] In addition, the Centers for Medicare & Medicaid Services (CMS) now publicly report process-of-care measures for quality indicators in acute myocardial infarction, heart failure and other disease processes across hospitals.[58]

Overall effectiveness of strategies

Several themes have emerged from studies examining strategies for improving the use of evidence-based medicine, many of which have been summarized in a series of systematic reviews and meta-analyses. In 1995, two systematic reviews were published that analyzed available data on strategies aimed at improving guideline use by providers, primarily through education-based interventions.[59,60] Both reviews found that no strategy consistently appeared to produce large or sustained benefits (i.e. no "magic bullet", according to the title of one article). Both systematic reviews also suggested that the most effective approaches were "active" and "multifaceted". Multifaceted refers to the simultaneous use of multiple strategies as an intervention (i.e. reminder systems combined with auditing and data feedback). In contrast, passive and simple strategies had little or no effect on changing behavior (i.e. a one-time dissemination of paper-based educational materials).

However, effects of more complex interventions applied at the provider level have not always been consistent. Audit and data feedback, for example, appeared to have a limited impact unless they were repetitively applied or coupled with other strategies. A more recent systematic review – actually a systematic review of 41 systematic reviews on interventions to change provider behavior – suggested that even those strategies that were determined to be effective have a largely modest impact on increasing the use of evidence-based medicine.[61] In this analysis, the median absolute improvements in recommended care varied from 6% to 14% across different types of interventions and there was great heterogeneity both across and within any specific intervention. Clinical reminders showed the greatest variation, with 14 cluster-randomized trials showing reported median effects of this intervention varying from -1.0% to 34.0%. This is not entirely unexpected. By necessity, strategies are tested in variable environments and sometimes across different providers or disease processes, making it likely that there would be inconsistent effects under these different circumstances. Finally, unlike the two prior systematic reviews, this latest study did not find significant improvements associated with the use of active and multifaceted interventions relative to other interventions.

The evidence base for organizational-, financial- and regulatory-level interventions has also shown mixed results. Case management programs in heart failure have been studied extensively but the impact of their utilization on clinical outcomes has shown large variation. In one recent meta-analysis, there were wide differences in the pre- and postdischarge components that were included. These varied from telephone follow-up to clinic follow-up to home visits. Duration of programs, time commitments and costs also differed. Not surprisingly, the effect of case management programs also varied, with studies suggesting anywhere from an approximately 50% relative risk reduction in repeat hospitalizations to no effect.[62] This heterogeneity was significant and has been implicated as a potential reason why case management programs may be underutilized in heart failure.[63]

Data exist that suggest that compensation systems for providers can impact on the use of evidence-based therapies. A market-level analysis of 56 medical groups affiliated with 15 integrated healthcare systems in the United States in 2001 found that compensation incentives and managed care pressures influenced the use of clinical guidelines, critical pathways and case or disease management programs by physicians.[64] A more recent example of financial-level interventions being pushed forward as a strategy for encouraging the adoption of evidence-based medicine is pay-for-performance programs introduced in the United States. While these programs all link changes in process of care and outcome measures to reimbursement, they vary substantially on where to apply the level of financial incentive and its size. In a recent systematic review of empirical studies that examined the relationship between financial incentives and quantitative measures of quality improvement, Petersen *et al* found that six studies focused on physician-level incentives, seven focused on provider groups, and two on healthcare system levels.[65] The majority of these studies did suggest improvements in process-of-care measures, most of which were targeted toward preventive services.

However, there was some evidence that unintended consequences also occurred, including adverse selection of patients (i.e. the avoidance of more severely ill patients) and less provider attention to aspects of care that are not subject to incentives. Furthermore, a recent analysis of the voluntary CRUSADE registry found no evidence that instituting a pay-for-performance program that was tied to bonus payments by CMS improved the use of evidence-based therapies in AMI using a composite measure.[66] Among the 54 hospitals within the pay-for-performance program, higher rates of improvement were noted relative to 446 control hospitals for two individual measures: aspirin use at discharge (odds ratio (OR), 1.31; 95% confidence interval (CI), 1.18–1.46) and smoking cessation counseling (OR, 1.50; 95% CI, 1.29–1.73). These mixed data, lack of suitable targets for measurement, and potential concerns about unintended consequences have pushed some to advocate for pay-for-participation programs, especially to improve quality for procedures.[67]

Regulatory-level interventions are being used more extensively even within loosely organized healthcare systems like those in the United States. As with other types of interventions, the data supporting regulatory-level interventions are mixed and heterogeneous. For example, public reporting of outcomes for hospitals and clinicians is a commonly used regulatory strategy although there are few empirical data supporting its use. In 2000, Marshall *et al* reviewed seven reporting systems in the United States (including the New York CABG reporting program) and found little evidence that consumers or physicians used (or trusted) the data, although hospitals appeared more responsive to it.[68] A more recent updated systematic review on the topic found increasing support that public reporting stimulates quality improvement efforts at the hospital level, but otherwise concluded that data on the impact of these programs remain scant.[69] As with pay-for-performance programs, however, there are challenges with selecting appropriate metrics to report and for public reporting to potentially lead to unintended consequences with the adverse selection of patients. A recent analysis of two large statewide PCI registries by Moscucci *et al* found that public reporting may have led clinicians to avoid PCI in higher-risk patients in New York as compared with Michigan.[70]

Similarly, the use of certificate-of-need (CON) programs as a regulatory-level intervention to improve quality has shown mixed results with potential improvements in utilization balanced by concerns of restricting access to specialists and specialized cardiovascular procedures. A recent study using data from the Medicare program suggested that mortality rates after CABG among beneficiaries were lower in states with certificate-of-need regulations, potentially due to the concentration of these procedures at higher-volume hospitals.[71] Furthermore, a separate analysis in the Medicare population suggested that although certificate-of-need regulations decrease the overall use of these procedures, these effects are negligible in those with strong clinical indications such as high-risk patients after AMI that require cardiac catheterization.[72]

Finally, expanding healthcare insurance and drug coverage to more individuals may also dramatically impact on the use of evidence-based therapies given that out-of-pocket spending is a significant barrier to utilization for patients. In one analysis based on a computer-based simulation model, expanding full coverage of medication benefits to insured patients after AMI would result in 1.1 fewer deaths and 13.1 fewer recurrent AMIs while saving insurers nearly $6000 in costs per patient.[73] However, the challenge of regulatory-level interventions like expanded drug coverage is that their likelihood of success depends strongly upon the political, social and cultural settings of a healthcare system.

Future directions

Improving the use of evidence-based medicine in cardiology remains an important but challenging goal for healthcare systems around the world. Three areas that will need to be addressed in the future relate to (1) the growing tension between the immediate need for quality improvement efforts and the time required to perform quality improvement science, (2) the development of stable funding sources and infrastructure for T3 translational research dedicated to moving evidence-based medicine generated at academic medical centers into clinical practice in the community, and (3) the creation of formal educational pathways for both individual and institutional providers that are dedicated to implementing quality improvement within their local environments.

Balancing quality improvement efforts and quality improvement science

Methodological approaches for assessing strategies for improving the use of evidence-based medicine have undergone substantial transformation as patient safety and quality improvement efforts have become increasingly emphasized over the last decade. Early study designs focused on case reports, case series and pre/post study designs. The primary goal of investigators was to rapidly report experiences with innovative strategies to allow for quick dissemination. However, more recent efforts have emphasized the need for a strong theoretical framework in designing interventions and implementing them within rigorous study designs where their impact can be accurately assessed. As stated eloquently by Shojania and Grimshaw in a recent review on this topic: "Strategies for implementing evidence-based medicine require an evidence base of their own".[18]

A recent article by Auerbach and colleagues has comprehensively summarized the arguments for and against rapid dissemination of interventions in quality improvement without an adequate scientific base of knowledge (Table 6.4).[74] Numerous examples exist where shortcomings in study designs have suggested large benefits for interventions that were subsequently overturned after more rigorous evaluations. For example, the recent AFFECT trial was a cluster randomized controlled trial that examined the effectiveness of hospital report cards generated by administrative data on process of care and outcome measures in AMI among 76 Canadian hospitals.[75] While the use of hospital report cards had been reported as successful in a number of observational studies, this carefully conducted study found no evidence supporting this approach. Rather than being seen as a 'negative' trial, the AFFECT trial provides important information on the limitations of report cards for benchmarking, which is critically important given the widespread dissemination of this type of intervention. A similar challenge has been raised in recent debates regarding the Institute for Healthcare Improvement's "100,000 Lives Campaign". This national campaign was clearly successful at galvanizing interest in patient safety at more than 3000 participating hospitals across the United States, but its true impact on outcomes remains controversial.[76,77]

In fact, Ting and colleagues[78] have argued that quality improvement science may benefit from following the same stepwise paradigm that has guided the development of scientific breakthroughs for the last several decades. Based on this framework, strategies in quality improvement should progress from preclinical, Phase I and II trials focused on feasibility at single centers toward larger and more definitive Phase III and IV trials that address broader implementation (e.g. the AFFECT trial).[79] This type of approach has been described in the United Kingdom Medical Research Council's research phases for complex interventions (e.g. case management programs for heart failure or strategies for increasing uptake of guidelines by clinicians) (Fig. 6.3).[79] Early research phases in this

Table 6.4 Arguments for and against the rapid dissemination of interventions in quality improvement (from Auerbach et al 2007[74])

Argument	Why proceeding quickly is critical	Why evaluation is critical
We cannot wait – the need to improve the quality of care is urgent	Thousands of patients are injured or killed each year by medical errors	The need to improved the treatment of many diseases is equally urgent, yet we demand rigorous evidence that a therapy works before recommending it widely
Any effort to improve quality is better than the current state of affairs	On balance, the harms of quality improvement are likely to be far less than those of the status quo	Knowledge of the harms and opportunity costs of quality improvement is important for an understanding of the net benefit to patients and healthcare systems, which is often small
Emulating successful organizations can speed effective improvement	Emulation and collaboration provide an efficient means of disseminating potentially effective solutions	Emulation and collaboration can incorrectly promote or even overlook interventions that have not worked
The effectiveness of some quality improvement strategies is obvious	Insistence on evidence may lead us to underuse interventions that are obviously effective	Even though many quality improvement practices have a simple rationale, they may be less effective than expected and can be difficult to implement fully
Innovation can be catalyzed by dissemination of strategies that have promise but are unproven	Preliminary data provide an important opportunity to speed innovation and improve care rapidly	Flawed, biased or incomplete data may lead to adoption of interventions that are ineffective or harmful
The framework of evidence-based medicine does not apply to quality improvement	The nature of quality improvement exempts it from the usual strategies of assessment	Given the complexity of quality and safety problems, the complexity of their causes, and how little we understand them, we should use rigorous study designs to evaluate them
Developing evidence in quality improvement is too costly	The resources and expertise required to evaluate quality and safety interventions rigorously make trails impractical, particularly when the field is moving so quickly	As compared with the large opportunity costs incurred by wide implementation of ineffective quality and safety strategies, investments in better evaluation would be small

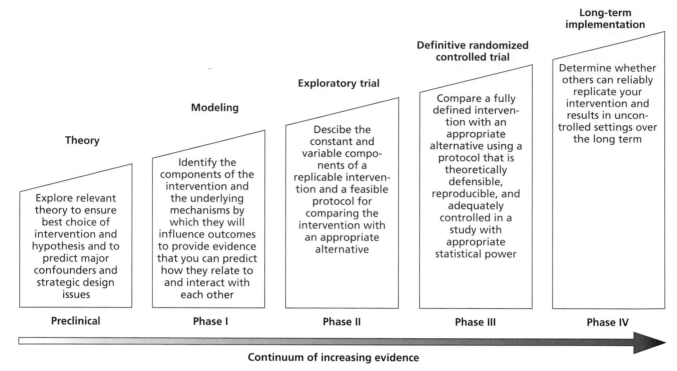

Figure 6.3 Sequential research phases for developing evidence in complex interventions. (From Campbell et al,[79] with permission.)

framework focus on establishing the 'efficacy' of quality improvement interventions in at least one setting and are designed using traditional methodologies from industrial quality improvement, the social sciences, cognitive psychology, human factors engineering, and organizational theory. All of these disciplines represent the 'basic sciences' of quality improvement. Later research phases examine the generalizability and long-term implementation of interventions aimed at quality improvement in larger and more diverse settings.

Funding and infrastructure for quality improvement science

The challenges associated with knowledge translation and quality improvement science are not unique to a particular healthcare system or country. Funding agencies worldwide that are involved in the biomedical and health sciences have a direct interest in ensuring that scientific breakthroughs are translated into clinical practice in their own local communities. For this to happen though, these agencies have recognized that they must play a more active and integral role in knowledge translation. Specific activities that these groups may use to ensure this include (1) requiring all grant proposals in clinical research to describe plans for knowledge translation and to use this as a criterion for funding and/or (2) explicitly increasing funding opportunities for research that is focused on developing new strate-

gies in quality improvement science. Funding agencies can also be instrumental in early dissemination by promoting findings through traditional (i.e. journals) and non-traditional (television) media sources. In a recent qualitative survey of 33 funding agencies across the world, knowledge translation was directly or indirectly referred to in 23 mission statements but relatively new to all these groups.[80] Moreover, funding agencies appeared to have widely differing views of what knowledge translation even meant, their requirements of researchers to participate in it, and how engaged the funding agencies should be in this process overall.[80]

One potential solution that has been widely discussed for expanding the infrastructure for quality improvement science is the development of practice-based research networks. The simple concept behind practice-based research networks is that our traditional notions of research need to move outside traditional academic environments into those clinical practice settings where the great majority of care is routinely delivered. There unfortunately is little infrastructure at this time for conducting research in these typically non-academic and outpatient environments. For these reasons, there has been great interest in providing resources to expand their development, particularly in the United States. Westfall and colleagues have pointed out how the NIH Roadmap supports practice-based research networks as part of its plan to re-engineer clinical research within the framework of the Clinical and Translational

Science Awards (CTSAs).[81] Of course, practice-based research networks do not only provide an infrastructure for examining interventions. They also have the advantage of supporting observational study designs to understand where practice gaps really exist in real-world settings.

Improving provider education in strategies for quality improvement

Optimizing the use of evidence-based medicine requires that individual and institutional providers will have the necessary skills to evaluate their own performance and to design tailored solutions that meet the needs of their local clinical practice. These issues become critical given that skills and knowledge may decline with the number of years physicians are out in practice.[82] Providers therefore must be life-long learners and continually improve their own knowledge base and training in quality improvement, but these areas have not been a traditional focus of training. In the past, formal training in quality improvement was uncommon during medical school or even postgraduate training. This has changed remarkably in recent years, though. Accreditation of postgraduate training programs in the United States is now tied to competency in systems-based practice and practice-based learning.[83] Even for physicians who have completed training and are actively in practice, recertification depends upon demonstrating knowledge in self-evaluation of practice performance.[84]

It is encouraging that a recent review of 39 studies on the effectiveness of teaching quality improvement to clinicians suggested that most appeared to apply established adult learning principles such as self-directed learning and reflection.[85] However, educational outcomes showed more consistent improvements than clinical outcomes which were rarely reported. Furthermore, while the majority of studies described providing teaching content to implement and evaluate local systems for changes, few taught about the larger healthcare system or patients' perspectives about the system. Further research is clearly needed to develop better methods for training providers in these skills as efforts to improve knowledge translation and quality improvement science expand in coming years.

Conclusion

Substantial developments have been made over the last several decades in our understanding of the role of evidence-based medicine in cardiology. However, while there has been an improved understanding of the basic mechanisms and treatments related to cardiovascular diseases, we have clearly fallen short in our ability to guide scientific breakthroughs into routine clinical practice. The practice gaps between "what we know" and "what we do" continue

to challenge policy makers and providers. Strategies to address these practice gaps through more effective knowledge translation continue to gain momentum, transforming from earlier approaches that relied on the passive diffusion of knowledge to recent efforts to incorporate information technology and systems engineering into a transformation of the healthcare delivery system. These strategies frequently utilize complex interventions that can be aimed at multiple levels of the healthcare delivery system. As these strategies move forward, there remain important challenges in the need to improve the evidence base for quality improvement science, to create stable funding and infrastructure for these efforts, and to improve provider education in this area.

References

1. Cutler DM, Rosen AB, Vijan S. The value of medical spending in the United States, 1960–2000. *N Engl J Med* 2006;**355**(9): 920–7.
2. Ford ES, Ajani UA, Croft JB *et al.* Explaining the decrease in U.S. deaths from coronary disease, 1980–2000. *N Engl J Med* 2007;**356**(23):2388–98.
3. Barker WH, Mullooly JP, Getchell W. Changing incidence and survival for heart failure in a well-defined older population, 1970–1974 and 1990–1994. *Circulation* 2006;**113**(6):799–805.
4. Roger VL, Weston SA, Redfield MM *et al.* Trends in heart failure incidence and survival in a community-based population. *JAMA* 2004;**292**(3):344–50.
5. Antman EM, Hand M, Armstrong PW *et al.* 2007 Focused update of the ACC/AHA 2004 guidelines for the management of patients with ST-elevation myocardial infarction: a report of the American College of Cardiology/American Heart Association Task Force on Practice Guidelines: developed in collaboration with the Canadian Cardiovascular Society endorsed by the American Academy of Family Physicians: 2007 Writing Group to Review New Evidence and Update the ACC/AHA 2004 Guidelines for the Management of Patients With ST-Elevation Myocardial Infarction, Writing on Behalf of the 2004 Writing Committee. *Circulation* 2008;**117**(2):296–329.
6. Anderson JL, Adams CD, Antman EM *et al.* ACC/AHA 2007 guidelines for the management of patients with unstable angina/non-ST-elevation myocardial infarction: a report of the American College of Cardiology/American Heart Association Task Force on Practice Guidelines (Writing Committee to Revise the 2002 Guidelines for the Management of Patients With Unstable Angina/Non-ST-Elevation Myocardial Infarction) developed in collaboration with the American College of Emergency Physicians, the Society for Cardiovascular Angiography and Interventions, and the Society of Thoracic Surgeons endorsed by the American Association of Cardiovascular and Pulmonary Rehabilitation and the Society for Academic Emergency Medicine. *J Am Coll Cardiol* 2007;**50**(7):e1–e157.
7. Nallamothu BK, Bradley EH, Krumholz HM. Time to treatment in primary percutaneous coronary intervention. *N Engl J Med* 2007;**357**(16):1631–8.

8. Hunt SA, Abraham WT, Chin MH *et al.* ACC/AHA 2005 guideline update for the diagnosis and management of chronic heart failure in the adult: a report of the American College of Cardiology/American Heart Association Task Force on Practice Guidelines (Writing Committee to Update the 2001 Guidelines for the Evaluation and Management of Heart Failure): developed in collaboration with the American College of Chest Physicians and the International Society for Heart and Lung Transplantation: endorsed by the Heart Rhythm Society. *Circulation* 2005;**112**(12):e154–235.

9. Hart RG. Atrial fibrillation and stroke prevention. *N Engl J Med* 2003;**349**(11):1015–16.

10. Hacke W, Donnan G, Fieschi C *et al.* Association of outcome with early stroke treatment: pooled analysis of ATLANTIS, ECASS, and NINDS rt-PA stroke trials. *Lancet* 2004;**363**(9411):768–74.

11. Smith SC, Allen J, Blair SN *et al.* AHA/ACC guidelines for secondary prevention for patients with coronary and other atherosclerotic vascular disease: 2006 update: endorsed by the National Heart, Lung, and Blood Institute. *J Am Coll Cardiol* 2006;**47**(10):2130–9.

12. McGlynn EA, Asch SM, Adams J *et al.* The quality of health care delivered to adults in the United States. *N Engl J Med* 2003;**348**(26):2635–45.

13. Balas EA, Boren SA. Managing clinical knowledge for health care improvement. In: *Yearbook of Medical Informatics 2000: Patient-centered Systems.* Stuttgart, Germany: Schattauer, **2000**:65–70.

14. Lenfant C. Clinical research to clinical practice – lost in translation? *N Engl J Med* 2003;**349**(9):868–74.

15. Eagle KA, Goodman SG, Avezum A *et al.* Practice variation and missed opportunities for reperfusion in ST-segment-elevation myocardial infarction: findings from the Global Registry of Acute Coronary Events (GRACE). *Lancet* 2002;**359**(9304):373–7.

16. Institute of Medicine. *Crossing the Quality Chasm: A New Health System for the 21st Century.* Washington, DC: National Academy Press, 2001.

17. Government of Canada, Canadian Institutes of Health Research. About Knowledge Translation – CIHR. Available at: www.cihr-irsc.gc.ca/e/29418.html.

18. Shojania KG, Grimshaw JM. Evidence-based quality improvement: the state of the science. *Health Aff* 2005;**24**(1):138–50.

19. Sackett DL, Rosenberg WM, Gray JA, Haynes RB, Richardson WS. Evidence based medicine: what it is and what it isn't. *BMJ* 1996;**312**(7023):71–2.

20. Eagle KA, Nallamothu BK, Mehta RH *et al.* Trends in acute reperfusion therapy for ST-segment elevation myocardial infarction from 1999 to 2006: we are getting better but we have got a long way to go. *Eur Heart J* 2008;**29**(5):609–17.

21. McNamara RL, Herrin J, Bradley EH *et al.* Hospital improvement in time to reperfusion in patients with acute myocardial infarction, 1999 to 2002. *J Am Coll Cardiol* 2006;**47**(1):45–51.

22. Xavier D, Pais P, Devereaux PJ *et al.* Treatment and outcomes of acute coronary syndromes in India (CREATE): a prospective analysis of registry data. *Lancet* 2008;**371**(9622):1435–42.

23. Petersen LA, Normand ST, Leape LL, McNeil BJ. Regionalization and the underuse of angiography in the Veterans Affairs Health Care System as compared with a fee-for-service system. *N Engl J Med* 2003;**348**(22):2209–17.

24. Ko DT, Wang Y, Alter DA *et al.* Regional variation in cardiac catheterization appropriateness and baseline risk after acute myocardial infarction. *J Am Coll Cardiol* 2008;**51**(7):716–23.

25. Fonarow GC, Yancy CW, Heywood JT, for the ADHERE Scientific Advisory Committee SG. Adherence to heart failure quality-of-care indicators in US hospitals: analysis of the ADHERE Registry. *Arch Intern Med* 2005;**165**(13):1469–77.

26. Kapral MK, Laupacis A, Phillips SJ *et al.* Stroke care delivery in institutions participating in the Registry of the Canadian Stroke Network. *Stroke* 2004;**35**(7):1756–62.

27. Komajda M, Follath F, Swedberg K *et al.* The EuroHeart Failure Survey programme – a survey on the quality of care among patients with heart failure in Europe. Part 2: treatment. *Eur Heart J* 2003;**24**(5):464–74.

28. Nieminen MS, Brutsaert D, Dickstein K *et al.* EuroHeart Failure Survey II (EHFS II): a survey on hospitalized acute heart failure patients: description of population. *Eur Heart J* 2006;**27**(22):2725–36.

29. Nieuwlaat R, Capucci A, Camm AJ *et al.* Atrial fibrillation management: a prospective survey in ESC member countries: the Euro Heart Survey on Atrial Fibrillation. *Eur Heart J* 2005;**26**(22):2422–34.

30. Nieuwlaat R, Capucci A, Lip GY *et al.* Antithrombotic treatment in real-life atrial fibrillation patients: a report from the Euro Heart Survey on Atrial Fibrillation. *Eur Heart J* 2006;**27**(24):3018–26.

31. Bhatt DL, Steg PG, Ohman EM *et al.* International prevalence, recognition, and treatment of cardiovascular risk factors in outpatients with atherothrombosis. *JAMA* 2006;**295**(2):180–9.

32. Sheifer SE, Escarce JJ, Schulman KA. Race and sex differences in the management of coronary artery disease. *Am Heart J* 2000;**139**(5):848–57.

33. Popescu I, Vaughan-Sarrazin MS, Rosenthal GE. Differences in mortality and use of revascularization in black and white patients with acute MI admitted to hospitals with and without revascularization services. *JAMA* 2007;**297**(22):2489–95.

34. Hernandez AF, Fonarow GC, Liang L *et al.* Sex and racial differences in the use of implantable cardioverter-defibrillators among patients hospitalized with heart failure. *JAMA* 2007;**298**(13):1525–32.

35. Lee DS, Tu JV, Juurlink DN *et al.* Risk-treatment mismatch in the pharmacotherapy of heart failure. *JAMA* 2005;**294**(10):1240–7.

36. Ko DT, Mamdani M, Alter DA. Lipid-lowering therapy with statins in high-risk elderly patients: the treatment-risk paradox. *JAMA* 2004;**291**(15):1864–70.

37. McAlister FA, Oreopoulos A, Norris CM *et al.* Exploring the treatment-risk paradox in coronary disease. *Arch Intern Med* 2007;**167**(10):1019–25.

38. Cabana MD, Rand CS, Powe NR *et al.* Why don't physicians follow clinical practice guidelines? A framework for improvement. *JAMA* 1999;**282**(15):1458–65.

39. Woolf SH. Practice guidelines: a new reality in medicine. III. Impact on patient care. *Arch Intern Med* 1993;**153**(23):2646–55.

40. Davis DA, Taylor-Vaisey A. Translating guidelines into practice. A systematic review of theoretic concepts, practical experience and research evidence in the adoption of clinical practice guidelines. *CMAJ* 1997;**157**(4):408–16.

41. Cook D, Giacomini M. The trials and tribulations of clinical practice guidelines. *JAMA* 1999;**281**(20):1950–1.

42. Freeman AC, Sweeney K. Why general practitioners do not implement evidence: qualitative study. *BMJ* 2001;**323**(7321). Available at: www.pubmedcentral.nih.gov/articlerender.fcgi?artid=59686

43. Kottke TE, Solberg LI, Brekke ML. Initiation and maintenance of patient behavioral change: what is the role of the physician? *J Gen Intern Med* 1990;**5**(5 suppl):S62–7.

44. Le May MR, So DY, Dionne R *et al.* A citywide protocol for primary PCI in ST-segment elevation myocardial infarction. *N Engl J Med* 2008;**358**(3):231–40.

45. Nallamothu BK, Bates ER, Wang Y, Bradley EH, Krumholz HM. Driving times and distances to hospitals with percutaneous coronary intervention in the United States: implications for pre-hospital triage of patients with ST-elevation myocardial infarction. *Circulation* 2006;**113**(9):1189–95.

46. Emanuel EJ, Fuchs VR. The perfect storm of overutilization. *JAMA* 2008;**299**(23):2789–91.

47. Dougherty D, Conway PH. The "3T's" road map to transform US health care: the "how" of high-quality care. *JAMA* 2008;**299**(19):2319–21.

48. Naylor CD. Putting evidence into practice. *Am J Med* 2002;**113**(2):161–3.

49. Blumenthal D, Kilo CM. A report card on continuous quality improvement. *Milbank Q* 1998;**76**(4):625–48.

50. Cochrane Effective Practice and Organisation of Care Group. Available at: www.epoc.cochrane.org/en/index.html.

51. Grimshaw J, Eccles M, Thomas R *et al.* Toward evidence-based quality improvement. Evidence (and its limitations) of the effectiveness of guideline dissemination and implementation strategies 1966–1998. *J Gen Intern Med* 2006;**21**(suppl 2):S14–20.

52. Lester WT, Grant RW, Octo Barnett G, Chueh HC. Randomized controlled trial of an informatics-based intervention to increase statin prescription for secondary prevention of coronary disease. *J Gen Intern Med* 2006;**21**(1):22–9.

53. Moscucci M, Rogers EK, Montoye C *et al.* Association of a continuous quality improvement initiative with practice and outcome variations of contemporary percutaneous coronary interventions. *Circulation* 2006;**113**(6):814–22.

54. Rich MW, Beckham V, Wittenberg C *et al.* A multidisciplinary intervention to prevent the readmission of elderly patients with congestive heart failure. *N Engl J Med* 1995;**333**(18):1190–5.

55. Laramee AS, Levinsky SK, Sargent J, Ross R, Callas P. Case management in a heterogeneous congestive heart failure population: a randomized controlled trial. *Arch Intern Med* 2003;**163**(7):809–17.

56. Steinbrook R. Public report cards – cardiac surgery and beyond. *N Engl J Med* 2006;**355**(18):1847–9.

57. Heart Surgery in United Kingdom. Available at: http://heartsurgery.healthcarecommission.org.uk/index.aspx.

58. Medicare.gov – Hospital Compare. Available at: www.hospitalcompare.hhs.gov/Hospital/Search/Welcome.asp?version=default&browser=Firefox%7C2%7C7CWinXP&language=English&defaultstatus=0&pagelist=Home.

59. Davis DA, Thomson MA, Oxman AD, Haynes RB. Changing physician performance. A systematic review of the effect of continuing medical education strategies. *JAMA* 1995;**274**(9):700–5.

60. Oxman AD, Thomson MA, Davis DA, Haynes RB. No magic bullets: a systematic review of 102 trials of interventions to improve professional practice. *CMAJ* 1995;**153**(10):1423–31.

61. Grimshaw JM, Shirran L, Thomas R *et al.* Changing provider behavior: an overview of systematic reviews of interventions. *Med Care* 2001;**39**(8 suppl 2):II2–45.

62. Whellan DJ, Hasselblad V, Peterson E, O'Connor CM, Schulman KA. Metaanalysis and review of heart failure disease management randomized controlled clinical trials. *Am Heart J* 2005;**149**(4):722–9.

63. Fonarow GC. Heart failure disease management programs: not a class effect. *Circulation* 2004;**110**(23):3506–8.

64. Shortell SM, Zazzali JL, Burns LR *et al.* Implementing evidence-based medicine: the role of market pressures, compensation incentives, and culture in physician organizations. *Med Care* 2001;**39**(7 suppl 1):I62–78.

65. Petersen LA, Woodard LD, Urech T, Daw C, Sookanan S. Does pay-for-performance improve the quality of health care? *Ann Intern Med* 2006;**145**(4):265–72.

66. Glickman SW, Ou F, DeLong ER *et al.* Pay for performance, quality of care, and outcomes in acute myocardial infarction. *JAMA* 2007;**297**(21):2373–80.

67. Birkmeyer NJ, Birkmeyer JD. Strategies for improving surgical quality – should payers reward excellence or effort? *N Engl J Med* 2006;**354**(8):864–70.

68. Marshall MN, Shekelle PG, Leatherman S, Brook RH. The public release of performance data: what do we expect to gain? A review of the evidence. *JAMA* 2000;**283**(14):1866–74.

69. Fung CH, Lim Y, Mattke S, Damberg C, Shekelle PG. Systematic review: the evidence that publishing patient care performance data improves quality of care. *Ann Intern Med* 2008;**148**(2):111–23.

70. Moscucci M, Eagle KA, Share D *et al.* Public reporting and case selection for percutaneous coronary interventions: an analysis from two large multicenter percutaneous coronary intervention databases. *J Am Coll Cardiol* 2005;**45**(11):1759–65.

71. Vaughan-Sarrazin MS, Hannan EL, Gormley CJ, Rosenthal GE. Mortality in Medicare beneficiaries following coronary artery bypass graft surgery in states with and without certificate of need regulation. *JAMA* 2002;**288**(15):1859–66.

72. Ross JS, Ho V, Wang Y *et al.* Certificate of need regulation and cardiac catheterization appropriateness after acute myocardial infarction. *Circulation* 2007;**115**(8):1012–19.

73. Choudhry NK, Avorn J, Antman EM, Schneeweiss S, Shrank WH. Should patients receive secondary prevention medications for free after a myocardial infarction? An economic analysis. *Health Aff* 2007;**26**(1):186–94.

74. Auerbach AD, Landefeld CS, Shojania KG. The tension between needing to improve care and knowing how to do it. *N Engl J Med* 2007;**357**(6):608–13.

75. Beck CA, Richard H, Tu JV, Pilote L. Administrative Data Feedback for Effective Cardiac Treatment: AFFECT, a cluster randomized trial. *JAMA* 2005;**294**(3):309–17.

76. Wachter RM, Pronovost PJ. The 100,000 Lives Campaign: a scientific and policy review. *Jt Comm J Qual Patient Saf* 2006;**32**(11):621–7.

77. Berwick DM, Hackbarth AD, McCannon CJ. IHI replies to The 100,000 Lives Campaign: a scientific and policy review. *Jt Comm J Qual Patient Saf* 2006;**32**(11):628–30.

78. Ting HH, Shojania KG, Montori VM, Bradley EH. Quality improvement: science and action. *Circulation* 2009;**119**(14):1962–74.

79. Campbell M, Fitzpatrick R, Haines A *et al.* Framework for design and evaluation of complex interventions to improve health. *BMJ* 2000;**321**(7262):694–6.

80. Tetroe JM, Graham ID, Foy R *et al.* Health research funding agencies' support and promotion of knowledge translation: an international study. *Milbank Q* 2008;**86**(1):125–55.

81. Westfall JM, Mold J, Fagnan L. Practice-based research – "Blue Highways" on the NIH roadmap. *JAMA* 2007;**297**(4):403–6.

82. Choudhry NK, Fletcher RH, Soumerai SB. Systematic review: the relationship between clinical experience and quality of health care. *Ann Intern Med* 2005;**142**(4):260–73.

83. Accreditation Council for Graduate Medical Education Outcome Project. Available at: www.acgme.org/outcome/comp/compFull.asp.

84. Overview/Guide. Improve your Practice With PIMs. American Board of Internal Medicine. Available at: www.abim.org/pims/default.aspx.

85. Boonyasai RT, Windish DM, Chakraborti C *et al.* Effectiveness of teaching quality improvement to clinicians: a systematic review. *JAMA* 2007;**298**(9):1023–37.

86. Jha AK, Li Z, Orav EJ, Epstein AM. Care in U.S. hospitals – the Hospital Quality Alliance program. *N Engl J Med* 2005;**353**(3):265–74.

87. Butler J, Arbogast PG, Daugherty J, Jain MK, Ray WA, Griffin MR. Outpatient utilization of angiotensin-converting enzyme inhibitors among heart failure patients after hospital discharge. *J Am Coll Cardiol* 2004;**43**(11):2036–43.

88. Wang Y, Wang QJ. The prevalence of prehypertension and hypertension among US adults according to the new joint national committee guidelines: new challenges of the old problem. *Arch Intern Med* 2004;**164**(19):2126–34.

7 The application of evidence-based medicine to employment fitness standards: the transportation industries with special reference to aviation

Michael Joy

Postgraduate Medical School, Surrey University, Guildford, Surrey, UK

Introduction

Medical standards are applicable to a number of occupational groups. Some of these are voluntary codes of practice, some statutory. The police and armed forces are examples, as is the offshore oil industry. Employers have a duty of care to protect employees from harm as well as guarding against medical conditions which may have a detrimental effect on performance in the workplace. Likewise, employees have an obligation to indicate any medical condition which might erode ability in the discharge of duty.

Medical standards exist for all transport modalities including roads, railways, shipping and in the air to protect both the individual as well as third parties. The development of these standards was initially empiric rather than evidence based. This no longer applies to aviation, and to some extent to road transport, both of which have based their fitness requirements on risk of event. As it is impossible in one short chapter to review the evidence base for the breadth of cardiologic standards across the workplace, it is intended to consider road and, more specifically air transport as examples of the application of evidence-based medicine (EBM) to achieve the twin goals of safety and good practice.

Passenger transportation does not have to be completely safe and the controling legislation does not require it to be so. It has to be "safe enough." It is self-evident that the good conduct of a means of transport requires it to be fit for purpose. Design, construction, maintenance and operation should be sound and reliable. This implies the need for regulation. The concept of safety criticality suggests that the consequences of failure of any aspect of the enve-lope need to be identified, minimized and tolerable in the operational environment. Sometimes systems are duplicated (redundant) but not always if a sufficiently low target failure rate can be achieved without. How, then, can these targets be identified and met?

People operate motor cars, railway trains and aircraft and may fail due to health or other considerations. This event rate, like the vehicles they operate, can be to some extent predetermined. Age makes a contribution. Decrement in human function or performance may be associated with sudden catastrophic failure or subtle, with gradual loss of efficiency. The safe operation of a system of transportation involves a level of medical fitness of those responsible for the lives of others.

The regulatory process

Operational standards (including medical standards) in civil aviation are agreed by international statute[1] and are implemented by national agencies (e.g.. the Civil Aviation Authority (CAA) in the UK). There may be additional supranational oversight (e.g.. the European Aviation Safety Agency (EASA)). There are also agreed European standards for the regulation of driving, including medical standards.[2,3] Medical fitness to fly and to drive has been swept up into the legal frameworks of the Western world, and elsewhere. Some medical conditions are inconsistent with driving or flying status and an adverse decision may terminate employment. Some cardiologic conditions such as coronary artery disease, on account of their large outcome databases, lend themselves to risk modeling. Others such as atrial fibrillation, due to symptomatic capriciousness, are more difficult. And there are orphans such as the long QT syndrome where risk stratification is based on slender outcome data, but where decisions still have to be taken. Third-party safety takes precedence but best practice is paramount to avoid the adoption of clinical courses of

Evidence-Based Cardiology, 3rd edition. Edited by S. Yusuf, J.A. Cairns, A.J. Camm, E.L. Fallen, and B.J. Gersh. © 2010 Blackwell Publishing, ISBN: 978-1-4051-5925-8.

action solely for the purpose of the preservation of employment. The need for good governance in the decision-making process requires no further emphasis.

Modes of transport and regulation

Regulation got off to an early start and in 2500 years BC the Cretans required maintenance and loading inspection of their ships, a practice which was revived in Europe in the Middle Ages. It was not until 1894 in the UK that the load line on a ship was made law in an attempt to reduce the number of vessels and crews lost from overloading. In 1930 international agreement was achieved. In Europe, the development of the European Union led to a harmonization process for all land (and air) based activities. This was to include competition, taxation (inevitably), safety and technical requirements, track rules and signaling, where appropriate. The endpoint was to be interoperability of road and rail across the continent. Currently 1.2 million lives are lost in road transport accidents each year, with some 0.5 billion injuries, worldwide. Although observational data are scarce, medical incapacitation accounts for only 0.1% of road traffic accidents of which some 25% may be attributed to cardiologic causes.[4] Historically, but with certain exceptions, the railways have had the best safety record on land.

The aviation environment

Aviation also has an impressive safety record and is tightly regulated. In 2006, 2.1 billion passengers were carried in some 35 million scheduled and non-scheduled flying hours for the loss of 863 passengers. The average sector length is now 2 hours. This has doubled in the last 30 years. Aviation is the only system of mass transportation that is regulated by international statute. All contracting states have treaty status with the International Civil Aviation Organization (ICAO), a safety directorate of the United Nations Organization. All are bound to maintain the standards in Annex 1 to the Convention on International Civil Aviation (ICAO Annex 1).[1] The Standards and Recommended Practices (SARPs) are promulgated in Annexes to the Convention and are regularly updated. The Standards are safety directed and obligatory. Recommended Practices are not so binding.

The ICAO cardiologic Standard is enshrined in eight brief paragraphs but may be interpreted by "accredited medical conclusion" to permit ongoing licensing provided flight safety will not be jeopardized. ICAO also publishes guidance material. In Europe and elsewhere, an operational multi-crew limitation (OML) may be imposed to prevent a pilot from flying on single-crew operations if the risk of medical (cardiologic) event is perceived as too high.

The Joint Airworthiness Authorities framework in Europe was set up in 1970, later becoming the Joint Aviation Authorities (JAA). The medical standards in the Joint Aviation Requirements FCL part 3 Medical[5] related guidance material were the first comprehensive approach, worldwide, to provide a written protocol. The cardiologic standards originated from four cardiologic workshops[6–9] specifically tasked to the interface with aviation. These have been amplified in the UK by a series of algorithms showing pathways of problem management which guide medical fitness and certification. This material has been adopted outside Europe but has no regulatory status elsewhere. The EASA[10] is the legally based successor to the JAA. Within the curtilage of this chapter, the terms *certificate* and *license* (to fly) are used synonymously whilst *fitness* indicates fitness to fly. The class 1 certificate relates to professional aircrew and the class 2 certificate to private pilots These are regulatory terms and should not be confused with classes of recommendations and levels of evidence as used in this book.

Aviation accident experience due to medical cause

Eighty percent of fatal aircraft accidents are attributable to "human factors." One-third of airline pilots admit to some level of incapacitation whilst on duty at some time during their career,[11] most commonly due to gastroenteritis. Significant medical cause incapacitation is rare, mainly because such events are rare in the population of pilot age (<65 years for professional pilots). Subtle incapacitation (see above) leading to error may be as important as complete incapacitation. It can be caused by illness, fatigue or the effects of medication. Routine medical scrutiny, which includes resting electrocardiography, identifies a few of those at increased risk of cardiologic mishap, allowing intervention, e.g. hypertension, diabetes. Alternatively, problems may present spontaneously, e.g. myocardial infarction, stroke. Notwithstanding, the UK license loss from cardiovascular cause remains low at <0.1%/thousand professional license holders per annum.

There were 29 airline accidents, worldwide, attributable to medical incapacitation during the years 1946–1985. There were five fatal accidents attributed to acute coronary events during the years 1961–1968.[12–14] In 1972 the HS Trident G-ARPI (known as Papa India) crashed 150 seconds into its flight when it stalled due to premature retraction of a leading edge lift device. This fatal error was attributed in part to incapacitation of the captain by an acute coronary event. One hundred and eighteen people died.[15]

In the aftermath of the Papa India disaster a number of initiatives were taken nationally and internationally. The ICAO required regular incapacitation training of multi-crew pilots; flight deck voice recorders were also mandated. Some well-travelled cardiologists were so shaken by the event that the American College of Cardiology[16] and the Royal College of Physicians of London[17] called for increased cardiologic scrutiny of pilots. This was to include exercise electrocardiography. But middle-aged otherwise fit males have a low probability of fatal/non-fatal coronary event and this recommendation was not evidence based in safety terms, nor justifiable in (Bayesian) terms of conditional probability. Had exercise electrocardiography been adopted it would have led to many more pilots being investigated for disease they did not have (false-positive responders) than those who did (true-positive responders). And, as an investigation for coronary artery disease, exercise electrocardiography is only 60–70% sensitive in the asymptomatic middle-aged male.

The Papa India disaster is the worst UK aviation accident to date. The pilot population at the time was relatively old and there was no crew training for recognition of incapacitation of a colleague. Following the accident, pilots were subsequently reviewed more rigorously but inconsistently as there were no agreed protocols of review. Since 1974, improved crew training, better cockpit resource management, better safety systems and better aircraft design have all contributed to the exceptional safety levels which are now being achieved in multi-crew (more than one pilot) airline operations. There have been almost no accidents/incidents attributable to pilot incapacitation in the 2/3 billion hours flown since, in spite of deaths and incapacitations which have continued to occur whilst aircrew are on their duty period.

Evidence-based medicine and workshops in aviation cardiology

Pre-empting Sackett et al[18] by nearly two decades, it was evident that there was a need for an authoritative overview of the evidence base on the presentation, natural history, outcome and impact of intervention on the common, and sometimes not so common, cardiologic conditions to make regulatory decisions more scientific, objective and fair. This led to the four workshops in aviation cardiology which took place between 1982 and 1998.[6–9] They followed the same pattern. Twenty-five cardiologists and epidemiologists who were leaders in their field, together with directly relevant specialists, were tasked to produce position papers on chosen topics. This resulted in one of the most comprehensive statements available on cardiologic problems and aircrew certification available at the time, or since.

Devereaux et al[19] produced a Venn diagrammatic model for the evolution of evidence-based clinical decisions. The key elements include research evidence, patient preferences and actions, the clinical state and circumstances, with clinical expertise being in the command or "overarching" position. In the regulatory environment an extra dimension is introduced. Transport safety is concerned with the probability of an incapacitating event in the operator but the decision to grant medical fitness is a binary one. The subject is either fit or unfit for the task with the exception of a detente where there is an OML. There are, therefore, potential conflicts between patient choice and the boundaries of regulation.

The regulator is not the pilot's physician and must play no part in clinical management. Certain clinical choices may deny subsequent fitness – the use of a mechanical valve in the management of aortic stenosis in a pilot, for example. The clinical indication for warfarin in this context is associated with fitness denial at present in Europe on account of the summative risk of bleeding from the treatment and the risk accruing from the underlying pathology. Thus although the thromboembolic rate of the tissue and mechanical valves in the aortic position is comparable, the risk of bleeding in the patient with an anticoagulated mechanical valve is significantly higher,[20] exceeding the target event rate (see below). The choice of a tissue valve may, however, be agreed between the patient and his/her cardiologist in spite of its long-term poorer performance[20] without pre-emption towards regaining flying status. This represents operation of the fourth dimension in Devereaux's Venn diagram. The decision to replace the valve will have been a clinical one,[21] assuming that the pilot with aortic stenosis was asymptomatic. Provided the UK CAA algorithm (Fig. 7.1), for example, can be subsequently navigated successfully, a favorable fitness statement should be possible.

The "1% rule" and best evidence

Although the workshop proceedings were to become manuals of regularly updated informal guidance material, their ground-breaking contribution was the evolution of what was to become known as the "1% rule." Credit is due to Tunstall-Pedoe[22,23] who related the chance of "failure" of a pilot in medical terms to the risk of failure of any major system in the aircraft. It is derived as follows: the industry target fatal accident rate for large jet aircraft is 1 in 10 million flying hours. Not more than 1 in 10 of such events should be due to a major system failure (i.e. the pilot) and not more than 1 in 10 of those due to failure of a subsystem (i.e. medical incapacity). This makes for an objective of 1 fatal accident in 1000 million hours from all-cause medical incapacitation.

This target will be met provided the all-cause crew medical failure rate does not exceed 1%/annum – the approximate cardiovascular mortality of a 66-year-old male in North West Europe. This is argued as follows: there

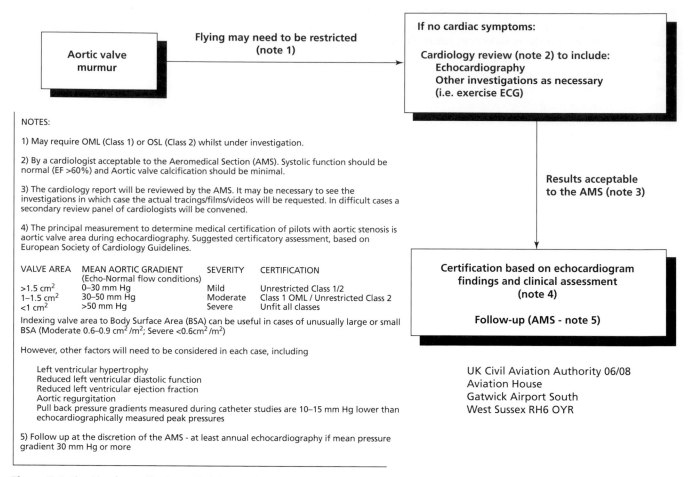

JAA Class 1/2 certification - Aortic valve stenosis

Aortic valve murmur

Flying may need to be restricted (note 1)

If no cardiac symptoms:

Cardiology review (note 2) to include:
Echocardiography
Other investigations as necessary
(i.e. exercise ECG)

Results acceptable to the AMS (note 3)

Certification based on echocardiogram findings and clinical assessment (note 4)

Follow-up (AMS - note 5)

NOTES:

1) May require OML (Class 1) or OSL (Class 2) whilst under investigation.

2) By a cardiologist acceptable to the Aeromedical Section (AMS). Systolic function should be normal (EF >60%) and Aortic valve calcification should be minimal.

3) The cardiology report will be reviewed by the AMS. It may be necessary to see the investigations in which case the actual tracings/films/videos will be requested. In difficult cases a secondary review panel of cardiologists will be convened.

4) The principal measurement to determine medical certification of pilots with aortic stenosis is aortic valve area during echocardiography. Suggested certificatory assessment, based on European Society of Cardiology Guidelines.

VALVE AREA	MEAN AORTIC GRADIENT (Echo-Normal flow conditions)	SEVERITY	CERTIFICATION
>1.5 cm^2	0–30 mm Hg	Mild	Unrestricted Class 1/2
1–1.5 cm^2	30–50 mm Hg	Moderate	Class 1 OML / Unrestricted Class 2
<1 cm^2	>50 mm Hg	Severe	Unfit all classes

Indexing valve area to Body Surface Area (BSA) can be useful in cases of unusually large or small BSA (Moderate 0.6–0.9 cm^2/m^2; Severe <0.6cm^2/m^2)

However, other factors will need to be considered in each case, including

Left ventricular hypertrophy
Reduced left ventricular diastolic function
Reduced left ventricular ejection fraction
Aortic regurgitation
Pull back pressure gradients measured during catheter studies are 10–15 mm Hg lower than echocardiographically measured peak pressures

5) Follow up at the discretion of the AMS - at least annual echocardiography if mean pressure gradient 30 mm Hg or more

UK Civil Aviation Authority 06/08
Aviation House
Gatwick Airport South
West Sussex RH6 OYR

Figure 7.1 Algorithm for certification to fly following the diagnosis of aortic stenosis. The cut-off points relate to the hierarchy of increasing risk assumed by reduction in valve area, and the prognostic implications of the presence of valvular calcification, left ventricular hypertrophy and the presence or absence of reduced left ventricular ejection fraction (**Class I**). Note that in the regulatory process, the terms "Class 1" and "Class 2" refer to the level of fitness assessment for professional and private aircrew respectively.

are 10 000 hours in a year (actually 8760 hours). If incapacitation occurs at 1% each year, the risk in any one hour will be 1 in 100 × 10 000 – 1 in 1 million. But there are two crew members and only 10% of the flight is critical (take off, climb out, approach and landing) and with adequate training (based on simulator data) only 1 in 100 such incidents will lead to an accident.

Thus the medical incapacitation *of one of the two crew members* should not lead to an accident more often than 1 in 1 million 1 in 10 × 1 in 100, i.e. 1 in 1 000 million hours. This coincides with the industry target for an unpredicted total loss which experience has shown to be realistic and appropriate. The chance of both pilots suffering medical incapacitation in the same hour will be the square of the individual risk (1 in 1 million × 1 in million – 1 × 10^{12}) which is extremely remote. The carriage of two pilots should, therefore, guarantee safety in all but the most adverse circumstances. In contrast, the single-pilot operation is uniquely vulnerable.[24,25]

In modeling the 1% rule, total cardiovascular mortality and coronary artery mortality were used as these are the most easily defined endpoints in the expression of cardiovascular risk. Co-morbid, non-lethal events, including stroke and unstable angina, will be 2–3 times as common but in the regulatory environment, screening by self-declaration following event will have removed some of this risk. Thus a 1% mortality in the general population is equivalent to a 1% event rate in the regulatory environment.[23]

Further development of the rule by Mitchell and Evans[26] has suggested that the target event rate could be relaxed to 2% *for multi-crew operations* without appreciable increase in risk to flight safety. This they based on a number of factors including reduced relative flight criticality brought about by longer flight duration and better equipment.

Furthermore, since the late 1970s, cardiovascular mortality in the UK has fallen 46%[27,28] in the under-65 year age group but in actuarial terms this risk reduction is "lost" in 3–4 years.[29,30] In other words a subject's "cardiologic age" at somatic age 64 years, now, is the equivalent of what it used to be at age 60, 25 years ago. Partly as a result of this, the age of professional pilot retirement from passenger-carrying operations has been increased from 60 to 65 years.

The impressive safety achievement in multi-crew operation is impossible in single-crew operations where the whole flight is critical in the context of pilot "failure" from any cause, including medical. In this environment the fatal accident rate due to failure by the single crew member will always be significantly worse than the medical incapacitation rate. The chance of being killed as a passenger in a single-pilot machine from any cause is likely to be one or two orders of magnitude ([mult]10–100) greater than in the multi-crew operation.

The foregoing arguments are predicated on the aviation environment but the principles are applicable elsewhere. In road and rail transportation, with a single crew operator, there may be sufficient warning of illness to permit safe conduct of a machine to a standstill. In rail transport the "dead man's handle" safety device is designed to stop the vehicle in the event of incapacitation of the driver. It is not universally fitted.

The 1% rule was evolved to define an appropriate cut-off point for denying multi-crew operational fitness to a pilot; it is not a yardstick for judging single crew fitness. In the context of coronary artery surgery, for example, if the predicted risk of event is <1%/annum, the pilot may be fit for multi-crew, but not single-crew operation. With the geometric increase in risk of occult coronary artery disease with age, it is not easy to determine placement of the risk cursor with its all-or-nothing impact on certification to fly. Doubling cardiovascular risk at age 60 years will be associated with a substantial increase in absolute risk when compared with age 40 years.[30]

Specific cardiologic issues in aircrew

Fitness to fly has evolved significantly over the years in tandem with the diagnostic, pharmacologic and interventional progress that has been made in medicine. The boundaries of fitness are under constant review as challenges to stretch the envelope in regulatory terms are made. The interface between regulation and cardiology is as broad as the specialty itself and for this reason only two of the most common cardiologic conditions will be considered in more detail – coronary artery disease and atrial fibrillation, whilst a third, rare, condition will also be examined. A fuller treatment of the subject is available.[31]

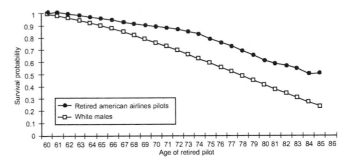

Figure 7.2 Survival probability curves of American Airline male pilots and an age- and sex-matched sample of the general population. (Reproduced with permission from the United States Federal Aviation Administration.[32])

Health maintenance

Of all occupational groups, aircrew are in one of the most favorable positions for health maintenance. Required as they are to pass regular medical examinations in order to maintain fitness (and thereby employment), it would be surprising if, as an occupational group, professional pilots did not enjoy a long retirement. Experience has shown this to be the case (Fig. 7.2). In the American Airlines study,[32] the median survival of pilots achieving age 60 in a sample of 2209 pilots and flight engineers was to age 83.8 years whilst that of age-matched white males was 78.2 years. This study is the only significantly robust one available although a number of other reports have suggested a similar effect. One from the UK contained limited data[33] and a similar one from Japan suggested increased longevity although the study was not sufficiently highly powered to estimate the survival benefit.[34]

Prevention of cardiovascular disease

If regular medical scrutiny is to be beneficial, the outcome must be acted upon, if indicated. There is abundant evidence that increased cardiovascular risk in terms of morbidity and mortality is present when one or more of the cardinal vascular risk factors is present. These include hypertension, increased total cholesterol, diabetes, smoking, obesity, sedentary lifestyle and the sometimes overlooked but increasingly powerful risk input of age. The European Health Charter[35,36] advocates the development and implementation of comprehensive health strategies and policies (**Class I**). This is to some extent enshrined in the new EASA requirements.[37]

A comprehensive review of the evidence and strategy for cardiovascular disease prevention is available[36] but in spite of this, it is not uncommon for a pilot in middle years to present with the signs of established hypertension, for example, when previously recorded levels have been within the normal range. There are a number of possible explanations including lack of awareness of, or a willingness to ignore, the importance and value of intervention in the preservation of cardiovascular health.

Coronary artery disease

Loss of license to fly from cardiovascular cause remains significant in the Western world in spite of the impressive fall in cardiovascular mortality. Neuropsychiatric problems are similarly important. The two most common cardiologic problem areas are coronary artery disease and the arrhythmias. Coronary artery disease, on account of its stealth, capricious presentation (often without diagnostic prodromal symptoms) and its ability to cause complete or subtle incapacitation, is important, notably in the single-crew operational environment. Increased chance of its presence can be calculated from risk algorithms but it remains what Rose has called the "prevention paradox" in that only three-fifths of subsequent events will occur in those in the top quintile of vascular risk. Purging high-risk asymptomatic individuals from the workforce has been attempted in the past, elsewhere, but was abandoned. In Europe, further investigation, particularly of single-crew operators, with exercise electrocardiography may be carried out and is routine at age 65 and 4 yearly thereafter. Although a pilot can be counselled on strategies of risk reduction, denial of fitness cannot be predicated on risk alone in the absence of evidence of disease although this has been attempted in certain states. It is possible to restrict such pilots to multi-crew operation but this appears difficult to apply consistently.

Coronary artery disease, unlike certain other cardiovascular disorders (such as thoracic aortic aneurysm), is not specifically disbarred under the European (EASA) rules. NPA 200817c: MED. B.005. (b)1 states "Applicants shall not possess any cardiovascular disorder which is likely to interfere with the safe exercise of the privileges of the applicable licence(s)."[37] The regulator, post hoc, is not as concerned with the first presentation of coronary disease as with its subsequent stability. In general terms the best-risk applicant will be asymptomatic, not receiving antianginal therapy, have no coronary obstruction >50% in any vessel unattended by percutaneous coronary intervention (PCI) or graft surgery, unless subtending a completed myocardial infarction (>30% in the proximal left anterior descending and left main stem vessels). Left ventricular function shall be good (ejection fraction >50%, however measured). Furthermore, the predicted risk of co-morbid MACE (major adverse cardiac event) has to be not more than that encompassing a mortality of the order of 1% per annum – see above. Finally, intervention against vascular risk factors present shall have been taken. This is a pretty tall order and some might question how durable the guiding principle of the 1% rule (recently relaxed to 2% per annum[26]) is in the

context of multiple stent implantation, in spite of concomitant pharmacologic intervention with statins and angiotensin-converting enzyme inhibitors (ACEI) for both their effect on outcome and their pleiotropic effect on plaque stability.[38,39]

Coronary artery disease lends itself to the mathematic modeling of risk on account of the massive amount of outcome data available. In the early days of recertification following coronary surgery, the validity of the step was underscored by Chaitman et al[40] who compared the survival of best-risk post coronary surgical patients with the profile of the pilot population who had undergone full revascularization, and who had normal or near normal left ventricular function, with a Framingham peer group. The surgical patients fared significantly better over a 5-year period. Under the circumstances it was both equitable and safe to allow fitness to fly (**Class I, Level C1**).

The postsurgical MACE rate is reassuringly flat 6 months later. The subsequent trajectory following stenting is less favorable than after coronary surgery.[41–45] The post-stent 12-month outcome in the recently published OLYMPIA data[42] using the Taxus stent "in the real world environment" was 4.5% for cardiac death, myocardial infarction and re-intervention alone. This is above what is tolerable in the aviation environment although some of the candidates in this study would have been excluded on the basis of age or co-existing pathology.

Figure 7.3 shows the rate of revascularization (for recurrent symptoms) following first intervention in the study of Hannan et al.[43] After the implantation of a drug-eluting stent in this comparative study of coronary artery surgery versus coronary stenting (PCI) for multi-vessel coronary artery disease, the 18-month repeat PCI rate was 28.4% versus 5.1% following coronary surgery (CABG) (P<0.001) although only one-quarter of interventions were for target vessel revascularization. This implies incomplete revascularization first time round, itself a reason for the denial of fitness status. It will also be noted that after the 6-month regulatory required waiting period, the revascularization rate has slowed but these data do not include other

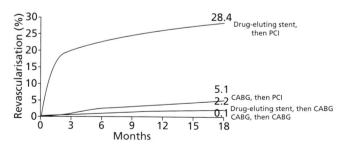

Figure 7.3 Revascularization following coronary artery surgery (CABG) and drug-eluting stenting (PCI). (Reproduced with permission from Hannan et al.[43])

MACE events. A similar increased need for reintervention following revascularization with a coronary stent when compared with bypass surgery was also noted by Serruys' group.[44,45]

Case history 1

The subject, JK, was a 57-year-old Air Traffic Control Officer (ATCO) who developed midsternal discomfort on first effort in cold weather. When guiding aircraft on the approach to London Heathrow airport at times of high traffic density he experienced similar symptoms and sought medical advice. He was normotensive (132/82) but there was a family history of coronary artery disease. He had smoked one pack of cigarettes a day until aged 40 and had a total cholesterol of 7.3 mmol/L. Exercise performance was limited by chest pain with diagnostic electrocardiographic change at 6 minutes 45 seconds of the Bruce treadmill protocol whilst subsequent coronary angiography confirmed the presence of proximal three-vessel coronary artery disease. Although the evidence is not recent, three controlled trials have shown the benefit of surgical revascularization in this context, versus medication, and the excellent outcome and low event rate in "best-risk" subjects[40,46] (**Level A**).

JK underwent quadruple bypass grafting including insertion of the left internal mammary artery into the anterior descending coronary artery. Six months later he was returned to duty having competed 11 minutes of the Bruce protocol without abnormality and having reduced his total cholesterol to 4.1 mmol/l with a statin.

Comment

Would a percutaneous intervention (coronary angioplasty/stenting) have been appropriate if technically feasible? At the preintervention conference it was agreed by the attending cardiologists that the percutaneous (PCI) approach was technically feasible. Inspection of the data, however, suggests that it is difficult to show a benefit both in survival terms as well as for MACE-free survival in this context.[47] In the COURAGE trial[47] which included 2287 subjects, the event rate for patients in the medically treated group was the same as in the angioplasty group over a mean of 4.6 years (the majority of the stents were bare metal). Composite death, myocardial infarction and stroke, together with hospitalization for acute coronary syndrome, was 20.0% in the PCI group and 19.5% in the medically treated group. Additionally, in the PCI group 21.1% had undergone further revascularization over the 4.6-year period (**Level A**). Such rates comfortably exceed the target event rate of 1–2% mortality with associated co-morbid events.

The event rate following stenting makes it less desirable than coronary artery surgery and there seems little reason to revise the earlier view of Webb-Peploe[48] that the procedure should be restricted in the aviation context to the reduction of not more than two lesions which should exclude the proximal left anterior descending and left main vessels (**Class I, Level A**).

Case history 2

The subject, DF, was a 53-year-old Airline Transport Pilot License (ATPL) holder who experienced indigestion-like symptoms whilst on a stopover in Hong Kong. He was asymptomatic on the return flight on which he acted as pilot in command. He sought medical advice when the symptoms recurred 2 weeks later. He was found to have borderline hypertension (156/88) and a total cholesterol of 6.4 mmol/L. He was a non-smoker and non-diabetic. He completed 8.1 minutes of the Bruce exercise protocol before being stopped by chest pain and diagnostic ST-T changes. Coronary angiography demonstrated proximal near obstruction of the right main vessel with non-flow limiting disease (30% stenosis) in the proximal left anterior descending coronary artery. The circumflex system showed early disease only.

As he was symptomatic, the right coronary artery was stented, the hypertension treated with an ACEI and the elevated cholesterol with a statin, both of which have been suggested to have a beneficial pleiotropic effect on atheromatous plaque stability.[38,39] Following a normal pharmacologic stress thallium myocardial perfusion scan (MPI) and an echocardiogram indicating well-preserved left ventricular function, he was assessed fit for multi-crew operation only, subject to annual review with exercise electrocardiography. Although there is no evidence of outcome benefit, either for coronary artery bypass grafting or coronary stenting in this clinical situation, the presence of symptoms and exercise-induced myocardial ischemia justifies the interventional approach, in addition to medication (**Class I, Level C2**). Six months later he was asymptomatic and had undergone a pharmacologic stress thallium MPI.[49,50] He was assessed fit for multi-crew operation subject to annual follow-up with exercise electrocardiography.

Comment

The current UK CAA algorithm for recertification to fly in the context of known coronary artery disease is shown in Figure 7.4 (**Class I**).

Atrial fibrillation

Atrial fibrillation is the most common sustained rhythm disturbance. In the Renfrew/Paisley study, its incidence was 0.4/1000 person-years in subjects aged 45–49 years rising to nearly 2.0/1000 person-years in subjects aged 60–64 years.[51] Twenty-five percent of males >40 years will develop the arrhythmia during their lifetime. Whereas the Renfrew population will not reflect the pilot population, it mirrors the Framingham experience[52] in terms of age-skewed prevalence. In Framingham the prevalence of atrial fibrillation appears to be increasing and was associated

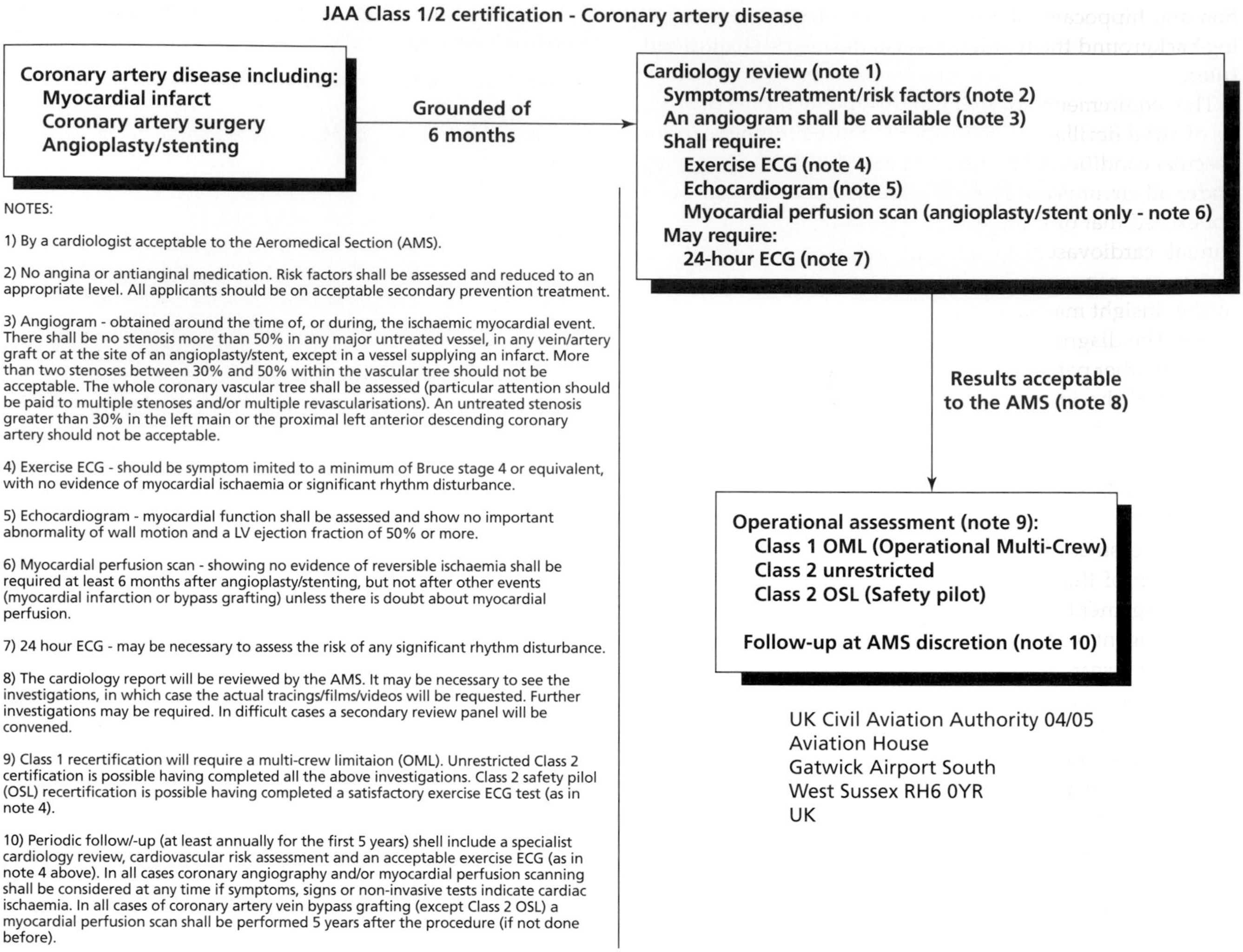

JAA Class 1/2 certification - Coronary artery disease

| Coronary artery disease including:
   Myocardial infarct
   Coronary artery surgery
   Angioplasty/stenting | → Grounded of
6 months → | Cardiology review (note 1)
  Symptoms/treatment/risk factors (note 2)
  An angiogram shall be available (note 3)
  Shall require:
    Exercise ECG (note 4)
    Echocardiogram (note 5)
    Myocardial perfusion scan (angioplasty/stent only - note 6)
  May require:
    24-hour ECG (note 7) |

Results acceptable to the AMS (note 8)

Operational assessment (note 9):
  Class 1 OML (Operational Multi-Crew)
  Class 2 unrestricted
  Class 2 OSL (Safety pilot)

Follow-up at AMS discretion (note 10)

UK Civil Aviation Authority 04/05
Aviation House
Gatwick Airport South
West Sussex RH6 0YR
UK

NOTES:

1) By a cardiologist acceptable to the Aeromedical Section (AMS).

2) No angina or antianginal medication. Risk factors shall be assessed and reduced to an appropriate level. All applicants should be on acceptable secondary prevention treatment.

3) Angiogram - obtained around the time of, or during, the ischaemic myocardial event. There shall be no stenosis more than 50% in any major untreated vessel, in any vein/artery graft or at the site of an angioplasty/stent, except in a vessel supplying an infarct. More than two stenoses between 30% and 50% within the vascular tree should not be acceptable. The whole coronary vascular tree shall be assessed (particular attention should be paid to multiple stenoses and/or multiple revascularisations). An untreated stenosis greater than 30% in the left main or the proximal left anterior descending coronary artery should not be acceptable.

4) Exercise ECG - should be symptom imited to a minimum of Bruce stage 4 or equivalent, with no evidence of myocardial ischaemia or significant rhythm disturbance.

5) Echocardiogram - myocardial function shall be assessed and show no important abnormality of wall motion and a LV ejection fraction of 50% or more.

6) Myocardial perfusion scan - showing no evidence of reversible ischaemia shall be required at least 6 months after angioplasty/stenting, but not after other events (myocardial infarction or bypass grafting) unless there is doubt about myocardial perfusion.

7) 24 hour ECG - may be necessary to assess the risk of any significant rhythm disturbance.

8) The cardiology report will be reviewed by the AMS. It may be necessary to see the investigations, in which case the actual tracings/films/videos will be requested. Further investigations may be required. In difficult cases a secondary review panel will be convened.

9) Class 1 recertification will require a multi-crew limitaion (OML). Unrestricted Class 2 certification is possible having completed all the above investigations. Class 2 safety pilol (OSL) recertification is possible having completed a satisfactory exercise ECG test (as in note 4).

10) Periodic follow/-up (at least annually for the first 5 years) shell include a specialist cardiology review, cardiovascular risk assessment and an acceptable exercise ECG (as in note 4 above). In all cases coronary angiography and/or myocardial perfusion scanning shall be considered at any time if symptoms, signs or non-invasive tests indicate cardiac ischaemia. In all cases of coronary artery vein bypass grafting (except Class 2 OSL) a myocardial perfusion scan shall be performed 5 years after the procedure (if not done before).

Figure 7.4 Algorithm for certification to fly following the diagnosis of coronary artery disease. Important issues are full revascularization and preservation of left ventricular function which powerfully predicts outcome.

with a fivefold increased risk of stroke overall. This and heart failure contributed to the excess mortality observed. In the Euro Heart survey of atrial fibrillation,[53] the mean age of the population was higher than the pilot population (65 +/− 14 years) and two-thirds had hypertension, one-third ischemic heart disease. It also complicated valvular heart disease (rheumatic mitral valve disease increases the risk of cerebral thromboembolism 10-fold), primary muscle disease as well as metabolic and other disorders. In about 25% of the population <65 years the arrhythmia may be "lone" and not associated with any demonstrable abnormality at presentation although genetic predisposition is attracting increasing attention.

Atrial fibrillation may be seen as an isolated self-limiting event in a normal subject following vomiting or alcoholic excess, for example. It may be conveniently divided into isolated (single episode sometimes with provocative cir-

cumstance), paroxysmal (self-terminating), persistent (persisting >1 week and until cardioversion) and permanent (immutable) forms. It may be completely asymptomatic, occasionally symptomatic and/or intolerable. It may cause distraction (subtle incapacitation) or syncope (complete incapacitation). It may be suppressed completely, partially or not at all by medication which may or may not give side effects. The potential for side effects (tremor and persistence of vision) of the class 1C antiarrhythmic agents (e.g. propafenone, flecainide) disbars them as a rule in the aviation but not road transport environment. Finally it is associated with an increased risk of cerebral thromboembolism, the incidence of which increases sharply with age, if hypertension, diabetes, heart failure or structural abnormality is present, or if previous thromboembolism has occurred. Even in the absence of stroke, atrial fibrillation is associated with memory impairment, cognitive dysfunction and hippocampal atrophy.[54,55] Against this unpromising background the regulator has to develop some ground rules.

The requirements for flying status following the diagnosis of atrial fibrillation are similar to those for other cardiovascular conditions. The applicant shall be free of symptoms under all circumstances and the predicted event rate shall not exceed that of the co-morbid event rate reflected by an annual cardiovascular mortality of 1%. Freedom from symptoms can only be determined at consultation but further insight may be obtained by exercise electrocardiography. The diagnosis *per se* does not disbar certification to fly but if other pathology co-exists it is likely to deny fitness in view of the increasing risk of thromboembolic stroke. The long-term outcome is not different whether the subject maintains sinus rhythm with the use of (permitted) therapeutic agents or remains in atrial fibrillation with rate control.[56,57]

The assessment of risk of cerebral thromboembolism and mitigation of the risk of stroke is a central component of the management of atrial fibrillation. The choice of an antiplatelet agent versus anticoagulation with warfarin has been well researched.[58,59] In European aviation, at present, warfarin and similar products such as phenindione are prohibited due to lack of reliability and risk of hemorrhage. In one review, the annual risk of bleeding in subjects receiving warfarin was identified as 0.6% (fatal), 3.0% (major) and 9.6% (minor), about five times the rate expected without warfarin.[60] The risk appears to be highest at the start of treatment, the first month bearing 10 times the risk of that a year later. Significant co-morbidity and age increase the risk whilst tight control of the INR between 2.0 and 3.0 reduces it. Warfarin reduced the thromboembolic risk in non-valvular atrial fibrillation by two-thirds[61] although the risk of cerebrovascular hemorrhage was doubled to 0.46%/annum. In the regulatory environment this risk has to be added to the uncovered stroke risk as well as to associated co-morbidity. A recent overview reports a relative risk reduction of 60% for all stroke (ischemic plus hemorrhagic).[62]

Aspirin is not contraindicated in fliers and its use reduced the risk of stroke by 21% in three trials[63] (**Level A**). The CHADS2 risk graticule was created by assigning one point each for the presence of congestive heart failure, hypertension, age >75 years and diabetes mellitus whilst two points were given for a history of stroke or transient ischemic attack.[64] It has proved superior to other models in the prediction of low and high risk of stroke. The crude annual stroke risk, on no treatment, for CHADS2 grade 0 is 1.2% and 2.8% for CHADS2 grade 1. Assuming the use of aspirin, lowest risk non-valvular atrial fibrillation, whether paroxysmal, persistent or permanent, is acceptable in aviation subject to the ability to fulfill the algorithm in Figure 7.5 (**Class I, Level A**).

Case history 3

The pilot was a normotensive 37-year-old Senior First Officer with no significant past medical history. He was receiving no medication and his alcohol intake was 10 units (8 g)/week. He presented with asymptomatic well-controlled atrial fibrillation at routine examination. His cardiovascular system was otherwise normal. He completed 13 minutes of the Bruce exercise protocol, achieving a maximum instantaneous heart rate of 230 beats/minute. His echocardiogram was normal and ambulatory monitoring revealed no significant other rhythm disturbance. There was no RR interval >3.0 s. As his atrial fibrillation was paroxysmal, he was asymptomatic and his thromboembolic risk judged to be acceptable (i.e. CHADS2 score 0), he was returned to flying. He was treated with aspirin and an OML was imposed to deny single-pilot operating privileges on smaller aircraft. He remained in paroxysmal atrial fibrillation for 4 years but for the last 7 has been in this rhythm permanently. Apart from atrial fibrillation, his resting and exercise electrocardiograms, and echocardiogram have remained normal.

Regulatory orphans and the long QT syndrome

As has been seen above, regulatory medical decision making evolves as the science of medicine moves forward. It must remain ethical and be fully justifiable.[65] The great majority of applicants will have no health issues and satisfy the requirements laid down. Most cardiologic problems are to some extent age related and have sufficient data in the literature for safe and fair fitness recommendations. Certain conditions such as the ion channelopathies are associated with an increased risk of ventricular tachycardia (torsades de pointes), syncope and sudden death (SCD) and are sufficiently newly described for the outcome database to be inadequate for fully informed judgment. In this circumstance either the pilot has to be made unfit (the easy option) or a best evidence view taken which relies to some extent on knowledge of the operational safeguards which exist.

Case history 4

The pilot was a 38-year-old asymptomatic normotensive airline captain who had previously undergone routine electrocardiography without comment having been passed. When he changed his employer, a computer-read recording correctly identified a prolonged QTcB (480 ms) – male normal </= 440 ms (see ECG 1, Fig. 7.6a). He underwent exercise electrocardiography which demonstrated non-sustained slow ventricular tachycardia on recovery (see ECG 2, Fig. 7.6b). A subsequent echocardiogram and magnetic resonance imaging were normal. Two repeat exercise electrocardiograms following treatment with a beta-blocking agent were normal. His 24-hour Holter recording, off treatment, showed no atrial or ventricular ectopic activity. The configuration of the ST segments and T waves, notably in V5 and V6, suggested the long QT2(a) variant.[66]

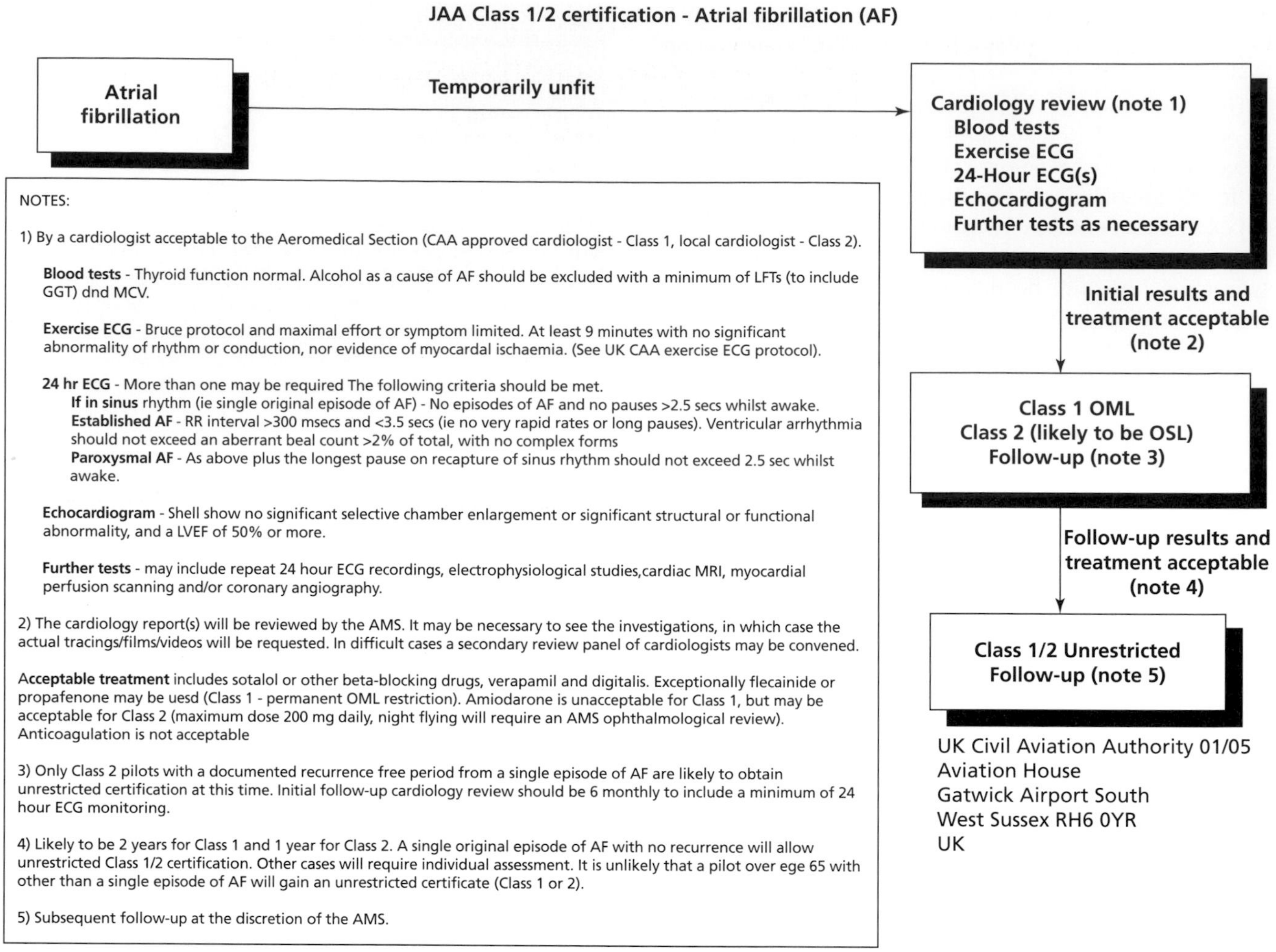

JAA Class 1/2 certification - Atrial fibrillation (AF)

```
┌──────────────┐     Temporarily unfit          ┌─────────────────────────────────┐
│   Atrial     │ ─────────────────────────────► │ Cardiology review (note 1)      │
│ fibrillation │                                │    Blood tests                  │
└──────────────┘                                │    Exercise ECG                 │
                                                │    24-Hour ECG(s)               │
                                                │    Echocardiogram               │
                                                │    Further tests as necessary   │
                                                └─────────────────────────────────┘
                                                              │
                                                  Initial results and
                                                  treatment acceptable
                                                       (note 2)
                                                              ▼
                                                ┌─────────────────────────────────┐
                                                │       Class 1 OML               │
                                                │   Class 2 (likely to be OSL)    │
                                                │      Follow-up (note 3)         │
                                                └─────────────────────────────────┘
                                                              │
                                                  Follow-up results and
                                                  treatment acceptable
                                                       (note 4)
                                                              ▼
                                                ┌─────────────────────────────────┐
                                                │   Class 1/2 Unrestricted        │
                                                │     Follow-up (note 5)          │
                                                └─────────────────────────────────┘
```

NOTES:

1) By a cardiologist acceptable to the Aeromedical Section (CAA approved cardiologist - Class 1, local cardiologist - Class 2).

Blood tests - Thyroid function normal. Alcohol as a cause of AF should be excluded with a minimum of LFTs (to include GGT) dnd MCV.

Exercise ECG - Bruce protocol and maximal effort or symptom limited. At least 9 minutes with no significant abnormality of rhythm or conduction, nor evidence of myocardial ischaemia. (See UK CAA exercise ECG protocol).

24 hr ECG - More than one may be required The following criteria should be met.
If in sinus rhythm (ie single original episode of AF) - No episodes of AF and no pauses >2.5 secs whilst awake.
Established AF - RR interval >300 msecs and <3.5 secs (ie no very rapid rates or long pauses). Ventricular arrhythmia should not exceed an aberrant beal count >2% of total, with no complex forms
Paroxysmal AF - As above plus the longest pause on recapture of sinus rhythm should not exceed 2.5 sec whilst awake.

Echocardiogram - Shell show no significant selective chamber enlargement or significant structural or functional abnormality, and a LVEF of 50% or more.

Further tests - may include repeat 24 hour ECG recordings, electrophysiological studies,cardiac MRI, myocardial perfusion scanning and/or coronary angiography.

2) The cardiology report(s) will be reviewed by the AMS. It may be necessary to see the investigations, in which case the actual tracings/films/videos will be requested. In difficult cases a secondary review panel of cardiologists may be convened.

Acceptable treatment includes sotalol or other beta-blocking drugs, verapamil and digitalis. Exceptionally flecainide or propafenone may be uesd (Class 1 - permanent OML restriction). Amiodarone is unacceptable for Class 1, but may be acceptable for Class 2 (maximum dose 200 mg daily, night flying will require an AMS ophthalmological review). Anticoagulation is not acceptable

3) Only Class 2 pilots with a documented recurrence free period from a single episode of AF are likely to obtain unrestricted certification at this time. Initial follow-up cardiology review should be 6 monthly to include a minimum of 24 hour ECG monitoring.

4) Likely to be 2 years for Class 1 and 1 year for Class 2. A single original episode of AF with no recurrence will allow unrestricted Class 1/2 certification. Other cases will require individual assessment. It is unlikely that a pilot over ege 65 with other than a single episode of AF will gain an unrestricted certificate (Class 1 or 2).

5) Subsequent follow-up at the discretion of the AMS.

UK Civil Aviation Authority 01/05
Aviation House
Gatwick Airport South
West Sussex RH6 0YR
UK

Figure 7.5 Algorithm for certification to fly following the diagnosis of atrial fibrillation. Only subjects with "lone" atrial fibrillation (no structural abnormality of the heart, no history of hypertension or diabetes and no metabolic cause) can be considered and then only if asymptomatic. The disturbance may be paroxysmal, persistent or permanent (see text). These are updated from time to time and reference needs to be made to the CAA website (Class I).

Comment

Over 300 mutations on seven genes (LQT1–7) have been described. Transmitted as autosomal dominant genes, all involve fast and slow activating delayed potassium repolarizing currents with the exception of the LQT3 which involves the SCN5A sodium encoding gene shared by the Brugada syndrome.[67] All are characterized by risk of ventricular tachycardia, syncope, cardiac arrest and sudden death. Data are incomplete and although the highest event rate seems to occur before adulthood,[68,69] the natural history of the condition remains to be fully characterized, particularly in later years. A recent review of some 18 500 UK Class certificate holders over a 10-year period revealed exactly 100 males in whom the QTcB exceeded the upper limit of normal (440 ms). All were asymptomatic and in only five the QTcB excoeded 480 ms. All were, and have remained, asymptomatic. All except one, an ATCO, retained their licenses, most with an OML endorsement.[70]

There are differences in presentation, LQT1 tending to occur with exercise, LQT2 with sudden arousal such as noise, and LQT3 at rest. There are also differences in response to treatment as the LQT2 variant may obtain less benefit from beta-blockade.[71] Ventricular tachycardia and aborted sudden death justify an implantable defibrillator. Excessive prolongation of the QTc (>500 ms) predicts events in LQT1 and 2 but not LQT3[68] and the locus of the mutation is also predictive.[71] The overall event rate is higher in LQT1 and 2 but the lethality of an event is higher in LQT3.[68,72] In due time, it is likely that genomic profiling of the individual will enable risk profiling with more confidence.

On an *ad hominem* basis, the regulatory issue is to balance the safety advantage of maintaining the flying status of a 10 000 hour pilot with the risk of an adverse cardiac event.

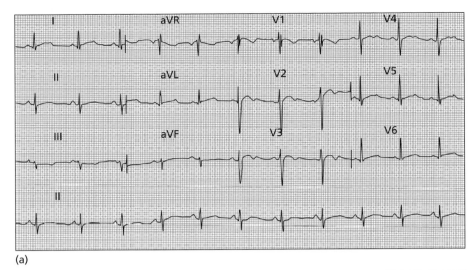

(a)

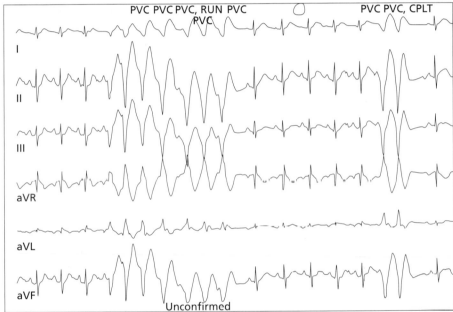

(b)

Figure 7.6 (a) The resting electrocardiogram of a 38-year-old airline captain with the LQT2 pattern and a QTcB of 480 ms. (b) Same patient: immediate postexercise non-sustained ventricular tachycardia.

Any prodromal event would deny certification, as would any subsequent event. Priori et al[68] suggested that the incidence of first cardiac arrest/sudden death <40 years in LQT2(a), before therapy. is 0.46%/year although the risk is not linear and data beyond 40 years are scant. This may be expressed as risk/hour – 0.00525% and for any arbitrary 6 minutes of flight criticality (i.e. during take off and landing),[26] 0.000525%. In the general population the annual incidence of sudden death in the age range 20–75 years is 0.1%/annum – 0.0011%/hour[73] but this will be age skewed and whatever additional burden the LQT proband carries, he/she will bear a cumulative additional age-related risk from coronary artery disease, for example. This additional increase in relative risk is not acceptable for an operational situation where the sole co-pilot could be inexperienced.

However, in certain long-haul operations, a third (sometimes a fourth) pilot is carried which would all but abolish the operational risk but for a very limited period. The regulatory authority was advised to consider the possibility of a limitation to heavy crew operation only, with an upper age cut-off, in the absence of further evidence of any event, of 60 years (**Class I, Level C2**).

Conclusion

The interface between evidence-based medicine and the regulatory environment reflects some of the most interesting and challenging problems in cardiology. Before regulation was based on scientific principles, fitness determination was arbitrary with implications both for safety and for the prosperity and well-being of the professional groups involved. Progress in cardiology should be matched by improved and enlightened attitudes to certification.

Note

Some of the material in this chapter relates to legally based requirements for medical fitness in the transportation industries. The statements and opinions are those of the author and have no regulatory standing. Those requiring further guidance should consult the relevant authority. The UK CAA algorithms (reproduced with permission) are regularly updated and are available at the web address provided at the end of the chapter.

References

1. *ICAO Annex 1 Personnel Licensing*, 10th edn. Montreal: ICAO, 2006. http://www.icao.int/icao/en/med/
2. *At a Glance Guide to the Current Medical Standards of Fitness to Drive*. http://www.dvla.gov.uk/media/pdf/medical/aagv1.pdf
3. European Parliament Fact Sheets 4.5.4. Road traffic and safety provisions. http://www.europarl.europa.eu/facts/4_5_4_en.ht
4. Joy M. Cardiovascular fitness to fly and to drive: an interface between cardiology and some statutory fitness requirements. In: Julian DG, Camm AJ, Fox KM, Hall RJC, Poole-Wilson PA, eds. *Diseases of the Heart*. London: Baillière Tindall, 1989;1574–606.
5. *Joint Aviation Requirements. JAR FCL part 3 Medical*. Hoofddorp: Joint Aviation Authorities; 1998. http://www.jaat.eu/licensing/licensing_jars.html
6. Joy M, Bennett G, eds. The First United Kingdom Workshop in Aviation Cardiology. *Eur Heart J* 1984;**5**(suppl A):1–164.
7. Joy M, Bennett G, eds. The Second UK Workshop in Aviation Cardiology. *Eur Heart J* 1988;**9**(suppl G):1–179.
8. Joy M, ed. The First European Workshop in Aviation Cardiology. *Eur Heart J* 1992;**13**(suppl H):1–175.
9. Joy M, ed. The Second European Workshop in Aviation Cardiology. *Eur Heart J* 1999;**1**(suppl D):D1–D131.
10. http://www.caa.co.uk/default.aspx?catid=620
11. DeJohn CA, Wolbrink AM, Larcher JG. *In-Flight Medical Incapacitation and Impairment of U.S. Airline Pilots: 1993 to 1998*. Washington, DC: Office of Aerospace Medicine, 2004.
12. Buley L. Incidence, causes and results of airline pilot incapacitation while on duty. *Aerospace Med* 1969;**40**:64–70.
13. Orlady H, Orlady LM. *Human Factors in Multi-Crew Flight Operations*. London: Ashgate, 1999.
14. Civil Aviation Authority. *World Airline Accident Summary*. CAP 479. Cheltenham: CAA, 1986.
15. Accidents Investigation Branch: Department of Trade and Industry. *Trident 1 G-ARPI. Report of the public enquiry into the causes and circumstances of the accident near Staines on 18 June 1972*. London: HMSO, 1973.
16. Eighth Bethesda Conference of the American College of Cardiology. Cardiovascular problems associated with aviation safety. *Am J Cardiol* 1975;**36**:573–620.
17. Cardiology Committee of the Royal College of Physicians of London. Cardiovascular fitness of airline pilots. *Br Heart J* 1978;**40**:335–50.
18. Sackett DL, Straus S, Richardson SR, Rosenberg W, Haynes RB. *Evidence-Based Medicine: how to Practice and Teach EBM*, 2nd edn. London: Churchill Livingstone, 2000.
19. Devereaux PJ, Haynes RB, Yusuf S. What is evidence based cardiology? In: Yusuf S, Cairns J, Camm J *et al*, eds. *Evidence-Based Cardiology*, 2nd edn. London: BMJ Books, 2003.
20. Hammermeister K, Sethi GK, Henderson WG *et al*. Outcomes 15 years after valve replacement with a mechanical versus bioprosthetic valve: final report of the Veterans Affairs Randomised Trial. *J Am Coll Cardiol* 2000;**32**:1152–58.
21. ESC. Guidelines on the management of valvular heart disease. *Eur Heart J* 2007; **28**: 230–68.
22. Tunstall-Pedoe H. Cardiovascular risk and risk factors in the context of aircrew certification. *Eur Heart J* 1992;**13**(suppl H):16–20.
23. Tunstall-Pedoe H. Acceptable cardiovascular risk in aircrew: introduction. *Eur Heart J* 1988;**9**(suppl G):9–11.
24. Accidents Investigation Branch: Department of Trade and Industry. *Piper PA-31–350 Navajo Chieftain G-BBJG. Report on the accident near Horsforth near Leeds Yorkshire on 6 December 1974*. London: HMSO, 1975.
25. AAIB Bulletin No. 1/2001. Ref: EW/200/6/5 – Category: 1.2. Farnborough: AAIB, 2001.
26. Mitchell SJ, Evans AD. Flight safety medical incapacitation risk of airline Pilots. *Aviat Space Environ Med* 2004;**75**:260–8.
27. Unal B, Critchley JA, Capewell S. Explaining the decline in coronary heart disease mortality in England and Wales between 1981 and 2000. *Circulation* 2004;**109**:1101–7.
28. http://www.heartstats.org/datapage.asp?id=722
29. Tyler A. How actuaries and underwriters look at risk. *Eur Heart J* 1988;**9**(suppl G):31–5.
30. Tunstall-Pedoe H. How cardiovascular risk varies with age, sex and coronary risk factors: do standard risk scores give an accurate perspective? *Eur Heart J* 1999;**1**(suppl D):D25–D31.
31. Joy M. Aviation cardiology. In: Ernsting J, Rainford DJ, eds. *A Textbook of Aviation Medicine*, 4th edn. London: Butterworth Heinemann, 2006.
32. United States Federal Aviation Administration. Report DOT/FAA/AM-95/5. Washington, DC: United States Federal Aviation Administration, 1995.
33. Irvine D, Davies DM. The mortality of British Airways pilots 1966–1989. *J Aviat Space Environ Med* 1992;**62**:276–9.
34. Kaji M, Tango T, Asukata I *et al*. Mortality experience of cockpit crew members from Japan Airlines. *J Aviat Space Environ Med* 1993;**63**:748–50.
35. Fourth Joint Task Force of the European Society of Cardiology and Other Societies on Cardiovascular Disease Prevention in Clinical Practice. European guidelines on cardiovascular disease prevention in clinical practice: executive summary. *Eur Heart J* doi:10.1093/eurheartj/ehm316
36. Fourth Joint Task Force of the European Society of Cardiology and Other Societies on Cardiovascular Disease Prevention in Clinical Practice. European guidelines on cardiovascular disease prevention in clinical practice. *Eur Heart J* 2007;**4**(suppl 2),
37. European Aviation Safety Agency. Notice of Proposed Amendment (NPA) No 200817c. AMCA to MED.B.005 Cardiovascular System. Cologne: European Aviation Safety Agency, 2008.

38. LaRosa JC. At the heart of the statin benefit. *J Am Col Cardiol* 2005;**46**:1863.

39. Koh KK, Quon MJ, Han SH *et al*. Vascular and metabolic effects of combined therapy with ramipril and simvastatin in patients with type 2 diabetes. *Hypertension* 2005;**45**:1088–93.

40. Chaitman BK, Davis KB, Dodge HT *et al*. Should airline pilots be eligible to resume flight status after coronary artery bypass surgery? A CASS registry study. *J Am Coll Cardiol* 1986;**8**:1318–24.

41. Bakhai A, Hill RA, Dundar Y, Dickson RC, Walley T. Percutaneous transluminal coronary angioplasty with stents versus coronary artery bypass grafting for people with stable angina or acute coronary syndromes. *Cochrane Database of Systematic Reviews* 2005, Issue 1. Art. No.: CD004588. DOI: 10.1002/14651858. CD004588.pub3.

42. Mendiz O, Thomas MR, Ahmed WH, Roy K, Mascioli S, OLYMPIA Investigators. *Eur Heart J* 2008;**29**(abstract supplement):517.

43. Hannan EL, Wu C, Walford G *et al*. Drug-eluting stents vs. coronary-artery bypass grafting in multivessel coronary disease. *N Engl J Med* 2008;**358**:331–41.

44. Serruys PW, Unger F, Sousa JE *et al*. Comparison of coronary-artery bypass surgery and stenting for the treatment of multivessel disease. *N Engl J Med* 2001;**344**:1117–24.

45. Serruys PW, Kutryk MJB, Ong ATL. Coronary artery stents. *N Engl J Med* 2006;**354**:483–95.

46. ACC/AHA. 2002 *Guideline Update for the Management of Patients with Chronic Stable Angina*. www.acc.org

47. Boden WE, O'Rourke RA, Teo KK *et al*. Optimal medical therapy with or without PCI for stable coronary disease. *N Engl J Med* 2007;**356**:1503–16.

48. Webb-Peploe MM. Late outcome following PTCA or coronary stenting: implications for certification to fly. *Eur Heart J* 1999;(suppl D):D67–77.

49. Hachamovitch R, Hayes S, Friedman JD *et al*. Determinants of risk and its temporal variation in patients with normal stress myocardial perfusion scans – what is the warranty period of a normal scan? *J Am Coll Cardiol* 2003;**41**:1329–40.

50. Iskandrian AS, Chae SC, Heo J, Stanberry CD, Wasserleben V, Cave V. Independent and incremental prognostic value of exercise single photon computed tomographic (SPECT) thallium imaging in coronary artery disease. *J Am Coll Cardiol* 1993;**22**:665–70.

51. Stewart S, Hart CL, Hole DJ *et al*. Population prevalence, incidence, and predictors of atrial fibrillation in the Renfrew/Paisley study. *Heart* 2001;**86**:516–21.

52. Kannel WB, Wolf PA, Benjamin EJ, Levy D. Prevalence, incidence, prognosis, and predisposing conditions for atrial fibrillation: population-based estimates. *Am J Cardiol* 1998;**82**:2N–9N.

53. Nieuwlaat R, Capucci A, Camm AJ *et al*. Atrial fibrillation management: a prospective survey in ESC member countries. Euro Heart Survey on Atrial Fibrillation. *Eur Heart J* 2005;**26**:2422–34.

54. Goette A, Braun-Dallaeus RC. Atrial fibrillation is associated with impaired cognitive function and hippocampal atrophy: silent cerebral ischaemia vs Alzheimers disease. *Eur Heart J* 2008;**29**:2067–9.

55. Knecht C, Oelschlager C, Duning T *et al*. Atrial fibrillation in stroke-free patients is associated with memory impairment and hippocampal atrophy.

56. Van Gelder IC, Hagens VE, Bosker HA *et al*. A comparison of rate control and rhythm control in patients with recurrent persistent atrial fibrillation. *N Engl J Med* 2002;**347**:1834–40.

57. Atrial Fibrillation Follow-up Investigation of Rhythm Management (AFFIRM) Investigators. A comparison of rate control and rhythm control in patients with atrial fibrillation. *N Engl J Med* 2002;**347**:1825–33.

58. Segal JB, McNamara R, Miller M, Powe N, Goodman SN, Robinson KA, Bass EB. Anticoagulants or antiplatelet therapy for non-rheumatic atrial fibrillation and flutter. *Cochrane Database of Systematic Reviews* 2006, Issue 3. Art. No.: CD001938. DOI: 10.1002/14651858.CD001938.pub2.

59. Gage BF, van Walraven C, Pearce L *et al*. Selecting patients with atrial fibrillation for anticoagulation. Stroke risk stratification in patients taking aspirin. *Circulation* 2004;**110**:2287–92.

60. Landefeld CS, Beyth RJ. Anticoagulant-related bleeding: clinical epidemiology, prediction, and prevention. *Am J Med* 1993;**95**: 315–28.

61. G AS, Hylek EM, Chang Y *et al*. Anticoagulation therapy for stroke prevention in atrial fibrillation. How well do randomised trials translate into clinical practice? *JAMA* 2003;**290**: 2685–92.

62. Hart RG, Pearce LA, Aguilare MI. Meta-analysis: antithrombotic therapy to prevent stroke in patients who have nonvalvular atrial fibrillation. *Ann Intern Med* 2007;**146**:857–67.

63. Laupacis A, Boysen G, Connolly S *et al*. The efficacy of aspirin in patients with atrial fibrillation: analysis of pooled data from 3 randomized trials. *Arch Intern Med* 1997;**157**:1237–40.

64. Gage BF, Waterman AD, Shannon W *et al*. Validation of clinical classification schemes for predicting stroke: results from the National Registry of Atrial Fibrillation. *JAMA* 2001;**285**: 2864–70.

65. Epstein AE, Miles WM, Benditt DG *et al*. Personal and public safety issues related to arrhythmias that may affect consciousness: implications for regulation and physician recommendations. A medical/scientific statement from the American Heart Association and the North American Society of Pacing and Electrophysiology. *Circulation* 1996;**94**:1147–66.

66. Zhang L, Timothy KW, Vincent M *et al*. Spectrum of ST-T wave patterns and repolarisation parameters in congenital long QT syndrome. *Circulation* 2000;**102**:2849–55.

67. Moss AJ, Kass RS. Long QT syndrome: from channels to cardiac arrhythmias. *J Clin Invest* 2005;**115**:2018–24.

68. Priori SG, Schwartz PJ, Napolitano C *et al*. Risk stratification in the long-QT syndrome. *N Engl J Med* 2003;**348**:1866–74.

69. Roden DM. Long-QT syndrome. *N Engl J Med* 2008;**358**:169–76.

70. Joy M. Certificatory aspects of the long QT syndrome (LQTS): a 10 year perspective. *Aviat Space Environ Med* 2004;**75**(suppl 1):C14–15.

71. Priori SG, Napolitano C, Schwartz PJ *et al*. Association of long QT syndrome loci and cardiac events among patients treated with beta-blockers. *JAMA* 2004;**292**:1341–4.

72. Zareba W, Moss AJ, Schwartz PJ *et al*. Influence of the genotype on the clinical course of the long-QT syndrome. *N Engl J Med* 1998;**339**:960–5.

73. Priori SG, Aliot E, Blomstrom-Lundqvist C *et al*. Task Force on Sudden Cardiac Death of the European Society of Cardiology. *Eur Heart J* 2001;**22**:1374–450.

Prevention of cardiovascular diseases

Salim Yusuf and John A Cairns, Editors

8 Global perspective on cardiovascular disease

K Srinath Reddy

All India Institute of Medical Sciences, New Dehli, India

Introduction

In the second half of the 20th century, cardiovascular diseases (CVD) became the dominant cause of global mortality and a major contributor to disease-related disability. At the beginning of the 21st century, this pattern has become even more pervasive as the CVD epidemic accelerates in many developing regions of the world, even as it retains its primacy as the leading public health problem in the developed regions.[1–9]

An estimated 17.5 million people died from cardiovascular diseases in 2005, representing 30% of all global deaths. Of these deaths, an estimated 7.6 million were due to coronary heart disease and 5.7 million were due to stroke. Over 80% of cardiovascular deaths took place in low- and middle-income countries and occurred equally in men and women.[1] The low- and middle-income countries contributed 83.8% of all CVD deaths and 88.5% of disability-adjusted life-years (DALY) loss attributed to CVD that year.

Around 9 million stroke cases were reported to occur in 2004. Large geographic differences exist in the burden of stroke as well as its case fatality rates globally. There is an increasing trend in the incidence of stroke in developing countries as opposed to the decreasing or stabilizing trend in developed countries. While coronary heart disease (CHD) was the dominant form of CVD in the developed countries, Latin America and India, stroke was the leading cause of cardiovascular deaths in sub-Saharan Africa and China. Epidemiologic studies in developing countries provide evidence that stroke mortality rates tend to be higher than coronary heart disease rates, and may be considerably higher than in developed countries.[1,2] In 2004, low- and middle-income countries contributed to 86.7% of global deaths due to cerebrovascular diseases. Hypertension and diabetes are more widely prevalent in stroke patients in developing countries as compared to developed countries.[3]

The rise and recent decline of the CVD epidemic in the developed countries have been well documented.[9–12] The identification of major risk factors through population-based studies and effective control strategies combining community education and targeted management of high-risk individuals have together contributed to the fall in CVD mortality rates (inclusive of coronary and stroke deaths) that has been observed in almost all industrialized countries. It has been estimated that, during the period 1965–90, CVD related mortality fell by 50% or so in Australia, Canada, France and the United States and by 60% in Japan.[8] Other parts of Western Europe reported more modest declines (20–25%).[9] The decline in stroke mortality has been more marked compared to the decline in coronary mortality. In the United States, the decline in stroke mortality commenced nearly two decades earlier than the decline in coronary mortality and maintained a sharper rate of decline.[11] During the period 1979–89, the age-adjusted mortality from stroke declined, in that country, by about one-third while the corresponding decline in coronary mortality was 22%.[11] In Canada, Japan, Switzerland and the United States, stroke mortality has declined by more than 50% in men and women aged 65–74 years since the 1970s.[12] In Japan, where stroke mortality outweighs coronary mortality, the impressive overall decline in CVD mortality is principally contributed by the former.

However, recent trends in some of the developed countries have provoked some concern. A flattening of age-adjusted mortality rates for major cardiovascular diseases in the USA has been reported since 1990, with an especially well-documented absence of a decline in stroke mortality since that year. This has been accompanied by an increase in mortality from congestive heart failure. Lack of decline in incidence of CHD and stroke, fall in the rate of decrease in cardiovascular risk factor levels and rising levels of obesity since 1990 have all been incriminated as factors

Evidence-Based Cardiology, 3rd edition. Edited by S. Yusuf, J.A. Cairns, A.J. Camm, E.L. Fallen, and B.J. Gersh. © 2010 Blackwell Publishing, ISBN: 978-1-4051-5925-8.

responsible for such a plateau effect on CVD mortality rates in USA over the past decade.[13]

Within Europe, there is a considerable variation in cardiovascular and all-cause mortality on both a national and a regional level. Mortality from both CHD and CVD has continuously been decreasing in most Western European countries over the last three decades. In most Central and Eastern European countries, on the other hand, cardiovascular mortality increased during the 1970s and 1980s and started to decline or stabilize in the early to mid-1990s. Despite the recent decrease, rates are considerably higher in most Central and Eastern European countries. With regard to cerebrovascular mortality rates, a different pattern is observed. Cerebrovascular mortality is reduced in the center of Western Europe, with the lowest national mortality rates in Switzerland, France, Norway, Spain, The Netherlands and Italy. Countries and regions with higher mortality rates surround this circle of reduced mortality such as the Central and East European Countries as well as some Mediterranean countries including Greece, Portugal and certain regions of Southern Spain and Italy.[14]

CHD, previously considered rare in sub-Saharan Africa, now ranks eighth among the leading causes of death in men and women. A wide variety of studies from Ethiopia, Ghana, Kenya, Nigeria, Tanzania and Zaire suggest that the incidence and prevalence of CVD is increasing, especially in urban and semi-urban areas.[15] This is the result of adverse behavioral and lifestyle changes associated with urbanization and epidemiologic transition.

Developing countries like China and India have experienced an epidemiologic transition in a much shorter time than many countries. Mortality analysis of China shows that deaths due to chronic diseases have increased as a proportion of all deaths, from 41.7% in 1973 to 74.1% in 2005, with CVD being a major contributor. China already has 177 million adults with hypertension.[16] An increasingly larger number are at risk of cardiovascular diseases because of smoking, dietary changes and reduced physical activity. In India, too, cardiovascular disease is now the leading cause of death, accounting for 29% of all deaths in 2005. The risk factors are also on the rise, as evidenced by a number of community surveys in different regions of the country. India is presently home to 40 million persons with diabetes and 118 million hypertensive individuals. These are projected to increase even further by 2025.[17]

Rheumatic heart disease (RHD) continues to be a burden in developing countries, although there is an overall decline in the incidence and deaths resulting from RHD. Of 12 million people currently affected by rheumatic fever and RHD, two-thirds are children between 5 and 15 years of age. There are around 300 000 deaths each year with 2 million people requiring repeated hospitalization and 1 million likely to require surgery in the next 5–20 years.[18]

Early age of CVD deaths in developing countries

Although the present high burden of CVD deaths is itself a reason for attention, a greater cause of concern is the early age of CVD deaths in developing countries compared to developed countries. Globally, more than 38% of CVD deaths occurred below the age of 70 years in 2002. Deaths from cardiovascular diseases in people younger than 70 years accounted for 21% of all deaths.[19] Age-specific CVD mortality rates for those between 35 and 64 years have increased many-fold between 1984 and 2002 in less developed countries. This kind of concentration of CVD deaths among people of working age (35–64 years) is not seen in industrialized nations. In India, China, Russia and Brazil, 30–40% of the CVD deaths occur in people of working age. The Philippines has over 50% of its CVD deaths in this age group, 8–10 times higher than the Western experience.[20]

South Asians have a greater prevalence of coronary risk factors than the rest of the world, and coronary artery disease often manifests at an early age.[21] Asians tend to have slimmer body build than Westerners, with less muscle mass and connective tissue than stockier subjects.[22] Further, Asian populations have a different fat distribution pattern from the Western population and are more prone to central obesity, even at low BMI levels.[23] Such considerations raise the possibility that the risks associated with adiposity at lower levels of BMI are greater in Asian population.

Epidemiologic transition and the evolution of the CVD epidemic

What is the "transition"?

The health status and dominant disease profile of human societies have been historically linked to the level of their economic development and social organization at any given stage. The shift from nutritional deficiencies and infectious diseases, as the major causes of death and disability, to degenerative disorders (chronic diseases like CVD, cancer, diabetes) has marked the economic ascent of nations as they industrialized. This shift has been called the epidemiologic transition.

The economic and social changes that propel this transition are related to a rise in per capita income, greater investments in public sanitation, housing and healthcare, assured availability of adequate nutrition and technologic advances in medical care. Life expectancy rises as causes of childhood and early adult mortality decline. This, in turn, leads to a decline in fertility. The age profile of the population changes from a pyramidal distribution dominated by the young to a columnar structure where adults and the elderly progressively expand their numbers. This has been described as the demographic transition. Since the disease profile is also linked to the age profile of the population, the health transition encompasses the effects of the epidemiologic and demographic transitions.

CVD profile at different stages of the epidemiologic transition

The model of epidemiologic transition originally described by Omran,[24] with three phases (the age of pestilence and famine, the age of receding pandemics;,the age of degenerative and man-made diseases), was later modified to include a fourth phase (the age of delayed degenerative diseases).[25] Life expectancy progressively increases from around 30 years in the first phase to over 70 years in the fourth phase. The shift to a dominant chronic disease profile occurs in the third phase. As the average life expectancy exceeds 50–55 years, the proportionate mortality due to CVD begins to exceed that of infectious diseases.[26]

The transition not only occurs between the broad disease categories but also within them. The disease profile within CVD alters at each phase of the epidemiologic transition. In the first phase (the age of pestilence and famine), CVD accounts for 5–10% of deaths.[26] The major causes of CVD are, however, related to infectious and nutritional deficiencies. Thus, RHD and cardiomyopathies (e.g. Chagas' disease) are the main CVD in this phase. Even as countries emerge from this phase, the residual burden of chronic valvular heart disease and congestive heart failure often remains for some period. These effects are still evident in sub-Saharan Africa and parts of South America and South Asia.[26]

In the second phase (the age of receding pandemics), the decline in infectious disease which accompanies socio-economic development ushers in changes in diet. As the subsistence nutrition changes to more complete diets, the salt content of the food increases. Hypertension and its sequelae (hypertensive heart disease and hemorrhagic stroke) now affect the population whose average age also has risen with increased life expectancy. Some residual burden of RHD and cardiomyopathies is also evident. These non-atherosclerotic diseases contribute to 10–35% of deaths. This pattern currently prevails in parts of Africa, North Asia, and South America.[26]

In the third phase (the age of degenerative and man-made disease), accelerated economic development and increased per capita incomes promote lifestyle changes in diet, physical activity, stress, and addictions. A diet rich in calories, saturated fat and salt is accompanied by reduced physical activity through increased use of mechanized transport and sedentary leisure time pursuits. The metabolic mismatch leads to obesity, increased blood lipids, diabetes, and elevated blood pressure. Tobacco consumption, especially cigarette smoking, starts as a pleasurable

pastime and turns into a severe addiction. These factors result in the onset of clinically manifest atherosclerotic vascular disease (CHD, atherosclerotic stroke, and peripheral vascular disease) at around 55 years of age. Such patterns first occur in the upper socio-economic classes who have disposable income to expend on rich diets, tobacco and transport vehicles. Several countries in South America and Asia currently manifest this pattern. As the epidemic advances further and involves all social strata, with homogenization of risk behaviors and risk factors across the population, the death toll of CVD rises to range between 35% and 65% of all deaths. This scenario is currently observed in Eastern Europe.

In the fourth phase (the phase of delayed degenerative disease), a number of changes occur in the society to modify risk behaviors and reduce risk factor levels in the population. Health research augments the knowledge of CVD risk factors. The desire to reduce the adverse impact of CVD on individuals as well as on society steers the community as well as the policymakers to apply this knowledge for disease prevention and health promotion. Community awareness through education, as well as its ability to exercise healthy choices through supportive regulatory measures, empowers its members to adopt healthier lifestyles. Saturated fat and salt consumption declines and leisure-time physical activity and exercise programs are avidly pursued. With concerns over the effects of active and passive smoking, tobacco consumption falls. Simultaneously, medical research makes available new technologies which are very effective in saving lives, modifying the course of disease, and reducing the levels of risk factors. All of these changes, in unison, delay the onset of disease, lower the age-standardized mortality rates and reduce the disability. The contribution of CVD to total mortality falls to 50% or below. These patterns are now established in most of North America, Western Europe, and New Zealand.[26]

Recent developments in some countries of Eastern Europe, with sharp declines in life expectancy and other health indices, led to a fifth phase of health transition being postulated.[7] In this stage of "social upheaval and health regression", the CVD spectrum too may witness a reversal with CHD and stroke occurring at younger ages, resulting in a fall in life expectancy, as in Russia. Further transition may also occur in the future, due to health impacts of global climate change and environmental degradation which can profoundly influence both infectious diseases and chronic diseases.

Variations in the transition

There are, however, variations on this theme. Even within Europe, for example, there is still a clear north-east to south-west gradient in mortality from CHD. With regard to the east–west gradient, dietary fat intake appears to play a major role. In Eastern Europe, higher consumption of saturated fat was reported during the 1980s and early 1990s. In Poland, changes in the dietary fat intake during the 1990s, leading to a more favorable ratio of polyunsaturated to saturated fat, were associated with a drop in mortality from CHD by approximately one-quarter. The attribution of single risk factors to regional variation may also vary depending on geographic location of the area of interest. For example, regional differences between Israel, Germany and Greece were found to be associated particularly with differences in blood pressure levels.[14]

The results of the Sino-MONICA study (1987–93) in China have shown large differences in the occurrence of coronary and stroke events, with higher rates in northern provinces and lower rates in southern provinces. This geographic difference in CVD mortality and incidence reflects underlying differentials in risk factor profiles (like hypertension and cholesterol levels).[27,28] Prevalence of CHD in the Japanese population remains lower than that in the US and other Western populations. However, lifestyle changes in recent decades have been accompanied by the increasing prevalence of hypercholesterolemia and diabetes, and recent data indicate an increase in prevalence of CHD.[29] The prevalence of lipid risk factors in younger Japanese people is now similar to that in the US.

The question of "arrested epidemiologic transition" is also raised with respect to some of the developing countries. If poverty continues to be a major problem for them, will they experience the CVD epidemic in its full fury or will the pre-transitional diseases of nutrition and infection continue to occupy the center stage? Even now, there is evidence that the social gradient has begun to reverse for risk factor levels and even for morbidity measures in some populations in the developing world.[5] Unless economic development is greatly stunted in some countries, it is likely that the model of epidemiologic transition will be applicable to most of the developing world.

The transition to the atherothrombotic phase of the epidemic may be preceded by a sharp fall in the burden of hemorrhagic strokes. The recent decline in CVD mortality reported from South Korea reflects such a fall in the contribution from hemorrhagic strokes, while thrombotic stroke and coronary heart disease burdens have just begun to rise.[30] The model of "health transition", while very useful, is not immutable and is likely to vary according to both levels of development and the nature of public health responses to social transition.

The model of health transition should also not lead to complacency regarding the high absolute burdens and early deaths in the developing countries. For example, even in a country in "early transition" like Tanzania, the stroke mortality rates in the age group of 15–59 years in rural and urban areas are 2–4 times higher than those in UK, in a similar age group.[31]

Early and late adopters

The pace of epidemiologic transition will vary both among countries and within countries. Usually lifestyle changes towards risk-prone behaviors occur first in the higher socio-economic groups and urban communities for whom the innovations of modernity are more easily accessible and affordable. As these innovations diffuse and become routinely available at prices amenable to mass consumption, the poorer sections and rural communities also join the CVD bandwagon. Soon the awareness of CVD risks as well as the economic independence to make healthy lifestyle choices in relation to diet and leisure time exercise (along with the greater ability to access healthcare) moves the "early adopters" in the affluent and urban strata into a reduced risk zone. The burden of CVD then is largely concentrated in the lower socio-economic groups and rural populations who continue to practice high-risk behaviors and display elevated risk factor levels.[24] These "late adopter" groups also will slowly alter their behaviors, lower their levels of risk and reduce their burden of CVD, as healthcare responses to the CVD epidemic become universally effective. The progressive reversal of CVD risk factors with increasing levels of urbanization is now evident in India.[32]

This is the evolutionary profile of the CVD epidemic, as evident from the analysis of mature epidemics in industrial nations and the advancing epidemics in the developing countries. Differences within countries and between countries, suggested by cross-sectional views at any point in this evolution, should not obscure the longitudinal perspective of an evolving epidemic in which most countries will traverse similar paths, albeit at different times determined by their pace of development. Global shifts in CVD risk factors and their reflection in global CVD trends indicate that all countries and communities have far more in common in terms of disease causation than the differences which demarcate them. The challenge of epidemiologic transition is not whether it will happen in the developing countries, but whether we can apply the available knowledge to telescope the transition and abbreviate phase three of the model in these countries.

Projections

The Global Burden of Diseases study estimates that annual mortality from non-communicable diseases will rise from an estimated 28.1 million deaths in 1990 to 49.7 million in 2020.[7] CVD, which accounts for a large proportion of these, will rise as a result of the accelerating epidemic in the developing countries. CHD will continue to be the leading cause of death in the world and, in terms of DALY lost, will rise from its fifth position in 1990 to top the DALY table in

Table 8.1 Global % change in CHD and stroke mortality 1990–2020

	CHD		Stroke	
	Men	**Women**	**Men**	**Women**
Developed countries	48	29	56	28
Developing countries	137	127	124	107
World	100	80	106	78

Adapted from Murray and Lopez.[4]

Table 8.2 Contribution of cardiovascular disease to DALY loss (percentage of total)

Region	**1990**	**2020**
World	10.85%	14.7%
Developed countries	25.7%	22.0%
Developing countries	8.9%	13.8%

Adapted from Murray and Lopez.[4]

2020.[7] Men as well as women in the developing countries will experience the largest rise in CHD and stroke mortality rates across the world (Table 8.1).

The profile of DALY loss attributable to CVD in 1990 in various regions of the world and the projected estimates for 2020 (Table 8.2) also indicate a large rise.[4] Among the developed countries, the sharp decline in the industrial nations is partly offset by the rise in the former socialist countries.

Deaths attributable to tobacco, a risk factor for CVD and other chronic diseases, are projected to rise from 3.0 million in 1990 to 8.4 million in 2020. The largest increases will be in India, China and other developing countries in Asia, where tobacco-attributable deaths will rise from 1.1 million to 4.2 million in 2020.[33]

These projections have been updated on the basis of substantial improvements in data availability and methods for dealing with incomplete and biased data (Table 8.3). According to the revised model, age-specific death rates for most chronic diseases are projected to decrease slightly at rates of around 0.5–1.0% per year in low- and middle-income countries. This is with the exceptions of lung cancer and chronic obstructive pulmonary disease (which are increasing because of the tobacco epidemic) and diabetes mellitus (which is increasing because of projected increases in the prevalence of overweight and obesity). Adverse trends for some risk factors like overweight and physical inactivity were probably more than offset in the selected countries by improved control of other risk factors like high

Table 8.3 Millions of projected deaths and DALYs for all chronic diseases as a proportion of deaths and DALYs for all causes in 23 selected low- and middle-income countries for 2005, 2010 and 2030

	2005	**2015**	**2030**
Deaths (all ages)	23.1 (61%)	27.2 (66%)	34.3 (71%)
Deaths in people younger than 70 years	11.2 (46%)	12.4 (50%)	13.7 (53%)
DALYs	496 (50%)	538 (55%)	597 (59%)

Adapted from Abegunde et al.[19]

blood pressure, high blood cholesterol and tobacco smoking and improved access to effective treatment interventions. Total deaths from cardiovascular diseases and diabetes are projected to rise to 14.3 million in 2015 and 17.3 million in 2030 in 23 selected low- and middle-income countries.[19] Just under half of these deaths will occur in people younger than 70 years compared to 27% in high-income countries.

Mechanisms which propel a cardiovascular disease epidemic in developing countries

Demographic changes due to the epidemiologic transition

A major public health challenge, identified by recent analyses of global health trends, is the projected rise in both proportional and absolute CVD mortality rates in the developing countries over the next quarter century. The reasons for this anticipated acceleration of the epidemic are many.[5] In the second half of the 20th century, most developing countries experienced a major surge in life expectancy. This was principally as a result of a decline in deaths occurring in infancy, childhood and adolescence and was related to more effective public health responses to perinatal, infectious and nutritional deficiency disorders and to improved economic indicators like per capita income and social indicators like female literacy in some areas. These demographic shifts have augmented the ranks of middle-aged and older adults. The increasing longevity provides longer periods of exposure to the risk factors of CVD, resulting in greater probability of clinically manifest CVD events. The concomitant decline of infectious and nutritional disorders (competing causes of death) further enhances the proportional burden due to CVD and other chronic lifestyle-related diseases.

The ratio of deaths due to pre-transitional diseases (related to infections and malnutrition) to those caused by post-transitional diseases (like CVD and cancer) varies among regions and between countries, depending on factors like the level of economic development and literacy as well as availability and access to healthcare. The direction of change towards a rising relative contribution of post-transitional diseases is, however, common to and consistent among the developing countries.[34] The experience of urban China, where the proportion of CVD deaths rose from 12.1% in 1957 to 35.8% in 1990, illustrates this phenomenon.[35]

Population expansion and aging

The aging of all populations heightens the importance of CVD both in people of working age and in those who are beyond working age. The world population is expected to rise from 5.71 billion in 1995 to 8.29 billion in 2025. By 2020, the median age of the population in much of the developing world will begin to approach that of the West. By 2040, the total number of people more than 65 years old in more developed countries will be only one-third of the number in less developed countries.[20]

While all the countries have experienced and will continue to experience a significant increase in population aged 65 and over, a difference is noted in "young" countries (those with a higher proportion of people aged less than 65 years). It will first produce a bulge of people of working age. Although overall dependency will fall, combined with changes in the demographic profile, this will result in a large number of adults potentially vulnerable to CVD. By 2020, the number of persons aged 65 years or above is projected to reach more than 690 million globally, with 460 million in the developing countries.[36] In India, for example, the population is expected to rise from 683.2 million in 1981 to somewhere between 1253.8 and 1480.5 million in 2021. Simultaneously, the proportion of adults aged 35 years or above will rise from 28.4% of the population to 42.4%.[37]

Increased standard of living leading to deleterious health behaviors

A third reason to arouse concern is that, if population levels of CVD risk factors rise as a consequence of adverse lifestyle changes accompanying industrialization and urbanization, the rates of CVD mortality and morbidity could rise even higher than the rates predicted solely by demographic changes. Both the degree as well as the duration of exposure to CVD risk factors would increase as a result of higher risk factor levels coupled with a longer life expectancy. Increase in body weight (adjusted for height), blood pressure and cholesterol levels in Chinese population samples aged 35–64 years, between the two phases of the Sino-MONICA study (1984–86, 1988–89) and the substantially higher levels of most CVD risk factors in urban popu-

lation groups compared to rural population groups in India, provide evidence of such trends.[35] The increasing use of tobacco in a number of developing countries will also translate into higher mortality rates of CVD, lung cancer and other tobacco-related diseases, while undesirable alterations in diet and physical activity are also impacting adversely on cardiovascular health.

In developing countries, risk factors often increase with rising incomes (hypertension and obesity). partly attributable to changing diet, that has more fats, salt and calories, and partly to increasing body weight and less exercise among the affluent.[20] The global availability of cheap vegetable oils and fats has resulted in greatly increased fat consumption among low-income countries in recent years.[38] The transition now occurs at lower levels of the gross national product than previously and is further accelerated by rapid urbanization. In China, for example, the proportion of upper-income persons who were consuming a relatively high-fat diet (>30% of daily energy intake) rose from 22.8% to 66.6% between 1989 and 1993. The lower and middle income groups also showed a rise (from 19% to 36.4% in the former and from 19.1% to 51.0% in the latter).[30] The Asian diet, traditionally high in carbohydrates and low in fat, has shown an overall decline in the proportion of energy from complex carbohydrates along with an increase in the proportion of fat.[38] The globalization of food production and marketing is also contributing to the increasing consumption of energy-dense foods that are poor in dietary fiber and several micronutrients.[39]

The rising tobacco consumption patterns in most developing countries contrast sharply with the overall decline in the industrial nations.[40] Recent projections from the World Health Organization suggest that by the year 2020 tobacco will become the largest single cause of death, accounting for 12.3% of global deaths.[33] India, China and countries in the Middle Eastern crescent will by then have tobacco contributing to more than 12% of all deaths. It is estimated from a recently conducted study in India that by 2010, the annual number of deaths from smoking will be about 1 million, 70% of which will occur in the middle age group. Also 20% of excess mortality among those resulting from cardiovascular diseases could be attributed to smoking alone.[41] Reports also indicate that the greatest increase in tobacco use between 1998 and 2005 occurred in persons between the ages of 15 and 24 years.[42]

Thrifty gene

A "programming" effect of factors promoting selective survival may also determine individual responses to environmental challenges and, thereby, the population differences in CVD. The "thrifty gene" has been postulated to be a factor in promoting selective survival, over generations, of persons who encountered an adverse environment of limited nutritional resources.[43] While this may have proved advantageous in surviving the rigours of a spartan environment over thousands of years, the relatively recent and rapid changes in environment may have resulted in a metabolic mismatch. Thus a salt-sensitive person whose forefathers thrived despite a limited supply of salt now reacts to a salt-enriched diet with high blood pressure. It has also been hypothesized that populations subjected to food scarcity have undergone selection of a gene which increases the efficiency of fat storage through an oversecretion of insulin in response to a meal. While this favors survival in a situation of low caloric availability, a current excess of caloric intake may lead to obesity, hyperinsulinemia, diabetes, and atherosclerosis. Similarly, an insulin-resistant individual whose ancestors may have survived because a lack of insulin sensitivity in the skeletal muscle ensured adequate blood glucose levels for the brain in daunting conditions of limited calorie intake and demanding physical challenges may now respond to a high-calorie diet and a sedentary lifestyle with varying degrees of glucose intolerance and hyperinsulinemia. While such mechanisms seem plausible, their contribution to the acceleration of the CVD epidemic in the developing countries remains speculative.

Maternal–fetal exposures as a cause of midlife CVD

A recently reported association which, if adequately validated by the tests of causation, may have special relevance to the developing countries is the inverse relationship between birth size and CVD in later life.[44–50] The "fetal origins hypothesis" states that adverse intrauterine influences like poor maternal nutrition lead to impaired fetal growth, resulting in low birth weight, short birth length, and a small head circumference. These adverse influences are postulated to also "program" the fetus to develop adaptive metabolic and physiologic responses which facilitate survival. These responses, however, may lead to disordered responses to environmental challenges as the child grows, with an increased risk of glucose intolerance, hypertension and dyslipidemia in later life, with adult CVD as a consequence. While an increasing body of global evidence for the hypothesis has been provided by observational studies, it awaits further evaluation for a causal role. The association of small birth size and "rebound adiposity" in early childhood, with adult-onset diabetes in an Indian cohort, lends credibility to the role that early life influences play in programmed susceptibility to adult metabolic and vascular diseases but the interaction with later environmental influences needs to be better studied.[51] If it does emerge as an important risk factor for CVD, the populations of developing countries will be at an especially enhanced risk because of the vast numbers of poorly nour-

ished infants who have been born in the past several decades. The steady improvement in child survival will lead to a higher proportion of such infants surviving to adult life when their hypothesized susceptibility to vascular disease may manifest itself.

Ethnic diversity

Although ethnic diversity in CVD rates, risk factor levels and risk factor interactions are evident from population studies, the extent to which genetic factors contribute is unclear. It is only after demographic profiles, environmental factors and possible programming factors are ascertained and adjusted for that differences in gene frequency or expression can be invoked as a probable explanation for interpopulation differences in CVD.[52] The extent to which chronic diseases, including CVD, occur within and amongst different populations is determined by genetic–environmental interaction which occurs in a wide and variable array, ranging from the essentially genetic to the predominantly environmental. This is perhaps best illustrated by the knowledge gained from studies in migrant groups, where environmental changes due to altered lifestyles are superimposed over genetic influences. These "natural experiments" have been of great value in enhancing the understanding of why CVD rates differ amongst ethnic groups. The classic Ni-Hon-San study of Japanese migrants revealed how blood cholesterol levels and CHD rates rose from Japan to Honolulu and further still to San Francisco, as Japanese communities in the three areas were compared.[53] Similarly, the Tokelau islanders who migrated to New Zealand had a higher risk of diabetes and were more obese compared to non-migrants.[54] The Boston-Irish Diet Heart Study, a study of the effects of Irish migration to USA, used sib comparison methodology and highlighted the role of key dietary factors attributable to relatively high burden of CHD.[55]

The experience gleaned from the study of South Asians, Chinese and Pima Indians further elucidates the complexities of ethnic variations in CHD.[56–58] The comparison of Afro-Caribbeans, South Asians and Europeans in UK brought out the sharp differences in central obesity, glucose intolerance, hyperinsulinemia and related dyslipidemia between the three groups despite similar profiles of blood pressure, body mass index and total plasma cholesterol.[59] Migrant studies have demonstrated a 1.1–3.8 CHD mortality ratio among migrants from the Indian subcontinent when compared to local populations.[60–62] However, urban-rural comparisons within India,[37] as well as migrant Indian comparison with their non-migrant siblings,[63] reveal large differences in these conventional risk factors. Thus, where the environment is common but gene pools differ, the non-conventional risk factors appear to be explanatory of risk variance, while when the same gene pool is confronted with different environments, the conventional risk factors stand out as being of major importance.

The extent to which ethnic diversity in response to CVD risk factors influences the course of the CVD epidemic in different developing countries remains to be studied. However, the experience of some of the migrant groups (e.g. South Asians) portends severe epidemics in the home countries as they advance in their transition.

Strategies to deal with the coronary epidemic

Risk factor

Decades of research, embracing evidence from observational epidemiology and clinical trials, have demonstrated that CHD is multifactorial in causation. The term "risk factor" was first used in the context of CHD.[64] A risk factor must fulfill the criteria of causality: strength of association (high relative risk or odds ratio), consistency of association (over many studies), temporal relationship (cause preceding the effect), dose–response relationship (the greater the exposure, the higher the risk), biologic plausibility, experimental evidence and, very importantly, evidence from human studies. Several such risk factors have been identified, ranging from the established "major" factors like smoking, elevated blood cholesterol and hypertension (conventional risk factors) to the recently investigated factors like homocysteine, lipoprotein A, apolipoprotein B, triglycerides, non-esterified fatty acids and C-reactive protein.

A major case–control study, involving 52 countries, has identified nine easily measured risk factors (smoking, lipids, hypertension, diabetes, obesity, diet, physical activity, alcohol consumption and psychosocial factors) that account for 90% of the risk of acute myocardial infarction (AMI). The INTERHEART study found that these risk factors are the same in almost every geographic region and every racial/ethnic group worldwide and are consistent in men and women. The strongest risk predictor was the apoB/apoA1 ratio (a more reliable marker of cholesterol risk), followed by current smoking. These two risk factors together predict 66.4% of all AMIs, worldwide. Five factors (smoking, lipids, hypertension, diabetes and abdominal obesity) accounted for 80% of the population-attributable risk. This landmark study provides the scientific basis for current intervention options even in countries where classic cohort studies have not been conducted to identify coronary risk factors.[65]

"Clinical" vs "prevention" norms

The need for making "clinical" decisions related to the management of these risk factors led to definition of thresh-old levels of risk and practice guidelines based on those. These "clinical norms" erroneously came to be identified, by health professionals as well as the community, to also represent the prevention norms. The former are defined by evidence of benefit exceeding risk when an intervention reduces a risk factor below a particular level (the net benefit being demonstrated in clinical trials specifically designed for that purpose). The latter, however, are usually identified from observational studies (long-term longitudinal prospective studies of large cohorts) and denote the optimal values of the risk factor at which the risk of developing disease is minimal.

The targeting of individuals is promoted by the "clinical" approach of healthcare providers who seek to identify persons at "high risk" of disease or its outcomes for intensive investigation and intervention. Thus thresholds are defined to categorize persons with "high cholesterol" or "high blood pressure" and implement individualized control strategies. Attention and action above this threshold often contrast with indifference and inertia below it.

As trial evidence is gathered, the clinical norms may progressively move towards the prevention norms, as in the case of cholesterol or hypertension where the thresholds for intervention have been lowered dramatically in the last decade. They may, however, remain higher than the prevention norms, since clinical trials may be conducted at a stage in the natural history where the risks of prior exposure may not be completely reversible and also because the intervention may itself be associated with some adverse effects. Thus the benefits of lowering a risk factor may appear less than those that may occur by preventing its rise in the first place.

The continuum of risk

It is clear that even though lifestyle disorders afflict some individuals, they arise from causes that are widespread in the population as a whole. Risk factors like cholesterol and blood pressure operate in a continuum of progressively increasing risk rather than through an all-or-none relationship suggested by cut-off values. For example, a systolic blood pressure (SBP) in the range 130–139 mmHg carries a higher risk than values in the range 120–129 mmHg for both heart attacks and strokes. While a SBP of 180 mmHg carries a much higher risk for an individual than 140 mmHg, the number of persons in any population who have SBP values in the range 130–139 mmHg is higher than those with values of 180 mmHg or higher. The Multiple Risk Factor Intervention Trial's (MRFIT) cohort study in the United States revealed that of all heart attacks which are attributable to SBP, 7.2% arise from the 0.9% segment of the population which represents the 180+ mmHg range, while 20.7% of all such heart attacks occur in the 22.8% segment of the population which has pressures in the range 130–139 mmHg[66] (Fig. 8.1). Similarly, 57% of all excess deaths

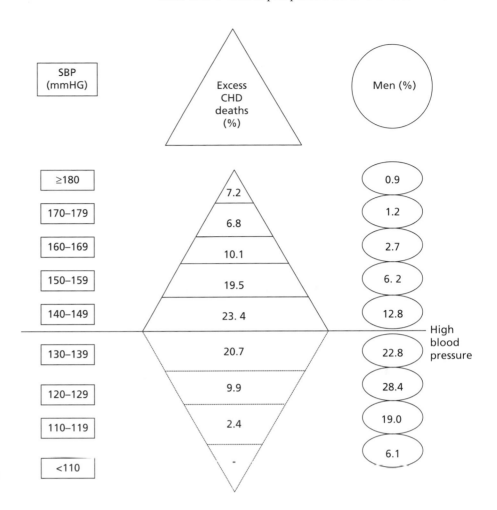

SBP (mmHG)	Excess CHD deaths (%)	Men (%)
≥180	7.2	0.9
170–179	6.8	1.2
160–169	10.1	2.7
150–159	19.5	6.2
140–149	23.4	12.8
130–139	20.7	22.8
120–129	9.9	28.4
110–119	2.4	19.0
<110	-	6.1

High blood pressure

Figure 8.1 The risk pyramid for blood pressure and coronary heart disease (CHD): baseline SBP and CHD death rates for men screened in MRFIT. (Adapted with permission from Stamler et al.[66])

attributable to diastolic blood pressure occur in the range 80–95 mmHg compared to only 15% which occur in the high range of 105–130 mmHg.

This dichotomy is also clearly seen in the Framingham Study on coronary risk factors.[66] People with a blood cholesterol level of 300 mg/dL run 3–5 times the risk of CHD as do people at a cholesterol level of 200 mg/dL. At cholesterol levels over 300 mg/dL, 90 out of 100 people developed the disease in the next 16–30 years of follow-up in Framingham. At cholesterol levels under 200 mg/dL, the rate was 20 out of 100 during the same period. However, more than twice as many people developed CHD with cholesterol levels under 200 mg% all their lives as did those with cholesterol levels over 300 mg%. This is because a 20% fraction of a 45% segment of the population is a much larger number than a 90% fraction of a 3–5% segment of the population.[67]

Thus, for most causal factors, there is a "risk pyramid". Those at the top of the pyramid are at the highest individual risk of disease but those at the lower levels of the pyramid account for the largest number of cases in the community because they constitute the largest segment of the population. Any approach which targets only those at the highest risk produces limited gains for the community, despite conferring definite benefits to the individuals in that category.

The concept that "sick individuals arise from sick populations" was propounded and proved by Geoffrey Rose.[68,69] He demonstrated that risk factor "distributions" throughout the population are predictive of disease burden in that community. The mean (average) levels of a risk factor across different populations correlate with the proportions of high-risk individuals in those populations, whatever the cut-off value is. Thus, as the average blood pressure value rises amongst populations, the proportion of hypertensive individuals also rises. In each population, there are groups who represent the extremes of the risk profile (very low risk versus very high risk). However, the proportion at "high risk" would be determined by the average value of that risk factor in the population. This in turn is dependent on the dominant behaviors that characterize the society at each stage of its development.

While Rose highlighted the importance of shifting the distribution at the level of any country's population, the principle is also relevant to the global population as a whole. With the developing countries acquiring higher levels of risk, the global distributions of blood pressure and cholesterol are shifting rightwards. Even if preventive measures succeed in reducing the risk levels in the developed countries, which have experienced high risk so far, global deaths due to CVD will continue to rise because the larger populations of the developing countries constitute the bulk of the distribution. Meaningful impact on global CVD will occur only when preventive measures effectively reduce the risk levels in the developing countries. We need to move the global bell curve of each risk factor leftwards.

Multiplicative risk

The process of identifying and estimating the independent risk associated with any single risk factor led to clinical and preventive strategies targeting it in isolation. However, observational studies like Framingham and MRFIT have clearly revealed that the co-existence of multiple risk factors confers a magnified risk which is multiplicative rather than merely additive. A smoker with modest elevations of cholesterol and diastolic or systolic blood pressure is at a greater risk of coronary death than a non-smoker with severe hypertension or marked hypercholesterolemia. In the MRFIT study, a non-smoker with SBP less than 118 mmHg and a total serum cholesterol level less than 182 mg% had a 20-fold lower risk of coronary death than a smoker with a SBP exceeding 142 mmHg and a serum cholesterol exceeding 245 mg% (age-adjusted CHD mortality of 3.09 vs 62.11, per 10 000 person-years). A smoker who has a SBP of 132–141 mmHg and a serum cholesterol of 203–220 mg% has a CHD mortality risk of 28.87 per 10 000 person-years, compared to a risk of 12.36 in a non-smoker with a SBP below 118 mmHg but with a serum cholesterol exceeding 245 mg%.[70]

The demonstration of such multiplicative risk has led to the concept of "comprehensive cardiovascular risk" or "total risk", quantifying an individual's overall risk of CVD resulting from the confluence of risk factors.[71] Both clinical and preventive strategies are veering away from unifactorial risk reduction to multifactorial risk modification, to reduce this overall risk in individuals as well as in populations.

Prevention

High-risk approach for prevention

Having recognized that environmental risk factors do not affect only a few individuals in isolation but are spread across populations, with a continuous rather than a threshold relationship to disease, how should that influence disease control strategies? The health policy debate, until recently, was on whether to focus the control strategies on individuals at the highest risk of disease (in view of their

markedly elevated risk factor levels) or on the population as a whole (aiming to achieve modest reductions in the risk of most members of that community). The high-risk approach aims at identifying persons with markedly elevated risk factors and, therefore, at the highest risk of disease.[66] These individuals are then targeted by interventions which aim to reduce the risk factor levels. If successful, the benefits to individuals are large, because the individual's risks are large. However, since the number of people in this high-risk category is proportionately much smaller than those in the moderate-risk group, the overall benefits to society are limited in terms of deaths or disability avoided.

"High-risk individuals can be defined as those aged between 40–79 years with a history of non-fatal coronary heart disease/cerebrovascular event or having an estimated absolute risk of dying from any cardiovascular event of 15% or more in the next 10 years. Absolute risk can be determined from country-specific risk charts that rely on easily measurable risk factors. (Fig. 8.2). For instance, the absolute risk chart given here was generated by categorizing simulated population according to sex, age, smoking status, systolic blood pressure and Body Mass Index. Countries can adopt different risk prediction strategies and the basic approach described here is only suggestive and not prescriptive. With more sophisticated algorithms that better target those at high risk, such as measurement of cholesterol/plasma glucose, both the costs and benefits can be expected to increase.[72]

Population approach for prevention

In contrast, the population approach aims at reducing the risk factor levels in the population as a whole, through community action.[68] Because there is a continuum of risk associated with most risk factors, this mass change will result in mass benefit across a wide range of risk. While individual benefits are relatively small, the cumulative societal benefits are large ("the prevention paradox"). The strategy is also behaviorally more appropriate. If the eating habits in the community alter towards preferred consumption of foods with lower saturated fat and salt content and a greater daily intake of fresh fruit and vegetables, even the high-risk individual on a prescribed diet will find a supportive ambience which does not mark him out as a deviant from social norms. If a new generation grows up in an environment where healthy behavior is considered common practice, its average blood cholesterol level may remain below 200 mg% rather than around 240 mg% and thus people will be at a lower risk than even the beneficiary of the high-risk strategy. However, the risks and benefits of such a strategy are less obvious to those in the moderate-risk range. The motivation for change is, therefore, not as strong as for those in the high-risk group. The gratification of achieving readily identifiable success in high-risk indi-

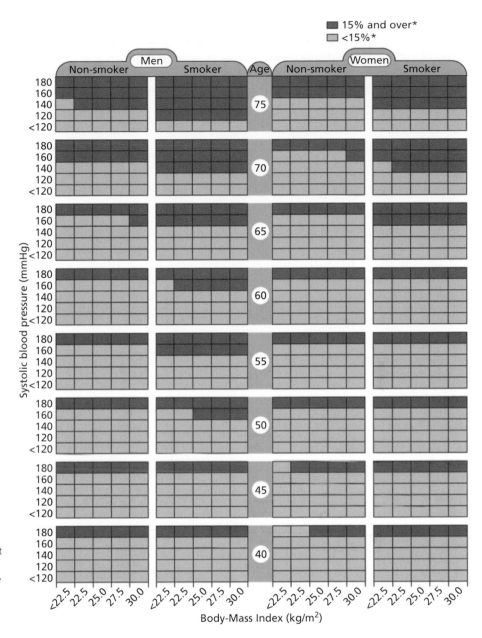

Figure 8.2 Example of an absolute risk chart using age, sex, smoking status, systolic blood pressure, and Body Mass Index. *Numbers are 10-year risk of fatal ischemic heart disease or cardiovascular events in Mexico. (Adapted from Lim et al.[72])

viduals, through drugs or other powerful interventions, is also denied to the physicians in the population strategy where the potential beneficiaries, though many, are faceless and nameless. Since such "anonymity of prevention" denies the pleasure of individual rescue acts, physician motivation for community counseling is neither strong nor sustained.[68] Policymakers can, however, ill afford to ignore the imperatives of investing in a population approach which will pay large long-term dividends in the control of lifestyle diseases. Health professionals too must recognize the benefits of this strategy to play a strong advocacy role for health-promoting behaviors in the community.

The impact of the population strategy is likely to be large, as suggested by an estimate that if every American had a diastolic blood pressure value which is a mere 2 mmHg lower than his or her present value, the number of heart attacks that could be prevented would exceed those that could be avoided by effectively treating every person with a diastolic pressure of 95 mmHg or higher. The corresponding benefit for preventing paralytic strokes would be 93% of those avoided by drug therapy.[73] Such blood pressure changes can be effectively achieved and sustained through modest reductions in weight and salt intake or through exercise.

The success of population strategies has been demonstrated both in developed countries (e.g. Finland) and in developing countries (e.g. Mauritius).[74,75] The North Karelia Project demonstrated large reductions in CVD mortality

(50.1% in males and 63.5% in females), CHD mortality (53.4% and 59.8%) and all-cause mortality (39.5% and 40.4%) during the 20 years intervention period. This resulted from a series of community-based strategies designed to change dietary behavior through media campaigns in collaboration with the food industry and agricultural policy changes. As people changed their behavior in terms of dietary preference, the food industry perceived new opportunities and developed products with less oil. Agriculturists developed a new type of rapeseed plant that grew well in the cold northern climate of Finland. This sold well and market proportion of unsaturated to saturated fats increased. Salt reduction was also adopted by food producers.[20]

Another example of a macroeconomic intervention that seems to have had an impact on CVD rates comes from Poland. The fall in heart disease deaths in 1992–94 coincided with a switch in Poland from consuming animal fats to vegetable fats. This resulted from a government decision to cut subsidies for animal fats and impose taxes, thus raising the price of animal fats to consumers and making vegetable oils more competitive. There followed a 23% decline in the availability of animal fats products and a 48% increase in the supply of vegetable fat products.[20]

In a comprehensive community-based project in China, notable outcomes included a reduction in the annual heart disease and stroke deaths among hypertensives from 1.6% to 0.8% between 2000 and 2002. An increase in the proportion of people participating in planned regular physical activity increased from 41% to 84% in the same period.[76] Yet another sodium intervention project (1989–92) demonstrated a significant net reduction in sodium intake among men in different educational and occupational groups. The mean systolic blood pressure decreased by 3 mmHg for the total population.[77] The Mauritius project included a government-led program that changed the main cooking oil from a predominantly saturated fat palm oil to soybean oil high in unsaturated fatty acids. Overall, total cholesterol concentration fell by 14% during the 5-year study (1987–92). These examples demonstrate the ability to change behavior through macroeconomic and health promotion interventions. However, evidence from other countries has yielded mixed results.[20]

Combining the strategies

These strategies are not mutually exclusive but are synergistic, complementary and necessary. The risks and benefits demonstrated in high-risk individuals serve to educate the community about risk factors, while the population approach makes it easier to achieve the desired level of lifestyle change in high-risk individuals. The population-based, lifestyle-linked risk reduction approach is particularly relevant in the context of the developing countries, where it is necessary to ensure that communities currently at low risk are protected from acquisition or augmentation

of risk factors ("primordial prevention"). This is true for adults in the rural regions of most developing countries as well as for children in all populations. It is also eminently applicable to moderate-risk groups in urban areas, where lifestyle-based risk modification will help avoid drug therapy, with its attendant economic and biologic costs. There will still be some people who need such pharmacologic or technologic interventions because of their high-risk status. However, their numbers too will decrease as the risk profile of the whole community gradually shifts.

Case management

Despite these preventive strategies, several individuals will manifest clinical disease because risks are not totally eliminated in the community or because genetic susceptibility is strongly expressed. The success of preventive efforts will reduce their number as well as delay the age of onset of clinical events. Those who develop disease will require optimal clinical care which can avert early death, reduce disability, and assure an adequate quality of life. This mandates early detection of disease and management.

Institution of emergency care and adequate treatment of established cases are also key points for enhancing the outcomes of any cardiovascular event. The GRACE study reveals substantial differences in the management of acute coronary syndrome (ACS) patients based on hospital type and geographic location.[78] However, with improved use of evidence-based pharmacologic and interventional therapies, significant reductions were observed in the rates of new heart failure and myocardial infarction cases at 6 months.[79] A prospective analysis of an ACS registry in India reveals that patients admitted to Indian hospitals have worse prognosis compared to developed countries. Most of the patients were poor and were less likely to get evidence-based treatments and there were delays in access to hospital and provision of affordable treatment that could have resulted in higher 30-day mortality.[80] For those who are at high risk, the individual-based strategies with the greatest accumulated evidence of effectiveness are drugs to prevent cardiovascular disease: blood pressure-lowering drugs, cholesterol-lowering drugs and aspirin. Although these are cost effective in low- and middle-income countries and are available in most markets, their current coverage in high-risk individuals remains low.[81] The contributory factors range from policymaker reluctance to fund provision of CVD drugs in primary healthcare to poor prescribing practices of healthcare providers.

CVD-related expenditure

In developed countries

Several studies in the industrialized world have attempted to estimate the direct healthcare costs of CVD and its clinically expressed risk factors. All have found CVD to be a major driver of rising healthcare costs. Thompson and Wolf in 2001 reviewed studies on the medical care cost burden of obesity. It was estimated to contribute between 2% and 7% of total health expenditures.[82] Annual direct health costs for coronary heart disease, stroke and hypertension in 1995 dollars were $50.8 billion, $18.1 billion and $15.6 billion respectively. It was also determined that half of the estimated annual healthcare costs of chronic diseases came from those aged 18–64 (productive years).[83]

Cost-effectiveness of population-wide approaches is sensitive to the cost of the intervention as well as the expected reduction in the indicators (like cholesterol level). In fact, the cost-effectiveness ratio ranged from being cost saving to $88 000 per life-year gained, depending on the percentage reduction. For example, a nationwide community intervention that expects a 4% reduction in total serum cholesterol and costs $5 per person every year could save more than $2 billion over 25 years.[84] When all the benefits of a nationwide intervention program, including blood pressure reductions and smoking cessation, were included, the results were favorable. Unfortunately, there is less cost information on physical activity interventions to determine their cost-effectiveness on a larger scale.

In developing countries

Healthcare costs for CVD in the developing world are likely to rise as prevalence rises and even if the rates plateau, costs are likely to become increasingly prohibitive as technologic options spread.[20] If nothing is done to reduce the risk of chronic disease, an estimated US$84 billion of economic production will be lost because of heart disease, stroke and diabetes in low- and middle-income countries between 2006 and 2015.[85]

Estimates from China indicate that hospital costs attributable to CVD conditions totaled over $9.6 billion in 1998, or nearly 20% of all hospital costs.[86] Healthcare expenditure increases with the location of the health facility, duration of stay in hospitals and type of health facility (government/private). Patient expenditures are 20% higher in urban than in rural areas, even where government facilities are the locus of care.[20] The effects of CVD on costs extend well beyond the health sector. A 1991 study in South Africa estimated that direct healthcare costs account for only 42% of the total costs for CVD. Hence, for every dollar spent on CVD by the health system, the South African economy pays another $1.38 due to CVD morbidity and mortality manifesting in disability and lost productivity costs.[87]

Cost-effectiveness analysis of multiple interventions in countries of low and middle income seems to be quite favorable. The intervention on salt reduction ranges from cost saving to $200 for each DALY averted across the range of estimates of the cost of the intervention as well as its range of effectiveness.[84] Juxtaposed with these population strategies, strategies involving multi-drug regimens to treat patients with high-risk cardiovascular disease also seem reasonable. All the results fall well under the Gross Domestic Product per head for each region, making them attractive options for scale-up.

Evidence to support action

The knowledge of cardiovascular risk factors continues to evolve, with continued investigation of putative risk factors through animal, human observational and experimental studies. However, there is sufficient information available on the role of major risk factors to enable effective measures for the prevention and control of CVD to be undertaken worldwide. While the application of the knowledge may have to be contextualized to match the sociodemographic profiles of different populations, the global evidence on the causation and prevention of CVD remains relevant to all populations.

The well-substantiated model of health transition enables the prediction of the emerging and anticipated course of the CVD epidemic across different regions of the world. This knowledge should be utilized to telescope the transition and shorten the phase of many mid-life deaths through effective prevention. Never before in human history have we been so clearly forewarned of our impending destiny and so effectively fore-armed to alter it. It is a challenge to human intellect and enterprise to move this knowledge into the arena of action, to reduce the global burden of CVD.

References

1. Cardiovascular disease. Fact sheet on chronic disease. Available at: www.healthinfo/global_burden_diseases/GBD_report-2004.
2. Ebrahim S, Smith GD. Exporting failure? Coronary heart disease and stroke in developing countries. *Int J Epidemiol* 2001;**30**: 201–5.
3. Feigin VL. Stroke epidemiology in the developing world. *Lancet* 2005;**365**:2160–1.
4. Murray CJL, Lopez AD. *The Global Burden of Disease: A Comprehensive Assessment of Mortality and Disability from Disease, Injuries and Risk Factors in 1990 and Projected to 2020*. Boston: Harvard University Press, 1996.
5. Reddy KS, Yusuf S. The emerging epidemic of cardiovascular disease in developing countries. *Circulation* 1998;**97**:596–601.
6. Howson CP, Reddy KS, Ryan TJ, Bale JR (eds). *Control of Cardiovascular Disease in developing countries. Research, development and Institutional Strengthening*. Washington, D.C.: National Academy Press, 1998.
7. Yusuf S, Reddy S, Ounppuu S, Anand S. Global burden of cardiovascular diseases. Part I: general considerations, the epidemiological transition, risk factors, and impact of urbanisation. *Circulation*. 2001;**104**:2746. Part II: variations in cardiovascular disease by specific ethnic groups and geographic regions and prevention strategies. *Circulation* 2001;**104**:2855.

8. American Heart Association. *2000 Heart and Stroke Statistical Update*. Dallas, TX: American Heart Association, 1999.
9. Lopez AD. Assessing the burden of mortality from cardiovascular disease. *Wld Hlth Stat Q* 1993;46:91–6.
10. Feinleib M, Ingster L, Rosenberg H, Maurer J, Singh G, Kochanek K. Time trends, cohort effects and geographic patterns in stroke mortality. United States. *Ann Epidemiol* 1993;3:458–65.
11. Whelton PK, Brancati FL, Appel LJ, Klag MJ. The challenge of hypertension and atherosclerotic cardiovascular disease in economically developing countries. *High Blood Press* 1995;4:36–45.
12. Marmot M. Coronary heart disease: rise and fall of a modern epidemic. In: Marmot M, Elliott P, eds. *Coronary Heart Disease Epidemiology. From Aetiology to Public Health.* Oxford: Oxford University Press, 1992, pp3–19.
13. Cooper, Cutler J, Desvigne-Nickens P *et al.* Trends and disparities in coronary heart disease in the United States. Findings of the National Conference on Cardiovascular Disease Prevention. *Circulation* 2000;102:3137–47.
14. Muller-Nordhorn J, Binting S, Roll S, Willich SN. An update on regional variation in cardiovascular mortality within Europe. *Eur Heart J* 2008;29:1316–26.
15. Mensah GA. Ischaemic heart disease in Africa. *Heart* 2008;94;836–43.
16. Yang G, Kong L, Zhao LC, Koplan JP. Emergence of chronic non communicable disease in China. *Lancet* 2008;372:1697–705.
17. Reddy KS. India wakes up to the threat of cardiovascular diseases. *J Am Coll Cardiol* 2007;50:1370–2.
18. Rheumatic fever and rheumatic heart disease. CVD Atlas 02. Rheumatic Heart Disease. Geneva: World Health Organization, 2002.
19. Abegunde DO, Mathers CD, Adam T, Ortegon M, Strong K. The burden and costs of chronic diseases in low-income and middle-income countries. *Lancet* 2007;370:1929–38.
20. A Race against time. The challenge of cardiovascular disease in developing economies. By the Trustees of Columbia University of New York. 2004.
21. Eagle K. Coronary artery disease in India: challenges and opportunities. *Lancet* 2008;371:1394–5.
22. Jee SH, Pastor-Barriuso R, Appel LJ, Suh I, Miller ER, Guallar E. Body mass index and incident ischemic heart disease in South Korean men and women. *Am J Epidemiol* 2005;162:42–8.
23. Hong JS, Yi SW, Kang HC, Ohrr H. Body Mass Index and mortality in South Korean men resulting from cardiovascular disease: a Kangwha Cohort Study. *Am Epidemiol* 2007;17: 622–7.
24. Omran AR. The epidemiologic transition: a key to the epidemiology of population change. *Millbank Mem Fund Q* 1971;49:509–38.
25. Olshansky SJ, Ault AB. The fourth stage of the epidemiologic transition: the age of delayed degenerative diseases. *Millbank Mem Fund Q* 1986;64:355–91.
26. Pearson TA, Jamison DT, Trejo-Gutierrez H. Cardiovascular disease, In: Jamison DT, ed. *Disease Control Priorities in Developing Countries.* New York: Oxford University Press, 1993, pp577–99.
27. Wu Z, Tao C, Zhao D, Wu G, Wang W, Liu J, Zeng Z, Wu Y. A collaborative study on trends and determinants in cardiovascular diseases in China, Part I: Morbidity and mortality monitoring. *Circulation* 2001;103:462.
28. Liu M, Wu B, Wang WZ, Lee LM, Zhang SH, Kong LZ. Stroke in China: epidemiology, prevention, and management strategies. *Lancet Neurol* 2007;6:456–64.
29. Kita ET. Coronary heart disease risk in Japan – an East/West divide? *Eur Heart J* 2004;6(suppl A);A8–A11.
30. Suh I. Cardiovascular mortality in Korea: a country experiencing epidemiologic transition. *Acta Cardiol* 2001;56:75–81.
31. Reddy KS, Prabhakaran D, Jeemon P, Thankappan KR, Joshi P, Chaturvedi V *et al.* Educational status and cardiovascular risk profile in Indians. *Proc Natl Acad Sci U S A* 2007;104:16263–8.
32. Unwin N, Setel P, Rashid S *et al.* Noncommunicable diseases in sub-Saharan Africa: where do they feature in the health research agenda? *Bull WHO* 2001;79:947–53.
33. World Health Organization. *Tobacco or Health: First Global Status Report.* Geneva: World Health Organization, 1996.
34. Bulatao RA, Stephens PW. *Global Estimates and Projections of Mortality by Cause 1970–2015. Pre-Working Paper 1007.* Washington, DC: Population Health and Nutrition Department, World Bank, 1992.
35. Yao C, Wu Z, Wu J. The changing pattern of cardiovascular diseases in China. *Wld Hlth Stat Q* 1993;46:113–18.
36. World Health Organization. *The World Health Report 1997.* Geneva: World Health Organization, 1997.
37. Reddy KS. Cardiovascular disease in India. *Wld Hlth Stat Q* 1993;46:101–7.
38. Drewnowski A, Popkin BM. The nutrition transition: new trends in the global diet. *Nutr Rev* 1997;55:31–43.
39. Lang T. The public health impact of globalisation of food trade. In: Shetty PS, McPherson K, eds. *Diet, Nutrition and Chronic Disease. Lessons from Contrasting Worlds.* Chichester: Wiley, 1997, pp173–87.
40. Peto R. Tobacco – the growing epidemic in China. *JAMA* 1996;275:1683–4.
41. Jha P, Jacob B, Gajalakshmi V, Gupta PC, Dhingra N, Kumar R *et al.* A nationally representative case control study of smoking and death in India. *N Engl J Med* 2008;358:1137–47.
42. International Institute for Population Sciences. *National Family Health Survey-3 (2005–6).* Mumbai, India: International Institute for Population Sciences, 2007. Available online at www.measuredhs.com.
43. Editorial. Thrifty genotype rendered detrimental by progress. *Lancet* 1989;ii:839–40.
44. Barker DJP, Martyn CN, Osmond C, Haleb CN, Fall CHD. Growth in utero and serum cholesterol concentrations in adult life. *BMJ* 1993;307:1524–7.
45. Martyn CN, Barker DJP, Jespersen S, Greenwald S, Osmond C, Berry C. Growth in utero, adult blood pressure and arterial compliance. *Br Heart J* 1995;73:116–21.
46. Law CM, Shiell AW. Is blood pressure inversely related to birth weight? The strength of evidence from a systematic review of the literature. *J Hypertens* 1996;14:935–41.
47. Joseph KS, Kramer MS. Review of evidence on fetal and early childhood antecedents of adult chronic disease. *Epidemiol Rev* 1996;18:158–74.
48. Eriksson JG, Forsen T, Tuomilehto J, Osmond C, Barker DJP. Early growth, adult income, and risk of stroke. *Stroke* 2000;31:869–74.
49. Eriksson JG, Forsen T, Tuomilehto J, Osmond C, Barker DJP. Fetal and childhood growth and hypertension in adult life. *Hypertension* 2000;36:790.

50. Eriksson JG, Forsen T, Tuomilehto J, Osmond C, Barker DJP. Early growth and coronary heart disease in later life: longitudinal study. *BMJ* 2001;**322**:949–53.

51. Bhargava SK, Sachdev HS, Fall C, Osmond C, Lakshmy R, Barker DJP et al. Relation of serial changes in childhood Body Mass Index to impaired glucose tolerance in young adulthood. *N Engl J Med* 2004;**350**:865–75.

52. Reddy KS, Coronary heart disease in different racial groups. In: Yusuf S, Wilhelmsen L, eds. *Advanced Issues in Prevention and Treatment of Atherosclerosis*. Surrey: Euromed Communications, 1996, pp47–60.

53. Robertson TL, Kato H, Rhoads GG et al. Epidemiologic studies of coronary heart disease and stroke in Japanese men living in Japan, Hawai and California. Incidence of myocardial infarction and death from coronary heart disease. *Am J Cardiol* 1977;**39**:239–49.

54. Ostbye T, Welby TJ, Prior IA, Salmond CE, Stokes YM. Type 2 (non-insulin-dependent) diabetes mellitus, migration and westernization: the Tokelau Island Migrant Study. *Diabetologia* 1989;**32**(8):585–90.

55. Kushi LH, Lew RA, Stare FJ, Ellison CR, El Lozy M et al. Diet and 20-year mortality from coronary heart disease. The Ireland–Boston Diet-Heart Study. *N Engl J Med* 1985;**312**(13):811–18.

56. Enas EA, Mehta JL. Malignant coronary artery disease in young Asian Indians: thoughts on pathogenesis, prevention and treatment. *Clin Cardiol* 1995;**18**:131–5.

57. Li N, Tuomilehto J, Dowse G et al. Prevalence of coronary heart disease indicated by electrocardiogram abnormalities and risk factors in developing countries. *J Clin Epidemiol* 1994;**47**:599–611.

58. Sievers ML, Nelson RG, Bennet PH. Adverse mortality experience of a southwestern American Indian community: overall death rates and underlying causes of death in Pima Indians. *J Clin Epidemiol* 1990;**43**:1231–42.

59. Chaturvedi N, McKeigue PM, Marmot MG. Relationship of glucose intolerance to coronary risk in Afro-Caribbeans compared with Europeans. *Diabetologia* 1994;**37**:765–72.

60. Wild SH, Fischbacher C, Brock A, Griffiths C, Bhopal R. Mortality from all causes and circulatory disease by country of birth in England and Wales 2001–2003. *J Public Health* 2007;**29**(2):191–8.

61. Palaniappan L, Wang Y, Fortmann SP. Coronary heart disease mortality for six ethnic groups in California, 1990–2000. *Ann Epidemiol* 2004;**14**(7):499–506.

62. Collins VR, Dowse GK, Cabealawa S, Ram P, Zimmet PZ. High mortality from cardiovascular disease and analysis of risk factors in Indian and Malanesian Fijians. *Int J Epidemiol* 1996;**25**:59–69.

63. Bhatnagar D, Anand IS, Durrington PN et al. Coronary risk factors in people from the Indian subcontinent living in West London and their siblings in India. *Lancet* 1995;**345**:404–9.

64. Kannel WB, Dawber TR, Kagan A, Revotskie N, Strokes J III. Factors of risk in the development of coronary heart disease – six-year follow-up experience. *Ann Intern Med* 1961;**55**:33–50.

65. Yusuf S, Hawken S, Ounpuu S, on behalf of the INTERHEART Study Investigators. Effect of potentially modifiable risk factors associated with myocardial infarction in 52 countries (the INTERHEART study): case-control study. *Lancet* 2004;**364**:937–52.

66. Stamler J, Stamler R, Neaton JD. Blood pressure, systolic and diastolic, and cardiovascular risks: US population data. *Arch Intern Med* 1993;**153**:598–615.

67. WHO Expert Committee. *Hypertension Control in Populations*. WHO Technical Report No 862. Geneva: World Health Organization, 1996.

68. Castelli WP, Anderson K, Wilson PW, Levy D. Lipids and risk of coronary heart disease. The Framingham Study. *Ann Epidemiol* 1992;**2**(1–2):23–8.

69. Rose G. Sick individuals and sick populations. *Int J Epidemiol* 1985;**14**:32–8.

70. Rose G, Day S. The population mean predicts the number of deviant individuals. *BMJ* 1990;**301**:1031–4.

71. Neaton JD, Kuller LH, Wentworth D, Borhani NO, for the Multiple Risk Factor Intervention Trial Research Group. Total and cardiovascular mortality in relation to cigarette smoking, serum cholesterol concentration, and diastolic blood pressure among black and white males followed for five years. *Am Heart J* 1984;**108**:759–69.

72. Lim SS, Gaziano TA, Gakidou E, Reddy KS, Farzadfar F, Lozano R, Rodgers A. Prevention of cardiovascular disease in high-risk individuals in low-income and middle-income countries: health effects and costs. *Lancet* 2007;**370**:2054–62.

73. Cook NR, Cohen J, Hebert PR, Taylor JO, Hennekens CH. Implications of small reductions in diastolic blood pressure for primary prevention. *Arch Intern Med* 1995;**155**:701–9.

74. Puska P, Tuomilehto J, Aulikki N, Enkki V. *The North Karelia Project. 20 Years Results and Experiences*. Helsinki: National Public Health Institute, 1995.

75. Dowsen GK, Gareeboo H, George K et al. Changes in population cholesterol concentrations and other cardiovascular risk factor levels after five years of non-communicable disease intervention programme in Mauritius. *BMJ* 1995;**311**:1255–9.

76. World Health Organization. *Preventing Chronic Diseases A Vital Investment*. Geneva: World Health Organization, 2005.

77. Tian HG, Guo ZY, Hu G, Yu SJ, Sun W, Pietinen P, Nissinen A. Changes in sodium intake and blood pressure ina community based intervention project in China. *J Hum Hypertens* 1995;**9**(12):959–68.

78. Fox KAA, Goodman SG, Klein W, Brieger D, Steg PG, Dabbous O, Avezum A. Management of acute coronary syndrome. Variations in practice and outcome. *Eur Heart J* 2002;**23**:1177–89.

79. Fox KA, Steg PG, Eagle KA, Goodman SG, Anderson FA, Granger CB et al. Decline in rates of death and heart failure in acute coronary syndromes, 1999–2006. *JAMA* 2007;**297**:1892–900.

80. Xavier D, Pais P, Devereaux PJ, Xie C, Prabhakaran D, Reddy KS et al. Treatment and outcomes of acute coronary syndromes in India (CREATE): a prospective analysis of registry data. *Lancet* 2008;**371**:1435–42.

81. Mendis S, Abegunde D, Yusuf S et al. WHO study on Prevention of REcurrences of Myocardial Infarction and StrokE (WHO-PREMISE). *Bull WHO* 2005;**83**:820–8.

82. Thompson D, Wolf AM. The medical care cost burden of obesity. *Obes Rev* 2001;**2**:189–97.

83. Hoffman C, Rice D, Sung H-Y. Persons with chronic conditions: their prevalence and costs. *JAMA* 1996;**276**:1473–9.

84. Gaziano TA, Galea G, Reddy KS. Scaling up interventions for chronic disease prevention: the evidence. *Lancet* 2007;**370**: 1939–46.

85. Beaglehole R, Ebrahim S, Reddy S, Voute J, Leeder S, on behalf of the Chronic Disease Action Group. Prevention of chronic diseases: a call to action. *Lancet* 2007;**370**:2152–7.

86. Zhou Y, Baker TD, Rao K, Li G. Productive losses from injury in China. *Inj Prev* 2003;**9**:124–7.

87. Pestana JA, Steyn K, Leiman A, Hartzenberg GM. The direct and indirect costs of cardiovascular disease in South Africa in 1991. *S Afr Med J* 1996;**86**:679–84.

Avoidance of worldwide vascular deaths and total deaths from smoking

Prabhat Jha,[1] Prem Mony,[1,2] James Moore[3] and Witold Zatonski[4]

[1] Centre for Global Health Research, St Michael's Hospital, University of Toronto, Canada
[2] St John's Research Institute, Bangalore, India
[3] Bill & Melinda Gates Foundation, New Dehli, India
[4] Maria Sklodowska-Curie Cancer Centre and Institute of Oncology, Warsaw, Poland

Introduction

Hundreds of millions of premature tobacco deaths could be avoided if effective interventions could be widely applied in all countries. Numerous studies from high-income countries, and a growing number from low- and middle-income countries, provide robust evidence that tobacco tax increases, timely dissemination of information about the health risks from smoking, restrictions on smoking in public and work places, comprehensive bans on advertising and promotion, and increased access to cessation therapies are effective in reducing tobacco use and its consequences. Cessation by the 1.1 billion current smokers is central to meaningful reductions in tobacco deaths over the next five decades. Reduced uptake of smoking by children would yield the benefits chiefly after 2050. Price and non-price interventions are, for the most part, highly cost effective.

This chapter begins with an overview of smoking trends and tobacco's health consequences, with a focus on cardiovascular disease mortality and morbidity from smoking. A review of the effectiveness of personal and population-level tobacco control interventions in reducing cardiovascular disease burden follows. Finally, the constraints to implementing tobacco control policies are discussed.

Smoking trends

Tobacco use, in both smoked and non-smoked forms, is common worldwide. This chapter focuses on smoked tobacco because smoked tobacco is more common, accounting for about 65–85% of all tobacco produced worldwide,[1]

Evidence-Based Cardiology, 3rd edition. Edited by S. Yusuf, J.A. Cairns, A.J. Camm, E.L. Fallen, and B.J. Gersh. © 2010 Blackwell Publishing, ISBN: 978-1-4051-5925-8.

and causes more disease and more diverse types of disease than does oral tobacco use.

Prevalence

A systematic review of 139 studies on adult smoking prevalence[2] found that over 1.1 billion people worldwide smoke, with about 82% of smokers residing in low- and middle-income countries. Table 9.1 provides an update of these estimates for the population in 2000. Globally, male smoking far exceeds female smoking, with a smaller gender difference in high-income countries. Smoking prevalence is highest in Eastern Europe and Central, Southern and Eastern Asia, where about 50% of all adults are smokers.

While overall smoking prevalence continues to increase in many low- and middle-income countries, many high-income countries have witnessed decreases, most clearly in men. A study in 36 mostly Western countries, from early 1980 to the mid-1990s, suggested that the decrease in smoking prevalence observed among men was due to the higher prevalence in younger age groups of those who have never smoked. Among women, there was little overall change in smoking prevalence because the increasing prevalence of smokers in younger age cohorts counterbalanced increasing cessation in older age groups.[3]

Cessation

Ex-smoking rates are a good measure of cessation at a population level. In some high-income countries, the prevalence rates of ex-smokers have increased over the past two to three decades. For example, in the United Kingdom, smoking prevalence among males over age 30 fell from 70% in the 1950s to 30% in 2000; female smoking prevalence fell from 40% to 20% over the same period. Much of the decrease arose from cessation. Today, there are twice as many ex-smokers as smokers among those currently aged 50 or over. Currently, 40% of the British male population is

Table 9.1 Estimated smoking prevalence (by gender) and number of smokers, 15 years of age and over, by World Bank Region, 2000

World Bank Region	Smoking prevalence (percent)			Total smokers	
	Males	Females	Overall	Millions	Percent of all smokers
East Asia and Pacific	63	5	34	429	38
Europe and Central Asia	56	17	35	122	11
Latin America and the Caribbean	40	24	32	98	9
Middle East and North Africa	36	5	21	37	3
South Asia	32	6	20	178	15
Sub-Saharan Africa	29	8	18	56	6
Low and middle income	49	8	29	920	82
High income	37	21	29	202	18

made up of former smokers.[4] Polish male cessation rates have also increased, partly due to control programs. One out of every four adult Polish males described himself as an ex-smoker.[5] In contrast, the prevalence of male ex-smokers in most developing countries is low: 10% in Vietnam, 5% in India, and 2% in China.[2,6,7] Even these low figures may be falsely elevated because they include people who quit either because they are too ill to continue or because of early symptoms of tobacco-related illness.[8]

The health consequences of smoking

The health consequences of smoking are often assumed to be widely understood. In fact, there is wide ignorance of the magnitude of tobacco hazards, in terms of individual health and population policy. Thus, the salient aspects of tobacco epidemiology are outlined in this section.

Key messages for the individual smoker

Over 50 years of epidemiology on smoking-related diseases have led to three key messages for individual smokers worldwide.[9,10]
• The eventual risk of death from smoking is high, with about one-half of long-term smokers eventually being killed by their addiction.
• These deaths involve a substantial amount of life-years foregone. At least half of all tobacco deaths occur at ages 35–69, losing about 20–25 years of life, compared to the life expectancy of non-smokers.
• Cessation works. Those adults who quit before middle age avoid almost all the excess hazards of continued smoking.
Globally, an estimated 1.6 million cardiovascular deaths were attributable to smoking in the year 2000; that is, 11% of all global cardiovascular deaths over the age of 30.[11] Detailed epidemiologic reviews of worldwide mortality

from smoking are found elsewhere.[7,12–16] The following discussion focuses on the consequences of smoking on adult cardiovascular mortality.

Key messages for heart health

The wealth of evidence linking smoking and cardiovascular disease points to three key messages pertaining to cardiovascular health.
• Heart attacks and strokes can strike suddenly and can be fatal if treatment is not sought immediately.
• Heart attacks and strokes are made more common by smoking.
• Quitting tobacco use reduces the chance of a heart attack or stroke, with benefits seen shortly after quitting.

Risks of cardiovascular disease from smoking

The relative risks of fatal and non-fatal heart disease associated with smoking from selected studies[7,15,17–20] are depicted in Table 9.2. Overall, the relative risk of non-fatal myocardial infarction is higher than that of fatal disease, and risks are higher for males and at younger ages.

Current mortality and disability from smoking

A recent update of indirect estimates of global tobacco mortality[21] estimated that in 2000 there were 5 million premature deaths caused by tobacco. About half (2.6 million) of these deaths were in low-income countries. Males accounted for 3.7 million deaths, or 72% of all tobacco deaths. About 60% of male and 40% of female tobacco deaths were of middle-aged persons (ages 35–69).

In high-income countries and former socialist economies, the 1 million middle-aged male tobacco deaths were largely composed of cardiovascular disease (0.45 million) and lung cancer (0.21 million). In contrast, in low-income countries, the leading causes of death among the 1.3 million male

Table 9.2 Tobacco use and cardiovascular disease risks in selected studies

Source[1]/setting/study design	Disease[3]	Study population (Age/Smoking status)	OR/RR (95% CI)[4] Overall	Males	Females
Fatal CVD					
1) ACS CPS-II[2] cited in Peto *et al*, 1992 USA; prospective study: 1 million participants	IHD[3] CeVD[3]			2.5 2.7	2.9 3.4
2) Liu *et al*, 1998 China; case–control study: 0.9 million deaths	CVD[3] (ICD-9: 390–415, 418–459)	35–69 yrs		1.2 (1.1–1.2)	1.0 (1.0–1.1)
3) Jha *et al*, 2008 India; case–control study: 152 000 participants	CVD[3] (1CD-10: I00-I99)	30–69 yrs		1.6 (1.5–1.8)[5]	1.7 (1.3–2.1)
Non-fatal CVD					
4) Parish *et al*, 1995 UK; case–control study: 46 315 participants	AMI[3]	30–39 yrs 40–49 yrs 50–59 yrs 60–69 yrs 70–79 yrs	6.3 4.7 3.1 2.5 1.9		
5) Rastogi *et al*, 2005 India; case–control study: 927 participants	AMI[3]	Current smokers Ever smokers Former smokers Never smokers		4.7 (3.2–6.9) 3.9 (2.8–5.6) 2.6 (1.6–4.3) 1.0	
6) Teo *et al*, 2006 52 countries; case–control study: 27 089 participants	AMI[3]	Smoking + chewing Current smoking Bidi smoking only Tobacco chewing only Ex-smoking Passive smoking	4.09 (2.98–5.61) 2.95 (2.77–3.14) 2.89 (2.11–3.96) 2.23 (1.41–3.52) 1.87 (1.55–2.24) 1.2–1.6		

[1] References: 7, 15, 17–20

[2] American Cancer Society – Second Cancer Prevention Study

[3] IHD, ischemic heart disease; CeVD, cerebral vascular disease; CVD, cardiovascular disease; AMI, acute myocardial infarction;

[4] OR/RR (95% CI), odds ratio/ relative risk (95% confidence interval)

[5] 99% confidence interval

tobacco deaths were cardiovascular disease (0.4 million), chronic obstructive pulmonary disease (0.2 million), other respiratory disease (chiefly tuberculosis, 0.2 million) and lung cancer (0.18 million). The specific numbers of deaths from tobacco and of total disability-adjusted life-years (DALYs) by gender are shown in Table 9.3.[21,22] Disability estimates are not discussed here; however, disability is highly correlated with mortality in most settings.

Cardiovascular mortality from smoking

Cardiovascular disease (CVD), which includes heart diseases and stroke, is the leading cause of death worldwide. Long a problem in high-income countries, CVD is now recognized as a global problem. CVD accounted for more

than one-quarter of all deaths worldwide in 2001, with four-fifths of those deaths occurring in low- and middle-income countries.

Of the 1.6 million cardiovascular deaths worldwide in the year 2000, 1.2 million were among men and 0.4 million among women. There were 0.9 million deaths in industrialized regions and 0.7 million deaths in the developing world. The proportion of adult cardiovascular deaths attributable to smoking was 17% for men and 5% for women.[11]

The estimated numbers of cardiovascular deaths attributable to smoking, disaggregated by region and sex, are depicted in Table 9.4. The proportions of total adult cardiovascular deaths attributable to smoking were generally

Table 9.3 Tobacco mortality and total disability-adjusted life years by gender and World Bank Region, 2000

World Bank Region	Tobacco deaths (thousands)		Total DALYs (thousands)	
	Males	Females	Males	Females
Low and middle income	2730	813	44044	13357
High income	929	548	12304	6866
World	3659	1361	56347	20222

DALYs, disability-adjusted life years
References: 21,22

highest in industrialized regions (12–22%), where smoking has been common for several decades. At the same time, the increase in smoking over the last quarter of the 20th century in a number of developing regions, including parts of Southeast Asia, Latin America and the Eastern Mediterranean, has resulted in ≥10% of all current adult cardiovascular deaths being attributable to smoking, the number being higher among men.[11]

Disease-specific patterns

Ezzati *et al*[11] have estimated the total cardiovascular mortality attributable to smoking for all adults aged 30 years and over by three clusters of cardiovascular diseases (CVD): ischemic heart disease (IHD), cerebrovascular disease (CeVD), and a cluster of "other cardiovascular diseases including heart failure". IHD accounted for the largest number of cardiovascular deaths attributable to smoking (870000 deaths; 54% of all smoking-attributable cardiovascular deaths) globally. This was similar in both developing and industrialized regions. The difference between the two regions, however, was that cerebrovascular disease was the second most common cause of deaths (30%) in developing countries while it was least common (22%) in industrialized countries.

Past and future trends in mortality

Future increases in tobacco deaths worldwide are expected to arise from increased smoking by males in developing countries, and by women worldwide. Such increases are a product of population growth and increased age-specific tobacco mortality rates, the latter relating to both smoking duration and the amount of tobacco smoked. Peto *et al*[23] have made the following calculation: if the proportion of young people taking up smoking continues to be about half of men and one-tenth of women, then there will be about 30 million new long-term smokers each year. As noted above, epidemiologic studies in developed and developing countries suggest that half of these smokers will eventually

die from smoking. However, conservatively assuming that "only" about one-third of smokers die as a result of smoking, then smoking will eventually kill about 10 million people a year. Thus, for the 25-year period from 2000–2025, there would be about 150 million tobacco deaths or about 6 million deaths per year on average; from 2025–2050, there would be about 300 million tobacco deaths, or about 12 million deaths per year.

Further estimations are more uncertain but based upon current smoking trends and projected population growth, from 2050–2100 there would be an additional 500 million tobacco deaths. These projections for the next three to four decades are comparable to retrospective and early prospective epidemiologic studies in China,[6,15,16] which suggest that annual tobacco deaths will rise to 1 million before 2010 and 2 million by 2025, when the young adult smokers of today reach old age. Similarly, results from a large retrospective study in India indicate that the annual number of deaths from smoking will be about 1 million during the 2010s, with about 70% (600000 among men and 100000 among women) occurring in middle age, rather than old age.[7] With other populations in Asia, Eastern Europe, Latin America, the Middle East and, less certainly, sub-Saharan Africa showing similar growth in population and age-specific tobacco death rates, the estimate of some 450 million tobacco deaths over the next five decades appears to be plausible. Almost all of these deaths will be among current smokers.

Benefits of tobacco cessation

Current tobacco mortality statistics reflect past smoking behavior, given the long delay between the onset of smoking and the development of disease. The prevention of a substantial proportion of these tobacco deaths before 2050 requires adult cessation. For example, halving the per capita adult consumption of tobacco by 2020 (akin to the declines in adult smoking in the United Kingdom) would avert about 180 million tobacco deaths. Continuing to reduce the percentage of children who start to smoke will prevent many deaths, but its main effect will be on mortality rates in 2050 and beyond (Fig. 9.1).[6,24–26]

There is substantial evidence that smoking cessation reduces the risk of death from tobacco-related diseases. Among doctors in the United Kingdom, those who quit smoking before the onset of major disease avoided most of the excess hazards of smoking.[10] The benefits of quitting were largest in those who quit before middle age (between ages 25 and 34 years), but were still significant in those who quit later (between ages 45 and 54 years).

Benefits of cessation on cardiovascular disease burden

Smoking cessation interventions have been identified to be effective in the general population of smokers for primary

Table 9.4 Estimated cardiovascular mortality attributable to smoking in 14 epidemiologic subregions of the world, 2000

Region-mortality stratum	Adult population (30 yrs +), millions		Smoking-attributable cardiovascular mortality		Proportion of total adult (30 yrs +) cardiovascular mortality, %		
	M	F	M	F	M	F	M + F
Developing countries							
AFR-D	41	43	10 000	3000	6	1	3
AFR-E	47	50	17 000	11 000	10	4	6
AMR-B	85	92	50 000	26 000	15	7	11
AMR-D	12	12	1000	500	3	1	2
EMR-B	25	22	22 000	6000	16	5	11
EMR-D	52	52	41 000	9000	12	3	8
SEAR-B	61	62	45 000	6000	18	2	10
SEAR-D	244	235	249 000	48 000	17	3	10
WPR-B	374	367	85 000	38 000	6	2	4
Industrialized countries							
AMR-A	91	98	91 000	126 000	23	21	22
EUR-A	125	137	135 000	66 000	23	7	13
EUR-B	50	54	121 000	38 000	27	7	16
EUR-C	63	80	282 000	55 000	35	5	17
WPR-A	47	51	22 000	19 000	16	10	12
World	**1317**	**1355**	**1171 000**	**451 500**	**17**	**5**	**11**

Mortality stratum: A indicates very low child mortality and very low adult mortality; B, low child mortality and low adult mortality; C, low child mortality and high adult mortality; D, high child mortality and high adult mortality; E, very high child mortality and very high adult mortality
Regions: AFR-Africa; AMR-America; EUR-Europe; EMR-Eastern Mediterranean; SEAR-South East Asian; WPR-Western Pacific
Countries: AFR-D: Algeria, Angola, Benin, Burkina Faso, Cameroon, Cape Verde, Chad, Comoros, Equitorial Guinea, Gabon, Gambia, Ghana, Guinea, Guinea-Bissau, Liberia, Madagascar, Mali, Mauritania, Niger, Nigeria, Sao Tome & Principe, Senegal, Seychelles, Sierra Leone, Togo. AFR-E: Botswana, Burundi, Central African Republic, Congo, Cote d'Ivoire, Congo, Eritrea, Ethiopia, Kenya, Lesotho, Malawi, Mozambique, Namibia, Rwanda, South Africa, Swaziland, Uganda, Tanzania, Zambia, Zimbabwe. AMR-A: Canada, Cuba, United States. AMR-B: Antigua, Argentina, Bahamas, Barbados, Belize, Brazil, Chile, Colombia, Costa Rica, Dominica, Dominican Republic, El Salvador, Grenada, Guyana, Honduras, Jamaica, Mexico, Panama, Paraguay, St. Kitts, St. Lucia, St. Vincent, Suriname, Trinidad & Tobago, Uruguay, Venezuela. AMR-D: Bolivia, Ecuador, Guatemala, Haiti, Nicaragua, Peru. EMR-B: Bahrain, Cyprus, Iran, Jordan, Kuwait, Lebanon, Libya, Oman, Qatar, Saudi Arabia, Syria, Tunisia, United Arab Emirates. EMR-D: Afghanistan, Djibouti, Egypt, Iraq, Morocco, Pakistan, Somalia, Sudan, Yemen. EUR-A: Andorra, Austria, Belgium, Croatia, Czech Republic, Denmark, Finland, France, Germany, Greece, Iceland, Ireland, Israel, Italy, Luxembourg, Malta, Monaco, Netherlands, Norway, Portugal, San Marino, Slovenia, Spain, Sweden, Switzerland, United Kingdom. EUR-B: Albania, Armenia, Azerbaijan, Bosnia, Bulgaria, Georgia, Kyrghyzstan, Poland, Romania, Slovakia, Tajikistan, Macedonia, Turkey, Turkmenistan, Uzbekistan, Yugoslavia. EUR-C: Belarus, Estonia, Hungary, Kazakhstan, Latvia, Lithuania, Moldova, Russia, Ukraine. SEAR-B: Indonesia, Sri Lanka, Thailand. SEAR-D: Bangladesh, Bhutan, North Korea, India, Maldives, Myanmar, Nepal. WPR-A: Australia, Brunei, Japan, New Zealand, Singapore. WPR-B: Cambodia, China, Cook Islands, Fiji, Kiribati, Laos, Malaysia, Marshall Islands, Micronesia, Mongolia, Nauru, Niue, Palau, Papua New Guinea, Philippines, South Korea, Samoa, Solomon Islands, Tongo, Tuvalu, Vanuatu, Vietnam.
Source: 11

prevention of heart disease. In a pooled cohort study of over 19 000 normal adults with a mean duration of follow-up of 13.8 years, it was noticed that people who stopped smoking had a decreased risk of myocardial infarction (hazard ratio (HR) 0.71, 95% confidence interval (CI) 0.59–0.85), after adjustment for other risk factors.[27]

Quitting smoking has also been found to be effective in patients with cardiovascular disease in the prevention of recurrence of further fatal and non-fatal cardiovascular events. Patients who quit smoking after successful percu-taneous coronary intervention were at lower risk for rein-farction and death than those who continued to smoke.[28] In those who had undergone coronary artery bypass grafting, it was associated with reduced long-term mortal-ity (relative risk (RR) 0.4–0.6) and need for repeat inter-ventions (RR 0.6–0.7).[29,30] Efficacy of tobacco cessation strategies in reducing subsequent cardiovascular mortality up to 50% has been shown in both hospital-based and clinic-based settings for smokers with coronary heart disease.[31–34]

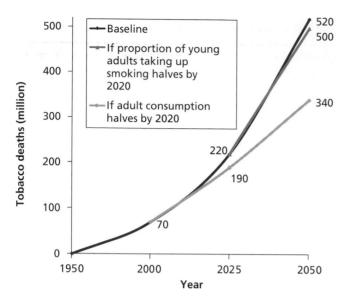

Figure 9.1 Tobacco deaths in the next 50 years under current smoking patterns. Note: Peto and others (1994) estimate 60 million tobacco deaths between 1950 and 2000 in industrial countries. This figure estimates an additional 10 million between 1990 and 2000 in developing countries. The figure also assumes no tobacco deaths before 1990 in developing countries and minimal tobacco deaths worldwide before 1950. Projections for deaths from 2000 to 2050 are based on Peto and Lopez, 2000[24,26].

Interventions to reduce demand for tobacco

Numerous studies, mostly from high-income countries, have examined the impact of interventions aimed at reducing the demand for tobacco products on smoking and other kinds of tobacco use. The small but growing number of studies from low- and middle-income countries provide useful lessons about differences in the impact of these interventions between these countries and high-income countries. The following is a review of the impact of price and non-price interventions to reduce demand for smoking, including a discussion of each intervention's impact on initiation and cessation.

Tobacco taxation

Well over 100 studies from high-income countries clearly demonstrate that increased taxes on cigarettes and other tobacco products lead to significant reductions in cigarette smoking and other tobacco use.[35] The reductions in tobacco use that result from higher taxes and prices reflect the combination of increased smoking cessation, reduced relapse, lower smoking initiation, and decreased consumption among continuing tobacco users.

Studies from the United States, United Kingdom, Canada, and many other high-income countries generally estimate that the price elasticity of cigarette demand ranges from –0.25 to –0.50, indicating that a 10% increase in cigarette prices will reduce overall cigarette smoking by 2.5–5.0%.[35,36] Estimates from a limited number of studies from low- and middle-income countries suggest a greater price elasticity of –0.8 in such countries. A recent study from India shows the "crowding-out" effect of tobacco expenditure and its implications on household resource allocation in India: tobacco-consuming households had lower per capita nutrition intake and also lower consumption of certain commodities such as milk, education, clean fuels, and entertainment.[37] Other studies using survey data have concluded that half or more of the effect of price on overall cigarette demand results from reducing the number of current smokers.[38,39] Higher taxes increase both the number of attempts at quitting smoking and the success of those attempts.[40,41] A study in the United States suggested that a 10% increase in price would result in 11–13% shorter smoking duration or a 3.4% higher probability of cessation.[40]

In the United States and the United Kingdom, increases in the price of cigarettes have had the greatest impact on smoking among the lowest income and least educated populations.[38,42] Furthermore, it was estimated that smokers in US households below median income level are four times more responsive to price increases than smokers in households above median income level. In general, estimates of price elasticity for low- and middle-income countries are about double those estimated for high-income countries, implying that significant increases in tobacco taxes in these countries would be effective in reducing tobacco use.

Restrictions on smoking

Over the past three decades, as the quantity and quality of information about the health consequences of exposure to passive smoking have increased, many governments, especially in high-income countries, have enacted legislation restricting smoking in a variety of public places and private worksites. In addition, increased awareness of the consequences of passive smoking exposure, particularly to children, has led many workplaces and households to adopt voluntary restrictions on smoking. While the intention of these restrictions is to reduce non-smokers' exposure to passive tobacco smoke, the policies also reduce smokers' opportunities to smoke. Additional reductions in smoking, especially among youth, will result from the changes in social norms that are introduced by adopting these policies.[43]

In Western populations, comprehensive restrictions on cigarette smoking have been estimated to reduce population smoking rates by 5–15%,[44,45] and can also lead to changes in social norms regarding smoking behavior, especially among youth. As with higher taxes, these restrictions reduce both the prevalence of smoking and cigarette consumption among current smokers. Smoking bans in workplaces generally reduce the quantity of cigarettes smoked by 5–25%, and reduce prevalence rates by up to 20%.[45] The no-smoking policies were most effective when strong social norms against smoking helped to make smoking restrictions self-enforcing.

Clean indoor air laws that ban smoking in public places may lead to significant reductions in the prevalence of smoking and cigarette consumption.[46] This may reduce the proportion of population exposed to environmental tobacco smoke which could in turn lead to a reduction in smoking-related diseases. For this and other reasons, many jurisdictions are implementing laws banning smoking in public places. Current interest in preventive cardiology is to examine whether enactment of legislation to require smoke-free workplaces and public spaces might be associated with a decline in hospital admissions for and deaths due to acute myocardial infarction. Some of the earliest and most robust evidence came from the California Tobacco Control Program in the last decade.[47] This program combined a 25 cent tax increase (20% of which went to pay for the tobacco control program) with an aggressive media campaign along with community-based interventions promoting clean indoor air policies. Since then there has been consistent evidence of the positive impact of clean air ordinances on cardiovascular health from North America and Europe where jurisdictions have gone smoke free. These offer non-randomized designs of before-and-after studies (some with concurrent control groups) to assess the efficacy of smoke-free policies to effectively reduce heart disease rapidly (Table 9.5).[47–54] Class of recommendation and level of evidence for these tobacco control interventions are shown using the grading schema as per the ACC/AHA (American College of Cardiology/American Heart Association) guidelines.[55]

Health information and counter-advertising

The 1962 report by the British Royal College of Physicians and the 1964 US Surgeon General's Report were landmark tobacco control events in high-income countries. These publications resulted in the first widespread press coverage of the scientific links between smoking and lung cancer. The reports were followed, in many countries, by policies requiring health warning labels on tobacco products, which were later extended to tobacco advertising.

Research from high-income countries indicates that these initial reports and the publicity that followed about the health consequences of smoking led to significant reductions in consumption, with initial declines of between 4% and 9%, and longer-term cumulative declines of 15–30%.[56,57] Efforts to disseminate information about the risks of smoking and

of other tobacco use in low- and middle-income countries have led to similar declines in tobacco use in these countries.[56] In addition, mass media anti-smoking campaigns, in many cases funded by earmarked tobacco taxes, have generated reductions in cigarette smoking and other tobacco usage.[56,58] Decreases in smoking prevalence were largest in Western countries where the public is constantly and consistently reminded of the dangers of smoking by extensive coverage of issues related to tobacco in the news media.[3]

In many low- and middle-income countries, there continues to be a lack of awareness of the risks of mortality and disease posed by smoking. For example, a national survey in China in 1996 found that 61% of smokers thought that tobacco did them "little or no harm".[59] In high-income countries, smokers are aware of the risks but a recent review of psychologic studies found that few smokers judge the size of these risks to be higher and more established than do non-smokers, and that smokers minimize the personal relevance of these risks.[60]

Bans on advertising and promotion

Cigarettes are among the most heavily advertised and promoted products in the world. In 2001, cigarette companies spent US$11.2 billion on advertising and promotion in the United States alone, the highest spending level reported to date.[61] Tobacco advertising efforts worldwide include traditional forms of advertising on television, radio, and billboards; in magazines and newspapers; favorable product placement; price-related promotions, such as coupons and multi-pack discounts; and sponsorship of highly visible sporting and cultural events.

Numerous econometric studies, mostly from the United States and the United Kingdom, have explored the relationship between cigarette advertising and promotional expenditure and cigarette demand. In general, these studies have resulted in mixed findings, with most studies concluding that advertising has, at most, a small positive impact on demand.[35,57] However, critics of these studies note that econometric methods, which estimate the impact of a marginal change in advertising expenditures on smoking, are ill suited for studying the impact of advertising.[57,61,62] Approaches employed by other disciplines, including survey research and experiments that assess reactions to and recall of cigarette advertising, do support the hypothesis that increases in cigarette advertising and promotion directly and indirectly increase cigarette demand and smoking initiation.[43,63] These studies conclude that cigarette advertising is effective in getting and retaining children's attention, with the strength of the association strongly correlated with current smoking behavior, smoking initiation, and smoking intentions.

Advertising and promotion bans on cigarette smoking should provide more direct evidence on the impact of

Table 9.5 Population tobacco interventions and impact on CVD disease burden

Reference[47-54]	Study design	Study setting and interventions	Impact on CVD mortality/morbidity (effect size)	Evidence
Fichtenberg & Glantz, 2000	Before and after study at multiple intervals	California tobacco control program (state-wide) pre-1989: no intervention 1989–1992: cigarettes surtax 1992–1997: weakening of laws through taxcuts	 California heart disease death rates comparable to rest of US pre-1989 Death rates 13% lower than expected Rose again but not as high as rest of US	**Class IIa, Level B**
Sargent and others, 2004	Before and after study	Helena, Montana Complete smoke ban for 6 months & then reversal	Significant drop in admissions for AMI by −16 admissions (95% CI = −31.7 to -0.3)	**Class IIa, Level B**
Barone-Adesi and others, 2006	Before and after study	Piedmont region in northern Italy Pre-ban period: October– December 2004 National laws banning smoking: Feb–Jun 2005	RR (95% CI) = 0.89 (0.81–0.98) in Piedmont region 11% reduction in admissions for AMI among those aged 60 years+ (Additional evidence: 8.9% drop in cigarette sales, 7.6% reduction in cigarette consumption, >90% drop in nicotine vapor phase concentration in pubs & discos)	**Class IIa, Level B**
Bartecchi and others, 2006	Before and after with control	Pueblo, Colorado, US (control: El Paso, Colo) Local smoke-free ordinance in Pueblo 1.5 yrs before ban & 1.5 yrs after ban	Drop in AMI hospital admissions RR (95% CI) = 0.73 (0.63–0.85) after ban in Pueblo RR (95% CI) = 0.97 (0.89–1.06) during same period in El Paso	**Class IIa, Level B**
Juster and others, 2007	Before and after study	New York state Smoking ban since year 2003	8% reduction in hospital admission for AMI in the year 2004 after the ban No reduction in stroke admission $56 million savings in direct healthcare costs	**Class IIa, Level B**
Seo & Torabi, 2007	Before and after with control	Monroe County, Indiana (control: Delaware) Local smoking ban	Significant drop in hospital admissions in Monroe Non-significant drop in hospital admissions in Delaware	**Class IIa, Level B**
Khuder and others, 2007	Before and after with control	Bowling Green, Ohio (control: Kent, Ohio) Clean indoor air ordinance 1999–2005	Drop in hospital admissions for AMI Drop by 39% after 1 year and 47% after 3 years in Bowling Green No significant change in Kent	**Class IIa, Level B**
Cesaroni and others, 2008	Before and after study	Rome, Italy City-wide ban in 2005	Drop in hospitalization for acute coronary events Reduction of 11.2% (95% CI = 6.9% to 15.3%) during 2005 compared to previous 4 years	

Table 9.6 Tobacco cessation interventions and impact on CVD disease burden

Reference[67,68]	Study design	Outcomes	Impact on CVD mortality/ morbidity	Evidence
Critchley & Capewell, 2004	Systematic review of 20 studies (12 603 patients)	Secondary prevention of heart disease; reduction in fatal & non-fatal myocardial infarction	36% reduction in mortality: RR (95% CI) = 0.64(0.58–0.71) Reduction in non-fatal MI: RR (95% CI) = 0.68 (0.55–0.80)	**Class I, Level A**
Wilson and others, Med 2000	Meta-analysis of 12 cohorts (5878 patients)	Reduction in mortality after acute myocardial infarction	46% reduction in mortality: RR (95% CI) = 0.54(0.46–0.62)	**Class I, Level A**

advertising.[58] One study using data from 22 high-income countries for the period 1970 through 1992 provides strong evidence that comprehensive bans on cigarette advertising and promotion lead to significant reductions in cigarette smoking. The study predicted that a comprehensive set of tobacco advertising bans in high-income countries could reduce tobacco consumption by over 6%, taking into account price and non-price control interventions.[64] However, the study concludes that partial bans have little impact on smoking behavior, given that the tobacco industry can shift its resources from banned media to other media that are not banned.

Smoking cessation treatments

Near-term reductions in smoking-related mortality depend heavily on smoking cessation. There are numerous behavioral smoking cessation treatments available, including self-help manuals, community-based programs, and minimal or intensive clinical interventions.[36] In clinical settings, pharmacologic treatments, including nicotine replacement therapies (NRT) and bupropion, have become much more widely available in recent years in high-income countries through deregulation of some NRTs from prescription to over-the-counter status.[36,65] The evidence is strong and consistent that pharmacologic treatments significantly improve the likelihood of quitting, with success rates two to three times those when pharmaceutical treatments are not employed.[36,65,66] The effectiveness of all commercially available NRTs seems to be largely independent of the duration of therapy, the setting in which the NRT is provided, regulatory status (over-the-counter versus prescribed), and the type of provider.[65] Over-the-counter NRTs without physician oversight have been used in many countries for a number of years with good success.

While successful in treating nicotine addiction, the markets for NRT and other pharmacologic therapies are more highly regulated and less affordable than are nicotine-containing tobacco products. Recent evidence indicates that the demand for NRT is related to economic factors, including price.[41] Policies that decrease the cost of NRT and increase availability, such as mandating private health insurance coverage of NRT, including NRT coverage in public health insurance programs, and subsidizing NRT for uninsured or underinsured individuals, would likely lead to substantial increases in the use of these products. Given the demonstrated efficacy of NRTs in treating smoking, these policies could generate significant increases in smoking cessation.

Over a hundred trials using NRT and nearly two dozen trials using bupropion have shown them to be safe and efficacious tobacco cessation interventions. A systematic review of 20 studies by the Cochrane group has shown a 36% reduction in crude relative risk of mortality for patients with CHD who quit compared to those who continued to smoke (RR 0.64, 95% CI 0.58–0.71).[67] A meta-analysis of 12 cohorts also revealed a 46% risk reduction (odds ratio (OR) 0.54, 95% CI 0.46–0.62) displaying consistency of effect across many regions of the world (Table 9.6).[68]

Effectiveness and cost effectiveness of tobacco control interventions

Using a static model of the cohort of smokers alive in 2000, we estimate the number of smoking-attributable deaths over the next few decades that could be averted by (a) price increases, (b) NRT, and (c) a package of non-price interventions other than NRT. Cost effectiveness of these policy interventions was calculated by weighing the approximate public sector costs against the years of healthy life saved, measured in DALYs. The details of this model have been published previously.[69]

Results of model projections

The following is an updated analysis, using higher price increases and a greater effectiveness for NRT. This analysis is conservative in its assumptions about effectiveness, and generous in its assumptions about the costs of tobacco control.

Potential impact of price increases

With a price increase of 33%, it is predicted that 22–65 million smoking-attributable deaths will be averted worldwide, which is approximately equivalent to 5–15% of all smoking-attributable deaths expected among those who smoke in 2000; see Table 9.7. Low- and middle-income countries account for about 90% of averted deaths. Total smoking-attributable deaths averted worldwide ranges from 33 million to 92 million for a 50% price increase and 46 million to 114 million for a 70% price increase. A 70% price increase would avert 10–26% of all smoking-attributable deaths worldwide.

Of the tobacco-related deaths that would be averted by a price increase, 80% would be male, reflecting the higher overall prevalence of smoking in men. The greatest relative impact of a price increase on deaths averted is among younger age cohorts. Note that these projections use conservative price increases. In certain countries, such as South Africa and Poland, recent tax increases have doubled the real price of cigarettes.[70]

Potential impact of nicotine replacement therapy

Provision of NRT with an effectiveness of 1% is predicted to result in the avoidance of about 3.5 million smoking-attributable deaths (Table 9.8). NRT of 5% effectiveness will have about five times the impact. Again, low- and middle-income countries would account for roughly 80% of the averted deaths. The relative impact of NRT (of 2.5% effectiveness) on deaths averted is 2–3% among individuals aged 15–59, and lower among those aged 60 and older (results not shown).

Potential impact of non-price interventions other than NRT

A package of non-price interventions, other than NRT, that decreases the prevalence of smoking by 2% is predicted to prevent about 7 million smoking-attributable deaths (more than 1.6% of all smoking-attributable deaths among those who smoked in 2000; see Table 9.8). A package of interventions that decreases the prevalence of smoking by 10% would have an impact five times greater. Low- and middle-

Table 9.7 Potential impact of price increases of 10%, 33%, 50%, and 70% on tobacco mortality by World Bank Region, 2000

World Bank Region	Smoking attributable deaths in millions	Change in number of deaths in millions					
		33% price increase		50% price increase		70% price increase	
		Low	High	Low	High	Low	High
Low and middle income (percent)	362	−19.7 (−5.4)	−56.8 (−15.7)	−29.8 (−8.2)	−79.2 (−21.9)	−41.7 (−11.5)	−98.2 (−27.1)
High income (percent)	81	−2.1 (−2.6)	−8.5 (−10.6)	−3.2 (−4.0)	−12.2 (−15.1)	−4.5 (−5.6)	−16.2 (−20.0)
World (percent)	443	−21.8 (−4.9)	−65.3 (−14.7)	−33.0 (−7.5)	−91.5 (−20.7)	−46.2 (−10.4)	−114.3 (−25.8)

Table 9.8 Potential impact of price increase of 33%, increased NRT use, and a package of non-price measures, 2000

World Bank Region	Smoking attributable deaths in millions	Change in number of deaths in millions					
		33% price increase		NRT effectiveness		Non-price intervention effectiveness	
		Low elasticity	High elasticity	1.0%	5.0%	2%	10%
Low and middle income (percent)	362	−19.7 (−5.4)	−56.8 (−15.7)	−2.9 (−0.8)	−14.3 (−4.0)	−5.7 (−1.6)	−28.6 (−7.9)
High income (percent)	81	−2.1 (−2.6)	−8.5 (−10.6)	−0.6 (−0.8)	−3.1 (−3.8)	−1.2 (−1.5)	−6.1 (−7.6)
World (percent)	443	−21.8 (−4.9)	−65.3 (−14.8)	−3.5 (−0.8)	−17.4 (−3.9)	−6.9 (−1.6)	−34.7 (−7.8)

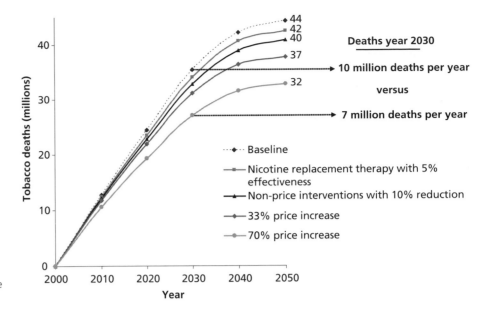

Figure 9.2 Potential impact of price increase, NRT use and a package of non-price interventions, 2000[22].

income countries would account for approximately four-fifths of quitters and averted deaths. The greatest relative impact of non-price interventions on deaths averted would be among younger age cohorts.

Figure 9.2 summarizes the potential impact of a set of independent tobacco control interventions, using 33% and 70% price increases (employing a high elasticity of –1.2 for low- and middle-income regions and –0.8 for high-income regions), a 5% effectiveness of NRT, and a 10% reduction from non-price interventions other than NRT. In this cohort of smokers alive in 2000, approximately 443 million are expected to die in the next 50 years in the absence of interventions. A substantial fraction of these tobacco deaths are avoidable with interventions. Price increases have the greatest impact on tobacco mortality, with the most aggressive price increase of 70% having the potential to avert almost one-quarter of all tobacco deaths. Even a modest price increase of 33% could potentially prevent 66 million tobacco deaths over the course of the next 50 year. While NRTs and other non-price interventions are less effective than price increases, they can still avert a substantial number of tobacco deaths (18 million and 35 million deaths, respectively). The greatest impact of these tobacco control interventions would occur after 2010, but a substantial number of deaths could be avoided even before that.

Note that no attempt has been made in this analysis to examine the impact of combining the various packages of interventions (for example, price increases with NRT, or NRT and other non-price interventions). Although a number of studies have compared the impact of price and non-price interventions, few empiric attempts have been made to assess how these interventions might interact. While price increases have been found in this analysis to

be the most cost-effective anti-smoking intervention, policy makers should use both price and non-price interventions to counter smoking. Non-price measures may be required to impact the most heavily dependent smokers, for whom medical and social support in stopping will be necessary. Furthermore, these non-price measures may be effective in increasing social acceptance and support of tobacco price increases.

Comprehensive tobacco control programs

In recent years, several governments, mostly in high-income countries, have adopted comprehensive programs to reduce tobacco use, often funded by earmarked tobacco tax revenues. These programs generally have similar goals for reducing tobacco use, including preventing initiation among youth and young adults, promoting cessation among all smokers, reducing exposure to passive tobacco smoke, and identifying and eliminating disparities among population subgroups.[43] Furthermore, these programs have one or more of four key components: community interventions engaging a diverse set of local organizations; counter-marketing and health information campaigns; program policies and regulations (such as taxes, restrictions on smoking, bans on tobacco advertising, and access to better cessation treatments); and surveillance and evaluation of potential issues, such as smuggling.[43,71] Programs have placed differing emphases on these four components, with substantial diversity among the types of activities supported within each component. Disaggregating current tobacco control program spending reveals that the greatest impact can be achieved through a focus on macro-level changes, such as policy change. Recent analyses from the United States and United Kingdom clearly indicate that these comprehensive efforts have been successful in reducing tobacco use and in improving public health.[42,43,72] In California, for example, the state's comprehensive tobacco control program has produced a rate of decline in tobacco use double that seen in the rest of the United States.[73]

Current estimates of the costs of implementing a comprehensive tobacco control program range from US$2.50 to US$10 per capita in the United States. The Centers for Disease Control and Prevention recommends spending US$6 to US$16 per capita for a comprehensive tobacco control program in the United States.[74] Canadian spending on tobacco control programs was approximately US$1.65 per capita in 1996.[75] At the highest recommending spending level (US$16 per capita) in the United States, annual funding for a comprehensive tobacco program would equal only 0.9% of US public spending, per capita, on health.

Evidence from the United States demonstrates that states with the greatest prevalence of smoking have a greater marginal impact with their tobacco control spending, suggesting that the potential gains from modest investments in comprehensive tobacco control measures are large. Each US$10 spent per capita on tobacco control annually has resulted in a 55% reduction (variation of 20–70%) in per capita cigarette consumption.[76] In the United States, US$10 translated into 0.03% of per capita GDP in 2003.

Conclusion

Worldwide, there are only two large and growing causes of death. One is HIV-1 infection and the other is tobacco. Tobacco is responsible for 10% of all deaths globally.[77] On current consumption patterns, about 1 billion people in the 21st century will be killed by their addiction to tobacco. There is strong evidence that tobacco tax increases, the dissemination of information about the health risks from smoking, restrictions on smoking in public places and workplaces, comprehensive bans on advertising and promotion, and increased access to cessation therapies are effective in reducing tobacco use. There is increasing evidence that they are also beneficial in reducing cardiovascular mortality and morbidity among both smokers and others. Reduction in tobacco use is at least partially responsible for the decrease of cardiovascular disease burden seen in the US.[78] Despite this evidence, these policies have been applied aggressively only in high-income countries, covering a small proportion of the world's smokers. Limited implementation of effective tobacco control for reducing cardiovascular disease burden in developing countries is due to political constraints as well as the lack

of awareness of the effectiveness and cost effectiveness of these interventions.

References

1. World Health Organization. *Tobacco or Heath: A Global Status Report*. Geneva: World Health Organization; 1997.
2. Jha P, Ranson MK, Nguyen SN, Yach D. Estimates of global and regional smoking prevalence in 1995 by age and sex. *Am J Public Health* 2002;**92**(6):1002–6.
3. Molarius A, Parsons RW, Dobson AJ *et al.* Trends in cigarette smoking in 36 populations from the early 1980s to the mid-1990s: findings from the WHO MONICA project. *Am J Public Health* 2001;**91**(2):206–12.
4. Peto R, Darby S, Deo H *et al.* Smoking, smoking cessation and lung cancer in the UK since 1950: combination of national statistics with two case-control studies. *BMJ* 2000;**321**(7257):323–9.
5. Zatonski W, Jha P. *The Health Transformation in Eastern Europe after 1990: A Second Look*. Warsaw: Marie Sklodowska-Curie Cancer Center and Institute of Oncology, 2000.
6. Jha P, Chaloupka FJ, eds. *Tobacco Control in Developing Countries*. Oxford: Oxford University Press, 2000.
7. Jha P, Jacob B, Gajalakshmi V *et al.* A nationally representative case-control study of smoking and death in India. *N Engl J Med* 2008;**358**(11):1137–47.
8. Martinson BC, O'Connor PJ, Pronk NP, Rolnick SJ. Smoking cessation attempts in relation to prior health care changes: the effect of antecedent smoking-related symptoms? *Am J Health Promot* 2003;**18**(2):125–32.
9. Peto R, Lopez A, Boreham J, Thun M. *Mortality from Smoking in Developed Countries*, 2nd ed. Oxford: Oxford University Press, 2003.
10. Doll R, Peto R, Boreham J, Sutherland I. Mortality in relation to smoking: 50 years' observation on male British doctors. *BMJ* 2004;**328**(7455):1519–28.
11. Ezzati M, Henley SJ, Thun MJ, Lopez AD. Role of smoking in global and regional cardiovascular mortality. *Circulation* 2005;**112**(4):489–97.
12. Gajalakshmi CK, Jha P, Ranson K, Nguyen S. Global patterns of smoking and smoking-attributable mortality. In: Jha P, Chaloupka FJ, eds. *Tobacco Control in Developing Countries*. Oxford: Oxford University Press, 2000.
13. Gajalakshmi V, Peto R, Kanaka TS, Jha P. Smoking and mortality from tuberculosis and other diseases in India: retrospective study of 43,000 adult male deaths and 35,000 controls. *Lancet* 2003;**362**(9883):507–15.
14. Gupta PC, Mehta HC. Cohort study of all-cause mortality amongst tobacco users in Mumbai, India. *Bull World Health Organ* 2000;**78**(7):877–83.
15. Liu BQ, Peto R, Chen ZM *et al.* Emerging tobacco hazards in China: 1. Retrospective proportional mortality study of one million deaths. *BMJ* 1998;**317**(7170):1411–22.
16. Niu SR, Yang GH, Chen ZM *et al.* Emerging tobacco hazards in China: 2. Early mortality results from a prospective study. *BMJ* 1998;**317**(7170):1423–4.
17. Peto R, Lopez AD, Boreham J *et al.* Mortality from tobacco in developed countries: indirect estimation from national vital statistics. *Lancet* 1992;**339**(8804):1268–78.

18. Parish S, Collins R, Peto R *et al.* Cigarette smoking, tar yields, and non-fatal myocardial infarction: 14,000 cases and 32,000 controls in the United Kingdom. The International Studies of Infarct Survival (ISIS) Collaborators. *BMJ* 1995;**311**(7003):471–7.

19. Rastogi T, Jha P, Reddy KS *et al.* Bidi and cigarette smoking and risk of acute myocardial infarction among males in urban India. *Tob Control* 2005;**14**(5):356–8.

20. Teo KK, Ounpuu S, Hawken S *et al.* Tobacco use and risk of myocardial infarction in 52 countries in the INTERHEART Study: a case-control study. *Lancet* 2006;**368**(9536):647–58.

21. Ezzati M, Lopez AD. Estimates of global mortality attributable to smoking in 2000. *Lancet* 2003;**362**(9387):847–52.

22. Jha P, Chaloupka FJ, Moore J *et al.* Tobacco addiction. In: Jamison DT, Breman JG, Measham AR, eds. *Disease Control Priorities in Developing Countries*, 2nd edn. New York: Oxford University Press, 2006;869–86.

23. Peto R, Lopez A, Boreham J *et al. Mortality from Smoking in Developed Countries, 1950–2000.* Oxford: Oxford University Press, 1994.

24. Peto R, Lopez AD. The future worldwide health effects of current smoking patterns. In: Koop EC, Pearson CE, Schwarz MR, eds. *Critical Issues in Global Health.* New York: Jossey-Bass, 2001.

25. Jha P, Chaloupka FJ. *Curbing the Epidemic: Governments and the Economics of Tobacco Control.* Washington, DC: World Bank, 1999.

26. Jha P, Chaloupka FJ. The economics of global tobacco control. *BMJ* 2000;**321**:358–61.

27. Godtfredsen NS, Osler M, Vestbo J *et al.* Smoking reduction, smoking cessation, and incidence of fatal and non-fatal myocardial infarction in Denmark 1976–1998: a pooled cohort study. *J Epidemiol Commun Health* 2003;**57**(6):412–16.

28. Hasdai D, Garratt KN, Grill DE *et al.* Effect of smoking status on the long-term outcome after successful percutaneous coronary revascularization. *N Engl J Med* 1997;**336**(11):755–61.

29. van Domburg RT, Meeter K, van Berkel DF *et al.* Smoking cessation reduces mortality after coronary artery bypass surgery: a 20-year follow-up study. *J Am Coll Cardiol* 2000;**36**(3):878–83.

30. Papathanasiou A, Milionis H, Toumpoulis I *et al.* Smoking cessation is associated with reduced long-term mortality and the need for repeat interventions after coronary artery bypass grafting. *Eur J Cardiovasc Prev Rehabil* 2007;**14**(3):448–50.

31. Thomson CC, Rigotti NA. Hospital- and clinic-based smoking cessation interventions for smokers with cardiovascular disease. *Prog Cardiovasc Dis* 2003;**45**(6):459–79.

32. Cole TK. Smoking cessation in the hospitalized patient using the transtheoretical model of behavior change. *Heart Lung* 2001;**30**(2):148–58.

33. Mohiuddin SM, Mooss AN, Hunter CB *et al.* Intensive smoking cessation intervention reduces mortality in high-risk smokers with cardiovascular disease. *Chest* 2007;**131**(2):446–52.

34. Tonstad S, Farsang C, Klaene G *et al.* Bupropion SR for smoking cessation in smokers with cardiovascular disease: a multicentre, randomised study. *Eur Heart J* 2003;**24**(10):946–55.

35. Chaloupka FJ, Hu TW, Warner KE *et al.* The taxation of tobacco products. In: Jha P, Chaloupka F, eds. *Tobacco Control in Developing Countries.* Oxford: Oxford University Press, 2000.

36. United States Department of Health and Human Services. *Reducing Tobacco Use. A Report of the Surgeon General.* Atlanta, GA: US Department of Health and Human Services, Public Health Service, Centers for Disease Control, Center for Chronic Disease Prevention and Health Promotion, Office on Smoking and Health, 2000.

37. John RM. Crowding out effect of tobacco expenditure and its implications on household resource allocation in India. *Soc Sci Med* 2008;**66**(6):1356–67.

38. Centers for Disease Control and Prevention. Response to increases in cigarette prices by race/ethnicity, income, and age groups – United States, 1976–1993. *MMWR* 1994;**43**(26):469–72.

39. Wasserman J, Manning WG, Newhouse JP *et al.* The effects of excise taxes and regulations on cigarette smoking. *J Health Econ* 1991;**10**(1):43–64.

40. Tauras JA. *The Transition to Smoking Cessation: Evidence from Multiple Failure Duration Analysis.* NBER Working Paper No. 7412. Cambridge, MA: National Bureau of Economic Research. 1999.

41. Tauras JA, Chaloupka FJ. The demand for nicotine replacement therapies. *Nicotine Tob Res* 2003;**5**(2):237–43.

42. Townsend JL, Roderick P, Cooper J. Cigarette smoking by socioeconomic group, sex, and age: effects of price, income, and health publicity. *BMJ* 1998;**309**(6959):923–6.

43. United States Department of Health and Human Services. *Preventing Tobacco Use amongst Young People. A Report of the Surgeon General.* Atlanta, GA: US Department of Health and Human Services, Public Health Service, Centers for Disease Control, Center for Chronic Disease Prevention and Health Promotion, Office on Smoking and Health, 1994.

44. Woolery T, Asma S, Sharp D. Clean indoor-air laws and youth access. In: Jha P, Chaloupka FJ, eds. *Tobacco Control in Developing Countries.* Oxford: Oxford University Press, 2000.

45. Levy DT, Friend K, Polishchuk E. Effect of clean indoor air laws on smokers: the clean air module of the SimSmoke computer simulation model. *Tob Control* 2001;**10**(4):345–51.

46. Fichtenberg CM, Glantz SA. Effect of smoke-free workplaces on smoking behaviour: systematic review. *BMJ* 2002;**325**(7357):188.

47. Fichtenberg CM, Glantz SA. Association of the California Tobacco Control Program with declines in cigarette consumption and mortality from heart disease. *N Engl J Med* 2000;**343**(24): 1772–7.

48. Sargent RP, Shepard RM, Glantz SA. Reduced incidence of admissions for myocardial infarction associated with public smoking ban: before and after study. *BMJ* 2004;**328**(7446):977–80.

49. Barone-Adesi F, Vizzini L, Merletti F, Richiardi L. Short-term effects of Italian smoking regulation on rates of hospital admission for acute myocardial infarction. *Eur Heart J* 2006;**27**(20): 2468–72.

50. Bartecchi C, Alsever RN, Nevin-Woods C *et al.* Reduction in the incidence of acute myocardial infarction associated with a city-wide smoking ordinance. *Circulation* 2006;**114**(14):1490–6.

51. Juster HR, Loomis BR, Hinman TM *et al.* Declines in hospital admissions for acute myocardial infarction in New York state after implementation of a comprehensive smoking ban. *Am J Public Health* 2007;**97**(11):2035–9.

52. Seo DC, Torabi MR. Reduced admissions for acute myocardial infarction associated with a public smoking ban: matched controlled study. *J Drug Educ* 2007;**37**(3):217–26.

53. Khuder SA, Milz S, Jordan T *et al.* The impact of a smoking ban on hospital admissions for coronary heart disease. *Prev Med* 2007;**45**(1):3–8.

54. Cesaroni G, Forastiere F, Agabiti N et al. Effect of the Italian smoking ban on population rates of acute coronary events. *Circulation* 2008;**117**(9):1183–8.

55. Methodology Manual for ACC/AHA Guideline Writing Committees – March 2009 update. American College of Cardiology Foundation and American Heart Association, Inc. Available at: http://www.americanheart.org/downloadable/heart/12378888766452009methodologyManualACCF_AHAGuidelineWritingCommittees.pdf (accessed on 17 June 2009).

56. Kenkel D, Chen L. Consumer information and tobacco use. In: Jha P, Chaloupka FJ, eds. *Tobacco Control in Developing Countries.* Oxford: Oxford University Press, 2000.

57. Townsend JL. Policies to halve smoking deaths. *Addiction* 1993;**88**(1):43–52.

58. Saffer H. Tobacco advertising and promotion. In: Jha P. Chaloupka FJ, eds. *Tobacco Control in Developing Countries.* Oxford: Oxford University Press, 2000.

59. Chinese Academy of Preventive Medicine. *Smoking in China: 1996 National Prevalence Survey of Smoking Pattern.* Beijing: China Science and Technology Press, 1997.

60. Weinstein ND. Accuracy of smokers' risk perceptions. *Ann Behav Med* 1998;**20**(2):135–40.

61. Federal Trade Commission. *Cigarette Report for 2001.* Washington, DC: Federal Trade Commission, 2003.

62. Chaloupka FJ, Tauras JA, Grossman M. The economics of addiction. In: Jha P, Chaloupka FJ, eds. *Tobacco Control in Developing Countries.* Oxford: Oxford University Press, 2000.

63. UK Department of Health. *Effect of Tobacco Advertising on Tobacco Consumption: A Discussion Document Reviewing the Evidence.* London: UK Department of Health, Economics and Operational Research Division, 1992.

64. Saffer H, Chaloupka FJ. Tobacco advertising: economic theory and international evidence. *J Health Econ* 2000;**19**(6):1117–37.

65. Novotny TE, Cohen JC, Yurekli A et al. Smoking cessation and nicotine-replacement therapies. In: Jha P, Chaloupka FJ, eds. *Tobacco Control in Developing Countries.* Oxford: Oxford University Press, 2000.

66. Raw M, McNeill A, West R. Smoking cessation: evidence-based recommendations for the healthcare system. *BMJ* 1999;**318**(7177): 182–5.

67. Critchley JA, Capewell S. Smoking cessation for the secondary prevention of coronary heart disease. *Cochrane Database of Systematic Reviews* 2003, Issue 4. Art. No.: CD003041. DOI: 10.1002/14651858.CD003041.pub2.

68. Wilson K, Gibson N, Willan A, Cook D. Effect of smoking cessation on mortality after myocardial infarction: meta-analysis of cohort studies. *Arch Intern Med* 2000;**160**(7):939–44.

69. Ranson MK, Jha P, Chaloupka FJ, Nguyen SN. Global and regional estimates of the effectiveness and cost-effectiveness of price increases and other tobacco control policies. *Nicotine Tob Res* 2002;**4**(3):311–19.

70. Guindon GE, Tobin S, Yach D. Trends and affordability of cigarette prices: ample room for tax increases and related health gains. *Tob Control* 2002;**11**(1):35–43.

71. World Health Organization. *WHO Framework Convention on Tobacco Control.* Geneva: World Health Organization, 2003.

72. Farrelly MC, Pechacek TF, Chaloupka FJ. The impact of tobacco control program expenditures on aggregate cigarette sales: 1981–2000. *J Health Econ* 2003;**22**(5):843–59.

73. Fichtenberg CM, Glantz SA. Smoke-free policies are an effective way to reduce heart disease rapidly. In: Marmot M, Elliott P, eds. *Coronary Heart Disease Epidemiology: From Aetiology to Public Health.* Oxford: Oxford University Press, 2005;792–804.

74. Centers for Disease Control and Prevention. *Best Practices for Comprehensive Tobacco Control Programs.* Atlanta, GA: US Department of Health and Human Services, Centers for Disease Control and Prevention, National Center for Chronic Disease Prevention and Health Promotion, Office on Smoking and Health, 1999.

75. Pechmann C, Dixon P, Layne N. An assessment of US and Canadian smoking reduction objectives for the year 2000. *Am J Public Health* 1998;**88**(9):1362–7.

76. Tauras JA, Chaloupka FJ, Farrelly MC et al. State tobacco control spending and youth smoking. *Am J Public Health* 2005;**95**(2): 338–44.

77. Mathers CD, Loncar D. Projections of global mortality and burden of disease from 2002 to 2030. *PLoS Med* 2006;**3**(11):e442.

78. National Institutes of Health, National Heart, Lung and Blood Institute. *Morbidity and Mortality: 2007 Chartbook on Cardiovascular Diseases.* Available at: www.nhlbi.nih.gov/resources/docs/07-chtbk.pdf.

10 Tobacco and cardiovascular disease: achieving smoking cessation in cardiac patients

Andrew Pipe

University of Ottawa Heart Institute, Ottawa, Canada

Introduction

Despite overwhelming evidence of the importance and effectiveness of smoking cessation in the prevention and management of heart disease, and the availability of effective cessation interventions it is, regrettably, still the case that smoking cessation has not figured prominently among the interventions provided by cardiologists. In part this may reflect the unfortunate and tragic persistence of outdated attitudes and perspectives: to the uninformed, smoking still remains a "habit" or "lifestyle choice" that can be addressed only by determination and the application of strong will. Some cardiologists may view the responsibility for smoking cessation as resting with others – typically the family physician. More likely, the lack of familiarity with the clinical principles of smoking cessation, a misperception of their efficacy and effectiveness, and a failure to appreciate the need for the systematic identification of smokers combined with the delivery of proven interventions may have contributed to an indifference to intervene in the cardiac setting.

It has been noted that it is difficult to identify any condition that is as prevalent, lethal and yet so prone to neglect as tobacco addiction.[1] One-half of all smokers will die prematurely as a consequence of their tobacco use.[2] In the United Kingdom it has been calculated that 40% of heart disease is attributable to smoking; the burden is similar in the USA and elsewhere in the developed world.[3–5] There can be no doubt of the causative role that tobacco addiction plays in the development and accentuation of cardiac and cardiovascular disease; the evidence is overwhelming and has been accumulating for decades.[6–7] Tobacco use is a principal contributor to the development of coronary artery disease (CAD), acute myocardial infarction (AMI), heart failure and the complications which inevitably follow. Deaths from coronary artery disease in smokers below the age of 45 exceed the mortality produced by any other tobacco-related disease.[8] Smoking cessation may have a greater effect on reducing mortality among smoking patients with CAD than any other intervention or treatment.[9] Sadly, tobacco use has been described as "reflecting a rare confluence of circumstances: (1) a highly significant health threat; (2) a disinclination among clinicians to intervene consistently; and (3) the presence of effective interventions".[10]

> "The rapidity and potency of risk reduction, as well as the other health-enhancing effects associated with smoking cessation, argue for the prioritization of smoking cessation in any program of secondary prevention of coronary disease."
>
> Forrester JS, Merz CNB, Bush TL *et al JACC* 1996;**27**:991–1006

In recent years the prevalence of smoking has declined in the developed world; regrettably rates of smoking in developing nations continue to rise and herald epidemics of tobacco-related disease for years to come. 100 million deaths resulted from tobacco use in the 20th century[11]; it has been estimated that one billion more will occur in the 21st.[12] A significant proportion of these deaths will occur as a result of the development of heart disease.

Cardiovascular physicians pride themselves on the degree to which their practices are based on carefully cultivated evidence derived from large, thoughtfully developed clinical trials which ultimately inform the development of practice guidelines. The evidence defining best practice for the treatment of smoking comes from several sources, principal among which are the influential guidelines that emerge regularly from the US Department of Health and Human Services.[10,13]

Smoking cessation is a very powerful and highly cost-efficient intervention.[14–16] The most recent recommendations

Evidence-Based Cardiology, 3rd edition. Edited by S. Yusuf, J.A. Cairns, A.J. Camm, E.L. Fallen, and B.J. Gersh. © 2010 Blackwell Publishing, ISBN: 978-1-4051-5925-8.

are clear and direct and have specific implications for all cardiologists and cardiovascular professionals: clinicians and health systems must "consistently identify and document tobacco use" among their patients and "treat every tobacco user seen in a healthcare setting"; clinicians should "offer every patient who uses tobacco ... the brief treatments shown to be effective"; and should encourage the "use of the numerous effective medications available for tobacco dependence".[10]

The pathophysiology of smoking and cardiovascular disease

Cigarette smoke contains nicotine, tar, and oxidant gases. Nicotine, the addictive constituent of tobacco, is delivered rapidly to the addiction centers of the brainstem when inhaled in tobacco smoke. Nicotine influences blood pressure and heart rate and, particularly in nicotine-naïve subjects, vasoconstriction. Carbon monoxide impairs the delivery of oxygen, while oxidant gases and their constituents play a major role in the initiation and progression of atheroma.[17]

Atheromatous lesions develop within a blood vessel as the consequence of a combination of pathophysiologic processes which impair vasomotor function, damage the vessel wall, accentuate the effects of elevated lipoproteins, and stimulate platelet aggregation and thrombosis. Cigarette smoking plays a distinct role in each of these processes. The constituents of cigarette smoke interfere with the availability of nitric oxide, thereby disrupting the normal vasomotor responses of the blood vessel wall; increase vascular inflammation, contributing to an accumulation of leukocytes on endothelial surfaces; promote the deposition of inflammatory and proinflammatory materials within the vessel wall; contribute to the elevation of total cholesterol and low-density lipoprotein cholesterol (LDL), and reduce levels of high-density lipoprotein cholesterol (HDL); increase the oxidation of LDL; accentuate platelet aggregation and adhesion; reduce the dissolution of thrombi; and contribute to plaque rupture.[7,18,19] Smoking also leads to elevated levels of carbon monoxide (CO), producing increased levels of carboxyhemoglobin and thereby reducing the blood's capacity to carry and release oxygen (Box 10.1).

Notwithstanding their increased risk of atherosclerosis, heart disease, and coronary events, smokers have been noted to demonstrate improved rates of survival following a myocardial infarction – the "smoker's paradox" – a phenomenon attributable to the younger age at which smokers experience acute coronary events, their more favorable coronary anatomy, and reduced levels of co-morbidity.[20,21]

Second-hand smoke (SHS) is a combination of exhaled *mainstream* smoke (15%) and the *sidestream* smoke pro-

BOX 10.1 The Perfect Storm: cigarette smoke contributes directly to the processes underlying the development of CAD

- Impairs nitric oxide activity
- Diminishes vasomotor responses
- Increases vascular inflammation
- Promotes deposition of inflammatory materials in vessel wall
- Oxidizes lipoproteins
- Accentuates platelet aggregation
- Reduces dissolution of thrombi
- Contributes to plaque rupture
- Increases carboxyhemoglobin levels

duced by an idling cigarette (85%).[18] SHS is harmful and also contributes to platelet activation and endothelial dysfunction, distorts lipoprotein profile, elevates levels of carboxyhemoglobin, accentuates inflammation and contributes to the progression of atherosclerosis.[22–24] Exposure to SHS has predictably deleterious effects on cardiac function; it results in a 30% elevation in the risk for coronary heart disease.[25–28] The ischemic stress of exercise is accentuated upon exposure to SHS which may precipitate anginal symptoms.[29,30] Second-hand smoke exposure has been estimated to cause 35000 excess cardiovascular events each year in the USA and is the third leading cause of preventable death[24] (**Class I, Level A**).

Smokeless tobacco, whose use has surged in North America in recent years, frequently produces levels of nicotine that are higher, and more sustained, than those seen with smoking. The use of these products is known to produce acute cardiovascular effects.[31] Blood pressure levels are influenced by the high sodium content of smokeless tobacco and the presence of its two pharmacologically active ingredients: nicotine and licorice.[32] Smokeless tobacco users are more likely to have elevated levels of both diastolic and systolic blood pressure,[33] and may have distorted lipoprotein profiles.[34] Insulin resistance and a higher prevalence of diabetes have been noted in smokeless tobacco users.[35,36] Physicians are advised to counsel users of smokeless tobacco products to quit.[37]

The benefits of smoking cessation

Smoking cessation confers distinct and immediate benefits to the smoker with cardiovascular disease. The elimination of exposure to mainstream tobacco smoke (and its multiplicity of toxic constituents) has a rapid impact on the reduction of those factors which contribute to the development and progression of atherosclerosis, removes the deleterious impact of smoking on established indices of cardiac performance, and eliminates the stimuli for clotting and thrombi formation central to the development of many acute cardiac conditions. The likelihood of sudden death, the propensity for myocardial infarction or re-infarction, the incidence of arrhythmia and an array of postinfarction complications, the adverse impact of smoking on myocardial contractility, and the progression of congestive heart failure (CHF) are all dramatically reduced following smoking cessation[9,38–42] (**Class I, Level A**). A very substantial, 36% relative risk reduction of mortality is experienced following smoking cessation in those with coronary artery disease; this intervention is more potent than other classic secondary preventive strategies (e.g. cholesterol treatment) which, arguably, have received far greater attention in recent years (Table 10.1, Fig. 10.1).[38] Quitting smoking produces a substantial, 30% decline in mortality in those with heart failure, a reduction of risk which equals or exceeds that produced by treatment with metoprolol, enalapril or spironolactone[42] (**Class I, Level A**).

Controling exposure to cigarette smoke

Elimination or reduction of exposure to second-hand smoke has a significant impact on the incidence of acute coronary events for the individual and for the community. Anginal thresholds are reduced upon exposure to second-hand smoke; the benefits to the cardiac patient of the elimination of smoking in the home and work environments are many[19,24,43] (**Class I, Level A**). Evidence continues to accumulate, from North America and Europe, of the beneficial effects of the introduction of smoke-free policies. There has been a distinct and clearly documented reduction in the incidence of acute myocardial infarctions in several cities following the introduction of bans on public smoking[44–48] (**Class I, Level B**). Cardiologists can play a significant role in supporting the introduction of such progressive public health policies.

Table 10.1 Reducing mortality in CHD: the benefits of smoking cessation are greater and accrue more rapidly in comparison to other important preventive interventions

Intervention	Reduction in mortality
Smoking cessation	36%
Statin therapy	29%
Beta-blockers	23%
ACE inhibitors	23%
Aspirin	15%

Source: adapted from Critchley JA, Capewell S. JAMA;2003;**290**: 86–97

Study	Ceased Smoking Patients, No.	Ceased Smoking Deaths, No.	Continued Smoking Patients, No.	Continued Smoking Deaths, No.	Weight, %	RR (95% CI)
Aberg et al,[41] 1983	542	110	443	142	8.3	0.63 (0.51–0.79)
Baughman et al,[51] 1982	45	9	32	14	1.8	0.46 (0.23–0.92)
Bednarzevski et al,[36] 1984	455	136	555	205	9.3	0.81 (0.68–0.97)
Burr et al,[39] 1992	665	27	521	41	3.5	0.52 (0.32–0.83)
Daly et al,[43] 1983	217	80	157	129	9.0	0.45 (0.37–0.54)
Greenwood et al,[19] 1995	396	64	136	29	4.5	0.76 (0.51–1.12)
Gupta et al,[37] 1993	173	56	52	24	4.9	0.70 (0.49–1.01)
Hallstrom et al,[46] 1986	91	34	219	104	6.1	0.79 (0.58–1.06)
Hasdai et al,[42] 1997	435	41	734	97	5.2	0.71 (0.50–1.01)
Hedback et al,[52] 1993	83	31	74	40	5.2	0.69 (0.49–0.98)
Herlitz et al,[50] 1995	115	20	102	31	3.2	0.57 (0.35–0.94)
Johansson et al,[7] 1985	81	14	75	27	2.6	0.48 (0.27–0.84)
Perkins and Dick,[47] 1985	52	9	67	30	2.1	0.39 (0.20–0.74)
Salonen,[45] 1980	221	26	302	60	4.0	0.59 (0.39–0.91)
Sato et al,[8] 1992	59	5	28	7	0.9	0.34 (0.12–0.97)
Sparrow and Dawber,[48] 1978	56	10	139	40	2.3	0.62 (0.33–1.15)
Tofler et al,[49] 1993	173	14	220	37	2.5	0.48 (0.27–0.86)
Van Domburg et al,[39] 2000	238	109	318	202	9.8	0.72 (0.61–0.78)
Vlietstra et al,[40] 1986	1490	223	2675	588	10.4	0.68 (0.59–0.85)
Voors et al,[44] 1996	72	26	95	37	4.4	0.93 (0.62–1.38)
Overall	5659	1044	6944	1884	100.0	0.64 (0.58–0.71)

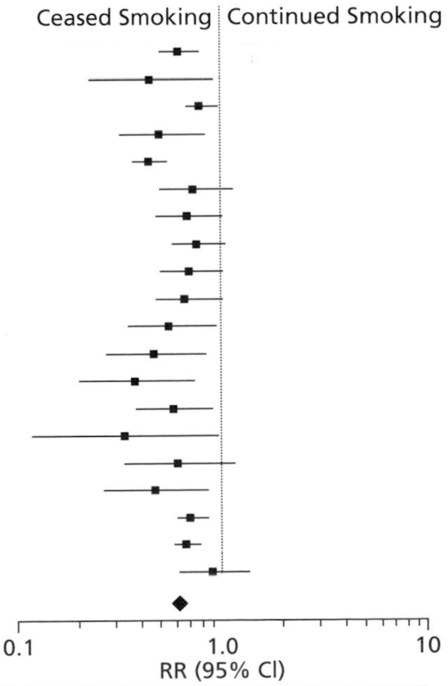

Figure 10.1 Pooled relative risks of mortality reduction when patients with CHD stop smoking: random effects meta-analysis of all 20 studies. The data show an overall 36% reduction in mortality associated with smoking cessation in patients with CHD. (Reproduced with permission from Critchley J, Capewell S. JAMA 2003;**290**(1):86–97.)

Nicotine addiction: the fundamental basis of smoking behavior

Minimal exposure to nicotine is all that is required to initiate the profound changes in neuroanatomy and neurophysiology that result in a brain, and a life, ordered and organized to ensure regular intake of nicotine. Only minimal exposure to nicotine via inhalation is necessary to produce addiction. Nicotine is arguably the most destructive of all the addictive drugs encountered in our society. It is the only drug which when used as intended will result in the premature death of one-half of all its users. The effects of nicotine on brain function, and ultimately behavior, are mediated via a number of nicotine receptors, principal among which is the $\alpha_4\beta_2$ nicotinic acetylcholine receptor (nAChR) located in the brainstem. This receptor is felt to be responsible for the initiation and preservation of the nicotine-addicted state.[49] Stimulation of nAChRs, principally the $\alpha_4\beta_2$ subtypes, results in a cascade of neurologic stimulation involving the mesolimbic system, culminating in the release of dopamine and other neurotransmitters in the nucleus accumbens region of the forebrain. Elevated levels of dopamine sustain addiction by producing pleasure, stimulation and mood modulation.[50]

In simple terms, the development of nicotine addiction can be seen as the requirement to maintain ongoing stimulation of nicotine receptors in order to ensure elevated levels of dopamine (Fig. 10.2). A cigarette is a drug delivery device which permits the rapid introduction of nicotine, titration of receptor stimulation, and dopamine release. As addiction develops, so does a degree of tolerance or desensitization at the receptor level which causes an increase in the absolute number of nicotine receptors. Smokers autotitrate their nicotine intake so as to maintain a personalized, idiosyncratic level of nicotine and comfort-maintaining levels of dopamine (Fig. 10.3).[51]

In the absence of nicotine intake, a withdrawal state quickly develops characterized by anxiety, irritation, frustration, depressed mood, lowered levels of concentration and restlessness.[52] As a consequence of the relative deficiency of dopamine that accompanies smoking cessation, a prominent symptom of withdrawal is "hedonic dysregulation" – a feeling that there is minimal or no pleasure in life and that no enjoyment accompanies previously rewarding activities.[53] Smoking cessation is often accompanied by the emergence of depressive symptoms and mood states. It is the discomfort and intensity of withdrawal, in association with the strongly conditioned behaviors, moods, and environmental factors associated with smoking, that can make this addiction so difficult to shed.[54] It is unlikely that non-smokers will ever in their lifetimes have to make the significant, complex life transformation that a smoker must undergo to become a non-smoker.

It is important that clinicians appreciate the difficulties associated with cessation. Unassisted, only a very small proportion of smokers, 3%, are able to remain abstinent from tobacco for a six-month period; most relapse within eight days.[55,56] Tobacco addiction should be viewed as a chronic relapsing addictive disorder requiring specific treatment for its elimination.

Most smokers understand the negative health consequences of their addiction, wish to stop smoking, and make at least one or two private attempts to stop smoking each

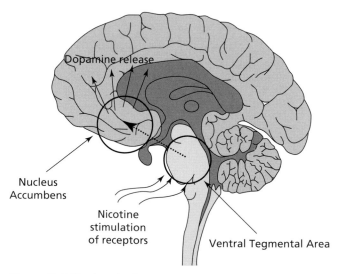

Figure 10.2 Nicotine stimulates receptors in the ventral tegmental area of the brainstem, causing the further stimulation, via the mesolimbic pathway, of regions in the nucleus accumbens of the forebrain, resulting in the release of dopamine. The brain rapidly adapts to the presence of increased levels of dopamine. Addiction quickly develops following minimal, repeated exposure to nicotine and the ensuing dopamine release.

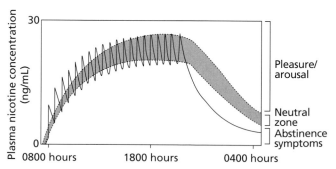

Figure 10.3 Smokers autotitrate nicotine intake to maintain plasma levels so as to accentuate "pleasure" and minimize "discomfort". As nicotine levels rise, "pleasure" is experienced; as levels fall below a certain threshold, "discomfort" in the form of withdrawal or craving symptoms is experienced. In the neutral zone comfort is achieved without accentuating arousal and discomfort is avoided as abstinence symptoms do not develop.(Adapted with permission from Benowitz NL. *Med Clin North Am* 1992;**76**:415–37.)

year – the overwhelming majority of which are unsuccessful.[57] Even in the face of compelling reasons for cessation, smoking cessation is difficult – following a myocardial infarction less than one-half of patients are able to stop smoking[58]; 17–40% of cardiac transplant recipients return to smoking at some point after their procedure.[59–62] "Brainstem trumps cerebral cortex": it is important to realize that admonitions and exhortations to smoking patients are likely to be of only limited assistance in addressing this tenacious addiction, one which mandates the ongoing application of more insightful, evidence-based treatment strategies.

It is now understood that there are genetic predispositions affecting receptor density, the rate of nicotine metabolism, the likelihood and tenacity of addiction, and the difficulty that may be experienced in attempting to shed it.[51,63–65] Individuals with certain psychiatric disorders, particularly schizophrenia and its related conditions, bipolar and other affective disorders, and substance abuse problems have a significantly increased likelihood of becoming smokers and a greater difficulty with cessation.[54,66–68] Such patients have a markedly reduced life expectancy, most of which is accounted for by tobacco-related diseases, principal among which is cardiovascular disease (**Class I, Level A**).

Smoking cessation: the fundamental preventive intervention

Smoking cessation should be the priority in the secondary prevention of cardiac disease[69] (**Class 1, Level A**). Sadly, there is evidence that physicians, particularly specialists, do not typically effectively address this preventive priority.[70] The substantial benefits of cessation for a cardiac patient occur rapidly; they equal or exceed those of other preventive therapies. It is important to ensure that a systematic approach is adopted in *every* professional environment (office, clinic, and inpatient settings) which permits the identification of a patient's smoking status; stimulates the delivery of clear, unambiguous, non-judgmental advice regarding the importance of quitting; prompts an offer of ongoing assistance with cessation; ensures familiarity with the prescription (and titration) of commonly used pharmacotherapies for cessation; and facilitates appropriate referral to other physicians, agencies or programs for follow-up where necessary or appropriate[10] (**Class I, Level A**).

The time-honored 5 As (**Ask** – about smoking status; **Advise** – about the importance of quitting; **Assess** – the readiness to quit; **Assist** – by providing effective medications and counseling; **Arrange** – for appropriate follow-up) have informed and influenced professional behavior for years. But not all elements need to be delivered personally,

separately or intensely. Some have suggested that we think of "Asking and Acting". Consistency is the hallmark of a successful intervention system and unless a systematic approach is adopted in every professional setting, the potential to dramatically enhance cardiac health for our patients and communities will be diminished.[1]

Counseling

The provision of supportive counseling has been a central element of recommended clinical approaches to cessation for many years. Many physicians have misconstrued this recommendation, assuming that it mandates the delivery of time-consuming interventions inappropriate for their practice, environment or skill-set. Contemporary recommendations clearly note that delivering minimal, strategic advice regarding enlisting the support of family and friends; the avoidance of social or environmental stimuli for smoking; compliance with medication; the importance of follow-up; and strategies for relapse management are as effective as more intense, sustained or highly structured behavioral treatments.[10,71] Strategic counseling can be efficiently provided and reinforced by other clinical staff, other physicians or via access to quit-lines or other community cessation programs, further enhancing cessation rates[72,73] (**Class I, Level A**).

Smoking cessation treatment should not be seen as a complex undertaking (the management of anticoagulation or the titration of lipid-lowering or hypertension medication can be far more involved and prolonged). The implementation of a systematized approach ensures effective use of time and resources and assures optimal outcomes in any population of smokers. Ensuring that office or institutional practices capture pertinent smoking information (e.g. at point of patient registration) and prompt an intervention (e.g. with a sticker, chart reminder or a prompt on an electronic medical record) means that clinician time can be used most appropriately. The provision of brief advice regarding smoking cessation by physicians has been demonstrated to produce an increase in cessation; the advice of nurses may enhance cessation rates; systems which support such behavior will only add to effectiveness.[74,75] It is also clear that the failure to involve a patient in supportive counseling does not detract from the ability of pharmacotherapy to significantly assist in achieving cessation.[10]

It has long been recognized that smoking cessation may induce or uncover depressive mood states or disorders[76,77] (**Class I, Level A**). Nicotine use is itself mood modulating as a consequence of its effect in producing changes in levels of dopamine and other transmitters. Smokers are more likely to have a history of depressive illness and may smoke because of the mood-enhancing properties of nicotine; quitting smoking may cause a re-emergence of those symptoms irrespective of the approach used in cessation.[78]

Those with a history of depression or other mood disorders or a history of depression in association with cessation may experience a return of those symptoms and should be so advised while being monitored normally as part of the cessation process.

The hospital

Given that many admitted cardiac patients are smokers (who will frequently begin to experience symptoms of nicotine withdrawal shortly after admission), the majority of whom know the reasons for quitting and wish to quit,[57] there is a unique opportunity in any hospital setting to provide specific, systematic assistance with cessation. Now a standard of care for the treatment of AMI and CHF in US settings, such programs can ensure the consistent delivery of a standardized protocol and enhance rates of cessation.[79,80] The delivery of an intensive smoking cessation intervention, including 12 weeks of follow-up and the provision of free pharmacotherapy to high-risk cardiovascular patients admitted to a coronary care unit, resulted in a dramatic reduction in readmission (relative risk reduction (RRR) = 44%) and all-cause mortality (RRR = 77%) over a 24-month period demonstrating the potential of hospital-based interventions for cessation (Fig. 10.4).[81] Smoking cessation interventions commenced in hospital settings, when coupled with at least one month's follow-up post discharge, demonstrate significant effectiveness in increasing the rate of cessation (Table 10.2)[82] (**Class I, Level A**).

Pharmacotherapy

The use of pharmacotherapy is the mainstay of successful cessation treatment. The benefits of pharmacotherapy are distinct and well documented (**Class I, Level A**). Physicians have access to 'three generations' of first-line pharmacotherapies, each of which has significant, proven efficacy when compared to placebo, in enhancing the likelihood of successful cessation: nicotine replacement therapy, bupropion, and varenicline (Table 10.3).

Nicotine replacement therapy (NRT)

All smokers seek to maintain a certain, personalized level of nicotine. In the absence of smoking, nicotine levels fall and stimulation of nicotinic receptors declines, resulting in a corresponding decline in the levels of dopamine and other neurotransmitters. The smoker will then begin to experience cravings and, in the absence of nicotine intake, the symptoms and discomfort of withdrawal emerge. The administration of amounts of nicotine sufficient to approach familiar levels of nicotine will eliminate craving and the symptoms of withdrawal, allowing a smoker to acquire and experience a repertoire of non-smoking behaviors leading to ultimate cessation. It has been recognized that the dose of NRT and duration of therapy may need to be titrated in order to meet the particular nicotine needs of an individual smoker. Very heavy smokers are unlikely to have their nicotine needs addressed by standard doses of NRT provided in a fixed-dose protocol. A history of heavy smoking, pronounced cravings in previous quit attempts or ongoing craving while using standard doses of NRT indicate that an increase in nicotine dose may be appropriate.

NRT is available in a variety of forms: patch, gum, inhaler/vaporizer, lozenge, and nasal spray. It is important to emphasize that a smoker will receive less nicotine, delivered slowly via the venous system, than they would obtain from continued smoking. At the same time, in contrast to smoking, there will be no arterial delivery of nicotine, carbon monoxide or any of the thousands of other compounds of tobacco smoke. Smokers are tolerant of the vasoactive properties of nicotine and the safety of NRT use in cardiac patients has been established in a variety of settings.[83–89] Many smokers will experience withdrawal symptoms shortly after admission to hospital; this has

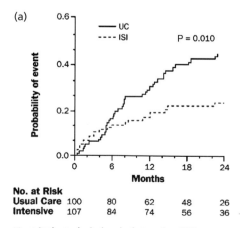

(a) Hospital readmission in intensive (ISI) vs usual care (UC) smoking cessation groups

No. at Risk					
Usual Care	100	80	62	48	26
Intensive	107	84	74	56	36

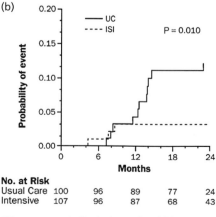

All-cause mortality in intensive (ISI) vs usual care (UC) smoking cessation groups

No. at Risk					
Usual Care	100	96	89	77	24
Intensive	107	96	87	68	43

Figure 10.4 A demonstration of the effect of an intensive in-hospital smoking cessation program for patients admitted with acute cardiovascular conditions. (a) Hospital readmission in intensive (ISI) vs usual care (UC) smoking cessation groups. (b) All-cause mortality in intensive (ISI) vs usual care (UC) smoking cessation groups. A dramatic reduction in readmission and all-cause mortality is observed over a 24-month follow-up period.(Adapted with permission from Mohuiddin SM *et al Chest* 2007;**131**:446–52.)

Table 10.2 The advantage of hospital-based smoking cessation programs

Review: Hospital smoking

Comparison: 01 Interventions for smoking cessation in patients hospitalized with cardiovascular disease

Outcome: 01 Smoking cessation for intervention versus control by intervention intensity

Study or sub-category	Treatment n/N	Control n/N	OR (fixed) 95% CI	Weight %	OR (fixed) 95% CI
01 Low Intensity					
Pelletier 1998	63/412	7/92		2.45	2.19 [0.97, 4.96]
Bolman 2002	103/334	110/401		17.50	1.18 [0.86, 1.62]
Hajek 2002	94/254	102/251		16.36	0.86 [0.60, 1.23]
Chouinard 2005	13/53	7/56		1.30	2.28 [0.83, 6.24]
Subtotal (95% CI)	1053	800		37.62	1.14 [0.92, 1.43]
Total events: 273 (Treatment), 226 (Control)					
Test for heterogeneity Chi^2 = 6.73, df = 3 (P = 0.08), I^2 = 55.4%					
Test for overall effect: Z = 1.20 (P = 0.23)					
02 Moderate Intensity					
Rigotti 1994	21/41	20/39		2.53	1.00 [0.41, 2.40]
Miller 1997	38/138	74/310		8.36	1.21 [0.77, 1.91]
Ortigosa 2000	26/42	31/45		2.89	0.73 [0.30, 1.78]
Subtotal (95% CI)	221	394		13.78	1.07 [0.74, 1.55]
Total events: 85 (Treatment), 125 (Control)					
Test for heterogeneity: Chi^2 = 1.01, df = 2 (P = 0.60), I^2 = 0%					
Test for overall effect: Z = 0.37 (P = 0.71)					
03 High Intensity					
Taylor 1990	47/72	20/58		1.95	3.57 [1.73, 7.39]
CASIS 1992	44/133	28/123		4.93	1.68 [0.96, 2.92]
De Busk 1994	92/131	64/121		5.02	2.10 [1.25, 3.52]
Miller 1997b	62/182	74/310		9.14	1.65 [1.10, 2.46]
Domelas 2000	28/54	16/46		2.11	2.02 [0.90, 4.53]
Quist-Paulsen 2003	57/115	44/120		5.50	1.70 [1.01, 2.86]
Reid 2003	49/125	46/127		7.02	1.14 [0.68, 1.89]
Froelicher 2004	64/134	55/132		7.33	1.28 [0.79, 2.08]
Chouinard 2005b	13/55	7/56		1.34	2.17 [0.79, 5.93]
Pedersen 2005	28/54	20/51		2.51	1.67 [0.77, 3.62]
Mohiuddin 2007	43/109	11/100		1.76	5.27 [2.53, 10.99]
Subtotal (95% CI)	1164	1244		48.60	1.81 [1.53, 2.15]
Total events: 527 (Treatment), 385 (Control)					
Test for heterogeneity: Chi^2 = 17.57, df = 10 (P = 0.06), I^2 = 43.1%					
Test for overall effect: Z = 6.77 (P < 0.00001)					
Total (95% CI)	2438	2438		100.00	1.46 [1.29, 1.66]
Total events: 885 (Treatment), 736 (Control)					
Test for heterogeneity; Chi^2 = 38.43, df = 17 (P = 0.002), I^2 = 55.8%					
Test for overall effect: Z = 5.84 (P < 0.00001)					

0.1 0.2 0.5 1 2 5 10
Favours control   Favours treatment

Adapted from Rigotti NA, Munafo MR, Stead LF. *Interventions for smoking cessation in hospitalised patients*. Cochrane Database Syst Rev, 2007(3).

Table 10.3 A comparison of the effectiveness of and abstinence rates from medications and combinations of medications compared to placebo at six months post quit date

Medication	Number of arms	Estimated odds ratio (95% CI)	Estimated abstinence rate (95% CI)
Varenicline (2 mg/day)	5	3.1 (2.5–3.8)	33.2 (28.9–37.8)
Nicotine nasal spray	4	2.3 (1.7–3.0)	26.7 (21.5–32.7)
Bupropion SR	26	2.0 (1.8–2.2)	24.2 (22.2–26.4)
Nicotine patch (6–14 weeks)	32	1.9 (1.7–2.2)	23.4 (21.3–25.8)
Patch (long-term; >14 weeks) + ad lib NRT (gum or spray)	3	3.6 (2.5–5.2)	36.5 (28.6–45.3)
Patch + bupropion SR	3	2.5 (1.9–3.4)	28.9 (23.5–35.1)
Patch + inhaler	2	2.2 (1.3–3.6)	25.8 (17.4–36.5)

Adapted from Fiore MC *et al. Treating Tobacco Use and Dependence: 2008 Update*. Rockville, MD: US Dept of Health and Human Services, Public Health Service, 2008.

particular relevance for the cardiac patient. The withdrawal syndrome is frequently manifested by unco-operative, belligerent or aggressive behavior; the provision of NRT in these circumstances can be of assistance in easing the discomfort of withdrawal and facilitating compliance with treatment, while accentuating the likelihood of successful cessation.

The effectiveness and safety of NRT have been extensively studied and documented, establishing it as a first-line choice for smoking cessation. NRT use will significantly enhance cessation when compared to placebo (nicotine patch, OR = 1.9; nicotine spray, OR = 2.3)[89] (**Class I, Level A**). All cardiac professionals should be adept in its use.

Bupropion

The serendipitous recognition that the administration of the antidepressant bupropion significantly increased spontaneous rates of smoking cessation led to clinical trials which ultimately validated the use of this drug as an aid to smoking cessation.[90–92] The development of a large evidence base has since confirmed the benefits of its use; like NRT, bupropion is now considered to be a first-line smoking cessation medication, effectively doubling the rate of smoking cessation when compared to placebo (OR = 2.0).[93] Its effectiveness is similar in both men and women[94] and has been specifically evaluated in the treatment of smokers with cardiovascular disease, where both its safety and effectiveness have been evident[95] (**Class I, Level A**).

It is well known that smoking cessation may unmask depression and that nicotine may have antidepressant effects.[96] It was assumed that bupropion would offer some benefit to those with a history of depression or those in whom smoking cessation unmasked a depressive state; this remains unproven.[91,93] Concerns have been expressed that antidepressants may worsen depression in those being treated for depression; warning statements to this effect have been added to labeling in the USA. Bupropion possesses noradrenergic and dopaminergic properties which were felt to be responsible for its effectiveness in smoking cessation; it is now recognized that it may also function as a nicotine antagonist.

There are known, dose-related side effects with bupropion. Insomnia, dry mouth and nausea are most commonly reported. When side effects occur, they frequently respond to a reduction in dose to 150 mg per day. Reduced dosing has not been associated with any significant decrease in smoking cessation effectiveness over a 12-month period.[97] Seizures, reported to occur in 1 in 1000 patients, are dose related. A history of seizures, anorexia, and recent withdrawal from other drugs of abuse are contraindications to the use of this drug. The usual dose of bupropion for smoking cessation is 150 mg bid, achieved by increasing doses in the days prior to a cessation attempt. Bupropion has been used simultaneously with NRT and demonstrated enhanced benefit in one study, though not in others.[98]

Varenicline

The realization that the leaves of the "Golden Rain" shrub (*Cytisus laburnum*) were used as a tobacco substitute during WWII prompted consideration of its use as an aid in combating tobacco dependence.[99] Smoking the leaves of this plant had been advised as a strategy to quit smoking.[100] In Eastern European countries, cytisine, the active ingredient of "Golden Rain", has been used for more than 40 years in smoking cessation. Cytisine stimulates nAChRs while blocking the ability of nicotine to do the same. Refinements of the molecular structure of cytisine have resulted in the creation of a new compound, varenicline, which binds avidly to the nicotine receptor, stimulates it only partially, and prevents nicotine binding. The result of this "partial agonist" and "antagonist" activity is diminished stimulation of the pathways leading to dopamine release, reduced levels of dopamine, and an elimination of the pleasurable sensations associated with smoking. An individual taking varenicline is less likely to crave a cigarette because of lessened but ongoing release of dopamine. Varenicline is almost completely excreted by the kidneys, and does not interact with commonly prescribed medications or the cytochrome P450 mechanisms.

Principal side effects of varenicline include nausea, insomnia and headache which diminish over time and are associated with low discontinuation rates. Persistent nausea may be addressed by reducing the dose to 0.5 mg twice daily; varenicline at this dose is still more efficacious than placebo.[101] The FDA and European Medicines Agency have warned prescribers and users of varenicline to monitor changes in behavior and mood due to postmarketing reports of depression, agitation and suicidal ideation and behavior in patients attempting smoking cessation with varenicline. No causal relationship has been determined.[102]

Varenicline is prescribed in stepped doses over a seven-day period to a dose of 1.0 mg twice a day, in order to minimize the development of nausea. Clinical trials have consistently demonstrated the superiority of varenicline for smoking cessation in comparison to placebo (OR = 3.2) and bupropion (OR = 1.66) when assessing continuous abstinence at 52 weeks[103] (**Class I, Level A**). Additional studies comparing varenicline to NRT and investigating its use in chronic obstructive airway disease (COPD) and CVD patients are under way.

Titration of pharmacotherapy

Evidence accumulates of the additional efficacy of modifying the dose of or prolonging the period of treatment with smoking cessation therapies. Thus NRT doses may be increased to achieve appropriate nicotine replacement levels, the dose of bupropion or varenicline may be reduced to control side effects, and consideration can be given to extending the initial period of treatment with all three therapies. It is likely that a willingness to use these medications in this manner will increase their effectiveness in clinical practice. It should be noted that the medication protocol producing the greatest effect on abstinence rates is long-term NRT in association with ad libitum NRT (Table 10.4).[10]

Other pharmacotherapy considerations

Combination therapies It is now recognized that combinations of pharmacotherapies may enhance the likelihood of cessation. In particular, combinations of NRT (patch plus inhaler, patch plus gum) may allow more accurate and precise titration of nicotine; a meta-analysis comparing the effectiveness of long-term patch use in association with either gum or inhaler showed the combination to be significantly more effective than patch alone (OR = 1.9).[10]

Largely on the basis of one study,[98] the combination of NRT with bupropion was also more effective than patch alone (OR = 1.3) (**Class I, Level A**).

Clonidine The antihypertensive clonidine has been shown to be effective in smoking cessation, approximately doubling cessation rates in comparison to placebo (OR = 2.1) (**Class I, Level A**). Its side effect profile, lack of approval for smoking cessation, and the need to establish a specific dosing regimen have limited its use. It is recommended as a second-line therapy whose use might be considered in patients unable to use preferred medications. When compared to the use of the NRT patch, it was not significantly more efficacious (OR = 1.1).[10]

Mecamylamine This medication has not been proven to be effective in smoking cessation in the two trials that have been performed and its use is not recommended.[10]

Nortriptyline A meta-analysis has demonstrated that the use of this antidepressant has consistently elevated rates of smoking cessation approximately twofold in comparison to placebo (OR = 2.34), but appears less effective than NRT patch use (OR = 0.9)[93] (**Class I, Level A**). This medication has not been approved for smoking cessation, has a distinct side effect profile, and is recommended only as a second-line therapy.[10]

Rimonabant This compound, a selective type 1 cannabinoid receptor antagonist, has been subjected to clinical trials which have suggested it may be of help in smoking cessation (OR = 1.61) in comparison to placebo but has not received approval for use as an aid to smoking cessation. Central cannabinoid receptors have been implicated in

Table 10.4 A comparison of the effectiveness of and abstinence rates using various medications relative to the nicotine patch

Medication	Number of arms	Estimated odds ratio (95% CI)
Nicotine patch (reference group)	32	1.0
Varenicline (2 mg/day)	5	1.6 (1.3–2.0)
Nicotine nasal spray	4	1.2 (0.9–1.6)
Bupropion SR	26	1.0 (0.9–1.2)
Patch (long-term; > 4 weeks) + NRT (gum or spray)	3	1.9 (1.3–2.7)
Patch + bupropion SR	3	1.3 (1.0–1.8)
Patch + inhaler	2	1.1 (0.7–1.9)

Adapted from Fiore MC *et al. Treating Tobacco Use and Dependence: 2008 Update.* Rockville, MD: US Dept of Health and Human Services, Public Health Service, 2008.

appetite control and in the development of dependence and habituation.[104]

Nicotine vaccine At least three nicotine vaccines are in development; there are challenges in associating the small nicotine molecule with a carrier (usually a virus). It is anticipated that a vaccine would induce and maintain significantly elevated levels of antibodies to nicotine, resulting in the production and persistence of nicotine–antibody complexes which are too large to cross the blood–brain barrier. Stimulation of brain nicotine receptors would not then be possible and the 'priming' role of minimal smoking in initiating a relapse would be eliminated.[105] Clinical trials continue.[105]

Other therapies

A variety of therapies have been suggested as being helpful in cessation and subjected to varying forms of evaluation. There is no evidence to support the use of hypnosis,[106] acupuncture, laser therapies[107] or nutritional strategies as being efficacious for smoking cessation.

Conclusion

Evidence continues to accumulate of the devastation wrought by tobacco and the important role it plays in the initiation and accentuation of heart disease. Stopping smoking in those who have cardiac disease produces clinical benefits that are substantial and accrue more rapidly than any other preventive intervention. Cardiovascular specialists can dramatically reduce the anticipated excess morbidity and mortality in their smoking patients to the extent that they are able to assist with cessation. The development and implementation, in every professional setting, of a systematic approach to the identification of all smokers; the provision of specific advice regarding, and assistance with, quitting; the prescription or provision of effective pharmacotherapies for cessation; and the organization of appropriate arrangements for follow-up will significantly enhance the quality of care provided to all patients and optimize the likelihood of cessation (Box 10.2). Smoking cessation is the most important and most cost-effective of all preventive interventions. The personal, unambiguous, and non-judgmental advice of a cardiologist consistently expressed at every patient visit emphasizing the relevance and primacy of cessation in managing a cardiac condition can have a significant impact on eventual rates of cessation.

The likelihood of cessation can be significantly increased by the use of one of three effective pharmacotherapies. All cardiac physicians should become familiar and proficient with the prescription and use of the first-line cessation

---

BOX 10.2 A systematic approach to smoking cessation

The essential elements of a systematic approach can be incorporated into office or clinic protocols, and hospital care maps. The introduction of a systematic approach will ensure that all smoking patients are identified and offered specific advice and assistance (including pharmacotherapy) in association with appropriate follow-up.

1. **Identification of Smoking Status:**
   - "Have you used any form of tobacco in the past six months?"
2. **Documentation:**
   - Smoking history (pack-years)
   - Previous cessation attempts
   - Time to first cigarette
3. **Counseling:**
   - Specific advice on benefits of quitting
   - Educational resources
   - Staff trained in delivery of cessation advice and assistance
4. **Pharmacotherapy:**
   - Available on formulary
   - Medical and nursing staff familiar with use
   - Treatment of withdrawal and initiation of smoking cessation
5. **Follow-up:**
   - Clinics, community resources, automated technologies

Adapted from Reid R, Pipe A, Quinlan B. Promoting smoking cessation during hospitalization for coronary artery disease. *Can J Cardiol* 2006;**22**(9):775–80.

---

therapies: nicotine replacement therapy (NRT), bupropion, and varenicline. In the hospital setting, the development and implementation of a systematic approach to the delivery of smoking cessation services to all admitted smokers can be expected to significantly increase the number of smokers who make quit attempts and achieve cessation success. Smoking cessation is a fundamental clinical responsibility of those treating smoking patients. The chances of cessation success are enhanced by "doing ordinary things extraordinarily well".[108]

References

1. Orleans CT. Increasing the demand for and use of effective smoking-cessation treatments reaping the full health benefits of tobacco-control science and policy gains in our lifetime. *Am J Prev Med* 2007; **33**(6):S340–S348.
2. Peto R *et al*. Mortality from Smoking in Developed Countries 1950–2000: Indirect Estimation from National Vital Statistics. Oxford: Oxford University Press, 1994.
3. Isles CG, Hole DJ, Hawthorne VM, Lever AF. Relation between coronary risk and coronary mortality in women of the Renfrew

and Paisley survey: comparison with men. *Lancet* 1992; **339**:702–6.

4. Armour BS *et al.* Annual smoking-attributable mortality, years of potential life lost and productivity losses – United States, 1997–2001. *MMWR* 2005;**54**:625–8.

5. Giovino GA. The tobacco epidemic in the United States. *Am J Prev Med* 2007;**33**(6S):S318–26.

6. Doll R, Peto R, Wheatley K, Gray R, Sutherland I. Mortality in relation to smoking: 40 years' observations on male British doctors. *BMJ* 1994;**309**:901–11.

7. *The Health Consequences of Smoking: A Report of the Surgeon General*. Atlanta, GA: US Department of Health and Human Services, Centers for Disease Control and Prevention, National Center for Chronic Disease and Health Promotion, Office on Smoking and Health, 2004.

8. Burns DM. Epidemiology of smoking-induced disease. *Prog Cardiovasc Dis* 2003;**46**:11–29.

9. Critchley J, Capewell S. Mortality risk reduction associated with smoking cessation in patients with coronary heart disease: a systematic review. *JAMA* 2003;**290**(1):1708–9.

10. Fiore MC *et al.* Treating Tobacco Use and Dependence: 2008 Update. Clinical Practice Guideline. Rockville, MD: US Dept of Health and Human Services, Public Health Service, 2008.

11. Mackay J, Erickson MP. The Tobacco Atlas. Geneva: World Health Organization, 2002.

12. Peto R, Lopez AD. The future worldwide health effects of current smoking patterns. In: Koop CE, Pearson DE, Schwarz MR, ed. Critical Issues in Global Health. San Francisco: Jossey-Bass, 2001.

13. Fiore M *et al.* Treating Tobacco Use and Dependence. Clinical Practice Guideline. Rockville, MD: US Department of Health and Human Services, Public Health Service, 2000.

14. Maciosek MV, Coffield AB, Edwards NM, Flottemesch TJ, Goodman MJ, Solberg LI. Priorities among effective clinical preventive services: results of a systematic review and analysis. *Am J Prev Med* 2006;**31**(1):52–61.

15. Solberg LI, Maciosek MV, Edwards NM, Khanchandani HS, Goodman MJ. Repeated tobacco-use screening and intervention in clinical practice: health impact and cost effectiveness. *Am J Prev Med* 2006;**31**(1):62–71.

16. Quist-Paulsen P, Lydersen S, Bakke PS, Gallefoss F. Cost effectiveness of a smoking cessation program in patients admitted for coronary heart disease. *Eur J Cardiovasc Prev Rehabil* 2006;**13**(2):274–80.

17. Tonstad S, Johnston JA. Cardiovascular risks associated with smoking: a review for clinicians. *Eur J Cardiovasc Prev Rehabil* 2006;**13**:507–14.

18. Ambrose J, Barua R. The pathophysiology of cigarette smoking and cardiovascular disease: an update. *J Am Coll Cardiol* 2004;**43**(10):1731–7.

19. Benowitz N. Cigarette smoking and cardiovascular disease: pathophysiology and implications for treatment. *Prog Cardiovasc Dis* 2003;**46**(1):91–111.

20. Metz L, Waters DD. Implications of cigarette smoking for the management of patients with acute coronary syndromes. *Prog Cardiovasc Dis* 2003;**46**(1):1–9.

21. Barbash GI, Reiner J, White HD *et al.* Evaluation of paradoxical beneficial effects of smoking in patients receiving thrombolytic therapy for acute myocardial infarction: mechanism of the "smoker's paradox" from the GUSTO-1 trial, with angiographic insights. *J Am Coll Cardiol* 1995;**26**:1222–9.

22. Celermajer DS, Adams MR, Clarkson P *et al.* Passive smoking and impaired endothelium-dependent arterial dilatation in healthy young adults. *N Engl J Med* 1996;**334**:150–4.

23. Valkonen M, Kuusi T. Passive smoking induces atherogenic changes in low-density lipoprotein. *Circulation* 1998;**97**:2012–16.

24. Barnoya J, Glantz SA. Cardiovascular effects of secondhand smoke: nearly as large as smoking. *Circulation* 2005;**111**:2684–98.

25. Law MR, Wald NJ. Environmental tobacco smoke and ischemic heart disease. *Prog Cardiovasc Dis* 2003;**46**(1):31–8.

26. Wells AJ. Heart disease from passive smoking in the workplace. *J Am Coll Cardiol* 1998;**31**(1):1–9.

27. He J, Vupputuri S, Allen K *et al.* Passive smoking and the risk of coronary heart disease: a meta-analysis of epidemiologic studies. *N Engl J Med* 1999;**340**:920–6.

28. National Cancer Institute. Health Effects of Exposure to Environmental Tobacco Smoke: The Report of the California Environmental Protection Agency. Smoking and Tobacco Control Monograph no. 10. Vol. NIH Pub. No. 99–4645. Bethesda, MD: US Department of Health and Human Services, National Institutes of Health, National Cancer Institute, 1999.

29. Aronow WS. Effect of passive smoking on angina pectoris. *N Engl J Med* 1978;**299**:21–4.

30. Leone A, Mori L, Bertanelli F, Fabiano P, Filippelli M. Indoor passive smoking: its effect on cardiac performance. *Int J Cardiol* 1991;**33**:247–51.

31. Benowitz NL, Porchet H, Sheiner L, Jacob P 3rd *et al.* Nicotine absorption and cardiovascular effects with smokeless tobacco use: comparison with cigarettes and nicotine gum. *Clin Pharmacol Ther* 1988;**44**:23–8.

32. Westman E. Does smokeless tobacco cause hypertension? *South Med J* 1995;**88**:716–20.

33. Bolinder GM, de Faire U. Ambulatory 24-h blood pressure monitoring in healthy, middle-aged smokeless tobacco users, smokers, and non-tobacco users. *Am J Hypertens* 1998; **11**:1153–63.

34. Tucker LA. Use of smokeless tobacco, cigarette smoking and hypercholesterolemia. *Am J Public Health* 1989;**79**:1048–50.

35. Persson PG, Carlsson S, Svanström L *et al.* Cigarette smoking, oral moist snuff use and glucose intolerance. *J Intern Med* 2000;**248**:103–10.

36. Eliasson M, Lundblad D, Hagg E. Cardiovascular factors in young snuff-users and cigarette smokers. *J Intern Med* 1991;**230**:103–10.

37. Gupta R, Gurm H, Bartholomew JR. Smokeless tobacco and cardiovascular risk. *Arch Intern Med* 2004;**164**:1845–9.

38. Critchley JA, Capewell S. Smoking cessation for the secondary prevention of coronary heart disease. *Cochrane Database of Systematic Reviews* 2003, Issue 4. Art. No.: CD003041. DOI: 10.1002/14651858.CD003041.pub2.

39. Hallstrom AP, Cobb LA, Ray R. Smoking as a risk factor for recurrence of sudden cardiac arrest. *N Engl J Med* 1986;**314**(5): 271–5.

40. Vlietstra RE, Kronmal RA, Oberman A, Frye RL, Killip T 3rd. Effect of cigarette smoking on survival of patients with angio-

graphically documented coronary artery disease. Report from the CASS registry. *JAMA* 1986;**255**(8):1023–7.

41. Peters RW, Brooks MM, Todd L, Liebson PR, Wilhelmsen L. Smoking cessation and arrhythmic death: the CAST experience. The Cardiac Arrhythmia Suppression Trial (CAST) Investigators. *J Am Coll Cardiol* 1995;**26**(5):1287–92.

42. Suskin N, Sheth T, Negassa A, Yusuf S. Relationship of current and past smoking to mortality and morbidity in patients with left ventricular dysfunction. *J Am Coll Cardiol* 2001;**37**:1677–82.

43. Pechacek TF, Babb S. How acute and reversible are the cardiovascular risks of secondhand smoke? *BMJ* 2004;**328**(7446):980–3.

44. Sargent RP, Shepard RM, Glantz SA. Reduced incidence of admissions for myocardial infarction associated with public smoking ban: before and after study. *BMJ* 2004;**328**(7446):977–80.

45. Bartecchi C, Alsever RN, Nevin-Woods C *et al.* Reduction in the incidence of acute myocardial infarction associated with a citywide smoking ordinance. *Circulation* 2006;**14**:1490–6.

46. Barone-Adesi F, Vizzini L, Merletti F, Richiardi L. Short term-effects of Italian smoking regulation on rates of hospital admission for acute myocardial infarction. *Eur Heart J* 2006;**27**:2468–72.

47. Cesaroni G, Forastiere F, Agabiti N *et al.* Effect of the Italian smoking ban on population rates of acute coronary events. *Circulation* 2008;**117**(9):1183–8.

48. Juster HR, Loomis BR, Hinman TM *et al.* Declines in hospital admissions for acute myocardial infarction in New York state after implementation of a comprehensive smoking ban. *Am J Public Health* 2007;**97**(11):2035–9.

49. Picciotto MR, Zoli M, Rimondini R *et al.* Acetylcholine receptors containing the beta-2 subunit are involved in the reinforcing properties of nicotine. *Nature* 1998;**391**:173–7.

50. Nestler EJ. Is there a common molecular pathway for addiction? *Nat Neurosci* 2005;**8**:1445–9.

51. Benowitz NL. Neurobiology of nicotine addiction: implications for smoking cessation treatment. *Am J Med* 2008;**121**(4A):S3-S10.

52. Diagnostic and Statistical Manual of Mental Disorders, 4th edn. Washington, DC: American Psychiatric Association, 1994.

53. Koob GF, Le Moal M. Drug abuse: hedonic homeostatic dysregulation. *Science* 1997;**278**:52–8.

54. Hughes JR. Clinical significance of tobacco withdrawal. *Nicotine Tob Res* 2006;**8**:153–6.

55. Hughes JR, Gulliver SB, Fenwick JW *et al.* Smoking cessation among self-quitters. *Health Psychol* 1992;**11**:331–4.

56. Hughes JR, Keely J, Naud S. Shape of the relapse curve and long-term abstinence among untreated smokers. *Addiction* 2004;**99**(1):29–38.

57. Hyland A, Borland R, Li Q *et al.* Individual-level predictors of cessation behaviours among participants in the International Tobacco Control (ITC) Four Country Survey. *Tob Control* 2006;**15**(suppl 3): iii83–94.

58. Rigotti NA, Singer DE, Mulley AG Jr, Thibault GE. Smoking cessation following admission to a coronary care unit. *J Gen Intern Med* 1992;**6**:305–11.

59. Nägele H, Kalmár P, Rödiger W, Stubbe HM. Smoking after heart transplant: an underestimated hazard? *Eur J Cardiothorac Surg* 1997;**12**:70–4.

60. Basile A, Bernazzali S, Diciolla F *et al.* Risk factors for smoking abuse after heart transplantation. *Transplant Proc* 2004;**36**:641–2.

61. Botha P, Peaston R, White K *et al.* Smoking after cardiac transplantation. *Am J Transplant* 2008;**8**:866–71.

62. Mehra MR, Uber PA, Prasad A, Scott RL, Park MH. Recrudescent tobacco exposure following heart transplantation: clinical profiles and relationship with athero-thrombosis risk markers. *Am J Transplant* 2005;**5**(5):1137–40.

63. Benowitz NL. The role of nicotine in smoking-related cardiovascular disease. *Prev Med* 1997;**26**(4):412–17.

64. Malaiyandi V, Lerman C, Benowitz NL *et al.* Impact of CYP2A6 genotype on pretreatment smoking behavior and nicotine levels from and usage of nicotine replacement therapy. *Mol Psychiatry* 2006;**11**(4):400–9.

65. Li MD. The genetic determinants of smoking related behaviour: a brief review. *Am J Med Sci* 2003;**326**(4):168–73.

66. Dalack GW, Healy DJ, Meador-Woodruff JH. Nicotine dependence in schizophrenia: clinical phenomena and laboratory findings. *Am J Psychiatry* 1998;**155**:1490–501.

67. Ziedonis D, Williams JM, Smelson D. Serious mental illness and tobacco addiction: a model program to address this common but neglected issue. *Am J Med Sci* 2003;**326**(4):223–30.

68. Lasser K, Boyd JW, Woolhandler S *et al.* Smoking and mental illness. A population-based prevalence study. *JAMA* 2000;**284**:2602–10.

69. Forrester JS, Merz CN, Bush TL *et al.* 27th Bethesda Conference: matching the intensity of risk factor management with the hazard for coronary disease events. Task Force 4. Efficacy of risk factor management. *J Am Coll Cardiol* 1996;**27**(5):991–1006.

70. Thorndike AN, Rigotti NA, Stafford RS, Singer DE. National patterns in the treatment of smokers by physicians. *JAMA* 1998;**279**(8):604–8.

71. Lancaster T, Stead LF. Individual behavioural counselling for smoking cessation. *Cochrane Database of Systematic Reviews* 2005, Issue 2. Art. No.: CD001292. DOI: 10.1002/14651858.CD001292.pub2.

72. Stead LF, Perera R, Lancaster T. Telephone counselling for smoking cessation. *Cochrane Database of Systematic Reviews* 2006, Issue 3. Art. No.: CD002850. DOI: 10.1002/14651858.CD002850.pub2.

73. Stead LF, Lancaster T. Group behaviour therapy programmes for smoking cessation. *Cochrane Database of Systematic Reviews* 2005, Issue 2. Art. No.: CD001007. DOI: 10.1002/14651858.CD001007.pub2.

74. Stead LF, Bergson G, Lancaster T. Physician advice for smoking cessation. *Cochrane Database of Systematic Reviews* 2008, Issue 2. Art. No.: CD000165. DOI: 10.1002/14651858.CD000165.pub3.

75. Rice VH, Stead LF. Nursing interventions for smoking cessation. *Cochrane Database of Systematic Reviews* 2008, Issue 1. Art. No.: CD001188. DOI: 10.1002/14651858.CD001188.pub3.

76. Grant BF, Hasin DS, Chou SP, Stinson FS, Dawson DA. Nicotine dependence and psychiatric disorders in the United States: results from the national epidemiologic survey on alcohol and related conditions. *Arch Gen Psychiatry* 2004;**61**(11):1107–15.

77. Hughes JR, Hatsukami DK, Mitchell JE, Dahlgren LA. Prevalence of smoking among psychiatric outpatients. *Am J Psychiatry* 1986;**143**(8):993–7.

78. Hughes JR. Effects of abstinence from tobacco: valid symptoms and time course. *Nicotine Tob Res*,2007;**9**(3):315–27.

79. Koplan KE, Regan S, Goldszer RC, Schneider LI, Rigotti NA. A computerized aid to support smoking cessation treatment for hospital patients. *J Gen Intern Med* 2008 **23**(8):1214–7.

80. Reid R, Pipe A, Quinlan B. Promoting smoking cessation during hospitalization for coronary artery disease. *Can J Cardiol* 2006;**22**(9):775–80.

81. Mohiuddin SM, Mooss AN, Hunter CB *et al.* Intensive smoking cessation intervention reduces mortality in high-risk smokers with cardiovascular disease. *Chest* 2007;**131**(2):446–52.

82. Rigotti N, Munafo' MR, Stead LF. Interventions for smoking cessation in hospitalised patients. *Cochrane Database of Systematic Reviews* 2007, Issue 3. Art. No.: CD001837. DOI: 10.1002/14651858.CD001837.pub2.

83. Tzivoni D, Keren A, Meyler S *et al.* Cardiovascular safety of transdermal nicotine patches in patients with coronary artery disease who try to quit smoking. *Cardiovasc Drugs Ther* 1998;**12**(3):239–44.

84. Mahmarian JJ, Moyé LA, Nasser GA *et al.* Nicotine patch therapy in smoking cessation reduces the extent of exercise-induced myocardial ischaemia. *J Am Coll Cardiol* 1997;**30**(1):125–30.

85. Hubbard R, Lewis S, Smith C *et al.* Use of nicotine replacement therapy and the risk of acute myocardial infarction, stroke, and death. *Tob Control* 2005;**14**(6):416–21.

86. Joseph A, Fu S. Safety issues in pharmacotherapy for smoking in patients with cardiovascular disease. *Prog Cardiovasc Dis* 2003;**45**(6):429–41.

87. Meine TJ, Patel MR, Washam JB, Pappas PA, Jollis JG. Safety and effectiveness of transdermal nicotine patch in smokers admitted with acute coronary syndromes. *Am J Cardiol* 2005;**95**(8).976–8.

88. Kimmel SE, Berlin JA, Miles C *et al.* Risk of acute first myocardial infarction and use of nicotine patches in a general population. *J Am Coll Cardiol* 2001;**37**(5):1297–302.

89. Stead LF, Perera R, Bullen C, Mant D, Lancaster T. Nicotine replacement therapy for smoking cessation. *Cochrane Database of Systematic Reviews* 2008, Issue 1. Art. No.: CD000146. DOI: 10.1002/14651858.CD000146.pub3.

90. Ferry LH, Burchette R. Evaluation of brupropion versus placebo for treatment of nicotine dependence. Abstracts of the 147th Annual Meeting of the American Psychiatric Association. Philadelphia: American Psychiatric Association, 1994.

91. Hurt RD, Sachs DP, Glover ED *et al.* A comparison of sustained-release bupropion and placebo for smoking cessation. *N Engl J Med* 1997;**337**(17):1195–202.

92. Jorenby DE, Leischow SJ, Nides MA *et al.* A controlled trial of sustained-release bupropion, a nicotine patch, or both for smoking cessation. *N Engl J Med* 1999;**340**(9):685–91.

93. Hughes JR, Stead LF, Lancaster T. Antidepressants for smoking cessation. *Cochrane Database of Systematic Reviews* 2007, Issue 1. Art. No.: CD000031. DOI: 10.1002/14651858.CD000031.pub3.

94. Scharf D, Shiffman S. Are there gender differences in smoking cessation, with and without bupropion? Pooled- and meta-analyses of clinical trials of Bupropion SR. *Addiction* 2004;**99**(11):1462–9.

95. Tonstad S, Farsang C, Klaene G *et al.* Bupropion SR for smoking cessation in smokers with cardiovascular disease: a multicentre, randomised study. *Eur Heart J* 2003;**24**(10):946–55.

96. Borrelli B, Niaura R, Keuthen NJB *et al.* Development of major depressive disorder during smoking-cessation treatment. *J Clin Psychiatry* 1996;**57**(11):534–8.

97. Swan GE, McAfee T, Curry SJ *et al.* Effectiveness of bupropion sustained release for smoking cessation in a health care setting: a randomized trial. *Arch Intern Med* 2003;**163**(19):2337–44.

98. Jorenby DE, Leischow SJ, Nides MA *et al.* A controlled trial of sustained-release bupropion, a nicotine patch, or both for smoking cessation. *N Engl J Med* 1999;**340**(9):685–91.

99. Seeger R. Cytisine as an aid for smoking cessation (in German). *Med Monatsschr Pharm* 1992;**15**:20–21.

100. Lickint F. Mdikamentöse Unterstützung der Tabakentwöhnung. *Therapiewoche* 1955–56;**6**:444–8.

101. Oncken C, Gonzales D, Nides M *et al.* Efficacy and safety of the novel selective nicotinic acetylcholine receptor partial agonist varenicline, for smoking cessation. *Arch Intern Med* 2006;**166**(15):1571–7.

102. Fagerstrom KO, Hughes J. Varenicline in the treatment of tobacco dependence. *Neuropsych DisTreat* 2008;**4**(2):353–63.

103. Cahill K, Stead LF, Lancaster T. Nicotine receptor partial agonists for smoking cessation. *Cochrane Database of Systematic Reviews* 2008, Issue 3. Art. No.: CD006103. DOI: 10.1002/14651858.CD006103.pub3.

104. Cahill K, Ussher MH. Cannabinoid type 1 receptor antagonists (rimonabant) for smoking cessation. *Cochrane Database of Systematic Reviews* 2007, Issue 4. Art. No.: CD005353. DOI: 10.1002/14651858.CD005353.pub3.

105. Maurer P, Bachmann MF. Vaccination against nicotine: an emerging therapy for tobacco dependence. *Expert Opin Investig Drugs* 2007;**16**(11):1775–83.

106. Abbot NC, Stead LF, White AR, Barnes J. Hypnotherapy for smoking cessation. *Cochrane Database of Systematic Reviews* 1998, Issue 2. Art. No.: CD001008. DOI: 10.1002/14651858.CD001008.

107. White AR, Rampes H, Campbell J. Acupuncture and related interventions for smoking cessation. *Cochrane Database of Systematic Reviews* 2006, Issue 1. Art. No.: CD000009. DOI: 10.1002/14651858.CD000009.pub2.

108. Reid RD, Quinlan B, Riley DL, Pipe AL. Smoking cessation: lessons learned from clinical trial evidence. *Curr Opin Cardiol* 2007;**22**(4):280–5.

11 Lipids and cardiovascular disease

Malcolm Law

Wolfson Institute of Preventive Medicine, London, UK

Introduction

Elevated serum cholesterol was the single most important cause of the 20th-century pandemic of ischemic heart disease, with the high-fat diet typical of many Western countries over the greater part of the 20th century extending more recently to non-Western countries. Modern cholesterol-lowering drugs (statins) can reduce risk more than any other single intervention.

Serum total and low-density lipoprotein cholesterol

Typical values of serum total and low-density lipoprotein (LDL) cholesterol in Western countries are high in comparison with those in agricultural and hunter-gatherer communities, because of the high saturated fat content of the Western diet. Average serum cholesterol concentrations (in men aged 45–60) are about 3–3.5 mmol/L in hunter-gatherer societies and rural China (where heart disease is rare), but over much of the 20th century they were about 5.0 mmol/L in Japan, 5.5 mmol/L in Mediterranean populations, and 6 mmol/L in the USA, Britain and Northern Europe.[1] Use of the term "normal" in reference to usual or average Western cholesterol values may therefore be misleading (we are all "high"). In recent years cholesterol levels in Japan have risen while those in the USA, Britain and Northern Europe have fallen a little. Average levels of LDL cholesterol are about 2 mmol/L lower than total cholesterol.[1]

Of the average total serum cholesterol in Western populations, two-thirds is LDL cholesterol and one-quarter is high-density lipoprotein (HDL) cholesterol. The atherogenic properties lie in the LDL fraction (sometimes measured as its carrier protein, apolipoprotein B, with which it is highly correlated). Many of the large epidemiologic studies and the earlier randomized trials measured only total serum cholesterol; total serum cholesterol has been used as a surrogate for LDL cholesterol. Fortuitously, the approximation is a good one. The absolute reduction in total serum cholesterol produced by diet and by most drugs (including statins[2–12]) is similar to the reduction in LDL cholesterol. Observational differences in total cholesterol between individuals in cohort studies are a little greater than the corresponding differences in LDL cholesterol, but this "surrogate dilution bias" can readily be corrected.[13] Much epidemiologic and clinical trial data are therefore available to estimate quantitatively the effect of lowering serum LDL cholesterol on the risk of ischemic heart disease.

Serum cholesterol and ischemic heart disease

For about two decades we have had evidence from genetics, animal studies, experimental pathology, epidemiologic studies and clinical trials indicating conclusively that elevated serum cholesterol is an important cause of ischemic heart disease and that lowering serum cholesterol reduces the risk.[14] Ten large randomized trials of statins, published over a 10-year period, have ensured that this is now widely accepted.[2–12] Three important practical questions arise: the nature of the dose–response relationship, the size of the effect, and the speed of the reversal of risk. To answer these questions, data from both cohort studies (or prospective observational studies) and randomized controlled trials are necessary: the two are complementary. Table 11.1 summarizes the advantages of each.

The nature of the dose–response relationship: is there a threshold?

A plot of ischemic heart disease mortality on total serum cholesterol in the Prospective Studies Collaboration (PSC)

Evidence-Based Cardiology, 3rd edition. Edited by S. Yusuf, J.A. Cairns, A.J. Camm, E.L. Fallen, and B.J. Gersh. © 2010 Blackwell Publishing, ISBN: 978-1-4051-5925-8.

meta-analysis of 61 cohort studies showed a near-perfect straight-line dose–response relationship linking *proportional* differences in ischemic heart disease mortality (the vertical axis uses a logarithmic scale) to absolute differences in serum cholesterol, across the range of cholesterol values in Western populations[15] (Fig. 11.1). Based on a

Table 11.1 Relative advantages of cohort studies and randomized trials in assessing the relation between serum cholesterol and ischemic heart disease

Objective	Advantage (comment)
Statistical power	Cohort studies (recorded seven times more ischemic heart disease events than the trials: 91 800 v 12 500[15,16])
Dose–response relationship	Cohort studies (observation across a wide range of cholesterol values, from 3 to 14 mmol/L)
Wide age range	Cohort studies (ischemic heart disease events at ages 35–89, but mostly 55–65 in trials)
Long-term effects of cholesterol differences	Cohort studies (the cholesterol differences between individuals observed at the start of the study will have been present for decades previously)
Short-term effects of cholesterol differences	Randomized trials (on recruitment serum cholesterol was the same in intervention and control groups)
Avoid bias	Randomized trials (not a major advantage – bias in cohort studies can be allowed for)

single (baseline) cholesterol measurement, there was a continuous straight-line relationship between baseline total cholesterol values of 3 mmol/L and 14 mmol/L, using the baseline cholesterol measurements to divide the cohort into subgroups. However, using a repeat measure to estimate the mean cholesterol of each subgroup ("usual total cholesterol"), thereby allowing for regression dilution bias, the straight-line relationship extended between usual cholesterol values of 4 and 9 mmol/L. The straight line establishes that there is no threshold below which a further decrease in serum cholesterol is not associated with a further decrease in risk of ischemic heart disease. The exponential relationship indicated by the straight line means that a given absolute difference in serum cholesterol concentration from *any* point on the cholesterol distribution is associated with a constant proportional difference in the incidence of ischemic heart disease.

The absence of a threshold has in the past been contentious. However, the cohort study evidence (itself conclusive)[15,16] is supported by subgroup analyses according to baseline cholesterol in a meta-analysis of randomized controlled trials showing similar proportional reduction in coronary heart disease (CHD) from all baseline levels,[17] by randomized trials showing a greater CHD risk reduction and a greater degree of coronary artery atheroma regression with more intensive than less intensive LDL cholesterol reduction (from 2.6 to 2.0 mmol/L),[18,19] by ecologic studies,[1,14] and by experimental data on the transfer of cholesterol from the blood into atheromatous lesions which exclude a threshold as low as 1 mmol/L.[20] People at higher

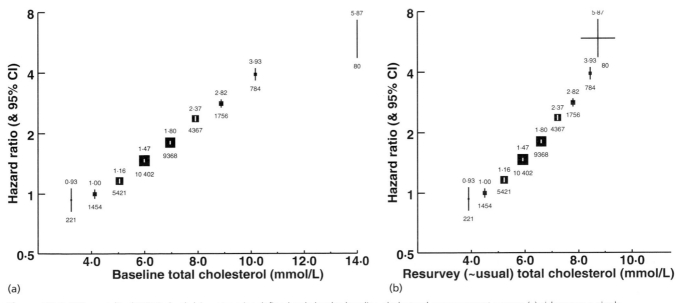

Figure 11.1 IHD mortality (33 853 deaths) in categories defined only by the baseline cholesterol measurement versus: (a) risk versus a single measurement of cholesterol – mean of baseline values in each group and (b) risk versus resurvey (usual) cholesterol – mean of first resurvey values in each group (approximating mean usual values). Reproduced with permission from Prospective Studies Collaboration.[15]

risk of an ischemic heart disease event should be offered a statin irrespective of their existing level of total or LDL cholesterol.

The size of the effect

Table 11.2 shows estimates of the long-term percentage decrease in the risk of an ischemic heart disease event according to age at event, from the Prospective Studies Collaboration. A reduction in total or LDL cholesterol of 1 mmol/L is associated with a decrease in risk of ischemic heart disease of about 61% at age 45, 46% at 55, 31% at 65, 20% at 75 and 17% at 85. Statins (for example, simvastatin 40 mg, atorvastatin 10 mg) reduce LDL cholesterol by 1.8 mmol/L;[16] from the dose–response relationship this would reduce the risk of ischemic heart disease events by about 60% on average in people aged 50–69 years.

Speed of reversal and consistency of observational and trial data

Efficacy of serum cholesterol reduction according to duration has been determined from the results of randomized trials by separate meta-analysis of all CHD events occurring in the first year of trials, all occurring in the second year of trials, etc.[16] Results are summarized in Table 11.2, applicable to age 60 (the average age of sustaining an ischemic heart disease event in the trials). The estimate of the long-term effect of cholesterol reduction, from the cohort studies (in which the cholesterol differences between individuals are longstanding), is also shown. The proportional reduction in risk increases continuously with the duration of the cholesterol reduction: there is relatively little effect

Table 11.2 PSC age-specific estimates of relative risk of ischemic heart disease for a 1 mmol/L lower total serum cholesterol,[15] and estimates adjusted for the surrogate dilution bias,[13] both for a 1 mmol/L lower LDL cholesterol

| Age | Relative risk estimate | | % reduction in ischemic heart disease |
	published	adjusted	
40–49 (45–54)	0.44	0.39	61%
50–59 (55–64)	0.58	0.54	46%
60–69 (65–74)	0.72	0.69	31%
70–79	0.82	0.80	20%
80–89	0.85	0.83	17%

(11% reduction) in the first year, but a 33% reduction by the third year and (from cohort studies) a 39% reduction in the long term. The similarity of the estimates of effect from the cohort studies and from the trial data from the third year onwards indicates that the reversal of risk is near maximal after two years – a surprisingly rapid effect.

The estimates of effect are similar in men and women, in people with and without previous ischemic heart disease, and for coronary death and non-fatal myocardial infarction.[15,17] Four randomized controlled trials have attained average LDL cholesterol reductions (treated minus placebo) exceeding 1.5 mmol/L (1.6 mmol/L on average).[16] In these four trials the average reduction in incidence of ischemic heart disease events from the third year onwards was 51% (95% confidence interval (CI) 42–58%, compared to an expected value from cohort studies of 55%).[16] Trial data therefore show directly that LDL cholesterol reductions attainable with statins reduce risk by over half. Importantly, most randomized trials of statins do not show their full potential for preventing ischemic heart disease events because of "contamination" – some patients allocated to the treated group leave the trial and stop taking the tablets, some patients allocated to the placebo group take statins, and the results are necessarily analyzed on an intention-to-treat basis. The randomized trials therefore confirm the dose–response relationship shown in the cohort studies (the greater the cholesterol reduction, the greater the reduction in heart disease events[16]) and confirm the estimates from the cohort studies in Table 11.2 of the long-term reduction in risk.

As a parallel to the observation that a few years are necessary before serum cholesterol reduction is fully effective, follow-up of the participants in one randomized trial after the trial had terminated showed that the protective effect persisted in previously treated patients for some years after the termination of the trial (LDL cholesterol was similar in the former treated and placebo groups during this follow-up period).[21]

Dietary fat and serum cholesterol

The relationship between dietary saturated fat and serum cholesterol is shown by the data from Japan and Britain in Table 11.3. This comparison is a useful one because dietary saturated fat differs greatly, yet dietary polyunsaturated fat and cholesterol are similar in the two countries, so the serum cholesterol difference is attributable to the saturated fat difference. As in other situations (salt and blood pressure, for example), the size of the association varies with age, yet there has been a tendency to generalize to older age groups the results of studies conducted in younger age groups. Many dietary trials, for example, have been conducted in people under 30. The few that have been

Table 11.3 Decrease in ischemic heart disease events for a cholesterol decrease of 1 mmol/L, according to duration of the cholesterol decrease, from randomized trials[16] and cohort studies[15]

	Duration of cholesterol difference	Decrease in risk (95% CI) of ischemic heart disease event	
Randomized trials:	1st year	11%	(4–18%)
	2nd year	24%	(17–30%)
	3rd–5th years	33%	(28–37%)
	≥6 years	36%	(26–45%)
Cohort studies:	decades	39%	(37–41%)

Table 11.4 Serum cholesterol and dietary saturated fat in Japan and Britain. Data compiled from national surveys in each country[1]

Age	Japan	Britain	Difference
Dietary saturated fat (% calories)			
All ages	6%	16%	10%
Serum cholesterol (mmol/L)			
20–29	4.5	5.0	0.5
30–39	5.0	5.6	0.6
40–49	5.1	6.0	0.9
50–59	5.2	6.2	1.0
60–69	5.0	6.2	1.2

conducted in people over 50 tend to support the above Japan–Britain comparison.[14] In older people a reduction in dietary saturated fat equivalent to 10% of calories will lower serum cholesterol by about 1 mmol/L, which in turn will reduce ischemic heart disease mortality in the long term by about 40%.

The chain lengths of saturated fatty acids influence the extent to which they increase blood cholesterol. Palmitic ($C_{16:0}$) and myristic ($C_{14:0}$) acids have the major effect, lauric acid ($C_{12:0}$) some effect, and stearic acid ($C_{18:0}$) and medium chain fatty acids have little or no effect.

Trans unsaturated fatty acids are also important: randomized trials show that they increase serum total and LDL cholesterol by about as much as these longer chain saturated fatty acids.[22,23] They are scanty in naturally occurring fats but are generated by the hydrogenation of vegetable oils for use as hardening agents in manufactured foods. They constitute 6–8% of dietary fat, or 2% of calories, in Western diets.

Naturally occurring *cis* unsaturated fatty acids reduce serum cholesterol by approximately half as much as longer chain saturated fatty acids increase it. Reduction in dietary cholesterol has a small effect on blood cholesterol concentration. Substitution of *cis* unsaturated for saturated fats in the Western diet is thus the most effective change in lowering the high levels of blood cholesterol in Western populations.

The reduction in serum total or LDL cholesterol that can easily be attained by individuals trying to alter their diet in isolation from family, friends and workmates is relatively small (about 0.3 mmol/L or 5%). A larger serum cholesterol reduction, about 0.6 mmol/L (10%), is realistic on a community basis, as the availability of palatable low-fat food increases when other family members or the community alter their diet, and the dietary change is perceived more positively. A reduction by about 7% of calories, a realistic target for a high-fat population, would lower serum cholesterol by 0.6 mmol/L, which in turn would reduce the mortality from ischemic heart disease at age 60 by 25–30%. Reductions in serum cholesterol of about 0.6 mmol/L through dietary change have occurred in entire Western communities, in the United States and Finland for example.[1] Measures that facilitate such a change include wider public education, labeling of foods sold in supermarkets, and the provision of information on the fat content of restaurant meals. Most important is the implementation of national and international policies on food subsidies that are linked to health priorities.

Serum cholesterol and circulatory diseases other than ischemic heart disease

Stroke

Cohort studies show a continuous dose–response relationship between serum cholesterol and ischemic stroke, similar to that with ischemic heart disease, but for hemorrhagic stroke (intracranial and subarachnoid) they show an *excess* risk at lower serum cholesterol levels.[15,16,24] These associations are particularly strong in cohort studies in which computed tomography (CT) scans or autopsy were used to distinguish ischemic and hemorrhagic strokes;[16,24] clinical criteria alone are unreliable and may result in misclassification. Cohort studies that do not distinguish the two types of stroke tend to show little or no association between cholesterol and stroke mortality, consistent with the two associations canceling each other out. Whether the association of lower cholesterol with hemorrhagic stroke is cause and effect is uncertain. It is more difficult to see how a spurious (non-causal) association with intracranial hemorrhage might arise through the disease (or predisposition to the disease) lowering serum cholesterol than was the case with depression and suicide or cancer. It is also difficult to see any mechanism by which the inverse association might be cause and effect, although experimental data lend some support to an interpretation of a causal effect of low cholesterol in that the endothelium of intracerebral arteries might be weaker at very low serum cholesterol levels.[25]

The randomized trials of serum cholesterol reduction, especially the statin trials, have shown a lower incidence of stroke (all types combined) in treated than control patients.[2–12] However, the strokes occurring in trials will mostly be ischemic strokes, for three reasons: they were mostly all non-fatal strokes (ischemic stroke has a lower case fatality than hemorrhagic stroke, and the cohort studies recorded total stroke), the trials tended to recruit patients in the upper half of the serum cholesterol distribution, where ischemic stroke will be more common because of its positive association with serum cholesterol, and many trials recruited patients with coronary artery disease on entry, in whom ischemic stroke will be more common than hemorrhagic. These observations can probably reconcile the reduction in the incidence of stroke in trials (where most of the strokes will have been ischemic) with the absence of an association between serum cholesterol and stroke mortality in cohort studies. Trials that distinguished ischemic from hemorrhagic stroke showed that the risk of ischemic stroke was significantly reduced by a statin,[16] but the trials recorded too few hemorrhagic strokes to confirm or refute the inverse association with cholesterol shown in cohort studies. Meta-analysis of the trials showed a 20% (95% CI 14–26%) reduction in all strokes and a 28% (20–35%) reduction in ischemic stroke for a 1 mmol/L reduction in LDL cholesterol.[16]

Even if the association between low cholesterol and hemorrhagic stroke were cause and effect, however, the increased mortality from hemorrhagic stroke at very low cholesterol concentrations is small compared to the lower mortality from ischemic heart disease and ischemic stroke. Patients who have had an ischemic stroke are at high risk of a recurrent event and should receive statins, as should patients with carotid artery disease and others at high risk. Patients who have had a hemorrhagic stroke should in general not receive statins.

Peripheral arterial disease

Observational data show an association between serum cholesterol and peripheral arterial disease.[26] Randomized trials show that statins reduce the incidence of intermittent claudication and, in patients with diagnosed peripheral arterial disease, increase pain-free walking time and reduce the need for surgical procedures.[27–29]

Abdominal aortic aneurysm

The pathology of this condition is complex, but abdominal aortic aneurysms are more common in people with coronary artery or peripheral arterial disease, and are associated with a higher serum LDL cholesterol and triglyceride and a lower HDL cholesterol. Moreover, aneurysms show a tendency to develop in atheromatous areas of the aorta. Randomized trial data on statins and aortic aneurysms are scanty, and the opportunity to conduct randomized trials has probably passed because statins and other therapy are now widely used in patients with abdominal aortic aneurysms too small for surgical resection and, whether or not they reduce the rate of expansion of such aneurysms, statins are indicated because of the increased risk of ischemic heart disease. It is unfortunate that the opportunity to conduct a trial, when statins were less widely used, was missed; a trial with aortic rupture as an endpoint would have been unrealistic but a small trial would have sufficed to show a reduced rate of aneurysmal expansion. A nonrandomized observational study showed that the rate of expansion of abdominal aortic aneurysms is about 40% lower in people who took statins than in those who did not.[30]

Other circulatory diseases

Cohort studies show a strong association between serum cholesterol and mortality from "circulatory diseases other than ischemic heart disease and stroke".[15] Deaths from peripheral arterial disease and abdominal aortic aneurysm are too infrequent to account for this. It will be attributable mainly to poorly certified ischemic heart disease: deaths certified due to atrial fibrillation, heart failure, myocardial degeneration and atherosclerosis, for example.

Safety of cholesterol reduction

The uncertainty concerning the excess mortality from hemorrhagic stroke at low serum cholesterol concentrations is unresolved. This apart, there are no material grounds for concern about hazard. Trials of "statin" drugs, particularly informative on safety because of the large reduction in serum cholesterol that they achieve, have resolved the issue of safety because they show no excess mortality from non-circulatory causes.[2–12,17] The excess mortality from cancer and accidents and suicide at very low serum cholesterol in observational studies is attributable to the cancer or depression lowering serum cholesterol, not the reverse.[25] Further reassurance on safety is provided by the condition of heterozygous familial hypobetalipoproteinemia, in which serum cholesterol levels are as low as 2–3 mmol/L. Life expectancy is prolonged because coronary artery disease is avoided, and no adverse effects from the low cholesterol are recognized[31,32] – an important natural experiment.

Statins as drugs are safe, with few adverse effects. Muscle disorders, particularly the rare complication of rhabdomyolysis, have received attention with the withdrawal from the market of cerivastatin and the 80 mg dose of rosuvastatin. With other statins, rhabdomyolysis is rare. The incidence is 3.4 per 100 000 person-years of statin use, an estimate derived from two cohort studies and supported by data from a meta-analysis of randomized controlled trials, with a case fatality of 10%.[33] The most important preventive measure is to avoid co-prescribing statins with gemfibrozil or with drugs that inhibit the CYP3A4 enzyme system (of which erythromycin and the azole antifungals are the most widely used).[33] Creatine kinase (CK) monitoring is ineffective; the elevated CK that characterizes rhabdomyolysis is a consequence of the disease, not a precursor of it. The incidence of lesser degrees of muscle pain and weakness, sufficient to consult a doctor but insufficient to warrant hospital admission (referred to as "myopathy" or other relatively non-specific terminology) is only about 11 per 100 000 person years, less common than is often thought.[33] Importantly, muscle symptoms are almost as common in the placebo groups as in the statin groups in randomized trials; most muscle symptoms occurring in people taking statins will not be attributable to the statin.[33] The evidence indicates that the incidence of liver disease and kidney disease is not increased by taking statins; it is likely that statins cause peripheral neuropathy but the incidence is rare (12 per 100 000 person-years) and the peripheral neuropathy generally reverses after the statin is stopped.[33]

Why was cholesterol reduction contentious?

It is perhaps surprising to recollect that for many years the issue of lipids and cardiovascular disease was seen as contentious and difficult to resolve. Unfavorable evidence was reported at regular intervals between the 1960s and the early 1990s. The earliest trials used toxic agents to lower serum cholesterol, notably estrogen (in men) and thyroxine. Some early trials were short in duration[34] and showed no reduction in risk, because little occurs in the first year after lowering cholesterol (see Table 11.3). Cross sectional studies of dietary saturated fat and serum cholesterol showed little or no relationship, an observation that was wrongly interpreted as indicating that lowering dietary saturated fat did not reduce cholesterol, until randomized trials established that it did. (The weak cross-sectional association arises because the inaccuracy in measuring individual dietary saturated fat is large in comparison to the small degree of variation between individu-

als in true saturated fat consumption.[35]) Clinicians were reluctant to accept that there was benefit in lowering average levels of serum cholesterol in high-risk patients: the notion that the average serum cholesterol in entire Western populations is high appeared counterintuitive. The issue of safety caused concern, as discussed above. Lastly, it has seemed inconsistent that serum cholesterol is a poor screening test yet an important cause of heart disease, as discussed below. All these issues are now satisfactorily resolved.

Triglycerides

Serum triglyceride concentration was associated with the risk of ischemic heart disease in many cohort studies, but the association is subject to confounding by serum LDL and HDL cholesterol, diabetes and other factors.[36,37] Whether an independent association exists is contentious. Very high serum levels of triglyceride caused by genetic defects (familial lipoprotein lipase deficiency, for example) are not associated with atheroma or coronary artery disease, and this observation, together with the potential for confounding in cohort studies, suggests that a material cause and effect relationship between serum triglyceride and heart disease is unlikely.

High-density lipoprotein (HDL) cholesterol

Cohort study data show an inverse association between HDL cholesterol (or apolipoprotein A1) and ischemic heart disease. The association is continuous across the range of values of HDL cholesterol in Western populations (0.9–1.7 mmol/L), with about a threefold difference in ischemic heart disease mortality across that range.[15] The association is similar in men and women but is age dependent; at age 40–49 the relative risk of ischemic heart disease was 1.63 for a 0.33 mmol/L lower usual HDL cholesterol.[15] The association is widely accepted as cause and effect; the threefold risk gradient, the continuous "dose–response" relationship and the observation that the association is independent of LDL cholesterol or any other evident source of confounding or bias support a causal interpretation. Moreover, a randomized trial of bezafibrate recorded a negligible change in LDL cholesterol but a significant increase in HDL cholesterol, and reported a 29% reduction in myocardial infarction ($P = 0.02$).[38] The higher HDL cholesterol in alcohol drinkers contributes to their lower risk of heart disease,[39] the lower HDL cholesterol in smokers contributes to their increased risk. Statins increase HDL cholesterol relatively little. Certain other cholesterol-lowering drugs (such as fibrates and niacin) increase HDL cholesterol more, but even in persons with relatively low HDL cholesterol the overall protective effect of these drugs is smaller because they reduce LDL cholesterol less, and so they should not be preferred to statins.

In a large randomized placebo-controlled trial the drug torcetrapib increased HDL cholesterol (by 0.9 mmol/L) and reduced LDL cholesterol (by 0.6 mmol/L), but surprisingly showed a 25% (95% CI 9–44%) excess risk of cardiovascular events and a 22% (−2–+52%) excess risk of major coronary events after one year.[40] The trial was terminated prematurely and plans to market torcetrapib were abandoned. The absence of a protective effect after one year might be explained if an increase in HDL cholesterol, as with a decrease in LDL cholesterol (see Table 11.3), showed little effect in the first year, and the excess cardiovascular mortality might, at least in part, be explained by the action of torcetrapib in increasing blood pressure (by 4.5 mmHg systolic/2.1 mmHg diastolic) and decreasing serum potassium.

Lipids as screening tests

Serum cholesterol reduction is important in reducing the risk of ischemic heart disease, but cholesterol and other lipids are poor population screening tests for ischemic heart disease. The reason for the apparent discrepancy is that the screening potential of a factor depends not only on the strength of its relationship with disease, but also on its variation in magnitude across individuals in a community. In the case of lipids, the high average values in Western societies place everyone at risk, and the variation between individuals is too small for use in population screening. By analogy, if everybody smoked between 15 and 25 cigarettes per day, cases of lung cancer would not cluster in the minority who smoked 25 cigarettes a day to the extent that those who smoked 15 or 20 could be ignored. Moreover, the Gaussian distribution of serum cholesterol means that many people have values around the average and few have relatively high values, so that most ischemic heart disease events will occur in people whose serum cholesterol is about average.

Among men aged 35–64, the 5% with the highest serum total cholesterol experience only about 12% of all deaths from ischemic heart disease – their risk is little more than double the population average.[36] The 5% of men with highest LDL cholesterol (or its carrier protein, apolipoprotein B) experience 17% of the heart disease deaths.[36] Including HDL cholesterol improves this poor detection by only about one percentage point. Lipids cannot identify a small minority of the population in whom the majority of future heart disease deaths will cluster. In a small proportion of the population, however, notably persons with familial

hypercholesterolemia, the absolute risk of death from ischemic heart disease at a young age is so great that it warrants identification and treatment of affected persons, even though the condition accounts for a fraction of all heart disease deaths in a population.

Appropriate policy

Because screening cannot identify a group who would *not* benefit from a reduction in dietary fat and serum cholesterol, such measures should be directed at the entire population. Serum cholesterol reductions of 0.6 mmol/L (10%), as discussed above, have occurred in entire Western communities, facilitated by health education, the wider availability of healthy food in restaurants and supermarkets, and a positive image of healthy eating. A reduction of 0.6 mmol/L is less likely when an individual attempts dietary change in isolation. The most important measures to lower cholesterol in healthy people therefore involve wider public education, encouragement of labeling of the nutrient content of foods, and the widespread availability of palatable low-fat foods.

Clinicians need to direct their activities towards high-risk patients, and the most important high-risk group are patients who have had a myocardial infarction or have known coronary artery disease. As a group, these patients face a risk of death from ischemic heart disease of about 5% per year (untreated), a risk that varies relatively little with age or sex. As in healthy people, serum cholesterol testing cannot identify a substantial group at either materially higher or materially lower than average risk of death. Also, the evidence strongly indicates that there is no threshold below which serum cholesterol reduction is not effective. It follows that serum cholesterol should be reduced in all such patients. Simvastatin 40 mg and atorvastatin 10 mg lowers serum cholesterol by 1.8 mmol/L (30%) and this will reduce mortality from heart disease by about 60% after two years, a substantially larger reduction in risk than can be achieved by any other single intervention. Other high-risk groups, including patients with an ischemic stroke, carotid artery disease and peripheral arterial disease and diabetics, should also receive statins routinely. Among people with no clinical history of vascular disease, the strongest risk marker is age. If coronary risk is computed in a person from measurements of risk factors that exclude age and some target is set (for example, 0.5% per year, 1% per year, 2% per year) almost all of us will cross that target at some age, and the age range across which most of us would cross it is relatively narrow. If the first clinical manifestation of ischemic heart disease (which could be death) is to be prevented, however, there is a case for everybody in Western populations to take a statin above some threshold of age or computed coronary risk.

Conclusion

The high levels of serum cholesterol found in Western populations are a major cause of the high mortality from ischemic heart disease and, to a lesser extent, stroke and other circulatory diseases. Realistic dietary change in a community can lower serum cholesterol by 0.6 mmol/L (10%) and reduce heart disease mortality by about 25–30%. Simvastatin and atorvastatin can lower cholesterol by

1.8 mmol/L (30%) and reduce the risk of heart disease death by about 60% from the third year onwards, and should be offered to all high-risk survivors. Despite the importance of lowering cholesterol, lipids are poor screening tests of individual risk, because the average risk is high and the range across a population is relatively narrow.

Key points

Serum cholesterol and ischemic heart disease

Grade A
- The effect of serum cholesterol reduction on ischemic heart disease mortality is large and important.
- There is little reduction in risk in the first year, but the expected reduction in risk is largely attained from the third year onwards.
- There is no threshold across the range of cholesterol values in Western countries below which reducing serum cholesterol reduction is not worthwhile.
- The greater the reduction in serum cholesterol, the greater the reduction in risk.
- Simvastatin and atorvastatin can lower cholesterol by 1.8 mmol/L (30%) and reduce the risk of heart disease death at age 60 by about 60% from the third year onwards; their use should be routine in people at higher risk.
- Realistic dietary change in a community can lower serum cholesterol by 0.6 mmol/L (10%) and reduce the risk of heart disease death by 25–30% at age 60. In an individual acting alone, the realistic change is half this.
- The proportional benefits are similar in men and women.

Serum cholesterol and other circulatory diseases
- Statins reduce the risk of ischemic stroke and peripheral arterial disease and should be used in high-risk patients.
- Cohort studies show excess mortality from hemorrhagic stroke at very low cholesterol levels. The interpretation is uncertain. The possible hazard, however, is greatly outweighed by the benefit of low mortality from heart disease at very low cholesterol levels.

Screening
- Lipids are poor screening tests for predicting heart disease death in an individual; it is not possible to identify a small minority in a community who will experience the majority of heart disease deaths.
- The 5% of men with highest total serum cholesterol experience only about 12% of heart disease deaths.
- In the extremity of the distribution, familial hypercholesterolemia is important to detect because the absolute risk of heart disease death at a young age is high, even though the condition accounts for only a small proportion of heart disease deaths.

References

1. Law MR, Wald NJ. An ecological study of serum cholesterol and ischaemic heart disease between 1950 and 1990. *Eur J Clin Nutr* 1994;**48**:305–25.
2. Scandinavian Simvastatin Survival Study Group. Randomised trial of cholesterol lowering in 4444 patients with coronary heart disease: the Scandinavian Simvastatin Survival Study (4S). *Lancet* 1994;**344**:1383–9.
3. West of Scotland Coronary Prevention Study (WOSCOPS) Group. Prevention of coronary heart disease with pravastatin in men with hypercholesterolaemia. *N Engl J Med* 1995;**333**: 1301–7.
4. Sacks FM, Pfeffer MA, Moye LA *et al.* The effect of pravastatin on coronary events after myocardial infarction in patients with average cholesterol levels: the Cholesterol and Recurrent Events (CARE) Trial. *N Engl J Med* 1996;**335**:1001–9.
5. The Long-Term Intervention with Pravastatin in Ischaemic Disease (LIPID) Study Group. Prevention of cardiovascular events and death with pravastatin in patients with coronary heart disease and a broad range of initial cholesterol levels. *N Engl J Med* 1998;**339**:1349–57.
6. Downs JR, Clearfield M, Weis S *et al.* Primary prevention of acute coronary events with lovastatin in men and women with average cholesterol levels: results of the Air Force/Texas Coronary Atherosclerosis Prevention Study (AFCAPS/TexCAPS). *JAMA* 1998;**279**:1615–22.
7. Heart Protection Study Collaborative Group. MRC/BHF Heart Protection Study of cholesterol lowering with simvastatin in 20536 high-risk individuals: a randomised placebo-controlled trial. *Lancet* 2002;**360**:7–22.
8. The Antihypertensive and Lipid-Lowering Treatment to Prevent Heart Attack Trial (ALLHAT-LLT). Major outcomes in moderately hypercholesterolemic, hypertensive patients randomized to pravastatin vs usual care. *JAMA* 2002;**288**:2998–3007.
9. PROspective Study of Pravastatin in the Elderly at Risk (PROSPER) Study Group. Pravastatin in elderly individuals at risk of vascular disease (PROSPER): a randomised controlled trial. *Lancet* 2002;**360**:1623–30.
10. Athyros VG, Papageorgiou AA, Mercouris BR *et al.* Treatment with atorvastatin to the National Cholesterol Educational Program goal versus 'usual' care in secondary coronary heart disease prevention: the GREek Atorvastatin and Coronary heart disease Evaluation (GREACE) Study. *Curr Med Res Opin* 2002;**18**:220–8.
11. Sever PS, Dahlöf B, Poulter NR *et al.* Prevention of coronary and stroke events with atorvastatin in hypertensive patients who have average or lower-than-average cholesterol concentrations, in the Anglo-Scandinavian Cardiac Outcomes Trial – Lipid Low-

ering Arm (ASCOT-LLA): a multicentre randomised controlled trial. *Lancet* 2003;**361**:1149–58.

12. Ridker PM, Danielson E, Fonseca FAH, *et al.* Rosuvastatin to prevent vascular events in men and women with elevated C-Reactive protein. *N Engl J Med* 2008;**359**:2195–207.

13. Law M, Wald N. Cholesterol, statins, and mortality. *Lancet* 2008;**371**:1161–2.

14. Law MR, Wald NJ, Thompson SG. By how much and how quickly does reduction in serum cholesterol concentration lower risk of ischaemic heart disease? *BMJ* 1994;**308**: 367–72.

15. Prospective Studies Collaboration. Blood cholesterol and vascular mortality by age, sex, and blood pressure: a meta-analysis of individual data from 61 prospective studies with 55 000 vascular deaths. *Lancet* 2007;**370**:1829–39.

16. Law MR, Wald NJ, Rudnicka AR. Quantifying effect of statins on low density lipoprotein cholesterol, ischaemic heart disease, and stroke: systematic review and meta-analysis. *BMJ* 2003;**326**:1423–7.

17. Cholesterol Treatment Trialists' (CTT) Collaborators. Efficacy and safety of cholesterol-lowering treatment: prospective meta-analysis of data from 90 056 participants in 14 randomised trials of statins. *Lancet* 2005;**370**:1829–39.

18. LaRosa JC, Grundy SM, Waters DD *et al.* Intensive lipid lowering with atorvastatin in patients with stable coronary disease. *N Engl J Med* 2005;**352**:1425–35.

19. Nissen SE, Tuzcu EM, Schoenhagen P *et al.* Effect of intensive compared with moderate lipid-lowering therapy on progression of coronary atherosclerosis. *JAMA* 2004;**291**:1071–80.

20. Smith EB, Slater RS. Relationship between low-density lipoprotein in aortic intima and serum-lipid levels. *Lancet* 1972;i:463–9.

21. Ford I, Murray H, Packard CJ, Shepherd J, Macfarlane PW, Cobbe SM, for the West of Scotland Coronary Prevention Study Group. Long-term follow-up of the West of Scotland Coronary Prevention Study. *N Engl J Med* 2007;**357**:1477–86.

22. Mensink RP, Katan MB. Effect of dietary *trans* fatty acids on high-density and low-density lipoprotein cholesterol levels in healthy subjects. *N Engl J Med* 1990;**323**:439–45.

23. Nestel P, Noakes M, Belling B *et al.* Plasma lipoprotein lipid and Lp[a] changes with substitution of elaidic acid for oleic acid in the diet. *J Lipid Res* 1992;**33**:1029–36.

24. Neaton JD, Blackburn H, Jacobs D *et al.* Serum cholesterol level and mortality findings for men screened in the multiple risk factor intervention trial. *Arch Intern Med* 1992;**152**:1490–500.

25. Law MR, Wald NJ, Wu T, Bailey A. Assessing possible hazards of reducing serum cholesterol. *BMJ* 1994;**308**:373–9.

26. Fowkes FGR, Housley E, Riemersma RA *et al.* Smoking, lipids, glucose intolerance, and blood pressure as risk factors for peripheral atherosclerosis compared with ischaemic heart disease in the Edinburgh Artery Study. *Am J Epidemiol* 1992;**135**:331–40.

27. Kjekshuj J, Pedersen TR, Pyorala K, Olsson AG. Effect of simvastatin on ischaemic signs and symptoms in the Scandinavian Simvastatin Survival Study (4S). *J Am Coll Cardiol* 1997;**29**(suppl A):75A.

28. Mohler ER, Hiatt WR, Creager MA. Cholesterol reduction with atorvastatin improves walking distance in patients with peripheral arterial disease. *Circulation* 2003;**108**:1481–6.

29. Heart Protection Study Collaborative Group. Randomized trial of the effects of cholesterol-lowering with simvastatin on peripheral vascular outcomes in 20,536 people with peripheral arterial disease and other high-risk conditions. *J Vasc Surg* 2007;**45**:653–4.

30. Schouten O, van Laanen JH, Hoersma E *et al.* Statins are associated with a reduced infrarenal abdominal aortic aneurysm growth. *Eur J Vasc Endovasc Surg* 2006;**32**:21–6.

31. Linton MF, Farese RV, Young SG. Familial hypobetalipoproteinemia. *J Lipid Res* 1993;**34**:521–41.

32. Glueck CJ, Gartside P, Fallat RW, Sielski J, Steiner PM. Longevity syndromes: familial hypobeta and familial hyperalpha lipoproteinemia. *J Lab Clin Med* 1976;**88**:941–57.

33. Law M, Rudnicka AR. Statin safety: a systematic review. *Am J Cardiol* 2006;**97**(suppl):52C–60C.

34. Frantz ID, Dawson EA, Ashman PL *et al.* Test of effect of lipid lowering by diet on cardiovascular risk. The Minnesota coronary survey. *Arteriosclerosis* 1989;**9**:129–35.

35. Jacobs DR, Anderson JT, Blackburn H. Diet and serum cholesterol. *Am J Epidemiol* 1979;**110**:77–87.

36. Wald NJ, Law M, Watt HC *et al.* Apolipoproteins and ischaemic heart disease: implications for screening. *Lancet* 1994;**343**: 75–9.

37. Pocock SJ, Shaper AG, Phillips AN. Concentrations of high density lipoprotein cholesterol, triglycerides, and total cholesterol in ischaemic heart disease. *BMJ* 1989;**298**:998–1002.

38. Tenenbaum A, Motro M, Fisman EZ, Tanne D, Boyko V, Behar S. Bezafibrate for the secondary prevention of myocardial infarction in patients with metabolic syndrome. *Arch Intern Med* 2005;**165**:1154–60.

39. Gaziano JM, Buring JE, Breslow JL *et al.* Moderate alcohol intake, increased levels of high-density lipoprotein and its subfractions, and decreased risk of myocardial infarction. *N Engl J Med* 1993;**329**:1829–34.

40. Barter PH, Caulfield M, Eriksson M *et al.* Effects of torcetrapib in patients at high risk for coronary events. *N Engl J Med* 2007;**357**:2109–22.

12 Use of lipid-lowering agents in the prevention of cardiovascular disease

R Alan Failor and Jeffrey L Probstfield
University of Washington, Seattle, WA, USA

Introduction

The primary purpose of this chapter is to review the evidence regarding plasma lipid-altering medications, their mechanisms of action, dosages and dosing schedules, effects on lipid and lipoprotein variables, adverse effects, and clinical uses. The 3-hydroxy-3-methylglutaryl-coenzyme A (HMG-CoA) reductase inhibitor agents (statins), which are highly effective LDL-C lowering agents, are reviewed, as are niacin, bile acid-sequestering agents (resins), fibrates, and ezetimibe. The evidence for cholesterol lowering in such subgroups as the elderly, women, diabetic patients, and those with small-dense LDL particles is also summarized.

Major trials have clearly demonstrated that decreases in low-density lipoprotein cholesterol (LDL-C) are associated with reductions in total mortality,[1-3] coronary heart disease (CHD) mortality,[1-3] fatal and non-fatal CHD as well as strokes.[1-4] Other major trials have also shown that lowering LDL-C can retard the progression of coronary artery atherosclerosis[5] and carotid atherosclerosis and may even cause their regression, as well as slowing the progression and occlusion of atherosclerosis in saphenous vein bypass grafts.[6] In both primary[2] and secondary[1,3] CHD prevention settings, decreases in total and cause-specific mortality have been demonstrated, and these benefits have been shown in subjects with elevated,[1,2] average,[4] and normal LDL-C levels. A brief review of the costs/1% LDL-C lowering/year and cost effectiveness concludes this chapter.

The National Cholesterol Education Program (NCEP) has been instrumental in developing and promulgating guidelines for initiating LDL-C lowering. These guidelines, developed on the basis of the patient's established baseline LDL-C and presence or absence of CHD or its risk factors, recommend treatment goals to attain desired levels of plasma LDL-C. To date, the NCEP has issued three Adult Treatment Panel (ATP) reports. ATP I emphasized primary prevention of CHD in persons with high (>160 mg/dL or 4.15 mmol/L) or borderline-high LDL levels (130–159 mg/dL or 3.18–4.15 mmol/L) and >2 risk factors for development of CHD. In ATP II, persons with established CHD were targeted for intensive lipid-lowering therapy.

ATP III, disseminated in 2001, identifies elevated LDL-C as the primary target of cholesterol-lowering therapy and maintains attention on intensive treatment of patients with CHD.[7] It expands the indications for intensive therapy to lower levels of cholesterol in clinical practice. A major new feature is that intensive LDL-C lowering treatment is a primary prevention measure for persons with multiple risk factors for developing CHD, as identified by the estimated 10-year CHD risk score developed from the Framingham data. ATP III sets the optimal LDL-C level as <100 mg/dL (2.60 mmol/L) and defines low HDL-C as <40 mg/dL (1.04 mmol/L) (previous cutpoint was <35 mg/dL (0.91 mmol/L)).[7]

In 2004, recommendations for modifications to footnote the ATP III LDL-C treatment algorithm were issued.[8] Based upon the results of five major clinical outcome trials completed since the ATP III guidelines were published, a therapeutic option of an LDL-C goal of <70 mg/dL (1.82 mmol/L) for those at very high risk was considered a reasonable clinical strategy. This more aggressive goal was also extended to those at high risk who have baseline LDL-C <100 mg/dL (2.60 mmol/L). In addition, it was recommended that those at high risk who also have high triglycerides, or low HDL-C levels, be considered for combination therapy of nicotinic acid or a fibrate along with an LDL-C lowering agent. When those at high risk, or moderately high risk, are treated with LDL-lowering therapy, it was recommended that the intensity of treatment be sufficient to achieve at least a 30–40% reduction in LDL levels.[8]

ATP III also recommends that persons with the metabolic syndrome – characterized by abdominal obesity, elevated blood pressure, insulin resistance, and athero-

Evidence-Based Cardiology, 3rd edition. Edited by S. Yusuf, J.A. Cairns, A.J. Camm, E.L. Fallen, and B.J. Gersh. © 2010 Blackwell Publishing, ISBN: 978-1-4051-5925-8.

genic dyslipidemia – elevated triglycerides, small LDL particles, and low HDL-C should be targeted for intensive therapeutic lifestyle modifications. Atherogenic dyslipidemia should be treated with lipid-altering agents.[7]

It has recently been demonstrated by the INTERHEART study that the Apo B to Apo A1 ratio will most completely capture the risk associated with dyslipidemia.[9] The role of

triglycerides as an independent risk factor for the development of atherosclerosis remains controversial. The risks and therapeutic benefits of treatment have been recently reviewed.[12]

Boxes 12.1–12.5 summarize the major new recommendations of ATP III and classifications of cholesterol levels.[7]

Use of individual lipid-altering agents

In this short,evidence-based overview, we focus on documented activities of known lipid- and lipoprotein-altering drugs on lipid and lipoprotein variables, and their related adverse effects. We identify those issues that remain more speculative as such. The interested reader is referred to the excellent and more complete reviews by Lousberg et al,[10] as well as the ATP III guidelines.[7]

BOX 12.1 New features of adult treatment panel III

- Focus on multiple risk factors
- Raises persons with diabetes without CHD, most of whom display multiple risk factors, to the risk level of CHD risk equivalent
- Uses Framingham projections of 10 year absolute CHD risk (that is, the percent probability of having a CHD event in 10 years) to identify certain patients with multiple (2+) risk factors for more intensive treatment
- Identifies persons with multiple metabolic risk factors (metabolic syndrome) as candidates for intensified therapeutic lifestyle changes
- Modifications of lipid and lipoprotein classification
- Identifies LDL-C <100 mg/dL (2.60 mmol/L) as optimal
- Raises categorical low HDL-C from <35 (0.91) to <40 mg/dL (1.04 mmol/L)
- Lowers the triglyceride classification cutpoints to give more attention to moderate elevations

Adapted from *Third Report of the National Cholesterol Education Program (NCEP) Expert Panel on detection, evaluation, and treatment of high blood cholesterol in adults (Adult Treatment Panel III)*[7]

BOX 12.2 ATP III classification of LDL, total and HDL cholesterol

LDL cholesterol:
<100 mg/dL (2.60 mmol/L) optimal
Near optimal/above optimal
Borderline high
High
≥190 mg/dL (4.94 mmol/L), very high

Total cholesterol:
<200 mg/dL (5.19 mmol/L), desirable
Borderline high
≥240 mg/dL (6.23 mmol/L), high

HDL cholesterol:
<40 mg/dL (1.04 mmol/L), low
≥60 mg/dL (1.56 mmol/L), high

Adapted from the *Third Report of the National Cholesterol Education Program (NCEP) Expert Panel on detection, evaluation, and treatment of high blood cholesterol in adults (Adult Treatment Panel III)*[7]

BOX 12.3 Major risk factors (exclusive of LDL cholesterol) that modify LDL goals*

- Cigarette smoking
- Hypertension (blood pressure >140/90 mmHg or on antihypertensive medication)
- Low HDL cholesterol (<40 mg/dL)[†]
- Family history of premature CHD (CHD in male first-degree relative <55 years; CHD in female first-degree relative <65 years)
- Age (men >45 years; women >55 years)

*Diabetes is regarded as a coronary heart disease (CHD) risk equivalent.
†HDL cholesterol >60 mg/dL (1.56 mmol/L) counts as a "negative" risk factor; its presence removes 1 risk factor from the total count.
Adapted from *Third Report of the National Cholesterol Education Program (NCEP) Expert Panel on detection, evaluation, and treatment of high blood cholesterol in adults (Adult Treatment Panel III)*[7]

BOX 12.4 Three categories of risk that modify LDL cholesterol goals

Risk category	LDL goal (mg/dL)
CHD and CHD risk equivalents	<100 (2.60 mmol/L)
Multiple (2+) risk factors*	<130 (3.38 mmol/L)
0–1 risk factor	<160 (4.16 mmol/L)

*Risk factors that modify the low density lipoprotein (LDL) goal are listed in BOX 12.3. CHD indicates coronary heart disease.
Adapted from *Third Report of the National Cholesterol Education Program (NCEP) Expert Panel on detection, evaluation, and treatment of high blood cholesterol in adults (Adult Treatment Panel III)*[7]

BOX 12.5 Recommendations for modifications to footnote the ATP III treatment algorithm for LDL-C

- Therapeutic lifestyle changes (TLC) remain an essential modality in clinical management. TLC has the potential to reduce cardiovascular risk through several mechanisms beyond LDL lowering.
- In high-risk persons, the recommended LDL-C goal is <100 mg/dL (2.60 mmol/L)

    An LDL-C goal of <70 mg/dL ((1.82 mmol/L) is a therapeutic option on the basis of available clinical trial evidence, especially for patients at very high risk (e.g. continued smoking).

  - If LDL-C is >100 mg/dL, an LDL-lowering drug is indicated simultaneously with lifestyle changes.
  - If baseline LDL-C is <100 mg/dL, institution of an LDL-lowering drug to achieve an LDL-C level <70 mg/dL is a therapeutic option on the basis of available clinical trial evidence.
  - If a high-risk person has high triglycerides or low HDL-C, consideration can be given to combining a fibrate or nicotinic acid with an LDL-lowering drug. When triglycerides are >200 mg/dL (2.26 mmol/L), non-HDL-C is a secondary target of therapy, with a goal 30 mg/dL (0.34 mmol/L) higher than the identified LDL-C goal. The risks and therapeutic benefits of treatment associated with elevated levels of triglycerides have recently been reviewed.[12]
- For moderately high-risk persons (2+ risk factors and 10-year risk 10–20%), the recommended LDL-C goal is <130 mg/dL (3.38 mmol/L); an LDL-C goal <100 mg/dL (2.60 mmol/L) is a therapeutic option on the basis of available clinical trial evidence. When LDL-C level is 100–129 mg/dL (2.60–3.38 mmol/L) at baseline or on lifestyle therapy, initiation of an LDL-lowering drug to achieve an LDL-C level <100 mg/dL (2.60 mmol/L) is a therapeutic option on the basis of available clinical trial evidence.

    New evidence suggests that the Apo B to Apo A1 ratio will most completely capture the risk associated with dyslipidemia.[9]
- Any person at high risk or moderately high risk who has lifestyle-related risk factors (e.g. obesity, physical inactivity, elevated triglyceride, low HDL-C or metabolic syndrome) is a candidate for TLC to modify these risk factors regardless of LDL-C level.
- When LDL-lowering drug therapy is employed in high-risk or moderately high-risk persons, it is advised that intensity of therapy be sufficient to achieve at least a 30–40% reduction in LDL-C levels.
- For people in lower risk categories, recent clinical trials do not modify the goals and cutpoints of therapy.

Adapted from Grundy et al.[8]

HMG-CoA reductase inhibitors (statins)

These agents have a powerful LDL-C lowering effect and those currently approved for use differ only in their dose–response curves and unit cost.

Mevastatin was first isolated in 1976 by Endo and colleagues as a natural product from *Penicillium* species. A related natural product, lovastatin, was approved by the FDA for cholesterol lowering in 1987. Subsequently, simvastatin, pravastatin, fluvastatin, atorvastatin, cerivastatin, and rosuvastatin were developed and approved for use in the US.[11] Cerivastatin was withdrawn later because of adverse effects.

Mechanism of action: lipid-altering effects

Brown et al demonstrated that lovastatin inhibits HMG-CoA reductase, the rate-limiting enzyme in cholesterol biosynthesis.[13] Statins occupy a portion of the binding site of HMG-CoA reductase, blocking access to the active site of the enzyme.[14] Total body cholesterol synthesis is reduced by at least 20%. Ultimately a critical reduction in cholesterol concentration occurs in the liver cell, leading to enhanced production of hepatic LDL receptors[15] and increased cellular uptake of LDL-C. Further, reduced very (V) LDL biosynthesis occurs via an effect upon hepatic Apo B secretion, as well as an increased rate of VLDL catabolism.

Pleiotropic effects

In addition to reducing cholesterol biosynthesis, other potential antiatherogenic mechanisms of action for the statins are under current, intense investigation but remain speculative. Pleiotropic effects of statins on the vascular system and the arterial walls – affecting endothelial function, inflammation, coagulation, plaque stabilization, and smooth muscle cell migration – have been identified.[16–18] The small GTP-binding protein, Rho, has membrane localization and may mediate the direct vascular effects of statins.

The PRINCE study provides clinical evidence of anti-inflammatory properties of a statin.[19] In this prospective, randomized, cohort study, pravastatin lowered levels of C-reactive protein (CRP), an inflammatory biomarker that is predictive of cardiovascular risk. Decreased CRP levels were seen as early as 12 weeks in pravastatin-treated participants ($P < 0.001$). Pravastatin lowered the median CRP level by 16.9% versus placebo ($P < 0.001$) at 24 weeks. The decreases occurred in both the primary and secondary prevention groups and regardless of sex, age, smoking, body mass index, baseline lipid levels, diabetes, and use of aspirin or hormone replacement therapy.[19]

Results of the PPP Project – a meta-analysis of three large, placebo-controlled, randomized trials including almost 20 000 patients and 102 559 person-years of follow-up – provide further clinical evidence that statins may be anti-inflammatory and/or antithrombotic. In particular, statins may be beneficial in reducing strokes.[20] Pooled data from two of the trials, CARE and LIPID, involving more than 13000 patients, showed a 22% reduction in total strokes and a 25% reduction in non-fatal stroke.[20] The third trial, WOSCOPS, had a smaller trend for reduction in total stroke. Pravastatin reduced the risk of non-hemorrhagic stroke over a wide range of lipid values in patients with documented CHD.[20]

In the MIRACL trial, atorvastatin (80 mg/day) reduced early recurrent ischemic events in patients with acute coronary syndromes.[21] The statin was initiated 24–96 hours after an acute coronary syndrome to over 3000 adults with unstable angina or non-Q-wave myocardial infarction (MI). In the atorvastatin group, 14.8% of patients had a primary endpoint (death, non-fatal acute MI, cardiac arrest with resuscitation or recurrent symptomatic myocardial ischemia requiring emergency rehospitalization) versus 17.4% in the placebo group ($P = 0.048$).[21] The MIRACL investigators suggest that patients with acute coronary syndromes begin statin therapy before hospital discharge, regardless of baseline LDL-C levels.

AVERT compared the efficacy of aggressive cholesterol-lowering therapy versus percutaneous transluminal coronary angioplasty in low-risk, stable patients with CHD. Aggressive lipid lowering was superior to angioplasty in patients with mild to moderate CHD. Atorvastatin was associated with a 36% reduction in ischemic events and a significant delay in time to first ischemic event.[22]

The CTT study, a meta-analysis of 14 randomized trials using statins in the prevention of CHD, found an approximate 1% reduction in coronary mortality and major vascular events for every 2 mg/dL reduction in LDL-C. These benefits were significant within the first year, but were greater in subsequent years. These results were consistent in all subgroups. There was no evidence that statins increased the incidence of cancer overall, or of any specific site.[23]

Dosage

The recommended dosages and described effects of these agents are shown in Table 12.1.[11]

Impact on lipid levels

All of these agents except atorvastatin and rosuvastatin will lower plasma total cholesterol by 20–40% and LDL-C by 25–45% at maximum approved doses. Triglycerides are reduced by 10–30%. HDL-C plasma levels are frequently increased by 5–10%, but the increases may be more modest or absent in patients with inherently low levels. Lp(a) levels are not affected.[11] Statin therapy alters small-dense LDL particles to a larger more buoyant form and also nor-

Table 12.1 Dose–response lipid and lipoprotein changes (% change)

Total dose (mg/d)	5	10	20	40	80
Total cholesterol reductions					
Lovastatin BID	19	24	29	34	
Simvastatin	19	23	28	31	36
Pravastatin		16	24	25	27
Fluvastatin			17	19	25
Atorvastatin		29	33	37	45
Rosuvastatin	24	40	34	40	
LDL cholesterol reductions					
Lovastatin BID	28	34	40	42	
Simvastatin	26	30	38	41	47
Pravastatin		22	32	34	37
Fluvastatin			22	25	35
Atorvastatin		39	43	50	60
Rosuvastatin	28	45	31	43	
Triglycerides					
Lovastatin BID	7	16	19	27	
Simvastatin	12	15	19	18	24
Pravastatin		15	11	24	19
Fluvastatin			12	14	19
Atorvastatin		19	26	29	37
Rosuvastatin	21	37	37	43	
HDL cholesterol					
Lovastatin BID	8	9	10		
Simvastatin	10	12	8	9	8
Pravastatin		7	2	12	13
Fluvastatin			3	4	7
Atorvastatin		6	9	6	5
Rosuvastatin	3	8	22	17	

From *Physicians' Desk Reference*[11]

malizes the responsiveness of coronary vessels to vasoactive stimulus.[18]

Atorvastatin and rosuvastatin are more powerful members of the statin class. At the maximal dose of 80 mg/day, atorvastatin has resulted in reductions in total cholesterol of 45–50%, LDL-C of up to 60%, triglycerides of 35–45%, and Apo B levels of 35–40%.[11] Changes in plasma levels of Lp(a) are small, and increases in HDL-C are inconsistent, but may reach 12%.[24] Rosuvastatin is the most recently approved statin and is the most powerful agent of the class on a per mg basis. It has a long half-life (20 hours) and is not metabolized by the cytochrome P450 3A4.[25] It has been shown to reduce LDL-C by up to 65%. Atorvastatin and rosuvastatin are somewhat more effective in lowering triglycerides than the other statins, and do so in a dose-dependent fashion.[26]

Part of the variability of the lipid response, and side effects of the statins, may be due to genetic differences in the rate of drug metabolism. The CYP2D6 phenotype can affect both lipid lowering and tolerability of simvastatin.[27] In addition, it has been shown that polymorphisms of the HMG-CoA reductase gene can affect lipid response to statin therapy.[28]

Adverse reactions

Overall adverse reactions occur in less than 2% of individuals. From 1% to 3% of persons taking a statin will have dose-related, elevated, hepatic enzyme levels.[29] While most studies document no abnormalities,[1,3,30] most abnormalities that do occur are seen within the first three months of treatment and require monitoring.[29] In patients who abuse alcohol, there is an increased risk of hepatic toxicity. An extremely low incidence of adverse events (not significantly different from placebo) has been documented over 5.5 years in the Heart Protection Study (HPS).[3]

Statins compete with other drugs for specific metabolic pathways of the cytochrome P450 system, whose enzymes act as a major catalyst for drug oxidation in the liver.[31] Lovastatin and simvastatin undergo extensive first-pass metabolism by CYP3A4, and caution is urged in using them with cyclosporin (a known inhibitor of CYP3A4), particularly when other inhibitors of the cytochrome P450 system, such as azole-derived antifungal drugs, erythromycin and clarithromycin, are in use, as well as nefazodone and many HIV protease inhibitors. Atorvastatin is also at least partially metabolized by this pathway. Fluvastatin is metabolized mostly by CYP2C9 and few drug–drug interactions have been noted. Pravastatin has less potential for drug interaction with other substrates, inhibitors or inducers of the CYP3A4 and CYP2C9 systems than the other statins because it is metabolized by sulfation, not the cytochrome system.[31]

About 10% of individuals taking statins may develop myalgias, but perhaps 90% of these symptoms are not related to statin therapy. Statin-induced myalgias and myopathy are most commonly associated with progressive, symmetric symptoms of the hip and shoulder girdles. Many of these patients report muscle pain without concomitant elevations of creatinine kinase (CK). Caution must be used in interpreting CK elevations as they can be increased due to even minor trauma or in sporting activities, and can be caused by other conditions such as hypothyroidism. However, one should consider discontinuing statin therapy if CK increases by more than threefold. Rare (less than 0.1%) and reversible increases of greater than 10-fold in CK levels have been described. The mechanism of muscle injury with statins remains poorly defined, although according to a recent publication it may be related to the HMG-CoA reductase mediated isoprenylation of muscle proteins.[32] Statin-associated myopathy, although rare, can progress to rhabdomyolysis.[33] This effect can be seen with any statin; however, cerivastatin was voluntarily withdrawn from the world market in 2001 because of an increased rate of rhabdomyolysis compared with other statins.

There are reports of statin use associated with a variety of other potential adverse effects including renal dysfunction, cognitive impairment, increased risk of cancer, peripheral neuropathy, a drug-induced lupus-like state, and cataracts. Despite extensive and widespread use of these agents, no report has established a causal relationship to the use of statins.

Clinical use

Although the biggest proportional reduction in LDL-C levels occurs at low doses, the clinical response to statins is dose dependent, and it appears to be independent of patient characteristics, such as age, gender, smoking status and initial lipid and lipoprotein levels.[34] ATP III calls for LDL-C lowering drug therapy in persons with CHD and CHD risk equivalents when the LDL-C is ≥130 mg/dL (3.38 mmol/L).[7] In persons with two or more risk factors for the development of CHD, ATP III suggests that lipid-lowering drug therapy also begin at LDL-C levels ≥130 mg/dL (3.38 mmol/L).[8] For those at very high risk, a more aggressive LDL-C goal of <70 mg/dL (1.82 mmol/L) is considered a therapeutic option. This goal should also be considered in those at high risk but with a baseline LDL-C level <100 mg/dL (2.60 mmol/L).[8]

ATP III also recommends that LDL-C be measured, either at admission or within 24 hours, in all patients hospitalized with a major coronary event.[7] Lipid-lowering drug therapy should be initiated at hospital discharge in a person with a coronary event or procedure if LDL-C is ≥130 mg/dL (3.38 mmol/L).[7] Treatment initiation at hospital discharge takes advantage of patients' likely higher motivation to comply with therapy at that time and may avoid the "treatment gap" that can occur if outpatient follow-up is less consistent.

Nicotinic acid

In the early 1950s Attschult noted profound reductions in plasma total cholesterol and triglyceride levels in association with use of nicotinic acid. Nicotinic acid has the most marked clinical effect on triglycerides and HDL,[35] and is the only lipid-altering agent to consistently lower Lp(a) plasma levels.[36] It also can alter small-dense LDL particles to larger, more buoyant forms.[36] A complete review of this agent has recently been published.[37]

Mechanism of action

Nicotinic acid's predominant effect on plasma lipid levels is to reduce production of VLDL particles, with subsequently reduced production of intermediate-density lipoprotein (IDL) and LDL particles. Nicotinic acid's major effect on VLDL metabolism results from inhibition of hormone-sensitive, lipase-induced lipolysis in adipose tissue, and decreased triglyceride esterification in the liver. It has recently been demonstrated that niacin exerts its effects by acting as a pharmacologic ligand for the adipocyte and macrophage G protein coupled receptor HM74.[39] The physiologic ligand for this receptor is beta-hydroxybutyrate.[40] Niacin increases HDL-C to a greater extent than other lipid treatment drugs, and this effect appears to be related to reduced Apo A-I clearance and increased production of Apo A-II.

Dosage

Crystalline nicotinic acid is available in 0.1 and 0.5 g tablets. There is a sustained-release form in dosages of 0.125, 0.25 and 0.5 g and the maximum daily dose is usually 3 g (Table 12.2). A new extended-release form of niacin has relatively mild hepatic effects, and can be taken at bedtime to lessen cutaneous flushing. Extended-release niacin is essentially equivalent to immediate-release niacin in increasing HDL-C. Newer agents that reduce flushing are in development.

Results

Regardless of the patient's clinical lipoprotein abnormality, dose-dependent reductions in total and LDL-C and plasma triglycerides have been achieved with use of nicotinic acid. HDL-C levels may increase 15–40%; the average increase is 25%, with increases commonly plateauing at a dosage between 1.5 and 3.0 g/d. Reductions in Lp(a) of 25–30% can be achieved.[41] As noted above, small-dense LDL particles become larger and more buoyant during nicotinic acid therapy.[42]

Adverse reactions

Even at very low doses (0.05–0.10 g), nicotinic acid often causes cutaneous flushing (>80%) and pruritus (50%). This effect is due to the subcutaneous release of prostaglandin D2 and is mediated by niacin's interaction with the G protein coupled receptor HM74 (as is its lipolytic effect, see above).[43] There is an ongoing search for agents that block this prostaglandin D2-mediated flushing. In individuals with a history of gout it can precipitate acute gouty attacks. Other frequently noted adverse effects are gastrointestinal symptoms (5–20%), liver enzyme elevations (3–10%, and

Table 12.2 Summary of effects of non-statin lipid-altering agents

Agent	Lipid/lipoprotein indication	Dosage and dosing	Response expected	Common adverse effects	Comments
Nicotinic acid	↑Triglyceride (TGs) ↑LDL-C ↓HDL-C ↑Lp(a)	1–3 g/d 6–8 g/d maximum Dose 3–4 admin/d	↓TGs 20–80% ↓LDL-C 25–40% ↑HDL-C 25% ↓Lp(a) 10–30%	Cutaneous flushing, pruritus, GI symptoms, "Flu-like" syndrome	Start low dose Advance slowly Relative contraindications: ↑FBS, ↑Liver function test (LFTs)
Bile acid sequestrants	↑LDL-C ↓HDL-C	4–24 g cholestyramine 5–30 g colestipol 2 admin/d, 1 at major meal	↓LDL-C 25–35% at maximum dose ↑TGs 15–20% ↑HDL-C 4–7%	GI symptoms	Premix, slow admin Alters absorption of other drugs, for example, glycosides, warfarin, etc. Contraindicated in hypertriglyceridemia
Fibric acid derivatives	↑TGs	Gemfibrozil 0.6 g/bid Fenofibrate 45 or 145 mg qd	↓LDL-C 10–20% ↓TGs 40–55% ↓HDL-C 15–20%	GI symptoms	Will ↑LDL-C in hypertriglyceridemic Patients Contraindicated in those with gallstones Marked dose alteration in those with chronic renal failure
Selective cholesterol absorption inhibitor	↓LDL-C ↑HDL-C	Ezetimibe 5 mg/d 10 mg/d	↓LDL-C 16–19% ↑HDL-C 3–3.5%	No common AEs shown to date	

more common with slow release prerparations), and uric acid increases (5–10%). The clinical picture of mild liver function abnormalities usually resolves with continued therapy or reduced doses.

Some 5–10% of patients taking nicotinic acid will have abnormal glucose tolerance tests or elevated fasting blood sugar levels due to nicotinic acid-induced insulin resistance.[44] A flu-like syndrome that can include hepatitis-like findings on liver biopsy, a secretory defect with profound decreases in LDL-C, decreases in HDL-C and a prothrombin time abnormality may occur. This clinical picture is dose dependent and resolves when the agent is stopped.[45] Blurred vision with macular edema occurs very rarely.

Clinical use

Many non-prescription forms of nicotinic acid are available in the US and are usually less expensive, but bioavailability may be a problem. Crystalline-form tablets are scored, which allows easy tailoring of the therapeutic regimen, e.g. 0.1 or 0.25 g/d as a starting dose. Dosing with the crystalline form requires three or four administrations a day. No regimen has been shown to be superior to multiples of 0.1 g crystalline tablets administered four times a day. Patients will have little or no effect from two administrations a day, unless using sustained-release preparations. Increases in the dosage are implemented every few days.[46] Clinicians commonly reduce the number of administrations to three times per day and use 0.5 g tablets starting with 0.25 g qd for the first week.

Nicotinic acid should always be taken with food, without hot drinks or alcoholic beverages. Dosages should be reduced or perhaps restarted if several successive doses are missed. Cutaneous flushing and pruritus will occur routinely if these precautions are not followed. If symptoms occur, they are the most severe during the first administration. Pretreatment with aspirin or ibuprofen may lessen cutaneous reactions.

Although nicotinic acid may profoundly alter glucose metabolism in some, many diabetic patients have had their lipid disorders successfully managed with this agent. A fasting blood sugar >115 mg/dL predicts subjects who will lose the acute insulin response with an intravenous glucose tolerance test. In patients who have a history of diabetes or glucose intolerance or are at increased risk of diabetes, it is prudent to follow blood sugars closely during initiation of nicotinic acid therapy.

Bile acid-sequestering agents (resins)
(see Table 12.2)

This class of agents was first developed for the treatment of cholestasis-related pruritus by Carey and Williams in 1960. Hashim and Van Itallie subsequently demonstrated that cholestyramine lowered plasma cholesterol and it has been in clinical use for 30 years. Other agents in this class are colestipol and the recently approved colesevelam.

Mechanism of action

The enterohepatic circulation of bile acids allows for only 6% or 7% of them to be excreted each day. These polymers have a molecular weight of over 10^6 and are not absorbed and function by binding bile acids in the gastrointestinal lumen. An increase in bile acid excretion causes an increased production of bile acids in the liver. This results in a relative depletion of cholesterol from the liver cells, thereby inducing inducing an increased level of hepatic LDL receptor activity.[47] The net effect is an increase in the catabolism of LDL-C and decreased plasma levels.

Dosage

Resins are dispensed in individual packets and are also available in a bulk formulation. Scoops, equivalent in size to the number of grams in one packet (cholestyramine, 4 g; colestipol, 5 g), are used to dispense from the parent container. Both of these agents are available in 1 g tablets. The newest resin, colesevelam, has a hydrogel tablet formulation.

Results

Resins are associated with significant reductions in plasma total and LDL-C and with small increases in plasma HDL-C levels.[48] Plasma triglycerides are inconsistently affected, but substantial increases may occur, if resins are used in those with already elevated plasma triglyceride levels.[49] In familial dysbetalipoproteinemia (type III or remnant removal disease) plasma triglyceride levels may increase by more than threefold.

Adverse reactions

No long-term adverse effects have been demonstrated.[48] Drugs that are highly charged, including the cardiac glycosides, the anticoagulant warfarin, diuretic agents, as well as thyroid hormone, will have their absorption affected[49] if taken in close proximity to resin administration. Concomitant warfarin and resin therapy may be extremely challenging. If a resin's effect on the absorption of a specific medication is not known, the resin should be taken at least four hours before or two hours after other medications. The absorption of fat-soluble vitamins may also be reduced.

Clinical use

The biggest proportional reduction in lipid levels occurs at low doses and in those who have moderately elevated levels of cholesterol. Careful selection of the vehicle and logistics used in resin administration will promote long-term patient adherence. Premixing with cold water (taking advantage of the resin's hygroscopic nature) and drinking the preparation slowly is by far the most frequent and successful method of administration. Still, some patients prefer mixing with a heavily textured juice. Pre-existing gastrointestinal symptoms should be addressed before resin therapy is started. Bloating, belching and increased flatus are related to rapid ingestion. Dyspepsia and increased stool consistency or frank constipation can be managed with increases in fluids or dietary fiber intake.

The newest agent in the resin class is colesevelam, which is a polymeric, high-potency, water-absorbing hydrogel with a non-systemic mechanism of action.[50] Based on data from approximately 1400 subjects, colesevelam reduced LDL-C by a median of 20%; the reduction is dose dependent. When combined with lovastatin, simvastatin or atorvastatin, colesevelam will reduce LDL-C levels by 8–16% over that seen with the statin alone.[50] Colesevelam has also been shown to increase HDL-C up to 9%; however, increases in triglycerides, as much as 25%, have also been reported.[50] Colesevelam does not cause constipation and is formulated as a tablet, which should eliminate palatability problems.[51] Colesevelam has been co-administered with digoxin, warfarin, sustained-release metoprolol and verapamil, quinidine and valproic acid, and no clinically significant effects on absorption were reported.[52]

Fibric acid derivatives (see Table 12.2)

The fibrates currently marketed in the US are gemfibrozil and fenofibrate for the treatment of hypertriglyceridemia. Fibrates available in other countries include bezafibrate, fenofibrate, ciprofibrate, beclafibrate, etiofibrate and clinofibrate. In a WHO study clofibrate was shown to reduce modestly ($P < 0.05$) all cardiovascular events. However, increases in non-cardiovascular morbidity and mortality and total mortality occurred.[53] In the Helsinki Heart Study, gemfibrozil was associated with a 35% reduction in MIs, particularly in those with elevated levels of plasma LDL-C and triglycerides and low levels of plasma HDL-C. Increases in non-cardiovascular deaths and no reduction in total mortality were observed,[54] leading to concerns about the use of fibrates. No fibrate trial has yet shown a significant decrease in total mortality.

Gemfibrozil has been shown to lower the risk of CHD and stroke in men with previous CHD, and low HDL-C and low LDL-C levels. In VA-HIT,[55] 2531 men with CHD (mean HDL-C 31.5 mg/dL and mean LDL-C 111 mg/dL) were randomized to receive gemfibrozil 1200 mg/day or placebo. There was a 22% reduction in CHD over five years.[55] A more recent VA-HIT analysis describes the effect on stroke. There were 134 confirmed strokes (90% ischemic), 76 and 58 in the placebo and gemfibrozil groups, respectively ($P = 0.03$). This is the first suggestion that stroke can be reduced with a form of lipid-altering therapy that has little effect on LDL-C. Risk reduction was evident after 6–12 months of gemfibrozil use. Adjusted for baseline variables, the relative risk reduction was 31%.[56] Attributing the reduction in CHD to a change in HDL-C levels has been questioned by some. Clearly the reduction in CHD may more properly be associated with changes in other lipoprotein particles[57] than with modest changes in HDL-C levels. The use of fenofibrate in type 2 diabetes mellitus has been assessed in the FIELD trial.

Mechanism of action

Decreased synthesis of VLDL with more efficient lipolysis and increased VLDL triglyceride catabolism has long been suggested as the mechanism of action of fibrates on lipid metabolism. Schoonjans *et al* offered direct evidence that fibrates and fatty acids work as ligands for a class of compounds called peroxisome proliferator-activated receptors (PPAR), of the nuclear receptor superfamily.[41] PPAR alpha partially mediates the inductive effects of fibrates on HDL-C levels by regulating the transcription of HDL apolipoproteins, Apo A-1 and Apo A-II. Four specific actions are noted:

• increased hydrolysis of plasma triglycerides due to induction of LPL and reduction of Apo-CIII expression
• stimulation of cellular fatty acid uptake and conversion to acyl-CoA derivatives due to increased expression of genes for fatty acid transport protein and acyl-CoA synthetase
• increased peroxisomal and mitochondrial beta-oxidation
• decreased synthesis of fatty acids and triglycerides with a concomitantly decreased production of VLDLs.

Gemfibrozil was associated with a greater reduction in clinical events than the change in lipid variable would predict.[55] This suggests that its effects on CHD are mediated by a different mechanism, possibly related to its effects on other lipoprotein particles. Fibrates also shift the size of LDL particles from smaller, denser forms to larger, more buoyant forms, which should be less atherogenic.

Results

In patients with familial combined hyperlipidemia, LDL-C levels may be reduced by fibrates but, particularly in those with elevated baseline levels of plasma triglycerides, there will almost uniformly be an increase in LDL-C levels as VLDL-C levels decrease. Gemfibrozil and clofibrate have similar impacts on lipids and lipoproteins. In patients with moderate to severe forms of hypertriglyceridemia, reductions in plasma triglycerides of 40–60% may occur with concomitant increases of 12–30% in HDL-C levels, but 100% increases in LDL-C may occur.[12]

Adverse reactions

Fibrates are associated with adverse effects in 5–10% of patients. Gastrointestinal side effects (5%) are the most common, but only rarely are these sufficient to warrant discontinuation of the medication. The increased incidence of hepatobiliary disease (particularly gallstones) occurs with all agents in this class.[58] Transient and dose-dependent minor alterations in several plasma biochemical values may occur. The effective non-toxic dose range is narrow, and at high doses fibrates may cause myositis or rhabdomyolysis, although the incidence of myositis may be specifically related to the concomitant use of statins and fibrates. They may potentiate the effects of oral anticoagulants and oral hypoglycemics.

Clinical use

The primary indication for the use of these agents has shifted to treatment of severe hypertriglyceridemia and more specifically familial dysbetalipoproteinemia or remnant removal disease. Long-term adverse effects on hepatobiliary function and the potential for increases in LDL-C levels, liver function tests and LDL-C levels must be monitored closely. Chronic renal failure requires a 50% reduction in gemfibrozil dose.[59]

Selective cholesterol absorption inhibitor

Ezetimibe is a novel cholesterol absorption inhibitor that selectively and potently inhibits intestinal absorption of dietary and biliary cholesterol without affecting the absorption of triglycerides or fat-soluble vitamins.[60] In a randomized, double-blind, placebo-controlled trial, ezetimibe at a dose of 10 mg/day reduced LDL-C by 17%.[61] Ezetimibe has been found to be effective when added to a statin, demonstrating essentially additive effects.[62] It is frequently used with a statin, allowing lower doses of the statin with the same LDL-C goal, which may be helpful in limiting muscle side effects. It is available in fixed combination with simvastatin.

Ezetimibe has been well tolerated in clinical trials.[61,63] When used alone, the incidence of transminase elevations or myopathy is similar to placebo. When used with a statin, the incidence of transaminase elevations is modestly higher than with a statin alone. There are rare reports of myalgia and rhabdomyolysis being associated with the use of ezetimibe, but a causal relationship has not been established. The fibrates have been shown to increase ezetimibe levels[64]

but the clinical significance is unknown. The combination has been used successfully, and safely.[65]

Reports (unpublished at present) for the ENHANCE study have raised questions about the usefulness of ezetimibe in a regimen with a statin for LDL lowering. To date, the reports on this trial using a surrogate outcome measure with limited power to assess clinical events suggest that we need further evaluation of this agent before we can form a definitive opinion about its effectiveness.

Novel agents

Policosanol is a phytochemical that is a mixture of higher primary aliphatic alcohols isolated from sugar cane wax.[66] At dosages of 10–20 mg/day, it decreased total-C by 17–21% and LDL-C by 21–29%, while raising HDL-C by 8–15%.[50] Policosanol appears to have an acceptable safety/tolerability profile.

Cholesterol ester transfer protein (CETP) inhibitors have generated much excitement due to their potential to raise HDL-C levels. These agents have been shown to decrease diet-induced atherosclerosis in rabbits, and to be very effective in raising HDL-C levels in humans.[67] However, there has been skepticism about the potential for benefit in reducing atherosclerotic complications based on the assertion that the HDL particles that result from CETP inhibition, although increased in numbers, are "dysfunctional" and unable to function appropriately in reverse cholesterol transport.[68]

Recent trials evaluating coronary atherosclerosis by intravascular ultrasound, and carotid intimal thickness by ultrasound demonstrated no benefit of a combination of atorvastatin plus the CETP inhibitor torcetrapib versus atorvastatin alone, and did demonstrate a significant increase in systolic blood pressure as well as HDL-C.[69,70] A large clinical trial of approximately 15 000 CHD patients randomized to atorvastatin or a combination of atorvastatin plus torcetrapib was prematurely terminated by the data and safety monitoring committee because of excess mortality ($P < 0.01$). In patients who received torcetrapib there was an increased risk of cardiovascular events (hazard ratio, 1.25, $P = 0.001$) and death from any cause (hazard ratio, 1.58, $P = 0.006$).[70] Whether these negative and adverse outcomes represent a class effect remains to be seen.

There are other means of attempting to utilize reverse cholesterol transport in the amelioration of atherosclerotic disease. Five weekly infusions of Apo A1 Milano complexed with phospholipids provided more benefit on atheroma regression assessed by intravascular ultrasound than 18 months of treatment with 80 mg/day of atorvastatin.[71] More recently, a trial of reconstituted HDL, administered as four weekly infusions in CHD patients, were compared to placebo by intravascular ultrasound. A 3.4%

reduction in total atheroma volume versus baseline was reported ($P < 0.001$), but no difference was seen versus the placebo group.[72]

Combination therapy

Combination drug therapy should be used when diet and single drug therapy do not reduce LDL-C to desired levels. Verification of adherence to and the efficacy of a prescribed regimen should be undertaken. Table 12.3 describes a stepped approach to combination therapy depending on the lipid or lipoprotein variable(s) that are the therapeutic objective. Reduction in LDL-C is the only alteration in lipid(s) or lipoprotein(s) that has been unequivocally demonstrated to reduce risks for CHD in clinical trials. Epidemiologic data demonstrate an increased risk associated with reduced levels of HDL-C,[41] increased plasma Lp(a) (usually in association with increased LDL-C levels) and, to a lesser extent, increased plasma triglyceride levels (usually in association with other risk factors).

Guidelines for selecting combination therapy

Practitioners should review four issues before adding other agents to initial diet and lipid-altering drug regimens.
• Document adherence to and efficacy of the initial regimen.
• Fasting hypertriglyceridemia is a relative contraindication to the use of bile acid-sequestering agents.
• Document the presence of chronic disease or chronic conditions which may be contraindications to the addition of other lipid-altering agents.
• Consider the total costs of a lipid-altering drug therapy regimen before the addition of each agent.

Efficacy of various combinations

Selected examples of maximum lipid and lipoprotein alterations are given in Table 12.4. Prior to the development of atorvastatin, the maximum lowering of LDL-C was demonstrated with a combination of lovastatin (40 mg/day), colestipol (30 g/day) and nicotinic acid (5.5 g/day) at 70%. Triglyceride reductions of 80% can be effected with nico-

tinic acid alone with little to be gained in efficacy by adding another agent. Lp(a) levels are affected substantially only by nicotinic acid. HDL-C can be consistently raised by 25% with nicotinic acid alone with little further gain by adding other agents.

Adverse effects

The important adverse effects of single agents are described in Table 12.2. The most serious interaction is seen when a statin drug is used in combination with ciclosporin and myopathy develops. While cessation of the statin allows symptomatic myopathy and elevated muscle enzymes to resolve, continued therapy at the same dose may lead to frank rhabdomyolysis. Statins have also been associated with myopathic syndromes in patients using erythromycin, niacin and gemfibrozil. Reduced levels of any statin should be used in transplant patients in association with niacin and gemfibrozil with careful monitoring of muscle enzyme levels. Erythromycin use is absolutely contraindicated in transplant patients already on ciclosporin and a statin.

Clinical use

Although single-drug therapy offers a simple regimen, combination therapy with low-dose statin and low-dose bile acid sequestrant has been investigated.[73,74] Since the largest portion of lipid alteration is effected at low doses of both of these classes of agents and they work by very different mechanisms, an additive or synergistic response may occur. Low-dose combinations provide a good clinical alternative for patients who have symptoms at higher statin dosages and for organ transplant patients. They also appear to be more cost effective than using a statin as a single agent. The combination of simvastatin and ezetimibe is available as a single tablet. It also is significantly more cost effective than using the individual agents in combination.

The newest resin, colesevelam, has been studied in combination with statins. Low-dose colesevelam and low-dose lovastatin were given to 135 hypercholesterolemic patients.[75] The combination lowered LDL-C by 34% and 32%. Both combinations were superior to either agent alone, and both decreased total-C by 21%. Neither combination treatment significantly changed HDL-C or

Table 12.3 Stepped approach to lipid medication-altering therapies

Elevated LDL-C	Elevated TG/LDL, decreased HDL-C	Elevated Lp(a)	Markedly elevated TGs
1. Statin	Niacin	Niacin	Fibrate/ niacin
2. Statin + resin/ezetimibe	Niacin + resin/ezetimibe		
3. ↑Statin + Resin/ezetimibe	Niacin + statin		
4. ↑Statin + Resin/ezetimibe + niacin	Niacin + fibrate + resin/ezetimibe		

Table 12.4 Efficacy of selected combination of hyperlipidemic drug therapy in modifying plasma concentrations of total, LDL and HDL cholesterol levels

Drug combination	% change			Reference
	Total	**LDL**	**HDL**	
Cholestyramine				
+niacin	−26	−32	+23	Angelin et al[94]
+lovastatin	−51	−61	+21	Leren et al[95]
+pravastatin	−36	−43	+18	Jacob et al[96]
Colestipol				
+niacin	−41	−48	+25	Packard et al[97]
+lovastatin	−45	−54	−2	Illingworth et al[98]
+niacin	−55	−66	+32	Malloy et al[99]
+simvastatin	−41	−50	+9	Simons et al[100]
+fenofibrate	−39	−54	+15	Heller et al[101]
Lovastatin				
+gemfibrozil	−34	−40	+7	Illingworth et al[102]
Simvastatin				
+gemfibrozil	−54	−58	+18	Feussner et al[103]
+ezetimibe	−49	−53	+8	McKenney et al[104]
Atorvastatin				
+colesevelam	−31	−48	+11	Hunninghake et al[105]
+niacin	−48	−49	+18	McKenney et al[104]
Ezetimibe				
+fenofibrate	−27	−36	−1.9	Bays et al[106]
+atorvastatin	−38	−55	−1.1	Bays et al[106]
+simvastatin	−35	−47	+9.3	Farnier et al[107]
+simvastatin + feno-ibrate	−38.7	−45.8	+18.7	Farnier et al[107]
Rosuvastatin + niacin	−47	−49	+20	McKenney et al[104]

triglycerides.[75] The resin was also studied alone or in combination with low-dose atorvastatin in hypercholesterolemic men and women. Combination therapy reduced LDL-C by 48%, but did not affect triglycerides.[76] All treatment groups had similar frequency of adverse effects and the combination was well tolerated.[76] Colesevelam, in combination with simvastatin, was given to 251 hypercholesterolemic patients in a randomized, double-blind,

placebo-controlled format. Among all combination treatment groups, the mean decrease in LDL-C was 42%; this exceeded the decrease with either simvastatin or colesevelam alone.[77]

Informed decisions about "gray zones"

Data have now accumulated on the use of lipid-lowering drugs in previously less well-studied subgroups such as the elderly, women, and diabetic patients. How and when should we use lipid-lowering drugs in the following groups?

The elderly

While some have suggested that risk attenuates for those who have hypercholesterolemia at older age, the absolute risk for developing CHD outcomes in the elderly over a short time interval is much higher than it is in younger individuals. Most new CHD events and most coronary deaths occur in persons older than 65 and a high LDL-C/low HDL-C level still has predictive power for development of CHD in an older person.[7]

WOSCOPS[2] (primary intervention, or PI) included patients up to the age of 64 years, 4S[1] (secondary intervention, or SI) up to the age of 70 years, Post-CABG[6] (SI) up to 74 years and CARE[4] (SI) previously provided limited data for those up to 75 years. All except Post-CABG showed benefit on CHD and CVD mortality. WOSCOPS and 4S showed benefit on total mortality, although statistical significance of the data from WOSCOPS was marginal. When data from WOSCOPS were pooled in the PPP, pravastatin significantly reduced relative risk of coronary events in older patients.[78]

The Heart Protection Study (HPS) enrolled over 20000 participants – including 5082 women, 3982 type 2 diabetic patients and 1263 elderly patients between the ages of 75 and 80 years. It also enrolled 3421 subjects with low baseline LDL-C levels, and follow-up lasted for 5.5 years.[3] Recently reported results show that a dose of 40 mg simvastatin once daily yielded striking results: 12% reduction in total mortality, 17% reduction in vascular mortality, 22% reduction in CHD events, 27% reduction in all strokes, and 16% reduction in non-coronary revascularizations.[3] Statin therapy appeared to be beneficial at all cholesterol levels – even in participants whose baseline levels were well below the currently recommended target levels of 100 mg/dL (2.60 mmol/L).[3]

The PROSPER trial randomized 5804 patients (men and women) aged 70–82 with a history of, or risk factors for, vascular disease to either 40 mg pravastatin or placebo.

There was a significant reduction in coronary death, non-fatal myocardial infarction or stroke (hazard ratio 0.81), but no decrease in all-cause mortality.[79]

The SAGE trial compared intensive and moderate statin therapy in patients age 65–85 with known CHD. Subjects were randomly assigned to 80 mg atorvastatin or 40 mg pravastatin. There was no difference in duration of ischemia on ambulatory monitoring at month 12, although there was a trend towards a reduction in the composite endpoint of major cardiovascular events in the intensive treatment group (hazard ratio (HR) 0.71) and a post hoc analysis demonstrated a significant reduction in mortality (HR 0.33).[80] In the TNT study, atorvastatin at 80 mg/day was compared to 10 mg/day in 10 001 patients with stable coronary heart disease. The more intensively treated group had a significantly reduced risk for major cardiovascular events in both those greater and those younger than 65 years of age. In a prespecified secondary analysis, those over 65 years of age were found to have a 2.3% absolute risk reduction, and a relative risk reduction of 19% for major cardiovascular events that favored the high-dose atorvastatin group.[81]

There appears to be ample evidence to support the use of lipid-lowering regimens in the secondary prevention of CHD in elderly individuals, while there are only limited data relevant to the use of lipid-lowering therapy in the primary prevention.

According to ATP III, "hard-and-fast" age restrictions do not appear to apply to the use of lipid-lowering drugs in elderly persons with established CHD.[7] For primary prevention, ATP III recommends therapeutic lifestyle changes, including low-fat diet, exercise, and weight loss if overweight, and LDL-lowering drugs if older persons are at increased risk because of multiple risk factors or advanced subclinical atherosclerosis.[7]

Women

The relationship between increases in plasma cholesterol and CHD exists for women at all ages. Based on recent secondary and primary prevention trials that did not convincingly show that hormone replacement therapy reduced CHD risk in postmenopausal women and did show benefits with statins, ATP III recommends a cholesterol-lowering drug over hormone replacement for CHD risk reduction in women.[10] The later onset of CHD in women should be factored into clinical decision making regarding cholesterol-lowering drugs.[7] In the PPP, pravastatin significantly reduced relative risk of coronary events in women.[20]

The first CHD primary prevention trial of statins to include women was the AFCAPS/TexCAPS trial.[53] Among 997 postmenopausal women who received either placebo or lovastatin (20–40 mg/day), statin therapy showed consistent but statistically insignificant decreases in first acute coronary major events and in all prespecified secondary endpoints.[53]

In HPS, 34% of subjects were women; male and female participants experienced similar reductions in risk.[3] In the CTT meta-analysis there was no significant difference in the vascular or mortality benefits of statin therapy in women versus men.[82]

Diabetic patients

Although aggressive control of blood glucose levels in type 2 diabetic patients reduces microvascular clinical outcomes, its effect on macrovascular disease outcomes remains unknown. The ACCORD study, currently in progress, may help answer this question.[38] Other traditional CHD risk factors are believed to increase dramatically the risk for clinical CHD events in these patients. Inherent in the diabetic disease process is an abnormality of lipoprotein lipase activity that is incompletely corrected by optimal glucose control. Any additional lipid and lipoprotein disorder(s) present in diabetic patients because of either inherited or secondary causes (obesity, alcohol consumption, etc.) accelerate atherosclerotic progression and increase the risk of clinical CHD events. Treatment of lipid disorders in diabetic patients with commensurate lowering of blood cholesterol levels suggests a similar treatment benefit in diabetic as in non-diabetic patients.[1,2,4,23]

The use of niacin in diabetic patients has not been recommended because of concerns about adverse effects on glycemic control. In ADMIT, however, niacin was given to diabetic patients in a prospective, randomized, placebo-controlled study enrolling 468 subjects, 125 of them with diabetes and diagnosed peripheral arterial disease.[44] Niacin was given at 3000 mg/day or to maximally tolerated dose, for up to 60 weeks. Niacin significantly increased HDL-C and decreased triglycerides and LDL-C in all participants ($P < 0.01$: niacin versus placebo for all). It modestly raised glucose levels in all participants while HbA_{1c} was unchanged from baseline through follow-up.[72] The ADMIT investigators conclude that lipid-modifying doses of niacin can be safely used in patients with diabetes and that niacin may be considered an alternative therapy in such patients who do not tolerate statins or in whom statins do not correct hypertriglyceridemia or low HDL-C levels.[44]

In CARE, 586 normocholesterolemic diabetic patients with CHD (14% of total sample) were given pravastatin or placebo for five years; there were 8% and 25% reductions respectively in absolute and relative risks of coronary events, and a 32% relative risk reduction in revascularization procedures.[53] In subjects who were not diabetic but who had impaired glucose tolerance, pravastatin also substantially lowered the risk of recurrent coronary events.[83] In PPP, pravastatin significantly reduced the relative risk of coronary events in diabetic patients.[78]

The HPS trial included 3980 persons with diabetes of whom 2930 had no CVD. As noted above, the event reductions seen with simvastatin occurred in diabetic patients as well. There was a 24% decrease in CVD and a 25% decrease in total CHD.[3] In the CTT meta-analysis, the vascular benefit of statin therapy was not significantly different in diabetic and non-diabetic subjects.[23] There were comparable reductions in all identified subgroups.

CARDS enrolled 2838 subjects with type 2 diabetes mellitus and without known cardiovascular disease. Participants were randomly assigned to receive 10 mg atorvastatin daily or placebo. The trial was stopped for early efficacy (median duration of follow-up of 3.9 years) as cardiovascular events were reduced by 37% in the atorvastatin group compared to placebo.[84] ASPEN had similar lipid inclusion criteria, although it included subjects with, and without, known CHD. After a median follow-up of four years there was no statistically significant reduction in the primary composite endpoint.[85] Adherence was a major confounding factor in ASPEN.

The FIELD trial randomly assigned 9795 type 2 diabetic patients to receive 200 mg micronized fenofibrate or placebo. Approximately a quarter of the patients had known prior cardiovascular disease. The fenofibrate was well tolerated as both monotherapy and in those who used it in combination with a statin. However, after a median follow-up of five years, a non-significant decrease in the modified primary outcome of coronary events was seen in the fenofibrate goup compared to the placebo (hazards ratio 0.89, 95% confidence interval (CI) 0.75–1.06). There was a non-significant increase in the original primary outcome of coronary mortality (HR 1.19, 95% CI 0.90–1.57), and a non-significant increase in all-cause mortality (HR 1.11, 95% CI 0.95–1.29).[86]

Peripheral vascular disease

In the Rancho Bernardo studies, patients with peripheral vascular disease had a several-fold increased risk of dying of CHD.[87] Greater than 80% of these individuals have CHD although some will manifest few symptoms. It is reasonable, but unsubstantiated, to treat these individuals as if they have CHD.

Small-dense LDL-C particles (phenotype B)

The entire population may be generally divided into two categories on the basis of the predominant LDL species present in plasma. People with a predominance of smaller, more dense LDL particles exhibit an increased propensity for oxidative susceptibility of these species. These individuals have a higher risk for CHD, which may be associated with changes in other plasma lipids, specifically an increase in triglycerides and reduced plasma levels of HDL. Alternatively, this pattern may be related to the insulin resistance syndrome, or syndrome X, which consists of impaired glucose tolerance, increased insulin levels, hypertension and abnormalities of coagulation factors. No trial of clinical outcomes and intervention on LDL subspecies has been done.

Key points for prevention of CHD/CVD

- Initiate LDL cholesterol-reducing therapy in individuals at increased risk of CHD. It is effective at reducing the incidence of CHD events in men and women and in ages up to at least 80 years of age **Class I, Level A**
- Initiation of LDL cholesterol-reducing therapy is cost effective in individuals above the age of 35.
- **Class I, Level A**
- Initiate LDL cholesterol-reducing therapy in individuals status post coronary artery saphenous vein bypass grafts. It extends the patency of such grafts. **Class I, Level A**
- In assessing CHD risk, the best single tool is the ApoB/ApoA1. **Class I, LevelA**
- Assess variables (NIDDM, hypertension, increased plasma triglycerides, low plasma HDL-C, small-dense LDL and increased PAI-1 levels) that are components of the so-called "insulin resistance syndrome". These variables appear to be a marker for individuals with small-dense LDLs. **Class II, Level C1**
- Assess plasma triglyceride and HDL-C levels in individuals with CHD. Although alteration in these levels has not been demonstrated conclusively to improve outcomes, there is a strong theoretical basis to support such intervention. **Class IIa, Level B**
- Consider initiation of appropriate therapy in high-risk individuals without initial determination of plasma lipid and lipoprotein levels, as treatment is effective even in those with low initial LDL levels. **Class I, Level A**
- Monitor LDL-C levels during treatment to assess for attainment of goals, and to monitor compliance. **Class I, Level C1**

Costs and cost effectiveness of lipid alterations for CHD prevention

True benefits for individuals and the public health have only been demonstrated for alteration of plasma LDL-C. One method for comparing the costs of cholesterol lowering is shown in Table 12.5 where the cost of the various statins is given in terms of the number of dollars per percentage of LDL-C lowering per year.

Until the release of results from the 4S study, reductions in CHD morbidity from plasma cholesterol-related CHD had been modest and reductions in CHD and total

Table 12.5 Comparative cost, dose and LDL-C lowering of statins

Agent	Dose (mg)	LDL-C b (%)[b] ↓	AWP ($/day)[c]	Cost/1%/LDLR ($/yr)
Lovastatin	10[a]	−21	1.36	23.63
	20	−24	2.37	36.04
Simvastatin	10[a]	−30	2.80	34.07
	80	−47	4.89	66.07
Pravastatin	20[a]	−32	3.27	37.29
	80	−37	4.79	47.29
Fluvastatin	20[a]	−22	2.53	41.97
	40	−24	2.53	38.47
Atorvastatin	10[a]	−39	3.03	28.35
	80	−60	4.32	26.16
Rosuvastatin	5[a]	−28	3.50	45.63
	10	−43	3.50	29.71

[a] Common starting dose, qd.
[b] From *Physicians' Desk Reference*[11]
[c] From *Red Book Update*. Montvale, NJ: Medical Economics Company; 2007
Cost/1%/LDLR was derived as cost/year/1% LDL reduction.

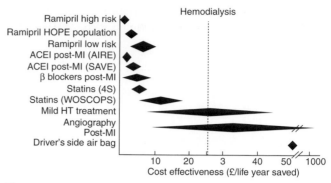

Figure 12.1 Comparison* of cost effectiveness of different strategies in prevention. * Estimates from previous studies are in 1994–1995 UK pounds. (Adapted from Malik *et al*[92].)

mortality had not been demonstrated. Since elevated plasma cholesterol is a major risk factor for CHD and is prevalent in Western countries, evaluation of the cost effectiveness of plasma cholesterol lowering is important because of the size of the potential population for intervention and the associated healthcare costs of what can be lifelong medical therapy. In a sensitivity analysis,[88] data from 4S demonstrate cost effectiveness of intervention for both men and women from 35 to 70 years and at plasma cholesterol levels above 213 mg/dL. The estimates of treatment costs for benefits observed in the 4S study indicate that treatment is cost effective in both men and women and at all plasma cholesterol levels between 213 and 309 mg/dL and with evidence of vascular disease.

A WOSCOPS economic analysis comparing pravastatin with dietary changes alone showed the economic efficiency of therapeutic intervention with a statin.[89] Caro *et al* used a generalized model of cardiovascular disease prevention and followed hypercholesterolemic men over a given time period to quantify the effect on cardiovascular diseases avoided. Over a broad range of inputs and regardless of country, cost-effectiveness ratios are below $35 000 per life-year gained. Pravastatin is cost effective in preventing CHD.[89] Based on US medical price levels and the clinical trial evidence up to 1998, Hay *et al* concluded that statin therapy is cost effective (that is, cost less than $50 000/year of life saved) in any patient with an annual CHD risk >1%, including those with previous CHD or diabetes.[90]

In a recent cost-effectiveness analysis of the VA-HIT trial, the cost per year of life gained with gemfibrozil was estimated. Using prices for gemfibrozil paid outside the VA

system (a lower price has been negoitiated by the VA), the cost of a quality-adjusted life-year saved by gemfibrozil ranged from $6300 to $17 000. This cost of a life-year saved is well below the threshold considered cost effective.[91]

Malik *et al*[92] provide a graphic demonstration of how cost effective statin therapy is versus other widely used therapies for CHD, such as ACE inhibitors, beta-blockers, and non-CV interventions, such as driver's side air bags (Fig. 12.1). The cost effectiveness threshold here is £25 000/year of life saved (US $50 000/year of life saved).

Future directions

The benefits of statins beyond the coronary vascular bed are now being intensively investigated. In addition to their lipid-lowering properties, statins demonstrate pleiotropic effects on many aspects of atherosclerosis, such as plaque thrombogenicity, cellular migration, endothelial function, and thrombotic tendency.[18] Whether or not these effects can be related to a decrease in progression of atherosclerosis or to reductions in acute coronary syndromes remains to be seen. Another area for more study is the benefit of moderate versus aggressive LDL lowering. For example, what are the risks and benefits of lowering LDL-C to 75 mg/dL compared to about 100 mg/dL? Heretofore, the major effort to ameliorate CHD through the treatment of lipid disorders has concentrated on LDL-C reduction. More recently, efforts to assess the benefits of manipulating HDL-C levels have intensified. The CETP inhibitors, although filled with promise, await further developments. It has recently been demonstrated that HDL-C levels are predictive of cardiovascular events in patients treated with statins, even in those with LDL-C levels less than 70 mg/dL.[93] Ongoing studies such as AIM-HIGH will help define potential benefits from treating low HDL-C levels. The increasing incidence of type 2 diabetes mellitus emphasizes the importance of delineating the most effective treatment strategies for diabetic dyslipidemia. Ongoing studies such as ACCORD should contribute to our understanding of this issue, although this will remain an important area for further study.

Conclusion

The HMG-CoA reductase inhibitors are an important advance in the treatment of CHD and there is compelling evidence that LDL-C lowering with these agents can decrease the risk of CHD events and total mortality in both primary and secondary prevention. In addition to their effects on LDL-C, statins have pleiotropic effects, which may affect the development and the occurrence of clinical events of atherosclerosis. Lipid-lowering therapy benefits the elderly, women, and diabetic patients, even if these individuals have normal LDL-C levels. Effective single and combination-agent regimens for intervention for other plasma lipid and lipoprotein variables are also available.

Key points for using lipid-altering agents

Document the diagnosis of hyperlipidemia.

Do the patient's current medications cause dyslipidemia or offer potential for drug interactions with hypolipidemic therapy?

Assess the total risk for CAD by considering all risk factors.

ALWAYS start the therapeutic regimen with diet and other lifestyle modifications. **Class I, Level C1**

The statins act as a class of agents, but possess different dose–response curves. Some may have substantial levels of adverse effects. **Class I, Level A**

The currently approved statins have powerful lipid-altering effects and a very low order of adverse effects. **Class I, Level A**

Nicotinic acid is a powerful agent which can be effective in many people, including some diabetic patients when used carefully. **Class I, Level A**

Nicotinic acid is the most effective of any agent on HDL-C levels and the only one with a substantial effect on Lp(a). **Class I, Level B**

Resin therapy can be effective for lowering LDL-C plasma levels with careful attention to details of dosing and administration, particularly when added to low-dose statin or low-dose niacin. **Class I, Level A**

Fasting hypertriglyceridemia is a relative contraindication to primary or combination resin therapy. **Class I, Level B**

Fibrates are effective agents for lowering triglyceride, particularly when extremely high, and moderately raising HDL-C levels, but changes in LDL-C levels need to be monitored. **Class I, Level A**

Consider direct and indirect costs before initiating primary lipid-altering therapy and with the addition of each agent to the regimen.

References

1. Scandinavian Simvastatin Survival Study Group. Randomized trial of cholesterol lowering in 4444 patients with coronary heart disease: the Scandinavian Simvastatin Survival Study (4S). *Lancet* 1995;**344**:1383–9.
2. Shepherd J, Cobbe SM, Ford I *et al* for the West of Scotland Coronary Prevention study Group. Prevention of coronary heart disease with pravastatin in men with hypercholesterolemia. *N Engl J Med* 1995;**333**:1301–7.
3. MRC/BHF. Heart Protection Study of cholesterol lowering with simvastatin in 20 536 high-risk individuals: a randomised placebo-controlled trial. *Lancet* 2002;**360**:7–22.
4. Sacks FM, Pfeffer MA, Moye LA *et al* for the Cholesterol and Recurrent Events Trial Investigators. The effect of pravastatin on coronary events after myocardial infarction in patients with average cholesterol levels. *N Engl J Med* 1996;**335**: 1001–9.
5. Brown G, Albers JJ, Fisher LD *et al*. Regression of coronary artery disease as a result of intensive lipid-lowering therapy in men with high levels of apolipoprotein B. *N Engl J Med* 1990;**323**:1289–98.
6. Post Coronary Artery Bypass Graft Trial Investigators. The effect of aggressive lowering of low-density lipoprotein cholesterol levels and low-dose anticoagulation on obstructive changes in saphenous-vein coronary-artery bypass grafts. *N Engl J Med* 1997;**336**:153–62.
7. Third Report of the National Cholesterol Education Program (NCEP) Expert Panel on detection, evaluation, and treatment of high blood cholesterol in adults (Adult Treatment Panel III). Executive summary. NIH Publication No. 01-3670 May 2001.
8. Grundy, SM, Cleeman, JI, Bairey Merz, CN *et al*. Implications of recent clinical trials for the National Cholesterol Education Program Adult Treatment Panel III Guidelines. *Circulation* 2004;**110**:227–39.
9. Yusuf, S, Hawken, S, Ounpuu, S *et al*. Effect of potentially modifiable risk factors associated with myocardial infarction in 52 countries (the INTERHEART study): case–control study. *Lancet* 2004;**364**:937.
10. Lousberg TR, Denham AM, Rasmussen JR. A comparison of clinical outcome studies among cholesterol-lowering agents. *Ann Pharmacother* 2001;**35**:1599–607.
11. Physicians' Desk Reference. Montvale, NJ: Medical Economics, 2007.
12. Brunzell, JD. Hypertriglyceridemia. *N Engl J Med* 2007;**357**: 1009.
13. Brown MS, Faust JR, Goldstein JL. Inhibition of 3-hydroxy-3-methylglutaryl coenzyme A reductase activity in human fibroblasts incubated with compactin (ML-236B), a competitive inhibitor of the reductase. *J Biol Chem* 1978;**253**:1121–8.
14. Istvan ES, Deisenhofer J. Structural mechanism for statin inhibition of HMG-CoA reductase. *Science* 2001;**292**:1160.
15. Brown MS, Goldstein JL. A receptor-mediated pathway for cholesterol homeostasis. *Science* 1986:**232**:34–47.
16. Corsini A, Bellosta S, Baetta R, Faumgalli R, Paoletti R, Bernini F. New insights into the pharmacodynamic and pharmacokinetic properties of statins. *Pharmacol Ther* 1999;**84**:413–28.
17. Farmer JA. Pleiotropic effects of statins. *Curr Atheroscler Rep* 2002;**2**:208–17.

18. Vaughan CJ, Gotto AM Jr, Basson CT. The evolving role of statins in the management of atherosclerosis. *J Am Coll Cardiol* 2000;**35**:1–10.

19. Albert MA, Danielson E, Rifai N, Ridker PM, for the PRINCE Investigators. Effects of statin therapy on C-reactive protein levels: the pravastatin inflammation/CRP evaluation (PRINCE): a randomized trial and cohort study. *JAMA* 2001;**286**:64–70.

20. Byington RP, Davis BR, Plehn JF *et al.* Reduction of stroke events with pravastatin: the Prospective Pravastatin Pooling (PPP) Project. *Circulation* 2001;**103**:387–92.

21. Schwartz GG, Olsson AG, Ezekowitz MD *et al.* Myocardial Ischemia Reductions with Aggressive Cholesterol Lowering (MIRACL) Investigators. Effects of atorvastatin on early recurrent ischemic events in acute coronary syndromes: the MIRACL study: a randomized controlled trial. *JAMA* 2001;**285**:1711–18.

22. Waters DD. Medical therapy versus revascularization: the atorvastatin versus revascularization treatment AVERT trial. *Can J Cardiol* 2000 Jan;**16**(suppl. A):11A–13A.

23. Cholesterol Treatment Trialists (CTT) Collaborators. Efficacy of statin therapy in people with diabetes: meta-analysis of data from 18,686 diabetic participants in 14 randomised trials of statins. *Lancet* 2008;**371**:117.

24. Farmer JA, Torre-Amione G. Comparative tolerability of the HMG-CoA reductase inhibitors. *Drug Saf* 2000;**23**:197–213.

25. Alderman JD, Pasternak RC, Sacks FM, Smith HS, Monrad S, Grossman W. Effect of modified, well tolerated niacin regimen on serum total cholesterol, high density lipoprotein cholesterol and the cholesterol to high density lipoprotein ratio. *Am J Cardiol* 1989;**64**:725–9.

26. Jones, PH, Davidson, MH, Stein, EA *et al.* Comparison of the efficiency and safety of of rosuvastatin vs atorvastatin, simvastatin, and pravastatin across doses.(STELLAR* Trial). *Am J Cardiol* 2003;**92**:152.

27. Mulder, AB, van Lijf, HJ, Bon, MA *et al.* Association of polymorphism in the cytochrome CYP2D6 and the efficiency and tolerability of simvastatin. *Clin Pharmacol Ther* 2001;**70**:546.

28. Chasman, DI, Posada, D, Subrahmanyan, L *et al.* Pharmacogenetic study of statin therapy and cholesterol reduction. *JAMA* 2004; **291**:2821.

29. Beaird SL. HMG-CoA reductase inhibitors: assessing differences in drug interactions and safety profiles. *J Am Pharm Assoc (Wash)* 2000;**40**:637–44.

30. Downs, JR, Clearfield, M, Weis, S *et al.* Primary prevention of acute coronary events with lovaststin in men and women with average cholesterol levels: results of AFCAPS/TEXCAPS, Air Force/Texas Coronary Atherosclerosis Prevention Study. *JAMA* 1998;**279**:1615.

31. Omar MA, Wilson JP, Cox TS. Rhabdomyolysis and HMG-CoA reductase inhibitors. *Ann Pharmacother* 2001;**35**:1096–107.

32. Schmitz G, Langmann T, Pharmacogenetics of cholesterol lowering therapy. *Vasc Pharmacol* 2006;**44**:75.

33. Shear CL, Franklin FA, Stinnett S *et al.* Expanded Clinical Evaluation of Lovastatin (EXCEL) study results: effect of patient characteristics on lovastatin-induced changes in plasma concentrations of lipids and lipoproteins. *Circulation* 1992;**85**:1293–303.

34. McTaggart F, Buckett L, Davidson R *et al.* Preclinical and clinical pharmacology of rosuvastatin, a new 3-hydroxy-3-methylglutaryl-coenzyme A reductase inhibitor. *Am J Cardiol* 2001;**87**:28B–32B.

35. Carlson LA, Hampsten A, Asplund A. Effects of hyperlipidemic drugs on serum levels of lipoprotein Lp(a) in hyperlipidemic subjects treated with nicotinic acid. *J Int Med* 1989;**226**:271–6.

36. Knopp RH. Evaluating niacin in its various forms. *Am J Cardiol* 2000;**86**:51L–56L.

37. Guyton JR, Bays HE. Safety considerations with niacin therapy. *Am J Cardiol* 2007;**99**(suppl):22C.

38. ACCORD Study Group. Action to Control Cardiovascular Risk in Diabetes (ACCORD) Trial: design and methods. *Am J Cardiol* 2007;**99**(suppl):21i.

39. Tunaru S, Kero J, Schaub A *et al.* PUMA-G and HM74 are receptors for nicotinic acid and mediate its antilipolytic effect. *Nat Med* 2003;**9**:352.

40. Taggert AK, Kero J, Gan X *et al.* (D)-beta-Hydroxybutyrate inhibits adipocyte lipolysis via the nicotinic acid receptor PUMAS-G. *J Biol Chem* 2005;**280**:26649.

41. Schoonjans K, Staels B, Auwrex J. Role of the peroxisome proliferator-activated receptors (PPAR), in mediating the effects of fibrates and fatty acids on gene expression. *J Lipid Res* 1996;**37**:907–25.

42. Superko HR, Krauss RM. Differential effects of nicotinic acid in subjects with different LDL subclass patterns. *Atherosclerosis* 1992;**95**:69–76.

43. Benyo C, Gille A, Kero J *et al.* GPR109A9PUMA-G(HM74A) mediates nicotinic acid induced flushing. *J Clin Invest* 2005; **115**:3634.

44. Elam MB, Hunninghake DB, Davis KB *et al.* Effect of niacin on lipid and lipoprotein levels and glycemic control in patients with diabetes and peripheral arterial disease: the ADMIT study: a randomized trial. Arterial Disease Multiple Intervention Trial. *JAMA* 2000;**284**:1263–70.

45. Patterson DJ, Dew EW, Gyorkey F, Graham DY. Niacin hepatitis. *South Med J* 1983;**76**:239–41.

46. Probstfield JL, Hunninghake DB. Nicotinic acid as a lipoprotein altering agent: therapy directed by the primary physician. *Arch Intern Med* 1994;**154**:1557–9.

47. Shepherd J, Packard CJ, Bicker S, Lawrie TD, Morgan HG. Cholestyramine promotes receptor-mediated low-density-lipoprotein catabolism. *N Engl J Med* 1980;**302**:1219–22.

48. Lipid Research Clinics Program. The Lipid Research Clinics Coronary Primary Prevention Trial results, I: reduction in the incidence of coronary heart disease. *JAMA* 1984;**251**:351–64.

49. Hunninghake DB. Bile acid sequestrants. In: Rifkind BM, ed. Drug Treatment of Hyperlipidemia. New York: Marcel Dekker, 1991.

50. Davidson MH, Dicklin MR, Maki KC, Kleinpell RM. Colesevelam hydrochloride: a non-absorbed, polymeric cholesterol-lowering agent. *Expert Opin Invest Drugs* 2000; **9**: 2663–71.

51. Aldridge MA, Ito MK. Colesevelam hydrochloride: a novel bile acid-binding resin. *Ann Pharmacother* 2001;**35**:898–907.

52. Donovan JM, Stypinski D, Stiles MR, Olson TA, Burke SK. Drug interactions with colesevelam hydrochloride, a novel, potent lipid-lowering agent. *Cardiovasc Drugs Ther* 2000;**14**:681–90.

53. Clearfield M, Downs JR, Weis S *et al.* Air Force/Texas Coronary Atherosclerosis Prevention Study (AFCAPS/TexCAPS): efficacy and tolerability of long-term treatment with lovastatin in women. *J Womens Health Gender Based Med* 2001;**10**:971–81.

54. Frick MJ, Elo O, Haapa K *et al.* Helsinki Heart Study: primary prevention trial with gemfibrozil in middle-aged men with dyslipidemia: safety of treatment, changes in risk factors, and incidence of coronary heart disease. *N Engl J Med* 1987;**317**:1237–45.

55. Bloomfield Rubin H, Robins S *et al.* Gemfibrozil for the secondary prevention of coronary heart disease in men with low levels of high density lipoprotein cholesterol. *N Engl J Med* 1999;**341**:410–18.

56. Bloomfield Rubin H, Davenport J, Babikiam V *et al* for the VA-HIT Study Group. Reduction in stroke with gemfibrozil in men with coronary heart disease and low HDL cholesterol: the Veterans Affairs HDL Intervention Trial (VA-HIT). *Circulation* 2001;**103**:2828–33.

57. Robins SJ, Collins D, Wittes JT *et al.* VA-HIT Study Group. Veterans Affairs High-Density Lipoprotein Intervention Trial. Relation of gemfibrozil treatment and lipid levels with major coronary events: VA-HIT: a randomized controlled trial. *JAMA* 2001;**285**:1585–91.

58. Palmer RH. Effects of fibric acid derivatives on biliary litogenicity. *Am J Med* 1987;**83**(suppl. 5B):37–43.

59. Goldberg AP, Sherrard DJ, Hass LB, Brunzell JD. Control of clofibrate toxicity in uremic triglyceride. *Clin Pharmacol Ther* 1977;**21**:317–25

60. Sudhop T, Lutjohann D, Kodal A *et al.* Inhibition of intestinal cholesterol absorption by ezetimibe in humans. *Circulation* 2002;**106**:1943.

61. Knopp RH, Gitter H, Truitt T *et al.* Effects of ezetimibe, a new cholesterol absorption inhibitor, on plasma lipids in patients with primary hypercholesterolemia. *Eur Heart J* 2003;**24**:729.

62. Davidson MH, McGarry T, Bettis R *et al.* Ezetimibe coadministered with simvastatin in patients with primary hypercholesterolemia. *J Am Coll Cardiol* 2002;**40**:2125.

63. Melani L, Mills R, Hassman D *et al.* Efficacy and safety of ezetimibe coadministered with simvastatin in patients with primary hypercholesterolemia: a randomized double blind, placebo controlled trial. *Eur Heart J* 2003;**24**:717.

64. Gustavson LE, Schweitzer SM, Burt DA *et al.*Evaluation of the potential for pharmokinetic interaction between fenofibrate and ezrtimibe:a phase I, open label, multiple dose, three-period crossover study in healthy subjects. *Clin Ther* 2006;**28**: 373.

65. McKenney JM, Farnier M, Lo KW *et al.* Safety and efficacy of long term coadministration of fenofibtate, and ezetimibe in patients with mixed hyperlipidemia. *J Am Coll Cardiol* 2006 **47**:1584.

66. Gouni-Berthold I, Berthold HK. Policosanol: clinical pharmacology and therapeutic significance of a new lipid-lowering agent. *Am Heart J* 2002;**143**:356–65.

67. Brousseau ME, Schafer EJ, Wolfe ML *et al.* Effects of an inhibitor of cholesterol ester transfer proteinon HDL cholesterol. *N Engl J Med* 2004;**350**:1505.

68. Hirano K, Yameshita S, Matsuzawa Y. Pros and cons of inhibiting cholesteryl ester transfer protein. *Curr Opin Lipidol* 2000;**11**:589.

69. Nissen SE, Tardif JC, Nicholls SJ *et al.* Effect of torcetrapib on carotid atherosclerosis in familial hypercholesterolemia. *N Engl J Med* 2007;**356**:1620.

70. Barter PJ, Caulfield M, Eriksson M *et al.* Effects of torcetrapib in patients at high risk for coronary events. *N Engl J Med* 2007;**357**:2109.

71. Nissen SE, Tsunada T, Tuzcu EM *et al.* Effect of recombinant Apo A1 Milano on coronary atherosclerosis in patients with acute coronary syndrome: a randomized controlled trial. *JAMA* 2003;**290**:2992.

72. Tardif JC, Gregoire J, L'allier PL *et al.* Effects of reconstituted high-density-lipoprotein infusions on coronary atherosclerosis: a randomized controlled trial. *JAMA* 2007;**297**:1675.

73. Simons LA, Simons J, Parfitt A. Successful management of primary hypercholesterolaemia with simvastatin and low-dose colestipol. *Med J Aust* 1992;**15**:455–59.

74. Jacob BG, Richter WO, Schwandt P. Long-term treatment (2 years) with the HMG CoA reductase inhibitors lovastatin or pravastatin in combination with cholestyramine in patients with severe primary hypercholesterolemia. *J Cardiovasc Pharmacol* 1993;**22**:396–400.

75. Davidson MH, Toth P, Weiss S *et al.* Low-dose combination therapy with colesevelam hydrochloride and lovastatin effectively decrease low-density lipoprotein cholesterol in patients with primary hypercholesterolemia. *Clin Cardiol* 2001;**24**: 467–74.

76. Hunninghake D, Insull W Jr, Toth Davidson D, Donovan JM, Burke SK. Coadministration of colesevelam hydrochloride with atorvastatin lowers LDL cholesterol additively. *Atherosclerosis* 2001;**158**:407–16.

77. Knapp JJ, Schrott H, Ma P *et al.* Efficacy and safety of combination simvastatin and colesevelam in patients with primary hypercholesterolemia. *Am J Med* 2001;**110**:352–60.

78. Sacks FM, Tonkin AM, Shepherd J *et al.* Effects of pravastatin on coronary disease events in subgroups defined by coronary risk factors: the Prospective Pravastatin Pooling Project. *Circulation* 2000;**102**:1893–900.

79. Shepard J, Blauw GJ, Murphy MB *et al.* Pravastatin in elderly individuals at risk of vascular disease (PROSPER): a randomized controlled trial. *Lancet* 2002;**360**:1623.

80. Deedwania P, Stone PH, Merz CN *et al.* Effects of intensive versus moderate lipid-lowering therapy on myocardial ischemia in older patients with coronary heart disease: results of the Study Assessing Goals in the Elderly (SAGE). *Circulation* 2007;**115**:700.

81. Wenger NK, Lewis SJ, Herrington DM *et al.* Outcomes of using high- or low-dose atorvastation in patients 65 years of age or older with stable coronary heart disease. *Ann Intern Med* 2007;**147**:1–9.

82. Cholesterol Treatment Trialists (CTT) Collaborators. Efficacy and safety of cholesterol-lowering treatment: prospective meta-analysis of data from 90,056 participants in 14 radomised trials of statins. *Lancet* 2005;**366**:1267–78.

83. Goldberg RB, Mellies MJ, Sacks FM *et al.* Cardiovascular events and their reduction with pravastatin in diabetic and glucose-intolerant myocardial infarction survivors with average cholesterol levels: subgroup analyses in the cholesterol and recurrent events (CARE) trial. The CARE Investigators. *Circulation* 1998;**98**:2513–19.

84. Colhoun HM, Betteridge DJ, Durrington PN *et al.* Primary prevention of cardiovascular disease with atorvastatin in type 2 diabetes on the Collaborative Atorvastatin Diabetes Study (CARDS): multicentre randomized placebo-controlled trial. *Lancet* 2004;**364**:685.

85. Knopp RH, d'Emden M, Smilde JG *et al.* Efficacy and safety of atorvastatin in the prevention of cardiovascular end points in subjects with type 2 diabetes: the Atorvastatin Study for Prevention of Coronary Heart Disease Endpoints in non-insulin-dependent diabetes mellitus (ASPEN). *Diabetes Care* 2006;**29**:1478.

86. Keech A, Simes RJ, Barter P *et al.* Effects of long term fenofibrate therapy on cardiovascular events in 9795 people with type 2 diabetes mellitus (the FIELD study): randomized controlled trial. *Lancet* 2005;**366**:1849.

87. Criqui MH, Langer RD, Fronek A *et al.* Mortality over a period of 10 years in patients with peripheral arterial disease. *N Engl J Med* 1992;**326**:381.

88. Weinstein MC, Stason WB. Foundations of cost effectiveness analysis for health and medical practices. *N Engl J Med* 1977;**296**:716–21.

89. Caro J, Klittich W, McGuire A *et al.* International economic analysis of primary prevention of cardiovascular disease with pravastatin in WOSCOPS. West of Scotland Coronary Prevention Study. *Eur Heart J* 1999;**20**:263–8.

90. Hay JW, Yu WM, Ashraf T. Pharmacoeconomics of lipid lowering agents for primary and secondary prevention of coronary artery disease. *Pharmacoeconomics* 1999;**15**:47–74.

91. Nyman JA, Martinson MS, Nelson D, the VA-HIT Study Group. Cost-effectiveness of gemfibrozil for coronary heart disease patients with low levels of high-density lipoprotein cholesterol: the Department of Veterans Affairs High-Density Lipoprotein Cholesterol Intervention Trial. *Arch Intern Med* 2002;**162**:177–82.

92. Malik IS, Bhatia VK, Kooner JS. Cost effectiveness of ramipril treatment for cardiovascular risk reduction. *Heart* 2001;**85**:539–43.

93. Barter P, Gotto AM, LaRosa JC *et al.* HDL cholesterol, very low levels of LDL cholesterol, and cardiovascular events. *N Engl J Med* 2007;**357**:1301.

94. Angelin B, Emarsson K. Cholesterol lowering effects of a combination of cholestyramine and niacin. *Atherosclerosis* 1981;**38**:33.

95. Leren TP, Johnson MH, Tuskinen OP. Cholestyramine in combination with the HMG CoA reductase inhibitor lovastatin: cholesterol lowering effects and tolerability. *Atherosclerosis* 1988;**73**:135.

96. Jacob BG, Richter WO, Schwandt P. Long term treatment (2 years) with the HMG coA reductase inhibitors lovastatin or pravastatin in combination with cholestyramine in patients with severe primary hypercholesterolemia. *J Cardiovas Pharmacol* 1993;**22**:396–400.

97. Packard CJ, Stewart JM, Morgan HG *et al.* Combined drug therapy for familial hypercholesterolemia. *Artery* 1980; **8**(4):281.

98. Illingworth DR, Phillipson BE, Rapp JH *et al.* Colestipol plus nicotinic acid in treatment of heterozygous familial hypercholesterolemia. *Lancet* 1981;**1**:296.

99. Malloy MJ, Kane JP, Kunitake ST *et al.* Complementarity of colestipol, niacin, and lovastatin in treatment of severe familial hypercholesterolemia. *Ann Int Med* 1987;**107**:616.

100. Simons LA, Simons J, Parfitt A. Successful management of primary hypercholesterolemia with simvastatin and low dose colestipol. *Med J Aust* 1992;**15**:455–59.

101. Heller FR, Desager JP, Harvengt C. Plasma lipid concentrations and lecithin:cholesterol acyltransferase activity in normolipidemic subjects given fenofibrate and colestipol. *Metab Clin Exp* 1981;**30**:67.

102. Illingworth DR. Fibric acid derivatives. In Rifkind BM, ed. *Drug Treatment of Hyperlipidemia.* New York: Marcel Dekker, Inc., 1991.

103. Feussner G, Eichenger M, Ziegler R. The influence of simvastatin alone, or in combination with gemfibrozil on plasma lipids and lipoproteins in patients with type III hyperlipoproteinemia. *Clin Invest* 1992;**70**:1027.

104. McKenney JM, Jones PH, Bays HE. Comparative effects on lipid levels of combination therapy with a statin and extended release niacin or ezetimibe versus a statin alone (the COMPELL study). *Atherosclerosis* 2007;**192**:432.

105. Hunninghake D, Insull W Jr Toth Davidson D *et al.* Coadministration of colesevelam hydrochloride with atorvastatin lowers LDL cholesterol additively. *Atherosclerosis* 2001;**158**;407.

106. Bays HE, Moore PB, Drehobi MA *et al.* Effectiveness and tolerability of ezetimibe in patients with primary hypercholesterolemia : pooled analysis of two phase II studies. *Clin Ther* 2001; **23**:1209.

107. Farnier M, Roth E, Gil-Extremera B *et al.* Efficacy and safety of the coadministration of ezetimibe/simvastatin with fenofibrate in patients with mixed hyperlipidemia. *Am Heart J* 2007;**153**:335.

13 Blood pressure and cardiovascular disease

Curt D Furberg,[1] Bruce M Psaty[2] and Elsayed Z Soliman[3]

[1] Division of Public Health Sciences, Wake Forest University School of Medicine, Winston-Salem, NC, USA
[2] Cardiovascular Health Research Unit, Departments of Medicine and Epidemiology, University of Washington, Seattle, WA, USA
[3] Epidemiological Cardiology Research Center (EPICARE), Wake Forest University School of Medicine, Winston-Salem, NC, USA

Definition and classification

The Seventh Report of the Joint National Committee on the Prevention, Detection, Evaluation, and Treatment of High Blood Pressure (JNC 7)[1] defines normal blood pressure (BP) as systolic blood pressure (SBP) below 120 mmHg and diastolic blood pressure (DBP) below 80 mmHg. Hypertension is defined as SBP 140 mmHg or greater and/or DBP 90 mmHg or greater. Individuals with SBP 140–159 mmHg and/or DBP 90–99 mmHg are classified as stage 1 hypertension while those at or above SBP 160 mmHg and/or DBP 100 mmHg constitute stage 2 hypertension.

A new category designated prehypertension has been added, and it is defined as SBP between 120 and 139 mmHg and DBP between 80 and 90 mmHg (Table 13.1). Prehypertension is a designation chosen to identify individuals at high risk for developing hypertension, so that both patients and clinicians are alerted to this risk and encouraged to intervene and prevent or delay the hypertension from developing. Individuals who are prehypertensive are not candidates for drug therapy based on their level of BP and should be firmly and unambiguously advised to practice lifestyle modification in order to reduce their risk of developing hypertension in the future. This classification does not stratify hypertensive individuals by the presence or absence of risk factors or target organ damage in order to make different treatment recommendations. Should either or both be present, JNC 7 suggests that all people with hypertension (stages 1 and 2) be treated. The treatment goal for individuals with hypertension and no other compelling conditions is <140/90 mmHg. The goal for individuals with prehypertension and no compelling indications is to lower BP to normal levels with lifestyle changes, and

prevent the progressive rise in BP using the recommended lifestyle modifications.

Impressive evidence has accumulated to warrant greater attention to the importance of SBP as a major risk factor for cardiovascular disease (CVD). Clinical trials have demonstrated that control of isolated systolic hypertension (ISH), defined as SBP ≥160 mmHg and DBP <90 mmHg, reduces total mortality, cardiovascular mortality, stroke, and heart failure.[2,3] A Clinical Advisory Statement[4] recommends that SBP should be the principal measure for the detection, evaluation, and treatment of hypertension in both middle-aged and older individuals.

Diagnosis and evaluation of hypertensive patients should include assessment of other cardiovascular risk factors or concomitant disorders that may affect prognosis and guide treatment (Box 13.1) and looking for identifiable causes of high BP. Identifiable causes of high BP include chronic kidney disease, coarctation of the aorta, Cushing's syndrome and other glucocorticoid excess states including chronic steroid therapy, drug-induced or drug-related hypertension, obstructive uropathy, pheochromocytoma, primary aldosteronism and other mineralocorticoid excess states, renovascular hypertension, sleep apnea, and thyroid or parathyroid disease.[1]

Prevalence

Hypertension affects 20–30% of the world's population.[5,6] When the new JNC 7 classification was applied to a nationally representative sample of US adults, it was found that in populations aged 20 or greater, an estimated 41.9 million men and 27.8 million women have prehypertension, 12.8 million men and 12.2 million women have stage 1 hypertension, and 4.1 million men and 6.9 million women have stage 2 hypertension.[7] A higher percentage of men than women have hypertension before age 45. From age 45 to age 54, the percentages of men and women with hypertension are similar. After that, a much higher percentage of

Evidence-Based Cardiology, 3rd edition. Edited by S. Yusuf, J.A. Cairns, A.J. Camm, E.L. Fallen, and B.J. Gersh. © 2010 Blackwell Publishing, ISBN: 978-1-4051-5925-8.

Table 13.1 JNC 7 blood pressure classification for adults aged 18 years and older*

Category	Systolic/diastolic (mmHg)
Normal	<120/80
Prehypertension	120–139/80–89
Hypertension	≥140/90
Stage 1	140–159/90–99
Stage 2	≥160/100

* The classification is based on the average of two or more properly measured, seated BP readings in individuals not taking antihypertensive drugs and not acutely ill. When systolic and diastolic BP fall into different categories, the higher category should be selected to classify the individual's BP status. For example, 160/92 mmHg should be classified as stage 2 hypertension. Isolated systolic hypertension is defined as SBP ≥140 mmHg and DBP <90 mmHg and staged appropriately. For example, 170/82 mmHg is defined as stage 2 isolated systolic hypertension.
Adapted from JNC 7[1]

BOX 13.1 Components for cardiovascular risk stratification in patients with hypertension

Major risk factors
Tobacco usage, particularly cigarettes
Dyslipidemia*
Diabetes mellitus*
Age older than 65 years for women, 55 years for men
Estimate glomerular filtration rate (GFR) <60 mL/min
Family history of cardiovascular disease: women under age 65 or men under age 55
Microalbuminuria
Obesity* (body mass index ≥30 kg/m^2)
Physical inactivity

Target organ damage/clinical cardiovascular disease
Left ventricular hypertrophy
Angina/prior myocardial infarction
Prior coronary revascularization
Heart failure
Stroke or transient ischemic attack
Chronic kidney disease
Peripheral arterial disease
Retinopathy

*Components of the metabolic syndrome
Adapted from JNC 7[1]

women have high BP than do men.[8] The age-related changes in BP explain the increase in overall prevalence of hypertension with age and the increase in the prevalence of ISH with advanced age. From 1988–1994 to 1999–2002, the prevalence of hypertension in adults increased from 35.8% to 41.4% among blacks, and it was particularly high among black women, at 44.0%. Prevalence among whites also increased from 24.3% to 28.1%.[9] Prevalence of prehypertension in African Americans is lower at older ages because of a higher prevalence of hypertension.[10]

Natural history

Hypertension is one of the major risk factors for cerebrovascular disease (stroke), coronary heart disease (acute myocardial infarction (MI) and angina pectoris), congestive heart failure, and chronic renal disease. The risk is directly associated with the BP level and with the presence of target organ manifestations and other cardiovascular risk factors. Ferrucci et al[11] calculated the cardiovascular risk score for each participant in the Systolic Hypertension in the Elderly Program (SHEP) using the multiple risk factor assessment equation.[12] This simple risk score is based on age, sex, total and high-density lipoprotein (HDL)-cholesterol, SBP, smoking, and diabetes. In the placebo group, the five-year rates of MI, stroke, and heart failure were progressively higher with higher quartiles of risk score in those who were free of cardiovascular disease at baseline. The *relative* event protection conferred by chlorthalidone-based treatment was similar across quartiles of risk. Thus, the *absolute* risk reduction increased by quartile of risk. This was reflected in a 2- to 10-fold lower "number needed to treat" (NNT) to prevent hypertensive complications in the highest-risk quartile (Fig. 13.1). The authors concluded that hypertensive patients with additional cardiovascular risk factors should be the prime candidates for antihypertensive treatment. Even in the absence of additional cardiovascular risk in individuals 40–70 years of age, each increment of 20 mmHg in SBP or 10 mmHg in DBP doubles the risk of CVD across the entire BP range from 115/75 to 185/115 mmHG.[13] The classification of "prehypertension" introduced by the JNC 7[1] recognizes this relationship and signals the need for increased education of healthcare professionals and the public health to reduce the BP levels in the general population.

The article by Franklin and colleagues[14] provides additional data on the natural history of BP ranges of 130–139 systolic or 80–89 diastolic (prehypertension as defined by the JNC 7). After adjustment for age and sex, the incidence of ISH per 100 person-years was 22.8 among individuals with BP 120/80 to 129/84 and 35.4 among individuals with BP 130/85 to 139/89, as opposed to only 6.6 among individuals with BP less than 120/80. Furthermore, 59% of subjects who developed ISH did not have diastolic hypertension at the baseline visit or at any other visit before ISH onset. These data provide further support to the argument that prehypertension, intended as the combination of normal plus high-normal BP categories, is a useful working definition in the setting of cardiovascular disease prevention because it identifies individuals at increased risk of

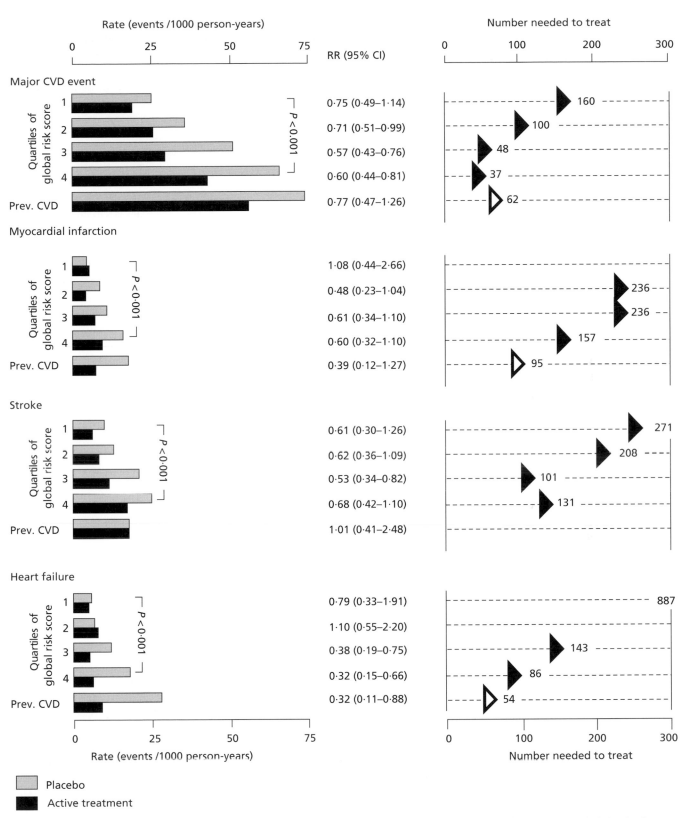

Figure 13.1 Rates of new cardiovascular events, relative risks (RR), and 95% confidence intervals and estimates of NNTs by quartile of global risk score for SHEP participants free of CVD. The fifth group of bars in each panel shows data for subjects with prevalent (prev.) CVD at baseline. (Adapted from Ferrucci et al.[11])

developing progressive vasculopathy with stiffening of the aorta and elastic arteries over time.

Burden

Worldwide prevalence estimates for hypertension may be as much as 1 billion individuals, and approximately 7.1 million deaths per year may be attributable to hypertension.[15] It has been identified as the leading risk factor for cardiovascular mortality, and is ranked third as a cause of disability-adjusted life-years.[16] From 1994 to 2004, the age-adjusted death rate from hypertension increased 25.2%, and the actual number of deaths rose 54.6%. The 2004 overall death rate from hypertension was 17.9%. Death rates were distributed as follows: 15.6% for white males, 49.9% for black males, 14.3% for white females, and 40.6% for black females.[17] Data from "Ambulatory care visits to physician offices, hospital outpatient departments, and emergency departments in the US" showed that the number of visits for essential hypertension was 45.3 million in 2002.[18] This is projected as an estimated direct and indirect cost of high BP in 2007 to be $66.4 billion.[17] Since as many as half of all hypertensives (defined as ≥140/90) remain untreated, the annual drug costs could easily double, unless we can change lifestyles more successfully or be more efficient in allocating resources.

Prevention of hypertension

Despite the established benefits of antihypertensive treatment, concerns are often raised about the prospect of use of antihypertensive drugs over decades by 25% or more of the adult population. All drugs have adverse effects and the cost of medical care for hypertension is considerable. Also, the 12-year follow-up of approximately 350 000 middle-aged men screened for the Multiple Risk Factor Intervention Trial shows that 32% of the coronary heart disease (CHD) deaths related to elevated BP occurred below the level at which drug treatment would be considered.[19]

The multifactorial etiology of hypertension is reflected by the large number of non-pharmaceutical approaches that have been tested.[20–22] Two types of populations have been examined. In individuals with above-optimal (prehypertension stage according to the JNC 7) but non-hypertensive BP levels, lifestyle interventions have been tested to determine their effect on BP. The outcome has been either BP reduction in short-term trials or prevention of BP elevation with age and reduction in the incidence of hypertension in long-term trials. Trials have also been conducted in hypertensive patients with the objective of determining the BP-lowering effects of various non-pharmacologic interventions. One rationale has been that the findings are likely to be generalizable to non-

hypertensive individuals. Another rationale has been to determine the efficacy of lifestyle modifications as definitive first-line or adjuvant therapy for hypertension. All treatment guidelines recommend lifestyle modifications as the first therapeutic approach in newly diagnosed, less severe hypertensive patients, with pharmacologic treatment to follow only in those who fail to respond adequately.

Cross-sectional or longitudinal observational studies have found the following factors to be associated with BP and prevalence or incidence of hypertension: adiposity, physical inactivity, alcohol consumption, high intake of sodium, low intake of potassium, magnesium, calcium, and certain types of dietary fiber, intake of certain macronutrients, and chronic stress.

Trial results on the efficacy of interventions for prevention of hypertension are summarized in Table 13.2. Based on literature reviews, including meta-analysis, evidence of efficacy is conclusive for weight loss, exercise, diets high in fruits and vegetables, reduction in alcohol and sodium intake, and potassium supplementation (**Level A**). A weight reduction of 10 lb (4.5 kg) can be expected to lower the BP by approximately 4/3 mmHg. Since exercise, as part of efforts to achieve caloric balance, influences weight, distinguishing an exercise effect on BP from the effect of weight loss can be difficult, but there is good evidence of BP reduction from fitness training.[23] Low-intensity/high-frequency activity appears as effective as or more effective than high-intensity exercise. A sodium reduction of 80–100 mmol/day induces an average BP reduction of 5/3 mmHg in hypertensives and 2/1 mmHg in non-hypertensives.[21] Similar BP effects were observed in trials that accomplished alcohol reductions of about 85% (a mean consumption of 3 drinks/day reduced to 3 drinks/week).[24]

The BP effects of lifestyle modifications are modest, but they appear to be additive under some circumstances.[25] A short-term study reported substantial BP reductions in adults given a diet rich in fruits, vegetables, and low-fat dairy foods, and reduced saturated and total fat.[26] A further reduction of SBP (2–8 mmHg) was observed when the sodium intake was reduced to below 100 mmol per day (2.4 g sodium or 6 g sodium chloride).[27–29] However, counseling, if required on an indefinite basis through a traditional clinical setting, may not be more cost effective than drugs. Therefore, interventions (such as reducing salt intake by modifying processed foods) that can potentially be accomplished on a population basis are attractive. The efficacy of supplementation with magnesium, fiber, fish oil or calcium has been judged to be limited or unproven at this time.[20] The trial findings are discordant and the effect sizes are small. Potassium supplementation (50–100 mmol KCl or equivalent increase from food) moderately reduces BP, especially in those who have a high sodium intake.[22]

In conclusion, long-term trials in individuals with high-normal BP have documented that sodium reduction,[21,25]

Table 13.2 Trial results on efficacy of interventions for primary prevention of hypertension

Intervention	References	Duration (months)	Change in targeted factors	Change in BP, mmHg (systolic/diastolic)
Sodium reduction	25	6	−50 mmol/day	−2.9/−1.6
	25	18	−43 mmol/day	−2.0/−1.2
	25	36	−40 mmol/day	−1.2/−0.7
	21	0.5–36	−76 mmol/day	−1.9/−1.1
Weight loss	30	6	−4.4 kg	−3.7/−2.7
	30	18	−2.0 kg	−1.8/−1.3
	30	36	−0.2 kg	−1.3/−0.9
Exercise	23	1–16	To 65% maximum exercise capacity	−2.1/−1.6
	31	1.5–7	30–90% of 1 repetition maximum	−3/−3
	32	0.7–24	Low–medium exercise intensity	−3.8/−2.6
Alcohol reduction	24	1.5	−2.6 drinks/day	−3.8/−1.4
	33	0.25–24	16–100% reduction in the daily consumption	−3.3/−2.0
Potassium increase	22	0.3–36	+46 mmol/day	−1.8/−1.0
Dietary pattern	26, 27	2	Increased fruit, vegetables, low fat dairy, protein, lower saturated fat, dietary cholesterol	−3.5/−2.1

weight loss,[30] exercise,[31,32] alcohol reduction,[24,33] and potassium supplementation[22] can reduce the incidence of hypertension by as much as half (**Level A**). The most impressive results are from a five-year trial of a multifactorial intervention.[34] The cumulative incidence of hypertension was 19.2% in the control group and 8.8% in the intervention group. The main factors contributing to this BP reduction were weight loss and sodium reduction.[25] Overweight adults with prehypertension appear to be prime candidates for this intervention. Lifestyle modification is an integral part of management of hypertension. The BP-lowering effects are on average modest. Some patients do not respond or are unable to modify their lifestyles, while others respond well. As a consequence, many patients do not have to be placed on antihypertensive drugs and, if they are, lower drug doses or fewer drugs may be required. The challenge is to sustain the lifestyle modifications.

Drug treatment

Placebo-controlled trials

Despite efforts at lifestyle modifications, most hypertensive patients require pharmacologic treatment. In the US, almost 25 million adults are currently taking antihypertensive medications.[17] This high level of drug use to treat an asymptomatic condition has been justified by the high population burden of major morbidity and mortality causally related to untreated hypertension, and by strong evidence of treatment efficacy and safety from large, long-term

clinical trials. In SHEP,[35] which enrolled older adults ≥60 years with isolated systolic hypertension (SBP ≥160 mmHg), the five-year event rates for the combined endpoints of CHD and stroke per 100 patients were 13.6 in the placebo group and 9.4 in the active group. The risk difference of 4.2% means that about 24 older adults need to be treated for five years in order to prevent one coronary or cerebrovascular event. It must be recognized that calculating the NNT in this manner from randomized clinical trials produces an underestimate for several reasons, chiefly the selection or self-selection of lower-risk patients into trials and the dilution of effects due to drop-in to active treatment by patients in the control group. For middle-aged populations, who are at lower risk, the NNT would be much higher. Because many people must receive therapy so that a few will benefit, even uncommon adverse effects may minimize or eliminate the BP-lowering benefits of antihypertensive therapy. Only with large, long-term trials such as SHEP can we be assured that the health benefits actually outweigh the health risks of particular therapies.

In a meta-analysis by Psaty et al,[36] the evidence from large, long-term, controlled clinical trials of antihypertensive therapy was reviewed. The 18 randomized trials included 48 220 patients followed for an average of about five years. Clinical trials were classified according to the primary treatment strategy. While most studies used more than one drug, the agents were generally used in a stepwise fashion, and it was usually easy to identify the first-line therapy.

Compared with controls, beta-blocker therapy was effective in preventing stroke and congestive heart failure

(Table 13.3). Similarly, high-dose diuretic therapy, which typically started with the equivalent of 50 mg/day of hydrochlorothiazide and often went to 100 mg/day, was associated with a reduced risk of stroke and heart failure. Despite lowering BP by an average of about 5–6 mmHg, neither beta-blocker therapy nor high-dose diuretic therapy demonstrated significant reduction of coronary disease events (**Level A**) (see Table 13.3).

Compared with controls, low-dose diuretic therapy prevented not only stroke and heart failure but also CHD and cardiovascular and total mortality (see Table 13.3). In contrast to high-dose diuretic therapy, the adverse metabolic effects of low-dose diuretic therapy are minimal. The safety and proven effectiveness make low-dose diuretic therapy the logical first-line pharmacologic treatment for hypertension. The JNC 7[1] appropriately identifies low-dose diuretics as preferred first-line agents in the treatment of hypertension (**Class I, Level A**).

It is not clear why low-dose diuretic therapy prevents CHD, but neither high-dose diuretic therapy nor beta-blocker therapy is associated with a reduced risk of coronary disease. The low-dose trials (see reference 36 for references) were conducted mainly in older adults while the high-dose trials were conducted largely in middle-aged adults. Evidence from observational studies suggests that, compared with low-dose diuretic therapy, high-dose diuretic therapy is associated with an increased risk of sudden death.[37] For high-dose diuretics, the most likely explanation for this increased risk of sudden death is the dose of the diuretics rather than the age of patients. Abrupt withdrawal of beta-blocker therapy is associated with an increased risk of MI in patients with high BP.[38] It is possible that withdrawal reactions from non-compliance with beta-blockers may have minimized the drugs' ability to prevent CHD in hypertensive patients, who generally represent a low-risk population group.

The findings for beta-blocker and high-dose diuretic therapy provide direct evidence that BP lowering alone is not adequate to predict the effect of an antihypertensive medication on important health outcomes. "In light of all previous cardiovascular trials …" Topol and colleagues remark, "surrogate endpoints cannot be considered authentic measures of true clinical efficacy and safety".[39] Evidence from individual comparative trials and meta-analyses of comparative trials strongly indicates that it matters how elevated BP is lowered (see below). Although average BP reductions are similar across different classes of drugs, important differences exist between these classes in terms of their effects on major morbid events, especially heart failure and acute MI.[40] Yet drug regulatory agencies currently approve antihypertensive medications primarily on the basis of their ability to lower BP.

A so-called network meta-analysis by Psaty et al[41] included trials through 2002. The database included 192 478 patients from 42 trials randomized to seven major treatment strategies, including placebo. For all major outcomes, low-dose diuretics were superior to placebo: coronary heart disease (CHD; relative risk (RR) 0.79; 95% confidence interval (CI) 0.69–0.92); congestive heart failure (CHF; RR 0.51; 95% CI 0.42–0.62); stroke (RR 0.71; 95% CI 0.63–0.81); cardiovascular disease events (RR 0.76; 95% CI 0.69–0.83); cardiovascular disease mortality (RR 0.81; 95% CI 0.73–0.92); and total mortality (RR 0.90; 95% CI 0.84–0.96). When the effects of low-dose diuretics on the six outcomes were compared to

Table 13.3 Meta-analysis of randomized, placebo-controlled clinical trials in hypertension according to first-line treatment strategy

Outcome drug regimen	Dose	Trials (n)	Events, active treatment/ control	RR (95% CI)
Stroke				
Diuretics	High	9	88/232	0.49 (0.39–0.62)
Diuretics	Low	4	191/347	0.66 (0.55–0.78)
Beta-blockers		4	147/335	0.71 (0.59–0.86)
HDFP	High	1	102/158	0.64 (0.50–0.82)
Coronary heart disease				
Diuretics	High	11	211/331	0.99 (0.83–1.18)
Diuretics	Low	4	215/363	0.72 (0.61–0.85)
Beta-blockers		4	243/459	0.93 (0.80–1.09)
HDFP	High	1	171/189	0.90 (0.73–1.10)
Congestive heart failure				
Diuretics	High	9	6/35	0.17 (0.07–0.41)
Diuretics	Low	3	81/134	0.58 (0.44–0.76)
Beta-blockers		2	41/175	0.58 (0.40–0.84)
Total mortality				
Diuretics	High	11	224/382	0.88 (0.75–1.03)
Diuretics	Low	4	514/713	0.90 (0.81–0.99)
Beta-blockers		4	383/700	0.95 (0.84–1.07)
HDFP	High	1	349/419	0.83 (0.72–0.95)
Cardiovascular mortality				
Diuretics	High	11	124/230	0.78 (0.62–0.97)
Diuretics	Low	4	237/390	0.76 (0.65–0.89)
Beta-blockers		4	214/410	0.89 (0.76–1.05)
HDFP	High	1	195/240	0.81 (0.67–0.97)

Trials (n) indicate number of trials with at least 1 endpoint of interest. Abbreviations: RR, relative risk; CI, confidence interval; HDFP, Hypertension Detection and Follow-up Program Study (5484 subjects in stepped care and 5455 in referred care). For these comparisons, the numbers of participants randomized to active therapy and placebo were 7768 and 12 075 for high-dose diuretic therapy; 4305 and 5116 for low-dose diuretic therapy; and 6736 and 12 147 for beta-blocker therapy. Because the Medical Research Council trial included two active arms, the placebo group is included twice in these totals, once for a diuretic comparison and again for beta-blocker comparison. The total numbers of participants randomized to active therapy and control therapy were 24 294 and 23 926, respectively.[36]

the other five active treatment strategies (beta-blockers, angiotensin-converting enzyme (ACE) inhibitors, calcium channel blockers (CCBs), alpha-blockers and angiotensin receptor blockers), diuretic treatment was significantly better for eight outcomes in the 30 possible comparisons. None of the remaining comparisons showed a statistically significant difference in favor of a comparator drug. This analysis provides compelling evidence that low-dose diuretics are the most effective first-line treatment for preventing the occurrence of cardiovascular disease morbidity and mortality.

Results from several long-term, placebo-controlled trials of the newer classes of antihypertensive agents have been published since 1997 (Table 13.4). A placebo-controlled trial of nitrendipine in ISH (Syst-Eur) found a statistically significant reduction in stroke risk and showed trends for reductions in risks of acute MI and congestive heart failure.[42] Two placebo-controlled trials in patients with type 2 diabetes and nephropathy, the Irbesartan Diabetic Nephropathy Trial (IDNT)[43] and the Reduction of Endpoints in NIDDM with the Angiotensin II Antagonist Losartan (RENAAL) Study,[44] investigated two different angiotensin II receptor blockers. The primary endpoint in both trials was a composite renal outcome defined as a doubling of serum creatinine, development of end-stage renal disease or death from any cause. The primary results were very similar: the composite renal outcome was lowered by 20% in IDNT by irbesartan and by 16% in RENAAL by losartan (P = 0.02 in both trials). IDNT also evaluated the effect of amlodipine, a calcium channel blocker, that did no better than placebo for the renal outcome (RR 1.04). In neither trial did the active treatments significantly reduce the risk of a composite cardiovascular outcome in comparison to the placebo controls.

The Perindopril Protection against Recurrent Stroke Study (PROGRESS) reported that ACE inhibitor-based treatment reduced the risk of stroke by 28% and the risk of total major vascular events by 26%.[45] Those receiving the combination of perindopril and the diuretic indapamide (56% of the population) benefited the most. In this subgroup, the mean reduction in BP was 12/5mmHg and the reduction in stroke risk was 43%. However, those assigned to perindopril alone experienced a small reduction in BP, 5/3mmHg, with no significant reduction in stroke risk.

In conclusion, placebo-controlled trials conducted through the early 1990s documented conclusively that low-dose diuretics and beta-blockers used as first-line drugs markedly reduce the devastating cardiovascular complications experienced by hypertensive patients. However, the role of beta-blockers as a first-line treatment has been challenged when compared to active treatment (see below) (**Level B**). The placebo-controlled trials have had two important consequences. First, they established low-dose diuretics as the proper control group for comparative trials. Second, they limited the opportunity for conducting long-term, placebo-controlled trials, since withholding active treatment generally became ethically unacceptable. Only in specific subgroups of hypertensive patients – for example, those with major co-morbidity such as nephropathy and cerebrovascular disease – were placebo-controlled designs considered acceptable. The focus of clinical research in hypertension has shifted from answering the question "Is BP lowering beneficial?" to asking "Does it matter how elevated BP is lowered?". The latter question requires comparative or active-controlled trials.

Active-controlled trials

Over the past decade, clinical trials of BP-lowering drugs shifted focus from placebo-controlled to actively controlled

Table 13.4 Clinical effects of newer antihypertensive agents from recent placebo-controlled trials

Trial	Study population	First-line treatment	Outcome	RR (95% CI)
Syst-Eur[42]	ISH	Nitrendipine	Stroke	0.58 (0.40–0.83)
			AMI	0.70 (0.44–1.09)
			Heart failure	0.71 (0.47–1.10)
IDNT[43]	Diabetic nephropathy	Irbesartan	Composite renal	0.80 (0.66–0.97)
			Composite CV	0.91 (0.72–1.14)
		Amlodipine	Composite renal	1.04 (0.86–1.25)
			Composite CV	0.88 (0.69–1.12)
RENAAL[44]	Diabetic nephropathy	Losartan	Composite renal	0.84 (0.72 0.98)
			Composite CV	0.90 (NA)
PROGRESS[45]	Stroke, TIA	Perindopril alone	Stroke	0.95 (0.77–1.19)
			Major vascular	0.96 (0.80–1.15)
		Perindopril + indapamide	Stroke	0.57 (0.46–0.70)
			Major vascular	0.60 (0.51–0.71)

CV, cardiovascular; TIA, transient ischemic attack.

designs. ALLHAT, initiated in 1994,[46] was one of the first major active-controlled or comparative outcome trials to examine whether the type of drug used to lower high BP matters. While the study hypotheses were formally two-sided, the primary interest was a test of superiority, with the overall objective being to determine whether each of three drugs from newer drug classes (ACE inhibitors, CCBs, and alpha-blockers), when used as first-line therapy, are superior to low-dose diuretics in reducing the risk of cardiovascular events. The alpha-blocker (doxazosin) arm was terminated early in 2000[47] for two reasons – a 25% excess of major cardiovascular events, primarily congestive heart failure, and a very small likelihood of observing that it is superior to low-dose diuretics in reducing major coronary events (Table 13.5). The fact that excess cardiovascular events with doxazosin occurred despite BP reduction that was similar to the diuretic group points to the importance of drug selection in the treatment of hypertension. In the other two arms of ALLHAT that continued until 2002,[48] chlorthalidone was as effective as ACE inhibitors or CCBs and was even superior in preventing one or more major forms of CVD (see Table 13.5). The low cost of diuretics represents a definite advantage over other drugs. Based on available data from placebo-controlled trials evaluating low-dose diuretics, major health outcomes for chlorthalidone and other thiazide-like drugs appear similar.[49] Hence, low-dose diuretics have emerged as first-line therapy for treatment of hypertension (**Level A**).

Unlike low-dose diuretics, the role of beta-blockers as treatment for primary hypertension has been challenged.[50] A preliminary analysis showed that atenolol was not very effective for treatment of hypertension.[51] To confirm that conclusion and to assess other beta-blockers, Lindholm et al[52] conducted a meta-analysis that included more data on atenolol and data on all other beta-blockers. Thirteen randomized controlled trials (n = 105 951) were included in their meta-analysis. Seven studies (n = 27 433) compared beta-blockers and placebo or no treatment. The relative risk of stroke was 16% higher for beta-blockers (95% CI 4–30%) than for other drugs. There was no difference for myocardial infarction. When the effect of beta-blockers was compared with that of placebo or no treatment, the relative risk of stroke was reduced by 19% for all beta-blockers (7–29%), about half of that expected from previous hypertension trials. There was no difference for myocardial infarction or mortality. These results raise questions about the appropriateness of beta-blockers as first-line therapy.

A meta-analysis of nine randomized comparative clinical trials of intermediate- and long-acting CCBs was conducted by Pahor et al.[53] The comparators were mostly low-dose diuretics, beta-blockers, and ACE inhibitors. The mean BP reduction was almost identical in the CCB and non-CCB groups. In the database that included nearly 120 000 person-years of treatment, use of CCBs was associated with approximately 25% excess rates of both congestive heart failure and acute MI ($P < 0.005$) (see Table 13.5). No differences were observed between the groups for stroke or all-cause mortality. When the database from a second meta-analysis[54] was used to examine the same question – CCBs versus non-CCBs – the results were similar and statistically significant.[55] In a similar type of meta-analysis, the benefit of ACE inhibitors was compared to that of non-ACE inhibitors, primarily CCBs in patients with diabetes.[56] The pooled analysis, supported subsequently by another trial,[57] strongly suggested that ACE inhibitors have advantages over non-ACE inhibitors in reducing the risk of acute myocardial infarction and major cardiovascular events, in spite of similar BP reduction in diabetic patients (see Table 13.5).

The evidence concerning the relevance of how elevated BP is lowered comes from two relatively recent trials with similar design in patients with nephropathy (see Table 13.5). The achieved BP levels were similar for the two therapies – amlodipine versus a drug blocking the renin–angiotensin system. In the AASK trial,[58] among patients with non-diabetic nephropathy, the amlodipine group was terminated early owing to a more rapid decline in renal function and a 60% higher risk of a composite renal outcome – renal disease progression, end-stage renal disease or death compared to the ramipril group. Amlodipine was also inferior to irbesartan in patients with diabetic nephropathy in IDNT.[43] The risk of the composite renal outcome was 32% higher in the amlodipine group compared to the irbesartan group. There was no group difference for a composite cardiovascular outcome.

In the LIFE trial[59] among patients with ECG-determined left ventricular hypertrophy, treatment with ARB (losartan) was more protective against a composite cardiovascular endpoint than treatment with a beta-blocker (atenolol) despite very similar BP reductions. In fact, the benefits were largely attributable to a protection against stroke and were particularly striking in the diabetic subgroup (see Table 13.5).

In the VALUE trial[60] 15 245 patients, aged 50 years or older with treated or untreated hypertension and high risk of cardiac events, were randomly assigned to either valsartan, an ARB drug, or amlodipine. The primary outcome of composite cardiovascular disease did not differ between treatment groups. Unequal reduction in BP initially might account for differences between groups in cause-specific outcomes. The findings emphasize the importance of prompt BP control in hypertensive patients at high CV risk (see Table 13.5).

In the Anglo-Scandinavian Cardiac Outcomes Trial (ASCOT),[61] high-risk patients were randomly assigned to amlodipine and perindopril or atenolol and bendroflumethiazide. Though not statistically significant, fewer individuals on the amlodipine-based regimen had a primary endpoint (non-fatal myocardial infarction and fatal CHD). However, this difference could be largely explained by the

Table 13.5 Clinical effects of newer antihypertensive agents from recent active-controlled trials and meta-analyses

Study	Study population	Treatment		Outcome	RR (95% CI)
		Study	Control		
ALLHAT[47]	Elderly, high-risk	Doxazosin	Chlorthalidone	CHD	1.03 (0.90–1.17)
				Total mortality	1.03 (0.90–1.15)
				Stroke	1.19 (1.01–1.40)
				Combined CVD	1.25 (1.17–1.33)
				CHF	2.04 (1.79–2.32)
				Coronary revasc.	1.15 (1.00–1.32)
ALLHAT[48]	Elderly, high-risk	Amlodipine	Chlorthalidone	CHD	0.98 (0.90–1.07)
				Total mortality	0.96 (0.89–1.02)
				Stroke	0.93 (0.82–1.06)
				Combined CVD	1.04 (0.99–1.09)
				CHF	1.38 (1.25–1.52)
				Coronary revasc.	1.09 (1.00–1.20)
ALLHAT[48]	Elderly, high-risk	Lisinopril	Chlorthalidone	CHD	0.99 (0.91–1.08)
				Total mortality	1.00 (0.94–1.08)
				Stroke	1.15 (1.02–1.30)
				Combined CVD	1.10 (1.05–1.16)
				CHF	1.19 (1.07–1.31)
				Coronary revasc.	1.10 (1.00–1.21)
Lindholm et al[52]	Primary hypertension	Beta-blockers	Non beta-blockers	AMI	1.02 (0.93–1.12)
				Stroke	1.16 (1.04–1.30)
				Total mortality	1.03 (0.99–1.08)
Pahor et al[55]	High risk	CCBs	Non-CCBs	CHF	1.25 (1.07–1.46)
				AMI	1.26 (1.11–1.43)
				Stroke	0.90 (0.80–1.02)
				Mortality	1.03 (0.94–1.13)
Pahor et al[56]*	Diabetics	Non-ACEIs, mostly CCBs	ACEIs	AMI	1.45 (1.12–1.89)
				Stroke	1.08 (0.80–1.43)
				CV event	1.20 (1.00–1.45)
				Mortality	1.08 (0.86–1.35)
AASK[58]	Non-diabetic nephropathy	Amlodipine	Ramipril	Composite renal	1.61 (1.15–2.27)
IDNT[43]	Diabetic nephropathy	Amlodipine	Irbesartan	Composite renal	1.32 (1.09–1.58)
				Composite CV	0.97 (0.76–1.23)
LIFE[59]	Diabetics	Losartan	Atenolol	Composite CV	0.76 (0.58–0.98)
				CV mortality	0.63 (0.42–0.95)
				Total mortality	0.61 (0.45–0.84)
VALUE[60]	High CV risk	Valsartan	Amlodipine	Composite CV	1.04 (0.94–1.15)
				Stroke	1.15 (0.98–1.35)
				MI	1.19 (1.02–1.38)
				CHF	0.89 (0.77–1.03)
				Total mortality	1.04 (0.94–1.14)
ASCOT[61]	High CV risk	Amlodipine ± perindopril	Atenolol ± bendroflumethiazide	Non-fatal MI	0.9 (0.79–1.02)
				Stroke	0.77 (0.66–0.89)
				CVD events	0.84 (0.78–0.90)
				Total mortality	0.89 (0.81–0.99)
				Diabetes incidence	0.7 (0.63–0.78)
ACCOMPLISH[62]	Elderly, high risk	Benazepril + amlodipine	Benazepril + hydrochlorothiazide	Composite CV	0.80 (0.72–0.90)

ACEIs, angiotensin-converting enzyme inhibitors; AMI, acute myocardial infarction; CCBs, calcium-channel blockers; CHD, coronary heart disease; CHF, congestive heart failure; CV, cardiovascular; CVD, cardiovascular disease.
*Updated to include reference 57.

difference in SBP in the two groups. The incidence of new-onset diabetes was also less on the amlodipine-based regimen (see Table 13.5). The Avoiding Cardiovascular Events through Combination Therapy in Patients Living with Systolic Hypertension (ACCOMPLISH) trial, reported that a combination of benazepril and amlodipine reduce a composite outcome of cardiovascular events compared to a combination of benazepril and hydrochlorothiazide by 19.6% in 3 years. The clinical relevance of the trial is limited by the fact that amlodipine was given in a full dose, while hydrochlorothiazide was given in half the recommend dose. It has been documented that chlorothalidone and hydrochlorothiazide have similar benefits,[49] but the effective dose of the latter is twice the that of the former.

In conclusion, these reports document that in certain circumstances it matters how elevated BP is lowered. In the reviewed trials, it appears that two types or classes of drugs, alpha-blockers and CCBs, are as effective as other antihypertensive agents in reducing SBP and DBP, but less effective in reducing the risk of heart failure (both classes) and MI (CCBs). In elderly high-risk hypertensive patients, doxazosin was less effective than chlorthalidone in reducing risk of congestive heart failure and stroke (**Level A**). There was no difference in risk of major coronary events. It is likely that these observations from ALLHAT apply to all alpha-blockers. Two-thirds of the heart failure cases were either hospitalized or fatal. Several sources of data[53–58] show that CCBs are inferior to other agents in reducing the hypertensive complications of congestive heart failure and acute MI. These findings may be especially relevant in patients with type 2 diabetes.[56,57] Since diuretics and ACE inhibitors are effective in the treatment and prevention of heart failure and most CCBs are not recommended in patients with this condition, these observations should not be surprising. In comparison with other antihypertensive drugs, the effect of beta-blockers is less than optimum, with a raised risk of stroke.[58] Hence, beta-blockers should not be first choice in the treatment of primary hypertension and should not be used as reference drugs in future randomized controlled trials of hypertension.

Some newer antihypertensive drugs

New classes of antihypertensive drugs and new drugs in the established classes have recently emerged. These include the aldosterone receptor blockers,[63] vasodilator beta-blockers (carvedilol, nevibolol, and celiprolol),[64] renin inhibitors (aliskiren),[65] endothelin receptor antagonists (bosantan, darusentan, sitaxsentan, and tezosentan),[66] and dual endopeptidase inhibitors (omapatrilat).[67] Only the specific aldosterone receptor blockers and the vasodilator beta-blockers appear to be promising in treating systemic hypertension in routine clinical practice.

Genetics, hypertension, and some potential drug–gene interactions

The phenotype of high BP represents a complex trait influenced by both genes and environment. Essential hypertension, generally mild to moderate elevations of BP in the population, has been associated with several genetic polymorphisms. Detection of such genetic polymorphisms have been adopted by many projects such as genome-wide scan for hypertension in sibships to identify possible hypertension loci on chromosomes (HyperGEN,[68] the BRIGHT study,[69] and the GENIHUSS study[70]). The National Millennium Project of Japan has already investigated 100 000 single nucleotide polymorphism markers in an attempt to identify genetic variations linked to the development of hypertension.[71] Polymorphism in the genes encoding for a number of substances has been found to be associated with hypertension; some of these include human atrial natriuretic peptide,[72] subunit of the epithelial Na+channel,[73] a-adducin,[74] beta 2- and beta 3-adrenoceptors,[75] cytochrome CYP1A1,[76] cytochrome CYP3A5,[77] ACE,[78] bradykinin B2 receptor,[79] aldosterone synthase (CYP11B2),[80] lipoprotein lipase,[81] angiotensin II type 2 receptor,[82] endothelin-2,[83] tyrosine hydroxylase,[84] and G(s) protein alpha-subunit.[85]

The genetic studies of hypertension are very important for understanding the biologic and molecular etiologies of high BP and, potentially, for the design of new drugs. The public health importance of variations in candidate genes for hypertension remains to be determined. While this work has enhanced our knowledge of molecular biology, the polymorphisms associated with essential hypertension, though some are common, tend to have small effects. As Corvol has aptly observed, "Most molecular variants lead to a low attributable risk in the population or a low individual effect at the individual level".[86]

Pharmacogenetics

The studies in molecular biology and genetics are occurring at a breath-taking pace. There are some studies that report the effectiveness of antihypertensive therapy based upon the genotype of selected patients. Amiloride was found to be effective as monotherapy in hypertensive patients with Thr594Met polymorphism in the epithelial sodium channel who have increased amiloride-sensitive sodium channel activity.[87] The therapeutic response to the ARB losartan was much greater in patients on the basis of AT1 receptor A1166C polymorphism.[88] The M235T polymorphism in the angiotensinogen gene was found to be an independent predictor of the BP response to ACE inhibition.[89] Polymorphism in the GNAS1 locus, encoding the G(s) protein alpha-subunit (FokI allele), was related to the BP response to beta-blockers.[90]

Single nucleotide polymorphisms in the angiotensinogen gene were associated with the BP-lowering response to atenolol.[90] However, correlations between gene polymorphism and high BP are not consistent and are often limited to a certain ethnicity[81] and sex,[83] and influenced by environmental factors. Studies have to show a health benefit, a reduction in cost or both before these genetic tests could be widely used.

In conclusion, it is too early to make any recommendation of a specific drug (class) for optimal treatment according to a patient's genotype.

Immunotherapy of hypertension

There are some recent developments in the area of immunotherapy of hypertension. In a small study, hypertensive patients responsive to an ACE inhibitor or ARB were given three or four injections of PMD3117, a vaccine based upon Ang I antigen, over a six-week period. The antibody titer rose from the second injection and peaked in six weeks, but it was not enough to influence BP. However, it blunted the fall in plasma renin after withdrawal of the ACE inhibitor or ARB and decreased aldosterone excretion significantly, indicating suppression of the RAS. The authors believe that much higher titers will be required to have an influence on BP.[91] Treatment of human hypertension with vaccines is feasible but is not likely to be available in the near future.

Cost effectiveness

Hypertension is a worldwide health problem that poses an increasing economic burden on health resources. Recent data suggest that 26.4% of the world adult population have hypertension, and the number is projected to increase to 29.2% by 2025.[92] The shift away from the less expensive, often generic diuretics and beta-blockers to the newer, generally more expensive ACE inhibitors, CCBs, alpha-blockers and angiotensin II blockers has been costly to society. Unfortunately, formal cost-effectiveness analyses are not possible for the newest antihypertensive agents because of the lack of data on effectiveness. Hence, it is predicted that future medical treatment of hypertension will be increasingly affected by cost considerations.

Although reducing high BP to lower levels is advisable in principle, economic factors either at the individual level or at the health system level become obstacles in achieving that goal. The question from a cost-effectiveness viewpoint is not whether treatment is effective, but whether the benefits justify the costs in light of competing healthcare needs. In the context of healthcare systems in which priorities are being established (fixed budgets), the prime candidates for antihypertensive drug treatment should be patients at high risk such as elderly patients, patients with moderate to severe hypertension, patients with other cardiovascular risk factors, and patients with target organ manifestations. These patient groups (among others) are at a higher risk of clinical hypertensive complications. Since clinical trials have demonstrated similar relative reductions in risk of stroke, acute MI, congestive heart failure, and mortality in low-risk compared to high-risk patients, the absolute benefit expressed as NNT to prevent one event or as number of events prevented per 100 patients treated is substantially greater in the high-risk groups described above.

Unanswered questions

- What is the optimal second-line drug to be added to low-dose diuretics if the BP is not controlled?
- What is the best method for risk stratification? How can we implement feasible and acceptable risk stratification in the clinical setting, thus allowing treatment decisions to be based on an individual's overall cardiovascular risk?
- What is the optimal achieved level of treated BP? Should the treatment goals be even lower than 140 mmHg (systolic) or 90 mmHg (diastolic) for certain high-risk subpopulations?
- Should the BP goal be <140 mmHg for elderly with ISH?
- What are the optimal method(s) for long-term lifestyle modifications?
- How can we best reduce the incidence of hypertension?
- Will genetic information improve the efficacy and safety of drug treatment with specific antihypertensive agents?

Key points

- In persons older than 50 years, SBP greater than 140 mmHg is a much more important cardiovascular disease (CVD) risk factor than DBP (**Level A**).
- The risk of CVD beginning at 115/75 mmHg doubles with each increment of 20/10 mmHg; individuals who are normotensive at age 55 have a 90% lifetime risk for developing hypertension (**Level A**).
- Individuals with a SBP of 120–139 mmHg or a DBP of 80–89 mmHg should be considered as prehypertensive and require health-promoting lifestyle modifications to prevent developing hypertension (**Class I, Level A**).
- Low-dose diuretics is the drug of choice in drug treatment for most patients with uncomplicated hypertension, either alone or combined with drugs from other classes. Certain high-risk conditions are compelling indications for the initial use of other antihypertensive drug classes (**Class I, Level A**).
- Most patients with hypertension will require two or more antihypertensive medications to achieve goal BP (<140/90 mmHg or <130/80 mmHg for patients with diabetes or chronic kidney disease) (**Level A**).
- Major differences in direct drug cost between low-dose diuretics and the newer and heavily promoted agents ought to be a strong incentive for use of the former (**Class I**).

Adapted from the JNC 7[1]

References

1. Chobanian AV, Bakris GL, Black HR *et al.* The Seventh Report of the Joint National Committee on Prevention, Detection, Evaluation, and Treatment of High Blood Pressure: the JNC 7 report. *JAMA* 2003;**289**:2560–72.

2. Kostis JB, Davis BR, Cutler J *et al.* Prevention of heart failure by antihypertensive drug treatment in older persons with isolated systolic hypertension. SHEP Cooperative Research Group. *JAMA* 1997;**278**:212–16.

3. Staessen JA, Thijs L, Fagard R *et al.* Predicting cardiovascular risk using conventional vs. ambulatory blood pressure in older patients with systolic hypertension. Systolic Hypertension in Europe Trial Investigators. *JAMA* 1999;**282**:539–46.

4. Izzo JL Jr, Levy D, Black HR. Importance of systolic blood pressure in older Americans. *Hypertension* 2000;**35**:1021–4.

5. Prospective Studies Collaboration. Age-specific relevance of usual blood pressure to vascular mortality: a meta-analysis of individual data for one million adults in 61 prospective studies. *Lancet* 2002;**360**:1903–13.

6. Asia Pacific Cohort Studies Collaboration. Blood pressure and cardiovascular disease in the Asia Pacific region. *J Hypertens* 2003;**21**:707–16.

7. Adnan I, Qureshi A, Fareed K *et al.* Prevalence and trends of prehypertension and hypertension in United States: National Health and Nutrition Examination Surveys 1976 to 2000. *Med Sci Monit* 2005;**11**:CR403–9.

8. National Center for Health Statistics. *Health, United States, 2005.* Hyattsville, MD: National Center for Health Statistics, 2005. Available at: www.cdc.gov/nchs/data/hus/hus05.pdf.

9. Hertz RP, Unger AN, Cornell JA, Saunders E. Racial disparities in hypertension prevalence, awareness and management. *Arch Intern Med* 2005;**165**:2098–104.

10. Greenlund KJ, Croft JB, Mensah GA. Prevalence of heart disease and stroke risk factors in persons with prehypertension in the United States, 1999–2000. *Arch Intern Med* 2004;**164**:2113–18.

11. Ferrucci L, Furberg CD, Penninx BWJH *et al.* Treatment of isolated hypertension is most effective in older patients with high-risk profile. *Circulation* 2001;**104**:1923–6.

12. Grundy SM, Pasternak R, Greenland P *et al.* Assessment of cardiovascular risk by use of multiple-risk-factor assessment equations: a statement for healthcare professionals from the American Heart Association and the American College of Cardiology. *Circulation* 1999;**100**:1481–92.

13. Lewington S, Clarke R, Qizilbash N *et al.* Age-specific relevance of usual blood pressure to vascular mortality: a meta-analysis of individual data for one million adults in 61 prospective studies. *Lancet* 2002;**360**:1903–13.

14. Franklin SS, Pio JR, Wong ND *et al.* Predictors of new-onset diastolic and systolic hypertension: the Framingham Heart Study. *Circulation* 2005;**111**:1121–7.

15. World Health Report 2002. *Reducing Risks, Promoting Healthy Life.* Geneva: World Health Organization, 2002. Available at: www.who.int/whr/2002/

16. Ezzati M, Lopez AD, Rodgers A, Vander Hoorn S, Murray CJ. Selected major risk factors and global and regional burden of disease. *Lancet* 2002;**360**:1347–60.

17. Rosamond W, Flegal K, Friday G. Report from the American Heart Association Statistics Committee and Stroke Statistics Subcommittee. *Circulation* 2007;**115**:e169–e71.

18. Schappert SM, Burt CW. Ambulatory care visits to physician offices, hospital outpatient departments and emergency departments: United States, 2001–2002. *Vital Health Stat* 2006;**159**:1–66.

19. Stamler J, Stamler R, Neaton J. Blood pressure, systolic and diastolic, and cardiovascular risks: US population data. *Arch Intern Med* 1993;**153**:598–615.

20. Cutler JA, Psaty BM, MacMahon S, Furberg CD. Public health issues in hypertension control: what has been learned from clinical trials. In: Laragh JH, Brenner BM, eds. *Hypertension: Pathophysiology, Diagnosis, and Management*, 2nd edn. New York: Raven Press, 1995.

21. Cutler JA, Follmann D, Allender PS. Randomized trials of sodium reduction: an overview. *Am J Clin Nutr* 1997;**65**:643S–51S.

22. Whelton PK, He J, Cutler JA *et al.* Effects of oral potassium on blood pressure. Meta-analysis of randomized controlled clinical trials. *JAMA* 1997;**277**:1624–32.

23. Fagard RH. Prescription and results of physical activity. *J Cardiovasc Pharm* 1995;**25**(suppl 1):S20–S27.

24. Puddey IB, Beilin LJ, Vandongen R, Rouse IL, Rogers P. Evidence for a direct effect of alcohol consumption on blood pressure in normotensive men: a randomized controlled trial. *Hypertension* 1985;**7**:707–13.

25. Trials of Hypertension Prevention Collaborative Research Group. Effects of weight loss and sodium reduction intervention on blood pressure and hypertension incidence in overweight people with high-normal blood pressure. *Arch Intern Med* 1997;**157**:657–70.

26. Appel LJ, Moore TJ, Obarzanek E *et al,* for the DASH Collaborative Research Group. A clinical trial of the effects of dietary patterns on blood pressure. *N Engl J Med* 1997;**336**:1117–24.

27. Sacks FM, Svetkey LP, Vollmer WM *et al.* Effects of blood pressure of reduced dietary sodium and the Dietary Approaches to Stop Hypertension (DASH) diet. *N Engl J Med* 2001;**344**:3–10.

28. Vollmer WM, Sacks FM, Ard J *et al.* Effects of diet and sodium intake on blood pressure: subgroup analysis of the DASH-sodium trial. *Ann Intern Med* 2001;**135**:1019–28.

29. Chobanian AV, Hill M. National Heart, Lung, and Blood Institute Workshop on Sodium and Blood Pressure: a critical review of current scientific evidence. *Hypertension* 2000;**35**:858–63.

30. Stevens VJ, Obazanek E, Cook NR *et al.* Long-term weight loss changes in blood pressure: results of the trials of hypertension prevention, phase II. *Ann Intern Med* 2001;**134**:1–11.

31. Kelley GA, Kelley KS. Progressive resistance exercise and resting blood pressure: a meta-analysis of randomized controlled trials. *Hypertension* 2000;**35**:838–43.

32. Whelton SP, Chin A, Xin X, He J. Effect of aerobic exercise on blood pressure: a meta-analysis of randomized, controlled trials. *Ann Intern Med* 2002;**136**:493–503.

33. Xin X, He J, Frontini MG, Ogden LG, Motsamai OI, Whelton PK. Effects of alcohol reduction on blood pressure: a meta-analysis of randomized controlled trials. *Hypertension* 2001;**38**:1112–17.

34. Stamler R, Stamler J, Gosch FC *et al.* Primary prevention of hypertension by nutritional-hygienic means: final report of a randomized, controlled trial. *JAMA* 1989;**262**:1801–7.

35. SHEP Cooperative Research Group. Prevention of stroke by antihypertensive drug treatment in older persons with isolated systolic hypertension: final results of the Systolic Hypertension in the Elderly Program (SHEP). *JAMA* 1991;**265**:3255–64.

36. Psaty BM, Smith NS, Siscovick DS *et al*. Health outcomes associated with antihypertensive therapies used as first-line agents: a systematic review and meta-analysis. *JAMA* 1997;**277**:739–45.

37. Siscovick DS, Raghunathan TE, Psaty BM *et al*. Diuretic therapy for hypertension and the risk of primary cardiac arrest. *N Engl J Med* 1994;**330**:1852–7.

38. Psaty BM, Koepsell TD, Wagner EH *et al*. The relative risk of incident coronary heart disease associated with recently stopping the use of beta-blockers. *JAMA* 1990;**263**:1653–7.

39. Topol EJ, Califf RM, van de Werf F *et al*. Perspectives on large-scale cardiovascular clinical trials for the new millennium. *Circulation* 1997;**95**:1072–82.

40. Furberg CD, Psaty BM, Pahor M, Alderman MH. Clinical implications of recent findings from the Antihypertensive and Lipid-Lowering Treatment to Prevent Heart Attack Trial (ALLHAT) and other studies of hypertension. *Ann Intern Med* 2001;**135**:1074–8.

41. Psaty BM, Lumley T, Furberg CD *et al*. Health outcomes associated with antihypertensive therapies used as first-line agents: a network meta-analysis. *JAMA* 2003;**289**:2534–44.

42. Staessen JA, Fagard R, Thijs L *et al*, for the Systolic Hypertension – Europe (Syst-Eur) Trial Investigators. Randomised double-blind comparison of placebo and active treatment for older patients with systolic hypertension. *Lancet* 1997;**350**:757–64.

43. Lewis EL, Hunsicker LG, Clarke WR *et al*. Renoprotective effect of the angiotensin-receptor antagonist irbesartan in patients with nephropathy due to type 2 diabetes. *N Engl J Med* 2001;**345**:851–60.

44. Brenner BM, Cooper ME, Zeeuw DD *et al*. Effects of losartan on renal and cardiovascular outcomes in patients with type 2 diabetes and nephropathy. *N Engl J Med* 2001;**345**:861–9.

45. PROGRESS Collaborative Group. Randomised trial of a perindopril-based blood-pressure-lowering regimen among 6105 individuals with previous stroke or transient ischemic attack. *Lancet* 2001;**358**:1033–41.

46. Davis BR, Cutler JA, Gordon DJ *et al*. Rationale and design for the Antihypertensive and Lipid Lowering Treatment to Prevent Heart Attack Trial (ALLHAT). *Am J Hypertens* 1996;**9**:342–60.

47. ALLHAT Officers and Coordinators for the ALLHAT Collaborative Research Group. Major cardiovascular events in hypertensive patients randomized to doxazosin vs chlorthalidone. The Antihypertensive and Lipid-Lowering Treatment to Prevent Heart Attack Trial (ALLHAT). *JAMA* 2000;**283**:1967–75.

48. ALLHAT Officers and Coordinators for the ALLHAT Collaborative Research Group. Major outcomes in high-risk hypertension patients randomized to angiotensin-converting enzyme inhibitor or calcium channel blocker vs diuretic: the ALLHAT trial. *JAMA* 2002;**288**:2981–97.

49. Psaty BM, Furberg CD. Meta-analysis of health outcomes of chlorthalidone-based vs nonchlorthalidone-based low-dose diuretic therapies. *JAMA* 2004;**292**:43–4.

50. Messerli FH, Beevers DG, Franklin SS, Pickering TG. Beta-blockers in hypertension – the emperor has no clothes: an open letter to present and prospective drafters of new guidelines for the treatment of hypertension. *Am J Hypertens* 2003;**16**:870–3.

51. Carlberg B, Samuelsson O, Lindholm LH. Atenolol in hypertension: is it a wise choice? *Lancet* 2004;**364**:1684–9.

52. Lindholm LH, Carlberg H, Samuelsson O. Should beta-blockers remain first choice in the treatment of primary hypertension? A meta-analysis. *Lancet* 2005;**366**:1545–53.

53. Pahor M, Psaty BM, Alderman MH *et al*. Health outcomes associated with calcium antagonists compared with other first-line antihypertensive therapies: a meta-analysis of randomized controlled trials. *Lancet* 2000;**356**:1949–540.

54. Blood Pressure Lowering Treatment Trialists' Collaboration. Effects of angiotensin-converting-enzyme inhibitors, calcium antagonists, and other blood-pressure-lowering drugs: results of prospectively designed overviews of randomized trials. *Lancet* 2000;**356**:1955–64.

55. Pahor M, Psaty BM, Alderman MH *et al*. Blood pressure-lowering treatment. *Lancet* 2001;**358**:152–3.

56. Pahor M, Psaty BM, Alderman MH *et al*. Therapeutic benefits of ACE inhibitors and other antihypertensive drugs in patients with type 2 diabetes. *Diabetes Care* 2000;**23**:888–92.

57. Lindholm LH, Hansson L, Ekbom T *et al*, for the STOP Hypertension-2 Study Group. Comparison of antihypertensive treatments in preventing cardiovascular events in elderly diabetic patients: results from the Swedish Trial in Old Patients with Hypertension-2. *J Hypertens* 2000;**18**:1671–6.

58. Agodoa LY, Appel L, Bakris GL *et al*. Effect of ramipril vs amlodipine on renal outcomes in hypertensive nephrosclerosis. A randomized controlled trial. *JAMA* 2001;**285**:2719–28.

59. Lindholm LH, Ibsen H, Dahlöf B *et al*. Cardiovascular morbidity and mortality in patients with diabetes in the Losartan Intervention For Endpoint reduction in hypertension study (LIFE): a randomized trial against atenolol. *Lancet* 2002;**359**:1004–10.

60. Julius S, Kjeldsen S, Weber M *et al*, for the VALUE trial group. Outcomes in hypertensive patients at high cardiovascular risk treated with regimens based on valsartan or amlodipine: the VALUE randomized trial. *Lancet* 2004;**363**:2022–31.

61. Dahlöf B, Sever P, Poulter N *et al*, for the ASCOT Investigators. Prevention of cardiovascular events with an antihypertensive regimen of amlodipine adding perindopril as required versus atenolol adding bendroflumethiazide as required, in the Anglo-Scandinavian Cardiac Outcomes Trial-Blood Pressure Lowering Arm (ASCOT-BPLA): a multicentre randomized controlled trial. *Lancet* 2005;**366**:895–906.

62. Jamerson K, Weber AW, Bakris GL *et al*. Benazepril plus amlodipine or hydrochlorothiazide for hypertension in high-risk patients. *N Engl J Med* 2008;**359**:2417–28.

63. Pratt-Ubunama MN, Nishizaka MK, Calhoun DA. Aldosterone antagonism: an emerging strategy for effective blood pressure lowering. *Curr Hypertens Rep* 2005;**7**:186–92.

64. Palazzuoli A, Calabria P, Verzuri MS *et al*. Carvedilol: something else than a simple beta-blocker? *Eur Rev Med Pharmacol Sci* 2002;**6**:115–26.

65. Sealey J, Laragh J. Aliskiren, the first renin inhibitor for treating hypertension: reactive renin secretion may limit its effectiveness. *Am J Hypertens* 2007;**20**:587–97.

66. Iqbal J, Sanghi R, Das SK. Endothelin receptor antagonists: an overview of their synthesis and structure activity relationship. *Mini Rev Med Chem* 2005;**5**:381–408.

67. Worthley MI, Corti R, Worthley SG. Vasopeptidase inhibitors: will they have a role in clinical practice? *Br J Clin Pharmacol* 2004;**57**:27–36.

68. North KE, Rose KM, Borecki IB *et al.* Evidence for a gene on chromosome 13 influencing postural systolic blood pressure change and body mass index. *Hypertension* 2004;**43**:780–84.

69. Caulfield M, Munroe P, Pembroke J *et al.* MRC British Genetics of Hypertension Study. Genome-wide mapping of human loci for essential hypertension. *Lancet* 2003;**361**:2118–23.

70. Benjafield AV, Wang WY, Speirs HJ *et al.* Genome wide scan for hypertension in Sydney sibships: the GENIHUSS Study. *Am J Hypertens* 2005;**18**:828–32.

71. Tabara Y, Kohara K, Nakura J *et al.* Hunting for hypertension genes: the National Millennium Project of Japan. *Am J Hypertens* 2005;**18**:262A.

72. Nannipieri M, Manganiello M, Pezzatini A *et al.* Polymorphisms in the hANP (human atrial natriuretic peptide) gene, albuminuria, and hypertension. *Hypertension* 2001;**37**:1416–22.

73. Persu A, Coscoy S, Houot AM *et al.* Polymorphisms of the [gamma] subunit of the epithelial Na+ channel in essential hypertension. *J Hypertens* 1999;**17**:639–45.

74. Bianchi G, Ferrari P, Staessen JA. Adducin polymorphism: detection and impact on hypertension and related disorders. *Hypertension* 2005;**45**:331–40.

75. Masuo K, Katsuya T, Fu Y *et al.* b2- and b3-adrenergic receptor polymorphisms are related to the onset of weight gain and blood pressure elevation over 5 years. *Circulation* 2005;**111**:3429–34.

76. Lancxa V, Alcantara P, Nogueira JB *et al.* The cytochrome P4501A1 T6325C polymorphism is associated with the risk of hypertension. *Am J Hypertens* 2005;**18**:110A.

77. Ho H, Pinto A, Hall SD *et al.* Association between the CYP3A5 genotype and blood pressure. *Hypertension* 2005;**45**:294–8.

78. Arnett DK, Davis BR, Ford CE *et al.* Pharmacogenetic association of the angiotensin-converting enzyme insertion/deletion polymorphism on blood pressure and cardiovascular risk in relation to antihypertensive treatment (GenHAT) Study. *Circulation* 2005;**111**:3374–83.

79. Fu Y, Katsuya T, Matsuo A *et al.* Relationship of bradykinin B2 receptor gene polymorphism with essential hypertension and left ventricular hypertrophy. *Hypertens Res* 2004;**27**:933–8.

80. Connell JM, Fraser R, MacKenzie SM *et al.* The impact of polymorphisms in the gene encoding aldosterone synthase (CYP11B2) on steroid synthesis and blood pressure regulation. *Mol Cell Endocrinol* 2004;**217**:243–7.

81. Yang W, Huang J, Ge D *et al.* Lipoprotein lipase gene is in linkage with blood pressure phenotypes in Chinese pedigrees. *Hum Genet* 2004;**115**:8–12.

82. Jin JJ, Nakura J,Wu Z *et al.* Association of angiotensin II type 2 receptor gene variant with hypertension. *Hypertens Res* 2003;**26**:547–52.

83. Sharma P, Hingorani A, Jia H *et al.* Quantitative association between a newly identified molecular variant in the endothelin-2 gene and human essential hypertension. *J Hypertens* 1999;**17**:1281–7.

84. Sharma P, Hingorani A, Jia H *et al.* Positive association of tyrosine hydroxylase microsatellite marker to essential hypertension. *Hypertension* 1998;**32**:676–82.

85. Jia H, Hingorani AD, Sharma P *et al.* Association of the G(s)alpha gene with essential hypertension and response to beta-blockade. *Hypertension* 1999;**34**:8–14.

86. Corvol P, Persu A, Gimenez-Roqueplo AP, Jeunemaitre X. Seven lessons from two candidate genes in human essential hypertension: angiotensinogen and epithelial sodium channel. *Hypertension* 1999;**33**:1324–31.

87. Swift PA, MacGregor GA. The epithelial sodium channel in hypertension: genetic heterogeneity and implications for treatment with amiloride. *Am J Pharmacogenomics* 2004;**4**:161–8.

88. Sookoian S, Castano G, Garcia SI *et al.* A1166C angiotensin II type 1 receptor gene polymorphism may predict homodynamic response to losartan in patients with cirrhosis and portal hypertension. *Am J Gastroenterol* 2005;**100**:636–4.

89. Hingorani AD, Jia H, Stevens PA *et al.* Renin angiotensin system gene polymorphisms influence blood pressure and the response to angiotensin converting enzyme inhibition. *J Hypertens* 1995;**13**:1602–9.

90. Kurland L, Liljedahl U, Karlsson J *et al.* Angiotensinogen gene polymorphisms: relationship to blood pressure response to antihypertensive treatment: results from the Swedish Irbesartan Left Ventricular Hypertrophy Investigation vs Atenolol (SILVHIA) Trial. *Am J Hypertens* 2004;**17**:8–13.

91. Brown MJ, Coltart J, Gunewardena K *et al.* Randomized double-blind placebo-controlled study of an angiotensin immunotherapeutic vaccine (PMD3117) in hypertensive subjects. *Clin Sci* 2004;**107**:167–73.

92. Kearney PM, Whelton M, Reynolds K, Muntner P, Whelton PK, He J. Global burden of hypertension: analysis of worldwide data. *Lancet* 2005;**365**:217–23.

14 Dysglycemia and the risk of cardiovascular events

Hertzel C Gerstein and Zubin Punthakee
McMaster University, Hamilton, Ontario, Canada

Introduction

Diabetes mellitus (DM) is diagnosed when plasma glucose levels rise above predefined thresholds. People diagnosed with DM have a high future risk of serious health consequences including cardiovascular events. Indeed, they develop cardiovascular disease approximately 15 years earlier than their non-diabetic counterparts[1] and have a cardiovascular risk up to fourfold higher than in people without DM.[1-4] The magnitude of this increased risk is progressively related to the degree of glucose elevation above normal. Moreover, this relationship is not restricted to people with DM and there is growing recognition that a progressive relationship exists between glucose levels and cardiovascular risk that begins at glucose levels well below the diagnostic thresholds for DM and that extends right into the diabetic range.[5] Thus, like low-density lipoprotein (LDL) cholesterol or systolic blood pressure, glycemia, as measured by fasting glucose level, postload glucose levels or HbA1c levels, is a progressive cardiovascular risk factor. Whether glucose lowering or prevention of the rise in glucose levels with time can reduce cardiovascular risk in people with various degrees of glucose elevation (i.e. impaired glucose tolerance, impaired fasting glucose, newly detected DM or established diabetes) is currently being actively studied.

What is diabetes and how common is it?

Diagnosis and classification

DM is a common chronic condition that is defined on the basis of high glucose levels, and that is an independent risk factor for a growing list of serious diseases including, but not limited to, blindness, renal failure, amputations, claudication, stroke, myocardial infarction, and premature death. It is diagnosed when there is evidence of persistently elevated glucose levels that are above specific thresholds or cutpoints (Table 14.1).[6] These thresholds were originally based on epidemiologic studies relating the risk of diabetic eye disease to the glucose level achieved two hours after drinking a 75 g oral glucose tolerance load.[7] People with higher levels were at high risk of diabetic retinopathy and nephropathy, whereas those with levels below this threshold were at low risk for these health consequences.[8,9]

Recent data have confirmed the general relevance of these thresholds for eye disease, and have shown that people with glucose levels below these thresholds have a lower (but not negligible) incidence of retinopathy.[10,11] More importantly, they have also highlighted the fact that these thresholds are not relevant to many of the other chronic consequences of DM that are listed in Table 14.2. Thus, as noted below, the risk of cardiovascular disease is progressively related to glucose levels extending from normal levels right into the DM range.

When the diagnostic thresholds for DM were established it was clear that many people had glucose levels that fell below the diabetic threshold but that were nevertheless still abnormal and could rise into the DM range with time. This led to the classification of impaired glucose tolerance (IGT) and impaired fasting glucose (IFG) which identified people at low risk for diabetic retinopathy and nephropathy but at very high risk for developing DM.[9] Table 14.1 summarizes the current diagnostic thresholds for IGT and IFG (sometimes referred to as "prediabetes") and Table 14.3 lists the relative risk and incidence of DM in people with these two dysglycemic states.[12] Of note, the American Diabetes Association has adopted lower thresholds for impaired fasting glucose (i.e. 5.6 mmol/L) to optimize its sensitivity and specificity for predicting future DM;[13] however, this lower threshold has not been adopted globally.[14]

Evidence-Based Cardiology, 3rd edition. Edited by S. Yusuf, J.A. Cairns, A.J. Camm, E.L. Fallen, and B.J. Gersh. © 2010 Blackwell Publishing, ISBN: 978-1-4051-5925-8.

Table 14.1 Diagnostic thresholds for diabetes, impaired glucose tolerance, and impaired fasting glucose

Classification	Random plasma glucose	Fasting plasma glucose	Two-hour postload plasma glucose[a]
Diabetes mellitus	≥11.1 mmol/L + classic signs & symptoms of hyperglycemia[b]	≥7.0 mmol /L[b]	≥11.1 mmol/L[b]
Impaired glucose tolerance	N/A	<7.0 mmol/L	≥7.8 and <11.1 mmol/L
Impaired fasting glucose (WHO)	N/A	≥6.1 and <7.0 mmol/L	N/A
Impaired fasting glucose (ADA)	N/A	≥5.6 and <7.0 mmol/L	N/A

WHO, World Health Organization; ADA, American Diabetes Association; [a]measured during a 75 g oral glucose tolerance test (OGTT); [b]must be confirmed on a subsequent day by any one of the three methods.

Table 14.2 Major chronic consequences of diabetes

Eye disease (cataracts, retinal disease)	Early death
Kidney disease (renal failure, nephropathy)	Ischemic heart disease
Nerve disease (sensory, motor)	Stroke
Foot disease (pain, ulceration, callus, infection)	Peripheral vascular disease
Lower limb amputation	Cognitive decline
Steatohepatitis and cirrhosis	Depression
Hip fractures	Connective tissue abnormalities
Imbalance and frailty	Erectile/sexual dysfunction

Table 14.3 Risk of diabetes and risk of death in "prediabetes"

Diagnostic category	Relative risk of future diabetes	Annual incidence of diabetes	Relative risk of death
Any impaired fasting glucose*	4.7 (2.5–6.9)	2–10%	1.2 (1.1–1.4)
Isolated impaired fasting glucose	7.5 (4.6–10.5)	2–10%	N/A
Impaired glucose tolerance	6.4 (4.9–7.8)	2–10%	1.3 (1.1–1.5)
Any impaired glucose tolerance	5.5 (3.1–7.9)	2–10%	N/A
Both impaired fasting glucose and impaired glucose tolerance	12.1 (4.3–20)	10–15%	N/A

Data are from a systematic overview and meta-analysis of prospective studies.[12]

*Defined as a fasting plasma glucose level ≥ 6.1 mmol/L (i.e. WHO criterion); N/A, not available.

Prevalence

The estimated prevalence of DM in 2003 was 5.1% of all adults in the world.[15] This prevalence has been rapidly rising and is currently reaching alarming proportions throughout much of the world. For example, in Ontario, Canada, the prevalence of DM rose from 5.2% of all adults in 1995 to 8.8% in 2005.[16] This prevalence rises with age, approaching 20% of all people over the age of 70 in Canada[16,17] and the USA.[18] It also varies with race and ethnicity, with the highest prevalence in people from aboriginal populations throughout the world, followed by those with South Asian, Middle Eastern, African and European ancestry.[15] In response to this epidemic, on December 20 2006 the United Nations formally recognized DM as a "chronic, debilitating and costly disease", which "poses severe risks for families, countries and the entire world" and encouraged countries "to develop national policies for the prevention, treatment and care of diabetes".

The prevalence of impaired glucose tolerance varies in a similar pattern; in most populations it is somewhat higher than the prevalence of diagnosed diabetes. Thus in 2003, the estimated prevalence of impaired glucose tolerance in the world was 8.2% of all adults.[15]

Etiology

DM emerges when an individual is unable to secrete sufficient pancreatic insulin to maintain normoglycemia in response to various glucose-raising stimuli (such as meals, stress, etc.) throughout the day. This may occur due to a number of causes.[19] Thus people with type 1 DM typically suffer from autoimmune damage to their beta cells and have minimal to absent insulin secretion. Conversely, people with type 2 DM or gestational DM may make abundant insulin; nevertheless, the absolute amount made is insufficient to maintain normal glucose homeostasis and to overcome whatever "insulin resistance" is present (due to obesity, inactivity or other factors). As insulin is the primary

Table 14.4 Etiologic classification of diabetes mellitus

Name	Characteristics	Etiology	Epidemiology
Type 1	Primarily due to pancreatic islet beta-cell destruction; prone to ketoacidosis	Autoimmune or idiopathic	~10% of people with diabetes; 0.2% of the general population
Type 2	Insufficient insulin secretion to compensate for resistance to insulin's effect	Strong familial component	~90% of people with diabetes; up to 10% of all adults
Gestational diabetes	Diabetes with onset or first recognition in pregnancy	Usually due to hormonal changes in pregnancy and usually resolves postpartum	~4% of pregnancies in the United States
Other specific types	Related to a genetic, congenital, pancreatic, endocrine, or infectious acquired disease, or drug induced	Examples include hemochromatosis, pancreatitis, hypercortisolemia	~2% of all patients with diabetes

Adapted from reference 6. Note that patients with any form of diabetes may require treatment with insulin at some stage of their disease. Use of insulin does not in itself classify the patient.

hormone that prevents hyperglycemia, by both inhibiting hepatic glucose production and facilitating glucose clearance by muscle, insufficient insulin quickly results in an elevated glucose level. The etiologic classification of DM and the associated characteristics and suspected causes of each type are listed in Table 14.4.

How much does dysglycemia increase cardiovascular risk?

Relative risk of cardiovascular disease with diabetes

People diagnosed with DM are two to four times more likely to suffer a cardiovascular (CV) event than people without a diagnosis of DM,[1–4] and people with DM develop cardiovascular disease approximately 15 years earlier than their non-diabetic counterparts.[1] Moreover, the relative risk is highest for young individuals, and is higher in women than in men. Thus, men and women aged 20–34 have a relative risk of myocardial infarction (MI) of 12 and 37.8 respectively, whereas by age 75 or older the risks are 1.86 and 2.41 respectively.[1] Figure 14.1 summarizes the incidence and risk of MI (Fig. 14.1a) and death (Fig. 14.1b) by sex and age group based on data from a population-based cohort of 9.4 million people (approximately 400 000 with diabetes) followed for six years from 1994 to 2000.[1] These findings are supported in a recent large meta-analysis of 37 prospective studies performed from 1966 to 2005, comprising 447 064 people followed for 4–36 years in five continents, which reported that compared to people without diabetes, the age-adjusted relative risk of fatal coronary heart disease was 3.69 and 2.16 in women and

men respectively; adjustment for other risk factors only modestly attenuated the risk to 3.12 and 1.99 respectively.[20] The fact that the high risk of cardiovascular disease in people with DM cannot be explained by the co-existence of other cardiovascular risk factors has focused attention on the factor that is pathognomonic of diabetes: the elevated glucose level.

Relationship of glycemia to cardiovascular disease in diabetes

Several prospective studies in people with DM have now clearly shown a graded relationship between HbA1c level and the incidence of cardiovascular outcomes. For example, the Wisconsin Epidemiologic Study of Diabetic Retinopathy followed a population-based sample of 1210 patients with DM presenting before the age of 30 and 1780 patients with DM presenting at or after the age of 30.[21] In both groups of subjects, 10-year mortality increased with the baseline glycated hemoglobin quartile. After controlling for other risk factors, a 1% increase in glycated hemoglobin was associated with a 10% (older onset subjects) to 18% (younger onset subjects) increase in the hazard of dying from ischemic heart disease. In an epidemiologic analysis of data from the United Kingdom Prospective Diabetes Study, a 1% higher HbA1c was associated with a 14% higher risk of death, a 14% higher risk of myocardial infarction and a 12% higher risk of stroke.[22] In another analysis of 1626 people with DM in the United States, a 1% higher HbA1c was associated with a 14% higher risk of myocardial infarction, fatal coronary heart disease or revascularization.[23] Finally, the best estimate of this relationship was reported in a recent meta-analysis of 10 prospective studies in which a 1% higher HbA1c was associated with an 18%

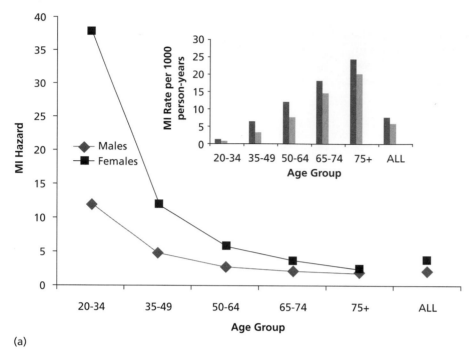

(a)

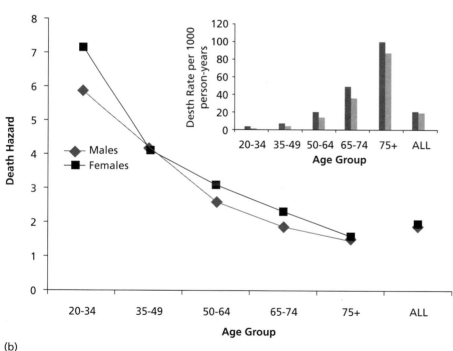

(b)

Figure 14.1 Myocardial infarction (MI) and death in men and women with diabetes. The hazard and rates (insert) of MI and death in men and women with diabetes in Ontario, Canada, between 1994 and 2000 by age range is shown in panels A and B respectively.[1] Data are from the cited article.

higher risk of coronary heart disease or stroke in people with type 2 diabetes; a similar relationship was noted in studies of people with type 1 DM.[24]

Relationship of glycemia to cardiovascular disease regardless of diabetes status

As noted above, prospective studies have consistently showed that the relationship between glucose levels and the subsequent risk of cardiovascular disease extends well below the diabetic threshold. For fasting glucose levels, a prospective 14-year study of 3458 non-diabetic men and women aged 40–70 with a fasting plasma glucose <7.8 mmol/L (140 mg/dL) reported that the age-adjusted ischemic heart disease mortality rates approximately doubled in men as the fasting glucose rose from 5 to 7 mmol/L (90–126 mg/dL), and tripled in women as the fasting glucose rose from 6 to 7.2 mmol/L (108–130 mg/

dL).[25] For postload glucose levels, a 10-year follow-up of 18050 non-diabetic male civil servants revealed up to a twofold increase in coronary heart disease and stroke mortality in subjects whose two hour postload capillary glucose value was greater than 5.4 mmol/L (97 mg/dL) compared to those with lower glucose levels; this increase was independent of age, smoking, blood pressure, cholesterol, and occupation.[26,27] Moreover, over a 33-year period, participants in this study had a 12% higher risk of coronary heart disease death per 1 mmol/L (18 mg/dL) higher two-hour glucose level (above 4.6 mmol/L or 83 mg/dL) after adjusting for several other cardiovascular risk factors.[28] Other cohort studies also subsequently showed a relationship between cardiovascular events and both fasting and postload glucose levels.[29]

In a 1998 systematic overview and meta-analysis of published cohort studies describing more than 1 million person-years of follow-up of mainly non-diabetic populations, the risk of cardiovascular disease increased continuously with fasting and postload glucose levels above 4.2 mmol/L (75 mg/dL).[30] In a more recent meta-analysis of several large prospective studies comprising more than 1 million person-years of follow-up of people with and without diabetes, a 1 mmol/L higher fasting glucose level was associated with a 20% higher risk of various cardiovascular outcomes.[31]

Prospective studies have also demonstrated a relationship between HbA1c and cardiovascular outcomes regardless of DM status. Thus, in a nine-year prospective study of 1326 people with no history of diabetes, the risk of myocardial infarction, fatal coronary heart disease or revascularization rose 68% per 1% point increase in the absolute HbA1c level, after accounting for other cardiovascular risk factors.[23] Moreover, in a six-year prospective study of 10232 people (243 with established diabetes) the age-adjusted risk of a cardiovascular disease event rose 30% per 1% point increase of HbA1c and 20% per 1% point increase of HbA1c after adjustment for many other risk factors.[32] These studies also suggest that the relationship between glucose and cardiovascular disease may be more marked in the prediabetes or early DM range than it is in people with established diabetes.

Therefore, glucose appears to be a continuous cardiovascular risk factor, similar to cholesterol or blood pressure in its dose–response relationship,[33,34] and dysglycemia rather than DM *per se* has been used to best capture this concept.[35,36] Thus people with dysglycemia alone are at risk for cardiovascular disease, people with dysglycemia and impaired glucose tolerance (IGT) are at higher risk for cardiovascular disease as well as DM, and people with DM are at even higher risk for cardiovascular disease as well as eye, kidney, and nerve disease (Fig. 14.2).

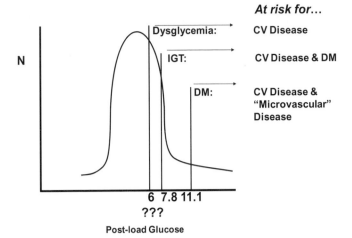

Figure 14.2 Frequency distribution of glucose levels in the general population. The significance of glucose as a risk factor for chronic disease depends on the level. Glucose levels above the diabetic threshold are associated with an increasing risk of cardiovascular and microvascular (e.g. retinal) disease, levels above the IGT threshold are associated with an increasing risk of diabetes, and elevated levels above some as yet undefined "dysglycemic" threshold are associated with an increasing risk of cardiovascular disease. CV, cardiovascular; DM, diabetes mellitus; IGT, impaired glucose tolerance.

Explanation of the dysglycemia–cardiovascular disease connection

Possible explanations for a glucose–cardiovascular disease relationship have been reviewed[5] and are summarized in Figure 14.3. They include:
- direct toxic effects of glucose
- decreased insulin effect due to reduced insulin secretion, reduced insulin action (i.e. insulin resistance)
- a genetic and/or environmental abnormality that predisposes individuals to both DM and cardiovascular disease; and
- a combination of these abnormalities.

Direct toxic effect of glucose

Glycation of a variety of proteins may directly promote cardiovascular disease.[37] Glycated albumin promotes albuminuria and endothelial cell dysfunction; glycated red cell membranes are less deformable; glycated LDL apoproteins are more susceptible than non-glycated LDL to uptake by scavenger cells (which would increase foam cell formation), oxidation, and increased platelet aggregation; glycated high-density lipoprotein (HDL) is less able to transport cholesterol; and glycated fibrin and platelet membranes adversely affect vascular homeostasis. Advanced glycation endproducts (AGE) also accumulate on vessel walls and in the vessel matrix, and may

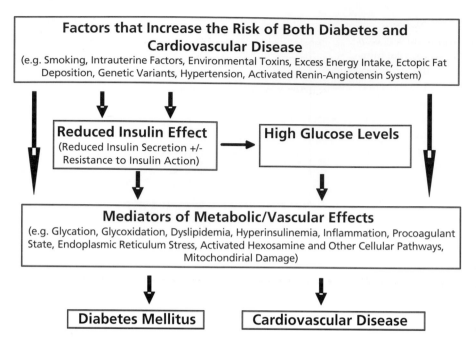

Figure 14.3 Possible explanations for the relationship between dysglycemia and cardiovascular disease. Insufficient insulin effect due to either reduced secretion, increased resistance or both leads to an elevated glucose level. Both the elevated glucose level and the reduced insulin effect may promote a variety of processes that in turn lead to both diabetes and cardiovascular disease. Antecedent factors may promote both diabetes and cardiovascular disease directly and/or by reducing insulin secretion or action, thereby increasing glucose levels.

adversely affect endothelial cell function and promote atherosclerosis.[38,39]

Glucose metabolism may also promote cellular damage. Excess glucose entry into cells may activate at least four different pathways implicated in atherosclerosis:[40,41]

• the polyol pathway, which depletes reduced glutathione (an intracellular antioxidant) and increases oxidative stress
• the hexosamine pathway, which promotes glycation of various intracelullar proteins, transcription of proinflammatory and prothrombotic signals, endoplasmic reticulum stress and apoptosis[42–48]
• the glyceraldehyde-3-phosphate pathway which increases protein kinase C and reactive oxygen species, and which increases formation of advanced glycation endproducts
• mitochondrial production of reactive oxygen species which may damage mitochondrial or cellular DNA.[41,47,49]

Decreased insulin effect

Glucose is the major stimulus for insulin secretion, which in turn prevents rises in glucose levels. Therefore an elevated glucose level implies a lack of sufficient insulin to maintain normoglycemia. Such a lack of *sufficient* insulin may occur in the presence of both low and high absolute levels of insulin, depending on the degree of insulin resistance. Indeed, the observation that apparently "normoglycemic" people with insulin resistance have slight glucose elevation[50] suggests that "insulin resistance" may represent a state of insufficient insulin effect, with hyperinsulinemia representing the pancreas' (unsuccessful) efforts at compensating for the reduced insulin effect. Such a possibility

may account for the association between hyperinsulinemia and markers of cardiovascular disease.[51,52] A number of observations support the possibility that insufficient (and not excess) insulin may be related to cardiovascular disease.

Patients with both type 1 DM (with no endogenous insulin secretion) and type 2 DM (who are not able to make sufficient insulin to maintain normoglycemia) are at high risk for cardiovascular disease.

Patients with cardiovascular disease have increased levels of proinsulin and split products[53,54] – a biochemical marker of a failing beta cell.

Insulin inhibits lipolysis and the lipolytic effect of stress hormones such as cortisol and catecholamines. Insufficient insulin effect therefore promotes free fatty acid flux which:

• reduces the effect of insulin at target tissues[55]
• promotes ectopic fat deposition in beta cells (which may damage them, further reducing insulin secretion)[56]
• promotes the synthesis of atherogenic lipoproteins[55,56]
• inhibit glycolysis and anaerobic ATP production in ischemic cardiac muscle.[57]

Insulin has anti-inflammatory properties[58] and reduces PAI-1 levels; therefore insulin insufficiency may promote inflammation and arterial thrombosis, thereby leading to atherosclerosis. Insufficient insulin may reduce ischemic preconditioning in heart muscle.[59] Insulin promotes endothelial nitric oxide synthesis and vasodilation, especially in response to ischemia[59]; insufficient insulin may therefore inhibit these effects.

Patients with insulinomas who are insulin resistant, hyperinsulinemic, and *hypoglycemic* have normal lipid profiles and blood pressure, and no clinical evidence of cardiovascular disease.[60] Studies of intensified insulin therapy in patients with type 1 DM taking multiple daily doses of insulin suggest a reduced and not an increased risk for cardiovascular events.[61]

Association with other risk factors

Both hyperglycemia and cardiovascular disease are associated with hypertension, smoking, excess energy intake, visceral/ectopic fat deposition, genetic variants, poor socioeconomic status, low birth weight, and intrauterine factors (see Fig. 14.3). As such, the observed association between dysglycemia and cardiovascular disease may be caused by one or more of these "proximal" risk factors or some other common antecedent such as an unrecognized environmental toxin. If true, these factors may directly cause both cardiovascular disease and DM and the association between dysglycemia and cardiovascular disease may be due to confounding with one or more of these proximal factors.[5]

All of the above

The most likely explanation for the link between dysglycemia and cardiovascular disease is some combination of the factors described above, that may together magnify each one's incremental effects.

Does glucose lowering reduce cardiovascular outcomes?

Glucose-lowering trials in people with diabetes

As of June 2008, several randomized controlled trials of intensive versus standard glucose lowering approaches have been completed in people with type 1 DM (in which different insulin regimens were used to lower glucose levels) and people with type 2 DM (in which different regimens of oral agents and/or insulin were used to lower glucose levels).

In **type 1** diabetes, the Diabetes Control and Complications Trial in 1441 relatively young people (mean age 27 years) studied the effect of an initial 6.5-year period of intensive insulin therapy targeting normoglycemia (which achieved a HbA1c of 7.4%) versus conventional insulin therapy (which achieved a HbA1c of 9.1%). No clear cardiovascular effect was detected at the end of the active treatment phase of the trial. Following this phase, 97% of the 1441 participants were followed passively for a further 11 years until at least 50 participants in the group originally allocated to standard therapy had a predefined cardiovascular outcome. During that time the HbA1c level in both groups was similar; nevertheless, by the end of passive

follow-up people who were allocated to the intensive group experienced a 42% (95% confidence interval (CI) 9–63%) reduction in a predefined cardiovascular composite outcome and a 57% (95% CI 12–79%) reduction in the first occurrence of non-fatal myocardial infarction, stroke or cardiovascular death.[61] Of note, adjustment for the 2% HbA1c difference between groups achieved in the active phase of the trial rendered the cardiovascular outcome difference non-significant. This suggests that the cardiovascular difference may be explained by the achieved HbA1c difference and strongly suggests that intensified insulin therapy targeting normoglycemia for at least six years reduces cardiovascular events in people with type 1 diabetes.

Several studies have now reported the effect of glucose-lowering in people with **type 2** diabetes. These studies include:
- the United Kingdom Prospective Diabetes Study (UKPDS) which recruited 3867 people with newly diagnosed DM at low cardiovascular risk and which tested the effect of intensive versus conventional glucose control starting with insulin, sulfonylurea or (in obese participants) metformin[62]
- the Action in Diabetes and Vascular Disease (ADVANCE) trial of 11 140 people with established DM (mean duration eight years) and high cardiovascular risk[63]
- the Veterans Administration Diabetes Trial (VADT) of 1791 people (mainly men) with established DM and high cardiovascular risk[64] (final report not published)
- the Action to Control Cardiovascular Risk in Diabetes (ACCORD) trial of 10 251 people with established DM (mean duration 10 years) and high cardiovascular risk[65]
- the Prospective Pioglitazone Clinical Trial in Macrovascular Events (PROACTIVE) study[66] which tested the effect of pioglitazone versus placebo in 5238 people with established DM (mean duration eight years) and high cardiovascular risk.

Table 14.5 lists the key characteristics and findings of these trials. These findings support several conclusions. First, they are consistent with the hypothesis that a glucose-lowering intervention may reduce cardiovascular outcomes in people with type 2 diabetes. The myocardial infarction trends favoring a 14% reduced risk in the UKPDS during 10 years of follow-up,[67] a 17% reduced risk in PROACTIVE during 2.9 years of follow-up[68] and the 24% reduction in ACCORD during 3.5 years of follow-up[65] all favor this possibility. This is also supported by the trends favoring a reduced risk of the composite cardiovascular outcomes in PROACTIVE, ACCORD, ADVANCE, and VADT. Unfortunately, the low cardiovascular event rate in the UKPDS (which recruited patients at low risk for cardiovascular events), the short follow-up of PROACTIVE, the truncated follow-up of the ACCORD study (due to the mortality signal discussed below), and the low power of the VADT study (due to overestimation of the event rate prior to

Table 14.5 Cardiovascular events and mortality in large outcome trials of glucose-lowering therapies

Study	N	Participants	Study duration	Median HbA1c contrast	Therapy tested	Relative risk reduction (95% CI)		
						MI	Primary CV outcome	Mortality
UKPDS[67,76]	3867	New DM	10 yrs	From 7.1% → 7.0% vs. 7.9%	Insulin or SU	16% (0, 29)	N/A	6% (−10, 20)
	753	Obese, new DM	10.7 yrs	From 7.2% → 7.4% vs. 8.0%	Metformin	39% (11, 59)	N/A	36% (9, 35)
PROACTIVE[68]	5238	DM [mult] 8 yrs High CV risk	2.9 yrs	From 7.9% → 6.9% vs. 7.5%	Pioglitazone	17% (−6, 35)	10% (−1, 20)	4% (−18, 22)
ACCORD[65]	10251	DM [mult] 10 yrs High CV risk	3.5 yrs	From 8.1% → 6.4% vs. 7.5%	Multiple therapies	24% (8, 38)	10% (−4, 22)	−22% (−1, −46)
ADVANCE[63]	11140	DM [mult] 8 yrs High CV risk	5 yrs	From 7.2% → 6.4% vs. 7.0%	SU + multiple therapies	2% (−23, 22)	6% (−6, 16)	7% (−6, 17)
VADT (ADA Presentation)	1791	DM [mult] 11.5 yrs High CV risk	6.3 yrs	From 9.5% → 6.9% vs. 8.4%	Multiple therapies	N/A	13% (−4, 27)	N/A

UKPDS, United Kingdom Prospective Diabetes Study; ACCORD, Action to Control Cardiovascular Risk in Diabetes; ADVANCE, Action in Diabetes and Vascular Disease; ADA, American Diabetes Association; DM, diabetes mellitus; Dx, diagnosis; MI, myocardial infarction; CVD, cardiovascular disease; SU, sulfonylurea; N/A, not available.

starting the study) reduced the ability of the currently completed studies to detect a benefit, even if one truly exists.

Second, participants most likely to benefit from a glucose-lowering intervention may be those with better glycemic control. The UKPDS, which studied people with newly diagnosed diabetes, and the ACCORD trial, which reported a clear reduction in the cardiovascular composite outcome exceeding 20% in participants whose baseline HbA1c level was less than 8% (see Table 14.5), both support this possibility. Third, the fact that the glycemic intervention in the ACCORD trial was stopped early after the Data Safety and Monitoring Board noted an absolute excess mortality of 0.3% and a relative excess of 22% ($P = 0.04$) suggests that a therapeutic strategy that attempts to intensively lower glucose levels to non-diabetic levels may cause harm within the first 2.5–3 years. The fact that the differences in mortality are small and were not observed in the other trials suggests that they could be related to the intensity of the intervention or participant characteristics, could represent an early adverse event of intensive glucose control in "poorly controlled" patients that may or may not persist, or could even be a chance finding.

Glucose-lowering trials in people with impaired glucose tolerance or impaired fasting glucose

As noted above, there is a progressive relationship between glycemia and cardiovascular risk that extends from normal levels right into the DM range. Moreover, this relationship may be more profound for people without established DM than for people with DM.[23,32] The possibility that glucose-lowering therapies may reduce cardiovascular events in people with IGT or IFG (sometimes called "prediabetes") was suggested by an analysis of data from a trial of acarbose to prevent DM in people with IGT.[69] Such an effect has not been seen in other prevention studies to date[70–73] which generally recruited people at low risk for cardiovascular outcomes, were short term, and reported few cardiovascular events. However, the recent finding that DM prevention with rosiglitazone also reduced a predefined renal outcome (albuminuria or a fall in the estimated glomerular filtration rate) in people with impaired glucose tolerance or impaired fasting glucose[74] is consistent with this possibility in light of the strong link between renal and cardiovascular disease.

The effect of glucose lowering in people with impaired glucose tolerance is currently being tested within two ongoing trials: the Nateglinide and Valsartan in Impaired Glucose Tolerance Outcomes Research (NAVIGATOR) trial (using nateglinide) and the Acarbose Cardiovascular Evaluation (ACE) trial (using acarbose). This possibility is also being assessed in the Outcome Reduction with an Initial Glargine Intervention (ORIGIN) trial in which 18% of participants did not have established DM at the time of randomization.[75]

Key points

Taken together, the body of research reviewed above supports a number of cardiovascular conclusions.

- Intensified insulin therapy targeting normoglycemia that is started while young reduces cardiovascular outcomes in people with type 1 diabetes.
- Metformin may reduce cardiovascular outcomes and mortality in newly diagnosed people with type 2 diabetes; these observations need replication.
- The effect of other specific glucose-lowering drugs on cardiovascular outcomes remains unknown.
- In people who start with poor glucose levels, intensive glucose lowering for a period of approximately 3.5 years that is achieved with a menu of medications and lifestyle approaches: a) does not clearly reduce cardiovascular outcomes; b) may reduce cardiovascular outcomes in people with lower glucose levels or less severe cardiovascular disease; and c) increases mortality. The cardiovascular and mortality effects of intensive glucose lowering after a longer follow-up period of at least five years are unclear and need to be established.
- The cardiovascular benefits and risks of DM prevention or of therapies that prevent the rise of glucose levels with time in people with impaired fasting glucose, impaired glucose tolerance or DM remain unknown.

Conclusion

Dysglycemia is clearly an independent risk factor for cardiovascular disease and there are a number of direct and indirect biologic pathways linking elevated glucose levels to cardiovascular disease.

Similar to dyslipidemia, in which ongoing studies are continuing to show the therapeutic value of reducing even minimally elevated lipid levels, therapies that reduce elevated glucose levels may reduce the risk of cardiovascular disease. However, they may also cause harm. As with other therapies, both benefits and risks may apply to specific drugs and to specific subsets of individuals and need to be carefully characterized. The ongoing ORIGIN, NAVIGATOR and ACE studies are clarifying these benefits and risks in people with early dysglycemia and several other cardiovascular risk factors.

These and other studies with newer classes of glucose-lowering drugs may provide novel ways of preventing cardiovascular disease in a growing number of individuals with dysglycemia. Until they are completed, cardiovascular prevention needs to focus on applying proven preventive therapies including blood pressure lowering with a variety of drugs, statin use, smoking cessation, and ACE inhibitor use.

References

1. Booth GL, Kapral MK, Fung K, Tu JV. Relation between age and cardiovascular disease in men and women with diabetes compared with non-diabetic people: a population-based retrospective cohort study. *Lancet* 2006;**368**(9529):29–36.
2. Kannel WB, McGee DL. Diabetes and cardiovascular disease. The Framingham study. *JAMA* 1979;**241**(19):2035–8.
3. Stamler J, Vaccaro O, Neaton JD, Wentworth D. Diabetes, other risk factors, and 12-yr cardiovascular mortality for men screened in the Multiple Risk Factor Intervention Trial. *Diabetes Care* 1993;**16**:434–44.
4. Goldbourt U, Yaari S, Medalie JH. Factors predictive of long-term coronary heart disease mortality among 10059 male Israeli civil servants and municipal employees. A 23 year mortality follow-up in the Israeli Ischemic Heart Disease Study. *Cardiology* 1993;**82**:100–21.
5. Punthakee Z, Werstuck GH, Gerstein HC. Diabetes and cardiovascular disease: explaining the relationship. *Rev Cardiovasc Med* 2007;**8**(3):145–53.
6. American Diabetes Association. Diagnosis and classification of diabetes mellitus. *Diabetes Care* 2008;**31**(suppl 1):S55–60.
7. National Diabetes Data Group. Classification and diagnosis of diabetes mellitus and other categories of glucose intolerance. *Diabetes* 1979;**28**:1039–57.
8. Report of the Expert Committee on the diagnosis and classification of diabetes mellitus. *Diabetes Care* 2003;**26**(suppl 1):S5–20.
9. Report of the Expert Committee on the Diagnosis and Classification of Diabetes Mellitus. *Diabetes Care* 1997;**20**(7):1183–97.
10. Diabetes Prevention Program Research Group. The prevalence of retinopathy in impaired glucose tolerance and recent-onset diabetes in the Diabetes Prevention Program. *Diabet Med* 2007;**24**(2):137–44.
11. Wong TY, Liew G, Tapp RJ et al. Relation between fasting glucose and retinopathy for diagnosis of diabetes: three population-based cross-sectional studies. *Lancet* 2008;**371**(9614):736–43.
12. Gerstein HC, Santaguida P, Raina P et al. Annual incidence and relative risk of diabetes in people with various categories of dysglycemia: a systematic overview and meta-analysis of prospective studies. *Diabetes Res Clin Pract* 2007;**78**(3):305–12.
13. Genuth S, Alberti KG, Bennett P et al. Follow-up report on the diagnosis of diabetes mellitus. *Diabetes Care* 2003;**26**(11):3160–7.
14. Ryden L, Standl E, Bartnik M et al. Guidelines on diabetes, pre-diabetes, and cardiovascular diseases: executive summary. The Task Force on Diabetes and Cardiovascular Diseases of the European Society of Cardiology (ESC) and the European Association for the Study of Diabetes (EASD). *Eur Heart J* 2007;**28**(1):88–136.
15. Secree R, Shaw J, Zimmet P. Diabetes and impaired glucose tolerance: prevalence and projections. In: Allgot B, Gan D, King H et al, eds. *Diabetes Atlas*, 2nd edn. Brussels: International Diabetes Federation, 2003: 17–71.
16. Lipscombe LL, Hux JE. Trends in diabetes prevalence, incidence, and mortality in Ontario, Canada 1995–2005: a population-based study. *Lancet* 2007;**369**(9563):750–6.

17. Public Health Agency of Canada. *Diabetes in Canada: Highlights from the National Diabetes Surveillance System 2004–2005.* Ottawa: Public Health Agency of Canada, 2005.

18. Centers for Disease Control and Prevention. *Prevalence of Diagnosed Diabetes by Age, United States, 1980–2005.* Available at: www.cdc.gov/diabetes/statistics/prev/

19. American Diabetes Association. Diagnosis and classification of diabetes mellitus. *Diabetes Care* 2007;**30**(suppl 1):S42–7.

20. Huxley R, Barzi F, Woodward M. Excess risk of fatal coronary heart disease associated with diabetes in men and women: meta-analysis of 37 prospective cohort studies. *BMJ* 2006; **332**(7533):73–8.

21. Moss SE, Klein R, Klein BEK, Meuer SM. The association of glycemia and cause-specific mortality in a diabetic population. *Arch Intern Med* 1994;**154**:2473–9.

22. Stratton IM, Adler AI, Neil HA *et al.* Association of glycaemia with macrovascular and microvascular complications of type 2 diabetes (UKPDS 35): prospective observational study. *BMJ* 2000;**321**(7258):405–12.

23. Selvin E, Coresh J, Golden SH, Brancati FL, Folsom AR, Steffes MW. Glycemic control and coronary heart disease risk in persons with and without diabetes: the atherosclerosis risk in communities study. *Arch Intern Med* 2005;**165**(16):1910–16.

24. Selvin E, Marinopoulos S, Berkenblit G *et al.* Meta-analysis: glycosylated hemoglobin and cardiovascular disease in diabetes mellitus. *Ann Intern Med* 2004;**141**(6):421–31.

25. Scheidt-Nave C, Barrett-Connor E, Wingard DL, Cohn BA, Edelstein SL. Sex differences in fasting glycemia as a risk factor for ischemic heart disease death. *Am J Epidemiol* 1991;**133**(6): 565–76.

26. Fuller JH, Shipley MJ, Rose G, Jarrett RJ, Keen H. Coronary-heart-disease risk and impaired glucose tolerance. The Whitehall study. *Lancet* 1980;**8183**:1373–6.

27. Fuller JH, Shipley MJ, Rose G, Jarrett RJ, Keen H. Mortality from coronary heart disease and stroke in relation to degree of glycemia: the Whitehall study. *BMJ Clin Res Ed* 1983;**287**(6396): 867–70.

28. Brunner EJ, Shipley MJ, Witte DR, Fuller JH, Marmot MG. Relation between blood glucose and coronary mortality over 33 years in the Whitehall Study. *Diabetes Care* 2006;**29**(1):26–31.

29. DECODE Study Group EDEG. Is the current definition for diabetes relevant to mortality risk from all causes and cardiovascular and noncardiovascular diseases? *Diabetes Care* 2003;**26**(3):688–96.

30. Coutinho M, Gerstein HC, Wang Y, Yusuf S. The relationship between glucose and incident cardiovascular events. A metaregression analysis of published data from 20 studies of 95,783 individuals followed for 12.4 years. *Diabetes Care* 1999;**22**(2): 233–40.

31. Lawes CM, Parag V, Bennett DA *et al.* Blood glucose and risk of cardiovascular disease in the Asia Pacific region. *Diabetes Care* 2004;**27**(12):2836–42.

32. Khaw KT, Wareham N, Bingham S, Luben R, Welch A, Day N. Association of hemoglobin A1c with cardiovascular disease and mortality in adults: the European prospective investigation into cancer in Norfolk. *Ann Intern Med* 2004;**141**(6):413–20.

33. Neaton JD, Wentworth D, MRFIT Research Group. Serum cholesterol, blood pressure, cigarette smoking, and death from coronary heart disease. Overall findings and differences by age for 316,099 white men. *Arch Intern Med* 1992;**152**(1):56–64.

34. Meigs JB, Nathan DM, Wilson PW, Cupples LA, Singer DE. Metabolic risk factors worsen continuously across the spectrum of nondiabetic glucose tolerance. The Framingham Offspring Study. *Ann Intern Med* 1998;**128**(7):524–33.

35. Gerstein HC, Yusuf S. Dysglycaemia and risk of cardiovascular disease. *Lancet* 1996;**347**(9006):949–50.

36. Canadian Diabetes Association Clinical Practice Guidelines Expert Committee. Canadian Diabetes Association 2003 Clinical Practice Guidelines for the Prevention and Management of Diabetes in Canada. *Can J Diabetes* 2003;**23**(suppl 2):S1–S152.

37. Yan SF, Yan SD, Herold K, Ramsamy R, Schmidt AM. Receptor for advanced glycation end products and the cardiovascular complications of diabetes and beyond: lessons from AGEing. *Endocrinol Metab Clin North Am* 2006;**35**(3):511–24, viii.

38. Goldin A, Beckman JA, Schmidt AM, Creager MA. Advanced glycation end products: sparking the development of diabetic vascular injury. *Circulation* 2006;**114**(6):597–605.

39. Jandeleit-Dahm K, Cooper ME. The role of AGEs in cardiovascular disease. *Curr Pharm Des* 2008;**14**(10):979–86.

40. Brownlee M. Biochemistry and molecular cell biology of diabetic complications. *Nature* 2001;**414**(6865):813–20.

41. Brownlee M. The pathobiology of diabetic complications: a unifying mechanism. *Diabetes* 2005;**54**(6):1615–25.

42. Han I, Kudlow JE. Reduced O glycosylation of Sp1 is associated with increased proteasome susceptibility. *Mol Cell Biol* 1997; **17**(5):2550–8.

43. Han I, Oh ES, Kudlow JE. Responsiveness of the state of O-linked N-acetylglucosamine modification of nuclear pore protein p62 to the extracellular glucose concentration. *Biochem J* 2000;**350** Pt 1:109–14.

44. Du XL, Edelstein D, Dimmeler S, Ju Q, Sui C, Brownlee M. Hyperglycemia inhibits endothelial nitric oxide synthase activity by posttranslational modification at the Akt site. *J Clin Invest* 2001;**108**(9):13418.

45. Du XL, Edelstein D, Rossetti L *et al.* Hyperglycemia-induced mitochondrial superoxide overproduction activates the hexosamine pathway and induces plasminogen activator inhibitor-1 expression by increasing Sp1 glycosylation. *Proc Natl Acad Sci USA* 2000;**97**(22):12222–6.

46. Werstuck GH, Khan MI, Femia G *et al.* Glucosamine-induced endoplasmic reticulum dysfunction is associated with accelerated atherosclerosis in a hyperglycemic mouse model. *Diabetes* 2006;**55**(1):93–101.

47. Robertson RP, Harmon J, Tran PO, Tanaka Y, Takahashi H. Glucose toxicity in beta-cells: type 2 diabetes, good radicals gone bad, and the glutathione connection. *Diabetes* 2003;**52**(3): 581–7.

48. Robertson RP, Harmon J, Tran PO, Poitout V. Beta-cell glucose toxicity, lipotoxicity, and chronic oxidative stress in type 2 diabetes. *Diabetes* 2004;**53**(suppl 1):S119–S124.

49. Nishikawa T, Edelstein D, Du XL *et al.* Normalizing mitochondrial superoxide production blocks three pathways of hyperglycaemic damage. *Nature* 2000;**404**(6779):787–90.

50. Stumvoll M, Tataranni PA, Stefan N, Vozarova B, Bogardus C. Glucose allostasis. *Diabetes* 2003;**52**(4):903–9.

51. Fontbonne A, Charles MA, Thibult N *et al.* Hyperinsulinemia as a predictor of coronary heart disease mortality in a healthy

population: the Paris Prospective Study, 15 year follow-up. *Diabetologia* 1991;**34**(5):356–61.

52. Ruige JB, Assendelft WJ, Dekker JM, Kostense PJ, Heine RJ, Bouter LM. Insulin and risk of cardiovascular disease: a meta-analysis. *Circulation* 1998;**97**(10):996–1001.

53. Bavenholm P, Proudler A, Tornvall P *et al.* Insulin, intact and split proinsulin, and coronary artery disease in young men. *Circulation* 1995;**92**(6):1422–9.

54. Haffner SM, Mykkanen L, Valdez RA *et al.* Disproportionately increased proinsulin levels are associated with the insulin resistance syndrome. *J Clin Endocrinol Metab* 1994;**79**(6):1806–10.

55. Lewis GF, Carpentier A, Adeli K, Giacca A. Disordered fat storage and mobilization in the pathogenesis of insulin resistance and type 2 diabetes. *Endocrin Rev* 2002;**23**(2):201–29.

56. Dubois M, Kerr-Conte J, Gmyr V *et al.* Non-esterified fatty acids are deleterious for human pancreatic islet function at physiological glucose concentration. *Diabetologia* 2004;**47**(3):463–9.

57. Lopaschuk GD. Metabolic abnormalities in the diabetic heart. *Heart Fail Rev* 2002;**7**(2):149–59.

58. Hansen TK, Thiel S, Wouters PJ, Christiansen JS, van den Berghe G. Intensive insulin therapy exerts antiinflammatory effects in critically ill patients and counteracts the adverse effect of low mannose-binding lectin levels. *J Clin Endocrinol Metab* 2003;**88**(3):1082–8.

59. Das UN. Insulin: an endogenous cardioprotector. *Curr Opin Crit Care* 2003;**9**(5):375–83.

60. Leonetti F, Iozzo P, Giaccari A, Buongiorno A, Tamburrano G, Andreani D. Absence of clinically overt atherosclerotic vascular disease and adverse changes in cardiovascular risk factors in 70 patients with insulinoma. *J Endocrinol Invest* 1993;**16**(11):875–80.

61. Nathan DM, Cleary PA, Backlund JY *et al.* Intensive diabetes treatment and cardiovascular disease in patients with type 1 diabetes. *N Engl J Med* 2005;**353**(25):2643–53.

62. UK Prospective Diabetes Study (UKPDS) Group. Intensive blood-glucose control with sulphonylureas or insulin compared with conventional treatment and risk of complications in patients with type 2 diabetes (UKPDS 33). *Lancet* 1998;**352**(9131):837–53.

63. ADVANCE Collaborative Group. Intensive blood glucose control and vascular outcomes in patients with type 2 diabetes. *N Engl J Med* 2008;**358**(24):2560–72.

64. Abraira C, Duckworth W, McCarren M *et al.* Design of the cooperative study on glycemic control and complications in diabetes mellitus type 2: Veterans Affairs Diabetes Trial. *J Diabetes Complications* 2003;**17**(6):314–22.

65. Action to Control Cardiovascular Risk in Diabetes Study Group. Effects of intensive glucose lowering in type 2 diabetes. *N Engl J Med* 2008;**358**(24):2545–59.

66. Dormandy JA, Charbonnel B, Eckland DJ *et al.* Secondary prevention of macrovascular events in patients with type 2 diabetes in the PROactive Study (PROspective pioglitAzone Clinical Trial In macroVascular Events): a randomised controlled trial. *Lancet* 2005;**366**(9493):1279–89.

67. UK Prospective Diabetes Study (UKPDS) Group. Intensive blood-glucose control with sulphonylureas or insulin compared with conventional treatment and risk of complications in patients with type 2 diabetes (UKPDS 33). *Lancet* 1998;**352**:837–53.

68. Dormandy J, Charbonnel B, Eckland DJA *et al.* Secondary prevention of macrovascular events in patients with type 2 diabetes in the PROactive Study (PROspective pioglitAzone Clinical Trial In macroVascular Events): a randomised controlled trial. *Lancet* 2005;**366**:1279–89.

69. Chiasson JL, Josse RG, Gomis R, Hanefeld M, Karasik A, Laakso M. Acarbose treatment and the risk of cardiovascular disease and hypertension in patients with impaired glucose tolerance: the STOP-NIDDM trial. *JAMA* 2003;**290**(4):486–94.

70. Gerstein HC, Yusuf S, Bosch J *et al.* Effect of rosiglitazone on the frequency of diabetes in patients with impaired glucose tolerance or impaired fasting glucose: a randomised controlled trial. *Lancet* 2006;**368**(9541):1096–105.

71. Knowler WC, Barrett-Connor E, Fowler SE *et al.* Reduction in the incidence of type 2 diabetes with lifestyle intervention or metformin. *N Engl J Med* 2002;**346**(6):393–403.

72. Ratner R, Goldberg R, Haffner S *et al.* Impact of intensive lifestyle and metformin therapy on cardiovascular disease risk factors in the diabetes prevention program. *Diabetes Care* 2005;**28**(4):888–94.

73. Ramachandran A, Snehalatha C, Mary S, Mukesh B, Bhaskar AD, Vijay V. The Indian Diabetes Prevention Programme shows that lifestyle modification and metformin prevent type 2 diabetes in Asian Indian subjects with impaired glucose tolerance (IDPP-1). *Diabetologia* 2006;**49**(2):289–97.

74. Dagenais GR, Gerstein HC, Holman R *et al.* Effects of ramipril and rosiglitazone on cardiovascular and renal outcomes in people with impaired glucose tolerance or impaired fasting glucose: results of the Diabetes REduction Assessment with ramipril and rosiglitazone Medication (DREAM) trial. *Diabetes Care* 2008;**31**(5):1007–14.

75. Origin Trial Investigators, Gerstein H, Yusuf S, Riddle MC, Ryden L, Bosch J. Rationale, design, and baseline characteristics for a large international trial of cardiovascular disease prevention in people with dysglycemia: the ORIGIN Trial (Outcome Reduction with an Initial Glargine Intervention). *Am Heart J* 2008;**155**(1):26–32.

76. UK Prospective Diabetes Study (UKPDS) Group. Effect of intensive blood glucose control with metformin on complications in overweight patients with type 2 diabetes (UKPDS 34). *Lancet* 1998;**352**:854–65.

15 Physical activity and exercise in cardiovascular disease prevention and rehabilitation

Ray W Squires

Mayo Clinic College of Medicine, Rochester, MN, USA

Introduction

A sedentary lifestyle has been established as a major modifiable coronary risk factor by the American Heart Association.[1] Unfortunately, approximately 70% of adults in the United States are sedentary or underactive, and almost one-half of America's young people aged 12–21 years are not physically active on a regular basis.[2] The reasons for this observation are closely related to industrialization, automation, and the resultant decreased requirement for occupational, household, and leisure-time physical activity in the past several decades. The need to walk, climb stairs, perform energy-requiring tasks around the home or engage in physical activity in the workplace has dramatically decreased for the vast majority of people. In the 21st century, individuals must make a conscious choice to be physically active.

The definitions of *physical activity, exercise* and *cardiorespiratory fitness* are important to the understanding of this chapter. The 1996 National Institutes of Health Consensus Conference on Physical Activity and Cardiovascular Health defined *physical activity* as "bodily movement produced by skeletal muscles that requires energy expenditure and produces health benefits".[3] Physical activity is informal in nature and structure and includes everyday activities such as walking or bicycling or stair climbing for transportation, as well as household or yard tasks, occupational tasks and low-intensity sports such as golf. Physical activity occurs within the structure of the requirements of usual daily living. Recently, energy expenditure due to changes in posture and movement associated with the routines of daily life, termed non-exercise activity thermogenesis (NEAT), was compared in lean and obese subjects.[4] Lean subjects expended an average of 350 kilocalories more each day in NEAT than did obese subjects, underscoring the importance of physical activity in coronary risk.

Exercise, also called exercise training, was defined as "planned, structured, and repetitive bodily movement done to improve or maintain one or more components of physical fitness".[3] It is characterized by periodic formal workouts involving sustained moderate- to high-intensity effort. It usually involves specific clothing, such as footwear, and equipment, as is present in fitness facilities, but is not an absolutely necessary part of the daily routine. It may involve sporting activities, such as basketball, racquet sports or soccer (non-American football).

Cardiorespiratory fitness (peak exercise oxygen uptake) is defined as the capacity to take in and process oxygen for the production of energy via aerobic metabolism for physical activity or exercise. This component of physical fitness is most closely associated with coronary risk. Cardiorespiratory fitness is directly influenced by the performance of habitual exercise training, but is also influenced by genetic potential,[5] age and gender, as well as by underlying chronic diseases that affect the cardiorespiratory systems, nervous system, blood and musculoskeletal system.

The goal of this chapter is to discuss the roles of physical activity and formal exercise in the prevention and rehabilitation (secondary prevention) of coronary heart disease (CHD). The following topics are included for this purpose:
- observational data concerning the relationship of occupational and leisure-time physical activity and exercise to coronary risk
- studies evaluating the relationship of cardiorespiratory fitness or change in cardiorespiratory fitness and coronary risk
- data addressing the results of exercise training in persons with established CHD with regard to disease progression and coronary events
- the risks of acute exercise
- potential mechanisms for the observed cardioprotective effects of physical activity and exercise training
- recommendations for physical activity and exercise training.

Evidence-Based Cardiology, 3rd edition. Edited by S. Yusuf, J.A. Cairns, A.J. Camm, E.L. Fallen, and B.J. Gersh. © 2010 Blackwell Publishing, ISBN: 978-1-4051-5925-8.

Observational studies in the prevention of coronary heart disease

Due to methodologic and ethical issues, there are no randomized trials of physical activity and exercise on clinical cardiovascular outcomes. Observational studies have been performed, however. An inherent limitation of observational data is selection bias. For example, individuals may be sedentary because of undetected pathology or physically active because of superior general health. However, investigations of either occupational or leisure time physical activity, exercise and coronary risk provide valuable information if the studies include large numbers of subjects.

Studies of occupational physical activity attempt to quantify the amount of physical activity that occurs during the performance of job duties. Most studies of this type report occupational physical activity by category, i.e. most active, moderately active, and least active. Because the requirement for occupational physical activity has decreased precipitously in the last several decades in developed countries, investigators have more recently turned attention to the relationship of leisure-time physical activity and exercise to coronary risk. This type of exercise is undertaken by people during discretionary time outside work, domestic tasks, and other routine activities of daily living.

Occupational physical activity

Multiple investigators have demonstrated an inverse relationship between the amount and intensity of job-related physical activity and coronary risk. The following three studies are illustrative of this finding.

A large population of US railroad workers (191 609 men, age range 30–64 years) was evaluated by Taylor and associates.[6] Occupational physical activity was determined by job class: sedentary clerks, more active switchmen, and most active section men. Potential confounding variables were not controlled. Death caused by atherosclerosis was more frequent for clerks (relative risk 2.03) and switchmen (relative risk 1.46) when compared with the more physically active section men.

Morris and colleagues studied 667 male London bus drivers and conductors (age range 30–69 years) for five years.[7] Physical activity on the job was assessed by specific work duties: drivers were sedentary whereas conductors moved about the double-decker buses collecting fares. The incidence of CHD was much lower for the more active conductors than for the drivers (age-adjusted relative risk 1.8).

Paffenbarger *et al* followed 6351 San Francisco longshoremen (35–74 years of age) for 22 years.[8] Physical activity was defined by specific job requirements and categorized as light (1.5–2.0 kcal/min, 1.3–1.8 metabolic equivalents (METs) for a 70 kg person), moderate (2.4–5.0 kcal/min, 2.0–4.3 METs) or heavy (5.2–7.5 kcal/min, 4.4–6.4 METs). Death attributable to CHD was inversely related with job energy expenditure (relative risk (RR) 1.8 for light and 1.7 for moderate, compared with heavy physical activity).

Leisure-time physical activity and exercise

Several studies have investigated the association between the amount and intensity of leisure-time physical activity or exercise and CHD endpoints. The most prominent investigation in this group is the Harvard Alumni Study of Paffenbarger and associates.[9] Beginning in 1962 and continuing until 1978, 16 936 men were followed for a variety of endpoints including first myocardial infarction (MI), cardiovascular death, and CHD death. An index of energy expenditure for physical activity and exercise in kcal/week was estimated for each subject based on self-reported physical activity, including number of blocks walked, stairs climbed, and participation in vigorous exercise. Among the findings of the study was an inverse relationship between the amount of habitual physical activity and/or exercise and first MI (age-adjusted relative risk 1.64 for men with <2000 kcal/week versus men with >2000 kcal/week). Interestingly, having participated in athletics as a young person was not associated with a lower risk unless there was evidence of current physical activity or exercise. After adjustment for age, smoking and hypertension, there remained a significant dose–response relationship. Figure 15.1 illustrates this dose–response relationship, as well as the cardioprotective advantage of vigorous exercise over less vigorous physical activity.

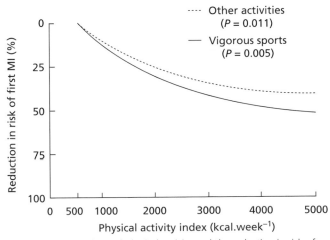

Figure 15.1 Exercise and physical activity and the reduction in risk of first myocardial infarction: the Harvard Alumni Study. (From Paffenbarger & Hyde[9].)

In 1977, a second physical activity and exercise questionnaire was administered to the Harvard Alumni Study cohort. A subgroup of 12516 survivors without documented CHD were followed until the end of 1993.[10] After adjustment for age and multiple well-established coronary risk factors, subjects who expended more than 1000 kcal/week experienced an approximately 20% lower coronary event rate than subjects who expended less than 1000 kcal/week. A third questionnaire was given to 7307 Harvard Alumni Study subjects in 1988, and included questions regarding the frequency and duration of each episode of physical activity and exercise.[11] Follow-up concluded at the end of 1993 and revealed that after adjustment for total energy expenditure, the duration of each episode of physical activity or exercise had no independent effect on coronary risk. As long as the total energy expenditure was similar, longer sessions of physical activity or exercise did not result in a greater risk reduction.

Morris and colleagues studied 17944 British male civil servants, aged 40–64 years, for an average of 8.5 years.[12] Baseline levels of physical activity and exercise were assessed by a unique 48-hour recall of leisure-time activities. Vigorous exercise was defined as an energy expenditure of at least 7.5 kcal/minute (6.4 METs for a 70 kg person). During follow-up, there were 1138 coronary events (fatal and non-fatal first MI). The age-adjusted relative risk of a coronary event for men reporting non-vigorous physical activity versus those reporting vigorous exercise was 2.2.

The Nurses' Health Study enrolled 72488 women, aged 40–65 years, who were initially free from CHD.[13] Habitual patterns of physical activity and exercise, including walking, cycling, jogging, swimming, racquet sports, calisthenics, aerobics, stairs climbed, and walking pace were collected in 1986 and subsequently updated in 1988 and again in 1992. After eight years of follow-up, 645 coronary events (MI, CHD death) occurred. There was a graded, inverse relationship between amount of physical activity or exercise and coronary events. The multivariate adjusted relative risk for the most physically active versus the least physically active quintile of the population was 0.66. Walking distance was inversely associated with risk. Vigorous exercise was associated with a 30–40% reduction in coronary events. Subjects who were initially sedentary and became more active during follow-up enjoyed a lower coronary risk than sedentary subjects who remained inactive.

The Women's Health Study included 39372 health professionals who were at least 45 years of age and free of CHD at enrollment.[14] Habitual levels of physical activity and exercise, including walking, pace of walking, flights of stairs climbed, and sporting pursuits were assessed. After an average follow-up interval of 5 years, 244 cases of CHD occurred (MI, coronary revascularization, CHD death). The multivariate adjusted relative risk for the most active

(>1500 kcal/week) versus the least active (<200 kcal/week) quartiles was 0.75. The time spent walking was more important in coronary risk reduction than was the pace of walking. For women with coronary risk factors such as obesity, cigarette smoking and dyslipidemia, physical activity and exercise were protective. Subjects who walked one hour per week experienced one half of the risk of subjects who did not walk.

Cardiorespiratory fitness and coronary death

When estimated with maximal graded exercise testing, cardiorespiratory fitness has been shown to be inversely related with cardiovascular risk. The following are examples of investigations, some that included both genders as well as younger and older subjects. An important limitation of these studies is that genetic potential plays a central role in cardiorespiratory fitness, independent of habitual exercise.[5]

Blair and associates studied patients of the Aerobics Center in Dallas, Texas, who had an initial evaluation including a maximal treadmill exercise test. Men (n = 10224) and women (n = 3120) were categorized by fitness level (low, moderate, high), based on treadmill exercise performance, and followed for an average of eight years.[15] The coronary death rate decreased dramatically with increasing fitness level for both genders (Table 15.1). However, there were relatively few coronary deaths in this population of rather young subjects (66 deaths in men, seven deaths in women). Blair also assessed the effects of improvement in cardiorespiratory fitness on coronary risk with subjects at the Aerobics Center.[16] A large cohort of men (n = 9777, age range 20–82 years) underwent two maximal treadmill exercise tests at a mean interval of 4.9 years. The subjects were followed for an average of 5.1 years. There were 87 cardiovascular deaths during follow-up. Relative to subjects who remained unfit, subjects who improved their fitness category experienced an age-adjusted relative risk of 0.48 (95% confidence interval (CI) 0.31–0.74).

A cohort of 1960 Norwegian men (age range 40–59 years) underwent maximal graded exercise testing and were followed for an average of 16 years.[17] Eighty-seven cardiovascular deaths occurred. After extensive statistical control of potential confounding factors, a strong inverse relationship between cardiorespiratory fitness and coronary risk was found. Compared with men in the lowest fitness quartile, the relative risks for quartiles 2, 3, and 4 were 0.59, 0.45, and 0.41, respectively.

Two studies involving all residents of Olmsted County, Minnesota, who underwent maximal treadmill exercise testing in the late 1980s provide additional insight into the relationship of cardiorespiratory fitness and coronary risk.

Table 15.1 Rates of coronary death by fitness level: the Aerobics Center Study (from Blair et al.[15])

N	Mean age	Follow-up
10224 ♂	41.5 years	8 years
3120 ♀	40.8 years	8 years

Fitness level	Coronary death rate per 10000 person-years	
	Male	Female
Low	24.6	7.4
Moderate	7.8	2.9
High	3.1	0.8

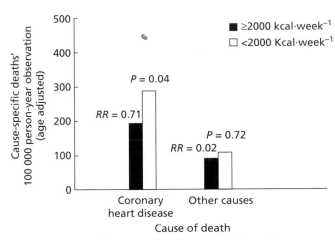

Figure 15.2 Physical activity and death rates in patients with coronary artery disease in the Harvard Alumni Study. (From Paffenbarger & Hyde[9].)

Roger and colleagues followed 1452 men and 741 women who had treadmill exercise tests in 1987 and 1988 for approximately six years.[18] Cardiovascular endpoints included cardiac death, non-fatal myocardial infarction, and congestive heart failure. A total of 160 cardiovascular endpoints occurred during follow-up (106 in men, 54 in women). After multivariate adjustment, peak treadmill workload in METs was the only variable associated with the outcome measures. For each 1 MET increment in cardiorespiratory fitness, cardiac events were reduced by 25%, with a similar effect for both genders. Using similar methods, Goraya and associates followed 3107 Olmsted County residents who underwent maximal treadmill exercise testing in 1987 to 1989 and were followed for a median of six years.[19] Both genders were included and 514 of the subjects were over 65 years of age. For each 1 MET increase in cardiorespiratory fitness, cardiovascular events were reduced by 14% and 18% for younger and older (>65 years) subjects, respectively.

Exercise training in established coronary disease

For patients with coronary heart disease, exercise training improves exercise capacity and symptoms. After three months of aerobic exercise training, peak oxygen uptake improves by 15–20%.[20] Symptoms of angina pectoris may be markedly improved by exercise training. Resistance training results in improvements in muscle strength and maintains muscle mass. There are also data available to demonstrate that physical activity and exercise training improve important clinical outcomes for patients with coronary heart disease. These data are the result of both observational and randomized controlled trials.

Observational data

In the Harvard Alumni Study, reviewed previously in this chapter, a subset of 782 subjects of the entire 16936-person cohort had documented coronary heart disease at the beginning of the study.[9] Over a follow-up interval of approximately 12 years, the more physically active subjects (those who expended more than 2000 kcal/week in leisure-time physical activity and exercise) experienced a 30% lower coronary event rate than less active subjects (Fig. 15.2). The beneficial effect of exercise persisted after statistical adjustment for smoking, blood pressure, body weight, family history of coronary heart disease and age.

In the British Regional Heart Study, 772 of the 5934 men in the cohort had documented coronary heart disease at the onset of the trial.[21] A baseline assessment of habitual physical activity, including intensity of activity, was performed. After five years of follow-up, 131 deaths had occurred (94 from cardiovascular disease). Compared with inactive subjects, persons who performed light, moderate or vigorous exercise experienced a substantially lower all-cause and cardiovascular mortality (Table 15.2). These results were similar for younger and older (>65 years of age) subjects.

Randomized trials

Kallio and colleagues randomized 301 men and 74 women with a history of myocardial infarction to a comprehensive rehabilitation program (exercise training, dietary and smoking cessation advice, psychosocial counseling) or to a control group.[22] Compared with the control group, the intervention group experienced an improvement in habitual physical activity, blood lipids and blood pressure. The three-year cumulative mortality was 18.6% in the intervention group versus 29.4% in the control group ($P = 0.02$). The

Table 15.2 Cardiovascular mortality by activity level in the British Regional Heart Study (from Wannamethee et al.[21])

Activity level	Cardiovascular mortality	
	Age-adjusted RR	*Fully adjusted RR
Inactive/occasional	1.00	1.00
Light	0.33	0.38
Moderate	0.39	0.50
Moderate to vigorous/ vigorous	0.49	0.61

* Adjusted for age, smoking, social class, self-rated health status, diabetes, and history of myocardial infarction and stroke.

difference was primarily the result of a reduction in the incidence of sudden cardiac death in the intervention group (5.8% versus 14.4%, $P < 0.01$). The rate of non-fatal reinfarction was similar for both groups.

Hamalainen and associates reported 10-year follow-up data for the same subjects.[23] No organized intervention occurred after the first three years of the study. At 10 years, the incidence of sudden cardiac death was less for the intervention group (12.8% versus 23.0%, $P = 0.01$). Cardiac mortality was also lower for intervention subjects (35.1% versus 47.1%, $P = 0.02$). The largest difference in mortality was observed during the first year of the investigation when beta-blocker use was similar for both groups.

Hambrecht et al randomized 101 men with stable coronary artery disease and exercise-induced myocardial ischemia to either percutaneous coronary intervention (PCI) or exercise training (20 minutes per day).[24] Medical therapy was similar for both groups. After one year, the investigators found that both treatment arms were equally effective in improving angina, although symptom improvement was more rapid for PCI. Exercise training was superior to PCI in the combined clinical endpoint of cardiac death, stroke, coronary bypass surgery, PCI, myocardial infarction and hospitalization for angina (event-free survival 88% exercise versus 70% PCI, $P < 0.02$).

Meta-analyses

Although there are many randomized controlled trials of cardiac rehabilitation including exercise training, no other studies besides the first two discussed above have provided evidence for a statistically significant reduction in mortality. Many of these trials have been plagued by insufficient numbers of subjects to achieve adequate statistical power and by subject drop-outs and cross-overs. Investigators have used meta-analysis to partially overcome these limitations and to determine pooled estimates of benefits.

In 1989, O'Connor and colleagues performed a meta-analysis of 22 randomized trials of exercise training and standard coronary risk factor intervention of varying intensity, resulting in a total sample of 4554 postmyocardial infarction patients.[25] Compared with control subjects, patients who were randomized to the exercise intervention experienced a reduction in total mortality, cardiovascular mortality, and fatal reinfarction of 20%, 22%, and 25%, respectively.

A more recent, expanded meta-analysis by Jolliffe and associates was published in the Cochrane Database.[26] The authors searched electronic databases for appropriate randomized trials from the earliest date until the end of 1998. They included studies with both genders, and included subjects with diagnoses of myocardial infarction, coronary bypass surgery, percutaneous revascularization, angina pectoris, and angiographically documented coronary atherosclerosis. All accepted trials used exercise training as a component of the intervention. Endpoints included mortality, morbidity, health-related quality of life and standard coronary risk factors. A total of 32 trials were included in their analysis, with 8440 subjects. A 31% reduction (relative risk 0.69) in cardiac mortality for intervention subjects was found. There was no effect on non-fatal myocardial infarction.

Exercise training in chronic heart failure

For patients with stable, compensated chronic heart failure (CHF), exercise training provides substantial benefits: improved exercise capacity, reduced symptoms, decreased evidence of neurohormonal activation, better quality of life and possibly improved mortality.[27] Early observational studies published in the 1970s and 1980s established the safety of exercise training for stable CHF patients and documented improvements in exercise capacity.[28]

More than 30 randomized controlled trials of exercise training in patients with CHF have been published, although the numbers of subjects in the trials were limited. A meta-analysis of the trials reported that the average improvement in VO_{2peak} after training was 17%.[29] Giannuzzi and colleagues randomized 90 patients with stable CHF to a six-month exercise program or a control group.[30] The exercise group demonstrated an improvement in exercise capacity as well as evidence of reverse cardiac remodeling with a decrease in end-diastolic and end-systolic volumes and a small increase in left ventricular ejection fraction.

ExTraMATCH was a collaborative meta-analysis which included nine parallel randomized controlled trials of exercise training in 801 CHF patients. With a mean follow-up of 705 days, there were 88 deaths in the exercise arm and 105 deaths in the control arm (hazard ratio 0.65, 95% confidence interval 0.46–0.92, $P = 0.015$)[31]. Additional studies with larger numbers of subjects are needed to fully assess the effects of exercise training on recurrent hospitalizations and mortality.

Recently, results from HF ACTION (Heart Failure: A Controlled Trial Investigating Outcomes of Exercise Training: 2331 subjects) were published.[32,33] After a median follow-up of 2.5 years and after adjustment for prognostic predictors, subjects in the exercise arm experienced a modest but significant reduction in both all-cause mortality and hospitalization. Although the improvement in VO$_2$ peak with training was modest, exercise subjects reported significant improvements in self-reported health status. Exercise training was found to be safe in these stable subjects with reduced ejection fraction.

Risks during acute exercise

Previous sections of this chapter have provided clear evidence for the cardioprotective effects of regular physical activity or exercise training. However, during an acute bout of exercise the risk of sudden cardiac death or myocardial infarction is transiently increased.[34] Acute exertion may trigger a cardiac event in a susceptible individual. Exercise-related cardiac events usually occur in persons with structural heart disease. Mittleman and colleagues interviewed 1228 survivors of acute myocardial infarction.[35] In approximately 5% of cases, heavy exertion apparently triggered the infarction.

The annual incidence of exercise-related cardiac arrest in previously healthy persons is 5.4/100 000.[34] The incidence is 56 times higher than that at rest for sedentary men and five times higher for physically active men.[36] The risk of myocardial infarction during exercise is 2–6 times higher than at rest.[34] Women experience a much lower risk of sudden death during exercise than do men.[37]

Even highly trained endurance athletes are not immune to exercise-associated cardiac death, although the risk is extremely low. In a survey of 215 413 marathon runners, four deaths were documented during running (prevalence of 0.002%).[38] Three of the four deaths were due to previously undetected coronary atherosclerosis.

Survey data from the 1980s and 1990s are available regarding the incidence of cardiac events in patients with coronary heart disease who exercise under supervision in cardiac rehabilitation programs.[39] The rates per 1 000 000 patient-hours of exercise for cardiac arrest, acute myocardial infarction and cardiac death were 8.6, 4.5 and 1.3, respectively.

Pathophysiologic mechanisms for exercise-related cardiac events

In young persons (<40 years of age), congenital cardiovascular abnormalities are generally responsible for exercise-related sudden death.[39] Examples of such abnormalities include the following.
• Hypertrophic cardiomyopathy
• Anomalous coronary artery anatomy

• Aortic stenosis
• Marfan's syndrome resulting in aortic rupture
• Mitral valve prolapse
• Arrhythmogenic right ventricular cardiomyopathy

For individuals older than 40 years, coronary artery disease is the most common pathologic finding. While not completely understood, the following are accepted as potential mechanisms for death during exertion in patients with coronary disease.

1 Hemodynamic stress may result in rupture and subsequent thrombus formation in a high-risk coronary plaque. Burke and associates reported autopsy evidence of this type of occurrence in 68% of cases of sudden cardiac death associated with exertion.[40] Acute exercise may increase platelet activation, thereby increasing risk of thrombus formation.[39] Plaque rupture and thrombosis may result in acute myocardial infarction, as well.

2 Myocardial ischemia is an important contributor to malignant ventricular arrhythmia. In patients with coronary atherosclerosis, an acute bout of exercise may cause constriction of diseased coronary segments, unlike the usual exertion-related vasodilation of healthy coronary arteries. This increases the likelihood of the development of ischemia. The reasons for this paradoxical coronary vasoconstriction include excessive sympathetic nervous system activation, endothelial dysfunction and platelet aggregation.[41]

3 Autonomic nervous system imbalance (autonomic dysfunction), with inappropriate activation of the sympathetic division and diminished parasympathetic activation, may result in ventricular arrhythmia independent of myocardial ischemia.[42]

How does habitual exercise decrease coronary risk?

The following discussion highlights some of the potential mechanisms for the cardioprotective effect of exercise.

Structural improvements in coronary arteries

Habitual physical activity and exercise may result in structural adaptations of the epicardial coronary arteries such as:
• increased cross-sectional area of the lumen[43]
• improved capacity for vasodilation, resulting from enhanced endothelial function[44]
• potential increased collateral circulation in patients with ischemic left ventricular dysfunction.[45]

Improvement in hypertension, blood lipids, obesity and depression

Observational data from the Harvard Alumni Study are consistent with the concept that habitual exercise appears to reduce the chances of developing hypertension.[46] Regular exercise may modestly lower blood pressure in hypertensive patients and in normal individuals by an average of 6–9 mm Hg for both systolic and diastolic pressures.[47]

Regular exercise results in modest improvements in the blood lipid profile. A meta-analysis revealed an average reduction in total cholesterol of 7–13 mg/dL, low-density lipoprotein cholesterol of 3–11 mg/dL, and triglycerides of 14–22 mg/dL.[48] High-density lipoprotein cholesterol increased by an average of 2 mg/dL. There is marked interindividual variability in the effect of exercise training on blood lipids.

Exercise, in adequate amounts, is effective as part of a comprehensive approach to reduce fat weight in obesity. McGuire and colleagues studied differences in obese subjects who were successful in maintaining an average 37 lb weight loss over seven years compared to subjects who were not.[49] The average number of weekly sessions of physical activity were higher (8.4 versus 5.5), as were the number of strenuous exercise sessions each week (2.8 versus 1.8), for subjects who maintained the weight loss. Exercise training reduces abdominal fat to a greater extent than gluteal or femoral fat in obese men.[50] In the Aerobics Center Longitudinal Study, over 5000 men and women underwent three treadmill exercise tests (between 1970 and 1994) and were followed for an average of 7.5 years.[51] Subjects who increased fitness from one treadmill test to the next, presumably by increasing habitual exercise, attenuated the usual age-related increase in body weight.

Symptoms of depression consistently improve with habitual physical activity and exercise.[52] Physically active persons appear to be at lower risk for the development of depression. In patients with documented coronary heart disease, exercise has been shown to improve anxiety, emotional distress, and depression.[20]

Metabolic syndrome

Patients with three or more of the following risk factors have the metabolic syndrome and a markedly increased coronary risk: abdominal obesity, elevated triglycerides, low high-density lipoprotein cholesterol, hypertension and impaired fasting blood glucose.[53] The causes of the metabolic syndrome for the overwhelming majority of patients are incorrect diet and too little physical activity. First-line therapy for the metabolic syndrome is increased physical activity and weight reduction.[54]

Impaired glucose metabolism and type 2 diabetes mellitus

Persons who perform exercise training have lower plasma insulin concentrations and improved insulin sensitivity compared with sedentary individuals.[55] With cessation of regular training, insulin concentration and sensitivity return to levels observed in sedentary persons.

Table 15.3 Weekly exercise amount and the risk of developing type 2 diabetes in the Nurses' Health Study, 1980–1996 (from Hu et al[56])

Weekly exercise duration	Relative risk
<0.5 h	1.0
0.5–1.9 h	0.89
2.0–3.9 h	0.87
4.0–6.9 h	0.83
≥7.0 h	0.71

Exercise and proper nutrition have been shown to improve glucose metabolism and to prevent the onset of type 2 diabetes mellitus. A one-year program of exercise and diet change resulted in an average weight loss of 10 kg and a decrease in fasting blood glucose and insulin concentrations.[49] In the Nurses' Health Study, subjects who performed more than 30 minutes of exercise per week experienced a much lower relative risk of developing diabetes over the 16 years of follow-up (Table 15.3).[56] The Diabetes Prevention Study was a randomized, controlled trial of an intervention of exercise and diet in 552 middle-aged men and women with impaired glucose tolerance but not type 2 diabetes mellitus.[57] After three years, intervention subjects had lost an average of 3–4 kg and experienced a 58% reduction in the incidence of diabetes (diabetes occurred in 11% of intervention subjects versus 23% of controls).

Autonomic nervous system dysfunction

Autonomic dysfunction, defined as a sustained increase in sympathetic activity and a decrease in parasympathetic activity, is associated with increased coronary risk and mortality.[42] Clinical indicators of autonomic dysfunction include: resting heart rate >90 beats/min, inability to achieve 85% of age-predicted maximal heart rate during graded exercise testing, abnormally slow heart rate recovery after maximal exercise (failure to decrease heart rate >12 beats/min during the first minute of recovery), and decreased heart rate variability (failure to change heart rate by ≥10 beats/min during one minute of slow deep breaths). Autonomic dysfunction may result in endothelial dysfunction, coronary vasospasm, left ventricular hypertrophy, and malignant ventricular arrhythmias. Exercise training results in a favorable decrease in sympathetic activity and an increase in parasympathetic tone in both healthy subjects[58] and in patients with coronary disease.[59]

Improved endothelial function

Endothelial dysfunction occurs in response to exposure to coronary risk factors and is an early and late player in

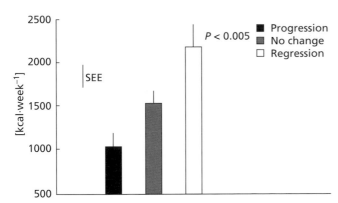

Figure 15.3 Energy expenditure per week and changes in angiographic coronary lesion morphology over one year. (From Hambrecht *et al.*[63])

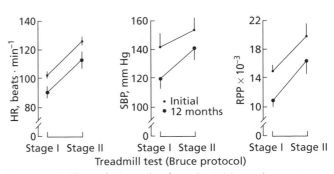

Figure 15.4 Effects of 12 months of exercise training on heart rate (HR), systolic blood pressure (SBP), and the rate pressure product (RPP) at stages I and II of the Bruce treadmill exercise testing protocol. All variables were significantly lower ($P < 0.01$) after training. (From Ehsani *et al.*[66])

atherogenesis.[60] The following abnormalities may result: impaired coronary vasodilation, increased vasospasm, increased permeability to lipoproteins and other blood constituents, and increased adhesion of platelets and glycoproteins. Endothelial dysfunction may result in reduced myocardial perfusion and plaque rupture, leading to acute coronary syndromes.[61] Exercise training improves measures of endothelial function (endothelial-dependent vasodilation) in patients with coronary atherosclerosis.[62]

Reduced progression of coronary atherosclerosis

Exercise training in sufficient amounts appears to slow the progression of, or even modestly reverse, coronary atherosclerosis. A one-year randomized controlled trial of supervised, moderate-intensity exercise and a low-fat diet without the use of lipid-lowering medications was performed in approximately 60 subjects.[63] Angiographically determined progression of disease occurred in 45% of controls and 10% of exercise subjects. A modest degree of regression of disease was found in 28% of exercisers versus 6% of controls. Figure 15.3 shows that partial regression of coronary atherosclerosis was present in patients who expended an average of at least 2200 kilocalories per week in exercise (approximately 5–6 hours of moderate-intensity exercise per week).

Decreased thrombosis risk

Acute exercise causes transient activation of the coagulation system, resulting in an increased risk of thrombosis.[64] However, habitual exercise training results in an overall decreased thrombotic risk by the following mechanisms:[65–67]

- reduced fibrinogen concentration
- reduced platelet aggregation

- decreased plasminogen activator inhibitor-1
- increased endogenous tissue plasminogen activator.

Improvement in myocardial ischemia

Exercise training may improve myocardial ischemia by decreasing myocardial demand and improving oxygen delivery to the heart.[68–70] As seen in Figure 15.4, after exercise training, at a standard submaximal exercise intensity the rate-pressure product is reduced resulting in a lower myocardial oxygen requirement. This enables the patient to perform a higher intensity of physical activity before exceeding the ischemic threshold.

The rate pressure product at the ischemic threshold is increased by exercise training, independent of changes in other risk factors or anti-ischemic medications, suggesting that myocardial blood supply has improved.[71] Exercise-induced myocardial ischemia, measured by exercise thallium perfusion imaging and without alteration in the rate pressure product, has been shown to improve substantially after training.[69,70]

Recommendations for types and amounts of physical activity and exercise for patients with cardiovascular diseases

Exercise training provides benefits not only for patients with coronary heart disease, but also for individuals with chronic heart failure, heart transplantation, and valvular replacement or repair.[72] The following types and amounts of physical activity and exercise training are recommended.[73]

- Physical activity: accumulate 30–60 minutes of moderate-intensity physical activity ≥5 days week; examples are walking for transportation, housework, yardwork, stair climbing, low-intensity games and sports
- Aerobic exercise training:
  3–5 sessions per week
  50–80% of exercise capacity

20–60 minutes

Walk, treadmill, cycle, row, stair climber, arm/leg ergometer, etc.

- Resistance training:

  2–3 sessions per week (non-consecutive days)

  10–15 repetitions to moderate fatigue

  1–3 sets of 8–10 different exercises for both the upper and lower body

  Calisthenics, elastic bands, hand weights, weight machines

Table 15.4 provides additional information regarding exercise program components for persons with and without cardiovascular disease.

Table 15.4 Exercise program components from the American College of Sports Medicine* for persons with and without cardiovascular (CV) disease

Persons without CV disease	Persons with CV disease
Warm-up: 5–10 minutes low-intensity, large muscle activity, low-intensity stretching	Same
Conditioning phase: endurance exercise, 20–60 minutes, 3–5 days/week, 55–90% maximal heart rate; resistance training, 1 + sets 3–20 repetitions to volitional fatigue, exercises for the major muscle groups, 2–3 days/week; flexibility exercises	*Supervised setting*: minimum of 6 sessions
	Intensity: moderate, below ischemic and anginal thresholds, systolic blood pressure <250 mmHg, diastolic blood pressure <115 mmHg
	Resistance training: begin 5 weeks after cardiac surgery or myocardial infarction, 3 weeks after percutaneous intervention; 1 set of 10–15 repetitions, exercises for the major muscle groups, perceived exertion "fairly light to somewhat hard"
Cool-down: 5 minutes low-intensity, large muscle activity, stretching exercises for the major muscle groups	Same

* American College of Sports Medicine. *ACSM's Guidelines for Exercise Testing and Prescription*, 7th edn. Philadelphia: Lippincott Williams and Wilkins, 2006.

Conclusion

The data presented in this chapter demonstrate that habitual exercise and physical activity are effective in reducing coronary risk. While an acute bout of exercise transiently increases the risk of a coronary event, the absolute risk is very small. The data for primary prevention are observational in nature, and randomized trials have not been performed due to logistical and ethical constraints. Occupational as well as leisure-time activities are cardioprotective. Cardiorespiratory fitness is inversely related to coronary risk. Investigations for secondary prevention include both observational studies and randomized trials. Individual trials were generally underpowered to detect differences in mortality and reinfarction, but meta-analyses have consistently demonstrated a protective effect of habitual physical activity and exercise training.

The data are consistent with the concept that the greater the total energy expenditure in physical activity or exercise, the lower the coronary risk. Most of the data suggest that higher intensity exercise is more protective than lower intensity activity.

The potential mechanisms responsible for the cardioprotective action of exercise and physical activity are not completely understood, but include improvement in classic coronary risk factors, reduction in autonomic nervous system and endothelial cell dysfunction, decreased thrombosis and increased fibrinolysis, less progression and possible modest regression of coronary atherosclerosis, and a reduction in myocardial ischemia. This information provides a solid evidence base for the use of exercise training and physical activity as part of a comprehensive approach to primary and secondary prevention of coronary heart disease.

Acknowledgment

Adapted from Squires RW, Hamm LF. Exercise and the coronary heart disease connection. In: American Association of Cardiovascular and Pulmonary Rehabilitation. *AACVPR Cardiac Rehabilitation Resource Manual*. Champaign, IL: Human Kinetics, 2006: 53–62.

References

1. Thompson PD, Buchner D, Pina IL *et al.* AHA scientific statement. Exercise and physical activity in the prevention and treatment of atherosclerotic cardiovascular disease. *Circulation* 2003; **107**:3109–16.
2. US Department of Health and Human Services. *Physical Activity and Health: A Report of the Surgeon General*. Atlanta, GA: US Department of Health and Human Services, Centers for Disease

Control and Prevention, National Center for Chronic Disease Prevention and Health Promotion, 1996.

3. Leon AS, ed. *Physical Activity and Cardiovascular Health: A National Consensus.* Champaign, IL: Human Kinetics, 1997:3–4.

4. Levine JA, Lanningham-Foster LM, McCrady SK *et al.* Interindividual variation in posture allocation: possible role in human obesity. *Science* 2005;**307**:584–6.

5. Bouchard C, Dione FT, Simoneau J, Boulay MR. Genetics of aerobic and anaerobic performances. In: Holloszy JO, ed. *Exercise and Sports Science Reviews.* Baltimore, MD: Williams and Wilkins, 1992: 27–58.

6. Taylor HL, Klepetar E, Keys A, Parlin W, Blackburn H, Puchner T. Death rates among physically active and sedentary employees of the railroad industry. *Am J Pub Health* 1962;**52**:1697–707.

7. Morris JN, Kagan A, Pattison DC, Gardner MJ, Raffle PAB. Incidence and prediction of ischemic heart disease in London busmen. *Lancet* 1966;**2**:553–9.

8. Paffenbarger RS, Hale WE. Work activity and coronary heart mortality. *N Engl J Med* 1975;**292**:545–50.

9. Paffenbarger RS, Hyde RT. Exercise in the prevention of coronary heart disease. *Prev Med* 1984;**13**:3–22.

10. Sesso HD, Paffenbarger RS, Lee IM. Physical activity and coronary heart disease in men: The Harvard Alumni Health Study. *Circulation* 2000;**102**:975–80.

11. Lee IM, Sesso HD, Paffenbarger RS. Physical activity and coronary heart disease risk in men: does the duration of exercise episodes predict risk? *Circulation* 2000;**102**:981–6.

12. Morris JN, Everitt MG, Pollard R, Chave SPW, Semmence AM. Vigorous exercise in leisure time: protection against coronary heart disease. *Lancet* 1980;**2**:1207–10.

13. Manson, JE, Hu FB, Rich-Edwards JW *et al.* A prospective study of walking as compared with vigorous exercise in the prevention of coronary heart disease in women. *N Engl J Med* 1999;**341**: 650–8.

14. Lee IM, Rexrode KM, Cook NR, Manson JE, Buring JE. Physical activity and coronary heart disease in women: is "no pain, no gain" passe? *JAMA* 2001;**285**:1447–54.

15. Blair SN, Kohl III HW, Paffenbarger RS, Clark DG, Cooper KH, Gibbons LW. Physical fitness and all-cause mortality: a prospective study of healthy men and women. *JAMA* 1989;**262**:2395–401.

16. Blair SN, Kohl III HW, Barlow CE, Paffenbarger RS, Gibbons LW, Macera CA. Changes in physical fitness and all-cause mortality: a prospective study of healthy and unhealthy men. *JAMA* 1995;**273**:1093–8.

17. Sandvik L, Erikssen J, Thaulow E, Erikssen G, Mundal R, Rodahl K. Physical fitness as a predictor of mortality among healthy, middle-aged Norwegian men. *N Engl J Med* 1993;**328**:533–7.

18. Roger VL, Jacobsen SJ, Pellika PA, Miller TD, Bailey KR, Gersh BJ. Prognostic value of treadmill exercise testing: a population-based study in Olmsted County, Minnesota. *Circulation* 1998; **98**:2836–41.

19. Goraya TY, Jacobsen SJ, Pellika PA *et al.* Prognostic value of treadmill exercise testing in elderly persons. *Ann Intern Med* 2000;**132**:862–70.

20. Ades PA. Cardiac rehabilitation and secondary prevention of coronary heart disease. *N Engl J Med* 2001;**345**:892–902.

21. Wannamethee SG, Shaper AG, Walker M. Physical activity and mortality in older men with diagnosed coronary heart disease. *Circulation* 2000;**102**:1358–63.

22. Kallio V, Hamalainen H, Hakkila J, Luurila OJ. Reduction in sudden deaths by a multifactorial intervention programme after acute myocardial infarction. *Lancet* 1979;**2**:1091–4.

23. Hamalainen H, Luurila OJ, Kallio V, Knuts LR, Arstila M, Hakkila J. Long-term reduction in sudden deaths after a multifactorial intervention programme in patients with myocardial infarction: 10-year results of a controlled investigation. *Eur Heart J* 1989;**10**:55–62.

24. Hambrecht R, Walther C, Mobius-Winkler S *et al.* Percutaneous coronary angioplasty compared with exercise training in patients with stable coronary artery disease: a randomized trial. *Circulation* 2004;**109**:1371–8.

25. O'Connor GT, Buring JE, Yusuf S *et al.* An overview of randomized trials of rehabilitation with exercise after myocardial infarction. *Circulation* 1989;**80**:234–44.

26. Jolliffe J, Rees K, Taylor RRS, Thompson DR, Oldridge N, Ebrahim S. Exercise-based rehabilitation for coronary heart disease. *Cochrane Database of Systematic Reviews* 2001, Issue 1. Art. No.: CD001800. DOI: 10.1002/14651858.CD001800.

27. McKelvie RS. Exercise training in patients with heart failure: clinical outcomes, safety, and indications. *Heart Fail Rev* 2008; **13**:3–11.

28. Squires RW. *Exercise Prescription for the High-Risk Cardiac Patient.* Champaign, IL: Human Kinetics, 1998: 123–51.

29. Smart N, Marwick TH. Exercise training for patients with heart failure: a systematic review of factors that improve mortality and morbidity. *Am J Med* 2004;**116**:693–706.

30. Giannuzzi P, Temporelli PL, Corra U, Tavassi L. Antiremodeling effect of long-term exercise training in patients with stable chronic heart failure: results of the Exercise in Left Ventricular Dysfunction and Chronic Heart Failure (ELVD-CHF) Trial. *Circulation* 2003;**108**:554–9.

31. ExTraMATCH Collaborative. Exercise training meta-analysis of trials with chronic heart failure (ExTraMATCH). *BMJ* 2004;**328**(7433):189.

32. O'Connor CM, Whellan DJ, Lee KL *et al.* Efficacy and safety of exercise training in patients with chronic heart failure. *JAMA* 2009;**301**:1439–50.

33. Flynn KE, Pina IL, Whellan DJ *et al.* Effects of exercise training on health status in patients with chronic heart failure. *JAMA* 2009;**301**:1451–9.

34. Thompson, PD, Moore GE. The cardiac risks of vigorous physical activity. In: Leon AS, ed. *Physical Activity and Cardiovascular Health: A National Consensus.* Champaign, IL: Human Kinetics, 1997: 137–42.

35. Mittleman MA, Maclure M, Tolfer GH, Sherwood JB, Goldberg RJ, Muller JE. Triggering of acute myocardial infarction by heavy physical exertion: protection against triggering by regular exertion. *N Engl J Med* 1993;**329**:1677–83.

36. Siscovick DS, Weiss NS, Fletcher RH, Lasky T. The incidence of primary cardiac arrest during vigorous exercise. *N Engl J Med* 1984;**311**:874–7.

37. Whang W, Manson JE, Hu FB *et al.* Physical exertion, exercise, and sudden cardiac death in women. *JAMA* 2006;**295**:1399–403.

38. Maron BJ, Polliac LC, Roberts WO. Risk for sudden death associated with marathon running. *J Am Coll Cardiol* 1996;**28**:428–31.

39. Thompson PD, Franklin BA, Balady GJ *et al.* Exercise and acute cardiovascular events: placing the risks into perspective. A scientific statement from the American Heart Association Council

on Nutrition, Physical Activity, and Metabolism and the Council on Clinical Cardiology. *Circulation* 2007;**115**:2358–68.

40. Burke AP, Farb A, Malcom GT, Liang YH, Smialek JE, Virmani R. Plaque rupture and sudden death related to exertion in men with coronary artery disease. *JAMA* 1999;**281**:921–6.

41. Hess OM, Buchi M, Kirkeeide R *et al.* Potential role of coronary vasoconstriction in ischemic heart disease: effect of exercise. *Eur Heart J* 1990;**II**(suppl B):58–64.

42. Curtis BM, O'Keefe JH. Autonomic tone as a cardiovascular risk factor: the dangers of chronic fight or flight. *Mayo Clin Proc* 2002;**77**:45–54.

43. Pellicia A, Spataro A, Granata J, Biffi A, Casselli G, Alabiso A. Coronary arteries in physiological hypertrophy: echocardiographic evidence of increased proximal size in elite athletes. *Int J Sports Med* 1990;**11**:120–6.

44. Haskell WL, Sims C, Myll J, Bortz WM, St Goar FG, Alderman EL. Coronary artery size and dilating capacity in ultradistance runners. *Circulation* 1993;**87**:1076–82.

45. Belardinelli R, Georgiou D, Ginzton L, Cianci G, Purcaro A. Effects of moderate exercise training on thallium uptake and contractile response to low-dose dobutamine in dysfunctional myocardium in patients with ischemic cardiomyopathy. *Circulation* 1998;**97**:553–61.

46. Paffenbarger RS, Wing AL, Hyde RT, Jung DL. Physical activity and incidence of hypertension in college alumni. *Am J Epidemiol* 1983;**117**:245–57.

47. Seals DR, Hagberg JM. The effect of exercise training on human hypertension: a review. *Med Sci Sports Exerc* 1984;**16**:207–15.

48. Tran ZV, Weltman A. Differential effects of exercise on serum lipid and lipoprotein levels seen with changes in body weight: a meta-analysis. *JAMA* 1985;**254**:919–24.

49. McGuire MT, Wing RR, Hill JO. Behavioral strategies of individuals who have maintained long-term weight losses. *Obes Res* 1999;**7**:334–41.

50. Ross R, Rissanen J, Pedwell H, Clifford J, Shragge P. Influence of diet and exercise on skeletal muscle and visceral adipose tissue in men. *J Appl Physiol* 1996;**81**:2445–55.

51. DiPietro L, Kohl III HW, Barlow CE, Blair SN. Improvements in cardiorespiratory fitness attenuate age-related weight gain in healthy men and women: the Aerobics Center longitudinal study. *Int J Obes* 1998;**22**:55–62.

52. Martinsen EW, Medhus A, Sandvik L. Effects of aerobic exercise on depression: a controlled study. *BMJ Clin Res Ed* 1985;**291**:109.

53. Ford ES, Giles WH, Dietz WH. Prevalence of the metabolic syndrome among US adults: findings from the third National Health and Nutrition Examination Survey. *JAMA* 2002;**287**:356–9.

54. Expert Panel on Detection, Evaluation, and Treatment of High Blood Cholesterol in Adults. Executive summary of the third report of the National Cholesterol Education Program (NCEP) expert panel on detection, evaluation, and treatment of high blood cholesterol in adults (Adult Treatment Panel III). *JAMA* 2001;**285**:2486–97.

55. Bjorntorp B, Fahlen M, Grimby G *et al.* Carbohydrate and lipid metabolism in middle-aged, physically well-trained men. *Metabolism* 1972;**21**:1032–44.

56. Hu FB, Manson JE, Stampfer MJ *et al.* Diet, lifestyle, and the risk of type 2 diabetes mellitus in women. *N Engl J Med* 2001;**345**:790–7.

57. Tuomilehto J, Lindstrom J, Eriksson JG *et al.* Prevention of type 2 diabetes mellitus by changes in lifestyle among subjects with impaired glucose tolerance. *N Engl J Med* 2001;**344**:1343–50.

58. Levy WC, Cerqueira MD, Harp GD *et al.* Effect of endurance exercise training on heart rate variability at rest in healthy young and older men. *Am J Cardiol* 1998;**82**:1236–41.

59. Tygesen H, Wettervik C, Wennerblom B. Intensive home-based exercise training in cardiac rehabilitation increases exercise capacity and heart rate variability. *Int J Cardiol* 2001;**79**:175–82.

60. Squires RW. Coronary atherosclerosis. In: American College of Sports Medicine. ACSM's Resource Manual for Guidelines for Exercise Testing and Prescription, 4th edn. Philadelphia: Lippincott Williams and Wilkins, 2001: 227–37.

61. Verma S, Anderson TJ. Fundamentals of endothelial function for the clinical cardiologist. *Circulation* 2002;**105**:546–9.

62. Hambrecht R, Wolf A, Gielen S *et al.* Effect of exercise on coronary endothelial function in patients with coronary artery disease. *N Engl J Med* 2000;**342**:454–60.

63. Hambrecht R, Niebauer J, Marburger C *et al.* Various intensities of leisure time physical activity in patients with coronary artery disease: effects on cardiorespiratory fitness and progression of coronary atherosclerotic lesions. *J Am Coll Cardiol* 1993;**22**:468–77.

64. Koenig W, Ernst E. Exercise and thrombosis. *Coronary Artery Dis* 2000;**11**:123–7.

65. Ernst E. Regular exercise reduces fibrinogen levels: a review of longitudinal studies. *Br J Sports Med* 1993;**27**:175–6.

66. Paramo JA, Olavide I, Barba J *et al.* Long-term cardiac rehabilitation program favorably influences fibrinolysis and lipid concentrations in acute myocardial infarction. *Haematologica* 1998;**83**:519–24.

67. Lehman M, Keul J. Physical activity and coronary heart disease: sympathetic drive and adrenaline-induced platelet aggregation. *Int J Sports Med* 1986;**7**(suppl 1):34–7.

68. Ehsani AA, Martin WH, Heath GW, Coyle EF. Cardiac effects of prolonged and intense exercise training in patients with coronary artery disease. *Am J Cardiol* 1982;**50**:246–54.

69. Schuler G, Schlierf G, Wirth A *et al.* Low-fat diet and regular, supervised physical exercise in patients with symptomatic coronary artery disease: reduction of stress-induced myocardial ischemia. *Circulation* 1988;**77**:172–81.

70. Todd IC, Bradnam MS, Cooke MB, Ballantyne D. Effects of daily high-intensity exercise on myocardial perfusion in angina pectoris. *Am J Cardiol* 1991;**68**:1593–9.

71. Laslett LJ, Paumer L, Amsterdam EA. Increase in myocardial oxygen consumption index by exercise training at the onset of ischemia in patients with coronary artery disease. *Circulation* 1985;**71**:958–62.

72. Williams MA, Ades PA, Hamm LF *et al.* Clinical evidence for a health benefit from cardiac rehabilitation: an update. *Am Heart J* 2006;**152**:835–41.

73. Balady GJ, Williams MA, Ades PA *et al.* Core components of cardiac rehabilitation/secondary prevention programs: 2007 update. A scientific statement from the American Heart Association Exercise, Cardiac Rehabilitation, and Prevention Committee; the Councils on Cardiovascular Nursing, Epidemiology and Prevention, and Nutrition, Physical Activity, and Metabolism; and the American Association of Cardiovascular and Pulmonary Rehabilitation. *Circulation* 2007;**115**:2675–82.

16 Psychosocial factors

Annika Rosengren

Sahlgrenska University Hospital, Goteborg, Sweden

Introduction

In the world of evidence-based medicine, psychosocial factors occupy a precarious position. With few exceptions, there are not many meta-analyses, systematic reviews, and randomized controlled trials of interventions. These designs yield a high level of evidence but such studies are mostly lacking in studies of psychosocial factors. Most data are purely descriptive and observational, derived from prospective cohort studies or case–control designs. There is a lack of consensus on the measurement and validation of psychosocial constructs, and a very real risk of publication bias. Even though psychosocial factors may be counted among the modifiable risk factors for cardiovascular disease, interventions, medical or otherwise, are only rarely investigated. Accordingly, the data available can be categorized as, at most, providing mid-range evidence.

This is not to say, however, that psychosocial factors are unimportant in the study of cardiovascular health. In contrast, there is a wealth of indicators that psychosocial factors may be at least as important as biologic factors as causes of cardiovascular disease.[1,2] In one of the few studies attempting to quantify population attributable risk of both psychosocial factors and biologic/lifestyle factors, a composite of stress (at home, at work, financial), low locus of control, life events and depression was found to have a population attributable risk of 32%, comparable to the effect of smoking.[3] Even so, the importance of psychosocial factors is still controversial and it has been argued, based on prospective data, that factors such as vital exhaustion, psychologic stress, and social class add little to the overall prediction of coronary heart disease.[4]

This chapter aims **to review the strength of the data on how** psychosocial factors can influence the disease processes in cardiovascular diseases, chiefly coronary heart disease (CHD). Factors investigated in the literature pertaining to the psychosocial area as causal factors for CHD are reviewed, as are the same factors with respect to prognosis in patients with established CHD. Finally, psychosocial intervention studies, which aim to improve prognosis in patients, are explored.

Potential mechanisms

Psychosocial risk factors affect disease processes via biobehavioral pathways, for example through unhealthy behaviors like smoking, inactivity or adverse dietary patterns with increased risk for obesity, hypertension and the metabolic syndrome, or through biologic characteristics like increased cardiovascular/neuroendocrine reactivity in response to acute or chronic stress, increased platelet activation, increased inflammatory cytokines or demonstrable progress in atherosclerosis. In patients with established cardiovascular disease, psychosocial factors can affect treatment adherence and lifestyle improvement.

Several studies indicate that adverse psychosocial factors are associated with higher levels of risk factors.[5-7] Chronic stress may be a contributory factor to a positive energy balance leading to obesity and to the metabolic syndrome, as prospective investigations in the Whitehall II cohort have shown.[8,9] However, associations between adverse risk factor patterns and psychosocial risk factors are not consistently found. For example, with respect to socioeconomic status, higher rates of current and ever smoking among less well-educated subjects were found in some but not all of 11 European countries investigated.[10] In a Swedish study high occupational status was associated with better lipid levels and lower blood pressure in women, but not men.[11]

By and large, two methods for investigating psychobiologic pathways are used: laboratory or clinical studies of acute physiologic stress responses, and observational

Evidence-Based Cardiology, 3rd edition. Edited by S. Yusuf, J.A. Cairns, A.J. Camm, E.L. Fallen, and B.J. Gersh. © 2010 Blackwell Publishing, ISBN: 978-1-4051-5925-8.

studies involving the effect of chronic or recurrent psychosocial stimuli on morphology or physiologic function. An extensive literature in this area exists and has been reviewed,[12] with the conclusion that disturbed psychobiologic reactivity as in, for example, lower socioeconomic status adults is present for some stimuli but not others, and interactions need to be studied. One investigation cited, relevant to this, is the study by Everson *et al* in which progression of carotid atherosclerosis over 4 years was greatest among middle-aged men who were high stress responders, and had also been exposed to the chronic stress of high work place demands.[13]

Several other studies pertaining to stress tests in relation to other psychosocial factors have been published. Prolonged impairment of *endothelial function* was demonstrated to occur in healthy men after a brief episode of mental stress, potentially representing a link between stress and the atherogenic process.[14] In 34 male survivors of acute myocardial infarction (AMI), *platelet activation* in response to a stress test was heightened in men who had stated acute negative emotion in the two hours before the event.[15] *Coronary flow velocity reserve* was significantly reduced in healthy men during and after a mental stress test.[16] A recent study investigating 22 healthy middle-aged men who underwent a mental stress test demonstrated significant changes in coagulation measures, indicating that stress may elicit a hypercoagulable state.[17] These data corroborate an extensive earlier review which critically reviewed 68 articles, investigating psychosocial factors in both experimental and observational settings, with the conclusion that associations between psychologic factors and several coagulation and fibrinolysis variables provide a plausible biobehavioral link to coronary artery disease.[18]

Several observational studies have also investigated associations between psychosocial factors and putative pathophysiologic mediators. A Dutch study in 109 male white-collar workers investigated *cardiovascular reactivity* in relation to effort–reward imbalance and overcommitment (including inability to unwind after work). High imbalance was associated with a higher heart rate during work and directly after work, a higher systolic blood pressure during work and leisure time, and a lower 24-hour vagal tone.[19]

Following the results of early animal studies on psychosocial influences on atherosclerosis,[20] a recent US cross-sectional study, which investigated the effect of psychosocial measures on *coronary calcification* using electron beam tomography in 783 middle-aged men and women, found that indicators of social isolation were independently associated with elevated risk for the presence of calcification,[21] whereas there was no independent association with socioeconomic status. However, in a study of 155 healthy women with measures of positive and negative affect/cognitions, coronary calcification was unrelated to these measures whereas there was evidence of associations of psychosocial

attributes with aortic calcification.[22] Depressive symptoms, anger, anxiety, and chronic stress burden were not associated with coronary calcification in asymptomatic adults.[23]

The effects of acute psychologic stress on circulating *inflammatory factors* in humans have been reviewed in a meta-analysis suggesting a modest increase in circulating inflammatory markers following laboratory-induced psychologic stress.[24] Additionally, in a recent overview, potential additional mechanisms for the association between stress and cardiovascular morbidity were extensively reviewed.[25]

Prospective studies

In a systematic review updated until 2001, aiming to assess the relative strength of the epidemiologic evidence for causal links between psychosocial factors and CHD incidence among healthy populations, and prognosis among CHD patients, over 100 prospective cohort studies were included.[26] A previous systematic review, by the same team of researchers, was published in 1999.[2] For inclusion, papers had to meet four quality criteria relating to design, size, psychosocial variable specification and outcomes. Only prospective studies were accepted and they had to include at least 500 participants (etiologic studies in healthy populations) or 100 participants (for prognosis in patients with established CHD). Psychosocial factors were included if they were reported in at least two eligible study populations. In this review, unspecified "stress" was not included because it was considered too vague to be informative. Valid outcomes were limited to fatal CHD, sudden cardiac death, non-fatal myocardial infarction (MI), incident angina, incident heart failure and all-cause mortality (for prognostic studies only). In the first review,[2] 65 papers were included while the updated review identified an additional 71 papers, of which 41 were published between 1998 and June 2001. The factors evaluated were type A behavior pattern and hostility, depression, anxiety and distress, and psychosocial work characteristics.

With respect to type *A behavior and hostility*, both eliciting much interest because of early positive reports from North American populations,[27,28] 18 prospective studies were included in the review. The majority (12/18) of the studies did not support type A/hostility as a risk factor, and the studies did not show hostility alone to be a risk factor either. Whether type A might predict incident CHD was again investigated in a more recent study in middle-aged men. Over a nine-year follow-up, there was no overall increased risk of CHD associated with any type A score, but further analysis showed an increase in risk over the first five-year period and a decreased risk between five and nine years, indicating that type A may be a potential trigger, rather than affecting the process of atherosclerosis.[29] Other personality types incude *type D personality*, a construct which has not been widely studied as a potential risk factor but which nevertheless has attracted attention. Type D personality is characterized by a propensity for experiencing negative emotions, while simultaneously inhibiting these emotions in social contacts with others.[30,31] Although potentially indicating worse prognosis in cardiac patients, there are no data to support that type D personality predicts cardiovascular events in healthy populations.

In a systematic search of the literature on *depression* and risk of CHD to May 2000, Rugulies identified 11 studies.[32] Depression was associated with a significant increased risk of CHD in seven of the 11 studies, with clinical depression a stronger and more consistent predictor than depressive mood. A subsequent systematic review by Kuper *et al* found 22 prospective studies which investigated the association between depression and CHD in healthy populations.[26] Roughly one-third found no clear association, with the rest finding moderate or strong effects. There was no apparent difference in strength of association between studies with shorter or longer follow-up, indicating that findings from studies with shorter follow-up were probably not confounded by early disease causing depression. In another, more recent systematic review of studies of depression as a risk factor for coronary disease in people without clinical evidence of prior heart disease and with at least four years follow-up, and which also controlled for other major coronary disease risk factors, 10 studies met inclusion criteria. Nine reported significantly increased risk, including two with mixed results; one study reported no increased risk. The combined overall relative risk of depression for the onset of coronary disease was 1.64.[33] Since this review appeared, additional studies have been published, further supporting depression as a risk factor for CHD.[34,35] A concept which is related to depression, but where there is little conclusive evidence for effects over and above depression, or pre-existing disease, is *vital exhaustion*.[36,37]

Anxiety and/or stress were investigated in eight studies identified by Kuper *et al*, with inconsistent results, and studies with longer follow-up less likely to find an association.[26] Other than these, the INTERHEART Study, the largest study reported so far, which used a case–control design in 11 119 patients with a first MI from 52 countries and 13 648 controls matched for age, sex, and region, found that stress was more commonly reported by cases than by controls.[38] Psychosocial stress during the previous 12 months was assessed with two single-item questions about stress at work and stress at home. In these questions stress was defined as feeling irritable or anxious, or as having disturbed sleep because of conditions at home or at work. Compared with controls, cases reported more frequent periods of stress at home during the previous 12 months as well as more frequent periods of stress at work.

This study is limited because of the retrospective case–control design, where cases were interviewed during hospitalization following an acute MI and were asked to report on psychosocial risks during the 12 months before the event. However, prospective studies using similar questions on self-perceived stress have also been performed, providing additional, albeit moderate, support for the contention that stress is related to CHD. One study, using the same question as in INTERHEART, found self-perceived stress to predict CHD as well as cardiovascular mortality over a 12-year follow-up period from baseline,[39] with an odds ratio of 1.7 for cardiovascular disease (CVD) death after adjustment for occupational class and other relevant risk factors, although the predictive power for CHD incidence waned after two decades.[40]

Number of work stressors has been associated with increased cardiovascular mortality in the Multiple Risk Factor Intervention Trial.[41] During a nine-year follow-up of 12 336 men, those with three or more work stressors had an increased risk of CVD death of 26%, while the experience of divorce increased risk by 33%. Similar results were observed in a large prospective study involving 281 cases in 73 424 Japanese men and women.[42] An extreme stressor, such as the death of a child, was associated with an increased risk of MI in parents, particularly for fatal MI.[43] Even so, there are also several studies with no or very limited relation between various measures of stress and CHD[44–46] and the concept of stress as an independent risk factor has also been criticized on the grounds that self-reported stress is related to health-related behaviors and largely due to confounding by socioeconomic position[47] or by a greater propensity to report symptoms and to be hospitalized.[48]

The review of studies on *work stress* presented a particular challenge because of the wide variety of measures and lack of standardization. However, of the 13 etiologic studies reviewed by Kuper *et al*, only three did not find a clear association, whereas 10 were moderately supportive, supportive for at least a subset or showed strong evidence for an effect of work stress on incidence of CHD.[26] Several studies have been added to the literature since this review. Within the Whitehall II Study, a ratio of high efforts to rewards predicted higher risk of CHD, though only modestly so.[49] In a multinational study of six European cohorts from four European countries (Belgium, France, Spain and Sweden) consisting of 21 111 middle-aged male subjects, the Karasek job strain model of psychologic demands was used.[50] This model emerged as a moderate but independent predictor of acute coronary events. Recent findings from the Framingham Offspring Study did not, however, support high job strain as a significant risk factor for CHD in men or women.[51] Possibly, effects for women differ from those for men, with recent prospective studies not showing a relation between job stress and CHD for women.[52,53]

Social supports and networks relate to the number and quality of a person's social contacts, including emotional support. Heterogeneous approaches have been used to measure this construct. The systematic review by Kuper *et al* included nine studies, with three not showing an association, four moderately supportive, and two strongly supportive.[26] In one of the latter, a subsequent follow-up found that both social integration and emotional support protected against CHD over an extended follow-up of 15 years.[54] In a prospective cohort study of 9011 British civil servants, negative aspects of close relationships were weakly but independently associated with future CHD events, including angina pectoris, over a 12-year follow-up period.[55] Further confirmation for the role of social support is provided in a review by Lett *et al*,[56] although more research is needed to determine which types of functional and structural support are most strongly related to outcome.

There is a large body of literature concerning *socioeconomic status (SES)* and coronary heart disease. A much-cited review published in 1993[57] indicated that there is a substantial body of evidence for a consistent relation between SES and the incidence and prevalence of cardiovascular disease, secular trends in cardiovascular mortality, survival with cardiovascular disease, and the prevalence of cardiovascular risk factors. By and large, more recent findings have not challenged these conclusions, at least not for Western populations.

There are several ways of measuring SES, with education, income, and occupational position most often used, but there is an increasing awareness that these variables cannot be used interchangeably.[58] In a study using Swedish and German register data, correlations between education, income, and occupational class were only low to moderate.[59] Which of these yielded the strongest effects on health depended on the type of health outcome in question. MI morbidity and mortality showed a mixed picture, with steeper gradients in the German than in the Swedish population. In mutually adjusted analyses each social dimension had an independent effect on each health outcome in both countries. The authors concluded that treating education, income, and occupational class as indicators of the same fundamental cause will understate their independent and distinct contributions to health.

Because there are differences in the distribution of risk factors, there has been a debate whether the effect of SES merely reflects these differences or whether there is an independent effect.[60,61] In addition, a relation between low SES and occupation has not been consistently observed in all populations. In one study in Europe a north–south gradient was observed, with CHD mortality strongly related to occupational class in England and Wales, Ireland, Finland, Sweden, Norway, and Denmark but not in France, Switzerland, and Mediterranean countries.[62] Ignoring SES

in risk factor estimation has been suggested to underestimate CVD risk in deprived people.[63]

Adverse socioeconomic circumstances in childhood may confer a greater risk for adult CVD. A recently published systematic review identified 40 studies, the majority of which found a robust inverse association between childhood circumstances and CVD risk, although findings sometimes varied among specific outcomes, socioeconomic measures, and sex.[64]

Psychosocial factors and prognosis in cardiovascular disease

Several literature reviews[2,65,66] have concluded that of various psychologic and social variables related to prognosis in CHD patients, the cumulative evidence is strongest for depression. Two recent systematic reviews have shown that, in people with established coronary heart disease, depression predicts an approximate twofold increase in all-cause mortality and cardiac mortality.[67,68] While not a formal meta-analysis, a narrative review paper summarizing a large number of studies found that depression confers a relative risk between 1.5 and 2.0 for the onset of CHD in healthy individuals, whereas depression in patients with existing CHD confers a relative risk between 1.5 and 2.5 for cardiac morbidity and mortality.[69]

However, studies have not consistently found this association.[70-72] In addition, these meta-analyses have been criticized on the grounds that they have not adequately considered the role of reverse causality, commenting that patients with severe CHD at baseline, and consequently worse prognosis, may be more likely to report depressive symptoms and that this may confound the association between depression and CHD prognosis. In a subsequent meta-analysis which sought to address these issues, 34 prognostic studies were identified, with a pooled relative risk of 1.80.[73] Adjustment for left ventricular function was done in only eight studies; this attenuated the relative risk from 2.18 to 1.53, a 48% reduction. Accordingly, almost half of the increased risk in patients with depression was accounted for by severity of CHD at baseline, suggesting an important role for reverse causality.

It has also been questioned whether the effect of depression assessed at different time periods may differ. A recent investigation seeking to investigate the long-term impact of depression on cardiac mortality after MI and to assess whether the timing of depression influences the findings found that depression was not associated with cardiac mortality, whether detected immediately before MI, 12 months after MI or at both time points.[74] The authors concluded that association between depression and post-MI mortality is complex, possibly being limited to depression immediately after MI, which they did not measure. Further, when comparing prognosis in patients post-MI with incident depression, as compared with ongoing or recurrent depressions, it was found that only patients with incident post-MI depression had an impaired cardiovascular prognosis.[75] However, despite these considerations, the available evidence suggests an independent prognostic role for depressive symptoms in patients with CHD.

With respect to personality traits, *type A/hostility* was not associated with an adverse prognosis in patients with CHD in the systematic review by Kuper *et al.*[26] In contrast, nonsystematic reviews have concluded that cardiac patients with *type D personality*, "a gloomy, anxious, and socially inept worrier",[30] are at increased risk for cardiovascular morbidity and mortality independent of cardiac risk factors. These conclusions were, however, based on comparatively few studies and most were derived from the same group of researchers. In addition, the extent to which the findings for type D personality are confounded by depression and other psychosocial factors is still unclear. Accordingly, more studies are needed to establish the role of type D personality as a negative prognostic factor in patients with CHD.

SES is usually not considered to be among the modifiable risk factors although low SES is often associated with an adverse lifestyle. Mortality from CHD has been associated with SES.[57,76] In comparison, far less is known about the effect of SES on prognosis after AMI. Associations between individual SES and long-term prognosis after AMI have been investigated.[77–79] In one US study of 3423 confirmed cases of AMI among metropolitan Worcester residents, a 30% higher death rate was estimated after AMI for patients living in census tracts with the most residents living below the poverty line compared with patients living in the wealthiest census tracts. Similarly, patients living in census tracts with the highest proportion of residents with less than a high school education experienced a 47% higher death rate than patients living in census tracts with the lowest proportion of residents with less than a high school education.[80] In one recent study of 3407 patients who were hospitalized for AMI in 53 large-volume hospitals in Canada, income was strongly and inversely correlated with two-year mortality rate. However, after adjustment for age and pre-existing cardiovascular events or conventional vascular risk factors, the effect of income was greatly attenuated, which suggests that the "wealth–health gradient" in cardiovascular mortality may be partially ameliorated by improved management of known risk factors.[81]

In one prospective study of women with CHD, level of marital stress, according to the Stockholm Marital Stress Scale, was associated with a higher risk of recurrent events.[82] Stress from family or work life may accelerate coronary disease processes in women, whereas relative protection may be obtained from a satisfactory job and a happy marriage. In a study of 80 female CHD patients who were evaluated for stress exposure and coronary atherosclerosis progression using serial quantitative coronary angiography, women with high stress from either family or work had significant disease progression over three years, whereas those with low stress had only slight progression.[83] One recent study found that a high level of anxiety in patients with documented chronic ischemic heart disease (IHD) constitutes a strong risk of subsequent myocardial infarction or death.[84]

The association of job strain with the risk of recurrent CHD events after a first MI has been documented in only two relatively small prospective studies whose findings were inconsistent.[82,85] However, in a recent prospective cohort study of 972 men and women who returned to work after a first MI, where a combination of high psychologic demands and low decision latitude was evaluated, chronic job strain was associated with a doubled risk of recurrent CHD which persisted in a multivariate model adjusted for 26 potentially confounding factors.[86]

Interventions

Stress management training aims to reduce stress and this, as well as other psychologic interventions, can form part of cardiac rehabilitation programs. A recent Cochrane review aimed to determine the effectiveness of psychologic interventions, in particular stress management interventions, on mortality and morbidity, psychologic measures, quality of life, and modifiable cardiac risk factors, in patients with coronary heart disease.[87] Randomized controlled trials of non-pharmacologic psychologic interventions until 2001, with a minimum follow-up of six months, were identified. Thirty six trials with altogether almost 13 000 patients were included. The quality of many trials was considered to be poor, with the majority not reporting adequate concealment of allocation or blinded assessment of outcome. Combining the results of all trials showed no strong evidence of effect on total or cardiac mortality, or revascularization. There was a reduction in the number of non-fatal reinfarctions in the intervention group but the two largest trials (comprising over a third of all randomized patients) were neutral, and there was statistical evidence of publication bias. The reviewers concluded that, overall, psychologic interventions showed no evidence of effect on prognosis with respect to total or cardiac mortality. Small reductions in anxiety and depression in patients were found. Trials which specifically considered stress management did not differ from the overall findings for all the trials. The authors considered that the poor quality of trials, heterogeneity observed between trials and significant publication bias made the pooled finding of a reduction in non-fatal myocardial infarction uncertain.

Psychologic treatment is sometimes a component of comprehensive cardiac rehabilitation, a broad class of interventions targeting lifestyle, for instance smoking, lack of exercise, poor eating habits, and often also psychologic distress. Most interventions use cognitive-behavioral interventions to reduce distress but the prognostic benefit of added psychologic treatment in cardiac rehabilitation programs is still in question. In a meta-analysis of 37 studies, the effects of psychoeducational (health education and stress management) programs for coronary heart disease patients were examined, with a suggested 34% reduction in cardiac mortality, a 29% reduction in recurrence of MI, and significant positive effects on blood pressure, cholesterol, body weight, smoking behavior, physical exercise, and eating habits.[88] However, the interventions used were highly heterogeneous and, in addition, studies with non-randomized designs were included. In a review from 2007, the authors identified 23 randomized trials of psychologic treatments which reported mortality data.[89] There was an overall beneficial effect on mortality for up to two years, but not thereafter. In addition, mortality benefits only applied to men, and for studies initiated at least two months after an event. Relaxation therapy, defined as teaching means to reduce tension, was reviewed, with relevant publications included in a meta-analysis, which, however, included non-randomized trials.[90] The most relevant findings were reduced heart rate, anxiety and angina. There were also reductions in cardiac events and in mortality, although the authors point out that there were few events.

Even though depression has been shown to be a negative prognostic factor in patients with IHD, it is at present not proven that *treatment of depression* helps improve survival. However, antidepressants have been demonstrated to be safe to use after an MI and effective in treating depression. The SADHART Study found sertraline to be a safe treatment for depression post-MI, but there was little difference in depression status between groups receiving sertraline and placebo after 24 weeks of treatment.[91] However, the effect of sertraline was greater in the patients with severe and recurrent depression. The study was not designed to assess the effects of treatment on cardiovascular prognosis, but severe cardiovascular events during the six-month treatment tended to be less frequent in the sertraline group.[91] In a randomized controlled trial (Enhancing Recovery in Coronary Heart Disease patients – ENRICHD) which examined the effect of cognitive behavior therapy, supplemented with a selective serotonin reuptake inhibitor when indicated, the intervention did not increase event-free survival.[92] Positive subgroup analyses have been reported from ENRICHD, but these findings require confirmation.[93,94] In a more recent substudy of the ENRICHD study the psychosocial intervention did not affect late mortality, but intervention patients whose depression did not improve were at higher risk for late mortality than were

patients who responded to treatment.[95] Additionally, in the Myocardial INfarction and Depression-Intervention Trial (MIND-IT) which sought to determine, using a randomized controlled design, whether antidepressant treatment for depression post-MI improved depression or cardiovascular prognosis, no differences were observed between intervention and control groups with respect to depression. The cardiac event rate was 14% among the intervention group and 13% among controls.[96]

Although *low levels of support* are associated with increased risk for CHD events, it is not clear what types of support are most associated with clinical outcomes in healthy persons and CHD patients.[56] Additionally, there is little scientific evidence about how, and how well, social support interventions work. Hogan *et al*, using a computerized search strategy, found 100 studies that evaluated the efficacy of a range of such interventions targeting a wide variety of problems.[97] Some of the studies using individual interventions through professionals targeted patients with ischemic heart disease, with positive effects on myocardial infarction recurrences and mortality. However, a similar intervention, which tried to replicate the results from earlier interventions, found that the supportive intervention had no survival impact.[98] Additionally, women in the treatment group had marginally higher cardiac and all-cause mortality than women in the control group. Neither of the two reviews found any conclusive evidence that interventions targeting social support improves outcome with respect to mortality or new events but, on the other hand, few studies have been specifically designed to answer this question.

Conclusions and directions for the future

Altogether, studies strongly suggest a role for psychosocial factors as causes and prognostic factors in cardiovascular disease. There are, however, several limitations to many studies in this area. A large proportion of the literature on psychosocial factors is derived from secondary analyses of data collected for other purposes, and accordingly, there is no means to keep track of analyses that have been done or which potentially could be performed. Accordingly, publication bias cannot be systematically evaluated. Further bias may occur after publication, where positive results may be more frequently cited than neutral or negative findings. Additionally, with few exceptions, data are derived from predominantly Caucasian, Western populations with very few data from other parts of the world, where most cases currently occur. Data from low- and middle-income countries and non-Western high-income countries are badly needed.

There is, so far, no or little evidence that any interventions targeting psychosocial factors improve prognosis in patients with cardiovascular disease, partly because of the heterogeneity, sometimes doubtful designs and non-optimal methodology of some studies. Equally, however, it is not possible to entirely dismiss potential beneficial prognostic effects on the basis of the data available. In the future, considerable attention needs to be given to methodologic and design issues, not least since the population sizes needed will require multicenter and probably multinational participation.

References

1. Rozanski A, Blumenthal JA, Davidson KW, Saab PG, Kubzansky L. The epidemiology, pathophysiology, and management of psychosocial risk factors in cardiac practice: the emerging field of behavioral cardiology. *J Am Coll Cardiol* 2005;**45**:637–51.

2. Hemingway H, Marmot M. Evidence based cardiology: psychosocial factors in the aetiology and prognosis of coronary heart disease. Systematic review of prospective cohort studies. *BMJ* 1999;**318**:1460–7.

3. Yusuf S, Hawken S, Ounpuu S *et al.* Effect of potentially modifiable risk factors associated with myocardial infarction in 52 countries (the INTERHEART study): case–control study. *Lancet* 2004;**364**:937–52.

4. Macleod J, Metcalfe C, Smith GD, Hart C. Does consideration of either psychological or material disadvantage improve coronary risk prediction? Prospective observational study of Scottish men. *J Epidemiol Community Health* 2007;**61**:833–7.

5. Brummett BH, Babyak MA, Siegler IC, Mark DB, Williams RB, Barefoot JC. Effect of smoking and sedentary behavior on the association between depressive symptoms and mortality from coronary heart disease. *Am J Cardiol* 2003;**92**:529–32.

6. Bonnet F, Irving K, Terra JL, Nony P, Berthezène F, Moulin P. Anxiety and depression are associated with unhealthy lifestyle in patients at risk of cardiovascular disease. *Atherosclerosis* 2005;**178**:339–44.

7. Bonnet F, Irving K, Terra JL, Nony P, Berthezène F, Moulin P. Depressive symptoms are associated with unhealthy lifestyles in hypertensive patients with the metabolic syndrome. *J Hypertens* 2005;**23**:611–17.

8. Brunner EJ, Chandola T, Marmot MG. Prospective effect of job strain on general and central obesity in the Whitehall II Study. *Am J Epidemiol* 2007;**165**:828–37.

9. Chandola T, Brunner E, Marmot M. Chronic stress at work and the metabolic syndrome: prospective study. *BMJ* 2006;**332**: 521–5.

10. Cavelaars AE, Kunst AE, Geurts JJ *et al.* Educational differences in smoking: international comparison. *BMJ* 2000;**320**:1102–7.

11. Manhem K, Dotevall A, Wilhelmsen L, Rosengren A. Social gradients in cardiovascular risk factors and symptoms of Swedish men and women: the Göteborg MONICA Study 1995. *J Cardiovasc Risk* 2000;**7**:359–68.

12. Steptoe A, Marmot M. The role of psychobiological pathways in socio-economic inequalities in cardiovascular disease risk. *Eur Heart J* 2002;**23**:13–25.

13. Everson SA, Lynch JW, Chesney MA *et al.* Interaction of workplace demands and cardiovascular reactivity in progression of carotid atherosclerosis: population based study. *BMJ* 1997; **314**:553–8.

14. Ghiadoni L, Donald AE, Cropley M *et al.* Mental stress induces transient endothelial dysfunction in humans. *Circulation* 2000; **102**:2473–8.

15. Strike PC, Magid K, Whitehead DL, Brydon L, Bhattacharyya MR, Steptoe A. Pathophysiological processes underlying emotional triggering of acute cardiac events. *Proc Natl Acad Sci* 2006;**103**:4322–7.

16. Hasegawa R, Daimon M, Toyoda T *et al.* Effect of mental stress on coronary flow velocity reserve in healthy men. *Am J Cardiol* 2005;**96**:137–40.

17. Zgraggen L, Fischer JE, Mischler K, Preckel D, Kudielka BM, von Känel R. Relationship between hemoconcentration and blood coagulation responses to acute mental stress. *Thromb Res* 2005;**115**:175–83.

18. von Känel R, Mills PJ, Fainman C, Dimsdale JE. Effects of psychological stress and psychiatric disorders on blood coagulation and fibrinolysis: a biobehavioral pathway to coronary artery disease? *Psychosom Med* 2001;**63**:531–44.

19. Vrijkotte TG, van Doornen LJ, de Geus EJ. Overcommitment to work is associated with changes in cardiac sympathetic regulation. *Psychosom Med* 2004;**66**:656–63.

20. Clarkson TB, Kaplan JR, Adams MR, Manuck SB. Psychosocial influences on the pathogenesis of atherosclerosis among nonhuman primates. *Circulation* 1987;**76**:I29–40.

21. Kop WJ, Berman DS, Gransar H *et al.* Social network and coronary artery calcification in asymptomatic individuals. *Psychosom Med* 2005;**67**:343–52.

22. Matthews KA, Owens JF, Edmundowicz D, Lee L, Kuller LH. Positive and negative attributes and risk for coronary and aortic calcification in healthy women. *Psychosom Med* 2006;**68**:355–61.

23. Diez Roux AV, Ranjit N, Powell L *et al.* Psychosocial factors and coronary calcium in adults without clinical cardiovascular disease. *Ann Intern Med* 2006;**144**:822–31.

24. Steptoe A, Hamer M, Chida Y. The effects of acute psychological stress on circulating inflammatory factors in humans: a review and meta-analysis. *Brain Behav Immun* 2007;**21**:901–12.

25. Brotman DJ, Golden SH, Wittstein IS. The cardiovascular toll of stress. *Lancet* 2007;**370**:1089–100.

26. Kuper H, Marmot M, Hemingway H. Systematic review of prospective cohort studies of psychosocial factors in the etiology and prognosis of coronary heart disease. *Semin Vasc Med* 2002;**2**:267–314.

27. Rosenman RH, Brand RJ, Sholtz RI, Friedman M. Multivariate prediction of coronary heart disease during 8.5 year follow-up in Western Collaborative Group Study. *Am J Cardiol* 1976;**37**:903–9.

28. Haynes SG, Feinleib M, Kannel WB. The relationship of psychosocial factors to coronary heart disease in the Framingham study: 3. Eight year incidence of coronary heart disease. *Am J Epidemiol* 1980;**111**:37–58.

29. Gallacher JE, Sweetnam PM, Yarnell JW, Elwood PC, Stansfeld SA. Is type A behavior really a trigger for coronary heart disease events? *Psychosom Med* 2003;**65**:339–46.

30. Sher L. Type D personality: the heart, stress, and cortisol. *QJM* 2005;**98**:323–9.

31. Pedersen SS, Denollet J. Type D personality, cardiac events, and impaired quality of life: a review. *Eur J Cardiovasc Prev Rehabil* 2003;**10**:241–8.

32. Rugulies R. Depression as a predictor for coronary heart disease. a review and meta-analysis. *Am J Prev Med* 2002;**23**:51–61.

33. Wulsin LR, Singal BM. Do depressive symptoms increase the risk for the onset of coronary disease? A systematic quantitative review. *Psychosom Med* 2003;**65**:201–10.

34. Empana JP, Jouven X, Lemaitre RN *et al.* Clinical depression and risk of out-of-hospital cardiac arrest. *Arch Intern Med* 2006;**166**:195–200.

35. Mykletun A, Bjerkeset O, Dewey M, Prince M, Overland S, Stewart R. Anxiety, depression, and cause-specific mortality: the HUNT Study. *Psychosom Med* 2007;**69**:323–31.

36. Prescott E, Holst C, Gronbaek M, Schnohr P, Jensen G, Barefoot J. Vital exhaustion as a risk factor for ischaemic heart disease and all-cause mortality in a community sample. A prospective study of 4084 men and 5479 women in the Copenhagen City Heart Study. *Int J Epidemiol* 2003;**32**:990–7.

37. Appels A. Exhaustion and coronary heart disease: the history of a scientific quest. *Patient Educ Couns* 2004;**55**:223–9.

38. Rosengren A, Hawken S, Ounpuu S *et al.* Association of psychosocial risk factors with risk of acute myocardial infarction in 11119 cases and 13648 controls from 52 countries (the INTERHEART study): case–control study. *Lancet* 2004;**364**:953–62.

39. Rosengren A, Tibblin G, Wilhelmsen L. Self-perceived psychological stress and incidence of coronary artery disease in middle-aged men. *Am J Cardiol* 1991;**68**:1171–5.

40. Wilhelmsen L, Lappas G, Rosengren A. Risk of coronary events by baseline factors during 28 years follow-up and three periods in a random population sample of men. *J Intern Med* 2004;**256**:298–307.

41. Matthews KA, Gump BB. Chronic work stress and marital dissolution increase risk of posttrial mortality in men from the Multiple Risk Factor Intervention Trial. *Arch Intern Med* 2002;**162**:309–15.

42. Iso H, Date C, Yamamoto A *et al.* Perceived mental stress and mortality from cardiovascular disease among Japanese men and women: the Japan Collaborative Cohort Study for Evaluation of Cancer Risk. *Circulation* 2002;**106**:1229–36.

43. Li J, Hansen D, Mortensen PB, Olsen J. Myocardial infarction in parents who lost a child: a nationwide prospective cohort study in Denmark. *Circulation* 2002;**106**:1634–9.

44. Moore L, Meyer F, Perusse M *et al.* Psychological stress and incidence of ischaemic heart disease. *Int J Epidemiol* 1999;**28**:652–8.

45. Macleod J, Davey Smith G, Heslop P, Metcalfe C, Carroll D, Hart C. Psychological stress and cardiovascular disease: empirical demonstration of bias in a prospective observational study of Scottish men. *BMJ* 2002;**324**:1247–51.

46. Ohlin B, Nilsson PM, Nilsson JA, Berglund G. Chronic psychosocial stress predicts long-term cardiovascular morbidity and mortality in middle-aged men. *Eur Heart J* 2004;**25**:867–73.

47. Heslop P, Smith GD, Carroll D, Macleod J, Hyland F, Hart C. Perceived stress and coronary heart disease risk factors: the contribution of socio-economic position. *Br J Health Psychol* 2001;**6**:167–78.

48. Metcalfe C, Davey Smith G, Macleod J, Heslop P, Hart C. Self-reported stress and subsequent hospital admissions as a result of hypertension, varicose veins and haemorrhoids. *J Public Health Med* 2003;**25**:62–8.

49. Kuper H, Singh-Manoux A, Siegrist J, Marmot M. When reciprocity fails: effort–reward imbalance in relation to coronary heart disease and health functioning within the Whitehall II study. *Occup Environ Med* 2002;**59**:777–84.

50. Kornitzer M, deSmet P, Sans S. Job stress and major coronary events: results from the Job Stress, Absenteeism and Coronary Heart Disease in Europe study. *Eur J Cardiovasc Prev Rehabil* 2006;**13**:695–704.

51. Eaker ED, Sullivan LM, Kelly-Hayes M, D'Agostino RB Sr, Benjamin EJ. Does job strain increase the risk for coronary heart disease or death in men and women? The Framingham Offspring Study. *Am J Epidemiol* 2004;**159**:950–8.

52. Kuper H, Adami HO, Theorell T, Weiderpass E. Psychosocial determinants of coronary heart disease in middle-aged women: a prospective study in Sweden. *Am J Epidemiol* 2006;**164**:349–57.

53. Lee S, Colditz G, Berkman L, Kawachi I. A prospective study of job strain and coronary heart disease in US women. *Int J Epidemiol* 2002;**31**:1147–53.

54. Rosengren A, Wilhelmsen L, Orth-Gomer K. Coronary disease in relation to social support and social class in Swedish men: a 15 year follow-up in the study of men born in 1933. *Eur Heart J* 2004;**5**:56–63.

55. De Vogli R, Chandola T, Marmot MG. Negative aspects of close relationships and heart diseae. *Arch Intern Med* 2007;**167**:1951–7.

56. Lett HS, Blumenthal JA, Babyak MA, Strauman TJ, Robins C, Sherwood A. Social support and coronary heart disease: epidemiologic evidence and implications for treatment. *Psychosom Med* 2005;**67**:869–78.

57. Kaplan GA, Keil JE. Socioeconomic factors and cardiovascular disease: a review of the literature. *Circulation* 1993;**88**:1973–98.

58. Braveman PA, Cubbin C, Egerter S *et al.* Socioeconomic status in health research: one size does not fit all. *JAMA* 2005;**294**: 2879–88.

59. Geyer S, Hemström O, Peter R, Vågerö D. Education, income, and occupational class cannot be used interchangeably in social epidemiology. Empirical evidence against a common practice. *J Epidemiol Community Health* 2006;**60**:804–10.

60. Yarnell J, Yu S, McCrum E *et al.* Education, socioeconomic and lifestyle factors, and risk of coronary heart disease: the PRIME Study. *Int J Epidemiol* 2005;**34**:268–75.

61. Lynch J, Davey Smith G, Harper S, Bainbridge K. Explaining the social gradient in coronary heart disease: comparing relative and absolute risk approaches. *J Epidemiol Community Health* 2006;**60**: 436–41.

62. Kunst AE, Groenhof F, Mackenbach JP. Mortality by occupational class among men 30–64 years in 11 European countries. EU Working Group on Socioeconomic Inequalities in Health. *Soc Sci Med* 1998;**46**:1459–76.

63. Woodward M, Brindle P, Tunstall-Pedoe H. Adding social deprivation and family history to cardiovascular risk assessment: the ASSIGN score from the Scottish Heart Health Extended Cohort (SHHEC). *Heart* 2007;**93**:172–6.

64. Galobardes B, Smith GD, Lynch JW. Systematic review of the influence of childhood socioeconomic circumstances on risk for cardiovascular disease in adulthood. *Ann Epidemiol* 2006;**16**: 91–104.

65. Rozanski A, Blumenthal JA, Kaplan J. Impact of psychological factors on the pathogenesis of cardiovascular disease and implications for therapy. *Circulation* 1999;**99**:2192–217.

66. Januzzi JL Jr, Stern TA, Pasternak RC, DeSanctis RW. The influence of anxiety and depression on outcomes of patients with coronary artery disease. *Arch Intern Med* 2000;**160**:1913–21.

67. Barth J, Schumacher M, Herrmann-Lingen C. Depression as a risk factor for mortality in patients with coronary heart disease: a meta-analysis. *Psychosom Med* 2004;**66**:802–13.

68. van Melle JP, de Jonge P, Spijkerman TA *et al.* Prognostic association of depression following myocardial infarction with mortality and cardiovascular events: a meta-analysis. *Psychosom Med* 2004;**66**:814–22.

69. Lett HS, Blumenthal JA, Babyak MA *et al.* Depression as a risk factor for coronary artery disease: evidence, mechanisms, and treatment. *Psychosom Med* 2004;**66**:305–15.

70. Dickens CM, McGowan L, Percival C *et al.* Lack of a close confidant, but not depression, predicts further cardiac events after myocardial infarction. *Heart* 2004;**90**:518–22.

71. Lane D, Carroll D, Ring C, Beevers DG, Lip GY. Do depression and anxiety predict recurrent coronary events 12 months after myocardial infarction? *QJM* 2000;**93**:739–44.

72. Mayou RA, Gill D, Thompson DR *et al.* Depression and anxiety as predictors of outcome after myocardial infarction. *Psychosom Med* 2000;**62**:212–19.

73. Nicholson A, Kuper H, Hemingway H. Depression as an aetiologic and prognostic factor in coronary heart disease: a meta-analysis of 6362 events among 146 538 participants in 54 observational studies. *Eur Heart J* 2006;**27**:2763–74.

74. Dickens C, McGowan L, Percival C *et al.* Depression is a risk factor for mortality after myocardial infarction: fact or artifact? *J Am Coll Cardiol* 2007;**49**:1834–40.

75. de Jonge P, van den Brink RH, Spijkerman TA, Ormel J. Only incident depressive episodes after myocardial infarction are associated with new cardiovascular events. *J Am Coll Cardiol* 2006;**48**:2204–8.

76. Smith GD, Hart C, Watt G, Hole D, Hawthorne V. Individual social class, area-based deprivation, cardiovascular disease risk factors, and mortality: the Renfrew and Paisley Study. *J Epidemiol Community Health* 1998;**52**:399–405.

77. Greenwood D, Packham C, Muir K, Madeley R. How do economic status and social support influence survival after initial recovery from acute myocardial infarction? *Soc Sci Med* 1995;**40**: 639–47.

78. Rao SV, Schulman KA, Curtis LH, Gersh BJ, Jollis JG. Socioeconomic status and outcome following acute myocardial infarction in elderly patients. *Arch Intern Med* 2004;**164**:1128–33.

79. Rasmussen JN, Rasmussen S, Gislason GH *et al.* Mortality after acute myocardial infarction according to income and education. *J Epidemiol Community Health* 2006;**60**:351–6.

80. Tonne C, Schwartz J, Mittleman M, Melly S, Suh H, Goldberg R. Long-term survival after acute myocardial infarction is lower in more deprived neighborhoods. *Circulation* 2005;**111**:3063–70.

81. Alter DA, Chong A, Austin PC *et al.* Socioeconomic status and mortality after acute myocardial infarction. *Ann Intern Med* 2006;**144**:82–93.

82. Orth-Gomér K, Wamala SP, Horsten M *et al.* Marital stress worsens prognosis in women with coronary heart disease: the Stockholm Female Coronary Risk Study. *JAMA* 2000;**284**: 3008–14.

83. Wang HX, Leineweber C, Kirkeeide R *et al.* Psychosocial stress and atherosclerosis: family and work stress accelerate progression of coronary disease in women. The Stockholm Female Coronary Angiography Study. *J Intern Med* 2007;**261**:245–54.

84. Shibeshi WA, Young-Xu Y, Blatt CM. Anxiety worsens prognosis in patients with coronary artery disease. *J Am Coll Cardiol* 2007;**49**:2021–7.

85. Theorell T, Perski A, Orth-Gomer K *et al.* The effects of the strain of returning to work on the risk of cardiac death after a first myocardial infarction before the age of 45. *Int J Cardiol* 1991;**30**: 61–7.

86. Aboa-Eboule C, Brisson C, Maunsell E *et al.* Job strain and risk of acute recurrent coronary heart disease events. *JAMA* 2007;**298**:1652–60.

87. Rees K, Bennett P, West R, Davey Smith G, Ebrahim S. Psychological interventions for coronary heart disease. *Cochrane Database of Systematic Reviews* 2004, Issue 2. Art. No.: CD002902. DOI: 10.1002/14651858.CD002902.pub2.

88. Dusseldorp E, van Elderen T, Maes S, Meulman J, Kraaij V. A meta-analysis of psychoeduational programs for coronary heart disease patients. *Health Psychol* 1999;**18**:506–19.

89. Linden W, Phillips MJ, Leclerc J. Psychological treatment of cardiac patients: a meta-analysis. *Eur Heart J* 2007;**28**:2972–84.

90. van Dixhoorn J, White A. Relaxation therapy for rehabilitation and prevention in ischaemic heart disease: a systematic review and meta-analysis. *Eur J Cardiovasc Prev Rehabil* 2005;**12**:193–202.

91. Glassman AH, O'Connor CM, Califf RM *et al.* Sertraline treatment of major depression in patients with acute MI or unstable angina. *JAMA* 2002;**288**:701–9.

92. Berkman LF, Blumenthal J, Burg M *et al.* Effects of treating depression and low perceived social support on clinical events after myocardial infarction: the Enhancing Recovery in Coronary Heart Disease Patients (ENRICHD) Randomized Trial. *JAMA* 2003;**289**:3106–16.

93. Schneiderman N, Saab PG, Catellier DJ *et al.* Psychosocial treatment within sex by ethnicity subgroups in the Enhancing Recovery in Coronary Heart Disease clinical trial. *Psychosom Med* 2004;**66**:475–83.

94. Taylor CB, Youngblood ME, Catellier D *et al.* Effects of antidepressant medication on morbidity and mortality in depressed patients after myocardial infarction. *Arch Gen Psychiatry* 2005;**62**:792–8.

95. Carney RM, Blumenthal JA, Freedland KE *et al.* Depression and late mortality after myocardial infarction in the Enhancing Recovery in Coronary Heart Disease (ENRICHD) study. *Psychosom Med* 2004;**66**:466–74.

96. Van Melle JP, de Jonge P, Honig A. Effects of antidepressant treatment following myocardial infarction. *Br J Psychiatry* 2007;**190**:460–6.

97. Hogan BE, Linden W, Najarian B. Social support interventions: do they work? *Clin Psychol Rev* 2002;**22**:381–440.

98. Frasure-Smith N, Lesperance F, Prince RH *et al.* Randomised trial of home-based psychosocial nursing intervention for patients recovering from myocardial infarction. *Lancet* 1997;**350**:473–9.

17 The social determinants of cardiovascular disease

Martin McKee[1] and Clara K Chow[2]
[1] London School of Hygiene and Tropical Medicine, London, UK
[2] Hamilton General Hospital, Hamilton, Ontario, Canada

Introduction

Research over the past four decades has greatly increased our understanding of the proximal determinants of cardiovascular disease, beginning with the pioneering work of Ancell Keys and his colleagues in the Seven Countries Study, which identified the role of cholesterol,[1] and progressing by means of international collaborations such as the MONICA project[2] to, most recently, the INTERHEART Study.[3] The last of these studies, which included subjects from 52 countries in all regions of the world, showed how nine risk factors (abnormal lipids, smoking, hypertension, diabetes, abdominal obesity, psychosocial factors, consumption of fruits, vegetables, and alcohol, and regular physical activity) could account for almost all the variation observed in myocardial infarction. Studies such as these provide an answer to the question "Why are some people healthy and others not?".[4] However, they raise the further question, first posed by Geoffrey Rose, of why some *populations* are healthy and others are not.[5] These risk factors are not distributed at random in the population but are geographically and socially patterned.

The consequence is that deaths from cardiovascular disease vary markedly among and within populations and their distribution is constantly changing. Beginning as a disease of the upper classes in industrialized countries, its subsequent increases among the lower classes would soon reverse the social gradient.[6] More recently, marked declines among those better off have not been seen among the poor, leading to a widening social gap.[7] The long-standing advantage enjoyed by countries in Southern Europe is now being eroded,[8] at a time when once very high rates in Nordic countries are falling rapidly. In the former Soviet Union death rates have fluctuated dramatically over the course of the past two decades, while remaining consistently very much higher than in Western Europe.[9]

It is also important to note, in a situation where medicine is increasingly dominated by the search for genetic explanations of disease, that levels of risk change when individuals move from one setting to another, elegantly described in studies of Japanese migrating to Hawaii and California.[10] The risk of cardiovascular disease is substantially influenced by the environment that the individual inhabits.

The reasons for some of the patterns that can be observed are either obvious or have been understood through research. Those living in the countries bordering the Mediterranean benefited from their geographical location and consequently their climate, which allowed them to produce the components now referred to as the Mediterranean diet, rich in fruit and vegetables and olive oil. Contemporary increases in mortality in some parts of Greece can plausibly be explained by a failure to reduce smoking rates. In Russia and its neighbors, the high cardiovascular mortality can be explained by, in addition to the traditional risk factors, the widespread practice of episodic heavy drinking, especially of surrogate products such as aftershaves.[11] coupled with weaknesses in the healthcare system and, especially, the management of hypertension.[12] Within societies, differences in smoking and diet, which are shaped by the environments that people inhabit, can also go some way to explaining social inequalities, and indeed some research has suggested that they may themselves be sufficient.[13]

However, there is an extensive body of research suggesting that psychosocial factors play a part. The largest of these studies, INTERHEART, found that those suffering a myocardial infarction were significantly more likely to have experienced stress at work or at home, financial stress or major life events in the past year. Put another way, those suffering several episodes of stress or permanent stress at work were more likely to suffer an infarction (respectively, odds ratios (OR) 1.38, 99% confidence interval (CI) 1.19–

Evidence-Based Cardiology, 3rd edition. Edited by S. Yusuf, J.A. Cairns, A.J. Camm, E.L. Fallen, and B.J. Gersh. © 2010 Blackwell Publishing, ISBN: 978-1-4051-5925-8.

Environment

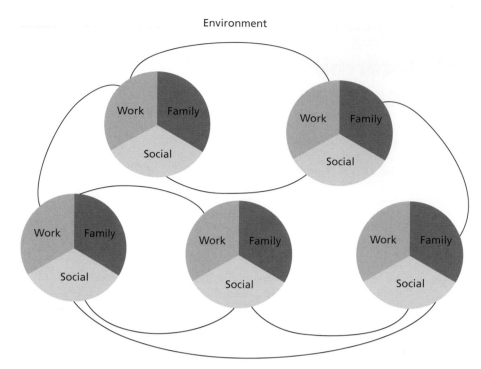

Figure 17.1 A simplified model of a community.

1.61, and OR 2.14, 99% CI 1.73–2.64), after adjustment for age, sex, geographic region, and smoking. The corresponding figures for several episodes or permanent stress at home were OR 1.52 (99% CI 1.34–1.72) and OR 2.12 (1.68–2.65). Severe financial stress and stressful life events in the past year showed similar associations (OR 1.33, 99% CI 1.19–1.48, and OR 1.48, 99% CI 1.33–1.64, respectively).[14]

This chapter begins from the intentionally simplified position that individuals inhabit three often overlapping communities, defined by their families, their work environment, and their social life. In each of these they have relations with other individuals. The roles that they fulfill and the relationships that they experience within each of these communities may impact on their risk of cardiovascular disease or their ability to survive it. Individuals also live within a larger community, where ties may be much looser but which surrounds them and whose environment is characterized by its physical, political, economic, social, and cultural attributes. This environment may impact on their risk of cardiovascular disease by virtue of the ease which it enables them to make healthy choices or constrains them from doing so. This framework is illustrated in Figure 17.1, with five individuals who are connected to each other through families, work, and social ties. Much of the rest of this chapter will focus on the evidence linking the nature and intensity of these connections, in these three domains, to cardiovascular disease, and on the way that the environment in which people live influences their degree of risk.

Family networks

The most intense social relationships are within the immediate family. There is considerable evidence that marriage is protective against cardiovascular disease, at least for men, who have been most intensively studied. Some research has been able to explain this on the basis of differences in risk factors.[15] Divorce is associated with taking up smoking or, among ex-smokers, relapsing, for both men and women.[16,17] In the Health Survey for England, single men and those with low social support were less likely to have hypertension adequately treated.[18] A small Israeli study found a more harmful pattern of lipids among divorced, separated or widowed women than in their married counterparts that was unexplained by age, smoking or physical activity.[19]

However, there is also considerable evidence that the excess risk associated with being unmarried persists after adjustment for conventional risk factors. In the British Regional Heart Study, single (never-married) men were at increased risk of dying from cardiovascular disease (relative risk (RR) 1.5, 95% CI 1.0–2.2) after adjustment for potentially confounding variables.[20] Men who were divorced or widowed at recruitment did not exhibit an increased risk but risk was greater among those who divorced during follow-up (RR 1.9, 95% CI 0.9–3.9), again unexplained by conventional risk factors. An increased risk associated with divorce was also found in the Multiple Risk

Factor Intervention Trial, which included men without evident cardiovascular disease at recruitment but who were at above-average risk on the basis of conventional risk factors.[21] In contrast, an analysis of the Whitehall Study found an excess risk of ischemic heart disease mortality associated with widowhood (RR 1.46, 95% CI 1.08–1.97). As it is possible that this could be associated with acute stress associated with bereavement, a subsequent analysis excluding deaths occurring in the first two years was undertaken, with the effect persisting.[22] In a cohort of over 90 000 Japanese men and women followed over 10 years, never-married men, compared with married men, were at a greater risk of cardiovascular mortality (RR 3.05, 95% CI 2.03–4.60) after adjustment for potentially confounding variables. Never-married women were also at greater risk, although less so than for men (RR 1.46, 95% CI 1.15–1.84). An increased risk was also seen among divorced and widowed men but not women.[23]

Some studies have also looked at the association between marital status and survival among those with established cardiovascular disease. Among men and women found to have significant disease at angiography, those who were unmarried and without a close confidant were more likely to die within three years than those who were married with a close confidant (OR 3.34, 95% CI 1.8–6.2).[24] Among those in the placebo arm of the Multicenter Diltiazem Post-infarction Trial, living alone was associated with an increased risk of major cardiac events, which included deaths and non-fatal myocardial infarction.[25] However, other research, in a German MONICA sample, found an increased risk of death among men living alone but not among women living alone, after adjustment for conventional risk factors,[26] with another study showing that men but not women living alone are also disadvantaged in terms of survival following myocardial infarction.[27]

Social networks

There has long been evidence that social networks are beneficial to health, with lower all-cause mortality observed in those engaging most frequently in activities such as cultural events.[28]

A few studies have looked at the effects of social networks on the incidence of myocardial infarction. A Swedish study following men over 15 years examined the association between incident coronary heart disease and two measures of social support: "emotional attachment" and "social integration". The hazard ratio (HR) for those in the highest quartile for social integration compared with the lowest was 0.45 (95% CI 0.24–0.84). The corresponding figure for emotional attachment was 0.58 (95% CI 0.37–0.91).[29] A cohort of over 13 000 Swedes, followed for three years, found that low social participation was significantly associ-

ated with first-time acute myocardial infarction, after adjustment for age, sex education, economic stress, daily smoking, physical activity and body mass index.[30] However, some other studies have not found an increased risk of incident disease in those with poor social networks.[31,32]

Other research has used mortality as an endpoint. For example, a study of approximately 30 000 male health professionals found that those defined as socially isolated men (not married, fewer than six friends or relatives, no membership in church or community groups) had a greater risk of cardiovascular disease mortality than those with the highest level of social networks at both four [32] and 10 years (relative risk. adjusted for a range of factors including traditional cardiovascular risk factors, 1.82, 95% CI 1.02–3.23).[33] In the Japanese Komo-Ise Study over 11 000 subjects were followed over seven years. Men who did not participate in hobbies, club activities or community groups had significantly higher relative risk of circulatory system mortality (RR 1.6), after adjustment for established risk factors.[34]

This seeming discordance between some of the evidence on incidence and the much more consistent finding with mortality has focused attention on how social networks may be more important in reducing case fatality than in preventing incident disease.[35] Participants in the Beta Blocker Heart Attack Trial who were socially isolated were twice as likely to die during three years of follow-up than those who were not after adjustment for conventional risk factors.[36] Those who scored highly on social isolation and on a measure of life stress (which included divorce, exposure to traumatic events, and financial difficulty) had an over fourfold increase in risk.

Participants in a population-based study in New Haven who were hospitalized with myocardial infarction were more likely to die in hospital and at up to one year if they had no social support. This result was consistent for men and women, at all ages, and regardless of the severity of disease. In a multivariate model adjusting for sociodemographic, psychosocial, and clinical factors, the excess risk (odds ratio) of mortality among those with no support compared to those with at least one source of support was 2.9 (95% CI 1.2–6.9).[37]

There is also some evidence that the nature of networks is important, with one study of patients undergoing coronary bypass grafting finding that those who were not members of voluntary organizations, including religious ones, or who do not draw support from faith, were seven times more likely to die.[38]

The preceding studies examined the networks that individuals inhabited. There is also a growing body of research looking at the characteristics of the communities in which individuals live. Some of this work employs the concept of social capital, a term that has been defined in a variety of ways.[39–41] However, the definitions are all characterized by notions that it relates to a community and not an individual and that its existence brings benefits that go beyond those who generate it. It is often measured by characteristics such as trust in others, perceived reciprocity, and density of membership in civic organizations.

Social capital can be assessed in a variety of ways. In one ecologic study, social surveys undertaken in 39 American states were used to obtain information on levels of trust and of membership of voluntary organizations, which were then related to state-level mortality from cardiovascular disease. Lower levels of both were associated with increased cardiovascular mortality, after adjusting for poverty.[42] Another study categorized Swedish neighborhoods in terms of violent crime and unemployment rates.[43] Residents aged 35–64 were followed up for a year. Those living in neighborhoods with higher levels of violent crime or unemployment had a higher incidence of coronary heart disease, affecting both men and women. For violent crime, the odds ratios were 1.75 (CI 1.37–2.22) and 1.39 (CI 1.19–1.63) for women and men, respectively. The corresponding figures for neighborhood unemployment were 2.05 (CI 1.62–2.59) and 1.50 (CI 1.28–1.75). These figures changed very little when a range of individual variables were included.

Finally, one study has examined prognosis. This used the Petris Social Capital Index, which characterizes neighborhoods according to level of employment in religious and community organizations.[44] Of almost 35 000 people in California previously admitted with acute coronary syndrome, the recurrence rate was lower in neighborhoods with higher scores on the index (after adjustment for medication, previous revascularization, and standard sociodemographic variables), but only among individuals living in poorer areas.

The work environment

An individual will only spend a relatively small proportion of their entire lives at work, perhaps 40 hours a week between the ages of 20 and 65. Yet, their experiences at work have a disproportionate impact on their lives, influencing how they spend their leisure time, their well-being in retirement, and their psychological well-being.

Interest in the potential impact of the work environment arose from research suggesting that observed social inequalities in cardiovascular disease could only partially be explained by the risk factors then being studied[45] (a more limited set of those included in more recent research such as the INTERHEART study).[3] It has grown in the light of concerns about the changing nature of work and, in particular, the greater insecurity of employment in many countries.

The literature on the health effects of the work environment is dominated by two explanatory models: the demand–control model and the effort–reward imbalance model. Both begin from the position that a work environment that provides opportunities for contributing in a meaningful way to the task in hand and which provides appropriate feedback is likely to be health enhancing while an environment that fails to do so may be health damaging. Two elements in particular have been highlighted. The first is self-efficacy or the belief that one can do what is asked of one.[46] An environment that encourages self-efficacy will allow those in it to make greatest use of their skills and to exercise control over their work. The second is self-esteem or feeling of one's own worth. An environment that encourages self-esteem will allow an individual to interact positively with others and obtain feedback following good performance. In contrast, repeated failure to recognize effort and success can be corrosive.

The demand–control model was developed in Sweden in the early 1980s.[47] In a study that combined a cohort and case–control design, those in what was described as "a hectic and psychologically demanding job" had an increased risk of developing cardiovascular disease and of dying from it, as had those in jobs where they had little discretion about how they did their work or how they scheduled it. The associations were especially marked among those with the least education and persisted after controlling for age, education, smoking, and overweight.

The demand–control model has been developed to include the extent to which the work environment encourages active learning, by which the worker can develop their self-efficacy, and some researchers have suggested inclusion of a third dimension, social support at work.[48] It has also been suggested that a high level of self-efficacy has effects that extend beyond the work environment into other aspects of the worker's life, including their involvement in social and cultural activities which, as the previous section showed, may itself be beneficial for health.[49]

The second, and complementary, model involves effort–reward imbalance.[50] It arises from the concept of social reciprocity, whereby individuals expect that their efforts will be rewarded appropriately. This may break down in a number of situations, such as where there are few alternative sources of employment, but can also arise in individuals who underestimate the demands placed upon them while overestimating their ability to cope.

Interpretation of the empiric evidence is complicated by the diverse range of measures employed to capture the work environment, the use of both objective measures and self-report, the use of both cohort[51] and case–control designs,[52] differing outcomes, and differences in the extent to which other risk factors are adjusted for. Much of the existing literature has been summarized in some recent systematic reviews.[53,54]

In brief, some of the earlier studies, prior to the generation of the theories described above, looked simply at job strain. Some found no effect[55] but others found a significant positive association, after adjustment for sociodemographic and biologic risk factors.[56]

Research on the demand–control model has also yielded conflicting results, with some finding a protective effect of high control and demand[57] while in others the findings were more equivocal[58] and others found that high demands increased risk with no effect for control.[59]

A number of empiric studies of the effort–reward imbalance model have also been undertaken,[60–63] with most finding a positive association between this form of psychologic stress and incident coronary heart disease or mortality, with odds or hazard ratios lying between 1.3 and 4.5, again after adjustment for sociodemographic and biologic risk factors.

Finally, some studies have found significant associations in one sex but not the other. While this could be due to chance, it should be noted that there is some evidence that different mechanisms may be at play, especially in relation to secretion of cortisol[64] (discussed further below).

Mechanisms and interpretation

Interpretation of these findings is complicated by the very diverse methods used. Thus, any conclusions must be surrounded by caveats. In particular, in many of the studies it is difficult to know whether all important confounders have been addressed. For example, one twin study found evidence that some of the measures often used in research on cardiovascular disease to assess psychological status were themselves partially inherited.[65] Conversely, care is needed when interpreting negative findings. Beyond the usual concerns about sample size and length of follow-up, no study has looked comprehensively across all three elements of the lives of subjects, including family, work, and social networks. It is entirely plausible that strong but unmeasured support in one area could overcome weaknesses in another. Thus, it has been suggested that the presence of high levels of social capital in Hawaii might explain why social isolation seems to exert little effect in that society.[31]

Yet while noting these caveats, theory-driven research that has adjusted for potential confounders does suggest that psychosocial factors play a role in the epidemiology of cardiovascular disease. In very general terms, those who have greater support, whether in their families or their broader social circle, or who have a work environment that is supportive, rewarding their efforts appropriately and giving them control, seem less likely to develop cardiovascular disease. The benefits of these relationships may be greater for those who have already developed disease and it is plausible that those with greater support would be more likely to access healthcare promptly.

This raises the question of what the biological mechanisms might be that can explain these findings. Research has focused on three mechanisms: the hypothalamic-pituitary-adrenal axis, inflammation, and coagulation. The available evidence does not suggest any major role for changes in lipid levels, which normally dominate discussion on the etiology of cardiovascular disease.[66]

It has been hypothesized that chronic stress, which may arise in many of the circumstances described above, may activate the hypothalamic-pituitary-adrenal axis. This has led to the concept of allostatic load, in which prolonged exposure to cortisol and noradrenaline leads to organ damage.[67] The evidence that psychosocial factors contribute to a high allostatic load is, however, inconsistent[68,69] and may differ in men and women. The precise mechanisms by which it might lead to cardiovascular disease are unclear although most commentators note an association with metabolic syndrome or hypertension.[70]

The second strand of evidence relates to inflammation, which is hypothesized to contribute to cardiovascular disease through its effects on endothelial function. Hence, one study found that endothelial dysfunction was associated with depression and improved by antidepressants.[71] The finding that some markers of inflammation are associated with a flat cortisol response provides a possible link with the first mechanism.[72] A number of different markers of inflammation have been studied, including heat shock protein 60,[72] C-reactive protein and interleukin 6.[73] High levels of C-reactive protein and interleukin 6 have both been associated with low socioeconomic position[73] and attitudes (cynical distrust).[74]

The third possible mechanism involves increased coagulability, as a result of elevated fibrinogen levels. These have been found to be associated with high work strain[75] and in men with low activity levels inside or outside the home and few social activities.[76] However, again the results are inconsistent, with evidence of differences between men and women.[77]

Finally, it is important to note that there have been a number of negative findings, including those where conventional risk factors were sufficient to explain observed social gradients and those that looked in detail at many of the putative factors but found no consistent associations.[78]

The broader environment

The previous sections have looked at influences on the development of and survival following cardiovascular disease after adjusting for conventional risk factors. However, it is also important to recognize that the levels of these risk factors are themselves shaped by the environment in which people live. A consideration of the social determinants of cardiovascular disease is incomplete without considering how the environment shapes their distribution within a population. This section will look at three of the major risk factors for cardiovascular disease: smoking, physical inactivity, and poor nutrition.

There is now extensive evidence of how smoking rates are influenced by prevailing social norms, which change over time and which can be modified by public policy. In some countries smoking is widespread and socially acceptable and individuals seeking a smoke-free environment will search in vain. Conversely, as in California, non-smoking has become the norm and those who wish to smoke must go into the open air. These norms can change rapidly, illustrated by the rapid acceptance of the ban on smoking in bars and restaurants in Ireland, something that many commentators had predicted would fail.

There is now a considerable volume of evidence, reviewed in detail elsewhere, about the effectiveness of policies designed to reduce smoking. A 10% increase in price, brought about through higher taxes, will reduce smoking by between 3% and 5%. The effect is greater among the young, those on low incomes, and light smokers. Bans on smoking in workplaces and leisure facilities are also effective, as are advertising bans and warnings on cigarette packs, ideally highly visible and accompanied by graphics. Limiting sales to those above a certain age has the potential to reduce smoking amongst adolescents but only if there are mechanisms to ensure effective compliance by retailers. These policies are synergistic, with the best results being achieved by a combination of measures.

The Tobacco Control Scale is an attempt to quantify the degree of implementation and to identify areas needing to be addressed. When applied to 30 European countries, it revealed wide diversity, with scores ranging from 26 out of 100 (Luxembourg) to 74 (Ireland).[79]

Smoking rates are also shaped by prevailing societal norms, which change over time. The Social Unacceptability Index is derived from survey data on individual attitudes towards smoking. Research in the United States has found that those states with higher values (and thus where smoking is less acceptable) have lower smoking rates independent of the price of cigarettes. A 10% increase in the index was associated with a 3.7% fall in consumption.[80]

The second major risk factor for cardiovascular disease is physical inactivity. Again, there is an extensive body of research showing how the environment can encourage or discourage physical activity. Environments supportive of physical activity are characterized by extensive footpaths and easy pedestrian access to shops and recreational areas,[81–84] attractive neighborhoods, and safe surroundings.[85] Such environments have been found, in a number of studies, to be associated with lower levels of obesity.[86–89]

As with smoking, it is possible to assess the extent to which environments encourage physical activity. Two approaches have been used: employing perceptions and objective measures. Perception-based measures are derived from surveys of how individuals view accessibility to facilities, opportunities for physical activity, safety, and aesthetics,[85,90] Objective measures involve systematic observation, increasingly involving use of satellite maps and geographic information systems.[91] These measure density of buildings or traffic, and distances to neighborhood facilities. These approaches have been employed to create a number of standardized instruments, such as the Neighborhood Walkability Scale,[85] the Built Environment Assessment Tool,[92] and the Urban Sprawl Index.[93] High levels of the last of these have been shown, in the USA, to correlate with the prevalence of obesity and hypertension.

The diet that an individual consumes is influenced by the resources that are available to them to purchase food and by the food that is available to them at an affordable price. Research in the USA has shown how healthier foods are less easily available in poor communities and those with large concentrations of African Americans and Hispanics, largely because the latter are served predominantly by convenience stores where much of what is sold is processed food.[94] In contrast, more affluent areas are better served by supermarkets, which stock large amounts of fresh fruit and vegetables. The Atherosclerosis Risk in Communities (ARIC) Study, which included over 10 000 participants in four American states, found that the presence of supermarkets was associated with a significantly lower prevalence of obesity and overweight (obesity prevalence ratio (PR) 0.83, 95% CI 0.75– 0.92; overweight PR 0.94, 95% CI 0.90–0.98), while the presence of convenience stores was associated with a higher prevalence (obesity PR 1.16, 95% CI 1.05–1.27; overweight PR 1.06, 95% CI 1.02–1.10).[95] These findings do, however, appear to be context specific. Thus, similar research from the United Kingdom and Australia found that those living in rich and poor areas had equal access to nutritious food and to supermarkets[96] and no independent association between neighborhood retail food provision and fruit and vegetable intake.[97]

Other research has looked at the role of fast-food outlets, given the high energy density and low price of many of their products. In North America, the density of fast-food outlets is highest in low-income neighborhoods[98] and a positive association has been found at state level between the density of these outlets and obesity.[99] In the United Kingdom, fast-food outlets are also concentrated in deprived areas[100] but in this case an association with obesity has not been found.[101] There are a number of possible explanations for these divergent results, including differing patterns of land use, social distance between income groups, and shopping patterns.

Finally, although the evidence base linking it to obesity and other cardiovascular risk factors is still somewhat limited, research on diet and physical activity has given rise to the concept of the *obesogenic environment*.[102] This concept, which has emerged from a wide range of disciplinary perspectives, is defined as "the sum of influences that the surrounding opportunities or conditions of life have on promoting obesity and individuals or populations".

Conclusion

The current state of knowledge on the social determinants of cardiovascular disease can be compared to a jigsaw in which only some of the pieces are in place. This is not surprising, given the complexity of the task. A recent report on obesity, which is only one of the risk factors for cardiovascular disease, by the UK government's Foresight program,[103] set out its known social determinants in a diagram with so many interconnecting lines that it has been described as looking like an upturned plate of spaghetti.

The researcher studying social determinants is confronted with a range of overlapping domains (family, work, and social) in which risk factors might act. The theoretical basis needed to develop standardized instruments is relatively recent and much of the available work uses very different measures. There may be differences between self-reported and objective measures. The influence of social risk factors is probably context dependent, as suggested by the finding that formally measured social isolation is less important in a society characterized by high levels of cohesion. It is difficult to account for confounding and this is anyway complicated by the possibility that some possible biologic confounders may lie along the same causal pathway as some psychosocial factors. Here, it is important to be aware of one study, among employees in Scottish factories, that found an implausible protective effect of stress, which was most marked for smoking-related cancers even after adjustment for smoking.[104] As the authors note, their finding was almost certainly due to undetected confounding but this is equally likely to occur in studies that produce the "expected" result.

So what, therefore, can be concluded from the available evidence? First, there is unambiguous evidence that the incidence and mortality from cardiovascular disease vary within populations, typically with higher rates in those who are materially disadvantaged. These differences cannot be explained by genetic factors (although this does not exclude some gene–environment interactions) and while differences in conventional risk factors, such as diet and smoking, clearly play a part, they do not seem able to explain all of the variation.

Although there are many studies with negative findings, there are sufficient that find that lack of family and social support and work characterized by high demands and low control, or high effort that is unrewarded, are associated with an increased risk of cardiovascular disease, with some evidence suggesting that the effects are greater for survival following the onset of disease than for incidence. It also seems that men lacking social support are more vulnerable than women. The mechanisms by which these characteristics lead to cardiovascular disease remain uncertain but the available evidence suggests that it may involve a combination of endothelial dysfunction and increased coagulability.

While the existing evidence is incomplete and there are some methodologic concerns, from a policy perspective it is important not to focus on cardiovascular disease in isolation. There is considerable evidence to link social isolation, job strain, and lack of control over one's life to a wide range of other adverse outcomes and, even if it was not possible to demonstrate any health effects, it is arguable that any policies that address these factors are intrinsically desirable.

References

1. Keys A, Menotti A, Karvonen MJ *et al.* The diet and 15-year death rate in the Seven Countries Study. *Am J Epidemiol* 1986;**124**(6):903–15.
2. Tunstall-Pedoe H, Kuulasmaa K, Mahonen M, Tolonen H, Ruokokoski E, Amouyel P. Contribution of trends in survival and coronary-event rates to changes in coronary heart disease mortality: 10-year results from 37 WHO MONICA project populations. Monitoring trends and determinants in cardiovascular disease. *Lancet* 1999;**353**(9164):1547–57.
3. Yusuf S, Hawken S, Ounpuu S *et al.* Effect of potentially modifiable risk factors associated with myocardial infarction in 52 countries (the INTERHEART study): case–control study. *Lancet* 2004;**364**(9438):937–52.
4. Evans RG, Barer ML, Marmor TR. *Why are Some People Healthy and Others Not? The Determinants of Health of Populations*. New York: A de Gruyter, 1994.
5. Rose G. *The Strategy of Preventive Medicine*. Oxford: Oxford University Press, 1992.
6. Marmot MG, Adelstein AM, Robinson N, Rose GA. Changing social-class distribution of heart disease. *BMJ* 1978;**2**(6145):1109–12.
7. Drever F, Whitehead M, eds. *Health Inequalities, Decennial Supplement, Series DS 15*. London: Office of National Statistics, 1997.
8. Hirte L, Nolte E, Mossialos E, McKee M. The changing regional pattern of ischaemic heart disease mortality in southern Europe: still healthy but uneven progress. *J Epidemiol Community Health* 2008;**62**(4):e4.
9. Leon DA, Chenet L, Shkolnikov VM *et al.* Huge variation in Russian mortality rates 1984–94: artefact, alcohol, or what? *Lancet* 1997;**350**(9075):383–8.
10. Marmot MG, Syme SL, Kagan A, Kato H, Cohen JB, Belsky J. Epidemiologic studies of coronary heart disease and stroke in Japanese men living in Japan, Hawaii and California:

prevalence of coronary and hypertensive heart disease and associated risk factors. *Am J Epidemiol* 1975;**102**(6):514–25.

11. Leon DA, Saburova L, Tomkins S *et al.* Hazardous alcohol drinking and premature mortality in Russia: a population based case–control study. *Lancet* 2007;**369**(9578):2001–9.

12. Andreev EM, Nolte E, Shkolnikov VM, Varavikova E, McKee M. The evolving pattern of avoidable mortality in Russia. *Int J Epidemiol* 2003;**32**(3):437–46.

13. Yarnell J, Yu S, McCrum E *et al.* Education, socioeconomic and lifestyle factors, and risk of coronary heart disease: the PRIME Study. *Int J Epidemiol* 2005;**34**(2):268–75.

14. Rosengren A, Hawken S, Ounpuu S *et al.* Association of psychosocial risk factors with risk of acute myocardial infarction in 11119 cases and 13648 controls from 52 countries (the INTERHEART study): case–control study. *Lancet* 2004;**364**(9438): 953–62.

15. Rosengren A, Wedel H, Wilhelmsen L. Marital status and mortality in middle-aged Swedish men. *Am J Epidemiol* 1989;**129**(1):54–64.

16. Nystedt P. Marital life course events and smoking behaviour in Sweden 1980–2000. *Soc Sci Med* 2006;**62**(6):1427–42.

17. Lee S, Cho E, Grodstein F, Kawachi I, Hu FB, Colditz GA. Effects of marital transitions on changes in dietary and other health behaviours in US women. *Int J Epidemiol* 2005;**34**(1): 69–78.

18. Shah S, Cook DG. Inequalities in the treatment and control of hypertension: age, social isolation and lifestyle are more important than economic circumstances. *J Hypertens* 2001;**19**(7): 1333–40.

19. Kushnir T, Kristal-Boneh E. Blood lipids and lipoproteins in married and formerly married women. *Psychosom Med* 1995;**57**(2):116–20.

20. Ebrahim S, Wannamethee G, McCallum A, Walker M, Shaper AG. Marital status, change in marital status, and mortality in middle-aged British men. *Am J Epidemiol* 1995;**142**(8):834–42.

21. Matthews KA, Gump BB. Chronic work stress and marital dissolution increase risk of posttrial mortality in men from the Multiple Risk Factor Intervention Trial. *Arch Intern Med* 2002;**162**(3):309–15.

22. Ben-Shlomo Y, Smith GD, Shipley M, Marmot MG. Magnitude and causes of mortality differences between married and unmarried men. *J Epidemiol Community Health* 1993;**47**(3):200–5.

23. Ikeda A, Iso H, Toyoshima H *et al.* Marital status and mortality among Japanese men and women: the Japan Collaborative Cohort Study. *BMC Public Health* 2007;**7**(147):73.

24. Williams RB, Barefoot JC, Califf RM *et al.* Prognostic importance of social and economic resources among medically treated patients with angiographically documented coronary artery disease. *JAMA* 1992;**267**(4):520–4.

25. Case RB, Moss AJ, Case N, McDermott M, Eberly S. Living alone after myocardial infarction. Impact on prognosis. *JAMA* 1992;**267**(4):515–19.

26. Kandler U, Meisinger C, Baumert J, Lowel H. Living alone is a risk factor for mortality in men but not women from the general population: a prospective cohort study. *BMC Public Health* 2007;**7**:335.

27. Schmaltz HN, Southern D, Ghali WA *et al.* Living alone, patient sex and mortality after acute myocardial infarction. *J Gen Intern Med* 2007;**22**(5):572–8.

28. Konlaan BB, Bygren LO, Johansson SE. Visiting the cinema, concerts, museums or art exhibitions as determinant of survival: a Swedish fourteen-year cohort follow-up. *Scand J Public Health* 2000;**28**(3):174–8.

29. Rosengren A, Wilhelmsen L, Orth-Gomer K. Coronary disease in relation to social support and social class in Swedish men. A 15 year follow-up in the study of men born in 1933. *Eur Heart J* 2004;**25**(1):56–63.

30. Ali SM, Merlo J, Rosvall M, Lithman T, Lindstrom M. Social capital, the miniaturisation of community, traditionalism and first time acute myocardial infarction: a prospective cohort study in southern Sweden. *Soc Sci Med* 2006;**63**(8):2204–17.

31. Reed D, McGee D, Yano K, Feinleib M. Social networks and coronary heart disease among Japanese men in Hawaii. *Am J Epidemiol* 1983;**117**(4):384–96.

32. Kawachi I, Colditz GA, Ascherio A *et al.* A prospective study of social networks in relation to total mortality and cardiovascular disease in men in the USA. *J Epidemiol Community Health* 1996;**50**(3):245–51.

33. Eng PM, Rimm EB, Fitzmaurice G, Kawachi I. Social ties and change in social ties in relation to subsequent total and cause-specific mortality and coronary heart disease incidence in men. *Am J Epidemiol* 2002;**155**(8):700–9.

34. Iwasaki M, Otani T, Sunaga R *et al.* Social networks and mortality based on the Komo-Ise cohort study in Japan. *Int J Epidemiol* 2002;**31**(6):1208–18.

35. Vogt TM, Mullooly JP, Ernst D, Pope CR, Hollis JF. Social networks as predictors of ischemic heart disease, cancer, stroke and hypertension: incidence, survival and mortality. *J Clin Epidemiol* 1992;**45**(6):659–66.

36. Ruberman W, Weinblatt E, Goldberg JD, Chaudhary BS. Psychosocial influences on mortality after myocardial infarction. *N Engl J Med* 1984;**311**(9):552–9.

37. Berkman LF, Leo-Summers L, Horwitz RI. Emotional support and survival after myocardial infarction. A prospective, population-based study of the elderly. *Ann Intern Med* 1992;**117**(12): 1003–9.

38. Oxman TE, Freeman DH Jr, Manheimer ED. Lack of social participation or religious strength and comfort as risk factors for death after cardiac surgery in the elderly. *Psychosom Med* 1995;**57**(1):5–15.

39. Coleman JS. *Foundations of Social Theory.* Cambridge, MA: Belknap Press of Harvard University Press, 1990.

40. Bourdieu P. The forms of capital. In: Richardson JG, ed. *The Handbook of Theory: Research for the Sociology of Education.* New York: Greenwood Press, 1986: 241–58.

41. Putnam RD, Leonardi R, Nanetti R. *Making Democracy Work: Civic Traditions in Modern Italy.* Princeton, NJ: Princeton University Press, 1993.

42. Kawachi I, Kennedy BP, Lochner K, Prothrow-Stith D. Social capital, income inequality, and mortality. *Am J Public Health* 1997;**87**(9):1491–8.

43. Sundquist K, Theobald H, Yang M, Li X, Johansson SE, Sundquist J. Neighborhood violent crime and unemployment increase the risk of coronary heart disease: a multilevel study in an urban setting. *Soc Sci Med* 2006;**62**(8):2061–71.

44. Scheffler RM, Brown TT, Syme L, Kawachi I, Tolstykh I, Iribarren C. Community-level social capital and recurrence of acute coronary syndrome. *Soc Sci Med* 2008;**66**(7):1603–13.

45. Marmot MG, Rose G, Shipley M, Hamilton PJ. Employment grade and coronary heart disease in British civil servants. *J Epidemiol Community Health* 1978;**32**(4):244–9.

46. Bandura A. *Social Foundations of Thought And Action: A Social Cognitive Theory*. Englewood Cliffs, NJ: Prentice-Hall, 1986.

47. Karasek R, Baker D, Marxer F, Ahlbom A, Theorell T. Job decision latitude, job demands, and cardiovascular disease: a prospective study of Swedish men. *Am J Public Health* 1981;**71**(7): 694–705.

48. Johnson JV, Hall EM. Job strain, work place social support, and cardiovascular disease: a cross-sectional study of a random sample of the Swedish working population. *Am J Public Health* 1988;**78**(10):1336–42.

49. Karasek R, Theorell T. *Healthy Work: Stress, Productivity, and the Reconstruction of Working Life*. New York: Basic Books, 1990.

50. Siegrist J. Adverse health effects of high-effort/low-reward conditions. *J Occup Health Psychol* 1996;**1**(1):27–41.

51. Kivimaki M, Leino-Arjas P, Luukkonen R, Riihimaki H, Vahtera J, Kirjonen J. Work stress and risk of cardiovascular mortality: prospective cohort study of industrial employees. *BMJ* 2002;**325**(7369):857.

52. Hallqvist J, Diderichsen F, Theorell T, Reuterwall C, Ahlbom A. Is the effect of job strain on myocardial infarction risk due to interaction between high psychological demands and low decision latitude? Results from Stockholm Heart Epidemiology Program (SHEEP). *Soc Sci Med* 1998;**46**(11):1405–15.

53. van Vegchel N, de Jonge J, Bosma H, Schaufeli W. Reviewing the effort–reward imbalance model: drawing up the balance of 45 empirical studies. *Soc Sci Med* 2005;**60**(5):1117–31.

54. Kuper H, Marmot M, Hemmingway H. Systematic review of prospective cohort studies of psychological factors in the aetiology and prognosis of coronary heart disease. In: Marmot M, Elliott P, eds. *Coronary Heart Disease Epidemiology. From Epidemiology to Public Health*. Oxford: Oxford University Press, 2005.

55. Reed DM, LaCroix AZ, Karasek RA, Miller D, MacLean CA. Occupational strain and the incidence of coronary heart disease. *Am J Epidemiol* 1989;**129**(3):495–502.

56. Haan MN. Job strain and ischaemic heart disease: an epidemiologic study of metal workers. *Ann Clin Res* 1988;**20**(1–2): 143–5.

57. Steenland K, Johnson J, Nowlin S. A follow-up study of job strain and heart disease among males in the NHANES1 population. *Am J Ind Med* 1997;**31**(2):256–60.

58. Alterman T, Shekelle RB, Vernon SW, Burau KD. Decision latitude, psychologic demand, job strain, and coronary heart disease in the Western Electric Study. *Am J Epidemiol* 1994;**139**(6): 620–7.

59. Netterstrom B, Kristensen TS, Sjol A. Psychological job demands increase the risk of ischaemic heart disease: a 14-year cohort study of employed Danish men. *Eur J Cardiovasc Prev Rehabil* 2006;**13**(3):414–20.

60. Lynch J, Krause N, Kaplan GA, Tuomilehto J, Salonen JT. Workplace conditions, socioeconomic status, and the risk of mortality and acute myocardial infarction: the Kuopio Ischemic Heart Disease Risk Factor Study. *Am J Public Health* 1997;**87**(4): 617–22.

61. Siegrist J, Peter R, Junge A, Cremer P, Seidel D. Low status control, high effort at work and ischemic heart disease: prospective evidence from blue-collar men. *Soc Sci Med* 1990;**31**(10):1127–34.

62. Bosma H, Peter R, Siegrist J, Marmot M. Two alternative job stress models and the risk of coronary heart disease. *Am J Public Health* 1998;**88**(1):68–74.

63. Kuper H, Singh-Manoux A, Siegrist J, Marmot M. When reciprocity fails: effort–reward imbalance in relation to coronary heart disease and health functioning within the Whitehall II study. *Occup Environ Med* 2002;**59**(11):777–84.

64. Kunz-Ebrecht SR, Kirschbaum C, Steptoe A. Work stress, socioeconomic status and neuroendocrine activation over the working day. *Soc Sci Med* 2004;**58**(8):1523–30.

65. Raynor DA, Pogue-Geile MF, Kamarck TW, McCaffery JM, Manuck SB. Covariation of psychosocial characteristics associated with cardiovascular disease: genetic and environmental influences. *Psychosom Med* 2002;**64**(2):191–203; discussion 204–5.

66. Jonsson D, Rosengren A, Dotevall A, Lappas G, Wilhelmsen L. Job control, job demands and social support at work in relation to cardiovascular risk factors in MONICA 1995, Goteborg. *J Cardiovasc Risk* 1999;**6**(6):379–85.

67. McEwen BS. Stress, adaptation, and disease. Allostasis and allostatic load. *Ann N Y Acad Sci* 1998;**840**:33–44.

68. Schnorpfeil P, Noll A, Schulze R, Ehlert U, Frey K, Fischer JE. Allostatic load and work conditions. *Soc Sci Med* 2003;**57**(4): 647–56.

69. Maselko J, Kubzansky L, Kawachi I, Seeman T, Berkman L. Religious service attendance and allostatic load among high functioning elderly. *Psychosom Med* 2007;**69**(5):464–72.

70. Tsutsumi A, Kayaba K, Tsutsumi K, Igarashi M. Association between job strain and prevalence of hypertension: a cross sectional analysis in a Japanese working population with a wide range of occupations: the Jichi Medical School cohort study. *Occup Environ Med* 2001;**58**(6):367–73.

71. Sherwood A, Hinderliter AL, Watkins LL, Waugh RA, Blumenthal JA. Impaired endothelial function in coronary heart disease patients with depressive symptomatology. *J Am Coll Cardiol* 2005;**46**(4):656–9.

72. Shamaei-Tousi A, Steptoe A, O'Donnell K *et al.* Plasma heat shock protein 60 and cardiovascular disease risk: the role of psychosocial, genetic, and biological factors. *Cell Stress Chaperones* 2007;**12**(4):384–92.

73. Hemingway H, Shipley M, Mullen MJ *et al.* Social and psychosocial influences on inflammatory markers and vascular function in civil servants (the Whitehall II study). *Am J Cardiol* 2003;**92**(8):984–7.

74. Ranjit N, Diez-Roux AV, Shea S *et al.* Psychosocial factors and inflammation in the multi-ethnic study of atherosclerosis. *Arch Intern Med* 2007;**167**(2):174–81.

75. Siegrist J, Peter R, Cremer P, Seidel D. Chronic work stress is associated with atherogenic lipids and elevated fibrinogen in middle-aged men. *J Intern Med* 1997;**242**(2):149–56.

76. Rosengren A, Wilhelmsen L, Welin L, Tsipogianni A, Teger-Nilsson AC, Wedel H. Social influences and cardiovascular risk factors as determinants of plasma fibrinogen concentration in a general population sample of middle aged men. *BMJ* 1990;**300**(6725):634–8.

77. Hirokawa K, Tsutsumi A, Kayaba K. Psychosocial job characteristics and plasma fibrinogen in Japanese male and female workers: the Jichi Medical School cohort study. *Atherosclerosis* 2008;**198**(2):468–76.

78. Dowd JB, Goldman N. Do biomarkers of stress mediate the relation between socioeconomic status and health? *J Epidemiol Community Health* 2006;**60**(7):633–9.

79. Joossens L, Raw M. The Tobacco Control Scale: a new scale to measure country activity. *Tob Control* 2006;**15**(3):247–53.

80. Alamar B, Glantz SA. Effect of increased social unacceptability of cigarette smoking on reduction in cigarette consumption. *Am J Public Health* 2006;**96**(8):1359–63.

81. De Bourdeaudhuij I, Sallis JF, Saelens BE. Environmental correlates of physical activity in a sample of Belgian adults. *Am J Health Promot* 2003;**18**(1):83–92.

82. Humpel N, Owen N, Iverson D, Leslie E, Bauman A. Perceived environment attributes, residential location, and walking for particular purposes. *Am J Prev Med* 2004;**26**(2):119–25.

83. Diez Roux AV, Evenson KR, McGinn AP *et al.* Availability of recreational resources and physical activity in adults. *Am J Public Health* 2007;**97**(3):493–9.

84. Sallis JF, Hovell MF, Hofstetter CR *et al.* Distance between homes and exercise facilities related to frequency of exercise among San Diego residents. *Public Health Rep* 1990;**105**(2):179–85.

85. Saelens BE, Sallis JF, Black JB, Chen D. Neighborhood-based differences in physical activity: an environment scale evaluation. *Am J Public Health* 2003;**93**(9):1552–8.

86. Boehmer TK, Hoehner CM, Deshpande AD, Brennan Ramirez LK, Brownson RC. Perceived and observed neighborhood indicators of obesity among urban adults. *Int J Obes (Lond)* 2007;**31**(6):968–77.

87. Mujahid MS, Roux AV, Shen M *et al.* Relation between neighborhood environments and obesity in the multi-ethnic study of atherosclerosis. *Am J Epidemiol* 2008;**167**(11):1349–57.

88. Giles-Corti B, Macintyre S, Clarkson JP, Pikora T, Donovan RJ. Environmental and lifestyle factors associated with overweight and obesity in Perth, Australia. *Am J Health Promot* 2003;**18**(1):93–102.

89. Joshu CE, Boehmer TK, Brownson RC, Ewing R. Personal, neighbourhood and urban factors associated with obesity in the United States. *J Epidemiol Community Health* 2008;**62**(3):202–8.

90. Huston SL, Evenson KR, Bors P, Gizlice Z. Neighborhood environment, access to places for activity, and leisure-time physical activity in a diverse North Carolina population. *Am J Health Promot* 2003;**18**(1):58–69.

91. Mujahid MS, Diez Roux AV, Morenoff JD, Raghunathan T. Assessing the measurement properties of neighborhood scales: from psychometrics to ecometrics. *Am J Epidemiol* 2007;**165**(8):858–67.

92. Araya R, Montgomery A, Rojas G *et al.* Common mental disorders and the built environment in Santiago, Chile. *Br J Psychiatry* 2007;**190**:394–401.

93. Ewing R, Schmid T, Killingsworth R, Zlot A, Raudenbush S. Relationship between urban sprawl and physical activity, obesity, and morbidity. *Am J Health Promot* 2003;**18**(1):47–57.

94. Morland K, Wing S, Diez Roux A, Poole C. Neighborhood characteristics associated with the location of food stores and food service places. *Am J Prev Med* 2002;**22**(1):23–9.

95. Morland K, Diez Roux AV, Wing S. Supermarkets, other food stores, and obesity: the atherosclerosis risk in communities study. *Am J Prev Med* 2006;**30**(4):333–9.

96. Macintyre S. Deprivation amplification revisited; or, is it always true that poorer places have poorer access to resources for healthy diets and physical activity? *Int J Behav Nutr Phys Act* 2007;**4**:32.

97. Powell LM, Slater S, Mirtcheva D, Bao Y, Chaloupka FJ. Food store availability and neighborhood characteristics in the United States. *Prev Med* 2007;**44**(3):189–95.

98. Reidpath DD, Burns C, Garrard J, Mahoney M, Townsend M. An ecological study of the relationship between social and environmental determinants of obesity. *Health Place* 2002;**8**(2):141–5.

99. Maddock J. The relationship between obesity and the prevalence of fast food restaurants: state-level analysis. *Am J Health Promot* 2004;**19**(2):137–43.

100. Cummins SC, McKay L, MacIntyre S. McDonald's restaurants and neighborhood deprivation in Scotland and England. *Am J Prev Med* 2005;**29**(4):308–10.

101. Macintyre S, McKay L, Cummins S, Burns C. Out-of-home food outlets and area deprivation: case study in Glasgow, UK. *Int J Behav Nutr Phys Act* 2005;**2**:16.

102. Swinburn B, Egger G, Raza F. Dissecting obesogenic environments: the development and application of a framework for identifying and prioritizing environmental interventions for obesity. *Prev Med* 1999;**29**(6 Pt 1):563–70.

103. Butland B, Jebb S, Kopleman P *et al. Foresight. Tackling Obesities: Future Choices – Project Report.* London: Government Office for Science, 2007.

104. Macleod J, Smith GD, Heslop P, Metcalfe C, Carroll D, Hart C. Are the effects of psychosocial exposures attributable to confounding? Evidence from a prospective observational study on psychological stress and mortality. *J Epidemiol Community Health* 2001;**55**(12):878–84.

18 Obesity

Raj S Padwal[1] and Arya M Sharma[2]
[1]University of Alberta Hospital, Edmonton, Alberta,Canada
[2]Royal Alexandra Hospital, Edmonton, Alberta, Canada

Introduction and historical perspective

Obesity is a highly prevalent and complex chronic disease that results from the accumulation of excessive adipose tissue. Hippocrates (ca. 460–370 BC) was one of the first to warn of the dangers of obesity when he wrote, "It is very injurious to health to take in more food than the constitution will bear, when, at the same time one uses no exercise to carry off this excess". In modern times, the continued rise in obesity prevalence occurring throughout the world[2] threatens to reverse gains made in prolonging life expectancy[3] and reducing the morbidity from coronary disease and other chronic health problems.[4] On a very simplistic level, the rapid rise of obesity in modern society can be thought of as the inevitable consequence of placing a population preselected for efficient fat storage into a sedentary environment of caloric overabundance. However, our understanding of how and why obesity develops is still incomplete, partly due to the complex interplay of socio-economic, behavioral, cultural, metabolic and genetic factors that contribute to the obesity epidemic.[5,6] Developing a clear understanding of these factors, reversing the rise in obesity prevalence and treating the multitude of associated obesity-related complications represents a challenge of considerable magnitude for current and future generations.

Nomenclature and definitions

Definitions of overweight and obesity in adults have varied over time.[7] Ideally, a health-oriented definition of obesity would be based on the amount of excess body fat that correlates with the weight-responsive health risk in a given

Evidence-Based Cardiology, 3rd edition. Edited by S. Yusuf, J.A. Cairns, A.J. Camm, E.L. Fallen, and B.J. Gersh. © 2010 Blackwell Publishing, ISBN: 978-1-4051-5925-8.

individual.[8] Body mass index (BMI), defined as weight in kilograms divided by height in meters squared (kg/m^2), is an easily obtained measure that is now widely used, as it has a high correlation with excess body fat or adiposity. However, BMI is not a measure of body fat and does not convey information on regional fat distribution. The latter is important, as it is now well established that central or visceral fat deposition is a major independent determinant of the metabolic and cardiovascular risk associated with increased body fat mass.[9-12] Recent evidence-based guidelines therefore recommend the use of both BMI and waist circumference in the assessment of overweight or obese patients.[5,6] Table 18.1 summarizes the current classification of overweight and obesity by BMI, waist circumference and associated disease risk. It should be noted that the waist circumference cut-off levels of 88 cm for women and 102 cm for men were primarily chosen because they correspond to BMI levels of $30 kg/m^2$ and not because validation studies have demonstrated these cut-off points to have greater discriminatory power in predicting obesity-related events.[5] In fact, lower, ethnic specific cut-off levels to predict disease risk have been recently proposed, particularly for Asian and South Asian populations, but these are preliminary and require further study and validation.[5]

Although there are benefits to the identification of cut-off points for monitoring overweight and obesity, it is important to realize that (as for other risk factors) health risks associated with increasing weight are part of a continuum, and individuals with BMI <$25 kg/m^2$ can have substantial weight-associated health problems (for example, impaired glucose tolerance, hypertension), whereas others may have no identifiable health problems at BMI levels significantly greater than $25 kg/m^2$. Individualized assessment of risk status and conditions associated with obesity must therefore form an integral part of patient assessment, before deciding on the potential benefits to be derived from weight management in an individual patient (Fig. 18.1).[5,6]

Table 18.1 Classification of overweight and obesity by body mass index (BMI), waist circumference, and associated disease risk[6]

	BMI, kg/m²	Disease risk* relative to normal weight and waist circumference	
		Men, 102 cm Women, 88 cm	Men, >102 cm Women, >88 cm
Underweight	<18.5	–	–
Normal†	18.5–24.9	–	Increased
Preobese	25.0–29.9	Increased	High
Obesity, class			
I	30.0–34.9	High	Very high
II	35.0–39.9	Very high	Very high
III	40	Extremely high	Extremely high

*Disease risk for type 2 diabetes, hypertension and cardiovascular disease.

– indicates that no risk at these levels of BMI was assigned.

†Increased waist circumference can also be a marker for increased risk even in persons of normal weight.

BOX 18.1 Health hazards associated with obesity

- Type 2 diabetes, prediabetes (impaired glucose tolerance, impaired fasting glucose)
- Hypertension
- Dyslipidemia
- Metabolic syndrome
- Cardiovascular disease: coronary artery disease, stroke, congestive heart failure, atrial fibrillation
- Non-alcoholic fatty liver disease
- Respiratory disease: sleep apnea, obesity-hypoventilation syndrome, restrictive lung disease
- Cancers, particularly gastrointestinal and reproductive
- Osteoarthritis
- Cholelithiasis
- Gastrointestinal reflux disease
- Infertility
- Venous stasis
- Frequent infections, including cellulitis and intertrigo
- Urinary incontinence
- Idiopathic intracranial hypertension
- Psychosocial: psychiatric disease (with severe obesity), reduced employment, increased absenteeism, limited mobility, discrimination, reduced quality of life

Incidence, natural history and prognosis

The worldwide prevalence of obesity is currently estimated at over 300 million individuals, with an additional 800 million people classified as overweight.[2] Approximately 40–70% of the adult population in industrialized countries and a substantial proportion in developing countries are now considered overweight or obese.[13] Particularly concerning is the disproportionately rapid rise in the prevalence of severe (Class III) obesity, currently estimated at 5% in the US.[14,15] Severely obese individuals are at much higher risk of developing obesity-related complications and premature death and use substantially more healthcare resources than those with milder degrees of obesity.[16]

Monogenic obesity syndromes such as congenital leptin deficiency present with early-onset severe childhood obesity but are extremely rare.[17] Most individuals have a polygenic and environmental cause for excess adipose tissue and develop obesity later in life, with the majority of women experiencing their largest amount of weight gain after pregnancy and men, after activity wanes in the second and third decades of life.[18] Slow, progressive weight gain is the general rule; due to the highly precise nature of body weight regulation, only a small positive daily caloric intake is needed to cause substantial weight gain over a long time period. For example, a weight gain of 9.1 kg (20 lbs) over a period of 30 years corresponds to an excess intake of only 0.3% of ingested calories.[19] Therefore, it is remarkably easy to gain weight and modest weight gain over the short term often remains unrecognized.

Obesity leads to a number of health hazards (Box 18.1), many of which develop only after decades spent in the obese state. The most significant risk associated with obesity is type 2 diabetes. Compared to individuals with a normal BMI level, the 10-year risk of developing diabetes is increased approximately 20-fold in individuals with a BMI of ≥35 kg/m².[20] Weight gain has also been associated with a significant increase in coronary risk. A weight increase of 15 kg after age 21 is associated with an increased coronary risk of 83% in women and 46% in men.[21] Ultimately, obesity diminishes life expectancy: a 40-year-old obese non-smoker can expect to die 6–7 years prior to a non-obese counterpart.[22] A meta-analysis of 57 observational studies involving nearly 900 000 participants demonstrated that mortality is lowest with BMI levels between 22.5–25 kg/m². Above this range, each 5 kg/m² increment in BMI was associated with a 30% higher overall mortality (HR 1.29; 95% CI, 1.27–1.32) and significant increases in cause-specific mortality (vascular, diabetic, renal, hepatic, neoplastic, and respiratory).[23]

Pathophysiology

Major factors associated with an increased risk of weight gain include low birth weight,[24] absence of history of breast feeding,[25] obesity in later childhood and adolescence,[26] pregnancy,[27] sedentary lifestyle,[28] obesity within a family member or close social contact,[26,29] smoking cessation,[30] and poor dietary restraint.[31]

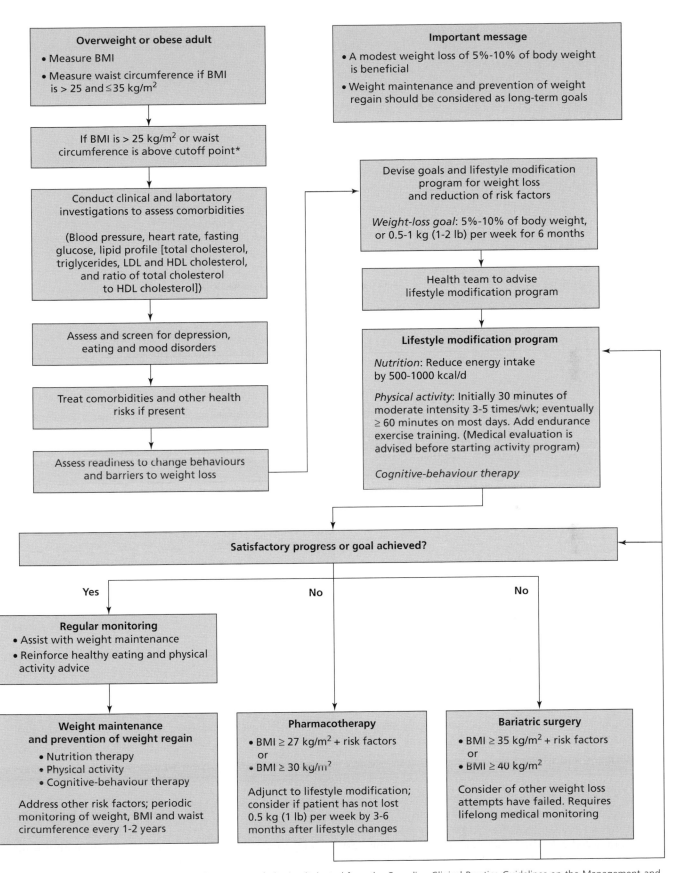

Overweight or obese adult
- Measure BMI
- Measure waist circumference if BMI is > 25 and ≤35 kg/m²

If BMI is > 25 kg/m² or waist circumference is above cutoff point*

Conduct clinical and labortatory investigations to assess comorbidities

(Blood pressure, heart rate, fasting glucose, lipid profile [total cholesterol, triglycerides, LDL and HDL cholesterol, and ratio of total cholesterol to HDL cholesterol])

Assess and screen for depression, eating and mood disorders

Treat comorbidities and other health risks if present

Assess readiness to change behaviours and barriers to weight loss

Important message
- A modest weight loss of 5%-10% of body weight is beneficial
- Weight maintenance and prevention of weight regain should be considered as long-term goals

Devise goals and lifestyle modification program for weight loss and reduction of risk factors

Weight-loss goal: 5%-10% of body weight, or 0.5-1 kg (1-2 lb) per week for 6 months

Health team to advise lifestyle modification program

Lifestyle modification program

Nutrition: Reduce energy intake by 500-1000 kcal/d

Physical activity: Initially 30 minutes of moderate intensity 3-5 times/wk; eventually ≥ 60 minutes on most days. Add endurance exercise training. (Medical evaluation is advised before starting activity program)

Cognitive-behaviour therapy

Satisfactory progress or goal achieved?

Yes   No   No

Regular monitoring
- Assist with weight maintenance
- Reinforce healthy eating and physical activity advice

Weight maintenance and prevention of weight regain
- Nutrition therapy
- Physical activity
- Cognitive-behaviour therapy

Address other risk factors; periodic monitoring of weight, BMI and waist circumference every 1-2 years

Pharmacotherapy
- BMI ≥ 27 kg/m² + risk factors
  or
- BMI ≥ 30 kg/m²

Adjunct to lifestyle modification; consider if patient has not lost 0.5 kg (1 lb) per week by 3-6 months after lifestyle changes

Bariatric surgery
- BMI ≥ 35 kg/m² + risk factors
  or
- BMI ≥ 40 kg/m²

Consider of other weight loss attempts have failed. Requires lifelong medical monitoring

Figure 18.1 Algorithm for the assessment and treatment of obesity. (Adapted from the Canadian Clinical Practice Guidelines on the Management and Prevention of Obesity.[5])

The mechanisms underlying the relationship between obesity and hypertension remain poorly understood. Several theories implicate increased sympathetic activity, sodium and volume retention, renal abnormalities, insulin resistance and, more recently, hyperleptinemia.[32,33]

Obesity predisposes towards type 2 diabetes primarily by increasing insulin resistance.[34] Hormones secreted by adipocytes (adipokines), such as tumor necrosis factor alpha (TNF-alpha[35]), are important promoters of inflammation and insulin resistance. Elevated free fatty acid levels, which are commonly found in the obese state, impair insulin secretion and enhance insulin resistance.[36]

Management

Achieving weight loss

Prior to or in conjunction with developing a treatment plan, one must assess and treat co-morbidities and determine barriers to weight loss including identifying readiness to change (see Fig. 18.1). In-depth explanation of these issues is beyond the scope of this chapter and the reader is referred to more detailed discussions.[5] Successful weight loss often requires the combination of multiple interventions and strategies, including diet, physical activity, behavior modification, pharmacotherapy and surgery (see Fig. 18.1). Because obesity is a chronic condition, all treatment, including pharmacotherapy, should be initiated with the expectation that, if successful, it will be continued over the long term.[5,6]

Goals of treatment

The primary goals of obesity treatment are to reduce body weight, maintain weight loss over the long term, improve obesity-related co-morbidity and increase quality of life.[5,6] Weight loss should be recommended for all patients with excess weight and obesity.[5,6] The initial recommended minimal weight loss target of 5–10% of baseline should be achieved gradually through a 500–1000 kcal/d (2092–4184 kJ/day) deficit, which should lower weight by 1–2 lbs per week in most individuals.[6] This degree of weight loss may appear trivial but is associated with improvements in obesity-related co-morbidities, as detailed below. The amount of weight loss and rate at which weight loss is achieved may be slower in patients with type 2 diabetes compared to non-diabetics.[6]

Lifestyle modification

With regard to dietary therapy, a review of 34 RCTs[6] concluded that an average weight loss of 8% can be obtained over six months with a 500–1000 kcal/day deficit diet, and that this weight loss is associated with a decrease in abdominal fat (**Class I, Level B**). An updated review of 41 randomized controlled trials (RCTs) of at least one year in duration found that counseling to reduce caloric intake and increase physical activity reduced weight by approximately 3–5 kg (**Class I, Level B**).[37] Treatment is more successful with intensive therapy (defined as follow-up more frequently than monthly) and with multimodal interventions (diet, exercise and/or behavioral therapy).[37] Dietary therapy generally produces the greatest amount of weight loss within the first year, with 50% of the weight initially lost regained within the first three years (**Class I, Level B**).[38]

Very low-calorie diets (VLCDs), generally involving the use of protein and dietary supplements and a caloric intake of 800 kcal/d or less, can produce greater initial weight losses than LCDs, but long-term (>1 year) weight loss appears to be only marginally higher than LCDs (**Class I, Level B**).[39] The most important element of dietary therapy appears to be caloric restriction. Varying dietary macronutrient composition (e.g. low carbohydrate, low fat or low glycemic index) does not result in materially greater amounts of weight loss (**Class I, Level B**).[40–42] Importantly, unless accompanied by physical activity, weight loss through dietary modification alone does not appear associated with an improvement in cardiorespiratory fitness as measured by maximum oxygen consumption.[6]

Physical activity alone does not appear to materially reduce weight but improves cardiorespiratory fitness, reduces abdominal fat and, in conjunction with dietary modification, assists with long-term weight maintenance (**Class I, Level B**).[6,43] A standard recommendation is that individuals engage in at least 30 minutes of moderate intensity physical activity 5–7 days per week. Individuals who achieve over 200 minutes of activity per week achieve greater weight loss than individuals performing 150 minutes per week or less.[5,44] There is also emerging evidence that accumulated, shorter bouts of activity throughout the day achieve the same health benefits as a single, longer activity session (**Class I, Level B**).[45]

There also appears to be additional value in behavioral therapy for selected patients as an adjunct to diet and exercise therapy.[6,37] Standard behavior modification techniques include self-monitoring and goal setting, modifying eating behaviors (e.g. slowing the rate of eating, controling where eating occurs, delaying gratification), stimulus control and reinforcement management.[5] In a meta-analysis of six short-term (<1 year) RCTs involving 467 overweight or obese adults, behavioral therapy resulted in 4.7 kg (95% confidence interval (CI) 4.5–4.9) greater weight loss compared to diet and exercise therapy alone (**Class I, Level B**).[46] There is a need for longer-term studies of behavioral therapy to confirm these findings.

Hypertension

A meta-analysis of 25 RCTs enrolling 4874 patients and with a mean follow-up duration of 66 weeks demonstrated that a net weight reduction of 5.1 kg (95% CI 4.3–6.0), by means of energy restriction, increased physical activity or both, reduced systolic blood pressure by 4.4 mmHg (95% CI 3.0–5.9) and diastolic blood pressure by 3.6 mmHg (95% CI 2.3–4.9). Blood pressure reductions were 1.1 mmHg (95% CI 0.7–1.4) systolic and 0.9 mmHg (95% CI 0.6–1.3) diastolic when expressed per kilogram of weight loss (**Class 1, Level B**).[47] A subsequent meta-analysis of 14 observational and randomized controlled studies with a duration of follow-up of two years or greater demonstrated that the blood pressure reductions associated with weight loss over the long term were about half that predicted by shorter term studies (**Class 1, Level B**).[48] In this analysis, for every 10 kg of weight loss, diastolic blood pressure was reduced by 4.6 mmHg and systolic blood pressure by 6.0 mmHg.

Which antihypertensive agent is best suited for the obese hypertensive patient? Current hypertension guidelines do not make specific recommendations on this issue, likely because of the lack of availability of high-quality data.[49] A 16-week study of 171 obese patients treated with felodipine/ramipril, verapamil/trandolapril or metoprolol/hydrocholorthiazide and randomized to sibutramine versus placebo found no significant difference in blood pressure control amongst the study arms (**Class I, Level B**).[50] Beta-blocker/thiazide therapy, however, was associated with a 2–3 kg incremental weight gain compared to the other antihypertensive combinations, which was likely due to the beta-blocker component.[51] In observational studies and post hoc/secondary analyses of RCTs, beta-blocker therapy and thiazide diuretics have been associated with an increased risk of type 2 diabetes whereas angiotensin-converting enzyme (ACE) inhibitors and angiotensin receptor blockers have been associated with a decreased risk (**Class I, Level B**).[52,53] However, a three-year randomized trial of 5269 patients at high-risk for type 2 diabetes found no significant effect of ramipril on the incidence of type 2 diabetes (hazard ratio (HR) 0.91, 95% CI 0.81–1.03) (**Class I, Level A**), although there was a significant increase in the proportion of individuals with impaired glucose tolerance (IGT) or increased fasting glucose (IFG) who regressed to normoglycemia.[54] These accumulated data, although not definitive, suggest that ACE inhibitor or angiotensin receptor blockers may be preferentially prescribed to control hypertension in obese patients at high risk for developing type 2 diabetes.

Diabetes

A large number of studies have documented the benefits of even moderate (5–10%) weight loss in improving metabolic control in diabetic patients.[5,6] However, the impact of weight reduction on the long-term incidence of diabetic complications and survival has not been demonstrated. Improvement in metabolic control depends more on the amount of weight loss, rather than on the method by which this is achieved. A 5 kg weight loss should decrease fasting plasma glucose levels in a diabetic individual by 1 mM or 18 mg/dL.[21] This is of a magnitude similar to that provided by many of the oral hypoglycemic agents. Although pharmacologic or surgical weight loss does not appear to improve glucose control beyond that achieved by lifestyle changes alone, both the degree of loss and the number of individuals achieving and maintaining weight loss are generally higher when lifestyle changes are combined with medication or surgery.[5,6]

Evidence from a meta-analysis of 10 randomized prospective trials indicates that lifestyle modification including modest weight reduction will markedly reduce the incidence of type 2 diabetes in high-risk individuals (HR 0.51, 95% CI 0.44–0.60) (**Class I, Level A**).[55] The best known of these trials, the Diabetes Prevention Program (DPP), employed a lifestyle intervention which aimed to reduce body weight by 7% and increase physical activity to at least 150 minutes per week in non-diabetic persons (mean BMI 34) with elevated fasting and postload plasma glucose concentrations. Over 2.8 years, this lifestyle intervention reduced the incidence by 58% compared with controls and was also significantly more effective than metformin in reducing diabetes incidence.[56] A large, 11.5-year RCT of 5145 patients with type 2 diabetes using the lifestyle intervention employed in the DPP trial is currently under way.[57] This study, known as the Look AHEAD (Action for Health in Diabetes) trial, is the first study to examine the impact of intentional weight loss through lifestyle modification on cardiovascular morbidity and mortality.

In contrast to metformin and acarbose, other antidiabetic medications, including sulfonylureas, thiazolidinediones and insulin, promote weight gain. Weight gain in patients with both type 1 and type 2 diabetes is associated with an increase in blood pressure and deterioration of metabolic control.[58,59] In a secondary analysis of the UK Prospective Diabetes Study, metformin was more effective than sulfonylureas or insulin in reducing diabetes-related endpoints and all-cause mortality.[60] Furthermore, metformin appears cost-saving when used as first-line pharmacologic therapy in overweight type 2 diabetics.[61]

Dyslipidemia

Lipid abnormalities in overweight and obese individuals are typically characterized by high triglycerides, increased small low-density lipoprotein (LDL) particles and low high-density lipoprotein (HDL) cholesterol levels.[5,62] In the presence of abdominal obesity, high serum triglycerides are commonly associated with a clustering of metabolic risk factors known as the metabolic syndrome (atherogenic lipoprotein phenotype, hypertension, insulin resistance, glucose intolerance, prothrombotic and proinflammatory states). Thus, in obese patients, elevated serum triglycerides are a marker for increased cardiovascular risk. The US National Cholesterol Education Program (NCEP) Adult Treatment Panel (ATP III) therefore recognizes the metabolic syndrome as a secondary target of risk reduction therapy, after the primary target, which is LDL cholesterol.[62]

Numerous studies document the short- and medium-term benefits associated with lifestyle modification on blood lipid levels.[63] Current evidence-based guidelines thus recommend weight reduction and increased physical activity as first-line therapies for all lipid and non-lipid risk factors associated with the metabolic syndrome.[5]

Pharmacotherapy

Antiobesity drug therapy can augment diet, physical activity and behavioral therapy to reduce weight and improve obesity-related co-morbidity[5,6] According to current guidelines, adjunctive drug treatment may be added in patients refractory to lifestyle modification alone who have a BMI level of 27–29.9 kg/m² and concomitant obesity-related risk factors (e.g. hypertension, dyslipidemia, type 2 diabetes) or a BMI level of 30 kg/m² or greater.[5,6] Drug therapy should be discontinued if 5% weight loss or improvement in obesity-related co-morbidity has not been achieved within the first 3–6 months.[64] Three antiobesity drugs are currently approved for long-term use (Table 18.2). Orlistat is a gastrointestinal lipase inhibitor that reduces enteral fat absorption by approximately 30%.[65] Sibutramine is a centrally acting monoamine (serotonin, norepinephrine and dopamine) reuptake inhibitor that primarily reduces hunger and increases satiety.[64] Rimonabant, the newest agent, is an endocannabinoid receptor blocker that reduces weight via a number of putative mechanisms including decreased appetite, increased satiety, enhanced thermogenesis and increased lipogenesis.[64] Orlistat and sibutramine have been approved by licensing authorities in most countries. Rimonabant was available in the European Union and other jurisdictions but has not been approved in North America (see below).

A meta-analysis of 16 orlistat, 10 sibutramine and four rimonabant weight loss and maintenance trials with follow-up periods of 1–4 years reported placebo-subtracted

Table 18.2 Medications approved for the long-term treatment of obesity

	Orlistat	Sibutramine	Rimonabant
Trade names	Xenical®	Reductil/Meridia®	Acomplia®
Mechanism of action	Lipase inhibitor	Monoamine reuptake inhibitor	Endocannabinoid receptor blocker
Dosage	120 mg 3 times/day prior to meals	5–15 mg/day	20 mg once daily
Cost (approximate UK price)	£40/month	£45/month	£55/month
Most frequent side effects	Flatulence with discharge, fecal urgency, fecal incontinence, steatorrhea, oily spotting, increased frequency of defecation, decreased absorption of fat-soluble vitamins	Dry mouth, headache, insomnia, constipation, anorexia, increase in heart rate, increase in blood pressure*	Nausea, depression, anxiety, insomnia, irritability, suicidal ideation, insomnia
Potential drug interactions	Reduction in absorption of ciclosporin and amiodarone	SSRIs, MAOIs, centrally active anorexants, sumatriptan, dihydroergotamine, dextromethorphan, meperidine, pentazocine, fentanyl, lithium, tryptophan	Metabolized by CYP 3A4 cytochrome system and may compete for metabolism with similar drugs
Contraindications	Chronic malabsorption syndromes, cholestasis	Uncontrolled hypertension, severe renal impairment, severe hepatic dysfunction, narrow-angle glaucoma, history of substance abuse, coronary artery disease, congestive heart failure, arrhythmias, stroke	Ongoing major depression or use of antidepressants, severe hepatic impairment, severe renal impairment, seizure disorders

*If there is a sustained increase in blood pressure or heart rate, either a reduction in the dose or discontinuation should be considered.

Table 18.3 Effect of orlistat, sibutramine and rimonabant on selected secondary cardiovascular risk factors

Parameter	Orlistat	Sibutramine	Rimonabant
LDL cholesterol (mmol/L)	−0.26 (−0.22 to −0.30)	NS	NS
Triglycerides (mmol/L)	NS	−0.18 (−0.07 to −0.30)	−0.24 (−0.17 to −0.34)
HDL cholesterol (mmol/L)	−0.03 (−0.01 to −0.04)	+0.04 (0.01 to 0.08)	+0.10 (0.08 to 0.11)
Systolic blood pressure	−1.6 (−0.9 to −2.2)	+1.7 (0.1–3.3)	−1.8 (−0.8 to −2.8)
Diastolic blood pressure	−1.4 (−0.8 to −2.1)	+2.4 (1.5–3.3)	−1.2 (−0.5 to −1.9)
A1C in patients with diabetes (%)	−0.38 (−0.18 to −0.59)	NS	−0.7 (−0.56 to −0.84)

weight reductions of 2.9 kg (95% CI 2.5–3.2 kg) with orlistat, 4.2 kg (95% CI 3.6–4.7 kg) with sibutramine and 4.7 kg (95% CI 4.1–5.3 kg) with rimonabant (**Class I, Level B**).[66] The number of patients achieving a 10% weight loss threshold was 12–21% higher with active therapy compared to placebo. Similarly, the number of patients achieving a 5% weight loss threshold was 21–33% greater and a significant reduction in waist circumference of 2–4 cm was noted. The major limiting factor in most studies was high attrition rates, averaging 30–40% across studies.[66] Such high drop-out rates limit the validity of these trials and the possibility that clinical efficacy was overestimated should be considered.

The three drugs have modest and somewhat differing effects on secondary cardiovascular risk factors (Table 18.3). Orlistat significantly improves glycemic control, reduces diabetes incidence in high-risk patients, reduces LDL cholesterol levels and improves blood pressure. Rimonabant and sibutramine improve triglyceride and HDL cholesterol profiles and rimonabant also lowers blood pressure.[66]

Orlistat, sibutramine and rimonabant also have differing major adverse effect profiles (see Table 19.2).[66] Orlistat increases the risk of gastrointestinal adverse effects (abdominal cramping, diarrhea, fecal incontinence) but appears devoid of serious systemic adverse effects. Small, dose-dependent increases in heart rate (3–5 bpm) and blood pressure (see Table 19.3) have been consistently noted with the use of sibutramine.[66] In some instances (1–5%) patients may experience a clinically significant rise in blood pressure (>10 mmHg). Nevertheless, weight reduction in hypertensive patients is often accompanied by a fall in both systolic and diastolic pressure, and several randomized controlled studies have shown that sibutramine can be used in overweight and obese patients with well-controlled hypertension.[66] Sibutramine therapy should be discontinued if a patient experiences an increase in resting heart rate of >10 bpm or uncontrolled hypertension develops. Similarly, treatment should be withdrawn in the event of previously well-controlled hypertension shifting to a

pattern of blood pressure >145/90 mmHg on two consecutive visits, or signs of progressive dyspnea, chest pain or ankle edema.

Rimonabant increases the risk of mood disorders (3% absolute increase in incidence (95% CI 2–5%)) and is contraindicated in patients with major depression or taking antidepressant medication.[66,67] A preliminary meta-analysis of all rimonabant trials (obesity, smoking cessation and other indications) by the Food and Drug Administration reported an increased risk of suicidality (OR 1.9, 95% CI 1.1–3.1).[68] Because of concern regarding this increased risk of mood disorders, rimonabant has recently been withdrawn from the market.[67] Until further data are available, we recommend that the drug not be prescribed in patients with any history of mood disorders.

Currently, there are no data demonstrating that anti-obesity drug therapy reduces mortality or major cardiovascular morbidity.[64] However, there is one large-scale study under way. The SCOUT (Sibutramine Cardiovascular OUTcomes) trial, a multicenter, double-blind, placebo-controlled randomized trial of over 10 000 obese and overweight patients, is evaluating the effect of sibutramine on myocardial infarction, stroke and cardiovascular mortality and is due to report in 2009.[69] The CRESCENDO (Comprehensive Rimonabant Evaluation Study of Cardiovascular ENDpoints and Outcomes) study, a double-blind, placebo-controlled randomized trial examining the impact of rimonabant on myocardial infarction, stroke and cardiovascular death in 17 000 centrally obese patients at high cardiovascular risk has been terminated.[70]

Surgery

Within the last decade, bariatric surgery has emerged as the preferred therapy for selected patients with medically refractory, moderate-to-severe obesity.[71,72] Surgery is currently indicated in patients with BMI levels of ≥40 kg/m² or BMI levels of 35–39.9 kg/m² with a major obesity-related

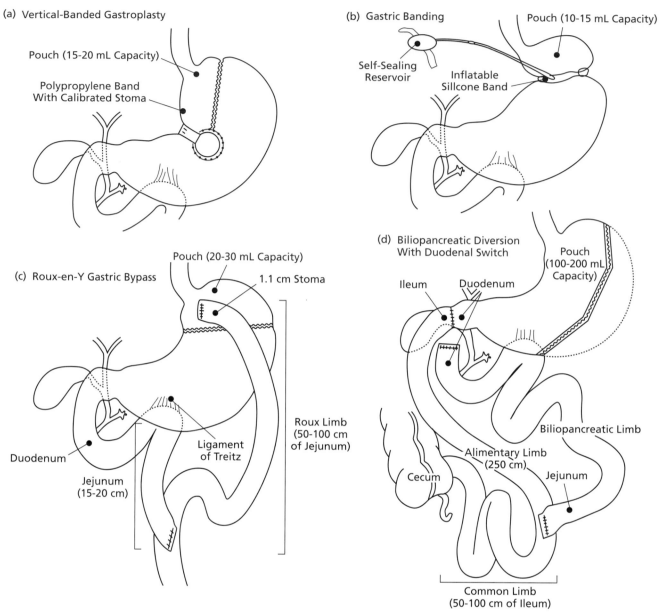

Figure 18.2 Types of bariatric surgery.[76] (a) Vertical-banded gastroplasty. A 15–20 mL upper gastric pouch empties into the remainder of the stomach through a calibrated stoma. (b) Gastric banding. A restrictive band is placed around the proximal stomach and gradually inflated over successive follow-up visits. (c) Roux-en-Y gastric bypass. A stapler fired across the cardia of the stomach creates a 20–30 mL pouch. The jejunum is divided distal to the ligament of Treitz with the distal end anastomosed to the upper stomach. (d) Biliopancreatic diversion with duodenal switch. A sleeve resection of the greater curvature of the stomach is performed. The first portion of the duodenum is divided and the proximal duodenum and approximately half of the length of the small intestine (biliopancreatic limb) is excluded from digestive continuity. The small bowel is divided approximately 300 cm above the ileocecal junction and the distal end is anastomosed to the first portion of the duodenum (alimentary limb). The distal end of the biliopancreatic limb is anastomosed the the ileum 50–100 cm proximal to the ileocecal junction.

co-morbidity (e.g. hypertension, diabetes, sleep apnea).[5,6] Surgery can substantially reduce weight, increase lifespan, markedly improve co-morbid conditions, and enhance quality of life (**Class I, Level C**). Physical domains of quality of life appear to demonstrate the greatest degree of improvement.[73]

The two major types of bariatric procedures are those that purely restrict gastric volume and those that, in addition to restricting gastric size, also bypass a portion of the small intestine (Fig. 18.2). Depending on the type of procedure performed, weight losses average 30–40% of initial body weight within the first several years of surgery (Table

Table 18.4 Weight loss and complications associated with bariatric procedures[71,72,87,89]

Surgery	Average Weight Loss (%)	Perioperative mortality	Perioperative complications	Longer-term postoperative complications
Purely restrictive (gastric banding, vertical banded gastroplasty)	25–30	0.1–0.4%	DVT/PE (1–3%); anastomotic leaks (1–5%); major wound infections (1–5%); major bleeding (0.5–1%); respiratory and cardiac complications (15%)	Symptomatic gallstone formation (up to 35%); vomiting/reflux (8–18%); band erosion (3%) or band slippage (2–14%) requiring reoperation (10–20%)
Roux-en-Y Gastric bypass	35	0.5 to 1.0%		Symptomatic gallstone formation (up to 35%); vomiting/reflux/dumping syndrome (10–15%); vitamin deficiencies (up to 50%); hernia (5–25%); anastomotic ulcers (1%); bowel obstruction (1%); stomal stenosis (6%); stricture (3–27%)
Biliopancreatic diversion	40			Dumping syndrome/vomiting/GI symptoms (38%); protein calorie malnutrition (3–5%); vitamin deficiency (30–50%)

18.4).[72] Weight losses are greater with combined restrictive/bypass procedures; however, perioperative mortality rates and complication rates are also higher compared to restrictive procedures alone. A laparoscopic (versus open) approach is generally preferred because of reduced lengths of stay, postoperative pain, tissue injury and perioperative morbidity.[74,75]

Restrictive procedures include gastric banding and vertical banded gastroplasty and involve banding or stapling the stomach to markedly restrict its size to about 15 mL (see Fig. 19.2). Vertical banded gastroplasty is not commonly performed because of poor long-term weight loss maintenance and/or a high incidence of gastrointestinal reflux and stenosis.[76] Combined restrictive/bypass procedures include Roux-en-Y gastric bypass and biliopancreatic diversion. Roux-en-Y gastric bypass is currently the most commonly performed procedure worldwide and restricts stomach capacity to about 30 mL.[77] Biliopancreatic diversion is less commonly performed and involves less restriction and more malabsorption. In both types of bypass procedures, biliopancreatic secretions in the bypassed intestinal limb do not mix with food until they enter the common limb at the point where the intestines have been rejoined. By increasing or decreasing the length of the common limb, the amount of malabsorption and weight loss is correspondingly decreased or increased.[76] In addition to restrictive and malabsorptive effects, emerging evidence suggests that favorable alterations in weight-regulating hormones such as ghrelin may contribute to the effectiveness of gastric bypass.[78] Reasons for choosing one bariatric procedure over another include patient preference, surgeon experience, the amount of weight loss targeted (bypass preferred if greater weight loss needed) and the desire for lower perioperative risk or future reversibility (banding preferred).

High-quality data from RCTs designed to examine the impact of surgery on cardiovascular morbidity or overall mortality are lacking.[79] The evidence base for bariatric surgery is, therefore, largely based upon observational data (controlled and uncontrolled retrospective and prospective cohorts and non-consecutive case series from selected centers).[71,72] Nevertheless, surgery is the only therapy associated with substantial, persistent long-term reductions in weight (averaging 33% after 2–3 years[72] and 18% after 10 years[80]), total mortality (29–89% reduction) and myocardial infarction (**Class I, Level C**).[81,82] The Swedish Obesity Study (SOS), a prospective cohort study of surgical cases and matched, medically treated controls, provides the most methodologically rigorous data to date, reporting a 15-year mortality rate of 5.0% in surgical patients and 6.3% in controls (HR 0.71, 95% CI 0.54–0.92).[82] In terms of medical co-morbidity, surgery is associated with resolution or improvement of type 2 diabetes, hypertension, dyslipidemia and sleep apnea in 70–90% of cases.[72] As important, surgery improves psychosocial functioning,[83] quality of life and physical function.[84,85] It should be recognized that, despite the substantial weight losses and improvements in health associated with bariatric surgery, most patients still remain significantly overweight or obese after their operation and, mortality rates in postsurgical patients who survive the immediate postoperative period are still 3–6-fold higher than age- and sex-matched controls in the general population.[86]

Potential complications of surgery can be divided into perioperative and longer term (see Table 19.4).[71,87] The risk of perioperative death is 0.5–1% for combined restrictive/bypass procedures and 0.1–0.4% for restrictive procedures alone.[71,72] Perioperative risks are highest in men, older patients (over 55–65 years), extremely obese patients (BMI >50 kg/m²) and patients with medical co-morbidities.[88,89]

Immediate postoperative complications occur in about 10% of individuals and include anastomotic leaks, venous thromboembolic disease, cardiorespiratory events and wound infections. Anastomotic leaks can present non-specifically with isolated postoperative tachycardia and a high index of suspicion is often required to make the correct diagnosis. Radiologic investigations are not reliably accurate and reoperation is required to confirm the diagnosis and repair the leak.

Longer-term complications may directly result from the weight loss achieved or may be procedure specific. Weight loss can promote gallstone formation, which is often treated prophylactically with ursodiol.[87] Furthermore, as weight is lost, a significant minority of patients will require extensive psychologic counseling and professional rehabilitation, and 30–40% of patients will require plastic surgical removal of excess skin.[90] Malabsorptive procedures increase the risk of nutrient deficiency (particularly iron, vitamin B12, calcium and vitamin D) and may result in dumping syndrome, manifesting as postprandial nausea, vomiting, diarrhea and vasomotor symptoms.[87] Dumping syndrome, commonly precipitated by eating high osmotic loads such as refined sugar, results from the rapid emptying of gastric pouch contents directly into the jejunum.[87,91] This is followed by compensatory insulin release and/or vagal stimulation due to intestinal distension from water following the solute load. Wernicke's encephalopathy due to thiamine deficiency is an uncommon complication of bariatric surgery, particularly in patients with persistent vomiting.[92] Patients undergoing purely restrictive procedures often experience postoperative nausea and vomiting (8–10%). Gastric banding may also be complicated by band slippage (6%) or erosion into surrounding structures (10%), often necessitating reoperation.[93]

Demand for bariatric surgery is increasing at an exponential rate. In the US, the annual number of procedures has risen eightfold over one decade to over 100 000 per year.[94] Despite this large increase, only 1% of eligible patients receive surgery annually in the US because the number of potential candidates is so great (estimated at 15 million in 2002[95]). The population eligible for surgery is disproportionately composed of ethnic minorities and individuals of low socioeconomic status,[96] yet surgery is most commonly performed in middle-aged women of moderate-to-high socioeconomic status and free of pre-existing cardiovascular disease.[72]

Because of the large gap between the potential demand for bariatric surgery and the capacity to perform such procedures, surgery will remain a risk-targeted approach for highly selected individuals. However, it is currently unclear how triaging should be performed. Certain patient subgroups, such as individuals with diabetes, clearly may benefit more from undergoing surgery but also are at higher risk for complications.[97] Surgery should only be performed at experienced, specialized centers, as complication rates are highest when surgeons perform fewer than 25 operations per year and medical centers perform fewer than 50 procedures per year.[88,89,98] Complication rates are lowest for surgeons performing more than 100 operations per year and hospitals performing more than 150 procedures per year.[99] Patients who have undergone surgery require lifelong medical surveillance.

Cardiovascular disease and mortality

Many observational studies of overweight and obese patients have demonstrated that intentional weight loss is associated with a reduction in cardiovascular disease and mortality,[100] but this area is not without controversy (**Class IIa, Level C**).[101] As mentioned above, there is a lack of high-quality RCT data demonstrating that intentional weight loss reduces hard cardiovascular outcomes and mortality. Further complicating matters is the fact that many studies demonstrating a beneficial effect of weight loss involve overweight and obese patients without pre-existing cardiovascular disease. When studies examine patients with pre-existing coronary disease or heart failure, overweight and mild obesity are often associated with a reduction in mortality compared to non-obese individuals.[102,103] Indeed, weight loss (albeit not intentional) in advanced heart failure is associated with increased mortality risk.[104] Whether these latter findings are a result of residual confounding, whether obesity is a marker of other favorable characteristics (e.g. absence of cachexia) or whether obesity is truly a protective factor is currently unknown. Notably, the association of obesity with reduced mortality has been reported in many chronic inflammatory diseases including chronic renal failure and HIV/AIDS.[102]

Overall, the favorable effects of weight loss on cardiovascular risk factors in overweight and obese patients imply that intentional weight loss will ultimately reduce cardiovascular morbidity and mortality. Furthermore, observational studies demonstrating that weight loss in severely obese patients undergoing bariatric surgery is associated with mortality reduction lend further credence to this conclusion. Data from trials such as Look AHEAD, SCOUT and CRESCENDO are urgently needed to provide more definitive evidence. It is our practice to routinely prescribe obesity treatment and weight loss to the vast majority of individuals with overweight and obesity, with the exception of patient populations in which weight loss clearly appears potentially detrimental (e.g. advanced heart failure). Indeed, one of the most important barriers to the treatment of obesity is the therapeutic inertia of healthcare professionals[105] and we do not wish to leave the reader with the impression that weight loss should not be attempted until hard outcome RCTs are available. The importance of obesity as a medical disease and a public health emergency cannot be overemphasized and demands aggressive action on the part of all involved, including all healthcare practitioners.

Conclusion

Obesity is a highly prevalent chronic disease and an important risk factor for cardiovascular morbidity and mortality. Weight loss programs should focus on achieving realistic initial weight loss goals (e.g. 5–10% of initial body weight) and should emphasize the need for weight maintenance. Weight reduction induced by lifestyle, pharmacologic or surgical measures has been shown to improve obesity-related co-morbidities and, in the case of lifestyle modification and surgery, has been associated with reductions in major morbidity and mortality in observational studies. Surgery is the only treatment that results in large amounts of weight loss and has become preferred therapy in medically refractory severely obese patients. Randomized controlled obesity studies with hard morbidity and mortality endpoints are still lacking but several are currently under way.

Key points

- BMI is the means most widely used to classify obesity. Measures of central adiposity, such as waist circumference, are also important predictors of obesity-related health risk.
- Obesity and overweight now affect 40–70% of adults in industrialized nations. Particularly concerning is the disproportionately rapid rise in the prevalence of severe obesity, which substantially increases the risk of obesity-related health complications.
- Important components of a comprehensive obesity treatment plan include assessing and treating co-morbidities, identifying readiness to change and barriers to weight loss, and setting realistic weight loss goals (initially 5–10% of initial body weight, which is sufficient to improve obesity-related co-morbidity).
- Weight loss should be recommended for all patients with a BMI ≥30 kg/m² and for those with a BMI ≥27 kg/m² with two or more obesity-related co-morbidities. Weight loss should be gradual (1–2 lbs/week), achieved through a 500–1000 kcal/d deficit diet.
- A multimodal lifestyle intervention (diet, exercise and behavioral modification) is preferred and reduces weight by approximately 3–5 kg after one year. Unfortunately, nearly 50% of the weight initially lost is typically regained within the first three years, emphasizing the importance of optimizing weight maintenance. Therefore, all treatment should be initiated with the expectation that, if successful, it will be continued over the long term.
- Calorie restriction is the most important component of dietary modification. Varying the proportions of macronutrients within the diet does not lead to materially greater amounts of weight loss.
- Individuals should perform at least 30 minutes of moderate-intensity physical activity 5–7 days per week. Exercise is primarily beneficial in assisting with weight maintenance.
- Lifestyle modification is particularly beneficial in improving blood pressure, glycemic control and lipid profiles. It is the most efficacious means to reduce diabetes incidence.
- Antiobesity drug therapy is indicated as an adjunct to lifestyle modification in patients with BMI levels of 27–29.9 kg/m² and concomitant obesity-related risk factors or BMI levels of 30 kg/m² or greater. Drug therapy should be discontinued if 5% weight loss or improvement in obesity-related comorbidity has not been achieved within the first 3–6 months.
- Orlistat (lipase inhibitor), sibutramine (adrenergic reuptake inhibitor) and rimonabant (endocannabinoid receptor antagonist) are the three antiobesity drugs with efficacy data of one year or greater.
- Compared to placebo, drug therapy significantly reduces weight by 3–5 kg, increases the proportion of patients achieving 5% and 10% weight loss thresholds, and reduces waist circumference. Each drug also has specific effects on cardiovascular risk factors.
- The major side effects are gastrointestinal for orlistat, hypertension for sibutramine and mood disorders for rimonabant.
- Bariatric surgery is currently indicated in patients with BMI levels of ≥40 kg/m² or BMI levels of 35–39.9 kg/m² with a major obesity-related co-morbidity. Surgery is the most efficacious treatment for severe obesity and substantially reduces weight, increases lifespan, reduces co-morbidity and increases quality of life.
- Gastric banding restricts the volume of the stomach to about 15 mL. Gastric bypass restricts stomach capacity to approximately 30 mL and bypasses a portion of the small intestine. Both procedures are preferentially performed laparoscopically to reduce morbidity, pain and lengths of stay.
- Perioperative mortality rates are 0.5–1.0% depending on the procedure. Perioperative morbidity occurs in about 10% of individuals. The major long-term complications are gastrointestinal in nature and vary according to the type of procedure performed. To minimize complications, surgery should be performed by experienced surgical teams and centers.
- Demand for bariatric surgery dramatically outstrips capacity. The optimal approach to selecting and triaging patients for surgery is currently unclear.
- High-quality RCT data demonstrating that intentional weight loss reduces mortality and cardiovascular morbidity are currently lacking but several trials are currently under way. With the exception of specific advanced disease states associated with cachexia and inflammation, the preponderance of evidence suggests that intentional weight loss is beneficial.

References

1. Haslam D. Obesity: a medical history. *Obes Rev* 2007;**8**(suppl 1):31–6.
2. Haslam D, James WPT. Obesity. *Lancet* 2005;**366**:1197–209.
3. Olshansky SJ, Passaro DJ, Hershow RC *et al.* A potential decline in life expectancy in the United States in the 21st century. *N Engl J Med* 2005;**352**:1138–45.
4. US Department of Health and Human Services. *The Surgeon General's Call to Action to Prevent and Decrease Overweight and Obesity.* Rockville, MD: US Department of Health and Human Services, Public Health Service, Office of the Surgeon General, 2001.
5. Lau DCW, Douketis JD, Morrison KM *et al.* 2006 Canadian clinical practice guidelines on the management and prevention of obesity in adults and children. *CMAJ* 2007;**176**(suppl 8):1–117.
6. National Heart, Lung, and Blood Institute, National Institutes of Health. *Clinical Guidelines on the Identification, Evaluation, and Treatment of Overweight and Obesity in Adults: The Evidence Report.* NIH Publication No. 98-4083. Bethesda, MD: National Institutes of Health, 1998.
7. Kuczmarski RJ, Flegal KM. Criteria for definition of overweight in transition: background and recommendations for the United States. *Am J Clin Nutr* 2000;**72**:1074–81.
8. Hubbard VS. Defining overweight and obesity: what are the issues? *Am J Clin Nutr* 2000;**72**:1067–8.
9. Lapidus L, Bengtsson C, Larsson B *et al.* Distribution of adipose tissue and risk of cardiovascular disease and death: a 12 year follow up of participants in the population study of women in Gothenburg, Sweden. *BMJ* 1984;**289**:1257–61.
10. Larsson B, Svardsudd K, Welin L *et al.* Abdominal adipose tissue distribution, obesity, and risk of cardiovascular disease and death: 13 year follow up of participants in the study of men born in 1913. *BMJ* 1984;**288**:1401–4.
11. Lean ME, Han TS, Seidell JC. Impairment of health and quality of life in people with large waist circumference. *Lancet* 1988;**351**:853–6.
12. Yusuf S, Hawken S, Ounpuu S *et al.* Obesity and the risk of myocardial infarction in 27,000 participants from 52 countries: a case-control study. *Lancet* 2005;**366**:1640–9.
13. International Obesity Task Force. Global obesity prevalence in adults. Available at: www.iotf.org/database/documents/GlobalPrevalenceofAdultObesity30thOctober07.pdf.
14. Ogden CL, Carroll MD, Curtin LR *et al.* Prevalence of overweight and obesity in the United States, 1999–2004. *JAMA* 2006;**295**:1549–55.
15. Sturm R. Increases in clinically severe obesity in the United States, 1986–2000. *Arch Intern Med* 2003;**163**:2146–8.
16. Hensrud DD, Klein S. Extreme obesity: a new medical crisis in the United States. *Mayo Clin Proc* 2006;**81**(suppl 10):S5–10.
17. Montague CT, Farooqi IS, Whitehead JP *et al.* Congenital leptin deficiency is associated with severe early-onset obesity in humans. *Nature* 1997;**387**:903–8.
18. Wing RR. Changing diet and exercise behaviors in individuals at risk of weight gain. *Obes Res* 1995;**3**:277–82.
19. Rosenbaum M, Leibel RL, Hirsch J. Obesity. *N Engl J Med* 1997;**337**(6):396–407.
20. Field AE, Coakley EH, Must A *et al.* Impact of overweight on the risk of developing common chronic diseases during a 10-year period. *Arch Intern Med* 2001;**161**:1581–6.
21. Anderson JW, Konz EC. Obesity and disease management: effects of weight loss on comorbid conditions. *Obes Res* 2001;**9**(suppl 4):326S–334S.
22. Peeters A, Barendregt JJ, Willekens F *et al.* Obesity in adulthood and its consequences for life expectancy: a life-table analysis. *Ann Intern Med* 2003;**138**:24–32.
23. Prospective Studies Collaboration. Body mass index and cause-specific mortality in 900 000 adults: collaborative analyses of 57 prospective studies. *Lancet* 2009;**373**:1083–96.
24. Jackson AA, Langley-Evans SC, McCarthy HD. Nutritional influences in early life upon obesity and body proportions. In: Ciba Foundation Symposium 201, ed. *The Origins and Consequences of Obesity.* Chichester: Wiley and Sons, 1996: 118.
25. Hediger ML, Overpeck MD, Kuczmarski RJ, Ruan WJ. Association between infant breastfeeding and overweight in young children. *JAMA* 2001;**285**:2453–60.
26. Whitaker RC, Wright JA, Pepe MS. Predicting obesity in young adulthood from childhood and parental obesity. *N Engl J Med* 1997;**337**:869–73.
27. Smith DE, Lewis CE, Caveny JL *et al.* Longitudinal changes in adiposity associated with pregnancy. The CARDIA Study. *JAMA* 1994;**271**:1747–51.
28. Prentice AM, Jebb SA. Obesity in Britain: gluttony or sloth? *BMJ* 1995;**311**:437–9.
29. Christakis NA, Fowler JH. The spread of obesity in a large social network over 32 years. *N Engl J Med* 2007;**357**:370–9.
30. Flegal KM, Troiano RP, Pamuk ER *et al.* The influence of smoking cessation on the prevalence of overweight in the United States. *N Engl J Med* 1995;**333**:1165–70.
31. Lawson OJ, Williamson DA, Champagne CM *et al.* The association of body weight, dietary intake, and energy expenditure with dietary restraint and disinhibition. *Obes Res* 1995;**3**:153–61.
32. Hall JE. Pathophysiology of obesity hypertension. *Curr Hypertens Rep* 2000;**2**:139–47.
33. Mark AL, Correia M, Morgan DA *et al.* State-of-the-art-lecture: obesity-induced hypertension: new concepts from the emerging biology of obesity. *Hypertension* 1999;**33**:537–41.
34. De Fronzo RA, Ferrannini E. Insulin resistance, a multifaceted syndrome responsible for NIDDM, obesity, hypertension, dyslipidemia and atherosclerotic cardiovascular disease. *Diabetes Care* 1991;**14**:173–94.
35. Hofmann C, Lorenz K, Braithwaite SS *et al.* Altered gene expression for tumor necrosis factor-alpha and its receptors during drug and dietary modulation of insulin resistance. *Endocrinology* 1994;**134**:264–70.
36. Boden G, Chen X. Effects of fat on glucose uptake and utilization in patients with NIDDM. *J Clin Invest* 1995;**96**:1261–8.
37. McTigue KM, Harris R, Hemphill B *et al.* Screening and interventions for obesity in adults: summary of the evidence for the U.S. Preventive Services Task Force. *Ann Intern Med* 2003;**139**:933–49.
38. Dansinger ML, Tatsioni A, Wong JB *et al.* Meta-analysis: the effect of dietary counseling for weight loss. *Ann Intern Med* 2007;**147**:41–50.
39. Saris WHM. Very-low-calorie diets and sustained weight loss. *Obes Res* 2001;**9**:295S–301S.

40. Nordmann AJ, Nordmann A, Briel M *et al*. Effects of low-carbohydrate vs low-fat diets on weight loss and cardiovascular risk factors: a meta-analysis of randomized controlled trials. *Arch Intern Med* 2006;**166**:285–93.

41. Thomas D, Elliott EJ, Baur L. Low glycaemic index or low glycaemic load diets for overweight and obesity. *Cochrane Database of Systematic Reviews* 2007, Issue 3. Art. No.: CD005105. DOI: 10.1002/14651858.CD005105.pub2.

42. Summerbell CD, Cameron C, Glasziou PP. Advice on low-fat diets for obesity. *Cochrane Database of Systematic Reviews* 2008, Issue 3. Art. No.: CD003640. DOI: 10.1002/14651858.CD003640.pub2.

43. Miller WC, Koceja DM, Hamilton EJ. A meta-analysis of the past 25 years of weight loss research using diet, exercise or diet plus exercise intervention. *Int J Obes Relat Metab Disord* 1997;**21**:941–7.

44. Jakicic JM, Marcus BH, Gallagher KI *et al*. Effect of exercise duration and intensity on weight loss in overweight, sedentary women: a randomized trial. *JAMA* 2003;**290**:1323–30.

45. Donnelly JE, Jacobsen DJ, Heelan KS *et al*. The effects of 18 months of intermittent vs. continuous exercise on aerobic capacity, body weight and composition, and metabolic fitness in previously sedentary, moderately obese females. *Int J Obes Relat Metab Disord* 2000;**24**:566–72.

46. Shaw KA, O'Rourke P, Del Mar C, Kenardy J. Psychological interventions for overweight or obesity. *Cochrane Database of Systematic Reviews* 2005, Issue 2. Art. No.: CD003818. DOI: 10.1002/14651858.CD003818.pub2.

47. Neter JE, Stam BE, Kok FJ *et al*. Influence of weight reduction on blood pressure: a meta-analysis of randomized controlled trials. *Hypertension* 2003;**42**:878–84.

48. Aucott L, Poobalan A, Smith WCS *et al*. Effects of weight loss in overweight/obese individuals and long-term hypertension outcomes: a systematic review. *Hypertension* 2005;**45**:1035–41.

49. Sharma AM, Pischon T, Engeli S, Scholze J. Choice of drug treatment for obesity-related hypertension: where is the evidence? *J Hypertens* 2001;**19**:667–74.

50. Scholze J, Grimm E, Herrmann D *et al*. Optimal treatment of obesity-related hypertension: the Hypertension-Obesity-Sibutramine (HOS) Study. *Circulation* 2007;**115**(15):1991–8.

51. Gress TW, Nieto FJ, Shahar E *et al*. Hypertension and antihypertensive therapy as risk factors for type 2 diabetes mellitus. *N Engl J Med* 2000;**342**:905–12.

52. Elliott WJ, Meyer PM. Incident diabetes in clinical trials of antihypertensive drugs: a network meta-analysis. *Lancet* 2007;**369**(9557):201–7.

53. Padwal R, Laupacis A. Antihypertensive therapy and incidence of type 2 diabetes. A systematic review. *Diabetes Care* 2007;**27**:247–55.

54. Dream Trial Investigators. Effect of ramipril on the incidence of diabetes. *N Engl J Med* 2006;**355**:1551–62.

55. Gillies CL, Abrams KR, Lambert PC *et al*. Pharmacological and lifestyle interventions to prevent or delay type 2 diabetes in people with impaired glucose tolerance: systematic review and meta-analysis. *BMJ* 2007;**334**:229.

56. Diabetes Prevention Program Research Group. Reduction in the incidence of type 2 diabetes with lifestyle intervention or metformin. *N Engl J Med* 2002;**346**:393–403.

57. Pi-Sunyer X, Blackburn G, Brancati FL *et al*. Reduction in weight and cardiovascular disease risk factors in individuals with type 2 diabetes: one-year results of the look AHEAD trial. *Diabetes Care* 2007;**30**:1374–83.

58. Diabetes Control and Complications Research Group. Weight gain associated with intensive therapy in the diabetes control and complications trial. *Diabetes Care* 1988;**11**:567–73.

59. Kanoun F, Ben AZ, Zouari B, Ben Khalifa F. Insulin therapy may increase blood pressure levels in type 2 diabetes mellitus. *Diabetes Metab* 2001;**27**:695–700.

60. UK Prospective Diabetes Study Group. Effect of intensive blood-glucose control with metformin on complications in overweight patients with type 2 diabetes (UKPDS 34). *Lancet* 1998;**352**:854–65.

61. Clarke P, Gray A, Adler A *et al*. Cost-effectiveness analysis of intensive blood-glucose control with metformin in overweight patients with type II diabetes (UKPDS No. 51). *Diabetologia* 2001;**44**:298–304.

62. National Heart, Lung, and Blood Institute. National Cholesterol Education Program (NCEP) Expert Panel on Detection, Evaluation, and Treatment of High Blood Cholesterol in Adults (Adult Treatment Panel III). *Executive Summary*. NIH publication No. 01–3670. Bethesda, MD: National Heart, Lung, and Blood Institute, 2001.

63. Dattiol AM, Kris-Etherton PM. Effects of weight reduction on blood lipids and lipoproteins: a meta-analysis. *Am J Clin Nutr* 1992;**56**:320–8.

64. Padwal RS, Majumdar SR. Drug treatments for obesity: orlistat, sibutramine, and rimonabant. *Lancet* 2007;**369**:71–7.

65. McNeely W, Denfield P. Orlistat. *Drugs* 1998;**56**.241–9.

66. Rucker D, Padwal R, Li SK *et al*. Long term pharmacotherapy for obesity and overweight: updated meta-analysis. *BMJ* 2007;**335**(7631):1194–9.

67. Christensen R, Kristensen P, Bartels E *et al*. Efficacy and safety of the weight-loss drug rimonabant: a meta-analysis of randomised trials. *Lancet* 2007;**370**:1706–13.

68. FDA Advisory Committee. *FDA Briefing Document: Zimulti (Rimonabant)*. NDA 21–888. Silver Spring, MD: FDA, 2007.

69. Torp-Pedersen C, Caterson I, Coutinho W *et al*. Cardiovascular responses to weight management and sibutramine in high-risk subjects: an analysis from the SCOUT trial. *Eur Heart J* 2007;**28**(23):2915–23.

70. CRESCENDO: Comprehensive rimonabant evaluation study of cardiovascular endpoints and outcomes, December 2005. Available at: www.clinicaltrials.gov/ct/show/NCT00263042?order=3.

71. Maggard MA, Shugarman LR, Suttorp M *et al*. Meta-analysis: surgical treatment of obesity. *Ann Intern Med* 2005;**142**:547–59.

72. Buchwald H, Avidor Y, Braunwald E *et al*. Bariatric surgery: a systematic review and meta-analysis. *JAMA* 2004;**292**:1724–37.

73. Livingston EH, Fink AS. Quality of life: cost and future of bariatric surgery. *Arch Surg* 2003;**138**:383–8.

74. Cottam DR, Nguyen NT, Eid GM, Schauer PR. The impact of laparoscopy on bariatric surgery. *Surg Endosc* 2005;**19**:621–7.

75. Livingston EH. Hospital costs associated with bariatric procedures in the United States. *Am J Surg* 2005;**190**:816–20.

76. Brolin RE. Bariatric surgery and long-term control of morbid obesity. *JAMA* 2002;**288**:2793–6.

77. Samuel I, Mason EE, Renquist KE *et al.* Bariatric surgery trends: an 18-year report from the International Bariatric Surgery Registry. *Am J Surg* 2006;**192**:657–62.

78. Cummings DE, Weigle DS, Frayo RS *et al.* Plasma ghrelin levels after diet-induced weight loss or gastric bypass surgery. *N Engl J Med* 2002;**346**:1623–30.

79. Courcoulas AP, Flum DR. Filling the gaps in bariatric surgical research. *JAMA* 2005;**294**:1957–60.

80. Sjöström L, Lindroos AK, Peltonen M *et al.* Lifestyle, diabetes, and cardiovascular risk factors 10 years after bariatric surgery. *N Engl J Med* 2004;**351**:2683–93.

81. Dixon J. Survival advantage with bariatric surgery: report from the 10th International Congress on Obesity. *Surg Obes Relat Dis* 2006;**2**:585–6.

82. Sjöström L, Narbro K, Sjöström CD *et al.* Effects of bariatric surgery on mortality in Swedish obese subjects. *N Engl J Med* 2007;**357**:741–52.

83. Herpertz SK, Wolf R, Langkafel AM. Does obesity surgery improve psychosocial functioning? A systematic review. *Int J Obes Relat Metab Disord* 1300; 2003 Nov;**27**(11):1300–14.

84. Karlsson J, Taft C, Rydén A *et al.* Ten-year trends in health-related quality of life after surgical and conventional treatment for severe obesity: the SOS intervention study. *Int J Obes Relat Metab Disord* 2007;**31**:1248–61.

85. Dixon JB, Dixon ME, O'Brien PE. Quality of life after lap-band placement: influence of time, weight loss, and comorbidities. *Obes Res* 2001;**9**:713–21.

86. Livingston EH. Obesity, mortality, and bariatric surgery death rates. *JAMA* 2007;**142**:923–8.

87. Abell TL, Minocha A. Gastrointestinal complications of bariatric surgery: diagnosis and therapy. *Am J Med Sci* 2006;**331**:214–18.

88. Flum DR, Dellinger EP. Impact of gastric bypass operation on survival: a population-based analysis. *J Am Coll Surg* 2004;**199**: 543–51.

89. DeMaria EJ. Bariatric surgery for morbid obesity. *N Engl J Med* 2007;**356**:2176–83.

90. Jacobs P, Ohinmaa A, Lier D *et al.* Costing of Alternative Interventions for the Treatment of Morbid Obesity. Alberta Health and Wellness Technical Report. Edmonton, Alberta, 2005.

91. Fujioka K. Follow-up of nutritional and metabolic problems after bariatric surgery. *Diabetes Care* 2005;**28**:481–4.

92. Berger JR. The neurological complications of bariatric surgery. *Arch Neurol* 2004;**61**:1185–9.

93. Suter M, Calmes J, Paroz A *et al.* A 10-year experience with laparoscopic gastric banding for morbid obesity: high long-term complication and failure rates. *Obes Surg* 2006;**16**: 829–35.

94. Steinbrook R. Surgery for severe obesity. *N Engl J Med* 2004;**350**:1075–9.

95. Flum DR, Khan TV, Dellinger EP. Toward the rational and equitable use of bariatric surgery. *JAMA* 2007;**298**:1442–4.

96. Livingston EH, Ko CY. Socioeconomic characteristics of the population eligible for obesity surgery. *Surgery* 2004;**135**:288–96.

97. Livingston EH. Development of bariatric surgery-specific risk assessment tool. *Surg Obes Relat Dis* 2007;**3**:14–20.

98. Nguyen NT, Paya M, Stevens CM *et al.* The relationship between hospital volume and outcome in bariatric surgery at academic medical centers. *Ann Surg* 2004;**240**:586–93.

99. Weller WE, Hannan EL. Relationship between provider volume and postoperative complications for bariatric procedures in New York State. *J Am Coll Surg* 2006;**202**:753–61.

100. Yang D, Fontaine KR, Wang C, Allison DB. Weight loss causes increased mortality: cons. *Obes Rev* 2003;**4**:9–16.

101. Sorensen TIA. Weight loss causes increased mortality: pros. *Obes Rev* 2003;**4**:3–7.

102. Kalantar-Zadeh K, Horwich TB, Oreopoulos A *et al.* Risk factor paradox in wasting diseases. *Curr Opin Clin Nutr Metab Care* 2007;**10**:433–42.

103. Romero-Corral A, Montori VM, Somers VK *et al.* Association of bodyweight with total mortality and with cardiovascular events in coronary artery disease: a systematic review of cohort studies. *Lancet* 2006;**368**:666–78.

104. Anker SD, Ponikowski P, Varney S *et al.* Wasting as independent risk factor for mortality in chronic heart failure. *Lancet* 1997;**349**:1050–3.

105. Manson JE, Skerrett PJ, Greenland P, Van Itallie TB. The escalating pandemics of obesity and sedentary lifestyle. A call to action for clinicians. *Arch Intern Med* 2004;**164**:249–58.

19 Ethnicity and cardiovascular disease

Clara K Chow, Sonia S Anand and Salim Yusuf
Hamilton General Hospital, Hamilton, Ontario, Canada

Introduction

Knowledge regarding the major risk factors for cardiovascular disease (CVD), which include elevated blood pressure, elevated cholesterol, cigarette smoking, and diabetes, have been derived from epidemiologic studies conducted primarily in white populations.[1] Globally, non-white populations constitute the majority of the world's population. Ethnicity-related CVD research compares and contrasts levels of known risk factors and new risk factors, effects of risk factors, efficacy of treatments and preventive strategies and healthcare utilization patterns to explore the reasons for differences in CVD rates among ethnic populations.[2] Such research can lead to specifically tailored CVD preventive strategies for different populations and therefore are of major public health importance.

General issues

Defining ethnic groups

The concept of race was based on the belief that members of a race were homogeneous with respect to biologic inheritance.[3] However, over the past 20 years, as our ability to unravel the genetic code has increased, little evidenc has arisen to support the contention that the historical "racial" divisions represent differences in genetic make-up.[3,4]

Ethnicity, on the other hand, is a term used to describe a group of people whose lifestyles are characterized by distinctive social and cultural traditions which are maintained within the group and passed on from generation to generation. Therefore ethnicity has both sociocultural and biologic components.[5] Given that variations in disease rates between populations may be explained by socio-economic, sociocultural, biologic, and genetic factors, classification by ethnic origin rather than race is desirable.[6]

Interpretation of studies in ethnic populations

The methodologic limitations of studies of ethnic populations must be recognized.[7] Mortality statistics often provide the first clues of differences in CVD rates between ethnic groups. Most developed countries have methods of collecting reliable mortality statistics.[8] However, in developing countries, these systems are less well organized and information on some selected populations may only be available from sample registration systems, community surveys and hospital admissions.

Worldwide patterns of disease

In 2001, 59% of the total global mortality was attributable to non-communicable diseases (NCD) such as CVD, cancer, and diabetes; this was 10% higher than estimates in 1990, and projected to rise to 69% by 2030.[9,10] Approximately 80% of global NCD mortality occurs in developing countries. In 2005 NCD accounted for about 61% of deaths, 50% of disease burden and 46% of premature death (deaths in people less than 70 years) in low- and middle-income countries (LMIC).[11] Coronary heart disease (CHD) and stroke are now the leading causes of deaths in LMIC. More than half of all cardiovascular deaths in LMIC occur among people aged 30 to 69 years, compared to about one-quarter in high-income countries (HIC).[12]

In most HIC, CVD rates are declining due to preventive strategies that target the most potent cardiovascular risk factors (CVRF). For example, tobacco use has declined in many HIC because of legislation and policy,[13] and the proportion of high-risk patients receiving evidence-based secondary prevention therapies has increased.[14] However, in LMIC increasing life expectancy associated with a decline in childhood and adult deaths from infections and coupled

Evidence-Based Cardiology, 3rd edition. Edited by S. Yusuf, J.A. Cairns, A.J. Camm, E.L. Fallen, and B.J. Gersh. © 2010 Blackwell Publishing, ISBN: 978-1-4051-5925-8.

Table 19.1 Trends in age-standardized (world population) death certification rates per 100 000 for coronary heart disease in all age groups in selected areas of the world 1965–1998[18]

Country	Men			Women		
	1965–9	1995–8	% Change	1965–9	1995–8	% Change
Belgium	155.0	79.8	−37.2	63.6	33.2	−36.5
Denmark	237.0	129.6	−45.3	121.9	62.0	−49.1
Greece	64.8	82.9	27.9	28.6	33.1	15.7
Poland	64.7	113.7	75.7	21.6	38.9	80.1
Russian Federation	NA	330.2	NA	NA	154.2	NA
Argentina	176.3	68.2	−61.3	88.9	27.1	−69.5
Canada	271.4	109.4	−59.7	130.7	54.2	−58.5
Mexico	43.8	76.6	74.9	29.7	50.5	70.0
USA	330.5	121.2	−63.3	166.0	67.1	−59.6
Japan	50.1	35.7	−28.7	27.5	17.5	−36.4

NA, not available.

with lifestyle changes secondary to rapid industrialization and urbanization have lead to increasing CVRF and CVD.

Differences in CVD mortality rates across countries are influenced by differences in the physical, social, political and cultural environment.[15] Ethnic variations in disease rates are closely tied to geographic patterns of disease. These geographic differences have provided many of the initial hypotheses of the association between lifestyle factors, which are strongly influenced by culture and ethnicity, and CVD. One of the first epidemiologic studies to highlight the variation in CHD rates between countries was the Seven Countries Study.[16] This study of 16 cohorts of men aged 49–59 years found substantial differences in CHD mortality between countries, for example very low rates in Japan and the Mediterranean countries and very high rates in Finland and the USA. Similarly, the WHO MONICA study in 26 countries[17] documented a more than 14-fold difference in CHD mortality among men and more than 11-fold differences in CHD mortality for women between countries. More recent data indicate that there is still wide variation across both space and time[18] (Table 19.1). The enduring differences in CHD rates across world regions have raised questions as to whether they are due to biologic factors, sociocultural factors, differences in environment or other risk factors.

Migrant groups

Observational studies have found that when members of a given ethnic group migrate to a new environment they often adopt new behaviors and risk factors and lose behaviors common to their native land. This suggests that environmental influences are very powerful factors in CVD causation. Conversely, despite different environments, similarities in disease rates within an ethnic group suggest an inherent propensity towards or protection from CVD that could be related to genetics. Comparing the mortality rates of long-settled migrants to the disease rates in their country of origin helps to establish the relative contribution of genetic and environmental influences to differences in mortality rates. The Ni-Ho-San Study of Japanese migrants to Hawaii and San Francisco revealed that changes in disease rates in this population likely reflected changing environmental influences.[19] The age-adjusted CHD mortality rate rose as the Japanese moved from Japan to Hawaii and California. More than half of the increase in CHD was attributable to different levels of conventional risk factors, as the US cohort had a higher fat diet and higher mean serum cholesterol compared to the Hawaii or Japan cohorts.[19] This suggests that the low rates of CHD mortality in Japan may be retained in Japanese migrants if they kept their risk factors at similar levels to those in Japan, which likely would require maintenance of their traditional lifestyle.

Specific ethnic groups

A major contribution to our understanding of ethnic variation in risk factors for CHD is the findings of the INTERHEART study. INTERHEART was a large case–control study involving about 14 000 cases of first myocardial infarction (MI) and 14 000 matched controls from 52 countries. It was designed to study the importance of conventional and emerging risk factors in different geographic regions and ethnic groups.[20] The principal findings of this study were that nine modifiable risk factors, including abnormal lipids, smoking, hypertension, diabetes, abdominal obesity, psychosocial factors, consumption of fruits and vegetables, alcohol intake and regular physical activity, account for more than 90% of the risk of MI worldwide, in both sexes, and at all ages, in all regions, and in all major ethnic groups. This study challenged the conventional belief that different ethnic groups had different CVRF and provided evidence that while the frequency of risk factors varied by ethnic group, the strength of association with MI was similar. Thus the differences in CVD rates across different regions and/or ethnic groups are attributable to the difference in distribution of established CVRF (Table 19.2).

The following sections review the CVD profile of seven major ethnic groups. Based on the best available data, we document their disease burden and changes in disease rates over time, and review common/influential CVD risk factors. We then discuss ethnic group-specific preventive strategies that need to be further developed or reinforced.

European origin (including North Americans)

People of European origin include those who originate from Northern Europe such as the Nordic countries and Germany, Western Europe including the United Kingdom and France, Southern Europe including Spain and Italy, and Eastern Europe (which includes the Slavic countries).

Disease burden

Differences in the age-standardized mortality rates (ASMR) vary widely between European populations, with the highest rates observed in Eastern Europe (e.g. Bulgaria, the Russian Federation) and the lowest in France and

Table 19.2 Population attributable risk associated with nine risk factors in males and females. Source: reference 20

Risk factor	Prevalence		OR (99% CI) adjusted for age, sex and smoking (OR 1)	PAR (99% CI)	OR (99% CI) adjusted additionally for all other risk factors (OR 2)	PAR 2 (99% CI)
	% Controls	% Cases				
Overall						
Current smoking*	26.76	45.17	2.95 (2.72,3.20)	–	2.87 (2.58,3.19)	–
Current + former smoking*	48.12	65.19	2.27 (2.11,2.44)	36.4 (33.9, 39.0)	2.04 (1.86,2.25)	35.7 (32.5,39.1)
Diabetes	7.52	18.45	3.08 (2.77,3.42)	12.3 (11.2,13.5)	2.37 (2.07,2.71)	9.9 (8.5,11.5)
Hypertension	21.91	39.02	2.48 (2.30,2.68)	23.4 (21.7,25.1)	1.91 (1.74,2.10)	17.9 (15.7,20.4)
Abd obesity (2 v 1)†	33.40	30.21	1.36 (1.24,1.48)	–	1.12 (1.01,1.25)	–
Abd obesity (3 v 1)†	33.32	46.31	2.22 (2.03,2.42)	33.7 (30.2, 37.4)	1.62 (1.45,1.80)	20.1 (15.3,26.0)
All psychosocial‡	–	–	2.51 (2.15,2.93)	28.8 (22.6,35.8)	2.67 (2.21,3.22)	32.5 (25.1,40.8)
Veg and fruits daily*	42.36	35.79	0.70 (0.64,0.77)	12.9 (10.0,16.6)	0.70 (0.62,0.79)	13.7 (9.9,18.6)
Exercise*	19.28	14.27	0.72 (0.65,0.79)	25.5 (20.1,31.8)	0.86 (0.76,0.97)	12.2 (5.5,25.1)
Alcohol intake*	24.45	24.01	0.79 (0.73,0.86)	13.9 (9.3,20.2)	0.91 (0.82,1.02)	6.7 (2.0,20.2)
ApoB/ApoA ratio(2 v 1)§	19.99	14.26	1.47 (1.28,1.68)	–	1.42 (1.22,1.65)	–
ApoB/ApoA ratio(3 v 1)§	20.02	18.05	2.00 (1.74,2.29)	–	1.84 (1.58,2.13)	–
ApoB/ApoA ratio(4 v 1)§	19.99	24.22	2.72 (2.38,3.10)	–	2.41 (2.09,2.79)	–
ApoB/ApoA ratio(5 v 1)§	20.00	33.49	3.87 (3.39,4.42)	54.1 (49.6,58.6)	3.25 (2.81,3.76)	49.2 (43.8,54.5)
All above Risk Factors combined¶	–	–	129.20* (90.24,184.99)	90.4 (88.1,92.4)*	129.20* (90.24,184.99)	90.4 (88.1,92.4)*

* The median waist /hip ratio was 0.93 in cases and 0.91 in controls ($P < 0.0001$), and the median ApoB/ApoA1 ratio was 0.85 in cases and 0.80 in controls ($P < 0.0001$). Percentage of controls with four or five factors positive is 2.2% compared with 29.2% in cases.

*PARs for smoking, abdominal obesity, and ApoB/ApoA1 ratio are based on a comparison of all smokers vs never, top two tertiles vs lowest tertile, and top four quintiles vs lowest quintile. For protective factors (diet, exercise, and alcohol), PARs are provided for the group without these factors.

† Top two tertiles vs lowest tertile.

‡ A model-dependent index combining positive exposure to depression, perceived stress at home or work (general stress), low locus of control, and major life events, all referenced against non-exposure for all five factors.

§ Second, third, fourth, or fifth quintiles vs lowest quintile.

¶ The model is saturated, so adjusted and unadjusted estimates are identical for all risk factors. The odds ratio of 129.20 is derived from combining all risk factors together, including current and former smoking vs never smoking, top two tertiles vs lowest tertile of abdominal obesity, and top four quintiles vs lowest quintile of ApoB/ApoA1. If, however, the model includes only current smoking vs never smoking, the top vs lowest tertile for abdominal obesity, and the top vs lowest quintile for ApoB/ApoA1, the odds ratio for the combined risk factors increases to 333.7 (99% CI 230.2–483.9).

Table 19.3 Age-standardized CVD mortality rates (45–74 years) in selected European countries, 2000[21]

Country	CHD mortality rates (men) SMR (95% CI)	CbVD mortality rates (men) SMR (95% CI)	CHD mortality rates (women) SMR (95% CI)	CbVD mortality rates (women) SMR (95% CI)
Switzerland	158 (149–167)	34 (30–38)	43 (39–48)	21 (17–24)
France	110 (103–118)	50 (44–55)	24 (21–28)	26 (22–29)
Sweden	239 (227–250)	65 (59–70)	75 (68–81)	38 (34–43)
Italy	147 (138–156)	64 (58–69)	43 (38–47)	37 (32–41)
Czech Republic	411 (396–426)	168 (159–177)	147 (138–153)	95 (88–101)
Romania	449 (433–465)	302 (289–314)	209 (199–220)	207 (196–217)
Bulgaria	404 (389–419)	361 (347–375)	157 (148–166)	220 (209–230)
Estonia	713 (693–733)	487 (471–504)	260 (248–271)	248 (237–260)

Switzerland (Table 19.3). In a recent update on regional variation in mortality rates across Europe, the rate ratio of dying from CHD between the countries with the highest mortality compared with the lowest mortality is 7.1 (95% confidence interval (CI) 6.6–7.6) for men (Latvia v France) and 9.9 (95% CI 8.5–11.5) for women (Estonia v France). There is still a clear north-east to south-west gradient in mortality from CHD.[21] For cerebrovascular disease (CbVD), the rate ratio is 14.5 (95% CI 12.7–16.4) for men (Estonia v Switzerland) and 12.0 (95% CI 10.2–14.1) for women (Estonia v Switzerland). With regard to CbVD, there appears to be a "green" circle of reduced mortality in the centre of Western Europe (France, northern Italy and Spain). Although in all countries the CVD mortality rates are much lower among women, substantial between-country differences persist. Over the past 30 years most European countries, the United States and Canada have experienced substantial declines in the CVD mortality rates.[22] However, the Eastern European countries, including Ukraine, the Russian Federation, Hungary, and the Czech Republic, continue to have among the highest rates of CHD and CbVD in the world, with a few showing a decline (Poland) and several showing an increase (Ukraine).[23,24]

Common risk factors

Throughout European populations the high rates of CVD are mainly attributable to high rates of a combination of risk factors including elevated serum cholesterol, elevated blood pressure, diabetes, diets high in saturated fat and smoking. More recently, high rates of overweight and obesity are likely to perpetuate the high rates of associated risk factors and disease. The epidemic of CVD in the Eastern European countries is in part related to high levels of smoking, diets high in animal fats, along with excessive alcohol consumption and social disparity.[25,26] Research to explain why the Italian and French populations remain

relatively "protected" from CHD has yielded numerous hypotheses. It is likely that dietary differences may explain the disparity. For example, the high consumption of olive oil and antioxidants may explain low CHD rates in Italy. In France, however, despite similar saturated fat consumption and levels of serum cholesterol, blood pressure and smoking, the CHD mortality rate remains low.[27] This immunity to CHD has been attributed to high consumption of wine which may offer cardioprotection by increasing HDL cholesterol levels, or by inhibiting postprandial hyperlipidemia and platelet aggregation.[28] Others believe the lower rate of CHD mortality may simply be due to a time lag as increases in consumption of animal fat and elevations in serum cholesterol have only occurred recently in France.[29]

Influential factors

CHD, like other epidemics, relates closely to social conditions and its prevalence appears to be more strongly related to the social and cultural conditions of a society than its genetic make-up. This is evidenced by the rapid decline in the rates of CHD in parallel to economic changes in the United States and Japan, and the increase in CHD rates in the Eastern European countries. These changes have occurred too quickly for changes in gene frequencies to have occurred.[26] Therefore, rather than explaining differences in CHD rates between populations largely on genetic differences, rapid changes in CHD rates can occur and are usually explained by changes in diet (including alcohol consumption) and smoking that are influenced by economics.

Special approaches to prevention

It is clear that major lifestyle changes, and vigilant treatment of risk factors, result in declines in CVD rates. In Finland, an impressive 60% reduction in CHD and stroke mortality was observed between 1972 to 1994, and it is estimated that approximately 75% of this decline can be explained by a substantial lowering of serum cholesterol by 13% (0.88 mmol/L) in men and 18% (1.19 mmol/L) in women, a lowering of diastolic blood pressure by 9% (6.6 mmHg) in men and 13% (12.2 mmHg) in women, and a significant reduction in smoking rates (30% in men) which have occurred as a result of individual and population-targeted interventions.[30]

In the USA, a 34% decline in CHD mortality occurred between 1980 and 1990. One-quarter of this decline is attributed to primary prevention efforts, such as decline in smoking due to effective policies,[13] and 29% is explained by secondary prevention efforts, such as treatments to lower cholesterol and blood pressure. Furthermore, 43% of this decline is attributed to improved medical and surgical management in patients with established CHD.[31] However, it is important to note that despite the general success in reducing CVRF in the US population, not all segments of society are benefiting equally and improvements may have slowed. Smoking and diabetes rates are particularly high among people with a lower socio-economic status. To further reduce CVD in the US, programs need to be targeted at these high-risk groups.

Population health interventions to reduce CVRF levels seem to be very effective in achieving long-term CVD prevention. In Finland the decline in CVRF and CVD was associated with the launch of the national demonstration project in North Karelia in the 1970s and with subsequent major national activities thereafter.[30] More recently in Poland, during the 1990s, a rapid decrease (about 25%) in CHD deaths in early middle age was observed. This sudden decline is attributed to rapid political and economic changes in Poland (and surrounding countries) that made fruit and vegetables more accessible and affordable and oppositely impacted foods of animal origin, which led to improved diets.[32] By contrast, a marked increase in death rates from CVD, accidents, violence, and infectious diseases has been observed in Russia over a relatively short time period, and is thought to be due to socio-economic upheaval.[33] Such examples substantiate the claim that societal factors contribute greatly to CVD burden.

Japanese

Disease burden

Mortality rates from CVD are much lower in Japan than Western countries.[23] Initial data from the Seven Countries study confirmed that the Japanese experience lower rates of CVD compared to Western populations.[16] The pattern of CVD in Japan also differs from Western populations, as they tend to experience relatively higher proportions of stroke (ASMR: M 79, F 41/100 000) and less CHD (ASMR: M 57, F 21/100 000).

Temporal trends

In parallel with a rise in economic prosperity, the CHD rates in Japan have declined like other OECD (Organization for Economic Co-operation and Development) countries. For CHD the ASMR decreased from 47/100 000 in 1995 to 42/100 000 in 1997 among males, and from 25 to 21/100 000 during the same time period among females.[23] Given the low rate of CHD in Japan, the life expectancy in Japan is among the highest in the world.[34] The mortality from stroke in Japan has also declined substantially since 1950.[26] Between 1995 and 1997, ASMR decreased for both men from 82/100 000 in 1995 to 79/100 000, and in women from 54/100 000 to 41/100 000 during the same time period. Low cholesterol levels and declining levels of blood pressure (due to reduction in salt intake and increased use of blood pressure-lowering treatments) and smoking (82.3% among men in 1965 to 45.5% in 2005) in a socially stable environment are probably responsible for the declines in CHD and stroke in Japan.[26,34,35]

Common risk factors

A review of CVRF in the Japanese population suggest that high blood pressure is a major determinant of CVD (particularly high rates of stroke), more so than cholesterol and cigarette smoking.[34] Low serum cholesterol related to a diet low in saturated fats is probably also an important contributing factor. Despite the fact that two-thirds of Japanese men smoke, CHD rates have remained unexpectedly low. Smoking rates and rates of hypertension are declining (prevalence of severe hypertension in men 60–69 years fell from 21% in 1965 to 4% in 1990), but the prevalence of type 2 (non-insulin dependent) diabetes in Japanese males and females is higher than rates in most Western countries. The National Nutrition Survey of 2000 reported that 22.6% (20.7–24.5) of men and 22.3% (20.7–23.9) of women aged 20 years and over had diabetes according to WHO 1999 criteria.[36] The same survey reported the prevalence of overweight (Body Mass Index (BMI) 25–29.9 kg/m²) to be 24.5% in men and the rates of obesity (30 kg/m²) as 2.3%. The corresponding rates in females were 17.8% and 3.4% respectively. Rates of obesity have increased in men over the last three decades but have been stable or decreased in women. In the last decade average BMI has increased in men by 0.45 kg/m² (0.42–0.47), but decreased in women by 0.08 (0.6–0.11) kg/m².[37] Therefore, obesity and type 2 diabetes appear to be emerging and may influence trends in CVD in the future for Japan.

Influential factors

Over the past 30 years blood pressure levels have declined in Japan due to primary prevention efforts.[38] However, "Westernization" of Japanese diets during this period likely explains the two- to threefold increase in glucose intolerance and type 2 diabetes, as well as obesity and more recently hypercholesterolemia.[34,39] Studies have documented that the average serum cholesterol concentration among Japanese has increased from 1980 to 1989, from age-adjusted total serum cholesterol levels of 4.84 to 5.22 mmol/L in men and from 4.91 to 5.24 mmol/L in women. These concerning trends combined with the substantial use of tobacco among Japanese males (59%) suggest that Japan may soon experience a rise in CVD.[34] Studies of Japanese migrant groups show they are susceptible to changing environments. Brazil-born Japanese had a higher proportion of fat in their diet (similar to the general Brazilian population) compared to Japan-born participants (first-generation migrants) and compared to data from Japan,[40] and this was associated with more adverse lipid profiles[41] and a higher prevalence of diabetes (also higher than the general Brazilian population).[42] Similar patterns have been observed in Japanese migrants to Hawaii and California.[19,43,44]

Special approaches to prevention/treatment

With increasing adoption of Western lifestyles in Japan,[38] the pattern of CVRF may become more and more like that of Western countries. A number of studies have shown the protective benefit of the traditional Japanese diet, particularly the Okinawan diet. People in Okinawa (South Island of Japan) enjoy the longest average life expectancy in Japan. Okinawans have less salt in their diet, low animal fat and marked soy bean and fish consumption.[45] Therefore, maintenance of traditional Japanese low-fat diets, high in soy, seaweed and green vegetables,[45] and control of cigarette smoking may be what Japan needs to focus on to prevent CVD.

Chinese

Disease burden

Although the overall mortality from CVD is less in China than in Western countries, CVD is the most common cause of death in China and Taiwan. When compared to Western populations, Chinese, like Japanese, experience higher stroke rates and lower rates of CHD. In urban China in 1999, the ASMR for CHD in men aged 35–74 was 106/100 000 and for women 71/100 000,[23] fivefold lower than the highest rates documented in the MONICA project from Europe.[23] In contrast, the ASMR for stroke in this period and age group was 217/100 000 in men and 147/100 000 in women.[23] CHD incidence in China is also relatively low (highest incidence reported in Sino-Monica 1987–1989 was 109/100 000 in men 35–64 years) whereas stroke incidence is high (highest incidence of stroke from the same study 553/100 000 for men 35–64 years). Hemorrhagic strokes are about two to three times more common in China compared to the West.[46] Only 6–12% of strokes in whites are reported as hemorrhagic compared to 25–30% of strokes among Chinese.[24]

Temporal trends

In parallel with increasing average life expectancy to 71.4 years in 2000 compared with 68.6 years a decade earlier,[47] death rates from CVD (particularly CHD) are increasing in China.[48] The proportion of all deaths due to CVD in China increased from 86/100 000 (12.8% of total death) in 1957 to 214/100 000 (35.8%) in 1990.[49] A recent study of a large representative cohort from China of 169 871 men and women 40 years and over found that CHD accounted for 22.5% and stroke for 21.3% of all deaths.[50] Although Japan has reported a decline in stroke mortality, the decline in stroke deaths in China has not been as striking. The relatively stable incident stroke levels may be due to the balance of falling rates of hemorrhagic stroke with rising rates of ischemic stroke and there is some evidence for this from Beijing and Shanghai where hemorrhagic stroke rates have fallen by 12.0% and 4.4% but ischemic stroke rates have increased by 5.0% and 7.7% respectively.[51]

Common risk factors

Data from the Sino-MONICA project (a 7-year study monitoring trends and determinants of CVD in geographically defined populations in different parts of China) indicate that mean blood pressure levels are high by international standards but total cholesterol and BMI are low.[52]

The rise in CVD in China is likely attributable to adverse changes in health behaviors such as falling levels of physical activity and dietary change associated with rapid urbanization. Risk factor levels are lower in rural compared to urban areas (Table 19.4). Amongst a representative sample of 15 540 Chinese adults, aged 35–74 years from the International Collaborative Study of Cardiovascular Disease in Asia, 78.1% and 21.8% of rural and urban residents, respectively, were physically active. Cigarette smoking is highly prevalent among Chinese males. Over 60% of men smoke and some evidence suggests rates are increasing.[53] Smoking rates among women are much lower, but about a third of smoking-related deaths in women are due to passive smoking.[54] While underweight is still a problem among some Chinese, the prevalence of overweight is increasing, particularly in urban areas.[55]

The strength of association of established CVRF (e.g. cholesterol, blood pressure, smoking, BMI) and CHD/stroke has been shown to be similar for populations from Chinese and Western populations in the APCSC (Asia Pacific Cohort Studies Collaboration).[56] The INTERHEART study included 3030 cases of first MI and 3056 controls from China and Hong Kong and indicates that the same risk factors that are responsible for CHD in other world regions explain the majority of CHD in China, as the nine INTERHEART risk factors explained 88.8% of the PAR for China and Hong Kong.[20] Thus in a study that modeled the impact of changes in risk factors and medical/surgical treatments on CHD mortality in Beijing between 1984 and 1999, most of the

Table 19.4 Cardiovascular risk factors levels in China from the INTERASIA China Study 2001

Factor	Population	Year	Men	Women
Smoking	National (Urban & rural)	2002	60.2%	6.9%
Smoking	National (Urban)[4]	1996	64.0%	~
Smoking	National (Rural)[4]	1996	68.4%	~
Hypertension[1]	National (Urban & rural)	2001	28.6%	25.8%
BMI 25–29	National (Urban)	2001	35.0%	32.6%
BMI 25–29	National (Rural)	2001	21.7%	24.6%
BMI ≥30	National (Urban)	2001	5.0%	2.2%
BMI ≥30	National (Rural)	2001	2.2%	4.9%
Waist adiposity[2]	National (Urban)	2001	27.3%	43.8%
Waist adiposity[2]	National (Rural)	2001	13.4%	36.6%
Total cholesterol	National (Urban)	2001	4.99 mmol/L	5.08 mmol/L
Total cholesterol	National (Rural)	2001	4.71 mmol/L	4.80 mmol/L
LDL cholesterol	National (Urban)	2001	3.02 mmol/L	3.06 mmol/L
LDL cholesterol	National (Rural)	2001	2.75 mmol/L	2.81 mmol/L
HDL – cholesterol	National (Urban)	2001	1.21 mmol/L	1.35 mmol/L
HDL – cholesterol	National (Rural)	2001	1.34 mmol/L	1.36 mmol/L
Diabetes[3]	National (Urban)	2001	7.9%	7.6%
Diabetes[3]	National (Rural)	2001	4.6%	5.5%

[1] SBP ≥ 140 and/or DBP ≥ 90 and/or on antihypertensive medication.
[2] Waist adiposity for men waist >90 cm and women waist >80 cm.
[3] Self-report diabetes or fasting plasma glucose ≥7.0 mmol/L.
From references 52, 61–65.

increase (~77% or 1397 additional deaths) was attributable to substantial rises in total cholesterol levels (more than 1 mmol/L), plus increases in diabetes and obesity.[57] Blood pressure decreased slightly, whereas smoking prevalence increased in men but decreased substantially in women. Changing levels of treatments seemed to have less impact; in 1999, medical and surgical treatments together prevented or postponed ~642 deaths, mainly from initial treatments for acute myocardial infarction (41%), hypertension (24%), angina (15%), secondary prevention (11%), and heart failure (10%).

Influential factors

Absolute rates of CVD are still lower in China and Chinese migrant populations. However, the burden of CVD is unlikely to have been fully realized in China. Smoking-related mortality and morbidity are climbing. A large national study in 1990 found that smoking was already causing about 12% of Chinese male mortality in middle age and predicted that this proportion would rise to about 33% by 2030.[58] China has the largest production and consumption of tobacco worldwide. It has witnessed a dramatic increase in tobacco consumption over the past two decades, with more than 34.8 million cartons of cigarettes being produced and 34.7 million sold annually. The continuous, rapid increase in the number of Chinese smokers is largely due to teenagers taking up smoking. The average daily consumption of tobacco per person in China rose from one cigarette in 1952 to 10 cigarettes in 1990.[59] Passive smoking as well as the effects of both indoor and outdoor air pollution are also likely to be important influencing factors for CVD in China in the future.[54] These together with the continuing high rates of hypertension and early evidence of effects of urbanization on health behaviors and subsequent falling levels of physical activity and increasing obesity and diabetes are concerning signs of what may come. In one urban cohort from China, acquisition of a motorized vehicle was associated with 80% higher odds of becoming obese.[60] Higher rates of CHD in Chinese populations with prolonged exposure to urban lifestyles such as in Singapore indicate that Chinese are not immune to the effects of CHD.

Migrant patterns

Data from Chinese migrants to Singapore and Mauritius provide evidence that exposure to urban environments leads to adverse risk factor profiles.[66,67] A comparison of rural Chinese in China to urban Chinese subjects living in Hong Kong and Australia found that despite a slightly better risk factor profile among the urban Chinese (based on HDL cholesterol and lower blood pressure), carotid intima media thickness (a measure associated with cardiovascular risk) was lower among the rural subjects (0.50 + 1.0 mmHg) than among urban subjects

$(0.56 + 0.12 \, \text{mmHg})$.[68] Together with urbanization, increased levels of metabolic risk factors and CHD in Chinese populations outside China may be due to cultural dietary differences such as the higher consumption of coconut and palm oil, mainly containing saturated fat, in Singapore.[69] Diabetes rates and mean serum cholesterol were also higher in Mauritius Chinese (5.5 mmol/L) than in Beijing Chinese (4.4 mmol/L), whereas the prevalence of hypertension and smoking was greater in Beijing.[66] Therefore, although the prevalence of hypertension and smoking may decline for these migrant populations, the rates of obesity, late-onset diabetes, elevated serum cholesterol, and CHD increase. However, Chinese migrants to the United States and Canada have lower rates of CHD relative to other migrant groups, and have low or similar rates of stroke, indicating they may still retain some level of protection from CVD compared to other populations.[44]

Approaches to prevention

Economic modernization in China is resulting in increased rates of CVRF common among Western populations becoming apparent in urban populations of China. This offers a major challenge for future prevention efforts in China as increasing populations are exposed to rapid urbanization. Important prevention strategies for the Chinese will include smoking cessation/prevention, maintenance of traditional Chinese lifestyles including diet (high in leafy green vegetables and fish, low in saturated fat) and regular physical activity to prevent continuing adverse changes in BMI, diabetes, serum cholesterol and blood pressure.

South Asians

South Asians include people who originate from India, Sri Lanka, Bangladesh, and Pakistan.

Disease burden

There are relatively few mortality studies from India as there is no uniform completion of death certificates and no centralized death registry for CVD.[70] However, the WHO and the World Bank data indicate that mortality attributable to CVD has increased in parallel with the expanding population in India, and now accounts for a large proportion of disability-adjusted life years (DALY). Of all deaths in 1990, approximately 25% were attributable to CVD, which is greater than the 10% due to diarrheal diseases, the 13% due to respiratory infections, and the 8% due to tuberculosis.[71] In 2006 the Global Burden of Disease Studies (GBDS) reported detailed cause of death estimates for the South Asian region based on 2001 data.[72] CHD was reported to be the number one cause of death in South Asia, accounting for 13.6% of all deaths, and CbVD was the fourth leading cause of death, accounting for 6.8% of all deaths.[72]

Temporal trends

In South Asia CHD is expected to rise in parallel with increasing life expectancy, increase in per capita income, and decline in infant mortality.[72,73] There are few direct measures of CHD incidence from India, which makes evaluation of trends difficult. However, indirect comparisons of studies in which CHD incidence was defined using ECG indicate that CHD incidence is probably increasing in India.[74]

Common risk factors

Historically most populations from South Asia have documented low levels of CVRF, particularly blood lipid levels, diabetes and hypertension. However, over the past several decades, the prevalence of these risk factors has increased, especially in urban areas.[75] For example, a recent survey of six major cities of India including 11 216 participants ≥20 years reported a diabetes prevalence of 12.1% and impaired glucose tolerance prevalence of 14.1%,[76] in contrast to rates of diabetes reported in urban studies in the 1970s of 1–3%.[77] There is also evidence that diabetes rates are increasing in rural areas. In comparison to the rates reported by the PODIS study (including 41 270 adults ≥25 years conducted between 1999 and 2002) of 1.9% in rural and 4.6% in urban areas, recent rural studies from select states report rates as high as 13%.[78,79] Similarly, rates of hypertension have increased from about 5% in urban areas in the 1960s to 12–15% in the 1990s.[80] Recent studies have also documented high rates of abdominal obesity in select urban and rural areas. In a survey of employees aged 20–59 years in a large industry near Delhi (n = 2935), 43% had central obesity (waist >90 cm) and the metabolic syndrome was present in 28–35% of individuals depending on the diagnostic criteria used.[81] In a survey of rural adults from Andhra Pradesh (n = 4535), the prevalence of central obesity (waist >90 cm in men, >80 cm in women) was 26.0% and the prevalence of metabolic syndrome ranged from 24.6% to 30.2% depending on the definitions used.[82]

Smoking rates are also high in India, particularly amongst men. Rural rates of smoking are higher than urban rates and may reflect socio-economic differences. In a cross-sectional survey (n = 19 973) of Indian industrial employees and family members from urban and peri-urban areas, tobacco use was significantly more prevalent in low versus high education groups (56.6% v 12.5%).[83] While previous evidence has indicated the possible importance of novel risk factors, such as higher levels of lipoprotein (a), homocysteine, fibrinogen, and plasminogen activator inhibitor (PAI-1),[84] in South Asian populations that may be driving the epidemic of CVD in South Asians, recent findings suggest otherwise. The INTERHEART study found protective factors were lower in South Asian controls than in controls from other countries (moderate- or high-intensity exercise, 6.1% v 21.6%; daily intake of fruits and vegetables,

26.5% v 45.2%; alcohol consumption once/wk, 10.7% v 26.9%). However, some harmful factors were more common in South Asians living in India than in individuals from other countries (elevated apoB/apoA-I ratio, 43.8% v 31.8%; history of diabetes, 9.5% v 7.2%). Similar relative associations were found in South Asians compared with individuals from other countries for the risk factors of current and former smoking, apoB/apoA-I ratio for the top versus lowest tertile, abdominal obesity as measured by the WHR for the top versus lowest tertile, history of hypertension, history of diabetes, psychosocial factors such as depression and stress at work or home, regular moderate- or high-intensity exercise, and daily intake of fruits and vegetables. Alcohol consumption was not found to be a risk factor for acute MI in South Asians, likely because the reported use of regular alcohol intake is low. The combined odds ratio (OR) for all nine risk factors was similar in South Asians (123.3, 95% CI 38.7–400.2) to individuals from other countries (125.7, 95% CI 88.5–178.4). The similarities in OR for the risk factors explained a high and similar degree of population attributable risk in both groups (85.8%, 95% CI 78.0–93.7%) versus 88.2% (95% CI 86.3–89.9%), respectively. When stratified by age, South Asians had more risk factors at ages younger than 60 years, which explained the younger mean age of MI in South Asians compared with other countries (Fig. 19.1).[85]

Influential factors

Urbanization of South Asian populations has influenced the rise in glucose intolerance, abdominal obesity, and its associated dyslipidemia (Table 19.5). This clustering of factors is also associated with impaired fibrinolysis, increased C-reactive protein, and enhanced thrombogenesis. Increasingly, data support the idea that elevations of glucose in the non-diabetic range which is prevalent among South Asians is associated with the development of atherosclerosis among South Asians.[86] Tobacco use, particularly indigenous forms, is also an important determinant of CVD in South Asian countries. Smoking rates are higher in rural men and women compared to their urban counterparts (Table 19.5). The INTERHEART study confirms previous indications that indigenous forms of tobacco use are also harmful. Smoking beedies alone was associated with increased risk (OR 2.89, 95% CI 2.11–3.96), similar to that associated with cigarette smoking. Chewing tobacco alone was associated with OR 2.23 (95% 1.41–3.52) and smokers who also chewed tobacco had the highest increase in risk (OR 4.09, 95% CI 2.98–5.61)[87] (Fig. 19.2).

Migrant patterns

Cross-sectional studies of CVRF in South Asians living in North America find a high prevalence of diabetes, impaired glucose tolerance, central obesity, elevated LDL choles-

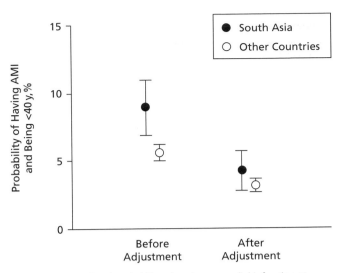

Figure 19.1 Predicted probability of acute myocardial infarction at a younger age in South Asians compared with individuals from other countries. (From Joshi, *JAMA* 2007;**297**:286–94 with permission.)

terol,[89] elevated triglycerides, and low HDL cholesterol.[90,91] The prevalence of impaired glucose tolerance and type 2 diabetes is four to five times higher in South Asian migrants than in Europeans by the age of 55 (20% v 4%).[90] The prevalence of diabetes in South Asians in the UK was 10–19%, 21% in Trinidad, 25% in Fiji, 22% in South Africa, 25% in Singapore, 20% in Mauritius, and 10% in Canada.[90,92]

Studies of South Asian migrants to countries such as the UK, South Africa, Singapore, and North America indicate that South Asians suffer between 1.5 and 4.0 times higher CHD mortality compared to other ethnic groups (Table 19.6).[89] Although the CHD mortality rate of South Asians compared to other populations remains high, a decline in CHD rates has been observed in most South Asian migrants over the past 10 years, although this decline has been less than that observed in the general population in most countries except Canada.[93,94]

A study which compared the risk profiles of urban South Asians living in the UK with their siblings living in India revealed that the UK cohort had a higher BMI (27 v 23), systolic BP (144 mmHg v 137 mmHg), total cholesterol (6.35 v 5.0 mmol/L), lower HDL cholesterol (1.14 v 1.27 mmol/L), and higher fasting glucose (5.4 v 4.6 mmol/L) compared to their siblings. Lp(a), which is mostly genetically determined, was similarly high in both groups.[103] These studies indicate that South Asians have a propensity for adverse changes in CVRF when they adopt urban and Westernized lifestyles, whether they live in India or abroad (Table 19.7).

Prevention strategies

Changes in the risk factor profiles of South Asians are attributable to changes in health behaviors associated with

Table 19.5 Urban–rural comparisons of CVD risk factors in India[88]

Cardiovascular risk factor comparisons in three age groups

Factor	Age (years)	Male		Female	
		Urban	Rural	Urban	Rural
Hypertension (%)	15–34	–	1.1	–	2.1
	35–54	38.2*	3.4	35.1*	9.5
	55 & above	47.5*	9.8	67.5*	16.8
Diabetes mellitus (%)	15–34	–	0.3	–	0.1
	35–54	6.2*	0.3	5.1*	1.7
	55 & above	10.9*	0.5	12.9	0
BMI 25 kg/m²& above	15–34	–	1.5	–	3.6
	35–54	34.1*	2.9	53.8*	9.1
	55 & above	41.0*	2.6	54.2*	4.7
Physically inactive	15–34	–	12.3	–	48.3
	35–54	47.2*	8.6	52.8*	39.4
	55 & above	40.4*	20.6	67.7*	57.6
Smoking – current (%)	15–34	–	49.2	–	3.3
	35–54	28.3	78.4	0.5*	26
	55 & above	17.3*	81.4	0.6*	47.1
Drinking alcohol	15–34	–	32.7	–	0
	35–54	49.3	46.6	0.2	0
	55 & above	39.7	30.9	0	0

Biochemical risk factors comparisons for people aged >35 years

Biochemical parameters	Urban		Rural	
	n	Mean	N	Mean
Total cholesterol (mmol/L)	96	4.73	90	4.06
HDL (mmol/L)	96	1.06	89	1.00
LDL (mmol/L)	96	2.82	89	2.35
Triglycerides (mmol/L)	96	1.85	90	1.51
Fasting serum insulin (uU/ml)	86	27.3	84	7.2
Post-glucose serum insulin (uU/ml)	85	52.7	87	20.4
Fasting plasma glucose (mmol/L)	95	4.96	90	5.52
Post-glucose load plasma glucose (mmol/L)	94	6.5	90	5.52

(–) City survey did not cover age group of <35 years.

*$P < 0.05$ for rural, town, city trend.

*Urban with reference to rural. HDL, high-density lipoprotein; LDL, low-density lipoprotein

urbanization, such as decreased physical activity and increased energy consumption which leads to obesity, abdominal obesity, and its harmful sequelae. The INTER-HEART study found that compared with individuals from other areas, native South Asians had significantly higher PARs associated with waist-to-hip ratio but lower PARs for history of hypertension and psychosocial stress. Therefore efforts to increase physical activity and improve diets are likely to lead to the greatest reduction in CHD.

Arabs

The term Arab refers to Semitic people who originate from the Middle East. Included in this region are the countries of Egypt, Saudi Arabia, Jordan, Iraq, Syria, Bahrain, Lebanon, Kuwait, Qatar, Yemen and the United Arab Emirates. People from Iran originate from the Middle East but are known as Persian and not typically included in the Arab ethnic group classification.

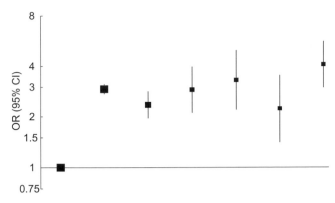

Figure 19.2 Risk of acute myocardial infarction associated with different tobacco use. (From Teo, *Lancet* 2006;**368**:647–58 with permission.)

Disease burden

Cardiovascular disease is the leading cause of death among Arabs living in the Middle East.[72] The high rates are likely secondary to rapid socio-economic development, urbanization, and improved survival in recent decades. The Global Burden of Disease report estimates that the acute MI rate among men and women in the Middle East was 139/100000 and 124/100000 respectively in 2000, which is an increase of 12% among men and 5% among women since 1990.[72]

Temporal trends

While national incidence and mortality data are not readily available for many Arab countries, one indication of the increase in CVD is the rise in hospital admission for CVD

Table 19.6 Standardized mortality ratios (SMR) (per 100000) for CHD in South Asians worldwide

Study (first author)	Country	Reference group	Age (yr)	Age SMR[a]
Wyndham[95] 1968–77	South Africa	Whites	15–64	300
Steinberg[96] 1968–85	South Africa	Whites	35–74	502
Baligadoo[97]	Mauritius	Europeans	40–45	260
Toumilehto[98] 1971–80	Fiji	Melanese	40–60+	350
Beckles[99] 1977–84	Trinidad	Blacks	35–69	260
Hughes[100] 1980–84	Singapore	Chinese	30–69	380
Hughes[100] 1980–84	Singapore	Malays	30–69	190
Adelstein[1/11] 1970–72	UK	Whites	20+	115
McKeigue[102] 1979–83	UK	Whites	20–64	160
Balarajan[93] 1979–83	UK	Whites	20–69	M:136, F:146
Sheth[94] 1979–83	Canada	Whites	35–74	M:122, F:139
Sheth[94] 1979–83	Canada	Chinese	35–74	M:329, F:344
Sheth[94] 1989–93	Canada	Whites	35–74	M:95, F:131
Sheth[94] 1989–93	Canada	Chinese	35–74	M:275, F:369

[a] Standardized mortality to reference indigenous population of 100.

Table 19.7 Comparison of South Asians from India and migrants in the UK[103]

	Indian subcontinent	Sibling migrants UK	Significance
Mean age (yr)	45.0	46.0	NS
Serum glucose (men) (mmol/L)	4.5	5.7	0.001
Serum glucose (women) (mmol/L)	4.7	5.1	0.05
Serum cholesterol (men) (mmol/L)	4.9	6.5	0.001
Serum cholesterol (women) (mmol/L)	5.1	6.2	0.001
HDL cholesterol (men) (mmol/L)	1.21	1.12	NS
HDL cholesterol (women) (mmol/L)	1.34	1.16	0.05
Serum Lp(a) (men) (mg/dL)	17.4	18.8	NS
Serum Lp(a) (women) (mg/dL)	18.9	20.4	NS
Systolic/diastolic blood pressure (men) (mmHg)	132/87	146/93	0.001/NS
Systolic/diastolic BP (women) (mmHg)	142/88	143/86	NS/NS
BMI (men)	22.9	26.8	0.001
BMI (women)	22.7	27.4	0.001

over time. In Egypt the proportion of hospital admissions due to CVD increased from 12% in 1970 to close to 40% in 1990.[104] In Saudi Arabia, CHD represented the leading cause of admissions in 1995.[105] In Oman during 1985–87 CHD and CbVD accounted for 30% of hospital deaths in the age group 15 years and above.[106]

Common risk factors

Cardiovascular risk factors are generally common in this region and are increasing in both urban and rural regions. Overweight (BMI 25–30) and obesity (BMI > 30) are highly prevalent in the Arabian Peninsula, and over half of all adults aged 40–69 years are either overweight or obese.[107] Obesity rates vary from 16% to 25% among men and from 17% to 43% among women. The perception that obesity is symbolic of prosperity may contribute to the higher rates of obesity observed in women.[108] Adverse lifestyles associated with socio-economic improvement and urbanization, such as diminished physical activity (with the availability of domestic help, private cars, popularity of television, etc.) and altered dietary patterns (increased fat and energy intakes), contribute to the high prevalence of obesity.[107] In a nationally representative sample from Bahrain rates of leisure time physical activity were low among all age and sex groups, though higher among men (30–49 years: 19.9%) than among women (30–49 years: 9.9%).[109]

High prevalence of type 2 diabetes is also observed in this region. In 1995 the prevalence of diabetes in the Middle East was approximately 6.3% and this is expected to increase to 8.2% by the year 2025.[110] In 1995, there was approximately twice the number of diabetics in urban compared to rural areas of the Middle East. By 2025 it is expected this ratio will increase dramatically, and there will be approximately 3.5 times the number of diabetics in urban compared to rural areas.[110] In Saudi Arabia in 2001, a national cross-sectional survey reported a diabetes (defined as fasting glucose ≥7.0 mmol/L) prevalence of 26.2% in men and 21.5% in women 30 years and over,[36] with similar levels reported at a similar time period in the United Arab Emirates (UAE) of 21.5% in men and 19.2% in women ≥20 years.[36]

The high prevalence of obesity and sedentary lifestyles may also be associated with high levels of hypertension in this region. National surveys have demonstrated high prevalence of hypertension in Oman (33.1%, up from 27%),[111] Egypt (26%),[112] and the UAE (37%).[113] In the UAE, 26% of hypertensive subjects were aware that they had high blood pressure, 41% were being treated for the disease, and only 19% were under control.[113] This high prevalence, coupled with low awareness and poor control, suggests the need for additional focus on prevention. Some studies also indicate significant levels of dyslipidemia and hypercholesterolemia in Saudi Arabia[114] and Syria.[115]

Smoking is typically more common among men than women for cultural reasons, and the prevalence varies markedly between countries within the region but increasing rates are seen amongst young females in some populations. In Jordan adult smoking rates for men are 50.5% and women 8.3%, but amongst 13–15 year males the rate is 36.5% and females 27.7% (Jordan Global Youth Tobacco Survey 2003).[36] In Saudi Arabia, the prevalence of smoking is 12% among men, compared to only 1% among women.[114] However, the increasing use of the "water pipe" has resulted in increased smoking among women. In Bahrain, approximately 46% of men and 30% of women reported smoking. Smoking is also common amongst youth in Bahrain with 33.5% of 13–15 year old males reporting current smoking in the Global Youth Tobacco Survey in 2001. Furthermore, women more often reported exposure to passive smoke (44%) compared to men (29%).[109] High levels of CVRF have also been observed in Arab migrant communities in the United States, with similar or higher levels of metabolic risk factors (diabetes and overweight) compared with NHANES III survey results.[116]

Influential factors

In comparison with European populations with similar degrees of obesity, Arabs experience more diabetes. This suggests that Arab people may have an increased genetic susceptibility to abdominal obesity (for example, the "thrifty gene"), which is expressed as glucose intolerance and excess abdominal fat in the face of an environment of abundant energy intake and relatively little physical activity.[117] Profound changes associated with rapid economic development and urbanization in much of this region which have occurred during the past 30 years are associated with the emergence of both obesity and diabetes, and this trend is expected to continue.

Approaches to prevention

Increased susceptibility to insulin resistance among Arabs suggests that control of obesity and diabetes is critical. Attention to lifestyle practices that promote obesity, such as sedentary lifestyles and increased energy intake, should be a focus. Cultural beliefs about overweight and obesity for both men and women must be understood in order to develop effective prevention strategies.[108] These directions have already been established in many countries of the Arabian Peninsula, and more recently in collaboration with the World Health Organization. Furthermore, tobacco use is high among some countries and increasing among some segments of society and effective prevention tactics should be introduced and maintained.

Hispanics

The term Hispanic includes Cuban Americans, Mexican Americans, and Puerto Rican Americans. There are approximately 35.3 million Mexican Americans living in the USA, and they comprise approximately 12.5% of the US population.[118] The majority of information on CVD in Hispanics has been derived from studies conducted among Mexican Americans.

Disease burden
Vital statistic data collected since the 1970s in the USA show that cardiovascular mortality has been lower in Hispanic men and women compared to non-Hispanic whites.[119] In findings from the National Health Interview Survey (NHIS) (1986–1994), Hispanics had ~20% lower all-cause, CHD and CVD mortality compared with whites in the United States. The Hispanic/white mortality ratio for CHD was 0.77 (95% CI 0.64–0.93) for men and 0.83 (95% CI 0.66–1.01) for women. The rate ratio for CVD (CHD and stroke) was 0.79 (95% CI 0.68–0.94) for men and 0.80 (95% CI 0.69–0.94) for women.[120]. However, given the lower all-cause mortality rate in Hispanics, the proportion of total deaths due to CHD or CVD was similar between the two populations for the same gender. For white men the proportion of deaths due to CHD was 29.7% and CVD for 44.7% compared to 28.1% and 43.2% among Hispanic men. Among white women, CHD accounted for 24.9% of deaths, CVD for 43.2% compared to 24.1% and 41% of deaths among Hispanic women.[120] The major weaknesses of vital statistics data to estimate mortality in Hispanics are misclassification (i.e. incorrectly assigning race to decedents) and underregistration. Most misclassified descendents are falsely reported as white Caucasians. Surveys of misclassification indicate that as many as 20% more deaths were Hispanic descendants than documented by death certificate. In contrast, the 1980 census undercounted Hispanics by as much as 8%. The aggregate effects of these errors are not known.

Cohort studies to date have found contradictory findings. The National Longitudinal Mortality Study followed up 700 000 respondents including 40 000 Hispanics from 1979 to 1987. Hispanics (≥25 years) had significantly lower CVD mortality than whites (standardized rate ratios: 0.65 for men, 0.80 for women).[121] However, in contrast the San Antonio Heart Disease Study of 1438 Mexican Americans and 921 non-Hispanic whites aged 45–64 years and followed for an average of 14.5 years found higher rates of CHD or CVD among Hispanics. The age- and gender-adjusted hazard ratio comparing Mexican Americans with non-Hispanic whites for all-cause mortality was 1.5 (95% CI 1.23–1.81), for CVD 1.70 (1.30–2.24) and for CHD 1.60 (1.09–2.36). After adjusting for all possible confounders including age, risk factors and socio-economic variables, the hazard ratios were all attenuated; for example, comparing Mexican Americans with non-Hispanic the hazard ratio for CHD mortality was 1.20 (95% CI 0.63–2.27).[122] The San Luis Valley Diabetes Cohort Study of 1862 Hispanics and non-Hispanic white participants found similar rates of CVD mortality in Hispanics and non-Hispanic whites.

The Corpus Christi Heart Project (CCHP), Texas, reported a greater incidence of MI in Mexican Americans compared to non-Hispanic whites over a 4-year period.[123] This population-based surveillance project conducted between 1988 and 1992 reported that age-adjusted incidence ratios comparing Mexican Americans to non-Hispanic whites were 1.52 (95% CI 1.28–1.80) and 1.25 (95% CI 1.10–1.42) among women and men respectively.[123] Although cross-sectional studies reveal a similar or lower prevalence of MI among Mexican Americans than non-Hispanic whites, the CCHP has reported a greater case-fatality rate following MI among Mexican Americans than non-Hispanic whites. Therefore a lower CHD prevalence in Mexican Americans does not necessarily reflect a lower incidence of CHD.

There are some data to suggest that all-cause mortality rates are higher amongst younger Hispanics. The Hispanic/white mortality ratios in the NHIS were 1.33, 0.92 and 0.76 among men aged 18–44, 45–64 and 65 and older respectively. Among women in the same age groups the Hispanic/white mortality ratios were 1.22, 0.75 and 0.70 respectively.[120] Hispanics under the age of 60 have a significantly elevated CbVD death rate compared to non-Hispanic whites (M 32 v 19, F 23 v 18 per 100 000 respectively). However, in older age categories the CbVD rate in Hispanics is substantially lower than whites (M 589 v 765, F 535 v 847 per 100 000).[23] Therefore, overall the CbVD death rate over 45 years of age in Hispanics is lower when compared to whites (M 115 v 147 and F 110 v 209 per 100 000).[23]

The data on CHD are conflicting but suggest that the burden of CHD is similar or greater compared to whites, and Hispanics have a higher case-fatality rate. For stroke it appears that Hispanics have lower incidence compared to whites.

Temporal trends
Although declines in CHD and CbVD mortality have occurred in Mexican Americans over the past 20 years, this decline has been less than that which has occurred among non-Hispanic whites.[23]

Common risk factors
Mexican Americans suffer a high prevalence of conventional CVRF such as smoking (42.5% in men and 23.8% in women), hypertension (17% men and 14% women), low HDL cholesterol (<0.90 mmol/L: 15.2% men and 5% women), elevated cholesterol (total cholesterol >6.2 mmol/L: 16.5% men and 16.5% women), diabetes (24%), physical inactivity (39%), and obesity (BMI >85th percentile: 30% men and 39% women). The San Antonio Heart Study reported that Mexican Americans had 2.5 times the prevalence of NIDDM compared to non-Hispanic whites as diagnosed by the oral glucose tolerance test.[122] They also observed that a socio-economic gradient within the

Hispanic population existed, with diabetes being more prevalent in the lower socio-economic groups.[124] Furthermore, Mexican Americans have higher blood concentrations of triglycerides and lower HDL cholesterol levels compared to non-Hispanic whites.[125]

Influential factors

A number of explanations have been put forward regarding the paradoxic findings of studies of Hispanic populations in the USA. The early studies which suggested that Hispanics have lower rates of CVD and CHD have been hypothesized to involve a "healthy migrant effect" – a diet that includes more fruits and vegetables, less chronic disease risk factor exposure before leaving their country of birth and health-preserving cultural psychosocial effects. It has also been suggested that some Hispanics may return to their country of birth when they retire or have a potentially fatal illness, especially those with a lower education, lower wages and fewer employment experiences. Selective out-migration would lead to underestimates of mortality, as would misclassification of deaths as discussed above. However, among long-settled Hispanics who adopt Western lifestyles, abdominal obesity and glucose intolerance appear to be the major factors for CHD among Mexican Americans.[119] Lower rates of smoking amongst older Mexican Americans compared with white Americans (11.9% v 15.4%)[126] and lower rates of smoking among Hispanic women compared with white women (12% v 28%) may contribute to lower rates of disease.[127] The greater mortality observed among Mexican Americans following MI in comparison to non-Hispanic whites is attributed in large part to the increased prevalence of diabetes. Findings from the San Antonio Heart Study also show that diabetic Mexican Americans not taking insulin treatment are at higher risk of fatal CVD compared with non-Hispanic white diabetics not using insulin.[122]

Latin America

While the above discussion has focused on Hispanics living in the USA, CVD is a major burden of disease in Latin America. In 2001, 28% of all deaths in Latin America were caused by CVD (GBD2001 http://www.dcp2.org/pubs/GBD/3/Table/3.B4). Latin America (LA) has also experienced major demographic, epidemiologic and nutritional transition in recent decades in an environment of increasing economic prosperity and urbanization. The Latin American region has exhibited a marked increase in the consumption of high-energy density foods (high in fats and sugars) and a decrease in physical activity, with rising trends of sedentary life among the urban population. The INTERHEART study recruited 1237 cases of AMI and 1888 controls from Argentina, Brazil, Colombia, Chile, Guatemala and Mexico. The most prevalent risk factor among controls was abdominal obesity; 48.6% of controls were in

the highest tertile compared with 31.2% in other countries participating in INTERHEART. Latin Americans had higher rates of current and former smoking (48.1% v 42%), dyslipidemia (42.0% v 32.0%) and hypertension (29.1% v 20.8%). Fruit and vegetables consumption and physical activity were, however, similar to other countries. Abdominal obesity was the most important risk factor in Latin Americans with an average population attributable risk for the region of 48.5%, followed by abnormal ratio of Apo B/Apo A-1 (40.8%) and smoking (38.4%).[128]

There is some evidence that CHD mortality rates are going down in some sectors of Latin America following the trends in the USA and Canada. CHD mortality fell by ~60% in the US and Canada and also fell by a similar amount in Argentina, but increased for some Latin America countries such as Costa Rica, Mexico and Venezuela for the period 1970 to 2000. The decline versus increase in rates by country and region is likely reflective of their various degrees of socio-economic transition and access to screening and treatment programs. Some of the decline may also be due to falling rates of smoking. Brazil reported smoking rates falling between 1989 and 2003 from 34.8% to 22.4%.[129] The rates of stroke also appear to be declining in most Latin American countries by approximately 30% compared to ~60% in USA and Canada (Table 19.8). The impact of rising obesity and sedentary habits on these regions in the future is, however, uncertain.

Approaches to prevention/treatment

Due to the discrepant data concerning the CHD mortality rates of Mexican Americans, despite their adverse risk factor profile, many researchers believe that they remain "protected" from CHD.[130] Clearly, the burden of CHD among Mexican Americans is considerable, and screening and modification of conventional CHD risk factors are necessary. Furthermore, primary prevention of obesity will be important to reduce the burden of type 2 diabetes in this group.

Aboriginal populations

Aboriginal populations or indigenous people generally refer to an ethnic group who inhabit the geographic region with which they have the earliest historical connections. For example, in Canada, Aboriginal people are the descendants of the original inhabitants of North America. (Indian and Northern Affairs Canada: http://www.ainc-inac.gc.ca/pr/info/info125_e.html) and include Indians (now known as First Nations people), Métis and Inuit. The focus of this next section is on Aboriginal populations of North America, but other indigenous populations such as the Aboriginals from Australia share a similar cardiovascular risk profile.

Table 19.8

(a) Trends in age-standardized (world population) death certification rates per 100000 for coronary heart disease in the Americas 1970–2000[22]

Country	Men			Women		
	1970–72	1998–2000	% Change	1970–72	1998–2000	% Change
Argentina	94.8	58.9	−38	69.3	38.0	−45
Brazil*	NA	85.5	−20Ψ	NA	61.7	−21Ψ
Chile*	91.1	62.8	−31	84.6	43.3	−49
Colombia*	61.7	47.1	−24	68.0	45.4	−33
Costa Rica	53.7	37.5	−30	52.7	34.1	−35
Cuba	63.7	53.0	−17	64.0	51.0	−20
Ecuador	39.1	35.4	−10	37.7	30.0	−20
Mexico	40.5	40.3	−1	42.6	36.6	−14
Puerto Rico	53.9	32.8	−39	46.3	25.6	−45
Venezuela	60.2	58.9	−2	56.6	49.8	−12
Canada	63.9	24.7	−61	54.1	22.2	−59
USA	73.9	27.7	−63	61.9	26.8	−57

*For Brazil 1986 was used for 1980 and 1995 for 2000; for Chile 1999 was used for 2000l and for Colombia 1972 was used for 1970, 1984 for 1980, 1991 for 1990, and 1999 for 2000

ΨChanges between 1995 and 1986.

NA, Not available

(b) Trends in age-standardized (world population) death certification rates per 100000 for cerebrovascular disease in the Americas 1970–2000

Country	Men			Women		
	1970–72	1998–2000	% Change	1970–72	1998–2000	% Change
Argentina	182.1	67.4	−63	89.2	28.3	−68
Brazil*	NA	88.1	−18Ψ	NA	51.4	−18Ψ
Chile*	110.9	74.1	−33	74.0	38.2	−48
Colombia*	94.9	93.4	−2	63.1	60.9	−3
Costa Rica	72.7	99.9	37	55.1	59.9	9
Cuba	138.8	123.3	−11	107.2	87.0	−19
Ecuador	32.5	36.7	13	22.4	21.2	−6
Mexico	42.2	82.0	94	28.4	53.9	90
Puerto Rico	142.6	95.9	−33	99.8	55.3	−45
Venezuela	119.7	136.4	14	75.2	78.5	4
Canada	267.1	97.9	−63	124.1	47.9	−61
USA	316.6	118.6	−63	157.4	67.2	−57

*For Brazil 1986 was used for 1980 and 1995 for 2000; for Chile 1999 was used for 2000l and for Colombia 1972 was used for 1970, 1984 for 1980, 1991 for 1990, and 1999 for 2000

ΨChanges between 1995 and 1986.

NA, Not available

Disease burden

Cardiovascular disease is the leading cause of death in North American Indian and Alaskan Native males and females. Although research in this ethnic group is limited, the Strong Heart Study,[131] which was initiated in 1988, studied 4549 American Natives aged 45–74 years from 13 tribes in the southern US. The prevalence estimates of definite MI in those aged 45–74 years was 2.8% in men without diabetes and 5.3% in men with diabetes, 0.4% in women without diabetes and 1.4% in women with diabetes. Data from the 2005 Behavioral Risk Factor Surveillance System (BRFSS) indicate that American Indian. Alaskan Natives report the highest prevalence of CHD (myocardial infarction or angina) of 11.2% compared to non-Hispanic whites (6.2%), African Americans (6.2%), Hispanics (6.9) and Asians (4.7%).[132] Similarly data from Canada indicate that Aboriginal people suffer higher rates of CHD compared to the general population.[92] There is little published information concerning the epidemiology of stroke in native populations. In the USA the stroke mortality rate under the age of 65 years is similar in Native Americans and white Americans, and substantially lower than rates in African Americans.[133] Over the age of 65, the stroke rate in Native Americans is reported to be approximately 40% lower than whites.[133] In Canada, CVD is the leading cause of death among Aboriginal peoples.[134] Although the CHD mortality rates among Aboriginal and Canadian males are similar, the CHD mortality among Aboriginal women is 61% higher compared with Canadian women. In addition, the stroke mortality rate is 44% and 93% higher among Aboriginal men and women respectively, compared with the general Canadian population.[134] However, all of the above data are based on studies conducted more than 10 years ago. More recent data from a prevalence study in Canada indicate a 2.5-fold higher rate of CVD among Aboriginal peoples compared with Canadians of European origin.[135] As more Aboriginal people give up their traditional lifestyles and adopt "urban" lifestyles, the prevalence of CVD and its risk factors is increasing.

Common risk factors

The common CVRF among Aboriginal people include obesity, abdominal obesity, diabetes, elevated blood pressure, low HDL cholesterol, and tobacco use. The prevalence of cigarette smoking is generally high and increasing among Aboriginal people but varies greatly between Aboriginal communities.[135] The prevalence of diabetes in the Strong Heart Study was an astounding 48% in the 45–64 year age group compared to approximately 5.5% in the US general population, and the prevalence of obesity was between 26% and 41%, with an average BMI of 31 and waist–hip ratio of 0.96 in men.[136] Interestingly, the prevalence of hypertension and elevated serum cholesterol among Aboriginal people appears to be lower when compared to the general US population. In Canada, however, the prevalence of hypertension requiring drug treatment, and elevated cholesterol requiring medication, was significantly increased among Aboriginal people compared to a similar sample of non-Aboriginal people.[135] In addition, the prevalence of low HDL cholesterol is greater in this group, as approximately 25% of Aboriginal people have HDL cholesterol values less than 0.90 mmol/L.[135] Canadian Aboriginal people also have a higher prevalence of CVD, atherosclerosis, glucose abnormalities, obesity, abdominal obesity, and tobacco use compared to European-origin Canadians. [135]

Influential risk factors

Obesity, diabetes, and tobacco use among Aboriginal people are the most influential risk factors for future CHD. Aboriginal people who are diabetic are two to four times more likely to suffer CVD than non-diabetic people.[135] In the Strong Heart Study other important risk factors for CHD included hypertension, obesity, and low HDL cholesterol.[136]

Approaches to disease prevention

Control of obesity through increased physical activity and lowering of energy consumption will continue to be the mainstay of prevention amongst Aboriginal people. In addition, provision of strong disincentives to tobacco use are necessary to prevent smoking initiation amongst young Aboriginals. Also the imbalance in socio-economic circumstances between Aboriginal and non-Aboriginal peoples must be addressed, as lower socio-economic status is clearly associated with adverse lifestyle practices, psychosocial stress, and CVD.

Black people of African origin

Disease burden

Cardiovascular disease mortality data from countries in sub-Saharan Africa (SSA) are limited, as only 1.1% of all deaths are registered with a central agency.[12] Data from other sources such as sample registries and small-scale population studies in 1990 indicate that the CHD mortality was 41/100 000.[137] These rates are considerably lower than those of whites and South Asians who live in Africa, as well as rates of most Western countries, which are on average five times higher. Even so, in SSA, the proportional mortality rate from CHD accounts for 26% of all deaths, and in the 60–70 year age group it is responsible for over 80% of all deaths.[12,137] First MI also appears to occur at an earlier age among people from SSA. In the INTERHEART study the mean age of presentation of first MI in SSA participants was 54.3 years (3.8 years earlier than the overall INTERHEART study). Men (53.2 years) presented at a younger age than women (56.4 years). Furthermore, the case-fatality rate of CHD is higher in SSA compared to Western countries, meaning that once an individual develops CHD in SSA, the probability of death in SSA is higher than in Western countries. This probably reflects the limited access to acute and chronic treatment strategies. Absolute numbers of strokes are also relatively low in SSA countries such as Zimbabwe (31/100 000 in 1997) and South Africa (101/100 000 in 1986) compared to the UK Oxford Vascular Study (145/100 000 in 2004) and the US North of Manhattan Stroke Study (223/100 000).[138] In-hospital stroke case fatality is high at 33%, and higher in hemorrhagic stroke (58%) compared to ischemic stroke (22%).[138]

Risk factors

The prevalence of most conventional CVRF is lower among blacks compared to other groups within Africa and the world, with the exception of hypertension and smoking among urban blacks.[139,140] Data from the WHO Inter-Health Program (a substudy of the MONICA project) assessed the risk factor profile of men and women aged 35–64 years from Tanzania.[140] The prevalence of smoking was 37% among men and 4% among women, the mean BMI was 21 in men, and 22 in women, the mean BP was 126/79 mmHg among men compared to 125/79 mmHg in women, the mean serum cholesterol was 4.1 mmol/L in men, and 4.3 mmol/L in women. When compared to the risk factor profile of other developing and developed countries, Tanzania's was more favorable, with the exception of smoking among men. Furthermore, the prevalence of multiple CVRF was low, as 65% of the population had no identifiable risk factors, 30% had a single risk factor, and only 5% had at least two risk factors, compared to 50%, 40%, and 10% in the USA.[140] The INTERHEART study found that the risk of MI increased with higher income and education in the black African group in contrast to findings from other African ethnic groups. Contrasting gradients in socio-economic class suggest that groups are at different stages of epidemiologic transition.[141] Although CHD rates among people of African origin remain relatively low, the data are limited and given the increased migration of blacks to urban centers[142] and a subsequent rise in the number of conventional CVRF, the rates of CHD and stroke are expected to rise.

Approaches to disease prevention

Regional analysis of 578 cases and 785 controls from nine SSA countries (80% from South Africa) in the INTERHEART study found that known CVRF accounted for approximately 90% of the MI observed in African populations, which was consistent with the overall INTERHEART study. However, a history of hypertension was associated with a higher MI risk in the black African group (OR 6.99, 95% CI 4.23–11.55) compared with the overall INTERHEART group (OR 2.48, 95% CI 2.30–2.68).[141] Thus prevention strategies to reduce the consumption of saturated fats and salt and control tobacco use and blood pressure are likely to be effective in these populations.

African Americans

African Americans comprise the largest non-white population in the USA and represent approximately 13% of the population.

Disease burden

Cardiovascular disease is the leading cause of death among African Americans, and the incidence of both CHD and stroke is higher in African Americans compared to white Americans. Mortality from both CHD and stroke has been noted to be higher in black compared to white Americans.[143,144] Sudden cardiac death rates have also been noted to be higher in black patients.[145] Although there has been a decline in mortality rates from CVD in both African Americans and white Americans over the past 30 years, these declines have been less marked in African Americans.[23]

Common risk factors

Compared to whites, African Americans develop high blood pressure at an earlier age, are more likely to develop hypertension over the life course, and appear to have a more severe type of hypertension.[116] The reason for black–white differences in hypertension prevalence likely involves a complex interaction between environmental response to diet and stress, and a potential genetic/physiologic difference such as differences in sodium/potassium excretion, perhaps linked to their origins in Africa. The prevalence of high cholesterol (>5.2 mmo/L) is similar or lower among African Americans compared with white Americans (47% v 54% in males, 51% v 53% in females)[23] and HDL cholesterol levels are generally higher. Smoking is more common among African American men (33% v 27%) compared with white men, but less common among African American women compared to white women.[23] Overweight and obesity are more common especially among African American women compared to white women (50% v 33%).[23] Physical activity is lower – 65% of African Americans report a sedentary lifestyle compared to about 56% of whites.[23] Diabetes rates are higher in African Americans compared to whites as demonstrated by NHANES II conducted from 1976 to 1980 in adults 20–74 years of age, which found that 9.9% of African Americans versus 6% of white Americans had type 2 diabetes.[23] The rate of diabetes is also increasing faster among African Americans, especially in women.[23] Although elevated levels of Lp(a) are found more often in African Americans than whites, whether or not elevated Lp(a) levels are related to an increased CHD risk among African Americans is unclear.[147]

However, even after consideration of these "biomedical" differences, an important determinant of persisting CVD among African Americans is the persisting differences in socio-economic status which translate into poorer access to medical services, less screening for risk factors and lower rates of coronary revascularization procedures.[148]

Influential factors

While hypertension is an important difference between black and white American people, at least 30% of the excess CHD mortality in blacks compared to whites can be accounted for by differences in socio-economic status.[148] In addition to poorer access to care, black Americans have worse outcomes from treatments. Black American CABG patients have significantly worse in-hospital mortality rates than other ethnic groups.[149]

Approaches to prevention/treatment

The rates of CHD among blacks in Africa are relatively low compared to the rates in most Western countries. However, in populations that have urbanized both within Africa and amongst migrant Africans to the West Indies and the USA, the rates of CVD are comparable to those of Western/European populations. As in other populations, conventional CVRF remain important but the dominant CVRF among people of African origin is hypertension and hence this needs to be specifically targeted for these populations. In the USA, the socio-economic disparity must be addressed to improve health outcomes for black groups. To ensure equal access to healthcare services overall changes in social policy are likely to be required at the national level.

Studies of multiple ethnic groups

Studies of diverse ethnic populations who reside in a single country and hence are exposed to a similar environment indicate that the pattern of CHD mortality in these groups initially resembles that of their home country. However, through the process of acculturation, prolonged exposure to new environmental factors results in similarities in CVRF and trends within multiethnic populations. However, comparative studies of ethnic groups within multiethnic countries (US and UK) suggest that certain ethnic groups are still relatively protected (e.g. Japanese, East Asians) and certain groups are more prone to CVD (e.g. black Africans, South Asians). This is likely due to a complex interaction of environment, sociocultural factors, behaviors and genetics.

Environmental contribution to ethnic and regional differences in cardiovascular disease

It is now apparent that most of the attributable risk for MI within populations from across the world can be ascribed to a limited number of risk factors.[20] What is less clear, however, is what shapes the distribution of risk factors between populations. There is now a growing body of evidence indicating that factors that describe our environment are likely to contribute to these differences.[15] These include: poor access to healthcare, a more toxic physical environment (e.g. less access to healthy food choices,[150] more fast food,[151] fewer opportunities for physical activity[152] more

exposure to air pollution), and less social support for those with disease.[153]

Genetic contribution to ethnic and regional differences in cardiovascular disease

Variation in risk factor levels across populations may also be genetically driven. Genetic factors have been shown to contribute to the development of certain risk factors. For example, many lipid abnormalities have genetic determinants and some have been shown to also predict clinical outcomes in patients with established CHD.[154] A number of possible mechanisms have been postulated, including that genetic variants could contribute to population differences in risk factors through:
- differences in allele frequency
- variation in gene expression
- epigenetic influences
- environmental interactions resulting in differences in gene expression.

Studies of different ethnic groups are ideally suited to understanding gene–environment interactions because they increase the range of allele frequencies and environmental exposures.[155]

Conclusion

Cardiovascular disease accounts for the largest percentage of deaths worldwide. To date, recognition and modification of the major CVRFs have led to declines in CVD rates in many OECD countries, although within many of these countries there remain high-risk groups as both ethnic and socio-economic disparities exist. Socio-economic development, urbanization, and increasing life expectancy have led to a progressive rise in CVD rates in developing countries such as India and China.

It is clear from the INTERHEART study that smoking, cholesterol and blood pressure are the major determinants of CVD globally, across all regions and across all ethnic groups. As populations urbanize, increasing levels of CVRF lead to an increasing burden of CVD for these populations. It seems that environment/social influences are implicated in these changing levels of CVRF. However, it is less clear what particular factors about our changing environment impact on population risk factors and how these interact with individual biologic and genetic factors. In the future a more detailed understanding of the interaction of environmental/social factors, human behaviors, individual risk factors and genetics will be needed to develop appropriate prevention strategies to decrease the global burden of cardiovascular disease.

Acknowledgments

CK Chow is supported through a Cottrell scholarship, Royal Australasian College of Physicians, and a Public Health (Sidney Sax) Overseas Fellowship co-funded by NHMRC and NHF of Australia. S Yusuf is supported by an endowed chair at the Heart and Stroke Foundation of Ontario.

References

1. Lenfant C. Task force on Research in Epidemiology and Prevention of Cardiovascular Diseases. *Circulation* 1994;**90**(6): 2609–17.
2. Anand SS. Using ethnicity as a classification variable in health research: perpetuating the myth of biological determinism, serving socio-political agendas, or making valuable contributions to medical sciences? *Ethn Health* 1999;**4**(4):241–4.
3. Littlefield A, Lieberman L, Reynolds L. Redefining race: the potential demise of a concept in physical anthropology. *Curr Anthropol* 1982;**23**:641–55.
4. Jackson FL. Race and ethnicity as biological constructs. *Ethn Dis* 1992;**2**(2):120–5.
5. Crews DE, Bindon JR. Ethnicity as a taxonomic tool in biomedical and biosocial research. *Ethn Dis* 1991;**1**(1):42–9.
6. Cooper R. A note on the biologic concept of race and its application in epidemiologic research. *Am Heart J* 1984;**108**(3 Pt 2):715–22.
7. Chaturvedi N, McKeigue PM. Methods for epidemiological surveys of ethnic minority groups. *J Epidemiol Community Health* 1994;**48**(2):107–11.
8. Lopez AD. Assessing the burden of mortality from cardiovascular diseases. *World Health Stat Q* 1993;**46**(2):91–6.
9. Lopez AD, Mathers CD, Ezzati M, Jamison DT, Murray CJ. Global and regional burden of disease and risk factors, 2001: systematic analysis of population health data. *Lancet* 2006; **367**(9524):1747–57.
10. Mathers CD, Loncar D. Projections of global mortality and burden of disease from 2002 to 2030. *PLoS Med* 2006;**3**(11):e442.
11. Abegunde DO, Mathers CD, Adam T, Ortegon M, Strong K. The burden and costs of chronic diseases in low-income and middle-income countries. *Lancet* 2007;**370**(9603):1929–38.
12. Murray C, Lopez A. *The Global Burden of Disease: A Comprehensive Assessment of Mortality and Disability from Disease, Injuries and Risk Factors in 1990 and Projected to 2020.* Boston: Harvard School of Public Health, 1996.
13. Levy DT, Nikolayev L, Mumford E. Recent trends in smoking and the role of public policies: results from the SimSmoke tobacco control policy simulation model. *Addiction* 2005;**100**(10): 1526–36.
14. DeWilde S, Carey IM, Richards N, Whincup PH, Cook DG. Trends in secondary prevention of ischaemic heart disease in the UK 1994 2005: use of individual and combination treatment. *Heart* 2008;**94**(1):83–8.
15. Chow CK, Lock K, Teo S, Subramanian SV, McKee M, Yusuf S. Environmental and societal influences acting on cardiovascular risk factors and disease at a population level: a review. *IJE* 2008;in press.
16. Menotti A, Keys A, Kromhout D, Blackburn H, Aravanis C, Bloemberg B et al. Inter-cohort differences in coronary heart disease mortality in the 25-year follow-up of the seven countries study. *Eur J Epidemiol* 1993;**9**(5):527–36.
17. Bothig S. WHO MONICA Project: objectives and design. *Int J Epidemiol* 1989;**18**(3 Suppl 1):S29–37.
18. Levi F, Lucchini F, Negri E, La Vecchia C. Trends in mortality from cardiovascular and cerebrovascular diseases in Europe and other areas of the world. *Heart* 2002;**88**(2):119–24.
19. Benfante R. Studies of cardiovascular disease and cause-specific mortality trends in Japanese-American men living in Hawaii and risk factor comparisons with other Japanese populations in the Pacific region: a review. *Hum Biol* 1992;**64**(6): 791–805.
20. Yusuf S, Hawken S, Ounpuu S, Dans T, Avezum A, Lanas F et al. Effect of potentially modifiable risk factors associated with myocardial infarction in 52 countries (the INTERHEART study): case-control study. *Lancet* 2004;**364**(9438):937–52.
21. Muller-Nordhorn J, Binting S, Roll S, Willich SN. An update on regional variation in cardiovascular mortality within Europe. *Eur Heart J* 2008;**29**(10):1316–26.
22. Rodriguez T, Malvezzi M, Chatenoud L, Bosetti C, Levi F, Negri E et al. Trends in mortality from coronary heart and cerebrovascular diseases in the Americas: 1970–2000. *Heart* 2006;**92**(4): 453–60.
23. WHO Statistical Information System. Geneva: WHO, 2008.
24. Thorvaldsen P, Asplund K, Kuulasmaa K, Rajakangas AM, Schroll M. Stroke incidence, case fatality, and mortality in the WHO MONICA project. World Health Organization Monitoring Trends and Determinants in Cardiovascular Disease. *Stroke* 1995;**26**(3):361–7.
25. Bobak M, Marmot M. Alcohol and mortality in Russia: is it different than elsewhere? *Ann Epidemiol* 1999;**9**(6):335–8.
26. Marmot M. Coronary heart disease: rise and fall of a modern epidemic. In: Marmot M, Elliot P, eds. *Coronary Heart Disease Epidemiology.* Oxford: Oxford University Press, 1995.
27. Artaud-Wild SM, Connor SL, Sexton G, Connor WE. Differences in coronary mortality can be explained by differences in cholesterol and saturated fat intakes in 40 countries but not in France and Finland. A paradox. *Circulation* 1993;**88**(6): 2771–9.
28. Criqui MH, Ringel BL. Does diet or alcohol explain the French paradox? *Lancet* 1994;**344**(8939–8940):1719–23.
29. Law M, Wald N. Why heart disease mortality is low in France: the time lag explanation. *BMJ* 1999;**318**(7196):1471–6.
30. Vartiainen E, Puska P, Jousilahti P, Korhonen HJ, Tuomilehto J, Nissinen A. Twenty-year trends in coronary risk factors in north Karelia and in other areas of Finland. *Int J Epidemiol* 1994;**23**(3):495–504.
31. Hunink MG, Goldman L, Tosteson AN, Mittleman MA, Goldman PA, Williams LW et al. The recent decline in mortality from coronary heart disease, 1980–1990. The effect of secular trends in risk factors and treatment. *JAMA* 1997;**277**(7): 535–42.
32. Zatonski WA, McMichael AJ, Powles JW. Ecological study of reasons for sharp decline in mortality from ischaemic heart disease in Poland since 1991. *BMJ* 1998;**316**(7137):1047–51.

33. Leon DA, Chenet L, Shkolnikov VM, Zakharov S, Shapiro J, Rakhmanova G et al. Huge variation in Russian mortality rates 1984–94: artefact, alcohol, or what? *Lancet* 1997;**350**(9075): 383–8.

34. Kitamura A, Iso H, Iida M, Naito Y, Sato S, Jacobs DR et al. Trends in the incidence of coronary heart disease and stroke and the prevalence of cardiovascular risk factors among Japanese men from 1963 to 1994. *Am J Med* 2002;**112**(2):104–9.

35. Ueshima H. Explanation for the Japanese paradox: prevention of increase in coronary heart disease and reduction in stroke. *J Atheroscler Thromb* 2007;**14**(6):278–86.

36. WHO Global Infobase Surf 2 Country Profiles. In: WHO, ed. *WHO Global InfoBase, 2005*. Geneva: WHO.

37. Yoshiike N, Kaneda F, Takimoto H. Epidemiology of obesity and public health strategies for its control in Japan. *Asia Pac J Clin Nutr* 2002;**11**(Suppl 8):S727–31.

38. Shimako M. The influence of changing lifestyles on health education and chornic disease prevention in Japan. In: Shetty P, Gopalan C, eds. *Diet, Nutrition and Chronic Disease, An Asian Perspective*. London: Smith-Gordon, 1998.

39. Ohmura T, Ueda K, Kiyohara Y, Kato I, Iwamoto H, Nakayama K et al. Prevalence of type 2 (non-insulin-dependent) diabetes mellitus and impaired glucose tolerance in the Japanese general population: the Hisayama Study. *Diabetologia* 1993;**36**(11): 1198–203.

40. Cardoso MA, Hamada GS, de Souza JM, Tsugane S, Tokudome S. Dietary patterns in Japanese migrants to southeastern Brazil and their descendants. *J Epidemiol* 1997;**7**(4):198–204.

41. Schwingel A, Nakata Y, Ito LS, Chodzko-Zajko WJ, Shigematsu R, Erb CT et al. Lower HDL-cholesterol among healthy middle-aged Japanese-Brazilians in Sao Paulo compared to Natives and Japanese-Brazilians in Japan. *Eur J Epidemiol* 2007;**22**(1): 33–42.

42. Ferreira SR, Iunes M, Franco LJ, Iochida LC, Hirai A, Vivolo MA. Disturbances of glucose and lipid metabolism in first and second generation Japanese-Brazilians. Japanese-Brazilian Diabetes Study Group. *Diabetes Res Clin Pract* 1996;**34**(Suppl): S59–63.

43. Ueshima H, Okayama A, Saitoh S, Nakagawa H, Rodriguez B, Sakata K et al. Differences in cardiovascular disease risk factors between Japanese in Japan and Japanese-Americans in Hawaii: the INTERLIPID study. *J Hum Hypertens* 2003;**17**(9):631–9.

44. Klatsky AL, Armstrong MA. Cardiovascular risk factors among Asian Americans living in northern California. *Am J Public Health* 1991;**81**(11):1423–8.

45. Yamori Y, Miura A, Taira K. Implications from and for food cultures for cardiovascular diseases: Japanese food, particularly Okinawan diets. *Asia Pac J Clin Nutr* 2001;**10**(2): 144–5.

46. Hong Y, Bots ML, Pan X, Hofman A, Grobbee DE, Chen H. Stroke incidence and mortality in rural and urban Shanghai from 1984 through 1991. Findings from a community-based registry. *Stroke* 1994;**25**(6):1165–9.

47. Liu L. Cardiovascular diseases in China. *Biochem Cell Biol* 2007;**85**(2):157–63.

48. Woo KS, Donnan SP. Epidemiology of coronary arterial disease in the Chinese. *Int J Cardiol* 1989;**24**(1):83–93.

49. Khor GL. Cardiovascular epidemiology in the Asia-Pacific region. *Asia Pac J Clin Nutr* 2001;**10**(2):76–80.

50. He J, Gu D, Wu X, Reynolds K, Duan X, Yao C et al. Major causes of death among men and women in China. *N Engl J Med* 2005;**353**(11):1124–34.

51. Jiang B, Wang WZ, Chen H, Hong Z, Yang QD, Wu SP et al. Incidence and trends of stroke and its subtypes in China: results from three large cities. *Stroke* 2006;**37**(1):63–8.

52. Wu Z, Yao C, Zhao D, Wu G, Wang W, Liu J et al. Sino-MONICA project: a collaborative study on trends and determinants in cardiovascular diseases in China, Part i: morbidity and mortality monitoring. *Circulation* 2001;**103**(3):462–8.

53. Yang G, Fan L, Tan J, Qi G, Zhang Y, Samet JM et al. Smoking in China: findings of the 1996 National Prevalence Survey. *JAMA* 1999;**282**(13):1247–53.

54. Gan Q, Smith KR, Hammond SK, Hu TW. Disease burden of adult lung cancer and ischaemic heart disease from passive tobacco smoking in China. *Tob Control* 2007;**16**(6):417–22.

55. Popkin BM, Paeratakul S, Ge K, Zhai F. Body weight patterns among the Chinese: results from the 1989 and 1991 China Health and Nutrition Surveys. *Am J Public Health* 1995;**85**(5): 690–4.

56. Zhang X, Patel A, Horibe H, Wu Z, Barzi F, Rodgers A et al. Cholesterol, coronary heart disease, and stroke in the Asia Pacific region. *Int J Epidemiol* 2003;**32**(4):563–72.

57. Critchley J, Liu J, Zhao D, Wei W, Capewell S. Explaining the increase in coronary heart disease mortality in Beijing between 1984 and 1999. *Circulation* 2004;**110**(10):1236–44.

58. Niu SR, Yang GH, Chen ZM, Wang JL, Wang GH, He XZ et al. Emerging tobacco hazards in China: 2. Early mortality results from a prospective study. *BMJ* 1998;**317**(7170):1423–4.

59. Zhang H, Cai B. The impact of tobacco on lung health in China. *Respirology* 2003;**8**(1):17–21.

60. Bell AC, Ge K, Popkin BM. The road to obesity or the path to prevention: motorized transportation and obesity in China. *Obes Res* 2002;**10**(4):277–83.

61. Gu D, Wu X, Reynolds K, Duan X, Xin X, Reynolds RF et al. Cigarette smoking and exposure to environmental tobacco smoke in China: the international collaborative study of cardiovascular disease in Asia. *Am J Public Health* 2004;**94**(11): 1972–6.

62. Reynolds K, Gu D, Whelton PK, Wu X, Duan X, Mo J et al. Prevalence and risk factors of overweight and obesity in China. *Obesity (Silver Spring)* 2007;**15**(1):10–18.

63. Gu D, Reynolds K, Wu X, Chen J, Duan X, Muntner P et al. Prevalence, awareness, treatment, and control of hypertension in China. *Hypertension* 2002;**40**(6):920–7.

64. He J, Gu D, Reynolds K, Wu X, Muntner P, Zhao J et al. Serum total and lipoprotein cholesterol levels and awareness, treatment, and control of hypercholesterolemia in China. *Circulation* 2004;**110**(4):405–11.

65. Gu D, Reynolds K, Duan X, Xin X, Chen J, Wu X et al. Prevalence of diabetes and impaired fasting glucose in the Chinese adult population: International Collaborative Study of Cardiovascular Disease in Asia (InterASIA). *Diabetologia* 2003;**46**(9): 1190–8.

66. Li N, Tuomilehto J, Dowse G, Alberti KG, Zimmet P, Min Z et al. Electrocardiographic abnormalities and associated factors in Chinese living in Beijing and in Mauritius. The Mauritius Non-Communicable Disease Study Group. *BMJ* 1992;**304**(6842): 1596–601.

67. Hughes K, Yeo PP, Lun KC, Thai AC, Sothy SP, Wang KW *et al.* Cardiovascular diseases in Chinese, Malays, and Indians in Singapore. II. Differences in risk factor levels. *J Epidemiol Community Health* 1990;**44**(1):29–35.

68. Woo KS, Chook P, Raitakari OT, McQuillan B, Feng JZ, Celermajer DS. Westernization of Chinese adults and increased subclinical atherosclerosis. *Arterioscler Thromb Vasc Biol* 1999; **19**(10):2487–93.

69. Zhang J, Kesteloot H. Differences in all-cause, cardiovascular and cancer mortality between Hong Kong and Singapore: role of nutrition. *Eur J Epidemiol* 2001;**17**(5):469–77.

70. Reddy KS. Cardiovascular diseases in India. *World Health Stat Q* 1993;**46**(2):101–7.

71. Chockalingam A, Balaguer-Vintro I, Achutti A, de Luna AB, Chalmers J, Farinaro E *et al.* The World Heart Federation's white book: impending global pandemic of cardiovascular diseases: challenges and opportunities for the prevention and control of cardiovascular diseases in developing countries and economies in transition. *Can J Cardiol* 2000;**16**(2):227–9.

72. Mathers CD, Salomon JA, Ezzati M, Begg S, Vander-Hoorn S, Lopez AD. *Global Burden of Disease and Risk Factors.* New York: Oxford University Press, 2006.

73. Lowy AG, Woods KL, Botha JL. The effects of demographic shift on coronary heart disease mortality in a large migrant population at high risk. *J Public Health Med* 1991;**13**(4):276–80.

74. Ahmad N, Bhopal R. Is coronary heart disease rising in India? A systematic review based on ECG defined coronary heart disease. *Heart* 2005;**91**(6):719–25.

75. Gupta R. Meta-analysis of prevalence of hypertension in India. *Indian Heart J* 1997;**49**(4):450.

76. Ramachandran A, Snehalatha C, Kapur A, Vijay V, Mohan V, Das AK *et al.* High prevalence of diabetes and impaired glucose tolerance in India: National Urban Diabetes Survey. *Diabetologia* 2001;**44**(9):1094–101.

77. Ramachandran A. Epidemiology of diabetes in India – three decades of research. *J Assoc Physicians India* 2005;**53**:34–8.

78. Chow CK, Raju PK, Raju R, Reddy KS, Cardona M, Celermajer DS *et al.* The prevalence and management of diabetes in rural India. *Diabetes Care* 2006;**29**(7):1717–18.

79. Chow CK. *Cardiovascular risk factor levels and cardiovascular risk estimation in a rural area of India.* Sydney: University of Sydney, 2007.

80. Gupta R. Trends in hypertension epidemiology in India. *J Hum Hypertens* 2004;**18**(2):73–8.

81. Prabhakaran D, Shah P, Chaturvedi V, Ramakrishnan L, Manhapra A, Reddy KS. Cardiovascular risk factor prevalence among men in a large industry of northern India. *Natl Med J India* 2005;**18**(2):59–65.

82. Chow CK, Naidu S, Raju K, Raju R, Joshi R, Sullivan D *et al.* Significant lipid, adiposity and metabolic abnormalities amongst 4535 Indians from a developing region of rural Andhra Pradesh. *Atherosclerosis* 2008;**196**(2):943–52.

83. Reddy KS, Prabhakaran D, Jeemon P, Thankappan KR, Joshi P, Chaturvedi V *et al.* Educational status and cardiovascular risk profile in Indians. *Proc Natl Acad Sci U S A* 2007;**104**(41): 16263–8.

84. Anand SS, Enas EA, Pogue J, Haffner S, Pearson T, Yusuf S. Elevated lipoprotein(a) levels in South Asians in North America. *Metabolism* 1998;**47**(2):182–4.

85. Joshi P, Islam S, Pais P, Reddy S, Dorairaj P, Kazmi K *et al.* Risk factors for early myocardial infarction in South Asians compared with individuals in other countries. *JAMA* 2007;**297**(3):286–94.

86. Gerstein HC, Pais P, Pogue J, Yusuf S. Relationship of glucose and insulin levels to the risk of myocardial infarction: a case-control study. *J Am Coll Cardiol* 1999;**33**(3):612–19.

87. Teo KK, Ounpuu S, Hawken S, Pandey MR, Valentin V, Hunt D *et al.* Tobacco use and risk of myocardial infarction in 52 countries in the INTERHEART study: a case-control study. *Lancet* 2006;**368**(9536):647–58.

88. Kumar R, Singh MC, Ahlawat SK, Thakur AS, Srivastava A, Sharma MK *et al.* Urbanization and coronary heart disease: a study of urban–rural differences in northern India. *Indian Heart J* 2006;**58**:126–30.

89. Enas EA, Yusuf S, Mehta JL. Prevalence of coronary artery disease in Asian Indians. *Am J Cardiol* 1992;**70**(9):945–9.

90. McKeigue PM, Shah B, Marmot MG. Relation of central obesity and insulin resistance with high diabetes prevalence and cardiovascular risk in South Asians. *Lancet* 1991;**337**(8738):382–6.

91. Joseph A, Kutty VR, Soman CR. High risk for coronary heart disease in Thiruvananthapuram city: a study of serum lipids and other risk factors. *Indian Heart J* 2000;**52**(1):29–35.

92. Anand SS, Yusuf S, Vuksan V, Devanesen S, Teo KK, Montague PA *et al.* Differences in risk factors, atherosclerosis, and cardiovascular disease between ethnic groups in Canada: the Study of Health Assessment and Risk in Ethnic groups (SHARE). *Lancet* 2000;**356**(9226):279–84.

93. Balarajan R. Ethnic differences in mortality from ischaemic heart disease and cerebrovascular disease in England and Wales. *BMJ* 1991;**302**(6776):560–4.

94. Sheth T, Nair C, Nargundkar M, Anand S, Yusuf S. Cardiovascular and cancer mortality among Canadians of European, south Asian and Chinese origin from 1979 to 1993: an analysis of 1.2 million deaths. *CMAJ* 1999;**161**(2):132–8.

95. Wyndham CH. Trends with time of cardiovascular mortality rates in the populations of the RSA for the period 1968–1977. *S Afr Med J* 1982;**61**(26):987–93.

96. Steinberg WJ, Balfe DL, Kustner HG. Decline in the ischaemic heart disease mortality rates of South Africans, 1968–1985. *S Afr Med J* 1988;**74**(11):547–50.

97. Baligadoo S, Manraj M, Krishnamoorthy R, Jankee S, Ramasawmy R. Genetic contribution to the height mortality from coronary disease in Indian Diaspora: case study of Mauritius. *Eur Heart J* 1994;**15**(162).

98. Tuomilehto J, Ram P, Eseroma R, Taylor R, Zimmet P. Cardiovascular diseases and diabetes mellitus in Fiji: analysis of mortality, morbidity and risk factors. *Bull World Health Organ* 1984;**62**(1):133–43.

99. Beckles GL, Miller GJ, Kirkwood BR, Alexis SD, Carson DC, Byam NT. High total and cardiovascular disease mortality in adults of Indian descent in Trinidad, unexplained by major coronary risk factors. *Lancet* 1986;**1**(8493):1298–301.

100. Hughes K, Lun KC, Yeo PP. Cardiovascular diseases in Chinese, Malays, and Indians in Singapore. I. Differences in mortality. *J Epidemiol Community Health* 1990;**44**(1):24–8.

101. Adelstein AM, Marmot MG, Bulusu L. Migrant studies in Britain. *Br Med Bull* 1984;**40**(4):315–19.

102. McKeigue PM, Marmot MG. Mortality from coronary heart disease in Asian communities in London. *BMJ* 1988;**297**(6653):903.

103. Bhatnagar D, Anand IS, Durrington PN, Patel DJ, Wander GS, Mackness MI *et al.* Coronary risk factors in people from the Indian subcontinent living in west London and their siblings in India. *Lancet* 1995;**345**(8947):405–9.

104. CAMPAS. *Annual Health Report for the Year 1990.* Cairo: CAMPAS, 1990.

105. Al Balla SR BE, Al Sekait M, Al Rasheed R. Pattern of adult admission into medical wards of King Khalid University Hospital, Riyad (1985–1990). *Saudi Med* 1993;**13**:8–13.

106. Drewnowski A, Darmon N, Briend A. Replacing fats and sweets with vegetables and fruits – a question of cost. *Am J Public Health* 2004;**94**(9):1555–9.

107. al-Mahroos F, al-Roomi K. Overweight and obesity in the Arabian Peninsula: an overview. *J R Soc Health* 1999;**119**(4): 251–3.

108. Treloar C, Porteous J, Hassan F, Kasniyah N, Lakshmanudu M, Sama M *et al.* The cross cultural context of obesity: an INCLEN multicentre collaborative study. *Health Place* 1999;**5**(4):279–86.

109. Musaiger AO, Al Roomi KA. Prevalence of risk factors for cardiovascular diseases among men and women in an Arab Gulf community. *Nutr Health* 1997;**11**(3):149–57.

110. King H, Aubert RE, Herman WH. Global burden of diabetes, 1995–2025: prevalence, numerical estimates, and projections. *Diabetes Care* 1998;**21**(9):1414–31.

111. Al Riyami AA, Afifi MM. Hypertension in Oman: distribution and correlates. *J Egypt Public Health Assoc* 2002;**77**(3–4): 383–407.

112. Ibrahim MM, Rizk H, Appel LJ, el Aroussy W, Helmy S, Sharaf Y *et al.* Hypertension prevalence, awareness, treatment, and control in Egypt. Results from the Egyptian National Hypertension Project (NHP). NHP Investigative Team. *Hypertension* 1995;**26**(6 Pt 1):886–90.

113. Yassin IM, Sherif ZB, Nizar F *et al.* Hypertension in UAE citizens – preliminary results of a prospective study. *Saudi J Kidney Dis Transplant* 1999;**10**:376–81.

114. Rahman Al-Nuaim A. High prevalence of metabolic risk factors for cardiovascular diseases among Saudi population, aged 30–64 years. *Int J Cardiol* 1997;**62**(3):227–35.

115. Maziak W, Rastam S, Mzayek F, Ward KD, Eissenberg T, Keil U. Cardiovascular health among adults in Syria: a model from developing countries. *Ann Epidemiol* 2007;**17**(9):713–20.

116. Hatahet W, Khosla P, Fungwe TV. Prevalence of risk factors to coronary heart disease in an Arab-American population in southeast Michigan. *Int J Food Sci Nutr* 2002;**53**(4):325–35.

117. Neel JV. The "thrifty genotype" in 1998. *Nutr Rev* 1999;**57**(5 Pt 2):S2–9.

118. US Bureau of the Census. *Census.* Washington, DC: US Bureau of the Census, 2000.

119. Becker TM, Wiggins C, Key CR, Samet JM. Ischemic heart disease mortality in Hispanics, American Indians, and non-Hispanic whites in New Mexico, 1958–1982. *Circulation* 1988;**78**(2):302–9.

120. Liao Y, Cooper RS, Cao G, Kaufman JS, Long AE, McGee DL. Mortality from coronary heart disease and cardiovascular disease among adult U.S. Hispanics: findings from the National Health Interview Survey (1986 to 1994). *J Am Coll Cardiol* 1997;**30**(5):1200–5.

121. Sorlie PD, Backlund E, Johnson NJ, Rogot E. Mortality by Hispanic status in the United States. *JAMA* 1993;**270**(20):2464–8.

122. Hunt KJ, Resendez RG, Williams K, Haffner SM, Stern MP, Hazuda HP. All-cause and cardiovascular mortality among Mexican-American and non-Hispanic White older participants in the San Antonio Heart Study – evidence against the "Hispanic paradox". *Am J Epidemiol* 2003;**158**(11):1048–57.

123. Gillum RF. Epidemiology of stroke in Hispanic Americans. *Stroke* 1995;**26**(9):1707–12.

124. Wei M, Valdez RA, Mitchell BD, Haffner SM, Stern MP, Hazuda HP. Migration status, socioeconomic status, and mortality rates in Mexican Americans and non-Hispanic whites: the San Antonio Heart Study. *Ann Epidemiol* 1996;**6**(4): 307–13.

125. Pappas G, Gergen PJ, Carroll M. Hypertension prevalence and the status of awareness, treatment, and control in the Hispanic Health and Nutrition Examination Survey (HHANES), 1982–84. *Am J Public Health* 1990;**80**(12):1431–6.

126. Sundquist J, Winkleby MA, Pudaric S. Cardiovascular disease risk factors among older black, Mexican-American, and white women and men: an analysis of NHANES III, 1988–1994. Third National Health and Nutrition Examination Survey. *J Am Geriatr Soc* 2001;**49**(2):109–16.

127. Finkelstein EA, Khavjou OA, Mobley LR, Haney DM, Will JC. Racial/ethnic disparities in coronary heart disease risk factors among WISEWOMAN enrollees. *J Women's Health (Larchmt)* 2004;**13**(5):503–18.

128. Lanas F, Avezum A, Bautista LE, Diaz R, Luna M, Islam S *et al.* Risk factors for acute myocardial infarction in Latin America: the INTERHEART Latin American study. *Circulation* 2007; **115**(9):1067–74.

129. Monteiro CA, Cavalcante TM, Moura EC, Claro RM, Szwarcwald CL. Population-based evidence of a strong decline in the prevalence of smokers in Brazil (1989–2003). *Bull World Health Organ* 2007;**85**(7):527–34.

130. Goff DC Jr, Ramsey DJ, Labarthe DR, Nichaman MZ. Greater case-fatality after myocardial infarction among Mexican Americans and women than among non-Hispanic whites and men. The Corpus Christi Heart Project. *Am J Epidemiol* 1994;**139**(5):474–83.

131. Howard BV, Lee ET, Cowan LD, Fabsitz RR, Howard WJ, Oopik AJ *et al.* Coronary heart disease prevalence and its relation to risk factors in American Indians. The Strong Heart Study. *Am J Epidemiol* 1995;**142**(3):254–68.

132. Neyer JR, Greenlund KJ, Denny CH, Keenan NL, Labarthe DR, Croft JB. Prevalence of Heart Disease – United States, 2005. *CDC MMWR weekly* 2007;**56**(6):113–19.

133. Gillum RF. The epidemiology of stroke in Native Americans. *Stroke* 1995;**26**(3):514–21.

134. Mao Y, Moloughney BW, Semenciw RM, Morrison HI. Indian Reserve and registered Indian mortality in Canada. *Can J Public Health* 1992;**83**(5):350–3.

135. Anand SS, Yusuf S, Jacobs R, Davis AD, Yi Q, Gerstein H *et al.* Risk factors, atherosclerosis, and cardiovascular disease among Aboriginal people in Canada: the Study of Health Assessment and Risk Evaluation in Aboriginal Peoples (SHARE-AP). *Lancet* 2001;**358**(9288):1147–53.

136. Welty TK, Lee ET, Yeh J, Cowan LD, Go O, Fabsitz RR *et al.* Cardiovascular disease risk factors among American Indians. The Strong Heart Study. *Am J Epidemiol* 1995;**142**(3): 269–87.

137. Murray CJ, Lopez AD. Alternative projections of mortality and disability by cause 1990–2020: Global Burden of Disease Study. *Lancet* 1997;**349**(9064):1498–504.

138. Connor MD, Walker R, Modi G, Warlow CP. Burden of stroke in black populations in sub-Saharan Africa. *Lancet Neurol* 2007;**6**(3):269–78.

139. Berrios X, Koponen T, Huiguang T, Khaltaev N, Puska P, Nissinen A. Distribution and prevalence of major risk factors of noncommunicable diseases in selected countries: the WHO Inter-Health Programme. *Bull World Health Organ* 1997;**75**(2):99–108.

140. Seedat YK. Ethnicity, hypertension, coronary heart disease and renal diseases in South Africa. *Ethn Health* 1996;**1**(4):349–57.

141. Steyn K, Sliwa K, Hawken S, Commerford P, Onen C, Damasceno A *et al.* Risk factors associated with myocardial infarction in Africa: the INTERHEART Africa study. *Circulation* 2005;**112**(23):3554–61.

142. Steyn K, Kazenellenbogen JM, Lombard CJ, Bourne LT. Urbanization and the risk for chronic diseases of lifestyle in the black population of the Cape Peninsula, South Africa. *J Cardiovasc Risk* 1997;**4**(2):135–42.

143. Popescu I, Vaughan-Sarrazin MS, Rosenthal GE. Differences in mortality and use of revascularization in black and white patients with acute MI admitted to hospitals with and without revascularization services. *JAMA* 2007;**297**(22):2489–95.

144. Howard G, Labarthe DR, Hu J, Yoon S, Howard VJ. Regional differences in African Americans' high risk for stroke: the remarkable burden of stroke for Southern African Americans. *Ann Epidemiol* 2007;**17**(9):689–96.

145. Gillum RF. Sudden coronary death in the United States: 1980–1985. *Circulation* 1989;**79**(4):756–65.

146. Geronimus AT, Bound J, Keene D, Hicken M. Black-white differences in age trajectories of hypertension prevalence among adult women and men, 1999–2002. *Ethn Dis* 2007;**17**(1):40–8.

147. Moliterno DJ, Jokinen EV, Miserez AR, Lange RA, Willard JE, Boerwinkle E *et al.* No association between plasma lipoprotein(a) concentrations and the presence or absence of coronary atherosclerosis in African-Americans. *Arterioscler Thromb Vasc Biol* 1995;**15**(7):850–5.

148. Geronimus AT, Bound J, Waidmann TA, Hillemeier MM, Burns PB. Excess mortality among blacks and whites in the United States. *N Engl J Med* 1996;**335**(21):1552–8.

149. Becker ER, Rahimi A. Disparities in race/ethnicity and gender in in-hospital mortality rates for coronary artery bypass surgery patients. *J Natl Med Assoc* 2006;**98**(11):1729–39.

150. Winkler E, Turrell G, Patterson C. Does living in a disadvantaged area mean fewer opportunities to purchase fresh fruit and vegetables in the area? Findings from the Brisbane food study. *Health Place* 2006;**12**(3):306–19.

151. Macdonald L, Cummins S, Macintyre S. Neighbourhood fast food environment and area deprivation – substitution or concentration? *Appetite* 2007;**49**(1):251–4.

152. Frank LD, Schmid TL, Sallis JF, Chapman J, Saelens BE. Linking objectively measured physical activity with objectively measured urban form: findings from SMARTRAQ. *Am J Prev Med* 2005;**28**(2 Suppl 2):117–25.

153. Chaix B, Rosvall M, Merlo J. Neighborhood socioeconomic deprivation and residential instability: effects on incidence of ischemic heart disease and survival after myocardial infarction. *Epidemiology* 2007;**18**(1):104–11.

154. Baroni MG, Berni A, Romeo S, Arca M, Tesorio T, Sorropago G *et al.* Genetic study of common variants at the Apo E, Apo AI, Apo CIII, Apo B, lipoprotein lipase (LPL) and hepatic lipase (LIPC) genes and coronary artery disease (CAD): variation in LIPC gene associates with clinical outcomes in patients with established CAD. *BMC Med Genet* 2003;**4**:8.

155. Zhang Q, Liu Y, Liu BW, Fan P, Cavanna J, Galton DJ. Common genetic variants of lipoprotein lipase and apolipoproteins AI-CIII that relate to coronary artery disease: a study in Chinese and European subjects. *Mol Genet Metab* 1998;**64**(3):177–83.

20 Fetal origins of coronary artery disease

Katherine M Morrison, Stephanie Atkinson and Koon K Teo

McMaster University and Hamilton Health Sciences, Hamilton, Ontario, Canada

Introduction

Although cardiovascular (CV) disease presents most commonly in middle-aged adults, it takes many years for the morphologic changes of atherosclerosis to develop and become manifest as clinical CV disease.[1,2] Several lines of evidence implicate exposures in fetal life as important determinants of obesity, type 2 diabetes, other CV risk factors and early development of the atherogenic process leading to CV disease. Maternal adiposity, particularly central body fat, and metabolic status at conception, maternal nutritional deprivation and smoking, and exposure of the fetus to an environment of maternal hyperglycemia, hypercholesterolemia, and diabetes, as well as size of the infant at birth, may be key initiating factors for later risk of CV disease (Fig. 20.1). Emerging evidence supports the concept that metabolic programming changes invoked during fetal development may be modified by exposures at other developmental stages in infancy and early childhood.

This chapter will focus on an evaluation of the evidence linking fetal factors to early risk indicators of CV disease to improve insight into the origins of CV disease and to explore how the risk factors at early stages of development can be amenable to modification. This knowledge can lead to effective prevention strategies throughout the life course.

Atherosclerosis development in youth

The earliest morphologic atherosclerotic change, the fatty streak, has been identified in the fetus and is present in many children by three years of age.[1] Progression of this collection of lipid-laden macrophages to an intermediate state (raised fatty streak), and eventually to fibrous plaques, occurs in the aorta of many youth by the second decade of life.[2-4] This development has been linked to the presence of established risk factors (elevated glucose and blood pressure, excessive weight, dyslipidemia and cigarette smoking) during childhood and adolescence. The prevalence of these risk factors is rising in youth, in part because of the sharp worldwide increases in childhood obesity. In the Pathobiological Determinants of Atherosclerosis in Youth (PDAY) Study and in a similar study in Japan, glycohemoglobin (a marker of dysglycemia), dyslipidemia, cigarette smoking and obesity were related to the extent of atherosclerosis found on postmortem examinations.[2,5,6] In the Bogalusa longitudinal study of CV risk factors in youth, the extent of atherosclerosis was also related to blood pressure, and to the clustering of CV risk factors by the second decade of life.[7] In addition to the traditional CV risk factors, maternal hypercholesterolemia also influences the development of atherosclerosis in children, independent of the child's blood cholesterol. This suggests that fetal exposure to hypercholesterolemia can influence atherosclerosis development in the offspring.[8] The evidence presented in this chapter highlights the fetal influences on the development of these CV risk factors in youth.

Non-invasive measures of vascular structure (carotid intima-media thickness or cIMT) and function (brachial flow-mediated dilation or FMD), employing ultrasound technology, are used in adults to delineate the extent of atherosclerosis[9-11] and predict future coronary artery disease risk.[12,13] In young adults followed since early life, childhood low-density lipoprotein (LDL) cholesterol level is an important determinant of cIMT, highlighting the importance of childhood risk factors in the development of adult CV disease. The potential of cIMT as a tool to non-invasively assess atherosclerosis in youth is supported by observations that cIMT is increased in adolescents with markedly elevated LDL cholesterol, and can be reduced by pharmacologic LDL cholesterol lowering in these subjects.[14] In addition, cIMT is also greater in adolescents with obesity

Evidence-Based Cardiology, 3rd edition. Edited by S. Yusuf, J.A. Cairns, A.J. Camm, E.L. Fallen, and B.J. Gersh. © 2010 Blackwell Publishing, ISBN: 978-1-4051-5925-8.

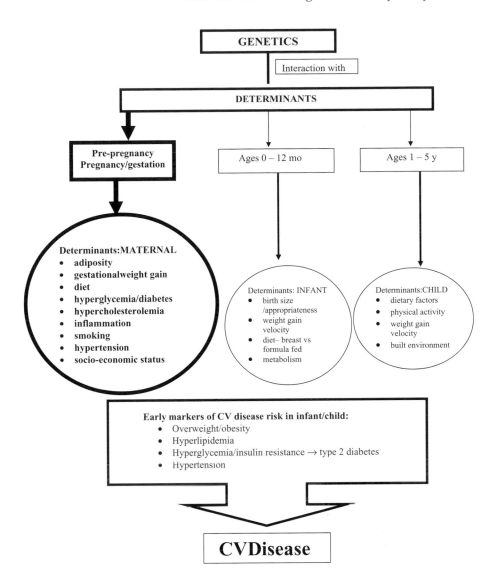

Figure 20.1 Determinants of risk of cardiovascular (CV) disease: focus on early life factors.

and type 1 diabetes.[15,16] cIMT and FMD have not yet been assessed in younger children in studying the effects of fetal influences, but may be potentially important tools. However, the clinical usefulness of cIMT is dependent on the resolution of the ultrasound equipment in imaging the thinner IMT in children and detection of excess thickness may not be reliable until after puberty.[17,18]

Fetal health and cardiovascular risk factors and disease: evidence from retrospective studies

The association between fetal health and adult CV disease was shown in early epidemiologic studies linking early childhood data (particularly birth weight) and adult mortality outcomes decades later. These studies provide the epidemiologic evidence that supports the hypothesis that fetal life is important in the development of atherosclerosis and CV disease in adulthood. For the most part, low birth weight was used as a surrogate marker of untoward fetal exposures, but as birth weight is linked to socioeconomic status (which may be reflected in maternal smoking, inadequate healthcare and suboptimal nutrition during pregnancy and which may also influence the child's health postnatally), the causal linkages between fetal health, birth outcome and later CV disease are difficult to clearly delineate.

Development of CV disease

The link between low birth weight and increased CV disease events in adults, first described in men in the United Kingdom,[19] has been reconfirmed in numerous studies, including a study of 15 000 Swedish men and women[20] in which 97% of the cohort was tracked at follow-up. Of the 7000 men born in 1915–29 and followed to 1995, risk of CV disease death was highest in those with a birth weight in the lowest quartile compared to the second, third and fourth quartiles (odds ratio (OR), 95% confidence interval (CI): 0.85, 0.71–1.02; 0.67, 0.53–0.84; 0.72, 0.51–1.02, respectively), even when corrected for gestational age and socioeconomic status at birth and in adulthood. This relationship was not evident in women in this study. In another study of US women, low birth weight was associated with lower self-reported CV disease events.[21] While suggestive, a wide gap in knowledge and information exists between low weight at birth and the subsequent development of CV disease many years later. One problem with these studies is that since CVD presents in mid to late adulthood, assessment of CV disease outcomes requires very long-term follow-up. Adequate follow-up of these cohorts is difficult and uncertainties can arise as to the validity of these findings.

Non-invasive assessment of vascular structure using B-mode ultrasound measuring the cIMT has been useful in identifying markers of atherosclerosis[9–11] which serve as surrogates for clinical CV disease in adults.[12,13] In a follow-up study of 347 adults aged 49–51 years, multiple health determinants at birth and throughout childhood and traditional CV risk factors in adulthood have been assessed. Although birth weight was inversely related to cIMT, this relationship was no longer significant when adult lifestyle was considered. Early childhood events explained only a small proportion of the variance in cIMT (2.2% in men, 2.0% in women) compared to adult lifestyle (3.4% in men and 7.6% in women) and biologic risk factors in adulthood (9.5% in men and 4.9% in women).[22]

The causality of the relationship between birth weight and CV disease has also been difficult to establish, as many retrospective historic cohorts were unable to correct for confounding factors including maternal smoking, maternal health and socioeconomic status. Conditions such as preeclampsia that result in lower birth weight are themselves associated with CV disease development in the mother, suggesting that conditions that influence the health of both the mother and baby may also confound the relationship of low birth weight[23,24] to subsequent CV risk in the fetus. Furthermore, the relative importance of fetal growth restriction relative to other postnatal factors in CV disease development has not been established. Offspring of mothers exposed to extreme undernutrition in the first trimester of pregnancy as a result of food restriction during extreme social upheaval had increased risk of coronary artery disease.[25] Suggested potential mechanisms for the influence of reduced fetal growth on adult CV disease include reduced or modified growth and development of the kidneys, vascular smooth muscle, endothelium, heart, pancreas, liver or increased activity of the hypothalamus-pituitary-adrenal axis leading to the development of hypertension, dysglycemia and obesity.

Development of CV risk factors

The observation of a possible relationship between birth weight and risk of subsequent adult CV disease has led to investigations of the relationship between CV risk factors and fetal environmental health. Exposures during the prenatal period of development are also associated with the development of obesity, CV risk factors and dysglycemia in childhood. The accumulation of these risk factors may underlie the increased CV disease risk identified in epidemiologic studies of historic cohorts. Aspects of maternal health including maternal obesity, glycemic environment, nutrition, cigarette smoking and hypercholesterolemia have been related to CV risk factors in the offspring. Furthermore, as with the development of CV disease, fetal growth patterns are also associated with metabolic disturbances. Although not a direct measure of CV disease, long-term follow-up of traditional CV risk factors from childhood to young adulthood affords an opportunity to examine CV risk in established cohorts who are now young adults, and in contemporary pediatric cohorts.

Effect of early growth patterns

In adults, both high and low birth weight have been linked to risk markers for chronic disease from early childhood. Fetal growth restraint, followed by rapid postnatal weight gain and early obesity, is thought to prime the metabolic and endocrine milieu for premature pathology, leading to early onset of chronic diseases such as obesity, hypertension and CV disease. Population and clinical studies demonstrate associations between low birth weight and risk for hypertension,[26,27] dysglycemia, insulin resistance[28–31] and central obesity in adulthood. Extreme maternal undernutrition during pregnancy has been linked with an increased risk of obesity, hypertension and dysglycemia in the adult offspring of exposed families during the Dutch famine during the Second World War.[25,32,33] In contrast, in a recent report, exposure to the Dutch famine was not associated with clustering of CV risk factors or metabolic syndrome,[34] and the offspring of mothers exposed to undernutrition during the WWII Leningrad siege showed no such predilection for increased CV risk factor development.[35]

The relationship between birth weight and adult blood pressure has been explored in several systematic reviews[36–38] and despite more than 80 published studies addressing this issue, the conclusions remain controversial. Though an inverse relationship between birth weight and adult blood pressure has been frequently reported, the magnitude of effect is smaller in larger studies (−1.9 mmHg/kg birth weight for studies with <1000 subjects compared to −0.6 mmHg/kg for studies with >3000 subjects). The discrepancy is in part related to the controversial practice of adjusting adult blood pressure for a factor along its causal pathway, adult body size, resulting in exaggerated findings.[39]

The relationship between birth weight and adult dysglycemia is more complex – described as J-shaped,[40] U-shaped[41] or inverse.[42] Thus, although highest risk is found in those with low and high birth weights in some studies, there is an inverse relation in others.[43] Interestingly, in the US Nurses' Study which initially reported a J-shaped relation, correction for adult BMI resulted in an inverse relationship, which was stronger in those with no family history of type 2 diabetes.[40] Type 2 diabetes results from both beta-cell dysfunction and insulin resistance, but the relative importance of these variables in individuals with low birth weight remains unclear. No consistent relationship between birth weight and insulin secretion has been identified[43] although it has been vigorously assessed in most studies. Animal studies suggest that nutritional compromise *in utero*, and low birth weight, may be associated with reduced pancreatic cell mass[44] but that reduced insulin sensitivity in muscle or adipocytes[45] may only be present concomitantly with accelerated postnatal growth.[46]

The influences of early programming on body composition in adulthood remain controversial. Low birth weight has been associated with central adiposity in some studies[47] but not others.[48] Most historic cohorts have relied on height, weight and body circumference measurements; few have assessed body fat directly. In several studies that have characterized body composition in adults with dual energy X-ray absorptiometry, a direct relationship between birth weight and lean mass was consistently shown, but inconsistent relationships to body fat were identified.[49]

Birth weight reflects the responses of the fetus to *in utero* conditions including maternal health, nutrition and placental function. Conditions that result in low birth weight, e.g. maternal smoking and pre-eclampsia, are associated with adiposity[50] and hypertension[51] respectively, in the adult offspring. Support for this comes from observations in animal studies of a relationship between low birth weight (due to nutrient restriction in the mother or restricted uteroplacental circulation) and increased adiposity and CV risk factor prevalence in the offspring.[52] It remains unclear, however, if the influence of cigarette smoking on adiposity and glucose homeostasis is a result of reduced growth or direct influence of the toxins in cigarette smoke. In an animal model, the offspring of animals exposed to nicotine during pregnancy showed evidence of impaired glucose tolerance[53] and loss of pancreatic beta-cell mass.[54] Critical windows of effect range from preimplantation to late pregnancy and proposed mechanisms include disturbances in the size and phenotype of organ systems, changes in biochemical thresholds for activity and changes in angiogenesis.[55]

Interestingly, patterns of accelerated fetal growth as seen in adolescent and adult offspring of mothers with diabetes or overweight are also associated with increased central adiposity, dysglycemia[56] and clustering of CV risk factors.[57]

Effect of glycemic status *in utero*

Maternal diabetes during pregnancy is consistently associated with greater adiposity and central deposition of body fat in the offspring.[28–30] Recently, impaired glucose tolerance (IGT) of pregnancy (often referred to as prediabetes) was also noted to increase risk of greater weight in the offspring.[58] Maternal diabetes also enhances the risk of dysglycemia in the offspring,[28–30,56] commencing as early as 1–4 years of age. This risk is enhanced in the offspring of mothers with diabetes during the pregnancy but not related to fathers with diabetes, suggesting that a glycemic environment during fetal life has a greater influence than genetic predisposition alone.[59] In the Pima Indian population who are at very high risk for the development of type 2 diabetes, prospective, longitudinal studies of offspring of mothers who eventually develop type 2 diabetes suggest a higher risk of dysglycemia if the mother developed type 2 diabetes prior to her pregnancy, i.e. if the offspring were exposed to a diabetic environment *in utero*.[60] Underscoring the importance of the glycemic environment is the finding that diabetes risk is greater in offspring of Pima mothers with a glycemic response to a glucose load in the upper "normal" range.[61] Although diagnostic cut-offs for dysglycemia are applied clinically, the glycemic response to a glucose load is a continuous relationship, which may have important implications in considering levels of risk. Outside the Pima population, the relationship of offspring health to maternal glycemic status in mothers without diabetes or prediabetes has not been reported.

In utero influence on cardiovascular risk factor development in childhood: evidence from contemporary prospective birth cohorts

In contrast to epidemiologic studies in historic cohorts which have provided important insights and generated hypotheses now being explored in studies, prospective assessment of the determinants for development of excess adiposity and CV risk factors allows consideration of potential confounding variables, and can reflect *in utero* effects in children reared in our current obesogenic environment. Fewer prospective studies are available as many are ongoing and the available data remain inconclusive. These contemporary birth cohorts exist or are being established in both developed (Australia, UK, Denmark, United States, Canada) and developing countries (India) (summarized in Table 20.1). Although adult CV disease cannot be assessed directly in childhood in these studies, markers of future CV disease including excess adiposity, dyslipidemia, dysglycemia and hypertension can be measured in childhood. Thus, examining the impact of fetal exposures on these CV risk factors in contemporary, prospective cohorts will assist in clarifying both pre- and postnatal influences on CV disease development.

Influence on body composition

Fetal influences on body size, adiposity and body composition have been assessed in several ongoing, prospective cohorts (see Table 20.1). In these cohorts, multiple determinants of body size in early childhood have emerged.[62] Important elements of maternal health including maternal gestational weight gain, maternal obesity and maternal cigarette exposure have emerged as determinants of body size in several studies. Paternal obesity is recognized as an important determinant in one study.[62] Postnatal factors including rapid weight gain in infancy, early childhood growth patterns, nutritional intake, sedentary activity levels and sleep patterns have been identified as important determinants of body size. In the single study that has reported body composition, rather than just body size, birth weight was directly related to lean mass and to total fat mass, but was unrelated to the ratio of lean mass to fat mass, raising questions about the role of the fetal environment in excess adiposity.[63] Thus, although birth weight and, by inference, fetal nutrition may have an influence on lean mass accretion, with smaller babies having less lean mass, the influence on fat mass development is less clear.

Although maternal diabetes during pregnancy is associated with greater risk of overweight or obesity in most studies identified in a recent review[64] and in a modern retrospective cohort,[65] a number of studies prospectively examining the development of adiposity have not reported on maternal glycemic status. In fact, few prospective cohorts have considered many identified confounding variables in examining the fetal and early childhood determinants of increased adiposity (see Table 20.1).

Influence on glycemia status

The influence of birth weight on dysglycemia in children has been investigated in three prospective cohort studies (see Table 20.1). Most studies investigated the influence of fetal exposures on insulin resistance although insulin secretion was estimated in one study. In a population of children followed from birth in Pune, India, insulin resistance was highest in those in the lowest quartile for birth weight and the upper quartile for BMI at eight years of age.[66] In the ALSPAC study, insulin resistance at eight years of age (n = 800) was most closely related to BMI at that age, and birth weight was related to insulin resistance only in the

heaviest group.[67] Among infants studied in New Zealand, reduced insulin sensitivity was identified in children 4–10 years of age who were born prematurely (both small for gestational age and appropriate for gestational age) compared to term born controls.[68]

Maternal diabetes (type 1 and 2) during pregnancy has consistently been related to increased prevalence of prediabetes and diabetes in the offspring, suggesting a role of *in utero* glycemia and not genetic predisposition to type 2 diabetes as the most important etiologic factor.[56,69,70] However, this relationship remains underinvestigated in contemporary prospective birth cohort studies.

Influence on blood pressure

Although body size during childhood is an important determinant of hypertension in youth, fetal factors including maternal gestational weight gain and cigarette smoke exposure *in utero* have also been identified as determinants. In longitudinal studies, elevated systolic blood pressure associated with maternal smoking persists until at least six years of age.[71]

Influence on clustering of metabolic risk factors

Clustering of risk factors including body mass index, blood pressure, dyslipidemia and glycemic status in childhood has been associated with fetal influences in prospective studies, though it remains underinvestigated (see Table 20.1). In one study, maternal smoking and postinfancy weight gain were identified as the most important predictors of multiple CV risk factors, and breast feeding for longer than four months (OR 0.6, 95% CI 0.37–0.97) was protective. In that study, heavy newborns born to mothers who smoked during pregnancy had a 14-fold increased risk of clustering of the CV risk factors at eight years of age. Unfortunately, this study was unable to account for the influence of maternal glycemic status, a factor shown to increase clustering of CV risk factors at 11 years of age in a smaller study.[57] In the latter study, those born with high birth weights to mothers with diabetes had a 3.6-fold greater risk of clustering of CV risk factors, while heavier babies born to mothers without diabetes had risk levels similar to offspring with normal birth weights.

Review of ongoing contemporary cohorts has identified several important fetal influences on increased adiposity and CV risk factor development in the offspring. Maternal weight gain, obesity, cigarette smoking and diabetes all appear to negatively influence the future CV and metabolic health of the offspring. While these outcomes are preliminary and need confirmation in future studies, they are all potentially preventable fetal exposures, and as such offer hope of future prevention interventions directed at early life.

Table 20.1 Fetal and early childhood influences on CV risk factor development in children: key findings from contemporary cohorts

Cohort (country)	N	Outcome	Age	Maternal factors			Birth weight	Infancy factors		Childhood factors	
				Smoking	Diabetes	Obesity		Wt gain	Breast fed	Nutrition	Wt gain
Influences on body size/adiposity											
Reilly et al[62] (UK)	5493	BMI > 95%	7	+1.8		+4.25	+1.05	+	−	+	+
Rogers et al[63] (UK)	6086	% body fat	9–10	Conf			+				
Rogers et al[63] (UK)	6086	fat: lean mass	9–10	Conf			−				
Oken et al[78,79] (SA)	1044/746	BMI	3	+	Conf	Conf	Conf	Conf	Conf	Conf	Conf
Dubois et al[80] (Canada)	1550	BMI > 95%	4.5	+1.8		+2	+	+3.9	−		
Influences on dysglycemia											
Bavdekar et al[81] (India)	477	HOMA-IR	8–9				+	+		+	+
Ong et al[67] (UK)	851	HOMA-IR / Insulin secretion	8				+	+		+	+
Jeffrey et al[82] (UK)	249	HOMA-IR	8		−	−	−	−	−	+	
Influences on hypertension											
Blake et al[71] (Australia)	702	SBP	6	+			+				
Oken et al[78,79] (USA)	970/746	SBP	3	+	Conf	Conf	Conf	Conf	Conf	Conf	Conf
Influences on clustering of CV risk factors*											
Huang et al[83] (Australia)	406	Cluster*	8	+1.8			+~		+0.6		+1.4
Boney et al[84] (USA)	179	MS**	11		−	+	+				
Bavdekar et al[8] (India)	477	HOMA-IR	8–9				+	−			+

'+, #', identified effect and OR where reported; '−', no significant effect; Conf, reported confounder; blank, variable not reported.

NOTES: Ong et al also reported significant effect of gestational weight gain; Dubois also reported effect of socioeconomic status; Boney et al reported OR of 3.6 for maternal diabetes + large for gestational age birth weight.

* Cluster of increased BMI, BP, serum triglyceride, serum glucose.

** BMI > 85th, increased BP, dyslipidemia, glucose intolerance.

~ U-shaped relation with birth weight – highest risk at lowest and highest birth weights.

Development of risk due to postnatal factors

The relative importance of prenatal versus postnatal growth on the development of CV disease and risk factors in adults has been controversial. The argument has been made that correction for adult weight has resulted in erroneous magnification of the influence of low birth weight on adult disease, and has minimized the potential role of postnatal factors. A systematic review of 21 studies confirmed the significant positive association between rapid infancy weight gain up to two years and obesity risk.[72] Further, as discussed above, numerous studies in youth suggest that low birth weight followed by accelerated growth in early life is closely related to the development of CV risk factors.[73] Many of the studies discussed conclude that postnatal growth is an important determinant of the development of CV risk factors, strongly suggesting that fetal effects are modulated in postnatal life. It is hypothesized that undernutrition *in utero* results in developmental changes in organ systems that are maladapted to an environment of plenty postnatally. For example, undernutrition *in utero* results in reduced pancreatic beta-cell number. In these offspring, in the face of increasing obesity postnatally, greater insulin requirements secondary to insulin resistance cannot be met, resulting in beta-cell failure and ultimately dysglycemia. Similar developmental changes in other organ systems including the renin-angiotensin system and liver are proposed to be maladapted to the current obesogenic environment.

Underlying mechanisms

As summarized in Figure 20.1, converging evidence from human and animal studies substantiate that a number of factors occurring before birth and in early childhood can profoundly alter subsequent CV disease risk. These factors interact with genetic predisposition. Interpretation of the relative influence of each of the fetal and early life factors on later CV disease risk must take into account adult health status and are modifiable by postnatal exposure to other factors.

While the mechanisms of programming in fetal life are not clear, the postulates center on the impact of the maternal nutritional and hormonal milieu on programming in the developing fetus and infant. Programming of organ growth (as discussed above) and of hypothalamic modification of appetite control, energy balance, altered metabolic rate and/or physical activity in the offspring[52,74] are emerging as important potential mechanisms. Several molecular mechanisms related to methylation status, sympathetic innervations and selective leptin resistance or programming of the mitochondrial and related genome have been proposed as the underlying processes involved in developmental programming.

Implications for primary prevention of cardiovascular disease

Evidence to date suggests that fetal life and early childhood are periods of increased sensitivity to exposures that may result in the development of CV risk factors in childhood, and CV disease in adulthood. Prenatal exposures, especially to maternal metabolic disturbances including malnutrition, cigarette smoking, dysglycemia and hypercholesterolemia, increase the risk of ill health in the offspring. Accelerated growth postnatally modifies these exposures. Although our current obesogenic environment appears to adversely influence these prenatal exposures, postnatal modification also affords an opportunity for primordial prevention efforts if introduced in children at high risk as identified by their prenatal exposures. Continued efforts are required to define the exposures and clarify our understanding of potential modifiable determinants of ill health in the offspring. While we await sufficient human data to develop evidence-based practice guidelines for intervention in women and their offspring at increased CV risk, messages regarding the risks of maternal ill health on pregnancy outcome and future health of the offspring are emerging.[75,76] These developments may afford new opportunities for primary prevention of CVD, such as that initiated by the NIH.[77] Although we should start thinking about preventive strategies based on our current understanding, we must recognize that, in spite of the promise, we do not yet have interventions that are proven effective in influencing these very early determinants of CV disease development.

References

1. Stary HC. Lipid and macrophage accumulations in arteries of children and the development of atherosclerosis. *Am J Clin Nutr* 2000;**72**(5 suppl):1297S-306S.
2. Imakita M, Yutani C, Strong JP *et al.* Second nation-wide study of atherosclerosis in infants, children and young adults in Japan. *Atherosclerosis* 2001;**155**(2):487–97.
3. McGill HC Jr, McMahan CA. Determinants of atherosclerosis in the young. Pathobiological Determinants of Atherosclerosis in Youth (PDAY) Research Group. *Am J Cardiol* 1998;**82**(10B): 30T–6T.
4. Strong JP. Natural history and risk factors for early human atherogenesis. Pathobiological Determinants of Atherosclerosis in Youth (PDAY) Research Group. *Clin Chem* 1995;**41**(1):134–8.
5. McGill HC Jr, McMahan CA, Malcolm GT, Oalmann MC, Strong JP. Relation of glycohemoglobin and adiposity to atherosclerosis in youth. Pathobiological Determinants of Atherosclerosis in

Youth (PDAY) Research Group. *Arterioscler Thromb Vasc Biol* 1995;**15**(4):431–40.

6. McGill HC Jr, McMahan CA, Zieske AW *et al.* Associations of coronary heart disease risk factors with the intermediate lesion of atherosclerosis in youth. The Pathobiological Determinants of Atherosclerosis in Youth (PDAY) Research Group. *Arterioscler Thromb Vasc Biol* 2000;**20**(8):1998–2004.

7. Berenson GS, Srinivasan SR, Bao W, Newman WP, Tracy RE, Wattigney WA. Association between multiple cardiovascular risk factors and atherosclerosis in children and young adults. The Bogalusa Heart Study. *N Engl J Med* 1998;**338**(23):1650–6.

8. Napoli C, Glass CK, Witztum JL, Deutsch R, D'Armiento FP, Palinski W. Influence of maternal hypercholesterolaemia during pregnancy on progression of early atherosclerotic lesions in childhood: Fate of Early Lesions in Children (FELIC) study. *Lancet* 1999;**354**(9186):1234–41.

9. Craven TE, Ryu JE, Espeland MA *et al.* Evaluation of the associations between carotid artery atherosclerosis and coronary artery stenosis. A case–control study. *Circulation* 1990;**82**(4):1230–42.

10. Crouse JR, III, Craven TE, Hagaman AP, Bond MG. Association of coronary disease with segment-specific intimal-medial thickening of the extracranial carotid artery. *Circulation* 1995;**92**(5):1141–7.

11. Pignoli P, Tremoli E, Poli A, Oreste P, Paoletti R. Intimal plus medial thickness of the arterial wall: a direct measurement with ultrasound imaging. *Circulation* 1986;**74**(6):1399–406.

12. Chambless LE, Folsom AR, Clegg LX *et al.* Carotid wall thickness is predictive of incident clinical stroke: the Atherosclerosis Risk in Communities (ARIC) study. *Am J Epidemiol* 2000;**151**(5):478–87.

13. Hodis HN, Mack WJ, LaBree L *et al.* The role of carotid arterial intima-media thickness in predicting clinical coronary events. *Ann Intern Med* 1998;**128**(4):262–9.

14. Wiegman A, Hutten BA, de Groot E *et al.* Efficacy and safety of statin therapy in children with familial hypercholesterolemia: a randomized controlled trial. *JAMA* 2004;**292**(3):331–7.

15. Singh TP, Groehn H, Kazmers A. Vascular function and carotid intimal-medial thickness in children with insulin-dependent diabetes mellitus. *J Am Coll Cardiol* 2003;**41**(4):661–5.

16. Tounian P, Aggoun Y, Dubern B *et al.* Presence of increased stiffness of the common carotid artery and endothelial dysfunction in severely obese children: a prospective study. *Lancet* 2001;**358**(9291):1400–4.

17. Davis PH, Dawson JD. Relationship between cardiovascular risk factors and carotid artery intimal-medial thickness. In: Lauer RM, Burns TL, Daniels SR, eds. *Pediatric Prevention of Atherosclerotic Cardiovascular Disease.* Oxford: Oxford University Press, 2006: 84–105.

18. Raitakari OT, Juonala M, Kahonen M *et al.* Cardiovascular risk factors in childhood and carotid artery intima-media thickness in adulthood: the Cardiovascular Risk in Young Finns Study. *JAMA* 2003;**290**(17):2277–83.

19. Barker DJ, Winter PD, Osmond C, Margetts B, Simmonds SJ. Weight in infancy and death from ischaemic heart disease. *Lancet* 1989;**2**(8663):577–80.

20. Leon DA, Lithell HO, Vagero D *et al.* Reduced fetal growth rate and increased risk of death from ischaemic heart disease: cohort study of 15 000 Swedish men and women born 1915- 29. *BMJ* 1998;**317**(7153):241–5.

21. Rich-Edwards JW, Stampfer MJ, Manson JE *et al.* Birth weight and risk of cardiovascular disease in a cohort of women followed up since 1976. *BMJ.* 1997;**315**:396–400.

22. Lamont D, Parker L, White M *et al.* Risk of cardiovascular disease measured by carotid intima-media thickness at age 49–51: lifecourse study. *BMJ* 2000;**320**(7230):273–8.

23. Davey SG, Hart C, Ferrell C *et al.* Birth weight of offspring and mortality in the Renfrew and Paisley study: prospective observational study. *BMJ* 1997;**315**(7117):1189–93.

24. Smith GD, Harding S, Rosato M. Relation between infants' birth weight and mothers' mortality: prospective observational study. *BMJ* 2000;**320**(7238):839–40.

25. Roseboom TJ, van der Meulen JH, Osmond C *et al.* Coronary heart disease after prenatal exposure to the Dutch famine, 1944–45. *Heart* 2000;**84**(6):595–8.

26. Gennser G, Rymark P, Isberg PE. Low birth weight and risk of high blood pressure in adulthood. *BMJ (Clin Res Ed)* 1988;**296**(6635):1498–500.

27. Leon DA, Johansson M, Rasmussen F. Gestational age and growth rate of fetal mass are inversely associated with systolic blood pressure in young adults: an epidemiologic study of 165,136 Swedish men aged 18 years. *Am J Epidemiol* 2000;**152**(7):597–604.

28. Pettitt DJ, Aleck KA, Baird HR, Carraher MJ, Bennett PH, Knowler WC. Congenital susceptibility to NIDDM: role of intrauterine environment. *Diabetes* 1988;**37**:622–8.

29. Pettitt DJ, Bennett PH, Saad MF, Charles MA, Nelson RG, Knowler WC. Abnormal glucose tolerance during pregnancy in Pima Indian women. Long- term effects on offspring. *Diabetes* 1991;**40**(suppl 2):126–30.

30. von Kries R, Kimmerle R, Schmidt JE, Hachmeister A, Bohm O, Wolf HG. Pregnancy outcomes in mothers with pregestational diabetes: a population-based study in North Rhine (Germany) from 1988 to 1993. *Eur J Pediatr* 1997;**156**(12):963–7.

31. Hovi P, Andersson S, Eriksson JG *et al.* Glucose regulation in young adults with very low birth weight. *N Engl J Med* 2007;**356**(20):2053–63.

32. Ravelli AC, Der Meulen JH, Osmond C, Barker DJ, Bleker OP. Obesity at the age of 50 y in men and women exposed to famine prenatally. *Am J Clin Nutr* 1999;**70**(5):811–16.

33. Ravelli AC, van der Meulen JH, Michels RP *et al.* Glucose tolerance in adults after prenatal exposure to famine. *Lancet* 1998;**351**(9097):173–7.

34. de Rooij Sr, Painter RC, Holleman F, Bossuyt PM, Roseboom TJ. The metabolic syndrome in adults prenatally exposed to the Dutch famine. *Am J Clin Nutr* 2007;**86**(4):1219–24.

35. Stanner SA, Yudkin JS. Fetal programming and the Leningrad Siege study. *Twin Res* 2001;**4**(5):287–92.

36. Huxley R, Neil A, Collins R. Unravelling the fetal origins hypothesis: is there really an inverse association between birthweight and subsequent blood pressure? *Lancet* 2002;**360**(9334):659–65.

37. Law CM, de Swiet M, Osmond C *et al.* Initiation of hypertension in utero and its amplification throughout life. *BMJ* 1993;**306**(6869):24–7.

38. Law CM, Shiell AW. Is blood pressure inversely related to birth weight? The strength of evidence from a systematic review of the literature. *J Hypertens* 1996;**14**:935–41.

39. Tu YK, West R, Ellison GT, Gilthorpe MS. Why evidence for the fetal origins of adult disease might be a statistical artifact: the

"reversal paradox" for the relation between birth weight and blood pressure in later life. *Am J Epidemiol* 2005;**161**(1):27–32.

40. Rich-Edwards JW, Colditz GA, Stampfer MJ *et al.* Birthweight and the risk for type 2 diabetes mellitus in adult women. *Ann Intern Med* 1999;**130**(4 Pt 1):278–84.

41. Pettitt DJ, Knowler WC. Long-term effects of the intrauterine environment, birth weight, and breast-feeding in Pima Indians. *Diabetes Care* 1998;**21**(suppl 2):B138-B141.

42. Hales CN, Barker DJ, Clark PM *et al.* Fetal and infant growth and impaired glucose tolerance at age 64. *BMJ* 1991;**303**(6809): 1019–22.

43. Newsome CA, Shiell AW, Fall CH, Phillips DI, Shier R, Law CM. Is birth weight related to later glucose and insulin metabolism? A systematic review. *Diabet Med* 2003;**20**(5):339–48.

44. Simmons RA, Templeton LJ, Gertz SJ. Intrauterine growth retardation leads to the development of type 2 diabetes in the rat. *Diabetes* 2001;**50**(10):2279–86.

45. Poore KR, Fowden AL. Insulin sensitivity in juvenile and adult Large White pigs of low and high birthweight. *Diabetologia* 2004;**47**(2):340–8.

46. Cottrell EC, Ozanne SE. Developmental programming of energy balance and the metabolic syndrome. *Proc Nutr Soc* 2007;**66**(2): 198–206.

47. Sachdev HS, Fall CH, Osmond C *et al.* Anthropometric indicators of body composition in young adults: relation to size at birth and serial measurements of body mass index in childhood in the New Delhi birth cohort. *Am J Clin Nutr* 2005;**82**(2): 456–66.

48. Sayer AA, Syddall HE, Dennison EM *et al.* Birth weight, weight at 1y of age, and body composition in older men: findings from the Hertfordshire Cohort Study. *Am J Clin Nutr* 2004;**80**(1): 199–203.

49. Wells JC, Chomtho S, Fewtrell MS. Programming of body composition by early growth and nutrition. *Proc Nutr Soc* 2007;**66**(3):423–34.

50. Toschke AM, Montgomery SM, Pfeiffer U, von Kries R. Early intrauterine exposure to tobacco-inhaled products and obesity. *Am J Epidemiol* 2003;**158**(11):1068–74.

51. Lawlor DA, Najman JM, Sterne J, Williams GM, Ebrahim S, Davey SG. Associations of parental, birth, and early life characteristics with systolic blood pressure at 5 years of age: findings from the Mater-University study of pregnancy and its outcomes. *Circulation* 2004;**110**(16):2417–23.

52. Nathanielsz PW, Poston L, Taylor PD. In utero exposure to maternal obesity and diabetes: animal models that identify and characterize implications for future health. *Obstet Gynecol Clin North Am* 2007;**34**(2):201–viii.

53. Holloway AC, Lim GE, Petrik JJ, Foster WG, Morrison KM, Gerstein HC. Fetal and neonatal exposure to nicotine in Wistar rats results in increased beta cell apoptosis at birth and postnatal endocrine and metabolic changes associated with type 2 diabetes. *Diabetologia* 2005;**48**(12):2661–6.

54. Bruin JE, Kellenberger LD, Gerstein HC, Morrison KM, Holloway AC. Fetal and neonatal nicotine exposure and postnatal glucose homeostasis: identifying critical windows of exposure. *J Endocrinol* 2007;**194**(1):171–8.

55. McMillen IC, Robinson JS. Developmental origins of the metabolic syndrome: prediction, plasticity, and programming. *Physiol Rev* 2005;**85**(2):571–633.

56. Silverman BL, Metzger BE, Cho NH, Loeb CA. Impaired glucose tolerance in adolescent offspring of diabetic mothers. Relationship to fetal hyperinsulinism. *Diabetes Care* 1995;**18**(5):611–17.

57. Boney CM, Verma A, Tucker R, Vohr BR. Metabolic syndrome in childhood: association with birth weight, maternal obesity, and gestational diabetes mellitus. *Pediatrics* 2005;**115**(3):e290–e296.

58. Hillier TA, Pedula KL, Schmidt MM, Mullen JA, Charles MA, Pettitt DJ. Childhood obesity and metabolic imprinting: the ongoing effects of maternal hyperglycemia. *Diabetes Care* 2007;**30**(9):2287–92.

59. Sobngwi E, Boudou P, Mauvais-Jarvis F *et al.* Effect of a diabetic environment in utero on predisposition to type 2 diabetes. *Lancet* 2003;**361**(9372):1861–5.

60. Dabelea D, Hanson RL, Lindsay RS *et al.* Intrauterine exposure to diabetes conveys risks for type 2 diabetes and obesity: a study of discordant sibships. *Diabetes* 2000;**49**(12):2208–11.

61. Franks PW, Looker HC, Kobes S *et al.* Gestational glucose tolerance and risk of type 2 diabetes in young Pima Indian offspring. *Diabetes* 2006;**55**(2):460–5.

62. Reilly JJ, Armstrong J, Dorosty AR *et al.* Early life risk factors for obesity in childhood: cohort study. *BMJ* 2005;**330**(7504):1357.

63. Rogers IS, Ness AR, Steer CD *et al.* Associations of size at birth and dual-energy X-ray absorptiometry measures of lean and fat mass at 9 to 10y of age. *Am J Clin Nutr* 2006;**84**(4):739–47.

64. Huang JS, Lee TA, Lu MC. Prenatal programming of childhood overweight and obesity. *Matern Child Health J* 2007;**11**(5): 461–73.

65. Gillman MW, Rifas-Shiman S, Berkey CS, Field AE, Colditz GA. Maternal gestational diabetes, birth weight, and adolescent obesity. *Pediatrics* 2003;**111**(3):e221–e226.

66. Bavdekar A, Yajnik CS, Fall CHD *et al.* Insulin resistance syndrome in 8-year-old Indian children. small at birth, big at 8 years, or both? *Diabetes* 1999;**48**:2422–9.

67. Ong KK, Petry CJ, Emmett PM *et al.* Insulin sensitivity and secretion in normal children related to size at birth, postnatal growth, and plasma insulin-like growth factor-I levels. *Diabetologia* 2004;**47**(6):1064–70.

68. Hofman PL, Regan F, Jackson WE *et al.* Premature birth and later insulin resistance. *N Engl J Med* 2004;**351**(21):2179–86.

69. Silverman BL, Rizzo TA, Cho NH, Metzger BE. Long-term effects of the intrauterine environment. The Northwestern University Diabetes in Pregnancy Center. *Diabetes Care* 1998;**21**(suppl 2):B142–B149.

70. Weiss PA, Scholz HS, Haas J, Tamussino KF, Seissler J, Borkenstein MH. Long-term follow-up of infants of mothers with type 1 diabetes: evidence for hereditary and nonhereditary transmission of diabetes and precursors. *Diabetes Care* 2000;**23**(7): 905–11.

71. Blake KV, Gurrin LC, Evans SF *et al.* Maternal cigarette smoking during pregnancy, low birth weight and subsequent blood pressure in early childhood. *Early Hum Dev* 2000;**57**(2):137–47.

72. Ong KK, Loos RJ. Rapid infant weight gain and subsequent obesity: systematic review and hopeful suggestions. *Acta Paediatr* 2006;**95**:904–8.

73. Ong KK, Dunger DB. Perinatal growth failure: the road to obesity, insulin resistance and cardiovascular disease in adults. *Best Pract Res Clin Endocrinol Metab* 2002;**16**(2):191–207.

74. Taylor PD, Poston L. Developmental programming of obesity in mammals. *Exp Physiol* 2007;**92**(2):287–98.

75. American College of Obstetricians and Gynecologists. ACOG Committee Opinion number 315, September 2005, Obesity in pregnancy. *Obstet Gynecol* 2005;**106**:671–5.

76. Scialli A. Teratology public affairs committee position paper: maternal obesity in pregnancy. *Birth Defects Res A Clin Mol Teratol* 2006;**76**:73–7.

77. National Institutes of Health. Guide to "It's Never Too Early to Prevent Diabetes. A Lifetime of Small Steps for a Healthy Family. Tip Sheet", 2008. Available at: www.ndep.nih.gov/campaigns/SmallSteps/SmallSteps_index.htm.

78. Oken E, Huh SY, Taveras EM, Rich-Edwards JW, Gillman MW. Associations of maternal prenatal smoking with child adiposity and blood pressure. *Obes Res* 2005;**13**(11):2021–8.

79. Oken E, Taveras EM, Kleinman KP, Rich-Edwards JW, Gillman MW. Gestational weight gain and child adiposity at age 3 years. *Am J Obstet Gynecol* 2007;**196**(4):322–8.

80. Dubois L, Girard M. Early determinants of overweight at 4.5 years in a population-based longitudinal study. *Int J Obes (Lond)* 2006;**30**(4):610–17.

81. Bavdekar A, Yajnik CS, Fall CH *et al.* Insulin resistance syndrome in 8-year-old Indian children: small at birth, big at 8 years, or both? *Diabetes* 1999;**48**(12):2422–9.

82. Jeffery AN, Metcalf BS, Hosking J, Murphy MJ, Voss LD, Wilkin TJ. Little evidence for early programming of weight and insulin resistance for contemporary children: EarlyBird Diabetes Study report 19. *Pediatrics* 2006;**118**(3):1118–23.

83. Huang RC, Burke V, Newnham JP *et al.* Perinatal and childhood origins of cardiovascular disease. *Int J Obes (Lond)* 2007;**31**(2):236–44.

84. Boney CM, Verma A, Tucker R, Vohr BR. Metabolic syndrome in childhood: association with birth weight, maternal obesity, and gestational diabetes mellitus. *Pediatrics* 2005;**115**(3):e290–e296.

21 Genetics of coronary heart disease

Michael S Cunnington and Bernard D Keavney

Institute of Human Genetics, Newcastle University, Newcastle upon Tyne, UK

Evidence for genetic susceptibility to coronary heart disease

Coronary heart disease is a complex phenotype which arises from the interaction of a number of risk factors including smoking, hyperlipidemia, hypertension, obesity, and diabetes. Epidemiologic studies have consistently indicated the importance of a family history of coronary heart disease (CHD) as an independent risk factor for disease. Perhaps the most frequently cited study in this regard is the 1994 report from the Swedish Twin Study.[1] That report included 21 004 individuals, of whom 2810 had fatal CHD. Among male twin pairs in which the first twin had died of CHD before the age of 55, the relative risk of fatal CHD in the second twin was 8.1 (95% confidence interval (CI) 2.7–24.5) for monozygotic (i.e. genetically identical) twins and 3.8 (95% CI 1.4–10.5) for dizygotic twins. Among female twin pairs in which the first twin had died of CHD before the age of 65, the relative risk of fatal CHD in the second twin was 15.0 (95% CI 7.1–31.9) for monozygotic twins and 2.6 (95% CI 1.0–7.1) for dizygotic twins. These results clearly indicate a significant genetic contribution to the risk of CHD death. A 2002 analysis of the same cohort, which at that time included 4007 CHD deaths and a follow-up time of up to 36 years, used more sophisticated statistical modeling approaches to conclude that the heritability of fatal CHD events was 57% for males and 38% for females.[2] By contrast with the earlier report from this study, it was suggested that there was persistence of the excess genetic risk of CHD death even into old age. A similar analysis among 7955 Danish twin pairs including 2476 CHD deaths reported a heritability of fatal CHD events of 53% for males and 58% for females, which is broadly concordant with the Swedish data.[3] Studies in the offspring of the original

Framingham Heart Study participants have shown strong evidence for association of parental cardiovascular disease with the risk of offspring cardiovascular disease, and for sibling–sibling association of cardiovascular disease even after multivariable adjustment for other measured risk factors. In these studies, the relative risk associated with parental or sibling cardiovascular disease was between 1.45 and 2.0.[4,5]

The INTERHEART case–control study identified nine modifiable risk factors (smoking, dyslipidemia, hypertension, diabetes, abdominal obesity, psychosocial factors, daily consumption of fruit and vegetables, regular alcohol consumption, and regular physical activity) which together predicted a very substantial proportion of the risk of a first myocardial infarction (MI) in populations derived from every inhabited continent.[6] Family history was also assessed as a risk factor in that study. After adjustment for age, sex, smoking and region of recruitment, a positive family history conferred an odds ratio (OR) for MI of 1.55 (95% CI 1.44–1.67). After additional adjustment for all of the nine most significant factors, the risk was reduced to 1.45 (95% CI 1.31–1.60), remaining significant.

Some studies have examined the heritability of quantitative phenotypes related to atherosclerotic disease, such as carotid intima-media thickness and arterial calcification in various sites;[7–9] substantial heritabilities have been found for these phenotypes (30–60%). These findings further substantiate the assertion that genes play a significant role in susceptibility to atherosclerosis and its consequences.

Genetic architecture of coronary heart disease susceptibility

While it is clear that there is a substantial genetic component to CHD susceptibility, the architecture of that component – in terms of the number of effects and their sizes – remains uncertain. Population genetic theory would predict that the

Evidence-Based Cardiology, 3rd edition. Edited by S. Yusuf, J.A. Cairns, A.J. Camm, E.L. Fallen, and B.J. Gersh. © 2010 Blackwell Publishing, ISBN: 978-1-4051-5925-8.

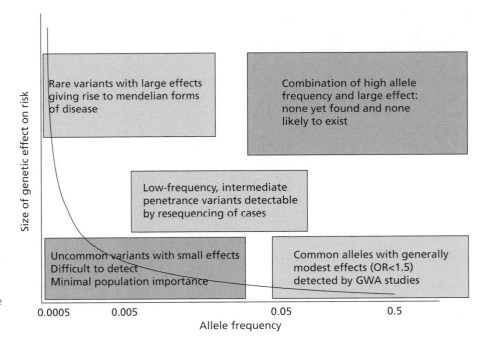

Figure 21.1 Effect size and allele frequency in populations. Both population genetic theory and empiric evidence suggest that the frequency of an allele will be inversely related to the size of its biologic effect (curve). Three general classes of detectable variants (boxes) can be distinguished; different approaches are needed to detect members of the different classes. GWA, genome-wide association.

size of the effect of an allele on a phenotype should vary inversely with its frequency: that is, alleles that are common in the population should have small biologic effects, while large effects should be confined to rare alleles. With relatively few exceptions, this prediction has been found to hold true both in humans and in experimental animals. Figure 21.1 illustrates this concept. Most of the successes in CHD genetics before 2007 were confined to the upper left-hand portion of the curve shown in Figure 21.1, where studies in families with Mendelian (single-gene) forms of CHD had revealed large-displacement alleles which substantially affected the function of particular genes and which were sufficient alone to confer very markedly increased risks of CHD (for example, LDL-receptor mutations which cause familial hypercholesterolemia). However, because these alleles are rare, each one possibly existing in only a handful of families worldwide, their individual contribution to the population burden of disease is modest. Common alleles which had only small effects on disease risk (conferring odds ratios of 1.2–1.5) would contribute far more significantly to the impact of disease in the population. Conversely, however, such alleles would not be expected to have great predictive value for individual patients.

CHD is, in evolutionary terms, a very recent disease. Moreover, even at the peak of the CHD epidemic that is now waning in most Western countries, deaths from CHD tended to occur at ages older than the best estimates of the average life expectancy throughout human history.[10,11] Therefore CHD, in common with many other degenerative diseases of later life, has almost certainly been invisible to

natural selection throughout our evolutionary history, as it would not have affected our ancestors' reproductive fitness. This implies that common variants (which tend to be evolutionarily ancient) with effects on CHD could have arisen and persisted by chance alone, although the effects of such variants would be expected to be small. It is an attractive hypothesis that variants with beneficial effects on conditions of greater evolutionary impact (for example, infectious disease or the ability to survive trauma) could have been selected for in our evolutionary history but have now "outlived their usefulness" in the toxic environmental setting of caloric abundance and limited physical activity. However, this has yet to be convincingly demonstrated for any variant.

In the last year, studies which have characterized common variation throughout the human genome in large numbers of CHD cases and controls have considerably clarified our understanding of the situation with respect to the contribution of such common variation to disease risk. One locus has been convincingly replicated in multiple studies thus far (even in relatively small studies), and it seems likely that this is the principal susceptibility locus existing in the genome. It is, however, clear that there remains a substantial "heritability gap" – that is, the fraction of the heritability of CHD that is accounted for by the existing confirmed candidate genes (such as variants in the apolipoprotein E gene) and the newly discovered alleles is far below the total calculated heritability of the condition. Among the possible explanations are that the rest of the heritability is due to very small effects of common alleles which lie beyond the resolution of even the largest association studies. Alternatively, the remaining heritability may be due to "low-frequency intermediate penetrance" variants, which would not have been captured by the existing genome-wide association studies but could nonetheless have significant effects on risk for those individuals who carry them. Some evidence in favor of the existence of such variants from systematic resequencing studies is described below; recent technologic innovations which have dramatically increased the speed and cost effectiveness of genome sequencing will enable systematic genome-wide evaluation of rare variants in the near future.

Mendelian disorders associated with coronary artery disease

A number of Mendelian disorders associated with premature CHD have been recognized, as summarized in Table 21.1. Such disorders explain only a very small proportion of CHD cases, but knowledge of them is important for a number of reasons. First, it allows the development of effective strategies for the detection, treatment and prevention of disease in affected individuals and families, which is particularly important as disease in these individuals often presents at a young age and follows an aggressive clinical course. Second, certain genes causing Mendelian forms of CHD have also been implicated in the risk of non-Mendelian CHD in the general population (see Table 21.1). Third, novel insights into the pathophysiologic mechanisms of disease gained through the study of Mendelian disorders may allow the identification of new biomarkers or targets for therapeutic intervention. Insights from investigations of familial hypercholesterolemia were important in the development of statins, and studies of apolipoprotein A-I (Apo A-I) deficiency have resulted in recent clinical trials of recombinant Apo A-I Milano for the treatment of CHD, as discussed below.

Familial hypercholesterolemia (FH) is the most common Mendelian disorder conferring CHD risk. It is an autosomal dominant condition caused by mutations in the low-density lipoprotein receptor (LDLR) gene, which disrupt the ability of the receptor to bind LDL at the cell membrane. Cellular uptake of LDL cholesterol is impaired, resulting in increased circulating levels of LDL cholesterol and stimulation of intracellular cholesterol synthesis.[12–15] Over 1000 mutations in the LDLR gene have been reported to be associated with the syndrome. Point mutations account for 91% of mutations (missenses, deletions, nonsenses, insertions and splice variants have all been described), and 9% are major rearrangements.[16] The heterozygote frequency of familial forms of hypercholesterolemia is around 1 in 500 in Western populations. The term familial hypercholesterolemia is usually used specifically for the syndrome associ-

ated with mutations in the LDLR gene, but similar phenotypes are associated with abnormalities of the APOB and PCSK9 genes. Detailed investigation of patients with "familial hypercholesterolemia" phenotypes demonstrated that 79.1% were due to LDLR mutations, with 5.5% due to APOB mutations, and 1.5% due to mutations in PCSK9.[17] Involvement of other genes may account for some of the remaining proportion.

FH heterozygotes have elevated circulating LDL cholesterol levels, typically in the range 190–465 mg/dL, and develop tendon xanthomas, corneal arcus and premature coronary artery disease often before the age of 50 years. Affected homozygotes are more severely affected, often with LDL cholesterol above 465 mg/dL, cutaneous xanthomas, and coronary disease which may present below the age of 30 years. Untreated, the risk of CHD in affected heterozygotes by age 60 years is approximately 50–85% for men and 30–55% for women.[18,19] The key elements of the clinical diagnostic criteria for FH are raised serum cholesterol, tendon xanthomas in the patient or a first-degree relative, and a dominant inheritance pattern of premature CHD or elevated cholesterol.[20] Opportunistic and cascade screening for relatives of affected individuals may be used in routine practice, as discussed below.

Apo A-I is the major protein constituent of high-density lipoprotein (HDL). Mutations in the APOA1 gene cause Apo A-I deficiency, which is an autosomal dominant disorder. Numerous mutations in the APOA1 gene have been reported, some of which lead to very low circulating HDL levels and increased risk of atherosclerosis.[21–23] However, a variant of Apo A-I (named Apo A-I Milano) identified in an Italian family in 1980 did not seem to be associated with increased CHD risk.[24] The pedigree carrying this mutation was traced to a village in northern Italy, revealing 33 heterozygous carriers of the mutation who had markedly reduced HDL (10–30 mg/dL), raised triglycerides but a lower, rather than higher, risk of atherosclerosis compared to the general population.[25,26] The Apo A-I Milano protein differs from native Apo A-I by the substitution of cysteine for arginine at position 173, which changes its properties and allows the formation of disulfide-linked homodimers and heterodimers with apoA-II.[27] Recombinant Apo A-I Milano complexed with a naturally occurring phospholipid has been manufactured to mimic the properties of nascent HDL, and studies in animal models of atherosclerosis showed that infusions of this complex rapidly reduced the lipid and macrophage content of atherosclerotic plaques.[28–31] A randomized double-blinded controlled trial of recombinant Apo A-I Milano therapy on coronary atherosclerosis in human subjects with acute coronary syndromes showed that intravenous infusion of the recombinant Apo A-I Milano complex at weekly intervals for five weeks significantly reduced coronary atheroma volume measured using intravascular ultrasound.[32] The

Table 21.1 Mendelian disorders involving coronary artery disease

Disorder	Inheritance	Affected genes	Consequences of gene mutation	Prevalence and clinical features
Familial hypercholesterolemia (OMIM# 143890)	Autosomal dominant	LDLR*	LDLR encodes the cell membrane LDL receptor. More than 1000 mutations have been reported in the LDLR gene, which disrupt the ability of the LDL receptor to bind and endocytose LDL.[16] This results in accumulation of LDL cholesterol in the circulation.	Heterozygote frequency 1/500. Heterozygotes have elevated circulating LDL levels, tendon xanthomas, corneal arcus, and premature CHD. Homozygotes more severely affected with higher LDL levels, cutaneous xanthomas, and CHD may present below the age of 30 years.
Familial defective Apo B (OMIM# 144010)	Autosomal dominant	APOB*	APOB encodes apolipoprotein B-100, which is the protein component of LDL. Apo B-100 is the major ligand for the LDL receptor and mediates binding of LDL to the receptor. 10 mutations reported in APOB, which reduce the binding affinity of Apo B-100 to the LDL receptor, resulting in impaired cellular uptake and processing of LDL.	Heterozygote frequency 1/1000. Elevated circulating LDL with phenotype very similar to FH, but slightly milder in some studies. Risk of premature CHD is lower than with FH, but remains substantially elevated.
Autosomal dominant hypercholesterolemia 3 (OMIM# 603776)	Autosomal dominant	PCSK9*	PCSK9 encodes proprotein convertase subtilisin/kexin type 9. The exact function of this glycoprotein is not well understood, but several gain-of-function mutations seem to be associated with a reduction in the number of LDL receptors at the cell surface.	Studied in several pedigrees. Phenotype similar to FH, but prevalence and variations in phenotype not yet well defined.
Autosomal recessive hypercholesterolemia (OMIM# 603813)	Autosomal recessive	ARH	ARH encodes LDL receptor adaptor protein 1 (LDLRRAP1). This interacts with the cytoplasmic domain of the LDL receptor and components of the clathrin endocytic machinery. Mutations lead to defective endocytosis of the LDL receptor.	Rare. Raised circulating LDL levels with phenotype similar to FH.
Apolipoprotein A-I (Apo A-I) deficiency (OMIM# 107680)	Autosomal dominant	APOA1*	APOA1 encodes Apo A-I, which is the major protein constituent of HDL. It mediates the interaction of HDL with cell surface receptors and other pathways. Mutations lead to very low circulating HDL levels.	Rare. Heterozygotes have low circulating HDL levels and some variants are associated with premature CHD risk[22,23] whilst others are not.[25] Homozygotes with certain mutations may have xanthomas or corneal opacities and early CHD.
Tangier disease (OMIM# 205400)	Autosomal recessive	ABCA1*	ABCA1 encodes ATP-binding cassette A1. This acts as a cholesterol efflux pump, involved in cellular cholesterol homeostasis and HDL formation. Mutations lead to lipid accumulation within cells, including macrophages, which produces characteristic clinical and histologic features.	Rare. Affected homozygotes usually have pathognomonic enlarged orange tonsils. HDL levels very low, with increased CHD risk. Other features include: hepatosplenomegaly, lymphadenopathy, thrombocytopenia, anemia, GI disturbance, neuropathy, corneal opacities. Heterozygotes have low HDL and increased CHD risk without the other clinical features.[117]

Continued on p. 272

Table 21.1 *Continued*

Disorder	Inheritance	Affected genes	Consequences of gene mutation	Prevalence and clinical features
Homocystinuria (OMIM# 236200)	Autosomal recessive	Cystathionine beta-synthase	Cystathionine beta-synthase is an enzyme in the methionine metabolism pathway. It catalyzes conversion of homocysteine and serine to cystathionine. Multiple loss-of-function mutations have been reported, producing high circulating homocysteine levels. The mechanisms leading to CHD are incompletely defined.	Worldwide 1/300000, in Ireland 1/65000.[118] Affected homozygotes have "marfanoid" skeletal abnormalities, developmental delay/mental retardation, ectopia lentis, osteoporosis, and thromboembolism. Untreated, 50% risk of thromboembolic vascular events (including CHD) by age 30 years.[119]
Autosomal dominant coronary artery disease 2 (OMIM# 610947)	Autosomal dominant	LRP6	LRP6 encodes LDL receptor related protein 6, which is related to the LDLR gene and acts as a co-receptor in the Wnt signaling pathway. Missense mutation associated with reduced Wnt signaling, raised LDL, and premature CHD.	Single Iranian pedigree. Elevated LDL, premature CHD and metabolic syndrome described in homozygotes and heterozygotes.[120]
Autosomal dominant coronary artery disease 1 (OMIM# 608320)	Autosomal dominant	Uncertain ?MEF2A	Genome-wide linkage analysis in a family with an autosomal dominant pattern of premature CHD identified chromosome 15q26 as a possible susceptibility locus.[121] Sequencing revealed a 21bp deletion in the MEF2A gene at this locus in affected individuals in that family, but analysis in other populations demonstrated that the 21bp MEF2A deletion did not co-segregate with CHD, suggesting it is not causative.[122] Other MEF2A mutations do not appear to be a common cause of CHD in Caucasians. The gene and mechanism remain to be elucidated.	Reported in isolated pedigrees. Premature CHD and MI.
Sitosterolemia (OMIM# 210250)	Autosomal recessive	ABCG5 ABCG8	ABCG5/8 encode ATP-binding cassette G5/G8. These limit intestinal absorption, and promote biliary excretion, of non-cholesterol sterols. Inactivating mutations lead to high levels of plasma sterols.	Rare. Affected homozygotes have high plasma sterol levels, xanthomas, and premature CHD.

OMIM#, National Center for Biotechnology Information Online Mendelian Inheritance in Man identifier (www.ncbi.nlm.nih.gov/sites/entrez?db=OMIM). *, genes for which variants have been shown to contribute to lipid/cardiovascular phenotypes in the general population. FH, familial hypercholesterolemia.

mechanism is uncertain, but may relate to an increase in reverse cholesterol transport from atheromatous lesions to the serum with subsequent hepatic removal. These investigations suggest that recombinant Apo A-I Milano, or drugs mimicking the effect of the mutation on lipoprotein trafficking, could be useful for the stabilization, and possibly even regression, of atheromatous plaque in the wider population with CHD.

Family-based studies of non-Mendelian coronary heart disease: genome-wide linkage analysis

Family-based linkage studies, which had delivered the identity of over 2000 genes for Mendelian conditions by 2005, have also been performed in many complex diseases, including CHD. In this approach, the inheritance of chromosomal segments is tracked through families which have multiple members affected with disease by typing markers spaced throughout the genome. Because the individuals involved in a family study are separated by few meioses, comparatively few markers are required to accurately identify the inheritance of each chromosomal segment genome-wide within a family (several hundred rather than the hundreds of thousands of markers required in genome-wide association studies). Segments that are shared more often than expected by chance among family members affected with disease can thus be identified; these segments may harbor genes which are involved in disease etiology. Most such studies in CHD were conceived in the early to mid 1990s, predating the vast expansion (by three orders of magnitude) in knowledge of genetic markers that made genome-wide association studies possible. Such studies were dogged by two intrinsic problems. First, although linkage is a very efficient approach to detect alleles of large effect (such as in the context of Mendelian disease), the power to detect alleles with small effects (odds ratios below about 2.0) is very low.[33] Second, even when a replicated linkage "hit" is obtained in a complex disease, the genomic region requiring investigation before a gene is identified remains very large, possibly containing hundreds of genes. As a result, there are relatively few examples where complex disease loci have been identified using this approach.

Several genome-wide linkage studies in CHD have been published,[34–40] but cross-study replication of identified loci has in general been lacking. Of these linkage studies, only one produced evidence in favor of a specific positional candidate gene, ALOX5AP, which encodes 5-lipoxygenase activating protein (FLAP).[38] FLAP is a necessary co-activator of the enzyme arachidonate 5-lipoxygenase (ALOX5) which synthesizes leukotriene A4 (LTA4), a short-lived mediator of inflammation. Variants in ALOX5AP were associated with a relative risk of MI of 1.8, and a relative risk of stroke of 1.67, in that study. These genetic findings have, however, not been consistently replicated in other studies, and the summary of the evidence to date suggests that the effect of the haplotypes studied, if it exists, is of a much smaller size than originally estimated.[41–46] Based on the initial genetic findings, a clinical trial was conducted to examine the effect of FLAP inhibition on levels of biomarkers associated with MI risk in 191 patients who had already suffered an MI and carried at-risk variants in FLAP.[47] The FLAP inhibitor led to suppression of plasma levels of leukotriene B4, myeloperoxidase, and C-reactive protein without any adverse events. This result suggests that clinical trials of agents inhibiting FLAP that are powered to detect differences in CHD endpoints would be of interest.

Single nucleotide polymorphisms and the human haplotype map

In the last 18 months genome-wide association (GWA) studies have delivered over a hundred new loci for upwards of 40 common diseases and continuous traits with a "complex" (that is, made up of multiple genetic effects) genetic architecture. The majority of such studies have been conducted in large numbers of unrelated cases of disease and controls, and at its simplest, the analysis consists of comparing the frequency of genotypes at a large number of genetic polymorphisms spaced throughout the human genome one by one in the cases and controls. The polymorphisms used in these analyses consist of single base alternatives in the genetic sequence, called single nucleotide polymorphisms (SNPs, usually pronounced "snips"). The large-scale sequencing studies conducted to complete the Human Genome Project established that SNPs were the most common type of human genetic variant, and that SNPs with a minor allele frequency of greater than 1% occurred on average every 300 bases throughout the human genome.

Consider an autosomal SNP which has as alternative alleles the nucleotides thymine (T) or adenine (A). A diploid individual has three possible genotypes: thymine/thymine (T/T), thymine/adenine (T/A) or adenine/adenine (A/A). If the frequency of these two alleles in the population were 80% T alleles and 20% A alleles, then the three genotype frequencies would be expected to be around 64%, 32%, and 4% respectively (since the frequency of each homozygote genotype would be expected to be the square of the frequency of the corresponding allele, and the heterozygote frequency twice the product of the two allele frequencies). Such a SNP would qualify as a "common variant" – though the cut-off is somewhat arbitrary, SNPs with minor allele frequencies greater than 5% are generally considered to be common. Common SNPs tend to be evolutionarily ancient, because rare variants have a much higher likelihood of being eliminated over time by the random selection of gametes that occurs from generation to generation. Alleles conferring susceptibility to common degenerative diseases of later life such as CHD may have persisted throughout evolution because they do not commonly affect fitness in the reproductive years and are therefore invisible to natural selection. Thus, genetic susceptibility to common disease might arise from a relatively small number of common variants in a particular susceptibility gene, as opposed to a large number of individually rare variants. This theory is known as the "common disease–common variant hypothesis". It is the main theoretical argument in favor of studying common SNPs for association with disease. From a practical point of view, rare SNPs with small effects on disease would be essentially impossible to detect in studies of a feasible size (see Fig. 21.1), and the technology to systematically investigate genes for rare SNPs, even of large effect, has until very recently been far behind that available for the investigation of common SNPs. Recent GWA studies of many diseases have convincingly shown that the common disease–common variant hypothesis is to an extent true, although even for diseases such as type 2 diabetes, in which a large number of susceptibility variants have been found, these together do not explain the bulk of the inherited propensity to disease.

A systematic discovery program for SNPs was implemented by the SNP Consortium, a public–private partnership formed in 1999. The consortium released 1.4 million SNPs into the public domain by 2001, and there are presently more than 7 million validated SNPs in public databases. This constitutes a fairly complete picture of human common SNP variation. However, simple knowledge of the SNPs did not make the task of assessing variation across the genome possible, since no platform exists that could type 7 million SNPs in each of a large number of cases and controls in a cost-effective manner. It was therefore necessary to additionally determine the relationships between the SNPs that had been discovered, in order to establish which SNPs gave redundant or substantially overlapping information about genetic variation in different regions of the genome, and establish a minimal set of SNPs that could be feasibly typed in case–control studies while retaining relatively full information. Such data were provided by the collaborative International Haplotype Map (HapMap) Project, which aimed to obtain detailed genome-wide information on patterns of common genetic variation in multiple world populations, suitable for association studies (www.hapmap.org).

Chromosomes in the present-day population are essentially mosaics which reflect the results of new mutations and genetic recombination on ancestral haplotypes (Fig. 21.2). When a SNP arises on a chromosome (since the per-base mutation rate at SNPs is low, most SNPs are thought to have arisen only once during evolution), initially the alleles present at all the surrounding pre-existing SNPs are strong predictors of genotype at the new SNP. As meiotic recombination occurs throughout the generations, the initially lengthy chromosomal segment containing strongly predictive genotypes will break down. Note that although in general terms more closely neighboring SNPs will be better predictors of each other's genotypes, the relationships cannot simply be derived mathematically; they must be empirically observed for each pair of SNPs of interest. The degree to which genotype at one SNP predicts genotype at a neighboring SNP is called "linkage disequilibrium", abbreviated "LD". For the purposes of association mapping it is most usefully measured by the correlation coefficient r^2 which varies between 0 in the case of two SNPs whose genotypes have no predictive value for each other, and 1 in the case of two SNPs that are perfect proxies

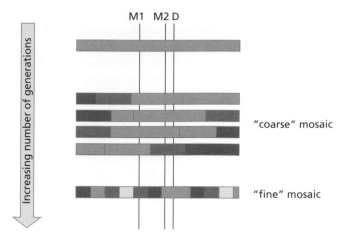

Figure 21.2 Decay of allelic association over time: chromosomes are mosaics. Consider a new disease susceptibility allele D arising on an ancestral chromosome (bar). In that generation, all the markers in the region including markers M1 and M2 will be correlated with D. Genetic recombination will break down the region of association over time, introducing new haplotypes into the region. If the mosaic is "coarse" (which is the case with the human genome) fewer markers are needed to tag each piece (or "haplotype block") of the mosaic: thus, M1 and M2 are both still good markers for D when the mosaic is coarse, but only M2 is a good marker after further time has elapsed and the mosaic is finer.

for each other (and therefore one of them is entirely redundant for association study purposes). r^2 is a useful measure because the power of an association study where the disease-causing variant is not directly observed varies inversely with r^2. Thus, if a study of 2000 cases and controls were required to have adequate power to detect an odds ratio of a particular size should the causative variant be directly typed, a study of 4000 would be required if the most closely correlated SNP that was typed had an r^2 of 0.5 with the untyped causative SNP.

The "grain" of the human genomic mosaic was a key factor in determining the feasibility of GWA studies (Fig. 21.2). If it had been very "fine", it might have been necessary to type most of the 10 million common SNPs to represent them all satisfactorily, and if relatively "coarse", typing of only a few hundred thousand SNPs might be sufficient. Some early studies[48] provided encouraging information that at the level of single genes, the mosaic was indeed quite coarse; subsequent studies in large genomic segments confirmed that this was more generally true,[49] and showed that the mean size of regions of strongly associated SNPs (also known as "haplotype blocks") is around 22 kb in populations of European or Asian ancestry, and 11 kb in populations of African ancestry.[50] These findings, among others, suggested that a substantial proportion of common variation genome-wide could indeed be characterized with several hundred thousand SNPs that were sufficiently well correlated with all the remaining untyped

SNPs that they could be considered to "tag" the untyped SNPs. In 2005 the Phase I HapMap reported data from around 1 million SNPs; in 2007, the Phase II HapMap containing data on 3 million SNPs covering most common variations in most of the human genome was made available.[51–53] This provided the necessary information to design experiments in which common variation either within candidate genes or genome-wide could be thoroughly assessed using a subset of "tag" SNPs. An excellent recent review provides more detailed information on the achievements of the HapMap.[54]

The key technologic advance required for the success of genome-wide association studies has been the development of "gene chips" able to assay up to 1 million SNPs chosen on the basis of the genomic knowledge from the HapMap. Currently such chips are available for less than 750 US dollars per sample, and the price is constantly falling even as the genomic coverage improves, in a situation analogous to that for computer microprocessors in recent years. The current "top of the range" products from the major manufacturers Illumina and Affymetrix tag 80–90% of genome-wide SNPs in non-African origin population at an r^2 of 0.8 or greater, although only around 66% of genome-wide SNPs are tagged at r^2 of 0.8 or greater in African origin populations in whom there is greater haplotype diversity.

Finally, large samples of well-characterized cases and controls have been required to render both reliable candidate–gene association studies and GWA studies feasible. Early work on CHD genetics in the 1990s clearly showed the potential for false-positive results in small samples; at that stage the problem was one of overoptimism, as investigators hoped to discover genetic effects much larger than those that (with the benefit of hindsight) appear to be present. In the initial stage of a GWA study, where up to 1 million SNPs may be typed, around 50000 SNPs would be expected to show statistical significance at the $P < 0.05$ level, most of these purely by chance. To avoid these false positives, extremely stringent levels of significance must be adopted (typically 5×10^{-7} or thereabouts). In order to obtain this level of significance for a SNP with a minor allele frequency of around 0.1, that confers an odds ratio of disease of about 1.3, 2000 cases and a similar number of controls are required. Within-study replication of associated SNPs in additional cohorts is considered an additional requirement to rule out the play of chance as a cause for the initial finding.

Candidate–gene association studies in coronary heart disease

In common with many other diseases, CHD has been the subject of large numbers of candidate–gene association studies that have examined many different genes. Nearly 1000 such published studies are currently in the Genetic Association Database, an archive of association studies in human complex diseases (http://geneticassociationdb.nih.gov). Conclusive identification of associated variants has been very rarely achieved. Several factors are likely to contribute to this. The prior probability of association of any particular SNP in any one of 20000 genes with a given disease is vanishingly small. Relevant pathophysiologic information that has led to the selection of a gene as a candidate (for example, its involvement in determining plasma levels of cholesterol) may increase the prior probability, but even so, it is certain that in this context $P < 0.05$, the conventionally accepted significance level for result reporting, does not represent secure evidence in favor of the involvement of that gene. Thus, most genetic associations initially reported with significance levels $0.01 < P < 0.05$ can reasonably be expected to be false. The majority of reported studies to date have been of insufficient size to robustly identify (i.e. with appropriately small P-values) the effects of small magnitude that would usually be expected for common SNPs. In a 2007 paper, Morgan and colleagues highlighted the replication problems in the field by typing 85 variants in 70 genes previously claimed to be associated with the risk of acute coronary syndrome, finding just one borderline significant ($P = 0.03$) association that was most likely due to the play of chance.[43] Although meta-analyses may, as in traditional epidemiology, assist in identifying true associations, a number of meta-analyses of genetic association studies have shown evidence for publication bias – the preferential reporting in the literature of small positive studies, whereas equally sized negative studies go unreported. This greatly complicates the interpretation of quantitative overviews of the published literature; statistical tests for publication bias are relatively insensitive, and the regular detection of publication bias in the field tends to undermine confidence that it is not present for a particular association even in the absence of statistical evidence. Results of several large-scale (that is, involving greater than 5000 cases of disease) meta-analyses are shown in Table 21.2. Of these, the most convincing evidence in favor of association is with the Apo E epsilon-2/epsilon-3/epsilon-4 isoform polymorphism. Apolipoprotein E is a ligand for receptors that clear remnants of chylomicrons and very low density lipoproteins; the three isoforms bind with different affinities and are associated with differences in levels of LDL-cholesterol. The recent GWA studies (see below) have not provided a great deal of additional evidence pertinent to this association because the two polymorphisms (Cys112Arg and Arg158Cys) that together define the isoform are not well "tagged" by the SNPs present on the genotyping chips used in studies to date.

Table 21.2 Candidate gene polymorphisms associated with CHD in large-scale meta-analyses (>5000 CHDcases)

Gene	Variant (rs number) and risk allele	Number of studies included	Number of CHD cases/controls	Relative risk (95% CI)	References
Cholesteryl ester transfer protein (CETP)	TaqIB (rs708272) –A allele	38	19035/32368	0.95 (0.92–0.99) per allele	123
	I405V (rs5882) –G allele	18	10313/32244	0.94 (0.89–1.00) per allele	123
	–629C>A (rs1800775) –A allele	17	11599/23185	0.95 (0.91–1.00) per allele	123
Apolipoprotein E (APOE)	ε2 isoform carrier	17	21331/47467	0.80 (0.70–0.90)	124
	ε4 isoform carrier	17	21331/47467	1.06 (0.99–1.13)	124
	ε4/ε4 homozygote	17	21331/47467	1.22 (1.08–1.38)	124
Angiotensin type 1 receptor (AGTR1)	+1166A/C (rs5186) –C allele	27	10180/17129	1.13 (1.04–1.23) per allele	125
Factor V	G1691A (rs6025) –A [Factor V Leiden]	60	15704/26686	1.17 (1.08–1.28) per allele	126
Prothrombin (factor II)	G20210A –A allele	40	11625/14462	1.31 (1.12–1.52) per allele	126
Plasminogen activator inhibitor (PAI-1)	[–675]4G/5G –4G allele	37	11763/13905	1.06 (1.02–1.10) per allele	126
Paraoxonase (PON1)	Q192R (rs662) –R allele	43	10106/11786	1.12 (1.07–1.16) per allele	127
Endothelial nitric oxide synthase (eNOS)	Glu298Asp –Asp/Asp homozygote	14	6036/6106	1.31 (1.13–1.51)	128
	Intron-4a –a/a homozygote	16	6212/6737	1.34 (1.03–1.75)	128
Apolipoprotein B (APOB)	SpIns/Del –DD homozygote	22	6007/5609	1.19 (1.05–1.35)	129
Methylene tetrahydrofolate reductase (MTHFR)	677C>T (rs1801133) –TT homozygote	40	11162/12758	1.16 (1.05–1.28)	130

Identification of lymphotoxin-alpha and galectin 2 by association study of 93 000 single nucleotide polymorphisms

The first report from an association study of CHD that typed many thousands of SNPs (although providing insufficient coverage to be classified as a true genome-wide association study) was published in 2002. Ozaki and colleagues examined almost 93 000 gene-based SNPs (mainly in exons, introns and flanking regions surrounding genes) in 14 000 genes, in 94 cases of MI and 658 controls.[55] Those SNPs showing a P-value for association of <0.01 were genotyped in a larger panel consisting of a total of 1133 cases with MI and 1006 controls. A susceptibility locus on chromosome 6p21 was identified, with maximal association found between MI and a five-SNP haplotype in the lymphotoxin-alpha (LTA) gene, which encodes a member of the tumor necrosis factor ligand family. Ozaki and colleagues then used molecular biologic techniques to identify novel proteins interacting with LTA, among which were galectin 2 (LGALS2), a sugar-binding lectin molecule of unknown function.[56] They identified SNPs in LGALS2 and tested them for association with CHD in a study of 2302 MI cases and 2038 controls. They found an odds ratio of 1.23 (95% CI 1.13–1.35; $Pp = 4.5 \times 10^{-6}$) for MI associated with genotype at a SNP in intron 1 (C3279T). The rare T allele appeared protective, and it was associated with a

halving of the transcriptional activity of the gene compared to the common allele. These studies identifying LTA and LGALS2 were large, rigorously conducted and included highly plausible functional data. It is therefore somewhat perplexing that the promising early results have not been successfully replicated in most other large studies.[44,57–63]

Genome-wide association studies of coronary heart disease endpoints

Four genome-wide association studies of CHD reported in 2007 demonstrated conclusive evidence for association between common SNPs in the same ~100 kb region on chromosome 9p21 and CHD risk.[64–67] Results of these studies are summarized in Table 21.3. The Wellcome Trust Case–Control Consortium (WTCCC) study examined around 400 000 SNPs in 1988 British Caucasians with a validated history of MI or coronary revascularization before the age of 66 years, and 3004 controls.[66] Associations were seen for SNPs across >100 kb in the 9p21 region, with the strongest association demonstrated for rs1333049 ($P = 1.8 \times 10^{-14}$). For this SNP the heterozygote odds ratio was 1.47 (95% CI 1.27–1.70) and the homozygote odds ratio was 1.90 (95% CI 1.61–2.24). 'Moderate' associations, defined as SNPs with a P-value greater than 5×10^{-7} but less than 1×10^{-5}, were reported for six other loci. Replication of the chromosome 9 locus was achieved in a subsequent paper which added

Table 21.3 Susceptibility loci identified in genome-wide association studies of CHD that have been successfully replicated in a separate cohort

Study	Phenotype	Total patients/ controls	SNPs on array	Locus/SNP.risk allele	Allele frequency		Relative risk (95% CI) heterozygote/ homozygote	P-value
					Controls	Cases		
WTCCC[66] and Samani[67]	CHD/MI	2863/4648	500 000	9p21/rs1333049/C	0.47	0.55	1.36 (1.27–1.46) per copy of risk allele	2.9×10^{-19}
				6q25.1/rs6922269/A	0.25	0.29	1.23 (1.15–1.33) per copy of risk allele	2.9×10^{-8}
	.			2q36.1/rs2943634/C	0.34	0.30	1.21 (1.13–1.30) per copy of risk allele	1.6×10^{-7}
Helgadottir[65]	MI/CHD	4587/12 767	305 000	9p21/rs2383207/G	0.492	0.548	1.25 (1.18–1.31) per copy of risk allele	2.0×10^{-16}
				9p21/rs10757278/G	0.453	0.517	1.28 (1.22–1.35) per copy of risk allele	1.2×10^{-20}
McPherson[64]	CHD	4306/20 119	100 000	9p21/rs10757274/G	0.487*	0.525*	1.18 (1.02–1.37)/1.29 (1.09–1.52)*	4×10^{-3}*
				9p21/rs2383206/G	0.505*	0.541*	1.26 (1.09–1.46)/1.26 (1.07–1.48)*	7×10^{-4}*

*Data from ARIC cohort only.

data from a cohort comprising 875 German Caucasians with MI before the age of 60 years and at least one family member with premature CHD, and 1644 controls, which had been genotyped using the same chip.[67] As shown in Table 21.3, two loci on chromosome 6 and chromosome 2 were also replicated in the German cohort. The combined analysis identified four additional loci potentially associated with CHD, one of which (chromosome 1p13.3) has subsequently been shown to be strongly associated with plasma LDL cholesterol. An analysis of 55 candidate genes previously reported to show association with CHD only confirmed association for two SNPs tagging a variant in the lipoprotein lipase gene in these cohorts.

Helgadottir and colleagues performed a similar study in 1607 Icelandic patients with MI (before age 70 years in males and 75 years in females) and 6728 controls, typed for around 300 000 genome-wide SNPs using the Illumina Hap300 chip.[65] The strongest association was found for three correlated SNPs in the same chromosome 9p21 region that was identified in the WTCCC study, each with P-values of approximately 1×10^{-6}. The association was replicated in four additional case–control cohorts. Combining data from all groups, allele G of the SNP rs10757278 showed the strongest association with MI, with an odds ratio of 1.28 (95% CI 1.22–1.35, $P = 1.2 \times 10^{-20}$) per allele.

In the third GWA study, McPherson and colleagues typed 100 000 SNPs in 322 cases of premature CHD and 312 controls, confirming positive results in a further 1658 cases and 9380 controls.[64] Two SNPs located within 20 kb of each other in the same region of chromosome 9p21 were signifi-

cantly associated with CHD. These two SNPs were validated in three additional independent cohorts (with varying inclusion parameters for defining CHD).

The chromosome 9p21 locus has thus shown a remarkably consistent association with CHD in GWA studies involving multiple Caucasian populations (Fig. 21.3). Subsequent reports have replicated the association in Japanese and Korean populations,[68] and in multiple additional Caucasian case–control series, confirmed by meta-analysis.[69–71] Fine mapping and detailed characterization of the locus were performed in a large case–control study of 4251 CHD cases and 4443 controls from four European populations by Broadbent and colleagues.[69] Analysis of 62 SNPs in the region identified a region of strong LD containing 14 SNPs that form four common haplotypes (cumulative frequency 89%), with the association of the linked SNPs at this locus a consequence of a perfect "yin–yang" pair of haplotypes spanning 53 kb.

At the time of writing, this field is rapidly evolving. As of February 2009, a number of subsequent GWA studies have provided strong evidence for several further loci, all of which have smaller effects than the chromosome 9p21 locus.[72–75]

The chromosome 9p21 region: mechanistic clues and candidate genes

The mechanism for the 9p21 association with CHD remains unclear at present; relationships between risk genotypes and other phenotypes have been explored to search for

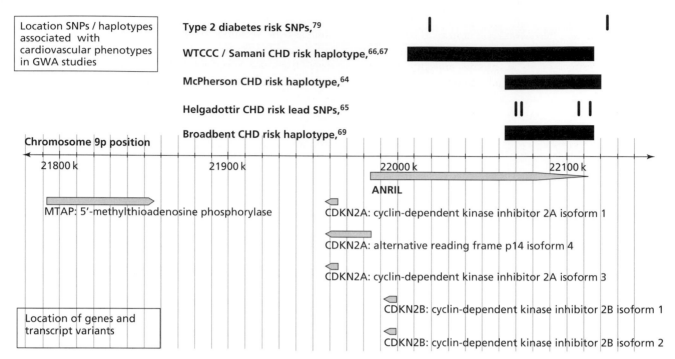

Figure 21.3 Position of the CHD risk SNPs/haplotypes and nearby genes at the chromosome 9p21 locus. Arrows denote genes or transcripts in the region, with the arrowhead pointing in the direction of transcription. Numbers designate base pairs along chromosome 9. The positions of lead SNPs/haplotypes associated with cardiovascular disease and diabetes at the chromosome 9p21 locus in GWA studies are represented by the bars in the top half of the figure. Figure adapted from www.hapmap.org.

mechanistic clues. Subgroup analyses in case–control studies have not demonstrated significant heterogeneity in the risk associated with genotype between patients who had presented with or without MI, suggesting that the genetic effect is not on plaque rupture but rather on atherosclerosis susceptibility. Nor has heterogeneity been demonstrated with regard to sex, age, and traditional risk factor status. Furthermore, no association between genotype and known risk factors for atherosclerosis has been demonstrated, suggesting the mechanism of the association is independent of any of these factors.[65,67,69,76]

GWA studies for type 2 diabetes mellitus published around the same time showed an association between diabetes and a chromosome 9p21 locus in some populations,[77–79] although this was not reported in other groups.[80,81] Diabetes is a major risk factor for CHD, associated with features such as vascular endothelial dysfunction and hyperlipidemia that are also important in atherogenesis, raising the prospect of a shared pathophysiologic mechanism for the two diseases. However, the most strongly associated SNP for type 2 diabetes in the region (rs10811661) lies beyond the linkage disequilibrium block that is strongly associated with CHD risk (see Fig. 22.3) and does not show association with CHD.[69,82] A second SNP (rs564398), associated with diabetes in a meta-analysis of 14586 cases,[79] which is not correlated with rs10811661, lies within the CHD-associated region described in the WTCCC study,

and shows moderate correlation ($0.28 < r^2 < 0.42$) with CHD-associated SNPs (see Fig. 21.3). rs564398 showed association with CHD in the study by Broadbent et al ($P = 4 \times 10^{-8}$), but once a marker of the CHD risk haplotype was included in the statistical model, this became non-significant ($P = 0.08$).[69] There is therefore no evidence for an effect of rs564398 on CHD risk independent of its association with the risk haplotype at the present time. However, insufficient numbers of people with and without CHD that are concordant and discordant for diabetes have been studied so far to enable a possible effect of rs564398 on both diabetes and CHD to be entirely ruled out.

A CHD risk SNP (rs10757278) from the chromosome 9p21 region has also been found to be significantly associated with abdominal aortic aneurysm (OR 1.31, P = 1.2×10^{-12}) and intracranial aneurysm (OR 1.29, P = 2.5×10^{-6}), although after excluding potentially confounding cases of known CHD, it was not significantly associated with peripheral arterial disease, ischemic stroke or diabetes in a study involving patients with multiple cardiovascular phenotypes.[82] This report showed that the effect of 9p21 variants on arterial disease is not solely confined to atherosclerotic conditions. Intracranial aneurysms typically present at a younger age than CHD, are commoner in females, and have non-atherosclerotic pathology. The identification of an association between the same variants and two different pathologic types of arterial disease suggests that the risk locus may be having its effect via a defect in the arterial ability to remodel in response to different types of stress, though this remains a conjecture at present. With respect to 9p21 variants and intermediate phenotypes related to coronary and cerebral atherosclerosis, two separate reports also found no association between CHD risk variants and carotid artery intima-media thickness, a marker of carotid vascular disease that is associated with both MI and stroke risk.[76,83]

A number of candidate genes potentially influencing the risk of CHD lie adjacent to the associated region (see Fig. 21.3). Functional studies to establish the influence of risk-associated SNPs on the transcription and activity of genes in the immediate region may enable one gene to be selected as the strongest candidate. The cell cycle checkpoint kinase genes CDKN2A and CDKN2B lie some 50 kb from the SNPs most associated with CHD (see Fig. 21.3). These tumor suppressor genes are involved in regulation of the cell cycle, aging, senescence and apoptosis, which are important factors in atherogenesis.[84,85] Resequencing of these genes in cases of MI has not identified variants explaining the genetic association in the region, though effects of the risk SNPs on regulation of these genes remain a plausible mechanism requiring further investigation.

The CHD risk haplotype overlaps with ANRIL, a gene first characterized in 2007 by investigators examining a deletion in a large melanoma-neural tumor syndrome family.[86] ANRIL encodes a large antisense non-coding RNA of presently unknown function. Such non-coding RNAs are believed to be involved in regulation of gene expression, through transcriptional and translational control mechanisms.[87] ANRIL has been shown to be widely expressed in different tissues, including heart, coronary smooth muscle, human monocyte-derived macrophages, carotid endarterectomy specimens, and abdominal aortic aneurysm samples.[69,86] The SNPs most strongly associated with CHD map to ANRIL introns and downstream sequences which could influence its expression, although no relationship between ANRIL expression and CHD risk has as yet been demonstrated.[69]

Somewhat more distant from the risk haplotype, the MTAP gene encodes methylthioadenosine phosphorylase, an enzyme that is involved in polyamine metabolism. It has been suggested that variants may influence plasma levels of homocysteine and folate, although a recent study reported no variation in these related to genotype of the CHD risk SNP rs10757274.[71]

It seems likely that the studies to date have identified on chromosome 9p21 the most important single association between common genetic variation and CHD present in the genome. However, individual GWA studies have only had adequate power (80%) to detect relative risks greater than about 1.5 at the stringent significance levels required for these analyses, and it is likely that further loci with smaller effects will be identified through larger studies or meta-analyses of existing datasets.[88,89] The potential health importance of particular loci, particularly with regard to drug discovery, is not predictable from the magnitude of the odds ratio: for example, variants of the KCNJ11 gene confer an odds ratio of only 1.2 for diabetes in genome-wide studies but this gene is the target for the sulfonyl-ureas, which have been a cornerstone of diabetes therapy for many years.[54,90,91] Meta-analyses should be facilitated by the recent development of genotype imputation algorithms which use the patterns of intermarker association in a set of common samples genotyped on two platforms to enable the combination of datasets typed on one or other platform.[92] It should also be noted that the genotyping chips used in studies so far do not have complete coverage of all common variants. The Affymetrix 500K chip used in the WTCCC and German studies tags only about 68% of HapMap SNPs in Caucasian populations at $r^2 > 0.8$; the Illumina HumanHap300 is somewhat better at about 77% but still incomplete.[51] Thus, additional genotyping to complete the representation of common genome-wide SNPs may yield additional loci in due course.

Genome-wide association studies of plasma lipids: new loci

Recent GWA studies investigating plasma lipoprotein concentrations as quantitative traits have produced convincing associations at a number of loci, many of which have been replicated in separate analyses.[92–97] These recent studies have confirmed over a dozen previously implicated loci and identified seven newly associated genes associated with HDL cholesterol, LDL cholesterol and triglyceride levels (Table 21.4). One of these studies examined the relationship between lipoprotein-associated SNPs and CHD risk in a combined cohort comprising the WTCCC sample and an expanded panel of British individuals. All of the alleles associated with LDL metabolism were more common in CHD cases than controls, with modest odds ratios of 1.04–1.29 per allele; the association was significant ($P < 0.05$) for eight of the 11 SNPs. These findings suggest that the newly identified loci are potential targets for novel therapies affecting lipoprotein levels and CHD risk.

"Mendelian randomization" studies: using genetics to identify causal emerging risk factors

As illustrated in the GWA studies of lipoproteins discussed above, it is now relatively straightforward to conduct GWA studies of intermediate traits potentially relevant to CHD

Table 21.4 Loci associated with lipid levels in genomewide association studies ($P < 10^{-6}$)

Trait	Locus	Nearest gene(s)	Largest effect size (mg/dL)
HDL cholesterol	16q13	CETP	4.12
	8p21	LPL	2.09
	15q21	LIPC	1.41
	18q21	LIPG/ACAA2	1.20
	1q42	GALNT2	1.11
	9q31	ABCA1	0.82
	16q22	LCAT	0.74
	12q24	MVK/MMAB	0.48
LDL cholesterol	19p13	LDLR	9.17
	19q13	APOE/C1/C4/C2	6.61
	1p13	CELSR2/PSRC1/SORT1	5.48
	2p24	APOB	4.89
	5q13	HMGCR	3.8*
	19p13	NCAN/CILP2/PBX4	3.32
	1p32	PCSK9	3.04
	3q13	B4GALT4	2.23
	6p21	B3GALT4	1.91
Triglycerides	11q23	APOA5/A4/C3/A1	25.82
	2p24	APOB	18.46*
	8p21	LPL	11.57
	2p23	GCKR/RBKS	8.59
	7q11	MLXIPL/BCL7B/TBL2	8.21
	1p31	ANGPTL3/DOCK7/ ATG4C	7.12
	8q24	TRIB1	6.42
	19p13	NCAN/CILP2/PBX4	6.10
	11q23	APOA1/C3/A4/A5/ ZNF259/ BUD13	5.68*
	1q42	GALNT2	4.25
	15q21–23	LIPC	3.62

* Estimated effect size in mg/dL obtained by multiplying the proportion of 1 standard deviation change reported by Kathiresan and colleagues[93] by the standard deviation of the lipid value from the MDC-CC cohort of that study.

the causality or otherwise of the intermediate trait in the disease process – an approach termed "Mendelian randomization".[98,99] The first large-scale application of this approach investigated the association between genotypes at the fibrinogen locus influencing plasma fibrinogen levels and the risk of MI.[100,101] In that study of around 5000 cases of MI and a similar number of controls, association between plasma fibrinogen level and MI risk was observed, as in many previous studies. Association was also found between polymorphisms in the promoter region of the beta-fibrinogen gene and plasma fibrinogen levels. The authors reasoned that if the relationship between plasma fibrinogen and MI were causal, the polymorphisms associated with fibrinogen level should show an association with MI risk that was commensurate with the associations between the polymorphisms on plasma fibrinogen, and between plasma fibrinogen and MI risk. No association between the SNPs typed and MI risk was observed, either in primary data or a literature-based meta-analysis of beta-fibrinogen SNPs and MI. This suggested that plasma fibrinogen did not play an important causal role in the risk of MI, but rather that the association observed was due to confounding or reverse causality.

Plasma levels of lipoprotein(a) have been known for many years to be highly genetically determined, with the major effect being due to a kringle IV type 2 size polymorphism in the Apo(a) gene. Plasma lipoprotein(a) levels are associated with MI risk, but the causal nature of the association has remained unclear. Recently, a "Mendelian randomization" approach involving 2800 cases and 37 000 controls showed consistent association between lipoprotein(a) levels and MI risk, and between kringle IV repeats and MI risk, suggesting the association is causal.[102] By contrast, a similar study involving 6500 MI cases, 2800 ischemic cerebrovascular disease cases, and over 35 000 controls did not suggest a causal association of C reactive protein with ischemic vascular disease.[103]

Genetic testing in coronary heart disease: ready for "prime time"?

The potential utility of genetic testing in predicting the risk of CHD and other serious conditions of later life is easily appreciated by scientists and the public alike. CHD, however, is a condition in which known and modifiable lifestyle factors play key roles. It could be argued that public health measures such as tobacco control, promotion of physical activity and healthy diet, and reducing salt consumption are likely to yield much more substantial reductions in CHD morbidity and mortality than genetic testing. Since there have not, as yet, been any loci discov-

susceptibility, and to test whether the association between genotype and intermediate trait translates to an association between genotype and disease. In the case of LDL cholesterol above, the disease–trait association is securely established through epidemiologic and randomized clinical trial data, so the disease–genotype association serves to validate the trait–genotype association. For emerging risk factors where the epidemiologically observed disease–trait association is not supported by randomized clinical trials (possibly because suitably specific agents are not available), the question can be posed somewhat differently to address

ered which modify the risk of non-Mendelian CHD to an extent that they would be considered useful in risk prediction, it remains unknown whether the reactions of patients at risk of CHD for genetic reasons would be to avoid lifestyle factors that further increased their risk or to take an attitude of "genetic determinism" that might if anything lead to adverse changes in their lifestyles.

For some of the monogenic disorders increasing CHD risk referred to above, genetic testing is already being applied in the clinical setting. In familial hypercholesterolemia, the most common such disorder with a population prevalence of 0.2%, there has been recent debate regarding the optimal strategy to deliver this service. Many patients with FH go untreated: only around 15% of the estimated 110 000 patients with FH in the UK are thought to be receiving treatment in lipid clinics[104] and up to 75% of patients with FH may be unrecognized prior to their first coronary event.[105] In The Netherlands and Iceland, both small countries with concentrated populations and well-supported government-funded programs, cascade screening for FH has proved very successful. The Dutch program is estimated to have found over a third of all cases to date, and is expected to achieve almost complete identification of cases by 2013.[106] The cascade screening strategy involves identification and mutation testing of all first-degree relatives of known cases in whom a mutation has been detected; of these relatives, 50% will be carriers of the same mutation. This optimizes the cost effectiveness of the approach by reserving the relatively costly genetic test for a group in which the prior probability of a positive result is substantial. Testing is then "cascaded" to the first-degree relatives of mutation-positive family members, and so on through the family. Cascade screening can also be carried out in families without identified FH mutations using gender- and age-specific LDL cholesterol criteria to diagnose FH, but in this situation there is a range of LDL-C concentration where the diagnosis remains unclear.

Recently, Wald and colleagues proposed an alternative approach based upon opportunistic screening of children for hypercholesterolemia at the time of their routine immunizations, arguing that in order for cascade screening to be optimally implemented, more index cases had to be identified.[107] Subsequent measurement of cholesterol in parents of hypercholesterolemic children was estimated by these authors to have power to detect around 96% of parents with FH, and thus potentially reduce the impact of FH in both generations of families where it was discovered. Such an approach raises many contentious issues including obtaining valid consent from the child, potential psychologic damage from screening, and the impact of false positives. However, in many healthcare settings it is unlikely that cascade screening will identify more than 50% of cases,

so novel approaches to case finding such as opportunistic childhood screening, screening of family practitioner records, and targeted screening of patients presenting with first MI or acute coronary syndrome will need to be considered and piloted. It is unlikely that a "one size fits all" approach will be effective across multiple healthcare systems.

Present knowledge about the genetic contribution to non-Mendelian CHD susceptibility does not argue in favor of genetic testing. Although population attributable fractions of up to 0.22 for genotype at SNPs in the chromosome 9p21 region have been claimed, it should be remembered that the case–control cohorts which have been used in studies to date have been specifically collected to be "genetically loaded" – that is, in general early-onset cases have been studied, with a preference for inclusion of families in whom there is an affected relative-pair. The generalizability of results regarding the relative magnitude of a genetic contribution to risk in such selected cohorts to the entire population at risk of CHD is questionable. From a practical point of view, the contribution of genotype at associated SNPs to the capacity to predict CHD in a representative population assessed for the "classic" CHD risk factors is perhaps the most important question. In a recent report, the chromosome 9p21 CHD risk SNP rs10757274 was typed in a prospective study of 2742 men aged 50–64 years old, who were free of CHD at baseline.[71] The report included 270 CHD events that had occurred during a 15-year follow-up period. Even in this relatively small number of cases, an effect of the SNP could be demonstrated ($P = 0.04$) with a per-allele effect size congruent with previous studies. The contribution of rs10757274 genotype to prediction of CHD risk was assessed using receiver operating characteristic (ROC) curves. The area under the ROC curve for the "classic" risk factors was 0.62 (95% CI 0.58–0.66), and this did not increase significantly when rs10757274 genotype was included. Simulations suggested that if 10 additional SNP genotypes of similar effect to rs10757274 could be identified, the area under the ROC curve could be increased to 0.76, a gain in predictive capacity which the authors judged to be potentially useful. However, it was noted that the proportion of individuals segregating multiple independently associated SNPs in any population would be low, limiting the likely clinical utility of such SNPs as predictors even if discovered. Moreover, the chromosome 9p21 locus is clearly the strongest common genetic risk factor for CHD that has been discovered so far, and it seems unlikely from currently available data that many further loci will be discovered that confer a similar level of risk.

In this context, perhaps the best hope for "personalized medicine" with regard to CHD risk prediction lies with the potential for discovery of low-frequency intermediate penetrance (LFIP) variants which, although contributing a small amount to the population attributable risk of disease, significantly impact an individual's personal risk.

Low-frequency intermediate penetrance variants: still largely unknown territory

Until recently, few studies had attempted to undertake systematic discovery of low-frequency variants (which we consider as those with allele frequencies 0.005–0.05 in the population) that may be involved in disease susceptibility. This is because such variants require gene sequencing to identify them directly; they cannot be indirectly inferred through association, as is possible with common variants. Sequencing using the Sanger method was too slow and costly to permit any but very limited studies of a handful of genes, which were conducted in major sequencing centers. Low-frequency variants might be expected to confer substantially higher disease odds ratios per allele than the 1.2–1.5 range generally observed in studies of common variation, as both theory and available data suggest that an inverse relationship between allele frequency and effect size will usually be the case (see Fig. 21.1). Depending on the size of the effect on risk and the allele frequency, variants with frequencies 0.005–0.05 could make significant contributions to familial risk. A hypothetical variant present in 1% of the population conferring an odds ratio of 3 for a disease with 5% population prevalence would have an insufficiently strong effect to result in Mendelian segregation in carrier families, but would also be too uncommon to have much chance of being detected in a GWA study despite its large effect size. Such a variant would, however, have a larger effect on familial risk than most of the risk alleles for any complex disease that have emerged from GWA studies to date.[84]

The PCSK9 gene provides the best example to date of the potential importance of LFIP variants in CHD risk. PCSK9 is a member of the proprotein convertase gene family and regulates the availability of LDL receptors on the cell surface; activating mutations reduce the number of receptors, while inactivating mutations result in a higher number (and thus a higher internalization of LDL cholesterol).[108] Activating mutations in PCSK9 give rise to autosomal dominant hypercholesterolemia.[109] Nonsense mutations which inactivate PCSK9 result in 30–40% lower plasma LDL levels, and are present in 3% of African Americans. Missense mutations with smaller effects on LDL (~15% lower) are present in a similar percentage of Caucasians. African American carriers of nonsense mutations have an 88% lower long-term CHD risk while European American carriers of missense mutations have a 47% lower CHD risk.[110] These differences in risk are larger than would have been predicted from trials that used statins to lower LDL,

presumably reflecting the additional benefit of lifelong lower LDL compared with LDL reduction initiated in middle life. These genetic results suggest that pharmacologic inhibition of PCSK9 may be a promising therapeutic strategy to achieve or enhance LDL lowering.

Most importantly for this discussion, the effects on risk conferred by the LFIP variants in PCSK9 are much larger than those associated with any common variant likely to be identified for CHD. If present for other genes, such substantial effects on risk would, by contrast with currently known common alleles, potentially be of interest in risk stratification. This would be true particularly if the intermediate trait affected by the gene were either unknown or not readily measurable (that is, unlike LDL cholesterol in the case of PCSK9), and if the rare allele effect were to increase, rather than to decrease risk. Novel resequencing technologies available within the last two years are now able to generate sequence data at over 200 times the speed of Sanger sequencing and a fraction of the cost, rendering systematic approaches to LFIP variants feasible.[111] Resequencing of several hundred individuals will be necessary to identify LFIP variants with security; in the first instance, such studies are likely to be targeted to those genes implicated in disease susceptibility either by GWA studies or findings in novel Mendelian families.

Pharmacogenetic studies in cardiovascular disease

Pharmacogenetic studies investigating the effect of common genetic variants on drug response or side effects are in general at an early stage, although robust information is available in the case of warfarin and statins. Warfarin dosage requirement is influenced by common variants in the vitamin K epoxide reductase (VKORC1) gene, which is a target of warfarin, and in the cytochrome P450-2C9 (CYP2C9) gene, which metabolizes warfarin. VKORC1 genotype has been estimated to explain around 30% of the variation in warfarin dose, and CYP2C9 genotype around 12% of the variation.[112] A recent GWA study confirmed the importance of these two genes, and found no additional large effects in a test sample of 181 patients and a replication cohort of 374 patients.[113] In August 2007, the US Food and Drug Administration decided that the labeling of warfarin should be modified to highlight the potential role of genetic information at the CYP2C9 and VKORC1 genes in prescribing decisions. However, it is as yet unclear whether routine incorporation of genotype data into dosing protocols when warfarin is commenced would be of substantial clinical benefit, particularly in relation to its cost.[114]

A recent genome-wide pharmacogenetic study of statin-induced myopathy typed around 300 000 SNPs in 85 subjects with myopathy and 90 controls, all taking

80 mg of simvastatin per day as part of a clinical trial (SEARCH) involving 12 000 participants.[115] A SNP in the SLCO1B1 gene, which encodes the hepatic transporter protein OATPB1, was strongly associated with myopathy ($P = 4 \times 10^{-9}$). The odds ratio among heterozygotes for the risk allele was 4.5 (95% CI 2.6–7.7) and in homozygotes it was 16.9 (95% CI 4.7–61.1). The frequency of the risk allele was 15%, and genotype was estimated to account for more than 60% of the risk of myopathy. The findings were confirmed in a second population drawn from a trial of 40 mg of simvastatin daily ($P = 0.004$). Variants in the SLCO1B1 gene have previously been shown to affect the blood levels of several different statins, so it is likely that the genetic effect will be present for other drugs within the class.[116] Among people taking 40 mg of simvastatin (or equivalent doses of other statins) or less, the incidence of myopathy is only around 1 in 10 000 cases per year, but it may be substantially increased at higher statin doses – for example, definite or incipient myopathy occurred in just under 1 in 60 patients taking 80 mg of simvastatin in the SEARCH study. These findings suggest that genotyping SLCO1B1 polymorphisms could be clinically useful in safety monitoring and tailoring of statin dosages, particularly among patients in whom high-dose statins are being considered.

Conclusion

The last 12 months have seen the emergence of robust results regarding the magnitude and nature of the contribution of common genetic variants to coronary heart disease risk. Four studies which systematically searched for variants associated with CHD risk throughout the human genome in large numbers of cases and controls all identified the same novel region of chromosome 9p. The association has been replicated in many follow-up studies and can be considered definite. The consensus estimate from these studies is that CHD risk is increased by between 20% and 30% per copy of the most strongly associated allele in the region that an individual carries, and the population attributable risk of CHD from this region has been estimated to be as high as 20%. The mechanism of the association is as yet unclear. Pooled analyses of multiple datasets may identify additional common alleles, which are likely to have smaller effects on risk than the chromosome 9p locus. In parallel with analyses of coronary disease endpoints, genome-wide association studies of plasma lipids in healthy populations have identified seven new loci with significant effects on HDL cholesterol, LDL cholesterol or triglycerides. New insights into the pathogenesis of CHD and the mechanisms of plasma lipoprotein metabolism are anticipated as a consequence of these recent discoveries. In addition to the technologic and knowledge advances that have rendered systematic studies of common genetic variants feasible, novel ultra-high throughput technologies will shortly render it possible to screen all coding genetic sequence in an individual at relatively low cost. This will enable the systematic investigation of lower frequency variants which may have higher odds ratios for disease than common alleles, and thus be of greater importance in delivering a useful genetic input to personalized assessments of CHD risk.

The challenges in this field are rapidly moving from identifying association signals to elucidating the mechanisms whereby the genes identified affect the risk of CHD. This will be a time-consuming endeavor, but a necessary prerequisite for the design of new therapeutic agents based on these genetic insights.

Glossary of genetic terms used

Alleles: Alternative variants of genetic sequence that can be found at the same chromosomal locus. Because human cells are diploid (having two copies of each chromosome), individuals have two alleles at each locus (which may be the same or different).

Autosomal: Pertaining to a non-sex chromosome (i.e. chromosomes 1–22 in humans, but not chromosomes X and Y).

Complex trait: Phenotype influenced by multiple genetic and environmental effects.

Dominant condition: Genetic disease where the presence of one abnormal allele is sufficient to cause the condition.

Exon: Part of a gene whose sequence appears in mature RNA and may encode a protein (i.e. the "coding" part of the gene).

Gene: A functional region of DNA, including sequence that is transcribed into RNA, regulatory elements, and also non-coding sequence that is removed during the formation of mature RNA (introns).

Genome: The total genetic information encoded by the DNA in a set of chromosomes.

Genotype: The combination of two alleles that represent an individual's genetic sequence at an individual locus.

Haplotype: The arrangement of alleles at a series of sites where variants exist along a chromosome.

Heterozygote: Individual with different alleles on the maternally and paternally inherited chromosomes at a particular chromosomal locus.

Homozygote: Individual with the same allele on the maternally and paternally inherited chromosomes at a particular chromosomal locus.

Intron: Part of a gene that is removed during the formation of mature RNA and which does not encode a protein (i.e. the "non-coding" part of the gene).

Linkage disequilibrium (LD): The association between alleles at two genetic markers. High LD means that genotype at one marker predicts genotype at the other marker (and therefore, only one may need to be typed in association studies).

Low-frequency intermediate penetrance variant: A genetic variant that is relatively uncommon (somewhat arbitrarily, the less frequent allele present on less than 5% of chromosomes in the population), but which has a moderate to large phenotypic effect.

Meiotic recombination: Exchange of genetic sequence between homologous chromosomes that occurs during gamete formation (meiosis).

Mendelian disease: A disease due to a single gene whose effects are sufficiently large that the disease and the abnormal allele co-segregate within carrier families.

Nucleotides: Purine and pyrimidine bases that make up the DNA sequence. There are four different nucleotides in DNA: adenine (A), cytosine (C), guanine (G), and thymine (T).

Polymorphism: Naturally occurring variation in the genetic sequence. Typically used for variants where the less frequent allele is present on at least 1% of chromosomes in the population.

Recessive condition: Genetic disease where the presence of two abnormal allele is required to cause the condition.

RNA: Ribonucleic acid. The nucleic acid into which DNA is transcribed; messenger RNA is subsequently translated into proteins, while other types of RNA have roles in regulating gene expression.

Single nucleotide polymorphism (SNP): A single base variation at a particular locus in the genetic sequence, where the less frequent allele is present on at least 1% of chromosomes in the population. Mostly biallelic, that is, two alternative nucleotides may be present at any given SNP. There are estimated to be approximately 10 million SNPs in the human genome, and they are the most common form of human genetic variation.

References

1. Marenberg ME, Risch N, Berkman LF, Floderus B, de Faire U. Genetic susceptibility to death from coronary heart disease in a study of twins. *N Engl J Med* 1994;**330**(15):1041–6.
2. Zdravkovic S, Wienke A, Pedersen NL, Marenberg ME, Yashin AI, De Faire U. Heritability of death from coronary heart disease: a 36-year follow-up of 20966 Swedish twins. *J Intern Med* 2002;**252**(3):247–54.
3. Wienke A, Holm NV, Skytthe A, Yashin AI. The heritability of mortality due to heart diseases: a correlated frailty model applied to Danish twins. *Twin Res* 2001;**4**:266–74.
4. Lloyd-Jones DM, Nam B-H, D'Agostino RB Sr *et al.* Parental cardiovascular disease as a risk factor for cardiovascular disease in middle-aged adults: a prospective study of parents and offspring. *JAMA* 2004;**291**(18):2204–11.
5. Murabito JM, Pencina MJ, Nam B-H *et al.* Sibling cardiovascular disease as a risk factor for cardiovascular disease in middle-aged adults. *JAMA* 2005;**294**(24):3117–23.
6. Yusuf S, Hawken S, Ounpuu S *et al.* Effect of potentially modifiable risk factors associated with myocardial infarction in 52 countries (the INTERHEART study): case–control study. *Lancet* 2004;**364**(9438):937–52.
7. Mayosi BM, Avery PJ, Baker M *et al.* Genotype at the -174G/C polymorphism of the interleukin-6 gene is associated with common carotid artery intimal-medial thickness: family study and meta-analysis. *Stroke* 2005;**36**(10):2215–19.
8. Peyser PA, Bielak LF, Chu JS *et al.* Heritability of coronary artery calcium quantity measured by electron beam computed tomography in asymptomatic adults. *Circulation* 2002;**106**(3):304–8.
9. O'Donnell CJ, Chazaro I, Wilson PWF *et al.* Evidence for heritability of abdominal aortic calcific deposits in the Framingham Heart Study. *Circulation* 2002;**106**(3):337–41.
10. Oeppen J, Vaupel JW. Broken limits to life expectancy. *Science* 2002;**296**(5570):1029–31.
11. Dumond DE. The limitation of human population: a natural history. *Science* 1975;**187**:713–21.
12. Brown MS, Goldstein JL. Familial hypercholesterolemia: defective binding of lipoproteins to cultured fibroblasts associated with impaired regulation of 3 hydroxy 3 methylglutaryl coenzyme A reductase activity. *Proc Natl Acad Sci USA* 1974;**71**(3):788–92.
13. Brown MS, Dana SE, Goldstein JL. Receptor dependent hydrolysis of cholesteryl esters contained in plasma low density lipoprotein. *Proc Natl Acad Sci USA* 1975;**72**(8):2925–9.
14. Goldstein JL, Brown MS. Familial hypercholesterolemia: identification of a defect in the regulation of 3 hydroxy 3 methylglutaryl coenzyme A reductase activity associated with overproduction of cholesterol. *Proc Natl Acad Sci USA* 1973;**70**(10):2804–8.
15. Brown MS, Goldstein JL. A receptor-mediated pathway for cholesterol homeostasis. *Science* 1986;**232**(4746):34–47.
16. Varret M, Abifadel M, Rabes JP, Boileau C. Genetic heterogeneity of autosomal dominant hypercholesterolemia. *Clin Genet* 2008;**73**(1):1–13.
17. Tosi I, Toledo-Leiva P, Neuwirth C, Naoumova RP, Soutar AK. Genetic defects causing familial hypercholesterolaemia: identification of deletions and duplications in the LDL-receptor gene and summary of all mutations found in patients attending the Hammersmith Hospital Lipid Clinic. *Atherosclerosis* 2007;**194**(1):102–11.
18. Slack J. Risks of ischaemic heart disease in familial hyperlipoproteinaemic states. *Lancet* 1969;**294**(7635):1380–2.
19. Stone NJ, Levy RI, Fredrickson DS, Verter J. Coronary artery disease in 116 kindred with familial type II hyperlipoproteinemia. *Circulation* 1974;**49**(3):476–88.
20. Marks D, Thorogood M, Neil HAW, Humphries SE. A review on the diagnosis, natural history, and treatment of familial hypercholesterolaemia. *Atherosclerosis* 2003;**168**(1):1–14.
21. von Eckardstein A. Differential diagnosis of familial high density lipoprotein deficiency syndromes. *Atherosclerosis* 2006;**186**(2):231–9.
22. Hovingh GK, Brownlie A, Bisoendial RJ *et al.* A novel apoA-I mutation (L178P) leads to endothelial dysfunction, increased

arterial wall thickness, and premature coronary artery disease. *J Am Coll Cardiol* 2004;**44**(7):1429–35.

23. Miller M, Aiello D, Pritchard H, Friel G, Zeller K. Apolipoprotein A-I(Zavalla) (Leu159-Pro): HDL cholesterol deficiency in a kindred associated with premature coronary artery disease. *Arterioscler Thromb Vasc Biol* 1998;**18**(8):1242–7.

24. Franceschini G, Sirtori CR, Capurso A. A-I(Milano) apoprotein. Decreased high density lipoprotein cholesterol levels with significant lipoprotein modifications and without clinical atherosclerosis in an Italian family. *J Clin Invest* 1980;**66**(5):892–900.

25. Gualandri V, Franceschini G, Sirtori CR. AI(Milano) apoprotein identification of the complete kindred and evidence of a dominant genetic transmission. *Am J Hum Genet* 1985;**37**(6):1083–97.

26. Sirtori CR, Calabresi L, Franceschini G et al. Cardiovascular status of carriers of the apolipoprotein Λ IMilano mutant : the Limone sul Garda Study. *Circulation* 2001;**103**(15):1949–54.

27. Weisgraber KH, Rall SC Jr, Bersot TP, Mahley RW, Franceschini G, Sirtori CR. Apolipoprotein A-IMilano. Detection of normal A-I in affected subjects and evidence for a cysteine for arginine substitution in the variant A- I. *J Biol Chem* 1983;**258**(4):2508–13.

28. Shah PK, Yano J, Reyes O et al. High-dose recombinant apolipoprotein A-IMilano mobilizes tissue cholesterol and rapidly reduces plaque lipid and macrophage content in apolipoprotein E-deficient mice: potential implications for acute plaque stabilization. *Circulation* 2001;**103**(25):3047–50.

29. Ameli S, Hultgardh-Nilsson A, Cercek B et al. Recombinant apolipoprotein A-I Milano reduces intimal thickening after balloon injury in hypercholesterolemic rabbits. *Circulation* 1994;**90**(4 I):1935–41.

30. Shah PK, Nilsson J, Kaul S et al. Effects of recombinant apolipoprotein A-I(Milano) on aortic atherosclerosis in apolipoprotein E-deficient mice. *Circulation* 1998;**97**(8):780–5.

31. Eberini I, Gianazza E, Calabresi L, Sirtori CR. ApoA-IMilano from structure to clinical application. *Ann Med* 2008;**40**(suppl 1):48–56.

32. Nissen SE, Tsunoda T, Tuzcu EM et al. Effect of recombinant ApoA-I Milano on coronary atherosclerosis in patients with acute coronary syndromes: a randomized controlled trial. *JAMA* 2003;**290**(17):2292–300.

33. Risch N, Merikangas K. The future of genetic studies of complex human diseases. *Science* 1996;**273**:1516–17.

34. Broeckel U, Hengstenberg C, Mayer B et al. A comprehensive linkage analysis for myocardial infarction and its related risk factors. *Nat Genet* 2002;**30**(2):210–14.

35. Wang Q, Rao S, Shen G-Q et al. Premature myocardial infarction novel susceptibility locus on chromosome 1P34–36 identified by genomewide linkage analysis. *Am J Hum Genet* 2004;**74**(2):262–71.

36. Hauser ER, Crossman DC, Granger CB et al. A genomewide scan for early-onset coronary artery disease in 438 families: the GENECARD Study. *Am J Hum Genet* 2004;**75**(3):436–47.

37. Harrap SB, Zammit KS, Wong ZYH et al. Genome-wide linkage analysis of the acute coronary syndrome suggests a locus on chromosome 2. *Arterioscler Thromb Vasc Biol* 2002;**22**(5):874–8.

38. Helgadottir A, Manolescu A, Thorleifsson G et al. The gene encoding 5-lipoxygenase activating protein confers risk of myocardial infarction and stroke. *Nat Genet* 2004;**36**(3):233–9.

39. Samani NJ, Burton P, Mangino M et al. A genomewide linkage study of 1,933 families affected by premature coronary artery disease: the British Heart Foundation (BHF) Family Heart Study. *Am J Hum Genet* 2005;**77**(6):1011–20.

40. Farrall M, Green FR, Peden JF et al. Genome-wide mapping of susceptibility to coronary artery disease identifies a novel replicated locus on chromosome 17. *PLoS Genet* 2006;**2**(5):e72.

41. Zee RYL, Cheng S, Hegener HH, Erlich HA, Ridker PM. Genetic variants of arachidonate 5-lipoxygenase-activating protein, and risk of incident myocardial infarction and ischemic stroke: a nested case-control approach. *Stroke* 2006;**37**(8):2007–11.

42. Girelli D, Martinelli N, Trabetti E et al. ALOX5AP gene variants and risk of coronary artery disease: an angiography-based study. *Eur J Hum Genet* 2007;**15**(9):959–66.

43. Morgan TM, Krumholz HM, Lifton RP, Spertus JA. Nonvalidation of reported genetic risk factors for acute coronary syndrome in a large-scale replication study. *JAMA* 2007;**297**(14):1551–61.

44. Koch W, Hoppmann P, Mueller JC, Schomig A, Kastrati A. No association of polymorphisms in the gene encoding 5-lipoxygenase- activating protein and myocardial infarction in a large central European population. *Genet Med* 2007;**9**(2):123–9.

45. Assimes T, Knowles J, Priest J et al. Common polymorphisms of ALOX5 and ALOX5AP and risk of coronary artery disease. *Hum Genet* 2008;**123**(4):399–408.

46. Linsel-Nitschke P, Götz A, Medack A et al. Genetic variation in the arachidonate 5-lipoxygenase-activating protein (ALOX5AP) is associated with myocardial infarction in the German population. *Clin Sci (Lond)* 2008;**115**(10):309–315.

47. Hakonarson H, Thorvaldsson S, Helgadottir A et al. Effects of a 5-lipoxygenase-activating protein inhibitor on biomarkers associated with risk of myocardial infarction: a randomized trial. *JAMA* 2005;**293**(18):2245–56.

48. Keavney B, McKenzie CA, Connell JM et al. Measured haplotype analysis of the angiotensin-I converting enzyme gene. *Hum Mol Genet* 1998;**7**(11):1745–51.

49. Daly MJ, Rioux JD, Schaffner SF, Hudson TJ, Lander ES. High-resolution haplotype structure in the human genome. *Nat Genet* 2001;**29**:229–32.

50. Gabriel SB, Schaffner SF, Nguyen H et al. The structure of haplotype blocks in the human genome. *Science* 2002;**296**(5576):2225–9.

51. International HapMap Consortium. International HapMap Project. *Nature* 2003;**426**(6968):789–96.

52. International HapMap Consortium. A second generation human haplotype map of over 3.1 million SNPs. *Nature* 2007;**449**(7164):851–61.

53. International HapMap Consortium. A haplotype map of the human genome. *Nature* 2005;**437**(7063):1299–320.

54. Manolio TA, Brooks LD, Collins FS. A HapMap harvest of insights into the genetics of common disease. *J Clin Invest* 2008;**118**(5):1590–605.

55. Ozaki K. Functional SNPs in the lymphotoxin-alpha gene that are associated with susceptibility to myocardial infarction. *Nat Genet* 2002;**32**:650–4.

56. Ozaki K, Inoue K, Sato H et al. Functional variation in LGALS2 confers risk of myocardial infarction and regulates lymphotoxin-alpha secretion in vitro. *Nature* 2004;**429**(6987):72–5.

57. Mangino M, Braund P, Singh R et al. LGALS2 functional variant rs7291467 is not associated with susceptibility to myocardial infarction in Caucasians. *Atherosclerosis* 2007;**194**(1):112–15.

58. Sedlacek K, Neureuther K, Mueller J et al. Lymphotoxin-α and galectin-2 SNPs are not associated with myocardial infarction in two different German populations. *J Mol Med* 2007;**85**(9): 997–1004.

59. Panoulas VF, Nikas SN, Smith JP et al. The lymphotoxin 252A>G polymorphism is common and associates with myocardial infarction in patients with rheumatoid arthritis. *Ann Rheum Dis* 2008:**67**(11):1550–6.

60. Asselbergs FW, Pai JK, Rexrode KM, Hunter DJ, Rimm EB. Effects of lymphotoxin-alpha gene and galectin-2 gene polymorphisms on inflammatory biomarkers, cellular adhesion molecules and risk of coronary heart disease. *Clin Sci* 2007;**112**(5):291–8.

61. Kimura A, Takahashi M, Choi BY et al. Lack of association between LTA and LGALS2 polymorphisms and myocardial infarction in Japanese and Korean populations. *Tissue Antigens* 2007;**69**(3):265–9.

62. Yamada A, Ichihara S, Murase Y et al. Lack of association of polymorphisms of the lymphotoxin a gene with myocardial infarction in Japanese. *J Mol Med* 2004;**82**(7):477–83.

63. Clarke R, Xu P, Bennett D et al. Lymphotoxin-alpha gene and risk of myocardial infarction in 6,928 cases and 2,712 controls in the ISIS Case-Control Study. *PLoS Genet* 2006;**2**(7):e107.

64. McPherson R, Pertsemlidis A, Kavaslar N et al. A common allele on chromosome 9 associated with coronary heart disease. *Science* 2007;**316**(5830):1488–91.

65. Helgadottir A, Thorleifsson G, Manolescu A et al. A common variant on chromosome 9p21 affects the risk of myocardial infarction. *Science* 2007;**316**(5830):1491–3.

66. Wellcome Trust Case Control Consortium. Genome-wide association study of 14,000 cases of seven common diseases and 3,000 shared controls. *Nature* 2007;**447**(7145):661–78.

67. Samani NJ, Erdmann J, Hall AS et al. Genomewide association analysis of coronary artery disease. *N Engl J Med* 2007;**357**(5): 443–53.

68. Hinohara K, Nakajima T, Takahashi M et al. Replication of the association between a chromosome 9p21 polymorphism and coronary artery disease in Japanese and Korean populations. *J Hum Genet* 2008;**53**(4):357–9.

69. Broadbent HM, Peden JF, Lorkowski S et al. Susceptibility to coronary artery disease and diabetes is encoded by distinct, tightly linked SNPs in the ANRIL locus on chromosome 9p. *Hum Mol Genet* 2008;**17**(6):806–14.

70. Schunkert H, Gotz A, Braund P et al. Repeated replication and a prospective meta-analysis of the association between chromosome 9p21.3 and coronary artery disease. *Circulation* 2008;**117**(13):1675–84.

71. Talmud PJ, Cooper JA, Palmen J et al. Chromosome 9p21.3 coronary heart disease locus genotype and prospective risk of CHD in healthy middle-aged men. *Clin Chem* 2008;**54**(3): 467–74.

72. Myocardial Infarction Genetics Consortium. Genome-wide association of early-onset myocardial infarction with single nucleotide polymorphisms and copy number variants. *Nat Genet* 2009;**41**(3):334–41.

73. Erdmann J, Groszhennig A, Braund PS, Konig IR, Hengstenberg C, Hall AS et al. New susceptibility locus for coronary artery disease on chromosome 3q22.3. *Nat Genet* 2009;**41**(3):280–2.

74. Tregouet D-A, Konig IR, Erdmann J, Munteanu A, Braund PS, Hall AS et al. Genome-wide haplotype association study identi-

fies the SLC22A3-LPAL2-LPA gene cluster as a risk locus for coronary artery disease. *Nat Genet* 2009;**41**(3):283–5.

75. Gudbjartsson DF. Sequence variants affecting eosinophil numbers associate with asthma and myocardial infarction. *Nat Genet* 2009;**41**:342–7.

76. Cunnington MS, Mayosi BM, Hall DH et al. Novel genetic variants linked to coronary artery disease by genome-wide association are not associated with carotid artery intima-media thickness or intermediate risk phenotypes. *Atherosclerosis* 2009;**203**:41–4.

77. Diabetes Genetics Initiative of Broad Institute of Harvard, Saxena R, Voight BF, Lyssenko V et al. Genome-wide association analysis identifies loci for type 2 diabetes and triglyceride levels. *Science* 2007;**316**(5829):1331–6.

78. Scott LJ, Mohlke KL, Bonnycastle LL et al. A genome-wide association study of type 2 diabetes in Finns detects multiple susceptibility variants. *Science* 2007;**316**(5829):1341–5.

79. Zeggini E, Weedon MN, Lindgren CM et al. Replication of genome-wide association signals in UK samples reveals risk loci for type 2 diabetes. *Science* 2007;**316**(5829):1336–41.

80. Salonen JT, Uimari P, Aalto J-M et al. Type 2 diabetes whole-genome association study in four populations: the DiaGen Consortium. *Am J Hum Genet* 2007;**81**(2):338–45.

81. Sladek R, Rocheleau G, Rung J et al. A genome-wide association study identifies novel risk loci for type 2 diabetes. *Nature* 2007;**445**(7130):881–5.

82. Helgadottir A, Thorleifsson G, Magnusson KP et al. The same sequence variant on 9p21 associates with myocardial infarction, abdominal aortic aneurysm and intracranial aneurysm. *Nat Genet* 2008;**40**(2):217–24.

83. Samani NJ, Raitakari OT, Sipila K et al. Coronary artery disease-associated locus on chromosome 9p21 and early markers of atherosclerosis. *Arterioscler Thromb Vasc Biol* 2008:**28**(9):1679–83.

84. Kim WY, Sharpless NE. The regulation of INK4/ARF in cancer and aging. *Cell* 2006;**127**(2):265–75.

85. Gil J, Peters G. Regulation of the INK4b-ARF-INK4a tumour suppressor locus: all for one or one for all. *Nat Rev Mol Cell Biol* 2006;**7**(9):667–77.

86. Pasmant E, Laurendeau I, Heron D, Vidaud M, Vidaud D, Bieche I. Characterization of a germ-line deletion, including the entire INK4/ARF locus, in a melanoma-neural system tumor family: identification of ANRIL, an ANTISENSE NONCODING RNA whose expression coclusters with ARF. *Cancer Res* 2007;**67**(8):3963–9.

87. Mattick JS, Makunin IV. Non-coding RNA. *Hum Mol Genet* 2006;**15**(suppl 1):R17–29.

88. McCarthy MI, Abecasis GR, Cardon LR et al. Genome-wide association studies for complex traits: consensus, uncertainty and challenges. *Nat Rev Genet* 2008;**9**(5):356–69.

89. Iles MM. What can genome-wide association studies tell us about the genetics of common disease? *PLoS Genet* 2008;**4**(2):e33.

90. Grant SFA, Hakonarson H. Recent development in pharmacogenomics: from candidate genes to genome-wide association studies. *Exp Rev Mol Diagn* 2007;**7**(4):371–93.

91. McCarthy MI. Progress in defining the molecular basis of type 2 diabetes mellitus through susceptibility-gene identification. *Hum Mol Genet* 2004;**13**:33–41.

92. Willer CJ, Sanna S, Jackson AU et al. Newly identified loci that influence lipid concentrations and risk of coronary artery disease. *Nat Genet* 2008;**40**(2):161–9.

93. Kathiresan S, Melander O, Guiducci C et al. Six new loci associated with blood low-density lipoprotein cholesterol, high-density lipoprotein cholesterol or triglycerides in humans. *Nat Genet* 2008;**40**(2):189–97.

94. Kooner JS, Chambers JC, Aguilar-Salinas CA et al. Genomewide scan identifies variation in MLXIPL associated with plasma triglycerides. *Nat Genet* 2008;**40**(2):149–51.

95. Wallace C, Newhouse SJ, Braund P et al. Genome-wide association study identifies genes for biomarkers of cardiovascular disease: serum urate and dyslipidemia. *Am J Hum Genet* 2008;**82**(1):139–49.

96. Saxena R, Voight BF, Lyssenko V et al. Genome-wide association analysis identifies loci for type 2 diabetes and triglyceride levels. *Science* 2007;**316**(5829):1331–6.

97. Sandhu MS, Waterworth DM, Debenham SL et al. LDL-cholesterol concentrations: a genome-wide association study. *Lancet* **371**(9611):483–91.

98. Katan MB. Apolipoprotein E isoforms, serum cholesterol, and cancer. *Lancet* 1986;**1**(8479):507–8.

99. Gray R, Wheatley K. How to avoid bias when comparing bone marrow transplantation with chemotherapy. *Bone Marrow Transplant* 1991;**7**(suppl 3):9–12.

100. Keavney B, Danesh J, Parish S et al. Fibrinogen and coronary heart disease: test of causality by 'Mendelian randomization'. *Int J Epidemiol* 2006;**35**(4):935–43.

101. Youngman LD, Keavney B, Palmer A et al. Plasma fibrinogen and fibrinogen genotypes in 4685 cases of myocardial infarction and in 6002 controls: test of causality by 'Mendelian randomization'. *Circulation* 2000;**102**(suppl II):31–2.

102. Kamstrup PR, Tybjaerg-Hansen A, Steffensen R, Nordestgaard BG. Genetically elevated lipoprotein(a) and increased risk of myocardial infarction. *JAMA* 2009;**301**(22):2331–9.

103. Zacho J, Tybjaerg-Hansen A, Jensen JS, Grande P, Sillesen H, Nordestgaard BG. Genetically elevated C-reactive protein and ischemic vascular disease. *N Engl J Med* 2008;**359**(18):1897–908.

104. Marks D, Thorogood M, Farrer JM, Humphries SE. Census of clinics providing specialist lipid services in the United Kingdom. *J Public Health* 2004;**26**(4):353–4.

105. Hamilton-Craig I. Case-finding for familial hypercholesterolemia in the Asia-Pacific region. *Semin Vasc Med* 2004;**4**(1):87–92.

106. Umans-Eckenhausen MAW, Defesche JC, Sijbrands EJG, Scheerder RLJM, Kastelein JJP. Review of first 5 years of screening for familial hypercholesterolaemia in the Netherlands. *Lancet* 2001;**357**(9251):165–8.

107. Wald DS, Bestwick JP, Wald NJ. Child–parent screening for familial hypercholesterolaemia: screening strategy based on a meta-analysis. *BMJ* 2007;**335**(7620):599.

108. Cameron J, Holla OL, Ranheim T, Kulseth MA, Berge KE, Leren TP. Effect of mutations in the PCSK9 gene on the cell surface LDL receptors. *Hum Mol Genet* 2006;**15**(9):1551–8.

109. Abifadel M, Varret M, Rabes JP et al. Mutations in PCSK9 cause autosomal dominant hypercholesterolemia. *Nat Genet* 2003;**34**(2):154–6.

110. Cohen JC, Boerwinkle E, Mosley TH Jr, Hobbs HH. Sequence variations in PCSK9, low LDL, and protection against coronary heart disease. *N Engl J Med* 2006;**354**(12):1264–72.

111. Wheeler DA, Srinivasan M, Egholm M et al. The complete genome of an individual by massively parallel DNA sequencing. *Nature* 2008;**452**(7189):872–6.

112. Wadelius M, Chen LY, Lindh JD et al. The largest prospective warfarin-treated cohort supports genetic forecasting. *Blood* 2008;[Epub ahead of print].

113. Cooper GM, Johnson JA, Langaee TY et al. A genome-wide scan for common genetic variants with a large influence on warfarin maintenance dose. *Blood* 2008;[Epub ahead of print].

114. Shurin SB, Nabel EG. Pharmacogenomics – ready for prime time? *N Engl J Med* 2008;**358**(10):1061–3.

115. SCG. SLCO1B1 variants and statin-induced myopathy – a genomewide study. *N Engl J Med* 2008;**359**(8):789–99.

116. König J, Seithel A, Gradhand U, Fromm M. Pharmacogenomics of human OATP transporters. *Naunyn-Schmiedeberg Arch Pharmacol* 2006;**372**(6):432–43.

117. Clee SM, Kastelein JJP, Van Dam M et al. Age and residual cholesterol efflux affect HDL cholesterol levels and coronary artery disease in ABCA1 heterozygotes. *J Clin Invest* 2000;**106**(10):1263–70.

118. Yap S. Classical homocystinuria: vascular risk and its prevention. *J Inherit Metab Dis* 2003;**26**:259–65.

119. Mudd SH, Skovby F, Levy HL. The natural history of homocystinura due to cystathionine beta-synthase deficiency. *Am J Hum Genet* 1985;**37**(1):1–31.

120. Mani A, Radhakrishnan J, Wang H et al. LRP6 mutation in a family with early coronary disease and metabolic risk factors. *Science* 2007;**315**(5816):1278–82.

121. Wang L, Fan C, Topol SE, Topol EJ, Wang Q. Mutation of MEF2A in an inherited disorder with features of coronary artery disease. *Science* 2003;**302**:1578–81.

122. Weng L. Lack of MEF2A mutations in coronary artery disease. *J Clin Invest* 2005;**115**:1016–20.

123. Thompson A, Di Angelantonio E, Sarwar N et al. Association of cholesteryl ester transfer protein genotypes with CETP mass and activity, lipid levels, and coronary risk. *JAMA* 2008;**299**(23):2777–88.

124. Bennet AM, Di Angelantonio E, Ye Z et al. Association of apolipoprotein E genotypes with lipid levels and coronary risk. *JAMA* 2007;**298**(11):1300–11.

125. Ntzani EE, Rizos EC, Ioannidis JPA. Genetic effects versus bias for candidate polymorphisms in myocardial infarction: case study and overview of large-scale evidence. *Am J Epidemiol* 2007;**165**(9):973–84.

126. Ye Z, Liu EH, Higgins JP et al. Seven haemostatic gene polymorphisms in coronary disease: meta-analysis of 66,155 cases and 91,307 controls. *Lancet* 2006;**367**(9511):651–8.

127. Wheeler JG, Keavney BD, Watkins H, Collins R, Danesh J. Four paraoxonase gene polymorphisms in 11212 cases of coronary heart disease and 12786 controls: meta-analysis of 43 studies. *Lancet* 2004;**363**(9410):689–95.

128. Casas JP, Bautista LE, Humphries SE, Hingorani AD. Endothelial nitric oxide synthase genotype and ischemic heart disease: meta-analysis of 26 studies involving 23028 subjects. *Circulation* 2004;**109**(11):1359–65.

129. Chiodini BD, Barlera S, Franzosi MG, Beceiro VL, Introna M, Tognoni G. APO B gene polymorphisms and coronary artery disease: a meta-analysis. *Atherosclerosis* 2003;**167**(2):355–66.

130. Klerk M, Verhoef P, Clarke R et al. MTHFR 677C→T polymorphism and risk of coronary heart disease: a meta-analysis. *JAMA* 2002;**288**(16):2023–31.

22 Molecular genetics of cardiovascular disorders

Ali J Marian[1] and Robert Roberts[2]

[1]Center for Cardiovascular Genetics, University of Texas Health Science Center, Houston, TX, USA
[2]University of Ottawa Heart Institute, Ottawa, Ontario, Canada

Introduction

The sequencing of the human genome is likely to be a landmark study of millennium proportions. The implications for cardiology from knowing the sequence of the human genome are many, but probably the most obvious is identifying the genes responsible for familial disorders. Abnormalities of the heart and blood vessels are number one among human birth defects occurring at about 1% of live births.[1,2] Genetic diagnosis and management are expected to be incorporated into the practice of a cardiologist by the end of this decade.[3] Knowing the etiology and understanding the pathogenesis of genetic disorders are most likely to improve the diagnosis, prevention and treatment of those disorders and in addition, provide fundamental insights into acquired disorders that simulate the phenotype. A good example is that of familial hypercholesterolemia in which there is a defective receptor for cell uptake of cholesterol.[4] The findings confirmed that the plasma cholesterol was a major factor in coronary artery disease and subsequently led to unraveling of the synthesis, transport and degradation of cholesterol.

The standard treatment today for coronary artery disease, both familial and acquired, includes the use of statins to lower plasma levels of low-density lipoprotein (LDL) cholesterol. It must be emphasized that practically all genetic disorders have an environmental component and the resulting phenotype is due to an interplay between the gene (genotype) and the environment (phenotype). Furthermore, for single gene disorders it is now recognized that some of the variability in the phenotype is also due to interplay between the causal mutations, environmental factors and the modifier genes.[5] An obvious example of the

importance of environmental factors is that of familial hypertrophic cardiomyopathy (FHCM). FHCM is a single gene disorder that is transmitted in an autosomal dominant pattern, giving rise to a phenotype of left ventricular hypertrophy.[6] The same genetic defect is present in the same abundance in the right and left ventricles yet the disease is seldom manifested in the right ventricle. This would imply that the high pressure of the left ventricle is an important stimulus in the pathogenesis of the phenotype of hypertrophy.

Genetic disorders are considered in three categories: chromosomal abnormalities, single gene disorders, and polygenic disorders. Chromosomal abnormalities are usually detected by the pediatric cardiologist in children while they are still very young. An example of an adult form of chromosomal abnormality would be Turner syndrome. In the last edition, we stated that the multigene disorders (e.g. coronary artery disease) are where the future must be but the technology had not yet arrived. The technology has now arrived and remarkable progress has been made in the past year.[7-9]

Mutations responsible for single gene disorders

Diseases due to an abnormality in a single gene are inherited in a predictable pattern termed Mendelian transmission. In single gene disorders, the responsible gene is both necessary and sufficient to induce the phenotype. Each individual has two copies of the gene, referred to as alleles, one from each parent. The odds of which of the two alleles from each parent is inherited are by chance alone, namely 50%. Genes are units of heredity that are transmitted independently to the next generation. Two genes separated on different chromosomes sort themselves independently through the process of cross-over between the chromosomes. The greater the distance between two loci, the more

Evidence-Based Cardiology, 3rd edition. Edited by S. Yusuf, J.A. Cairns, A.J. Camm, E.L. Fallen, and B.J. Gersh. © 2010 Blackwell Publishing, ISBN: 978-1-4051-5925-8.

likely they are to be separated during genetic transmission. A given disease may be due to multiple mutations in the same gene (allele heterogeneity) or to a single or multiple mutations in two or more genes (locus heterogeneity). It is important to keep in mind, however, that within any one family the gene and the mutation responsible for the disease are the same and only rarely would two genes be transmitted for the same disease. Mutations involving only a single nucleotide are known as point mutations and are responsible for 70% or more of all adult single gene disorders (Table 22.1). A point mutation may be due to substitution of one nucleotide for another (missense mutation) or it may change the amino acid to a stop signal (nonsense), which will truncate the protein (truncated mutant); or it may eliminate a stop signal so the protein is elongated (elongated mutant). Nucleotides may be deleted or added which will result in a different reading from left to right and the gene may be read entirely differently, resulting in a non-functioning product (frameshift).

Table 22.1 Cardiac diseases with an identified genetic locus or gene

Cardiomyopathies	Chromosomal locus
Hypertrophic cardiomyopathy	1q32, 3p21, 11q11, 12q23, 14q12, 15q22, 19p13, 15q11, 14q1, 4q26–27
Dilated cardiomyopathy without conduction defects	1q32, 6q1, 9q12, 10q24, 15q1, 2q31
Dilated cardiomyopathy with conduction defects	1q1, 3p22, 6q23
Arrhythmogenic right ventricular cardiomyopathy	1q12, 2q32, 14q12, 14q23, 3p23, 1q42
Mitochondrial cardiomyopathies	Mitochondrial DNA
Cardiac septal defects	
Holt–Oram syndrome	12q2
Di George syndrome	22q
Noonan syndrome	12q
Aortic diseases	
Aneurysms	11q23–24
Supravalvular aortic disease	9q
Marfan syndrome	15q
Conduction disorder	
Familial heart block	19q13, 1q32
Ventricular arrhythmias	
Long QT syndrome	3p21, 4q25, 7q35, 11p15, 21q22, 17q23
Brugada syndrome	3p21
Idiopathic VT	3p21

Patterns of inheritance of single gene disorders

Autosomal dominant disorders are so named because the disease occurs despite a mutation in only one of the alleles. Males and females are equally affected with about 50% of the offspring expected to have the defective gene (Fig. 22.1). The following features are characteristic of autosomal dominant inheritance:

- each affected individual has at least one affected parent
- 50% of the offspring will have the defective gene
- normal children of an affected individual bear only normal offspring
- males and females are equally affected
- both sexes are equally likely to transmit the abnormal allele to male and female offspring and therefore, male-to-male transmission occurs
- vertical transmission through successive generations occurs
- it is typical for autosomal dominant disorders to have delayed age of onset and variable clinical expression.

Autosomal dominance is the predominant form of inheritance in adult cardiovascular disorders and examples would be FHCM and long QT syndrome.

Autosomal recessive inheritance, in contrast, requires both alleles to be defective and thus both parents must have the defective gene. The following features are characteristic of autosomal recessive inheritance:

- generally the parents are clinically normal heterozygotes
- alternate generations are affected with no vertical transmission
- both sexes are affected with equal frequency
- each offspring of heterozygous carriers has a 25% chance of being affected, a 50% chance of being an unaffected carrier and a 25% chance of inheriting only normal alleles.

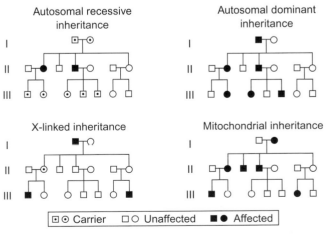

Figure 22.1 Mendellian patterns of inheritance. Indicates carrier, unaffected and affected patterns of inheritance.

If one parent is homozygous and the other is heterozygous, the pattern is changed, with 50% being affected and 50% being carriers.

Examples of autosomal recessive disorders affecting the heart include Jervell and Lang-Nielson long QT syndrome and Pompe's disease.

X-linked inherited disorders are caused by genes located on the X chromosome. Since a female has two X chromosomes, she may carry either one mutant allele or two mutant alleles; the trait may therefore display dominant or recessive expression. Since males have only a single X chromosome, they are likely to display the full syndrome whenever they inherit the abnormal gene from their mother. Hence, the terms *X-linked dominant* and *X-linked recessive* apply only to the expression of the gene in females. Since males must pass on their Y chromosome to all male offspring, they cannot pass on mutant X alleles to their sons; therefore, no male-to-male transmission of X-linked disorders can occur. All females receiving a mutant X chromosome are thus carriers and those who become affected clinically are usually homozygous for the defective gene. The characteristic features of X-linked inheritance are as follows:

• no male-to-male transmission
• all daughters of affected males are carriers
• sons of carrier females have a 50% risk of being affected and daughters have a 50% chance of being carriers
• affected homozygous females occur only when an affected male and a carrier female have children
• the pedigree pattern in X-linked recessive traits tends to be oblique because of the occurrence of the trait in the sons of normal carrier sisters of affected males.

Examples of X-linked disorders of the heart include X-linked cardiomyopathy, Barth's syndrome and muscular dystrophy.

Another uncommon inheritance pattern is that of mitochondrial abnormalities. The mitochondrion has its own genome of about 37 genes contained in 16K of DNA in a single circular chromosome. Most of the disorders involve oxidative phosphorylation and are usually evident very early in life. Phenotypes due to mitochondrial DNA mutations are transmitted by maternal inheritance only since the ovum has mitochondria but the sperm does not. The characteristic features of mitochondrial inheritance of disease include:

• equal frequency and severity of disease for each sex
• transmission through females only, with offspring of affected males being unaffected
• all offspring of affected females may be affected
• extreme variability of expression of disease within a family
• phenotypes may be age dependent
• organ mosaicism is common.

An example of mitochondrial inherited cardiac disease is the cardiomyopathy of Kearns–Sayre syndrome.

Family history and inherited cardiovascular disorders

Identification of a disease segregating in a particular family is determined from the family history. Obtaining a careful family history has not hitherto been an emphasis for the cardiologist. Recognizing the importance of family history in single gene disorders and also in family cluster disorders such as atherosclerosis and hypertension must be a foremost part of the history and physical examination. Certain ethnic groups may direct specific testing such as for hemoglobinopathies in populations from the Mediterranean or sickle cell disease in the African American. The first individual to be recognized to have the disease is usually referred to as the proband. Once a proband is recognized, information should be collected on all first-, second- or third-degree relatives. The information should include medical problems, pregnancies and information on those individuals related to the family who are deceased. Frequently, it is important to pursue miscarriages, birth defects and other factors that may appear to be unrelated. A pedigree should be constructed analogous to those shown in Figure 23.1, to determine the pattern of inheritance.

Genetic counseling

Once it has been established that there is a familial disease, it is important to provide information to the individual or parents appropriate to the education of the individual. Every attempt must be made to explain the disease so that important issues are understood by the individual. An attempt must be made to outline the diagnosis, prognosis if known, and mode of transmission together with a discussion of the psychologic and social issues. It is also important in young couples to emphasize the mode of transmission and their chances of passing on the disease as well as the availability of prenatal diagnosis if appropriate. The information must be provided in a non-judgmental and unbiased manner. The family must be able to make a decision with respect to their religion, social and cultural backgrounds. It is sometimes frustrating for the counselor but personal bias must be avoided. Sometimes the issues are extremely sensitive and the options must be presented with concern and compassion but still remaining non-directional.

Single gene cardiovascular disorders

These diseases cover a wide spectrum from structural defects such as familial atrial septum to functional defects such as long QT syndrome (see Table 22.1). For most of these diseases, the chromosomal location (locus) has been mapped but the gene has not yet been identified. However, diseases such as the cardiomyopathies, particularly FHCM, have undergone major investigations with elucidation of the pathogenesis. Animal models of human FHCM have been developed and therapies have been evaluated. There is considerable progress in the identification of genes responsible for ventricular arrhythmias, particularly the long QT and Brugada syndromes. It is still premature to manage these disorders based on their genetic etiology. This is in part because genetic screening is not available and the populations studied are not yet adequately characterized to provide generalized approaches to treatment. A few of these disorders will be discussed to indicate our progress in improving diagnosis, prevention and treatment. The discussion also indicates the trends for the future when most of these genes will be identified and data become available on the pathogenesis and prognosis as they relate to the specific molecular defects.

Long QT syndrome

Several mutations have been identified in cardiac ion channels (sodium, potassium and calcium channel genes) responsible for long QT syndrome (LQT) which predisposes to ventricular arrhythmias and sudden death. Since the initial locus identified was on chromosome 11, seven loci have been mapped and six genes identified (see Table 22.1). Several mutations have been identified in the sodium channel gene SCN5A.[10–12] The long QT-associated mutations in SCN5A are associated with increased sodium flux and prolonged depolarization. The mechanism for the arrhythmias is believed to be an imbalance between the inward and outward currents during the plateau of the action potential. Most of the mutations in the sodium channel appear to be gain of function. The pattern of inheritance is most frequently autosomal dominant although a rare recessive form has also been identified.

Several mutations have also been noted in potassium channels, which decrease potassium flux through a loss of function.[11,12] These mutations appear to have a dominant negative effect. Rarely, the QT syndrome is inherited in an autosomal recessive manner and may be associated with deafness (e.g. the Jervell and Lang–Nielsen syndromes). This observation led to the recognition that the inward potassium current is necessary for endolymph production in the inner ear.[13] There is extensive phenotypic variability among these various genes and mutations and within the same family there are many modifiers yet to be recognized to properly interpret genotype/phenotype correlations.

Mutations are claimed to have some prognostic significance. In general, patients with LQT1 due to the KVLQT1 gene and LQT2 due to HERG have a higher risk of cardiac events than patients with LQT3 due to SCN5A.[14] The latter,

despite causing fewer events, has a relatively higher mortality, which indicates higher lethality of the events. The first line of therapy in patients with LQT1 is beta-blockers. Preliminary data suggest LQT3 patients might benefit from Na^{+1} channel blockers, such as mexiletine, but long-term data are not available yet (**Class IIb**).

A new syndrome has been described associated with shortening of the QT interval on the ECG and clinically with syncope and sudden death. This syndrome, referred to as the short QT syndrome, is due to mutations in the SCN5A gene.[15]

Another form of cardiac channelopathy is idiopathic ventricular fibrillation. The ECG may be normal although some individuals have an associated electrocardiographic abnormality, including ST segment elevation in V1–3 together with right bundle branch block, referred to as Brugada syndrome.[16–18] Mutations responsible for this disease have been linked to SCN5A with dominant inheritance. There is at present no proven mechanism for the ventricular arrhythmia but it is believed to be due to heterogeneity between the epicardium and endocardium during repolarization which leads to re-entry.

Brugada syndrome

The ECG pattern is characteristic of this syndrome, consisting of right bundle branch block and ST segment elevation in V1–3 and sudden death at a young age.[19]

SCN5A was identified as the first and, thus far, the only causal gene for Brugada syndrome in 1998.[20] Over 60 different mutations in SCN5A have been identified that collectively account for approximately 25% of all cases with Brugada syndrome. As in many other genetic disorders, Brugada syndrome also exhibits locus heterogeneity, and a second locus on chromosome 3 has been mapped.[21] However, the causal gene has not yet been identified. The only treatment is an implantable cardioverter-defibrillator (ICD). Once a case is identified, it is recommended the family be screened for the mutation. SCN5A mutations induce a large spectrum of phenotypes, including Brugada syndrome, long QT syndrome (LQT3), isolated progressive cardiac conduction defect, idiopathic ventricular fibrillation, and sudden unexpected death syndrome (SUDS).[22]

Familial atrial fibrillation

Atrial fibrillation is the most common cardiac arrhythmia with a prevalence of 6% over the age of 65 years.[23] The chance of developing atrial fibrillation over age 40 years is about 25% in men and women.[24] Atrial fibrillation accounts for about one-third of all strokes and 30% of all patients with atrial fibrillation have a family history of the disease.[25] In 1997, Brugada et al identified the first locus on chromosome 10q22–24 in a Spanish family.[26] Since that time, seven

Table 22.2 Genetic loci responsible for atrial fibrillation

Locus	Gene	Mode of inheritance	Effect on function
10q22	–	AD	
11p15	KCNQ1	AD	Gain of function
21q22	KCNE2	AD	Gain of function
11q13	KCNE3	AD	
17q23	KCNJ2	AD	Gain of function
12p13	KCNA5	AD	
1q21	GJA5	AD	
6q14–16	–	AD	
5p13	–	AR	

loci have been mapped and five genes identified: *KCNQ1, KCNE2, KCNE3, KCNJ2, KCNA5* (Table 22.2). All of the genes identified encode a potassium channel subunit. The mechanism of action by which these genes induce atrial fibrillation is shortening of the action potential duration and shortening of the atrial effective refractory period. The consistency of the mechanism of action suggests the development of therapy specifically targeted to prevent these molecular events.

The most recent finding is that of somatic mutations in the connexin 40 gene.[27] This gene (*CJA5*) encodes for the gap junction protein connexin 40, which is involved in electrical conduction in the myocardium. The mutation was identified through genetic screening of human atrial samples obtained from patients with atrial fibrillation undergoing cardiac surgery for valvular or other diseases. In addition to monogenic diseases, there is the observation that patients with structural heart disease are predisposed to atrial fibrillation by inherited DNA polymorphisms.[28] The recent development of chips with hundreds of thousands of SNPs, enabling genome-wide scans will, over the next few years, elucidate those SNPs that predispose to atrial fibrillation. Within the next decade, one can expect most of the genes responsible for atrial fibrillation and those SNPs that confer predisposition to be identified and therapies will be developed based on an individual's genomic profile.

Wolf–Parkinson-White syndrome

A gene responsible for an uncommon form of Wolff–Parkinson-White syndrome (WPW) was shown to be *AMPK*.[29,30] Several mutations in *AMPK* have since been identified[31–33] as inducing WPW which is associated with hypertrophic cardiomyopathy and conduction disorders along with a high incidence of atrial fibrillation. It appears that *AMPK* induces abnormalities in glycogen which leads to all three phenotypes: WPW, conduction disturbance and hypertrophic cardiomyopathy. A genetic animal model of

WPW expressing the *AMPK* gene has been developed which should elucidate pathogenesis and suggest potential therapies.[34]

Familial hypertrophic cardiomyopathy (HCM)

Clinical and pathologic features of HCM

HCM is an autosomal dominant disease defined by cardiac hypertrophy in the absence of an increased external load (primary hypertrophy). Patients with HCM exhibit protean clinical manifestations ranging from minimal or no symptoms to severe heart failure and sudden cardiac death (SCD). The majority of patients with HCM are asymptomatic or mildly symptomatic. The clinical manifestations often do not develop until the third or fourth decades of life. HCM is a relatively benign disease with an estimated annual mortality rate of <0.7% in the adult population.[35] However, SCD is often the first and tragic manifestation of HCM in the young.[36] HCM is the most common cause of SCD in young competitive athletes, accounting for approximately one-third of all SCD.[36]

The main pathologic features of HCM include myocyte hypertrophy and disarray, interstitial fibrosis and, to a lesser extent, thickening of the media of intramural coronary arteries. While hypertrophy and fibrosis are the common responses of the heart to all forms of injury, myocyte disarray is considered the pathologic hallmark of HCM.[37] Cardiac hypertrophy and interstitial fibrosis are the major determinants of mortality and morbidity in HCM.[38–40] In those with mild or no cardiac hypertrophy, myocyte disarray is associated with the risk of SCD.[41]

Molecular genetics

HCM is a genetic disease with an autosomal dominant mode of inheritance. Family history of HCM is present in approximately half of all index cases (familial HCM) and the remainder are sporadic. *Sporadic* means offspring of parents of whom neither has the mutant gene or the disease. Presumably, the mother was exposed shortly after conception (12–24 hours) to a mutagen (EG radiation) that induced in the embryo a mutation that causes HCM. The mutation, albeit *de novo*, in the affected offspring will transmit the mutation and disease to their offspring in the same pattern as familial. HCM usually is due to mutations in any of at least 12 contractile sarcomeric proteins (Table 22.3). Recently, a new gene (*MY0Z2* or myozenin 2) was identified as being responsible for HCM.[42] The gene encodes a Z disk protein and thus expands the spectrum of the causal genes to include those encoding the Z disk proteins. Over 500 mutations in 12 genes have been identified.[9]

Genotype/phenotype correlations

Genotype/phenotype correlation studies suggest that causal mutations affect the magnitude of cardiac hypertrophy and

Table 22.3 Causal genes for HCM: genes coding for sarcomeric proteins

Gene	Symbol	Locus	Frequency	Predominant mutations
β-Myosin heavy chain	MYH7	14q12	~30%	Missenses
Myosin binding protein-C	MYBPC3	11p11.2	~30%	Splice junction and insertion/deletion
Cardiac troponin T	TNNT2	1q32	~5%	Missenses
Cardiac troponin I	TNNI3	19p13.2	~5%	Missense and deletion
α-Tropomyosin	TPM1	15q22.1	<5%	Missenses
Essential myosin light chain	MYL3	3p21.3	<5%	Missenses
Regulatory myosin light chain	MYL2	12q23–24.3	<5%	Missense and 1 truncation
Cardiac α-actin	ACTC	15q11	<5%	Missense mutations
Titin	TTN	2q24.1	<5%	Missense mutations
Telethonin (Tcap)	TCAP	17q2	Rare	Missense mutations
Myozenin 2	MYOZ2	4q26	1:250	Missense mutations
α-Myosin heavy chain	MYH6	14q1	Rare	Missense and rearrangement mutations, (association)
Cardiac troponin C	TNNC1	3p21.3–3p14.3	Rare	Missense mutations (association)
Cardiac myosin light peptide kinase	MYLK2	20q13.3	Rare	Point mutations (association)
Caveolin 3	CAV3	3p25	Rare	Point mutations (association)
Phospholamban	PLN	6p22.1	Rare	Point mutations (association)

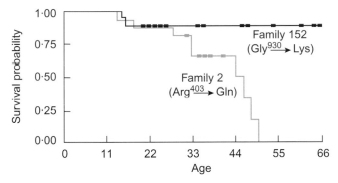

Figure 22.2 Stratification of risk according to mutation. Shown here are two different mutations in the βMHC gene. The mutation in Family 152 is associated with essentially normal lifespan while Family 2 has a mean lifespan of about 28 years. This emphasizes the potential prognostic significance of individual mutations.

the risk of SCD (Fig. 22.2). Mutations in the beta-myosin heavy chain (MyHC) are generally associated with an early onset and more extensive hypertrophy and a higher incidence of SCD.[43,44] In contrast, mutations in the myosin-binding protein C (MyBP-C) are associated with a low penetrance, relatively mild hypertrophy, late onset of clinical manifestations and a low incidence of SCD.[44-46] Mutations in cTnT are usually associated with a mild degree of hypertrophy but more extensive disarray and a high incidence of SCD.[41,47,48] Mutations in alpha-tropomyosin are generally associated with a benign phenotype and mild left ventricular hypertrophy. However, a phenotype of mild hypertrophy and high incidence of SCD also has been described.[49] Mutations

in essential and regulatory myosin light chains have been associated with mid-cavity obstruction in HCM and skeletal myopathy in some[50] but not in others.[51] Mutations in titin[52] and alpha actin[53-55] have been observed in a small number of families.

Despite the observed associations between severity of the phenotype and the causal mutations, there is considerable variability in phenotypic expression of HCM among affected members, even among those who have identical causal mutations. Overall, the results of genotype/phenotype correlation studies have been subject to a large number of confounding factors, such as the small size of the families, small number of families with identical mutations due to low frequency of each mutation, influence of modifier genes,[56] influence of non-genetic factors and rarely homozygosity for causal mutations and compound mutations.[20,57,58] Correlations in the small number of patients studied suggest prognostic stratification by the mutations but caution must be exercised until larger studies are performed (see Fig. 22.2).

Pathogenesis of HCM

The initial defects induced by the mutant sarcomeric proteins are diverse. They comprise impaired acto-myosin interaction and cardiac myocyte contractile performance, altered Ca^{+2} sensitivity, reduced ATPase activity, sarcomere dysgenesis, altered subcellular localization and altered stoichiometry of the sarcomeric protein.[59] However, despite the diversity of the initial defects, the final phenotype is hypertrophy, fibrosis, and disarray. We have proposed that a common link between the initial defect and the final phenotype is impaired cardiac myocyte contractile function,[60] which increases myocyte stress and leads to activation of stress-responsive intracellular signaling kinases and trophic factors. Release of trophic factors activates the transcription machinery, leading to cardiac hypertrophy, interstitial fibrosis and other histologic and clinical phenotypes of HCM.[60] Accordingly, myocyte hypertrophy and disarray, interstitial fibrosis and thickening of the media of intramural coronary arteries are considered "secondary" phenotypes and thus, potentially reversible. In addition, the severity of the phenotype is affected by factors other than the causal genes, i.e. the environmental factors and the modifier genes. In support of this hypothesis, we have shown that stress-responsive signaling kinases ERK1/2 are activated in the heart of transgenic animal models of HCM and that cardiac hypertrophy and interstitial fibrosis could be reversed or attenuated by pharmacologic interventions, discussed later.

Dilated cardiomyopathy (DCM)

Genetics of DCM

Dilated cardiomyopathy (DCM) is a primary disease of the myocardium diagnosed by a decreased left ventricular ejection fraction (<0.45) and an increased left ventricular cavity size (end-diastolic diameter >$2.7 cm/m^2$). Clinical features of DCM are those of heart failure, including syncope, cardiac arrhythmias and SCD. The etiology of DCM is diverse and a family history of DCM is present in approximately half of all index cases.[61–63] Thus, in such cases DCM is considered a familial disease. The remainder have no family history of DCM and thus DCM is considered sporadic. A significant number of patients with DCM and their affected relatives are asymptomatic and are mistakenly considered as normal unless subjected to clinical and genetic investigation.[60] Familial DCM is commonly inherited as an autosomal dominant disease,[61] which clinically manifests during the third and fourth decades of life. X-linked and autosomal recessive patterns of inheritance also occur, which may manifest early, often during the second decade of life. The mode of transmission is matrilineal when DCM occurs because of mutations in the mitochondrial DNA. DCM also occurs in conjunction with the triplet repeat syndromes and follows their pattern of inheritance.

DCM is an extremely heterogeneous disease (Table 22.4). Despite the diversity of the causal genes and mutations, the vast majority of them encode for proteins that are either components of the myocardial cytoskeleton or support it. Therefore, DCM is considered a disease of cytoskeletal proteins. Given the diversity of causal genes and mutations, it is not surprising that each causal gene accounts for a very small fraction of familial DCM and none predominates.

Collectively, the mapped genes account for approximately half of all familial DCM cases and in a significant number of families, while the chromosomal loci have been mapped, the causal genes remain unidentified. The gene encoding cardiac alpha-actin (*ACTC1*) was the first causal gene identified for familial DCM with an autosomal dominant mode of inheritance.[64] The authors proposed that defects in the cytoskeletal proteins could cause DCM by impairing the transmission of contractile force.[64] Mutations in two additional components of the sarcomere, namely the beta-myosin heavy chain and cardiac troponin T, were found in patients with DCM.[65] As discussed earlier, mutations in *ACTC1*, *MYH7* and *TNNT2* are also known to cause HCM. These findings suggest that the topography of the mutations within the sarcomeric proteins and the modifier genes plays a significant role in determining the ensuing clinical phenotype. Mutations in the cytoskeletal proteins delta sarcoglycan,[66] metavinculin and dystrophin[45] are also known to cause DCM. Mutations in alpha-sarcoglycan (adhalin) cause an autosomal recessive form of DCM that occurs in conjunction with limb-girdle muscular dystrophy. An intriguing causal gene for familial DCM is the lamin A/C gene,[67–69] which encodes a nuclear envelope protein. The observed phenotype resulting from mutations in the rod domain of lamin A/C is progressive conduction disease, atrial arrhythmias, heart failure and SCD. Finally, mutations in the intermediary filament desmin and its associated protein alpha/B-crystallin have been identified in patients with DCM.[70–72] Often such mutations lead to a phenotype of cardiac and skeletal myopathy, referred to as desmin-related myopathy.[71] Collectively, these findings suggest that mutations affecting the integrity of the cytoskeleton can cause DCM. Genotype/phenotype correlations are not yet available in a systematic study.

Pathogenesis of DCM

Mutations in cardiac alpha-actin, beta-myosin heavy chain, cardiac troponin T and other cytoskeletal proteins impart a dominant-negative effect on transmission of the contractile force to the extracellular matrix proteins.[64] Mutations in the dystrophin gene lead to decreased expression level of dystrophin, a major cytoskeletal protein in skeletal and cardiac muscles. Decreased expression of dystrophin impairs efficient mechanical coupling and myocyte shortening. In X-linked DCM, the severity of the clinical phenotype correlates inversely with the expression level of dystrophin. The pathogenesis of DCM resulting from mutations in desmin and alpha/B-crystallin involves deposition of desmin and alpha/B-crystallin aggregates in the myocardium. The molecular pathogenesis of DCM caused by mutations in lamin A/C or emerin remains largely unknown. It is likely that lamin A/C is also involved in maintaining the integrity of the cytoskeleton. The pathogenesis of cardiomyopathies in patients with the triplet

Table 22.4 Genetic causes of dilated cardiomyopathy

Gene	Symbol	Locus	Frequency	Phenotypes
Cardiac α actin	ACTC	15q11–14	Low	DCM or HCM based on topography of the mutation and probably genetic background
β-myosin heavy chain	MYH7	14q11–13	Low	DCM or HCM based on topography of the mutation and probably genetic background
Cardiac troponin T	TNNT2	1q32	Low	DCM or HCM based on topography of the mutation and probably genetic background
δ Sarcoglycan	SGCD	5q33–34	Low	DCM
β-Sarcoglycan	SGCB	4q12	Autosomal dominant	
Dystrophin	DMD	Xp21	Low	X-linked DCM
Lamin A/C	LMNA	1p21.2	Low	DCM and conduction defect
				Emery Driefus muscular dystrophy, Lipodystrophy (Dunnigan variety)
Taffazin (G4.5)	TAZ	Xq28	Low	DCM, ventricular non-compaction, skeletal myopthay, mitochondrial abnormalities
Desmin	DES	2q35	Low	Desmin-related myopathies
αB-crystallin	CRYAB	11q35	Low	Desmin-related myopathy
Desmoplakin	DSP	6p23–25	Low	Recessive DCM
Muscle LIM protein	MLP (CSPR3)	11q15.1	Low	Autosomal dominant
Cypher/ZASP (LIM domain binding 3)	LDB3	10q22.3–q23.2	Low	Familial and sporadic
Telethonin (T-cap)	TCAP	17q12	Low	
?	?	1q32	?	
?	?	2q14–22	?	DCM + Conduction defect
?	?	2q31	?	
?	?	3p22–25	?	DCM + Conduction defect
?	?	6q23–24	?	DCM + Hearing loss
?	?	9q13–22	?	DCM + Conduction defect + Adult onset limb girdle dystrophy
?	?	10q21–23	?	DCM + MVP

repeats syndrome is also unclear. Expansion of the CTG (CUG in mRNA) repeats in the 3′ untranslated region of the myotonin protein kinase gene could lead to unstable mRNA and decreased expression of the protein. It is also possible that proteins that bind to CUG repeats may be necessary for proper transcription, splicing, translation, and nuclear transport of mRNAs of cardiac genes.

Arrhythmogenic right ventricular cardiomyopathy (ARVC)

ARVC is the primary abnormality of the myocardium characterized by a progressive loss of myocytes, fatty infiltration and replacement fibrosis, which occur predominantly in the right ventricle.[73] ARVC, also referred to as arrhythmogenic right ventricular dysplasia, often manifests as ventricular arrhythmias originating from the right ventricle. A characteristic electrocardiographic pattern is the presence of an epsilon wave and less characteristic findings are depolarization/repolarization abnormalities in the right precordial leads. The age of onset of the disease is variable but commonly ARVC manifests with minor arrhythmias during adolescence, which progress to serious ventricular arrhythmias during the third and fourth decades of life, leading to SCD. In Italy, ARVC is a relatively common cause of SCD in the young.[74] Gradual fibro-fatty infiltration of the myocardium leads to regional and global right ventricular dysfunction and, less frequently, left ventricle failure. In advanced stages, both ventricles are involved and heart failure is the predominant manifestation.

Several loci for ARVC have been mapped, including loci on 14q23-q24 (ARVD1),[75] 1q42-q43 (ARVD2),[76] 14q12-q22 (ARVD3),[77] 2q32-q32.3 (ARVD4),[78] 3p23 (ARVD5),[79] and 10p14-p12 (ARVD6).[80] The causal gene for ARVC2 with its locus on chromosome 1q42-q43 has been identified as the cardiac ryanodine receptor gene (RYR2).[81] Mutations in the RYR2 gene in four independent families with ARVC have been identified.[81] However, the phenotype may be a phenocopy of catecholaminergic polymorphic ventricular tachycardia and not true ARVC. Mutations in DSP, JUP, PKP2 and DSG2, encoding the desmosomal proteins desmoplakin (DP), plakoglobin (PG), plakophilin 2 (PKP2) and desmoglein 2 (DSG2), have been identified.[82–86] Mutations in *PKP2* appear to be the most common, accounting for approximately 20% of the cases.[83,86] Mutations in *DSG2* and *DSP* each account for approximately 10–15% of the cases of ARVC.[86] Most mutations cause a frameshift and hence are expected to lead to premature termination of the proteins. The only treatment is an ICD to prevent sudden cardiac death. Mechanistic studies suggest suppression of the canonical Wnt signaling through beta-catenin by nuclear plakoglobin or plakophilin 2 as the mechanism responsible for myocyte apoptosis and fibro-fatty replacement of the myocardium.[87]

The causal gene for an autosomal recessive form of ARVC, palmoplantar keratoderma, and peculiar woolly hairs (Naxos syndrome), is *JUP*, which encodes plakoglobin.[88] Plakoglobin is also a desmosome protein and, along with desmoplakin, anchors intermediate filaments to desmosomes. The phenotype was described first in a family from the island Naxos in Greece and was mapped to 17q21.

Integration of genetics into routine clinical management

Single gene disorders, many of which are already known, could theoretically be tested for multiple mutations. However, such testing has not yet been incorporated into clinical management. This is due to many reasons: medical insurance is not available to offset the cost; certain ethical, social and legal issues await federal policies; and for many disorders, the screening technology is not yet available. There are also other issues (e.g. penetrance and expressivity) that confound the interpretation of genetic data even when a mutation is known. Penetrance refers to the percentage of individuals with the mutant gene who will develop the disease. Most genes are not 100% penetrant and the onset of the disease further confounds the diagnosis since it is often age dependent. These problems are of greater concern when the pattern of inheritance is dominant. Expressivity refers to the variability of clinical manifestations. In some individuals with the mutant gene, the phenotype is only partially represented which poses the problem of a causal relationship.

Despite the lack of availability of clinical genetic testing, screening of first-degree relatives and other family members should be encouraged.[89] Once a DNA-based diagnosis of HCM is known within a family, clinical screening including history, physical examination, 12-lead ECG and two-dimensional echocardiography should be performed on individuals who are 12 years of age or older. In general, individuals do not develop hypertrophy until puberty when there is a significant growth spurt. Individuals affected should be re-evaluated every 12–18 months. Individuals within the family who do not have evidence of

HCM should be screened every five years. There is some debate as to whether at age 25 or 30, if there is no evidence of the disease, screening should be discontinued; however, since certain genes do not have onset until middle age or later, until genetic testing has been performed, clinical assessment should continue. In the meantime, it is suggested that individuals of suspected HCM families undergo genetic testing through either a research laboratory or one of the independent private laboratories. In addition, genetic testing is sometimes necessary to exclude other causes of hypertrophy such as lysosomal enzyme abnormalities.

Polygenic or complex disorders

There is ample evidence from dizygotic and monozygotic twins as well as endemic populations to indicate that diseases such as coronary artery disease (CAD) and hypertension have a significant genetic predisposition.[90] It is estimated that genetic predisposition accounts for over 50% of risk in patients with coronary artery disease and an even greater component in those with premature heart disease.[91] Despite the success with single gene disorders, there has been very little progress with the common chronic diseases such as coronary artery disease and hypertension. In single gene disorders, a single gene responsible for the disease is inherited in a Mendelian pattern (i.e. passed from parents to their children). Families with these diseases can be analyzed for the genetic anomaly using a few hundred DNA markers (spanning the genome at 10 million base pair intervals). Using a process referred to as genetic linkage analysis, researchers can determine which markers are present in affected individuals versus normals and map the location of the gene. While genetic linkage analysis is useful for single gene disorders within an affected family, this approach cannot be used for complex common diseases such as CAD and hypertension.

Twenty diseases account for about 89% of all deaths in the world, with cardiovascular disease accounting for over 40%.[92] In contrast to single gene disorders, genetic predisposition contributing to these diseases is due to multiple genes, with some contributing as little as 5% risk. The more appropriate and sensitive method to detect genes and other genomic alterations responsible for multigene disorders is referred to as a case–control association study.[93] In this type of study, the genomes of large populations of unrelated individuals with a chronic disease are compared to another large population without the disease, and the pool of genetic differences between the two is identified. These genetic differences are then assessed in independent populations to determine whether the association remains significant (referred to as replication). This method is best performed with a genome-wide scan that uses hundreds of thousands of DNA markers that span the entire human genome. While the need for these genome-wide scans has been recognized for some time, they have not been feasible because of the availability of too few DNA markers and the prohibitive cost of genotyping large populations.[93] In the meantime researchers pursued a less expensive and less time-consuming method referred to as the candidate gene approach. This consisted of selecting one gene at a time and determining whether one or more forms of that gene are more common in diseased versus normal individuals. Several genes were claimed to be associated with disease, but recent studies[94] indicate that essentially none have been confirmed in independent populations.

New technology

The DNA of the human genome consists of 3.3 billion bases, the sequence of which was determined in 2003 by the Human Genome Project. This sequence is 99.9% identical in all humans, meaning the DNA sequence which carries the genetic differences varies by only one-tenth of 1% or about 3 million bases. Most of these variations are referred to as single nucleotide polymorphisms (SNPs) since ≥80% are due to substitutions of single bases (nucleotides) scattered throughout the genome. On average, each genome has one SNP per 1000 base pairs. The remaining 15–20% of variation is due to differing patterns of repetitive sequences, and deletion or addition of nucleotides, referred to as copy number variation (CNV). These SNPs and CNVs account for all human variation such as height, weight and susceptibility for, or protection against, disease.[95] Utilizing the SNPs as DNA markers, it was possible to generate platform arrays of millions of markers that could be used to search the entire genome for genes that predispose to chronic disease. This makes it possible to perform what are now referred to as genome-wide association (GWA) studies. Commercial platforms utilizing millions of DNA markers are currently available. With markers spaced across the genome at intervals averaging 1000 to 6000 base pairs, it is possible to detect genes that contribute even modestly to the disease. This is the newest technology evolving to map the location of the genes predisposing to chronic disease.[96]

Success is already evident from genome-wide case–control association studies. Results from these studies are beginning to appear, with promising implications. Recently, three independent groups using the GWA approach discovered the same genetic variation at chromosome 9p21 that results in a significantly increased risk of heart disease in Caucasians.[96] The risk of this genetic variation is independent of all known risk factors such as cholesterol, high blood pressure and diabetes. Several genes have also been identified in other chronic diseases including diabetes, Crohn's disease and prostate cancer.[97]

Coronary artery disease

Identifying the genes responsible for several single gene disorders affecting cholesterol metabolism has contributed significantly to our understanding of the pathogenesis and treatment of CAD (e.g familial hypercholesterolemia). However, as indicated previously, progress until recently has been minimal. Most of the research utilized the candidate gene approach and none of these genes have been replicated in independent populations and so remain suspect.[94] The list of candidate genes in Table 22.5 may be discarded as the results of the GWA studies become available. Two examples, namely *ABCA1* and *CYBA*, are discussed briefly. Plasma levels of high-density lipoprotein (HDL) cholesterol and its apolipoprotein A1 (apo-A1) are under tight control of genetic factors, which are largely unknown. Mutations in the ATP binding cassette transporter (*ABCA1*) gene in patients with Tangier disease[98] have very low plasma levels of HDL-C and apo-A1 and an increased risk of coronary atherosclerosis. This suggests a major role for the ABCA1 protein in regulating plasma HDL-C and apo-A1 levels and thus the risk of atherosclerosis.[99] Several studies have reported an association between plasma HDL-C levels and SNPs in *ABCA1*.[100–102]

A second example is the *CYBA* gene located on 16q24, which is involved in maintaining the delicate balance between oxidation and reduction (redox) in the vessel wall. *CYBA* codes for p22^{phox} protein, which is a component of the plasma membrane-associated enzyme NADPH oxidase. NADPH oxidase is the most important source of superoxide anion, the precursor to a variety of potent oxidants, in intact vessel walls. p22^{phox} in conjunction with gp91 forms a membrane-bound heterodimeric protein referred to as flavocytochrome b$_{558}$. The latter is considered the redox center of the NADPH oxidase. The p22^{phox} protein is essential for the assembly and activation of the NADPH oxidase and plays a major role in NADPH-dependent O_2^- production in the vessel wall. There are several genetic variants of p22^{phox} including a 242C/T transition that results in replacement of histidine by tyrosine at amino acid position 72 (H72Y), a potential heme-binding site. We determined the association of the 242C/T variants with severity and progression of coronary atherosclerosis and response to treatment with a statin in a well-characterized cohort of Lipoprotein Coronary Atherosclerosis Study population.[103] In the placebo group, subjects with the mutation had 3–5-fold greater loss in mean minimum lumen diameter (MLD) and lesion-specific MLD than those without. Progression was also more and regression less common in those with the mutation.

As indicated previously, GWA studies are likely to identify many genes predisposing to CAD in the very near future. The first major locus has been identified on chromosome 9p21.[96] The mechanism whereby this DNA region of 58 K base pairs predisposes to CAD remains to be

Table 22.5 Selected candidate genes for coronary atherosclerosis and myocardial infarction

Gene	Locus	Polymorphism	Allele	Function
Vascular homeostasis				
ACE	17q23	I/D	D	↑ACE
AGT	1q42	M235T	T	↑AGT
AT1	3q22	C1166A	AA	Unknown
ENOS	7q35–36	A/b	a	Unknown
		Gln298Asp	Asp	?
Hemostatic factors				
β-Fibrinogen	4q2	G-453A	A	↑Fibrinogen
PAI-1	7q21.3–22	4G/5G	4G	↑PAI-1
GpIIb/IIIa	17q21.32	PI A1/A2 (T/C)PIA2	?	
Factor V	1q25–25	Arg506Gln	Gln	Resistance to APC
Factor VII	13q34	Arg353Gln	Arg	↓VII
Thrombomodulin	20p1	GG-9/-10AT	AT	?
Lipids and associated factors				
Paraxoxonase	7q21–22	A/B (Gln92Arg)	B (Arg)	↑activity
LPL	8p22	Asn291Ser	Ser	↓HDL, ↑TG
		Asp9Asn	Asn	↓HDL, ↑TG
		Gly188Glu	Glu	↓HDL, ↑TG
Hepatic lipase	15	Various mutations		↓HDL
LDLr	19p13.3	Various mutations		↑LDL
ApoE, (& C1, CII)	19q13.2	E2/E3/E4	E4	↑LDL, ↑VLDL
ApoAI-CIII-AIV	11q23	Various mutations	–	↓HDL, ↑TG
ApoB100	2p24	Various mutations		↑LDL, ↑VLDL
Apo(a)	6q26	KIV repeats		↑Lp(a)
CETP	16q22	Few mutations		↓HDL
LCAT	16q22	Few mutations		↓HDL
Metabolic factors				
MTHFR	1p36.3	C677T	T	↑Homocysteine
CBS	21q22.3	Various mutations	–	↑Homocysteine

ACE, angiotensin-converting enzyme; AGT, angiotensinogen; AT1, angiotensin II receptor 1; PAI-1, plasminogen activator inhibitor-1; GpIIb-IIIa, glycoprotein IIb-IIIa; eNOS, endothelial nitric oxide synthase; LPL, lipoprotein lipase; MTHFR, methylenetetrahydrofolate reductase; LCAT, lecithin cholesteryl acyltransferase; CETP, cholesteryl ester transfer protein; LDLr, low-density lipoprotein receptor; CBS, cysthathionine β synthase; HDL, high-density cholesterol; VLDL, very low-density cholesterol.

determined. Nevertheless, in the Ottawa Heart Genome Study, 23 000 Caucasians were genotyped and the heterozygous form was present in 50% and the homozygous form in about 25%. The relative risk for CAD is increased 40% by the homozygous form and 15–20% by the heterozygous form. The overall population risk is estimated to be about 10%. The 9p21 region was independently confirmed for increased risk of myocardial infarction by the Icelandic group in over 17 000 Caucasians with a similar gene frequency.[104] This was followed by further confirmation in a population of 5000 by the Wellcome Trust Case Control Consortium.[105] Thus, the 9p21 region has been confirmed as a significant risk factor for CAD, in over 45 000

Caucasians, and appears to be statistically independent of known risk factors. It does not appear to be a risk factor in African Americans and remains to be determined in other ethnic groups such as the Indian and Chinese populations.

Hypertension

Hypertension is among the top three or four most common diseases throughout the world. It is an independent risk factor for cardiac morbidity and mortality. It is a major stimulus for cardiac hypertrophy, which in itself significantly increases susceptibility for SCD. Hypertension, as indicated previously, is primarily a polygenic disease. There are likely to be multiple genes that increase susceptibility for developing hypertension. These genes interact with the environment and the onset of hypertension is usually age dependent with 20–30% of the population being hypertensive in their elderly years. The susceptibility genes remain elusive but with the new ability to perform GWA studies, it is expected that many of these genes predisposing to hypertension will be identified in the next 5–10 years.

Geller and his associates recently identified a family with early onset of hypertension.[106] The disease segregates as a dominant Mendelian disorder. A mutation was identified in the mineralocorticoid receptor. The patient had severe hypertension, decreased plasma renin activity, serum aldosterone and no other underlying cause for hypertension. The mutation was a missense mutation in which leucine was substituted for serine at codon 810. The mutation is in the domain of the receptor that binds to the hormone. Normally, 21-hydroxyl group steroids are necessary to activate this receptor. In contrast, the receptor with the mutation seems to activate itself and does not require 21-hydroxyl stimulation. The potent antagonist spironolactone, which would block mineralocorticoid activity in normal individuals, acts as an agonist in individuals with this mutation, causing hypertension and further activating mineralcorticoid activity. This is quite a drastic and unexpected change for the mutation to not only have a positive effect but change the receptor to respond to hormones and drugs opposite to its normal response. Another important observation occurred in pregnancy, in which about 6% of individuals develop hypertension and may proceed to preeclampsia. It was noted that progesterone, which normally does not activate the mineralcorticoid receptor, does so in individuals with the mutation. This has significant implications in pregnancy since progesterone levels are normally increased 100-fold and thus, women with this mutation would be expected to develop hypertension. Furthermore, treatment with spironolactone would increase the hypertension and may precipitate pre-eclampsia. Two of the carriers in this family had undergone pregnancies all complicated by hypertension. It is also of note that while pregnant, these women had decreased serum potassium and aldosterone levels in keeping with the expected abnormal response induced by the mutation. While this is not part of the polygenic causes for hypertension, it emphasizes the pathogenetic mechanism involved with hypertension and clearly has improved the treatment of this condition which is particularly important in pregnancy. It is hoped that other Mendelian disorders causing hypertension will be identified since although they form a very small percentage of the etiology of hypertension, compared to polygenic forms, they could have significant implications for prevention and treatment.[106]

Genetics and future therapy

Once the gene responsible for a disease is identified, it is usually possible through genetic animal models to determine the function as well as the pathogenesis of the disease. Genetic animal models of human FHCM have been developed both in mice and in the rabbit.[107–109] In the mouse, expression of Arg 403, known to cause human FHCM, exhibits myocyte and myofibrillar disarray, impaired cardiac function and extensive fibrosis. However, there is very little hypertrophy. Expression of this same mutation, Arg 403, in the rabbit is associated with a phenotype that is virtually identical to that observed in human FHCM.[109] This may be because the rabbit has beta-MHC as the predominant myosin in the heart, as is found in human myocardium, whereas the mouse heart has alpha-MHC. In the transgenic rabbit, there is myocyte disarray, impaired systolic and diastolic function, extensive interstitial fibrosis and extensive septal and posterior wall hypertrophy. There is also a significant incidence of sudden death. Utilizing these two models, the pathogenesis of FHCM has been considerably elucidated. It does appear that impaired contractility due to the inherited defect in the beta-MHC leads to impaired contractility,[60] which in turn is associated with disarray and upregulation of several growth factors that stimulate fibroblast proliferation with increased matrix formation, myocyte hypertrophy and further disarray.[60] It has been shown in human FHCM that several growth factors are upregulated[60] and the pathology is that of fibrosis and hypertrophy. Recognizing that fibrosis and hypertrophy are secondary phenotypes would imply that, with appropriate therapy, there could be attenuation, prevention or even regression of these phenotypes.

A randomized placebo-controlled study was performed in the mouse model with 12 transgenic mice receiving placebo, 12 receiving losartan and 12 controls.[110] This study showed that despite a fully developed phenotype of disarray and fibrosis, there was essentially a reversal of the phenotype to normal after about six weeks of therapy. TGF-beta, which is known to be a stimulus of fibroblastic activity and collagen deposition, also returned to control levels. It is thus likely that TGF-beta is a major mediator of fibrosis in the mouse. In the rabbit model, a similar randomized placebo-controlled study[111] was performed with simvastatin. After 12 weeks of therapy, this model showed a 37% reduction in hypertrophy and fibrosis with significant improvement in ventricular function. The mechanism whereby simvastatin induces regression of hypertrophy and fibrosis is most likely due to the inhibition of isoprenylation of signaling proteins. This process is necessary to induce growth of the cardiac myocytes and/or fibroblasts. In similar studies spironolactone was also shown to reverse the HCM phenotype in the mouse.[112] Most recently, in similar placebo-controlled studies, atorvastatin was shown to prevent the development of the HCM phenotype, when given prior to puberty in the transgenic rabbit.[113]

These studies are very exciting and provide compelling evidence for an appropriate clinical study in humans. We are even more excited about these results since all of these drugs have been shown to be safe as they have been taken by millions of patients for other reasons. These animal models provide the potential to identify other targets for development of new therapies but clearly losartan, simvastatin, atorvastatin and spironolactone can be evaluated in the near future. It is of note that FHCM in humans usually does not present prior to puberty and thus, there is at least a 10–12 year window in those positive for the mutation in which appropriate therapy could prevent or modulate the rate of development of the phenotype of fibrosis and hypertrophy. There is also, of course, the possibility that one can inhibit the fibrosis separately, which would lead to more specific therapy for the treatment of the disease in humans. It is an example of how one can work from the bedside to the bench in identifying the gene and then back to the bedside, having developed therapies in animal models that can be evaluated in clinical trials.

We are also interested in a novel diagnostic means for the preclinical diagnosis of FHCM. In the transgenic rabbit model of human FHCM induced by expression of the Arg 403 mutation, tissue Doppler velocities of the myocardium were assessed. It was observed that rabbits positive for the mutation, despite having no hypertrophy, exhibited impaired tissue Doppler velocities. These animals developed hypertrophy and the full phenotype but not until several months later.[114] Tissue Doppler velocities were evaluated in patients with FHCM, those positive for a mutation but without any clinical features and controls.[115] Thirteen patients positive for mutations but without hypertrophy or any other clinical phenotype exhibited decreased myocardial tissue velocity. We compared these findings with controls and patients with a clinical phenotype of FHCM. Tissue Doppler imaging had a sensitivity of 85% and specificity of 90% in individuals without other clinical findings. These findings have been confirmed by other investigators[116] and hopefully will be used to initiate therapy for prevention and possibly for screening athletes. The combination of effective therapy in animal models and a non-invasive test for preclinical diagnosis in patients offers great promise for the future. It is hoped clinical trials will be initiated in the near future for HCM, the most common cause of sudden cardiac death in the young.

Acknowledgment

This work is supported in part by grants from the Canadian Foundation for Innovation #NA6120, Canadian Institutes of Health Research #165041, the National Heart, Lung, and Blood Institute, Specialized Centers of Research P50-HL42267–01, R01HL68884 and a Clinician-Scientist Award from Burroughs Wellcome Fund.

References

1. Hoffman JIE. Incidence of congenital heart disease: II. Prenatal incidence. *Pediatr Cardiol* 1995;**16**:155–65.
2. Berko BA, Swift M. X-linked dilated cardiomyopathy. *N Engl J Med* 1987;**316**:1186–91.
3. Roberts R. A perspective: the new millennium dawns on a new paradigm for cardiology – molecular genetics. *J Am Coll Cardiol* 2000;**36**(3):661–7.
4. Brown MS, Goldstein JL. A receptor-mediated pathway for cholesterol homeostasis. *Science* 1986;**232**:34–47.
5. Daw EW, Shete S, Lu Y *et al.* A demonstration of oligogenic simultaneous segregation and linkage analysis to map modifier loci: two new hypertrophic cardiomyopathy loci. *Genetic Epidemiol* 2005;**29**(3):241.
6. Cao H. Nuclear lamin A/C R482Q mutation in Canadian kindreds with Dunnigan-type familial partial lipodystrophy. *Hum Mol Genet* 2000;**9**:109–12.
7. Roberts R, Stewart AFR, Wells G, Williams K., Kavaslar N, McPherson R. Identifying genes for coronary artery disease – an idea whose time has come. *Can J Cardiol* 2007;**23**:7–15.
8. Roberts R., Stewart AFR. Personalized medicine: a future prerequisite for the prevention of coronary artery disease. *Am Heart J* 2006;**4**(3):222–7.
9. Marian AJ, Roberts R. The molecular genetic basis for hypertrophic cardiomyopathy. *J Mol Cell Cardiol* 2001;**33**(4):655–70.
10. Keating MT, Sanguinetti MC. Molecular and cellular mechanisms of cardiac arrhythmias. *Cell* 2001;**104**:569–80.
11. Wang Q, Shen J, Splawski I *et al.* SCN5A mutations associated with an inherited cardiac arrhythmia, long QT syndrome. *Cell* 1995;**80**:805–11.
12. Dumaine R, Wang Q, Keating MT *et al.* Multiple mechanisms of Na+ channel-linked long-QT syndrome. *Circ Res* 1996;**78**:916–24.
13. Kimua A, Harada H, Park J-E *et al.* Mutations in the cardiac troponin I gene associated with hypertrophic cardiomyopathy. *Nat Genet* 1997;**16**:379–82.
14. Zareba W, Moss AJ, Schwartz PJ *et al.* Influence of the genotype on the clinical course of the long-QT syndrome. *N Engl J Med* 1998;**339**:960–5.
15. Gussak I, Brugada P, Brugada J *et al.* Idiopathic short QT interval: a new clinical syndrome? *Cardiology* 2000;**94**:99–102.
16. Chen Q, Kirsch GE, Zhang D *et al.* Genetic basis and molecular mechanism for idiopathic ventricular fibrillation. *Nature* 1998;**392**(6673):293–6.
17. Antzelevitch C. The Brugada syndrome: ionic basis and arrhythmia mechanisms. *J Cardiovasc Electrophysiol* 2001;**12**:268–72.
18. Brugada R, Roberts R. Brugada syndrome: why are there multiple questions to a simple answer? *Circulation* 2001;**104**:3017–19.
19. Chandra M, Rundell VL, Tardif J-C *et al.* Ca(2+) activation of myofilaments from transgenic mouse hearts expressing R92Q

mutant cardiac troponin T. *Am J Physiol Heart Circ Physiol* 2007;**280**:H705–H713.

20. Jeschke B, Uhl K, Weist B *et al.* A high risk phenotype of hypertrophic cardiomyopathy associated with a compound genotype of two mutated beta-myosin heavy chain genes. *Hum Genet* 1998;**102**:299–304.

21. Tardiff JC, Factor SM, Tompkins BD *et al.* A truncated cardiac troponin T molecule in transgenic mice suggests multiple cellular mechanisms for familial hypertrophic cardiomyopathy. *J Clin Invest* 1998;**101**:2800–11.

22. Van Driest SL, Jaeger MA, Ommen SR *et al.* Comprehensive analysis of the beta-myosin heavy chain gene in 389 unrelated patients with hypertrophic cardiomyopathy. *J Am Coll Cardiol* 2004;**44**(3):602–10.

23. Feinberg WM, Blackshear JL, Laupacis A, Kronmal R, Hart RG. Prevalence, age distribution, and gender of patients with atrial fibrillation. Analysis and implications. *Arch Intern Med* 1995;**155**(5):469–73.

24. Lloyd-Jones DM, Larson MR, Beiser A *et al.* Lifetime risk of developing coronary heart disease. *Lancet* 1999;**353**:89–92.

25. Wolf PA, Abbott RD, Kannel WB. Atrial fibrillation: a major contributor to stroke in the elderly: the Framingham Study. *Arch Intern Med* 1987;**147**:1561–4.

26. Brugada R, Tapscott T, Czernuszewicz GZ *et al.* Identification of a genetic locus for familial atrial fibrillation. *N Engl J Med* 1997;**336**:905–11.

27. Gollob MH, Jones DL, Krahn AD *et al.* Somatic mutations in the connexin 40 gene (GJA5) in atrial fibrillation. *N Engl J Med* 2006;**354**(25):2677–88.

28. Roberts R. Mechanisms of disease: genetic mechanisms of atrial fibrillation. *Nat Clin Pract* 2006;**3**(4):276–82.

29. Gollob MH, Green MS, Tang A *et al.* Identification of a gene responsible for familial Wolff-Parkinson-White syndrome. *N Engl J Med* 2001;**344**(24):1823–64.

30. Gollob MH, Roberts R. AMP activated protein kinase and familial Wolff-Parkinson-White syndrome: new perspectives on heart development and arrhythmogenesis. *Eur Heart J* 2002;**23**(9):679–81.

31. Gollob MH, Seger JJ, Gollob TN *et al.* Novel PRKAG2 mutation responsible for the genetic syndrome of ventricular preexcitation and conduction system disease with childhood onset and absence of cardiac hypertrophy. *Circulation* 2001;**104**(25):3030–3.

32. Arad M, Benson DW, Perez-Atayde A *et al.* Constitutively active AMP kinase mutations cause glycogen storage disese mimicking. *Clin Invest* 2002;**109**:357–62.

33. Blair E, Redwood CS, Ashrafian H *et al.* Mutations in the gamma(2) subunit of AMP-activated protein kinase cause hypertrophic cardiomyopathy: evidence for the central role of energy comp disease pathogenesis. *Hum Mol Genet* 2001;**10**(11):1215–20.

34. Sidhu J, Yadavendra S, Rajawat YS *et al.* Transgenic mouse model of ventricular preecitation and atrioventricular reentrant tachycardia induced by an AMP-activated protein kinase loss-of-function mutation responsible for Wolff-Parkinson-White syndrome. *Circulation* 2005;**111**:21–9.

35. Cannan CR, Reeder GS, Bailey KR, Melton LJ, III, Gersh BJ. Natural history of hypertrophic cardiomyopathy. A population-based study, 1976 through 1990. *Circulation* 1995;**92**:2488–95.

36. Maron BJ, Shirani J, Poliac LC, Mathenge R, Roberts WC, Mueller FO. Sudden death in young competitive athletes. Clinical, demographic, and pathological profiles. *JAMA* 1996;**276**:199–204.

37. Maron BJ, Anan TJ, Roberts WC. Quantitative analysis of the distribution of cardiac muscle cell disorganization in the left ventricular wall of patients with hypertrophic cardiomyopathy. *Circulation* 1981;**63**:882–94.

38. Shirani J, Pick R, Roberts WC, Maron BJ. Morphology and significance of the left ventricular collagen network in young patients with hypertrophic cardiomyopathy and sudden cardiac death. *J Am Coll Cardiol* 2000;**35**(1):36–44.

39. Spirito P, Bellone P, Harris KM, Bernabo P, Bruzzi P, Maron BJ. Magnititude of left ventricular hypertrophy and risk of sudden death in hypertrophic cardiomyopathy. *N Engl J Med* 2000;**342**:1778–85.

40. Varnava AM, Elliott PM, Baboonian C, Davison F, Davies MJ, McKenna WJ. Hypertrophic cardiomyopathy; histopathological features of sudden death in cardiac troponin T disease. *Circulation* 2001;**104**:1380–4.

41. Varnava AM, Elliott PM, Mahon N, Davies MJ, McKenna WJ. Relation between myocyte disarray and outcome in hypertrophic cardiomyopathy. *Am J Cardiol* 2001;**88**:275–9.

42. Osio A, Tan L, Chen SN *et al.* Myozenin 2 is a novel gene for human hypertrophic cardiomyopathy. *Circ Res* 2007;**100**(6):766–8.

43. Niimura H, Bachinski LL, Sangwatanaroj S *et al.* Mutations in the gene for cardiac myosin-binding protein C and late-onset familial hypertrophic cardiomyopathy. *N Engl J Med* 1998;**338**(1248):1257.

44. Charron P, Dubourg O, Desnos M *et al.* Genotype-phenotype correlations in familial hypertrophic cardiomyopathy. A comparison between mutations in the cardiac protein-C and the beta-myosin heavy chain genes. *Eur Heart J* 1998;**19**:139–45.

45. Arbustini E, Diegoli M, Morbini P *et al.* Prevalence and characteristics of dystrophin defects in adult male patients with dilated cardiomyopathy. *J Am Coll Cardiol* 2000;**35**:1760–8.

46. Cohn JN, Franciosa JA, Francis GS *et al.* Effect of short-term infusion of sodium nitroprusside on mortality rate in acute myocardial infarction complicated by left ventricular failure. *N Engl J Med* 1982;**306**:1129–35.

47. Watkins H, McKenna WJ, Thierfelder L *et al.* Mutations in the genes for cardiac troponin T and a-tropomyosin in hypertrophic cardiomyopathy. *N Engl J Med* 1995;**332**:1058–64.

48. Hackel DB, Reimer KA, Ideker RE *et al.* Comparison of enzymatic and anatomic estimates of myocardial infarct size in man. *Circulation* 1984;**70**:824–35.

49. Karibe A, Tobacman LS, Strand J *et al.* Hypertrophic cardiomyopathy caused by a novel a-tropomyosin mutation (V95A) is associated with mild cardiac phenotype, abnormal calcium binding to troponin and myosin cycling, and a poor prognosis. *Circulation* 2001;**103**:65–71.

50. Poetter K, Jiang H, Hassenzadeh S *et al.* Mutations in either the essential or regulatory light chains of myosin are associated with a rare myopathy in human heart and skeletal muscle. *Nat Genet* 1996;**13**:63–9.

51. Flavigny J, Richard P, Isnard R *et al.* Identification of two novel mutations in the ventricular regulatory myosin light chain gene

(MYL2) associated with familial and classical forms of hypertrophic cardiomyopathy. *J Mol Med* 1998;**76**:208–14.

52. Satoh M, Takahashi M, Sakamoto T, Hiroe M, Marumo F, Kimura A. A structural analysis of the titin gene in hypertrophic cardiomyopathy: identification of a novel disease gene. *Biochem Biophys Res Commun* 1999;**262**:411–17.

53. Morgensen J, Klausen C, Pedersen AK *et al.* a-cardiac actin is a novel disease gene in familial hypertrophic cardiomyopathy. *J Clin Invest* 1999;**103**(10):R39–R43.

54. Olson TM, Doan TP, Kishimoto NY, Whitby FG, Ackerman MJ, Fananapazir L. Inherited and de novo mutations in the cardiac actin gene causing hypertrophic cardiomyopathy. *J Mol Cell Cardiol* 1999;**32**:1687–94.

55. Roberts R, Sobel BE. Creatine kinase isoenzymes in the assessment of heart disease. *Am Heart J* 1978;**95**:521–8.

56. Marian AJ. Modifier genes for hypertrophic cardiomyopathy. *Curr Opin Cardiol* 2002;**17**(3):242–52.

57. Ho CY, Lever HM, DeSanctis R, Farver CF, Seidman JG, Seidman CE. Homozygous mutation in cardiac troponin T: implications for hypertrophic cardiomyopathy. *Circulation* 2000;**102**:1950–5.

58. American Heart Association. Heart Facts 1983. Dallas, TX: American Heart Association, 1982.

59. Marian AJ, Salek L, Lutucuta S. Molecular genetics and pathogenesis of hypertrophic cardiomypathy. *Minerva Med* 2001;**92**: 435–51.

60. Marian AJ. Pathogenesis of diverse clinical and pathological phenotypes in hypertrophic cardiomyopathy. *Lancet* 2000;**355**: 58–60.

61. Mestroni L, Rocco C, Gregori D *et al.* Familial dilated cardiomyopathy: evidence for genetic and phenotypic heterogeneity. *J Am Coll Cardiol* 1999;**34**:181–90.

62. Kasper EK, Agema WRP, Hutchins GM, Deckers JW, Hare JM, Baughman KL. The causes of dilated cardiomyopathy: a clinicopathological review of 673 consecutive patients. *J Am Coll Cardiol* 1994;**23**:586–90.

63. Kirshenbaum LA, Schneider MD. The cardiac cell cycle, pocket proteins, and p300. *TCM* 1995;**5**(6):230–5.

64. Olson TM, Michels VV, Thibodeau SN, Tai Y-S, Keating MT. Actin mutations in dilated cardiomyopathy, a heritable form of heart failure. *Science* 1998;**280**:750–2.

65. Kamisago M, Sharma SD, DePalma SR *et al.* Mutations in sarcomere protein genes as a cause of dilated cardiomyopathy. *N Engl J Med* 2000;**343**:1688–96.

66. Tsubata S, Bowles KR, Vatta M *et al.* Mutations in the human delta-sarcoglycan gene in familial and sporadic dilated cardiomyopathy. *J Clin Invest* 2000;**106**(5):655–62.

67. Fatkin D, MacRae C, Sasaki T *et al.* Missense mutations in the rod domain of the lamin A/C gene as causes of dilated cardiomyopathy and conduction-system disease. *N Engl J Med* 1999;**341**:1715–24.

68. Bonne G, Di Barletta MR, Varnous S *et al.* Mutations in the gene encoding lamin A/C cause autosomal dominant Emery-Dreifuss muscular dystrophy. *Nat Genet* 1999;**21**:285–8.

69. Roberts R. Editorial: the two out of three criteria for the diagnosis of infarction – is it passe? *Chest* 1984;**86**:511–13.

70. Li D, Tapscoft T, Gonzalez O *et al.* Desmin mutation responsible for idiopathic dilated cardiomyopathy. *Circulation* 1999;**100**(5): 461–4.

71. Perng MD, Muchowski PJ, Van Den IJ *et al.* The cardiomyopathy and lens cataract mutation in alphaB-crystallin alters its protein structure. *J Biol Chem* 1999;**274**:33235–43.

72. Hamer A, Vohra J, Hunt D, Sloman G. Prediction of sudden death by electrophysiologic studies in high risk patients surviving acute myocardial infarction. *Am J Cardiol* 1982;**50**:223–9.

73. Corrado D, Fontaine G, Marcus FI *et al.* Arrhythmogenic right ventricular dysplasia/cardiomyopathy: need for an international registry. Study Group on Arrhythmogenic Right Ventricular Dysplasia/Cardiomyopathy of the Working Groups on Myocardial and Pericardial Disease and Arrhythmias of the European Society of Cardiology and of the Scientific Council on Cardiomyopathies of the World Heart Federation. *Circulation* 2000;**101**(11):E101–E106.

74. Corrado D, Basso C, Thiene G *et al.* Spectrum of clinicopathologic manifestations of arrhythmogenic right ventricular cardiomyopathy/dysplasia: a multicenter study. *J Am Coll Cardiol* 1997;**30**:1512–20.

75. Rampazzo A, Nava A, Buja G *et al.* The gene for arrhythmogenic right ventricular cardiomyopathy maps to chromosome 14q23-q24. *Hum Mol Genet* 1994;**3**:959–62.

76. Rampazzo A, Nava A, Erne P *et al.* A new locus for arrhythmogenic right ventricular cardiomyopathy (ARVD2) maps to chromosome 1q42-q43. *Hum Mol Genet* 1995;**4**:2151–4.

77. Severini GM, Krajinovic M, Pnamonti B *et al.* A new locus for arrhythmogenic right ventricular dysplasia on the long arm of chromosome 14. *Genomics* 1996;**31**:193–200.

78. Rampazzo A, Nava A, Miorin M *et al.* ARVD4, a new locus for arrhythmogenic right ventricular cardiomyopathy, maps to chromosome 2 long arm. *Genomics* 1997;**45**:259–63.

79. Ahmad F, Li D, Karibe A *et al.* Localization of a gene responsible for arrhythmogenic right ventricular dysplasia to chromosome 3p23. *Circulation* 1998;**98**:2791–5.

80. Li D, Ahmad F, Gardner MJ *et al.* The locus of a novel gene responsible for arrhythmogenic right ventricular dysplasia characterized by early onset and high penetrance maps to chromosome 10p12-p14. *Am J Hum Genet* 2000;**66**:148–56.

81. Tiso N, Stephan DA, Nava A *et al.* Identification of mutations in the cardiac ryanodine receptor gene in families affected with arrhythmogenic right ventricular cardiomyopathy type 2 (ARVD2). *Hum Mol Genet* 2001;**10**:189–94.

82. McKoy G, Protonotarios N, Crosby A *et al.* Identification of a deletion in plakoglobin in arrhythmogenic right vetricular cardiomyopathy with palmoplantar keratoderma and woolly hair (Naxos disease). *Lancet* 2000;**355**:2119–24.

83. Gerull B, Heuser A, Wichter T *et al.* Mutations in the desmosomal protein plakophilin-2 are common in arrhythmogenic right ventricular cardiomyopathy. *Nat Genet* 2005;**36**(11):1162–4.

84. Norgett EE, Hatsell SJ, Carvajal-Huerta L *et al.* Recessive mutation in desmoplakin disrupts desmoplakin-intermediate filament interactions and causes dilated cardiomyopathy, woolly hair and keratoderma. *Hum Mol Genet* 2000;**9**:2761–6.

85. Alcalai R, Metzger S, Rosenheck S *et al.* A recessive mutation in desmoplakin causes arrhythmogenic right ventricular dysplasia, skin disorder, and woolly hair. *J Am Coll Cardiol* 2003;**42**:319–27.

86. Pilichou K, Nava A, Basso C *et al.* Mutations in desmoglein-2 gene are associated with arrhythmogenic right ventricular cardiomyopathy. *Circulation* 2006;**113**(1171):1179.

87. Garcia-Gras E, Lombardi R, Giocondo MJ *et al.* Suppression of canonical Wnt/beta-catenin signaling by nuclear plakoglobin recapitulates phenotype of arrhythmogenic right ventricular cardiomyopathy. *J Clin Invest* 2006;**116**(7):2012–21.

88. McKoy G, Protonotarios N, Crosby A *et al.* Identification of a deletion in plakoglobin in arrhythmogenic right ventricular cardiomhopathy with palmoplantar keratoderma and woolly hair (Naxos disease). *Lancet* 2000;**355**:2119–24.

89. Garg V, Kathiriya IS, Barnes R *et al.* GATA4 mutations cause human congenital heart defects and reveal an interaction with TBX5. *Nature* 2003;**424**(6947):443–7.

90. Risch N. Linkage strategies for genetically complex traits. II. The power of affected relative pairs. *J Genet Hum* 1990;**46**: 229–41.

91. Chan L, Boerwinkle E. Gene–environment interactions and gene therapy in atherosclerosis. *Cardiol Rev* 1994;**2**(3):130–7.

92. Chronic Disease Prevention Alliance of Canada. Available from: http://www.cdpac.ca accessed on 28 April 2009.

93. Hirshhorn JN, Daly MJ. Genome-wide association studes for common diseases and complex traits. *Nat Rev Genet* 2005;**6**:95–108.

94. Pare G, Serre D, Brisson D *et al.* Genetic analysis of 103 candidate genes for coronary artery disease and associated phenotypes in a founder population reveals a new association between endothelin-1 and high-density lipoprotein cholesterol. *Am Hum Genet* 2007;**80**(4):673–82.

95. Farh KK-H, Grimson A, Jan C *et al.* The widespread impact of mammalian microRNAs on mRNA repression and evolution. *Science* 2005;**310**(5755):1817–21.

96. McPherson R, Pertsemlidis A, Kavaslar N *et al.* A common allele on chromosome 9 associated with coronary heart disease. *Science* 2007;**316**:1488–91.

97. Couzin J, Kaiser J. Genome-wide association. Closing the net on common disease genes. *Science* 2007;**316**(5826):820–2.

98. Rust S, Rosier M, Funke H *et al.* Tangier disease is caused by mutations in the gene encoding ATP-binding cassette transporter 1. *Nat Genet* 1999;**22**(4):352.

99. Clee SM, Kastelein JJ, Van Dam M *et al.* Age and residual cholesterol efflux affect HDL cholesterol levels and coronary artery disease in ABCA1 heterozygotes. *J Clin Invest* 2000;**106**(10): 1263–70.

100. Lutucuta S, Ballantyne CM, Elghannam H, Gotto A, Marian AJ. Novel polymorphisms in promoter region of ATP binding cassette transporter gene and plasma lipids, severity, progression, and regression of coronary atherosclerosis and response to therapy. *Circ Res* 2001;**88**(9):969–73.

101. Frikke-Schmidt R, Nordestgaard BG, Jensen GB, Tybjaerg-Hansen A. Genetic variation in ABC transporter A1 contributes to HDL cholesterol in the general population. *J Clin Invest* 2004;**114**(9):1343–53.

102. Cohen JC, Kiss RS, Pertsemlidis A *et al.* Multiple rare alleles contribute to low plasma levels of HDL cholesterol. *Science* 2004;**305**(5685):869–72.

103. Cahilly C, Ballantyne CM, Lim DS, Gotto A, Marian AJ. A variant of p22(phox), involved in generation of reactive oxygen species in the vessel wall, is associated with progression of coronary atherosclerosis. *Circ Res* 2000;**86**(4):391–5.

104. Helgadottir A, Thorleifsson G, Manolescu A *et al.* A common variant on chromosome 9p21 affects the risk of myocardial infarction. *Science* 2007;**316**(5830):1491–3.

105. Wellcome Trust Control Consortium. Genome-wide association study of 14,000 cases of seven common diseases and 3,000 shared controls. *Nature* 2007;**447**(7145):661–78.

106. Geller DS, Farhi A, Pinkerton CA. Activating mineralcorticoid receptor mutation in hypertension exacerbated by pregnancy. *Science* 2000;**289**:119–223.

107. Seidman CE. Hypertrophic cardiomyopathy: from man to mouse. *J Clin Invest* 2000;**106**:S9-S13.

108. Oberst L, Zhao G, Park J-T *et al.* Expression of a human hypertrophic cardiomyopathy mutation in transgenic mice impairs left ventricular systolic function, detected by 178Ta radionucleide angiography, which precedes hisological changes. *J Am Coll Cardiol* 1999;**33**:3A.

109. Marian AJ, Wu Y, Lim D-S *et al.* A transgenic rabbit model for human hypertrophic cardiomyopathy. *J Clin Invest* 1999;**104**: 1683–92.

110. Lim DS, Lutucuta S, Bachireddy P *et al.* Angiotensin II blockade reverses myocardial fibrosis in a transgenic mouse model of human hypertrophic cardiomyopathy. *Circulation* 2001;**103**(6): 789–91.

111. Patel R, Nagueh SF, Tsybouleva N *et al.* Simvastatin induces regression of cardiac hypertrophy and fibrosis and improves cardiac function in a transgenic rabbit model of human hypertrophic cardiomyopathy. *Circulation* 2001;**104**:r27–r34.

112. Tsybouleva N, Zhang L, Chen S *et al.* Aldosterone, through novel signaling proteins, is a fundamental molecular bridge bridge between the genetic defect and the cardiac phenotype of hypertrophic cardiomyopathy. *Circulation* 2004;**109**:r59–r66.

113. Senthil V, Chen SN, Tsybouleva N *et al.* Prevention of cardiac hypertrophy by atorvastatin in a transgenic rabbit model of human hypertrophic cardiomyopathy. *Circ Res* 2005;**97**(3): 285–92.

114. Nagueh SF, Kopelen H, Lim DS, Zoghbi WA, Quinones MA, Roberts R. Tissue Doppler imaging consistently detects myocardial contraction and relaxation abnormalities, irrespective of cardiac hypertrophy, in a transgenic rabbit model of human hypertrophic cardiomyopathy. *Circulation* 2000;**102**:1346–50.

115. Nagueh SF, Bachinski LL, Meyer D *et al.* Tissue Doppler imaging consistently detects myocardial abnormalities in patients with hypertrophic cardiomyopathy and provides a novel means for an early diagnosis before and independently of hypertrophy. *Circulation* 2001;**104**(2):128–30.

116. Ho CY, Sweitzer NK, McDonough B *et al.* Assessment of diastolic function with doppler tissue imaging to predict genotype in preclinical hypertrophic cardiomyopathy. *Circulation* 2002;**105**:2992–7.

23 Diet and cardiovascular disease

K Srinath Reddy

All India Institute of Medical Sciences, New Dehli, India

Introduction

Diet, as regularly consumed, and the nutrients supplied by it are major determinants which initiate and influence the course of atherothrombotic vascular disease.[1] It is estimated that up to 30% of deaths from coronary heart disease (CHD), a major form of cardiovascular disease (CVD), are due to unhealthy diets.[2] Identification of increased or decreased risk associated with dietary patterns or specific nutrients, in a methodologically rigorous manner, should lay the scientific foundation for general dietary recommendations to populations as well as specific nutritional interventions in individuals at high risk of CVD.

Methodologic issues in the study of causal associations

Issues related to study design

Studies investigating the influence of diet on CVD or cardiovascular risk factors have employed a wide variety of study designs: ecologic studies within and across populations, cross-sectional surveys, case–control studies (*de novo* or nested), cohort studies, community-based demonstration projects, randomized clinical trials and before/after type of metabolic studies. These differ widely in terms of their ability to (a) identify, avoid and adjust for confounding, (b) establish a temporal relationship of cause preceding the effect, (c) minimize bias, (d) provide a wide range of exposure, (e) ascertain composite endpoints, including fatal outcomes, (f) evaluate population-attributable risk, and (g) yield generalizable results.

Clinical trials, if well designed, provide the best framework for studying associations, as the results are relatively

Evidence-Based Cardiology, 3rd edition. Edited by S. Yusuf, J.A. Cairns, A.J. Camm, E.L. Fallen, and B.J. Gersh. © 2010 Blackwell Publishing, ISBN: 978-1-4051-5925-8.

free from bias and confounding. However, they often evaluate interventions which are relatively short term and introduced late in the natural history of disease and may not reflect the effects of long-term differences in dietary exposures. Genetics now offers an alternative approach through "Mendelian randomization". This approach takes into account that genotypic differences in the metabolism of food ingredients may cause lifelong differences in exposure to food components and their metabolites or to purported risk factors, and may thus establish causality without the need for prolonged follow-up.[3,4]

A related issue is the use of experimental animals. Although these are often referred to as "animal models", their validity in predicting outcomes in humans is unclear. Lipid metabolism especially is species specific, as exemplified by the lack of efficacy of cholesterol-lowering statin drugs in many animal species, including monkeys.[5] Experiments in animals are therefore best reserved for elucidating mechanisms, and cannot be used to argue that a particular food will have a particular effect on cardiovascular disease in humans.

Issues involving outcome variables

These principally relate to a choice between disease endpoints and intermediate variables and the type of variables which are selected for study. Ideally, disease-related endpoints are preferable since they clearly demonstrate the benefits or risks of dietary exposures. With an exposure such as diet, effects may extend beyond cardiovascular outcomes. The need to evaluate impact of diet on total mortality and major co-morbidities, therefore, becomes important. Dietary exposures which influence thrombotic pathways may have opposite effects on the risk of hemorrhagic stroke and thrombotic stroke. The need to differentiate the types of stroke in outcome evaluation is, therefore, clear and has important implications for populations which differ in their stroke profiles.

Intermediate variables have been frequently utilized in studies evaluating the association of dietary constituents or dietary patterns to CVD. Most often, these are risk factors like blood pressure or plasma lipids. However, similar changes in total plasma cholesterol may be associated with variable effects on levels of LDL cholesterol and HDL cholesterol and on the ratio of total to HDL cholesterol. The impact on risk of atherosclerotic CVD may thus vary. The 25-year follow-up experience of the Seven Countries Study revealed that while the increase in relative risk of CHD for comparable levels of plasma cholesterol elevation was similar across diverse populations, the absolute risk of CHD varied widely at the same level of plasma cholesterol, possibly due to other dietary and non-dietary influences.[6] Dietary changes may also influence LDL particle size differentially, and also the level of plasma triglycerides, with variable net effects on the atherogenicity of the plasma lipid pool. Such limitations were clearly illustrated in a study by Rudel et al[7] in which monkeys fed monounsaturated fat had similar lowering of LDL cholesterol as monkeys fed polyunsaturated fat but developed atherosclerosis equivalent to those fed saturated fat. In monkeys fed monounsaturated fatty acids, there was an enrichment of cholesteryl oleate in plasma cholesteryl esters, which correlated with coronary artery cholesteryl ester concentration.[8] Plasma lipids, as intermediate variables, could not also explain the degree of cardiovascular protection conferred by the Mediterranean diet in the Lyon Diet Heart Study.[9] While studies of intermediate variables (e.g. cholesterol levels) are useful in identifying mechanistic pathways of diet, there is a need for methodologically strong studies which relate dietary patterns or dietary interventions to hard endpoints such as total mortality and combined fatal and non-fatal cardiovascular events.

Issues involving exposure variables

These involve the type of exposure selected for study, the methods of measurement employed as well as the duration and dose of exposure. First, the types of dietary exposure assessed for associations with CVD have varied from specific nutrients (such as saturated fat) to dietary items (such as fish) to food groups (such as fruit and vegetables) to dietary patterns (such as the Mediterranean diet or Adventist diet) and composite dietary interventions (e.g. the DASH diet). A reductionist approach has inherent limitations in the area of diet, because multiple interactions among many nutrients are likely to determine the physiologic effects and pathologic outcomes much more than the individual effects of an isolated nutrient. Multicomponent dietary exposures, however, render identification of mechanistic causal pathways difficult to elucidate. While this frustrates efforts to develop and market specific food supplements or nutriceuticals, interests of public health are likely to be better served by a causal enquiry exploring the connections of food patterns and food components to cardiovascular health.

Second, the strengths and limitations of various methods of collecting accurate food consumption data are well recognized.[10] Questionnaire methods of ascertaining information related to habitual food intake pose problems of validity and reproducibility even within well-defined populations but these problems are likely to be magnified when such instruments are applied across different cultures. Even if the nutrient composition of self-reported diets is accurately estimated, different cooking methods may alter the final bio-availability of those nutrients as actually consumed. The need for valid and reproducible biomarkers is, therefore, important when studies of specific nutrients are proposed. For example, adipose tissue fatty acid composition is a suitable biomarker for habitual type of dietary fat intake.[11] There may, however, be technical and financial constraints which limit the use of such biomarkers in large epidemiologic studies.

Third, a causal enquiry needs to recognize the lag time effect, wherein a long period of exposure to dietary variables is required before effect is evident on outcome variables Short-term studies may be incapable of identifying true effects even when they exist. This is clearly illustrated by trials evaluating the effect of sodium restriction on blood pressure, where benefit was demonstrated only in trials in which the duration of exposure was at least 5 weeks.[12] The dose of exposure is another critical variable, where many of the nutrients are physiologic requirements at a certain level but may pose risk of cardiovascular dysfunction and disease at other levels. The relationships may vary from linear to J-shaped or threshold, for different variables.

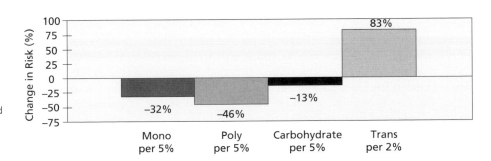

Figure 23.1 Change in CHD risk associated with replacement of saturates by other fats (Nurses' Health Study). (Reproduced with permission from Hu et al[21].)

Issues related to diet as an independent variable

Unhealthy dietary behaviors often occur in association with other unhealthy behaviors such as physical inactivity and smoking. Furthermore, unhealthy dietary practices such as high consumption of saturated fats, salt and refined carbohydrates as well as low consumption of fruit and vegetables tend to cluster together. In contrast, persons who habitually adopt one healthy dietary practice are more likely to adopt other healthy dietary habits as well as practice regular physical activity and abstinence from smoking. Dietary behaviors may also reflect patterns influenced by social class and may be influenced by stress levels. Dissociating the specific effects of individual dietary components from other dietary components, physical activity levels and other behaviors becomes difficult outside the setting of a randomized controlled clinical trial. In observational studies, the question arises whether some dietary practices are merely a surrogate for other dietary practices or lifestyles such as physical activity, or for a composite of multiple health behaviors.

The effects of diet on multiple cardiovascular risk factors, ranging from body weight to blood lipids and blood pressure to thrombotic mechanisms, also pose the question of when and how far to adjust for these variables in evaluating the relationship of diet to CVD. Since many of these are intermediate variables linking diet to CVD, adjustment to exclude their effect would underestimate the effect of diet. However, such variables are also influenced by factors other than diet.

Nutrients and cardiovascular disease

Willett defined a good diet by using a score based on low trans fat, high polyunsaturated fat, low glycemic load, high cereal fiber, fish twice a week or more, and high folic acid.[13]

Dietary fats

The relationship between dietary fats and CVD, especially CHD, has been extensively investigated, with strong and consistent associations emerging from a wide body of evidence accrued from animal experiments, as well as observational studies, clinical trials and metabolic studies conducted in diverse human populations. The relationship of dietary fat to CVD was initially considered to be mediated mainly through the atherogenic effects of plasma lipids (total cholesterol, lipoprotein fractions and triglycerides). The effects of dietary fats on thrombosis and endothelial function as well as the relationship of plasma and tissue lipids to the pathways of inflammation have been more recently understood.[11,14] Similarly the effects of

dietary fats on blood pressure have also become more evident through observational and experimental research.

Cholesterol in the blood and tissues is derived from two sources: diet and endogenous synthesis. Dairy fat and meat are major sources. Egg yolk is particularly rich in cholesterol but, unlike dairy and meat, does not provide saturated fatty acids. Dietary cholesterol raises plasma cholesterol levels.[15] Although both HDL and LDL increase, the effect on the total/HDL ratio is still unfavorable, but small.[16] Observational evidence on an association of dietary cholesterol intake with cardiovascular disease is contradictory.[17,18] The upper limit for dietary cholesterol intake has been prescribed, in most guidelines, to be 300 mg/day. However, since there is no requirement for dietary cholesterol, it is advisable to keep the intake as low as possible.[14] If intake of dairy fat and meat is controlled, there would be no need for a severe restriction of additional egg yolk intake.

Fatty acids are grouped into three classes – saturated fatty acids (SFA), monounsaturated fatty acids (MUFA) and polyunsaturated fatty acids (PUFA). SFA and MUFA can be synthesized in the body and hence are not dietary essentials. PUFA are essential fatty acids, since they cannot be synthesized in the body.

Saturated fatty acids (SFAs) as a group raise total and LDL cholesterol, but individual SFAs have different effects.[11,19] Myristic and lauric acids have greater effect than palmitic acid, but the latter is more abundant in food supply. The plasma cholesterol-raising effects of these three SFAs is higher when combined with high-cholesterol diets. Stearic acid has not been shown to elevate blood cholesterol and is rapidly converted to oleic acid (OA) *in vivo*. Metabolic (feeding) studies demonstrate a marked elevation of both HDL and LDL cholesterol induced by SFA diets.[20,21] Replacement of saturated fatty acids by polyunsaturated fat reduces the total to HDL cholesterol ratio but replacement by carbohydrates does not. Also, tropical fats rich in lauric acid (C-12) raise total cholesterol strongly, but because of their specific effect on HDL, the ratio of total to HDL cholesterol falls. Thus effects on blood lipids can be variable, depending on which blood lipids are studied, and we need data on actual outcomes to determine the true effects of fats on coronary heart disease.[22]

The relationship of dietary saturated fat to plasma cholesterol levels and to CHD was graphically demonstrated by the Seven Countries Study involving 16 cohorts, in which saturated fat intake explained 73% of the total variance in CHD across these cohorts.[23] In the Nurses' Health Study,[21] the effect of saturated fatty acids was much more modest, especially if saturates were replaced by carbohydrates. The most effective replacement for saturated fatty acids in terms of CHD outcome is by polyunsaturated fatty acids, i.e. linoleic acid. This agrees with the outcome of large randomized clinical trials, in which replacement of saturated and trans fats by polyunsaturated vegetable oils effectively lowered coronary heart disease risk.[24]

Trans fatty acids (t-FAs) are geometric isomers of unsaturated fatty acids that assume a saturated fatty acid-like configuration. Partial hydrogenation, the process used to create t-FAs, also removes essential fatty acids such as linoleic acid and alpha-linolenic acid. Metabolic studies have demonstrated that t-FAs render the plasma lipid profile even more atherogenic than SFAs, by not only elevating LDL cholesterol to similar levels but also decreasing HDL cholesterol.[25] As a result, the ratio of LDL cholesterol to HDL cholesterol is significantly higher with a t-FA diet (2.58) than with a SFA diet (2.34) or an oleic acid diet (2.02). Evidence that intake of t-FAs increases the risk of CHD initially became available from large population-based cohort studies in the US[26,27] and was corroborated in an elderly Dutch population.[28] Levels of t-FAs in a biochemical analysis of replicated baseline food composites correlated with the risk of coronary death in the cohorts of the Seven Countries Study. Most trans fatty acids are contributed by industrially hardened oils, but the dairy and meat fats of ruminants are also a source. Eliminating t-FAs from the diet would be an important public health strategy to prevent cardiovascular disease. Since these agents are commercially introduced into the diet, policy measures related to the food industry would be required along with public education. Trans fatty acids have been eliminated from retail fats and spreads in a large part of the world, but deep-fat fried fast foods and baked goods are a major and increasing source.[29]

The only nutritionally important *monounsaturated fatty acid* (MUFA) is oleic acid, which is abundant in olive and canola oils and also in nuts. The epidemiologic evidence related to MUFAs and CHD is derived from studies on the Mediterranean diet, as well as from the Nurses' Health Study and other similar studies, which investigated the association and controlled for confounding factors.[30] MUFAs have been shown to lower blood glucose and triglycerides in type 2 diabetics and may decrease susceptibility of LDL to oxidative modification.

Polyunsaturated fatty acids (PUFAs) are derived from dietary linoleic acid (LA) (n-6 PUFAs) and dietary alpha linolenic acid (ALNA) (n-3 PUFAs). The important n-6 PUFAs are arachidonic acid (AA) and dihomogammalinolenic acid (DHGLA), while the important n-3 PUFAs are eicosapentaenoic acid (EPA) and docosahexaenoic acid (DHA). Eicasanoids derived from AA have opposing metabolic properties to those derived from DHA. A balanced intake of n-6 and n-3 PUFAs is, therefore, essential for health.

The biologic effects of n-3 PUFAs are wide ranging, involving lipids and lipoproteins, blood pressure, cardiac function, arterial compliance, endothelial function, vascular reactivity and cardiac electrophysiology as well as potent antiplatelet and anti-inflammatory effects, including reduced neutrophil and monocyte cytokine production.[11,31] DHA appears to be more responsible for the beneficial effects of fish and fish oils on lipids and lipoproteins, blood pressure, heart rate variability, and glycemic control, in comparison to EPA, while a mixture of DHA and EPA significantly reduced platelet aggregation in comparison to ALNA *in vitro*.[11,32] The very-long chain n-3 polyunsaturated fatty acids powerfully lower serum triglycerides, but they raise LDL cholesterol.[33] Therefore, their effect on coronary heart disease is probably mediated through pathways other than cholesterol.

Much of the epidemiologic evidence related to n-3 PUFAs is derived from the study of fish consumption in populations or interventions involving fish diets in clinical trials. Fish oils were, however, used in the GISSI study of 11 300 survivors of myocardial infarction.[34] In this factorial design, fish oil (1 g/day) and vitamin E (300 mg/day) were compared, alone and in combination, to placebo. After 3.5 years of follow-up, the fish oil group had a statistically significant 20% reduction in total mortality, 30% reduction in cardiovascular death and 45% decrease in sudden death. While most published studies do not indicate that dietary n-3 PUFAs prevent restenosis after percutaneous coronary angioplasty or induce regression of coronary atherosclerosis, one study reported that occlusion of aortocoronary venous bypass grafts was reduced after 1 year by daily ingestion of 4 g fish oil concentrate.[35]

The Lyon Diet Heart Study incorporated an n-3 fatty acid (alpha-linolenic acid) into a diet altered to develop a Mediterranean diet intervention.[9] In the experimental group plasma ALNA and EPA increased significantly and the trial reported a 70% reduction in cardiovascular mortality at 5 years in its initial report. Total cholesterol and LDL cholesterol were identical in the experimental and control groups, suggesting that thrombotic and perhaps arrhythmic events may have been favorably influenced by n-3 PUFAs. Since the diet altered many other variables, such as fiber and antioxidants (by increasing fruit and vegetable consumption), direct attribution of benefits to n-3 PUFAs becomes difficult to establish.

The effect of different fatty acids on cardiac arhythmias has been an area of great interest. Diets rich in saturated fatty acids increase the risk of ventricular fibrillation and sudden cardiac death in primates. A population-based case–control study, using biomarkers, revealed a modest association of trans fatty acids in general and a strong association of trans isomers of linoleic acid in particular with primary cardiac arrest in humans.[36] Several studies in different animal models, primate and rodent, have shown that n-3 PUFAs are protective against cardiac arrhythmias, especially ventricular fibrillation.[37] It has been suggested that the fall in CHD mortality in the USA and Australia since 1967 is probably attributable to an increase in polyunsaturate fat consumption in both countries since 1960.[38]

The decline in CHD mortality in the Zutphen cohort has similarly been attributed to a decreased consumption, over time, of trans fatty acids.[28]

The proportions of SFAs, MUFAs and PFAs as constituents of total fat intake and total energy consumption have engaged active attention, in view of the strong relationship of these fatty acids to the risk of CVD, especially CHD. The reduction of SFAs in the diet has been widely recommended, but its replacement remains an area of debate as to whether the place of reduced SFAs should be taken by MUFAs, PUFAs or carbohydrate. In a meta-analysis of studies on the effect of various dietary fats on blood lipids, the negative effect of dietary trans fat was about twice that of saturated fat on a calorie-for-calorie basis.[39] Dietary trans fats have additional adverse effects, including increased serum triglyceride and lipoprotein (a) levels and adverse effects on endothelial function.[40,41] Both MUFA and PUFA improve the lipoproteins profile, although polyunsaturated fatty acids are somewhat more effective. In view of this, recent US dietary recommendations suggested that SFAs should be reduced to 7–8%, MUFAs should be increased to 13–15% and PUFAs raised to 7–10% of daily energy, with the total fat contributing no more than 30% of all calories consumed.[30,42] These may need to be adjusted for populations who consume lower quantities of total fat, so as to ensure an adequate intake of MUFAs and PUFAs even under those circumstances.

The total quantity of fat consumed, as a proportion of daily energy intake, has not shown a relation to CVD that is independent of the SFAs content. It has been argued that the type of fats consumed is far more important than the total amount of fat consumed.[43] The compatibility of high-fat Mediterranean diets (with total fat contributing >30% of calories) with coronary protection has also been cited as supportive evidence. While the emphasis on the type of fat is well placed, it must be recognized that high-fat diets are also high in energy. Whether this contributes substantially to overweight is a subject of much debate.[44] The Strong Heart Study examined the association between dietary fat

intake and CHD incidence in American Indians.[45] Participants (n = 2938) were followed for a mean (±SD) of 7.2 ± 2.3 years. In the age group of 47–59 years, those in the highest quartile of intake of total fat, saturated fatty acids or monounsaturated fatty acids had higher CHD mortality than did those in the lowest quartile (hazard ratio (95% CI): 3.57 (1.21–10.49), 5.17 (1.64–16.36), and 3.43 (1.17–10.04), respectively) after confounders were controlled for. These associations were not observed for those aged 60–79 years. Based on these strong independent risk associations, it would be prudent to reduce fat intake early in life to reduce the risk of dying from CHD.

Enhancing the nutritional quality of dietary fat consumption, to provide greater cardiovascular protection, may be attempted by decreasing the sources of saturated fats and eliminating trans fatty acids in the diet, increasing the consumption of foods containing unsaturated fatty acids (both MUFAs and PUFAs) and decreasing dietary cholesterol consumption. Figure 23.2 provides a breakdown of different types of fats in the commonly consumed edible fats/oils.[46]

Carbohydrates

The relationship of dietary carbohydrates to CVD appears to be mediated through indirect mechanisms: contribution to total energy and its effect on overweight and obesity; influence on central obesity; effects on plasma lipids, especially triglycerides, and effects on glycemic control. The balance between carbohydrates and fat as sources of energy as well as the fiber component of the diet are also areas of interest when considering this relationship. In feeding experiments, an increase in dietary energy from carbohydrates is usually associated with a moderate increase in fasting plasma triglyceride levels in the first few weeks but these return to near original levels eventually. Epidemiologically, high carbohydrate intakes are associated with low plasma cholesterol and variable plasma triglyceride concentrations.[47]

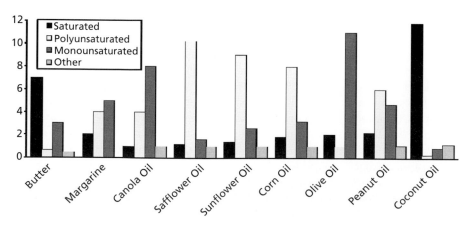

Figure 23.2 Breakdown of fat types in various fats and oils. (Reproduced with permission from Steckel[46].)

High-carbohydrate diets appear to reduce HDL cholesterol levels and increase the fraction of small dense LDL, both of which may impact adversely on vascular disease. This dyslipidemic pattern is consistent with the elevation of plasma triglycerides. There is as yet no clear evidence that the risk of CVD is altered independently by the carbohydrate levels in the diet. The glycemic index of foods might also be a determinant of the extent to which carbohydrates can influence the glycemic status. Carbohydrate diets with high glycemic index might adversely impact on glucose control, with associated changes in plasma lipids.[48,49]

Liu *et al*[50] first reported a positive association between a higher dietary glycemic load (GL) and risk of CHD in the Nurses' Health Study (NHS). Buelens *et al*[51] report a similar association between GL and risk of CVD in the EPIC (European Prospective Investigation into Cancer and Nutrition) cohort. The analysis included 15714 women aged 49–70 years without diabetes or CVD at baseline. During 9 years of follow-up, 556 incident cases of major CVD events were documented. After adjusting for CVD risk factors and dietary fat and fiber, the investigators found a significant association between dietary GL and increased risk of CVD (risk ratio comparing extreme quartiles = 1.47, 95% confidence interval (CI) 1.04–2.09, *P* for trend = 0.03). In both the NHS and EPIC cohorts, the increased risk was more pronounced among overweight and obese women compared with normal-weight women.

It is mainly the amount and the type of carbohydrate consumed that will increase a person's risk of developing cardiovascular disease, increased weight or type 2 diabetes. Non-refined carbohydrates, rich in dietary fiber, like wholegrains, fruit, vegetables and legumes, reduce the risk of heart disease. The greater risk of heart disease is associated with eating patterns high in refined carbohydrates, such as confectionery, cakes, biscuits, pastries and high-sugar drinks and fruit juice drinks. Limiting the amount of carbohydrate from foods containing refined carbohydrates is important for weight management and thus lowering the risk for heart disease.

Dietary fiber

Dietary fiber is a heterogeneous mixture of polysaccharides and lignin that cannot be degraded by the endogenous enzymes of vertebrate animals.[53] Water-soluble fibers include pectins, gums, mucilages and some hemicelluloses. Insoluble fibers include cellulose and other hemicelluloses. Most soluble fibers reduce plasma total and LDL cholesterol concentrations, as reported by several trials.[54] Pectins, psyllium, gums, mucilages, algal polysaccharides and some hemicelluloses lower total and LDL cholesterol levels without affecting HDL cholesterol, the reductions in total cholesterol being usually in the range of 5–10%. Human

---

BOX 23.1 Recommendations by the National Heart Foundation, Australia[52]

There is good evidence in the scientific literature to indicate that:
- there is no significant association between the total carbohydrate intake and the risk of developing cardiovascular disease
- eating patterns with a high glycemic load raise blood triglyceride levels, increasing the risk of cardiovascular disease
- eating patterns high in soluble fiber lower blood LDL cholesterol levels, reducing the risk of CVD
- total carbohydrate intake has no effect on insulin sensitivity or the risk of developing type 2 diabetes

There is moderate evidence in the scientific literature to indicate that:
- consuming dietary fiber from cereals (particularly wholegrains) and fruit is associated with a lower risk of cardiovascular disease
- eating patterns low in refined carbohydrates are associated with a lower risk of developing type 2 diabetes

---

experiments have clearly shown that oat fiber tends to lower plasma total and LDL cholesterol but wheat fiber does not. Rice bran and barley may also lower cholesterol.[55] Fiber consumption predicted insulin levels, weight gain and cardiovascular risk factors like blood pressure, plasma triglycerides, LDL and HDL cholesterol and fibrinogen more strongly than other dietary components in the CARDIA cohort study of young adults.[56] However, fiber intake may be confounded with many other determinants of cardiovascular health.

Between 1996 and 2001, five very large cohort studies in the USA, Finland and Norway all reported that subjects consuming relatively large amounts of wholegrain cereals have significantly lower rates of CHD.[55,57] High intake of fiber from cereal sources was associated with a reduced risk of CHD in the Nurses' Health Study[57] and was inversely associated with the risk of hypertension in the Health Professionals Follow-up Study.[58]

There are no randomized controlled trials evaluating the effects of wholegrain consumption on CHD events. However, numerous reviews have examined wholegrain intakes and the risk of CHD.[59–62] Others have linked wholegrain consumption to lowered risk of diabetes and obesity in men[63] and women.[64] Both diabetes and overweight are risk factors for early-onset CHD and there is the possibility that modifying their risk could mediate some of the protective effects of wholegrains.[60] Lowering of plasma total and LDL cholesterol has been shown in male and female

Hispanic Americans.[65] In contrast, Davy et al[66] did not find a significant reduction in total or LDL cholesterol but demonstrated a lowering of more atherogenic small, dense LDL particles by oat bran relative to wheat cereal in sedentary, overweight American men.

Thus, the large body of prospective data provides convincing evidence for a protective effect of wholegrains against CHD. Available evidence supports a recommendation for consumption of about 15 g /1000 kcal of fiber.[54] Since some of the reported benefits may have arisen from other dietary components occurring in association with fiber in natural foods, dietary consumption of high-fiber foods should be recommended rather than isolated fiber. Addition of oat bran may be considered, where necessary, to supplement natural foods in order to attain the recommended dietary intake.

Antioxidants

The oxidation of LDL by oxygen free radicals results in the unregulated uptake of modified LDL by macrophages in arterial walls, accelerating the atherosclerotic process. Antioxidant nutrients, which can directly scavenge free radicals, include alpha-tocopherol (vitamin E isomer) and ascorbic acid (vitamin C), which have shown antioxidant activity both *in vitro* and *in vivo*, as well as beta-carotene (a provitamin A carotenoid) which has displayed antioxidant activity *in vitro*.[67] These mechanisms suggested that increased dietary intake or supplementation of these nutrients would be protective against atheroslerotic vascular disorders. This was supported by evidence from observational studies for vitamin E and beta-carotene, but results of clinical trials employing supplements have been disappointing.

Observational cohort data suggest a protective role for carotenoids. The randomized trials, in contrast, reported a moderate adverse effect of beta-carotene supplementation, with a relative increase in the risk of cardiovascular death of 12% in a meta-analysis of four trials.[68] Cancer risk was also increased.

Several large cohort studies showed significant reductions in the incidence of cardiac events in men and women taking high-dose vitamin E supplements.[67] However, the HOPE trial, a definitive clinical trial relating vitamin E supplementation to cardiovascular outcomes, revealed no effect of vitamin E supplementation (at 400 IU/day, for a mean follow-up of 4.5 years) on MI, stroke or death from cardiovascular causes in men or women.[69] Other trials also failed to demonstrate a cardioprotective effect of vitamin E supplements.[70] A recent meta-analysis also showed no evidence of a protective effect of antioxidant or B vitamin supplements on the progression of atherosclerosis.[71]

Flavonoids are polyphenolic antioxidants which occur in a variety of foods of vegetable origin, such as tea, onions and apples. Data from several prospective studies indicate an inverse association of dietary flavonoids with coronary heart disease.[65] A benefit on stroke risk has also been reported.[66] However, confounding may be a major problem and may explain conflicting results of observational studies on flavonoids and coronary heart disease. Fruits and vegetables also contain other phytochemicals that may have protective properties, including isothiocyanates and indoles (found in cruciferous vegetables), sulfides (found in onions and garlic), terpenes (found in citrus oils) and phytoestrogens.[54] The overall health benefit of flavonoid consumption is unproven, and their intake in the form of fortified foods or supplements should not be encouraged.[72]

Systematic reviews[73,74] appraising large amounts of epidemiologic and observational evidence suggest that flavonoids in chocolates may lower the risk of CHD mortality. Crude approximations suggest that eating 50 g of dark chocolate per day may reduce one's risk of CVD by 10.5% (95% CI 7.0–13.5%). However, these estimates were based on results from studies of short duration, extrapolated to long-term CVD outcomes. Long-term randomized feeding trials, beyond short-term studies of CVD risk factor intermediates, are warranted to investigate the impact of chocolate consumption on cardiovascular outcomes.

Phenolics in red wine were shown to be able to inhibit the oxidation of LDL *in vitro* and this was suggested as an explanation of the "French paradox".[75] The Zutphen study, an epidemiologic study in The Netherlands, suggested an inverse correlation between the incidence of CHD and stroke and the dietary intake of flavonoids, especially quercetin.[76]

Green tea polyphenols have been studied extensively as CVD chemopreventive agents. A population-based prospective cohort study (the Ohsaki Study) examined the association between green tea consumption and mortality from CVD, cancer and all causes with 40 530 persons in Miyagi Prefecture, in northern Japan.[77] Green tea consumption was inversely associated with mortality from CVD and this inverse association was more pronounced in women ($P = 0.08$ for interaction with sex). Kuriyama[78] reviewed the association between green tea or green tea extracts and CVD risk profiles and reported that more than half of the trials have demonstrated the beneficial effects of green tea on CVD risk profiles. These results suggest a plausible mechanism for the beneficial effects of green tea.

Sesso et al[79] determined whether the intake of lycopene or tomato-based foods is associated with the risk of CVD in a prospective cohort of 39 876 middle-aged and older women initially free of CVD and cancer. They found that the dietary lycopene was not strongly associated with the risk of CVD. However, some inverse associations for CVD, noted for higher levels of tomato-based products, particularly tomato sauce and pizza, suggested that dietary lycopene or other phytochemicals consumed as oil-based tomato products could confer cardiovascular benefits.

The conflict between diet-based observational studies and clinical trials employing supplements may arise because of one or more explanatory factors: confounding, interactions/synergistic activity (among antioxidants; with other nutrients), isomers with differing activity in food compared to supplements, other associated protective elements in natural foods (e.g. flavonoids, phytoestrogens) and/or temporal dissociation of antioxidant blood levels from fat intake in meals, when administered as once-daily pills. While the failure of pill supplementation does not necessarily exclude protective effects of dietary antioxidants, current evidence does not support supplementation of any of these antioxidant vitamins for prevention of CHD. However, intake of their primary food resources, especially fruit and vegetables, may be encouraged.

Folate

The relationship of folate to CVD has been mostly explored through its effect on homocysteine (HCY), which has been incriminated as an independent risk factor for CHD and probably stroke.[80–83] Folic acid is required for the methylation of homocysteine to methionine. Reduced plasma folate has been strongly associated with elevated plasma homocysteine levels and folate supplementation has been demonstrated to decrease those levels.[84] However, the role of homocysteine as an independent risk factor for CVD has been subject to debate, in view of the data from several prospective studies which did not find this association to be independent of other risk factors.[85] Furthermore, clinical trials such as the Norwegian Vitamin Trial (NORVIT),[86] Vitamin Intervention for Stroke Prevention (VISP)[87] and HOPE-2[88] showed that, even though vitamin supplementation reduced HCY levels, there was no significant effect on cardiovascular risk. It has also been suggested that elevation of plasma HCY is a consequence and not a cause of atherosclerosis, wherein impaired renal function due to atherosclerosis raises plasma HCY levels.[89] At present, we cannot recommend the use of vitamin supplementation to reduce CVD risk.

Minerals: blood pressure and cardiovascular disease

Sodium

High blood pressure (HBP) is a major risk factor for CHD and both forms of stroke (ischemic and hemorrhagic). The relative risk of CVD for both systolic and diastolic blood pressures operates in a continuum of increasing risk for rising pressure but the absolute risk of CVD is considerably modified by co-existing risk factors.[90] Of the many risk factors associated with high blood pressure, the dietary exposure most investigated has been daily sodium consumption. It has been studied extensively in animal experimental models, in epidemiologic studies, controlled clinical trials and in population studies on restricted sodium intake.[90] Salt or sodium intake has been directly correlated with mean blood pressure levels and prevalence of hypertension in many populations. Comprehensive epidemiologic evidence was provided by the INTERSALT Study[91,92] which investigated the relationship of 24-hour urinary electrolyte excretion to blood pressure in 52 population groups across 32 countries, using standardized methodology to provide comparable data. In adults aged 20–59 years, there was a significant positive relationship between urinary sodium excretion and blood pressure across the 52 population samples. Further, it was also observed that in four of these populations in whom the mean 24-hour urinary sodium excretion was lower than 100 mmol/day, systolic blood pressure did not rise with age.[93]

The effects on blood pressure levels of increased sodium consumption accompanying urbanization were demonstrated in the Kenyan Luo Migration Study wherein rural farmers who traditionally consumed a low-salt diet were observed to have an elevation of blood pressure when they migrated to an urban environment. These migrants exhibited blood pressure levels higher than rural controls and comparable to levels observed in Western populations.[94] This rise in blood pressure was related to an increase in salt consumption and a reduced dietary intake of potassium. An overview of observational data in populations suggested that a difference in sodium intake of 100 mmol/day could be associated with average differences in systolic blood pressure of 5 mmHg at age 15–19 years and 10 mmHg at 60–69 years.[95] Diastolic blood pressures are reduced by about half as much, but the association increases with age and the magnitude of the initial blood pressure. It was estimated that a universal reduction in dietary intake of salt by 50 mmol/day would lead to a 50% reduction in the number of people requiring antihypertensive therapy, a 22% reduction in number of deaths due to strokes and a 16% reduction in number of deaths from coronary heart disease.[95]

A cohort study in Finland prospectively followed 1173 men and 1263 women aged 25–64 years, with complete data on 24-hour urinary sodium excretion and cardiovascular risk factors.[96] The hazard ratios for CHD, CVD and all-cause mortality, associated with a 100 mmol increase in 24-hour urinary sodium excretion, were 1.51 (95% CI 1.14–2.00), 1.45 (1.14–1.84) and 1.26 (1.06–1.50) respectively, in both men and women. The frequency of acute coronary events, but not acute stroke events, rose significantly with increasing sodium excretion. Disaggregated analyses revealed significant risk ratios in men only and revealed that sodium predicted mortality in men who were overweight. Despite the limitations of such subgroup analyses, the overall association of increasing sodium excretion with CVD and all-cause mortality further supports the evidence linking increased sodium intake to adverse cardiovascular health outcomes.

Several clinical intervention trials, conducted to evaluate the effects of dietary salt reduction on blood pressure levels in hypertensive and normotensive individuals, have been systematically reviewed.[12,97] Many of the earlier trials were of limited size and short duration and were deficient in statistical power. Based on an overview of 32 methodologically adequate trials (22 in hypertensive subjects and 12 in normotensive persons), Cutler *et al*[12] concluded that a daily reduction in intake of sodium by 70–80 mmol was associated with a lowering of blood pressure in both hypertensive and normotensive individuals, with systolic and diastolic blood pressure reductions of 4.8/1.9 mmHg in the former and 2.5/1.1 mmHg in the latter. Clinical trials have also demonstrated the sustained blood pressure lowering effects of sodium restriction in infancy,[98] as well as in the elderly in whom it provides a useful non-pharmacologic therapy.[99] In a 3-year study of salt restriction by Cook *et al*,[100] the Trials of Hypertension Prevention (TOHP), Phase II, participants had a decrease in systolic blood pressure (1.3 mmHg, $P = 0.02$) that corresponded with a significant dose-dependent reduction in sodium excretion. The Trial of Nonpharmacologic Interventions in the Elderly (TONE) was the first multicenter clinical trial of sufficient size and duration to show that lifestyle modifications can be used to control high blood pressure in older people. In elderly participants, sodium restriction resulted in mean reductions of 4.3 mmHg ($P < 0.001$) and 2.0 mmHg ($P = 0.001$) in systolic and diastolic blood pressure, respectively.[101]

The effect of a multi-component lifestyle intervention that includes the combination of sodium restriction, the DASH diet, weight loss and regular aerobic exercise was evaluated in the Diet, Exercise, and Weight Loss Intervention Trial (DEW-IT).[102] After 9 weeks, systolic and diastolic blood pressures were decreased by 12.1 mmHg ($P < 0.001$) and 6.6 mmHg ($P < 0.001$) respectively in the intervention participants compared with those in the control group. In subjects with above optimal blood pressure, the PREMIER trial showed that those in the "established recommendations" or "established + DASH diet" intervention groups had significant weight loss and reduction in sodium intake; both groups achieved greater reductions in systolic and diastolic blood pressure than did patients in the "advice only" group.[103]

The results of the low sodium – DASH diet trial[104] further strengthen the conclusion that reduction of daily sodium intake, through salt-restricted diets, lowers blood pressure effectively and is additive to the benefits conferred by the DASH diet. This trial revealed that low-sodium diets, with 24-hour sodium excretion levels around 70 mmol/day, are effective and safe. Sodium consumption has also been linked to the presence of left ventricular hypertrophy and restricted sodium intake has been demonstrated to result in regression of this important indicator of cardiovascular risk.[105,106] Of three population studies on restriction of salt, two (the Portuguese Salt Trial and the Tianjin trial in China) revealed significant reductions in blood pressure in the intervention group, while the third (the Belgian Salt Intervention Trial) did not reveal success because of difficulties in reducing salt consumption.[107–109] Animal models as well as ecologic associations derived from the INTERSALT study suggest a direct relationship between sodium consumption and the risk of stroke, though the methodology employed in these studies is not strong.[109,110]

Based on the observational and trial data so far available, it would be justified to recommend a salt intake of less than 5 g/day.[104] Such advice would be appropriate even in tropical climates, as sodium homeostasis regulates sodium excretion in sweat and urine without adverse effects under such conditions.

Potassium

Cardioprotective effects of dietary potassium have been hypothesized as the basis for low CVD rates in populations consuming "primitive" diets and in vegetarians in industrialized cultures.[111] The INTERSALT study provided evidence of an inverse association between urinary potassium excretion and blood pressure levels, across diverse populations.[91] Migrant studies also revealed a rise in blood pressure when diets changed to a lower potassium and higher sodium intake.[94]

A protective effect of potassium on blood pressure was suggested by clinical studies reporting that severe short-term potassium restriction induces salt sensitivity in normotensive humans,[112] as well as the blood pressure lowering effect of potassium supplements to the diet (ranging from 24 to 104 mmol/day) in hypertensive subjects.[111] Whelton *et al* concluded, from a meta-analysis of randomized controlled trials, that potassium supplements reduced mean blood pressures (systolic/diastolic) by 1.8/1.0 mmHg in normotensive subjects and 4.4/2.5 mmHg in hypertensive subjects.[113] An increase in dietary intake of potassium, from approximately 60 to 80 mmol/day, was shown to be inversely and significantly related to the incidence of stroke mortality in women.[114]

While dietary potassium has been shown to have protective effects on blood pressure and CVD, there is no evidence to suggest that long-term potassium supplements should be administered for cardiovascular protection. Supplemental potassium has the potential for toxicity and adequate dietary intake of potassium, though foods rather than supplements should be the preferred pathway for

For sodium
Reducing dietary sodium is associated with a fall in blood pressure in hypertensive and normotensive individuals. This is supported by good evidence in the scientific literature to indicate that:
- a reduction in dietary sodium from 140 to 100 mmol/day is associated with a fall in systolic blood pressure of 2 mmHg from an average systolic blood pressure of 135 mmHg
- a reduction in dietary sodium from 140 to 65 mmol/day is associated with a fall in systolic blood pressure of 7 mmHg from an average systolic blood pressure of 135 mmHg
- a reduction in dietary sodium of approximately 75 mmol/day is associated with a fall in systolic blood pressure of 4–5 mmHg in hypertensive individuals (baseline systolic blood pressure = 140 mmHg) and a fall in systolic blood pressure of 2 mmHg in normotensive individuals (baseline systolic blood pressure <120 mmHg).

There is moderate evidence in the scientific literature to indicate that:
- high dietary sodium intake is associated with increased stroke incidence, and mortality from coronary heart disease and cardiovascular disease.

For potassium
Increasing dietary potassium is associated with a fall in blood pressure in hypertensive and normotensive individuals. This is supported by good evidence in the scientific literature to indicate that:
- an increase in dietary potassium intake of approximately 54 mmol/day is associated with a fall in systolic blood pressure of 4–8 mmHg in hypertensive individuals (baseline systolic blood pressure = 140 mmHg) and a fall in systolic blood pressure of 2 mmHg in normotensive individuals (baseline systolic blood pressure <120 mmHg).

There is moderate evidence in the scientific literature to indicate that:
- High potassium intake is associated with decreased stroke mortality.

For Sodium/Potassium ratio
There is weak evidence in the scientific literature to indicate that:
- Blood pressure responsiveness to increased dietary potassium intake is greater in subjects with high sodium intake
- Blood pressure responsiveness to decreased sodium intake is greater in subjects with low potassium intake

cardiovascular potential. The beneficial effects of fruit and vegetables recommend their regular use in daily diets at a level that should assure an adequate intake of dietary potassium.

Calcium and magnesium

A meta-analysis of studies involving calcium supplements reveals modest effects on blood pressure. The estimated blood pressure reduction was 2.1 mmHg for systolic blood pressure and 1.1 mmHg for diastolic blood pressure.[116] There is weak evidence in the scientific literature to indicate that an increase in calcium intake reduces the risk of ischemic stroke.[115]

A review of 29 studies of magnesium was inconclusive due to methodologic problems but suggested that there was no negative association of blood pressure with magnesium.[117] There is presently no evidence to recommend public health or clinical interventions involving the use of these minerals for cardiovascular protection in populations or individuals, other than in the form of a balanced diet providing an adequate daily intake.

Food items and food groups

Fruits and vegetables

While the consumption of fruit and vegetables has been widely believed to promote good health, evidence related to their protective effect has only been presented in recent years.[118–120] A systematic review reported that nine of 10 ecologic studies, two of three case–control studies and six of 16 cohort studies found a significant protective association for coronary heart disease with consumption of fruit and vegetables or surrogate nutrients.[120] For stroke, three of five ecologic studies and six of eight cohort studies found a significant protective association.[120]

A 5-year follow-up study of 39876 female health professionals[121] observed a significant inverse association between fruit and vegetable intake and CVD risk. For increasing quintiles of total fruit and vegetable intake, the relative risks were 1.0, 0.78, 0.72, 0.68 and 0.68. After excluding participants with a self-reported history of diabetes, hypertension or high cholesterol at baseline, the multivariate adjusted relative risk was 0.45 when extreme quintiles were compared (95% CI 0.22–0.91). In a 12-year follow-up of 15220 male physicians in United States,[122] men who consumed at least 2.5 servings of vegetables/day were observed to have an adjusted relative risk of 0.77 for coronary heart disease, compared with men in the lowest category (<1 serving per day). Combining analyses of data from two large prospective cohort studies of women and men respectively, Joshipura et al[123] reported that overall fruit and vegetable consumption were inversely related to the risk of ischemic stroke after adjusting for confounders. Assessed as a continuous trend, an increment of one serving/day was associated with 6% lower risk of ischemic stroke among men and women combined. When analyzed separately for the type of fruit and vegetables, the lowest risks were observed for high consumption of cruciferous vegetables such as Brussels sprouts, cabbage and cauliflower, green leafy vegetables, citrus fruits, vitamin C-rich fruits and vegetables.

The effects of increased fruit and vegetable consumption on blood pressure, alone or in combination with a low-fat diet, were assessed in the DASH trial.[124] While the combination diet was more effective in lowering blood pressure, the fruit and vegetable diet also lowered the blood pressure in comparison to the control diet (2.8 mmHg systolic and 1.1 mmHg diastolic). Such reductions, while seeming modest at the individual level, would result in a substantial reduction in population-wide risk of CVD by shifting the blood pressure distribution.

As per a recent review by Winkler,[125] the nature of the relationship does not appear to follow a strict dose–response pattern, but generally does show additional risk reduction with increases in fruit and vegetable intake (Table 23.1).

The bulk of evidence supports an inverse association between fruit and/or vegetable consumption and CHD. Fruits and vegetables, being low in energy, sodium, saturated fat and total fats, bring about a reduction in obesity, blood pressure and serum lipids as a result of replacing "less healthy" alternative foods in the diet. Thus the benefits of a plant-based diet, rich in fruit and vegetables, may derive from protective phytonutrients, high fiber content and replacement value of substitution for atherogenic or obesogenic foods, all contributing in concert.

Fish

Most, but not all, population studies have shown that fish consumption in populations is associated with a reduced risk of CHD.[126–128] A systematic review concluded that the discrepancy in the studies may be due to differences in the populations studied, with only high-risk individuals benefiting from increasing their fish consumption.[128] It was estimated that, in high-risk populations, an optimum fish intake estimated at 40–60 g/day would lead to approximately a 50% reduction in death from coronary heart disease. In the Diet and Reinfarction Trial, 2-year mortality was reduced by 29% in survivors of a first myocardial infarction receiving advice to consume fatty fish at least twice a week.[129] While the protective effects of fish on CHD are principally mediated by n-3 PUFAs, the contribution of other constituents of fish cannot be ruled out. The effect of dietary fish on the risk of stroke has been investigated in cohort studies, with conflicting results on the risk of ischemic stroke.[130,131] An ecologic study reported that fish consumption is associated with a reduced risk of death from all causes as well as CHD and stroke mortality, using data from 36 countries.[132]

In addition to the Nurses' Health Study[133] and the Health Professionals Follow-up Study,[134] other prospective cohort studies[135,136] also exhibited an inverse association between increasing omega-3 consumption and the risk of stroke. In multivariate analyses, tuna, broiled or baked fish consumption was inversely associated with total stroke ($P = 0.04$) and ischemic stroke ($P = 0.02$). There was a 13% lower risk of ischemic stroke with an intake of 1–3 times per week (relative risk (RR) 0.87), a 27% lower risk with an intake of 1–4 times per week (RR 0.73) and 30% lower risk with intake of five or more times per week (RR 0.70), compared with an intake of less than once per month.[135]

Omega-3 can reduce the incidence of atrial fibrillation (AF) in the elderly[137] and in patients undergoing coronary bypass surgery.[138] In a randomized, double-blind, placebo-controlled study of 65 patients with cardiac arrhythmias without coronary heart disease or heart failure, Singer et al[139] supplemented patients with 3 g daily fish oil or olive oil over 6 months. In the fish oil group, the incidence of atrial and ventricular premature complexes was reduced by 47% and 68% respectively; couplets were reduced by 72% and triplets entirely disappeared. Other studies[140–142] also support a preventive role of omega-3s in arrhythmias and sudden death.

Two meta-analyses[143,144] further support an inverse association between omega-3 and CHD. He et al[143] assessed 222 364 individuals with an average 11.8 years of follow-up. The pooled multivariate RRs for CHD mortality were 0.89 for fish intake 1–3 times per month, 0.85 for once per week, 0.77 for 2–4 times per week and 0.62 for five or more times per week. Each 20 g/day increase in fish intake corroborated to a 7% lower risk of CHD mortality (P for trend = 0.03). Whelton et al[144] conducted a meta-analysis of 19 observational studies (14 cohort and five case–control). Fish consumption versus little to no fish consumption was associated with a RR of 0.83 ($P < 0.005$) for fatal CHD and 0.86 ($P < 0.005$) for total CHD.

Hooper et al[145] reported no benefit of omega-3 in relation to total or CV mortality in a meta-analysis. The inclusion of the Diet and Reinfarction Trial-2,[146] which reported an increase in sudden death with fish and fish oil intake, contributed substantial heterogeneity to the meta-analysis. The results are also at variance with DART-1, in which fish or fish oil supplementation decreased mortality by 29% over a 2-year period.[147] The omission of the DART-2 trial from the analysis provided an overall RR of death of 0.83 (CI 0.75–0.91) with no significant heterogeneity.

Thus, convincing evidence exists that supplemental omega-3 fatty acids in relatively high doses of about 1 g per day modestly reduce blood pressure and triglycerides but, to date, this has not resulted in a consistent reduction in CVD risk in well-designed randomized controlled trials.[148–150]

Table 23.1 Summary of findings related to association between consumption of fruits and vegetables and outcomes related to coronary heart disease

Study	#	Location	Design	Size	Duration	Incidence/mortality	Fruits & vegetables	Fruit only	Vegetables only	Subgroup analysis
WHS	1	US	cohort	39876 women	5 years	I	inv +	inv*	inv, ns	inv*
NHS & HPS	2	US	cohort	84251 women	8 years	I	inv*	inv*	inv*	inv*
				42158 men		I	inv +	N/A	N/A	N/A
NHANES/NHEFS	3	US	cohort	9608 adults	16.6 years	M	inv*	N/A	N/A	inv*
HFS	4	UK	cohort	10741 adults	18–24 years	M	N/A	inv*	N/A	inv*
ARIC	5	US	cohort	11940 adults	11 years	M	inv*	N/A	N/A	inv*
KIHD	6	Finland	cohort	2641 men	12,8 years	I	inv*	N/A	N/A	inv, ns
Odyssey	7	US	cohort	6151 adults	13 years	M	inv*	inv, ns	N/A	inv*
BLSA	8	US	cohort	501 men	18 years	M	inv*	N/A	inv*	inv*
PHS	9	US	cohort	15220 men	12 years	I	N/A	N/A	inv*	inv*
INTERHEART	10	52 countries	case-control	15152 cases	N/A	I[a]	inv*	N/A	N/A	inv*
				14820 controls						
Pamplona Hospital Study	11	Spain	case-control	171 cases	N/A	I[a]	N/A	inv*	inv +	n/a
				171 controls						
India Multi-center Study	12	India	case-control	350 cases	N/A	I[a]	N/A	pos*	inv*	inv*
				700 controls (women)						
Three Italian Case-Control Studies	13	Italy	case-control	1713 cases	N/A	I[a]	N/A	N/A	inv*	
				2317 controls						
TOTAL – cohort studies						5 incidence	8/8 inv	4/4 inv	4/4 inverse	7/7 inverse
						4 mortality	8/8 significant	3/4 significant	3/4 significant	6/7 significant
TOTAL – case-control						4 incidence	1/1 inv	1/2 inv	3/3 inverse	2/2 inverse
						0 mortality	1/1 significant	2/2 significant	3/3 significant	2/2 significant
TOTAL – all studies						9 incidence	9/9 inv	5/6 inv	7/7 inverse	8/8 inverse
						4 mortality	9/9 significant	5/6 significant	6/7 significant	7/8 significant

WHS = Women's Health Study; NHS = Nurses' Health Study; HPS = Health Professionals' Study; HFS = Health Food Shoppers Study; ARIC = Atherosclerosis Risk in Communities Study;
KIHD = Kuopio Ischemic Heart Disease Study; BLSA = Baltimore Longitudinal Study of Ageing; PHS = Physician's Health Study
I = incidence; M = Mortality
+ = statistically significant in some strata but not highest;
* = statistically significant in highest stratum or per serve; ns = not statistically significant; N/A = not assessed
[a] these case-control studies included incident cases of non-fatal MI only; deceased cases were not included
Source: Winkler 2006[125]

Nuts

Five large epidemiologic studies have, thus far, demonstrated that frequent consumption of nuts was associated with decreased risk of CHD, the best known among them being the Adventist Health Study.[151–154] The RR ranged from 0.43 to 0.82 for subjects who consumed nuts more than five times/week compared to those who never consumed nuts. An inverse dose–response relationship was demonstrated between the frequency of nut consumption and the risk of CHD, in men and women. Most of these studies considered nuts as a group, combining many types of nuts.

The effect of specific nuts on lipid and lipoprotein endpoints was evaluated in several clinical studies. The nuts studied to date include walnuts, almonds, legume peanuts, macadamia nuts, pecans and pistachio nuts.[151] Collectively, these clinical studies indicate that inclusion of nuts in a lipid-lowering diet has favorable effects, but do not provide unequivocal evidence of an additive effect of nuts to the effects of a low saturated fat diet *per se*. The fatty acid profile of nuts (high in unsaturated fatty acids and low in saturated fatty acids) contributes to cholesterol lowering by altering the fatty acid composition of the diet as a whole. Nuts are also a rich source of dietary fiber. It must, however, be recognized that the high fat content of nuts makes them high in calorie content and advice to include nuts in the diet must be tempered in accordance with the desired energy balance. While further research is needed to characterize the independent protective effects of nuts against CVD and identify the mechanisms of such protection, available evidence suggests that nuts should be recommended as part of an energy-appropriate healthy diet which is intended to reduce the risk of CHD.

In 2003, the FDA approved two qualified health claims for nuts, one for nuts in general and another for walnuts.[155] The approved language is as follows: "'Scientific evidence suggests but does not prove that eating 1.5 oz (42 g) per day of most nuts, as part of a diet low in saturated fat and cholesterol, may reduce the risk of heart disease". This health claim language was consumer tested and found to be ranked significantly higher than the FDA generic claim for clarity and understandability. In order for a food to qualify for the health claim, the product must contain 11 g or more of whole or chopped nuts per reference amount customarily consumed (a standardized serving size). Any nuts labeled with the claim must contain no more than 4 g saturated fat per 50 g. Eligible nuts for the claim include almonds, hazelnuts, peanuts, pecans, some pine nuts, pistachio nuts, and walnuts.[156,157]

Soy

Several trials indicate that intake of soy has a beneficial effect on plasma lipids.[158,159] A composite analysis of 38 clinical trials found that an average consumption of 47 g of soy protein a day led to a 9% decline in total cholesterol and a 13% decline in LDL cholesterol in subjects free of CHD.[158] The benefit of soy consumption was associated with baseline cholesterol levels, such that those with the highest cholesterol levels derived the maximum benefit (subjects with total cholesterol >335 mg/dL showed a 19% reduction in total and 24% reduction in LDL cholesterol). Cholesterol lowering of this magnitude could potentially reduce the risk for CHD by 20–40%.

Soy is rich in isoflavones, compounds that are structurally and functionally similar to estrogen. Several animal experiments suggest that intake of these isoflavones may provide protection against CHD[160] but human data on efficacy and safety are still awaited. Naturally occurring isoflavones, isolated with soy protein, reduced the plasma concentrations of total and LDL cholesterol without affecting the concentrations of triglycerides or HDL cholesterol in mildly hypercholesterolemic individuals, in a casein-controlled clinical trial.[161]

A very large amount of soy protein, more than half the daily protein intake, may lower LDL cholesterol by a few percentage points when it replaces dairy protein or a mixture of animal proteins.[162] The evidence favors soy protein rather than soy isoflavones as the responsible nutrient. No benefit is evident on HDL cholesterol, triglycerides, lipoprotein (a) or blood pressure. Thus, the direct cardiovascular health benefit of soy protein or isoflavone supplements is minimal at best. For this reason, use of isoflavone supplements in food or pills is not recommended. In contrast, soy products such as tofu, soy butter, soy nuts or some soy burgers should be beneficial to cardiovascular and overall health because of their high content of polyunsaturated fats, fiber, vitamins, and minerals, and low content of saturated fat. Using these and other soy foods to replace foods high in animal protein that contain saturated fat and cholesterol may confer benefits to cardiovascular health.[163] Soy protein also may be used to increase total dietary protein intake and to reduce carbohydrate or fat intake.

Garlic

Zhang *et al*[164] reported that gender might affect the action of garlic on plasma cholesterol and glucose levels of normal subjects. A systematic review of the effectiveness of garlic as an antihyperlipidemic agent included 10 studies and found that in six studies garlic was effective in reducing serum cholesterol levels. The average drop in total cholesterol was 9.9%, LDL 11.4%, and triglycerides 9.9%.[165] Other direct cardioprotective effects of garlic in humans have also been reported, such as a decrease in unstable angina,[166] an increase in the elastic property of blood vessels,[167] and a decrease in peripheral arterial occlusive disease.[168] In addition, garlic has been shown to increase peripheral blood flow in healthy subjects[169] while inhibiting the progression of coronary calcification in patients receiving statin therapy.[170] Rahman and Lowe[171] concluded in their review that although garlic appears to hold promise in reducing parameters associated with cardiovascular disease, more in-depth and well-designed studies are required.

Dairy products

Milk and milk products are important contributors to dietary fat and can be high in saturated fat and cholesterol. They are also sources of minerals like potassium, magnesium and calcium. Milk protein has been implicated in a study reporting elevated levels of antibodies to milk protein in patients with myocardial infarction in comparison with healthy controls.[172] Dairy consumption has been correlated positively, in an ecologic study, with blood cholesterol as well as coronary mortality. Milk consumption correlates positively with coronary mortality rates in 43 countries and with myocardial infarction in 19 regions of Europe.[173,174] In contrast, a population-based study in men of Japanese ancestry in Honolulu reported a reduced risk of ischemic stroke in older middle-aged men, which could not be explained by the intake of dietary calcium.[175]

On the basis of presently available evidence, reduced intake of high-fat dairy foods should be recommended for cardiovascular protection. Whether milk or milk products modified to substantially lower the content of saturated fat are associated with an increase or decrease in cardiovascular risk cannot be commented upon at present. They formed a component of the DASH diet which significantly lowered blood pressure and may be considered as part of a composite dietary advice.

Alcohol

Alcohol is both a nutrient supplying 29 kJ/g and a drug that is a central nervous system depressant.[176] The relationship of alcohol to overall mortality and cardiovascular mortality has generally been J-shaped, when studied in Western populations in whom the rates of atherothrombotic vascular disorders are high.[177–181] The protective effect of moderate ethanol consumption is primarily mediated through its effect on the risk of CHD, as supported by more than 60 prospective studies.[178] A consistent coronary protective effect has been observed for consumption of 1–2 drinks per day of an alcohol-containing beverage but heavy drinkers have higher total mortality than moderate drinkers or abstainers, as do binge drinkers. Moderate alcohol consumption (up to two drinks per day) has also been associated with a reduced risk of ischemic stroke in men and women.[182] Long-term heavy alcohol consumption (>60 g/day) increases an individual's risk for all stroke subtypes.

Several mechanisms for the cardioprotective effects of alcohol have been proposed: increase in plasma HDL cholesterol; reduced platelet aggregation or clotting; enhanced fibrinolysis; phenolic constituents of some alcoholic beverages acting as antioxidants or platelet inhibitors.[183] Genetic variations which slow alcohol metabolism have been shown to increase HDL cholesterol and reduce the risk of myocardial infarction.[4] Based on current evidence, the benefit of moderate alcohol consumption seems to be a generic effect regardless of the type of beverage.[184] While the specific advantages of red wine over other alcoholic beverages are unproven, the claimed beneficial effects of flavonoids on lipoprotein oxidation are available from grape juice as from wine.[185]

Certain subgroups have a lower risk of coronary heart disease associated with alcohol intake. These include postmenopausal women and men over the age of 45 years.[186] In these groups, light and moderate drinking of alcohol has consistently been associated with lower risk of coronary heart disease.[187–189]

A systematic review of ecologic, case–control and prospective studies concluded that all alcoholic drinks were linked with a lower risk of coronary heart disease.[190] However, beyond three drinks per day for men and two per day for women, the disadvantages of alcohol consumption rapidly outweigh the advantages.[191] This is especially true for those at low risk of death from coronary heart disease. In younger populations, drinking larger amounts of alcohol in one session is associated with injuries and cardiovascular heart disease mortality.[192]

The possible beneficial effects of moderate ethanol consumption must be weighed against the deleterious effects of high intake, including increased risk of hypertension, cardiomyopathy and hemorrhagic stroke. Alcohol consumption, in excess of three drinks per day, is associated with a rise in blood pressure and plasma triglyceride levels. Reduction or cessation of alcohol consumption is a widely recommended measure for non-pharmacologic therapy of hypertension, in many international guidelines. The recommendations related to alcohol should be made in accordance with the cultural practices of the populations and the clinical profile of individuals, with advice to avoid excess in all cases. The optimal intake, for cardiovascular protection, depends on age, gender, presence of other risk factors or associated diseases and on the intake of folic acid. However, it is generally recommended to be about two drinks a day for men and one a day for women.

Eggs

Eggs are unique because of their high cholesterol content. Major effects on atherosclerosis are observed in experimental animals but extrapolation to humans is doubtful. A large observational study suggested that there was no increase in the risk of CHD up to one egg per day (except in a diabetic subgroup), in the US population.[193] In terms of global recommendations, it may still be prudent to limit the intake to 3–4 eggs/week. With all the trimmings, a three-white egg omelet is almost indistinguishable by taste from an omelet enriched with 600 mg cholesterol, and the whites-only omelet also remains a very good source of protein, riboflavin, and selenium.[194]

Djoussé and Gaziano[195] have calculated an adjusted hazard ratio of 1.41 for all-cause mortality over a 20-year span in 21 327 Harvard-educated male physicians who ate ≥1 egg/day. It is important that a pattern of less frequent intake did not influence risk. However, if diabetes was co-existent in these healthcare professionals, a trend existed across a broader range of egg consumption. The egg intake pattern in this study population was extremely low: only 8% of participants were eating ≥1 egg/day. For comparison, 36% of the men in the Framingham Study[196] and 37% of men in a Japanese study[197] with similar outcome assessments ate ≥1 egg/day. However, in both these cohorts, there was no association between egg consumption and myocardial infarction, CVD death or all-cause mortality. Yet, this much higher consumption pattern may has confounded a graded effect that occurred at lower egg intakes.

Data from the most recent National Health and Nutritional Examination Survey (NHANES III, 1988–94) were utilized by Song and Kerver[198] to compare the nutritional quality indicators of diets that contained eggs (USDA food grouping system) with those that did not. In this cross-sectional and population-based study, egg consumption made important nutritional contributions to the American diet and was not associated with high serum cholesterol concentrations.

Dietary patterns and composite dietary interventions

The Mediterranean diet

The traditional Mediterranean diet has been described to have eight components:
1 high monounsaturated-to-saturated fat ratio
2 moderate ethanol consumption
3 high consumption of legumes
4 high consumption of cereals (including bread)
5 high consumption of fruits
6 high consumption of vegetables
7 low consumption of meat and meat products
8 moderate consumption of milk and dairy products.[118]
Most of these are found in many diets. The characteristic component is olive oil, and many equate a Mediterranean diet with consumption of olive oil.

Based on ecologic comparisons, Keys *et al*[199] hypothesized that a traditional Mediterranean diet conferred protection against CVD and several other disorders, principally because of a low saturated fat content. Three prospective population studies in Greece, Denmark and Australia provided supportive evidence of protective effects on overall mortality.[200] However, this traditional form of Mediterranean diet has not been tested in controlled clinical trials.

A secondary prevention trial of dietary intervention in survivors of a first recent myocardial infarction, which aimed to study the cardioprotective effects of a Mediterranean type of diet, actually left out its most characteristic component, olive oil.[201] This diet was designed to supply <35% of energy as fat, <10% of energy as saturated fat, <4% of energy as linoleic acid (n-6) and >0.6% of energy as alpha-linolenic acid (n-3). The main fat source was rapeseed oil. Vegetables and fruits were also increased in the diet. Two major biologic factors were modified by the intervention: plasma levels of alpha-tocopherol and ascorbic acid were elevated and plasma n-3 fatty acids increased, along with a decrease in n-6 fatty acids. Other biologic mediators of altered risk, like flavonoids, folate and minerals like potassium, were probably altered but not measured. While the initial publication reported a 70% reduction in recurrence of myocardial infarction and cardiac death, the 4-year follow-up study reported a 72% reduction in cardiac death and non-fatal myocardial infarction. The risk of overall mortality was lowered by 56%.[9]

In the Mediterranean Diet, Cardiovascular Risks and Gene Polymorphisms (Medi-RIVAGE) study, the effects of a Mediterranean-type diet (Med group) or a low-fat diet (low-fat group) on risk factors were evaluated in 212 volunteers (men and women) with moderate risk factors for cardiovascular disease. After a 3-month intervention, both diets significantly reduced cardiovascular disease risk factors to an overall comparable extent.[202]

Vegetarian diets

A reduced risk of CVD has been reported in populations of vegetarians living in affluent countries[203–205] and in case–control comparisons in developing countries.[206] Reduced consumption of animal fat and increased consumption of fruit, vegetables, nuts and cereals may underlie such a protective effect. However, vegetarian diets *per se* need not be healthful.[205] If not well planned, they can contain a large amount of refined carbohydrates and trans fatty acids while being deficient in the levels of vegetable and fruit consumption. The composition of the vegetarian diet should, therefore, be defined in terms of its cardioprotective constituents rather than endorsing the "vegetarian" label as an omnibus category.

"Prudent" versus "Western" patterns

Using factor analysis on a 131-item food frequency questionnaire, Hu *et al* identified two major dietary patterns at baseline in 44 875 men followed up for 8 years in the Health Professionals Follow-up Study.[207] The "prudent" pattern was characterized by higher intake of vegetables, fruit, legumes, wholegrains, fish and poultry whereas the "Western" pattern was characterized by higher intake of red meat, processed meat, refined grains, sweets and dessert, French fries and high-fat dairy products. After adjustment for age and other coronary risk factors, relative risks, from the lowest to the highest quintiles of the prudent pattern score, were 1.0, 0.87, 0.79, 0.75 and 0.70. In contrast, the relative risks across increasing quintiles of the Western pattern were 1.0, 1.21, 1.36, 1.40 and 1.64. These associations persisted in subgroup analyses according to cigarette smoking, Body Mass Index and parental history of myocardial infarction.

Japanese diet

The traditional Japanese diet has attracted much attention because of the highest life expectancy and low CHD mortality rates among the Japanese.[208] This diet is low in fat and sugar and includes soy, seaweeds, raw fish and a predominant use of rice. It has been high in salt, but salt consumption has recently been declining in response to Japanese Health Ministry guidelines. There is also a recent trend towards increased fat consumption and plasma cholesterol levels have risen, and their effects on CHD and CVD mortality rates need to be watched.

DASH diets

The effects of composite dietary interventions on blood pressure levels, in "normotensive" and "hypertensive" individuals, were studied in well-designed clinical trials.[104,124] The initial dietary intervention, used in the Dietary Approaches to Stop Hypertension (DASH) trial, involved a diet that emphasized fruits, vegetables and low-fat dairy products and included wholegrains, poultry, fish and nuts while reducing the amounts of red meat, sweets and sugar-containing beverages. Two variants of the intervention diet were used: a fruit and vegetables (F-V) diet and a low fat F-V (DASH) diet. The latter was designed to lower the intake of total and saturated fat as well as dietary cholesterol. In comparison with a "typical" diet in the United States, both intervention diets lowered blood pressure but the DASH diet was more effective in substantially reducing systolic and diastolic blood pressures, both in people with and those without hypertension.[104] The DASH diet was also demonstrated to be effective as first-line therapy in individuals with stage I isolated systolic hyper-

tension (i.e. with a systolic blood pressure of 140–159 mmHg and a diastolic blood pressure below 90 mmHg), with 78% of those on the DASH diet reducing their systolic blood pressure to <140 mmHg, in comparison to 24% in the control group.[209] The DASH diet resulted in lowering plasma levels of total cholesterol and LDL cholesterol but these changes were also accompanied by a reduction in HDL cholesterol levels.[210] While the Framingham risk score improved as a result of the impact on total and LDL cholesterol as well as blood pressure, the impact of the associated reduction in HDL cholesterol needs to be assessed.

The DASH trial was followed by a well-designed factorial trial combining the DASH diet with high, intermediate and low levels of sodium consumption and measuring the effects on blood pressure, in comparison to a control diet typical of the United States, administered with similar graded variations in the sodium content.[124] Within each assigned group (DASH v typical), participants ate foods with high, intermediate and low levels of sodium for 30 consecutive days each, in random order. Reduction in sodium intake, at each level, resulted in significant lowering of systolic and diastolic blood pressures in both DASH and control groups. The fall was, however, maximal when the DASH diet was modified to reduce the sodium content. As compared with the control diet with a high sodium level, the DASH diet with a low sodium level led to a mean systolic blood pressure that was 7.1 mmHg lower in participants without hypertension and 11.5 mmHg lower in participants with hypertension (Fig. 23.3). There was also a −4.5 mmHg difference in the mean diastolic pressure level, between the low sodium-DASH diet phase and the high sodium-control diet phase of the trial.

The effects of the low sodium-DASH diet have great potential for application in both population-based and individual focused strategies for prevention and control of high blood pressure and associated CVD. Adoption of the low sodium-DASH diet, by populations at large, is

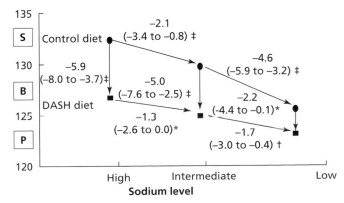

Figure 23.3 Effect of the low sodium DASH diet on systolic blood pressure.

likely to be safe and beneficial in shifting the population distributions of blood pressure (and plasma cholesterol) towards lower levels of cumulative risk of CVD in those populations. Similarly, this diet will also provide an effective non-pharmacologic therapeutic intervention in the clinical management of individuals identified to be at increased risk of CVD because of high blood pressure and associated risk factors.

Implications for policy

Diet and nutrition play a critical role in the causation of major CVDs and, along with physical activity, influence many of the biologic variables that mediate the risk of those diseases. There is, therefore, an opportunity to alter the direction and dimensions of the global CVD epidemic through policy interventions (at the local, national and global levels), which promote the availability, affordability and acceptability of health-promoting diets and restrain the marketing and consumption of unhealthy foods.

Currently available evidence strongly indicates that cardiovascular health is heavily influenced by the quality of dietary fat and the quantity of fruits and vegetables as well as salt consumed daily. While several other food items also contribute to enhanced or decreased risk of CVD, these remain the principal determinants of diet-related CVD risk. Whether derived from controlled clinical trials or an ecologic study of reasons for the sharp decline in coronary mortality in Poland since 1991, the evidence suggests that dietary changes can substantially alter the risk of CVD.[211,212] Policies must, therefore, address these directly and decisively.

These measures must encompass a wide range of educational as well as regulatory measures, acting through price and non-price mechanisms. That success in reducing CVD risk factor levels as well as CVD mortality is achievable through such measures that influence usual diet patterns is clear from the experience of developed countries.[213] Developing countries like Mauritius too have shown that population levels of CVD risk factors can be altered by a combination of community education and regulatory inter-

---

BOX 23.3 Dietary recommendations for cardiovascular health

- A low intake of saturated fatty acids (SFAs): less than 7% of daily energy intake (within these limits, intake of foods rich in myristic and palmitic acids should be especially reduced). Edible fat intake need not exceed 40 g and total fat intake should be limited to levels at which fat will provide no more than 20% of total energy. The use of ghee (clarified butter) should be restricted to special occasions and should not be a regular daily feature.
- A very low intake of trans fatty acids (hydrogenated oils and fats): less than 1% of daily energy intake.
- Adequate intake of polyunsaturated fatty acids (PUFAs): 6–10% of daily energy intake, with an optimal balance of n-6 PUFAs and n-3 PUFAs at 5–8% and 1–2% levels of daily energy intake, respectively.
- Intake of monounsaturated fatty acids (MUFAs) to make up the rest of daily energy intake from fats, with daily total fat intake ranging between 15% and 30% of daily energy intake (this may be based on current levels of population consumption in different regions and modified in accordance with age, activity and goals of body weight).
- While there is no evidence that links the quantity of dietary fat to CVD, independent of the effects of fat composition and unhealthy weight gain, there are concerns over potential excess energy consumption associated with an unrestricted fat intake. These support a recommendation that fat intake should not exceed 30% of daily energy intake. However, in very active groups with healthy dietary practices and stable healthy weight, fat intake may go up to 35% of energy.
- Dietary cholesterol consumption should be restricted to less than 300 mg per day, mainly through the restriction of dairy fats.
- Daily intake of fresh fruit and vegetables (including berries, green leafy and cruciferous vegetables and legumes), in an adequate quantity (400–500 g per day), is recommended to reduce the risk of CHD, stroke and high blood pressure.
- Restrict daily salt (sodium chloride) intake to less than 5 g per day. This should take into account total sodium intake from all dietary sources. Minimize other forms of sodium consumption such as as through food additives or preservatives, such as monosodium glutamate (MSG). Potassium intake should be at a level which will keep the sodium:potassium ratio close to 1, i.e. at daily potassium intake levels of 70–80 mmol per day. This may be achieved through adequate daily consumption of fruits and vegetables. Such a balance may also be obtained through use of potassium-enriched low-sodium salt substitutes.
- The consumption of fish and other marine foods should provide over 200 mg per day of docosahexaenoic acid (DHA) and eicosapentaenoic acid (EPA).
- Regular low to moderate consumption of alcohol (that is 1–2 drinks per day) is protective against CHD. Concerns about other cardiovascular and health risks associated with alcohol consumption (including stroke, hypertension and some cancers) do not favor a general recommendation for its use.

Source: Adapted from WHO Expert Consultation on Diet and Prevention of Chronic Diseases 2002: www.who.int/hpr/nutrition/ExpertConsultationGE.htm

ventions related to the price of edible oils.[214] Measures to influence the quality of dietary fat (as well as the total quantity) consumed must address the elimination of trans fats and reduction of saturated fats from the daily diet. Governments must work with the food industry to influence production, processing, pricing and labeling of food products so that these goals can be met. Consumer education must be enhanced so that informed choices can be made, even as the availability of healthier foods is promoted through such measures. As market economy becomes a globally pervasive economic model, it must be recognized that markets are not autonomous entities and should be molded, for public good, by consumer consciousness as well as enlightened regulatory measures.

Recent initiatives in different regions of the world offer models for such policy interventions. The agreement between the food industry and the food standard authorities of UK, to progressively reduce the salt content in processed foods, is yielding results in terms of reduced salt consumption by the population.[215] The ban on trans fats in the restaurants of New York and for processed foods in Denmark exemplifies nutrition regulation in the interests of public health.[216] Food labeling, ranging from display of nutrient composition to "traffic lights" signals indicating the health-related nutrient profile of food products, is being practiced or proposed by an increasing number of countries. Voluntary or legally imposed restrictions on advertising of high-energy/low-nutrient beverages and foods to young people ("advertising code") are also on the anvil in the European Union. The WHO's Global Strategy on Diet and Physical Activity and Health (DPAS) provides guidelines for multisectoral policies which countries should implement to prevent CVD and other chronic diseases.[217] Policy interventions such as these do not as yet have the evidence of evaluated implementation to support them. However, the weight of scientific evidence which links salt, trans fats and refined sugars to high risk of CVD and other health disorders should be adequate to initiate such policies.

As these policies are progressively implemented, rigorous evaluation must be conducted to assess their impact. As Louis Pasteur exhorted his research students, "Keep your enthusiasm but let strict verification be its constant companion".

References

1. Reddy KS. Cardiovascular diseases in the developing countries: dimensions, determinants, dynamics and directions for public health action. *Public Health Nutr* 2002;**5**:231–7.
2. Lichtenstein AH, Appel LJ, Brands M, Carnethon M, Daniels S, Franch HA *et al.* Diet and Lifestyle Recommendations Revision 2006 A scientific statement from the American Heart Association Nutrition Committee. *Circulation* 2006;**114**:82–96.
3. Clayton D, McKeigue PM. Epidemiological methods for studying genes and environmental factors in complex diseases. *Lancet* 2001;**358**(9290):1356–60.
4. Hines LM, Stampfer MJ, Ma J *et al.* Genetic variation in alcohol dehydrogenase and the beneficial effect of moderate alcohol consumption on myocardial infarction. *N Engl J Med* 2001;**344**: 549–55.
5. Krause BR, Princen HMG. Lack of predictability of classical animal models for hypolipidemic activity: a good time for mice? *Atherosclerosis* 1998;**140**:15–24.
6. Verschuren WMM, Jacobs DR, Bloemberg BPM *et al.* Serum total cholesterol and long-term coronary heart disease mortality in different cultures: twenty-five year follow-up of the Seven Country Study. *JAMA* 1995;**274**:131–6.
7. Rudel LL, Parks JS, Sowyer JK. Compared with dietary mono unsaturated and saturated fat, poly unsaturated fat protects African green monkeys from coronary artery arteriosclerosis. *Arterioscler Throm Vasc Biol* 1995;**15**:2101–10.
8. Rudel LL, Hains JL, Sowyer JK *et al.* Hepatic origin of cholesteryl oliate in coronary artery arteriosclerosis in African green monkeys: enrichment by dietary mono unsaturated fat. *J Clin Invest* 1997;**100**:74–83.
9. De Lorgeril M, Salen P, Martin JL *et al.* Mediterranean diet, traditional risk factors, and the rate of cardiovascular complications after myocardial infarction: final report of Lyon Diet Heart Study. *Circulation* 1999;**99**:779–85.
10. Willett WC. *Nutritional Epidemiology*. New York: Oxford University Press, 1990.
11. Kris-Etherton P, Daniels SR, Eckel RH *et al*, for the Nutrition Committee of the American Heart Association. Summary of the Scientific Conference on Dietary Fatty Acids and Cardiovascular Health. *Circulation* 2001;**103**:1034–9.
12. Cutler JA, Follmann D, Allender PS. Randomized trials of sodium reduction: an overview. *Am J Clin Nutr* 1997;**65**(suppl 2):643S–651S.
13. Willett W. Concepts and controversies on diet: stop recommending low-fat diets! *Permanente J* 2003;**7**(3):24–33.
14. Ghafoorunissa. Dietary lipids and heart disease – the Indian context. *Natl Med J India* 1994;**7**:270–5.
15. Hopkins PN. Effects of dietary cholesterol on serum cholesterol: a meta-analysis and review. *Am J Clin Nutr* 1992;**55**: 1060–70.
16. Weggemans RM, Zock PL, Katan MB, Dietary cholesterol from eggs increases the ratio of total cholesterol to high- density lipoprotein cholesterol in humans: a meta-analysis. *Am J Clin Nutr* 2001;**73**:885–91.
17. Stamler JS, Shekelle RB. Dietary cholesterol and human coronary heart disease. *Arch Pathol Lab Med* 1988;**112**:1032–40.
18. Hu F, Stampfer MJ, Rimm EB *et al.* A prospective study of egg consumption and risk of cardiovascular disease in men and women. *JAMA* 1999;**281**:1387–94.
19. Grundy S, Vega GL. Plasma cholesterol responsiveness to saturated fatty acids. *Am J Clin Nutr* 1998;**47**:822–4.
20. Katan MJ, Zock PL, Mensink RP. Dietary oils, serum lipoproteins and coronary heart disease. *Am J Clin Nutr* 1995;**61**(suppl): 1368S–73S.
21. Hu F, Stampfer MJ, Manson JE *et al.* Dietary fat intake and the risk of coronary heart disease in women. *N Engl J Med* 1997;**337**:1491–9.

22. Assmann G, Schulte H. Relation of high-density lipoprotein cholesterol and triglycerides to incidence of atherosclerotic coronary artery disease (the PROCAM experience). *Am J Cardiol* 1992;**70**:733–7.

23. Kromhout D, Menotti A, Bloemberg B et al. Dietary saturated and trans fatty acids and cholesterol and 25-year mortality from coronary heart disease: the Seven Countries Study. *Prev Med* 1995;**24**:308–15.

24. Mensink RP, Katan MB. Effect of dietary fatty acids on serum lipids and lipoproteins – a meta-analysis of 27 trials. *Arterioscler Thromb* 1992;**12**:911–19.

25. Ascherio A, Katan MB, Zock PL, Stampfer MJ, Willett WC. Trans fatty acids and coronary heart disease. *N Engl J Med* 1997;**340**:1994–8.

26. Willett WC, Stampfer MJ, Manson JE et al. Intake of trans fatty acids and risk of coronary heart disease among women. *Lancet* 1993;**341**:581–5.

27. Ascherio A, Rimm EB, Giovannucci EL et al. Dietary fat and risk of coronary heart disease in men: cohort follow up study in the United States. *BMJ* 1996;**313**:84–90.

28. Oomen CM, Ocke MC, Feskens EDM et al. Association between trans fatty acid intake and 10-year risk of coronary heart disease in the Zutphen Elderly Study: a prospective population-based study. *Lancet* 2001;**357**:746–51.

29. Katan MB. Trans fatty acids and plasma lipoproteins. *Nutr Rev* 2000;**58**:188–91.

30. Kris-Etherton PM. Monosaturated fatty acids and risk of cardiovascular disease. *Circulation* 1999;**100**:1253–8.

31. Mori TA, Beilin LJ. Long-chain omega 3 fatty acids, blood lipids and cardiovascular risk reduction. *Curr Opin Lipidol* 2001;**12**:11–17.

32. Mori TA, Bao DQ, Burke V et al. Purified eicosapentaenoic acid and docosahexaenoic acid have differential effects on serum lipids and lipoproteins, LDL-particle size, glucose and insulin, in mildly hyperlipidaemic men. *Am J Clin Nutr* 2000;**71**:1085–94.

33. Harris WS. n-3 fatty acids and serum lipoproteins: human studies. *Am J Clin Nutr* 1997;**65**: 1645S–1654S.

34. GISSI Prevenzione Investigators. Dietary supplementation with n-3 polyunsaturated fatty acids and vitamin E after myocardial infarction: results of the GISSI Prevenzione Trial. Gruppo Italiano per lo Studio della Sopravvivenza nell'Infarto Miocardico. *Lancet* 1999;**354**:447–55.

35. Von Schacky C. n-3 fatty acids and the prevention of coronary atherosclerosis. *Am J Clin Nutr* 2000;**71**(1 suppl): 224S–227S.

36. Lemaitre RN, King IB, Raghunathan TE et al. Cell membrane trans-fatty acids and the risk of primary cardiac arrest. *Circulation* 2002;**105**:697–701.

37. McLennan PL, Abeywardena MY, Charnock JS. Dietary fish oil prevents ventricular fibrillation following coronary artery occlusion and reperfusion. *Am Heart J* 1998;**116**: 709–17.

38. Hetzel BS, Charnock JS, Dwyer T, McLennan PL. Fall in coronary heart disease mortality in U.S.A. and Australia due to sudden death: evidence for the role of polyunsaturated fat. *J Clin Epidemiol* 1989;**42**:885–93.

39. Katan MB, Zock PL, Mensink RP. Effects of fats and fatty acids on blood lipids in humans: an overview. *Am J Clin Nutr* 1994;**60**(6 suppl):1017S–1022S.

40. Katan MB, Mensink R, Van Tol A et al. Dietary trans-fatty acids and their impact on plasma lipoproteins. *Can J Cardiol* 1995; 11(suppl G):36G–38G.

41. de Roos NM, Bots ML, Katan MB. Replacement of dietary saturated fatty acids by trans-fatty acids lowers serum HDL cholesterol and impairs endothelial function in healthy men and women. *Arterioscler Thromb Vasc Biol* 2001;**21**(7):1233–7.

42. Grundy SM. What is the desirable ratio of saturated, polyunsaturated, and monounsaturated fatty acids in the diet? *Am J Clin Nutr* 1997;**66**(suppl):988S–990S.

43. Grundy SM. The optimal ratio of fat-to-carbohydrate in the diet. *Annu Rev Nutr* 1999;**19**:325–41.

44. Willett WC. Dietary fat plays a major role in obesity. *Obesity Rev* 2002;**3**:59–68.

45. Xu J, Eilat-Adar S, Loria C, Goldbourt U, Howard BV, Fabsitz RR et al. Dietary fat intake and risk of coronary heart disease: the Strong Heart Study. *Am J Clin Nutr* 2006;**84**:894–902.

46. Steckel M, 1996–2007. Available at: www.spinalhealth.net/fats.html.

47. Truswell AS. Food carbohydrates and plasma lipids – an update. *Am J Clin Nutr* 1994;**59**(suppl):710S–8S.

48. Jenkins DJA, Jenkins AL, Wolever TMS et al. Low glycemic index: lente carbohydrates and physiological effects of altered food frequency. *Am J Clin Nutr* 1994;**59**(suppl):706S–9S.

49. Liu S, Willet WC, Stampfer MJ et al. A prospective study of dietary glycemic load, carbohydrate intake, and risk of coronary heart disease in US women. *Am J Clin Nutr* 2000;**71**:1455–61.

50. Liu S, Willett WC, Stampfer MJ et al. A prospective study of dietary glycemic load, carbohydrate intake, and risk of coronary heart disease in US women. *Am J Clin Nutr* 2000;**71**:1455–61.

51. Beulens JWJ, de Bruijne LM, Stolk RP et al. High dietary glycaemic load and glycemic index increase risk of cardiovascular disease among middle-aged women: a population-based follow-up study. *J Am Coll Cardiol* 2007;**50**:14–21.

52. National Heart Foundation of Australia. Position statement: carbohydrates, dietary fibre, glycaemic index/load and cardiovascular disease. 2006. Available at: www.heartfoundation.com.au.

53. Marlett JA. Content and composition of dietary fiber in 117 frequently consumed foods. *J Am Diet Assoc* 1992;**92**:175–86.

54. Shikany JM, Ala B, White GL. Dietary guidelines for chronic disease prevention. *South Med J* 2000;**93**:1138–51.

55. Truswell AS. Cereal grains and coronary heart disease. *Eur J Clin Nutr* 2002;**56**:1–14.

56. Ludwig DS, Pereira MA, Kroenke CH et al. Dietary fiber, weight gain, and cardiovascular risk factors in young adults. *JAMA* 1999;**282**:1539–46.

57. Liu S, Stampfer MJ, Hu FB et al. Whole grain consumption and the risk of coronary heart disease: from the Nurses' Health Study. *Am J Clin Nutr* 1999;**70**:412–19.

58. Rimm EB, Ascherio A, Giovannucci E et al. Vegetable, fruit and cereal fiber intake and risk of coronary heart disease among men. *JAMA* 1996;**275**:447–51.

59. Anderson JW. Whole grains protect against atherosclerotic cardiovascular disease. *Proc Nutr Soc* 2003;**62**:135–42.

60. Jacobs DR, Gallaher DD. Whole grain intake and cardiovascular disease: a review. *Curr Atheroscler Rep* 2004;**6**:415–23.

61. Richardson DP. Wholegrain health claims in Europe. *Proc Nutr Soc* 2003;**62**:161–9.

62. Topping D. Relationship Between Whole Grain Intake and Risk of Coronary Heart Disease. Food Standards Australia New Zealand: Diet-disease Relationship Review 2006. http://www.foodstandard.gov.au

63. Koh-Banerjee P, Franz M, Sampson L, Liu S, Jacobs DR Jr, Spiegelman D *et al.* Changes in whole-grain, bran, and cereal fibre consumption in relation to 8-y weight gain among men. *Am J Clin Nutr* 2004;**80**:1237–45.

64. Liu S, Willett WC, Manson JE, Hu FB, Rosner B, Colditz G. Relation between changes inintakes of dietary fibre and grain products and changes in weight and development of obesity among middle-aged women. *Am J Clin Nutr* 2003;**78**:920–7.

65. Karmally W, Montez MG, Palmas W *et al.* Cholesterol-lowering benefits of oat-containing cereal in Hispanic Americans. *J Am Diet Assoc* 2005;**105**:967–70.

66. Davy BM, Davy KP, Ho RC, Beske SD, Davrath LR, Melby CL. High-fiber oat cereal compared with wheat cereal consumption favorably alters LDL-cholesterol subclass and particle numbers in middle-aged and older men. *Am J Clin Nutr* 2002;**76**:351–8.

67. Rimm EB, Stampfer MJ. Antioxidants for vascular disease. *Med Clin North Am* 2000;**84**:239–49.

68. Ness AR. Commentary: beyond beta-carotene – antioxidants and cardiovascular disease. *Int J Epidemiol* 2001;**30**:143–4.

69. Yusuf S, Dagenais G, Pogue J, Sleight P. Vitamin E supplementation and cardiovascular events in high-risk patients. The Heart Outcomes Prevention Evaluation Study Investigators. *N Engl J Med* 2000;**345**:154–60.

70. Collaborative Group of the Primary Prevention Project (PPP). Low-dose aspirin and vitamin E in people at cardiovascular risk: a randomized trial in general practice. *Lancet* 2001;**357**:89–95.

71. Bleys J, Miller ER, Pastor-Barriuso R, Appel LJ, Guallar E. Vitamin-mineral supplementation and the progression of atherosclerosis: a meta-analysis of randomized controlled trials *Am J Clin Nutr* 2006;**84**:880–7.

72. Halliwell B. Dietary polyphenols: good, bad, or indifferent for your health? *Cardiovasc Res* 2007;**73**:341–7.

73. Ding EL, Hutfless SM, Ding X, Girotra S. Chocolate and prevention of cardiovascular disease: a systematic review. *Nutr Metab (Lond)* 2006;**3**:2–14.

74. Florescu M. Chocolate and prevention of cardiovascular disease: a systematic review. *J Clin Med* 2006;**1**(3):84.

75. Szmitko PE, Verma S. Antiatherogenic potential of red wine: clinician update. *Am J Physiol Heart Circ Physiol* 2005;**288**:H2023–30.

76. Hertog MGL, Feskens EJM, Hollman PCH, Katan MB, Kromhout D. Dietary antioxidant flavonoids and risk of coronary heart disease. The Zutphen Elderly Study. *Lancet* 1993;**342**:1007–11.

77. Kuriyama S, Shimazu T, Ohmori K, Kikuchi N, Nakaya N, Nishino Y *et al.* Green tea consumption and mortality due to cardiovascular disease, cancer, and all causes in Japan – the Ohsaki Study. *JAMA* 2006;**296**(10):1255–65.

78. Kuriyama S. The relation between green tea consumption and cardiovascular disease as evidenced by epidemiological studies. *J Nutr* 2008;**138**:1548S–1553S.

79. Sesso HD, Gaziano JM, Liu S, Buring JE. Flavonoid intake and the risk of cardiovascular disease in women. *Am J Clin Nutr* 2003;**77**:1400–8.

80. Stampfer MJ, Malinow MR, Willett WC *et al.* A prospective study of plasma homocysteine and risk of myocardial infarction in US physicians. *JAMA* 1992;**268**:877–81.

81. Selhub J, Jacques PF, Bostom AG *et al.* Association between plasma homocysteine concentrations and extracranial carotid-artery stenosis. *N Engl J Med* 1995;**332**:286–91.

82. Stampfer MJ, Malinow MR, Willett WC *et al.* A prospective study of plasma homocysteine and risk of myocardial infarction in US physicians. *JAMA* 1992;**268**:877–81.

83. Welch GN, Loscalzo J. Homocysteine and atherothrombosis. *N Engl J Med* 1998;**338**:1042–50.

84. Brouwer IA, van Dusseldorp M, Thomas CM *et al.* Low dose folic acid supplementation decreases plasma homocysteine concentrations: a randomized trial. *Am J Clin Nutr* 1999;**69**:99–104.

85. Scott JM. Homocysteine and cardiovascular risk. *Am J Clin Nutr* 2000;**72**:333–4.

86. Bonaa KH. NORVIT: randomized trial of homocysteine-lowering with B-vitamins for secondary prevention of cardiovascular disease after acute myocardial infarction. Program and Abstracts from the European Society of Cardiology Congress 2005, September 3–7.

87. Toole JF, Malinow MR, Chambless LE *et al.* Lowering homocysteine in patients with ischemic stroke to prevent recurrent stroke, myocardial infarction, and death. The Vitamin Intervention for Stroke Prevention (VISP) randomized controlled trial. *JAMA* 2004;**291**:565–75.

88. Lonn E, Yusuf S, Arnold MJ, for the Heart Outcomes Prevention Evaluation (HOPE) 2 Investigators. Homocysteine lowering with folic acid and B vitamins in vascular disease. *N Engl J Med* 2006;**354**(15):1567–77.

89. Guttormsen AB, Ueland PM, Svarstad E, Refsum H. Kinetic basis of hyperhomocysteinemia in patients with chronic renal failure. *Kidney Int* 1997;**52**:495–502.

90. Gibbs CR, Lip GYH, Beevers DG. Salt and cardiovascular disease: clinical and epidemiological evidence. *J Cardiovasc Risk* 2000;**7**:9–13.

91. INTERSALT Cooperative Research Group. INTERSALT: an international study of electrolyte excretion and blood pressure. Results for 24 hr urinary sodium and potassium excretion. *BMJ* 1988;**297**:319–28.

92. Elliott P, Stamler J, Nicholas R *et al*, for the INTERSALT Cooperative Research Group. INTERSALT revisited: further analyses of 24 hr sodium excretion and blood pressure within and across populations. *BMJ* 1996;**312**:1249–1253.

93. Mancilha Carvalho JJ, Baruzzi RG, Howard PF *et al.* Blood pressure in four remote populations in the Intersalt study. *Hypertension* 1989;**14**:238–46.

94. Poulter NK, Khaw KT, Hopwood BEC, Mugambi M, Peart WS, Rose G *et al.* The Kenyan Luo migration study: observations on the initiation of a rise in blood pressure. *BMJ* 1990;**300**:967–72.

95. Law MR, Frost MD, Wald NJ. By how much does salt reduction lower blood pressure? III. Analysis of data from trials of salt reduction. *BMJ* 1991;**302**:819–24.

96. Tuomilehto J, Jousilahti P, Rastenyte D, Moltchanov V, Tanskanen A, Pietinen P, Nissinen A. Urinary sodium excretion and

cardiovascular mortality in Finland: a prospective study. *Lancet* 2001;**357**:848–51.

97. Law MR, Frost CD, Wald NJ III. Analysis of data from trials of salt reduction. *BMJ* 1991;**302**:819–24.

98. Geleijnse JM, Hofman A, Witteman JC, Hazebroek AA, Valkenburg HA, Grobbee DE. Long-term effects of neonatal sodium restriction on blood pressure. *Hypertension* **1997**;29: 913–17. (Published erratum in Hypertension 1997;29:1211.)

99. Whelton PK, Appel LJ, Espeland MA *et al.* Sodium reduction and weight loss in the treatment of hypertension in older persons – a randomized controlled Trial of Nonpharmacologic Interventions in the Elderly (TONE). TONE Collaborative Research Group. *JAMA* 1998;**279**:839–46.

100. Cook NR, Kumanyika SK, Cutler JA, Whelton PK. Dose-response of sodium excretion and blood pressure change among overweight, nonhypertensive adults in a 3-year dietary intervention study. *J Hum Hypertens* 2005;**19**:47–54.

101. Appel LJ, Espeland MA, Easter L, Wilson AC, Folmar S, Lacy CR. Effects of redcued sodium intake on hypertension control in older individuals. Results from the Trial of Nonpharmacological Interventions in the Elderly (TONE). *Arch Intern Med* 2001;**161**(5):685–93.

102. Miller ER, Erlinger TP, Young DR, Jehn M, Charleston J, Rhodes D *et al.* Results of the Diet, Exercise, and Weight Loss Intervention Trial (DEW-IT). *Hypertension* 2002;**40**:612–18.

103. Lien LF, Brown AJ, Ard JD, Loria C, Erlinger TP, Feldstein AC *et al.* Effects of PREMIER lifestyle modifications on participants with and without the metabolic syndrome. *Hypertension* 2007; **50**:609–16.

104. Sacks FM, Svetkey LP, Vollmer WM *et al.* Effects on blood pressure of reduced dietary sodium and the Dietary Approaches to Stop Hypertension (DASH) Diet. *N Engl J Med* 2001;**344**:3–10.

105. Schmieder RE, Messerli FH, Garavaglia GE, Nunez BD. Dietary salt intake. A determinent of cardiac involvement in essential hypertension. *Circulation* 1988;**78**:951–6.

106. Forte JG, Miguel JM, Miguel MJ *et al.* Salt and blood pressure: a community trial. *J Hum Hypertens* 1989;**3**:179–84.

107. Tian HG, Guo ZY, Hu G *et al.* Changes in sodium intake and blood pressure in a community-based intervention project in China. *J Hum Hypertens* 1995;**9**:959–68.

108. Staessen J, Bulpitt CJ, Fagard R *et al.* Salt intake and blood pressure in the general population: a controlled intervention trial in two towns. *J Hypertens* 1988;**6**:965–73.

109. Tobian L, Hanlon S. High sodium chloride diets injure arteries and raise mortality without raising blood pressure. *Hypertension* 1990;**15**:900–3.

110. Xie JX, Sasaki S, Joossens JV, Kesteloot H. The relationship between urinary cations obtained from the INTERSALT study and cerebrovascular mortality. *J Hum Hypertens* 1992;**6**:17–21.

111. Young DB, Lin H, McCabe RD. Potassium's cardiovascular protective mechanisms. *Am J Physiol* 1995;**268**:R825–R837.

112. Krishna GG, Miller E, Kapoor S. Increased blood pressure during potassium depletion in normotensive men. *N Engl J Med* 1989;**320**:1177–82.

113. Whelton PK, He J, Cutler JA *et al.* Effects of oral potassium on blood pressure: meta-analysis of randomized controlled clinical trials. *JAMA* 1996;**275**:1016–22.

114. Khaw KT, Barrett-Connor E. Dietary potassium and stroke associated mortality. *N Engl J Med* 1987;**316**:235–40.

115. National Heart Foundation of Australia. Summary of evidence statement on the relationships between dietary electrolytes and cardiovascular disease, October 2006. Available at: www.heart-foundation.com.au.

116. Griffith LE, Guyatt GH, Cook RJ *et al.* The influence of dietary and non-dietary calcium supplementation on blood pressure. An updated meta-analysis of randomized controlled trials. *J Hypertens* 1999;**12**:84–92.

117. Mizushima S, Cuppauccio FP, Nichols R, Elliott P. Dietary magnesium intake and blood pressure: a qualitative overview of the observational studies. *J Hum Hypertens* 1998;**12**:447–53.

118. Nestle M. Animal v. plant foods in human diets and health: is the historical record unequivocal? *Proc Nutr Soc* 1999;**58**: 211–18.

119. Law MR, Morris JK. By how much does fruit and vegetable consumption reduce the risk of ischaemic heart disease? *Eur J Clin Nutr* 1998;**52**:549–56.

120. Ness AR, Powles JW. Fruit and vegetables, and cardiovascular disease: a review. *Int J Epidemiol* 1997;**26**:1–13.

121. Liu S, Manson JE, Lee I-M *et al.* Fruit and vegetable intake and risk of cardiovascular disease: the Women's Health Study. *Am J Clin Nutr* 2000;**72**:922–8.

122. Liu S, Lee I-M, Ajani U *et al.* Intake of vegetables rich in carotenoids and risk of coronary heart disease in men: the Physicians' Health Study. *Int J Epidemiol* 2001;**30**:130–5.

123. Joshipura KJ, Ascherio A, Manson JF *et al.* Fruit and vegetable intake in relation to risk of ischemic stroke. *JAMA* 1999;**282**: 1233–9.

124. Appel LJ, Moore TJ, Obarzanek E *et al.* A clinical trial of the effects of dietary patterns on blood pressure. *N Engl J Med* 1998;**336**:1117–24.

125. Winkler E, Newman B. Food Standards Australia New Zealand Diet – Disease Relationship Review. Dietary fruit and vegetable intake and risk of coronary heart disease. Report July 2000. http://www.foodstandard.gov.au

126. Kromhout D, Bosschieter EB, de Lezenne Coulander C. The inverse relation between fish consumption and 20 year mortality from coronary heart disease. *N Engl J Med* 1985;**312**: 1205–9.

127. Daviglus ML, Stamler J, Orencia AJ *et al.* Fish consumption and the 30-year risk of fatal myocardial infarction. *N Engl J Med* 1997;**336**:1046–53.

128. Marckmann P, Gronbaek M. Fish consumption and coronary heart disease mortality. A systematic review of prospective cohort studies. *Eur J Clin Nutr* 1999;**53**:585–90.

129. Burr ML, Fehily AM, Gilbert JF *et al.* Effects of changes in fat, fish and fibre intakes on death and myocardial reinfarction: diet and reinfarction trial (DART). *Lancet* 1989;**2**:757–61.

130. Gillman MW, Cupples LA, Millen BE *et al.* Inverse association of dietary fat with development of ischaemic stroke in men. *JAMA* 1997;**278**:2145–50.

131. Orenica AJ, Daviglus ML, Dyer AR *et al.* Fish consumption and stroke in men. *Stroke* 1996;**27**:204–9.

132. Zhang J, Sasaki S, Amano K, Kesteloot H. Fish consumption and mortality from all causes, ischaemic heart disease and stroke: an epidemiological study. *Prev Med* 1999;**28**:520–9.

133. Iso H, Rexrode KM, Stampfer MJ, Manson JE, Colditz GA, Speizer FE *et al.* Intake of fish and ω3 and risk of stroke in women. *JAMA* 2001;**285**(3):304–12.

134. He K, Rimm EB, Merchant A, Rosner BA, Stampfer MJ, Willett WC, Ascherio A. Fish consumption and risk of stroke in men. *JAMA* 2002;**288**(24):3130–6.

135. Mozaffarian D, Longstreth WT, Lemaitre RN, Manolio TA, Kuller LH, Burke GL, Siscovick DS. Fish consumption and stroke risk in elderly individuals: the cardiovascular health study. *Arch Intern Med* 2005;**165**(2):200–6.

136. Erkkila AT, Lichtenstein AH, Mozaffarian D, Herrington DM. Fish intake is associated with a reduced progression of coronary artery atherosclerosis in postmenopausal women with coronary artery disease. *Am J Clin Nutr* 2004;**80**(3):626–32.

137. Mozzaffarian D, Psaty BM, Rimm EB, Lemaitre RN, Burke GL, Lyles MF *et al.* Fish intake and risk of incident atrial fibrillation. *Circulation* 2004;**110**(4):368–73.

138. Calo L, Bianconi L, Colivicchi F, Lamberti F, Loricchio ML, de Ruvo E *et al.* N-3 fatty acids for the prevention of atrial fibrillation after coronary artery bypass surgery: a randomized, controlled trial. *J Am Coll Cardiol* 2005;**45**(10):1723–8.

139. Singer P, Wirth M. Can n-3 PUFA reduce cardiac arrhythmias? Results of a clinical trial. *Prostaglandins Leukotrienes Essential Fatty Acids* 2004;**71**(3):153–9.

140. Christensen JH, Riahi S, Schmidt EB, Molgaard H, Kirstein Pedersen A, Heath F *et al.* n-3 Fatty acids and ventricular arrhythmias in patients with ischaemic heart disease and implantable cardioverter defibrillators. *Europace* 2005;**7**(4):338–44.

141. Leaf A, Albert CM, Josephson M, Steinhaus D, Kluger J, Kang JX *et al.* Prevention of fatal arrhythmias in high-risk subjects by fish oil n-3 fatty acid intake. *Circulation* 2005;**112**(18):2762–8.

142. Raitt MH, Connor WE, Morris C, Kron J, Halperin B, Chugh SS *et al.* Fish oil supplementation and risk of ventricular tachycardia and ventricular fibrillation in patients with implantable defibrillators: a randomized controlled trial. *JAMA* 2005;**293**(23):2884–91.

143. He K, Song Y, Daviglus ML, Liu K, Van Horn L, Dyer AR. Greenland P. Accumulated evidence on fish consumption and CHD mortality: a meta-analysis of cohort studies. *Circulation* 2004;**109**(22):2705–11.

144. Whelton SP, He J, Whelton PK, Muntner P. Meta-analysis of observational studies on fish intake and CHD. *Am J Cardiol* 2004;**93**(9):1119–23.

145. Hooper L, Harrison RA, Summerbell CD, Moore H, Worthington HV, Ness A, Capps N, Davey Smith G, Riemersma R, Ebrahim S. Omega 3 fatty acids for prevention and treatment of cardiovascular disease. *Cochrane Database of Systematic Reviews* 2004, Issue 4. Art. No.: CD003177. DOI: 10.1002/14651858. CD003177.pub2.

146. Burr ML, Ashfield-Watt PAL, Dunstan FDJ *et al.* Lack of benefit of dietary advice to men with angina: results of a controlled trial. *Eur J Clin Nutr* 2003;**57**:193–200.

147. Burr ML, Fehily AM, Gilbert JF, Rogers S, Holliday RM, Sweetnam PM *et al.* Effects of changes in fat, fish, and fibre intakes on death and myocardial reinfarction: Diet And Reinfarction Trial (DART). *Lancet* 1989;**2**(8666):757–61.

148. Balk EM, Lichtenstein AH, Chung M, Kupelnick B, Chew P, Lau J. Effects of omega-3 fatty acids on serum markers of cardiovascular disease risk: a systematic review. *Atherosclerosis* 2006;**189**(1):19–30.

149. Hooper L, Thompson RL, Harrison RA, Summerbell CD, Ness AR, Moore HJ *et al.* Risks and benefits of omega 3 fats for mortality, cardiovascular disease, and cancer: systematic review. *BMJ* 2006;**332**(7544):752–60.

150. Mozaffarian D, Rimm EB. Fish intake, contaminants, and human health: evaluating the risks and the benefits. *JAMA* 2006;**296**(15):1885–99.

151. Kris-Etherton PM, Zhao G, Binkoski AE *et al.* The effects of nuts on coronary heart disease risk. *Nutr Rev* 2001;**59**:103–11.

152. Fraser GE, Sabate J, Beeson WL, Strahan TM. A possible protective effect of nut consumption on risk of coronary heart disease. The Adventist Health Study. *Arch Intern Med* 1992;**152**:1416–24.

153. Fraser GE, Lindsted KD, Beeson WL. Effect of risk factor values on lifetime risk of and age at that first coronary event. The Adventist Health Study. *Am J Epidemiol* 1995;**142**:746–58.

154. Hu FB, Stamfer MJ. Nut consumption and risk of coronary heart disease: a review of epidemiologic evidence. *Curr Atherosclero Rep* 1999;**1**:204–9.

155. Office of Nutritional Products, Labeling and Dietary Supplements, Food and Drug Administration. Qualified health claims: letter of enforcement discretion – nuts and coronary heart disease (docket No 02P20505), July 14, 2007. Available at: www. cfsan.fda.gov/;dms/qhcnuts2.html.

156. Ternus M, McMahon K, Lapsley K, Johnson G. Qualified health claim for nuts and heart disease prevention: development of consumer friendly language. *Nutr Today* 2006;**41**:62–6.

157. King JC, Blumberg JB, Ingwersen L, Jenab M, Tucker KL. Tree nuts and peanuts as components of a healthy diet. *J Nutr* 2008;**138**:1736S–40S.

158. Anderson JW, Smith BM, Washnok CS. Cardiovascular and renal benefits of dry bean and soybean intake. *Am J Clin Nutr* 1999;**70**(suppl):S464–74.

159. Third International Symposium on the role of soy in preventing and treating chronic disease. *J Nutr* 2000;**130**(suppl):S653–711.

160. Anthony MS, Clarkson TB, Bullock BC. Soy protein versus soy phitoestrogens (isoflavones) in the prevention of coronary artery atherosclerosis of cynomolgus monkeys (abstract). *Circulation* 1996;**94**(suppl 1):1–265.

161. John R, Crouse III, Morgan T *et al.* Randomized trial comparing the effect of casein with that of soy protein containing varying amounts of isoflavones on plasma concentrations of lipids and lipoproteins. *Arch Intern Med* 1999;**159**:2070–6.

162. Sacks FM, Lichtenstein A, Horn LV, Harris W, Kris-Etherton P, Winston M. Soy protein, isoflavones, and cardiovascular health: an American Heart Association Science Advisory for Professionals From the Nutrition Committee. *Circulation* 2006;**113**:1034–44.

163. Yeung J, Yu T. Effects of isoflavones (soy phyto-estrogens) on serum lipids: a meta-analysis of randomized controlled trials *Nutr J* 2003;**2**:15–23.

164. Zhang XH, Lowe D, Giles P, Fell S, Connock MJ, Maslin DJ. Gender may affect the action of garlic oil on plasma cholesterol and glucose levels of normal subjects. *J Nutr* 2001;**131**:1471–8.

165. Alder R, Lookinland S, Berry JA, Williams M. A systematic review of the effectiveness of garlic as an antihyperlipidemic agent. *J Am Acad Nurse Pract* 2003;**15**:120–9.

166. Li G, Shi Z, Jia H, Ju J, Wang X, Xia Z *et al.* A clinical investigation on garlicin injection for the treatment of unstable angina pectoris and its actions on plasma endothelin and blood sugar levels. *J Trad Chin Med* 2000;**20**:243–6.

167. Breithaupt-Grogler K, Ling M, Boudoulas H, Belz GG, Heiden M, Wenzel E, Gu LD. Protective effect of chronic garlic intake

on elastic properties of aorta in the elderly. *Circulation* 1997;**96**:2649–55.

168. Kiesewetter H, Jung F, Jung EM, Mroweitz C, Koscielny J, Wenzel E. Effect of garlic on platelet aggregation in patients with increased risk of juvenile ischaemic attack. *Eur J Clin Pharmacol* 1993;**45**:333–6.

169. Anim-Nyame N, Sooranna SR, Johnson MR, Gamble J, Steer PJ. Garlic supplementation increases peripheral blood flow: a role for interleukin-6? *J Nutr Biochem* 2004;**15**:30–6.

170. Budoff MJ, Takasu J, Flores FR, Niihara Y, Lu B, Lau BH *et al.* Inhibiting progression of coronary calcification using Aged Garlic Extract in patients receiving statin therapy: a preliminary study. *Prev Med* 2004;**39**:985–91.

171. Rahman K, Lowe GM. Garlic and cardiovascular disease: a critical review. *J Nutr* 2006;**136**:736S–740S.

172. Davies DF, Rees BW, Davies PT. Cow's milk antibodies and coronary heart disease. *Lancet* 1980;**1**(8179):1190–1.

173. Law MR, Wald N. An ecological study of serum cholesterol and ischaemic heart disease between 1850 and 1990. *Eur J Clin Nutr* 1994;**48**(5):305–25.

174. Seely S. Diet and coronary disease. A survey of mortality rates and food consumption statistics of 24 countries. *Med Hypoth* 1981;**7**:907–18.

175. Abbott RD, Curb JD, Rodriguez BL *et al.* Effect of dietary calcium and milk consumption on risk of thromboembolic stroke in older middle aged men. *Stroke* 1996;**27**:813–18.

176. Gaziano JM, Buring JE, Breslow JL *et al.* Moderate alcohol intake, increased levels of high-density lipoprotein and its subfractions, and decreased risk of myocardial infarction. *N Engl J Med* 1993;**329**:1829–34.

177. Rehm J, Bondy S. Alcohol and all cause mortality: an overview. *Novartis Foundation Symp* 1998;**216**:223–32.

178. Gaziano JM, Godfried S, Hennekens CH. Alcohol and coronary heart disease trends. *Cardiovasc Med* 1996;**329**:1829–34.

179. Maclure M. Demonstration of deductive meta-analysis: ethanol intake and risk of myocardial infarction. *Epidemiol Rev* 1993;**15**:328–51.

180. Moore RD, Pearson T. Moderate alcohol consumption and coronary artery disease: a review. *Medicine* 1986;**65**:242–67.

181. Sacco RL, Elkind M, Boden-Albala B *et al.* The protective effect of moderate alcohol consumption on ischemic stroke. *JAMA* 1999;**281**:53–60.

182. Gaziano JM, Buring JE, Brestlow JL *et al.* Moderate alcohol intake increased levels of high-density lipoprotein and its subfractions, and decreased risk of myocardial infarction. *N Engl J Med* 1993;**329**:1829–34.

183. Gaziano JM, Hennekens CH, Godfried SL *et al.* Type of alcoholic beverage and risk of myocardial infarction. *Am J Cardiol* 1999;**83**:52–7.

184. Miyagi Y, Miwa K, Inoue H. Inhibition of human low-density lipoprotein oxidation by flavonoids in red wine and grape juice. *Am J Cardiol* 1997;**80**:1627–31.

185. Hu FB, Stampfer MJ, Rimm EB *et al.* A prospective study of egg consumption and risk of cardiovascular disease in men and women. *JAMA* 1999;**281**(15):1387–94.

186. Ministry of Health, New Zealand. *Food and Nutrition Guidelines for Healthy Adults: A Background Paper.* 2003. Available at: www.moh.govt.nz/moh.nsf/f872666357c511eb4c25666d000c8888/fe468ceed06b0771cc256cd600709490?OpenDocument.

187. Marmot M, Brunner E. Alcohol and cardiovascular disease: the status of the U shaped curve. *BMJ* 1991;**303**:565–8.

188. Maclure M. Demonstration of deductive meta-analysis: ethanol intake and risk of myocardial infarction. *Epidemiol Rev* 1993;**15**:328–51.

189. Shaper AG, Wannamethee G, Walker M. Alcohol and coronary heart disease: a perspective from the British Regional Heart Study. *Int J Epidemiol* 1994;**23**:482–94.

190. Rimm EB, Williams P, Fosher K, Criqui M, Stampfer MJ. Moderate alcohol intake and lower risk of coronary heart disease: meta-analysis of effects on lipids and haemostatic factors. *BMJ* 1999;**319**:1523–8.

191. Cowie MR. Alcohol and the heart. *Br J Hosp Med* 1997;**57**(9):457–60.

192. Jurgen R, Greenfield T, Rogers J. Average volume of alcohol consumption, patterns of drinking, and all-cause mortality: results from the US National Alcohol Survey. *Am J Epidemiol* 2001;**153**:64–71.

193. Trichopoulou A, Kouris-Blazos A, Vassilakou T *et al.* The diet and survival of elderly Greeks; a link to the past. *Am J Clin Nutr* 1995;**61**(suppl):1346S–1350S.

194. Eckel RH. Egg consumption in relation to cardiovascular disease and mortality the story gets more complex *Am J Clin Nutr* 2008;**87**:799–800.

195. Djoussé L, Gaziano JM. Egg consumption in relation to cardiovascular disease and mortality: the Physicians' Health Study. *Am J Clin Nutr* 2008;**87**:964–9.

196. Dawber TR, Nickerson RJ, Brand FN, Pool J. Eggs, serum cholesterol, and coronary heart disease. *Am J Clin Nutr* 1982;**36**:617–25.

197. Nakamura Y, Okamura T, Tamaki S *et al.* Egg consumption, serum cholesterol, and cause-specific and all-cause mortality: the National Integrated Project for Prospective Observation of Non-communicable Disease and Its Trends in the Aged, 1980 (NIPPON DATA80). *Am J Clin Nutr* 2004;**80**:58–63.

198. Song WO, Kerver JM. Nutritional contribution of eggs to American diets. *J Am Coll Nutr* 2000;**19**(suppl):556S–62S.

199. Keys A, Menotti A, Karvonen MJ *et al.* The diet and 15-year death rate in the Seven Countries Study. *Am J Epidemiol* 1986;**124**:903–15.

200. Trichopoulou A, Vasilopoulou E. Mediterranean diet and longevity. *Br J Nutr* 2000;**84**(suppl-2):S205–S209.

201. De Lorgeril M, Renaud S, Mamelle N *et al.* Mediterranean alpha-linolenic acid-rich diet in secondary prevention of coronary heart disease. *Lancet* 1994;**343**:1454.

202. Vincent-Baudry S, Defoort C, Gerber M, Bernard M, Verger P, Helal O *et al.* The Medi-RIVAGE study: reduction of cardiovascular disease risk factors after a 3-mo intervention with a Mediterranean-type diet or a low-fat diet *Am J Clin Nutr* 2005;**82**:964–71.

203. Rimm EB, Ascherio A, Giovannucci E *et al.* Vegetable, fruit, and cereal fiber intake and risk of coronary heart disease among men. *JAMA* 1996;**275**:447.

204. Gilman MW, Cupples LA, Gagnon DJ *et al.* Protective effect of fruits and vegetables on development of stroke in men. *JAMA* 1995;**273**:1113–17.

205. Willett WC. Convergence of philosophy and science: the Third International Congress on Vegetarian Nutrition. *Am J Clin Nutr* 1999;**70**(suppl):434S–8S.

206. Pais P, Pogue J, Gerstein H, Zachariah E *et al.* Risk factors for acute myocardial infarction in Indians: a case–control study. *Lancet* 1996;**348**:358–63.

207. Hu FB, Rimm EB, Stampfer MJ *et al.* Prospective study of major dietary patterns and risk of coronary heart disease in men. *Am J Clin Nutr* 2000;**72**:912–21.

208. Shimamoto T, Komachi Y, Inada H *et al.* Trends for coronary heart disease and stroke and their risk factors in Japan. *Circulation* 1989;**79**:503–15.

209. Moore TJ, Conlin PR, Ard J, Svetkey LP for the DASH Collaborative Research Group. DASH (Dietary Approaches to Stop Hypertension) Diet is effective treatment for stage 1 isolated systolic hypertension. *Hypertension* 2001;**38**:155–8.

210. Obarzanek E, Sacks FM, Vollmer WM *et al.* Effects on blood lipids of a blood pressure-lowering diet: the Dietary Approaches to Stop Hypertension (DASH) Trial. *Am J Clin Nutr* 2001;**74**:80–9.

211. Truswell AS. Review of dietary intervention studies: effect on coronary events and on total mortality. *Aust N Z J Med* 1994;**24**:98–106.

212. Zatonski WA, McMichael AJ, Powles JW. Ecological study of reasons for sharp decline in mortality for ischaemic heart disease in Poland since 1991. *BMJ* 1998;**317**:678.

213. Pietinen P, Vartianinen E, Seppanen R *et al.* Changes in diet in Finland from 1972 to 1992: impact on coronary heart disease risk. *Prev Med* 1996;**25**:243–50.

214. Dowsen GK, Gareeboo H, George K *et al.* Changes in population cholesterol concentrations and other cardiovascular risk factor levels after five years of non-communicable disease intervention programme in Mauritius. *BMJ* 1995;**311**: 1255–9.

215. Cappuccio FP. Salt and cardiovascular disease. *BMJ* 2007;**334**; 859–60.

216. www.nyc.gov/html/doh/downloads/pdf/cardio/cardio-transfat-bro.pdf

217. World Health Organization. *Global Strategy on Diet, Physical Activity and Health.* Geneva: WHO, 2004. Available at: www.who.int/dietphysicalactivity.

24 Integrating approaches to prevention of cardiovascular disease

David A Wood and Kornelia Kotseva

Cardiovascular Medicine, National Heart and Lung Institute, Imperial College, London, UK

Introduction and historical perspective

Cardiovascular diseases (CVD), of which coronary heart disease (CHD) is the most common, are the major causes of death in middle-aged and older people in most developed countries and in many developing countries.[1-3] Cardiovascular diseases result in substantial disability worldwide and contribute in large part to the escalating costs of healthcare, especially with an increasing aging population,[4] and are predicted to be the leading cause of death and disability-adjusted life-years by 2020.[5] A significant proportion of cardiovascular morbidity and mortality could be prevented through population strategies, and by making cost-effective clinical interventions accessible and affordable, both for people with established disease and for those at high risk of developing cardiovascular disease.[6,7]

This chapter is about integrating clinical approaches to prevention of cardiovascular disease for those with established atherosclerotic disease (secondary prevention) and those who are asymptomatic but at high risk of developing the disease (primary prevention).

The World Heart and Stroke Forum (WHSF) Guidelines Task Force of the World Heart Federation (WHF) recommends that every country develop a national policy on CVD prevention.[8] This national policy should set priorities for public health and clinical interventions appropriate to the country, and be the foundation for developing national evidence-based clinical guidelines on CVD prevention.

While the causes of CVD are common to all parts of the world, the approaches to cardiovascular prevention at a societal or individual level will differ between countries for cultural, social, medical, and economic reasons. Although national guidelines will share common principles of CVD prevention – the need for patient priorities, absolute risk

Evidence-Based Cardiology, 3rd edition. Edited by S. Yusuf, J.A. Cairns, A.J. Camm, E.L. Fallen, and B.J. Gersh. © 2010 Blackwell Publishing, ISBN: 978-1-4051-5925-8.

thresholds for treatment and treatment targets – they may differ in terms of the organization of preventive cardiology, risk factor treatment thresholds and targets, and the availability and use of cardioprotective medications.

Nomenclature and definitions

The World Health Organization report on prevention of coronary heart disease describes three strategies for prevention,[1] which still apply today but for all atherosclerotic cardiovascular disease. These three strategies complement each other:

• a 'population' strategy – for altering, in the entire population, the lifestyle and environmental factors, and their social and economic determinants, that are the underlying causes of the mass occurrence of CVD

• a 'high-risk' strategy – identification of individuals at high risk of developing the disease, and action to reduce their risk factor levels

• secondary prevention – prevention of disease progression and recurrent cardiovascular events in patients with clinically established coronary or other atherosclerotic disease.

The *secondary prevention* strategy addresses those who have survived the development of symptomatic atherosclerotic disease – acute coronary syndromes, angina, transient cerebral ischemia, stroke, peripheral arterial disease – with the object of reducing the risk of recurrent cardiovascular events, improving quality of life and life expectancy. However, it is necessarily limited to survivors. The first manifestation of CVD can be sudden collapse and death, e.g. ventricular fibrillation in the context of acute myocardial infarction. In addition, among those who survive the initial ischemic insult, the resulting tissue damage may be so great that secondary prevention offers little gain. This is because prognosis is largely determined by the extent of cardiac or cerebral damage. Therefore, a high-risk primary prevention strategy is required.

The *high-risk* strategy identifies those asymptomatic individuals in the population who are apparently well but at high multifactorial risk of developing CVD, with the object of reducing their total CVD risk through lifestyle, risk factor and therapeutic management. However, its overall impact on the burden of disease in the population is limited because it only targets those at highest risk whereas the burden of CVD arises in those at modest risk where medical interventions are not appropriate.

Therefore, a *population* strategy, which tackles the major determinants of cardiovascular diseases at a societal level, is paramount and without such a strategy, these diseases will remain a major cause of ill health and premature death, regardless of the fact that secondary prevention and high-risk strategies do reduce cardiovascular morbidity and mortality for individuals.

Incidence, natural history, and prognosis

Secondary prevention

The first clinical presentation of atherosclerotic disease is with sudden death or, more commonly, a non-fatal event, principally of the coronary arteries, cerebral arteries or peripheral arteries. Whatever the affected arterial territory, the pathology of the disease is the same and is usually ubiquitous. Although the acute management will differ according to the affected arterial territory, the ways of preventing a recurrence are common to all manifestations of atherosclerosis – lifestyle (smoking cessation, eating a healthy diet and being physically active), the management of other risk factors (blood pressure, lipids and glucose) and the use of cardioprotective drugs, some of which have specific clinical indications, e.g. beta-blockers following myocardial infarction, based on evidence from randomized controlled trials.

All patients with atherosclerotic cardiovascular disease should be eligible for a comprehensive prevention program. Traditionally, such programs have focused on patients with coronary disease, especially those following myocardial infarction or revascularization, usually by cardiac surgery. Yet the benefits of prevention demonstrated in those who have had a myocardial infarction are as likely to be achieved in patients with angina pectoris, stroke or other atherosclerotic disease. So the new challenge is to provide preventive cardiology programs for all atherosclerotic disease patients.

High-risk strategy

Primary prevention of CVD in individuals has traditionally focused on single risk factors, such as "hypertension", rather than multiple risk factors or the total risk approach and as a consequence, the potential benefits of total CVD

risk reduction have not been achieved. Although there is a continuous relationship between blood pressure and the risk of developing CVD, the higher the blood pressure, the higher the risk. The term "hypertension" dichotomizes this distribution into those with a blood pressure consistently greater than a specified level, e.g. 140/90 mmHg, and those with a blood pressure less than this level which is commonly referred to as "normal". The level of blood pressure defining "hypertension" is not based on the epidemiology of blood pressure and cardiovascular risk, but is rather deduced from randomized controlled trials which have shown evidence of benefit through reducing blood pressure in those with levels above, say, 140/90 mmHg. The consequence of this approach is that someone with a blood pressure of 142/92 mmHg is considered to be "hypertensive" and therefore receives blood pressure-lowering therapy, but another person of the same age and sex with a blood pressure of 138/88 mmHg is considered to be "normotensive" and therefore requires no treatment. Yet the total risk of developing CVD is not just a function of blood pressure but of all the cardiovascular risk factors taken together which are associated with a given level of blood pressure. This is called total cardiovascular risk. This term is used to describe the probability of a person developing an atherosclerotic cardiovascular event over a defined period of time.

The concept of total CVD risk assessment and management was first advanced by Jackson in 1993 in the context of treating "hypertension"; namely, the indication for treating blood pressure was not just a function of the blood pressure level but rather the absolute CVD risk, based on a combination of all risk factors, of which blood pressure was just one component.[9] This was followed in 1994 and 1998 by the Joint European Societies' recommendations which applied this principle of total coronary risk assessment to the management of all risk factors: blood pressure, lipids and diabetes.[10,11] The European CHD risk charts, developed from a concept pioneered by Anderson,[12] used age, sex, smoking status, blood cholesterol and SBP to estimate the 10 year risk of a first fatal or non-fatal coronary heart disease event. There were separate European charts for those with and without diabetes.

The importance of estimating total CVD risk before making a decision to intervene medically is illustrated in Figure 24.1. The figure illustrates that in a middle-aged man who is a non-smoker with a blood pressure of 120 mmHg, the absolute risk of developing fatal CVD progressively increases as the total cholesterol to HDL-cholesterol ratio rises from 3.0 to 7.0. However, at every level of this lipid ratio the absolute risk for a man of the same age who smokes cigarettes and has raised blood pressure is substantially higher. In fact, the chances of such a man developing CVD with a lipid ratio of 3.0 is actually higher than a lipid ratio of 7.0 in a non-smoking man with lower blood pressure. Although women are usually, age for age, at lower absolute risk of CVD than men, this advantage is lost at any level of the lipid ratio if the woman is a smoker with raised blood pressure.

The third and fourth editions of the Joint European Societies Guidelines published in 2003 and 2007[13,14] introduced

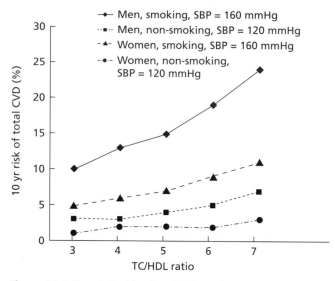

Figure 24.1 The relationship of total cholesterol/HDL cholesterol ratio to 10-year fatal CVD events in men and women aged 60 years with and without risk factors, based on a risk function derived from the SCORE project. (Reproduced with permission from Graham et al.[2])

a new system for cardiovascular risk estimation called SCORE (Systematic Coronary Risk Estimation), based on data from 12 European prospective cohort studies: 205,178 subjects with 2.7 million years of follow-up and 7934 cardiovascular deaths.[15] Two charts were produced: one for high-risk regions and the other for low-risk regions of Europe (Figs 24.2, 24.3). SCORE estimates the 10-year risk of a first fatal atherosclerotic event, whether heart attack, stroke, aneurysm of the aorta or other fatal manifestation of atherosclerotic disease. All ICD (International Classification of Diseases) codes that could be due to atherosclerosis are included. One advantage of a risk score based on mortality is that it can be recalibrated if good-quality, up-to-date mortality and risk factor prevalence data are available for a country. The SCORE CVD mortality charts have been recalibrated for a number of European countries: Germany, Greece, Poland, Spain, Sweden, Cyprus, Bosnia/Herzegovina and Russia. The electronic, interactive version of SCORE, called HEARTSCORE, is available from the European Society of Cardiology (www.escardio org/heartscore).

A 10-year CVD risk of 5% or more (red zone) for fatal events was defined in the 2003 Joint European Societies guidelines as high risk, and people at this level of risk should receive a professional lifestyle intervention and, if appropriate, drug therapies to reduce total CVD risk. Although an individual's treatment should be guided by their total CVD risk, the physician also needs to

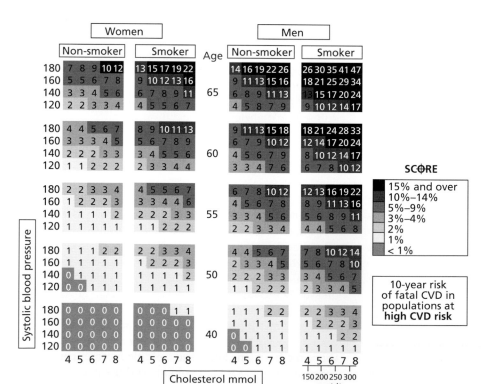

Figure 24.2 SCORE chart: 10-year risk of fatal CVD in populations at high CVD risk based on the following risk factors: age, gender, smoking, systolic blood pressure and total cholesterol. (Reproduced with permission from Graham et al.[2])

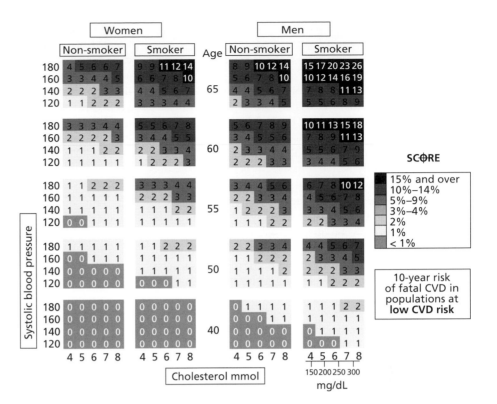

Figure 24.3 SCORE chart: 10-year risk of fatal CVD in populations at low CVD risk based on the following risk factors: age, gender, smoking, systolic blood pressure and total cholesterol. (Reproduced with permission from Graham *et al.*[2])

take account of other factors, e.g. co-morbidity and life expectancy, before committing a person to lifelong therapies.

In 2007 the WHO developed CVD risk prediction charts because equations derived from Caucasian populations are not necessarily valid to predict CVD risk in low- and middle-income countries.[1] The Comparative Risk Assessment (CRA) Project, conducted by the WHO and described in the 2002 World Health Report, determined the burden of disease attributable to selected major risk factors, including smoking, Body Mass Index, high blood pressure, and high blood cholesterol.[16] This project involved the standardized collection and assessment of risk factor prevalences by WHO epidemiologic subregion. Estimates of relative risk per unit increase in continuous risk factors, i.e. per mmHg for systolic blood pressure, were determined from the CRA project largely from prospective cohort studies. Absolute risk of a cardiovascular event was determined by scaling individual relative risk to population incidence rates of cardiovascular disease (coronary heart disease and stroke), estimated from the Global Burden of Disease Study. The probability of a cardiovascular event was extrapolated to a 10-year period. The new WHO/International Society of Hypertension (ISH) risk prediction charts are based on these data and there are charts with and without cholesterol, and for patients with and without diabetes.

In summary, the great strength of the total risk approach is that it provides a rational means of making decisions about intervening in a targeted way, thereby making best use of resources available to reduce cardiovascular risk. The traditional approach focused on single risk factors as if they were "diseases" and this way of thinking is still being promoted with the use of terms such as "pre-hypertension" or "pre-diabetes". Many in the medical profession are reluctant to change from a unifactorial to a total risk approach because of their traditional medical training. The total risk approach also runs counter to the special interests of some professional societies, which focus on single risk factors, and the pharmaceutical industry and regulatory authorities which license drugs for single clinical indications. This unifactorial approach leads to people being labelled as "high risk" and for many this will be incorrect, leading to inappropriate use of drug therapies. In contrast, the total risk approach identifies that section of the population at highest risk of developing CVD. Such individuals have the most to gain from lifestyle and medical interventions to reduce their cardiovascular risk. So CVD risk scoring moves the focus of identification and treatment from individual risk factors to multiple risk factors. The intensity of interventions can then be matched to the level of total CVD risk. Research is required to validate the WHO regional risk prediction charts for each national population, and to confirm that using risk stratification methods in low- and middle-income countries results in benefits for both patients and the population as a whole.

Management

Secondary prevention

Cardiac rehabilitation traditionally focused on physical rehabilitation but this specialty has gradually evolved into more comprehensive professional lifestyle programs – smoking cessation, making healthy food choices and becoming physically active – based on behavioral models of change. Risk factor management in terms of controling blood pressure, lipids and glucose to defined targets, and the use of cardioprotective drug therapies, is also now integral to this approach. Finally, the psychosocial and vocational support required to help patients lead as full a life as possible is also provided. This evolution in cardiac rehabilitation is reflected in the current WHO definition.[17]

"The rehabilitation of cardiac patients is the sum of activities required to influence favorably the underlying cause of the disease, as well as the best possible physical, mental and social conditions, so that they may, by their own efforts, preserve or resume when lost, as normal a place as possible in the community. Rehabilitation cannot be regarded as an isolated form of therapy but must be integrated with the whole treatment of which it forms only one facet."

The original definition[18] was changed in 1993 with the addition of the following words: "to influence favorably the underlying cause of the disease"– in short, all aspects of CVD prevention.

The overall preventive objective for patients who present with symptoms of coronary artery disease – stable angina, unstable angina or acute MI – is to reduce the risk of a further non-fatal event or death from cardiovascular disease. Cardiac rehabilitation was originally provided only for patients recovering from a myocardial infarction (MI) and those who had coronary artery bypass graft (CABG) surgery (or other forms of cardiac surgery). With the more recent emphasis on influencing the underlying causes of atherosclerotic disease, patients presenting with all forms of coronary artery disease, including unstable and stable angina, are now being included together with those who have other forms of atherosclerotic disease (e.g. transient cerebral ischemia or peripheral arterial disease) in cardiovascular prevention and rehabilitation programs. By addressing all aspects of lifestyle and risk factor management, and prescribing cardioprotective drug therapies, the risk of future cardiovascular events can be reduced in all these patients as evidenced by the meta-analyses.

The scientific evidence from randomized controlled trials shows that exercise-based cardiac rehabilitation of coronary patients reduces both total and cardiac mortality.

The main objective of the Cochrane systematic reviews and meta-analyses,[19] last updated in 2004,[20] was to determine the effectiveness of exercise only, or exercise as part of a comprehensive cardiac rehabilitation programme, on total and CHD mortality, morbidity, health-related quality of life (HRQoL) and modifiable cardiac risk factors of patients with coronary heart disease. The last review also addressed previous concerns regarding the applicability of this evidence to routine clinical practice. Trials with 6 or more months of follow-up were included if they assessed the effects of exercise training alone or in combination with psychologic or educational interventions. Altogether, 48 trials with a total of 8940 patients were included. Cardiac rehabilitation compared with usual care was associated with reduced all-cause mortality (odds ratio (OR) 0.80; 95% confidence interval (CI) 0.68–0.93) and cardiac mortality (OR 0.74; 95% CI 0.61–0.96) (**Class I, Level A**). There was no difference in recurrent myocardial infarction, CABG or PTCA (**Class IIb, Level B**) (Table 24.1).

At follow-up the proportion of patients who reported smoking was significantly reduced with cardiac rehabilitation (OR 0.64; 95% CI 0.50–0.83) (**Class IIa, Level B**). There was a significantly greater reduction in systolic blood pressure for those in cardiac rehabilitation (weighted mean difference, −3.2 mmHg; 95% CI −5.4 to −0.9 mmHg) but no difference in diastolic blood pressure (**Class IIa, Level B**). There was also a significantly greater reduction in total cholesterol concentration (weighted mean difference, −0.37 mmol/L (−14.3 mg/dL); 95% CI −0.63 to −0.11 mmol/L (−24.3 to −4.2 mg/dL)) and triglyceride concentration (weighted mean difference, −0.23 mmol/L (−20.4 mg/dL); 95% CI −0.39 to −0.07 mmol/L (−34.5 to −6.2 mg/dL)) for those in cardiac rehabilitation, but no difference in low-density or high-density lipoprotein concentrations (**Class IIa, Level B**). With the exception of smoking, the other risk factor changes in favor of intervention were rather small, and therefore would have had a limited impact on clinical events. So the reduction in total and cardiac mortality

Table 24.1 Pooled odds ratios (OR) and 95% confidence intervals (CI) for total and cardiac mortality, recurrent myocardial infarction, CABG and PTCA in patients with CHD randomly assigned to evidence-based cardiac rehabilitation versus usual care[20]

Clinical outcomes	Treatment n/N	Control n/N	OR (95% CI)
Total mortality	326/4295	381/4137	0.80 (0.68–0.93)
Cardiac mortality	211/2706	267/2665	0.74 (0.61–0.90)
Recurrent myocardial infarction	203/2416	214/2331	0.79 (0.57–1.09)
CABG	101/1556	120/1581	0.87 (0.65–1.16)

observed in this meta-analysis can be largely attributed to lifestyle changes: increased physical activity, healthier diets and smoking cessation.

Importantly, this meta-analysis showed no difference in mortality between exercise-only cardiac rehabilitation and comprehensive cardiac rehabilitation. The effect of cardiac rehabilitation on total mortality was independent of coronary heart disease diagnosis, type of cardiac rehabilitation, dose of exercise intervention or duration of follow-up. Health-related quality of life improved to similar levels with cardiac rehabilitation and usual care.

The contribution of secondary prevention programs, with or without exercise, was evaluated in two related systematic reviews and meta-analyses,[21,22] the most recent in 2005.[22] This meta-analysis included 63 randomized trials (21 295 patients with coronary disease), including 51 trials that were not included in the first review (limited to literature published before 1999 and excluding any studies with exercise components) and 26 trials that were not included in Taylor's review of cardiac rehabilitation (limited to literature published before 2003 and including few "individual counseling" programs). The summary risk ratio was 0.85 (95% CI 0.77–0.94) for all-cause mortality (Table 24.2), but this result improved over time from a risk ratio of 0.97 (95% CI 0.82–1.14) at 12 months to 0.53 (95% CI 0.35–0.81) at 24 months (**Class I, Level A**). The summary risk ratio was 0.83 (95% CI 0.74–0.94) for recurrent myocardial infarction over a median follow-up of 12 months (**Class I, Level A**). The effects on mortality and myocardial infarction were similar for programs that included both exercise and risk factor education, or risk factor education without exercise, or for exercise alone. Thirty-five trials reported effects on cardiovascular risk factors and although summary effects are not reported in this review, the effect sizes were generally considered to be small to moderate (**Class IIb, Level B**). Of the 27 trials that assessed the use of cardioprotective medications, eight demonstrated statistically significantly better application of at least one therapy in the intervention patients, three demonstrated better prescribing in intervention but not achieving statistical significance, and 11 did not demonstrate any appreciable difference between intervention and control patients (**Class IIb, Level B**). Quality of life was not formally evaluated overall but effect sizes in the individual trials were reported to be generally small.

Importantly, this distinction between "cardiac rehabilitation" and "secondary prevention" is artificial and any comparisons based on these rather arbitrary classifications will usually be confounded. In "exercise-only" trials people are free to adopt a healthier diet and stop smoking. In "secondary prevention" trials, without a supervised exercise component, people are free to exercise. What these meta-analyses really demonstrate, from different perspectives depending on trials included, are the overall benefits of an integrated multidisciplinary and multifactorial approach to reducing

Table 24.2 Risk ratios (RR) and 95% confidence intervals (CI) for total mortality and recurrent myocardial infarction for secondary prevention programs without exercise, with exercise and exercise only[22]

	Treatment n/N	Control n/N	RR (95% CI)
All-cause mortality			
Program without exercise	364/4598	417/4604	0.87 (0.76–0.99)
Program with exercise	223/2404	242/2251	0.88 (0.74–1.04)
Exercise-only program	72/1165	101/1120	0.72 (0.54–0.95)
Overall	659/8167	760/7975	0.85 (0.77–0.94)
Recurrent myocardial infarction			
Program without exercise	194/2787	221/2742	0.86 (0.72–1.03)
Program with exercise	198/2075	230/1922	0.62 (0.44–0.87)
Exercise-only program	77/1124	99/1073	0.76 (0.57–1.01)
Overall	469/5986	550/5737	0.83 (0.74–0.94)

cardiovascular risk and cardiovascular and all-cause mortality. The relative and absolute contributions in such comprehensive programs of their individual components – smoking cessation, diet, physical activity, lowering blood pressure, cholesterol and glucose – to reducing cardiovascular and total mortality are not known from these meta-analyses, and data quality from many trials is either incomplete or inadequate for such analyses to be performed. As many of the postmyocardial cardiac rehabilitation trials were undertaken before the modern management of acute coronary disease, e.g. primary PTCA and thrombolysis, and the introduction of cardioprotective medications such as antiplatelet therapies, beta-blockers, ACE inhibitors and ARBs, some calcium channel blockers and statins, the added value of such programs to current practice is also not known. However, it is likely that relative reductions in risk achieved by cardiovascular prevention and rehabilitation, principally through lifestyle changes from these early randomized controlled trials, will still apply to coronary and other atherosclerotic disease patients even though they are now, because of modern treatments, at lower absolute risk of recurrent disease and death.

Unfortunately, risk factor management in patients with CHD in Europe is far from optimal. Surveys of preventive cardiology practice such as EUROASPIRE I, II and III show a considerable gap between evidence-based guidelines and the lifestyle, risk factor and therapeutic management of patients with coronary disease.[23–27] Over a period of 12 years there are adverse time trends in smoking (higher rates in younger patients <50 years, especially among women), in the prevalence of obesity and central obesity which are both increasing, no change in the prevalence of raised blood pressure, and an increasing prevalence of diabetes. Only lipid management has improved, and improved

Table 24.3 Time trends in the prevalence (%) of risk factors in patients with CHD in Europe: comparison between EUROASPIRE I, II and III in eight countries by survey, country, diagnosis and gender[26]

Survey	Smoking[1]			Obesity[2]			Central obesity[3]			Raised blood pressure[4]			Elevated total cholesterol[5]			Reported diabetes mellitus		
	EA I %	EA II %	EA III %	EA I %	EA II %	EA III %	EA I %	EA II %	EA III %	EA I %	EA II %	EA III %	EA I %	EA II %	EA III %	EA I %	EA II %	EA III %
Risk factor prevalence	20.3	21.2	18.2	25.0	32.6	38.0	42.2	53.0	54.9	58.1	58.3	60.9	94.5	76.7	46.2	17.4	20.1	28.0
Overall significance§	P = 0.64			P = 0.0006			P = 0.0001			P = 0.49			P < 0.0001			P = 0.004		

[1] Self-reported smoking or >10 ppm carbon monoxide in breath; [2] BMI ≥30 kg/m^2; [3] Waist circumference ≥88 cm for women or ≥102 cm for men; [4] Systolic blood pressure ≥140 mmHg and/or diastolic blood pressure ≥90 mmHg for non-diabetics and systolic blood pressure ≥130 mmHg and/or diastolic blood pressure ≥80 mmHg for diabetics; [5] Total cholesterol ≥4.5 mmol/L; § Adjusted for differences in distribution of age and diagnostic category.

Table 24.4 EUROASPIRE III: prevalence (%) of CHD risk factors and use of cardioprotective medication in patients with CHD in 22 countries in Europe[27]

Current smoking[1] %	Obesity[2] %	Increased waist circum-ference[3] %	Raised blood pressure[4] %	Elevated TC[5] %	Diabetes mellitus[6] %	Anti-platelets %	Beta-blockers %	ACE inhibitors/ ARB %	Calcium channel blockers %	Statins %	Anti-coagulants %
17.2	35.3	52.7	56.0	51.1	34.8	90.5	79.8	70.9	24.5	78.1	5.6

[1] Self-reported and/or CO in breath >10 ppm; [2] BMI ≥30 kg/m^2; [3] Waist circumference ≥102 cm for men and ≥88 cm for women; [4] Systolic blood pressure ≥140 mmHg and/or diastolic blood pressure ≥90 mmHg (systolic blood pressure ≥130 mmHg and/or diastolic blood pressure ≥80 mmHg in patients with diabetes); [5] Serum total cholesterol ≥4.5 mmol/L; [6] Self-reported and/or fasting plasma glucose ≥7.0 mmol/L.

substantially, due to the huge increase in prescriptions of statins[26] (Table 24.3). In the most recent EUROASPIRE III survey of 13,935 coronary patients from 22 countries, there is evidence of considerable potential to further reduce cardiovascular risk in this patient population, as many are still not achieving the recommended lifestyle and risk factor targets defined in the European guidelines[27] (Table 24.4). In Europe only about a third of coronary patients receive any form of cardiac rehabilitation, with considerable variation between European regions.[28] Patients with other clinical manifestations of atherosclerotic CVD receive little or no systematic preventive and rehabilitative care. The majority of coronary patients in the EUROASPIRE II survey were not advised to follow a cardiac rehabilitation program, and less than a third of all patients attended such a program.[28] The traditions and practice of cardiac rehabilitation in Europe differ substantially between countries, ranging from intensive residential rehabilitation through to ambulatory hospital, community- and home-based programs. They also differ in their patient populations, staffing, management protocols, duration and follow-up. According to EUROASPIRE II, whatever form of cardiac rehabilitation was provided for the coronary patients who reported

attending such programs, the majority still did not achieve the lifestyle, risk factor and therapeutic goals[28] (Table 24.5). In addition, the families of patients with premature CHD are not systematically followed up, with fewer than one in 10 first-degree relatives having a cardiovascular risk assessment as a consequence of premature disease developing in their family[29] (Table 24.6).

Primary prevention

In primary prevention the evidence for multiple risk factor interventions is less strong. Primary prevention programs in many countries attempt to reduce mortality and morbidity due to CHD through risk factor modification. It is widely believed that multiple risk factor intervention using counseling and educational methods is efficacious and cost-effective and should be expanded. The effects of multiple risk factor intervention for reducing cardiovascular risk factors, mortality from CHD and total mortality among adults without clinical evidence of established cardiovascular disease have been assessed in Cochrane reviews and meta-analyses on two occasions, in 1997[30] and 2006.[31] Intervention studies using counseling or education to modify

Table 24.5 EUROASPIRE II: prevalence of risk factors according to participation in a cardiac rehabilitation program in patients with CHD in 15 countries in Europe[28]

Current smoking[1]		Obesity[2]		Raised BP[3]		Raised cholesterol[4]		Diabetes[5]	
No CRP %	CRP %	No CRP %	CRP %	No CRP %	CRP %	No CRP %	CRP %	No CRP %	CRP %
22.4	18.7	33.0	28.2	51.4	48.8	60.2	55.0	20.6	17.6
$P < 0.001^6$		$P = 0.02^6$		$P = 0.001^6$		$P < 0.001^6$		$P = 0.20^6$	

[1] Self-reported and/or CO in breath >10 ppm; [2] BMI ≥30 kg/m²; [3] SBP/DBP ≥140/90 mmHg; [4] Total cholesterol ≥5 mmol/L ; [5] Self-reported and/or fasting plasma glucose ≥7.0 mmol/L. [6] Significance of differences in prevalences between CR and No CR groups adjusted for center, diagnostic category, gender and age.

Table 24.6 EUROASPIRE II: screening for risk factors in relatives of patients with premature CHD[29]

	Siblings	Children
Prevalence of CHD (%)	9.9	1.5
Screening because of CHD in the family (%)	11.1	5.6
Index patient CABG (%)	16.5	8.6
Index patient PTCA (%)	9.9	4.1
Index patient AMI (%)	7.5	6.2
Index patient ischemia (%)	5.9	3.4

Table 24.7 Peto odds ratios (POR) and 95% confidence intervals (CI) for total mortality and CHD mortality in multiple risk factor interventions versus control[31]

	Treatment n/N	Control n/N	POR (95% CI)
Total mortality	3466/62267	4622/62900	0.96 (0.92–1.01)
Coronary heart disease mortality	1234/62267	1639/62900	0.96 (0.89–1.04)
Non-fatal myocardial infarction[+]	NR	NR	1.01 (0.93–1.10)

NR, not reported.
[+] WHO factories; Gotheborg Study, Oslo Study only.

more than one cardiovascular risk factor in adults from general populations, occupational groups, or high-risk groups were identified. Trials of less than 6 months duration were excluded. A total of 39 trials were found in the 2006 meta-analysis, more than double the 18 trials identified for the original review. Ten out of the 39 trials reported total mortality or coronary heart disease mortality as outcomes. However, only four of these trials were sufficiently large to have meaningful power to address these disease endpoints. In the 10 trials with clinical event endpoints, the pooled effects suggest that multiple risk factor intervention has no effect on mortality (Table 24.7). The pooled OR for total and CHD mortality were 0.96 (95% CI 0.92–1.01) and 0.96 (95% CI 0.89–1.04) respectively (**Class IIb, Level B**). However, there was evidence of statistical heterogeneity in the pooled OR for total mortality, but not for CHD mortality. Three hypertension trials (Hypertension, Detection and Follow-up Program, Johns Hopkins Hypertension Trial and Swedish RIS) reported significant reductions in total mortality, and this is most likely due to the benefits of effective antihypertensive therapy in these trials. Removal of these three trials reduced the heterogeneity for total mortality. Importantly, there was a significant interaction between

intervention and level of CHD risk at baseline, which indicated that trials recruiting higher risk patients were more likely to demonstrate clinical benefits. An important caveat to these results is that a small, but potentially important, benefit of treatment (about a 10% reduction in CHD mortality) may have been missed.

This apparent lack of effect on coronary and total mortality overall reflects a modest reduction in smoking and small changes in blood pressure and lipids, the latter due to limited drug treatment in these trials. The odds of reduction in smoking prevalence was 20% (95% CI 8–31%) with substantial heterogeneity (**Class IIb, Level B**). Validation of reported smoking habit with biochemical measures suggests that this improvement may be overestimated. Changes in systolic (SBP) and diastolic (DBP) blood pressure were small. The weighted mean differences between intervention and control were −3.6 mmHg (95% CI −3.9 to −3.3 mmHg) for SBP and for DBP −2.8 mmHg (95% CI −2.9 to −2.6 mmHg) (**Class IIb, Level B**). Exclusion of those trials in which a high proportion of subjects were on pharmacologic treatment resulted in smaller but still statistically significant net reductions in blood pressure: SBP −2.7 mmHg (95% CI −3.9 to −3.3) and DBP − 1.7 mmHg

Table 24.8 EUROASPIRE III: prevalence (%) of CHD risk factors and use of cardioprotective medication in patients at high cardiovascular risk in 12 countries in Europe*

Current smoking[1] %	Obesity[2] %	Increased waist circum-ference[3] %	Raised blood pressure[4] %	Elevated TC[5] %	Diabetes mellitus[6] %	Anti-platelets %	Beta-blockers %	ACE inhibitors/ ATRB %	Calcium channel blockers %	Diuretics %	Statins %
16.9	43.5	61.6	70.8	78.9	38.6	22.0	31.2	55.7	24.0	33.8	39.9

[1] Self-reported and/or CO in breath >10 ppm; [2] BM I ≥30 kg/m²; [3] Waist circumference ≥102 cm for men and ≥88 cm for women; [4] Systolic blood pressure ≥140 mmHg and/or diastolic blood pressure ≥90 mmHg (systolic blood pressure ≥130 mmHg and/or diastolic blood pressure ≥80 mmHg in patients with diabetes); [5] Serum total cholesterol ≥4.5 mmol/L; [6] Self-reported and/or fasting plasma glucose ≥7.0 mmol/L.
* www.escardio.org/congresses/esc2008/congress-reports/Pages/4480-4481-wood-ryden.aspx

(95% CI −2.0 to −1.5). Blood cholesterol concentrations showed a small but highly significant fall of −0.07 mMol/L (95% CI −0.8 to −0.06 mMol/L) between intervention and control (**Class IIb, Level B**). There was also substantial heterogeneity in this analysis. Several trials made substantial use of lipid-lowering drugs but exclusion of these trials did not make any difference to the overall pooled difference observed. Risk factor net changes were strongly correlated with initial level of smoking, diastolic (but not systolic) blood pressure and blood cholesterol. Those studies with the highest baseline smoking prevalence, diastolic blood pressure and blood cholesterol levels demonstrated larger intervention-associated falls in these risk factors. In some studies, outcomes may have been overestimated because of regression to the mean effects, lack of intention-to-treat analyses, habituation to blood pressure measurement, and use of self-reports of smoking. One important observation from this meta-analysis was that interventions using personal or family counseling and education, with or without pharmacologic treatments, appear to be more effective at achieving risk factor reduction and consequent reductions in mortality.

In contrast, numerous single risk factor trials using drug therapies to lower blood pressure and lipids have shown comparable reductions in CVD risk that would be predicted from the epidemiologic relationships.[32–38] Therefore, if multifactorial interventions were to achieve the same treatment effects as those demonstrated in unifactorial trials, a substantial reduction in total CVD risk would be expected. The challenge is to integrate management through a multidisciplinary multifactorial program.

In primary prevention the gap between evidence-based guidelines and clinical practice is even greater than that seen for coronary patients. The EUROASPIRE III survey of primary prevention in 12 countries showed that in 5687 patients being treated for blood pressure, dyslipidemia or diabetes there is even greater potential to further reduce cardiovascular risk. (www.escardio.org/congresses/esc2008/congress-reports/Pages/4480-4481-wood-ryden.

aspx). A large majority of such patients are not achieving the recommended lifestyle and risk factor targets defined in the European guidelines (Table 24.8).

Yet it is possible to further reduce this gap between guidelines and practice by providing a comprehensive program of preventive care, as demonstrated by the European Society of Cardiology EUROACTION project (www.escardio.org/euroaction). This cluster randomized controlled trial of a nurse-managed preventive cardiology program for coronary (hospital) and high-risk (primary care) patients showed that they, and their families, were more likely to make healthy changes to their diet and physical activity levels, and to have their blood pressure and other risk factors managed more effectively compared to usual care.[39,40]

The EUROACTION Preventive Cardiology Program in hospital and general practice

The object of EUROACTION was to demonstrate whether a professional multidisciplinary preventive cardiology program could help more patients and their families achieve the lifestyle, risk factor and therapeutic goals defined in the European prevention guidelines. The EURO-ACTION program was set up in eight countries and 24 hospital and general practice centers in the context of a matched pair cluster randomized controlled trial.[39]

In the hospitals, cardiologists and nurses recruited eligible patients and their families. After a multidisciplinary assessment of lifestyle, risk factors, and drug treatment by a nurse, dietitian and physiotherapist, couples attended at least eight sessions, one every week, in which they were individually assessed by each member of the team. The patients and their partners then attended a group workshop and a supervised exercise class. The cardiologists initiated and uptitrated the cardioprotective drugs and nurses monitored risk factors and adherence to drug treatments at each session. At 16 weeks, patients and their partners were reassessed by the whole team and a report was sent to their family doctors.

In the general practice centers, family doctors and nurses recruited patients and their families. The program started with the same nurse assessment of lifestyle, risk factors, and drug treatment as for the hospital patients but was then open ended. At each visit (one every week), couples were assessed by the nurse, who led the group workshops, and by the family doctors responsible for drug treatment. Patients and partners did not have supervised exercise classes.

Patients and partners in hospital and general practice were provided with a personal record card for lifestyle and risk factor targets, together with family support packs (www.escardio.org/euroaction).

The EUROACTION preventive cardiology program reduced the risk of cardiovascular disease compared with usual care mainly through lifestyle changes by families, who together made healthier food choices and became more physically active (**Class I, Level A**) (Table 24.9). These lifestyle changes led to some weight loss in both groups of patients and, for high-risk patients, there was also a significant reduction in central obesity. Blood pressure control was improved in both groups of patients and for those with coronary heart disease this was achieved without the use of additional antihypertensive drugs. Control of blood cholesterol concentrations improved in both groups of patients and significantly so in high-risk patients because of increased use of statins. Overall, the use of all cardioprotective drugs was substantially higher in the hospital compared to the primary care program. However, for high-risk patients in the EUROACTION program, ACE inhibitors and statins were both prescribed more frequently compared to usual care.

Although these results are encouraging for the multidisciplinary approach, there is still scope for further improvement. The smoking cessation intervention based on advice reduced relapse in patients with coronary heart disease, but had no impact on smoking high-risk patients. Despite protocol recommendation to use smoking cessation therapies, these were hardly used at all because of cost. Although the same protocol for risk factor management was used in hospital and general practice, use of blood pressure and lipid-lowering drugs was more conservative in general practice. As a consequence, most of the high-risk patients did not achieve lipid targets. Diabetes care could have been improved if the intervention nurses had taken responsibility for diabetes management.

EUROACTION is a contemporary example of an integrated approach to cardiovascular disease prevention which incorporated several important principles. By setting up this program in busy general hospitals and general practices, it is possible to generalize the results to the management of all coronary and high-risk patients in everyday clinical practice. Integrating initial diagnosis and management with continued preventive care in the same healthcare facility is likely to increase and maintain participation in the program. In the EUROASPIRE survey only a third of coronary patients attended cardiac rehabilitation, whereas two-thirds joined the EUROACTION hospital program and nine out of 10 eligible high-risk patients participated in primary care. EUROACTION addressed all the priority patient groups for cardiovascular prevention and made no distinction between symptomatic coronary disease (secondary prevention) and those at high risk (primary prevention). All these patients are at high risk of cardiovascular disease and need professional lifestyle support and risk factor management. It was a family-centered program involving patients' partners and other family members because of the evidence of concordant lifestyle within families and concordance for change.[41,42] Patients making the greatest changes had partners making similar changes. In addition, first-degree relatives of patients with premature atherosclerotic disease are at increased CVD risk so it is appropriate to offer lifestyle and risk factor management to the whole family, not just the patient.

In summary, the EUROACTION demonstration project in preventive cardiology showed that standards of preventive care in general hospitals and general practices across Europe can be improved. This nurse-managed, multidisciplinary, family-based, ambulatory program achieved healthier lifestyles and improvements in other risk factors for patients with coronary heart disease, those at high risk of developing cardiovascular disease, and their partners by comparison with those in usual care. EUROACTION is a model of preventive cardiology, successfully implemented and objectively assessed, which can be used in routine clinical practice. To achieve the beneficial effects of the EUROACTION program, we need to go beyond specialized cardiac rehabilitation services and provide local preventive cardiology programs, appropriately adapted to the medical, cultural, and economic setting of a country.

The Polypill concept

The concept of combining drugs (aspirin, beta-blocker, angiotensin converting enzyme inhibitors and statins) that have been proven to reduce major vascular events in secondary prevention into a combination tablet was suggested by Yusuf.[43] Such a combination pill could theoretically lead to a 75% relative risk reduction in vascular events. Combining these drugs into a single pill could enhance adherence (both physician and patient), reduce costs and increase affordability, and thereby assist in reducing the treatment gap. Wald and Law[44] expanded this concept to primary prevention (all >55 years) irrespective of the levels of risk factors on the grounds that most individuals in urban societies have elevated risk factors and that age alone is a sufficiently important risk factor. They hypothesized that use of a polypill which includes half doses of three antihyper-

Table 24.9 EUROACTION: proportions of coronary and high-risk patients and partners achieving the European lifestyle, risk factor and therapeutic targets for CVD prevention at 1 year[40]

Proportion n (%) achieving European targets at 1 year*	Hospital				General practice			
	Coronary patients		Partners		High-risk patients		Partners	
	INT	UC	INT	UC	INT	UC	INT	UC
Not smoking**	57.9 P = 0.06	47.1	32.3 P = 0.13	17.5	73.5 P = 0.89	72.3	85.0 P = 0.07	79.4
Saturated fat <10% of total energy***	55.1 P = 0.009	40.3	60.0 P = 0.31	42.1	NA	NA	NA	NA
Oily fish ≥3x/week	16.5 P = 0.04	8.2	10.6 P = 0.71	7.5	11.1 P = 0.13	6.0	19.6 P = 0.054	6.9
Fish ≥20 g/day	79.0 P = 0.62	66.9	77.8 P = 0.68	63.3	82.6 P = 0.07	66.5	80.9 P = 0.26	65.6
Fruit and vegetables ≥400 g/day	72.0 P = 0.004	35.2	72.0 P = 0.002	36.5	78.4 P = 0.005	38.8	76.9 P = 0.002	54.4
Physical activity ≥30 minutes, ≥4x/week	53.8 P = 0.002	19.6	40.8 P = 0.06	26.6	50.3 P = 0.01	22.1	44.4 P = 0.03	24.6
BMI <25 kg/m²	27.2 P = 0.20	20.7	38.3 P = 0.26	33.8	27.6 P = 0.85	22.0	29.3 P = 0.52	32.3
Weight loss ≥5% in patients with BMI ≥25 kg/m² at initial assessment	19.5 P = 0.28	13.2	NA Na	NA	16.5 P = 0.005	6.8	NA Na	NA
Ideal waist circumference (men <94 cm; women <80 cm)	30.9 P = 0.11	21.5	27.9 P = 0.10	25.8	23.2 P = 0.10	15.2	27.2 P = 0.45	24.7
BP <140/90 mmHg (<130/85 in those with diabetes)	65.3 P = 0.04	55.2	67.0 P = 0.21	63.0	57.6 P = 0.03	40.5	71.2 P = 0.03	53.2
BP <140/90 mmHg in patients without diabetes	71.9 P = 0.04	60.0	Numbers too small		66.8 P = 0.04	48.4	Numbers too small	
BP <130/85 mmHg in patients with diabetes	36.2 P = 0.26	32.8	Numbers too small		38.4 P = 0.04	19.0	Numbers too small	
TC <5 mmol/L	77.5 P = 0.23	70.8	34.7 P = 0.60	33.0	35.8 P = 0.64	295 (31.5)	33.2 P = 0.0.76	30.2
LDL-C <3 mmol/L	80.7 P = 0.07	74.0	42.9 P = 0.48	40.1	44.8 P = 0.17	35.2	39.4 P = 0.71	37.5
HbA1c <7% (in those with diabetes)	60.6 P = 0.29	50.0	54.6 Numbers too small	44.4	79.9 P = 0.12	65.4	83.3 Numbers too small	31.3
Antiplatelet therapy	93.2 P = 0.28	92.2	13.5 P = 0.45	14.4	13.4 P = 0.19	10.2	14.4 P = 0.35	9.1
Beta-blockers	76.4 P = 0.16	80.1	17.0 P = 0.79	17.1	17.4 P = 0.91	15.7	18.8 P = 0.43	12.4
ACE inhibitors	52.4 P = 0.26	56.2	16.3 P = 0.92	10.5	29.4 P = 0.02	19.5	12.1 P = 0.84	11.0
Statins	85.7 P = 0.04	80.1	19.1 P = 0.38	15.0	37.7 P = 0.03	22.1	22.0 P = 0.23	15.4

*The difference in percentages were calculated by combining the country-specific differences using a random effect meta-analysis (REML estimation); **Hospital: patients at goal as a proportion of the target population (self-reported smoking in the month prior to the index event); Primary care: proportion of patients not smoking at final assessment; ***Random subsample only; NA: not available; INT, intervention; UC; usual care.

tensive agents, a statin and folic acid (to lower homocysteine levels) could reduce coronary heart disease by 80% and stroke by 88%, with few adverse effects. While the use of a polypill in secondary prevention is likely to be more readily acceptable as each component is already recommended in this population, the use of the polypill in individuals with no CVD and selected solely on age is controversial. At present there is only one trial of the polypill that has been published.[45] The Indian Polypill Study (TIPS)[15] evaluated 8 different drug (combination) regimens and demonstrated that the polypill was well tolerated, but that the degree of reduction of BP and LDL was substantially lower (by about half) than the projections of Wald and Law. Using the observed decreases in risk factors, the TIPS investigators projected that a polypill could reduce the risk of myocardial infarction by about 50%, and that of stroke by about 60%. These estimates require validation in large and long term randomized trials, and at least two such trials in primary prevention are underway.

Summary

An integrated approach to prevention of cardiovascular disease is required for all eligible patients in everyday clinical practice. The WHO describes strategies for secondary and primary prevention of atherosclerotic disease in order to reduce the risk of cardiovascular events, improve quality of life and life expectancy.

In a meta-analysis of cardiac rehabilitation compared with usual care, all-cause mortality was reduced (OR 0.80; 95% CI 0.68–0.93), as was cardiac mortality (OR 0.74; 95% CI 0.61–0.96) (**Class I, Level A**). There was no difference in recurrent myocardial infarction, CABG or PTCA (**Class IIb, Level B**). At follow-up, the number of patients who reported smoking was also reduced in the cardiac rehabilitation group (OR 0.64; 95% CI 0.50–0.83) (**Class IIa, Level B**) and there were significant reductions in systolic blood pressure, total cholesterol and triglyceride concentration (**Class IIa, Level B**). With the exception of smoking, other risk factor changes were rather small so the observed reduction in total and cardiac mortality can be largely attributed to lifestyle changes. The contribution of secondary prevention programs, with or without exercise, was also evaluated in a separate meta-analysis. All-cause mortality was reduced with a risk ratio (RR) of 0.85 (95% CI 0.77–0.94) and this benefit improved over time with a RR of 0.53 (95% CI 0.35–0.81) at 24 months (**Class I, Level A**). Recurrent myocardial infarction was also reduced with a RR of 0.83 (95% CI 0.74–0.94) over a median follow-up of 12 months (**Class I, Level A**). The effects of these programs on other cardiovascular risk factors were also considered to be moderate to small (**Class IIb, Level B**). Importantly, total mortality and myocardial infarction reductions were similar for programs

Table 24.10 Integrated approach to lifestyle, risk factor and therapeutic management for secondary and primary prevention of cardiovascular disease

	Patients with atherosclerotic cardiovascular disease	Asymptomatic patients at high multifactorial risk of developing CVD
Lifestyle		
Smoking habit	All smokers should be advised and supported by a physician or other health professional to stop smoking completely (**Class I, Level A**)	
	Therapeutic support with (i) nicotine replacement therapies or (ii) buproprion or (iii) nicotine receptor antagonist, should be offered to all smokers (**Class I, Level B**)	
Diet	A dietitian or trained health professional should formally assess nutrient intake of patients and their partners and then advise on healthy food choices which achieve the following:	
	Total intake of fat ≤30% of total daily energy intake (**Class I, Level A**)	
	Intake of saturated fats to ≤10% of total daily energy intake (**Class I, Level A**)	
	Replacement of saturated fats with monounsaturated or polyunsaturated fats (**Class I, Level A**)	
	Reduction of daily salt intake to less than 5 g per day (**Class I, Level A**)	
	Daily intake of fresh fruit and vegetables, as well as wholegrains and pulses, to at least 400 g per day (**Class IIa, Level C**)	
	Consumption of fish and other marine foods to provide >200 mg per day of eicosapentaenoic (EPA) and docosahexanaenoic (DHA) fatty acids (**Class I, Level A**)	
	Reduction of the intake of dietary cholesterol to <300 mg per day (**Class IIa, Level C**)	
	Reduction of alcohol to <14 units/week (in women) and <21 units/week (in men) (**Class IIa, Level C**)	
Physical activity	An exercise specialist or trained health professional should formally assess physical activity of patients and their partners and then advise on specific activities which achieve the following: regular moderate-intensity activity (e.g. brisk walking) lasting at least 30 minutes per day on at least 5 days of the week (**Class I, Level A**)	

Continued on p. 340

Table 24.10 *Continued*

	Patients with atherosclerotic cardiovascular disease	Asymptomatic patients at high multifactorial risk of developing CVD
Other risk factors		
Body weight and distribution	A dietitian or other health professional should measure height, weight and waist circumference. All individuals who are overweight or obese should be encouraged to lose weight through a combination of a reduced-energy diet and increased physical activity (**Class I, Level B**) The targets for BMI and waist circumference are: BMI: <25 kg/m^2 (Caucasians); <23 kg/m^2 (Asians) Waist circumference: Caucasians: men <94 cm; women <80 cm Asians: men <90 cm; women <80 cm	
Blood pressure	Blood pressure should be measured regularly by a health professional The decision to start blood pressure-lowering medication depends not only on the blood pressure levels but also on total CVD risk Lifestyle advice should be given to all patients with elevated blood pressure Individuals with established CVD, people at high multifactorial risk and individuals with particularly elevated blood pressure, or lesser degree of raised blood pressure with target organ damage, should be given blood pressure-lowering therapy (**Class I, Level A**)	
Lipids Total cholesterol LDL cholesterol	Fasting lipids (total cholesterol, HDL cholesterol and triglycerides) should be measured regularly by a health professional The decision to start lipid-lowering medication depends not only on the lipid levels but also on total CVD risk Lifestyle advice should be given to all patients with dyslipidemia Individuals with established CVD, people at high multifactorial risk, individuals with particularly elevated total and LDL cholesterol should be given a statin or other LLD (if statin is contraindicated) (**Class I, Level A**)	
Glucose Fasting plasma glucose	Fasting plasma glucose should be measured on at least three separate occasions and if the FPG is >6.0 mmol/L (>110 mg/dL) an oral glucose tolerance test (OGTT) should be performed. Glycated hemoglobin (HbA1c) should be checked in all patients with DM Patients with dysglycemia or DM require professional dietary advice and oral hypoglycemic +/– insulin medication (**Class I, Level A**) ACE inhibitors/ARBs and statins are recommended to reduce cardiovascular risk (**Class I, Level A**)	
Cardioprotective drug therapies		
Antiplatelet drugs	Aspirin 75 mg/daily (**Class I, Level A**)	Aspirin 75 mg/daily (**Class IIa, Level B**)
Beta-blockers	All people following myocardial infarction (**Class I, Level A**) People with heart failure or LV dysfunction (**Class I, Level A**) For angina to relieve the symptom of myocardial ischemia (**Class I, Level A**)	As an antihypertensive therapy (ACE inhibitors, calcium channel blockers and diuretics are preferred as the first- and second-line antihypertensive therapies) (**Class IIa, Level A**)
ACE inhibitors/ARBs	Treatment of heart failure or left ventricular dysfunction (**Class I, Level A**) To reduce blood pressure for secondary prevention (**Class IIa, Level B**)	To reduce blood pressure for primary prevention (**Class I, Level A**)
Statins	All patients with established CVD to reduce TC and LDL cholesterol to target (**Class I, Level A**)	All high-risk people for primary prevention (**Class I, Level A**)
Anticoagulants	Consider in: large anterior MI, left ventricular aneurysm, paroxysmal tachyarrhythmia, severe heart failure to reduce the risk of thromboembolic event (**Class II, Level B**)	
Blood relatives	First-degree relatives of patients with premature atherosclerotic disease (men <55 years and women <65 years) should be screened for cardiovascular risk factors, including fasting lipids. The genetic disorder of familial hypercholesterolemia (FH) should be considered when interpreting lipid results in these family members (**Class IIa, Level C**)	If total cholesterol is > or equal to 8.0 mmol/L consider screening first-degree relatives for FH (**Class IIa, Level C**)

that included exercise and risk factor education, or risk factor education without exercise, or exercise alone. So the distinction between "cardiac rehabilitation" and "secondary prevention" is artificial and comparisons based on crude program definitions are usually confounded. What these meta-analyses really demonstrate are the overall benefits of an integrated multidisciplinary and comprehensive multifactorial approach to reducing cardiovascular risk, cardiovascular events and all-cause mortality.

In primary prevention those programs undertaking multifactorial interventions have not achieved the same clinical outcomes as those seen for single risk factor interventions. In a meta-analysis the pooled OR for total and CHD mortality were 0.96 (95% CI 0.92–1.01) and 0.96 (95% CI 0.89–1.04) respectively (**Class IIb, Level B**). A small but potentially important treatment benefit (about a 10% reduction in CHD mortality) may have been missed. There was a modest reduction in smoking (the odds of reduction in smoking prevalence was 20% (95% CI 8–31%)) (**Class IIb, Level B**) with only small changes in blood pressure and lipids. Importantly, it is the use of drugs or not which largely explains differences in treatment effect between unifactorial (almost entirely drugs) and multifactorial (lifestyle and limited drugs) trials in primary prevention. A multidisciplinary and comprehensive multifactorial approach to primary prevention, combining a professional lifestyle intervention and appropriate drug management of other major risk factors, will have a greater beneficial impact on clinical outcomes.

A nurse-managed multidisciplinary, comprehensive multifactorial, preventive cardiology program (EUROACTION) for coronary and high-risk patients and their families across Europe achieved healthier lifestyles and better control of blood pressure and other risk factors, with more effective use of cardioprotective drug therapies (**Class I, Level A**). EUROACTION is only one model of preventive cardiology, successfully implemented and objectively assessed, which is generalizable to everyday clinical practice. At present, lifestyle and risk factor standards set by prevention guidelines are not achieved by a majority of patients, as evidenced by EUROASPIRE and other surveys, and only a minority access professional preventive cardiology programs. To achieve the clinical benefits of a multidisciplinary, comprehensive multifactorial, prevention program, we need to integrate professional lifestyle interventions with effective risk factor management and evidence-based drug therapies, appropriately adapted to the medical, cultural, and economic setting of a country.

References

1. World Health Organization. *Prevention of Cardiovascular Disease: Guidelines for Assessment and Management of Total Cardiovascular Risk*. Geneva: WHO, 2007.

2. Graham I, Atar D, Borch-Johnsen K *et al.* European Guidelines on Cardiovascular Disease Prevention in Clinical Practice: Fourth Joint Task Force of the European Society of Cardiology and Other Societies on Cardiovascular Disease Prevention in Clinical Prevention in Clinical Practice. *Eur J Cardiovasc Prev Rehabil* 2007;**14**(suppl 2):S1–S113.

3. Allender S, Scharbotough P, Peto V, Rayner M, Leal J, Luengo-Fernández R, Gray A. *European Cardiovascular Disease Statistics: 2008 Edition*. London: British Heart Foundation, 2008.

4. Leal J, Luengo-Fernández R, Gray A, Petersen S, Rayner M. Economic burden of cardiovascular diseases in the enlarged European Union. *Eur Heart J* 2006;**27**:1610–19.

5. Lopez A, Mathers CD, Ezzati M, Jamison D, Murray C. Global and regional burden of disease and risk factors, 2001: systematic analysis of population health data. *Lancet* 2006;**367**:1747–57.

6. Manuel DG, Lim J, Tanuseputro P *et al.* Revisiting Rose: strategies for reducing coronary heart disease. *BMJ* 2006;**332**: 659–62.

7. World Health Organization. *Prevention of recurrent heart attacks and strokes in low and middle income populations. Evidence-based recommendations for policy makers and health professionals*. Geneva: WHO, 2003.

8. Smith S, Jackson R, Pearson T *et al.* Principles for national and regional guidelines on cardiovascular disease prevention: a scientific statement from the World Heart and Stroke Forum. *Circulation* 2004;**109**:3112–21.

9. Jackson R, Barham P, Bills J *et al.* Management of raised blood pressure in New Zealand: a discussion document. *BMJ* 1993;**307**: 107–10.

10. Pyörälä K, De Backer G, Graham I, Poole-Wilson PA, Wood D. Prevention of coronary heart disease in clinical practice. Recommendations of the Task Force of the European Society of Cardiology, European Atherosclerotic Society and European Society of Hypertension. *Eur Heart J* 1994;**15**:1300–31.

11. Wood D, De Backer G, Faergeman D, Graham I, Mancia G, Pyörälä K. Prevention of coronary heart disease in clinical practice. Recommendations of the Second Joint Task Force of European and other Societies on coronary prevention. *Eur Heart J* 1998;**19**:1434–503.

12. Anderson KM, Wilson PW, Odell PM, Kannel WB. An updated coronary risk profile. A statement for health professionals. *Circulation* 1991;**83**:356–62.

13. De Backer G, Ambrosioni E, Bort-Johnsen K *et al.* European guidelines on cardiovascular disease prevention in clinical practice. Third Joint Task Force of European and other Societies on Cardiovascular Disease Prevention in Clinical Practice. *Eur J Cardiovasc Prev Rehab* 2003;**10**(suppl 1):S1–S78.

14. Graham I, Atar D, Borch-Johnsen K *et al.* European Guidelines on Cardiovascular Disease Prevention in Clinical Practice: Fourth Joint Task Force of the European Society of Cardiology and Other Societies on Cardiovascular Disease Prevention in Clinical Prevention in Clinical Practice (Constituted by representatives of nine societies and by invited experts). *Eur J Cardiovasc Prev Rehabil* 2007;**14**(Suppl 2): S1–S113. Executive summary: *Eur J Cardiovasc Prev Rehabil* 2007; **14** (Suppl 2): E1–E40; *Eur Heart J* 2007;**28**:2375–414.

15. Conroy RM, Pyörälä K, Fitzgerald AP *et al.* Estimation of ten-year risk of fatal cardiovascular disease in Europe: the SCORE project. *Eur Heart J* 2003;**24**:987–1003.

16. World Health Organization. *The World Health Report 2002: reducing risks, promoting healthy life.* Geneva: WHO, 2002.

17. World Health Organization. *Needs and Priorities in Cardiac Rehabilitation and Secondary Prevention in Patients with Coronary Heart Disease.* WHO Technical Report Series 831. Geneva: WHO, 1993.

18. World Health Organization. *Report on a Seminar, Noordwijk aan Zee. The Rehabilitation of Patients with Cardiovascular Diseases.* Copenhagen: WHO, Regional Office for Europe, 1969.

19. Jolliffe J, Rees K, Taylor RRS, Thompson DR, Oldridge N, Ebrahim S. Exercise-based rehabilitation for coronary heart disease. *Cochrane Database of Systematic Reviews* 2001, Issue 1. Art. No.: CD001800. DOI: 10.1002/14651858.CD001800.

20. Taylor R, Brown A, Ebrahim S *et al.* Exercise based rehabilitation for patients with coronary heart disease: systematic review and meta-analysis of randomized controlled trials. *Am J Med* 2004;**116**:682–92.

21. McAlister FA, Lawson FME, Teo KK, Armstrong PW. Randomised trials of secondary prevention programmes in coronary heart disease: systematic review. *BMJ* 2001;**323**:957–62.

22. Clark AM, Hartling L, Vandermeer B, McAlister FA. Meta-analysis: secondary prevention programs for patients with coronary artery disease. *Ann Intern Med* 2005;**143**:659–72.

23. EUROASPIRE Study Group. EUROASPIRE. A European Society of Cardiology survey of secondary prevention of coronary heart disease: principal results. *Eur Heart J* 1997;**18**: 1569–82.

24. EUROASPIRE Study Group. Lifestyle and risk factor management and use of drug therapies in coronary patients from 15 countries. Principal results from EUROASPIRE II. Euro Heart Survey Programme. *Eur Heart J* 2001;**22**:554–72.

25. EUROASPIRE Study Group. Clinical reality of coronary prevention guidelines: a comparison of EUROASPIRE I and II in nine countries. *Lancet* 2001;**357**:995–1001.

26. Kotseva K, Wood D, De Backer G, De Bacquer D, Pyorala K, Keil U, on behalf of EUROASPIRE study Group. Cardiovascular prevention guidelines – the clinical reality: a comparison of EUROASPIRE I, II and III surveys in 8 European countries. *Lancet* 2009;**372**:929–40.

27. Kotseva K, Wood D, De Backer G, De Bacquer D, Pyorala K, Keil U, on behalf of EUROASPIRE study Group. EUROASPIRE III: A survey on the lifestyle, risk factors and use of cardioprotective drug therapies in coronary patients from twenty two European countries. EUROASPIRE Study Group. *Europ J Cardiovasc Prev Rehabilitation* 2009;**16**:121–37.

28. Kotseva K, Wood D, De Bacquer D *et al*, on behalf of the EUROASPIRE II Study Group. Cardiac rehabilitation for coronary patients: lifestyle, risk factor and therapeutic management. Results from the EUROASPIRE II survey. *Eur Heart J* 2004;**6**(suppl J):J17–J26.

29. De Sutter J, De Bacquer D, Kotseva K *et al*, on behalf of the EUROASPIRE II Study Group. Screening of family members of patients with premature coronary heart disease. Results from the EUROASPIRE II family survey. *Eur Heart J* 2003;**24**:249–57.

30. Ebrahim S, Davey Smith G. Systematic review of randomised controlled trials of multiple risk factor interventions for preventing coronary heart disease. *BMJ* 1997;**314**:1666–74.

31. Ebrahim S, Beswick A, Burke M, Davey Smith G. Multiple risk factor interventions for primary prevention of coronary heart disease. *Cochrane Database of Systematic Reviews* 2006, Issue 4. Art. No.: CD001561. DOI: 10.1002/14651858.CD001561.pub2.

32. Critchley JA, Capewell S. Smoking cessation for the secondary prevention of coronary heart disease. *Cochrane Database of Systematic Reviews* 2003, Issue 4. Art. No.: CD003041. DOI: 10.1002/14651858.CD003041.pub2.

33. Blood Pressure Lowering Treatment Trialists' Collaboration. Effects of different blood pressure-lowering regimens on major cardiovascular events: results of prospectively designed overviews of randomised trials. *Lancet* 2003;**362**:1527–45.

34. Blood Pressure Lowering Treatment Trialists' Collaboration. Effects of different blood pressure-lowering regimens on major cardiovascular events in individuals with and without diabetes mellitus. *Arch Intern Med* 2005;**165**:1410–19.

35. Blood Pressure Lowering Treatment Trialists' Collaboration. Effects of different regimens to lower blood pressure on major cardiovascular events in older and younger adults: meta-analysis of randomised trials. *BMJ* 2008;**336**:1121–3.

36. Law MR, Wald NJ, Thompson SG. By how much and how quickly does reduction in serum cholesterol concentration lower risk of ischaemic heart disease? *BMJ* 1994;**308**:367–72.

37. Law MR, Wald NJ, Rudnicka AR. Quantifying effect of statins on low density lipoprotein cholesterol, ischaemic heart disease, and stroke: systematic review and meta-analysis. *BMJ* 2003;**326**: 1423–9.

38. Cholesterol Treatment Trialists' (CTT) Collaboration. Efficacy and safety of cholesterol-lowering treatment: prospective meta-analysis of data from 90 056 participants in 14 randomised trials of statins. *Lancet* 2005;**366**:1267–78.

39. Wood DA, Kotseva K, Jennings C *et al.* EUROACTION: a European Society of Cardiology demonstration project in preventive cardiology. A cluster randomised controlled trial of a multi-disciplinary preventive cardiology programme for coronary patients, asymptomatic high risk individuals and their families. Summary of design, methodology and outcomes. *Eur Heart J* 2004;**6**(suppl J):J3–J15.

40. Wood DA, Kotseva K, Connolly S *et al*, on behalf of the EURO-ACTION Study Group. EUROACTION: a European Society of Cardiology demonstration project in preventive cardiology. A paired cluster randomised controlled trial of a multi-disciplinary family based preventive cardiology programme for coronary patients and asymptomatic high risk individuals. *Lancet* 2008;**371**:1999–2012.

41. Wood DA, Roberts TL, Campbell M. Women married to men with myocardial infarction are at increased risk of coronary heart disease. *J Cardiovasc Risk* 1997;**4**:7–11.

42. Pyke SD, Wood DA, Kinmonth AL, Thomson SG. Change in coronary risk and coronary risk factor levels in couples following lifestyle intervention. The British Family Heart Study. *Arch Fam Med* 1997;**6**:354–60.

43. Yusuf S. Two decades of progress in preventing vascular disease. *Lancet* 2002;**360**:2–3.

44. Wald NJ, Law MR. A strategy to reduce cardiovascular disease by more than 80%. *BMJ* 2003;**326**:1419.

45. The Indian Polycap Study (TIPS), Yusuf S, Pais P, Afzal R, Xavier D, Teo K, Eikelboom J, Sigamani A, Mohan V, Gupta R, Thomas N. Effects of a polypill (Polycap) on risk factors in middle-aged individuals without cardiovascular disease (TIPS): a phase II, double-blind, randomised trial. *Lancet* 2009; **373**(9672): 1341–51.

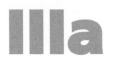

IIIa Stable coronary artery disease

John A Cairns and Bernard J Gersh, Editors

25 Medical management of stable coronary artery disease

William E Boden

Division of Cardiovascular Medicine, State University of New York at Buffalo; Buffalo General Hospital, Buffalo, NY, USA

Introduction

Angina pectoris accounts for approximately 6.5 million of the 13 million cases of coronary heart disease (CHD) prevalence in the United States. The economic burden of symptomatic angina and CHD is great, with aggregate direct and indirect costs approximating $150 billion per year.[1] Stable angina refers to discomfort in the chest, neck, arms, and jaws that is precipitated typically by physical activity or emotional stress and is relieved by rest or nitroglycerin. It usually occurs in patients with obstruction of one or more of the coronary arteries though some patients presenting with angina may have normal coronary arteries. Impaired microvascular perfusion related in part to obstructive plaque formation causes a mismatch between myocardial oxygen demand and supply which contributes to development and progression of angina.[2,3]

Despite the unabated growth in percutaneous coronary intervention (PCI) and coronary artery bypass graft (CABG) surgery for treating symptomatic CHD, the prevalence of angina pectoris in the US continues to increase. Inability to tolerate full doses of antianginal agents, limitations due to adverse effects from combinations of medications, intolerance or tachyphylaxis to various antianginal agents, such as nitrates, and persistent ischemia despite revascularization[4] have emphasized a need for more aggressive approaches to management of persistent as well as recurring angina. Drug therapy for stable angina includes antianginal and anti-ischemic agents that improve the "quality" of life and vasculoprotective agents that increase the "quantity" of life.[5] Aspirin, beta-blockers, angiotensin-converting enzyme (ACE) inhibitors and statins are recognized as vasculoprotective agents while beta-blockers also prevent or reduce ischemia. By contrast, long-acting nitrates, calcium channel blockers (CCBs) and newer agents such as ranolazine are anti-ischemic, but have not been shown to provide vasculoprotection.[3]

Epidemiology

Chronic stable angina is the major symptomatic presentation in about 50% of CHD patients.[5,6] There is a growing prevalence of chronic ischemia and angina due to residual coronary artery disease (CAD) after PCI and CABG. Of the 1620 consecutive NHLBI dynamic registry patients who underwent PCI, 26% continued to report angina despite more than one antianginal medication.[7] In the ARTS trial, patients were randomized to PCI or CABG for symptom relief. Despite optimal revascularization nearly 80% of the patients in the PCI group and 60% in the CABG group continued to experience angina and required antianginal medications.[4] Thus increased revascularization has led to increasing residual ischemia, and an increasing need for medical therapy.

Patients continue to experience persistent ischemia and angina despite traditional drug therapy. A significant percentage of patients have relative intolerance to full doses of nitrates, CCB and beta-blockers, and despite use of traditional agents, patients reported having two anginal episodes per week on average.[3] Combinations of beta-blockers and CCBs have similar depressive effects on blood pressue (BP), heart rate (HR) and AV nodal conduction, thus limiting maximal dosage of each of the medications. Thus improved treatment of recurring ischemia and angina remains an important therapeutic goal.

Definition and classification

Chronic stable angina pectoris is often predictable and is classically manifest as substernal or precordial chest discomfort that typically occurs after physical activity,

Evidence-Based Cardiology, 3rd edition. Edited by S. Yusuf, J.A. Cairns, A.J. Camm, E.L. Fallen, and B.J. Gersh. © 2010 Blackwell Publishing, ISBN: 978-1-4051-5925-8.

emotional stress or both. The site of discomfort is usually retrosternal but may radiate to neck, arms or jaw. Classic (typical) angina presents as a sensation in the chest of squeezing, heaviness or pressure, which usually lasts up to 15 minutes and abates when the stressor is gone, the patient rests or uses sublingual nitroglycerin. Chest discomfort that occurs during rest or at night has been described in patients with chronic stable angina, although this is generally more typical of unstable angina or acute coronary syndrome. Anginal equivalents such as exertional dyspnea, sweating, excessive fatigue, and fainting are common in women and in the elderly. Atypical presentations are more common in women who may report variable pain thresholds, inframammary pain, palpitations or sharp stabbing pain. Patient with diabetes and dysautonomia may present with atypical pain, dyspnea or no symptoms ("silent myocardial ischemia"). Classification of the severity of the angina is useful in management of chronic angina (Box 25.1).[3,8]

Pathophysiology

A disparity between the metabolic demands of the myocardium during exertion (as a consequence of increasing contractility, heart rate and systolic wall stress) and the inability to supply incremental coronary blood flow (CBF) due to narrowed epicardial coronary arteries in the face of increased myocardial oxygen demand is the principal factor in developing angina pectoris in CHD.[9] Increases in heart rate precipitated by adrenergic stresses, such as physical or emotional stress, sexual activity, or physiologic stresses such as arrhythmias, thyrotoxicosis or infection may precipitate so-called "demand angina".[9] CBF is the most important determinant of myocardial oxygen supply. Numerous factors influence the epicardial and subendocardial blood flow. Limitations of CBF may be due to atherosclerosis in either the epicardial or coronary microvasculature. In the epicardial coronary arteries, as coronary atherosclerosis progresses, there is progressive plaque deposition in the wall of the artery. As atherosclerosis worsens, the plaque may cause hemodynamic obstruction to CBF and may result in angina.[3] Typically, coronary luminal narrowings less than 70% of cross-sectional area

may not elicit either spontaneous or exercise-induced angina or ischemia, since the microvasculature (coronary resistance vessels) has the capacity to dilate and increase subendocardial perfusion in response to increasing demand. Such dilation, however, generally becomes maximized when coronary stenoses exceed 70% which, in turn, will trigger either spontaneous or exercise-induced anginal episodes. Symptomatic angina usually occurs about 25–30 seconds after onset of the ischemic cascade.[10] Approximately one-half of all stable CAD patients experience episodes of silent myocardial ischemia.

Endothelial dysfunction and coronary vasomotor control are important determinants of myocardial oxygen supply. Impaired smooth muscle relaxation has been suggested as a marker for atherosclerosis. In the WISE study, attenuation of coronary flow reserve was observed with intracoronary adenosine, suggesting impaired vascular smooth muscle relaxation.[11] In patients with CAD, there is loss of endothelium-dependent vasodilation and increased sensitivity to catecholamine-induced vasoconstriction.[12] This may become manifest in patients as "variable threshold angina" due to superimposed dynamic obstruction secondary to vasoconstriction of narrowed atherosclerotic vessels.

There is accumulating evidence that implicates coronary microcirculatory dysfunction in CHD patients with angina pectoris, including wide variability in effort tolerance over time, a large scatter or overlap between stenosis severity and coronary flow reserve, and variability in clinical outcomes after initial successful PCI. Approximately 25% of biomarker-positive ACS patients exhibit no flow-limiting stenosis at coronary angiography, but may display plaque fissuring or erosion with microvascular embolization.[13]

Medical management of myocardial ischemia

Comprehensive management of myocardial ischemia involves antianginal (anti-ischemic) agents and vasculoprotective agents. Antianginal therapies with nitrates, beta-blockers and CCBs are useful for symptom management. Vasculoprotective therapy includes lifestyle changes and pharmacologic therapy with antiplatelet therapy, ACE inhibitors (ACE-I), and statins which, in the aggregate, reduce progression of atherosclerosis, stabilize atherosclerotic plaque, and decrease the risk of thrombosis in patients with chronic stable angina.

Lifestyle changes

Intensive multifactorial risk reduction has been shown to reduce the rate of coronary luminal narrowing and decrease hospitalizations for cardiac events.[14] Patients with chronic stable angina who are receiving medical therapy should be encouraged to exercise as tolerated by their symptoms. Regular exercise may promote "ischemic preconditioning" and provide protection during recurring bouts of ischemia. A trial comparing PCI with graded, regular aerobic exercise in patients with single-vessel CAD showed that 20 minutes of daily exercise was associated with improved maximal myocardial O_2 uptake, lower costs, and fewer rehospitalizations for angina pectoris as compared with PCI during a 1-year follow-up.[15] All patients should be encouraged to enroll in a comprehensive cardiac rehabilitation program. A diet low in saturated fat, and with appropriate restriction of excessive carbohydrate consumption (especially in patients with diabetes mellitus (DM) or insulin resistance) is encouraged.[5] Epidemiologic studies have also consistently demonstrated the benefits associated with modest alcohol intake, which may reduce progression of CAD and lower the likelihood of developing coronary events.[5] Vigorous efforts at smoking cessation and weight control should be encouraged in all patients.[5] In patients with DM, strict control of blood sugar (with a target HbA1C less than 7%) and control of blood pressure (target less than 120–130/80 mmHg) may reduce the rate of secondary events.[5]

Adjunctive pharmacologic therapy

Antiplatelet agents

Aspirin and clopidogrel are the common antiplatelet agents that have been used in the secondary prevention of cardiovascular disease. In high-risk patients with CHD, the use of aspirin was associated with a significantly reduced risk of non-fatal MI, non-fatal stroke and vascular death by 22%.[16] In patients with chronic stable angina, use of aspirin was associated with significant reduction in proinflammatory markers and high-sensitivity C-reactive protein (hs-CRP) levels.[17] Long-term aspirin at a dose of 81–325 mg is recommended in all patients with stable angina who do not exhibit aspirin allergy or evidence of aspirin resistance,[5] in which cases clopidogrel may be substituted. The use of clopidogrel alone was slightly superior to aspirin, and associated with 8.7% relative reduction in vascular death, ischemic stroke and myocardial infarction in the large CAPRIE study.[18]

Dual antiplatelet therapy has been well studied in patients with acute coronary syndrome (ACS) and those undergoing PCI. In the CHARISMA trial,[19] over 15 000 patients with clinically evident cardiovascular disease or multiple risk factors were randomized to receive clopidogrel (75 mg) with low-dose aspirin (75–162 mg daily) or placebo plus low-dose aspirin. The combination of clopidogrel plus aspirin was not significantly more effective than aspirin alone in reducing the composite primary endpoint of MI, stroke or death from cardiovascular causes among patients with stable CHD or multiple cardiovascular risk factors. There was a strong suggestion of benefit in patients with established vascular disease and symptomatic atherothrombosis (prespecified secondary endpoint), but alternatively, a suggestion of harm in asymptomatic patients with multiple risk factors and no demonstrable heart or vascular disease.

ACE inhibitors

The role of ACE-I in patients with left ventricular dysfunction has been well documented.[20–22] ACE-I improve survival in patients with symptomatic and asymptomatic heart failure, improve heart function after MI, and have provided renal protection in patients with renal insufficiency, especially diabetics. The use of ACE-I is a **Class I, Level A** recommendation in stable angina patients with diabetes, previous MI and those with evidence of left ventricular systolic dysfunction, generally defined as an ejection fraction <40%.[5] Treatment with quinapril improved endothelial function in patients who did not have severe hyperlipidemia or heart failure.[23] The Heart Outcomes Prevention and Evaluation (HOPE) trial showed that ramipril reduced cardiovascular death, MI and stroke in patients with vascular disease in the absence of heart failure.[22] However, the Prevention of Events with Angiotensin Converting Enzyme Inhibition (PEACE) trial showed that in patients with stable heart disease and preserved left ventricular function receiving standard therapy, trandolapril did not add any incremental mortality benefit.[24]

Controversy exists over the best ACE-I to use in patients with CAD. Tissue-specific agents such as quinapril, ramipril, perindopril and trandolapril may have high lipophilicity and better ACE binding capability. It is postulated that these tissue specific ACE-I are able to penetrate the endothelial wall better and achieve better degrees of ACE inhibition that may impede atherogenesis, although this remains an unsettled question clinically. In patients who are unable to tolerate ACE-I, angiotensin receptor-blocking agents (ARBs) may be used. ARBs have been shown to be as effective as ACE-I in high-risk patients.[25–27]

Statins

Multiple randomized controlled trials of both primary and secondary prevention have convincingly demonstrated the clinical benefit of statins in reducing death, MI and stroke. The role of statins in patients with cardiovascular disease continues to evolve, with more and more aggressive efforts to lower low-density lipoprotein (LDL) cholesterol to levels <70 mg/d (1.82 mmol/L) in high-risk CHD patients (those who are post-MI, ACS patients, diabetics, and those with prior stroke or peripheral arterial disease). Epidemiologic studies have shown a consistent and positive relationship between LDL cholesterol and the risk of coronary heart disease.[28] Statins have emerged as the most widely prescribed medication for lowering LDL cholesterol. The reduction in LDL cholesterol with statins ranges from 30% to 60%. The benefits of statins may at least partly be explained by the reduction in LDL cholesterol. Statins generally do not cause a significant increase in high-density lipoprotein (HDL) cholesterol or a reduction in serum triglyceride levels, with the possible exception of rosuvastatin. They have been shown to promote plaque stabilization in ACS patients,[29] improve endothelial dysfunction, and elicit regression of atherosclerotic plaques.[30] The anti-inflammatory effects of statins are reflected in the reduction seen in C-reactive protein levels.[31] These benefits have translated clinically into significant reductions in total mortality, rates of fatal and non-fatal MI, stroke, and the need for myocardial revascularization procedures in patients with stable CAD.[32,33] Lipid reduction with statins has been shown to reduce the progression of atherosclerosis not only in native vessels, but also in graft vessels after CABG surgery.[34] Intensive lowering of lipids (LDL <70 mg/dL) as compared to moderate lipid reduction (LDL <100 mg/dL) has been demonstrated to result in less progression of atheroma burden in the coronary arteries.[35] Trials of lower LDL cholesterol levels in patients with stable CAD and angina have demonstrated the benefits of statins and the need to lower the targets for LDL cholesterol for secondary prevention. These trials form the basis of the NCEP guidelines for LDL cholesterol to less than 100 mg/dL in high-risk patients and less than 70 mg/dL for very high-risk patients (e.g. diabetes).[36] Higher doses of statins may increase the incidence of adverse effects. Intensive lipid lowering with 80 mg of atorvastatin daily is associated with greater incidence of elevated serum aminotransferases as compared to 10 mg of atorvastatin daily.[37] The risk of muscle injury is increased with higher doses of statins as well as with the concomitant use of fibrates, which may be used in CAD patients with mixed dyslipidemia (high LDL-C and triglyceride levels).

The role of HDL-C is being increasingly recognized because of the strong inverse relationship between low levels of HDL-C and the risk of developing cardiac events. There are abundant epidemiologic data to support the observation that a low HDL-C level is a strong, independent predictor of CHD risk, with levels less than 35 mg/dL associated with an eightfold higher risk than HDL-C levels above 65 mg/dL.[38] Raising the level of HDL-C has been shown to reduce coronary event rates in primary and secondary prevention. Based on growing clinical evidence, patients should be treated to achieve HDL-C of 40 mg/dL in men and 50 mg/dL in women.[39] Combination therapy with a statin and extended-release niacin may offer the best strategy for controlling mixed dyslipidemia characterized by increased LDL-C and reduced HDL-C levels, and may optimize cardiovascular rate reduction in patients with CHD.[40,41]

Inhibition of cholesterol absorption

Ezetimibe is the first member of a class of agents that inhibits the absorption of cholesterol from the intestine.[42,43] Ezetimibe co-administered with statins produces inhibition of both cholesterol synthesis and intestinal cholesterol absorption, resulting in complementary effects that lower LDL-C.[44,45] Co-administration of ezetimibe with a statin results in approximately a 18–24% greater reduction of LDL-C, beyond the LDL-C reduction attributable to the statin alone.[46,47] Accordingly, the percentage of patients who can reach their risk-appropriate NCEP goal is considerably higher when ezetimibe is added to LDL-C-reducing therapy, especially statins.[42,47]

Recent data have shown that ezetimibe also leads to significantly greater reductions in CRP in combination with statins; in one study, reductions on CRP ranged from 26% to 44% across background simvastatin doses of 10–80 mg as compared with 4–20% reductions with simvastatin alone at the same doses. Thus, with both greater LDL-C and CRP reductions, the percentage of patients who reach LDL-C <70 mg/dL in conjunction with CRP <2 mg/dL[17] is nearly doubled when ezetimibe is added. In the recent Vytorin Versus Atorvastatin (VYVA) trial, the combination ezetimibe/simvastatin approximately doubled the rates of achieving this degree of lowering of LDL-C and CRP across the approved dose ranges.[44] This promises to be an important component of combination dyslipidemic therapy, although definitive clinical outcomes data are presently lacking until the ongoing IMPROVE-IT Trial is completed and published.

Anti-ischemic/antianginal therapy

Beta-blockers

Beta-blockers have a **Class 1, Level A** recommendation for the initial therapy of patients with prior MI.[5] However, there is a paucity of prospectively acquired data in patients without prior MI and, in such patients, the ACC/AHA recommendation for chronic stable angina is **Class I, Level B**. Beta-blockers reduce heart rate and contractility and reduce myocardial oxygen demand. Reduction in heart rate increases the diastolic filling time during which nutritive coronary flow occurs, enhancing myocardial tissue perfusion. Beta-blockers limit increases in heart rate during exercise and are particularly effective in exercise-induced angina. Beta-blockers may be non-selective (e.g. propranolol), cardioselective (e.g. atenolol, metoprolol),[48] with intrinsic sympathomimetic effect (e.g. pindolol, acebutolol) or with alpha-blocking activity (e.g. labetolol, carvedilol).[49,50] All of the beta-blockers, including those with combined alpha and beta receptor blockade, have been studied for treatment of stable angina.[51,52] Beta-blockers have been shown to improve survival in patients with previous MI, primary angioplasty for acute ST segment

Table 25.1 Dosage of beta-blockers

Beta-blockers	Dosage	Conditions that may limit use
Propranolol	80–240 mg	Asthma
Metoprolol short acting	50–150 mg twice daily	Severe bradycardia
		AV block
Metoprolol long acting	100–300 mg once daily	Severe depression
		Raynaud's syndrome
Atenolol	25–100 mg once daily	Sick sinus syndrome

Table 25.2 Dosage of calcium channel blockers

Calcium channel blockers	Dose	Conditions that limit use
Nifedipine, sustained release	30–90 mg once daily	AV block
		Bradycardia
Amlodipine	2.5–10 mg once daily	Heart failure
Verapamil, short acting	40–120 mg 2–3 times/ day	Left ventricular dysfunction
Verapamil, sustained release	180–240 mg once/ twice daily	Sinus node dysfunction
Diltiazem, sustained release	120–480 mg once daily	

elevation MI, and patients with heart failure secondary to left ventricular systolic dysfunction. There have been no randomized trials showing survival benefit or reduction in rates of coronary events in patients with only stable angina. Hence, the doses of beta-blockers must be titrated so as to increase exercise tolerance and reduce symptoms of angina while avoiding unwanted side effects (Table 25.1). All beta-blockers are equally effective in alleviating angina pectoris, although optimal doses may vary. Prominent side effects of beta-blockers include bradycardia, bronchoconstriction, fatigue, depression, impotence, and worsening of peripheral vascular disease. Despite concerns about their side effects, beta-blockers can be safely used in many patients with chronic obstructive pulmonary disease or peripheral arterial disease. Beta-blockers may be combined with nitrates and CCBs. The combination of beta-blockers and nitrates is more effective than either agent alone.[53,54] Caution should be used when combining beta-blockers with verapamil and diltiazem due to additive negative inotropic and chronotropic effects and the risk of AV block.

Calcium channel blockers

A variety of calcium channel blockers have been studied in the long-term treatment of chronic stable angina. Calcium channel blockers block the entry of calcium into the myocardial and vascular smooth muscle cells and promote both coronary and peripheral vasodilation. Dihydropyridines (e.g. nifedipine, amlodipine, nicardipine) have a proportionately greater effect on vascular smooth muscle and are particularly effective in reducing systemic arterial blood pressure. Results of a meta-analysis indicated that the use of these drugs for hypertension does not increase morbidity and mortality.[55] Verapamil and diltiazem affect conduction through the AV node and have a negative chronotropic action.

All calcium channel blockers have been shown to be effective in the treatment of chronic stable angina.[56,57] Dihydropyridines reduce the frequency of anginal episodes, improve exercise duration and reduce the need for nitroglycerin. Verapamil, diltiazem and short-acting nifedipine

are effective in vasospastic (Prinzmetal's) angina.[58] Short-acting nifedipine is associated with an increased incidence of cardiovascular events and is not recommended for patients with unstable angina or ACS.[59] On the other hand, verapamil, diltiazem and long-acting dihydropyridines (e.g. amlodipine, extended-release nifedipine) have been shown to be safe and effective in treating stable angina.

Nitrates

Nitroglycerin was the first medication to be used for angina more than 150 years ago. Nitrates reduce myocardial oxygen demand by increasing venous capacitance, thus decreasing LV volume (preload). Nitrates dilate coronary arteries and favorably enhance subendocardial perfusion.[60] Sublingual nitroglycerin has been used to treat the acute onset of anginal symptoms as well as prophylactically to minimize or prevent anginal symptoms when these agents are administered in advance of the known offending activity. Isosorbide dinitrate and its active metabolite, isosorbide mononitrate, are used as an oral preparation for the treatment of angina.[61] Extended-release preparations like isosorbide mononitrate and transdermal nitrate patches offer the convenience of once-daily regimens. None of the nitrate regimens provides 24-hours antianginal prophylaxis due to the development of nitrate tolerance.[62] Prevention of tolerance requires an intermittent dosing strategy with a nitrate-free interval of 8–12 hours. A combination of nitrates with hydralazine, folic acid and antioxidants like vitamin E may reduce the development of nitrate tolerance.[63,64] Carvedilol, with its antioxidant, alpha- and beta-blocking effect, may be a useful combination with nitrates.[65] Nitrates are generally well tolerated, with facial flushing and headache being the most common side effects. Severe hypotension may occur if nitrates are used within 24 hours of phosphodiesterase inhibitors (sildenafil, tadalafil, vardenafil).

Table 25.3 Dosage of nitrates

Nitrates	Dosage	Conditions that limit use
Isosorbide dinitrate, short acting	20–60 mg once daily	Severe aortic stenosis
Isosorbide dinitrate, sustained release	60–120 mg once daily	Hypertrophic obstructive cardiomyopathy
Isosorbide mononitrate, short acting	20 mg twice daily	Caution in patients using medications for erectile dysfunction
Isosorbide mononitrate, sustained release	60–120 mg once daily	
Nitroglycerin patch	0.4–0.6 mg	

Combination of antianginal medications

Combinations of antianginal drugs may be used if symptoms persist. Beta-blockers and nitrates may be more effective than nitrates or beta-blockers alone.[53] Similarly, the combination of beta-blockers with dihydropyridines was more effective for improving exercise duration and was better tolerated than either alone.[66] No data exist on the efficacy of using more than two drugs. Certain drug combinations should be avoided because of the potential for adverse effects including hypotension or bradycardia. Newer agents may offer additional pharmacologic benefit in combination with traditional antianginal medications without the risk of adverse effects.

Newer agents in angina and myocardial ischemia management

Despite intensive escalation of antianginal therapy, including combinations of beta-blockers, long-acting nitrates and calcium channel blockers, some patients continue to experience persistent or refractory angina, and there are now newer mechanistic approaches to optimize pharmacologic management of myocardial ischemia. Additionally, an improved understanding of ischemia mechanisms has prompted new therapeutic approaches towards the treatment of stable angina. The mechanisms of action of these newer drugs are complementary to those of the traditional antianginal medications.

Ranolazine

First approved by the FDA in early 2006, ranolazine is a late sodium (Na^+) current inhibitor that has an antianginal and anti-ischemic effect without eliciting any change in the heart rate, blood pressure or rate-pressure (double) product.[67,68]

Myocardial ischemia causes an exaggerated, enhanced late inward Na^+ current, which leads to intracellular sodium overload which, in turn, leads to intracellular calcium overload, resulting in increased diastolic LV stiffness as well as electrical instability. The ischemia-associated diastolic stiffness compresses the intramyocardial vessels, leading to reduced coronary blood flow and the exacerbation of myocardial ischemia. Ranolazine prevents the abnormal increase in the late inward sodium current, and thereby prevents the "downstream" consequences of ischemic left ventricular stiffness and compression of intramyocardial blood vessels which, in turn, reduces myocardial ischemia.[67]

In chronic stable angina patients, ranolazine monotherapy significantly improved total exercise duration, time to angina onset and time to ST depression as compared to placebo.[69] There was no significant increase in the heart rate or blood pressure at rest or with exercise. Ranolazine significantly improved exercise duration and anginal symptoms when added to standard antianginal therapy, which included beta-blockers, diltiazem or amlodipine.[70] Added to maximum-dose amlodipine (10 mg daily), ranolazine reduced anginal frequency and nitroglycerine consumption.[71] Of note, those patients with the most frequent angina (>4.5 episodes/week) experienced the greatest benefit from the addition of ranolazine, suggesting that these patients may have more severe or prolonged ischemia-associated myocardial dysfunction and consequent hypoperfusion, a pathophysiologic state most likely to benefit from the unique mechanism of action of ranolazine.

Ranolazine also appears to be effective in patients with and without diabetes. A *post hoc* analysis of diabetic patients in the CARISA trial reported not only a reduction in the mean number of anginal episodes per week, but also a reduction in the HbA1c levels by 0.72 from the baseline.[72]

As a result of its multiple effects on transmembrane ion currents (both late inward Na^+ current and the inward potassium (K^+) rectifier current), ranolazine slightly prolongs the QT (~6 ms on average) with no clinical sequelae and no reported instances to date of torsades de pointes.[73] There was also no associated effect of QT dispersion. The use of ranolazine was not associated with early after depolarization (EAD) or increased dispersion of ventricular repolarization. Ranolazine can be used in combination with all CCBs, beta-blockers or nitrates. Dosing should be initiated at 500 mg bid and increased to maximum dose of 1000 mg bid based on clinical symptoms. Dizziness and nausea were the most common side effects, mostly at high doses.

Potent inhibitors of CYP3A (e.g. macrolides, protease inhibitors) increase levels of ranolazine and prolong the QTc interval, and thus should not be co-administered with ranolazine. Ranolazine can be used as add-on therapy in patients with chronic stable angina who have not achieved an adequate response with other antianginal agents but is now approved as first-line therapy for chronic angina.

The recently published MERLIN trial[74] demonstrated in over 6500 patients that ranolazine therapy was safe and well tolerated, even in high-risk patients following an acute coronary syndrome treated with a wide variety of concomitant anti-ischemic therapies. While this study did not show that ranolazine was superior to placebo in reducing the composite primary endpoint of death, MI or recurrent myocardial ischemia, ranolazine was shown to significantly reduce the secondary endpoint of recurrent myocardial ischemia in this population of ACS patients.

Fasudil

Rho kinase in the myocardial cell triggers vasoconstriction through accumulation of phosphorylated myosin. Animal models of coronary artery spasm have shown that Rho kinase inhibitors effectively suppress vasoconstriction. Fasudil, an orally available Rho kinase inhibitor, increased the time to >1 mm ST segment depression and improved exercise duration.[75] Fasudil did not affect the heart rate or blood pressure and was well tolerated.

Trimetazidine

Trimetazidine is a metabolic modulator and partial fatty acid oxidation inhibitor that has proven to be beneficial for combination therapy in patients with stable angina. Oxygen requirements of glucose pathways are lower than the free fatty acid (FFA) pathway. During ischemia, oxidized FFA levels rise which, in turn, blunt the glucose pathway. Trimetazidine inhibits beta-oxidation and shifts the equilibrium towards increased use of glucose, thus improving oxygen utilization. Trimetazidine in combination with long-acting nitrates or beta-blockers has been shown to decrease the number of anginal attacks per week.[76]

Ivabradine

The I_f current is an inward Na^+/K^+ current that activates pacemaker cells of the sinoatrial (SA) node. Ivabradine is a novel, specific heart rate-lowering agent that acts on SA node cells by selectively inhibiting pacemaker I_f current in a dose-dependent manner. It slows the diastolic depolarization slope of the SA node cells and reduces HR during rest and exercise in animals and human volunteers. Ivabradine at 7.5 mg bid and 10 mg bid was non-inferior to atenolol 100 mg daily for all exercise parameters. Sinus bradycardia occurred in 2.2% (ivabradine 7.5 mg), 5.4% (ivabradine 10 mg) and 4.3% in the atenolol group. Results from the INITIATIVE study suggest that I_f current inhibition with ivabradine may be as effective as beta-blockade in the treatment of stable angina.[77] A recent placebo-controlled multicenter trial of ivabradine in stable ischemic heart disease (BEAUTIFUL trial) did not show long-term clinical event reduction but improved angina.

Nicorandil

This drug activates the ATP-sensitive K^+ channels, which play an important role in ischemic preconditioning and promote dilation of the coronary resistance arterioles. Its nitrate moiety dilates epicardial coronary vessels and systemic veins. The addition of nicorandil to standard antianginal therapy was associated with a significant improvement in CAD death, non-fatal MI or unplanned hospital admission for cardiac chest pain.[78]

Non-pharmacologic antianginal approaches

Non-pharmacologic antianginal strategies include enhanced external counterpulsation (EECP), transmyocardial laser revascularization (TMR) and spinal cord stimulation (SCS). EECP promotes coronary collateral formation and may improve endothelial function. EECP has been shown to reduce the frequency and severity of angina in randomized trials.[79] TMR involves making laser channels into the myocardium and promotes angiogenesis. TMR improves angina class in patients with class IV anginal symptoms.[80] Both EECP and TMR are FDA approved for the treatment of chronic stable angina. In addition, SCS improves release of endogenous opiates, redistributes myocardial blood flow and decreases neurotransmission of painful stimuli. In patients with class III and IV angina, SCS may provide equivalent symptom relief to CABG.[81]

Role of myocardial revascularization

Revascularization includes PCI (i.e. balloon angioplasty and stenting) and CABG surgery which have both been shown to improve symptoms in patients with angina. Revascularization has not been shown to improve survival in patients with chronic angina and normal left ventricular function, except for those with left main coronary disease.[82–84] Several trials have compared cardioprotective medical therapy with PCI. In patients with Canadian Cardiovascular Society (CCS) class I or II stable angina, aggressive medical therapy, including lifestyle modification, vasculoprotective agents and revascularization (if symptoms worsen), results in similar rates of death and MI as with PCI.[85,86]

The Clinical Outcomes Utilizing Revascularization and Aggressive Drug Evaluation (COURAGE) trial was a multicenter study of patients with documented myocardial ischemia and angiographically confirmed single- or multivessel coronary artery disease who were randomized to a strategy of PCI plus intensive medical therapy or intensive medical therapy alone.[87] Lifestyle modification included smoking cessation, moderately intensive exercise five times per week and dietary fat less than 30% of daily calories. Aggressive medical therapy goals included target BP of less than 130/85 mmHg, LDL 60–85 mg/dL and HDL >40 mg/dL. The primary outcome during long-term follow-up included all-cause mortality and non-fatal MI. A total of 2287 patients with objective evidence of myocardial ischemia and significant CAD from 50 US and Canadian centers were enrolled between 1999 and 2004; 1149 patients were assigned to PCI with optimal medical therapy and 1138 to optimal medical therapy alone.

The baseline characteristics of the patients were similar in the two groups, the median duration of angina prior to randomization was 26 months (mean six episodes per week), 58% of patients had CCS class II or III angina and 2168 patients (95%) had objective evidence of myocardial ischemia. Among patients who underwent myocardial perfusion imaging at baseline, 90% had either single (23%) or multiple (67%) reversible defects from inducible ischemia. There was a high usage rate of multiple, evidence-based therapies post randomization and during follow-up, which was comparable in both study arms. At the 5-year follow-up visit, 70% of subjects achieved an LDL <85 mg/dL (2.21 mmol/L: (median 71 ± 1.3 mg/dL; 1.84 ± 0.03 mmol/L), 65% and 94% achieved systolic and diastolic blood pressure targets of <130 mmHg and <85 mmHg, respectively, and 45% of diabetics achieved a HgbA1C ≤7.0%.

The primary outcome (death from any cause or non-fatal MI) occurred in 19.0% of the PCI group and 18.5% of the medical therapy group (unadjusted hazard ratio 1.05; 95% confidence interval (CI) 0.87–1.27; $P = 0.62$). For the pre-specified secondary outcome of death, non-fatal MI or stroke, the event rate was 20.0% in the PCI group and 19.5% in the medical therapy group (hazard ratio 1.05; 95% CI 0.87–1.27; $P = 0.62$). The rates of hospitalization for ACS were 12.4% in the PCI group and 11.8% in the medical therapy group (hazard ratio 1.07; 95% CI 0.84–1.37; $P = 0.56$), and adjudicated MI rates were 13.2% and 12.3%, respectively (hazard ratio 1.13; 95% CI 0.89–1.43; $P = 0.33$). For death alone, the rates were 7.7% and 8.3% (hazard ratio 0.87; 95% CI 0.65–1.16). For stroke alone, the rate was 2.1% in the PCI group and 1.8% in the medical therapy group (hazard ratio 1.56; 95% CI 0.80–3.04; $P = 0.19$).

Over the 7 years of follow-up, 21% of the PCI patients had additional revascularization as compared with 33% of the medical therapy patients (hazard ratio 0.61; 95% CI 0.51–0.72; $P < 0.001$). The median time to first (or repeat) revascularization was approximately 11 months; in the first year 10.5% and 16.5% of patients in the PCI and optimal medical therapy groups, respectively, required revascularization. In the initial PCI group, 77 patients subsequently underwent CABG, as compared with 81 patients in the medical therapy group. At 5 years, 74% of the PCI patients and 72% of the medical therapy patients were free of angina ($P = \text{ns}$).

There was no significant interaction ($P < 0.01$) between treatment effect and any predefined subgroup variable. When subgroup variables were included in a multivariate analysis, the hazard ratio for treatment was essentially unchanged (1.09; 95% CI 0.90–1.33; $P = 0.77$).

Recommended initial management approach in stable coronary artery disease patients with angina

The COURAGE trial demonstrated the profound impact of intensive medical therapy and lifestyle intervention on mitigating clinical events in both randomized arms of the trial during long-term follow-up. A recent meta-analysis[88] which evaluated 4 trials (including COURAGE) of bare metal stent vs. optimal medical therapy in patients with stable coronary artery disease, was entirely consistent with the findings in COURAGE. Among stable CAD patients with chronic angina, *optimal medical therapy as an initial management strategy is both safe and effective*. Simply stated, CAD is a systemic problem that requires systemic treatment. Flow-limiting lesions cause angina and ischemia but may not necessarily be the lesions predisposing to death, MI, and ACS. Optimal medical therapy (OMT) is directed toward stabilizing so-called vulnerable plaques that are frequently mild angiographically and non-obstructive, such that OMT should rightfully be regarded as the preferred therapeutic approach to reducing clinical events in patients with chronic coronary syndromes and as complementary to focal revascularization approaches directed toward angina and ischemia relief, if needed. Achieving and maintaining multiple treatment targets may be a difficult challenge, but is well worth the effort.

Lifestyle changes of regular aerobic exercise, smoking cessation, dietary intervention, and weight maintenance should be instituted (**Class I, Level B**). Control of blood pressure (**Class I, Level A**), elevated blood sugar in diabetics (**Class I, Level B**), and secondary goals of lipid control (**Class I, Level A**) should be achieved. Antiplatelet agents are to be used in all patients (**Class I, Level A**). Vasculoprotective agents including ACE-I and statins should also be prescribed to all patients with chronic angina (**Class I, Level A**). Beta-blockers are recommended as the initial therapy for patients with prior MI (**Class I, Level A**) and, despite the absence of randomized trials demonstrating clinical event reduction in CAD patients without MI, are widely prescribed for chronic stable angina patients and are effective for relieving angina and abolishing or attenuating ischemia (**Class I, Level B**). Short-acting nitrates are used for acute anginal episodes (**Class I, Level C**). Calcium channel blockers and long-acting nitrates can be used if beta-blockers are not tolerated or contraindicated (**Class I, Level B**). Combinations of anti-anginal drugs may be used if symptoms of angina persist (**Class I, Level B**) (Figure 25.1). Beta-blockers plus nitrates may be more effective than either alone. Similarly, the combination of beta-blockers with dihydropyridines was more effective for improving exercise duration and was better tolerated than either alone. Newer agents like ranolazine

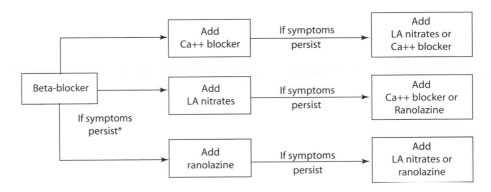

Figure 25.1 Algorithm for treatment of stable coronary artery disease.

*Depending on clinical characteristics and absence of a contraindication

offer additional antianginal effect without additive side effects.

Coronary angiography and the possibility of revascularization should be considered in patients with impaired left ventricular function, angina refractory to maximal medical therapy, symptomatic multivessel disease or high-risk features on stress testing[82–84] (**Class I, Level A**). Advanced age, diffuse disease, poor distal targets, lack of suitable conduits and co-morbid conditions that increase perioperative complications may be barriers to revascularization necessitating medical therapy.[89] In addition, CAD progression is a major reason for postrevascularization angina.[90]

Conclusion

Evidence-based OMT has been shown to significantly reduce the rates of anginal symptoms, death or MI in stable CAD patients, and should be considered the foundation of contemporary management. CAD is fundamentally a systemic vascular disease process that may ultimately lead to ACS when non-flow limiting vulnerable plaques rupture. Revascularization is a "focal" approach to stenotic coronary segments that alleviates angina but does not reduce the overall burden of vascular disease. PCI has not been shown, to date, to reduce the rates of death or MI in non-ACS patients, whether drug-eluting or bare metal stents are employed. A "focal" approach to CAD management, as well as a "systemic" approach with intensive, multifaceted medical therapy and lifestyle intervention, should be viewed as complementary and additive treatment strategies, and should be regarded as the optimal overall approach to contemporary CAD management.

References

1. Thom T *et al.* Heart disease and stroke statistics – 2006 update: a report from the American Heart Association Statistics Committee and Stroke Statistics Subcommittee. *Circulation* 2006;**113**(6): e85–151.

2. Panting JR *et al.* Abnormal subendocardial perfusion in cardiac syndrome X detected by cardiovascular magnetic resonance imaging. *N Engl J Med* 2002;**346**(25):1948–53.

3. Abrams J. Clinical practice. Chronic stable angina. *N Engl J Med* 2005;**352**(24):2524–33.

4. Serruys PW *et al.* Comparison of coronary-artery bypass surgery and stenting for the treatment of multivessel disease. *N Engl J Med* 2001;**344**(15):1117–24.

5. Fraker TD, Fihn SD, Gibbons RJ *et al.* 2007 chronic angina focused update of the ACC/AHA 2002 guidelines for the management of patients with chronic stable angina. *Circulation* 2007;**116**:2762–72.

6. Pepine CJ *et al.* Characteristics of a contemporary population with angina pectoris. TIDES Investigators. *Am J Cardiol* 1994; **74**(3):226–31.

7. Holubkov R *et al.* Angina 1 year after percutaneous coronary intervention: a report from the NHLBI Dynamic Registry. *Am Heart J* 2002;**144**(5):826–33.

8. Sangareddi V, Chockalingam A, Gnanavelu G, Subramaniam T, Jagannathan V, Elangovan S. Canadian Cardiovascular Society classification of effort angina: an angiographic correlation. *Coron Artery Dis* 2004;**15**:111–14.

9. O'Rourke RA, Schlaut RC, Douglas JS. Diagnosis and management of patients with chronic ischemic heart disease. In: Hurst's, *The Heart*, 10th edition, pp. 1207–1236. McGrain-Hill, 2001.

10. Cohn PF, Fox KM, Daly C. Silent myocardial ischemia. *Circulation* 2003;**108**(10):1263–77.

11. Shaw LJ *et al.* The economic burden of angina in women with suspected ischemic heart disease: results from the National Institutes of Health – National Heart, Lung, and Blood Institute-sponsored Women's Ischemia Syndrome Evaluation. *Circulation* 2006;**114**(9):894–904.

12. Maseri A, Lanza GA, Sanna T. Coronary blood flow and myocardial ischemia. In: Hurst's, *The Heart*, 10th edition, pp. 1109–1130. McGrain-Hill, 2001.

13. Handberg E *et al.* Impaired coronary vascular reactivity and functional capacity in women: results from the NHLBI Women's Ischemia Syndrome Evaluation (WISE) Study. *J Am Coll Cardiol* 2006;**47**(3 suppl):S44–9.

14. Haskell WL *et al.* Effects of intensive multiple risk factor reduction on coronary atherosclerosis and clinical cardiac events in

men and women with coronary artery disease. The Stanford Coronary Risk Intervention Project (SCRIP). *Circulation* 1994; **89**(3):975–90.

15. Hambrecht R *et al.* Percutaneous coronary angioplasty compared with exercise training in patients with stable coronary artery disease: a randomized trial. *Circulation* 2004;**109**(11): 1371–8.

16. Antithrombotic Trialists Collaboration. Collaborative meta-analysis of randomised trials of antiplatelet therapy for prevention of death, myocrdial infarction and stroke in high risk patients. *BMJ* 2002;**324**:71–86.

17. Ridker PM. C-reactive protein levels and outcomes after statin therapy. *N Engl J Med* 2005;**352**:20–8.

18. CAPRIE Steering Committee. A randomised, blinded, trial of Clopidogrel versus Aspirin in Patients at Risk of Ischaemic Events (CAPRIE). *Lancet* 1996;**348**(9038):1329–39.

19. Bhatt DL *et al.* Clopidogrel and aspirin versus aspirin alone for the prevention of atherothrombotic events. *N Engl J Med* 2006;**354**(16):1706–17.

20. Pfeffer MA *et al.* Effect of captopril on mortality and morbidity in patients with left ventricular dysfunction after myocardial infarction. Results of the Survival And Ventricular Enlargement trial. The SAVE Investigators.[see comment]. *N Engl J Med* 1992;**327**(10):669–77.

21. SOLVD Investigators. Effect of enalapril on survival in patients with reduced left ventricular ejection fractions and congestive heart failure. *N Engl J Med* 1991;**325**(5):293–302.

22. Yusuf S *et al.* Effects of an angiotensin-converting-enzyme inhibitor, ramipril, on cardiovascular events in high-risk patients. The Heart Outcomes Prevention Evaluation Study Investigators. *N Engl J Med* 2000;**342**(3):145–53.

23. Mancini GBJ, Henry GC, Macaya C *et al.* Angiotensin converting enzyme inhibition with quinapril improves endothelial vasomotor dysfunction in patients with coronary artery disease: the TREND Trial. *Circulation* 1996;**94**:258–65.

24. Braunwald E *et al.* Angiotensin-converting-enzyme inhibition in stable coronary artery disease. *N Engl J Med* 2004;**351**(20): 2058–68.

25. Pfeffer MA *et al.* Valsartan, captopril, or both in myocardial infarction complicated by heart failure, left ventricular dysfunction, or both. *N Engl J Med* 2003;**349**(20):1893–906.

26. Dickstein K, Kjekshus J, OPTIMAAL Steering Committee of the OPTIMAAL Study Group. Effects of losartan and captopril on mortality and morbidity in high-risk patients after acute myocardial infarction: the OPTIMAAL randomised trial. Optimal Trial in Myocardial Infarction with Angiotensin II Antagonist Losartan. *Lancet* 2002;**360**(9335):752–60.

27. ONTARGET Investigators. Telmisartan, ramipril, or both in patients at high risk for vascular events. *N Engl J Med* 2008;**358**:1547–59.

28. Pekkanen J *et al.* Ten-year mortality from cardiovascular disease in relation to cholesterol level among men with and without preexisting cardiovascular disease. *N Engl J Med* 1990;**322**(24): 1700–7.

29. Cannon CP *et al.* Intensive versus moderate lipid lowering with statins after acute coronary syndromes. *N Engl J Med* 2004; **350**(15):1495–504.

30. Corti R *et al.* Effects of lipid-lowering by simvastatin on human atherosclerotic lesions: a longitudinal study by high-resolution,

noninvasive magnetic resonance imaging. *Circulation* 2001; **104**(3):249–52.

31. Ridker PM *et al.* C-reactive protein levels and outcomes after statin therapy.[see comment]. *N Engl J Med* 2005;**352**(1): 20–8.

32. Pedersen TR *et al.* Randomised trial of cholesterol lowering in 4444 patients with coronary heart disease: the Scandinavian Simvastatin Survival Study (4S). *Atherosclerosis* 2004;**5**(3):81–7.

33. Cholesterol Treatment Trialists' (CTT) Collaborators. Efficacy and safety of cholesterol-lowering treatment: prospective meta-analysis of data from 90,056 particpants in 14 randomised trials of statins. *Lancet* 2005;**371**:1267–78.

34. Post Coronary Artery Bypass Graft Trial Investigators. The effect of aggressive lowering of low-density lipoprotein cholesterol levels and low-dose anticoagulation on obstructive changes in saphenous-vein coronary-artery bypass grafts. *N Engl J Med* 1997;**336**(3):153–62.

35. Nissen SE *et al.* Effect of intensive compared with moderate lipid-lowering therapy on progression of coronary atherosclerosis: a randomized controlled trial. *JAMA* 2000;**291**(9):1071–80.

36. Grundy SM *et al.* Implications of recent clinical trials for the National Cholesterol Education Program Adult Treatment Panel III Guidelines. *J Am Coll Cardiol* 2004;**44**(3):720–32.

37. LaRosa JC *et al.* Intensive lipid lowering with atorvastatin in patients with stable coronary disease.[see comment]. *N Engl J Med* 2005;**352**(14):1425–35.

38. Gordon T *et al.* High density lipoprotein as a protective factor against coronary heart disease. The Framingham Study. *Am J Med* 1977;**62**(5):707–14.

39. Elam MB *et al.* Effect of niacin on lipid and lipoprotein levels and glycemic control in patients with diabetes and peripheral arterial disease: the ADMIT study: a randomized trial. Arterial Disease Multiple Intervention Trial. *JAMA* 2000;**284**(10): 1263–70.

40. Gordon DJ, Probstfield JL, Garrison RJ *et al.* High-density lipoprotein cholesterol and cardiovascular disease. Four prospective American studies. *Circulation* 1989;**79**:8–15.

41. Brown BG, Zhao XQ, Chait A *et al.* Simvastatin and niacin, antioxidant vitamins, or the combination for the prevention of coronary disease. *N Engl J Med* 2001;**345**:1583–92.

42. Sudhop T, Lutjohann D, Kodal A *et al.* Inhibition of intestinal cholesterol absorption by ezetimibe in humans. *Circulation* 2002;**106**:1943–8.

43. Kosoglou T, Meyer I, Veltri EP et al. Pharmacodynamic interaction between new selective cholesterol absorption inhibitor ezetimibe and simvastatin. *Br J Clin Pharmacol* 2002;**54**:309–19.

44. Ballantyne CM, Abate N, Yuan Z *et al.* Dose-comparison study of the combination of ezetimibe and simvastatin (Vytorin) versus atorvastatin in patients with hypercholesterolemia: the VYVA Study. *Am Heart J* 2005;**149**:464–73.

45. Ballantyne CM, Blazing MA, King TR *et al.* Efficacy and safety of ezetimibe co-administered with simvastatin compared with atorvastatin in adults with hypercholesterolemia. *Am J Cardiol* 2004;**93**:1487–94.

46. Pearson TA, Denke MA, McBride PE *et al.* A community-based, randomized trial of ezetimibe added to statin therapy to attain NCEP ATP III goals for LDL cholesterol in hypercholesterolemic patients: the ezetimibe add-on to statin for effectiveness (EASE) trial. *Mayo Clin Proc* 2005;**80**:587–95.

47. Bays HE, Ose L, Fraser N *et al.* A multicenter, randomized, double-blind, placebo-controlled, factorial design study to assess the lipid-altering capacity and safety profile of the ezetimibe/simvastatin tablet compared with ezetimibe and simvastatin monotherapy in patients with primary hypercholesterolemia. *Clin Ther* 2004;**26**: 758–73.

48. Jackson G *et al.* Atenolol: once-daily cardioselective beta blockade for angina pectoris. *Circulation* 1980;**61**(3):555–60.

49. Weiss R *et al.* Effectiveness of three different doses of carvedilol for exertional angina. Carvedilol-Angina Study Group. *Am J Cardiol* 1998;**82**(8):927–31.

50. Kaski JC *et al.* Efficacy of carvedilol (BM 14,190), a new beta-blocking drug with vasodilating properties, in exercise-induced ischemia. *Am J Cardiol* 1985;**56**(1):35–40.

51. Furberg B *et al.* Comparison of the new beta-adrenoceptor antagonist, nadolol, and propranolol in the treatment of angina pectoris. *Curr Med Res Opin* 1978;**5**(5):388–93.

52. Jackson G *et al.* Comparison of atenolol with propranolol in the treatment of angina pectoris with special reference to once daily administration of atenolol. *Br Heart J* 1978;**40**(9): 998–1004.

53. Waysbort J, Meshulam N, Brunner D. Isosorbide-5-mononitrate and atenolol in the treatment of stable exertional angina. *Cardiology* 1991;**79**(suppl 2):19–26.

54. Krepp HP. Evaluation of the antianginal and anti-ischemic efficacy of slow-release isosorbide-5-mononitrate capsules, bupranolol and their combination, in patients with chronic stable angina pectoris. *Cardiology* 1991;**79**(suppl 2):14–18.

55. Alderman MH, Cohen H, Roque R *et al.* Effect of long-acting and short-acting calcium antagonists on cardiovascular outcomes in hypertensive patients. *Lancet* 1997;**349**:594–8.

56. Weiner DA, Klein MD. Verapamil therapy for stable exertional angina pectoris. *Am J Cardiol* 1982;**50**(5):1153–7.

57. Subramanian VB *et al.* Calcium channel blockade as primary therapy for stable angina pectoris. A double-blind placebo-controlled comparison of verapamil and propranolol. *Am J Cardiol* 1982;**50**(5):1158–63.

58. Chahine RA *et al.* Randomized placebo-controlled trial of amlodipine in vasospastic angina. Amlodipine Study 160 Group.[see comment]. *J Am Coll Cardiol* 1993;**21**(6):1365–70.

59. Furberg CD, Psaty BM, Meyer JV. Nifedipine. Dose-related increase in mortality in patients with coronary heart disease. *Circulation* 1995;**92**(5):1326–31.

60. Kaski JC *et al.* Improved coronary supply: prevailing mechanism of action of nitrates in chronic stable angina. *Am Heart J* 1985;**110**(1 Pt 2):238–45.

61. Abrams J. Nitroglycerin and long-acting nitrates in clinical practice. *Am J Med* 1983;**74**(6B):85–94.

62. Thadani U. Nitrate tolerance, rebound, and their clinical relevance in stable angina pectoris, unstable angina, and heart failure. *Cardiovasc Drug Ther* 1997;**10**(6):735–42.

63. Gogia H *et al.* Prevention of tolerance to hemodynamic effects of nitrates with concomitant use of hydralazine in patients with chronic heart failure. *J Am Coll Cardiol* 1995;**26**(7):1575–80.

64. Gori T *et al.* Folic acid prevents nitroglycerin-induced nitric oxide synthase dysfunction and nitrate tolerance: a human in vivo study. *Circulation* 2001;**104**(10):1119–23.

65. Watanabe H *et al.* Preventive effects of carvedilol on nitrate tolerance – a randomized, double-blind, placebo-controlled comparative study between carvedilol and arotinolol. *J Am Coll Cardiol* 1998;**32**(5):1201–6.

66. Leon MB *et al.* Combination therapy with calcium-channel blockers and beta-blockers for chronic stable angina pectoris. *Am J Cardiol* 1985;**55**(3):69B–80B.

67. Belardinelli L, Shryock JC, Fraser H. Inhibition of the late sodium current as a potential cardioprotective principle: effects of the late sodium current inhibitor ranolazine. *Heart* 2006;**92**(suppl 4):iv6–iv14.

68. Nash DT, Nash SD. Ranolazine for chronic stable angina. *Lancet* 2008;**372**:1335–41.

69. Chaitman BR *et al.* Anti-ischemic effects and long-term survival during ranolazine monotherapy in patients with chronic severe angina. *J Am Coll Cardiol* 2004;**43**(8):1375–82.

70. Chaitman BR *et al.* Effects of ranolazine with atenolol, amlodipine, or diltiazem on exercise tolerance and angina frequency in patients with severe chronic angina: a randomized controlled trial. *JAMA* 2004;**291**(3):309–16.

71. Stone PH, Gratsiansky NA, Blokhin A *et al.* Antianginal efficacy of ranolazine when added to maximal treatment with a conventional therapy: the efficacy of ranolazine in chronic angina (ERICA) trial. *J Am Coll Cardiol* 2006;**48**:566–75.

72. Timmis AD, Chaitman BR, Crager M. Effects of ranolazine on exercise tolerance and HbA1c in patients with chronic angina and diabetes. *Eur Heart J* 2006;**27**(1):42–8.

73. Antzelevitch C *et al.* Electrophysiological effects of ranolazine, a novel antianginal agent with antiarrhythmic properties. *Circulation* 2004;**110**(8):904–10.

74. Morrow DA, Scirica BM, Karwatowska-Prokopczuk E *et al.* Effects of ranolazine on recurrent cardiovascular events in patients with non-ST-segment elevation acute coronary syndromes: the MERLIN-TIMI 36 randomized Trial. *JAMA* 2007;**297**: 1775–83.

75. Vicari RM *et al.* Efficacy and safety of fasudil in patients with stable angina: a double-blind, placebo-controlled, phase 2 trial. *J Am Coll Cardiol* 2005;**46**(10):1803–11.

76. Chazov EI *et al.* Trimetazidine in angina combination therapy – the TACT study: trimetazidine versus conventional treatment in patients with stable angina pectoris in a randomized, placebo-controlled, multicenter study. *Am J Therapeutics* 2005;**12**(1):35–42.

77. Tardif JC *et al.* Efficacy of ivabradine, a new selective I(f) inhibitor, compared with atenolol in patients with chronic stable angina. *Eur Heart J* 2005;**26**(23):2529–36.

78. Group IS. Effect of nicorandil on coronary events in patients with stable angina: the Impact Of Nicorandil in Angina (IONA) randomised trial. *Lancet* 2002;**359**(9314):1269–75.

79. Bonetti PO *et al.* Enhanced external counterpulsation improves endothelial function in patients with symptomatic coronary artery disease. *J Am Coll Cardiol* 2003;**41**(10):1761–8.

80. Allen KB *et al.* Comparison of transmyocardial revascularization with medical therapy in patients with refractory angina. *N Engl J Med* 1999;**341**(14):1029–36.

81. Mannheimer C *et al.* Electrical stimulation versus coronary artery bypass surgery in severe angina pectoris: the ESBY study. *Circulation* 1998;**97**(12):1157–63.

82. Rihal CS *et al.* Indications for coronary artery bypass surgery and percutaneous coronary intervention in chronic stable angina: review of the evidence and methodological considerations. *Circulation* 2003;**108**(20):2439–45.

83. Hoffman SN *et al*. A meta-analysis of randomized controlled trials comparing coronary artery bypass graft with percutaneous transluminal coronary angioplasty: one- to eight-year outcomes. *J Am Coll Cardiol* 2003;**41**(8):1293–304.

84. Berger PB, Sketch MH Jr, Califf RM. Choosing between percutaneous coronary intervention and coronary artery bypass grafting for patients with multivessel disease: what can we learn from the Arterial Revascularization Therapy Study (ARTS)? *Circulation* 2004;**109**(9):1079–81.

85. Hueb W *et al*. The Medicine, Angioplasty, or Surgery Study (MASS-II): a randomized, controlled clinical trial of three therapeutic strategies for multivessel coronary artery disease: one-year results. *J Am Coll Cardiol* 2004;**43**(10):1743–51.

86. Bucher HC *et al*. Percutaneous transluminal coronary angioplasty versus medical treatment for non-acute coronary heart disease: meta-analysis of randomised controlled trials. *BMJ* 2000;**321**(7253):73–7.

87. Boden WE, O'Rourke RA, Teo KK *et al*. Optimal medical therapy with or without PCI for stable coronary artery disease. *N Engl J Med* 2007;**356**:1503–16.

88. Trikalinos TA, Alsheikh-Ali AA, Tatsioni A, Nallamothu BK, Kent DM. Percutaneous coronary interventions for non-acute coronary artery disease: a quantitative 20-year synopsis and a network meta-analysis. *Lancet* 2009;**373**:911–18.

89. Alderman EL *et al*. Native coronary disease progression exceeds failed revascularization as cause of angina after five years in the Bypass Angioplasty Revascularization Investigation (BARI).[see comment]. *J Am Coll Cardiol* 2004;**44**(4):766–74.

90. Mannheimer C *et al*. The problem of chronic refractory angina; report from the ESC Joint Study Group on the Treatment of Refractory Angina. *Eur Heart J* 2002;**23**(5):355–70.

Percutaneous intervention

David A Wood, Rohit Khurana and Christopher E Buller
University of British Columbia, Vancouver, British Columbia, Canada

Introduction

Percutaneous coronary intervention (PCI) has been the most commonly employed coronary revascularization strategy for almost 20 years. In patients with chronic stable angina, the goals of PCI include the relief of angina and ischemia as well as preventing the progression and complications of coronary artery disease (CAD). This chapter describes the principles and evidence basis for coronary intervention technologies and reviews historic and contemporary trials that have compared PCI with medical therapy in stable CAD.

Principles and historic overview

Myocardial ischemia arises principally from an imbalance between myocardial oxygen requirements and supply. Coronary flow reserve (CFR) describes the normal physiologic capacity to increase coronary blood flow (hyperemia) in response to heightened downstream demand through dilation of coronary resistance vessels (principally precapillary arterioles). By definition, hemodynamically significant stenoses in upstream epicardial coronary arteries are those that diminish CFR by preventing physiologic hyperemia, leading to the potential for regional myocardial ischemia. The threshold for ischemia is determined substantially by the severity of the epicardial stenosis, but is also modulated by factors such as collateral flow, myocardial viability and blood oxygen content. Successful PCI alleviates the offending epicardial stenosis, thereby preventing ischemia through partial or complete normalization of CFR.

Dotter and Judkins first proposed the concept of transluminal angioplasty in peripheral arteries in 1964.[1]

Thirteen years later, Gruntzig performed the first balloon angioplasty of a stenotic coronary artery in a conscious human.[2,3] The ability of balloon angioplasty to enlarge the vessel lumen and relieve stenosis was originally attributed to compression of the atheromatous plaque.[3] However, luminal improvement immediately following balloon or stent-based PCI is actually the result of plaque displacement. Luminal stretching (barotrauma) leads to fracture of the intimal plaque and partial disruption of the media and adventitia, allowing enlargement of the lumen by increasing overall vessel diameter.[4] Elastic vessel recoil, post-traumatic neointimal proliferation, and positive (favorable) or negative remodeling of the treated segment determine the final healed result which stabilizes 4–6 months following intervention.

Balloon-based percutaneous transluminal coronary angioplasty (PTCA) became widely disseminated in the 1980s. As equipment design and operator experience improved, PTCA was progressively employed in higher risk patients and in more challenging anatomy, including longer lesions, bifurcations, total occlusions and multivessel disease.[5] The technique remained limited, however, by dissection and thrombosis of the treated vessel (threatened or actual abrupt closure) requiring emergency CABG in 3–5% of patients, and by restenosis of the treated segment in 20–30% of patients. A variety of novel devices were developed to solve these problems; however, only coronary stenting has demonstrated improved procedural safety and late clinical outcomes when rigorously compared to balloon angioplasty alone (see below).

Compared to balloon angioplasty alone, modern metallic stents nearly eliminate elastic recoil and compress or seal planes of barotrauma-induced disruption, thereby preventing propagation of dissection and reducing the stimuli for thrombosis that lead to abrupt vessel closure. While metallic stents prevent negative vessel remodeling, they also prevent positive remodeling and have no beneficial effect on neointimal proliferation. Thus bare metal stents have reduced, but by no means eliminated, restenosis. Active antiproliferative drug coatings employed on drug-eluting

Evidence-Based Cardiology, 3rd edition. Edited by S. Yusuf, J.A. Cairns, A.J. Camm, E.L. Fallen, and B.J. Gersh. © 2010 Blackwell Publishing, ISBN: 978-1-4051-5925-8.

stents substantially prevent neointimal proliferation and have reduced restenosis rates to below 10%. Bare metal or drug-eluting stents are now used in more than 95% of PCI cases, with procedural success rates greater than 98% and emergency CABG rates less than 1% in most institutions.[6] Balloon angioplasty is now most often used to dilate a vessel prior to stent deployment in order to enhance visualization of the target segment, improve stent deliverability, and ensure calcified vessels yield to dilation forces. Balloon angioplasty, often at high pressures (14–24 atmospheres), is also employed to further expand the stent and vessel following initial stent deployment. This technique is intended to ensure optimum lumen dimensions and complete apposition of stent struts to the vessel wall, and is associated with a reduced incidence of restenosis and stent thrombosis.[6] Stand-alone balloon angioplasty (no stent) is now reserved for specific circumstances: small-caliber vessels (<2.5 mm), side branch treatment at bifurcations, distal bypass graft anastomotic lesions, select cases of focal in-stent restenosis, and in patients unable to tolerate dual antiplatelet therapy.

Percutaneous coronary intervention technology

PCI systems share three basic components: a guiding catheter that provides stable access to the coronary ostium; a steerable guidewire that is advanced distal to the stenosis and acts as a rail for delivering a variety of therapeutic devices; and a non-elastomeric balloon (with or without a mounted stent) for dilating the physiologically significant epicardial stenosis (Fig. 26.1).

A number of diagnostic and guiding catheters have been developed for coronary arteriography. To allow passage of balloons and other devices, early thick-walled guiding catheters were constructed from large 10 and 11 F tubes that demanded correspondingly large-caliber arterial sheaths with their attendant bleeding risks. Modern guide catheters allow most cases to be completed through 6 F or smaller vascular access sheaths, thereby reducing bleeding risk and enabling radial or femoral artery access (see below).

Modern guidewires combine atraumatic tip softness with precise torque control for steering, graduated support for device delivery, and improved radiographic visibility. Lubricated hydrophilic coatings are employed on specialty wires for tortuous or critically stenotic segments. Stiffer tip designs with different shaft and taper characteristics are now available for crossing chronic total occlusions (CTOs). The large selection of modern guidewires has improved procedural success in a wide range of challenging anatomic substrates.

The cross-sectional profiles of modern angioplasty balloon catheters and stent delivery systems have also decreased substantially while their flexibility has increased. Together with myriad other design improvements, modern balloon catheters and stent delivery systems can readily be made to pass through marked tortuosity and to access distal arterial segments. These improvements may also reduce trauma, endothelial injury and associated plaque progression in coronary segments proximal to the target lesion, though these benefits have not been clearly demonstrated.

Vascular access

A variety of vascular approaches are available for PCI. The right and left femoral arteries are the most commonly used access sites. Although Sones first introduced a cutdown approach for the brachial artery for diagnostic coronary angiography, this approach has been supplanted by percutaneous radial artery access. Access site selection currently depends on operator and patient preference, anticoagulation status, body habitus, and the presence of significant peripheral vascular disease (PVD).

Small trials suggest a transradial approach is preferred in patients with morbid obesity.[7,8] The recent Agostoni *et al* meta-analysis included 12 randomized trials (n = 3224)

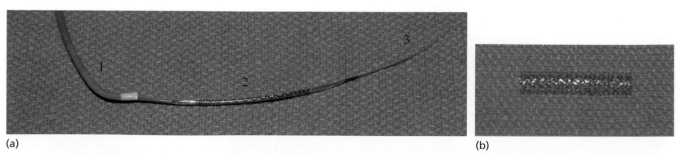

(a)   (b)

Figure 26.1 (a) Photograph of a guiding catheter that provides stable access to the coronary ostium (1), a non-elastomeric balloon (with a mounted stent) (2) for dilating physiologically significant epicardial stenosis, and a steerable guidewire (3) that is advanced distal to the stenosis and acts as a rail for delivering a variety of therapeutic devices. (b) Expanded 5.0 × 32 mm bare metal stent.

comparing the transradial and transfemoral approach.[9] The risk of major adverse cardiac events (MACE) was similar for both the radial and femoral approach (odds ratio (OR) 0.92, 95% confidence interval (CI) 0.57–1.48; $P = 0.7$). Radial access was associated with a significantly lower rate of entry site complications and bleeding (OR 0.20, 95% CI 0.09–0.42; $P = 0.0001$) but a higher rate of procedural failure (OR 3.30, 95% CI 1.63–6.71; $P = 0.001$). The multicenter OASIS-7/CURRENT trial is enrolling patients and will help clarify the importance of access site selection in PCI.

Technology and pharmacology trials of percutaneous coronary intervention in stable coronary artery disease

Bare metal stents

Balloon-expandable metallic stents were the first advance to reduce restenosis, reduce acute complications and provide superior medium-term clinical outcomes when compared to balloon angioplasty alone.

BENESTENT-1 and STRESS were early pivotal trials comparing bare metal stents (BMS) with balloon angioplasty[10,11] in simple, short coronary stenoses. Elective Palmaz-Schatz stenting was compared to balloon angioplasty and the results provided the evidence base for FDA approval in 1994 for the prevention of restenosis in *de novo* lesions. Both studies showed improved initial angiographic results using quantitative coronary angiography (QCA), larger postprocedural minimal luminal diameters (MLD), fewer residual dissections, and decreased clinical and angiographic restenosis at six months. In BENESTENT-1 (n = 520), the mean (±SD) MLD immediately after the procedure were 2.48 ± 0.39 mm in the stent group and 2.05 ± 0.33 mm in the angioplasty group; at follow-up, the diameters were 1.82 ± 0.64 mm in the stent group and 1.73 ± 0.55 mm in the angioplasty group ($P = 0.09$), which correspond to rates of restenosis (diameter of stenosis (DS) >50%) of 22% and 32%, respectively ($P = 0.02$). In STRESS (n = 410), the mean (±SD) MLD immediately after the procedure were 2.49 ± 0.43 in the stent group and 1.99 ± 0.47 mm in the angioplasty group ($P < 0.001$). At six months, the patients with stented lesions continued to have a larger luminal diameter (1.74 ± 0.60 vs 1.56 ± 0.65 mm, $P = 0.007$) and a lower rate of restenosis (DS 31.6% vs 42.1%, $P = 0.046$). TOSCA-1 was the largest stent versus balloon trial in complex coronary stenoses (non-acute occlusions).[12] Stenting again resulted in larger mean six-month MLD (1.48 versus 1.23 mm, $P < 0.01$) and a reduced binary angiographic restenosis rate (55% versus 70%, $P < 0.01$).

Bare metal stents were initially limited by stiffness, modest radial strength and inconsistencies in paving which restricted their utility in complex anatomy. Numerous design iterations by stent manufacturers lead to second-, third- and fourth-generation stents that incorporated substantially improved stent flexibility (both before and after stent deployment), superior radial strength and paving, thinner struts, enhanced radiographic visibility, and innovative metallurgy. However, newer trials employed noninferiority designs to compare different types of bare metal stents, making it difficult to confirm or quantify the effects of improved stent designs.

Two meta-analyses have been published comparing stenting with balloon angioplasty. Brophy *et al* identified a total of 29 trials involving 9918 patients (Figs 26.2, 26.3).[13] No overall difference between strategies of routine coronary stenting versus routine balloon angioplasty was observed for death or myocardial infarction outcomes (odds ratio 0.90, 95% CI 0.72–1.11) or the need for coronary artery bypass surgery (odds ratio 1.01, CI 0.79–1.31). However, nearly all trials allowed or encouraged early cross-over to stenting for patients experiencing balloon angioplasty failure due to marked recoil, dissection and threatened or actual abrupt closure, a design feature that almost certainly obscured from the primary intention-to-treat analyses an important safety advantage provided by stents. Coronary stenting did reduce the rate of restenosis by half (odds ratio 0.52, CI 0.37–0.69) and the need for repeated balloon angioplasty by 40% (odds ratio 0.59, CI 0.50–0.68]). Al Suwaidi *et al* performed a separate meta-analysis of 23 trials and reached similar conclusions.[14]

Clinical trials comparing routine stenting to routine balloon angioplasty enrolled anatomically and clinically selected patients. Outcomes in real-world practice including patients with complex stenoses, multivessel disease and a typical burden of co-morbidity were described in a population-based analysis from Canada.[15] After adjustment, this analysis showed the adoption of routine bare

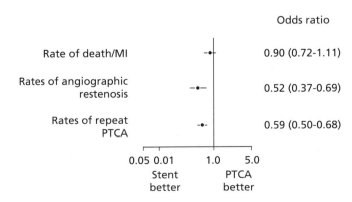

Figure 26.2 Meta-analysis of stents versus conventional balloon angioplasty on rate of death or MI, angiographic restenosis, and repeat PTCA. MI, myocardial infarction; PTCA, percutaneous transluminal coronary angioplasty. (From Brophy *et al*.[13])

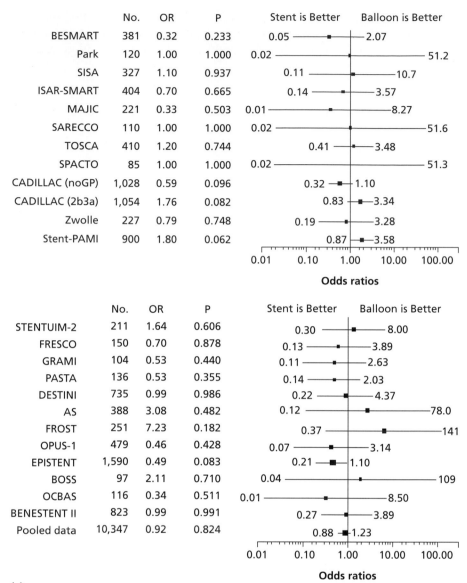

	No.	OR	P	Stent is Better	Balloon is Better
BESMART	381	0.32	0.233	0.05 —■—	2.07
Park	120	1.00	1.000	0.02 ——	51.2
SISA	327	1.10	0.937	0.11 —■—	10.7
ISAR-SMART	404	0.70	0.665	0.14 —■—	3.57
MAJIC	221	0.33	0.503	0.01 —■—	8.27
SARECCO	110	1.00	1.000	0.02 ——	51.6
TOSCA	410	1.20	0.744	0.41 —■—	3.48
SPACTO	85	1.00	1.000	0.02 ——	51.3
CADILLAC (noGP)	1,028	0.59	0.096	0.32 —■—	1.10
CADILLAC (2b3a)	1,054	1.76	0.082	0.83 —■—	3.34
Zwolle	227	0.79	0.748	0.19 —■—	3.28
Stent-PAMI	900	1.80	0.062	0.87 —■—	3.58

Odds ratios (0.01 0.10 1.00 10.00 100.00)

	No.	OR	P	Stent is Better	Balloon is Better
STENTUIM-2	211	1.64	0.606	0.30 —■—	8.00
FRESCO	150	0.70	0.878	0.13 —■—	3.89
GRAMI	104	0.53	0.440	0.11 —■—	2.63
PASTA	136	0.53	0.355	0.14 —■—	2.03
DESTINI	735	0.99	0.986	0.22 —■—	4.37
AS	388	3.08	0.482	0.12 —■—	78.0
FROST	251	7.23	0.182	0.37 —■—	141
OPUS-1	479	0.46	0.428	0.07 —■—	3.14
EPISTENT	1,590	0.49	0.083	0.21 —■—	1.10
BOSS	97	2.11	0.710	0.04 —■—	109
OCBAS	116	0.34	0.511	0.01 —■—	8.50
BENESTENT II	823	0.99	0.991	0.27 —■—	3.89
Pooled data	10,347	0.92	0.824	0.88 ■ 1.23	

Odds ratios (0.01 0.10 1.00 10.00 100.00)

(a)

Figure 26.3 Evaluation of the Effects of routine stenting versus conventional PTCA on death and reinfarction. (a) Effects on death; (b) effects on reinfarction. AS, Angioplasty or Stent; BENESTENT, Belgian Netherlands Stent Study; BESMART, Bestent in Small Arteries; BOSS, Balloon Optimization versus Stent Study; CADILLAC, Controlled Abciximab and Device Investigation to Lower Late Angioplasty Complications; DESTINI, Doppler Endpoint Stenting International Investigation; EPISTENT, Evaluation of Platelet IIb/IIIa Inhibitor for Stenting; FRESCO, Florence Randomized Elective Stenting in Acute Coronary Occlusions; FROST, French Optimal Stenting Trial; GRAMI, Gianturco-Roubin in Acute Myocardial Infarction; ISAR-SMART, Intracoronary Stenting or Angioplasty for Restenosis Reduction in Small Arteries; MAJIC, Mayo-Japan Investigation for Chronic Total Occlusion; OCBAS, Optimal Coronary Balloon Angioplasty With Provisional Stenting Versus Primary Stent; OPUS, Optimum Percutaneous Transluminal Coronary Angioplasty Compared With Routine Stent Strategy; OR, odds ratio; PASTA, Primary Angioplasty Versus Stent Implantation in Acute Myocardial Infarction; SARECCO, Stent or Angioplasty after Recanalization of Chronic Coronary Occlusions; SISA, Stenting in Small Arteries; SPACTO, Stent versus Percutaneous Angioplasty in ChronicTotal Occlusion; Stent-PAMI, Stent Primary Angioplasty in MI; STENTUIM, Immediate Coronary Angioplasty with Elective Wiktor Stent Implantation Comparedwith Conventional Balloon Angioplasty in Acute Myocardial Infarction; TOSCA, Total Occlusion Study of Canada; other abbreviations as in Fig. 27.2. (From Brophy et al.[13])

metal stenting was associated with a 28% reduction in target vessel revascularization and 21% reduction in major adverse cardiac events. Clinical results and outcomes with bare metal stents have continued to improve with the development of more flexible and thin-strut stent designs[16] and widespread adoption of modern antithrombotic and antiplatelet therapies administered during and after stent insertion (see below).

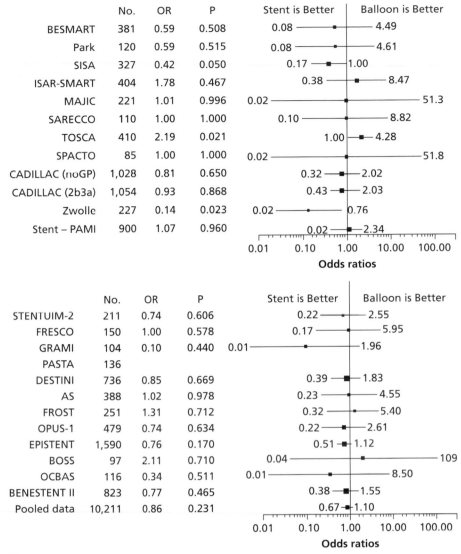

	No.	OR	P	Stent is Better	Balloon is Better
BESMART	381	0.59	0.508	0.08 ——■—	4.49
Park	120	0.59	0.515	0.08 ——■—	4.61
SISA	327	0.42	0.050	0.17 —■—	1.00
ISAR-SMART	404	1.78	0.467	0.38 ——■—	8.47
MAJIC	221	1.01	0.996	0.02 ——■—	51.3
SARECCO	110	1.00	1.000	0.10 ——■—	8.82
TOSCA	410	2.19	0.021	1.00 —■—	4.28
SPACTO	85	1.00	1.000	0.02 ——■—	51.8
CADILLAC (noGP)	1,028	0.81	0.650	0.32 —■—	2.02
CADILLAC (2b3a)	1,054	0.93	0.868	0.43 —■—	2.03
Zwolle	227	0.14	0.023	0.02 ——■—	0.76
Stent – PAMI	900	1.07	0.960	0.02 —■—	2.34

0.01　0.10　1.00　10.00　100.00

Odds ratios

	No.	OR	P	Stent is Better	Balloon is Better
STENTUIM-2	211	0.74	0.606	0.22 ——■—	2.55
FRESCO	150	1.00	0.578	0.17 ——■—	5.95
GRAMI	104	0.10	0.440	0.01 ———■—	1.96
PASTA	136				
DESTINI	736	0.85	0.669	0.39 —■—	1.83
AS	388	1.02	0.978	0.23 ——■—	4.55
FROST	251	1.31	0.712	0.32 ——■—	5.40
OPUS-1	479	0.74	0.634	0.22 —■—	2.61
EPISTENT	1,590	0.76	0.170	0.51 —■—	1.12
BOSS	97	2.11	0.710	0.04 ———■——	109
OCBAS	116	0.34	0.511	0.01 ——■—	8.50
BENESTENT II	823	0.77	0.465	0.38 —■—	1.55
Pooled data	10,211	0.86	0.231	0.67 —■—	1.10

0.01　0.10　1.00　10.00　100.00

Odds ratios

Figure 26.3 *Continued*

(b)

Drug-eluting stents (DES)

Although BMS constituted an important advance over balloon angioplasty alone, restenosis due to neointimal overgrowth continues to pose a significant clinical challenge particularly when it is diffuse, proliferative or occlusive.[17] In a multicenter cross-sectional registry describing the burden of in-stent restenosis in the immediate pre-DES era, approximately 7% of all cardiac catheterization procedures performed involved patients with restenosis of one or more bare metal stents.[18] Local delivery of potent antiproliferative drugs via DES has proven an efficacious technology. At the time of writing, four DES device are approved for coronary use in Europe or North America. In order of regulatory approval, these are the Cypher™ (sirolimus eluting, Cordis, Miami Lakes, FL), Taxus™ (paclitaxel

eluting, Boston Scientific, Boston, MA), Endeavor™ (zotarolimus eluting, Medtronic, Minneapolis, MN) and XienceV™ (everolimus eluting, Abbott Vascular, Santa Clara, CA). All are composed of a balloon-expandable metallic stent with an adherent polymer that serves as the reservoir for the antiproliferative drug. The drugs elute and diffuse into peri-stent vascular tissue in the weeks following stent deployment where, to a variable degree, they inhibit mitosis of smooth muscle cells that are the primary cellular constituent of restenotic neointimal tissue.

Multiple surrogates have been used to evaluate BMS and DES efficacy. In addition to the quantitative angiographic measures of lumen dimensions and binary restenosis, "ischemia driven" target lesion or target vessel revascularization (TLR or TVR) and clinical restenosis are commonly employed clinically relevant endpoints. Angiographic and clinical restenosis rates after BMS implantation typically exceed 20% and 10% respectively, with rates more than doubling in certain patient subsets. Risk factors for restenosis include small reference vessel diameter, long lesion or stent length, and medically treated diabetes mellitus.[19] A small minimal stent cross-sectional area on intravascular ultrasound (IVUS) imaging also predicts restenosis (see below).[20] In contrast, clinical and angiographic restenosis rates are less than 10% in multiple DES series.[21-28]

SIRIUS[21] and TAXUS IV[22] were pivotal trials that demonstrated decreased clinical and angiographic restenosis with drug-eluting versus bare metal stents. Although TLR dramatically decreased, there was again no difference in death or myocardial infarction. In SIRIUS, the mean in-segment (stent plus 5 mm margins) MLD of the sirolimus-coated Bx Velocity stent at 240 days was 2.15 ± 0.61 mm vs 1.60 ± 0.72 mm ($P < 0.001$) for the bare metal stent with a restenosis rate (DS >50%) of 8.9 versus 36.3% (I < 0.01). In

TAXUS IV, the mean in-segment MLD of the paclitaxel-coated Express stent at nine months was 2.03 ± 0.55 mm versus 1.68 ± 0.61 mm ($P < 0.001$) for the bare metal stent with a restenosis rate of 7.9 versus 26.6% ($P < 0.001$).

Two non-inferiority trials have demonstrated similar MLD and restenosis rates with the remaining commercially marketed DES: ENDEAVOR-3 compared zotralimus-eluting and sirolimus-eluting stents and SPIRIT-3 compared everolimus-eluting and paclitaxel-eluting stents.

The widespread adoption of DES reduced restenosis and decreased the need for subsequent procedures compared to BMS.[23-28b] Stone et al performed a pooled analysis of four double-blind trials in which 1748 patients were randomly assigned to receive either sirolimus-eluting stents or BMS and five double-blind trials in which 3513 patients were randomly assigned to receive either paclitaxel-eluting stents or BMS (Figs 26.4, 26.5).[23] The four-year rates of stent thrombosis were 1.2% in the sirolimus stent group versus

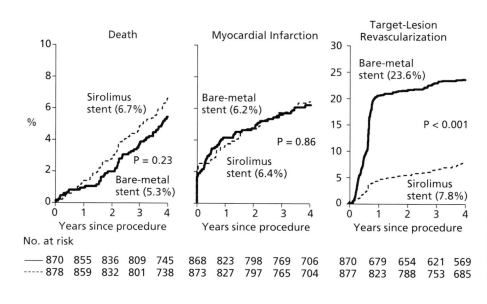

Figure 26.4 Analysis of randomized trials of sirolimus versus BMS on death, MI, and TLR. BMS, bare metal stents; MI, myocardial infarction; TLR, target lesion revascularization. (From Stone et al.[23])

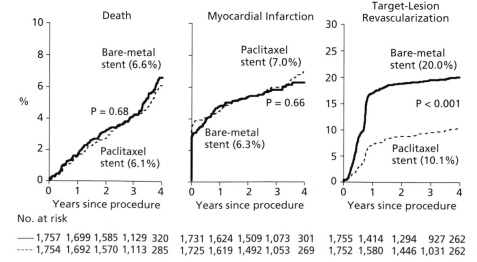

Figure 26.5 Analysis of randomized trials of paclitaxel versus BMS on death, MI, and TLR. Abbreviations as in Fig. 27.4. (From Stone et al.[23])

0.6% in the BMS group ($P = 0.20$) and 1.3% in the paclitaxel stent group versus 0.9% in the BMS group ($P = 0.30$). However, after one year, there were five episodes of stent thrombosis in patients with sirolimus-eluting stents versus none in patients with BMS ($P = 0.025$) and nine episodes in patients with paclitaxel-eluting stents versus two in patients with BMS ($P = 0.028$). The four-year rates of target lesion revascularization were markedly reduced in both the sirolimus stent and the paclitaxel stent group, as compared with the BMS groups. The rates of death or MI did not differ significantly between the groups that received DES or BMS.

The decreased restenosis rates with DES may come at a price. Although the on-label randomized controlled trials failed to detect an increase in late stent thrombosis with DES, large off-label real-world registries have produced conflicting results. It appears that the increased late stent thrombosis observed with DES may be offset by decreased restenosis-driven myocardial infarctions over time. Large, multicenter trials powered to address these questions are ongoing. Currently, the data as a whole support the following conclusions.[29]

- DES significantly reduce restenosis compared with BMS.
- Overall stent thrombosis rates are low and occur with both BMS and DES.
- The timing of stent thrombosis appears to vary, with DES more likely to be associated with late and very late stent thrombosis. Cessation of clopidogrel appears to be an important but not universal precipitating factor.
- In the carefully selected and monitored patient populations enrolled in the randomized trials leading to FDA approval, there was no difference in death or MI during follow-up.
- The optimal duration of dual antiplatelet therapy with clopidogrel remains uncertain.

Atherectomy

Plaque volume is a predictor of restenosis.[30] The directional atherectomy catheter gained FDA approval in 1990 and allowed cutting and removal of coronary plaque in a controlled ("directional") manner. It was hypothesized that plaque removal, by avoiding barotrauma and reducing plaque volume, would incite a less vigorous neointimal response and restenosis. However, increased rates of myocardial infarction, death, and major complications without a significant reduction in restenosis were found in adequately powered randomized trials, leading to abandonment of this technology.[31–33]

Rotational atherectomy (Rotablator™, Boston Scientific, Boston, MA) is a debulking procedure employing a rapidly rotating diamond-tipped abrasive burr (160000–180000 rpm). The device pulverizes calcified atherosclerotic plaque into tiny particles intended to pass through the microcirculation and be removed by the reticuloendothelial system. Unfortunately, sludging of particles can result in obstruction of the microcirculation with an increased risk of ischemia and non-Q wave myocardial infarction.[34–36] Its use is primarily limited, therefore, to removal of superficial calcium that may otherwise prevent lumen and vessel expansion.

Intravascular ultrasound (IVUS)

Since the introduction of IVUS to interventional cardiology in 1988, it has gained acceptance as both a research tool and

---

BOX 26.1 Intravascular imaging ultrasound (IVUS) (modified from 2005 ACC/AHA/SCAI guideline update for percutaneous coronary intervention)

Class IIa indications

IVUS is reasonable for the following:

- Assessment of the adequacy of deployment of coronary stents, including the extent of stent apposition and determination of the minimum luminal diameter within the stent. (**Level B**)
- Determination of the mechanism of stent restenosis (inadequate expansion versus neointimal proliferation) and to enable selection of appropriate therapy (vascular brachytherapy versus repeat balloon expansion). (**Level B**)
- Evaluation of coronary obstruction at a location difficult to image by angiography in a patient with a suspected flow-limiting stenosis. (**Level C**)
- Assessment of a suboptimal angiographic result after PCI. (**Level C**)
- Establishment of the presence and distribution of coronary calcium in patients for whom adjunctive rotational atherectomy is contemplated. (**Level C**)
- Determination of plaque location and circumferential distribution for guidance of directional coronary atherectomy. (**Level B**)

Class IIb indications

IVUS may be considered for the following:

- Determination of the extent of atherosclerosis in patients with characteristic anginal symptoms and a positive functional study with no focal stenoses or mild CAD on angiography. (**Level C**)
- Preinterventional assessment of lesional characteristics and vessel dimensions as a means to select an optimal revascularization device. (**Level C**)
- Diagnosis of coronary disease after cardiac transplantation. (**Level C**)

Class III indications

- IVUS is not recommended when the angiographic diagnosis is clear and no interventional treatment is planned. (**Level C**)

a clinical modality useful for clarifying epicardial coronary anatomy when the angiographic interpretation is unclear or ambiguous. IVUS can provide not only high spatial resolution images of the vessel lumen and stent, but also detailed and potentially useful information about plaque and arterial wall characteristics.

Despite an extensive literature validating the precision and intraprocedural utility of IVUS, data supporting the ability of this technology to improve clinical outcomes are few. The CLOUT trial evaluated IVUS-guided balloon angioplasty.[37] IVUS use resulted in a larger mean MLD, from 1.95 to 2.21 mm ($P < 0.0001$), and a larger luminal area from 3.2 to 4.5 mm^2 ($P < 0.0001$). Periprocedural complication rates and six-month restenosis rates were nevertheless similar. The SIPS trial (n = 269) compared IVUS-guided versus angiographically guided balloon angioplasty with bailout stenting where appropriate.[38] There was a significant improvement in TLR in the IVUS optimized group at two-year follow-up (17% vs 29%; $Pp < 0.05$).

Subsequent IVUS-guided stent trials have demonstrated that minimum stent area (MSA), as measured by IVUS, is a predictor of late angiographic and clinical restenosis.[39] However, the conflicting findings of small IVUS-guided stent optimization trials have been rationalized by the differing angiographic procedural endpoints in the IVUS-guided arms, as well as the disparate adjunctive medical treatment strategies employed (see below).

Recent concerns with late stent thrombosis with DES have fuelled speculation that the mechanism may be related to incomplete stent apposition against the arterial wall.[40–42] Using IVUS to guide DES deployment and thereby ensure adequate stent expansion and complete stent–vessel wall apposition has therefore been advocated in anatomically complex target lesions, but large randomized long-term studies that evaluate clinical outcomes after procedures with and without IVUS are needed to confirm this hypothesis. Presently there are no randomized or compelling outcome data that support the contention that routine IVUS during PCI improves clinical results.

Pressure wire

The ratio of the mean coronary artery pressure distal to a stenosis to the mean aortic pressure during maximal vasodilation (maximal hyperemia) is called the fractional flow reserve (FFR).[43] Comparisons with differing stress testing modalities in patients with stable coronary artery disease revealed that in 45 consecutive patients, the sensitivity of FFR for the identification of reversible ischemia was 88%, the specificity 100%, the positive predictive value 100%, and the negative predictive value 88%. A 0.014 inch pressure sensor-tipped coronary angioplasty guidewire is advanced across a stenosis, and the absolute distal pressure is recorded at rest and at maximal hyperemia induced by

> **BOX 26.2** Coronary artery pressure and flow: use of fractional flow reserve and coronary vasodilatory reserve (modified from 2005 ACC/AHA/SCAI guideline update for percutaneous coronary intervention)
>
> **Class IIa indications**
> Reasonable to use intracoronary physiologic measurements (IVUS, pressure wire) in the assessment of the effects of intermediate coronary stenoses (30–70% luminal narrowing) in patients with anginal symptoms. Coronary pressure or Doppler velocimetry may also be useful as an alternative to performing noninvasive functional testing (e.g. when the functional study is absent or ambiguous) to determine whether an intervention is warranted. (**Level B**)
>
> **Class IIb indications**
> - Intracoronary physiologic measurements may be considered for the evaluation of the success of PCI in restoring flow reserve and to predict the risk of restenosis. (**Level C**)
> - Preinterventional assessment of lesional characteristics and vessel dimensions as a means to select an optimal revascularization device. (**Level C**)
> - Intracoronary physiologic measurements may be considered for the evaluation of patients with anginal symptoms without an apparent angiographic culprit lesion. (**Level C**)
>
> **Class III indications**
> - Routine assessment with intracoronary physiologic measurements such as Doppler ultrasound or fractional flow reserve to assess the severity of angiographic disease in patients with a positive, unequivocal noninvasive functional study is not recommended. (**Level C**)

intracoronary or intravenous infusion of adenosine. The ischemic threshold value of FFR is <0.75 and current indications are listed in Box 26.2.

The appropriateness of intervening on stable coronary artery lesions of intermediate severity and without functional obstruction using pressure wire criteria was assessed in the DEFER study.[44] In 325 patients scheduled for PCI of an intermediate stenosis, FFR was measured prior to the planned intervention. If the FFR was ≥0.75, patients were randomly assigned to deferral (Defer group, n = 91) or PCI (Perform group, n = 90). If FFR was <0.75, PCI was performed as planned and these patients were followed up as the reference group (Reference group, n = 144). At five years, event-free survival was not different between the Defer and Perform groups (80% and 73% respectively; $P = 0.52$), but was significantly worse in the reference group (63%; $P = 0.03$). The composite rate of cardiac death and acute myocardial infarction in the Defer, Perform, and Reference groups was 3.3%, 7.9%, and 15.7%, respectively ($P = 0.21$ for Defer vs Perform group; $P = 0.003$ for the Reference vs both other groups). The risk that a hemodynamically non-significant stenosis (FFR ≥0.75) would cause death or myocardial infarction in patients with stable CAD was <1% per year and was not decreased by stenting.

The efficacy of the pressure wire in multivessel disease was recently assessed in the large multicenter FAME study.[45] Before randomization, lesions requiring PCI were identified on the basis of their angiographic appearance. In 1005 randomized patients, those assigned to angiography-guided PCI had drug-eluting stents placed in all indicated lesions. Those assigned to FFR-guided PCI underwent stenting of indicated lesions only if the FFR was 0.80 or less. The 1-year rate of death, nonfatal myocardial infarction, and repeat revascularization was 18.3% (91 patients) in the angiography group and 13.2% (67 patients) in the FFR group ($P = 0.02$). Seventy-eight percent of the patients in the angiography group were free from angina at 1 year versus 81% of the patients in the FFR group ($P = 0.20$). Like IVUS, routine or selected use of the pressure wire has not yet been demonstrated to improve long-term clinical outcomes.

Adjunctive pharmacology trials

PCI results in de-endothelialization and deep arterial injury that exposes luminal blood to tissue factor and other highly thrombotic molecules. Moreover, the artificial surfaces on catheters, guidewires and implanted metallic stents are themselves thrombogenic. Because thrombosis at the site of PCI can lead to catastrophic ischemic complications, periprocedural administration of antiplatelet and anticoagulant drugs is integral to PCI success and safety. Through intensive and rigorous study, antithrombotic agents and strategies have evolved rapidly over the past three decades.

Aspirin

Aspirin has been universally used in all forms of coronary heart disease for decades, based upon clinical trials performed in a wide variety of clinical settings and presentations.[46] Its specific role in PCI for preventing peri- and postprocedural ischemic events was demonstrated in a randomized controlled trial performed in the balloon angioplasty era. The active treatment comprised an oral aspirin/dipyridamole combination (330/75 mg) given three times daily, beginning 24 hours prior to PCI. Among the 376 randomized patients, there were 16 periprocedural Q-wave myocardial infarctions – 13 in the placebo group and three in the active drug group (6.9% vs 1.6%, $P = 0.0113$).[47] Aspirin has since been standard therapy before and after coronary intervention of all types, and has provided background antiplatelet therapy for all interventional clinical trials testing new antithrombotic regimens, devices and strategies.

The optimal daily dosage of aspirin with a reliable effect in PCI is uncertain. In the USA, 325 mg is common, while in Europe 100 mg or 75 mg is accepted. Higher doses (over 100 mg) are associated with more, predominantly gastrointestinal, side effects but have not been convincingly demonstrated to provide greater long-term protection from thrombotic or ischemic events. *Post hoc* analysis of the PCI-CURE trial examining patients undergoing BMS placement reported an increased risk of bleeding on long-term higher-dose aspirin (162–325 mg) compared to lower dose (75–100 mg).[48] On the other hand, clinically relevant inhibition of platelet aggregation requires 95% blockade of TXA_2 synthesis,[49] a level often not reached for 48 hours after initiating daily oral dosages of 75 mg. The OASIS-7/CURRENT trial is presently enrolling patients in a randomized comparison of ASA 81 mg versus 325 mg administered in combination with clopidogrel.

Thienopyridines

Ticlopidine was the first agent in this class to be widely used as an oral adjunct to ASA and heparin during and after PCI. The STARS trial randomized 1653 patients undergoing native coronary artery stenting, including elective procedures for stable CAD, and demonstrated that a combination of aspirin and ticlopidine was superior to an anticoagulation regimen in preventing subacute stent thrombosis at 30 days.[50] The benefit was obtained at the expense of increased bleeding complications (mostly access site related), but this trial formed the basis for modern ASA/thienopyridine combination therapy after PCI. Later trials, such as CLASSICS[51] and TOPPS,[52] demonstrated non-inferiority of clopidogrel vs ticlopidine, in combination with aspirin, for patients undergoing elective stenting. A meta-analysis of randomized and registry comparisons of ticlopidine and clopidogrel post stenting showed clopidogrel to be associated with a lower adverse cardiac event rate (2.1% versus 4.0%, $P = 0.001$) and mortality (0.48% versus 1.09%, $P = 0.001$) at 30 days.[53] These data, together with poor GI tolerance and infrequent but serious blood dyscrasias (neutropenia in ~2% of patients and rare cases of agranulocytosis), have resulted in abandonment of ticlopidine except for those intolerant of clopidogrel.[54]

The omnipresence of clopidogrel in contemporary PCI trials and guidelines (Box 26.3) has led to its routine use for patients in North America and Europe.[55] The duration of clopidogrel therapy was evaluated in the CREDO trial and demonstrated that optimal benefit was achieved by continuing 75 mg daily for 12 months post PCI in stable patients.[56] Clopidogrel in combination with aspirin conferred a 3% absolute risk reduction in the combined risk of death, MI or stroke ($P = 0.02$) when compared to aspirin alone. The timing and dosage of clopidogrel loading prior to PCI for patients not chronically treated appear to influence PCI outcome. *Post-hoc* analysis of the CREDO trial suggested that loading with oral clopidogrel 300 mg at least 15 hours pre-procedure was associated with the lowest adjusted risk of thrombotic and ischemic events. The ISAR-REACT trial showed that for patients at low-to-intermediate risk for early ischemic complications after elective PCI, pretreat-

BOX 26.3 Oral antiplatelet therapy (modified from 2007 focused update of the ACC/AHA/SCAI 2005 guideline update for percutaneous coronary intervention)

Class I indications
- Patients already taking daily long-term aspirin therapy should take 75 mg to 325 mg of aspirin before PCI is performed. (**Level A**)
- Patients not already taking daily long-term aspirin therapy should be given 300 mg to 325 mg of aspirin at least 2 hours and preferably 24 hours before PCI is performed. (**Level C**)
- After PCI, in patients without allergy or increased risk of bleeding, aspirin 162 mg to 325 mg daily should be given for at least 1 month after BMS implantation, 3 months after sirolimus-eluting stent implantation, and 6 months after paclitaxel-eluting stent implantation, after which daily long-term aspirin use should be continued indefinitely at a dose of 75 mg to 162 mg. (**Level B**)
- A loading dose of clopidogrel, generally 600 mg, should be administered before or when PCI is performed. (**Level C**) In patients undergoing PCI within 12–24 hours of receiving fibrinolytic therapy, a clopidogrel oral loading dose of 300 mg may be considered. (**Level C**)
- For all post-PCI stented patients receiving a DES, clopidogrel 75 mg daily should be given for **at least 12 months** if patients are not at high risk of bleeding. For post-PCI patients receiving a BMS, clopidogrel should be given for a minimum of 1 month and **ideally up to 12 months** (unless the patient is at increased risk of bleeding; then it should be given for a minimum of 2 weeks). (**Level B**)

Class IIa indications
- If clopidogrel is given at the time of procedure, supplementation with GP IIb/IIIa receptor antagonists can be beneficial. (**Level B**)
- For patients with an absolute contraindication to aspirin, it is reasonable to give a 300–600 mg loading dose of clopidogrel, administered at least 6 hours before PCI, and/or GP IIb/IIIa antagonists, administered at the time of PCI. (**Level C**)
- In patients for whom the physician is concerned about risk of bleeding, a lower dose of 75 mg to 162 mg of aspirin is reasonable during the initial period after stent implantation. (**Level C**)

Class IIb indications
- Continuation of clopidogrel therapy beyond 1 year may be considered in patients undergoing DES placement. (**Level C**)

ment with a 600 mg loading dose of clopidogrel was not associated with a measurable clinical benefit, irrespective of increasing the pretreatment interval beyond 2–3 hours or adjunctive treatment with abciximab.[57] The ARMYDA-2 trial showed reduced periprocedural marker elevation and MI in patients who were given a 600 mg clopidogrel loading dose rather than 300 mg.[58] The large CURRENT/OASIS 7 trial is testing a low dose (300 mg loading dose, followed by 75 mg/day maintenance therapy) versus high dose (600 mg loading dose, followed by 150 mg/day for a week and then 75 mg/day thereafter) clopidogrel regimen and a low (81 mg) versus high-dose (325 mg) ASA regimen and is powered to examine clinical events at 30 days.

The optimal loading and maintenance dose of clopidogrel to achieve rapid, predictable and sustained platelet inhibition is further confounded by interindividual variability. Platelet aggregation and expression of activation-dependent receptor expression in patients undergoing elective PCI treated with clopidogrel 300 mg orally followed by 75 mg daily has been found to vary widely.[59] Using a cut-off of <10% absolute change in aggregation to define clopidogrel resistance, the prevalence was 50–60% at 2 h, ~30% at 1 and 5 days and ~15% at 30 days post PCI. However, point-of-care platelet function assays are neither readily available nor well correlated to clinical outcomes; thus most centers have adopted a standard regimen of 600 mg loading dose followed by 75 mg maintenance dose.

The optimum duration of clopidogrel therapy following PCI, especially after DES implantation, is uncertain. Pivotal trials leading to approval of contemporary DES devices required ASA plus clopidogrel for at least three months after PCI. Late stent thrombosis was infrequent, but most patients were anatomically simple and the majority were treated with clopidogrel for at least six months. Subsequent recognition of late and very late DES thrombosis as infrequent but life-threatening events linked to anatomic or procedural complexity and associated with clopidogrel withdrawal has led to guideline revisions calling for one year's therapy after DES insertion. Recently published recommendations aimed at reducing the incidence of late DES thrombosis emphasize patient education regarding the hazards of premature clopidogrel discontinuation.[60] However, there is no randomized trial to directly inform optimum duration of therapy.

Prasugrel is a new, potent platelet $P2Y_{12}$ receptor inhibitor, and in combination with aspirin performed favorably against clopidogrel in a large trial of ACS patients undergoing PCI.[61] Overall, major adverse cardiac events were reduced (9.9% versus 12.1%, $P < 0.001$) but at the expense of increased serious bleeding. At the time of writing, prasugrel is not commercially available.

Glycoprotein IIb/IIIa receptor blockers

Three glycoprotein IIb/IIIa receptor inhibitors (GPI) have been evaluated in PCI clinical trials that included patients with stable CAD. These are abciximab, derived from a chimeric murine monoclonal antibody, and the synthetic peptides eptifibatide and tirofiban. Only abciximab and eptifibatide remain in frequent use. Both were evaluated with background aspirin and heparin.

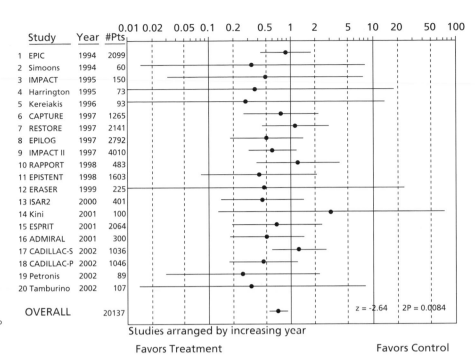

Study	Year	#Pts
1 EPIC	1994	2099
2 Simoons	1994	60
3 IMPACT	1995	150
4 Harrington	1995	73
5 Kereiakis	1996	93
6 CAPTURE	1997	1265
7 RESTORE	1997	2141
8 EPILOG	1997	2792
9 IMPACT II	1997	4010
10 RAPPORT	1998	483
11 EPISTENT	1998	1603
12 ERASER	1999	225
13 ISAR2	2000	401
14 Kini	2001	100
15 ESPRIT	2001	2064
16 ADMIRAL	2001	300
17 CADILLAC-S	2002	1036
18 CADILLAC-P	2002	1046
19 Petronis	2002	89
20 Tamburino	2002	107
OVERALL		20137

z = -2.64   2P = 0.0084

Studies arranged by increasing year

Favors Treatment   Favors Control

Figure 26.6 Improved 30-day mortality in GP IIb/IIIa inhibition arm of trials. (Adapted from Karvouni et al.[65])

The utility of abciximab in non-emergent PCI was evaluated in the EPIC, EPILOG, and EPISTENT trials.[62–64] EPIC enrolled 2099 patients deemed to be at high risk for ischemic complications of PCI and demonstrated that abciximab administered as a bolus plus infusion reduced the primary 30-day endpoint of death, MI or urgent intervention by 35%, compared to placebo or to abciximab bolus alone. EPILOG extended this experience into lower risk elective PCI procedures, and tested abciximab in combination with reduced-dose heparin. The trial was terminated early for efficacy after enrollment of 2792 patients (4800 planned). Greater than 50% relative reduction in death or MI, and in death, MI or urgent intervention was observed at 30 days in both abciximab arms (standard dose or reduced dose heparin) when compared to placebo. Major bleeding was numerically least frequent with the combination of abciximab and reduced dose heparin (2.0% versus 3.1% placebo versus 3.5% abciximab plus standard dose heparin, P = NS). EPISTENT compared three PCI strategies: balloon angioplasty plus abciximab, stenting plus placebo, or stenting plus abciximab, and employed the reduced dose heparin regimen from EPILOG. The primary endpoint of death, MI or urgent revascularization was observed in 10.8% of those assigned stent plus placebo, 6.9% of those assigned balloon angioplasty plus abciximab and in 5.5% of those assigned stent plus abciximab (P < 0.001). Many of the endpoints in these trials were small periprocedural myocardial infarctions. However, a subsequent meta-analysis of abciximab PCI trials demonstrated that abciximab significantly reduced death; this quelled much of the criticism that had focused on endpoint definition[65] (Fig. 26.6).

In summary, abciximab has been demonstrated to reduce early ischemia, abrupt vessel closure, subacute thrombosis, and MI, but late target vessel revascularization events (due to restenosis) are not affected.[66] As with any therapeutic intervention, the greatest benefit is likely observed in the highest risk patients.

IMPACT-II, the initial Phase III evaluation of eptifibatide, randomly assigned 4010 patients undergoing non-emergent balloon angioplasty to eptifibatide 135 μg/kg bolus followed by 24-hour infusions of 0.5 or 0.75 μg/kg/min, or placebo.[67] No statistically significant reduction in the primary endpoint of death, MI, emergency revascularization or bailout stenting was observed. Pharmacodynamic studies, however, suggested that eptifibatide dosing may have been inadequate in IMPACT II. This led to the development of the ESPRIT trial that compared a double bolus regimen followed by a larger 2.0 μg/kg/min infusion for 18–24 hours to placebo in 2064 patients undergoing elective stenting.[68] Thienopyridine-pretreated patients were excluded. The primary endpoint was the composite of death, MI, urgent target vessel revascularization and bailout GPI use within 48 hours. The trial was terminated early due to efficacy, with significant endpoint reduction in the eptifibatide arm (6.6% versus 10.5%, P = 0.0015) and durable benefit to six months. As with the abciximab trials, many events in ESPRIT were small periprocedural myocardial infarctions.

Proven regimens with abciximab and eptifibatide depended upon administration of a prolonged intravenous infusion that required nursing time, may have contributed to bleeding, and delayed hospital discharge. Because length of hospitalization substantially impacts cost, shorter duration abciximab and eptifibatide regimens have recently been studied. Following uncomplicated PCI, the BRIEF trial demonstrated that eptifibatide infusion can be safely abbreviated to ≤2 h, without compromising efficacy compared to the standard 18-h regimen, with less major bleeding.[69]

Pivotal trials testing GPI use in non-emergent PCI were performed in the 1990s before clopidogrel pretreatment was routine practice. The incremental benefit of GPI use in patients pretreated with both aspirin and clopidogrel was addressed in the ISAR-REACT series of randomized, placebo-controlled trials. For patients undergoing elective PCI and at low to intermediate risk for thrombotic complications, abciximab did not provide incremental benefit after 600 mg clopidogrel pretreatment. This contrasted with results in a higher risk patient group defined by presentation with non-ST elevation myocardial infarction (STEMI) (ISAR-REACT 2) where abciximab, in addition to periprocedural unfractionated heparin (UFH), conferred a 25% relative risk reduction in 30-day major adverse cardiac event rate compared to placebo (8.9% versus 11.9%, P = 0.03), without compromise in safety, and with benefit maintained at one year.[70,71] The CLEAR PLATELETS 1b trial evaluated the effect of combining eptifibatide with clopidogrel loading (300 or 600 mg) versus clopidogrel loading alone on myonecrotic and inflammatory marker release in 120 patients after elective stenting.[72] The combination regimen reduced the release of CK-MB, myoglobin, troponin-I and CRP (P < 0.01 for each parameter). The clinical translation of the attenuated release of these markers suggests that more potent platelet inhibition is beneficial.

Periprocedural anticoagulant
Unfractionated and low molecular weight heparin Use of a potent anticoagulant during PCI has been standard therapy since coronary balloon angioplasty was first described. Until recently, unfractionated heparin (UFH) has been unchallenged as the most commonly employed agent for this indication. Large placebo-controlled trials demonstrating the need for UFH during PCI were never performed. Anecdotal experience from PCI performed without heparin or other anticoagulant, sometimes by medical error, suggest a high incidence of acute coronary thrombosis in its absence.

Attention has been paid to heparin dosing during PCI. In the balloon angioplasty era, heparin was commonly administered as a non-weight adjusted high dose bolus of 10 000–12 000 units. When combined with concurrent practices that included larger bore arterial sheaths (8 F) and delayed sheath removal, arterial access site bleeds were common.[62] Contemporary heparin dosing is dependent on whether there is concurrent GPI administration.[68,73] In those patients without GPI, sufficient UFH should be given during PCI to maintain an activated clotting time (ACT) of 300 seconds. A weight-adjusted heparin bolus (70–100 IU/kg) is usually used to achieve the target anticoagulation

and supplemented as necessary with boluses of 2000–5000 IU. The UFH bolus should be reduced to 50–70 IU/kg in the presence of GPI to achieve an ACT of 200 seconds. Postprocedural UFH infusions are not recommended.

Compared to UFH, low-molecular weight heparins (LMWH) display more consistent protein and cellular binding, resulting in greater biovailability and less interpatient variability with respect to potency and clearance. Other potential advantages of LMWH relevant to PCI include a low incidence of heparin-induced thrombocytopenia, freedom from activated partial thromboplastin time (APTT) monitoring, and avoidance of need to switch antithrombotic agents in acute coronary syndrome (ACS) patients medically stabilized with subcutaneous LMWH.[74] The safety and efficacy of intravenous LMWH (enoxaparin; 1 mg/kg) in elective PCI were validated in the NICE-1 trial.[75] STEEPLE was the largest trial directly comparing a LMWH (enoxaparin) to UFH in elective PCI.[76] Patients were randomly assigned to one of two bolus doses of intravenous enoxaparin (0.5 mg/kg or 0.75 mg/kg) or to UFH (70–100 IU/kg or 50–70 IU/kg bolus) with or without a GPI. Concerns arose that the lower enoxaparin dose was associated with higher mortality due to thrombotic complications. The overall mortality rate of 1.0% in the 0.5 mg/kg enoxaparin group was twice that expected for patients undergoing elective PCI, especially patients at low risk for complications. This observation was argued to be directly treatment related rather than a chance effect. Another confounding factor with this trial is that interpretation of the primary endpoint, the incidence of major or minor bleeding not related to coronary artery bypass grafting, varied depending on the bleeding index used. The authors employed unique definitions of major and minor bleeds that had not been shown to have prognostic import. Reanalysis of the results using TIMI bleeding criteria showed no significant differences in bleeding rates between the enoxaparin and UFH groups, whereas the GUSTO index demonstrated superiority of the lower dose enoxaparin regimen. A meta-analysis incorporating 11 trials among patients undergoing elective PCI demonstrated similar efficacy between LMWH and UFH with respect to all-cause mortality and major adverse cardiac events (P = 0.93).[77] A significant reduction in major bleeding risk with LMWH compared with UFH (P = 0.002) and a trend towards a reduction in minor bleeds (P = 0.24) were also apparent.

There are currently two strategies guiding the use of LMWH (with or without concomitant GPI) for PCI:[78] UFH may substituted for LMWH prior to angiography and coronary intervention if the last LMWH dose was given more than 8–12 hours before the procedure, or alternatively, LMWH may be safely continued as the sole anticoagulant throughout the PCI without switching to UFH.

Hirudin/bivalirudin In REPLACE-2, the direct thrombin inhibitor bivalirudin[79] was compared to UFH plus planned

GPI, using a non-inferiority design in a diverse population undergoing PCI.[80] Elective cases comprised 56% of enrollment. The primary endpoint was a composite of death, MI, urgent revascularization or in-hospital major bleeding at 30 days and occurred in 9.2% of the bivalirudin cohort compared with 10% patients in the UFH plus GPI group ($P = 0.32$). In hospital major bleeding was significantly reduced by bivalirudin (2.4% versus 4.1%, $P < 0.001$), with the results driven by access site-related complications and gastrointestinal bleeds.

High-risk patients undergoing PCI have also been evaluated in several important trials including HELVITCA,[81] HAS[82] and ACUITY.[83] Together, these trials suggest that direct antithrombin inhibitors reduce acute thrombotic complications and bleeding when compared to heparin. This evidence has led to the incorporation of bivalirudin into the latest AHA/ACC guidelines for routine interventional practice (Box 26.4).

Fonadaparinux

Fondaparinux is an indirect factor Xa inhibitor with proven superiority to standard therapies for the prevention of venous thrombosis, the safety and efficacy of which were piloted in the ASPIRE trial in patients who underwent elec-

tive or urgent PCI for ACS.[84] Concerns regarding inadequate protection against lesion-related or catheter-related thrombus first surfaced with fondaparinux-treated patients in ASPIRE. The subsequent and much larger OASIS-5 trial randomized ACS patients to either fondaparinux or enoxaparin treatment.[85] After additional reports of catheter thrombus with fondaparinux, the protocol was amended to encourage open-label administration of supplemental UFH for fondaparinux-treated patients undergoing PCI. With this hybrid strategy, subcutaneous fondaparinux (2.5 mg/day for ≤8 days) was non-inferior to subcutaneous enoxaparin (1 mg/kg twice daily, once daily in those with renal dysfunction) in reducing death or ischemic events at nine days, with efficacy being maintained for up to six months. Major bleeding occurred in fewer fondaparinux recipients, resulting in a benefit/risk balance favoring fondaparinux. Importantly, catheter thrombus was more common with fondaparinux than with enoxaparin (0.9% versus 0.4%), but this complication was largely prevented by the addition of UFH at the time of PCI, with no increase in the bleeding rate.

Strategic trials of percutaneous coronary intervention versus medical therapy in stable coronary artery disease

Insofar as ischemia due to coronary stenosis is a defining feature of coronary artery disease ("ischemic heart disease"), the prevention of ischemia through the relief of coronary stenoses with PCI would at first appear to offer self-evident potential for improving long-term outcomes. At least in the case of patients with chronic ischemia, demonstrating such a benefit has been conspicuously difficult. The degree to which this reflects the biology of chronic ischemic heart disease versus limitations in trial design and power, populations enrolled, advances in medical therapy, and the PCI technologies and techniques employed remains a matter of some debate.

Historic trials

A Comparison of Angioplasty with Medical Therapy in the Treatment of Single-Vessel Coronary Artery Disease (ACME)[86] randomly assigned 212 patients with stable, single-vessel CAD and exercise-induced myocardial ischemia to coronary balloon angioplasty or medical therapy alone. Angioplasty resulted in a greater proportion of patients free from angina at six months (64% versus 46%, $P < 0.01$) and greater objective improvement in treadmill exercise duration (2.1 versus 0.5 minutes; $P < 0.0001$) compared to medical therapy alone. These results were obtained despite a high rate of PCI failure (20%) and in an era that predated modern interventional or medical therapies. A subsequent trial from the ACME group enrolled 328 patients with double-vessel disease and was reported in

1997.[87] Patients with double-vessel disease, treated with balloon angioplasty versus medical therapy, experienced comparable improvement in exercise duration (+1.2 versus +1.3 min, respectively, $P = 0.89$), freedom from angina (53% and 36%, respectively, $P = 0.09$) and improvement of overall quality of life score (+1.3 versus +4.4, respectively, $P = 0.32$) at six months compared with baseline. This contrasts with greater advantages favoring PTCA by these criteria in patients with single-vessel disease ($P = 0.0001$ to 0.02). Trends present at six months persisted at late follow-up. Patients undergoing double-vessel dilation had less complete initial revascularization (45% versus 83%) and greater average stenosis of worst lesions at 6 months (74% versus 56%). Likewise, patients with double-vessel disease showed less improved myocardial perfusion imaging (59% versus 75%). Neither trial was powered to show differences in myocardial infarction or death.

The largest prospective trial of balloon angioplasty versus medical therapy was the multicenter Randomized Intervention Treatment of Angina (RITA) 2 trial.[88] Most of the patients had mild symptoms (80% Canadian Cardiovascular Society (CCS) class 0 to II), 60% had single-vessel CAD, and one-third had two-vessel disease. The primary endpoint of death or myocardial infarction occurred in 6.3% (32 patients) of the balloon angioplasty group and 3.3% (17 patients) of the medical therapy group (absolute difference 3.0%, 95% CI 0.4–5.7; $P = 0.02$). The combined rates of death, myocardial infarction, and non-protocol revascularization were similar at three years. Angina pectoris, treadmill exercise time and quality of life measures improved significantly in both groups. The subgroup of patients with baseline angina CCS class II or worse, however, appeared to derive incremental benefit from PCI that included a lower incidence of angina, longer treadmill exercise times, greater improvements in physical functioning, vitality, and general health at three months and one year. By three years, however, this advantage was lost, likely due in part to cross-over PCI rescue of the most symptomatic medically assigned patients (cross-over rate 27%).[89]

The Atorvastatin Versus Revascularization Treatment (AVERT) trial[90] enrolled 341 patients with low-risk CAD (99% of patients had stable CCS class 0 to II angina) in a randomized trial of controversial design comparing percutaneous revascularization plus usual medical care to medical care that included high-dose atorvastatin. Overall, 166 patients in the angioplasty group underwent the assigned procedure (with a total of 213 treated lesions). Concomitant stenting was used in 64 of the lesions. Though a greater proportion of the PCI group had improved angina (54% versus 41%, $P = 0.009$), fewer cardiac events (cardiac death or arrest, revascularization, stroke or worsening angina) developed in the atorvastatin group (21% PCI versus 13% atorvastatin, $P = 0.048$). The potentially complementary combination of PCI and high-dose statin therapy was not tested.

The ACIP (Asymptomatic Cardiac Ischemia Pilot) study examined 558 patients with silent ischemia who were judged angiographically suitable for revascularization.[91] Three treatment strategies were tested: angina-guided drug therapy (n = 183), ischemia-guided drug therapy (n = 183) or revascularization by angioplasty or bypass surgery (n = 192). Two-year total mortality was 6.6% in the angina-guided strategy, 4.4% in the ischemia-guided strategy, and 1.1% in the revascularization strategy ($P < 0.02$). Of the 92 undergoing PTCA, two-year event rates were mortality 1.1% (one patient); death or MI 5.5% (five patients); and death, MI or recurrent hospitalization 31.7% (29 patients). The corresponding rates for the 78 patients undergoing CABG were respectively 0%, 2.7% (two patients) and 12.9% (10 patients). Death or myocardial infarction was 12.1% in the angina-guided strategy, 8.8% in the ischemia-guided strategy, and 4.7% in the revascularization strategy ($P < 0.04$). Recurrent hospitalization was also reduced by the strategy of revascularization. ACIP was a pilot study which was not planned to have sufficient statistical power to detect differences in clinical outcomes. The difference in two-year mortality between the angina-guided and revascularization strategies is based on only 14 deaths (12 in the angina-guided strategy and 2 in the revascularization strategy). The results for death or non-fatal MI are based on only 31 events (22 in the angina-guided strategy and nine in the revascularization strategy). Although the dramatic differences seen produced a statistically significant result, there are too few events to allow for reliable assessment of effect size.

Bucher et al performed a systematic review of six randomized clinical trials that enrolled 1904 patients (from 1979 to 1998) with stable, predominantly single-vessel CAD and generally normal left ventricular function, assigned to balloon angioplasty plus medication versus medication alone.[92] The AVERT trial, with the limitations discussed above, contributed the second largest pool of patients. Routine PTCA resulted in significant improvement in angina (risk ratio (RR) 0.70, 95% CI 0.50–0.98); however, patients assigned to PTCA required CABG more frequently (RR 1.59, 95% CI 1.09–2.32). No differences in death (RR 1.32, 95% CI 0.65–2.70) or myocardial infarction (RR 1.42, 95% CI 0.90–2.25) were observed. The review did not include enough patients for informative estimates of the effect of angioplasty on myocardial infarction, death, or subsequent revascularization.

A more recent meta-analysis by Katritsis et al that considered 11 trials (1987–2001) including 2950 patients concluded that a strategy of routine PTCA performed in patients with stable symptoms, predominantly single-vessel CAD and normal left ventricular function does not prevent death, myocardial infarction or the need for subsequent revascularization when compared with routine medical treatment (Fig. 26.7).[93] By random effects, the risk

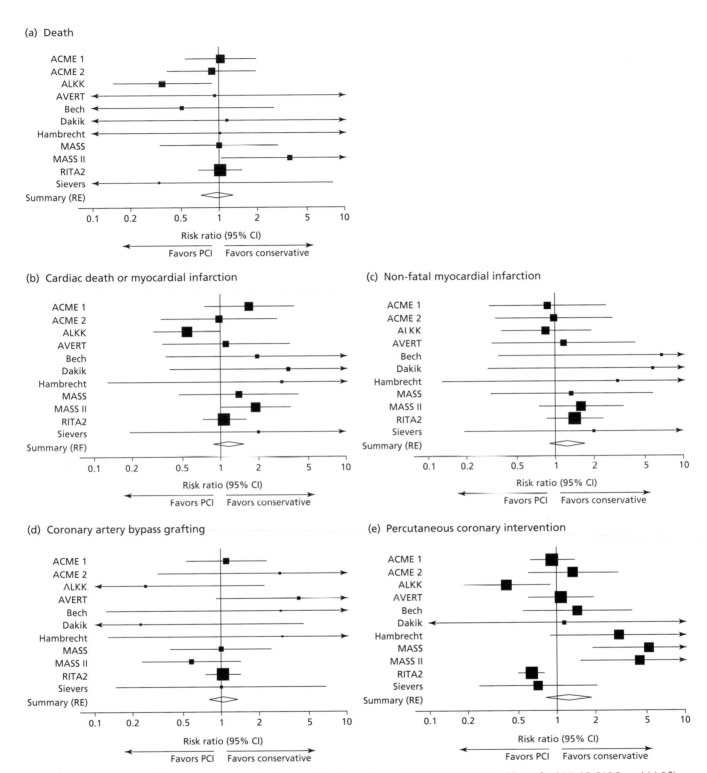

Figure 26.7 Comparison of PCI vs conservative medical treatment for (a) death, (b) cardiac death or any MI, (c) non-fatal MI, (d) CABG, and (e) PCI during follow-up. Each study is shown by name along with point estimate of risk ratio and respective 95% CIs. In each panel, size of box denoting point estimate in each study is proportional to weight of study. Also shown are summary risk ratio and 95% CIs according to Der Simonian and Laird random effects (RE) model. Meta-analysis of studies on the effect of PCI versus medical therapy. (From Katritsis et al.[93])

ratios (95% CI) for the PCI versus conservative treatment arms were for mortality 0.94 (0.72–1.24), cardiac death or myocardial infarction 1.17 (0.88–1.57), non-fatal myocardial infarction 1.28 (0.94–1.75), CABG 1.03 (0.80–1.33), and PCI 1.23 (0.80–1.90). A possible survival benefit was seen for PCI only in trials of patients who had a relatively recent myocardial infarction (RR 0.40, 95% CI 0.17–0.95). Except for PCI during follow-up, there was no significant between-study heterogeneity for any outcome. A large proportion of patients again came from the RITA-2 and AVERT trials.

Current era trials

Two recent trials of PCI versus medical therapy have focused attention on the appropriate use of PCI in stable CAD: MASS (Medicine, Angioplasty, or Surgery Study)-2 trial[94] and the COURAGE (Clinical Outcomes Utilizing Revascularization and Aggressive DruG Evaluation) trial.[95]

The MASS-2 study assigned 611patients (enrolled between 1995 and 2000) with limited multivessel CAD, stable angina, and preserved ventricular function to CABG (n = 203), PCI (n = 205) or medical therapy (n = 203). The one-year survival rates were 96.0% for CABG, 95.6% for PCI, and 98.5% for medical therapy (P = NS). The rates for one-year survival free of Q-wave MI were 98% for CABG, 92% for PCI, and 97% for medical therapy. After one-year follow-up, 8.3% of medical therapy patients and 13.3% of PCI patients underwent additional revascularization procedures, compared with only 0.5% of CABG patients. At one-year follow-up, 88% of the patients in the CABG group, 79% in the PCI group, and 46% in the medical therapy group were free of angina (P < 0.0001).

The COURAGE study compared an initial management strategy of percutaneous coronary intervention and optimal medical management (PCI) to optimal medical therapy (OMT) alone in patients with stable CAD.[95] Between 1999 and 2004, 1149 patients were assigned to PCI and 1138 to OMT. Baseline characteristics included: 43% of patients had either no angina or only class 1 angina, 30% of patients had single-vessel disease, the ejection fraction was approximately 61% in both groups, and DES were not routinely available. Balloon angioplasty (no stent) was used in 6% of those assigned PCI, and DES were employed in fewer than 3%. Neither glycoprotein inhibitors nor thienopyridine pretreatment was provided routinely. PCI was judged angiographically unsuccessful in 7%.

There were 211 primary events (death from any cause and non-fatal MI) in the PCI group and 202 events in the medical therapy group. The 4.6-year cumulative primary-event rates were 19.0% in the PCI group and 18.5% in the medical therapy group (hazard ratio (HR) for the PCI group 1.05; 95% CI 0.87–1.27; P = 0.62). There were no significant differences between the PCI group and the medical therapy group in the composite of death, MI, and stroke (20.0%

versus 19.5%; HR 1.05; 95% CI 0.87–1.27; P = 0.62); hospitalization for ACS (12.4% versus 11.8%; HR 1.07; 95% CI 0.84–1.37; P = 0.56) or MI (13.2% versus 12.3%; HR 1.13; 95% CI 0.89–1.43; P = 0.33). These results were not unexpected given the low-risk baseline characteristics of the enrolled population, low overall mortality, and the results of prior CABG versus medicine trials demonstrating the futility of CABG for prolonging survival in similar cohorts.[96]

COURAGE documented symptomatic benefits attributable to routine PCI, but these were modest. A significantly larger proportion of PCI-assigned patients were angina free during most of the follow-up period, though the two arms converged in this regard. At five years, 74% of patients in the PCI group and 72% of those in the medical therapy group were free of angina (P = 0.35). Routine PCI also resulted in a lower rate of non-protocol revascularization during follow-up (21.1% versus 32.6%; HR 0.60; 95% CI 0.51–0.71; P < 0.001). Critics of the study note that larger differences in metrics of symptom burden may have been buffered by several factors, including the enrolment of many patients with mild or no angina at entry, enrollment bias toward medical responders, unusually intensive medical follow-up and treatment, relatively high PCI failure rates, infrequent use of DES, and cross-over to PCI in one-third of those assigned OMT. A recent meta-analysis of trials of BMS vs optimal medical therapy, including the COURAGE trial, found similar results.

A substudy of COURAGE enrolled 314 patients evaluated with centrally analyzed quantitative SPECT myocardial perfusion imaging before treatment and again 6–18 months after enrollment.[97] The observed reduction in ischemic myocardium was significantly greater with PCI (−2.7%; 95% CI −1.7% to −3.8%) than with OMT (−0.5%; 95% CI −1.6–0.6%; P < 0.0001). The difference favoring routine PCI was most marked amongst patients with moderate to severe pretreatment ischemia in whom 78% experienced significant ischemia reduction with PCI versus 52% with OMT (P = 0.007). Patients with ischemia reduction had lower unadjusted risk for death or myocardial infarction (P = 0.037 [risk-adjusted P = 0.26]), particularly if baseline ischemia was moderate to severe (P = 0.001 [risk-adjusted P = 0.08]).

Overall, the strategy of PCI as a routine or frequent component of therapy to reduce major cardiac events in patients with stable symptomatic or silent ischemia has not been adequately tested. Trials performed to date have significant limitations with respect to populations studied, procedural success, pharmacology and technology, and statistical power to detect differences in long-term mortality. The degree to which the results of these trials can be generalized to contemporary cardiology practice is therefore limited. Moreover, widespread application of PCI for symptom relief may, at this stage, make performing a definitive trial difficult or impossible. Trials comparing PCI to medical therapy in high-risk patient groups may still be feasible and could provide important insights. For example, the recent BARI 2D trial performed in patients with type 2 diabetes and stable coronary artery disease, found no difference in major outcomes between PCI and optimal medical therapy.[97a] Existing and ongoing trials comparing PCI to CABG in cohorts already known to benefit from CABG are discussed in Chapter 30.

Conclusions: elective percutaneous coronary intervention versus medical therapy (Boxes 26.5 and 26.6)

- Among patients with medically refractory angina pectoris, PCI is indicated for symptom improvement (**Class I**).
- In the absence of symptoms or myocardial ischemia, PTCA is not indicated merely for the presence of an anatomic stenosis (**Class I**).
- Electively placed stents are superior to balloon angioplasty for reducing the need for repeat procedures (**Class I**).
- DES are superior to BMS for reducing the need for repeat procedures (**Class I**).
- PCI is reasonable for patients with recurrent stenosis after PTCA, a large area of viable myocardium at risk or high-risk criteria on non-invasive testing (**Class II**).

Future directions and challenges

A variety of anatomic circumstances present unique challenges during PCI. These include aorto-ostial lesions, chronic total occlusions (CTOs), bifurcation lesions, and saphenous vein grafts (SVGs). Numerous prospective, randomized trials published over the past 10 years have compared elective stenting to balloon angioplasty under various conditions. These studies have enrolled patients with various lesion types, including elective procedures for single discrete lesions in vessels of 3 mm or larger,[10,11,98–106] restenosis lesions after previous balloon angioplasty,[107] lesions of saphenous vein grafts.[108] small-caliber vessels[109–112] and chronic total occlusions.[12,113–118] BMS implantation decreases the need for target vessel revascularization in these challenging anatomic substrates.

Aorto-ostial lesions extend proximal to the coronary ostia into the aortic wall where abundant elastic fibers contribute to elastic recoil and poor outcome after balloon angioplasty.[119] By resisting recoil, stents maintain significantly larger lumens and lower the risk of restenosis in aorto-ostial lesions. Preliminary data suggest DES may further improve outcomes.[120] SVGs remain a challenging problem. Following bypass graft surgery, approximately 5–10% of patients per year develop recurrent angina and by 10 years almost 50% of SVGs are occluded.[16] Although

---

BOX 26.5 Patients with asymptomatic ischemia or CCS class I or II angina

Class IIa indications

- PCI is reasonable in patients with asymptomatic ischemia or CCS class I or II angina and with 1 or more significant lesions in 1 or 2 coronary arteries suitable for PCI with a high likelihood of success and a low risk of morbidity and mortality. The vessels to be dilated must subtend a moderate to large area of viable myocardium or be associated with a moderate to severe degree of ischemia on noninvasive testing. (**Level B**)
- PCI is reasonable for patients with asymptomatic ischemia or CCS class I or II angina, and recurrent stenosis after PCI with a large area of viable myocardium or high-risk criteria on non-invasive testing. (**Level C**)
- Use of PCI is reasonable in patients with asymptomatic ischemia or CCS class I or II angina with significant left main CAD (greater than 50% diameter stenosis) who are candidates for revascularization but are not eligible for CABG. (**Level B**)

Class IIb indications

- The effectiveness of PCI for patients with asymptomatic ischemia or CCS class I or II angina who have 2- or 3-vessel disease with significant proximal LAD CAD who are otherwise eligible for CABG with 1 arterial conduit and who have treated diabetes or abnormal LV function is not well established. (**Level B**)
- PCI might be considered for patients with asymptomatic ischemia or CCS class I or II angina with non-proximal LAD CAD that subtends a moderate area of viable myocardium and demonstrates ischemia on non-invasive testing. (**Level C**)

Class III indications

- PCI is not recommended in patients with asymptomatic ischemia or CCS class I or II angina who do not meet the criteria as listed under the class II recommendations or who have 1 or more of the following:
  - Only a small area of viable myocardium at risk (**Level C**)
  - No objective evidence of ischemia. (**Level C**)
  - Lesions that have a low likelihood of successful dilation. (**Level C**)
  - Mild symptoms that are unlikely to be due to myocardial ischemia. (**Level C**)
  - Factors associated with increased risk of morbidity or mortality. (**Level C**)
  - Left main disease and eligibility for CABG. (**Level C**)
  - Insignificant disease (less than 50% coronary stenosis). (**Level C**)

From ACC/AHA/SCAI 2005 Guideline Update for Percutaneous Coronary Intervention.[6]

BOX 26.6 Patients with CCS Class III angina

Class IIa indications
- It is reasonable that PCI be performed in patients with CCS class III angina and single-vessel or multivessel CAD who are undergoing medical therapy and who have 1 or more significant lesions in 1 or more coronary arteries suitable for PCI with a high likelihood of success and low risk of morbidity or mortality(**Level B**)
- It is reasonable that PCI be performed in patients with CCS class III angina with single-vessel or multivessel CAD who are undergoing medical therapy with focal saphenous vein graft lesions or multiple stenoses who are poor candidates for reoperative surgery. (**Level C**)
- Use of PCI is reasonable in patients with CCS class III angina with significant left main CAD (greater than 50% diameter stenosis) who are candidates for revascularization but are not eligible for CABG. (**Level B**)

Class IIb indications
- PCI may be considered in patients with CCS class III angina with single-vessel or multivessel CAD who are undergoing medical therapy and who have 1 or more lesions to be dilated with a reduced likelihood of success. (**Level B**)
- 2PCI may be considered in patients with CCS class III angina and no evidence of ischemia on non-invasive testing or who are undergoing medical therapy and have 2- or 3-vessel CAD with significant proximal LAD CAD and treated diabetes or abnormal LV function. (**Level B**)

Class III indications
- PCI is not recommended for patients with CCS class III angina with single-vessel or multivessel CAD, no evidence of myocardial injury or ischemia on objective testing, and no trial of medical therapy, or who have 1 of the following:
  - Only a small area of myocardium at risk. (**Level C**)
  - All lesions or the culprit lesion to be dilated with morphology that conveys a low likelihood of success. (**Level C**)
  - A high risk of procedure-related morbidity or mortality. (**Level C**)
  - Insignificant disease (less than 50% coronary stenosis). (**Level C**)
  - Significant left main CAD and candidacy for CABG. (**Level C**)

From ACC/AHA/SCAI 2005 Guideline Update for Percutaneous Coronary Intervention.[6]

DES may improve outcomes, the need for repeat revascularization is often driven by progressive disease in other segments within the same vein graft.

Clinical and angiographic rates of restenosis are high following recanalization and treatment of CTOs with either balloon angioplasty or BMS. Initial results suggest improved angiographic restenosis rates with DES; definitive results are expected with publication of TOSCA-4 (personal communication, D. Kandzari and C. Buller). A reliable technology for navigating and crossing total coronary occlusions in the first place, however, is urgently needed. CTOs resistant to crossing with current guidewires remain a frequent source of medically refractory angina and a common reason for CABG.

Atherosclerosis frequently develops at branch points and thus more than 20% of lesions treated with PCI involve bifurcations.[121] For lesions that have atherosclerotic involvement of both the main and side branch, a decision as to whether to undertake a provisional approach (in which the side branch is stented only if treatment of the main branch results in compromised flow) or dual stent strategy (in which both main and side branches are treated with DES devices *de novo*) is required. Although a complete discussion of bifurcation stenting is beyond the scope of this chapter, observational studies show the dual stent strategy is associated with higher risk of stent thrombosis[122] and a provisional strategy was shown to be safe and effective in the randomized NORDIC trial.[123] Dedicated-design bifurcation stents are currently under development and clinical investigation but have yet to be demonstrated superior. Technology that provides predictable and durable treatment of the left main coronary artery and its bifurcation or trifurcation point is required before PCI can be legitimately compared to CABG in this important subset.

References

1. Dotter CT, Judkins MP. Transluminal treatment of arteriosclerotic obstruction: description of a new technique and a preliminary report of its application. *Circulation* 1964;**30**:654.
2. Gruntzig A. Transluminal dilatation of coronary-artery stenosis. *Lancet* 1978;**1**:263.
3. Gruntzig AR, Senning A, Siegenthaler WE. Nonoperative dilatation of coronary-artery stenosis: percutaneous transluminal coronary angioplasty. *N Engl J Med* 1979;**301**:61–8.
4. Sandborn TA, Faxon DP, Haudenschild C *et al.* The mechanism of transluminal angioplasty: evidence for formation of aneurysms in experimental atherosclerosis. *Circulation* 1983;**68**:1136.
5. Detre K, Holubkov R, Kelsey S *et al*, for the Coinvestigators of the NHLBI PTCA Registry. Percutaneous transluminal coronary angioplasty in 1985–1986 and 1977–1981. *N Engl J Med* 1988;**318**:265–270.
6. ACC/AHA/SCAI. 2005 Guideline update for percutaneous coronary intervention. A report of the American College of Cardiology/American Heart Association Task Force on Practice Guidelines (ACC/AHA/SCAI Writing Committee to Update the 2001 Guidelines for Percutaneous Coronary Intervention). *J Am Coll Cardiol* 2006;**47**:1–121.
7. Cooper C, El-Shiekh R, Cohen D *et al.* Effect of transradial access on quality of life and cost of catheretrization: a randomized comparison. *Am Heart J* 1999;**138**:430–6.

8. McNulty P, Ettinger S, Field J *et al.* Cardiac catheterization in morbidly obese patients. *Catheter Cardiovasc Interv* 2002;**56**: 174–7.

9. Agostoni P, Biondi-Zoccai G, De Benedictis ML *et al.* Radial versus femoral approach for percutaneous coronary diagnostic and interventional procedures: systematic overview and meta-analysis of randomized trials. *J Am Coll Cardiol* 2004;**44**:349–56.

10. Serruys PW, de Jaegere P, Kiemeneij F *et al.* A comparison of balloon-expandable-stent implantation with balloon angioplasty in patients with coronary artery disease. Benestent Study Group. *N Engl J Med* 1994;**331**:489–95.

11. Fischman DL, Leon MB, Baim DS *et al.* A randomized comparison of coronary-stent placement and balloon angioplasty in the treatment of coronary artery disease. Stent Restenosis Study Investigators. *N Engl J Med* 1994;**331**:496–501.

12. Buller CE, Dzavik V, Carere RG *et al.* Primary stenting versus balloon angioplasty in occluded coronary arteries: the Total Occlusion Study of Canada (TOSCA). *Circulation* 1999;**100**: 236–42.

13. Brophy JM, Belisle P, Joseph L. Evidence for use of coronary stents. A hierarchical Bayesian meta-analysis. *Ann Intern Med* 2003;**138**:777–86.

14. Al Suwaidi J, Holmes DR Jr, Salam AM *et al.* Impact of coronary artery stents on mortality and nonfatal myocardial infarction: metaanalysis of randomized trials comparing a strategy of routine stenting with that of balloon angioplasty. *Am Heart J* 2004;**147**:815–22.

15. Rankin JM, Spinelli JJ, Carere RG *et al.* Improved clinical outcome after widespread use of coronary-artery stenting in Canada. *N Engl J Med* 1999; **341**:1957–65.

16. Stone GS. Coronary stenting. In: *Grossman's Cardiac Catheterization, Angiography, and Intervention*, 7th edn. Philadelphia: Lippincott Williams and Wilkins, 2006.

17. Mehran R, Dangas G, Abizaid AS *et al.* Angiographic patterns of in-stent restenosis: classification and implications for long-term outcome. *Circulation* 1999;**100**:1872–8.

18. Pate GE, Lee M, Humphries K *et al.* Characterizing the spectrum of in-stent restenosis: implications for contemporary treatment. *Can J Cardiol* 2006; **22**:1223–9.

19. Ho KK, Senerchia C, Rodriquez O *et al.* Predictors of angiographic restenosis after stenting: pooled analysis of 1197 patients with protocol-mandated angiographic follow-up from five randomized stent trials. *Circulation* 1998;**98**:362–8.

20. Morino Y, Honda Y, Okura H *et al.* An optimal diagnostic threshold for minimal stent area to predict target lesion revascularization following stent implantation in native coronary lesions. *Am J Cardiol* 2001;**88**:301–3.

21. Moses JW, Leon MB, Popma JJ *et al.* Sirolimus-eluting stents versus standard stents in patients with stenosis in a native coronary artery. *N Engl J Med* 2003;**349**:1315–23.

22. Stone GW, Ellis SG, Cox DA *et al.* A polymer-based, paclitaxel-eluting stent in patients with coronary artery disease. *N Engl J Med* 2004;**350**:221–31.

23. Stone GW, Moses JW, Ellis SG *et al.* Safety and efficacy of sirolimus and paclitaxel-eluting coronary stents. *N Engl J Med* 2007;**356**:998–1008.

24. Spaulding C, Daemen J, Boersma E, Cutlip DE, Serruys PW. A pooled analysis of data comparing sirolimus-eluting stents with baremetal stents. *N Engl J Med* 2007;**356**:989–97.

25. Kastrati A, Mehilli J, Pache J *et al.* Analysis of 14 trials comparing sirolimus-eluting stents with bare-metal stents. *N Engl J Med* 2007;**356**:1030–9.

26. Lagerqvist B, James SK, Stenestrand U *et al.* Long-term outcomes with drug-eluting stents versus bare metal stents in Sweden. *N Engl J Med* 2007;**356**:1009–19.

27. Mauri L, Hsieh W, Massaro JM *et al.* Stent thrombosis in randomized clinical trials of drug-eluting stents. *N Engl J Med* 2007;**356**:1020 9.

28. Holmes DR Jr, Kereiakes DJ, Laskey WK *et al.* Thrombosis and drug-eluting stents: an objective appraisal. *J Am Coll Cardiol* 2007;**50**:109–18.

28a. James SK, Stenestrand U, Lindback J *et al.* for the SCAAR Study Group. Long-term safety and efficacy of drug-eluting versus bare-metal stents in Sweden. *N Engl J Med* 2009;**360**:1933–45.

28b. Stone GW, Lansky AJ, Pocock SJ *et al.* for the HORIZONS-AMI Trial Investigators. Paclitaxel-eluting stents versus bare-metal stents in acute myocardial infarction. *N Engl J Med* 2009;**360**: 1949–59.

29. Holmes DR Jr, Gersh BJ, Whitlow P *et al.* Percutaneous coronary intervention for chronic stable angina: a reassessment. *J Am Coll Cardiol Intv* 2008;**1**:34–43.

30. Prati F, Dimarco C, Moussa I *et al.* In-stent neointimal proliferation correlates with the amount of residual plaque burden outside the stent: an intravascular ultrasound study. *Circulation* 1999;**99**:1011–14.

31. Elliott JM, Berdan LG, Holmes DR *et al.* One-year follow-up in the Coronary Angioplasty Versus Excisional Atherectomy Trial (CAVEAT I). *Circulation* 1995;**91**:2158–66.

32. Holmes DR Jr, Topol EJ, Califf RM *et al.* A multicenter, randomized trial of coronary angioplasty versus directional atherectomy for patients with saphenous vein bypass graft lesions. CAVEAT-II Investigators. *Circulation* 1995;**91**:1966–74.

33. Stankovic G, Colombo A, Bersin R *et al.* Comparison of directional coronary atherectomy and stenting versus stenting alone for the treatment of de novo and restenotic coronary artery narrowings. *Am J Cardiol* 2004;**93**:953–8.

34. Reifart N, Vandormael M, Krajcar M *et al.* Randomized comparison of angioplasty of complex coronary lesions at a single center. Excimer Laser, Rotational Atherectomy, and Balloon Angioplasty Comparison (ERBAC) Study. *Circulation* 1997;**96**:91–8.

35. Reisman M, Harms V, Whitlow P *et al.* Comparison of early and recent results with rotational atherectomy. *J Am Coll Cardiol* 1997;**29**:353–7.

36. MacIsaac AI, Bass TA, Buchbinder M *et al.* High speed rotational atherectomy: outcome in calcified and noncalcified coronary artery lesions. *J Am Coll Cardiol* 1995;**26**:731–6.

37. Stone GW, Hodgson JM, St Goar FG *et al.* Improved procedural results of coronary angioplasty with intravascular ultrasound-guided balloon sizing: the CLOUT Pilot Trial. Clinical Outcomes With Ultrasound Trial (CLOUT) Investigators. *Circulation* 1997;**95**:2044–52.

38. Frey AW, Hodgson JM, Muller C *et al.* Ultrasound-guided strategy for provisional stenting with focal balloon combination catheter: results from the randomized Strategy for Intracoronary Ultrasound-guided PTCA and Stenting (SIPS) trial. *Circulation* 2000;**102**:2497–502.

39. de Jaegere P, Mudra H, Figulla H *et al.* Intravascular ultrasound-guided optimized stent deployment. Immediate and 6

months clinical and angiographic results from the Multicenter Ultrasound Stenting in Coronaries Study (MUSIC Study). *Eur Heart J* 1998;**19**:1214–23.

40. Windecker S, Meier B. Late coronary stent thrombosis. *Circulation* 2007;**116**:1952–65.

41. Serruys PW, Degertekin M, Tanabe K *et al.* Intravascular ultrasound findings in the multicenter, randomized, double-blind RAVEL (RAndomized study with the sirolimus-eluting VElocity balloon-expandable stent in the treatment of patients with de novo native coronary artery Lesions) trial. *Circulation* 2002;**106**:798–803.

42. Hong MK, Mintz GS, Lee CW *et al.* Late stent malapposition after drug-eluting stent implantation: an intravascular ultrasound analysis with long-term follow-up. *Circulation* 2006;**113**: 414–19.

43. Pijls NH, De Bruyne B, Peels K *et al.* Measurement of fractional flow reserve to assess the functional severity of coronary-artery stenoses. *N Engl J Med* 1996;**334**:1703–8.

44. Pijls NH, van Schaardenburgh P, Manoharan G *et al.* Percutaneous coronary intervention of functionally nonsignificant stenosis: 5-year follow-up of the DEFER Study. *J Am Coll Cardiol* 2007;**49**:2105–11.

45. Tonino PA, De Bruyne, Pijls NH *et al.* for the FAME study investigators. Fractional flow reserve versus angiography for guiding percutaneous coronary intervention. *N Engl J Med* 2009;**360**:213–24.

46. Antiplatelet Trialists' Collaboration. Collaborative overview of randomised trials of antiplatelet therapy I: Prevention of death, myocardial infarction, and stroke by prolonged antiplatelet therapy in various categories of patients. *BMJ* 1994;**308**: 81–106.

47. Schwartz L, Bourassa MG, Lespérance J *et al.* Aspirin and dipyridamole in the prevention of restenosis after percutaneous transluminal coronary angioplasty. *N Engl J Med* 1988;**318**: 1714–9.

48. Mehta SR, Yusuf S, Peters RJ *et al.* Effects of pretreatment with clopidogrel and aspirin followed by long-term therapy in patients undergoing percutaneous coronary intervention: the PCI-CURE study. *Lancet* 2001;**358**:527–33.

49. Reilly IA, Fitzgerald GA. Inhibition of thrmboxane formation in vivo and ex vivo: implications for therapy with platelet inhibitory drugs. *Blood* 2000;**68**:180–6.

50. Leon MB, Baim DS, Popma JJ *et al.* A clinical trial comparing three antithrombotic-drug regimens after coronary-artery stenting. Stent Anticoagulation Restenosis Study Investigators. *N Engl J Med* 1998;**339**:1665–71.

51. Bertrand ME, Rupprecht HJ, Urban P *et al.* Double-blind study of the safety of clopidogrel with and without a loading dose in combination with aspirin compared with ticlopidine in combination with aspirin after coronary stenting: the clopidogrel aspirin stent international cooperative study (CLASSICS). *Circulation* 2000;**102**:624–9.

52. Muller C, Buttner HJ, Petersen J *et al.* A randomized comparison of clopidogrel and aspirin versus ticlopidine and aspirin after the placement of coronary-artery stents. *Circulation* 2000; **101**:590–3.

53. Bhatt DL, Bertrand ME, Berger PB *et al.* Meta-analysis of randomized and registry comparisons of ticlopidine with clopidogrel after stenting. *J Am Coll Cardiol* 2002;**39**:9–14.

54. Lubbe DF, Berger PB. The thienopyridines. *J Interv Cardiol* 2002;**15**:85–93.

55. King SB 3rd, Smith SC Jr, Hirshfeld JW Jr *et al.* 2007 Focused Update of the ACC/AHA/SCAI 2005 Guideline Update for Percutaneous Coronary Intervention: a report of the American College of Cardiology/American Heart Association Task Force on Practice Guidelines: 2007 Writing Group to Review New Evidence and Update the ACC/AHA/SCAI 2005 Guideline Update for Percutaneous Coronary Intervention, Writing on Behalf of the 2005 Writing Committee. *Circulation* 2008;**117**:261–95.

56. Steinhubl SR, Berger PB, Mann JT *et al.* Early and sustained dual oral antiplatelet therapy following percutaneous coronary intervention: a randomized controlled trial. *JAMA* 2002;**288**: 2411–20.

57. Kandzari DE, Berger PB, Kastrati A *et al.* Influence of treatment duration with a 600-mg dose of clopidogrel before percutaneous coronary revascularization. *J Am Coll Cardiol* 2004;**44**: 2133–6.

58. Patti G, Colonna G, Pasceri V *et al.* Randomized trial of high loading dose of clopidogrel for reduction of periprocedural myocardial infarction in patients undergoing coronary intervention: results from the ARMYDA-2 (Antiplatelet therapy for Reduction of MYocardial Damage during Angioplasty) study. *Circulation* 2005;**111**:2099–106.

59. Gurbel PA, Bliden KP, Hiatt BL *et al.* Clopidogrel for coronary stenting: response variability, drug resistance, and the effect of pretreatment platelet reactivity. *Circulation* 2003;**107**:2908–13.

60. Grines CL, Bonow RO, Casey DE Jr *et al.* Prevention of premature discontinuation of dual antiplatelet therapy in patients with coronary artery stents: a science advisory from the American Heart Association, American College of Cardiology, Society for Cardiovascular Angiography and Interventions, American College of Surgeons, and American Dental Association, with representation from the American College of Physicians. *Circulation* 2007;**115**:813–18.

61. Wiviott SD, Braunwald E, McCabe CH *et al.* Intensive oral antiplatelet therapy for reduction of ischaemic events including stent thrombosis in patients with acute coronary syndromes treated with percutaneous coronary intervention and stenting in the TRITON-TIMI 38 trial: a subanalysis of a randomised trial. *Lancet* 2008;**371**:1353–63.

62. EPIC Investigators. Use of a monoclonal antibody directed against the platelet glycoprotein IIb/IIIa receptor in high-risk coronary angioplasty. *N Engl J Med* 1994;**330**:956–61.

63. EPILOG Investigators. Platelet glycoprotein IIb/IIIa receptor blockade and low-dose heparin during percutaneous coronary revascularization. *N Engl J Med* 1997;**336**:1689–96.

64. Topol EJ, Mark DB, Lincoff AM *et al.* Outcomes at 1 year and economic implications of platelet glycoprotein IIb/IIIa blockade in patients undergoing coronary stenting: results from a multicentre randomised trial. EPISTENT Investigators. Evaluation of Platelet IIb/IIIa Inhibitor for Stenting. *Lancet* 1999;**354**: 2019–24.

65. Karvouni E, Katritsis DG, Ioannidis JP. Intravenous glycoprotein IIb/IIIa receptor antagonists reduce mortality after percutaneous coronary interventions. *J Am Coll Cardiol* 2003;**41**:26–32.

66. Stone GW, Grines CL, Cox DA *et al.* Comparison of angioplasty with stenting, with or without abciximab, in acute myocardial infarction. *N Engl J Med* 2002;**346**:957–66.

67. Tcheng JE, Harrington RA, Kottke-Marchant K *et al.* Multi-center, randomized, double-blind, placebo-controlled trial of the platelet integrin glycoprotein IIb/IIIa blocker Integrelin in elective coronary intervention. IMPACT Investigators. *Circulation* 1995;**91**:2151–7.

68. ESPRIT Investigators. Novel dosing regimen of eptifibatide in planned coronary stent implantation (ESPRIT): a randomised, placebo-controlled trial. *Lancet* 2000;**356**:2037–44.

69. Fung A, Saw J, Starovoytov A *et al.* Abbreviated infusion of eptifibatide after successful coronary intervention: the BRIEF-PCI randomized trial. *J Am Coll Cardiol* 2009;**53**:837–45.

70. Kastrati A, Mehilli J, Neumann FJ *et al.* Abciximab in patients with acute coronary syndromes undergoing percutaneous coronary intervention after clopidogrel pretreatment: the ISAR-REACT 2 randomized trial. *JAMA* 2006;**295**:1531–8.

71. Ndrepepa G, Kastrati A, Mehilli J *et al.* One-year clinical outcomes with abciximab versus placebo in patients with non-ST-segment elevation acute coronary syndromes undergoing percutaneous coronary intervention after pre-treatment with clopidogrel: results of the ISAR-REACT 2 randomized trial. *Eur Heart J* 2008;**29**:455–61.

72. Gurbel PA, Bliden KP, Tantry US. Effect of clopidogrel with and without eptifibatide on tumor necrosis factor-alpha and C-reactive protein release after elective stenting: results from the CLEAR PLATELETS 1b study. *J Am Coll Cardiol* 2006;**48**:2186–91.

73. Lincoff AM, Bittl JA, Kleiman NS *et al.* Comparison of bivalirudin versus heparin during percutaneous coronary intervention (the Randomized Evaluation of PCI Linking Angiomax to Reduced Clinical Events [REPLACE]-1 trial. *Am J Cardiol* 2004;**93**:1092–6.

74. White HD, Kleiman NS, Mahaffey KW *et al.* Efficacy and safety of enoxaparin compared with unfractionated heparin in high-risk patients with non-ST-segment elevation acute coronary syndrome undergoing percutaneous coronary intervention in the Superior Yield of the New Strategy of Enoxaparin, Revascularization and Glycoprotein IIb/IIIa Inhibitors (SYNERGY) trial. *Am Heart J* 2006;**152**:1042–50.

75. Kereiakes DJ, Grines C, Fry E *et al.* Enoxaparin and abciximab adjunctive pharmacotherapy during percutaneous coronary intervention. *J Inv Cardiol* 2001;**13**:272–8.

76. Montalescot G, White HD, Gallo R *et al.* Enoxaparin versus unfractionated heparin in elective percutaneous intervention. *N Engl J Med* 2006;**355**:1006–17.

77. Dumaine R, Borentain M, Bertel O *et al.* Intravenous low-molecular-weight heparins compared with unfractionated heparin in percutaneous coronary intervention: quantitative review of randomized trials. *Arch Intern Med* 2007;**167**:2423–30.

78. Wong GC, Giugliano RP, Antman EM. Use of low-molecular-weight heparins in the management of acute coronary artery syndromes and percutaneous coronary intervention. *JAMA* 2003;**289**:331–42.

79. Lepor NE. Anticoagulation for acute coronary syndromes: from heparin to direct thrombin inhibitors. *Rev Cardiovasc Med* 2007;**8**:S9–17.

80. Lincoff AM, Bittl JA, Harrington RA *et al.* Bivalirudin and provisional glycoprotein IIb/IIIa blockade compared with heparin and planned glycoprotein IIb/IIIa blockade during percutaneous coronary intervention: REPLACE-2 randomized trial. *JAMA* 2003;**289**:853–63.

81. Serruys PW, Herrman JP, Simon R *et al.* A comparison of hirudin with heparin in the prevention of restenosis after coronary angioplasty. Helvetica Investigators. *N Engl J Med* 1995;**333**:757–63.

82. Bittl JA, Strony J, Brinker JA *et al.* Treatment with bivalirudin (Hirulog) as compared with heparin during coronary angioplasty for unstable or postinfarction angina. Hirulog Angioplasty Study Investigators. *N Engl J Med* 1995;**333**:764–9.

83. Stone GW, McLaurin BT, Cox DA *et al.* Bivalirudin for patients with acute coronary syndromes. *N Engl J Med* 2006;**355**:2203–16.

84. Mehta SR, Steg PG, Granger CB *et al.* Randomized, blinded trial comparing fondaparinux with unfractionated heparin in patients undergoing contemporary percutaneous coronary intervention: Arixtra Study in Percutaneous Coronary Intervention: a Randomized Evaluation (ASPIRE) Pilot Trial. *Circulation* 2005;**111**:1390–7.

85. Mehta SR, Granger CB, Eikelboom JW *et al.* Efficacy and safety of fondaparinux versus enoxaparin in patients with acute coronary syndromes undergoing percutaneous coronary intervention: results from the OASIS-5 trial. *J Am Coll Cardiol* 2007;**50**:1742–51.

86. Parisi AF, Folland ED, Hartigan P. A comparison of angioplasty with medical therapy in the treatment of single-vessel coronary artery disease. Veterans Affairs ACME Investigators. *N Engl J Med* 1992;**326**:10–16.

87. Folland ED, Hartigan PM, Parisi AF. Percutaneous transluminal coronary angioplasty versus medical therapy for stable angina pectoris: outcomes for patients with double-vessel versus single-vessel coronary artery disease in a Veterans Affairs cooperative randomized trial. Veterans Affairs ACME Investigators. *J Am Coll Cardiol* 1997;**29**:1505–11.

88. RITA-2 Trial Participants. Coronary angioplasty versus medical therapy for angina: the second Randomised Intervention Treatment of Angina (RITA-2) trial. *Lancet* 1997;**350**:461–8.

89. Pocock SJ, Henderson RA, Clayton T *et al.* Quality of life after coronary angioplasty or continued medical treatment for angina: three-year follow-up in the RITA-2 trial. Randomized Intervention Treatment of Angina. *J Am Coll Cardiol* 2000;**35**:907–14.

90. Pitt B, Waters D, Brown WV *et al.* Aggressive lipid-lowering therapy compared with angioplasty in stable coronary artery disease. Atorvastatin versus Revascularization Treatment Investigators. *N Engl J Med* 1999;**341**:70–6.

91. Davies RF, Goldberg AD, Forman S *et al.* Asymptomatic Cardiac Ischemia Pilot (ACIP) study 2-year follow-up: outcomes of patients randomized to initial strategies of medical therapy versus revascularization. *Circulation* 1997;**95**:2037–43.

92. Bucher HC, Hengstler P, Schindler C *et al.* Percutaneous transluminal coronary angioplasty versus medical treatment for non-acute coronary heart disease: meta-analysis of randomised controlled trials. *BMJ* 2000;**321**:73–7.

93. Katritsis DG, Ioannidis JP. Percutaneous coronary intervention versus conservative therapy in nonacute coronary artery disease: a metaanalysis. *Circulation* 2005;**111**:2906–12.

94. Hueb W, Soares PR, Gersh BJ *et al.* The Medicine, Angioplasty, or Surgery Study (MASS-II): a randomized, controlled clinical trial of three therapeutic strategies for multivessel coronary artery disease: one-year results. *J Am Coll Cardiol* 2004;**43**:1743.

95. Boden WE, O'Rourke RA, Teo KK *et al.* Optimal medical therapy with or without PCI for stable coronary disease. *N Engl J Med* 2007;**356**:1503–16.

96. Alderman EL, Fisher LD, Litwin P *et al.* Results of coronary artery surgery in patients with poor left ventricular function. *Circulation* 1983;**68**:785–95.

96a. Trikalinos TA, Alsheikh-Ali AA, Tatsioni A, Nallamothu BK, Kent DM. Percutaneous coronary interventions for non-acute coronary artery disease: a quantitative 20-year synopsis and a network meta-analysis. *Lancet* 2009;**373**:911–18.

97. Shaw LJ, Berman DS, Maron DJ *et al.* Optimal medical therapy with or without percutaneous coronary intervention to reduce ischemic burden: results from the Clinical Outcomes Utilizing Revascularization and Aggressive Drug Evaluation (COURAGE) trial nuclear substudy. *Circulation* 2008;**117**: 1283–91.

97a. The BARI 2D Study Group. A randomized trial of therapies for type 2 diabetes and coronary artery disease. *N Engl J Med* 2009;**360**:2503–15.

98. Versaci F, Gaspardone A, Tomai F, Crea F, Chiariello L, Gioffre PA. A comparison of coronary-artery stenting with angioplasty for isolated stenosis of the proximal left anterior descending coronary artery. *N Engl J Med* 1997;**336**:817–22.

99. George CJ, Baim DS, Brinker JA *et al.* One-year follow-up of the Stent Restenosis (STRESS I) Study. *Am J Cardiol* 1998;**81**:860–5.

100. Kiemeneij F, Serruys PW, Macaya C *et al.* Continued benefit of coronary stenting versus balloon angioplasty: five-year clinical follow-up of Benestent-I trial. *J Am Coll Cardiol* 2001;**37**: 1598–603.

101. Serruys PW, van Hout B, Bonnier H *et al.* Randomised comparison of implantation of heparin-coated stents with balloon angioplasty in selected patients with coronary artery disease (Benestent II). *Lancet* 1998;**352**:673–81.

102. Betriu A, Masotti M, Serra A *et al.* Randomized comparison of coronary stent implantation and balloon angioplasty in the treatment of de novo coronary artery lesions (START): a four-year follow-up. *J Am Coll Cardiol* 1999;**34**:1498–506.

103. Lincoff AM, Califf RM, Moliterno DJ *et al.* Complementary clinical benefits of coronary-artery stenting and blockade of platelet glycoprotein IIb/IIIa receptors. Evaluation of Platelet IIb/IIIa Inhibition in Stenting Investigators. *N Engl J Med* 1999;**341**:319–27.

104. EPISTENT Investigators. Randomised placebo-controlled and balloon-angioplasty-controlled trial to assess safety of coronary stenting with use of platelet glycoprotein-IIb/IIIa blockade. Evaluation of Platelet IIb/IIIa Inhibitor for Stenting. *Lancet* 1998;**352**:87–92.

105. Eeckhout E, Stauffer JC, Vogt P, Debbas N, Kappenberger L, Goy JJ. Comparison of elective Wiktor stent placement with conventional balloon angioplasty for new-onset lesions of the right coronary artery. *Am Heart J* 1996;**132**:263–8.

106. Witkowski A, Ruzyllo W, Gil R *et al.* A randomized comparison of elective high-pressure stenting with balloon angioplasty: six-month angiographic and two-year clinical follow-up. On behalf of AS (Angioplasty or Stent) trial investigators. *Am Heart J* 2000;**140**:264–71.

107. Erbel R, Haude M, Hopp HW *et al.* Coronary-artery stenting compared with balloon angioplasty for restenosis after initial balloon angioplasty. Restenosis Stent Study Group. *N Engl J Med* 1998;**339**:1672–8.

108. Savage MP, Douglas JS Jr, Fischman DL *et al.* Stent placement compared with balloon angioplasty for obstructed coronary bypass grafts. Saphenous Vein De Novo Trial Investigators. *N Engl J Med* 1997;**337**:740–7.

109. Park SW, Lee CW, Hong MK *et al.* Randomized comparison of coronary stenting with optimal balloon angioplasty for treatment of lesions in small coronary arteries. *Eur Heart J* 2000; **21**:1785–9.

110. Kastrati A, Schomig A, Dirschinger J *et al.* A randomized trial comparing stenting with balloon angioplasty in small vessels in patients with symptomatic coronary artery disease. ISAR-SMART Study Investigators. Intracoronary Stenting or Angioplasty for Restenosis Reduction in Small Arteries. *Circulation* 2000;**102**:2593–8.

111. Koning R, Eltchaninoff H, Commeau P *et al.* Stent placement compared with balloon angioplasty for small coronary arteries: in-hospital and 6-month clinical and angiographic results. *Circulation* 2001;**104**:1604–8.

112. Doucet S, Schalij MJ, Vrolix MC *et al.* Stent placement to prevent restenosis after angioplasty in small coronary arteries. *Circulation* 2001;**104**:2029–33.

113. Sirnes PA, Golf S, Myreng Y *et al.* Stenting in Chronic Coronary Occlusion (SICCO): a randomized, controlled trial of adding stent implantation after successful angioplasty. *J Am Coll Cardiol* 1996;**28**:1444–51.

114. Rubartelli P, Niccoli L, Verna E *et al.* Stent implantation versus balloon angioplasty in chronic coronary occlusions: results from the GISSOC trial. Gruppo Italiano di Studio sullo Stent nelle Occlusioni Coronariche. *J Am Coll Cardiol* 1998;**32**:90–6.

115. Hancock J, Thomas MR, Holmberg S, Wainwright RJ, Jewitt DE. Randomised trial of elective stenting after successful percutaneous transluminal coronary angioplasty of occluded coronary arteries. *Heart* 1998;**79**:18–23.

116. Sievert H, Rohde S, Utech A *et al.* Stent or angioplasty after recanalization of chronic coronary occlusions? (The SARECCO Trial.) *Am J Cardiol* 1999;**84**:386–90.

117. Hoher M, Wohrle J, Grebe OC *et al.* A randomized trial of elective stenting after balloon recanalization of chronic total occlusions. *J Am Coll Cardiol* 1999;**34**:722–9.

118. Lotan C, Rozenman Y, Hendler A *et al.* Stents in total occlusion for restenosis prevention. The multicenter randomized STOP study. The Israeli Working Group for Interventional Cardiology. *Eur Heart J* 2000;**21**:1960–6.

119. Kereiakes DJ. Percutaneous transcatheter therapy for aorto-ostial stenoses. *Cathet Cardiovasc Diagn* 1996;**38**:292–300.

120. Jain SP, Liu MW, Dean LS *et al.* Comparison of balloon angiography versus debulking devices versus stenting in right coronary artery ostial lesions. *Am J Cardiol* 1997;**79**:1334–8.

121. Louvard Y, Lefevre T, Morice MC. Percutaneous coronary intervention for bifurcation coronary disease. *Heart* 2004;**90**:713–22.

122. Colombo A, Moses JW, Morice MC *et al.* Randomized study to evaluate sirolimus-eluting stents implanted at coronary bifurcation lesions. *Circulation* 2004;**109**:1244–9.

123. Steigen TK, Maeng M, Wiseth R *et al.* Randomized study on simple versus complex stenting of coronary artery bifurcation lesions: The Nordic Bifurcation Study. *Circulation* 2006;**114**: 1955–61.

27 Surgical coronary artery revascularization

Morgan L Brown and Thoralf M Sundt III
Mayo Clinic, Rochester, MN, USA

Introduction and historic perspective

Throughout its development, coronary artery bypass grafting (CABG) has been studied extensively through randomized trials, prospective registries, and retrospective studies. It is arguably one of the most studied procedures in medicine. Despite improvements in medical therapies and percutaneous interventions, CABG remains an important therapy for millions of patients every year. Pioneering methods to restore blood supply to ischemic myocardium included placement of a pectoralis muscle flap on abraded pericardium by Beck in 1935,[1] direct implantation of the internal thoracic artery (ITA) onto the myocardium in 1950 by Vineberg,[2,3] and "myocardial acupuncture" in 1965 by Sen.[4] Direct revascularization was possible after the development of the cardiopulmonary bypass (CPB) machine by Gibbon[5] which, along with cardioplegia, allowed the heart to be stopped and the coronary arteries opened safely. In 1958, Longmire reported an ITA to coronary anastomosis after an unsuccessful coronary atherectomy.[6] Goetz performed the first successfully planned CABG using a metal connector in 1960, with angiographic patency confirmed two weeks after operation.[7] The first saphenous vein was used as a graft in 1962 by Sabiston.[8] Kolessov, a Russian surgeon, was credited with the first successful planned sutured ITA to coronary artery anastomosis in 1964.[9]

After the development of coronary angiography at the Cleveland Clinic in 1957, the elective treatment of coronary atherosclerosis began to grow.[10] The first large-scale series of CABG procedures were published between 1968 and 1970 demonstrating the success of CABG and ensuring its place in the treatment of coronary artery disease (CAD).[11–15] Over the ensuing three and a half decades, the procedure has been refined with a decline in mortality rate below

2.5% currently.[16] Curiously, one of the most recent developments is a return to "off-pump" techniques obviating the need for CPB, the very technologic innovation arguably most responsible for the widespread adoption of CABG.

Incidence, natural history, and prognosis

Given the clinical importance of the condition, the incidence, natural history, and prognosis of CAD in general are covered in detail elsewhere in this volume. Still, it is worth emphasizing that in contrast to percutaneous techniques, surgical revascularization has been definitively shown to improve five-year survival among patients with multivessel disease.[17–19] This may be due to the ability of CABG to protect against future culprit lesions (Fig. 27.1).[20]

Management

Coronary artery bypass grafting versus medical management

The American Heart Association and American College of Cardiology have developed comprehensive guidelines (Box 27.1) describing the indications for CABG based on patient symptom status and angiographic features of CAD.[21] These guidelines are based on the best available evidence; however, many of the classic studies have limitations. Most patients in the CABG versus medical management trials were younger than 65 years of age, 80% had a left ventricular (LV) ejection fraction of ≥50%, and the majority of patients were men. Thus, patients enrolled in these trials were generally low risk from the standpoint of both the risk of performing the procedure and the risk of the natural history of the disease itself. Furthermore, the surgical patients did not routinely receive arterial bypass conduits nor did they receive routine aspirin postoperatively, both

Evidence-Based Cardiology, 3rd edition. Edited by S. Yusuf, J.A. Cairns, A.J. Camm, E.L. Fallen, and B.J. Gersh. © 2010 Blackwell Publishing, ISBN: 978-1-4051-5925-8.

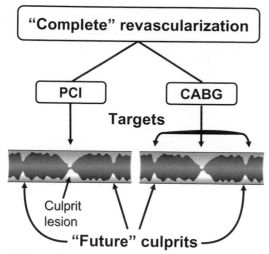

Figure 27.1 PCI is targeted at a specific culprit lesion. CABG protects against future culprit lesions by bypassing much of a coronary artery including both culprit and "future culprit" lesions. The dark shading indicates the residual lumen. (Reproduced with permission from Elsevier Ltd. Opie LH, Commerford PJ, Gersh BJ. *Lancet* 2006;**367**:69–78.)

of which may be expected to positively impact graft patency. Of course, they also underwent surgical procedures without current myocardial protection strategies which may be expected to reduce perioperative risk. Equally, it must be said that among the patients who received medical therapy alone, there was no routine aspirin, beta-blockade or lipid-lowering therapy, nor were angiotensin-converting enzyme (ACE) inhibitors routinely prescribed. Despite these major limitations, these studies are remarkably consistent in their primary findings and their conclusions continue to be supported by recent studies, suggesting that they remain generalizable to current practice.

The Coronary Artery Surgery Study (CASS),[22] the Veterans Administration (VA) Co-operative Study Group,[23,24] the European Coronary Surgery Study (ECSS),[25,26] and several other smaller randomized trials[27–30] conducted between 1972 and 1984 provide outcome data comparing medical and surgical therapy. The relative benefits of CABG over medical therapy on survival are greatest in patients at highest risk of complications of their disease as defined by the severity of angina and/or ischemia, the number of diseased vessels, and the presence of LV dysfunction[31] (Fig. 27.2). The survival advantage of surgery over medicine has not been demonstrable among patients with single-vessel disease.[32–34] It should be emphasized, however, that these trials involved primarily patients with moderate chronic stable angina. These conclusions may, therefore, not necessarily apply to patients with unstable angina or to patients with more severe degrees of chronic

stable angina in whom the area of myocardium at risk may be higher.

A meta-analysis[31] of the seven randomized trials cited above demonstrated a survival benefit at five, seven and 10 years for surgically treated patients at highest risk of death due to their disease and among those at moderate risk, but no evidence of a survival benefit for those patients at lowest risk, as defined by a modified version of the Veterans Administration Risk Score[23] and a stepwise risk scoring system.[31] These scoring systems used a combination of both clinical and angiographic variables including angina class, history of hypertension, history of myocardial infarction, depressed ejection fraction (<50%), and a proximal left anterior descending (LAD) lesion >50%. Nonrandomized studies have also demonstrated a beneficial effect of surgery on survival of patients with multivessel disease and severe ischemia regardless of LV function.[35–38]

The more recent randomized trials of CABG versus medical therapy also support a strategy of revascularization among patients with symptomatic angina. The Trial of Invasive versus Medical therapy in Elderly (TIME) enrolled elderly (>70 y) patients with chronic symptomatic CAD. The incidence of major adverse events (death, non-fatal myocardial infarction (MI) or hospitalization) was lower (19% vs 49%, $P < 0.0001$) and angina relief was greater (anginal class decreased by 2 vs 1.3, $P < 0.0001$), and all measures of quality of life ($P < 0.05$ for SF36 score, Duke activity score, and Rose score) were superior for those undergoing coronary angiography and surgical revascularization than in those randomized to an initial trial of medical therapy without angiography.[39] In the Asymptomatic Cardiac Ischemia Pilot (ACIP) trial, patients with anatomy amenable to CABG were randomized to anti-ischemic therapy directed at relief of angina, to drug therapy guided by non-invasive measures of ischemia, or to revascularization by CABG or percutaneous coronary interventions (PCI).[40] At two years, mortality was 6.6% in the angina-guided group, 4.4% in the ischemia-guided group, and 1.1% in the revascularization group ($P < 0.02$). At two years of follow-up, the rates of death or MI were 12.1%, 8.8%, and 4.7% respectively ($P < 0.04$). In the recent BARI 2D trial performed in patients with type 2 diabetes and stable coronary artery disease, by 5 years of follow-up there were fewer major cardiovascular events among CABG patients than among those receiving only optimal medical therapy.[40a]

Early concern over high operative mortality in patients with decreased LV systolic function has been replaced by the realization that the survival benefit to these patients is particularly great with surgical revascularization compared with medical therapy. Thus, LV dysfunction in patients with documented ischemia is now considered an important indication for CABG[21,22,35,41,42] with operative mortality rates as low as 4.6%.[43] Evidence that hibernating or stunned myocardium regains contractile function

BOX 27.1 American College of Cardiology/American Heart Association Guidelines published in 2004 outline the indications for coronary artery bypass grafting.[21] This box summarizes guidelines for asymptomatic or mild angina and stable angina.

Asymptomatic or mild angina

Class I
- Significant left main coronary artery stenosis. (**Level A**)
- Left main equivalent: ≥70% stenosis of the proximal LAD and proximal left circumflex artery. (**Level A**)
- Three-vessel disease. (Survival benefit is greater in patients with abnormal LV function, e.g. LVEF <50% and/or large areas of demonstrable myocardial ischemia.) (**Level C**)

Class IIa
- Proximal LAD stenosis with one- or two-vessel disease. (Becomes a Class I if extensive ischemia is documented by non-invasive study and/or LVEF <50%.) (**Level A**)

Class IIb
- One- or two-vessel disease not involving the proximal LAD. (If a large area of viable myocardium and high-risk criteria are met on non-invasive testing, this recommendation becomes Class I.) (**Level B**)

Stable angina

Class I
- Significant left main coronary artery stenosis. (**Level A**)
- Left main equivalent: ≥70% stenosis of the proximal LAD and proximal left circumflex artery. (**Level A**)
- Three-vessel disease. (Survival benefit is greater when LVEF <50%.) (**Level A**)
- Two-vessel disease with significant proximal LAD stenosis and either LVEF <50% or demonstrable ischemia on no-ninvasive testing. (**Level A**)

- One or two-vessel CAD without significant proximal LAD stenosis but with a large area of viable myocardium and high-risk criteria on non-invasive testing. (**Level B**)
- Disabling angina despite maximal non-invasive therapy, when surgery can be performed with acceptable risk. If angina is not typical, objective evidence of ischemia should be obtained. (**Level B**)

Class IIa
- Proximal LAD stenosis with one-vessel disease. (This recommendation becomes Class I if extensive ischemia is documented by non-invasive study and/or LVEF <50%). (**Level A**)
- One- or two-vessel CAD without significant proximal LAD stenosis but with a moderate area of viable myocardium and demonstrable ischemia on non-invasive testing. (**Level B**)

Class III
- One- or two-vessel disease not involving significant proximal LAD stenosis, patients who have mild symptoms that are unlikely to be due to myocardial ischemia, or who have not received an adequate trial of medical therapy and have only a small area of viable myocardium or have no demonstrable ischemia on non-invasive testing. (**Level B**)
- Patients with angina who have borderline coronary stenoses (50–60% diameter in locations other than the left main coronary artery) and no demonstrable ischemia on non-invasive testing. (**Level B**)
- CABG is not recommended for patients with stable angina who have insignificant coronary stenosis (<50% diameter reduction). (**Level B**)

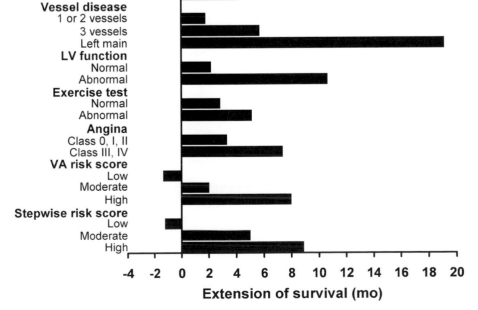

Figure 27.2 After 10 years of follow-up, CABG extends survival in most moderate- and high-risk subgroups when compared to medical management. Patients were classified into low, moderate, and high risk using the formula: (0.015 × age) + (0.56 × presence of class III/IV angina) + (0.35 × history of myocardial infarction) + (0.62 × abnormal ejection fraction) + (0.53 × proximal lesion of >50% in LAD). (Reproduced with permission from Elsevier Ltd. Yusuf S, Zucker D, Passamani E *et al. Lancet* 1994;**344**:563–70.)

following effective revascularization[44,45] has prompted expansion of the indications for surgical revascularization among patients with severe LV dysfunction to encompass most patients, including those who would otherwise be considered candidates for cardiac transplantation.

Apart from affording a survival benefit, CABG is indicated for the relief of angina pectoris and improvement in quality of life. Between 80% and 90% of patients who are symptomatic on medical therapy become symptom free following CABG. This benefit extends to low-risk patients for whom survival benefit from surgery is not likely.[31] Relief of symptoms appears to relate to both the completeness of revascularization and maintenance of graft patency, with the benefit of CABG diminishing with time. Recurrence of angina following CABG surgery occurs at rates of 3–20% per year.[46–49] Although enhanced survival is reported when an ITA graft is used to the LAD, there is no significant difference in postoperative freedom from angina when compared to venous grafts.[50] This may be due to occurrence of ischemia due to diseases in the vein grafts used to targets other than the LAD or ischemia due to progression of native disease.

Unfortunately, few patients experience an advantage in work rehabilitation with surgery as compared with medical management. Generally, employment declines in both groups and is determined nearly as much by socioeconomic factors such as age, preoperative unemployment, and type of job, as by type of therapy or clinical factors such as postoperative angina.[51–53] Notably, surgical revascularization has not been shown to reduce the incidence of non-fatal events such as MI, although this may be due to perioperative infarctions which offset the lower incidence of infarction in follow-up.[36,54]

Coronary artery bypass grafting versus percutaneous interventions

This topic is discussed in Chapter 28.

Techniques

On-pump and off-pump coronary artery bypass grafting

The current results of conventional on-pump CABG (ONCAB) are excellent. Perioperative mortality rates as reported to the Society of Thoracic Surgeons (STS) database have demonstrated a consistent decline despite an increasing patient risk profile (Fig. 27.3).[55] In 2005, the unadjusted mortality rate for isolated primary CABG in the STS database was 2.2% and the median hospital length of stay was only five days.[16] In return, the operation provides durable relief from angina pectoris and improves long-term survival.

ONCAB comes at a physiologic price, however, as CPB causes trauma to red cells and platelets while inducing a generalized inflammatory response and activation of the cytokine, coagulation, and fibrinolytic cascades.[56] Nonpulsatile flow may have adverse effects on end-organ function[57] and cannulation for arterial inflow may cause embolization of either air or calcium. Despite these risks, ONCAB became the predominant method of surgical revascularization through the 1980s.[58]

While the techniques and technologies to perform ONCAB were being refined, including the introduction of biocompatible surfaces and centrifugal pumps,[59] interest in off-pump (OPCAB) techniques persisted among a small number of surgeons. In the early 1990s, observational studies were published[60–63] demonstrating good outcomes using OPCAB techniques. These data, along with a drive to make procedures less invasive by avoiding the known adverse effects of CPB, stimulated the development of cardiac stabilizing and positioning devices which have simplified OPCAB procedures.

Unfortunately, despite initial enthusiasm, it has been difficult to prove unequivocal superiority of OPCAB to ONCAB. As a general statement, retrospective studies have tended rather consistently to demonstrate benefit of OPCAB, while prospective randomized studies have not. This may be in part due to the tendency of randomized trials to enroll low-risk patients and observational studies to include higher-risk patients. When mainly low-risk patients are enrolled, demonstration of differences between any two therapies – OPCAB vs ONCAB or PCI vs CABG – becomes very difficult, as adverse events are infrequent and large numbers of patients are required for differences between treatments to reach statistical significance. Statistically significant differences are more likely to be demonstrable in observational trials thanks to the inclusion of high-risk patients.

Differences in mortality have been demonstrated by some investigators but not others. Randomized trials such

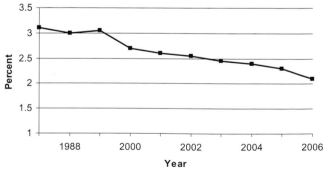

Figure 27.3 The Society of Thoracic Surgeons database demonstrates a decreasing unadjusted operative mortality for patients undergoing isolated CABG procedures. This is despite increasing numbers of high-risk patients undergoing CABG. http://www.sts.org/sections/stsnationaldatabase/publications/executive/article.html.

as Octopus,[64,65] SMART,[66,67] PRAGUE-4,[68,69] and others[70–73] found no difference in survival. In an observational study of more than 68 000 patients, Racz and colleagues found no difference in risk-adjusted mortality between OPCAB and ONCAB.[74] In a large propensity-matched cohort, however, Mack *et al* demonstrated a difference in adjusted mortality (2.2% vs 3.7%, $P < 0.001$) favoring OPCAB.[75] Apparent differences in mortality have also been demonstrated among specific high-risk subgroups. In a retrospective study of patients with a low ejection fraction (≤30%), OPCAB had a lower risk-adjusted mortality rate (1.47% vs 4.13%; $P < 0.001$).[76] Puskas *et al* demonstrated that OPCAB was associated with a significant reduction in death (odds ratio (OR) 0.39, $P = 0.001$) when compared to ONCAB in a cohort of 7740 women.[66,67] An important subgroup of patients with CAD are those with renal failure. In an analysis of patients with end-stage renal disease (ESRD), OPCAB was associated with an operative mortality of 1.7%, whereas the mortality rate of ONCAB was 10-fold higher (17.2%, $P = 0.003$).[77] At late follow up, however, the OPCAB group of patients with ESRD had an increased late mortality when compared to the ONCAB group (38.1% vs 19% annual mortality, $P = 0.03$). This somewhat surprising result may be due to the lower number of mean grafts per patient in the OPCAB group (2.4 ± 1.0 vs 3.3 ± 0.9, $P < 0.001$).[77]

Apart from mortality, a number of retrospective studies have shown a benefit to OPCAB with regard to morbidity, including lower need for blood products, less reoperation for bleeding, and less renal failure,[74,75] although the results of randomized trials have varied. Puskas reported results of the SMART study in 2003, in which patients randomized to OPCAB received fewer units of blood and cardiopulmonary bypass was an independent predictor of blood transfusion (OR 2.42, $P = 0.007$).[66] The reduction in blood transfusion rates was also reported in both the BHACAS trial and by Khan *et al*[72] but was not found to be different between OPCAB and ONCAB in other studies.[69,70] In the SMART trial, postoperative length of stay was shorter in the OPCAB group by one day ($P = 0.005$)[66] but in both the PRAGUE-4 study[68,69] and others,[70,72,73] no differences in hospital stay were observed between OPCAB and ONCAB.

There has been heightened awareness of neurocognitive changes occurring after CABG surgery. While this is a "soft" endpoint and defined by complex neurocognitive testing, the degree of public concern is justifiably great. It is arguable that a reduction in either neurologic decline or stroke would be the greatest benefit of OPCAB surgery. Unfortunately, this has been difficult to prove. A small randomized study demonstrated a dramatic superiority in cognitive outcomes at one week after OPCAB surgery.[78] Conversely, a randomized study of 60 patients demonstrated no difference in cognitive function after three months in OPCAB and ONCAB patients.[79] The largest pro-

spective randomized study performed to address this question was the Octopus Study which enrolled 281 low-risk patients randomized to OPCAB or ONCAB. There was no difference in cognitive outcomes at five years after surgery ($P > 0.99$).[64,65] Interpretation of these data is made more difficult by the variability in neurocognitive testing, the impact of other factors on testing outcomes such as depression, and the anticipated decline in neurocognitive function with aging, particularly among patients with advanced atherosclerotic disease. Indeed, similar changes in neurocognitive function have been identified after PCI.[80] Furthermore, the majority of individuals demonstrating neurocognitive changes early after cardiac surgery experience a return to baseline by three months.[81]

While subject to underrecognition on clinical grounds, the endpoint of stroke is at least in some regards more clearly objective than that of neurocognitive decline. Hopes that OPCAB would reduce the incidence of this endpoint have also been largely unmet. Multiple small studies have been reported with results on both sides of the argument. In two different meta-analyses, however, the incidence of stroke following OPCAB surgery was not statistically significantly reduced in comparison with ONCAB.[82,83] Similarly, there has been no difference in stroke in most randomized trials.[66–69,72,74] Arguments have been made that, as is the case for the issue of operative mortality, differences in stroke rate have not been demonstrable in these relatively small studies due to the low-risk nature of the populations studied. This notion is supported by the results of a recent analysis of 49 830 patients in the New York State Registry in which a lower incidence of stroke was demonstrable in OPCAB patients (adjusted OR 0.70, 95% confidence interval (CI) 0.57–0.86) (84). Unfortunately, most surgeons still place a clamp on the ascending aorta to perform proximal anastomoses for vein grafts when performing OPCAB. The operation is, therefore, not truly "no touch" with respect to the likely culprit source of cerebral embolic material, and it has been argued that the incidence of stroke after CABG may be determined more by the amount of aortic manipulation and less by the use of CPB.[85]

Technically, OPCAB is more difficult to perform than ONCAB. This was particularly true in the early experience, and is still true today despite the introduction of a variety of stabilizing and positioning devices that facilitate anastomoses on the beating heart. Accordingly, in almost every study, the number of grafts performed off-pump is less than the number performed in the ONCAB control group. The quality of the anastomoses performed on the beating heart is also questioned by some. A meta-analysis of seven trials of patients undergoing OPCAB demonstrated a lower rate of complete revascularization (relative risk (RR) 0.959) and lower graft patency than patients undergoing traditional on-pump grafting (standardized mean difference

−0.164).[86] Others argue that this is a manifestation of inadequate institutional and surgeon experience, as centers with extensive experience in OPCAB have reported similar numbers of grafts to those performed in ONCAB.[66]

Thus, while there is some controversy over the benefits of OPCAB over ONCAB, there is general agreement among surgeons that, in experienced hands, OPCAB can be performed with mortality rates at least similar to, if not lower than, those for ONCAB procedures. There is likely a lower rate of transfusion and may well be a lower risk of renal failure with OPCAB. A reduction in stroke likely depends upon complete avoidance of aortic manipulation. There may be particular benefit with regard to morbidity among high-risk patients such as women and the elderly (**Class IIa, Level B**). Utilization of the technique has stabilized in the United States at approximately 20%.[16]

Left anterior small thoracotomy procedure

There was some interest in the use of limited anterior small thoracotomy (LAST) procedures during the early years of OPCAB. This procedure was also called minimally invasive direct coronary artery bypass grafting (MIDCAB), and was applicable for revascularization of the LAD with the left ITA (LITA). It was argued that the small thoracotomy allowed for preservation of chest wall integrity while improving cosmesis due to the smaller incision. The procedure proved technically demanding, however, with an increased risk of injury to the LITA during harvesting and lower anastomotic patencies when compared to a full sternotomy approach[87] (**Class IIb, Level C**). The chest wall incisions proved painful for the patients as well, indeed more so than a full sternotomy, and lung herniation was also a problem, dampening enthusiasm for the procedure. Furthermore, with advances in stent technology, the enthusiasm of cardiologists to refer patients for single-vessel bypass grafting waned. Currently, the principal application of the LAST procedure is in hybrid procedures involving surgical revascularization of the LAD artery and coronary stenting of the circumflex and right coronary arteries.[88,89]

Robotics

Efforts to apply robotic and endoscopic techniques to perform CABG are ongoing. Robotics have been applied to every aspect of the procedure, ranging from mechanical stabilization of the endoscopic cameras to actual closed-chest, port-assisted ITA harvesting. Perhaps the most challenging aspect has been the robotic coronary artery anastomosis, a necessary step to accomplish the ultimate goal of totally endoscopic coronary artery bypass or TEACAB.[90–93] The main limiting factors include the difficulty with coronary artery anastomoses without using mechanical connectors and difficulty accessing the posterior aspects of the heart. Thus far clinical experience is small and there are no data concerning long-term graft patency rates. As technology improves, this may find a role in the future (**Class IIb, Level C**).

Conduits

The choice of conduit is dictated by three features: the anatomy of the CAD, the projected patency of various conduits, and conduit availability. Conduits are not all created equal, and their choice can have an important impact on long-term results. This must be kept in mind when evaluations of the ultimate role of surgical CABG are made.

Arterial conduits

Although the first conduits used were venous, due to their ready availability and favorable handling characteristics, a number of visionary individuals explored the use of arterial conduits almost from the inception of CABG. Theoretically, arterial conduits should have a number of advantages over venous conduits, including inherent structural characteristics adapted to higher, pulsatile pressures and an ability to autoregulate to meet increasing oxygen demand. Fortuitously, the most convenient of these, the internal thoracic artery (ITA), is particularly resistant to atherosclerosis. However, both arterial and venous grafts are limited by the target native coronary artery anatomy, as competitive flow and poor run-off may limit patency.

Internal thoracic arteries The left ITA (LITA) should be used preferentially to graft the LAD artery (**Class I, Level C**). The durability of the LITA to the LAD has been demonstrated repeatedly to be superb, with angiographic patency rates as high as 96–98% at one year, 88–95% at 10 years, and 88% at 15 years.[44,94–96] This compares with saphenous veins anastomosed to the LAD which demonstrate patencies of 79% at two years.[97] The use of the LITA has been shown to increase late survival when compared to saphenous vein grafts.[44,98,99] Use of the LITA has also been shown to be associated with lower operative mortality, even in the elderly, perhaps as a reflection of superior patency even in the immediate postoperative period.[100–102] Some reports have also shown a decrease in subsequent MI and reoperation.[44,103]

The right internal thoracic artery (RITA) has similarly good patency rates when compared to the LITA when grafted to the LAD. The patency of both arteries, however, is dependent on the territory to which it is anastomosed. Tatoulis *et al* have reported on over 2000 arterial conduits, with overall RITA patency of 96% patency at five years, 81% at 10 years, and 65% at 15 years.[96] Patency was best when the RITA was anastomosed to the LAD and worst when anastomosed to the right coronary artery territory. An adverse effect of competitive flow was also apparent, with optimal patencies obtained when the native coronary artery had obstructive disease greater than 70–90%.[96,104]

Accordingly, the RITA should be utilized as an alternative conduit to the LAD in patients who have appropriate anatomy (**Class IIa, Level C**).

These findings have lead to the use of both right and left (bilateral) internal thoracic arteries (BITA). Large observational studies have shown slightly lower reoperative and reintervention rates in patients who receive two internal thoracic arteries (ITA).[105–107] It has been more difficult to demonstrate a clear survival benefit for BITA grafting. A large retrospective study from the Cleveland Clinic, however, has demonstrated seven-, 10-, 15-, and 20-year survival to be 87%, 78%, 58%, and 37% in patients who received one internal mammary compared to 89%, 81%, 67%, and 50% in patients who received BITA ($P < 0.001$).[108,109] However, retrospective comparisons such as this are subject to selection bias (despite propensity matching), as it was likely younger healthier patients were more likely to receive BITA grafting. A slightly increased risk of mediastinitis has been noted in diabetics[110] but this has been refuted in other studies,[111,112] particularly when the arteries are taken in a skeletonized fashion (the artery is isolated from its surrounding veins and other tissues).[113,114] BITA are used mainly in younger patients in whom long-term patency is especially important (**Class IIa, Level C**).

Radial artery The radial artery was first employed by Carpentier early in the experience with CABG; however, early experience suggested high graft occlusion and graft spasm in this artery.[115] Subsequently, a number of grafts thought to be occluded at early study were found to be patent at late angiography,[116] stimulating renewed interest. The randomized Radial Artery Patency Study (RAPS) demonstrated increased patency of radial arteries at one year when compared to venous grafts (91.8% vs 86.4 %, $P = 0.009$).[117] Occlusion or stenosis of the radial artery was more likely in native vessels with <90% stenoses. However, in patients with peripheral vascular disease, radial arteries had a poorer patency when compared to venous grafts.[118] Radial arteries may also be used as part of a composite graft with the LITA to achieve a total arterial grafting strategy (Fig. 27.4). In composite grafts, radial arteries can achieve statistically similar patencies to the LITA when anastomosed to critically stenosed targets in the left coronary artery system.[119,120] The radial artery is generally harvested from the forearm of the non-dominant hand in patients with an intact palmar arch and various vasodilators are used to decrease spasm intraoperatively and postoperatively. Radial arteries can be used as an alternative to venous grafting (**Class IIa, Level B**).

Other arterial conduits Other arterial conduits have been proposed including the inferior gastroepiploic artery (IEA) and right gastroepiploic artery (GEA). The GEA is most frequently anastomosed to the posterior descending artery

and GEA grafts have a reported one-, five- and 10-year patency rate of 91–93%, 80%, and 62%.[121–124] Patency of the GEA improves as the severity of coronary artery lesions increases in native coronary arteries, much like the radial artery. Previous gastric resection, GEA instrumentation or documented mesenteric vascular insufficiency are contraindications to its use. GEA use has generally been superseded by the radial artery, as the GEA has limited long-term

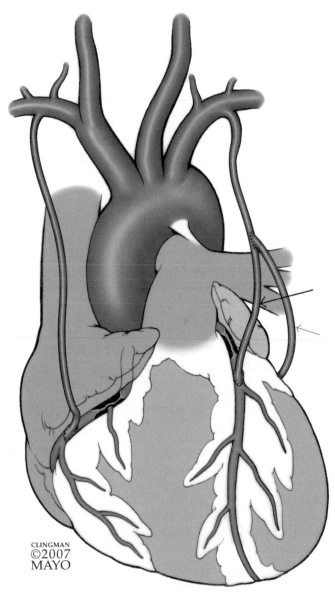

CLINGMAN
©2007
MAYO

Figure 27.4 Both arterial and venous conduits may be used to form composite grafts which allow for a reduction in the number of proximal anastomoses. Composite grafts may increase late conduit patency due to increased distal run-off. The black arrow demonstrates a composite ("Y") graft made up of a LIMA (large, dark arrow) and a venous graft (smaller, light arrow). (Reproduced with permission of Mayo Foundation for Medical Education and Research. All rights reserved.)

data, frequent spasm, potential for intra-abdominal complications, and size mismatch with the native coronary arteries (**Class IIb, Level C**).

Other arterial conduits have been proposed in patients who have limited conduit availability. Use of the ulnar, left gastric, splenic, thoracodorsal, and lateral femoral circumflex arteries has been reported.[125–127] As these conduits do not have proven long-term patencies, they should not be considered preferable to venous grafts and should be generally used only when other conduits are unavailable (**Class IIb, Level C**).

Venous conduits

Greater saphenous veins The saphenous vein continues to be commonly used due to its accessibility, versatility, and availability of both early and late results (**Class IIa, Level B**). The greater saphenous vein has two recognized modes of failure. Early failure is generally a technical problem, due to anastomotic problems, kinking of the graft, poor run-off or progression of native CAD. At one year, approximately 75–80% of veins will remain angiographically patent.[128] Late failure of vein grafts is usually due to progression of atherosclerotic disease of the graft itself. Freedom from graft failure at five and 10 years is approximately 60% and 40%, respectively.[129]

These vein graft patency estimates were produced before many routine medical therapies such as early aspirin administration and lipid-lowering therapy,[130–133] which may increase late vein patency (**Class IIa, Level B**). A trial is under way to determine if aspirin and clopidogrel may further decrease intimal hyperplasia of vein grafts when compared to aspirin alone.[134] Newer therapies are also in development, and the recent PREVENT IV trial tested the impact of edifoligide, an inhibitor of E2F transcription factors, on short-term vein patency. Unfortunately, no benefit was found as the graft failure rate was 45.2% in the edifoligide group and 46.3% in the placebo group at one year ($P = 0.66$), although longer follow-up may be required to demonstrate benefit of this novel therapy.[135]

With increasing frequency, saphenous veins are harvested using a minimally invasive endoscopic technique (**Class IIa, Level B**). Despite concerns regarding the potential of increased trauma during harvesting, there appears to be little evidence of damage.[136–139] The advantages of endoscopic harvest include decreased wound complications and improved cosmetic results. The three- and six-month patency rates were similar to open harvest in two small randomized studies.[140,141] However, there are no data on long-term patency, which may be when intimal damage is most apparent with accelerated atherosclerosis of the vein grafts.

Alternative venous conduits The lesser saphenous and cephalic veins, as well as cryopreserved homologous vein grafts and glutaraldehyde-treated homologous vein grafts, have poor patencies in comparison to the greater saphenous vein.[142,143] These alternative conduits should only be used in the absence of any other conduit material (**Class III, Level C**).

Endarterectomy

Coronary endarterectomy may be performed in combination with bypass grafting in patients with diffuse CAD for whom no acceptable site for distal anastomosis can be found. The operative mortality rate is in most series approximately twofold greater than that of patients who undergo CABG, but this may be a reflection of greater co-morbidities in these patients.[144] It is generally accepted that the graft patency rate is less when the target has been endarterectomized when compared to direct grafting; however, it is not prohibitive.[145] Therefore, endarterectomy remains a valuable tool in selected patients who have some of the most severe CAD (**Class IIb, Level C**).

Conclusion

Surgical coronary artery bypass grafting continues to evolve. There have been novel developments in both CABG and medical management which have enabled good survival and quality of life for patients with CAD. With greater understanding of which patients derive the greatest benefit from surgical revascularization, CABG will continue to be an important modality in the treatment of CAD. In stable angina, surgical revascularization remains indicated according to AHA/ACC guidelines for left main CAD, left main equivalent CAD, and triple-vessel disease (**Class I**). Also, proximal LAD disease with either a depressed ejection fraction (<35%) or documented ischemia, proximal LAD disease with two-vessel disease and a large territory of myocardium at risk, and disabling angina despite maximal non-invasive therapy are also Class I indications. Furthermore, Class II indications in stable angina include proximal LAD stenosis with one-vessel disease and one- or two-vessel disease with a documented moderate amount of myocardium at risk and demonstrable ischemia.

References

1. Beck CS. The development of a new blood supply to the heart by operation. *Ann Surg* 1935;**102**:801–13.
2. Vineberg AM, Miller WD. An experimental study of the physiological role of an anastomosis between the left coronary circulation and the left internal mammary artery implanted in the left ventricular myocardium. *Surg Forum* 1950;294–9.

3. Vineberg A, Miller G. Internal mammary coronary anastomosis in the surgical treatment of coronary artery insufficiency. *Can Med Assoc J* 1951;**64**:204–10.

4. Sen PK, Udwadia TE, Kinare SG, Parkular GB. Transmyocardial acupuncture: a new approach to myocardial revascularization. *J Thorac Cardiovasc Surg* 1965;**50**:181–9.

5. Gibbon JH Jr. Application of a mechanical heart and lung apparatus to cardiac surgery. *Minn Med* 1954;**37**:171–85.

6. Longmire WP Jr, Cannon JA, Kattus AA. Direct-vision coronary endarterectomy for angina pectoris. *N Engl J Med* 1958;**259**:993–9.

7. Goetz RH, Rohman M, Haller JD, Dee R, Rosenak SS. Internal mammary-coronary artery anastomosis. A nonsuture method employing tantalum rings. *J Thorac Cardiovasc Surg* 1961;**41**:378–86.

8. Sabiston DC Jr, Ross RS, Criley JM, Gaertner RA, Neill CA, Taussig HB. Surgical management of congenital lesions of the coronary circulation. *Ann Surg* 1963;**157**:908–24.

9. Kolessov VI. Mammary artery-coronary artery anastomosis as method of treatment for angina pectoris. *J Thorac Cardiovasc Surg* 1967;**54**:535–44.

10. Sones FM Jr. Cine-coronary arteriography. *Ohio Med* 1962;**58**:1018–19.

11. Favaloro RF, Effler DB, Groves LK, Fergusson DJ, Lozada JS. Double internal mammary artery-myocardial implantation. Clinical evaluation of results in 150 patients. *Circulation* 1968;**37**:549–55.

12. Favaloro RG, Effler DB, Groves LK, Suarez EL. Surgery for coronary arteriosclerosis. Clinical experience in 1,500 operated patients. *Presa Med Argent* 1968;**55**:1019–26.

13. Favaloro RG, Effler DB, Groves LK, Sheldon WC, Riahi M. Direct myocardial revascularization with saphenous vein autograft. Clinical experience in 100 cases. *Dis Chest* 1969;**56**:279–83.

14. Johnson WD, Felmma RJ, Lepley D, Ellison EH. Extended treatment of severe coronary artery disease: a total surgical approach. *Ann Surg* 1969;**170**:460–70.

15. Favaloro R. Indirect revascularization of the myocardium implantation of internal mammary artery; direct myocardial revascularization with grafting of the saphenous vein (indications, surgical technique, immediate and late results). *Fracastoro* 1970;**63**:725–39.

16. www.sts.org/documents/pdf/Spring2007Executive Summary.pdf. Executive summary.

17. Hoffman SN, TenBrook JA, Wolf MP, Pauker SG, Salem DN, Wong JB. A meta-analysis of randomized controlled trials comparing coronary artery bypass graft with percutaneous transluminal coronary angioplasty: one- to eight-year outcomes. *J Am Coll Cardiol* 2003;**41**:1293–304.

18. Rihal C, Raco D, Gersh B, Yusuf S. Indications for coronary artery bypass surgery and percutaneous coronary intervention in chronic stable angina. *Circulation* 2003;**108**:2439–45.

19. Hannan EL, Racz MJ, Walford G *et al.* Long-term outcomes of coronary-artery bypass grafting versus stent implantation. *N Engl J Med* 2005;**26**:2174–83.

20. Opie LH, Commerford PJ, Gersh BJ. Controversies in stable coronary artery disease. *Lancet* 2006;**267**:69–78.

21. Eagle KA, Guyton RA, Davidoff R *et al.* American College of Cardiology; American Heart Association. ACC/AHA 2004 guideline update for coronary artery bypass graft surgery: a report of the American College of Cardiology/American Heart Association Task Force on Practice Guidelines (Committee to Update the 1999 Guidelines for Coronary Artery Bypass Graft Surgery). *Circulation* 2004;**110**:e340–437.

22. CASS Principal Investigators. Coronary Artery Surgery Study (CASS). A randomized trial of coronary artery bypass surgery; survival data. *Circulation* 1983;**68**:939–50.

23. Veterans Administration Coronary Artery Bypass Surgery Cooperative Study Group. Eleven-year survival in the Veterans Administration Randomized Trial of Coronary Bypass Surgery for Stable Angina. *N Engl J Med* 1984;**311**:1333–9.

24. Murphy ML, Hultgren HN, Detre K, Thomsen J, Takaro T. Treatment of chronic stable angina: a preliminary report of survival data of the randomized Veterans Administration Cooperative Study. *N Engl J Med* 1977;**297**:621–7.

25. Varnauskas E, European Coronary Surgery Study Group. Twelve-year follow-up of survival in the randomized European Coronary Surgery Study. *N Engl J Med* 1988;**319**:332–7.

26. European Coronary Surgery Study Group. Prospective randomized study of coronary artery bypass surgery in stable angina pectoris: second interim report. *Lancet* 1980;**2**:491–5.

27. Norris RM, Agnew TM, Brandt PWT *et al.* Coronary surgery after recurrent myocardial infarction: progress of a trial comparing surgical and nonsurgical management for asymptomatic patients with advanced coronary disease. *Circulation* 1981;**63**:785–92.

28. Mathur VS, Guinn GA. Prospective randomized study of the surgical therapy of stable angina. *Cardiovasc Clin* 1977;**8**:131–44.

29. Kloster FE, Kremkau EL, Ritzmann LW, Rahimtoola SH, Rosch J, Kanarek PH. Coronary bypass for stable angina: a prospective randomized study. *N Engl J Med* 1979;**300**:149–57.

30. National Cooperative Study Group. Unstable angina pectoris: National Cooperative Study Group to compare surgical and medical therapy: II. In-hospital experience and initial follow-up results in patients with one, two and three vessel disease. *Am J Cardiol* 1978;**42**:839–48.

31. Yusuf S, Zucker D, Peduzzi P *et al.* Effect of coronary artery bypass graft surgery on survival: overview of ten-year results from randomized trials by the Coronary Artery Bypass Graft Surgery Trialist Collaboration. *Lancet* 1994;**344**:563–70.

32. Alderman EL, Bourassa MG, Cohen LS *et al.* Ten-year follow-up of survival and myocardial infarction in the randomized Coronary Artery Surgery Study. *Circulation* 1990;**82**:1629–46.

33. Hueb WA, Bellotti G, de Oliveira SA *et al.* The Medicine, Angioplasty, or Surgery Study (MASS): a prospective, randomized trial of medical therapy, balloon angioplasty, or bypass surgery for single proximal left anterior descending artery stenoses. *J Am Coll Cardiol* 1995;**26**:1600–5.

34. Goy JJ, Eeckhout E, Burnand B *et al.* Coronary angioplasty versus left internal mammary artery grafting for isolated proximal left anterior descending artery stenosis. *Lancet* 1994;**343**:1449–53.

35. Kaiser GC, Davis KB, Fisher LD *et al.* Survival following coronary artery bypass grafting in patients with severe angina pectoris (CASS): an observational study. *J Thorac Cardiovasc Surg* 1985;**89**:513–24.

36. Myers WO, Schaff HV, Fisher LD *et al.* Time to first new myocardial infarction in patients with severe angina and three-vessel disease comparing medical and early surgical therapy: a CASS Registry study of survival. *J Thorac Cardiovasc Surg* 1988;**95**:382–9.

37. Mock MB, Ringqvist I, Fisher LD *et al.* Survival of medically treated patients in the Coronary Artery Surgery Study (CASS) registry. *Circulation* 1982;**66**:562–8.

38. Harris PJ, Harrell FE Jr, Lee KL, Behar VS, Rosati RA. Survival in medically treated coronary artery disease. *Circulation* 1979;**60**:1259–69.

39. TIME Investigators. Trial of invasive versus medical therapy in elderly patients with chronic symptomatic coronary-artery disease (TIME): a randomized trial. *Lancet* 2001;**358**:951–7.

40. Davies RF, Goldberg AD, Forman S *et al.* Asymptomatic Cardiac Ischemia Pilot (ACIP) study two-year follow-up: outcomes of patients randomized to initial strategies of medical therapy versus revascularization. *Circulation* 1997;**95**:2037–43.

40a. The BARI 2D Study Group. A randomized trial of therapies for type 2 diabetes and coronary artery disease. *N Engl J Med* 2009;**360**:2503–15.

41. Kirklin JW, Naftel DC, Blackstone EH, Pohost GM. Summary of a consensus concerning death and ischemic events after coronary artery bypass grafting. *Circulation* 1989;**79**:181–91.

42. Weintraub WS, Jones EL, King SB 3rd *et al.* Changing use of coronary angioplasty in coronary bypass surgery in the treatment of chronic coronary artery disease. *Am J Cardiol* 1990;**65**:183–8.

43. Appoo J, Norris C, Merali S *et al.* Long-term outcome of isolated coronary artery bypass surgery in patients with severe left ventricular dysfunction. *Circulation* 2004;**110**:II13–17.

44. DeNofrio D, Loh E. Myocardial viability in patients with coronary artery disease and left ventricular dysfunction: transplantation or revascularization? *Curr Opin Cardiol* 1996;**11**:394–402.

45. Schinkel AF, Bax JJ, Poldermans D, Elhendy A, Ferrari R, Rahimtoola SH. Hibernating myocardium: diagnosis and patient outcomes. *Curr Probl Cardiol* 2007;**32**:375–410.

46. Van Brussel BL, Plokker HW, Ernst SM *et al.* Venous coronary artery bypass surgery. A 15-year follow-up study. *Circulation* 1993;**88**:II87–92.

47. Bergsma TM, Grandjean JG, Voors AA, Boonstra PW, den Heyer P, Ebels T. Low recurrence of angina pectoris after coronary artery bypass graft surgery with bilateral internal thoracic and right gastroepiploic arteries. *Circulation* 1998;**97**:2402–5.

48. Alderman EL, Kip KE, Whitlow PL *et al.* Bypass Angioplasty Revascularization Investigation. Native coronary disease progression exceeds failed revascularization as cause of angina after five years in the Bypass Angioplasty Revascularization Investigation (BARI). *J Am Coll Cardiol* 2004;**44**:766–74.

49. Ogus TN, Basaran M, Selimoglu O, Yildirim T, Ogus H, Ozcan H, Us MH. Long-term results of the left anterior descending coronary artery reconstruction with left internal thoracic artery. *Ann Thorac Surg* 2007;**83**:496–501.

50. Loop FD, Lytle BW, Cosgrove DM *et al.* Influence of the internal-mammary-artery graft on 10-year survival and other cardiac events. *N Engl J Med* 1986;**314**:1–6.

51. Boulay FM, David PP, Bourassa MG. Strategies for improving the work status of patients after coronary artery bypass surgery. *Circulation* 1982;**66**:III43–9.

52. Bradshaw PJ, Jamrozik K, Gilfillan IS, Thompson PL. Return to work after coronary artery bypass surgery. *Heart Lung Circ* 2005;**14**:191–6.

53. Sellier P, Varaillac P, Chatellier G *et al.* Investigators of the PERISCOP Study. Factors influencing return to work at one year after coronary bypass graft surgery: results of the PERISCOP study. *Eur J Cardiovasc Prev Rehabil* 2003;**10**:469–75.

54. VA Coronary Artery Bypass Surgery Cooperative Study Group. Eighteen-year follow-up in the Veterans Affairs Cooperative Study of Coronary Artery Bypass Surgery for stable angina. *Circulation.*1992;**86**:121–30.

55. Ferguson TB Jr, Jammill BG, Peterson ED, DeLong ER, Grover F, STS National Database Committee. A decade of change – risk profiles and outcomes for isolated coronary artery bypass grafting procedures, 1990–1999: a report from the STS National Database Committee and the Duke Clinical Research Institute. *Ann Thorac Surg* 2002;**73**:480–9.

56. Pintar T, Collard CD. The systemic inflammatory response to cardiopulmonary bypass. *Anesthesiol Clin North Am* 2003;**21**:453–64.

57. Ji B, Undar A. An evaluation of the benefits of pulsatile versus nonpulsatile perfusion during cardiopulmonary bypass procedures in pediatric and adult cardiac patients. *ASAIO J* 2006;**52**:357–61.

58. Elahi MM, Khan JS. Revascularization with off-pump coronary artery surgery: what appears new is actually the old rediscovered. *Card Revasc Med* 2007;**8**:52–9.

59. Rubens FD, Mesana T. The inflammatory response to cardiopulmonary bypass: a therapeutic overview. *Perfusion* 2004;**19**:S5–12.

60. Benetti FJ, Naselli G, Wood M, Geffner L. Direct myocardial revascularization without extracorporeal circulation. Experience in 700 patients. *Chest* 1991;**100**:312–16.

61. Buffolo E, de Andrade CS, Branco JN, Teles CA, Aguiar LF, Gomes WJ. Coronary artery bypass grafting without cardiopulmonary bypass. *Ann Thorac Surg* 1996;**61**:63–6.

62. Pfister AJ, Zaki MS, Garcia JM *et al.* Coronary artery bypass without cardiopulmonary bypass. *Ann Thorac Surg* 1992;**54**:1085–91.

63. Atkins CW, Boucher CA, Pohost GM. Preservation of interventricular septal function in patients having coronary artery bypass grafts without cardiopulmonary bypass. *Am Heart J* 1984;**107**:304–9.

64. Van Dijk D, Spoor M, Hijman R *et al.* Octopus Study Group. Cognitive and cardiac outcomes 5 years after off-pump vs on-pump coronary artery bypass graft surgery. *JAMA* 2007;**297**:701–8.

65. Nathoe HM, van Dijk D, Jansen EW *et al.* Octopus Study Group. A comparison of on-pump and off-pump coronary bypass surgery in low-risk patients. *N Engl J Med* 2003;**348**:394–402.

66. Puskas JD, Williams WH, Duke PG *et al.* Off-pump coronary artery bypass grafting provides complete revascularization with reduced myocardial injury, transfusion requirements, and length of stay: a prospective randomized comparison of two hundred unselected patients undergoing off-pump versus conventional coronary artery bypass grafting. *J Thorac Cardiovasc Surg* 2003;**125**:797–808.

67. Puskas JD, Williams WH, Mahoney EM *et al.* Off-pump vs conventional coronary artery bypass grafting: early and 1-year

graft patency, cost, and quality-of-life outcomes: a randomized trial. *JAMA* 2004;**291**:1841–9.

68. Widimsky P, Straka Z, Stros P *et al.* One-year coronary bypass graft patency: a randomized comparison between off-pump and on-pump surgery angiographic results of the PRAGUE-4 trial. *Circulation* 2004;**110**:3418–23.

69. Straka Z, Widimsky P, Jirasek K *et al.* Off-pump versus on-pump coronary surgery: final results from a prospective randomized study PRAGUE-4. *Ann Thorac Surg* 2004; **77**:789–93.

70. Gerola LR, Buffolo E, Jasbik W *et al.* Off-pump versus on-pump myocardial revascularization in low-risk patients with one or two vessel disease: perioperative results in a multicenter randomized controlled trial. *Ann Thorac Surg* 2004;**77**:569–73.

71. Karolak W, Hirsch G, Buth K, Legare JF. Medium-term outcomes of coronary artery bypass graft surgery on pump versus off pump: results from a randomized controlled trial. *Am Heart J* 2007;**153**:689–95.

72. Khan NE, De Souza A, Mister R *et al.* A randomized comparison of off-pump and on-pump multivessel coronary-artery bypass surgery. *N Engl J Med* 2004;**350**:21–8.

73. Angelini GD, Taylor GC, Reeves BC, Ascione R. Early and midterm outcome after off-pump and on-pump surgery in Beating Heart Against Cardioplegic Arrest Studies (BHACAS 1 and 2): a pooled analysis of two randomized controlled trials. *Lancet* 2002;**259**:1194–9.

74. Racz MJ, Hannan EL, Isom OW *et al.* A comparison of short- and long-term outcomes after off-pump and on-pump coronary artery bypass graft surgery with sternotomy. *J Am Coll Cardiol* 2004;**43**:557–64.

75. Mack MJ, Brown PP, Kugelmass AD *et al.* Current status and outcomes of coronary revascularization 1999 to 2002: 148,396 surgical and percutaneous procedures. *Ann Thorac Surg* 2004;**77**(3):766–8.

76. Dewey TM, Herbert MA, Prince SL *et al.* Avoidance of cardiopulmonary bypass improves early survival in multivessel coronary artery bypass patients with poor ventricular function. *Heart Surg Forum* 2004;**7**:45–50.

77. Dewey TM, Herbert MA, Prince SL *et al.* Does coronary artery bypass graft surgery improve survival among patients with end-stage renal disease? *Ann Thorac Surg* 2006;**81**:591–8.

78. Diegeler A, Hirsch R, Schneider F *et al.* Neuromonitoring and neurocognitive outcome in off-pump versus conventional coronary bypass operation. *Ann Thorac Surg* 2000;**69**:1162–6.

79. Lloyd CT, Ascione R, Underwood MJ, Gardner F, Black A, Angelini GD. Serum S-100 protein release and neuropsychologic outcome during coronary revascularization on the beating heart: a prospective randomized study. *J Thorac Cardiovasc Surg* 2000;**119**:148–54.

80. Hlatky MA, Bacon C, Boothroyd D *et al.* Cognitive function 5 years after randomization to coronary angioplasty or coronary artery bypass graft surgery. *Circulation* 1997;**96**:II11–14.

81. McKhann GM, Grega MA, Borowicz LM *et al.* Is there cognitive decline 1 year after CABG? Comparison with surgical and nonsurgical controls. *Neurology* 2005;**65**:991–9.

82. Takagi H, Tanabashi T, Kawai N, Umemoto T. Off-pump surgery does not reduce stroke compared with on-pump surgery does not reduce stroke, compared with results of on-pump coronary artery bypass grafting: a meta-analysis of randomized clinical trials. *J Thorac Cardiovasc Surg* 2007; **134**:1059–60.

83. Cheng DC, Bainbridge D, Martine JE, Novick RJ, Evidence-Based Perioperative Clinical Outcomes Research Group. Does off-pump coronary artery bypass reduce mortality, morbidity, and resource utilization when compared with conventional coronary artery bypass? A meta-analysis of randomized trials. *Anesthesiology* 2005;**102**:188–203.

84. Hannan EL, Wu C, Smith CR *et al.* Off-pump versus on-pump coronary artery bypass graft surgery: differences in short-term outcomes and in long-term mortality and need for subsequent revascularization. *Circulation* 2007;**116**:1145–52.

85. Lev-Ran O, Braunstein R, Sharony R *et al.* No-touch aorta off-pump coronary surgery: the effect on stroke. *J Thorac Cardiovasc Surg* 2005;**129**:307–13.

86. Lim E, Drain A, Davies W, Edmonds L, Rosengard BR. A systematic review of randomized trials comparing revascularization rate and graft patency of off-pump and conventional coronary surgery. *J Thorac Cardiovasc Surg* 2006;**132**: 1409–13.

87. Diegeler A, Matin M, Kayser S *et al.* Angiographic results after minimally invasive coronary artery bypass grafting using the minimally invasive direct coronary bypass grafting (MIDCAB) approach. *Eur J Cardiothorac Surg* 1999;**15**:680–4.

88. Cisowski M, Morawski W, Drzewiecki J *et al.* Integrated minimally invasive direct coronary artery bypass grafting and angioplasty for coronary artery revascularization. *Eur J Cardiothorac* 2002;**22**:261–5.

89. Wittwer T, Cremer J, Boonstra P *et al.* Myocardial "hybrid" revascularization with minimally invasive direct coronary artery bypass grafting combined with coronary angioplasty: preliminary results of a multicentre study. *Heart* 2000;**83**:58–63.

90. Mack MJ. Minimally invasive cardiac surgery. *Surg Endosc* 2006;**20**:S488–92.

91. Kiaii B, McClure RS, Stitt L *et al.* Prospective angiographic comparison of direction endoscopic, and telesurgical approaches to harvesting the internal thoracic artery. *Ann Thorac Surg* 2006;**82**:624–8.

92. Argenziano M, Kat M, Bonatti J *et al.* TECAB Trial Investigators. Results of the prospective multicenter trial of robotically assisted totally endoscopic coronary artery bypass grafting. *Ann Thorac Surg* 2006;**81**:1666–74.

93. Srivastava S, Gadsalli S, Agusala M *et al.* Use of bilateral internal thoracic arteries in CABG through lateral thoracotomy with robotic assistance in 150 patients. *Ann Thorac Surg* 2006;**81**:800–6.

94. Barner HB, Standeven JW, Reese J Twelve-year experience with internal mammary artery for coronary artery bypass. *J Thorac Cardiovasc Surg* 1985;**90**:668–75.

95. Barner HB, Barnett MG. Fifteen- to twenty-one-year angiographic assessment of internal thoracic artery as a bypass conduit. *Ann Thorac Surg* 1994;**57**:1526–8.

96. Tatoulis J, Buxton BF, Fuller JA. Patencies of 2127 arterial to coronary conduits over 15 years. *Ann Thorac Surg* 2004;**77**:93–101.

97. Lytle BW, Loop FD, Thurer RL, Groves LK, Taylor PC, Cosgrove DM. Isolated left anterior descending coronary atherosclerosis: long-term comparison of internal mammary artery and venous autografts. *Circulation* 1980;**61**:869–74.

98. Cameron A, Kemp HG Jr, Shimomura S *et al.* Aortocoronary bypass surgery: a 7-year follow-up. *Circulation* 1979;**60**:9–13.

99. Zeff RH, Kongtahworn C, Iannone LA *et al.* Internal mammary artery versus saphenous vein graft to the left anterior descending coronary artery: prospective randomized study with 10-year follow-up. *Ann Thorac Surg* 1988;**45**:533–6.

100. Edwards FH, Clark RE, Schwartz M. Impact of internal mammary artery conduits on operative mortality in coronary revascularization. *Ann Thorac Surg* 1994;**57**:27–32.

101. Leavitt BJ, O'Connor GT, Olmstead EM *et al.* Use of the internal mammary artery graft and in-hospital mortality and other adverse outcomes associated with coronary artery bypass surgery. *Circulation* 2001;**103**:507–12.

102. Ferguson TB Jr, Hammill BG, Peterson ED, DeLong ER, Grover FL, for the STS National Database Committee. A decade of change – risk profiles and outcomes for isolated coronary artery bypass grafting procedures, 1990–1999: a report from the STS National Database Committee and the Duke Clinical Research Institute. Society of Thoracic Surgeons. *Ann Thorac Surg* 2002;**73**:480–9.

103. Cameron A, Kemp HG Jr, Green GE. Bypass surgery with the internal mammary artery graft: 15 year follow-up. *Circulation* 1986;**74**:III30–6.

104. Sabik JF 3rd, Lytle BW, Blackstone EH, Houghtaling PL, Cosgrove DM. Comparison of saphenous vein and internal thoracic artery graft patency by coronary system. *Ann Thorac Surg* 2005;**79**:544–51.

105. Stevens LM, Carrier M, Perrault LP *et al.* Influence of diabetes and bilateral internal thoracic artery grafts on long-term outcome for multivessel coronary artery bypass grafting. *Eur J Cardiothorac Surg* 2005;**27**:281–8.

106. Ioannidis JP, Galanos O, Katritsis D *et al.* Early mortality and morbidity of bilateral versus single internal thoracic artery revascularization: propensity and risk modeling. *J Am Coll Cardiol* 2001;**37**:521–8.

107. Endo M, Nishida H, Tomizawa Y, Kasanuki H. Benefit of bilateral over single internal mammary artery grafts for multiple coronary artery bypass grafting. *Circulation* 2001;**104**:2164–70.

108. Lytle BW, Cosgrove DM, Loop FD, Borsh J, Goomastic M, Taylor PC. Perioperative risk of bilateral internal mammary artery grafting: analysis of 500 cases from 1971 to 1984. *Circulation* 1986;**74**:III37–41.

109. Lytle BW, Blackstone EH, Sabik JF, Houghtaling P, Loop FD, Cosgrove DM. The effect of bilateral internal thoracic artery grafting on survival during 20 postoperative years. *Ann Thorac Surg* 2004;**78**:2005–12.

110. Savage EB, Grab JD, O'Brien SM *et al.* Use of both internal thoracic arteries in diabetic patients increases deep sternal wound infection. *Ann Thorac Surg* 2007;**83**:1002–6.

111. Svensson LG, Mumtaz MA, Blackstone EH *et al.* Does use of a right internal thoracic artery increase deep wound infection and risk after previous use of a left internal thoracic artery? *J Thorac Cardiovasc Surg* 2006;**131**:609–13.

112. Stevens LM, Carrier M, Perrault LP *et al.* Influence of diabetes and bilateral internal thoracic artery grafts on long-term outcome for multivessel coronary artery bypass grafting. *Eur J Cardiothorac Surg* 2005;**27**:281–8.

113. Peterson MD, Borger MA, Rao V, Peniston CM, Feindel CM. Skeletonization of bilateral internal thoracic artery grafts lowers the risk of sternal infection in patients with diabetes. *J Thorac Cardiovasc Surg* 2003;**126**:1314–19.

114. Hirose H, Amano A, Takanashi S, Takhashi A. Skeletonized bilateral internal mammary artery grafting for patients with diabetes. *Interact Cardiovasc Thorac Surg* 2003;**2**:287–92.

115. Carpentier A, Guermonprez JL, Deloche A, Frechette C, DuBost C. The aorta to coronary radial artery bypass graft: a technique avoiding pathological chances in grafts. *Ann Thorac Surg* 1973;**16**:111–21.

116. Acar C, Farge A, Chardigny C *et al.* Use of the radial artery for coronary artery bypass. A new experience after 20 years. *Arch Mal Coeur Vaiss* 1993;**86**:1683–9.

117. Desai ND, Cohen EA, Naylor CD, Fremes SE, Radial Artery Patency Study Investigators. A randomized comparison of radial-artery and saphenous-vein coronary bypass grafts. *N Engl J Med* 2004;**351**:2302–9.

118. Desai ND, Naylor CD, Kiss A *et al.* Radial Artery Patency Study Investigators. Impact of patient and target-vessel characteristics on arterial and venous bypass graft patency: insight from a randomized trial. *Circulation* 2007;**115**:684–91.

119. Maniar HS, Sundt TM, Barner HB *et al.* Effect of target stenosis and location on radial artery graft patency. *J Cardiothorac Surg* 2002;**123**:45–52.

120. Barner HB, Sundt TM, Bailey M, Zang Y. Midterm results of complete arterial reascularization in more than 1,000 patients using an internal thoracic artery/radial artery T graft. *Ann Surg* 2001;**234**:447–453.

121. Suma H, Isomura T, Horii T, Sato T. Late angiographic results of using the risk gastroepiploic artery as a graft. *J Thorac Cardiovasc Surg* 2000;**120**:496–8.

122. Suma H, Tanabe H, Takahashi A *et al.* Twenty years experience with the gastroepiploic artery graft for CABG. *Circulation* 2007;**11**:I118–91.

123. Buxton BF, Chan AT, Dixit AS, Eizenberg N, Marshall RD, Raman JS. Ulnar artery as a coronary bypass graft. *Ann Thorac Surg* 1998;**65**:1020–4.

124. Kim KB, Cho KR, Choi JS, Lee HJ. Right gastroepiploic artery for revascularization of the right coronary territory in off-pump total arterial revascularization: strategies to improve patency. *Ann Thorac Surg* 2006;**81**:2135–41.

125. Moro H, Ohzeki H, Hayashi JI *et al.* Evaluation of the thoracodorsal artery as an alternative conduit for coronary bypass. *J Thorac Cardiovasc Surg* 1997;**45**:277–9.

126. Mueller DK, Blakeman BP, Pickleman J. Free splenic artery used in aortocoronary bypass. *Ann Thorac Surg* 1993;**55**:162–3.

127. Schamun CM, Duran JC, Rodriguez JM *et al.* Coronary revascularization with the descending branch of the lateral femoral circumflex artery as a composite arterial graft. *J Thorac Cardiovasc Surg* 1998;**116**:870–1.

128. Campeau L, Enjalbert M, Lesperance J, Vaislic C, Grondin CM, Bourassa MG. Atherosclerosis and late closure of aortocoronary saphenous vein grafts: sequential angiographic studies at 2 weeks, 1 year, 5 to 7 years and 10 to 12 years after surgery. *Circulation* 1983;**68**:SII–1.

129. Campeau L, Enjalbert M, Lesperance J *et al.* The relation of risk factors to the development of atherosclerosis in saphenous-

vein bypass grafts and the progression of disease in the native circulation: a study 10 years after aortocoronary bypass surgery. *N Engl J Med* 1984;**311**:1329–32.

130. Chesebro JH, Fuster V, Elveback LR *et al.* Effect of dipyridamole and aspirin on late vein-graft patency after coronary bypass operations. *N Engl J Med* 1984;**310**:209–14.

131. Goldman S, Copeland J, Moritz T *et al.* Starting aspirin therapy after operation: effects on early graft patency. *Circulation* 1991;**84**:520–6.

132. Blankenhorn DH, Nessim SA, Johnson RL. Beneficial effects of combined colestipol-niacin therapy on coronary atherosclerosis and coronary venous bypass grafts. *JAMA* 1987;**257**:323.

133. Domanski MJ, Borkowf CB, Campeau L *et al.* Prognostic factors for atherosclerosis progression in saphenous vein grafts: the postcoronary artery bypass graft (Post-CABG) trial. Post-CABG Trial Investigators. *J Am Coll Cardiol* 2000;**36**:1877.

134. Kulik A, Le May M, Wells GA, Mesana TG, Ruel M. The Clopidogrel After Surgery for Coronary Artery Disease (CASCADE) randomized controlled trial: clopidogrel and aspirin versus aspirin alone after coronary bypass surgery. *Curr Control Trials Cardiovasc Med* 2005;**6**:15.

135. Alexander JH, Hafley G, Harrington RA *et al.* PREVENT IV Investigators. Efficacy and safety of edifoligide, an E2F transcription factor decoy, for prevention of vein graft failure following coronary artery bypass graft surgery: PREVENT IV: a randomized controlled trial. *JAMA* 2005;**294**:2446–54.

136. Black EA, Guzik TJ, West NE *et al* Minimally invasive saphenous vein harvesting: effects on endothelial and smooth muscle function. *Ann Thorac Surg* 2001;**71**:1503–7.

137. Fabricius AM, Diegeler A, Doll N, Weidenbach H, Mohr FW. Minimally invasive saphenous vein harvesting techniques:

138. Griffith GL, Allen KB, Waller BF *et al.* Endoscopic and traditional saphenous vein harvest: a histologic comparison. *Ann Thorac Surg* 2000;**69**:520–3.

139. Lancey RA, Cuenoud H, Nunnari JJ. Scanning electron microscopic analysis of endoscopic versus open vein harvesting techniques. *J Cardiovasc Surg (Torino)* 2001;**42**:297–301.

140. Yun KL, Wu Y, Aharonian V *et al.* Randomized trial of endoscopic versus open vein harvest for coronary artery bypass grafting: six-month patency rates. *J Thorac Cardiovasc Surg* 2005;**129**:496–503.

141. Perrault LP, Jeanmart H, Bilodeau L *et al.* Early quantitative coronary angiography of saphenous vein grafts for coronary artery bypass grafting harvested by means of open versus endoscopic saphenectomy: a prospective randomized trial. *J Thorac Cardiovasc Surg* 2004;**127**:1402–7.

142. Stoney WS, Alford WC Jr, Burrus GR, Glassford DM Jr, Petracek MR, Thomas CS Jr. The fate of arm veins used for aorta-coronary bypass grafts. *J Thorac Cardiovasc Surg* 1984;**88**:522–6.

143. Wijnberg DS, Boeve WJ, Ebels T *et al.* Patency of arm vein grafts used in aorto-coronary bypass surgery. *Eur J Cardiothorac Surg* 1990;**4**:510–13.

144. Tiruvoipati R, Loubani M, Lencioni M, Ghosh S, Jones PW, Patel RL. Coronary endarterectomy: impact on morbidity and mortality when combined with coronary artery bypass surgery. *Ann Thorac Surg* 2005;**79**:1999–2003.

145. Singhal AK, Sundt TM 3rd. Coronary endarterectomy: the choice of tactics is dictated by the lay of the land *Ann Thorac Surg* 2006;**81**:1178–9.

28 Comparisons of percutaneous coronary intervention and coronary artery bypass grafting

Arashk Motiei, Thoralf M Sundt III and Charanjit S Rihal

Mayo Clinic, Rochester, MN, USA

Introduction

Coronary artery bypass grafting (CABG) and percutaneous coronary intervention (PCI) are the most commonly performed major procedures in the world today. Since their introduction, these procedures have been increasingly used for the treatment of coronary artery disease (CAD). In the United States, according to National Center for Health Statistics estimates, nearly 427 000 CABG and 1.2 million PCI procedures were performed in 2004.[1] It is estimated that these interventions account for a significant proportion of healthcare expenditures, with the estimated direct and indirect costs of CAD for 2007 being $151.6 billion.[1] The immediate risks inherent in these procedures need to be balanced against the expected benefits. Sound clinical judgment and decision making with respect to revascularization options in patients who have CAD require detailed knowledge of both the evidence in support of these procedures and the specific patient subsets that are likely to derive the most benefit.

In general, the broad indications for myocardial revascularization are to:
- improve prognosis (probability of survival)
- improve symptoms
- potentially prevent non-fatal events, such as myocardial infarction (MI), arrhythmias or heart failure.

Over the past four decades, a considerable volume of literature from prospective randomized clinical trials and large national databases has been published on the application and comparisons of various revascularization strategies. These data have helped in formulating well-defined indications for and the selection of appropriate revascularization methods. However, because of rapid growth and refinements in revascularization techniques and technologies, the optimal method of revascularization for numerous patients continues to be a subject of intense debate. In this chapter, we summarize the data from clinical trials and databases, with a view to developing a conceptual framework that allows the application of this information to clinical practice.

The effectiveness of coronary artery bypass graft surgery versus medical therapy (see also Chapter 27)

The early randomized trials of the 1970s first established CABG as an effective treatment for angina pectoris. These small, prospective, randomized controlled trials included the European Coronary Surgery Study (ECSS),[2,3] the Veterans Administration Coronary Artery Bypass Surgery Cooperative Study (VA)[4] and the Coronary Artery Surgery Study (CASS).[5,6] The trials compared CABG with medical therapy in patients who had stable angina. In a collaborative meta-analysis,[3] the primary patient information on 2649 patients enrolled in the evaluated trials was combined to assess outcomes at five and 10 years. Overall, CABG improved survival across all patients by 4.3 months at 10-year follow-up ($P = 0.003$). Because of the perioperative mortality rate associated with CABG, the mortality rate at one year was not significantly different between the groups, and a net benefit in favor of CABG was not observed for 2–3 years. At 5–7 years, the advantage with CABG increased before it narrowed again at 10–12 years (Fig. 28.1). A significant heterogeneity of treatment effect was observed among various angiographic and clinical subsets. The patients who seemed to derive the most benefit were those with left main CAD (n = 174) (relative risk (RR) 0.32; $P = 0.004$), multivessel disease (RR 0.58; $P < 0.001$), and one- or two-vessel disease with proximal left anterior descending coronary artery (LAD) involvement (RR 0.58; $P = 0.05$). Although the relative benefits were similar

Evidence-Based Cardiology, 3rd edition. Edited by S. Yusuf, J.A. Cairns, A.J. Camm, E.L. Fallen, and B.J. Gersh. © 2010 Blackwell Publishing, ISBN: 978-1-4051-5925-8.

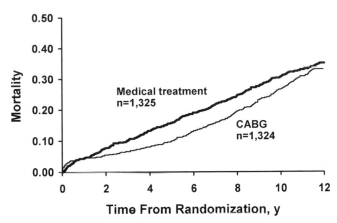

Figure 28.1 Comparison of mortality rates of all studies in meta-analysis of trials of coronary artery bypass grafting (CABG) versus medical treatment. (Reproduced with permission from Yusuf et al[3])

regardless of left ventricular (LV) function, the absolute benefit was greater in patients with abnormal LV ejection fraction (EF) because of the higher risk of death in this group. Absolute mortality benefits were also greater among patients with evidence of myocardial ischemia as manifested by severe anginal symptoms or an abnormal exercise test (Table 28.1).

It has been established that, in regard to symptomatic improvement, surgically treated patients have a higher likelihood of staying symptom free than medically treated patients, and use less antianginal medication than medically treated patients at five years.[7] However, at 10 years, these differences are not statistically significant. It should be noted, however, that a high degree of cross-over from medical treatment to surgical treatment by 10 years may account for these findings.

In the application of these results to patient care in the current era, several limitations of the trials must be recognized. These early trials tended to include low-risk patients of whom only 20% had an EF of less than 50%. Furthermore, almost all patients were male and between 40 and 60 years of age. Only one trial (CASS) included women and, in this trial, medical therapy was limited to nitrates and beta-blockers. At the time of these trials, aspirin and lipid-lowering agents were not routinely prescribed for patients with CAD. In CASS, only 14% of patients received an internal mammary artery (IMA) graft.[8] The profound impact of these grafts on survival is now well documented.[9,10] The limited use of IMA grafts is a critical limitation of earlier trials of CABG. Also, patients with severe LV dysfunction were excluded from most of the randomized controlled trials. Data on this patient group are largely based on observational studies. In their meta-analysis of randomized trials, Yusuf et al[3] found that 40% of the patients assigned to medical therapy in the trials had had surgery by 10 years. These cross-overs in treatment tended to occur in the subgroups at highest risk. Therefore, the true benefits

of surgery, particularly in the high-risk groups, are likely underestimated. In the recent BARI 2D trial performed in patients with type 2 diabetes and stable coronary artery disease, by 5 years of follow-up there were fewer major cardiovascular events among CABG patients than among those receiving only optimal medical therapy.[40a]

Patients older than 75 years are increasingly undergoing CABG, and population-based rates estimates are higher than for patients younger than 75 years.[2,11] Despite this profile of increasing risk, operative mortality rates have continued to decline.[12] Since the early trials, advances have been substantial in the medical, percutaneous, and surgical management of CAD. Beta-blocker use is now more widespread, and the introduction of newer antiplatelet agents, statins, and angiotensin-converting enzyme inhibitors has revolutionized the medical management of these patients. Percutaneous revascularization techniques are common and continue to evolve with improved technology, experience, and the use of drug-eluting stents (DES) and adjuvant antiplatelet therapies. The operative and perioperative management of patients who undergo bypass surgery has also improved with increased use of arterial grafting, less invasive procedures, and improved attention to secondary prevention. Although the main messages obtained from the early trials are still relevant today, estimates of the degree of risks and benefits are likely to be different today from those suggested by these studies.

The effectiveness of percutaneous coronary intervention

Since the introduction of percutaneous transluminal coronary angioplasty (PTCA) in the 1970s as a treatment for single-vessel CAD, it has become one of the most commonly performed procedures. During the past three decades, PTCA procedures have been applied to multivessel CAD and even to left main CAD. Initial trials of PTCA compared balloon angioplasty with medical therapy. However, with the advent of coronary artery stents, subsequent studies saw an increasing use of these devices.

Balloon angioplasty versus medical therapy
(see also Chapter 26)

A meta-analysis of six prospective, randomized clinical trials comparing balloon angioplasty with medical therapy included 1904 patients with nonacute CAD.[13,14] Among the low-risk patients with symptomatic CAD (Canadian Cardiovascular Society (CCS) angina class II or greater; average mortality rate <1% per year), balloon angioplasty clearly provided superior control of angina pectoris, although it was associated with an increased need for subsequent CABG. There was no significant impact on subsequent

Table 28.1 Results of subgroups with medical therapy and with coronary artery bypass grafting (CABG) at five years

Subgroup	Overall numbers		Medical treatment mortality rate, %	Odds ratio (95% CI)	P for CABG surgery vs medical treatment	P for interaction
	Deaths	Patients				
Vessel disease						
One vessel	21	271	9.9	0.54 (0.22–1.33)	0.18	0.19
Two vessels	92	859	11.7	0.84 (0.54–1.32)	0.45	
Three vessels	189	1341	17.6	0.58 (0.42–0.80)	<0.001	
Left main artery	39	150	36.5	0.32 (0.15–0.70)	0.004	
No LAD disease						
One or two vessels	50	606	8.3	1.05 (0.58–1.90)	0.88	0.06
Three vessels	46	410	14.5	0.47 (0.25–0.89)	0.02	
Left main artery	16	51	45.8	0.27 (0.08–0.90)	0.03	
Overall	112	1067	12.3	0.66 (0.44–1.00)	0.05	
LAD disease present						
One or two vessels	63	524	14.6	0.58 (0.34–1.01)	0.05	0.44
Three vessels	143	929	19.1	0.61 (0.42–0.88)	0.009	
Left main artery	22	96	32.7	0.30 (0.11–0.84)	0.02	
Overall	228	1549	18.3	0.58 (0.43–0.77)	0.001	
LV function						
Normal	228	2095	13.3	0.61 (0.46–0.81)	<0.001	0.90
Abnormal	115	549	25.2	0.59 (0.39–0.91)	0.02	
Exercise test status						
Missing	102	664	17.4	0.69 (0.45–1.07)	0.10	0.37
Normal	60	585	11.6	0.78 (0.45–1.35)	0.38	
Abnormal	183	1400	16.8	0.52 (0.37–0.72)	<0.001	
Severity of angina						
Class 0, I, II	178	1716	12.5	0.63 (0.46–0.87)	0.005	0.69
Class III, IV	167	924	22.4	0.57 (0.40–0.81)	0.001	

CI, confidence interval; LAD, left anterior descending artery; LV, left ventricular. Modified from Yusuf et al,[3] with permission.

death, MI or subsequent balloon angioplasty. These data suggested that balloon angioplasty was indicated when the desired level of anginal relief and physical activity could not be achieved with medical therapy alone and that prophylactic balloon angioplasty could not be recommended for the treatment of CAD in the absence of angina or ischemia.[14] However, most of these studies were undertaken before 1997. Balloon angioplasty was plagued by restenosis, with a need for repeat procedures in up to 34% of patients at one year.[15]

Bare metal stents

The high incidence of restenosis after balloon angioplasty was initially addressed with the introduction of bare metal stents (BMS). Introduced for the treatment of coronary dissections after balloon angioplasty, BMS were rapidly adopted by clinicians for routine use during balloon angioplasty, thus leading to immediate improvements in procedural safety and success. In particular, the rate of emergency CABG decreased from about 5% to less than 1%, and angiographic success became routine and independent of lesion morphologic factors[16] (Fig. 28.2). The short-term therapeutic effects of these stents have been evaluated in several trials,[17,18] and although restenosis was significantly decreased, it continued to be a substantial clinical problem.[17] In a meta-analysis based on 29 trials involving 9918 patients, there was no evidence of a difference between routine coronary stenting and standard PTCA in terms of deaths or MI (odds ratio (OR) 0.90, 95% confidence interval (CI) 0.72–1.11) or the need for CABG (OR 1.01, CI 0.79–1.31). Coronary stenting decreased both the rate of restenosis (OR 0.52, CI 0.37–0.69) and the need for repeated PTCA (OR 0.59, CI 0.50–0.68).[19] It is important to note that these trials did not include higher-risk lesions treatable with stenting but not with PTCA alone.

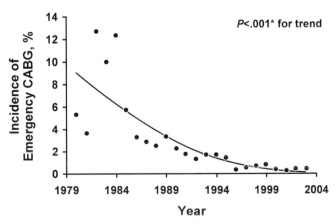

Figure 28.2 Incidence of emergency coronary artery bypass grafting (CABG) over time after percutaneous coronary intervention procedures, 1979–2004. *Armitage test for trend. (Reproduced with permission from Yang et al[16])

Several studies have compared PCI performed with or without stents with medical therapy in patients who have stable CAD. A meta-analysis of 11 randomized controlled trials of PCI versus medical therapy included a total of 2950 patients with non-acute CAD.[20] The use of stents in the trials of this meta-analysis was variable (range, 30–100%). There was no substantial difference between initial PCI and initial medical strategies with regard to mortality rate, cardiac death, fatal MI or non-fatal MI[20] (Fig. 28.3).

The most recent comparison of PCI and medical therapy was the Clinical Outcomes Utilizing Revascularization and Aggressive Drug Evaluation (COURAGE) trial.[21] The investigators randomly assigned 2287 patients with stable CAD to receive either optimal medical therapy alone or PCI with optimal medical therapy on the basis of carefully selected clinical and angiographic criteria. At a median follow-up of 4.6 years, the cumulative frequency of the primary endpoint of death or non-fatal MI was 19.0% in the PCI group and 18.5% in the medical therapy group ($P = 0.62$).

In conclusion, PCI and medical therapy appear to lead to similar outcomes in rates of death and MI in patients with stable CAD. PCI with BMS is consistently associated with lower rates of angina and subsequent revascularization compared with medical therapy. In patients who have characteristics similar to those of patients enrolled in the randomized controlled trials, either strategy, medical therapy or PCI, is appropriate.

Drug-eluting stents

Despite the introduction of BMS, the chief limiting factor of percutaneous revascularization continued to be restenosis. Consequently, numerous agents have been used as stent coatings in the hope of preventing thrombosis, neointimal proliferation, and subsequent restenosis. Currently, all FDA-approved DES are a device-polymer-drug combination. Several randomized clinical trials have found that these stents are efficacious in decreasing the rates of restenosis and revascularization.[22–37]

In a meta-analysis of 19 randomized controlled trials that included 8987 patients and compared DES with BMS, the overall mortality rate was not significantly different between the treatment groups (0.9% with DES vs 1.2% with BMS; $P = 0.92$).[38] The overall adjusted rate for angiographic restenosis was 10.6% in the DES group versus 31.8% in the BMS (control) group ($P < 0.001$) (Fig. 28.4). The overall adjusted rate for angiographic target-lesion revascularization was 6.2% in the DES group versus 16.6% in the control group ($P < 0.001$). The Q-wave MI-adjusted percentage was 1.1% with DES versus 0.8% with BMS ($P = 0.33$).

There has been a tendency to regard restenosis as a benign process. However, emerging data seem to challenge

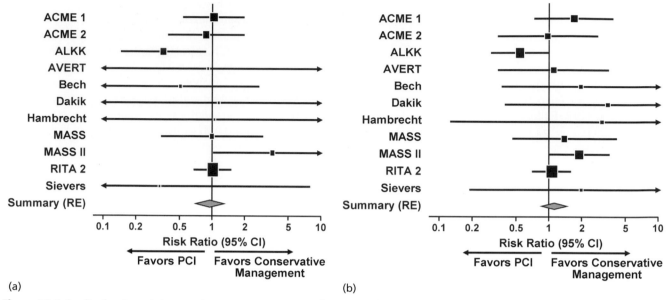

Figure 28.3 Results of meta-analysis comparing percutaneous coronary intervention (PCI) with conservative management. (a) Death. (b) Cardiac death or myocardial infarction. ACME, Angioplasty Compared to Medicine Evaluation; ALKK, Working Group of Leading Hospital Cardiologists; AVERT, Atorvastatin Versus Revascularization Treatment; CI, confidence interval; MASS, Medicine, Angioplasty or Surgery Study; RE, random effects; RITA, Randomized Intervention Treatment of Angina. (Reproduced with permission from Katritsis and Ioannidis.[32])

this notion, largely because a substantial fraction of patients who have restenosis present with acute coronary syndromes. In a study of 4503 consecutive patients treated with at least one BMS, 667 patients had 836 occurrences of clinical restenosis.[39] The cumulative incidence of at least one restenosis was 9.6% at one year, 13.9% at five years, and 18.1% at 10 years. Among all patients, the 10-year incidence of restenosis according to mode of presentation was stable angina in 9.0%, unstable angina in 7.4%, MI in 2.1%, and other unstable presentations, such as decompensated heart failure or ventricular arrhythmia, in 0.4%. Among 87 patients with an MI presentation of restenosis, non-ST segment elevation MI (NSTEMI) was seen in 87% and ST segment elevation MI (STEMI) was seen in 13%. Presentation of MI with restenosis was associated with a significantly greater mortality risk than either a presentation of MI with no restenosis (hazard ratio (HR) 2.37, 95% CI 1.72–3.27; $P < 0.001$) or a non-MI presentation of restenosis (HR 2.42, 95% CI 1.68–3.47; $P < 0.001$). Interestingly, there was no significant difference in long-term survival among patients with no restenosis compared to patients with a non-MI presentation of restenosis (HR 0.99, 95% CI 0.85–1.14; $P = 0.85$).

Safety

There have been recent concerns about the long-term safety of DES. However, recent pooled analyses of the trials of

sirolimus-eluting stents and paclitaxel-eluting stents show no difference in the long-term rates of death, MI or stent thrombosis.[40–42] In one analysis, the risk of stent thrombosis increased after one year with the use of a DES.[43] This did not translate into an increased frequency of death or of MI. Data from the Swedish Coronary Angiography and Angioplasty Registry (SCARR)[44] seemed to suggest an increased incidence of both death and MI on long-term follow-up of patients with DES. More recent data from SCARR showed no differences in death or MI.[45] In the clinical trials, the enrolled subjects were patients with PCI who were at relatively low risk.

A 2006 review of patient data in the American College of Cardiology (ACC) National Cardiovascular Data Registry found that 24% of procedures involving DES were for off-label indications (i.e. STEMI, in-stent restenosis, saphenous vein graft stenosis, and chronic total occlusion).[46] Of the 3323 patients in the Evaluation of Drug-eluting Stents and Ischemic Events (EVENT) registry, 1817 (54.7%) patients had at least one off-label characteristic on the basis of FDA-approved indications for sirolimus- and paclitaxel-eluting stents. During the index hospitalization, the composite clinical outcome occurred in 198 (10.9%) patients in the off-label group and 76 (5.0%) patients in the on-label group (adjusted OR 2.32, 95% CI 1.75–3.07; $P < 0.001$). At one year, the composite clinical outcome occurred more often in the off-label group (309 (17.5%) patients) than in the on-label group

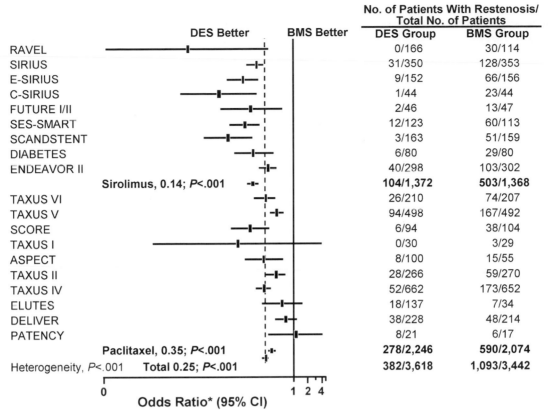

	No. of Patients With Restenosis/ Total No. of Patients	
	DES Group	**BMS Group**
RAVEL	0/166	30/114
SIRIUS	31/350	128/353
E-SIRIUS	9/152	66/156
C-SIRIUS	1/44	23/44
FUTURE I/II	2/46	13/47
SES-SMART	12/123	60/113
SCANDSTENT	3/163	51/159
DIABETES	6/80	29/80
ENDEAVOR II	40/298	103/302
Sirolimus, 0.14; P<.001	**104/1,372**	**503/1,368**
TAXUS VI	26/210	74/207
TAXUS V	94/498	167/492
SCORE	6/94	38/104
TAXUS I	0/30	3/29
ASPECT	8/100	15/55
TAXUS II	28/266	59/270
TAXUS IV	52/662	173/652
ELUTES	18/137	7/34
DELIVER	38/228	48/214
PATENCY	8/21	6/17
Paclitaxel, 0.35; P<.001	**278/2,246**	**590/2,074**
Heterogeneity, P<.001 Total 0.25; P<.001	**382/3,618**	**1,093/3,442**

Figure 28.4 Angiographic restenosis found in meta-analysis of trials comparing the drug-eluting stent (DES) with the bare metal stent (BMS). ASPECT, Asian Paclitaxel-eluting Stent Clinical Trial; C-SIRIUS, Canadian Sirolimus-coated Balloon-expandable Stent in the Treatment of Patients With De Novo Native Coronary Artery Lesions; DELIVER, Non-polymer-based Paclitaxel-coated Coronary Stents for the Treatment of Patients With De Novo Coronary Lesions; DIABETES, Diabetes and Sirolimus-eluting Stent Trial; ELUTES, European Evaluation of Paclitaxel-eluting Stent; ENDEAVOR, Randomized, Controlled Trial of the Medtronic Endeavor Drug (ABT-578)-eluting Coronary Stent System Versus the Taxus Paclitaxel-eluting Coronary Stent System in De Novo Native Coronary Artery Lesions; E-SIRIUS, European Sirolimus-coated Balloon-expandable Stent in the Treatment of Patients with De Novo Native Coronary Artery Lesions; FUTURE, First Use to Underscore Reduction in Restenosis With Everolimus; PATENCY, Paclitaxel-coated Logic Stent for the Cytostatic Prevention of Restenosis; RAVEL, Randomized Study With Sirolimus-coated BX Velocity Balloon-expandable Stent in the Treatment of Patients with De Novo Native Coronary Lesions; SCANDSTENT, Randomized Multicentre Comparison of Sirolimus Versus Bare Metal Stent Implantation in Complex Coronary Lesions; SCORE, Study to Compare Restenosis Rate Quest and Quads QP2; SES-SMART, Randomized Comparison of a Sirolimus-eluting Stent and a Standard Stent in the Prevention of Restenosis in Small Coronary Arteries; SIRIUS, Sirolimus-eluting Balloon-expandable Stent in the Treatment of Patients With De Novo Native Coronary Artery Lesions; TAXUS, Treatment of De Novo Coronary Disease Using a Single Paclitaxel-eluting Stent. *OR 0.25 (95% CI 0.22–0.29); P < 0.001. (Modified with permission from Roiron et al[38])

(131 (8.9%) patients) (adjusted HR 2.16, 95% CI 1.74–2.67; P < 0.001). In-stent thrombosis also occurred more frequently among patients in the off-label group than among patients in the on-label group during the initial hospitalization (8 (0.4%) patients vs 0 patients) and at one year (29 (1.6%) patients vs 13 (0.9%) patients) (adjusted HR 2.29, 95% CI 1.02–5.16; P = 0.05).[47]

A higher prevalence of complex interventions that use DES in subsets of patients at relatively higher risk will in all likelihood translate into increased event rates in DES subgroups in registry studies. For all these high-risk groups, compared to low-risk groups, event rates are increased after any treatment. The available data on the use of DES in specific complex subsets of patients and lesions seem to suggest that these stents may be superior to BMS in these circumstances.[48,49] Randomized clinical trials are needed to fully define the role of DES in such patient groups.[50]

Comparisons of percutaneous coronary intervention versus coronary artery bypass graft

Considerable controversy has existed, and continues to exist, about the relative benefits of PTCA compared with CABG as initial treatment strategies. Up to 15 randomized trials comparing PCI, with or without stents, with CABG have been published and were reviewed extensively by both Eagle *et al*[51] and Hoffman *et al*.[52] Recently, the 10-year results of the Bypass Angioplasty Revascularization Investigation (BARI), the largest of the randomized trials of PTCA versus CABG, were published.[52] In this trial, 1829 symptomatic patients with multivessel CAD were randomly assigned to initial treatment with PTCA or CABG and were observed for an average of 10.4 years. The 10-year survival was 71.0% for the PTCA group and 73.5% for the CABG group ($P = 0.18$). At 10 years, the PTCA group had substantially higher subsequent revascularization rates than the CABG group (76.8% vs 20.3%; $P < 0.001$), but angina rates for the two groups were similar. In the subgroup of patients with no treated diabetes mellitus, survival rates were nearly identical for the PTCA group compared with the CABG group (77.0% vs 77.3%; $P = 0.59$). In the subgroup with treated diabetes, the group assigned CABG had higher survival rates than the group assigned PTCA (57.8% vs 45.5%; $P < 0.03$).

Another recent publication comparing CABG, PCI, and medical therapy was based on the five-year outcomes of the Medicine, Angioplasty or Surgery Study-II (MASS-II)[53,54] which randomly assigned 611 patients with stable angina to medical therapy, PCI or CABG. Medical therapy included aspirin, angiotensin-converting enzyme inhibitors, beta-blockers, and statins. At five-year follow-up, the primary endpoints had occurred in 21.2% of patients who underwent CABG compared with 32.7% of patients treated with PCI and 36% of patients who received medical therapy alone ($P < 0.003$).

The paired treatment comparisons of the primary endpoints showed no difference between PCI and medical therapy (RR 0.93, 95% CI 0.67–1.30) and a significant protective effect of CABG compared with medical therapy (RR 0.53, 95% CI 0.36–0.77). The cumulative survival rate was 88.4% for PCI, 92.1% for CABG and 87.7% for medical therapy; the survival rates were not significantly different. Additional interventions were performed for 32.2% of the PCI patients, 24.2% of the medically treated patients, and 3.5% of the surgically treated patients ($P < 0.03$). Non-fatal MI occurred in 11.2% of the PCI group, 15.3% of the medically treated group, and 8.3% of the CABG group ($P < 0.79$). It is important to note, however, that the degree of revascularization achieved in the PCI group and the CABG group differed. Although 74% of all intended vessels were grafted in the surgical cases, only 41% of cases in the PCI group were completely revascularized. Adjunctive pharmacotherapy with clopidogrel and glycoprotein IIb/IIIa inhibitors was not utilized. Although stenting was performed in at least one vessel in 72% of cases, BMS were used. Because of these considerations, and even though this trial suggests a relative inferiority of PCI as a treatment strategy, the argument could be made that the results are not applicable to the current setting.

Since the advent of coronary stenting, several trials have compared stents with CABG in patients with multivessel disease. The Arterial Revascularization Therapy Study (ARTS)[56] randomly assigned 1205 patients with multivessel disease to PCI with stents or to CABG. At five years, the mortality rate was 8.0% in the stent group and 7.6% in the CABG group ($P = 0.83$). Among 208 diabetic patients, the mortality rate was 13.4% in the stent group and 8.3% in the CABG group ($P = 0.27$) (see section on diabetic patients, below). Overall, freedom from death, stroke or MI was not significantly different between the stent group (18.2%) and the surgical group (14.9%) ($P = 0.14$). The incidence of repeat revascularization was significantly higher in the stent group than in the CABG group (30.3% vs 8.8%; $P < 0.001$). The rate of composite event-free survival (freedom from cardiovascular and cerebrovascular events) was 58.3% in the stent group and 78.2% in the CABG group ($P < 0.0001$).

Two additional trials showed the superiority of CABG in terms of fewer repeat revascularization procedures. In the multicenter Stent or Surgery (SoS) trial,[57] based on 988 patients, the primary endpoint of repeat revascularization occurred in 21% of the patients in the stent group versus 6% of those in the surgical group ($P < 0.001$). In the Argentine Randomized Trial: Coronary Angioplasty Versus Coronary Bypass Surgery in Multivessel Disease-II (ERACI-II),[58] 450 patients with multivessel disease were randomly assigned to undergo either PCI or CABG. At five years, there were no significant differences in the rate of death from all causes between the CABG and PCI arms (11.5% vs 7.1%; $P < 0.19$). There also were no significant differences in the incidence rates of new non-fatal MI between the PCI and CABG groups (2.8% vs 6.2%; $P < 0.13$). However, the incidence of repeat revascularization was 28.4% in the PCI group and 7.2% in the CABG group ($P < 0.001$). Of note, none of these trials included patients treated with DES, which have been shown to decrease the rate of repeat revascularization.

In a recent meta-analysis based on 23 randomized controlled trials, in which 5019 patients were randomly assigned to PCI and 4944 to CABG, the difference in subsequent survival rates with PCI versus CABG was less than 1% over 10 years of follow-up.[59] Survival did not differ between the PCI group and the CABG group for patients with diabetes mellitus in the six trials that reported on this subgroup. Procedure-related strokes were more common after CABG than after PCI (1.2% vs 0.6%; $P = 0.002$). Angina relief was greater after CABG than after PCI, with absolute risk differences ranging from 5% to 8% at 1–5 years ($P < 0.001$). Angina was relieved at five years in 79% of PCI patients and 84% of CABG patients. Repeat revascularization was more common after PCI than after CABG (absolute risk difference 24% at one year and 33% at five years; $P < 0.001$); the absolute rates at five years were 46.1% after balloon angioplasty, 40.1% after PCI with stents, and 9.8% after CABG. In the observational studies, the HR for death favored PCI among patients with the least severe disease and CABG among those with the most severe disease.

It should be noted that these trials did not include patients who were considered to be at high risk for an adverse outcome with surgical treatment. Data comparing surgical intervention with PCI in this subgroup of patients are limited. The Angina With Extremely Serious Operative Mortality Evaluation (AWESOME) study enrolled 454 patients of high surgical risk at 16 Veterans Affairs hospitals.[60] This five-year, multicenter, randomized clinical trial was designed to compare long-term survival among patients with medically refractory myocardial ischemia and a high risk of adverse outcomes who were assigned to either a CABG or a PCI strategy, which could include stents. At 36 months, the survival rates in both groups were similar (79% with CABG vs 80% with PCI).

For treatment of patients with single-vessel CAD, the trial most relevant to clinical practice was the Stenting Versus Internal Mammary Artery (SIMA) trial,[61] in which 121 patients with isolated LAD disease were randomly assigned to BMS or CABG with the left IMA. At 2.4 years, patients assigned to stenting had experienced more revascularization procedures than patients who were surgically treated (31% vs 7%). Mortality rates did not differ between the two groups.

In summary, these trials have shown that CABG tends to give better relief of angina with less need for repeat procedures than does PCI. However, with PCI, initial costs are lower, complications occur less frequently, and patients are able to return to work earlier. Because of the greater need for reinterventions, patients who have PCI generate direct costs over the long term that are similar to those of patients who have CABG. Long-term survival rates also tend to be similar with the two forms of treatment. This similarity appears to hold true for diabetic patients, as well as the patients described earlier in this chapter.

It must be recognized that the patients enrolled in such trials are not always representative of the global population of patients with CAD; therefore, the results of such trials are not necessarily applicable to the general population of patients. Indeed, only 5% of screened patients with multivessel disease were enrolled in these trials, and patients with left main disease were excluded. Registry studies have provided valuable information about the relative benefits of medical therapy, PCI, and CABG, particularly for the global population of patients with CAD. In general, these studies have yielded results that are congruent with the findings of the randomized trials.

Jones *et al*[62] reviewed the Duke University Medical Center database of 9263 patients with CAD who underwent PCI (n = 2924), CABG (n = 3890) or medical therapy (n = 2449) only. Patients were observed for a mean of 5.3 years. The anatomic severity of the coronary artery stenoses best defined the survival benefit from CABG and PCI versus medical treatment. All patients with single-vessel disease, except those with proximal LAD stenosis of 95% or greater, benefited from PCI compared with CABG. All patients with three-vessel disease and those with two-vessel disease and proximal LAD stenosis of 95% or greater were best treated by CABG.

A recently published study based on the New York State PCI and CABG registries examined the outcomes of 37 212 patients who had undergone CABG and 22 102 patients who had undergone PCI with stenting.[63] The adjusted HR for the long-term risk of death after CABG relative to stent implantation was 0.64 (95% CI 0.56–0.74) for patients with three-vessel disease with involvement of the proximal LAD and 0.76 (95% CI 0.60–0.96) for patients with two-vessel disease with involvement of the non-proximal LAD. Additionally, the three-year rates of revascularization were considerably higher in the stenting group compared to the CABG group (7.8% vs 0.3% for subsequent CABG; 27.3% vs 4.6% for subsequent PCI). However, 85% of patients with multivessel disease underwent CABG. Therefore, only those patients who had specific reasons not to undergo bypass surgery underwent PCI. Such reasons may have included high surgical risk, poor target vessels, and patient refusal. This clearly leads to a substantial selection bias. The superior results observed with CABG in such studies seem to derive from more frequent complete revascularization. In a subsequent publication assessing patients with PCI who received stents, the authors compared long-term mortality rates and subsequent revascularization among patients with complete versus incomplete revascularization. After adjustment for these baseline differences, the data show that patients who received incomplete revascularization were significantly more likely to die at any time (adjusted HR 1.15, 95% CI 1.01–1.30) than patients who received complete revascularization. Patients with total occlusions and a total of two vessels with incomplete revascularization were at higher risk compared with patients who received complete revascularization (HR 1.36, 95% CI 1.12–1.66).

Given that the advantage of CABG seems to be driven largely by a decreased frequency of revascularization procedures, there is great interest in comparisons of CABG with PCI using DES. The ARTS-II registry is a non-randomized comparison of contemporary PCI with historic controls from the ARTS-I in patients with multivessel CAD (n = 607 patients).[64] The primary endpoint of the study was major adverse cardiovascular and cerebrovascular events (MACCEs), including death, cerebrovascular event, MI, and revascularization at one year. The event-free survival was 89.5% in ARTS-II compared with 88.5% in the ARTS-I CABG registry. Survival free from reintervention was 91.5% in ARTS-II compared with 95.9% in the ARTS-I CABG registry. There were no differences in terms of death, cerebrovascular event, MI, and repeat CABG between the ARTS-I patients who received BMS, the ARTS-II patients who received DES, and the ARTS-I patients who had CABG. However, a significantly higher revascularization rate was seen in the ARTS-I stent group. These observations suggest that DES may significantly improve outcomes in patients with multivessel disease.

The current relevance of the trials mentioned above is limited because of the use of non-contemporary PCI techniques. In recent years, progress has been made in surgical revascularization. The impact on mortality rate of an IMA graft to the LAD is clear.[65] On the basis of studies demonstrating superior outcomes with bilateral IMA grafts[10] and complete arterial revascularization, surgeons are increasingly using additional arterial conduits. Even among those surgeons using venous conduits, long-term outcomes are improving with the routine use of pharmacologic agents for secondary prevention.[66] Furthermore, off-pump techniques likely reduce operative risks in some subsets of patients.[67]

Currently, at least four randomized clinical trials are comparing DES with CABG in multivessel or left main disease.[68] The Synergy Between PCI With Taxus Drug-eluting Stent and Cardiac Surgery (SYNTAX) trial[68a] was based in multiple centers in Europe and the United States and enrolled 1800 patients. The primary outcome of 12-month MACCEs was significantly higher in the PCI group (17.8%, vs. 12.4% for CABG; P = 0.002), mainly because of an increased rate of repeat revascularization (13.5% vs. 5.9%, P < 0.001). The rates of death and myocardial infarction were similar between the two groups, whereas stroke was more frequent with CABG (2.2% vs. 0.6% with PCI; P = 0.003). At least three trials of PCI with DES versus CABG are being conducted in diabetic patients and are discussed below.

In the decision about revascularization for a patient, many factors must be taken into consideration, including the patient's age, coronary anatomy, extent of stenoses, co-morbidities, LV function and, to some degree, preference. In addition, the technical suitability for either PCI or CABG and the urgency of the procedure must be considered. The importance of such an approach was highlighted by data from the BARI registry, where physician-selected procedures resulted in excellent outcomes. The mortality rates at seven years were similar for PTCA (13.9%) and

CABG (14.2%) (P = 0.66) before and after adjustment for baseline differences between patients selected for PTCA versus those selected for CABG (adjusted RR 1.02; P = 0.86).[69] Both PCI and CABG provide good relief of symptoms in most patients who are appropriately selected. These procedures need to be considered as complementary, and many patients will undergo both of these techniques of revascularization during their lifetime.

Coronary artery bypass graft versus percutaneous coronary intervention in diabetic patients

The prevalence of diabetes mellitus in the United States is increasing rapidly, mirroring the rapid rise in obesity. In 1999, 4.9% of the US population were estimated to have diabetes; by 2002, this percentage had increased to 6.3%.[70–72] Of individuals older than 60 years, 18.3% are estimated to be diabetic. These demographic changes are almost certainly related to the aging of the US population, a sedentary lifestyle, poor diet, and obesity. This alarming increase in prevalence of diabetes has important consequences related to CAD and its management, and for society as a whole.

For persons with type 1 diabetes, the mortality rate from cardiovascular disease is four times that of the general population[73] and, by age 55 years, one-third of these patients will have died of CAD.[74] For persons with type 2 diabetes, the incidence of atherosclerosis is estimated to be 2–3 times that of the general population.[75] The risk of an acute MI for persons with diabetes is 20% over seven years, with a hospital mortality rate that is 1.5–2.0 times higher than that for people without diabetes.[76] Moreover, persons with diabetes who have an MI are more likely to experience congestive heart failure, cardiogenic shock, recurrent ischemia, and reinfarction and eventually have a poorer survival rate.[77]

The observed poorer clinical outcomes among diabetic patients with CAD are likely due to multiple factors, including co-existent renal disease, hypertension, peripheral vascular disease and the aggressive nature of the CAD itself. Compared with persons who do not have diabetes, diabetic people are more likely to have left main disease,[78–82] multivessel disease, diffuse disease with smaller luminal diameters, and a larger number of lipid-rich plaques, which are more prone to rupture.[83] Persons with diabetes who have CAD represent a special high-risk subset of patients in whom very aggressive treatment strategies are warranted.

Indications for coronary revascularization in patients with diabetes are generally the same as for non-diabetic patients and include symptom improvement, left main disease, three-vessel disease (particularly with decreased LV function), and severe angina. However, diabetic patients are more likely to be asymptomatic than non-diabetic patients, with significant myocardial ischemia. In the absence of angina, progression of ischemia with decreased LV function may occur, and this ischemia may explain, in part, the ultimate poorer prognosis in diabetic patients. The Asymptomatic Cardiac Ischemia Pilot (ACIP) study, including patients with and without diabetes, showed that, in the absence of angina, coronary revascularization was beneficial in selected patients.[84] Overall, when therapy was directed by the onset of subsequent angina, the mortality rate at two years was 6.6% in patients with known CAD. Patients who received revascularization in the absence of angina but as guided by the presence of ischemia had a mortality rate at two years of 1.1%. Because of the asymptomatic nature of CAD in many persons with diabetes, an aggressive approach should be adopted in these patients to detect myocardial ischemia and to advise subsequent revascularization.

According to the 10-year outcomes of the BARI trial and in the subgroup with treated diabetes, the group assigned CABG had a higher survival rate than the group assigned PTCA (57.8% vs 45.5%; $P < 0.03$).[53] Similar findings showing a trend toward improved results with CABG compared with PCI for diabetic patients were also observed in the Emory Angioplasty Versus Surgery Trial (EAST)[85] (the eight-year mortality rate with CABG was 24.5%; with PCI, 39.9%). As mentioned previously, the patients in ARTS who had diabetes and underwent stenting had a mortality rate of 13.4% at five years compared with 8.3% in those who underwent CABG.[69] Within the stent group, diabetic patients had a significantly higher mortality rate than non-diabetic patients. In the meta-analysis reported by Hoffman *et al*, patients with multivessel disease and diabetes had a survival advantage at four years with CABG compared with PCI.[52]

These observations were further put into perspective in the BARI registry, where the mode of revascularization was determined by physician preference. In this registry, patients who were sicker and at higher risk were preferentially referred for CABG, whereas those with lesser degrees of CAD often underwent PCI. During follow-up, diabetic patients in the BARI registry had equal survival rates (74%) whether treated with PCI or with CABG.[69] Interestingly, in a recent meta-analysis comparing PCI with CABG, survival did not differ between PCI and CABG for patients with diabetes in the six trials that reported on this subgroup.[59]

The better survival results observed with CABG than with PCI seem to result from both the use of arterial grafting and the extent of revascularization. The improved survival rate seen in diabetic patients who underwent CABG was contingent on the presence of an IMA graft to the LAD (seven-year survival rate, 83.2%; for IMA graft, n = 140), whereas long-term survival of patients treated with saphenous vein grafts was similar to that of patients treated with balloon angioplasty.[86] Patients with an IMA graft had a dramatic reduction in the mortality rate after subsequent MI compared with patients who did not receive an IMA graft. Further data from the BARI trial indicated that diabetic patients appeared to have more complete revascularization and less jeopardized myocardium at risk after CABG compared with diabetic patients who received revascularization with PCI. Diabetic patients also had increased rates of restenosis after PCI compared with non-diabetic patients, whereas graft patency in those who underwent CABG (venous and arterial) was not influenced by diabetes status.[87] These data suggest that the survival advantage of CABG in diabetic patients may result from a more complete and more durable revascularization than that achieved by PCI.

A meta-analysis of eight randomized controlled trials of DES versus BMS in diabetic patients showed that target lesion revascularization occurred in 22.9% of patients treated with BMS and 7.5% of patients treated with DES. These data indicate a 66% decrease in the need for target lesion revascularization with DES compared with BMS ($P < 0.001$).[88] Therefore, interest has grown in comparisons of DES with CABG in diabetic patients.

The Future Revascularization Evaluation in Patients With Diabetes Mellitus: Optimal Management of Multivessel Disease (FREEDOM) study is enrolling diabetic patients with multivessel disease, in a randomized controlled trial of PCI with DES versus CABG. The target enrollment is 2400 patients; the primary endpoint is the composite of non-fatal infarction, stroke, and death due to all causes. The minimum planned follow-up is three years.

The Department of Veterans Affairs has approved funding for a similar trial that will randomly assign CABG or PCI to patients with diabetes mellitus who have both a hemoglobin A1c level of greater than 7 and angiographically significant disease with involvement of the anterior wall and one or more other territories. The minimum planned follow-up for this trial is two years. Another trial in diabetic patients is the Coronary Artery Revitalization in Diabetes (CARDia) trial, based in the United Kingdom and Ireland. This trial is making a comparison between PCI with both DES and abciximab and CABG in patients with multivessel disease or complex single-vessel disease. The primary endpoint is the composite of death, non-fatal MI, and a cerebrovascular accident at one year.

The BARI 2D trial[10a] focused on earlier revascularization and the use of insulin sensitizing therapies. In the PCI stratum, there was no difference in major vascular events between those randomized to PCI vs those to optimal medical therapy. However, in the CABG stratum, there were significantly fewer major vascular events among those randomized to CABG vs. those to optimal medial therapy.

On the basis of the data presented herein, CABG is the best revascularization procedure for most diabetic patients with multivessel disease. In the near future, ongoing trials comparing DES with CABG will help define the role of PCI in the management of these patients.

Conclusions and recommendations

The following recommendations summarize the points of care for revascularization of patients with chronic stable angina.
- Revascularization by means of CABG or PCI is indicated in patients with chronic stable angina refractory to medical therapy (**Class I, Level A**).
- Patients at moderate to high risk for adverse outcomes with medical therapy should be treated with CABG. Such patients include those with left main or multivessel disease; two-vessel disease with involvement of the proximal LAD; LV dysfunction; and diabetes mellitus (**Class I, Level A**).
- For single-vessel disease, both PCI and CABG are effective, but repeat revascularization is required more frequently after PCI than after CABG. However, given the increased initial morbidity and hospitalization with CABG, most patients with single-vessel disease should be treated with PCI (**Class I, Level B**).
- For patients with left main CAD, CABG is indicated (**Class I, Level A**).
- In patients with two-vessel disease and significant proximal LAD involvement and either LV dysfunction or demonstrable ischemia on stress testing, CABG is indicated (**Class I, Level A**).
- For multivessel CAD that is potentially amenable to therapy with either PCI or CABG, a distinction should be made between diabetic patients and non-diabetic patients, and an assessment of LV function should be completed. For diabetic patients and patients with LV dysfunction, CABG is the superior therapy and is the preferred mode of revascularization (**Class I, Level A**). For non-diabetic patients with preserved LV function, the choice of a revascularization strategy has to weigh the initial morbidity associated with CABG against the higher risk of subsequent repeat revascularization and attendant repeat hospitalizations associated with PCI. In this circumstance, a decision is best made by taking the patient's preferences into account after an extensive discussion of the risks, benefits, advantages, and disadvantages of both procedures (**Class I, Level C**).

References

1. Rosamond W, Flegal K, Friday G *et al.* American Heart Association Statistics Committee and Stroke Statistics Subcommittee. Heart disease and stroke statistics: 2007 update: a report from the American Heart Association Statistics Committee and Stroke Statistics Subcommittee. *Circulation* 2007;**115**:e69–171. Erratum in: *Circulation* 2007;**115**:e172.

2. Varnauskas E. Twelve-year follow-up of survival in the randomized European Coronary Surgery Study. *N Engl J Med* 1988;**319**:332–7.

3. Yusuf S, Zucker D, Peduzzi P *et al.* Effect of coronary artery bypass graft surgery on survival: overview of 10-year results from randomised trials by the Coronary Artery Bypass Graft Surgery Trialists Collaboration. *Lancet* 1994;**344**:563–70. Erratum in: *Lancet* 1994;**344**:1446.

4. Veterans Administration Coronary Artery Bypass Surgery Cooperative Study Group. Eleven-year survival in the Veterans Administration randomized trial of coronary bypass surgery for stable angina. *N Engl J Med* 1984;**311**:1333–9.

5. Coronary Artery Surgery Study (CASS). A randomized trial of coronary artery bypass surgery. Quality of life in patients randomly assigned to treatment groups. *Circulation* 1983;**68**:951–60.

6. Hlatky MA, Califf RM, Harrell FE Jr, Lee KL, Mark DB, Pryor DB. Comparison of predictions based on observational data with the results of randomized controlled clinical trials of coronary artery bypass surgery. *J Am Coll Cardiol* 1988;**11**:237–45.

7. Rogers WJ, Coggin CJ, Gersh BJ *et al.* Coronary Artery Surgery Study (CASS). Ten-year follow-up of quality of life in patients randomized to receive medical therapy or coronary artery bypass graft surgery. *Circulation* 1990;**82**:1647–58.

8. Myers WO, Davis K, Foster ED, Maynard C, Kaiser GC. Surgical survival in the Coronary Artery Surgery Study (CASS) registry. *Ann Thorac Surg* 1985;**40**:245–60.

9. Loop FD, Lytle BW, Cosgrove DM *et al.* Influence of the internal-mammary-artery graft on 10-year survival and other cardiac events. *N Engl J Med* 1986;**314**:1–6.

10. Pick AW, Orszulak TA, Anderson BJ, Schaff HV. Single versus bilateral internal mammary artery grafts: 10-year outcome analysis. *Ann Thorac Surg* 1997;**64**:599–605.

10a. The BARI 2D Study Group. A randomized trial of therapies for type 2 diabetes and coronary artery disease. *N Engl J Med* 2009;**360**:2503–15.

11. Gerber T, Rihal CS, Sundt TM 3rd *et al.* Coronary revascularization in the community: a population-based study, 1990 to 2004. *J Am Coll Cardiol* 2007;**50**:1223–9.

12. Ferguson TB Jr, Hammill BG, Peterson ED, DeLong ER, Grover FL, STS National Database Committee, Society of Thoracic Surgeons. A decade of change: risk profiles and outcomes for isolated coronary artery bypass grafting procedures, 1990–1999: a report from the STS National Database Committee and the Duke Clinical Research Institute. *Ann Thorac Surg* 2002;**73**:480–9.

13. Bucher HC, Hengstler P, Schindler C, Guyatt GH. Percutaneous transluminal coronary angioplasty versus medical treatment for non-acute coronary heart disease: meta-analysis of randomised controlled trials. *BMJ* 2000;**321**:73–7.

14. Rihal CS, Raco DL, Gersh BJ, Yusuf S. Indications for coronary artery bypass surgery and percutaneous coronary intervention in chronic stable angina: review of the evidence and methodological considerations. *Circulation* 2003;**108**:2439–45.

15. Pocock SJ, Henderson RA, Rickards AF *et al.* Meta-analysis of randomised trials comparing coronary angioplasty with bypass surgery. *Lancet* 1995;**346**:1184–9.

16. Yang EH, Gumina RJ, Lennon RJ, Holmes DR Jr, Rihal CS, Singh M. Emergency coronary artery bypass surgery for percutaneous

coronary interventions: changes in the incidence, clinical characteristics, and indications from 1979 to 2003. *J Am Coll Cardiol* 2005;**46**:2004–9.

17. Fischman DL, Leon MB, Baim DS *et al.* Stent Restenosis Study Investigators. A randomized comparison of coronary-stent placement and balloon angioplasty in the treatment of coronary artery disease. *N Engl J Med* 1994;**331**:496–501.

18. Serruys PW, de Jaegere P, Kiemeneij F *et al.* Benestent Study Group. A comparison of balloon-expandable-stent implantation with balloon angioplasty in patients with coronary artery disease. *N Engl J Med* 1994;**331**:489–95.

19. Brophy JM, Bilisle P, Joseph L. Evidence for use of coronary stents: a hierarchical bayesian meta-analysis. *Ann Intern Med* 2003;**138**:777–86.

20. Katritsis DG, Ioannidis JP. Percutaneous coronary intervention versus conservative therapy in nonacute coronary artery disease: a meta-analysis. *Circulation* 2005;**111**:2906–12.

21. Boden WE, O'Rourke RA, Teo KK *et al.* COURAGE Trial Research Group. Optimal medical therapy with or without PCI for stable coronary disease. *N Engl J Med* 2007;**356**:1503–16.

22. Morice MC, Serruys PW, Sousa JE *et al.* RAVEL Study Group. Randomized study with the sirolimus-coated Bx velocity balloon-expandable stent in the treatment of patients with de novo native coronary artery lesions. A randomized comparison of sirolimus-eluting stent with a standard stent for coronary revascularization. *N Engl J Med* 2002;**346**:1773–80.

23. Holmes DR Jr, Leon MB, Moses JW *et al.* Analysis of 1-year clinical outcomes in the SIRIUS trial: a randomized trial of a sirolimus-eluting stent versus a standard stent in patients at high risk for coronary restenosis. *Circulation* 2004;**109**:634–40.

24. Schofer J, Schlüter M, Gershlick AH *et al.* E-SIRIUS Investigators. Sirolimus-eluting stents for treatment of patients with long atherosclerotic lesions in small coronary arteries: double-blind, randomised controlled trial (E-SIRIUS). *Lancet* 2003; **362**:1093–9.

25. Schampaert E, Cohen EA, Schlüter M *et al.* C-SIRIUS Investigators. The Canadian study of the sirolimus-eluting stent in the treatment of patients with long de novo lesions in small native coronary arteries (C-SIRIUS). *J Am Coll Cardiol* 2004;**43**: 1110–15.

26. Kelbaek H, Helqvist S, Thuesen L *et al.* SCANDSTENT Investigators. Sirolimus versus bare metal stent implantation in patients with total coronary occlusions: subgroup analysis of the Stenting Coronary Arteries in Non-Stress/Benestent Disease (SCANDSTENT) trial. *Am Heart J* 2006;**152**:882–6.

27. Gruberg L. DIABETES Trial Substudy: sirolimus-eluting stent implantation in very small vessels of diabetic patients. c2005. Available from: www.medscape.com/viewarticle/523055.

28. Grube E, Silber S, Hauptmann KE *et al.* TAXUS I: six- and twelve-month results from a randomized, double-blind trial on a slow-release paclitaxel-eluting stent for de novo coronary lesions. *Circulation* 2003;**107**:38–42.

29. Colombo A, Drzewiecki J, Banning A *et al.* TAXUS II Study Group. Randomized study to assess the effectiveness of slow- and moderate-release polymer-based paclitaxel-eluting stents for coronary artery lesions. *Circulation* 2003;**108**:788–94.

30. Stone GW, Ellis SG, Cox DA *et al.* TAXUS-IV Investigators. A polymer-based, paclitaxel-eluting stent in patients with coronary artery disease. *N Engl J Med* 2004;**350**:221–31.

31. Gruberg L. TAXUS-V De Novo: clinical and angiographic results of the taxus stent in complex lesions. c2005. Available from: www.medscape.com/viewarticle/501427.

32. Park SJ, Shim WH, Ho DS *et al.* A paclitaxel-eluting stent for the prevention of coronary restenosis. *N Engl J Med* 2003;**348**: 1537–45.

33. Lansky AJ, Costa RA, Mintz GS *et al.* DELIVER Clinical Trial Investigators. Non-polymer-based paclitaxel-coated coronary stents for the treatment of patients with de novo coronary lesions: angiographic follow-up of the DELIVER clinical trial. *Circulation* 2004;**109**:1948–54.

34. Stone GW, Ellis SG, Cox DA *et al.* TAXUS-IV Investigators. One-year clinical results with the slow-release, polymer-based, paclitaxel-eluting TAXUS stent: the TAXUS-IV trial. *Circulation* 2004;**109**:1942–7.

35. Stone GW, Ellis SG, Cannon L *et al.* TAXUS V Investigators. Comparison of a polymer-based paclitaxel-eluting stent with a bare metal stent in patients with complex coronary artery disease: a randomized controlled trial. *JAMA* 2005;**294**: 1215–23.

36. Gruberg L. TAXUS VI: a randomized trial of moderate-rate-release, polymer-based, paclitaxel-eluting stent for the treatment of longer lesions: 9-month clinical results. c2004. Available from: www.medscape.com/viewarticle/482822.

37. Ardissino D, Cavallini C, Bramucci E *et al.* SES-SMART Investigators. Sirolimus-eluting vs uncoated stents for prevention of restenosis in small coronary arteries: a randomized trial. *JAMA* 2004;**292**:2727–34.

38. Roiron C, Sanchez P, Bouzamondo A, Lechat P, Montalescot G. Drug eluting stents: an updated meta-analysis of randomised controlled trials. *Heart* 2006;**92**:641–9.

39. Doyle B, Rihal CS, O'Sullivan CJ *et al.* Outcomes of stent thrombosis and restenosis during extended follow-up of patients treated with bare-metal coronary stents. *Circulation* 2007;**116**:2391–8.

40. Spaulding C, Daemen J, Boersma E, Cutlip DE, Serruys PW. A pooled analysis of data comparing sirolimus-eluting stents with bare-metal stents. *N Engl J Med* 2007;**356**:989–97.

41. Mauri L, Hsieh WH, Massaro JM, Ho KK, D'Agostino R, Cutlip DE. Stent thrombosis in randomized clinical trials of drug-eluting stents. *N Engl J Med* 2007;**356**:1020–9.

42. Kastrati A, Mehilli J, Pache J *et al.* Analysis of 14 trials comparing sirolimus-eluting stents with bare-metal stents. *N Engl J Med* 2007;**356**:1030–9.

43. Stone GW, Moses JW, Ellis SG *et al.* Safety and efficacy of sirolimus- and paclitaxel-eluting coronary stents. *N Engl J Med* 2007;**356**:998–1008.

44. Lagerqvist B, James SK, Stenestrand U *et al.* SCAAR Study Group. Long-term outcomes with drug-eluting stents versus bare-metal stents in Sweden. *N Engl J Med* 2007;**356**:1009–19.

45. James SK, Stenestrand U, Lindbäck *et al.* Long-term safety and efficacy of drug-eluting versus bare-metal stents in Sweden. *N Engl J Med* 2009;**360**:1933–45.

46. Rao SV, Shaw RE, Brindis RG *et al.* Patterns and outcomes of drug-eluting coronary stent use in clinical practice. *Am Heart J* 2006;**152**:321–6.

47. Win HK, Caldera AE, Maresh K *et al.* EVENT Registry Investigators. Clinical outcomes and stent thrombosis following off-label use of drug-eluting stents. *JAMA* 2007;**297**:2001–9.

48. Spaulding C, Henry P, Teiger E *et al.* TYPHOON Investigators. Sirolimus-eluting versus uncoated stents in acute myocardial infarction. *N Engl J Med* 2006;**355**:1093–104.

49. Menichelli M, Parma A, Pucci E *et al.* Randomized trial of Sirolimus-Eluting Stent Versus Bare-Metal Stent in Acute Myocardial Infarction (SESAMI). *J Am Coll Cardiol* 2007;**49**: 1924–30.

50. Stone GW, Laasky LJ, Pocock SJ *et al.* Paclitaxol eluting stents versus bare metal stents in acute myocardial infarction. *N Engl J Med* 2009;**360**:1946–59.

51. Eagle KA, Guyton RA, Davidoff R *et al.* ACC/AHA 2004 guide update for coronary artery bypass graft surgery: a report of the American College of Cardiology/American Heart Association Task Force on Practice Guidelines (Committee to Update the 1999 Guidelines for Coronary Artery Bypass Graft Surgery). Circulation 2004;**110**:e340–437. Erratum in: *Circulation* 2005;**111**:2014.

52. Hoffman SN, TenBrook JA, Wolf MP, Pauker SG, Salem DN, Wong JB. A meta-analysis of randomized controlled trials comparing coronary artery bypass graft with percutaneous transluminal coronary angioplasty: one- to eight-year outcomes. *J Am Coll Cardiol* 2003;**41**:1293–304.

53. BARI Investigators. The final 10-year follow-up results from the BARI randomized trial. *J Am Coll Cardiol* 2007;**49**:1600–6.

54. Hueb W, Lopes NH, Gersh BJ *et al.* Five-year follow-up of the Medicine, Angioplasty or Surgery Study (MASS II): a randomized controlled clinical trial of 3 therapeutic strategies for multivessel coronary artery disease. *Circulation* 2007; **115**:1082–9.

55. King SB III. Five-year follow-up of the Medicine, Angioplasty or Surgery Study (MASS-II): prologue to COURAGE. *Circulation* 2007;**115**:1064–6.

56. Serruys PW, Ong AT, van Herwerden LA *et al.* Five-year outcomes after coronary stenting versus bypass surgery for the treatment of multivessel disease: the final analysis of the Arterial Revascularization Therapies Study (ARTS) randomized trial. *J Am Coll Cardiol* 2005;**46**:575–81.

57. SoS Investigators. Coronary artery bypass surgery versus percutaneous coronary intervention with stent implantation in patients with multivessel coronary artery disease (the Stent or Surgery trial): a randomised controlled trial. *Lancet* 2002; **360**:965–70.

58. Rodriguez AE, Baldi J, Fernández Pereira C *et al.* ERACI II Investigators. Five-year follow-up of the Argentine randomized trial of coronary angioplasty with stenting versus coronary bypass surgery in patients with multiple vessel disease (ERACI II). *J Am Coll Cardiol* 2005;**46**:582–8.

59. Bravata DM, Gienger AL, McDonald KM *et al.* Systematic review: the comparative effectiveness of percutaneous coronary interventions and coronary artery bypass graft surgery. *Ann Intern Med* 2007;**147**:703–16.

60. Morrison DA, Sethi G, Sacks J *et al.* Angina With Extremely Serious Operative Mortality Evaluation (AWESOME), Investigators of the Department of Veterans Affairs Cooperative Study #385. Percutaneous coronary intervention versus coronary artery bypass graft surgery for patients with medically refractory myocardial ischemia and risk factors for adverse outcomes with bypass: a multicenter, randomized trial. *J Am Coll Cardiol* 2001;**38**:143–9.

61. Goy JJ, Kaufmann U, Goy-Eggenberger D *et al.* A prospective randomized trial comparing stenting to internal mammary artery grafting for proximal, isolated de novo left anterior coronary artery stenosis: the SIMA trial. Stenting vs Internal Mammary Artery. *Mayo Clin Proc* 2000;**75**:1116–23.

62. Jones RH, Kesler K, Phillips HR III *et al.* Long-term survival benefits of coronary artery bypass grafting and percutaneous transluminal angioplasty in patients with coronary artery disease. *J Thorac Cardiovasc Surg* 1996;**111**:1013–25.

63. Hannan EL, Racz MJ, Walford G *et al.* Long-term outcomes of coronary-artery bypass grafting versus stent implantation. *N Engl J Med* 2005;**352**:2174–83.

64. Serruys P. ARTS-II trial. Presented at the American College of Cardiology. Orlando, FL 2005.

65. Cameron A, Davis KB, Green G, Schaff HV. Coronary bypass surgery with internal-thoracic-artery grafts: effects on survival over a 15-year period. *N Engl J Med* 1996;**334**:216–19.

66. Arora R, Sowers JR, Saunders E, Probstfield J, Lazar HL. Cardioprotective strategies to improve long-term outcomes following coronary artery bypass surgery. *J Card Surg* 2006; **21**:198–204.

67. Noora J, Puskas JD. Off-pump coronary artery bypass grafting through sternotomy: for whom? *Curr Opin Cardiol* 2006;**21**: 573–7.

68. King SB III. Coronary artery bypass graft versus percutaneous coronary intervention: status of the trials. *J Intervent Cardiol* 2006;**19**(5 suppl):S3–7.

68a. Surreys PW, Morice M-C, Koppetein AP *et al.* Percutaneous coronary intervention versus coronary-artery bypass grafting for severe coronary artery disease. *N Engl J Med* 2009;**360**: 961–72.

69. Feit F, Brooks MM, Sopko G *et al.* BARI Investigators. Long-term clinical outcome in the Bypass Angioplasty Revascularization Investigation Registry: comparison with the randomized trial. *Circulation* 2000;**101**:2795–802.

70. Boyle JP, Honeycutt AA, Narayan KM *et al.* Projection of diabetes burden through 2050: impact of changing demography and disease prevalence in the U.S. *Diabetes Care* 2001; **24**:1936–40.

71. Mokdad AH, Ford ES, Bowman BA *et al.* Diabetes trends in the U.S.: 1990–1998. *Diabetes Care* 2000;**23**:1278–83.

72. Flaherty JD, Davidson CJ. Diabetes and coronary revascularization. *JAMA* 2005;**293**:1501–8.

73. Krowlewski AS, Kosinski EJ, Warram JH *et al.* Magnitude and determinants of coronary artery disease in juvenile-onset, insulin-dependent diabetes mellitus. *Am J Cardiol* 1987;**59**:750–5.

74. Krolewski AS, Warram JH, Rand LI, Kahn CR. Epidemiologic approach to the etiology of type I diabetes mellitus and its complications. *N Engl J Med* 1987;**317**:1390–8.

75. Kannel WB. Lipids, diabetes, and coronary heart disease: insights from the Framingham Study. *Am Heart J* 1985; **110**:1100–7.

76. Stone PH, Muller JE, Hartwell T *et al.* MILIS Study Group. The effects of diabetes mellitus on prognosis and serial left ventricular function after acute myocardial infarction: contribution of both coronary disease and diastolic left ventricular dysfunction to the adverse prognosis. *J Am Coll Cardiol* 1989;**14**:49–57.

77. Savage MP, Krolewski AS, Kenien GG, Lebeis MP, Christlieb AR, Lewis SM. Acute myocardial infarction in diabetes mellitus

and significance of congestive heart failure as a prognostic factor. *Am J Cardiol* 1988;**62**(10 Pt 1):665–9.

78. Mak KH, Moliterno DJ, Granger CB *et al.* GUSTO-I Investigators. Global utilization of streptokinase and tissue plasminogen activator for occluded coronary arteries. Influence of diabetes mellitus on clinical outcome in the thrombolytic era of acute myocardial infarction. *J Am Coll Cardiol* 1997;**30**:171–9.

79. Waller BF, Palumbo PJ, Lie JT, Roberts WC. Status of the coronary arteries at necropsy in diabetes mellitus with onset after age 30 years: analysis of 229 diabetic patients with and without clinical evidence of coronary heart disease and comparison to 183 control subjects. *Am J Med* 1980;**69**:498–506.

80. Lemp GF, Vander Zwaag R, Hughes JP *et al.* Association between the severity of diabetes mellitus and coronary arterial atherosclerosis. *Am J Cardiol* 1987;**60**:1015–19.

81. Ledru F, Ducimetière P, Battaglia S *et al.* New diagnostic criteria for diabetes and coronary artery disease: insights from an angiographic study. *J Am Coll Cardiol* 2001;**37**:1543–50.

82. Goraya TY, Leibson CL, Palumbo PJ *et al.* Coronary atherosclerosis in diabetes mellitus: a population-based autopsy study. *J Am Coll Cardiol* 2002;**40**:946–53.

83. Moreno PR, Murcia AM, Palacios IF *et al.* Coronary composition and macrophage infiltration in atherectomy specimens from patients with diabetes mellitus. *Circulation* 2000;**102**:2180–4.

84. Davies RF, Goldberg AD, Forman S *et al.* Asymptomatic Cardiac Ischemia Pilot (ACIP) study two-year follow-up: outcomes of patients randomized to initial strategies of medical therapy versus revascularization. *Circulation* 1997;**95**:2037–43.

85. King SB III, Kosinski AS, Guyton RA, Lembo NJ, Weintraub WS. Eight-year mortality in the Emory Angioplasty versus Surgery Trial (EAST). *J Am Coll Cardiol* 2000;**35**:1116–21.

86. Detre KM, Lombardero MS, Brooks MM *et al.* Bypass Angioplasty Revascularization Investigation Investigators. The effect of previous coronary-artery bypass surgery on the prognosis of patients with diabetes who have acute myocardial infarction. *N Engl J Med* 2000;**342**:989–97.

87. Schwartz L, Kip KE, Frye RL, Alderman EL, Schaff HV, Detre KM, Bypass Angioplasty Revascularization Investigation. Coronary bypass graft patency in patients with diabetes in the Bypass Angioplasty Revascularization Investigation (BARI). *Circulation* 2002;**106**:2652–8.

88. Boyden TF, Nallamothu BK, Moscucci M *et al.* Meta-analysis of randomized trials of drug-eluting stents versus bare metal stents in patients with diabetes mellitus. *Am J Cardiol* 2007;**99**:1399–402.

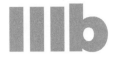

Acute coronary syndromes

John A Cairns and Bernard J Gersh, Editors

29 Non-ST segment elevation acute coronary syndromes: unstable angina and non-ST segment elevation myocardial infarction

Pierre Theroux[1] and John A Cairns[2]
[1] Montreal Heart Institute, Montreal, Quebec, Canada
[2] University of British Columbia, Vancouver, British Columbia, Canada

Introduction and historic perspective

The rapid evolution of the understanding, definition and management of acute myocardial ischemic syndromes constitutes a major milestone of modern cardiology. The widely used terminology of "acute coronary syndromes" (ACS) highlights the specific pathophysiologic mechanisms that distinguish unstable angina (UA), non-ST segment elevation myocardial infarction (NSTEMI), and ST segment elevation myocardial infarction (STEMI) from stable coronary artery disease.[1] Pathologic studies have documented the presence of intracoronary thrombus on a ruptured or fissured complex atherosclerotic plaque in 95% of patients with unstable angina who have developed sudden cardiac death.[2-4] These plaques are rich in lipids and inflammatory cells and possess a thin cap that makes them prone to rupture.[5] At autopsy, the thrombi may be of various ages and at multiple sites; they typically overlie stenotic lesions of only moderate severity; platelet aggregates in the distal small intramyocardial arteries and microscopic foci of necrosis are often found as well.

DeWood documented by angiography that the very early stage of STEMI was consistently associated with a completely occlusive thrombus.[6] Subsequent studies focused on the characteristics of culprit lesions associated with ACS, visualized using a variety of methods including angiography, intravascular angioscopy, ultrasound, and thermography. It became recognized that the active plaque was often not unique, suggesting a more diffuse inflammatory state. These concepts led to a new era of research in cell biology and clinical investigation supported by emerging technologies and methodologically sophisticated clinical research, providing a foundation for our current evidence-based approaches to therapy.

New dimensions and definitions

The definitions of ACS encompass various aspects of the disease including epidemiology, prognosis, clinical manifestations, pathophysiology, and therapeutic options. Their delineation has led to improved understanding of the mechanisms and manifestation of plaque activation, and has opened new therapeutic perspectives. Professional practice guidelines for the management of UA and NSTEMI were first published in 1979, jointly by the American College of Cardiology and the American Heart Association and independently by the European Society of Cardiology. They were subsequently updated in 2002 and 2007 to incorporate algorithms for rapid diagnosis, risk stratification, patient triage, and therapy.[1,7] Large registries[8-10] monitor national and international adherence to guidelines and their performance in various hospital settings as well as their impact on quality of care and prognosis. CRUSADE has been succeeded by the American College of Cardiology's NCDR-ACTION Registry™ (Acute Coronary Treatment and Intervention Outcomes Network), which collects data from hundreds of hospitals across the US into one unified platform with standardized clinical data elements to facilitate benchmarking outcomes, and to analyze treatment regimens.[11] Such initiatives are leading the way in the monitoring and evaluation of quality of care and are facilitating the systematic application of guidelines.

From a clinical perspective, a fundamental aspect of an acute coronary syndrome is the recognition of a change in the pattern of ischemic symptoms to one of increased severity. In the absence of evidence of causative extracoronary factors, such symptoms may signal a rapid progression in the severity of the coronary artery disease. As this

Evidence-Based Cardiology, 3rd edition. Edited by S. Yusuf, J.A. Cairns, A.J. Camm, E.L. Fallen, and B.J. Gersh. © 2010 Blackwell Publishing, ISBN: 978-1-4051-5925-8.

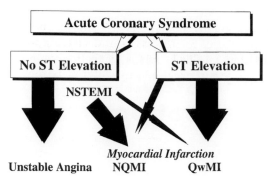

Figure 29.1 Nomenclature of acute coronary syndromes (ACS). The spectrum of clinical conditions that range from unstable angina to non-Q wave MI and Q-wave MI is referred to as acute coronary syndrome. Patients with ischemic discomfort may present with or without ST segment elevation on the ECG. Most patients who present with non-ST segment elevation ACS will eventually be classified as having unstable angina or non-Q wave MI. The distinction between these two diagnoses is ultimately made based on the presence or absence of a cardiac marker detected in the blood. Only a minority of patients with non-ST elevation ACS will develop a Q-wave MI. Most patients with ST segment elevation ACS will evolve to develop a Q-wave MI, although some may evolve to a non-Q wave MI or may occasionally resolve without myocardial necrosis. (Adapted with permission from Anderson JL, Adams CD, Antman EM et al.[1])

Table 29.1 Clinical presentation of non-ST segment elevation acute coronary syndrome

New-onset angina	New-onset angina of at least CCS class III in severity[12]
	I. Angina at strenuous, rapid or prolonged exertion.
	II. Slight limitation of ordinary activity, e.g. angina occurs on walking or climbing stairs rapidly.
	III. Marked limitation of of ordinary activity; angina occurs on walking 1–2 blocks on level or climbing 1 flight of stairs in normal conditions at normal pace.
	IV. Inability to perform any physical activity without discomfort; anginal syndrome may be present at rest.
Increasing (crescendo) angina	Angina that has become distinctly more severe, more frequent, longer in duration, or lower in threshold (that is, increased by greater than or equal to 1 CCS class to at least CCS class III severity)
Rest angina	Angina occurring at rest and prolonged, usually >20 minutes
Early post-MI ischemia	Ischemic chest pain recurrent within 30 days after MI

situation may demand immediate attention, any healthcare professional should be able to make a diagnosis of possible ACS on first seeing the patient. The term "acute coronary syndrome" has thus become a working diagnosis which facilitates rapid access to diagnostic and therapeutic procedures. It provides a logical framework within which to categorize and risk stratify patients who present with a constellation of clinical symptoms compatible with acute myocardial ischemia. It also encourages consistent diagnostic terminology and patient selection for clinical trials and epidemiologic studies. The working diagnosis of ACS is based upon clinical and ECG characteristics which guide immediate management. The subsequent clinical course and appropriate laboratory tests will lead to a final diagnosis which could be ST segment elevation myocardial infarction (STEMI), non-ST segment elevation myocardial infarction (NSTEMI), unstable angina, stable angina or another cardiac or non-cardiac condition (Fig. 29.1).

Clinical diagnosis

Table 29.1 summarizes the clinical manifestations and Figure 29.1 provides current nomendature for ACS. An immediate 12-lead ECG must be obtained, and repeated when the pattern of pain changes, to detect ST elevation or new left bundle branch block (LBBB) indicative of evolving STEMI and the need for immediate reperfusion

therapy.[13] In the absence of ST segment elevation, the working diagnosis becomes a non-ST segment elevation acute coronary syndrome, the likelihood of which is increased by the presence of ST segment depression and/or T-wave inversion on the ECG.[1] An elevated cardiac troponin T or I level then indicates an evolving NSTEMI, while normal values point to unstable angina. If troponin assays are not available, the best alternative is CK-MB measured by mass assay.

The availability of troponins T and I has increased the sensitivity of the diagnosis of myocardial infarction and has sharpened the distinction between unstable angina and myocardial infarction.[1] Troponin measurements allow the detection of cell necrosis and myocardial infarction in up to 30% of patients who would otherwise be diagnosed as having unstable angina based on normal CK-MB blood values, ultimately improving patient care and outcomes.[13] On the other hand, although highly sensitive and specific for myocardial cell necrosis, cardiac troponins are not specific for cell death related to ischemia resulting from coronary artery disease. The latest expert consensus document for a universal definition of myocardial infarction[14] lists the potential causes of troponin elevation outside the context of ischemia; some of them are commonly found in the age range of patients with an ACS, e.g. congestive heart failure, aortic valve disease, tachy or brady arrhythmias, renal failure, and pulmonary embolism. Myocardial infarction is defined as myocardial cell death due to prolonged myocardial ischemia. Myocardial infarction may be diagnosed when a rise and/or fall of cardiac biomarkers (preferably troponin) is detected, with at least one value above the 99th percentile of the upper reference limit, together with evidence of myocardial ischaemia with at least one of: i) symptoms of ischaemia; ii) ECG changes indicative of new ischemia (new ST-T changes or new LBBB); iii) development of pathologic Q-waves in the ECG; or iv) imaging evidence of new loss of viable myocardium or new regional wall motion abnormality. Detection of a rising and/or falling pattern of troponin is needed to distinguish MI from elevated background levels; but this pattern is not absolutely required for the diagnosis of MI in a patient presenting >24 hours after the onset of symptoms because troponin values may remain elevated for 7–14 days following the onset of symptoms. Thus, troponin elevation is an indicator of MI, usually STEMI when there is ST segment elevation or a left bundle branch block and NSTEMI when there is not. True posterior or high lateral MIs can be electrocardiographically silent. Furthermore, the absence of ST segment shifts on the admission ECG does not rule out an acute coronary syndrome. Serial ECGs are required and cardiac markers must be measured 6–9 hours after the onset of pain when the first determination is negative. A negative work-up may not totally exclude ACS or even coronary artery disease and the need for treatment, but generally does confer a favorable prognosis.

A quick appraisal of the patient's demographics, risk factors, cardiac and non-cardiac antecedents, and medications is mandatory for decision making. The characteristics of chest pain and associated symptoms complement the evaluation of disease severity. Thus new-onset angina, crescendo or progressive angina, pain at rest, nocturnal pain, prolonged pain, and recurrent ischemia after myocardial infarction carry increasingly worse prognoses. Although the Canadian Cardiovascular Classification[12] was designed to describe the severity of stable exertional angina, in practice it is often applied to describe angina of sufficient progression and severity to warrant the designation of ACS.

Incidence, natural history and prognosis

There were 4 497 000 visits to US emergency departments (EDs) with a primary diagnosis of cardiovascular disease (CVD) in 2003.[15] The National Center for Health Statistics reported 1 565 000 hospitalizations for primary or secondary diagnosis of an ACS in 2004, 669 000 with UA and 896 000 with MI.[15] Statistics on NSTE-ACS are less reliable than those of STEMI because the diagnostic criteria have been evolving over time, with the introduction of more sensitive and specific criteria allowing the identification of

more patients with the diagnosis but limiting the hospitalization to higher-risk patients. On the other hand, the absolute incidence of STEMI has been decreasing for various reasons that are likely related to better control of risk factors and use of drugs effective in primary prevention.[16] Reperfusion therapy and antithrombotic therapy have also dramatically reduced the short- and long-term mortality and morbidity associated with STEMI. Such is not the case in NSTEMI, which is often associated with more risk factors, including older age, and with a more advanced and diffuse atherosclerotic process. Accordingly, NSTEMI is now associated with a worse prognosis than STEMI past the acute phase. The average age of a person having a first heart attack is now 65.8 years for men and 70.4 years for women; 43% of ACS patients of all ages are women.[15]

Epidemiologic data using the WHO MONICA criteria for the diagnosis of Q-wave MI showed a more than 30% decrease in the mortality rates from Q-wave MI between 1975 and 1995, two-thirds of this decline being attributable to reduced incidence and one-third to decreased hospital mortality.[17-20] The ENACT registry, which included 3092 patients from 29 European countries in the mid-1990s, showed that the distribution of admission diagnosis was unstable angina/NSTEMI in 46%, myocardial infarction in 39%, and suspected ACS in 14%, with no regional differences across Europe.[21] In the more recent Global Registry of Acute Coronary Events (GRACE) that collected data from 10 693 patients across North and South America, Australia, New Zealand, and Europe between 1999 and 2001, two-thirds of admitted patients had unstable angina/non-ST segment elevation ACS and one-third STEMI.[22] This ratio is reversed in India, with its low socio-economic status.[23]

In an epidemiologic study of 5832 residents from metropolitan Worcester, Massachusetts, the annual incidence of Q-wave MI between 1975 and 1997 decreased from 171 per 100 000 population to 101 per 100 000 compared with an increase from 62 to 131 per 100 000 for non-Q wave MI.[24] The hospital mortality for Q-wave MI in the registry declined from 24% to 14%, but that of non-Q wave MI remained constant at 12%. Similarly in the GRACE registry, the risk-adjusted hospital deaths declined between 1999 and 2006 by 18% in STEMI and 0.7% in NSTEMI.[25] It appears that despite impressive declines in the incidence and in-hospital and long-term mortality rates of Q-wave MI, the incidence of non-Q wave MI has been stable or increasing with mortality rates that have changed little over the last decade. Part of these data in NSTEMI might be explained by the wide use of troponin resulting in higher sensitivity and specificity for the diagnosis, and selective hospitalization of higher risk patients.

The natural history of UA/NSTEMI is difficult to assess given the increasingly effective therapeutic interventions introduced over the last 2–3 decades in parallel with better diagnostic and risk stratification tools. Treatment now targets multiple facets of the disease, combining drugs and interventions. Early studies have shown a 10-fold increase in the short-term risk of an event in patients with unstable angina compared with patients with stable angina, and several-fold more compared with individuals with risk factors but no known coronary disease. Recent randomized trials have shown an impressive decrease in MI and death. Prior to the routine prescription of bed rest, nitrates and beta-blockers for unstable angina, the one-month rate of MI was in the range of 40%, and of death, 25%.[26] By the 1970s these rates had fallen to about 10% and 2%. In 1979–80, a study of all patients hospitalized with unstable angina in Hamilton, Canada, over a period of one year noted showed in-hospital and one-year mortalities rates of 1.5% and 9.2% respectively.[27] By the time of the studies with heparin in the late 1980s, study inclusion criteria had shifted toward patients at somewhat higher risk with some trials limiting enrollment to patients with NSTEMI. The rates of the composite outcome of death or non-fatal myocardial infarction by five days were then about 10%.[28,29] They fell to about 4% with the addition of heparin to aspirin, and further with enoxaparin and the glycoprotein IIb/IIIa antagonists. The event rates at 30 days in recent trials with new antithrombotic therapies and an invasive management strategy are shown in Figure 29.2.[30–41] The risk of the disease is highest in the first few days, decreases over the following weeks and months, and eventually becomes similar to the prognosis of patients with stable angina. The long-term prognosis is influenced by the severity of the underlying disease. In the OASIS registry, the incidence of events was 10% at

one month and increased steadily in the following two years to reach more than 20% after 24 months (Fig. 29.3), and was still higher in diabetic patients and in patients with previously known coronary artery disease.[42] In the GUSTO-II study, the in-hospital mortality rate was highest, as expected, in patients with STEMI; however, increasing mortality during follow-up in patients with ST segment depression exceeded that of patients with ST elevation after six months, reaching 8.7% vs 6.8% (Fig. 29.4).[43]

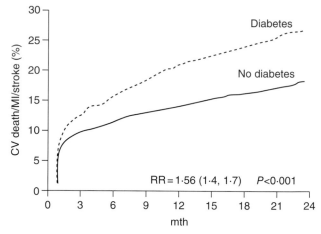

Figure 29.3 Kaplan–Meier event curves for diabetic and non-diabetic patients for total cardiovascular death, MI, stroke, and new onset of congestive heart failure during a 24-month follow-up period after an episode of non-ST segment elevation ACS. (Data from the OASIS Registry study reproduced with permission from Malmberg et al.[42])

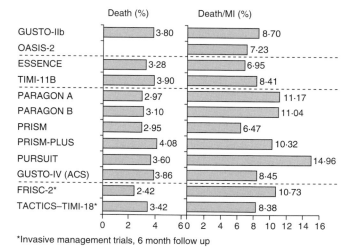

*Invasive management trials, 6 month follow up

Figure 29.2 Rates of death and of death or myocardial infarction in contemporary trials that evaluated new antithrombotic drugs and routine invasive treatment strategy in patients with non-ST segment elevation ACS. Data are the average of events in the intervention and control groups. The interventions resulted in a reduction in rates of death ranging from –5% to 36% and in rates of death or myocardial infarction ranging from –8% to 27%.[29–40]

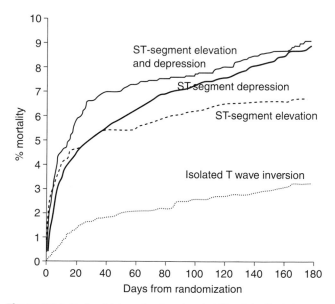

Figure 29.4 Kaplan–Meier estimates of probability of death at six months by ECG changes at admission. The event rate was highest in-hospital in patients with ST segment elevation MI. However, by six months, mortality in patients with ST depression exceeded that of patients with ST elevation. (Data from the GUSTO-II study, reproduced with permission from Savonitto et al.[43])

The empiric concept that NSTEMI represents an unresolved ACS at risk of completion, likely due to an underlying disease process that remains active, appears to be correct for a significant number of patients. This is supported by data showing that markers of inflammation and of activation of coagulation may remain elevated months past the acute phase of an episode of ACS.[44,45]

Risk stratification

A gradient in risk exists in ACS from relatively benign to severe; accordingly, patient management should be guided by clinical risk stratification. The high-risk features for death and ischemic events present at admission, or developing rapidly, have been identified in many registries and clinical trials. Registry studies look at a broad spectrum of patients with acute chest pain and are likely to provide more "real-world" data[22,24,42] while clinical trials enroll more selected and homogeneous populations predefined by entry criteria, collect data prospectively, and often include innovative substudies to test new hypotheses. The two approaches are complementary.

Cardiac risk factors are strong predictors of the presence and prognostic of coronary artery disease, but are generally not useful for the diagnosis of an ACS and its associated risk.[46] Angiographic predictors of a future episode of ACS are a known high extent score of the disease defined by the number of coronary artery segments showing a stenosis whatever its severity.[47] On the other hand, the occurrence of an ACS is a strong indicator that the severity of an obstructive lesion has progressed significantly.[48] Many parameters influence prognosis, some related to the acute thrombotic events, others to the extent and severity of the underlying disease, and still others to co-morbidities.

The clinical evaluation, the 12-lead ECG, and the troponin T or I blood levels are powerful and now standard first-line instruments for risk evaluation. These are included in risk scores, are part of recommended treatment algorithms, and are used as entry criteria in clinical trials to identify the high-risk patients. There are, however, other strong demographic and clinical predictors of prognosis that impact on the prognosis of UA and that should now also be considered in risk stratification. These are mainly older age, left ventricular function, and co-morbid conditions, particularly renal failure and diabetes. Bleeding has recently emerged as a strong prognostic factor; it is largely iatrogenic as a result of aggressive treatment.

Clinical features

In the evaluation of prognosis, the physician is first oriented by symptoms, recognizing an increasingly severe prognosis from new angina, to progressive angina, rest angina, and prolonged chest pain, further worsened if ischemic episodes are accompanied by hemodynamic or electrical instability and if they are recurrent despite optimal medical therapy.[1] It is important to recognize that women, the elderly, and the diabetic patient are more likely to have atypical presentations, because the prognosis with atypical symptoms at the time of an infarction can be worse than that of patients with more typical symptoms.[49] Women enrolled in clinical trials are in general older than men and have more risk factors such as diabetes and hypertension. The proportion of women with ST segment elevation is less than in men but their prognosis is then worse. Women who present with NSTE-ACS less often have an elevation of the cardiac markers and have a better prognosis. The odds ratio (OR) for infarction and death in the GUSTO-IIb study in women compared to men was 0.65 (95% confidence interval (CI) 0.49–0.87; $P = 0.003$),[50] and in the non-invasive strategy arm of the FRISC-II study was 0.64 (95% CI 0.43–0.97; $P = 0.03$).[51] Coronary angiography in general revealed less severe coronary artery disease among women than men.[51]

Diabetes

Diabetes has become a major determinant of risk as its prevalence has reached epidemic proportions. It is present in 20–25% of patients enrolled in trials in ACS. Diabetes increases morbidity and mortality in the setting of ACS and after percutaneous interventions and coronary artery bypass grafting. In the OASIS registry, diabetes was an important and independent predictor of two-year mortality (relative risk (RR) 1.57; 95% CI 1.38–1.81; $P < 0.001$), as well as of cardiovascular death, new myocardial infarction, stroke, and new congestive heart failure.[42] The relative risk of death in diabetic women was significantly higher than in diabetic men (RR 1.98 and 1.28 respectively). Diabetic patients without known prior cardiovascular disease had the same event rates for all outcomes as non-diabetic patients with previous vascular disease (see Fig. 29.3). In a subgroup analysis of patients enrolled in 11 independent TIMI Group clinical trials from 1997 to 2006 that included 62 036 patients (46 577 with STEMI and 15 459 UA/NSTEMI), 17.1% had diabetes.[52] The unadjusted 30-day mortality rates were significantly higher among patients with diabetes than those without for both UA/NSTEMI (2.1% vs 1.1%, $P < 0.001$) and STEMI (8.5% vs 5.4%, $P < 0.001$), as were the odds ratios adjusted for baseline characteristics and management (1.78; 95% CI 1.24–2.56 and 1.40, 95% CI 1.24–1.57 respectively). The hazard ratio (HR) for one-year mortality after UA/NSTEMI was 1.65; 95% CI 1.30–2.10) and after STEMI (HR 1.22; 95% CI 1.08–1.38). By one year following ACS, patients with diabetes presenting with UA/NSTEMI had a risk of death that

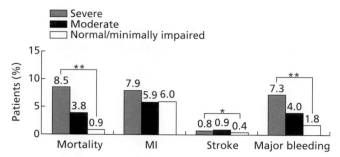

Figure 29.5 Hospital outcomes according to degree of renal impairment for the subgroup of patients with non-ST-elevation myocardial infarction/unstable angina from the GRACE Registry. *P < 0.05 across all categories of renal function; **P < 0.0001 across all categories of renal function. (Reproduced with permission from Santopinto et al.[59].)

approached that of patients without diabetes presenting with STEMI (7.2% vs 8.1%).

Depression may also have a negative impact on prognosis. In a study of 430 patients with NSTE-ACS, depression predicted the endpoint of cardiac death or non-fatal MI, with an adjusted odds ratio of 6.73 (95% CI 2.43–18.64; P < 0.001) after controlling for other significant prognostic factors that included baseline ECG, left ventricular ejection fraction, and number of diseased coronary vessels.[53]

Chronic kidney disease

Chronic kidney disease (CKD) is associated with a higher risk of cardiovascular and all-cause mortality.[54–56] It is also a marker of impaired prognosis in patients with coronary artery disease or with a myocardial infarction, and in patients with an ACS (Fig. 29.5) or undergoing coronary angiography. These cross-interactions are likely linked to a high incidence of traditional risk factors in CKD, mainly diabetes and high blood pressure, and also of non-traditional risk factors such a proinflammatory state, a prothrombotic state, and hyperhomocysteinemia. Complicating these issues, CKD is associated with a higher bleeding risk (see Fig. 29.5); the more severe the dysfunction, the higher is the bleeding risk.[57] Routine calculation of the estimated creatinine clearance rate by the Cockcroft–Gault method or of the estimated glomerular filtration rate (GRF) by the Modification of Diet in Renal Disease (MDRD) formula is strongly recommended over the simple measure of plasma creatinine levels.[58] Cystatin C is also emerging as a valid marker of GFR.[59]

The 12-lead ECG

Current information on the prevalence of ECG abnormalities is difficult to obtain, in part because the ECG and other diagnostic criteria used to select patients for clinical registries are often less homogeneous and rigorous than those used for clinical studies. In the TIMI-III Registry of 1416 patients enrolled because of unstable angina or non-Q wave MI,[60] ST segment deviation ≥1 mm was present in 14.3% of patients, isolated T-wave inversion in 21.9%, and LBBB in 9.0%. By one-year follow-up, death or MI had occurred in 11% of patients with ST segment depression, 6.8% of patients with isolated T-wave inversion, and in 8.2% of those with no ECG changes. ST segment depression 0.5 mm or more and LBBB were significant predictors of death and MI, with rates of 16.3% and 22.9%, respectively. The ECG is not infrequently confounded by LBBB, left ventricular hypertrophy, paced rhythm or other derangements. In the PARAGON-A study, these confounders were associated with near doubling in the one-year mortality rates (12.6% versus 6.5%). Among the 12142 patients enrolled in the GUSTO-II trial with symptoms at rest within 12 hours of admission and ischemic ECG changes, 22% had T-wave inversion, 28% ST segment elevation, 35% ST segment depression, and 15% ST segment elevation and depression.[43] The 30-day rates of death or myocardial reinfarction were 5.5%, 9.4%, 10.5%, and 12.4% respectively (P < 0.001). The cumulative rates of death in this study are shown in Figure 29.4.

There is a gradient of increasing risk of death or myocardial infarction in hospital and up to one year, from nonspecific ECGs to T-wave inversion to ST segment depression including confounding ST-T changes. Such a gradient exists from ST segment depression >0.05 mm, to >1 mm, to >2 mm, to ≥2 mm, and to depression in more than two contiguous leads.[61] The prognostic value of ST segment depression extends to four years following hospital discharge.[62] Special attention is required for patients showing deep T-wave inversions in leads V1 through V6 and in leads I and AVL on the admission or on subsequent ECGs even in the absence of symptoms; the changes are quite specific for the presence of significant disease in the proximal left anterior coronary artery and are predictive of a high risk of progression to an infarction that can be massive; when the T-wave inversions spare leads I and AVL, the mid-LAD is more often the site of the culprit lesion.[63] Similarly, ST segment elevation in lead AVR associated with ST-T changes in other leads can be a marker of left main disease and severe three-vessel disease. The two last criteria deserve special attention.

The importance of recording the 12-lead ECG during chest pain must be emphasized. The detection of ST segment depression during pain has diagnostic and prognostic value.[64] Occasionally, transient ST segment elevation will be detected in association with a critical dynamic coronary artery stenosis due to spasm or thrombus formation, or with small vessel disease. ST segment shifts during pain occurring on medical management indicate refractory ischemia, an endpoint commonly used in clinical trials. Such refractory ischemia predicts near tripling of adjusted one-year mortality.[65]

Biomarkers

Markers of necrosis

Elevation of serum troponin follows the ischemic insult by six hours, as does CK-MB; with newer assays, troponin elevation may be detected earlier. Myoglobin can be useful as an early and sensitive marker of necrosis as it rises within two hours after the onset of pain to peak within 4–6 hours; however, it is non-specific and mandates confirmation of the cardiac origin by elevation of CK-MB or troponin. CK-MB is a valid second choice to troponin when determined by a mass assay. The measurement of ancillary markers such as total CK, AST, ALT is unnecessary and can be misleading.

In contrast to CK-MB and myoglobin, cardiac troponins T and I are not normally detectable in the peripheral blood and therefore provide an exquisitely sensitive and specific marker of cardiomyocyte necrosis. The necrosis is usually of ischemic origin, but there are multiple causes of myocardial necrosis other than MI. Only one elevated value is required for the diagnosis of myocardial infarction as long as the patient presents within 24h after the onset of compatible symptoms. Otherwise, such as in patients with renal failure, the diagnosis of acute MI requires the demonstration of a rising and/or falling pattern against the background value.

Multiple studies have validated the prognostic value of an elevation in the serum troponin levels.[66] Figure 29.6 depicts the results of a clinical trial of a study of patients consulting in the emergency department for acute chest pain;[18] the 30-day rate of death or myocardial infarction was highest in patients with elevated troponin T or troponin I levels, intermediate in patients with ST segment depression, and lowest in patients with normal troponin levels. The higher the elevation in troponin levels,[67] the worse the prognosis, but even small elevations are associated with a significantly impaired prognosis.[68] In the FRISC study, among patients with a non-ST segment elevation ACS, the risk of myocardial infarction or cardiac death at six months was respectively 4.3%, 10.5%, and 16.1% in patients within the first, second, and third tertile of maximal elevation of troponin during the first 24 hours.[69,70]

A meta-analysis among patients with unstable angina, including 12 reports with troponin T and nine with troponin I, demonstrated a risk ratio for the occurrence of myocardial infarction at 30 days of 4.2 (95% CI 2.7–6.4; $P < 0.001$) for troponin I and of 2.7 (95% CI 2.1–3.4; $P < 0.001$) for troponin T.[71] A second meta-analysis included 18 982 patients with unstable angina from 21 studies and showed odds of death or myocardial infarction at 30 days of 3.44 (95% CI 2.94–4.03; $P < 0.00001$) for the total population of troponin-positive patients, 2.86 (95% CI 2.35–3.47; $P < 0.0001$) for patients with ST segment elevation, 4.93 (95% CI 3.77–6.45; $P < 0.0001$) for patients with non-ST segment elevation, and 9.39 (95% CI 6.46–13.67; $P < 0.0001$) for patients with unstable angina.[72] A third meta-analysis included seven clinical trials and 19 cohort studies. The odds of mortality among 11 963 patients with positive troponin T or I was 3.1 (5.2% versus 1.6%). The discriminative value of elevated troponin levels was greater in cohort studies than in clinical trials: 8.4% versus 0.7% (OR 8.5) for troponin I, and 11.6% versus 1.7% (OR 5.1) for troponin T.[73]

Determination of troponin levels has many utilities. Elevated levels in the setting of NSTE-ACS strongly suggest the presence of an active intracoronary thrombotic process that is associated with small foci of myocardial necrosis, likely because of distal embolization of thrombotic material originating from the culprit lesion. Beyond providing a highly sensitive and specific test for the diagnosis of myocardial infarction, any elevation provides important prognostic information in acute coronary syndromes. Patients with troponin elevation are also more likely to profit from therapy with a Gp IIb/IIIa antagonist,[74] from a low molecular weight heparin,[75] and from interventional procedures.[76] Some have recently questioned the prognostic significance of the very small elevation of troponin that can be detected with the new generations of ultrasensitive tests.

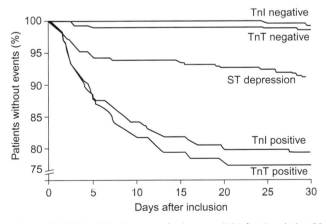

Figure 29.6 Risk of death or non-fatal myocardial infarction during 30 days of follow-up by troponin T (TnT) and I (TnI) levels, elevation (positive) or no elevation (negative), and ST segment depression on the ECG. The risk for myocardial infarction and death increases with increasing serum troponin concentrations and may be 20% in 30 days and 25% within six months in patients with the highest troponin levels. (Reproduced with permission from Hamm and Braunwald.[70])

Markers of inflammation

Consistent with excessive plaque inflammation as the main trigger to plaque rupture and thrombus formation, a wide range of markers of inflammation are found to be elevated in ACS. These include acute phase proteins (C-reactive protein, serum amyloid A protein, fibrinogen), soluble adhesion molecules (sVCAM-1, sICAM-1, E-selectin, P-selectin), proinflammatory cytokines (interleukin-6, TNF-alpha, interleukin-18), degradation enzymes (myeloperoxidase, matrix metalloproteinases, placenta-associated plasma protein-A), and markers of thrombosis (D-dimers, F1.2), oxidative stress (myeloperoxidase), inflammation (CD40 ligand), and of immune system activation (neopterin).

C-reactive protein (CRP) is a non-specific but highly sensitive marker of an inflammatory state. It is produced by the liver upon stimulation by interleukin-6, which is induced by TNF-alpha, IL-1, IL-18, platelet-derived growth factor, antigens, and endotoxins. As CRP half-life is 19 hours, blood levels are determined mainly by rates of production, These can be very high in inflammatory and infectious disease, and in the acute phase of a large infarction where they rise within six hours and peak at 48 hours. In NSTEMI, the elevation precedes that of markers of myocardial necrosis in patients who had previous progressive angina, but not in patients without.[77] The early levels may thus be less useful for risk evaluation; on the other hand, levels obtained after 24–48 hours can represent a transient non-specific acute phase reaction caused by the ongoing cell necrosis. and inconsistently predict future events. Elevated levels at a later time and before hospital discharge are found in up to 40–50% of patients and are associated with high rates of late cardiac events, including death/MI/ recurrent ischemia at 12 months,[78] death/MI at six months[79,80] and up to two years,[81] and death at 36 months.[82] In the CAPTURE trial of 447 patients, CRP levels >10 mg/L did not predict mortality or myocardial infarction at 72 hours in contrast to elevated troponin T levels, but did predict death or MI at six months (18.9% compared to 9.5%), independently of the troponin status.[80] Of interest, high levels of neopterin levels have been linked with the presence of multiple active inflammatory plaques.[83]

The assessment of CRP levels is not currently part of the recommendations of various guidelines. The cut-off points that best predict early and late prognosis as well as the ideal timing for blood sampling remain to be better defined and no study has yet documented that a treatment specific for CRP has improved prognosis. In one study, PCI or CABG had little effect on the one-year excess of recurrent ischemic events in patients with NSTE-ACS and high CRP levels. Elevated CRP levels are associated with increased risk of restenosis and acute complications after PCI,[84,85] and with an increased risk of new ischemic events up to eight years after CABG.[86] The JUPITER trial was designed to determine whether long-term treatment with rosuvastatin (20 mg orally od) would reduce the rate of first major cardiovascular events, defined as the combined endpoint of cardiovascular death, stroke, myocardial infarction, hospitalization for unstable angina, or arterial revascularization

among individuals with LDL-C levels <130 mg/dL (3.36 mmol/L) at high vascular risk because of an enhanced inflammatory response as indicated by hsCRP levels ≥2 mg/L.[87] The trial was terminated prematurely upon the recommendation of the DSMB because early efficacy.

Beta-type natriuretic peptides

Beta-type natriuretic peptides are cardiac neurohormones released in response to ventricular myocyte stretch; proBNP is enzymatically cleaved to the N-terminal proBNP (NTproBNP) and subsequently to BNP. The value of assessing BNP was first shown for the diagnosis and evaluation of heart failure. Since then, large data sets have documented a high predictive value independent of conventional risk factors and other biomarkers in patients with STEMI and with UA/NSTEMI.[88,89] This predictive value extends to early and late blood sampling. Increasing levels are associated with proportionally higher short- and long-term mortality rates. In the GUSTO-IV trial of 6809 patients, the one-year mortality rates by increasing quartiles were 1.8%, 3.9%, 7.7%, and 19.2%, respectively (P < 0.001). (Fig. 29.7) This prognostic value was independent of a previous history of HF and of clinical or laboratory signs of LV dysfunction on admission or during hospital stay. A previous study had shown that this prognostic value was applicable to patients with unstable angina, STEMI, and particularly NSTEMI. The exact reasons for this selective predictive value in ACS are not clear but likely relate to larger zones of ischemic myocardium associated with necrosis and stunning and is in line with the impaired prognosis shown with modest depression of LVEF.[90] Current guidelines do not recommend routine determination of natriuretic factors

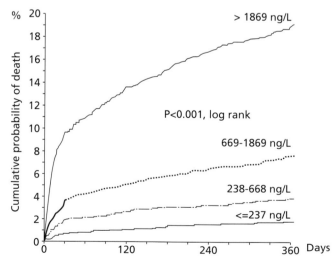

Figure 29.7 Patients with acute coronary syndromes without ST segment elevation in GUSTO-IV. Kaplan–Meier survival curves regarding probability of death during 1 year for patient strata, according to quartiles of NT-proBNP. (Reproduced with permission from James et al[89].)

because elevations would be unlikely to prompt the use of specific evidence-based therapies, and the prognostic value lies more in long-term than in short-term outcomes. It is stated as a class II recommendation, however, that natriuretic factors may be measured to supplement the assessment of global risk in patients with suspected ACS.[1] They should also be used if another indication exists.

Multiple markers and panels of markers

The mechanisms of ACS are highly complex and involve many pathophysiologic cascades with numerous interactions between them. Many studies have shown that a multimarker approach will improve the prognostic value. In the TIMI-11A study of 630 patients with a non-ST segment elevation ACS, the risk of death at 14 days was highest with elevated troponin T and CRP, intermediate when either marker was elevated, and lowest when both were normal (CRP < 1.55 mg/L).[91] In the GUSTO study, levels of NT-proBNP, troponin (Tn) T, CRP, heart rate, and creatinine clearance, in addition to ST segment depression, correlated independently with one-year mortality, but NT-proBNP was the marker with the strongest relation.[89] In contrast, only troponin T, creatinine clearance, and ST segment depression were independently related to future MI. The combination of NT-proBNP and creatinine clearance provided the best prediction, with a one-year mortality of 25.7% with both markers in the top quartile vs 0.3% with both markers in the bottom quartile. The cumulative benefit of using TnI, CRP and BNP was demonstrated in substudies of two large clinical trials[92] (Fig. 29.8). Multimarker measurement is not recommended at the present time since the cost/benefit ratio would be low in the absence of a prospectively validated scenario. Troponin assessment is a must – another marker and the only one recommended for routine use. BNP or NT-proBNP could be useful in some patients for a more global evaluation and CRP as well.

The near future will see the introduction of growing numbers of markers to help delineate the complex and dynamic pathophysiology of cardiovascular diseases and tailor treatment selection to specific patient needs. These will include clusters of blood markers tracking various pathophysiologic pathways, cell membrane markers, the genome and proteome, and molecular probes for tissue imaging.

Risk scores

Prognosis can be predicted by various clinical, ECG, and laboratory parameters. Accordingly, predictive models have been derived from various databases by applying multiple regression analyses to identify independent predictors of prognosis. However, the results of such analyses are influenced by the characteristics of the test populations

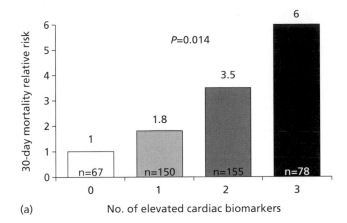

(a)

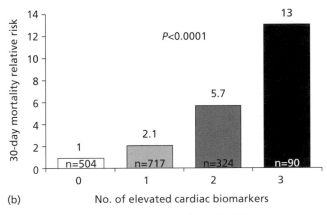

(b)

Figure 29.8 Relative 30-day mortality risks in OPUS-TIMI 16 (a) and TACTICS-TIMI 18 (b) in patients stratified by the number of elevated cardiac biomarkers. (Reproduced with permission from Sabatine *et al*[92].)

and by the baseline data collected. The GUSTO, TIMI and PURSUIT scores[93] were developed from the databases of large clinical trials of NSTE-ACS, whereas the GRACE score was built on registry data acquired across the entire spectrum of ACS. The TIMI score excluded patients with planned revascularization within 24h and those at high bleeding risk from enoxaparin treatment (including significant renal dysfunction); it looked at the rates of death/MI and recurrent ischemia requiring an intervention by 14 days. Renal failure was an exclusion criterion in the PURSUIT trial, and the outcome of death or MI was assessed at 30 days. The GRACE score was shown to be useful to predict death or MI at one year and death at six months and four years.[94,95] It can be measured at admission, to assess the risk of death or death or MI from admission to discharge or to six months, or at hospital discharge to evaluate the risk to six months or to one year. These scores all add to the prognostic value of biomarkers and the ECG and are useful to identify patients who will most benefit from more aggressive medical and invasive treatment.[96]

Age is a strong predictor in all scores. The TIMI score can be readily and simply assessed at admission or shortly thereafter by calculating the sum of seven independent

Score	TIMI (7 points)		GRACE (Odds Ratio, score)		Others
History	1. Age > 65 yrs	1	1. Age	1.7 / 10Y	
	2. > 3 risk factors	1			GUSTO
	FHx. HTN. DM.				
	Smoking. ↑Chol				PURSUIT
	History of CAD				
	3. Known CAD	1			
	4. AAS < 7 days	1			
Presentation	5. Severe angina <24H	1	2. Heart rate	1.3 / 30-beat/min ↑	
	6. ↑cardiac markers	1	3. Systolic BP	1.4 / 20 mm Hg ↓	
	7. ST shift ≥ 0.5 mm	1	4. ↑markers	1.6	
			5. Heart failure	2.0 / class	
			6. Cardiac arrest	4.3	
			7. ST deviation	2.4	
			8. serum creatinine	1.2 / 88.4 μmol/L	

Figure 29.9 Risk scores used in UA/NSTEMI. The components of the TIMI and GRACE scores are shown in detail. Each component in the TIMI score counts for 1. Odds ratios are given for the components of the GRACE score. Algorithms to calculate these scores can be easily downloaded from the Web for use in bedside devices.

predictors, allowing discrimination of a 10-fold difference in risk through 14 days (Fig. 29.9). The PURSUIT and GRACE scores added an important dimension of LV function and the GRACE score a component of chronic renal disease.

Pathophysiology

This section will focus on the mechanisms of acute coronary syndromes that are the most relevant with respect to management. Interested readers are referred to more exhaustive reviews.[5,97] The culprit lesion becomes clinically manifest only with the development of an obstruction severe enough to impede coronary blood flow at rest, or when it is the site of a thrombotic occlusion shedding thromboembolic material into the distal coronary circulation. Therefore, the active plaque is clinically detected only at an advanced stage of the underlying disease. Further, the concept of a single active plaque has been challenged. Pathologic studies have shown multiple rupture sites and thrombi at multiple sites often associated with platelet aggregates in small intramyocardial arteries and microscopic foci of necrosis.[4,98,99] An angiographic study in 253 patients with an acute myocardial infarction documented that complex and ruptured plaques could be found in 40% of patients and that these were associated with a 10-fold increase in the risk of a recurrent ACS.[100]

Atherosclerosis is the substrate for ACS. The severity of atherosclerosis underlying an episode of an acute coronary syndrome is highly variable, ranging from absence of significant stenoses to the presence of left main disease in 5–10% of patients, and single-, double- or three-vessel disease in respectively 20%, 30%, and 40%.[101] A severely obstructive lesion containing a variable amount of dynamic thrombus over a plaque is most often identified, providing a rationale for coronary revascularization. On inspection and histologic analyses, the culprit lesion is clearly distinct from the stable plaque which is most often of only moderate severity, with an inner core rich in cholesterol and cholesterol esters and a thin fibrous cap, poor in connective tissue and smooth muscle cells.[5] At microscopy, the culprit lesion is rich in monocyte-macrophages, mast cells, lymphocytes, and neutrophils. Biologically, it is extremely active, with an intense inflammatory reaction marked by heterotypic cell-to-cell interactions and activity of proinflammatory cytokines, matrix-degrading metalloproteinases, and growth factors.[97] This culprit lesion is the site of a rupture or fissure, occurring most often at the shoulder region of the plaque. The endothelial disruption is overlain by a thrombus extending variably within the lumen of the artery and the vessel wall.[5] A number of intravascular imaging technologies have allowed description of the culprit lesion in the living man, including intravascular angioscopy, ultrasound (IVUS), thermography (recording plaque temperature), optical coherence tomography (OCT) (generating images from backscattered reflections of infrared light), intravascular spectroscopy, and magnetic resonance imaging-based approaches.[102]

Thrombus formation is triggered by tissue factor (TF), which is expressed by lipid-laden macrophages in the core of the atherosclerotic plaque and diseased endothelium. When exposed to the circulating blood, TF binds circulating factor VIIa (FVIIa). The complex triggers the proximal coagulation cascade by activating factor IX and X within the tenase complex. Factor X forms a quaternary complex with TF-FVIIa and tissue factor pathway inhibitor (TFPI) to limit the generation of TF-FVIIa and the thrombogenic stimulus. The thrombus will progress, however, when large enough amounts of FXa are produced. FXa is pivotal in the coagulation cascade. It converts prothrombin to thrombin within the prothrombinase complex. Thrombin has multiple pathophysiologic effects, converting fibrinogen to fibrin, activating factor XIII, which cross-links fibrin, and amplifying its own generation by activation of factors V, VIII, and XI on the platelet surface. It is the most potent platelet agonist _in vivo_, acting mainly through the thrombin protease-activated receptor type 1 (PAR-1). Additional thrombin receptors in human platelets are PAR-4 and GP Ib-IX-V. Platelet activation is promptly associated with an outside translocation of the inner anionic phospholipid layer of platelets, providing a membrane surface well suited to the assembly of coagulation factors and thrombus formation and growth. Circulating platelets also promptly adhere to the damaged endothelium through receptor–ligand interactions. Gp Ib/IX recognizes von Willebrand factor present in large quantities in the subendothelium, and Gp Ia/IIa recognizes collagen. Platelet adhesion and other local agonists produce intracellular signaling that increases cytosolic Ca^{2+} content and induces shape change, release of potent vasoactive, proaggregant and procoagulant substances, and activation of Gp IIb/IIIa receptors.[5] Activated Gp IIb/IIIa receptors recognize and bind the RGD sequence of various moieties, particularly fibrinogen, resulting in platelet cross-bridging and aggregation. P-selectin, CD40L, and other compounds secreted by activated platelets attract leukocytes, linking mechanisms of thrombosis and inflammation.

The mainstay of immediate therapy in ACS is the control of the thrombotic activity to prevent its rapid progression to occlusion or distal microembolization of thrombotic material. The best results have been achieved with combinations of antiplatelet and anticoagulant therapy consistent because of the contributions to arterial thrombosis of both platelet activation/aggregation and intravascular coagulation.

Management

The goals of treatment in ACS are to control ischemia, decrease the substantial early risk of myocardial infarction and death, and prevent recurrences of the syndrome. These objectives can be collectively regrouped under the terms stabilization or passivation of culprit lesions during the acute phase, and secondary prevention of the underlying atherosclerosis thereafter. They are best achieved acutely by judicious use of anti-ischemic therapy, antithrombotic agents, and reperfusion procedures, then by a program of risk factor control. There are no clear boundaries between these two phases. Treatment is generally guided by risk evaluation based on patient demographics, clinical presentation, the 12-lead ECG, troponin levels, and other patient characteristics associated with an enhanced risk (Table 29.2). Risk stratification is an ongoing process that must be repeatedly updated during the hospital stay and follow-up after discharge.

Initial measures (generally Class I, Level C)

Patient's response to symptoms
The patient may first consult with family or colleagues, may visit a medical clinic, doctor's office or emergency department, or may call a healthcare provider, optimally 911. Rapid access to the emergency cardiac care system increases the likelihood of prehospital care and prompt prehospital recording of a 12-lead ECG, and rapid transport to an appropriate center for prompt optimal therapy.

Medical triage
Patients are further evaluated in an emergency department where blood levels of biomarkers of infarction are obtained. Patients with milder symptoms such as new onset of

Table 29.2 Determinants of prognosis of non-ST segment elevation ACS

Confirming high-risk ACS	Clinical pattern of pain
	ST-T ischemic changes
	Troponin T or I elevation
	Hemodynamic or electrical instability
	Recurrent ischemia
	Previous aspirin use
Other cardiovascular	Left ventricular dysfunction
	Congestive heart failure
	Previous myocardial infarction
	Previous CABG
	Extensive coronary or vascular disease
	Provocative testing
Other non-cardiac	Older age
	Bleeding
	Diabetes
	Chronic renal failure
	Depression
Biomarkers	BNP, NTpro-BNP
	CRP
	Other markers (e.g. MCP-1, IL-6, MPO)

angina and/or mild exacerbation of previously stable angina, stable hemodynamics, no angina at rest, no ECG changes and normal serial troponin levels can be further triaged by provocative testing before discharge or as an outpatient soon after discharge. If coronary artery disease (CAD) is suspected, educational material is provided and initial treatment is instituted and re-evaluated at subsequent follow-up. Patients at intermediate risk might go to a coronary care unit (CCU), an intermediate care unit or to a regular ward depending on the availability of facilities and the specific level of risk. High-risk patients should go to the CCU for prompt treatment and are considered for urgent coronary angiography.

General measures

Ischemia at rest or low threshold activity mandates measures to minimize myocardial oxgen demand, including rest in bed or a recliner chair and stool softeners. Emotional distress is minimized by judicious control of the environment, supportive medical and nursing care, limitation and education of visitors, provision for restful sleep, and the control of ischemic pain whenever present with nitrates, intravenous narcotics and other specific anti-ischemic agents as appropriate. Morphine (1–5 mg IV to be repeated if needed) is a useful adjunct, although a note of caution has been raised, by a finding in a large observational registry, of a higher adjusted likelihood of death in patients administered morphine (OR 1.41, 95% CI 1.26–1.57).[103] A randomized trial may be warranted. Oxygen is administered to patients with cyanosis or respiratory distress or if finger pulse oximetry reveals an SaO_2 under 90%. Attention is indicated to detect depressive symptoms which may adversely affect prognosis independently of other predictors.[53]

Anti-ischemic therapy

Nitroglycerin

Nitroglycerin remains a mainstay of angina therapy. It is converted to nitric oxide to cause endothelium-independent vasodilation of capacitance veins (resulting in decreased venous return and preload) and of arterioles (resulting in a reduction in blood pressure and afterload). Together these effects strikingly reduce wall stress and myocardial oxygen demand. Myocardial oxygen delivery may be enhanced if small coronary arteries are concomitantly dilated and no coronary steal occurs. The decrease in myocardial oxygen demand is partly offset by reflex increases in heart rate and contractility, which can be counteracted by adequate beta-blockade.

Nitroglycerin (NTG) is given as a sublingual tablet, by oral or sublingual spray or as an intravenous bolus for the immediate relief of chest pain; long-acting oral or transdermal nitrates or nitroglycerin intravenous infusion are useful to prevent recurrent angina, and to rapidly control blood pressure during the acute phase. Intravenous NTG may be initiated at a rate of $10\,\mu g$ per min through continuous infusion via non-absorbing tubing and increased by $10\,\mu g$ increments every 3–5 min until there is some relief of symptoms or blood pressure response, or headache occurs which is not promptly controlled by acetaminophen. In general, systolic blood pressure should not be titrated to less than 110 mmHg in previously normotensive patients or to more than 25% below the starting mean arterial blood pressure if hypertension was present.

To minimize the rapid tolerance which occurs with nitroglycerin, a drug-free interval of 6–12 hours a day is generally recommended. This may be undesirable in unstable patients in whom tolerance can be attenuated by reducing the infusion rate once chest pain and blood pressure are under control and increasing the rate subsequently if needed. A ceiling dose of $200\,\mu g$ per min is empirically advised although prolonged (2–4 weeks) infusion at rates of $300–400\,\mu g$ per min has not resulted in increased methemoglobin levels.[104]

Nitroglycerin should be avoided in patients with initial systolic blood pressure less than 90 mmHg and in patients with marked bradycardia or tachycardia. Pre-existing hypovolemia is common in the elderly and may predispose to nitroglcerin-induced hypotension. Side effects include headache and hypotension. Hypotension associated with inappropriate bradycardia, reflecting vagal stimulation, may be corrected by Trendelenburg positioning and volume administration or the administration of atropine or glycopyrrolate. Even though the half-life of NTG is short, exacerbation of ischemic changes following abrupt cessation of intravenous NTG has been described[105] and a graded reduction in the intravenous dose is advisable.

The phosphodiesterase-5 inhibitors used for the treatment of erectile dysfunction decrease the biodegradation of cyclic guanosine monophosphate (cGMP) whereas organic nitrates also increase levels of cGMP by activating guanylate cyclase. Synergistic decreases of both systolic and diastolic pressure can result in an excessive fall in blood pressure which has been associated with profound hypotension, MI, and even death. The duration of the interaction is variable depending on the half-life of the various drugs. It is advised not to administer nitrates for 4–6 half-lives after the use of a phophodiesterase-5 inhibitor (24 hours for sildenafil and vardenafil and 48 hours for tadalafil). A recent study of healthy individuals suggested that the sildenafil–nitroglycerin interaction could be gone after four hours.[106] The presence of even trace amounts of nitrates could have deleterious effects in combination with a PDE-5 inhibitor, and the administration of sildenafil or another PDE-5 inhibitor to a patient who has taken a nitrate in the preceding 24 hours is contraindicated, as is the administration of any nitrate within 24–48 hours of the administration of a PDE-5 inhibitor. In general, PDE-5 inhibitors should be avoided altogether in patients who require nitroglycerin for treatment of their angina.[107] Most studies of nitrates in unstable angina were small, employed case series or case–control designs, and dose regimens varied considerably.[108] Many issues such as nitrate tolerance were not addressed. Partial relief of anginal episodes was usually achieved, occasionally relief was complete, and absence of benefit was infrequent. Thus, the widespread use of oral, topical, and IV nitrates in unstable angina is based upon reasonable extrapolation from pathophysiologic observations, case series, evidence of modest reduction of mortality in acute MI,[109–111] and extensive clinical experience using regimens developed in careful clinical studies[111] (**Class I, Level C**).

Beta-blockers and calcium antagonists

Based on their effectiveness in the treatment of stable angina, beta-blockers were widely used for the management of unstable angina in the absence of objective evidence for their efficacy. As the calcium channel blockers became available and their effectiveness for the control of stable angina was demonstrated, they also began to be used for the management of unstable angina, and therapeutic trials generally focused on comparisons of beta-blockers and various calcium antagonists. A small randomized and placebo-controlled trial of 126 patients hospitalized with unstable angina showed similar protective effects with nifedipine and the combination of propranolol/isosorbide dinitrate to prevent recurrent chest pain during an evaluation period of 14 days.[112] It was noted that the propranolol/isosorbide combination was more effective than nifedipine in patients not taking beta-blockers prior to admission, whereas nifedipine was more effective among patients already on beta-blockade. In the subsequent HINT study,[113] 338 patients not receiving beta-blocker on admission were randomly allocated, double blind, to nifedipine, metoprolol, both or neither. Metoprolol was significantly more effective than nifedipine ($P < 0.05$) in preventing acute MI or recurrent angina with ST change. The 177 patients already on a beta-blocker at admission were randomly allocated, double blind, to nifedipine or placebo, and nifedipine was superior ($P > 0.05$). In a trial of patients receiving "optimal" doses of nitrates and nifedipine who were then randomized to the addition of either propranolol or placebo,[114] propranolol was effective. In another study in patients who had failed maximum treatment with propranolol and long-acting nitrates and were then randomized to the addition of nifedipine or placebo, nifedipine was effective ($P > 0.03$).[115]

Diltiazem was compared to propranolol in a randomized single-blind study of patients hospitalized for angina accompanied by ECG abnormalities and occurring in a crescendo pattern, at rest or following MI.[116] Chest pain frequency was significantly reduced by both regimens, and there was no difference in efficacy. In another study, patients with rest angina were randomized to diltiazem or propranolol in maximum tolerated doses.[117] The agents were equally effective in reducing the frequency of daily anginal episodes, but in the subgroup with angina only at rest, diltiazem was efficacious whereas propranolol was not. The Multicenter Diltiazem Postinfarction Trial Research Group randomly assigned 2466 patients with a non-W wave MI to diltiazem (240 mg daily) or placebo for 12–52 months (mean 25). Mortality rates were nearly identical among the two treatment groups. First recurrent cardiac events (death from cardiac causes or non-fatal reinfarction) were 11% fewer in the diltiazem group (202 vs 226; HR 0.90; 95% CI 0.74–1.08). A significant ($P = 0.0042$) bidirectional interaction between diltiazem and pulmonary congestion was observed on X-ray examination. In patients without pulmonary congestion, diltiazem was associated with a reduced number of cardiac events (HR 0.77; 95% CI 0.61–0.98); in patients with pulmonary congestion, diltiazem was associated with an increased number of cardiac events (HR 1.41; 95% CI 1.01–1.96). A similar pattern was observed with respect to the ejection fraction, dichotomized at 0.40.[118] A retrospective analysis of the DAVIT trial with verapamil suggested the same detrimental effect on mortality rates in patients with LV dysfunction.[119] Small placebo-controlled trials of verapamil demonstrated statistically significant reductions in the frequency of ischemic pain, but longer-term follow-up showed a relatively high incidence of AMI and death.[120] Yusuf et al[121] examined five trials involving about 4700 patients with threatened MI who were placed on intravenous beta-blocker followed by oral therapy for about a week. There was a modest 13% reduction in the risk of development of MI in this group. Although a meta-analysis of verapamil[122] therapy indicated a favorable effect on outcomes, the Yusuf meta-analysis found no overall reduction of death and non-fatal MI with calcium antagonists among patients with unstable angina.[121]

Altogether these trials suggest that patients not receiving a beta-blocker or a calcium antagonist prehospitalization may benefit from a beta-blocker, diltiazem or verapamil. However, the the meta-analytic data for benefit of beta-blockers but not calcium antagonists and the evidence for improved long-term outcomes with beta-blocker therapy among survivors of myocardial infarction[121] and those with chronic ischemia, support beta-blockers over rate-limiting calcium antagonists as the first-choice therapy in patients with unstable angina (**Class I, Level A**). Patients at high risk may benefit from initial intravenous beta-blocker, followed by an oral regimen (**Class I, Level C**). Diltiazem or verapamil are suitable alternatives for patients with a contraindication to beta-blocker therapy (**Class I, Level C**). A short-acting dihydropyridine without a beta-blocker is contraindicated as it can increase the incidence of MI[123] (**Class III, Level A**). A long-acting dose preparation or an agent with an intrinsically long half-life such as amlodipine appears to be preferable, but there has been no rigorous assessment (**Class I, Level C**). Patients already receiving a beta-blocker can benefit from the addition of a calcium antagonist to prevent recurrent angina (**Class I, Level A**). Beta-blockers, diltiazem and verapamil should be avoided in patients with severe LV dysfunction (**Class III**).

Among patients with variant angina, characterized by recurrent ischemic episodes occurring mainly at rest and in the early morning hours and accompanied by transient ST segment elevation, randomized, placebo-controlled, double-blind trials of verapamil,[124–126] diltiazem,[127–129] and nifedipine[130–132] have demonstrated the efficacy of each of these agents in reduction of angina frequency. Several comparisons of calcium antagonists to beta-blockers have demonstrated greater efficacy with the calcium antagonists.[125,126,130] These agents, along with nitrates, are regarded as the therapy of choice for variant angina (Class I, Level A), although there are few direct comparative data with long-acting nitrates.

Ranolazine

This is a piperazine derivative approved for the control of angina in patients with chronic stable angina who have failed to respond to prior angina therapy with beta-blockers, calcium channel blockers or nitrates.[133] It is contraindicated in patients with pre-existing QT interval prolongation. Patients with moderate to severe hepatic impairment and those taking CYP3A4 inhibitors should be closely monitored for adverse effects, including QT prolongation. Ranolazine has no effects on heart rate and blood pressure. Although the exact mechanism of action is unknown, it acts as a partial fatty acid oxidase inhibitor to shift adenosine triphosphate (ATP) production away from fatty acid oxidation to more oxygen-efficient glucose oxidation during periods of myocardial ischemia. It also inhibits the inward late sodium current during cardiac repolarization, leading to a reduction in intracellular sodium and calcium overload, and a decrease in the inotropic state and myocardial oxygen demand.

In the recent MERLIN TIMI 36 trial,[134] 6560 patients with unstable angina/NSTEMI were randomized within 48 hours of ischemic symptoms and subsequently followed up for a median of 348 days. The drug was first administered intravenously, then orally. The primary efficacy endpoint of cardiovascular death, MI, or recurrent ischemia did not differ between ranolazine and placebo. However, recurrent ischemia was less frequent with ranolazine (13.9% versus 16.1% with placebo, $P = 0.03$). Side effects were unfrequent, including QTc prolongation which required a reduction in the dose of intravenous drug in 0.9% receiving ranolazine and 0.3% receiving placebo. There was no difference in the rates of documented symptomatic arrhythmias or of mortality in the two groups. The risk of clinically significant arrhythmias on Holter monitoring was reduced by 11% ($P < 0.001$) in the patients assigned to ranolazine.

Antithrombotic therapy

Antithrombotic therapy is a cornerstone in the management of ACS. It reduces the incidence of death and myocardial infarction whether patients are managed by medical therapy only or by the addition of invasive therapy. Antithrombotic effects are enhanced with combined inhibition of platelets and of the coagulation process, but the risk of hemorrhage is increased. Thrombolytic therapy is beneficial in ST segment elevation ACS but contraindicated in non-ST segment elevation ACS.[135]

Antiplatelet therapy

Whereas aspirin remains the gold standard of antiplatelet therapy, an armamentarium of new agents acting on different aspects of platelet function has been developed.[136] Antiplatelet agents evaluated in ACS include aspirin, dipyridamole, prostacyclin, sulfinpyrazone, inhibitors of thromboxane synthase and/or its receptor, ticlopidine, clopidogrel, prasugrel and the intravenous and oral Gp IIb/IIIa antagonists. The various drugs can be classified first by their site of action on the main steps of platelet function from adhesion to activation and aggregation, and secondarily by their specific effects at each step. Adhesion can be inhibited by agents under development which act mainly on von Willebrand factor and its ligand, Gp 1b/IX. Activation can be inhibited by agents acting on intracellular calcium mobilization such as dypiridamole, and by agents inhibiting more specific activation pathways. Aspirin blocks the thromboxane pathway and the thienopyridines block the $P2Y_{12}$ ADP-receptor pathways. Gp IIb/IIIa antagonists occupy the receptor to prevent fibrinogen binding and platelet aggregation.

Aspirin Four clinical trials with differing designs and aspirin dosages have shown statistically significant improvements in major clinical outcomes among patients with non-ST segment elevation ACS. The Veterans Administration Study included 1338 men with unstable angina randomly allocated within 72 hours of admission to ASA 324 mg or placebo.[137] The rate of death or myocardial infarction was reduced from 10.1% to 5.0% (RR 49%, $P = 0.0005$) over a 12-week treatment period. In the Canadian Multicenter Trial, 555 patients (73% men) with unstable angina were randomized before hospital discharge to aspirin (325 mg four times daily), sulfinpyrazone (200 mg four times daily), placebo, or both drugs.[138] Aspirin reduced the outcome of death or myocardial infarction at two years from 17% to 8.6% (RR 49.2%; $P = 0.008$) by efficacy analysis and by 30% ($P = 0.072$) by intention-to-treat analysis, and the outcome of death was reduced by 71% ($P = 0.004$) and 43.4% ($P = 0.035$) respectively. Sulfinpyrazone had no significant effect or interaction with aspirin. In the Montreal study, 479 patients were randomized during the acute phase of disease to aspirin (325 mg bid), heparin, both or neither in a 2×2 factorial design.[29] Aspirin reduced the risk of death or myocardial infarction at six days from 6.3% to 2.6%, a 63% risk reduction ($P = 0.04$). The RISC study randomized 945 patients to aspirin (80 mg daily), intravenous heparin, both or placebos.[28] Endpoints were assessed in 796 patients meeting the entry criteria. Aspirin, compared to no aspirin, reduced the rate of death or MI at five days from 5.8% to 2.6% ($P = 0.033$), at seven days from 13.4% to 4.3% ($P = 0.0001$), and at 30 days from 17.1% to 6.5% ($P = 0.0001$). Overviews of these trials[1,7] have shown a reduction of death or MI from 12.5% to 6.4% ($P = 0.0005$) and a NNT of 17.

The most recent meta-analysis by the Antiplatelet Trialists' Collaboration reviewed 287 studies involving 135000 patients in comparisons of antiplatelet therapy versus control and 77000 patients in comparisons of different antiplatelet regimens.[139] Antiplatelet therapy reduced the outcome of any serious vascular event by 22%, non-fatal MI by 34%, non-fatal stroke by 25%, and vascular mortality by 15%. Aspirin was the most widely studied antiplatelet drug. The absolute benefit of aspirin increases with the inherent risk of the condition for which it is prescribed, and is substantial in patients with a non-ST segment elevation ACS.[139]

The mechanism accounting for the benefit of aspirin in ACS is its acetylation of platelet cyclo-oxygenase-1 (COX-1), which is irreversible and saturable at low doses and blocks the formation of thromboxane A2. The APT meta-analysis found the risk reductions did not vary significantly among aspirin doses ranging from 75 to 1500 mg per day, although the benefits appeared to be less for doses under 75 mg per day.[139] The risk of bleeding appears to rise when daily dose exceeds 200 mg.[140] A loading dose of 150–365 mg (non-enteric coated and chewed) is recommended followed by doses of 75–162 mg daily (**Class I, Level A**). Atherosclerotic vascular events have a variety of pathophysiologic origins, only some of which are responsive to aspirin, and yet the term "aspirin resistance" is often used to describe failure of aspirin to prevent vascular events in some patients. A more appropriate descriptive term might be "aspirin treatment failure" with aspirin resistance being considered as a subcategory in which there is a failure of aspirin to inhibit TXA2 production.[141] Aspirin resistance might result from non-compliance, inadequate dose, poor absorption or rapid metabolism (particularly at low doses), steric interference with aspirin's access to the active site of COX-1 by ibuprofen or naproxyn and possibly genetic polymorphisms of the COX-1 gene. Other possibilities include aspirin-insensitive TXA_2 production catalyzed by COX-2 in inflammatory cells and immature platelets or by COX-1 in immature platelets. To define aspirin resistance as a failure to inhibit TXA_2 production, specific and reliable assays such as serum TXB_2 or possibly urinary 11-dehydro-TxB_2 must be employed. Currently the recommendations from expert panels and societies are to avoid testing platelet function in an attempt to assess the clinical antiplatelet effect of aspirin in individual patients[1,7,142] (**Class I, Level C**).

Other agents acting on the cyclo-oxygenase pathway The inhibition of prostacyclin (PGI_2) generation by low-dose aspirin does not appear to limit its protective effects significantly, and a study of the infusion of prostacyclin in unstable angina patients resulted in no benefit.[143] The thromboxane synthase inhibitors and/or receptor antagonists investigated so far were not shown to be superior or inferior to aspirin.

ADP receptor antagonists There are three subtypes of purinergic receptors on platelets: P2Y1 receptors are involved in platelet aggregation, P2Y12 receptors in stabilization of platelet aggregates, and the precise roles of ion-gated P2X1 receptors are still being evaluated. Currently available ADP receptor blockers, classified as thienopyridines and non-thienopyridines, target P2Y12. The thienopyridines

(ticlopidine, clopidogrel, and prasugrel) are all prodrugs whose metabolites inhibit P2Y12 irreversibly. Because of its greater safety and ease of administration, clopidogrel has largely replaced ticlopidine, although the latter is still used in some countries and may be useful in some patients allergic to clopidogrel, although cross-reactions are possible. The prasugrel metabolite is produced more rapidly than that of clopidogrel, resulting in a more rapid and complete receptor inhibition and fewer non-responders.[144]

Newer non-thienopyridines which are direct and reversible inhibitors of the P2Y12 receptor have improved dose–response profiles. Cangrelor is administered intravenously and can fully inhibit P2Y12; its effect is immediate with a half-life of 3–5 minutes, allowing full receptor recovery within 30 minutes after discontinuation of the infusion. The drug is currently being investigated in the CHAMPION PLATFORM and CHAMPION-PCI trials.[145] Ticangrelor (AZD6140) is administered orally. Its onset of action is within two hours with peak effect at approximately two hours; its offset is approximately after 12 hours but significant inhibition is still present after 24 hours. Using a twice-daily dosing regimen, the DISPERSE and DISPERSE-2 clinical studies demonstrated more potent and consistent platelet aggregation inhibition as compared with clopidogrel, with an increase in minor but not in major bleeding.[146,147] The PLATO trial compared the drug to clopidogrel in patients with ACS with continuing admisistration for up to one year; results are expected for early 2009. PRT060128, a non-thienopyridine inhibitor of P2Y12 that can be administered both intravenously and orally, allowing seamless transition from IV to oral administration, is at an early stage of investigation.

Many placebo-controlled trials of ticlopidine in unstable angina and in the secondary prevention of stroke found risk reductions in the same range of those observed in aspirin trials,[148] while a direct comparison among patients with prior stroke found that ticlopidine was superior to aspirin.[149] Clopidogrel 75 mg/day was compared to aspirin 325 mg/day in the CAPRIE trial,[150] which randomized 19 185 patients with atherosclerotic vascular disease manifested as recent ischemic stroke, recent myocardial infarction, or symptomatic peripheral vascular disease. The annual risk of ischemic stroke, myocardial infarction, or vascular death during a follow-up of 1–3 years was reduced by 8.7% from 5.83% to 5.32% by clopidogrel ($P = 0.043$). The risk reductions (RR) were 23.8% ($P = 0.00028$) in patients enrolled because of peripheral vascular disease and 7.3% in patients enrolled because of stroke, but there was a risk increase of 5.03% ($P = 0.66$) in patients enrolled because of a myocardial infarction. In two randomized trials of ticlopidine versus clopidogrel added to aspirin among patients receiving stents, there were no significant differences in major vascular outcomes.[151,152] However, clopidogrel has supplanted ticlopidine, because of its lower incidence of GI

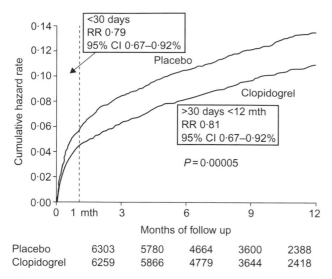

Placebo   6303   5780   4664   3600   2388
Clopidogrel   6259   5866   4779   3644   2418

Figure 29.10 Cumulative hazard rates for the outcome of cardiovascular death, non-fatal myocardial infarction, or stroke during the 12 months of the CURE study with the use of clopidogrel versus placebo on a background of aspirin in all patients. The results demonstrate sustained benefit of clopidogrel from the time of randomization through to the end of the study. (Reproduced with permission from the CURE Investigators.[152])

side effects and freedom of serious hematologic and hepatic toxicity, and once-daily dose regimen.[150]

In the CURE trial,[153] 12562 patients were randomized within 24 hours after the onset of NSTE-ACS to receive clopidogrel (300mg bolus, 75mg daily) or placebo in addition to aspirin 160–360mg daily for 3–12 months. The primary composite outcome of cardiovascular death, non-fatal MI, or stroke occurred in 9.3% of patients in the clopidogrel group and 11.4% in the placebo group (RR 0.80; 95% CI 0.72–0.90; $P < 0.001$) (Fig. 29.10). Clopidogrel also reduced the rates of in-hospital severe ischemia and of revascularization, the need for fibrinolytic therapy or intravenous Gp IIb/IIIa-receptor antagonists, and the occurrence of heart failure. The benefits became apparent within a few hours of beginning treatment and increased throughout the follow-up period to one year. These benefits were homogeneous among all secondary endpoints, subgroup analyses, and patients at low, medium, and high risk, enhancing the clinical relevance of the trial. There were benefits even among patients without ST segment depression and those without elevation of cardiac markers, in contrast to trials of enoxaparin and the GP IIb/IIIa antagonists in which benefits were apparent only among high-risk patients. There were significantly more patients with major bleeding in the clopidogrel group than in the placebo group (3.7% versus 2.7%; RR 1.38; $P = 0.001$), but there was no excess in life-threatening bleeding (2.2% versus 1.8%; $P = 0.13$) or hemorrhagic stroke (0.1% versus 0.1%). The risk of major bleeding was increased in patients undergoing CABG surgery within the

first five days of stopping clopidogrel (9.6% versus 6.3%, RR 1.53; $P = 0.06$) but not when CABG was performed after five days (4.4% versus 5.3%).

The CURE trial focused mainly on medical management, but revascularization was performed during the initial admission in 23% of the patients, among whom 4.5% of clopidogrel patients had cardiovascular death, myocardial infarction, or urgent target vessel revascularization within 30 days of PCI, compared with 6.4% in placebo patients (RR 0.70, 95% CI 0.50–0.97, $P = 0.03$). Long-term administration of clopidogrel after PCI was associated with a lower rate of cardiovascular death, myocardial infarction, or any revascularization ($P = 0.03$), and of cardiovascular death or myocardial infarction ($P = 0.047$).[154] Clopidogrel is generally recommended at a daily dose of 75mg, preceded by a loading dose of 300mg in ACS, as in the CURE regimen, but if the angiogram is required urgently, the loading dose is generally increased to 600mg to achieve faster platelet inhibition; these doses are generally well tolerated.[155]

The CURRENT trial has tested higher doses of clopidogrel and of aspirin in a 2×2 factorial design in NSTE-ACS undergoing PCI; the high dose of clopidogrel is a 600mg loading dose and 150mg daily dose for one month; the high dose of aspirin is a 300mg loading dose and 300–325mg daily for one month. There are currently no provisions in the various treatment guidelines for the so-called clopidogrel poor or non-responders.

Prasugrel was recently directly compared with clopidogrel in the TRITON TIMI-38 trial.[156] The trial enrolled 13608 patients, 10074 with unstable angina or NSTEMI with ischemic symptoms within the previous 72 hours, a thrombolysis in myocardial infarction (TIMI) risk score ≥3 and ST segment deviation ≥1mm or elevated cardiac biomarker, and 3534 with STEMI within 12 hours after onset of symptoms if primary PCI was planned or within 14 days after receiving medical treatment. Coronary anatomy had to be known and suitable for PCI before randomization with the exception of planned primary PCI in STEMI or coronary anatomy already known to be suitable for PCI (very rarely encountered) in which case pretreatment with the study drug was permitted for up to 24 hours before PCI. On a background of aspirin, a loading dose of prasugrel 60mg or clopidogrel 300mg was administered after randomization and until one hour after leaving the catheterization laboratory followed by maintenance doses of 10mg and 75mg daily for 6–15 months (median 14.5 months). Prasugrel significantly reduced the primary endpoint of cardiovascular death, non-fatal myocardial infarction, or non-fatal stroke at three days from 5.6% in the clopidogrel group to 4.7% (HR 0.82; 95% CI 0.71–0.96; $P = 0.01$). From three days to the end of the study, the endpoint was reduced from 6.9% to 5.6% (HR 0.80; 95% CI 0.70–0.93; $P = 0.003$) largely in relation with a reduction in myocardial infarction. The benefits of prasugrel extended to other prespecified endpoints, without significant interactions with patient characteristics or subgroups, including the entry diagnosis of UA/NSTEMI or NSTEMI and the use of a GPIIb/IIIa antagonists.

Excess bleeding occurred with prasugrel: major non-CABG related bleeding in 2.4% vs 1.32% with clopidogrel (95% CI 1.03–1.68; P = 0.03), and life-threatening bleeding from randomization to day 3 (0.4% vs 0.3%; HR 1.38; 95% CI 0.79–2.41; P = 0.26) and from day 3 to the end of the study (1.0% vs 0.6%; HR 1.60; 95% CI 1.05–2.44; P = 0.03) for a total of 1.4%, vs 0.9% at the end of the study (HR 1.52; 95% CI 1.08–2.13; P = 0.01). More patients treated with prasugrel (2.5%, vs 1.4% of patients treated with clopidogrel; P < 0.001) discontinued the study drug owing to adverse events related to hemorrhage. The combination of non-CABG related TIMI major or minor hemorrhage occurred also more frequently (HR 1.31; 95% CI 1.11–1.56; P = 0.002). Fatal TIMI major bleeding occurred in 0.4% and 0.1% of patients respectively (P = 0.002) and intracranial hemorrhage in 19 patients (0.3%) receiving prasugrel and 17 patients (0.3%) receiving clopidogrel (P = 0.74). Among the few patients who underwent CABG, the rate of TIMI major bleeding was also in excess with prasugrel (13.4% vs 6 3.2%, HR 4.73; 95% CI 1.90–11.82; P < 0.001).

A series of *post hoc* exploratory analyses were conducted to identify the subgroups of patients with no favorable net clinical benefit or with net harm, taking into account death from any cause, non-fatal myocardial infarction, non-fatal stroke and non-CABG related non-fatal TIMI major bleeding. Three such subgroups emerged: 1. patients with previous stroke or transient ischemic attack (n = 518) had net harm from prasugrel (HR 1.54; 95% CI 1.02–2.32; P = 0.04); 2. patients ≥75 years of age had no net benefit (HR 0.99; 95% CI 0.81–1.21; P = 0.92); and 3. patients weighing <60 kg had no net benefit (HR 1.03; 95% CI 0.69–1.53; P = 0.89). Patients with a history of stroke showed a strong trend toward a greater rate of TIMI major bleeding (P = 0.06), including intracranial hemorrhage in six patients (2.3%) in the prasugrel group, as compared with none in the clopidogrel group (P = 0.02).

Analogous to aspirin's specificity for the TXA_2 pathway, clopidogrel's specificity for the PGY_{12} receptor limits its effectiveness to the the prevention of vascular events which arise from activation of this receptor. Accordingly, the term "clopidogrel resistance" should be reserved for those phenomena which may impede clopidogrel's capacity to reduce the action of the $P2Y_{12}$ pathway.[157] These include inadequate dosing, poor absorption, drug competition for the P450 enzymes, and polymorphisms of these enzymes, the $P2Y_{12}$ receptor or of other platelet receptors. The standard test for clopidogrel resistance has been the assessment of platelet aggregation in platelet-rich plasma or whole blood following activation with ADP, but this test is not specific for clopidogrel. The platelet vasodilator-stimulated phosphoprotein-phosphorylation assay using flow cytometry is the most promising available assay[158] but as for aspirin, it is recommended that no test of platelet function should be performed in the attempt to assess the clinical antiplatelet effect of clopidogrel in individual patients.[1,7,139] Prasugrel might be a preferable alternative therapy for those patients who are truly clopidogrel resistant.

Gp IIb/IIIA-receptor blockers Three Gp IIb/IIIa antagonists are approved for IV use: abciximab, eptifibatide, and tirofiban. Abciximab is a Fab fragment of a chimeric monoclonal antibody that binds the RGD and dodecapeptide recognition sequences of the receptor. The plasma half-life of the drug is approximately 10 minutes but the biologic half life extends to 6–12 hours. Abciximab has strong affinity for the receptor and receptor occupancy persists weeks after drug exposure, although platelet aggregation progressively returns to normal within 12–24 hours. Abciximab is not specific for the Gp IIb/IIIa integrin, also inhibiting the vitronectin receptor ($\alpha v\beta 3$) on the endothelium and smooth muscle cell and the MAC-1 ($\alpha m\beta 2$) integrin on neutrophils and monocytes. The clinical relevance of occupancy of these receptors involved in cell proliferation and leukocyte activation respectively remains ill defined. Eptifibatide is a cyclic heptapeptide derived from the structure of barbourin in the venom of the pigmy rattlesnake, possessing a KGD sequence recognized by the receptor. Tirofiban is a non-peptide mimetic of the RGD sequence. The half-life of the two small molecules is approximately two hours. After drug discontinuation, there is 50% recovery of receptor occupancy and platelet aggregation within four hours and nearly 100% within eight hours. These drugs have no special affinity for the receptor and receptor occupancy parallels blood levels.

Many trials have documented the efficacy of abciximab in reducing periprocedural MI and the need for urgent revascularization when it is administered in the cardiac catheterization laboratory before a revascularization procedure and continued for 12 hours thereafter.[159,160] In the c7E3 Fab Antiplatelet Therapy in Unstable Refractory angina (CAPTURE)[161] trial involving 1265 patients with refractory unstable angina, abciximab was administered after identification at previous angiography of a culprit lesion suitable for coronary angioplasty. The procedures were performed 20–24 hours later and abciximab was continued for one hour after the procedure. Abciximab, compared with placebo, reduced the rate of death and myocardial infarction by 30 days from 15.9% to 11.3% (P = 0.012). In a comparison trial, abciximab was shown to be significantly superior to tirofiban in preventing complications associated with urgent or elective stent placement.[162] The doses of tirofiban that were used just before the procedure in this study are now known to have been suboptimal to achieve adequate receptor inhibition.[163] Contrasting with the benefits observed in percutaneous intervention and in stent implantation trials, the GUSTO-IV trial failed to show a benefit of abciximab in the medical management of patients with a non-ST segment elevation ACS. In this trial, 7800 patients with chest pain and either ST segment depression or raised troponin T or I concentrations were randomly assigned placebo, an abciximab bolus and 24 h infusion, or an abciximab bolus and 48 h infusion.[39] The primary outcome of death or myocardial infarction 30 days after randomization occurred in 8.0% of patients on placebo, 8.2% of patients on 24 h abciximab, and 9.1% of patients on 48 h abciximab (OR 1.0 between placebo and 24 h abciximab, and 1.1 (95% CI 0.94–1.39) for difference between placebo and 48 h abciximab). The lack of benefit with abciximab was consistent in most subgroups investigated including, remarkably, patients with elevated troponin T or I, although they were at a high risk of subsequent events.

Tirofiban was investigated in two ACS trials. In one, tirofiban alone with placebo heparin versus heparin with placebo tirofiban resulted in an early benefit at 72 hours that was not sustained, however, after 30 days.[32] The second trial compared the combination of tirofiban with heparin to heparin alone. The combination reduced the occurrence of the primary endpoint of death, myocardial infarction or refractory ischemia at seven days by 32% ($P = 0.004$) and of death or myocardial infarction by 43% ($P = 0.006$).[37] The gain appeared early and was sustained after six months.

Many trials were performed with eptifibatide. In the PURSUIT trial, 9461 patients with a non-ST segment elevation ACS were randomized to eptifibatide or placebo; the rate of death or myocardial infarction after 30 days was reduced by 10% with eptifibatide (14.2% versus 15.7%, $P = 0.042$).[36] In the placebo-controlled ESPRIT trial, eptifibatide used at higher doses with a double bolus injection significantly reduced the event rate associated with coronary stenting to an extent similar to that observed with abciximab.[164] Altogether, these trials show efficacy of abciximab and eptifibatide in reducing event rates in percutaneous coronary interventions and of tirofiban and eptifibatide in non-ST segment elevation ACS. The benefits were additive to those of aspirin and of heparin.

Several meta-analyses found a benefit of intravenous Gp IIb/IIIa antagonist therapy in patients with an ACS. One meta-analysis published in 1999, before the confounding results of GUSTO-IV appeared, included the data from the CAPTURE, PURSUIT, and PRISM-PLUS trials, and showed event rates of 2.5% with treatment and 3.8% with placebo during the period of medical management and of 4.9% and 8.0% respectively in the 48 hours that followed PCI in the subgroups of patients who underwent a procedure (RR reduction 34%, $P < 0.001$). An early benefit of Gp IIb/IIIa inhibitors during medical treatment was then documented, and a larger benefit when PCI was performed on drug therapy.[165] A second meta-analysis with individual data on

31 402 patients from six trials not mandating coronary angiography except for the PRISM-PLUS, and that included GUSTO-IV,[33,166] showed reduced odds of death or MI at 30 days of 9% (10.8% versus 11.8%; OR 0.91; 95% CI 0.84–0.98; $P = 0.015$) with the Gp IIb/IIIa antagonists. The relative treatment benefit matched patients' risk. Benefit was present in both males and females when the baseline troponin levels were elevated but only in males when normal. A third meta-analysis examined more specifically the subset of 6458 diabetic patients enrolled in the six trials. In these patients, the Gp IIb/IIIa inhibitors reduced the mortality at 30 days from 6.2% to 4.6% (OR 0.74; 95% CI 0.59–0.92; $P < 0.007$) with a statistically significant interaction between treatment and diabetic status ($P = 0.036$). Mortality at 30 days among the 1279 who underwent PCI was reduced from 4.0% to 1.2% (OR 0.30; 95% CI 0.14–0.69; $P < 0.002$).[167] A significant risk reduction in 30-day mortality was observed in another meta-analysis that included 20 186 patients (0.9 vs 1.3%, OR 0.73, 95% CI 0.55–0.96, $P = 0.024$).[168]

The overall management of ACS, including the use of antithrombotic therapy, has changed markedly since these early trials and meta-analyses were performed. First, the early invasive approach is undertaken earlier, shortening to a few hours the time between admission and cardiac catheterization and reducing the risk of an early event; second, bare metal or drug-eluting stents are routinely deployed, improving blood flow and reducing shear-induced platelet aggregation and stent thrombosis; third, clopidogrel and new anticoagulants (e.g. enoxaparin, bivaluridin, and fondaparinux) are widely used. As clopidogrel yielded 20% risk reductions over the use of aspirin alone, the need for an agent that blocks the GPIIb/IIa receptors become less critical. Thus a recent randomized placebo-controlled trial in stable patients undergoing PCI and prescribed a loading dose of 600 mg of clopidogrel in addition to aspirin was associated with such a low frequency of early complications that the use of abciximab offered no clinically measurable benefit at 30 days.[169] A second trial that used the same study design and included stable diabetic patients also failed to show a benefit of abciximab.[170] A third trial conducted by the same group of investigators enrolled 2022 ACS patients managed invasively, and all administered aspirin and the same loading dose of clopidogrel at least two hours prior to the procedure.[171] The primary endpoint of death, MI, or urgent target vessel revascularization within 30 days was reached in 90 patients (8.9%) assigned to abciximab vs 120 patients (11.9%) assigned to placebo (RR 0.75; 95% CI 0.58–0.97; $P = 0.03$). All the benefit occurred among patients with elevated troponin levels (RR 0.71; 95% CI 0.54–0.95; $P = 0.02$ vs RR 0.99; 95% CI 0.56–1.76 with normal troponin levels). The benefits were maintained at one year as the primary outcome was reached in 23.3% of abciximab patients and 28.0% of placebo patients (RR 0.80; 95% CI 0.67–0.95,

$P = 0.012$), and the incidence of death or MI in 11.6% and 15.3% (RR 0.74, 95% CI 0.59–0.94, $P = 0.015$) respectively.[172] The risk of major and minor bleeding as well as need for transfusion was the same in the abciximab and placebo groups.

Many studies and registry data have, however, showed a significant increase in the risk of bleeding with Gp IIb/IIIa antagonists that not only neutralized the benefits of the drug but could result in harm, particularly among elderly and female patients. In the GRACE registry,[173] mortality rates with LMWH were lower than with UFH, among patients not treated with Gp IIb/IIIa inhibitors, whether they had PCI (OR 0.45; 95% CI 0.21–0.98) or not (OR 0.77; 95% CI 0.63–0.94); there was excess bleeding in LMWH-treated patients who had PCI. Elderly patients (>75 years) who were manged medically with Gp IIb/IIIa antagonists had a very high bleeding risk with both LMWH and UFH. The issue of excess bleeding in women was explored among 32601 patients in the CRUSADE registry, 18436 of whom were treated with a Gp IIb/IIIa antagonist. Major bleeding was defined as a hematocrit drop ≥0.12, need for transfusion or intracranial bleeding; it was adjusted for clinical factors and antithrombotic dose. Gp IIb/IIIa inhibitor dose was defined as excessive if not reduced when creatinine clearance was <50 mL/min for eptifibatide or <30 mL/min for tirofiban. Women in general had higher rates of major bleeding than men with a Gp IIb/IIa antagonist (15.7% vs 7.3%; $P < 0.0001$) or without (8.5% vs 5.4%;$P<0.0001$). Women who received Gp IIb/IIIa inhibitors were more likely to receive excessive doses than men (46.4% versus 17.2%, adjusted OR 3.81, $P < 0.0001$). Excess dosing was associated with increased risk of bleeding in women (OR 1.72, 95% CI 1.30–2.28) and in men (OR 1.27, 95% CI 0.97–1.66), but risk attributable to dosing was much higher in women (25.0% versus 4.4%).[174]

Another current issue with Gp IIb/IIIa antagonists is the optimal timing of administration, whether routine upfront at admission or deferred until after coronary angiography and before angioplasty. This issue was examined in the 9207 patients enrolled in the ACUITY-Timing trial[175] and is now being tested in the very large EARLY-ACS trial.[176] In the former, upfront was a mean of 1.3 hours and deferred was a mean of 13.1 hours, showing that PCI was performed very early. Deferred use resulted in less 30-day major bleeding by the ACUITY definition (4.9% vs 6.1%, $P = 0.009$); by the TIMI criteria, rates of major bleeding were not reduced but those of minor bleeding were, and rates of transfusion were less (2.3% vs. 3%, $P = 0.05$). Ischemic events, however, did not meet the criterion for non-inferiority (7.9% vs 7.1%, $P = 0.04$) mainly due to an excess unplanned revascularization (2.8 vs 2.1%, $P = 0.03$). The net clinical outcome at 30 days assessed by the composite of death/MI/unplanned revascularization/major bleeding) was the same (11.7%) in each group.

Oral Gp IIb/IIIa antagonists In an attempt to extend the benefit of intravenous Gp IIb/IIIa antagonists to the subacute and chronic phases of the disease, orally active inhibitors were developed. Four different agents – xemilofiban, orbofiban, sibrafiban and latrofiban – were investigated in five large trials. No single trial showed a benefit in reducing ischemic events and two were prematurely interrupted because of excess mortality. A meta-analysis of four of these trials totaling 33326 patients showed a statistically significant increase in mortality with therapy (OR 1.37; $P = 0.001$) and trends to more MI. There was a twofold increase in the rate of major bleeding and a high rate of less severe bleeding leading to study drug discontinuation.[177] The trials have provided a lesson on the validity of evidence-based medicine, as they ended by trying to find why they were toxic. Contrasting with the IV agents used as infusion, the oral agents have rapid on and off binding to the receptor with the potential of reactivation of the disease at trough levels; they further bind the inactivated receptors, resulting in outside-to-inside signaling and paradoxic platelet activation.

PAR antagonists A new class of antiplatelet agents is emerging targeting the platelet protease-activated receptor (PAR-1). Thrombin is the most potent platelet agonist *in vivo*. Its effects on platelets (as well as on endothelial cells and leukocytes) are uniquely blocked by these agents, without affecting its conversion of fibrinogen to fibrin and fibrin clot formation, creating the potential for greater efficacy and less bleeding. PAR antagonists are now in clinical investigation, some in advanced Phase III trials.

Anticoagulants

Anticoagulants evaluated during the acute phase of non-ST segment elevation ACS include unfractionated heparin (UFH), low-molecular weight heparins (LMWH), direct thrombin inhibitors and the pentasaccharide fondaparinux. New and promising agents such as r-tissue factor pathway inhibitor, r-protein C, and other specific inhibitors of factor Xa are under investigation (Fig. 29.11). Documentation of reactivation of the disease following the discontinuation of heparin[178,179] and persisting prothrombotic activity past the acute phase have led to the evaluation of long-term therapy with coumadin and the LMWHs.

Unfractionated and low molecular weight heparins Unfractionated heparin, low molecular weight heparins, and the pentasaccharides inhibit coagulation factors by greatly enhancing the physiologic properties of circulating antithrombin, with differential effects on factor Xa and thrombin related to the molecular weight of the various heparins (Fig. 29.12).[180] In the study by Theroux *et al* of 479 patients, the incidence of fatal and non-fatal myocardial infarction was reduced from 7.5% to 1.2% (RR 85%; $P = 0.007$) with

Sites of Action Of New Anticoagulants

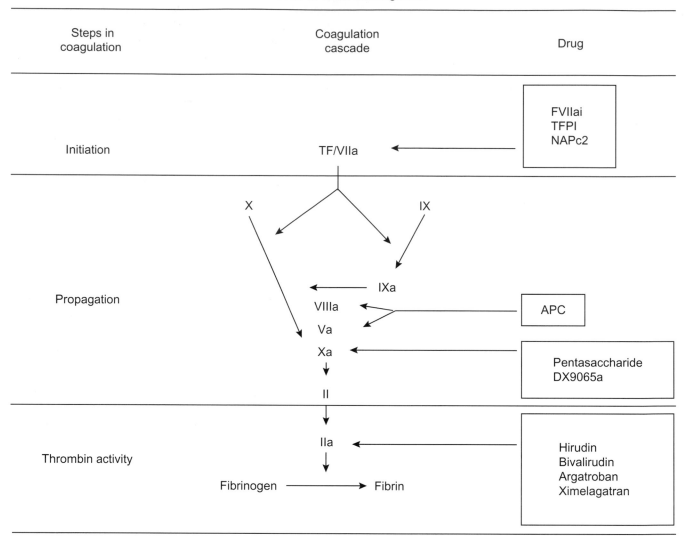

Figure 29.11 The coagulation cascade and sites of action of new anticoagulants. Initiation of coagulation is triggered by the tissue factor/factor VIIa complex (TF/VIIa), which activates factor IX (IX) and factor X (X). Activated factor IX (IXa) propagates coagulation by activating factor X in a reaction that utilizes activated factor VIII (VIIIa) as a co-factor. Activated factor X (Xa), with activated factor V (Va) as a co-factor, converts prothrombin (II) to thrombin (IIa). Thrombin then converts fibrinogen to fibrin. Active site-blocked VIIa (VIIai) competes with VIIa for TF, whereas tissue factor pathway inhibitor (TFPI) and nematode anticoagulant peptide (NAPc2) target VIIa bound to TF. Synthetic pentasaccharide and DX-9065a inactivate Xa, activated protein C (APC) inactivates Va and VIIIa, and hirudin, bivalirudin, argatroban, and ximelagatran target thrombin. (Reproduced with permission from Weitz and Buller.[179])

unfractionated heparin compared with placebo, and of recurrent refractory ischemia from 19.7% to 9.6% (RR 51%; $P = 0.02$).[30] In the RISC study, which enrolled 945 men, the combination of aspirin and heparin resulted in a significant risk reduction in death and myocardial infarction at five days.[29] In the FRISC study, 1506 patients were randomized to subcutaneous dalteparin twice daily for six days followed by once a day for 35–45 days or placebo.[181] During the first six days the rate of death or MI was reduced with dalteparin (1.8% versus 4.8%; RR 0.37; 95% CI 0.20–0.68). Survival analysis showed a risk of reactivation and reinfarction when the dose was decreased; the benefit persisted at 40 days but not at 4–5 months.[151] A meta-analysis of 12 trials that compared unfractionated heparin or a low molecular weight heparin to placebo in a total of 17157 patients showed an odds ratio for myocardial infarction or death during the short term (up to seven days) of 0.53 (95% CI 0.38–0.73; $P = 0.0001$) in favor of the anticoagulant.[182] These results validate the use of unfractionated heparin or of a LMWH in combination with aspirin in patients with a non-ST segment elevation ACS.

Low molecular weight heparins present distinct advantages over unfractionated heparin. They can be administered subcutaneously once or twice a day. They bind

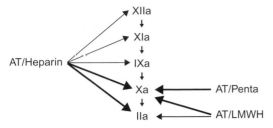

Figure 29.12 Antithrombin (AT)-mediated inhibition of coagulation factors. The complex heparin/AT inhibits especially factor Xa and thrombin (IIa) and also factor XIIa, factor XIa, and factor IXa. The shorter saccharide chains contained in the low molecular weight heparins (LMWH) allow more selective inhibition of factor Xa than factor IIa. The unique pentasaccharide chain of fondaparinux allows highly specific inhibition of factor Xa. (Adapted with permission from Hirsh et al.[180])

plasma proteins and endothelial cells less avidly than unfractionated heparin, resulting in more predictable anticoagulation, with no need for monitoring. The ratio of inhibition factor Xa/thrombin is greater. Low molecular weight heparins also stimulate platelets less and are less often associated with heparin-induced thrombocytopenia.

Four trials have directly compared a LMWH with unfractionated heparin. No advantages were observed with dalteparin in a trial involving 1482 patients[183] and with nadroparin in a trial of 3468 patients.[184] Enoxaparin was shown to be superior to unfractionated heparin in the two trials that evaluated the drug. In the ESSENCE trial, enoxaparin, 1 mg/kg administered twice daily for 48 hours to eight days (median 2.6 days) in 3171 patients, reduced the composite outcome of death, MI or recurrent angina by 16.2% at 14 days (16.6% versus 19.8%; $P = 0.019$), and by 19% at 30 days (19.8% versus 23.3%; $P = 0.017$) compared to unfractionated heparin. The rate of death was unaffected, but the rate of myocardial infarction was reduced by 29% (3.2% versus 4.5%; $P = 0.06$) at 14 days, and by 26% (3.9% versus 5.2%) at 30 days ($P = 0.08$).[31] The TIMI-11B trial showed in 3910 patients a reduction in the composite outcome of death, myocardial infarction or refractory ischemia requiring an urgent revascularization from 16.6% to 14.2% at 14 days ($P = 0.04$) and from 19.6% to 17.3% at 43 days ($P = 0.06$).[38] A meta-analysis of trials that directly compared any LMWH to unfractionated heparin showed no statistically significant difference in the odds of death or MI (OR 0.88; 95% CI 0.69–1.12; $P = 0.34$). On the other hand, a combined analysis of the data from ESSENCE and TIMI-11B showed a statistically significant reduction in the rate of death or myocardial infarction in favor of enoxaparin.[185]

Fondaparinux A synthetic pentasaccharide which selectively binds antithrombin III, causing rapid and predictable inhibition of factor Xa. OASIS-5[186] randomized 20 078 patients with NSTE-ACS to fondaparinux (2.5 mg SC, once

daily) or enoxaparin (1 mg/kg SC, twice daily) within 24 h of onset of symptoms. Fondaparinux was not inferior to enoxaparin in terms of the primary outcome (death, MI, or refractory ischemia at nine days) (5.8% vs 5.7%; HR 1.01; 95% CI 0.90–1.13) with a markedly lower rate of major bleeding at nine days (2.2% versus 4.1%; HR 0.52; $P < 0.001$). Fondaparinux was associated with significantly fewer deaths at 30 days (2.9% versus 3.5%; HR 0.83; 95% CI 0.71–0.97; $P = 0.02$) and at 180 days (5.8% versus 6.5%; HR 0.89; 95% CI 0.80–1.00; $P = 0.05$). A concern in the management of patients undergoing PCI is that of catheter thrombosis with fondaparinux, necessitating supplementary UFH administration during the procedure. The drug is now approved for the prevention of deep vein thrombosis in a variety of clinical settings, pulmonary embolus, and in Europe for patients with ACS not expected to undergo early PCI.

Direct thrombin inhibitors These drugs are potent anticoagulants that directly inhibit thrombin, require no co-factor for their effects (see Fig. 29.11) and have a highly predictable response. Hirudin, now produced by recombinant technology, and bivalirudin, a synthetic agent, are bivalent, binding to both the active site and the fibrinogen-binding exosite of thrombin, whereas the low-molecular weight thrombin inhibitors argatroban, efegatran and inogatran bind only to the active site.[179]

Hirudin in a dose of 0.2 mg/kg bolus with infusion of 0.1 mg/kg/h was used in the GUSTO-IIb, which enrolled 12 142 patients, two-thirds of them with a non-ST segment elevation ACS and one-third with ST segment elevation MI,[30] and in the TIMI-9B trial, which enrolled 3002 patients with ST segment elevation MI.[187] Among patients with no ST segment elevation in GUSTO-IIb, the composite endpoint of death or MI at 30 days occurred in 8.3% of the patients on hirudin and in 9.1% of patients on heparin (OR 0.90; 95% CI 0.78–1.06; $P = 0.22$); at 24 h, the risk of death or MI was significantly lower in the patients who received hirudin (2.1% versus 1.3%; $P = 0.001$). The OASIS pilot study suggested a greater benefit with an intermediate dose of 0.4 mg/kg bolus and 0.15 mg/kg/h infusion.[188] This dose was used in the large OASIS-2 trial, which randomized 10 141 patients with NSTE-ACS to UFH (5000 IU bolus plus 15 U/kg/h) or recombinant hirudin for 72 h.[37] The primary endpoint of cardiovascular death or new MI at seven days was reduced with hirudin from 4.2% to 3.6% ($P = 0.064$); there was an excess of major bleeds requiring transfusions (1.2% versus 0.7%; $P = 0.014$). A meta-analysis of the GUSTO-IIb, TIMI-9B, OASIS pilot and OASIS-2 showed that the risk of death or MI at 35 days was significantly reduced with hirudin compared with heparin (RR 0.90; $P = 0.015$).[41]

A meta-analysis of 35 970 patients in 11 trials of hirudin, bivalirudin, and low-molecular weight antithrombins in

ACS and PCI showed an overall reduction in the risk of death or MI at the end of the treatment period with the direct antithrombins (4.3% versus 5.1%; OR 0.85; 95% CI 0.77–0.94; $P = 0.001$) and after 30 days (7.4% versus 8.2%; OR 0.91; 95% CI 0.84–0.99; $P = 0.02$).[189] The benefit was restricted to hirudin and bivalirudin; hirudin increased the risk of major bleeding compared with heparin but bivalirudin reduced it.[189] No further studies were performed with hirudin because of this excess bleeding. Bivalirudin, a less potent and reversible antithrombin, was further evaluated in the context of PCI, in the ACUITY trial. There were 13 819 patients with moderate- or high-risk NSTE-ACS randomized to UFH or enoxaparin plus a Gp IIb/IIIa inhibitor, bivalirudin plus a Gp IIb/IIIa inhibitor, or bivalirudin alone.[190] The composite efficacy endpoint (death, MI or unplanned revascularization for ischemia) occurred in 7.8% of bivalirudin patients and 7.3% of heparin plus abciximab patients (RR 1.08; 95% CI 0.93–1.24; $P = 0.32$) with rates of bleeding of 3.0% and 5.7% respectively (RR 0.53; 95% CI 0.43–0.65; $P < 0.001$). This reduced rate of bleeding resulted in a significant net clinical benefit of bivalirudin. Previous trials with bivalirudin had used a similar non-inferiority design comparing the drug alone to the combination in stable patients undergoing PCI[191] and in ST segment elevation MI patients undergoing primary PCI.[192] These also generally showed non-significant trends to more ischemic events and a significant reduction in bleeding with bivaluridin alone, resulting in a significant net clinical benefit when combining the efficacy and safety endpoints. Hirudin, bivalirudin, and argatroban are approved for use in patients with heparin-induced thrombocytopenia. Hirudin is also approved for the prevention of deep vein thrombosis in patients undergoing orthopedic surgery, and bivalirudin for use in the cath lab during PCI in stable patients. The FDA expressed concerns, however, with the results of the ACUITY trial in patients with NSTE-ACS and those of the HORIZON trial in STEMI, and did not approve bivalirudin for these indications.

Long-term anticoagulation Prolonged administration of LMWH and of warfarin has been evaluated to prolong the benefit of anticoagulants past the acute phase and prevent reactivation of the disease. In the ATACS trial, 214 patients were randomized to ASA alone or the combination of ASA plus UFH followed by warfarin. At 14 days, there was a reduction in the composite outcome of death, MI, and recurrent ischemia with the combination therapy (27.0% versus 10.5%; $P = 0.004$). In a small randomized pilot study of 57 patients allocated to warfarin or placebo in addition to ASA, there was less progression and more regression in the severity of the culprit lesion after a few weeks of treatment with warfarin. The OASIS pilot study[188] compared a fixed dosage of 3 mg of warfarin with a moderate dose titrated to an international normalized ratio (INR) of 2 to 2.5 administered for seven months. Low-intensity warfarin had no benefit, whereas the moderate-intensity regimen reduced the risk of death, MI or refractory angina by 58% and the need for rehospitalization for unstable angina by 58%. These results were not reproduced in the larger OASIS-2 trial[37] which randomized 3712 patients to the moderate-intensity regimen. The rate of cardiovascular death, MI or stroke after five months was 7.65% with the anticoagulant and 8.4% without ($P = 0.37$). The authors suggested that poor compliance with treatment in some countries could have explained the negative results. A meta-analysis of 30 randomized studies published between 1960 and July 1999 among patients with CAD showed that high-intensity and moderate-intensity anticoagulation were effective in reducing MI and stroke but increased the risk of bleeding. In the presence of aspirin, low-intensity anticoagulation was not superior to aspirin alone, while moderate- to high-intensity anticoagulation and aspirin versus aspirin alone appeared promising with a modest increase in bleeding risk.[193]

In FRISC-II, dalteparin was administrated double-blind for three months following five days of open-label administration. A significant reduction in rates of death, MI, and revascularization was observed after 30 days (3.1% versus 5.9%; RR 0.53; $P = 0.02$) and three months (29.1% versus 33.4%; $P = 0.03$), which was not sustained at six months.[183] A meta-analysis of prolonged use of LMWH for up to tjree months after hospital discharge showed no consistent benefit (OR 0.98; 95% CI 0.81–1.17; $P = 0.80$) but an excess risk of major bleeding (OR 2.26; 95% CI 1.63–3.14; $P < 0.0001$).[182]

Most modern trials that have compared a novel anticoagulant to UFH have used the former for the duration of hospitalization but the latter for only about 48 hours. In these trials, the novel anticoagulant benefit generally appeared after 24–72 h, suggesting that the longer duration of therapy could account for the benefit. A Phase II pilot study of ximelagatran, an orally active direct thrombin inhibitor, suggested a benefit of prolonged therapy with the drug initiated after an acute myocardial infarction[194] but the subsequent development was discontinued because of liver toxicity. A similar study is now being conducted with dagibatran, an orally active direct thrombin inhibitor with a better safety profile.

Summary of treatment recommendations for antiplatelet and anticoagulant drugs
The ACC/AHA recommends that all patients should receive aspirin (150–325 mg load, 75–162 mg maintenance) (**Class I, Level A**) and an anticoagulant (**Class I, Level A**), as soon as the diagnosis of NSTE-ACS appears likely or definite.

With invasive management, acceptable anticoagulant options include UFH or enoxaparin (**Class I, Level A**) or fondaparinux or bivalrudin (**Class I, Level B**). In addition, either clopidogrel (600 mg load, 75 mg maintenance) or a IIb/IIIa inhibitor should be started as soon as possible and before angiography (**Class I, Level A**), and both may be indicated if there is a delay to angiography, there are high risk features present or chest discomfort recurs (**Class IIa, Level B**). Generally eptifibatide or tirofiban is the preferred IIb/IIIa inhibitor, although abciximab is a reasonable choice if there is no appreciable delay to angiography and PCI is likely (**Class IIa, Level B**). If significant coronary artery disease is found on angiography, aspirin should be continued indefinitely in all patients (**Class I, Level A**). Clopidogrel should be continued for at least one month (**Class I, Level A**), and ideally for up to one year (**Class I, Level B**); prolonged use is more important if a DES is implanted. UFH may be discontinued within 48 h of cessation of chest discomfort (**Class I, Level A**), enoxaparin and fondaparinux should be maintained for the duration of the hospital stay (up to eight days) (**Class I, Level A**). UFH and LMWH may be discontinued shortly following uncomplicated PCI, bivalirudin may be either stopped or continued at reduced doses for 72 h and tirofiban and eptifibatide may be continued for 12–24 h (**Class I, Level B**). If the patient is to have CABG, antithrombotic agents should ideally be discontinued at the following times prior to surgery: clopidogrel 5–7 days, a IIb/IIIa inhibitor 4 h, enoxaparin 12–24 h, fondaparinux 24 h and bivalrudin 3 h (**Class I, Level B for all**).

With conservative, management, acceptable anticoagulant options include UFH, enoxaparin or fondaparinux (**Class I, Level A**), although enoxaparin or fondaparinux are preferred (**Class I, Level B**) and clopidogrel (load and maintenance) should be started (**Class I, Level A**). Eptifibatide or tirofiban may be added if there are high-risk features or chest discomfort recurs (**Class IIa, Level B**). Aspirin should be continued indefinitely in all patients (**Class I, Level A**). Clopidogrel should be continued for at least one month (**Class I, Level A**), and ideally for up to one year (**Class I, Level B**). Enoxaparin and fondaparinux should be maintained for the duration of the hospital stay (up to eight days) (**Class I, Level A**), while if UFH was used, it should be discontinued within 48 h of cessation of chest discomfort (**Class I, Level A**). If a IIb/IIIa inhibitor was used it should be discontinued within 12 h of the cessation of chest discomfort (**Class I, Level B**).

The ESC recommends, in all patients without contraindications, immediate aspirin (160–325 mg load, 75–100 mg maintenance), clopidogrel (300 mg load, 75 mg maintenance) and anticoagulation.

With invasive management, UFH (**Class I, Level C**), enoxaparin (**Class IIa, Level B**) or bivalirudin (**Class I, Level B**) should be started immediately. The loading dose of clopidogrel should be 600 mg (**Class I, level A**). Whichever anticoagulant is chosen, it should be maintained during the PCI. If fondaparinux has been chosen, additional standard doses of UFH (50–100 IU/kg bolus) are required during PCI (**Class IIa, Level C**). In high-risk patients not pretreated with a GP IIb/IIIa inhibitor, abciximab is recommended immediately following angiography (**Class I, Level A**), whereas if tirofiban or eptifibatide was begun prior to angiography, it should be maintained during and after PCI (**Class IIa, Level B**). Anticoagulation can be stopped within 24 h after an invasive procedure (**Class IIa, Level C**). Aspirin should be continued indefinitely (**Class I, Level A**), and clopidogrel for 12 months unless there is an excessive risk of bleeding (**Class I, Level A**).

With conservative management, or prior to a decision about invasive manangement, fondaparinux is recommended (**Class I, Level A**). In patients at intermediate to high risk, particularly those with elevated troponins, ST depression or diabetes, either eptifibatide or tirofiban is recommended in addition to oral antiplatelet agents and anticoagulant (**Class IIa, Level A**). Fondaparinux, enoxaparin or other LMWH may be maintained up to hospital discharge. Aspirin should be continued indefinitely (**Class I, Level A**), and clopidogrel for 12 months unless there is an excessive risk of bleeding (**Class I, Level A**).

Coronary reperfusion procedures

There is a strong rationale for early reperfusion in patients with NSTE-ACS, given the thrombotic pathophysiology, although fibrinolytic therapy is harmful.[135,195] A number of randomized trials have been conducted in the context of 15 years of increasing procedural experience, technologic improvements in revascularization procedures and the development of new antiplatelet and anticoagulant regimens. Two general approaches have emerged from reviews of these studies.

• Routine early *invasive management* whereby patients receive optimal medical therapy with the addition of either (a) urgent angiography/revascularization (as quickly as possible after hospital presentation) for clinically unstable presentations or (b) early angiography/revascularizataion (within a few hours) as part of a standard approach to managment of NSTE-ACS.

• Routine early *conservative management* ("selective invasive therapy"), whereby patients receive optimal medical therapy, with angiography/revascularization reserved for those who cannot be medically stabilized or in whom objective evidence of significant ischemia is provoked in the subacute phase.

TIMI-3B randomized 1473 patients with NSTE-ACS to early invasive versus early conservative therapy. The primary outcome of death, MI or an unsatisfactory symptom-limited exercise stress test performed at six weeks occurred in 16.2% of patients assigned to the early invasive strategy versus 18.1% of patients assigned to the early conservative strategy (NS). The average length of initial hospitalization, the incidence of rehospitalization within six weeks, and days of rehospitalization were all decreased in the early invasive group.[195] VANQWISH randomized 920 patients with NSTEMI on the basis of CK-MB elevation within 72 hours of admission. More patients in the early invasive group experienced inhospital death (21 versus 6; $P = 0.007$) or a composite of death or MI (36 versus 15; $P = 0.004$); statistically significant differences persisted at one year and a trend towards higher mortality was still observed at two years.[196] The clinical applicability of the results was questioned on the basis of the high mortality associated with CABG; no mortality was seen with PCI.

More recently, the FRISC-II study enrolled 2457 patients with chest pain within the previous 48 hours plus either (a) ST or T-wave changes or (b) elevated troponin T or CK-MB.[40] All patients received dalteparin in addition to aspirin in the first five days and were thereafter randomized to placebo or continued dalteparin administration for three months. Coronary angiography was done within the first seven days in 96% of patients in the invasive arm and in 10% in the non-invasive arm, and revascularization was performed within the first 10 days in 71% and 9% of patients respectively. After six months there was a decrease in the composite endpoint of death or MI in the invasive group (9.4% versus 12.1%; RR 0.78; 95% CI 0.62–0.98; $P < 0.031$). At one year the mortality rate in the invasive strategy group was 2.2% compared with 3.9% in the non-invasive strategy group ($P = 0.016$).[197] The frequencies of symptomatic angina and readmission were halved by the invasive strategy. It was concluded that patients who first received an average of six days of treatment with LMWH, ASA, nitrates, and beta-blockers have a better outcome at six months.

TACTICS-TIMI 18 enrolled 2220 patients with NSTE-ACS characterized by ST-T changes suggestive of ischemia, elevated levels of cardiac markers, or a history of coronary artery disease.[198] All patients received aspirin, heparin, and tirofiban. Patients were randomized to invasive therapy (routine coronary angiography at a median of 22h and revascularization as appropriate) or ongoing medical therapy. The primary outcome of death, non-fatal MI or rehospitalization for an acute coronary syndrome at six months was 15.9% with use of the early invasive strategy and 19.4% with use of the conservative strategy (OR 0.78; 95% CI 0.62–0.97; $P = 0.025$). The rate of death or non-fatal MI at six months was similarly reduced (7.3% versus 9.5%; OR 0.74; 95% CI 0.54–1.00; < 0.05).

RITA 3[199] enrolled 1810 patients with NSTE-ACS who were all managed with optimal medical therapy and randomized to angiography (median two days), followed by PCI or CABG as appropriate, or to ongoing medical therapy. Of the PCI patients, 88% received a stent and 25% a GP IIb/IIIa inhibitor. The relative risk of death or non-

fatal MI at one year in the invasive group was 0.91 ($P = 0.58$), while that of death, non-fatal MI or refractory angina was 0.66 ($P = 0.001$). A meta-analysis of these five large trials and two smaller trials found that the incidence of death or non-fatal MI in the invasive group was 12.2% versus 14.4% in the conservative group (OR 0.82, 95% CI 0.72–0.93, $P < 0.001$).[200]

ISAR-COOL[201] was designed to determine whether prolonged antithrombotic pretreatment might improve the outcomes of patients undergoing routine invasive management. There were 410 patients enrolled with symptoms of unstable angina plus either ST segment depression or elevation of cardiac troponin T. All patients received UFH, aspirin, clopidogrel and tirofiban and were randomized to early (<6h) or delayed (3–5 days) angiography/revascularization. The principal outcome of death or non-fatal MI by 30 days occurred in 5.9% of the early invasive group versus 11.6% of the delayed invasive group (RR 0.51, $P = 0.04$). The most recent such large study, ICTUS,[202] enrolled 1200 patients with accelerated angina or angina at rest accompanied by an elevated troponin plus either ischemic ECG changes or a history of coronary artery disease. They all received aspirin, enoxaparin, clopidogrel and a statin and were randomized to invasive therapy (addition of abciximab, routine angiography at a median of 23h, with 88% of PCI patients receiving a stent) or to a selective invasive strategy with angiography/revascularization reserved for those with refractory angina, instability or significant ischemia on predischarge exercise testing. The composite outcome of death, non-fatal MI or rehospitalization within one year occurred in 22.7% of the early invasive group versus 21.2% of the selective invasive group (RR 1.07, $P = 0.33$). Mortality was no different, whereas in the early invasive group MI was more frequent and rehospitalization less frequent.

A meta-analysis of trials performed in the current era of the use of stents and GP IIb/IIIa agents found that two-year mortality was 4.9% in the early invasive group versus 6.5% in the conservative therapy group (RR 0.75, 95% CI 0.63–0.90, $P = 0.001$).[203] A Cochrane systematic overview[204] confirmed earlier findings of trends toward increased hospital mortality and non-fatal MI in the early invasive group, but statistically significant reductions at all subsequent follow-up intervals out to 2–5 years. This overview also confirmed earlier evidence for the independent contributions to risk and the likelihood of observing a benefit of early invasive therapy among patients with ST segment depression or troponin elevation, or both. However, the authors stressed the importance of making an assessment of global risk (PURSUIT, TIMI, GRACE risk scores).

A more recent collaborative meta-analysis[205] of eight trials involving 7075 men and 3075 women found one-year composite outcome of death, MI or rehospitalization with ACS was 21.1% in the invasive group versus 25.9% in the conservative group (OR 0.78; 95% CI 0.61–0.98) (Fig. 29.13). The OR was significant in men (OR 0.73, 95% CI 0.55–0.98) but not in women (OR 0.81, 95% CI 0.65–1.01). Among biomarker-positive women, the OR was 0.67 (95% CI 0.50–0.88) but among biomarker-negative women the OR was 0.94 (95% CI 0.61–1.44). Among biomarker-positive men, the OR was 0.56 (95% CI 0.46–0.67) while among biomarker-negative men the OR was 0.72 (95% CI 0.51–1.01). As in previous meta-analyses, the rates of death or non-fatal MI were higher in the invasive group during the index hospitalization, but by one year they were significantly less in this group.

An early invasive strategy is recommended for patients with refractory angina or hemodynamic or electrical instability (**Class I, Level B**) and for those who have a relatively high risk of clinical events as predicted by a positive bio-marker assay, ST segment changes or a high risk score according to the TIMI scale or equivalents (**Class I, Level A**). This recommendation is equally applicable to men and women. A conservative strategy is recommended for women who are stabilized and remain biomarker negative (**Class IIa, Level A**). Either early invasive or conservative therapy is a reasonable option for men who are stabilized and remain biomarker negative (**Class IIa, Level A**).

Cell protection

Cell necrosis remains a significant problem in patients with UA/NSTEMI as close to 50% of patients have some degree of necrosis at admission and 5–15% develop a new MI within a few weeks. Reperfusion procedures are also frequently associated with MI which impacts on prognosis; there is a correlation between subsequent mortality and elevation of blood markers of necrosis, particularly CK-MB, even within the range of only one and three times normal.[206] Measures that could prevent or limit the progression of myocardial cell ischemia to necrosis might optimize the benefit to be derived from other treatment strategies. These protective measures have been investigated mainly in evolving STEMI. Although often effective in animal models, none of these interventions was sufficiently convincing in human studies to be incorporated in routine management, including Na^+/H^+ exchanger inhibition to prevent accumulation of calcium within the ischemic cell,[207] antibodies against leukocyte integrins and against the cytokine tissue necrosis factor alpha (TNF-alpha)[208] and pexelizumab, a monoclonal antibody against C5 blocking formation of the terminal complement and excessive inflammatory reactions.[209] So far, adenosine has been the only agent that could reduce infarct size in subgroups of patients with an anterior myocardial infarction successfully reperfused and lead to a non-statistically significant reduction in the endpoint of death or new heart failure.[210]

Although beta-blockers were shown in a meta-analysis to be of moderate benefit to prevent myocardial infarction in patients with threatened myocardial infarction,[121] many large randomized clinical trials have documented their efficacy in reducing death following MI and guidelines have advised their use, a recent randomized trial of IV followed by oral metoprolol among patients with acute MI showed no reduction of in-hospital mortality and recommended that beta-blockers be reserved for those patients not at risk of heart failure or cardiogenic shock.[211]

Plaque passivation

Control of inflammatory processes associated with plaque degradation and resulting in plaque rupture and thrombus formation could be an effective management strategy for ACS, but since there are no means to easily and reliably identify vulnerable plaques, administration of such a therapy prior to the clinical manifestations of ACS is not practicable. On the other hand, secondary preventive measures initiated during the acute phase and continued at hospital discharge are effective and practical. PCI, including stenting, is very effective acutely, possibly by interrupting some of the processes implicated in the disease. A 48-hour course of methylprednisone in a small pilot study in patients with unstable angina was ineffective to prevent ischemic events and even accelerated their manifestations.[212]

Statins and ACE inhibitors can promote plaque stabilization by so-called pleiotropic effects that include anti-inflammatory, antioxidant, anti-cell proliferative and anticoagulant properties.[213] Many trials and registries have shown that statins started early after an ACS, even at admission, are well tolerated, effective in reducing LDL cholesterol, and possibly protective against ischemic events associated with interventions. In pooled observational data of 20 809 ACS patients enrolled in clinical trials, the presence of lipid-lowering therapy at hospital discharge was associated with a 56% reduction in risk of mortality at one month ($P = 0.001$).[214] A Swedish registry of 5528 AMI survivors reported a one-year mortality of 9.3% in the 14 071 patients who had no statin at hospital discharge and 4.0% in the 5528 patients with a statin.[215] The MIRACL study[216] randomized 3086 patients with no interventions anticipated within 24–96 hours of hospitalization to high-dose atorvastatin or placebo. At 16 weeks, the primary outcome of death, non-fatal MI, resuscitated cardiac arrest or worsening angina requiring urgent revascularization was 14.8% in treated patients and 17.4% in placebo patients (RR 0.84; $P = 0.048$). More recently, the PROVE-It trial[217] randomized 4162 patients within 10 days of an ACS to pravastatin 40 mg daily or atorvastatin 80 mg daily to determine if the then standard therapy to lower LDL-C to the recommended goal of 100 mg/dL was as effective in preventing further coronary events as more aggressive therapy that lowered LDL-C to 70 mg/dL. The rate of the primary endpoint

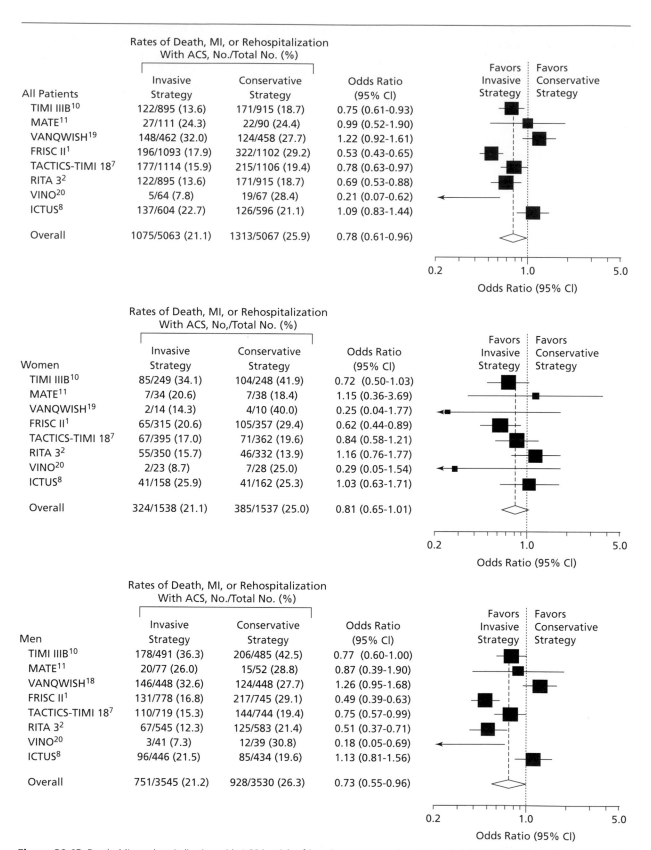

Figure 29.13 Death, MI or rehospitalization with ACS in trials of invasive vs conservative strategy in NSTE-ACS. ACS, acute coronary syndromes; CI, confidence interval; MI, myocardial infarction; NSTE, non-ST segment elevatlion. Size of data markers is wieghted based on the inverse variance. (Reproduced with permission from O'Donaghue *et al*[205].)

(death from any cause, MI, documented UA requiring hospitalization, PTCA or coronary bypass surgery, or stroke) was reduced by 16% after a mean follow-up of 24 months from 26.3% in the pravastatin group to 22.4% in the atorvastatin group (P = 0.005). Early initiation of statin therapy also increases the likelihood that patients will continue to comply with statin therapy and results in a greater percentage of patients using a statin after one year.[218]

Subacute therapy

The subacute and longer term management of patients who undergo urgent, early or selective angiography/revascularization is generally similar to, although more aggressive than, that of patients undergoing PCI or CABG for stable angina (see Chapters 26–28). Nitroglycerin can be discontinued rapidly in patients successfully managed with an invasive strategy and in those whose acute ischemia resolves quickly and who remain stable with no recurrence of ischemic pain for about 24–48 hours. Beta-blockers should be continued indefinitely. If a rate-limiting calcium antagonist was chosen because of contraindications to a beta-blocker, although there is no rigorous evidence for long-term benefit in terms of major cardiovascular outcomes, it is reasonable to continue it. If large doses of beta-blocker or calcium antagonists, or combined therapy, were required for control of the ischemic episodes, judicious decrements of intensity are likely to be appropriate once the patient is fully mobilized. Those patients found to be at relatively low risk, based upon a variety of prognostic factors and non-invasive testing, may be promptly discharged on medical therapy with careful long-term follow-up (**Class I, Level A**).

Whether or not the patient undergoes revascularization, aspirin should be continued indefinitely, based upon the evidence from the initial trials of aspirin for unstable angina[137,138] demonstrating ongoing benefit for up to two years, consistent with evidence in survivors of MI and patients with stable angina[139] (**Class I, Level A**). Clopidogrel should be started on admission, and continued for at least 9–12 months, in conjunction with aspirin whether the patient has been treated medically or invasively (**Class I, Level A**). The one-year duration of administration is particularly important in patients who have received a DES and likely in diabetics as well[219] (**Class I, Level B**). For those patients intolerant of aspirin, clopidogrel alone is indicated (**Class I, Level A**). Among patients receiving medical therapy only, fondaparinux, LMWH or UFH is indicated (**Class I, Level A**) and should be sustained for at least 48 hours following the resolution of acute ischemic episodes and preferably until hospital discaharge[149] (**Class I, Level B**). In patients being managed non-invasively, fondaparinux and LMWHs appear to be at least as efficacious as UFH, and may be preferable in terms of ease of use, less bleeding and cost–benefit considerations (**Class IIa, Level B**). Fondaparinux causes less bleeding than LMWH (**Level A**). Intravenous Gp IIb/IIIa receptor antagonists should be added only in the early hospital phase in particularly unstable patients, with eptifibatide or tirofiban being the preferred agents (**Class IIb, Level B**) and should be discontinued within 48 hours of resolution of acute ischemic episodes.

The long-term use of an ACE inhibitor is likely to be beneficial in all patients who have experienced NSTE-ACS[220] (**Class I, Level A**). An angiotensin receptor blocker should be substituted for patients with ACE-I intolerance (**Class I, Level A**). A statin should be commenced early in hospital, regardless of the LDL-C, and should be continued indefinitely with a target LDL-C <2.0 (**Class I, Level A**). Early attention to optimal management of coronary risk factors (**Class I**) blood pressure (**Level A**), smoking (**Level B**), diabetes (Level B), weight (Level B), and exercise (**Level B**) is mandatory for all patients with NSTE-ACS, including those who have undergone revascularization, with the expectation of limiting progression of disease in non-revascularized vessels and in areas of percutaneous intervention and bypass conduits. The HPS study showed benefit independently of initial cholesterol levels.[221] Recent evidence indicates that tight control of glucose in patients with type 2 diabetes may reduce the risk of death following MI and among patients with newly detected type 2 diabetes.[222–224]

The recurrence of an unstable phase of coronary artery disease or poor symptomatic control in patients being managed on medical therapy generally mandates reconsideration of the option of angiography/revascularization (**Class I, Level B**) or, if not feasible, augmented or alternative medical therapy (**Class I, Level C**).

Conclusion

The underlying pathophysiology of NSTE-ACS is most often the rupture of a vulnerable atherosclerotic plaque followed by the development of an overlying subtotally occlusive, platelet-rich thrombus. The symptoms are usually those of angina at rest, of new onset or with a pattern of increasing severity. Management should be focused initially on preventing death and MI (patient recognition of symptoms, activation of the 911 system, and expeditious management in the ambulance and emergency room), relieving ischemic symptoms (bed rest, nitrates, beta-blockers/calcium antagonists) and resolving coronary thrombosis (aspirin, clopidogrel, an anticoagulant (a choice of UFH, LMWH, bivalirudin or fondaparinux) and Gp IIb/IIIa antagonists). Immediate and ongoing risk stratification must govern the pace, intensity and extent of therapy. Angiography and revascularization (PCI or CABG) as appropriate should be undertaken urgently for patients in whom ischemic symptoms are severe, progressive and/or accompanied by hemodynamic instability. Patients who are stabilized quickly should be managed by a strategy of early invasive therapy if they are at higher risk. For men at intermediate or low risk the management strategy may be either early invasive or selective invasive, whereas for women in the lower risk categories the management strategy should be selective invasive. Aspirin should be started immediately and continued indefinitely; clopidogrel should be started early unless there is a high likelihood of CABG, and continued for at least a year. A beta-blocker (or calcium antagonist), initially used to control ischemic symptoms, should generally be continued indefinitely unless the patient undergoes revascularization. Most patients should begin an ACE inhibitor (or ARB if there is ACE intolerance), and all should begin a statin in hospital and continue indefinitely. Optimal management of coronary risk factors and ongoing follow-up are indicated for all patients whether or not they undergo revascularization.

References

1. Anderson JL, Adams CD, Antman EM et al. ACC/AHA 2007 guidelines for the management of patients with unstable angina/non ST-elevation myocardial infarction: a report of the American College of Cardiology/American Heart Association Task Force on Practice Guidelines. Circulation 2007;116: e148–304.
2. Davies MJ, Thomas A. Thrombosis and acute coronary artery lesions in sudden cardiac ischemic death. N Engl J Med 1984;310:1137–40.
3. Davies M, Thomas A, Knapman P, Hangartner R. Intramyocardial platelet aggregation in patients with unstable angina suffering sudden ischaemic cardiac death. Circulation 1986; 73:418–27.
4. Falk E. Unstable angina with fatal outcome: dynamic coronary thrombosis leading to infarction and/or sudden death: autopsy evidence of recurrent mural thrombosis with peripheral embolization culminating in total coronary occlusion. Circulation 1985;71:699–708.
5. Theroux P, Fuster V. Acute coronary syndromes: unstable angina and non-Q-wave myocardial infarction. Circulation 1998;97:1195–206.
6. DeWood MA, Spores J, Notske R et al. Prevalence of total coronary occlusion during the early hours of transmural myocardial infarction. N Engl J Med 1980;303:897–902.
7. Bassand JP, Hamm CW, Ardissino D et al. Guidelines for the diagnosis and treatment of non-ST segment elevation acute coronary syndromes. Eur Heart J 2007;28:1598–660.
8. http://www.escardio.org/knowledge/ehs/
9. Fox KAA, Goodman SG, Klein W et al., for the GRACE Investigators. Management of acute coronary syndromes. Variations in practice and outcome: findings from the Global Registry of Acute Coronary Events (GRACE). Eur Heart J 2002;23:1177–89.
10. Hoekstra SW, Pollack CV, Roe MJ et al. Improving the care of patients with non-ST-elevation acute coronary syndrome in the emergency department. The CRUSADE initiative. Acad Emerg Med 2002;9:1146–55.
11. http://www.ncdr.com/webncdr/ACTION/default.aspx
12. Campeau L. Letter: Grading of angina pectoris. Circulation 1976;54:522–23.
13. Antman EM, Hand M, Armstrong PW et al. 2007 focused update of the ACC/AHA 2004 guidelines for the management of patients with ST-elevation myocardial infarction: a report of the American College of Cardiology/American Heart Association Task Force on Practice Guidelines. J Am Coll Cardiol 2008;51:210–47.
14. Thygesen K, Alpert JS, White HD. Universal definition of myocardial infarction. J Am Coll Cardiol 2007;50:2173–95.
15. Rosamond W, Flegal K, Friday G et al. Heart disease and srtroke statistics – 2007 update: a report from the American Heart Association Statistics Committee and Stroke Statistics Subcommittee. Circulation 2007;115:e69–171.
16. Gibbons RJ, Abrams J, Chatterjee K et al. ACC/AHA 2002 guideline update for the management of patients with chronic stable angina. Circulation 2003;107:149–58.
17. Bata IR, Gregor RD, Eastwood BJ, Wolf HK. Trends in the incidence of acute myocardial infarction between 1984 and 1993 – The Halifax County MONICA Project. Can J Cardiol 2000;16:589–95.
18. Volmink JA, Newton JN, Hicks NR, Sleight P, Fowler GH, Neil HA. Coronary event and case fatality rates in an English population: results of the Oxford myocardial infarction incidence study. The Oxford Myocardial Infarction Incidence Study Group. Heart 1998;80:40–4.
19. Madsen M, Rasmussen S, Juel K. [Acute myocardial infarction in Denmark. Incidence development and prognosis during a 20-year period]. Ugeskr Laeger 2000;162:5918–23.
20. van der Pal-de Bruin KM, Verkleij H, Jansen J, Bartelds A, Kromhout D. The incidence of suspected myocardial infarction in Dutch general practice in the period 1978–1994. Eur Heart J 1998;19:429–34.
21. Fox KA, Cokkinos DV, Deckers J, Keil U, Maggioni A, Steg G. The ENACT study: a pan-European survey of acute coronary syndromes. European Network for Acute Coronary Treatment. Eur Heart J 2000;21:1440–9.
22. Goldberg RJ, Steg PG, Sadiq I et al. Extent of, and factors associated with, delay to hospital presentation in patients with acute coronary disease (the GRACE registry). Am J Cardiol 2002;89:791–6.
23. Xavier D, Pais P, Devereaux PJ et al. CREATE registry investigators. Treatment and outcomes of acute coronary syndromes in India (CREATE): a prospective analysis of registry data. Lancet 2008;371:1435–42.
24. Furman MI, Dauerman HL, Goldberg RJ, Yarzebski J, Lessard D, Gore JM. Twenty-two year (1975 to 1997) trends in the incidence, in-hospital and long-term case fatality rates from initial Q-wave and non-Q-wave myocardial infarction: a multihospital, community-wide perspective. J Am Coll Cardiol 2001; 37:1571–80.
25. Fox KAA, Steg PG, Eagle KA et al. Decline in rates of death and heart failure in acute coronary syndromes, 1999–2006. JAMA 2007;297:1892–900.

25. Cairns JA, Fantus IG, Klassen GA. Unstable angina pectoris. *Am Heart J* 1976;**92**:373–86.

26. Cairns J, Singer J, Gent M *et al.* One-year mortality outcomes of all coronary and intensive care units with acute myocardial infarction, unstable angina or other chest pain in Hamilton, Canada, a city of 375 000 people. *Can J Cardiol* 1989;**5**:239–46.

27. RISC Group. Risk of myocardial infarction and death during treatment with low-dose aspirin and intravenous heparin in men with unstable coronary artery disease. *Lancet* 1990;**226**:827–30.

28. Theroux P, Ouimet H, McCans J *et al.* Aspirin, heparin or both to treat unstable angina. *N Engl J Med* 1988;**336**: 827–30.

29. Global Use of Strategies to Open Occluded Coronary Arteries (GUSTO) IIb Investigators. A comparison of recombinant hirudin with heparin for the treatment of acute coronary syndromes. *N Engl J Med* 1996;**335**:775–82.

30. Cohen M, Demers C, Gurfinkel EP *et al.* A comparison of low molecular-weight heparin with unfractionated heparin for unstable coronary artery disease. Efficacy and Safety of Subcutaneous Enoxaparin in Non-Q-Wave Coronary Events Study Group. *N Engl J Med* 1997;**337**:447–52.

31. Platelet Receptor Inhibition for Ischemic Syndrome Management in Patients Limited by Unstable Signs and Symptoms (PRISM) Study Investigators. A comparison of aspirin plus tirofiban versus aspirin plus heparin for unstable angina. *N Engl J Med* 1998;**338**:1498–505.

32. Platelet Receptor Inhibition in Ischemic Syndrome Management in Patients Limited by Unstable Signs and Symptoms (PRISM-PLUS) Study Investigators. Inhibition of the platelet glycoprotein IIb/IIIa receptor with tirofiban in unstable angina and non-Q-wave myocardial infarction. *N Engl J Med* 1998;**338**: 1488–97.

33. PARAGON Investigators. International, randomized, controlled trial of lamifiban (a platelet glycoprotein IIb/IIIa inhibitor), heparin, or both in unstable angina. Platelet IIb/IIIa Antagonism for the Reduction of Acute Coronary Syndrome Events in a Global Organization Network. *Circulation* 1998;**97**:2386–95.

34. Mahaffey KW, Roe MT, Dyke CK *et al.* Misreporting of myocardial infarction end points: results of adjudication by a central clinical events committee in the PARAGON-B trial. Second Platelet IIb/IIIa Antagonist for the Reduction of Acute Coronary Syndrome Events in a Global Organization Network Trial. *Am Heart J* 2002;**143**:242–8.

35. PURSUIT Investigators. Inhibition of platelet glycoprotein IIb/IIIa with eptifibatide in patients with acute coronary syndromes. Platelet Glycoprotein IIb/IIIa in Unstable Angina: Receptor Suppression Using Integrilin Therapy. *N Engl J Med* 1998;**339**: 436–43.

36. Organisation to Assess Strategies for Ischemic Syndromes (OASIS-2) Investigators. Effects of recombinant hirudin (lepirudin) compared with heparin on death, myocardial infarction, refractory angina, and revascularisation procedures in patients with acute myocardial ischaemia without ST elevation: a randomized trial. *Lancet* 1999;**353**:429–38.

37. Antman EM, McCabe CH, Gurfinkel EP *et al.* Enoxaparin prevents death and cardiac ischemic events in unstable angina/non-Q-wave myocardial infarction: results of the thrombolysis in myocardial infarction (TIMI) 11B trial. *Circulation* 1999;**100**: 1593–601.

38. GUSTO IV-ACS Investigators. Effect of glycoprotein IIb/IIIa receptor blocker abciximab on outcome in patients with acute coronary syndromes without early coronary revascularisation: the GUSTO IV-ACS randomized trial. *Lancet* 2001;**357**: 1915–24.

39. FRISC II Investigators. Invasive compared with non-invasive treatment in unstable coronary-artery disease: FRISC II prospective randomized multicenter study. *Lancet* 1999; **354**:708–15.

40. Cannon CP, Weintraub WS, Demopoulos LA *et al.* Comparison of early invasive and conservative strategies in patients with unstable coronary syndromes treated with the glycoprotein IIb/IIIa inhibitor tirofiban. *N Engl J Med* 2001; **344**: 1879–87.

41. Malmberg K, Yusuf S, Gerstein HC *et al.* Impact of diabetes on long-term prognosis in patients with unstable angina and non-Q-wave myocardial infarction: results of the OASIS (Organization to Assess Strategies for Ischemic Syndromes) Registry. *Circulation* 2000;**102**:1014–19.

42. Savonitto S, Ardissino D, Granger CB *et al.* Prognostic value of the admission electrocardiogram in acute coronary syndromes. *JAMA* 1999;**281**:707–13.

43. Bogaty P, Poirier P, Simard S, Boyer L, Solymoss S, Dagenais GR. Biological profiles in subjects with recurrent acute coronary events compared with subjects with long-standing stable angina. *Circulation* 2001;**103**:3062–8.

44. Bahit MC, Granger CB, Wallentin L. Persistence of the prothrombotic state after acute coronary syndromes: implications for treatment. *Am Heart J* 2002;**143**:205–16.

45. Jayes RL Jr, Beshansky JR, D'Agostino RB, Selker HP. Do patients' coronary risk factor reports predict acute cardiac ischemia in the emergency department? A multicenter study. *J Clin Epidemiol* 1992;**45**:621–6.

46. Moise A, Theroux P, Taeymans Y *et al.* Clinical and angiographic factors associated with progression of coronary artery disease. *J Am Coll Cardiol* 1984;**3**:659–66.

47. Moise A, Theroux P, Taeymans Y *et al.* Unstable angina and progression of coronary atherosclerosis. *N Engl J Med* 1983;**309**:685–9.

48. Sheifer SE, Manolio TA, Gersh BJ. Unrecognized myocardial infarction. *Ann Intern Med* 2001;**135**:801–11.

49. Hochman JS, Tamis JE, Thompson TD *et al.* Sex, clinical presentation, and outcome in patients with acute coronary syndromes. Global Use of Strategies to Open Occluded Coronary Arteries in Acute Coronary Syndromes IIb Investigators. *N Engl J Med* 1999;**341**:226–32.

50. Lagerqvist B, Safstrom K, Stahle E, Wallentin L, Swahn E. Is early invasive treatment of unstable coronary artery disease equally effective for both women and men? FRISC II Study Group Investigators. *J Am Coll Cardiol* 2001;**38**:41–8.

51. Donahoe SM, Stewart GC, McCabe CH *et al.* Diabetes and mortality following acute coronary syndromes. *JAMA* 2007;**298**:765–75.

52. Lesperance F, Frasure-Smith N, Juneau M, Theroux P. Depression and 1-year prognosis in unstable angina. *Arch Intern Med* 2000;**160**:1354–60.

53. Santopinto JJ, Fox KA, Goldberg RJ *et al.* Creatinine clearance and adverse hospital outcomes in patients with acute coronary syndromes: findings from the global registry of acute coronary events (GRACE). *Heart* 2003;**89**:1003–8.

54. Anavekar NS, McMurray JJ, Velazquez EJ *et al.* Relation between renal dysfunction and cardiovascular outcomes after myocardial infarction. *N Engl J Med* 2004;**351**:1285–95.

55. Hemmelgarn BR, Southern DA, Humphries KH, Culleton BF, Knudtson ML, Ghali WA. Refined characterization of the association between kidney function and mortality in patients undergoing cardiac catheterization. *Eur Heart J* 2006;**27**:1191–7.

56. Kirtane AJ, Piazza G, Murphy SA *et al.* Correlates of bleeding events among moderate- to high-risk patients undergoing percutaneous coronary intervention and treated with eptifibatide: observations from the PROTECT-TIMI-30 trial. *J Am Coll Cardiol* 2006; **47**:2374–9.

57. Moore MA, Pennathur S, Smith GL, Wilson PW. Detection of chronic kidney disease in patients with or at increased risk of cardiovascular isease: a science advisory from the American Heart Association Kidney and Cardiovascular Disease Council; the Councils on High Blood Pressure Research, Cardiovascular Disease in the Young, and Epidemiology and Prevention; and the Quality of Care and Outcomes Research Interdisciplinary Working Group: Developed in Collaboration With the National Kidney Foundation. *Hypertension* 2006;**48**:751–5.

58. Santopinto JJ, Fox KAA, Goldberg RJ *et al.*, on behalf of the GRACE Investigators. Creatinine clearance and adverse hospital outcomes in patients with acute coronary syndromes: findings from the global registry of acute coronary events (GRACE). *Heart* 2003;**89**:1003–8.

59. Cannon CP, McCabe CH, Stone PH *et al.* The electrocardiogram predicts one-year outcome of patients with unstable angina and non-Q wave myocardial infarction: results of the TIMI III Registry ECG Ancillary Study. Thrombolysis in Myocardial Ischemia. *J Am Coll Cardiol* 1997;**30**:133–40.

60. Kaul P, Fu Y, Chang WC *et al.* Prognostic value of ST segment depression in acute coronary syndromes: insights from PARAGON-A applied to GUSTO-IIb. *J Am Coll Cardiol* 2001; **38**:64–71.

61. Hyde TA, French JK, Wong CK *et al.* Four-year survival of patients with acute coronary syndromes without ST segment elevation and prognostic significance of 0.5-mm ST segment depression. *Am J Cardiol* 1999;**84**:379–85.

62. de Zwaan C, Bär FW, Janssen JHA *et al.* Angiographic and clinical characteristics of patients with unstable angina showing an ECG pattern indicating critical narrowing of the proximal LAD coronary artery. *Am Heart J* 1989;**117**:657–65.

63. Cohen M, Hawkins L, Greenberg S, Fuster V. Usefulness of ST segment changes in >2 leads on the emergency room electrocardiogram in either unstable angina pectoris or non-Q-wave myocardial infarction in predicting outcome. *Am J Cardiol* 1991;**67**:1368–73.

64. Armstrong PW, Fu Y, Chang WC *et al.* Acute coronary syndromes in the GUSTO-IIb trial. Prognostic insights and impact of recurrent ischemia. *Circulation* 1998;**98**:1860–8.

65. Hamm CW, Ravkilde J, Gerhardt W *et al.* The prognostic value of serum troponin T in unstable angina. *N Engl J Med* 1992;**327**:146–50.

66. Antman EM, Tanasijevic MJ, Thompson B *et al.* Cardiac-specific troponin I levels to predict the risk of mortality in patients with acute coronary syndromes. *N Engl J Med* 1996;**335**:1342–9.

67. Lindahl B, Venge P, Armstrong P *et al.* Troponin-T 0.03 μg/l is the most appropriate cut-off level between high and low risk

acute coronary syndrome patients: prospective verification in a large cohort of placebo patients from the GUSTO-IV ACS study. *J Am Coll Cardiol* 2001;**37**(suppl A):326A.

68. Lindahl B, Venge P, Wallentin L. Relation between troponin T and the risk of subsequent cardiac events in unstable coronary artery disease. The FRISC study group. *Circulation* 1996; **93**:1651–7.

69. Hamm CW, Braunwald E. A classification of unstable angina revisited. *Circulation* 2000;**102**:118–22.

70. Olatidoye AG, Wu AH, Feng YJ, Waters D. Prognostic role of troponin T versus troponin I in unstable angina pectoris for cardiac events with meta-analysis comparing published studies. *Am J Cardiol* 1998;**81**:1405–10.

71. Ottani F, Galvani M, Nicolini FA *et al.* Elevated cardiac troponin levels predict the risk of adverse outcome in patients with acute coronary syndromes. *Am Heart J* 2000;**140**:917–27.

72. Heidenreich PA, Alloggiamento T, Melsop K, McDonald KM, Go AS, Hlatky MA. The prognostic value of troponin in patients with non-ST elevation acute coronary syndromes: a meta-analysis. *J Am Coll Cardiol* 2001;**38**:478–85.

73. Hamm CW, Heeschen C, Goldmann B *et al.* Benefit of abciximab in patients with refractory unstable angina in relation to serum troponin T levels. c7E3 Fab Antiplatelet Therapy in Unstable Refractory Angina (CAPTURE) Study Investigators. *N Engl J Med* 1999;**340**:1623–9.

74. Morrow DA, Antman EM, Tanasijevic M *et al.* Cardiac troponin I for stratification of early outcomes and the efficacy of enoxaparin in unstable angina: a TIMI-11B substudy. *J Am Coll Cardiol* 2000;**36**:1812–17.

75. Morrow DA, Cannon CP, Rifai N *et al.* The TACTICS-TIMI 18 Investigators. Ability of minor elevations of troponins I and T to predict benefit from an early invasive strategy in patients with unstable angina and non-ST elevation myocardial infarction: results from a randomized trial. *JAMA* 2001;**286**:2405–12.

76. Liuzzo G, Biasucci LM, Gallimore JR *et al.* Enhanced inflammatory response in patients with pre-infarction unstable angina. *J Am Coll Cardiol* 1999;**34**:1696–703.

77. Biasucci LM, Liuzzo G, Grillo RL *et al.* Elevated levels of C-reactive protein at discharge in patients with unstable angina predict recurrent instability. *Circulation* 1999;**99**:855–60.

78. Toss H, Lindahl B, Siegbahn A *et al.* Prognostic influence of increased fibrinogen and C-reactive protein levels in unstable coronary artery disease. FRISC Study Group. Fragmin during Instability in Coronary Artery Disease. *Circulation* 1997; **96**:4204–10.

79. Heeschen C, Hamm CW, Bruemmer J *et al.* Predictive value of C-reactive protein and troponin T in patients with unstable angina: a comparative analysis. CAPTURE Investigators. Chimeric c7E3 AntiPlatelet Therapy in Unstable angina REfractory to standard treatment trial. *J Am Coll Cardiol* 2000;**35**:1535–42.

80. Haverkate F, Thompson SG, Pyke SD *et al.* Production of C-reactive protein and risk of coronary events in stable and unstable angina. European Concerted Action on Thrombosis and Disabilities Angina Pectoris Study Group. *Lancet* 1997;**349**:462–6.

81. Lindahl B, Toss H, Siegbahn A *et al.* Markers of myocardial damage and inflammation in relation to long-term mortality in unstable coronary artery disease. FRISC Study Group. Fragmin during Instability in Coronary Artery Disease. *N Engl J Med* 2000;**343**:1139–47.

82. Goldstein JA, Demetriou D, Grienes CJ *et al.* Multiple complex coronary plaques in patients with acute myocardial infarction. *N Engl J Med* 2000;**343**:915–22.

83. Buffon A, Liuzzo G, Biasucci LM *et al.* Preprocedural serum levels of C-reactive protein predict early complications and late restenosis after coronary angioplasty. *J Am Coll Cardiol* 1999;**34**:1512–21.

84. Chew DP, Bhatt DL, Robbins MA *et al.* Incremental prognostic value of elevated baseline C-reactive protein among established markers of risk in percutaneous coronary intervention. *Circulation* 2001;**104**:992–7.

85. Milazzo D, Biasucci LM, Luciani N *et al.* Elevated levels of C-reactive protein before coronary artery bypass grafting predict recurrence of ischemic events. *Am J Cardiol* 1999;**84**:459–61.

86. Ridker PM on behalf of the JUPITER Study Group. Rosuvastatin in the primary prevention of cardiovascular disease among patients with low levels of low-density lipoprotein cholesterol and elevated high-sensitivity C-reactive protein: rationale and design of the JUPITER trial. *Circulation* 2003;**108**:2292–7.

87. de Lemos JA, Morrow DA, Bentley JH *et al.* The prognostic value of B-type natriuretic peptide in patients with acute coronary syndromes. *N Engl J Med* 2001;**345**:1014–21.

88. James SK, Lindahl B, Siegbahn A *et al.* N-terminal pro-brain natriuretic peptide and other risk markers for the separate prediction of mortality and subsequent myocardial infarction in patients with unstable coronary artery disease: a Global Utilization of Strategies To Open occluded arteries (GUSTO)-IV substudy. *Circulation* 2003;**108**:275–81.

89. Bosch X, Theroux P. Left ventricular ejection fraction to predict early mortality in patients with non-ST segment elevation acute coronary syndromes. *Am Heart J* 2005;**150**:215–20.

90. Morrow DA, Rifai N, Antman EM *et al.* C-reactive protein is a potent predictor of mortality independently of and in combination with troponin T in acute coronary syndromes: a TIMI 11A substudy. Thrombolysis in Myocardial Infarction. *J Am Coll Cardiol* 1998;**31**:1460–5.

91. Sabatine MS, Morrow DA, de Lemos JA *et al.* Multimarker approach to risk stratification in non-ST elevation acute coronary syndromes: simultaneous assessment of troponin I, C-reactive protein, and B-type natriuretic peptide. *Circulation* 2002;**105**:1760–3.

92. de Araujo Goncalves P, Ferreira J *et al.* TIMI, PURSUIT, and GRACE risk scores: sustained prognostic value and interaction with revascularization in NSTE-ACS. *Eur Heart J* 2005;**26**:865–72.

93. Eagle KA, Lim MJ, Dabbous OH *et al.*, for the GRACE investigators. A validated prediction model for all forms of acute coronary syndrome. Estimating the risk of 6-month postdischarge death in an international registry. *JAMA* 2004;**291**:2727–33.

94. Tang EW, Wong CK, Herbison P. Global Registry of Acute Coronary Events (GRACE) hospital discharge risk score accurately predicts long-term mortality post acute coronary syndrome. *Am Heart J* 2007;**153**:29–35.

95. Antman EM, Cohen M, Bernink PJ *et al.* The TIMI risk score for unstable angina/non-ST elevation MI: a method for prognostication and therapeutic decision-making. *JAMA* 2000; **284**:835–42.

96. Libby P, Ridker PM, Maseri A. Inflammation and atherosclerosis. *Circulation* 2002;**105**:1135–43.

97. Arbustini E, Bello BD, Morbini P *et al.* Plaque erosion is a major substrate for coronary thrombosis in acute myocardial infarction. *Heart* 1999;**82**:269–72.

98. Frink RJ. Chronic ulcerated plaques: new insights into the pathogenesis of acute coronary disease. *J Invas Cardiol* 1994;**6**:173–85.

99. Goldstein JA, Demetriou D, Grines CL, Pica M, Shoukfeh M, O'Neill WW. Multiple complex coronary plaques in patients with acute myocardial infarction. *N Engl J Med* 2000; **343**:915–22.

100. TIMI IIIA Investigators. Early effects of tissue-type plasminogen activator added to conventional therapy on the culprit coronary lesion in patients with ischemic cardiac pain at rest. Results of the Thrombolysis in Myocardial Ischemia (TIMI IIIA) Trial. *Circulation* 1993;**87**:38–52.

101. Honda Y, Fitzgerald PJ. Frontiers in intravascular imaging technologies. *Circulation* 2008;**117**:2024–37.

102. Meine TJ, Roe MT, Chen AY *et al.* Association of intravenous morphine use and outcomes in acute coronary syndromes: results from the CRUSADE Quality Improvement Initiative. *Am Heart J* 2005;**149**:1043–9.

103. *Physicians' Desk Reference*, 53rd edn. Mountvale, NJ: Medical Economic Co, 1999: 1331.

104. Figueras J, Lidon R, Cortadellas J. Rebound myocardial ischaemia following abrupt interruption of intravenous nitroglycerin infusion in patients with unstable angina at rest. *Eur Heart J* 1991;**12**:405–11.

105. Kloner RA. Cardiovascular effects of the 3 phosphodiesterase-5 inhibitors approved for the treatment of erectile dysfunction. *Circulation* 2004;**110**:3149–55.

106. Cheitlin MD, Hutter AM Jr, Brindis RG *et al.* Use of sildenafil (Viagra) in patients with cardiovascular disease. *Circulation* 1999;**99**:168–77.

107. Orlander R. Use of nitrates in the treatment of unstable and variant angina. *Drugs* 1987;**33**:131–9.

108. Jugdutt BL, Warnica JW. Intravenous nitroglycerin therapy to limit myocardial infarction size, expansions and complications. Effective timing, dosage and infarct location. *Circulation* 1988;**78**:906–20.

109. ISIS-4. A randomized factorial trial assessing early oral captopril, oral mononitrate, and intravenous magnesium sulphate in 58050 patients with suspected myocardial infarction. *Lancet* 1995;**345**:669–85.

110. Gruppo Italiano per lo Studio della Sopravvivenze nell'Infarto Miocardico. GISSI-3: effects of lisinopril and trandermal glyceryl trinitrate single and together on 6-week mortality and ventricular function after acute myocardial infarction. *Lancet* 1994;**343**:1115–22.

111. Muller JE, Turi ZG, Pearle DL *et al.* Nifedipine and conventional therapy for unstable angina pectoris: a randomized, double-blind comparison. *Circulation* 1984;**69**:728–39.

112. The Netherlands Interuniversity Nifedipine/Metropolol Trial (HINT) Research Group. Early treatment of unstable angina in the coronary care unit: a randomized, double-blind, placebo controlled comparison of recurrent ischemia in patients treated with nifedipine or metropolol or both. *Br Heart J* 1986;**73**:331–7.

113. Gottlieb SO, Weisfeldt M, Ouyang P *et al.* Effect of the addition of propranolol to therapy with nifedipine for unstable angina

pectoris. A randomized, double-blind, placebo-controlled trial. *Circulation* 1986;**73**:331–7.

114. Gerstenblith G, Ouyang P, Achuff SC *et al.* Nifedipine in unstable angina: a double-blind, randomized trial. *N Engl J Med* 1982;**306**:885–9.

115. Theroux P, Taeymans Y, Morrissette D, Bosch Y, Pelletier GB, Waters DD. A randomized study comparing propranolol and diltiazem in the treatment of unstable angina. *J Am Coll Cardiol* 1985;**5**:717–22.

116. Andre-Fouet X, Usdin JP, Gayet CH *et al.* Comparison of short-term efficacy of diltiazem and propranolol in unstable angina at rest. A randomized trial in 70 patients. *Eur Heart J* 1983;**4**:691–8.

117. Gibson RS, Boden WE, Theroux P *et al.* Diltiazem and reinfarction in patients with non-Q-wave myocardial infarction. Results of a double-blind, randomized, multicenter trial. *N Engl J Med* 1986;**315**:423–9.

118. Hansen JF, Hagerup L, Sigurd B *et al.* Cardiac event rates after acute myocardial infarction in patients treated with verapamil and trandolapril versus trandolapril alone. Danish Verapamil Infarction Trial (DAVIT) Study Group. *Am J Cardiol* 1997;**79**:738–41.

119. Scheidt S, Frishman WH, Packer M, Parodi O, Subramanian VB. Long-term effectiveness of verapamil in stable and unstable angina pectoris. One-year follow-up of patients treated in placebo-controlled double-blind randomized clinical trials. *Am J Cardiol* 1982;**50**:1185–90.

120. Yusuf S, Wittes J, Friedman L. Overview of results of randomized clinical trials in heart disease. II. Unstable angina, heart failure, primary prevention with aspirin, and risk factor modification. *JAMA* 1988;**260**:2259–63.

121. Pepine CJ, Faich G, Makuch R. Verapamil use in patients with cardiovascular disease: an overview of randomized trials. *Clin Cardiol* 1998;**21**:633–41.

122. Furberg CD, Psaty BM, Meye JV. Nifedipine. Dose-related increase in mortality in patients with coronary heart disease. *Circulation* 1995;**92**:1326–31.

123. Johnson SM, Mauritson DR, Willerson JT, Hillis LD. A controlled trial of verapamil for Prinzmetal's variant angina. *N Engl J Med* 1981;**304**:862–66.

124. Capucci A, Bracchetti D, Carini GC, DiCio G, Maresta A, Magnani B. Propranolol versus verapamil in patients with unstable angina. In: Zanchetti A, Krikler DM, eds. Calcium Antagonism in Cardiovascular Therapy. Experience with Verapamil. Amsterdam: Excerpta Medica, 1981.

125. Parodi O, Simoneti I, Michelassi C *et al.* Comparison of verapamil and propranolol therapy for angina pectoris at rest. A randomized, multiple-crossover, controlled trial in the coronary care unit. *Am J Cardiol* 1986;**57**:899–906.

126. Rosenthal SJ, Ginsburg R, Lamb IH, Baim DS, Schroeder JS. Efficiacy of diltiazem for control of symptoms of coronary artery spasm. *Am J Cardiol* 1980;**46**:1027–32.

127. Pepine CJ, Feldman RL, Whittle J, Curry RC, Conti GR. Effect of diltiazem in patients with variant angina. A randomized double-blind trial. *Am Heart J* 1981;**101**:719–25.

128. Schroeder JS, Feldman RL, Giles TD *et al.* Multiclinic controlled trial of diltiazem for Prinzmetal's variant angina. *JAMA* 1982;**72**:227–32.

129. Tilmant PY, LaBlanche JM, Thieuleux FA, Dupuis BA, Bertrand ME. Detrimental effect of propranolol in patients with coronary

130. Previtali M, Salerno J, Tavazzi L *et al.* Treatment of angina at rest with nifedipine: a short-term controlled study. *Am J Cardiol* 1980;**45**:825–30.

131. Ginsburg R, Lab IH, Schroeder JS, Hu M, Harrison DC. Randomized double-blind comparison of nifedipine and isosorbide dinitrate therapy in variant angina pectoris due to coronary artery spasm. *Am Heart J* 1982;**103**:44–8.

132. Chaitman B. Ranolazine for the treatment of chronic angina and potential use in other cardiovascular conditions. *Circulation* 2006;**113**:2462–72.

133. Morrow DA, Scirica BM, Karwatowska-Prokopczuk E *et al.*, MERLIN-TIMI 36 Trial Investigators. Effects of ranolazine on recurrent cardiovascular events in patients with non-ST-elevation acute coronary syndromes: the MERLIN-TIMI 36 randomized trial. *JAMA* 2007;**297**:1775–83.

134. Fibrinolytic Therapy Trialists' (FTT) Collaborative Group. Indications for fibrinolytic therapy in suspected acute myocardial infarction: collaborative overview of early mortality and major morbidity results from all randomized trials of more than 1000 patients. *Lancet* 1994;**343**:311–22.

135. Theroux P. Thrombosis in coronary artery disease: its pathophysiology and control. *Dialogues Cardiovasc Med* 2002;**7**: 3–18.

136. Lewis HD, Davis JW, Archibald DG *et al.* Protective effects of aspirin against myocardial infarction and death in men with unstable angina. *N Engl J Med* 1983;**313**:396–403.

137. Cairns JA, Gent M, Singer J *et al.* Aspirin, sulfinpyrazone, or both in unstable angina. *N Engl J Med* 1985;**313**: 1369–75.

138. Antithrombotic Trialists' Collaboration. Collaborative meta-analysis of randomized trials of antiplatelet therapy for prevention of death, myocardial infarction, and stroke in high-risk patients. *BMJ* 2002;**324**:71–86.

139. Patrono C, Coller B, Dalen JE *et al.* Platelet-active drugs. The relationships among dose, effectiveness, and side effects. *Chest* 2001;**119**:39S–63S.

140. Hankey GJ, Eikelboom JW. Aspirin resistance. *Lancet* 2006;**367**:606–17.

141. Patrono C, Rocca B. Drug insight: aspirin resistance – fact or fashion? *Nature Clin Prac* 2007;**4**:42–50.

142. Theroux P, Latour JG, Diodati J *et al.* Hemodynamic, platelet, and clinical response to prostacycline in unstable angina pectoris. *Am J Cardiol* 1990;**65**:1084–9.

143. Wiviott SD, Trenk D, Frelinger AL *et al.* Prasugrel compared with high loading- and maintenance-dose clopidogrel in patients with planned percutaneous coronary intervention: the Prasugrel in Comparison to Clopidogrel for Inhibition of Platelet Activation and Aggregation-Thrombolysis in Myocardial Infarction 44 trial. *Circulation* 2007;**116**:2923–32.

144. http://clinicaltrials.gov/ct/show/NCT00305162.

145. Storey RF, Husted S, Harrington RA *et al.* Inhibition of platelet aggregation by AZD6140, a reversible oral P2Y12 receptor antagonist, compared with clopidogrel in patients with acute coronary syndromes. *J Am Coll Cardiol* 2007;**50**:1852–6.

146. Cannon CP, Husted S, Harrington RA *et al.* Safety, tolerability, and initial efficacy of AZD6140, the first reversible oral adenosine diphosphate receptor antagonist, compared with clopidogrel, in patients with non-ST segment elevation acute coronary

arterial spasm countered by combination with diltiazem. *Am J Cardiol* 1983;**52**:230–3.

syndrome: primary results of the DISPERSE-2 trial. *J Am Coll Cardiol* 2007;**50**:1844–51.

147. Balsano F, Rizzon P, Violi F *et al.* Antiplatelet treatment with ticlopidine in unstable angina. *Circulation* 1990;**82**:17–26.

148. Gent M, Blakely JA, Easton JD *et al.* The Canadian American Ticlopidine Study (CATS) in thromboembolic stroke. *Lancet* 1989;**1**:1215–20.

149. CAPRIE Steering Committee. A randomized, blinded, trial of clopidogrel versus aspirin in patients at risk of ischaemic events (CAPRIE). *Lancet* 1996;**348**:1329–39.

150. Muller C, Buttner HJ, Petersen J, Roskamm H. A randomized comparison of clopidogrel and aspirin versus toclopidine and aspirin after the placement of coronary-artery stents. *Circulation* 2000;**101**:590–3.

151. Bertrand ME, Ruppreccht HJ, Urban P, Gerschlick AH, CLAS-SICS Investigators. Double-blind study of the safety of clopidogrel with and without a loading dose of in combination with aspirin after soronary stenting: the clopidogrel aspirin stent international cooperative study (CLASSICS). *Circulation* 2000;**102**:624–9.

152. Yusuf S, Zhao F, Mehta SR, Chrolavicius S, Tognoni G, Fox KK. Effects of clopidogrel in addition to aspirin in patients with acute coronary syndromes without ST segment elevation. *N Engl J Med* 2001;**345**:494–502.

153. Mehta SR, Yusuf S, Peters RJ *et al.* Effects of pretreatment with clopidogrel and aspirin followed by long-term therapy in patients undergoing percutaneous coronary intervention: the PCI-CURE study. *Lancet* 2001;**358**:527–33.

154. von Beckerath N, Taubert D, Pogatsa-Murray G, Schomig E, Kastrati A, Schomig A. Absorption, metabolization, and antiplatelet effects of 300-, 600-, and 900-mg loading doses of clopidogrel: results of the ISAR-CHOICE (Intracoronary Stenting and Antithrombotic Regimen: Choose Between 3 High Oral Doses for Immediate Clopidogrel Effect) Trial. *Circulation* 2005;**112**:2946–50.

155. Wiviott SD, Braunwald E, McCabe CH *et al.* Prasugrel versus clopidogrel in patients with acute coronary syndromes. *N Engl J Med* 2007;**357**:2001–15.

156. Cairns JA, Eikelboom J. Clopidogrel resistance: more grist for the mill. *J Am Coll Cardiol* 2008;**51**:1935–7.

157. Aleil B, Ravanat C, Cazenave JP, Rochoux G, Heitz A, Gachet C. Flow cytometric analysis of intraplatelet VASP phosphorylation for the detection of clopidogrel resistance in patients with ischemic cardiovascular diseases. *J Thromb Haemost* 2005;**3**:85–92.

158. EPIC Investigators. Use of a monoclonal antibody directed against the platelet glycoprotein IIb/IIIa receptor in high-risk coronary angioplasty. *N Engl J Med* 1997;**336**: 1689–96.

159. EPISTENT Investigators. Randomized placebo-controlled and balloon-angioplasty-controlled trial to assess safety of coronary stenting with use of platelet glycoprotein-IIb/IIIa blockade. Evaluation of Platelet IIb/IIIa Inhibitor for Stenting. *Lancet* 1998;**352**:87–92.

160. CAPTURE Investigators. Randomized placebo-controlled trial of abciximab before and during coronary intervention in refractory unstable angina: the CAPTURE trial. *Lancet* 1997;**349**:1429–35.

161. Topol EJ, Moliterno DJ, Herrmann HC *et al.* Comparison of two platelet glycoprotein IIb/IIIa inhibitors, tirofiban and abcix-imab, for the prevention of ischemic events with percutaneous coronary revascularization. *N Engl J Med* 2001;**344**:1888–94.

162. RESTORE Investigators. Randomized Efficacy Study of Tirofiban for Outcomes and REstenosis. Effects of platelet glycoprotein IIb/IIIa blockade with tirofiban on adverse cardiac events in patients with unstable angina or acute myocardial infarction undergoing coronary angioplasty. *Circulation* 1997;**96**:1445–53.

163. O'Shea JC, Hafley GE, Greenberg S *et al.* Platelet glycoprotein IIb/IIIa integrin blockade with eptifibatide in coronary stent intervention: the ESPRIT trial: a randomized controlled trial. *JAMA* 2001;**285**:2468–73.

164. Boersma E, Akkerhuis KM, Theroux P, Califf RM, Topol EJ, Simoons ML. Platelet glycoprotein IIb/IIIa receptor inhibition in non-ST-elevation acute coronary syndromes early benefit during medical treatment only, with additional protection during percutaneous coronary intervention. *Circulation* 1999;**100**:2045–8.

165. Boersma E, Harrington RA, Moliterno DJ *et al.* Platelet glycoprotein IIb/IIIa inhibitors in acute coronary syndromes: a meta-analysis of all major randomized clinical trials. *Lancet* 2002;**359**:189–98.

166. Roffi M, Chew DP, Mukherjee D *et al.* Platelet glycoprotein IIb/IIIa inhibitors reduce mortality in diabetic patients with non-ST segment-elevation acute coronary syndromes. *Circulation* 2001;**104**:2767–71.

167. Kong DF, Hasselblad V, Harrington RA *et al.* Meta-analysis of survival with platelet glycoprotein IIb/IIIa antagonists for percutaneous coronary interventions. *Am J Cardiol* 2003;**92**:651–5.

168. Kastrati A, Mehilli J, Schuhlen H *et al.* Intracoronary Stenting and Antithrombotic Regimen-Rapid Early Action for Coronary Treatment Study Investigators. A clinical trial of abciximab in elective percutaneous coronary intervention after pretreatment with clopidogrel. *N Engl J Med* 2004;**350**:232–8.

169. Mehilli J, Kastrati A, Schuhlen H *et al.* Intracoronary stenting and antithrombotic regimen: is abciximab a superior way to eliminate elevated thrombotic risk in diabetes (ISAR-SWEET) study Investigators? *Circulation* 2004;**14**:3627–35.

170. Kastrati A, Mehilli J, Neumann FJ *et al.* Abciximab in patients with acute coronary syndromes undergoing percutaneous coronary intervention after clopidogrel pretreatment: the ISAR-REACT 2 randomized trial. *JAMA* 2006;**295**:1531–8.

171. Ndrepepa G, Kastrati A, Mehilli J *et al.* One-year clinical outcomes with abciximab versus placebo in patients with non-ST segment elevation acute coronary syndromes undergoing percutaneous coronary intervention after pre-treatment with clopidogrel: results of the ISAR-REACT 2 randomized trial. *Eur Heart J* 2008;**29**:455–61.

172. Brieger D, Van de Werf F, Avezum A *et al.* GRACE Investigators. Interactions between heparins, glycoprotein IIb/IIIa antagonists, and coronary intervention. The Global Registry of Acute Coronary Events (GRACE). *Am Heart J* 2007;**153**(6): 960–9.

173. Alexander KP, Chen AY, Newby LK *et al.* Sex differences in major bleeding with glycoprotein IIb/IIIa inhibitors: results from the CRUSADE (Can Rapid risk stratification of Unstable angina patients Suppress ADverse outcomes with Early implementation of the ACC/AHA guidelines) initiative. *Circulation.* 2006;**114**(13):1380–7.

174. Stone GW, Bertrand ME, Moses JW *et al.* Routine upstream initiation vs deferred selective use of glycoprotein IIb/IIIa inhibitors in acute coronary syndromes. The ACUITY Timing trial. *JAMA* 2007;**297**:591–602.

175. Giugliano RP, Newby LK, Harrington RA *et al.* The early glycoprotein IIb/IIIa inhibition in non-ST segment elevation acute coronary syndrome (EARLY ACS) trial: a randomized placebo-controlled trial evaluating the clinical benefits of early front-loaded eptifibatide in the treatment of patients with non-ST segment elevation acute coronary syndrome – study design and rationale. *Am Heart J* 2005;**149**:994–1002.

176. Chew DP, Bhatt DL, Sapp S, Topol EJ. Increased mortality with oral platelet glycoprotein IIb/IIIa antagonists. A meta-analysis of phase III multicenter randomized trials. *Circulation* 2001;**103**:201–6.

177. Theroux P, Waters D, Lam J, Juneau M, McCans J. Reactivation of unstable angina after the discontinuation of heparin. *N Engl J Med* 1992;**327**:141–5.

178. Weitz JI, Buller HR. Direct thrombin inhibitors in acute coronary syndromes. Present and future. *Circulation* 2002;**105**:1004–11.

179. Hirsh J, Anand SS, Halperin JL, Fuster V. Guide to anticoagulant therapy. Heparin: a statement for healthcare professionals from the American Heart Association. *Circulation* 2001;**103**:2994–3018.

180. Fragmin during Instability in Coronary Artery Disease (FRISC) Study Group. Low-molecular-weight heparin during instability in coronary artery disease. *Lancet* 1996;**347**:561–8.

181. Eikelboom JW, Anand SS, Malmberg K, Weitz JI, Ginsberg JS, Yusuf S. Unfractionated heparin and low-molecular weight-heparin in acute coronary syndrome without ST elevation: a meta-analysis. *Lancet* 2000;**355**:1936–42.

182. Klein W, Buchwald A, Hillis SE *et al.* Fragmin in unstable coronary artery disease study: comparison of low-molecular weight-heparin with unfractionated heparin acutely and with placebo for 6 weeks in the management of unstable coronary artery disease. *Circulation* 1997;**96**:61–8.

183. FRAXIS Study Group. Comparison of two treatment durations (6 days and 14 days) of a low molecular weight heparin with a 6-day treatment of unfractionated heparin in the initial management of unstable angina or non-Q-wave myocardial infarction: FRAXIS (FRAXiparine in Ischaemic Syndrome). *Eur Heart J* 1999;**20**:1553–62.

184. Antman EM, Cohen M, Radley D *et al.* Assessment of the treatment effect of enoxaparin for unstable angina/non-Q-wave myocardial infarction. TIMI 11B-ESSENCE meta-analysis. *Circulation* 1999;**100**:1602–8.

185. Yusuf S, Mehta SR, Chrolavicious S *et al.* Comparison of fondaparinux and enoxaparin in acute coronary syndromes. *N Engl J Med* 2006;**354**:1464–76.

186. Antman EM. Hirudin in acute myocardial infarction. Thrombolysis and Thrombin Inhibition in Myocardial Infarction (TIMI) 9B trial. *Circulation* 1996;**94**:911–21.

187. Organization to Assess Strategies for Ischemic Syndromes (OASIS) Investigators. Comparison of the effects of two doses of recombinant hirudin compared with heparin in patients with acute myocardial ischemia without ST elevation: a pilot study. *Circulation* 1997;**96**:769–77.

188. Direct Thrombin Inhibitor Trialists' Collaborative Group. Direct thrombin inhibitors in acute coronary syndromes: principal results of a meta-analysis based on individual patients' data. *Lancet* 2002;**359**:294–302.

189. Stone GW, McLaurin BT, Cox DA *et al.* Bivalirudin for patients with acute coronary syndrome. *N Engl J Med* 2006;**355**:2203–16.

190. Lincoff AM, Bittl JA, Harrington RA *et al.* Bivalirudin and provisional glycoprotein IIb/IIIa blockade compared with heparin and planned glycoprotein IIb/IIIa blockade during percutaneous coronary intervention: REPLACE-2 randomized trial. *JAMA* 2003;**289**:853–63.

191. Stone GW, Witzenbichler B, Guagliumi G *et al.* Bivalirudin during primary PCI in acute myocardial infarction. *N Engl J Med* 2008;**358**:2218–30.

192. Anand SS, Yusuf S. Oral anticoagulant therapy in patients with coronary artery disease: a meta-analysis. *JAMA* 1999;**282**:2058–67.

193. Wallentin L, Wilcox RG, Weaver WD *et al*, ESTEEM Investigators. Oral ximelagatran for secondary prophylaxis after myocardial infarction: the ESTEEM randomised controlled trial. *Lancet* 2003;**362**:789–97.

194. TIMI IIIB Investigators. Effects of tissue plasminogen activator and a comparison of early invasive and conservative strategies in unstable angina and non-Q-wave myocardial infarction: results of the TIMI IIIB Trial. Thrombolysis in Myocardial Ischemia. *Circulation* 1994;**89**:1545–56.

195. Boden WE, O'Rourke RA, Crawford MH *et al.* Outcomes in patients with acute non-Q-wave myocardial infarction randomly assigned to an invasive as compared with a conservative management strategy. Veterans Affairs Non-Q-Wave Infarction Strategies in Hospital (VANQWISH) Trial Investigators. *N Engl J Med* 1998;**338**:1785–92.

196. Wallentin L, Lagerqvist B, Husted S *et al.* Outcome at one year after an invasive compared with a non-invasive strategy in unstable coronary artery disease: the FRISC II invasive randomized trial. *Lancet* 2000;**356**:9–16.

197. Cannon CP, Weintraub WS, Demopouluos LA *et al.* Comparison of early invasive and conservative strategies in patients with unstable coronary syndromes treated with the glycoprotein IIb/IIIa inhibitor tirofiban. *N Engl J Med* 2001;**344**:1879–87.

198. Fox KA, Poole-Wilson P, Clayton TC *et al.* 5-year outcome of an interventional strategy in non-ST-elevation acute coronary syndrome: the British Heart Foundation RITA 3 randomised trial. *Lancet* 2005;**366**:914–20.

199. Mehta SR, Cannon CP, Fox KA *et al.* Routine versus selective invasive strategies in patients with acute coronary syndromes: a collaborative meta-analysis of randomized trials. *JAMA* 2005;**293**:2908–17.

200. Neumann FJ, Kastrati A, Pogatsa-Murray G *et al.* Evaluation of prolonged antithrombotic pretreatment ("cooling-off" strategy) before intervention in patients with unstable coronary syndromes: a randomized controlled trial. *JAMA* 2003;**290**:1593–9.

201. de Winter RJ, Windhausen F, Cornel JH *et al.* Early invasive versus selectively invasive management for acute coronary syndromes. *N Engl J Med* 2005;**353**:1095–104.

202. Bavry AA, Kumbhani DJ, Rassi A, Bhatt DL, Askari AT. Benefit of early invasive therapy in acute coronary syndromes: a meta-analysis of contemporary randomized clinical trials. *J Am Coll Cardiol* 2006;**48**:1319–25.

203. Hoenig MR, Doust J, Aroney CN, Scott IA. Early invasive versus conservative strategies for unstable angina & non-ST-elevation myocardial infarction in the stent era. *Cochrane Database of Systematic Reviews* 2006, Issue 3. Art. No.: CD004815. DOI: 10.1002/14651858.CD004815.pub2.

204. O'Donoghue M, Boden WE, Braunwald E *et al.* Early invasive versus onservative treatment strategies in women and men with unstable angina and non-ST segment elevation myocardial infarction. A meta-analysis. *JAMA* 2008;**300**:71–80.

205. Tardiff BE, Califf RM, Tcheng JE *et al.* Clinical outcomes after detection of elevated cardiac enzymes in patients undergoing percutaneous intervention. IMPACT-II Investigators. Integrilin (eptifibatide) to Minimize Platelet Aggregation and Coronary Thrombosis-II. *J Am Coll Cardiol* 1999; **33**:88–96.

206. Theroux P, Chaitman BR, Danchin N *et al.* Inhibition of the sodium-hydrogen exchanger with cariporide to prevent myocardial infarction in high-risk ischemic situations. Main results of the GUARDIAN trial. Guard During Ischemia Against Necrosis (GUARDIAN) Investigators. *Circulation* 2000;**102**: 3032–8.

207. Baran KW, Nguyen M, McKendall GR *et al.* Double-blind, randomized trial of an anti-CD18 antibody in conjunction with recombinant tissue plasminogen activator for acute myocardial infarction: limitation of myocardial infarction following thrombolysis in acute myocardial infarction (LIMIT AMI) study. *Circulation* 2001;**104**:2778–83.

208. Armstrong PW, Granger CB, Adams PX *et al.* Pexelizumab for acute ST-elevation myocardial infarction in patients undergoing primary percutaneous coronary intervention: a randomized controlled trial. *JAMA* 2007;**297**:43–51.

209. Ross AM, Gibbons RJ, Stone GW, Kloner RA, Alexander RW. A randomized, double-blinded, placebo-controlled multicenter trial of adenosine as an adjunct to reperfusion in the treatment of acute myocardial infarction (AMISTAD-II). *J Am Coll Cardiol* 2005;**45**:1775–80.

210. COMMIT (Clopidogrel and Metoprolol in Myocardial Infarction Trial) Collaborative Group. Early intravenous then oral metoprolol in 45852 patients with acute myocardial infarction: Randomised placebo-controlled trial. *Lancet* 2005;**366**:1622–32.

211. Azar RR, Rinfret S, Theroux P *et al.* A randomized placebo-controlled trial to assess the efficacy of anti-inflammatory therapy with methylprednisolone in unstable angina (MUNA trial). *Eur Heart J* 2000;**21**:2026–32.

212. Davignon J, Mabile L. Mechanisms of action of statins and their pleiotropic effects. *Ann Endocrinol (Paris)* 2001;**62**:101–12.

213. Aronow HD, Topol EJ, Roe MT *et al.* Effect of lipid-lowering therapy on early mortality after acute coronary syndromes: an observational study. *Lancet* 2001;**357**:1063–8.

214. Stenestrand U, Wallentin L. Early statin treatment following acute myocardial infarction and 1-year survival. *JAMA* 2001;**285**:430–6.

215. Schwartz GG, Olsson AG, Ezekowitz MD *et al.* Myocardial Ischemia Reduction with Aggressive Cholesterol Lowering (MIRACL) Study Investigators. Effects of atorvastatin on early recurrent ischemic events in acute coronary syndromes: the MIRACL study: a randomized controlled trial. *JAMA* 2001;**285**:1711–18.

216. Cannon CP, Braunwald E, McCabe CH *et al*, for the Pravastatin or Atorvastatin Evaluation and Infection Therapy-Thrombolysis in Myocardial Infarction 22 Investigators: Intensive versus moderate lipid lowering with statins after acute coronary syndromes. *N Engl J Med* 2004;**350**:1495–504.

217. Fonarow GC, Gawlinski A, Moughrabi S, Tillisch JH. Improved treatment of coronary heart disease by implementation of a Cardiac Hospitalization Atherosclerosis Management Program (CHAMP). *Am J Cardiol* 2001;**87**:819–22.

218. Brar SS, Kim J, Brar SK *et al.* Long-term outcomes by clopidogrel duration and stent type in a diabetic population with de novo coronary artery lesions. *J Am Coll Cardiol* 2008;**51**:2220–7.

219. Yusuf S, Sleight P, Pogue J, Bosch J, Davies R, Dagenais G. Effects of an angiotensin-converting-enzyme inhibitor, ramipril, on cardiovascular events in high-risk patients. The Heart Outcomes Prevention Evaluation Study Investigators. *N Engl J Med* 2000,**342**.145–53.

220. Heart Protection Study Collaborative Group. MRC/BHF Heart Protection Study of cholesterol lowering with simvastatin in 20/536 high-risk individuals: a randomised placebo-controlled trial. *Lancet* 2002;**360**:7–22.

221. Malmberg K, Ryden L, Efendic S *et al.* Randomized trial of insulin-glucose infusion followed by subcutaneous insulin treatment in diabetic patients with acute myocardial infarction (DIGA-MI study): effects on mortality at 1 year. *J Am Coll Cardiol* 1995;**26**:57–65.

222. American Diabetes Association. Standards of medical care for patients with diabetes mellitus (position statement). *Diabetes Care* 1999;**22**(suppl 1):S32–41.

223. UK Prospective Diabetes Study Group. Tight blood pressure control and risk of macrovascular and microvascular complications in type 2 diabetes: UKPDS 38. *BMJ* 1998;**317**:703–13.

30 Early prehospital management of ST elevation myocardial infarction

Robert C Welsh and Paul W Armstrong

University of Alberta, Edmonton, Alberta, Canada

Introduction

Over the last three decades, major advances have occurred in the treatment of patients with ST elevation myocardial infarction (STEMI) that have significantly enhanced our knowledge and understanding. A commensurate improvement in outcomes has ensued. Despite this burgeoning knowledge and a multi-pronged investment in both the content and process of STEMI care, important care gaps exist. These include a significant proportion of patients not treated with reperfusion therapy, inadequate patient triage, delayed time to reperfusion, suboptimal utilization of appropriate adjunctive medical therapy, subsequent underutilization of cardiac rehabilitation programs, and failure to undertake lifestyle modifications.

Time to initiation of reperfusion remains a critical factor pivotal to modulating STEMI patient outcomes. Clinical evidence and guidelines have defined key parameters necessary to achieve optimal time to reperfusion once patients establish first medical contact.[1-3] In Figure 30.1 the specific temporal segments are outlined and include time from medical presentation to acquisition of the first 12-lead ECG, first ECG until completion of patient assessment and confirmation of diagnosis, and time from diagnosis to reperfusion therapy. Contemporary STEMI guidelines indicate that time from first medical contact to initiation of fibrinolysis should be 30 minutes or less and within 90 minutes to first balloon inflation in the case of mechanical reperfusion.[1,2,4]

Rich and often unrealized opportunities exist, prior to arrival at hospital, to limit STEMI patient morbidity and mortality by enhancing early management via the prehospital emergency medical system (EMS). The initial early activation of EMS depends upon appropriate recognition of symptoms or circumstances, which must be coupled with timely and appropriate responses from affected individuals, often assisted by family members, friends, coworkers or bystanders. Unfortunately, utilization of EMS remains suboptimal with many STEMI patients presenting to the hospital using personal transportation. Despite dedicated public education strategies, little impact on this behavior has ensued. Advanced prehospital STEMI management which expedites patient assessment, diagnosis, triage, and treatment has been successful in various health systems worldwide, including over two decades of experience in France and Ireland. These prehospital STEMI treatment protocols are most effective when operating within an integrated system-wide regional reperfusion program which includes continuous quality improvement.

Patient symptom recognition, public education strategies and activation of the prehospital emergency medical system

The American College of Cardiology (ACC) and American Heart Association (AHA) guidelines, with a current focused update, have encouraged the reduction of total ischemic time to less than two hours.[1,2,4] Unfortunately it has been consistently demonstrated that patient delay in seeking medical attention is the major limitation to realizing this goal and time to reperfusion remains suboptimal. Within clinical trials greater than 50% of reperfusion delay occurs prior to first medical contact; an even longer delay is evident within "real-world" registry data.[5-8] Addressing patient delay requires understanding the patient's perception, interpretation, and action as well as the influence of other factors modulating behaviors (Fig. 30.2).

Specific patient demographic factors have been identified which affect the duration of symptoms prior to seeking medical advice (Table 30.1). Older patients and women have consistently been shown to delay seeking medical

Evidence-Based Cardiology, 3rd edition. Edited by S. Yusuf, J.A. Cairns, A.J. Camm, E.L. Fallen, and B.J. Gersh. © 2010 Blackwell Publishing, ISBN: 978-1-4051-5925-8.

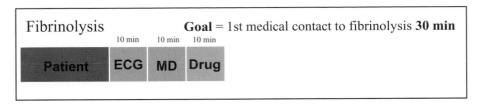

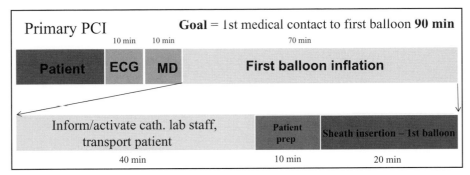

Figure 30.1 Understanding time to treatment: pharmacologic and mechanical reperfusion. Understanding process of care and associated temporal delay required to deliver reperfusion therapy facilitates healthcare providers' ability to achieve goal times and develop appropriate systematic interventions. Upon arrival in the catheterization laboratory the patient is prepared for the procedure and the interventional cardiologist achieves arterial access and undertakes diagnostic coronary angiography. If the anatomy is consistent with PCI, appropriate equipment is prepared and anticoagulant therapy administered prior to crossing the specific lesion and achieving first balloon inflation; the total process typically requires 30 minutes. Therefore, it is essential that systematic interventions are implemented to expedite activation of the interventional cardiologist and catheterization laboratory personnel as well as patient transportation from the emergency department such that the time from confirmed diagnosis to arrival in the laboratory is abbreviated to 40 minutes or less.

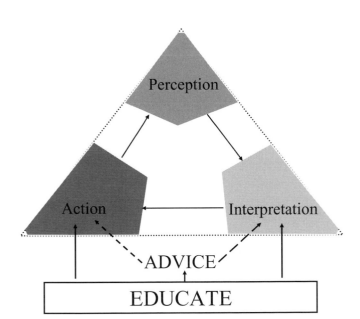

Figure 30.2 Understanding time to reperfusion – patient delay. When a person perceives a novel or recurrent sensation (such as chest pressure) their interpretation is influenced by the severity of the symptom as well as a host of factors influenced by past experience and education. Seeking advice from friends, family, co-workers or bystanders regarding the interpretation of the symptom as well as appropriate action required may occur. Education influences the personal interpretation of symptoms and appropriate action as well as the advice that may be offered from others.

Table 30.1 Demographic factors associated with patient delay

	GRACE (3693)	Worcester (3837)	NRMI (364 131)	Minnesota (2409)
Age	↑	↑	↑	↑
Female gender	↑	X	↑	↑
Race	X	X	↑	X
Angina	↑	↑	↑	X
Prior heart failure	↑	X	X	↑
Diabetes	↑	↑	↑	X
Prior myocardial infarction	↓	X	↓	X
Hypertension	↑	X	↑	↑
Prior CABG	NS	X	X	↓
Prior PCI	↓	X	↓	↓

CABG, coronary artery bypass grafting; PCI, percutaneous coronary intervention; ↑, factor associated with increased delay from symptom onset to medical presentation; ↓, factor associated with decreased delay; NS, no significant relationship demonstrated; X, factor not reported.

Table 30.2 Situational factors associated with patient delay

	GRACE (3693)	Worchester (3837)	NRMI (364 131)	Minnesota (2409)
Shock	↓	X	↓	X
Chest pain	↓	X	X	↑
Diaphoresis	↓	X	X	X
Dyspnea	↑	X	X	X
Time of day (off hrs)	↑	↑	X	↑
Ambulance transport	↓	X	X	X

↑, factor associated with increased delay from symptom onset to medical presentation; ↓, factor associated with decreased delay; NS, no significant relationship demonstrated; X, factor not reported.

Table 30.3 Systematic review of interventions to reduce delay in patients with suspect AMI

Design	Author, year	Country	Duration	Outcomes
RCTs	Meischke 1997	USA	7 week	No effect
	Luepker 2000	USA	18 month	No effect
CT	Rowley 1982	England	32 month	Increased call to MD
Before and after	Mitic 1984	Canada	8 week	Increased prehosp delay
	Ho 1989	USA	2 month	No effect
	Moses 1991	USA	24 month	No effect
	Rustige 1992	Germany	9 month	No effect
	Belt 1993	Australia	1 week	No effect
	Blohm 1994	Sweden	14 month	Reduced prehosp delay
	Gaspoz 1996	Switzerland	12 month	Reduced prehosp delay
	Maeso-Madronero 2000	Germany	6 month	Reduced prehosp delay

RCTs, randomized controlled trial; CT, controlled trial; Before and after, analysis prior to and following the intervention.[66]

attention until later in the course of their symptoms.[8–11] Ironically, patients with known past medical diagnoses with increased risk of cardiovascular events have also prolonged delay, including those with prior angina, hypertension, diabetes mellitus, and congestive heart failure.[8–11] Patients with prior percutaneous coronary revascularization and prior acute myocardial infarction appear to present after less symptomatic delay.[8,9,11]

A host of situation-specific factors have also been shown to modulate time from symptom onset to medical presentation (Table 30.2). The most consistent of these are linked to severity of symptoms at presentation, especially those of cardiogenic shock or resuscitated arrhythmia presenting earlier.[8,9] Longer delays in presentation also occur outside regular working hours or on weekends and holidays.[8,10,11]

Psychosocial factors also influence patient delay. These include misinterpretation of symptoms and denial of their importance. Female STEMI patients are known to deny or misinterpret their symptoms since they are conditioned to interpret acute myocardial infarction as a "male" disease.[8,9,11–13] There are also significant socioeconomic factors related to the cost of healthcare, particularly activation of the prehospital EMS which has additional associated cost implications in many countries.[14]

Remarkably, in industrialized nations, only 50% of patients with symptoms suggestive of acute myocardial infarction activate the prehospital EMS. This figure is staggering and tragic considering the evidence indicating that ambulance assistance leads to shortened time to definitive care and diminishes the potential individual patient and population hazards with self-transportation of patients at risk of hemodynamic compromise and dysrhythmia.

Although they are logical, dedicated educational programs that have attempted to increase appropriate utilization of EMS and decrease reperfusion delay through enhanced patient response have typically met with limited

success (Table 30.3). Within the United States, the Rapid Early Action for Coronary Treatment (REACT) trial randomized 20 cities, matched for community size and patient demographics, to receive an 18-month educational intervention.[15] The premises of this program were that: (1) time to treatment was currently excessive; (2) patient response accounted for the majority of delay; and (3) dedicated community educational intervention would improve knowledge and decrease patient-related delay. Central educational themes were promulgated, aimed at early symptom recognition and rapid response by calling 911 if symptoms suggestive of myocardial ischemia persisted for more than 15 minutes. This interventional strategy focused on: (1) community organizations including health professionals and other leaders; (2) public education to develop general awareness of acute myocardial infarction symptoms, the presence of heart disease in females, and appropriate action through MI survival plans, bystander response, and the importance of calling 911; (3) professional education including focused discussions with physicians, nurses, cardiac rehabilitation, emergency department and ambulance staff through academic detailing, continuing health education events and special seminars; and (4) education of patients with a past history of coronary artery disease or significant cardiovascular disease risk factors. Each community involved in these programs had a local office with two staff to organize events and promote the program. Despite enhancing awareness and increasing utilization of EMS, this intensive educational program, which was associated with an annual cost between $156 000 and $294 000 per 100 000 person community, did not demonstrate a reduction from symptom onset to first medical presentation in STEMI patients.[15,16] Paradoxically greater utilization of EMS occurred in patients with symptoms determined to be non-cardiac.

Although these results are discouraging and highlight the limitation of current educational strategies to reduce patient treatment delay, enhancing awareness of those with established disease or other risks remains a legitimate goal. Future campaigns to shorten patient delay are likely to be more effective if they address psychosocial and behavioral impediments to action, are sustained rather than short term, and focus on those patients and families at highest risk, including those with known coronary heart disease.

Prehospital diagnosis of ST elevation myocardial infarction

During the acute phase of STEMI, patients may experience a diverse range of symptoms varying from classic crushing retrosternal chest discomfort with typical associated symptoms, to isolated dyspnea, syncope, malaise, and neurologic impairment. In elderly patients, females, diabetics, and those taking non-steroidal anti-inflammatory drugs (NSAIDs), symptoms may be subtle or absent and such patients are known to be at increased risk of suffering "silent myocardial infarctions".[17-22] This reality makes recognition of patients with STEMI challenging for frontline medical personnel in emergency departments as well as in the prehospital environment.

EMS programs typically have a system of triage to be implemented at the time of a 911 call, which are based upon key symptoms communicated from patients or their families, including chest discomfort, shortness of breath, syncope, and other indicators of potential myocardial ischemia. In some centers, this involves physician participation to prioritize prehospital response to appropriate patients with mobilization of advance care mobile intensive care units. In other regions where prehospital care is delivered by non-physician paramedical staff, preliminary triage may also be undertaken to facilitate the activation of advanced cardiac life support (ACLS) units capable of delivering advanced prehospital cardiac care.

On arrival at a scene where symptoms compatible with myocardial infarction are recognized or confirmed, rapid completion of a prehospital 12-lead ECG is a key factor in determining diagnosis and guides subsequent therapy. It has been shown that prehospital 12-lead ECGs can be expeditiously completed with reliable lead placement and provide high-quality diagnostic tracings.[23,24] Furthermore, provision of a prehospital 12-lead ECG adds little incremental prehospital delay, i.e. a 1–10 minute increase in prehospital on-scene time.[24-27]

Various approaches to 12-lead ECG interpretation have been employed within the prehospital environment. When an experienced physician is present, onsite interpretation is feasible; if not, opportunities exist for either ECG remote transmission for physician interpretation or computer-assisted interpretation by paramedical staff. Evidence demonstrates that well-trained paramedics can efficiently use the 12-lead ECG to guide early treatment. Although this has been proven effective in a research environment, more widespread implementation carries the potential for over-, under- and inappropriate diagnosis of STEMI, and robust evaluations of the success of such programs are warranted.

Remote prehospital 12-lead ECG interpretation requires appropriate technology at both ends of the transmission, the immediate availability of an experienced physician, and a system of communication between the physician and prehospital paramedics with the attendant liability of system failure at multiple levels. Transmission of all prehospital 12-lead ECGs for remote interpretation is impractical given that only about 5% of such patients, i.e. those identified with symptoms possibly related to myocardial infarction, have confirmed evidence of STEMI.[28] Preliminary paramedic ECG interpretation has been effectively employed in several regions for selective transmission of the prehospital 12-lead ECG. In a single-center analysis, greater than 70% of all STEMI patients were correctly identified by prehospital paramedic teams following modest training in STEMI patient identification and 12-lead ECG interpretation.[22] Even within the setting of a prehospital fibrinolysis trial, where stringent inclusion and exclusion criteria are employed, paramedic EMS staff correctly identified and enrolled 46% of all STEMI patients.

In conjunction with completion of the prehospital 12-lead ECG, prehospital paramedical staff can effectively and thoroughly complete prehospital reperfusion checklists to determine eligibility for reperfusion. Thereafter, prehospital reperfusion can be administered or patients can be triaged to centers capable of achieving expedited mechanical or pharmacologic reperfusion.

Prehospital management of ST elevation myocardial infarction

In patients with a likely or confirmed diagnosis of STEMI, implementation of contemporary guidelines should be considered prior to hospital arrival to minimize patient distress, morbidity, and mortality, especially those with demonstrated time dependency (Table 30.4)[1,2,4] Prehospital

Table 30.4 ACC/AHA guidelines for management of STEMI relevant to the prehospital environment

Procedure or therapy	Class	Level of evidence
911 – dispatch recommend ASA (in absence of contraindications)[1]	IIa	C
Paramedics perform prehospital 12-lead ECG[1]	IIa	B
Complete prehospital reperfusion check list[1]	IIa	C
Defibrillation (hemodynamically significant dysrhythmia)[1]	I	A
ASA 162–325 mg (chew and swallow – in absence of CI)[1]	I	C
Oxygen – hypoxia[1]	I	B
Oxygen – 1st six hours to all confirmed STEMI[1]	IIa	C
NTG SL with ongoing ischemic discomfort[1] 0.4 mg × 3 does every 5 min	I	C
NTG IV for relief of ongoing ischemic discomfort or to manage significant hypertension or pulmonary edema[1]	I	C
NTG contraindicated:[1]	III	C
BP < 90		
HR < 50		
HR > 100		
RV MI		
Recent administration of a phosphodiesterase inhibitor[1]	III	B
Morphine sulfate is the analgesic of choice (2–4 mg IV with increments of 2–8 mg IV repeated at 5–15 min. intervals)[4]	I	C
Beta-blocker therapy[4]		
Oral initiated in first 24 hours without contraindications	I	B
Intravenous is reasonable to administer for the management of hypertension without contraindications	IIa	B
Contraindications for early beta-blocker therapy: 1) signs of heart failure, 2) evidence of low output state, 3) increase risk of cardiogenic shock, and 4) other relative contraindications	III	A
Prehospital fibrinolysis[1]	IIa	B
Prehospital destination protocols for primary PCI[1,4]		
Expected time from first medical contact to balloon inflation is less than 90 min (with experienced interventional cardiologists present)	I	A
Cardiogenic shock <75 years	I	A
Contraindication to fibrinolysis	I	B
Cardiogenic shock ≥75 years	IIa	B

EMS teams managing patients with STEMI should be capable of advanced cardiac life support techniques to address hemodynamic and electrical instability as well as respiratory compromise. Synchronized cardioversion, defibrillation or percutaneous pacing can be employed to treat malignant arrhythmias. In the setting of symptomatic hypotension, intravenous fluid resuscitation is standard and intravenous inotropes can be administered when appropriate medical supervision exists.

Oxygen and respiratory support

Supplemental oxygen is administered to patients with oxygen saturation less than 90%. There is experimental evidence that oxygen administration may limit ischemic myocardial injury; therefore even in uncomplicated myocardial infarction this may be an effective strategy.[29] It has become ubiquitous to administer oxygen to virtually all patients with symptoms suggestive of myocardial ischemia.

In patients with cardiopulmonary compromise, such as pulmonary edema, severe congestive heart failure, cardio-

genic shock or presumed mechanical complications of STEMI, advanced respiratory support may be required. This may include bag, valve and mask with oral airway or endotracheal intubation to provide adequate oxygenation and ventilation.

Analgesia

It is the expectation that patients with STEMI will receive reperfusion therapy although not all will be candidates; continuing pain relief is required in either case. Although retrospective data have raised concerns about potential adverse events from morphine in patients with non-STEMI, this has not been the case with STEMI patients.[30] Therefore, administration of morphine sulfate (2–4 mg IV with increments of 2–8 mg IV repeated at 5–15 minute intervals) is the analgesic of choice for management of pain associated with STEMI. This should be undertaken judiciously in patients with hemodynamic or respiratory instability.

In the STEMI patient population treated within the EXTRACT TIMI 25 trial, an increased risk of death, reinfarction, heart failure or shock was demonstrated in those taking NSAIDs within seven days of enrollment.[31] Although not as pertinent to the prehospital environment, there is a known increased risk of cardiovascular events among patients taking COX-2 inhibitors and other NSAIDs; therefore, patients who are taking these agents at the time of STEMI should discontinue them immediately.

Nitroglycerin

In the setting of ongoing ischemic discomfort, sublingual nitroglycerin should be administered (0.3–0.4 mg) every five minutes up to a maximum of three doses or until symptoms are relieved. If prehospital infusion pumps are available, intravenous nitroglycerin is indicated for relief of refractory ischemic symptoms, to control hypertension or manage pulmonary congestion. Nitroglycerin should not be administered with: hypotension (systolic blood pressure <90 mmHg), significant bradycardia, suspected right ventricular infarction, or in patients who have received a phosphodiesterase inhibitor to treat erectile dysfunction within 24 hours.

Beta-blockers

Administration of intravenous and oral beta-blockers has been encouraged in the early period following diagnosis of STEMI, based upon evidence acquired largely in the pre-reperfusion era. The COMMIT-Metoprolol Trial allocated 45 852 patients within 24 hours of diagnosis of STEMI to receive metoprolol administered as three doses of 5 mg IV in the first 15 minutes followed by 200 mg/day orally or matching placebo.[32] This strategy did not improve the primary endpoint and was associated with an excess risk of cardiogenic shock of 11 per 1000 treated with the incidence increased in patients with age >70 years, systolic blood pressure <120 mmHg, presenting heart rate >110/min or congestive heart failure as measured by Killip class >I. These results underscore the potential risk of administering intravenous or aggressive oral beta-blockers in the prehospital setting.

Antithrombotic agents

Because of the potential benefits of early ASA (aspirin) use, its limited risk and low cost, it is reasonable for prehospital care providers to administer it to all patients with symptoms suggestive of STEMI in the absence of contraindications. In fact, ASA 162–325 mg to chew should be initiated remotely by 911 dispatchers to non-ASA allergic patients with symptoms suspicious for STEMI while awaiting arrival of EMS.

Although not extensively investigated, additional antiplatelet agents could be considered for administration in the prehospital environment. Clinical and pharmacody-namic evidence indicates some delay in the onset of action of clopidogrel following oral administration.[33] Although not yet supported by evidence in clinical guidelines, administration of this agent in the prehospital environment seems logical in STEMI patients in whom early percutaneous coronary intervention is intended. Since a proportion of patients may require urgent coronary artery bypass grafting, this strategy requires definitive investigation prior to widespread implementation. The early utilization of intravenous glycoprotein IIb/IIIa receptor blockers and the host of novel oral antiplatelet agents in current development require assessments in the prehospital environment to clarify their risk and benefit.

Clear evidence supports the importance of appropriate and adequate anticoagulation in conjunction with pharmacologic reperfusion to sustain coronary patency. In the setting of mechanical reperfusion, the optimal antithrombin (e.g. unfractionated heparin, low molecular weight heparin, bivalirudin, fondaparinux) and dose remain unclear. Very early administration of an antithrombin in the setting of mechanical reperfusion currently lacks supportive evidence. Despite this, prehospital administration with seamless transition to the cardiac catheterization laboratory and in-hospital care seems reasonable.

Pharmacologic or mechanical reperfusion

The optimal choice of reperfusion therapy is best determined by assessing the time from symptom onset to first medical contact, the estimated baseline patient risk, location and extent of myocardial ischemia, and predicted percutaneous coronary intervention (PCI)-related delay (measured as the interval between initiation of fibrinolysis and the first balloon inflation). The decision is further influenced by regional staff, resources, hospital protocols, and physician and patient bias (Table 30.5). Although primary PCI is considered the reperfusion strategy of choice, it is clear that this advantage is time dependent and limited to specific patient populations. The DANAMI II trial has shown that the benefit of primary PCI is limited to a minority of patients, i.e. the 25% at highest risk as measured by TIMI risk score ≥ 5 (n = 393, three-year mortality primary PCI 25.3% vs fibrinolysis 36.2%, $P = 0.02$).[34] Of the 1134 patients with a TIM I risk score <5, three-year mortality for primary PCI was 8.0% vs 5.6% for fibrinolysis (P = ns).[34] Regardless of the form of reperfusion, rapid diagnosis and intervention are crucial for effective early management. Unfortunately, the polarizing debate over the advantage of primary PCI versus fibrinolysis has had a potentially negative impact on optimizing time to reperfusion for all STEMI patients.

The use of EMS in itself has been associated with expedited evaluation in the emergency department, wider use of acute reperfusion therapy, and earlier pharmacologic or mechanical reperfusion.[35–40] Opportunities to improve

Table 30.5 ACC/AHA guidelines for choice of reperfusion strategy[1]

Fibrinolysis generally preferred	Invasive strategy generally preferred
Early presentation (≤3 h from sx onset and delay to invasive strategy)	Skilled PCI lab available with surgical back-up (med contact to balloon <90 min)
Invasive strategy not an option (cath lab not available, no vasc access, lack of skilled PCI lab)	High risk from STEMI (cardiogenic shock, Killip class ≥3)
Delay to invasive strategy (door-to-balloon, door-to-needle) >1 h; first medical contact to balloon >90 min)	Contraindication to lysis (including increased bleeding/ICH risk) Late presentation (>3 h) Diagnosis in doubt

reperfusion delay utilizing prehospital EMS can be considered in four tiers of response and action. Tier one utilizes the prehospital 12-lead ECG to expedite in-hospital care upon arrival in the emergency department. Tier two employs the prehospital 12-lead ECG in conjunction with reperfusion screening checklists to facilitate activation of in-hospital response prior to arrival in the emergency department. Tier three utilizes these resources with communication to a remote physician or through implementation of predefined standardized protocols to deliver patients to the most appropriate center to provide expedited reperfusion, including bypass of community hospitals for mechanical reperfusion when appropriate. Tier four utilizes these resources in conjunction with an integrated treatment program whereby prehospital fibrinolysis can be administered or direct transportation to a cardiac catheterization laboratory occurs to reduce treatment delay and optimize patient outcomes.

The ACC/AHA guidelines for the treatment of STEMI suggest that "it is reasonable that all ACLS providers perform and evaluate 12-lead ECGs routinely in chest pain patients suspected of STEMI" (**Class IIa, Level C**).[1] Having a 12-lead ECG available to the in-hospital team upon the patient's arrival in the emergency department is associated with reduction in treatment delay to fibrinolysis by approximately 10 minutes and to primary PCI by approximately 20 minutes.[41,42] In combination with a prehospital reperfusion checklist addressing patient eligibility for reperfusion, communication of this information to the receiving emergency department may further facilitate care. After confirmation of the diagnosis by in-hospital emergency department staff, these patients may receive expedited in-hospital reperfusion.

Creation of regional cardiac destination hospitals capable of rapid cardiac catheterization and primary PCI delivered by experienced interventional cardiologists has been proposed as a means of improving outcomes in STEMI patients.[43,44] This strategy reduces time to treatment by 30–50 minutes.[45–47] In centers without prehospital confirmation of the diagnosis, i.e. tier two prehospital system, sig-

nificant financial and personnel strain may result from misdiagnosis based upon the paramedic-interpreted ECG and deployment of the cardiac catheterization team. Hence in one study of this issue, inappropriate activation of the catheterization laboratory occurred in 35% of patients with suspected STEMI (n = 1335) diagnosed in the emergency department as assessed by the following three criteria: no culprit coronary artery (14%), no significant coronary artery disease (9.5%), and negative cardiac biomarker results (11.2%).[48] Although the frequency of this phenomenon has not been determined in the prehospital environment, it is improbable that paramedical EMS staff would achieve better results than emergency physicians.

Fibrinolytic therapy of STEMI significantly improves mortality rates; treatment within six hours of the onset of symptoms leads to a reduction in mortality between 26–65 per 1000 patients treated which has been extensively documented.[49] Randomized trials of prehospital versus in-hospital fibrinolysis demonstrate a one-hour reduction in treatment delay with improved patient mortality (1.7% absolute reduction, odds ratio (OR) 0.83, 95% confidence interval (CI) 0.70–0.98).[50] Furthermore, prehospital STEMI patients tend to present sooner: in the two largest contemporary trials utilizing prehospital fibrinolysis, the median time to treatment was approximately two hours, comparing favorably with contemporary trials of in-hospital fibrinolysis (which includes ambulance or self-transportation patients).[51,52] These data provide a powerful impetus for healthcare systems to implement such programs.

Prehospital fibrinolysis has been validated in over two decades of clinical experience and research has demonstrated that this can be achieved in diverse health regions with variable population density, past experience with prehospital fibrinolysis, and the presence or absence of a physician in the prehospital environment.[53,54] Paramedics have been shown to be competent to complete on-scene assessment, record and transmit the 12-lead ECG for remote physician oversight, obtain informed consent and administer fibrinolytic therapy.[54] Prehospital fibrinolysis can be achieved rapidly with no evidence of adverse events in those managed by the paramedical prehospital personnel. Although the clinical experience and enhanced training of physicians in the prehospital setting may represent the ideal situation, trials and the wealth of clinical experience worldwide have demonstrated the efficacy, safety, and feasibility of paramedic-based prehospital fibrinolysis. The ACC/AHA STEMI guidelines recommend prehospital fibrinolysis as a reasonable alternative when "1) physicians are present in the ambulance; or 2) in well-organized EMS systems with full-time paramedics capable of acquiring prehospital 12-lead ECG and preliminary interpretation with initiation and ongoing training, direct medical oversight, and a medical director with training and experience in STEMI management; and an ongoing continuous quality improvement program".[1]

Although successful in various regions, fully integrated advanced prehospital management of STEMI, i.e. tier four, has not been consistently employed across the globe. Such programs are based upon individualized patient triage utilizing available evidence as outlined by current guidelines (see Table 30.5) which recommend pharmacologic reperfusion in situations where mechanical reperfusion is not feasible within the appropriate time frame of 60 minutes of PCI-related delay. This opportunity is critical: (1) when the catheterization laboratory is occupied; (2) in periods of high traffic in urban regions or during adverse weather conditions which are common throughout many populous regions; and (3) during periods where hospital overcrowding has led to emergency room diversions of patients. With the majority of prehospital STEMI patients presenting early after symptom onset, expedited prehospital fibrinolysis can achieve excellent patient outcomes. In patients with contraindications to fibrinolysis or in the minority with high-risk clinical characteristics such as hypotension, cardiogenic shock or pulmonary edema, direct triage to a prehospital activated cardiac catheterization laboratory expedites mechanical reperfusion. Additionally a fully integrated system minimizes the need for "lights and sirens" transportation, which has been linked to vehicular accidents and excess risk to patients, ambulance personnel, and innocent bystanders.[55,56]

Mechanical co-intervention subsequent to prehospital fibrinolysis

Following prehospital fibrinolysis, direct triage of selected patients to the catheterization laboratory should be undertaken to expedite care and enhance outcomes. This should be considered in high-risk clinical scenarios including:
- cardiogenic shock (<75 years old; **Class I, Level B**, and ≥75 years old; **Class IIa, Level B**)
- severe congestive heart failure (**Class I, Level B**)
- hemodynamically compromising ventricular arrhythmias (**Class I, Level C**).[4]

Following full-dose fibrinolysis, coronary angiography with intent to perform PCI should be considered in patients failing to achieve reperfusion clinically (**Class IIa, Level C**) and in those with persistent ST elevation (<50% resolved after 90 minutes following initiation of fibrinolysis) and at least a moderate area of myocardium at risk (**Class IIa, Level B**). These recommendations are based upon a 50% reduction in the combined clinical endpoint of death, repeat myocardial infarction, cerebral vascular accident or severe heart failure within six months comparing rescue PCI (15.3%), conservative management (29.8%) or repeat administration of fibrinolysis (31%) in patients failing to achieve ECG evidence of reperfusion (<50% reduction in ST elevation) within 90 minutes of initial fibrinolysis.[57] In certain circumstances, optimal patient care may include observation for successful reperfusion in a community hospital emergency department with the EMS team on standby, thereby expediting transfer to a catheterization laboratory for rescue PCI (required in approximately 30% of patients).[51,58,59]

Facilitated PCI, where patients are routinely taken directly to the catheterization laboratory following administration of reduced-dose fibrinolysis, has been implemented in certain regions when patients are unable to achieve primary PCI within acceptable time intervals.[60–62] Although this strategy may appear attractive, large-scale clinical trials have failed to demonstrate enhanced patient outcomes with either full-dose or reduced-dose fibrinolysis followed by PCI.[63,64] A planned reperfusion strategy using full-dose fibrinolysis followed by immediate PCI has been discouraged in the recent ACC/AHA focused STEMI update (**Class III, Level B**).[4]

Integration of prehospital strategies in a system-wide reperfusion program

Expansion and enhancement of prehospital diagnosis, triage, treatment, and initiation of definitive reperfusion strategies in the prehospital environment provides a key opportunity to improve STEMI patient outcomes. For such programs to be successful over the long term, it is essential that they be integrated and supported by a system-wide reperfusion protocol. If prehospital teams are linked to such regional reperfusion programs, seamless integration of patient care may occur. If such programs are not fully supported, the sustainability of prehospital reperfusion strategies would be significantly hampered. Communication and continuous quality improvement programs with engagement of all partners within the healthcare team, including hospital and regional administration, physicians, nurses, and paramedical staff, are essential (Fig. 30.3).

Within a system-wide reperfusion program, establishing clear guidelines and empowering experienced decision makers to implement best care for individual patients are required. This should include identifying high-risk patient populations suitable for early reperfusion, linked to appropriate triage to tertiary care centers for risk stratification and interventional management as required. Dedicated assessment of the success of reperfusion following pharmacologic therapies with aggressive rescue PCI may also improve patient outcomes. In the future, computer-based dynamic modeling may facilitate aligning patient risk with choice of therapy as well as subsequent destination hospital. Such dynamic modeling must be an ongoing process, with reassessment of risk in the early hours after initiation of therapies guiding subsequent investigation and management.

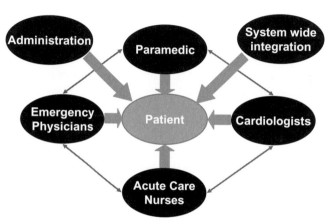

Figure 30.3 Reflections on STEMI care; success through co-operation. Within the healthcare system all stakeholders from paramedics to administrative staff must adopt a patient-centered focus to deliver base care to each patient.

Conclusion

This chapter has discussed key opportunities that exist to limit STEMI patient morbidity and mortality by enhancing early management via the prehospital emergency medical system (EMS). Advanced prehospital STEMI management which expedites patient assessment, diagnosis, triage, and treatment has been successfully implemented. Empowering adequately trained paramedic teams to administer life-saving therapy such as fibrinolysis in the prehospital environment deserves a high international priority.

Although this chapter has focused on STEMI patients and the enhancement of their care through advanced prehospital management, the importance of early diagnosis, triage and treatment is not unique to these patients. The development of prehospital STEMI protocols can be seen as the initial template from which to advance care in other acute cardiovascular diseases (Fig. 30.4).[65] This could include high-risk NSTEMI with implementation of early pharmacologic therapy and prehospital triage to appropriate tertiary care centers for early angiography. Early implementation of therapy in stroke and survivors of cardiac arrest may also be linked to improved outcomes following these potentially devastating events. Opportunities will continue to expand as technology continues to advance, with enhanced diagnostic and therapeutic capability across the spectrum of cardiovascular disease.

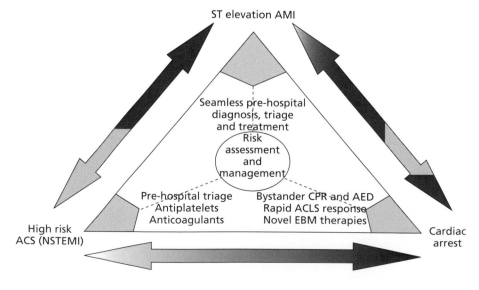

Figure 30.4 Opportunities in prehospital cardiovascular care. Opportunities provided by enhanced prehospital cardiovascular care move beyond the scope of this chapter focused on ST elevation myocardial infarction (STEMI) and include non-ST elevation acute coronary syndromes (ACS), cardiac arrest (sudden death), and a host of other cardiovascular disease.[65] The capacity of prehospital teams to assess and manage patient risk with rapid initiation of evidence-based treatments and triage to appropriate medical institution portends optimal medical treatment. ACLS, advance cardiac life support; AED, automated external defibrillator; CPR, cardiopulmonary resuscitation; EBM, evidence-based medicine.

References

1. Antman EM, Anbe DT, Armstrong PW *et al* ACC/AHA guidelines for the management of patients with ST elevation myocardial infarction: a report of the American College of Cardiology/American Heart Association Task Force on Practice Guidelines (Committee to Revise the 1999 Guidelines for the Management of patients with acute myocardial infarction). *J Am Coll Cardiol* 2004; **44**(3):E1-E211.

2. Armstrong PW, Bogaty P, Buller CE, Dorian P, O'Neill BJ. The 2004 ACC/AHA Guidelines: a perspective and adaptation for Canada by the Canadian Cardiovascular Society Working Group. *Can J Cardiol* 2004; **20**(11):1075–9.

3. Nallamothu BK, Bates ER. Percutaneous coronary intervention versus fibrinolytic therapy in acute myocardial infarction: is timing (almost) everything? *Am J Cardiol* 2003; **92**(7):824–6.

4. Antman EM, Hand M, Armstrong PW *et al* 2007 Focused update of the ACC/AHA 2004 Guidelines for the Management of Patients With ST elevation Myocardial Infarction. A report of the American College of Cardiology/American Heart Association Task Force on Practice Guidelines. *Circulation* 2008; **117**(2):296–329.

5. GUSTO Investigators. An international randomized trial comparing four thrombolytic strategies for acute myocardial infarction. *N Engl J Med* 1993; **329**(10):673–82.

6. Davies C, Christenson J, Campbell A *et al* Fibrinolytic therapy in acute myocardial infarction: time to treatment in Canada. *Can J Cardiol* 2004; **20**(8):801–5.

7. Van de Werf F, Adgey J, Ardissino D *et al* Single-bolus tenecteplase compared with front-loaded alteplase in acute myocardial infarction: the ASSENT-2 double-blind randomised trial. *Lancet* 1999; **354**(9180):716–22.

8. Goldberg RJ, Steg PG, Sadiq I *et al* Extent of, and factors associated with, delay to hospital presentation in patients with acute coronary disease (the GRACE registry). *Am J Cardiol* 2002; **89**(7):791–6.

9. Goldberg RJ, Gurwitz JH, Gore JM. Duration of, and temporal trends (1994–1997) in, prehospital delay in patients with acute myocardial infarction: the second National Registry of Myocardial Infarction. *Arch Intern Med* 1999; **159**(18):2141–7.

10. Goldberg RJ, Yarzebski J, Lessard D, Gore JM. Decade-long trends and factors associated with time to hospital presentation in patients with acute myocardial infarction: the Worcester Heart Attack study. *Arch Intern Med* 2000; **160**(21):3217–23.

11. Gurwitz JH, McLaughlin TJ, Willison DJ *et al* Delayed hospital presentation in patients who have had acute myocardial infarction. *Ann Intern Med* 1997; **126**(8):593–9.

12. Finnegan JR Jr, Meischke H, Zapka JG *et al* Patient delay in seeking care for heart attack symptoms: findings from focus groups conducted in five U.S. regions. *Prev Med* 2000; **31**(3):205–13.

13. Meischke H, Yasui Y, Kuniyuki A, Bowen DJ, Andersen R, Urban N. How women label and respond to symptoms of acute myocardial infarction: responses to hypothetical symptom scenarios. *Heart Lung* 1999; **28**(4):261–9.

14. Meischke H, Ho MT, Eisenberg MS, Schaeffer SM, Larsen MP. Reasons patients with chest pain delay or do not call 911. *Ann Emerg Med* 1995; **25**(2):193–7.

15. Luepker RV, Raczynski JM, Osganian S *et al* Effect of a community intervention on patient delay and emergency medical service use in acute coronary heart disease: the Rapid Early Action for Coronary Treatment (REACT) trial. *JAMA* 2000; **284**(1):60–7.

16. Goff DC Jr, Mitchell P, Finnegan J *et al* Knowledge of heart attack symptoms in 20 US communities. Results from the Rapid Early Action for Coronary Treatment Community Trial. *Prev Med* 2004; **38**(1):85–93.

17. Davis TM, Fortun P, Mulder J, Davis WA, Bruce DG. Silent myocardial infarction and its prognosis in a community-based cohort of Type 2 diabetic patients: the Fremantle Diabetes Study. *Diabetologia* 2004; **47**(3):395–9.

18. Ellenberger L. Silent myocardial infarction. *Postgrad Med* 1990; **87**(5):32.

19. Lundblad D, Eliasson M. Silent myocardial infarction in women with impaired glucose tolerance: the Northern Sweden MONICA study. *Cardiovasc Diabetol* 2003; **2**:9.

20. O'Sullivan JJ, Conroy RM, MacDonald K, McKenna TJ, Maurer BJ. Silent ischaemia in diabetic men with autonomic neuropathy. *Br Heart J* 1991; **66**(4):313–15.

21. Schweizer W. Silent myocardial infarction. *Geriatrics* 1968; **23**(1):96–8.

22. Welsh RC, Travers A, Senaratne M, Williams R, Armstrong PW. Feasibility and applicability of paramedic-based prehospital fibrinolysis in a large North American center. *Am Heart J* 2006; **152**(6):1007–14.

23. Aufderheide TP, Hendley GE, Thakur RK *et al* The diagnostic impact of prehospital 12-lead electrocardiography. *Ann Emerg Med* 1990; **19**(11):1280–7.

24. Grim P, Feldman T, Martin M, Donovan R, Nevins V, Childers RW. Cellular telephone transmission of 12-lead electrocardiograms from ambulance to hospital. *Am J Cardiol* 1987; **60**(8):715–20.

25. Aufderheide TP, Keelan MH, Hendley GE *et al* Milwaukee Prehospital Chest Pain Project phase I: feasibility and accuracy of prehospital thrombolytic candidate selection. *Am J Cardiol* 1992; **69**(12):991–6.

26. Giovas P, Papadoyannis D, Thomakos D *et al* Transmission of electrocardiograms from a moving ambulance. *J Telemed Telecare* 1998; **4**(suppl 1):5–7.

27. Karagounis L, Ipsen SK, Jessop MR *et al* Impact of field-transmitted electrocardiography on time to in-hospital thrombolytic therapy in acute myocardial infarction. *Am J Cardiol* 1990; **66**(10):786–91.

28. Weaver WD, Cerqueira M, Hallstrom AP *et al* Prehospital-initiated vs hospital-initiated thrombolytic therapy. The Myocardial Infarction Triage and Intervention Trial. *JAMA* 1993; **270**(10):1211–16.

29. Maroko PR, Radvany P, Braunwald E, Hale SL. Reduction of infarct size by oxygen inhalation following acute coronary occlusion. *Circulation* 1975; **52**(3):360–8.

30. Meine TJ, Roe MT, Chen AY *et al* Association of intravenous morphine use and outcomes in acute coronary syndromes: results from the CRUSADE Quality Improvement Initiative. *Am Heart J* 2005; **149**(6):1043–9.

31. Antman EM, Morrow DA, McCabe CH *et al* Enoxaparin versus unfractionated heparin with fibrinolysis for ST elevation myocardial infarction. *N Engl J Med* 2006; **354**(14):1477–88.

32. Chen ZM, Pan HC, Chen YP *et al* Early intravenous then oral metoprolol in 45,852 patients with acute myocardial infarction: randomised placebo-controlled trial. *Lancet* 2005; **366**(9497): 1622–32.

33. Steinhubl SR, Berger PB, Brennan DM, Topol EJ. Optimal timing for the initiation of pre-treatment with 300 mg clopidogrel before percutaneous coronary intervention. *J Am Coll Cardiol* 2006; **47**(5):939–43.

34. Thune JJ, Hoefsten DE, Lindholm MG *et al* Simple risk stratification at admission to identify patients with reduced mortality from primary angioplasty. *Circulation* 2005; **112**(13):2017–21.

35. Brown AL, Mann NC, Daya M *et al* Demographic, belief, and situational factors influencing the decision to utilize emergency medical services among chest pain patients. Rapid Early Action for Coronary Treatment (REACT) study. *Circulation* 2000; **102**(2):173–8.

36. Canto JG, Zalenski RJ, Ornato JP *et al* Use of emergency medical services in acute myocardial infarction and subsequent quality of care: observations from the National Registry of Myocardial Infarction 2. *Circulation* 2002; **106**(24):3018–23.

37. Goff DC Jr, Feldman HA, McGovern PG *et al* Prehospital delay in patients hospitalized with heart attack symptoms in the United States: the REACT trial. Rapid Early Action for Coronary Treatment (REACT) Study Group. *Am Heart J* 1999; **138**(6 Pt 1):1046–57.

38. Hedges JR, Feldman HA, Bittner V *et al* Impact of community intervention to reduce patient delay time on use of reperfusion therapy for acute myocardial infarction: rapid early action for coronary treatment (REACT) trial. REACT Study Group. *Acad Emerg Med* 2000; **7**(8):862–72.

39. Lambrew CT, Bowlby LJ, Rogers WJ, Chandra NC, Weaver WD. Factors influencing the time to thrombolysis in acute myocardial infarction. Time to Thrombolysis Substudy of the National Registry of Myocardial Infarction-1. *Arch Intern Med* 1997; **157**(22):2577–82.

40. Swor R, Anderson W, Jackson R, Wilson A. Effects of EMS transportation on time to diagnosis and treatment of acute myocardial infarction in the emergency department. *Prehosp Disaster Med* 1994; **9**(3):160–4.

41. Canto JG, Rogers WJ, Bowlby LJ, French WJ, Pearce DJ, Weaver WD. The prehospital electrocardiogram in acute myocardial infarction: is its full potential being realized? National Registry of Myocardial Infarction 2 Investigators. *J Am Coll Cardiol* 1997; **29**(3):498–505.

42. Curtis JP, Portnay EL, Wang Y *et al* The prehospital electrocardiogram and time to reperfusion in patients with acute myocardial infarction, 2000–2002: findings from the National Registry of Myocardial Infarction-4. *J Am Coll Cardiol* 2006; **47**(8):1544–52.

43. Califf RM, Faxon DP. Need for centers to care for patients with acute coronary syndromes. *Circulation* 2003; **107**(11):1467–70.

44. Henry TD, Atkins JM, Cunningham MS *et al* ST-segment elevation myocardial infarction: recommendations on triage of patients to heart attack centers: is it time for a national policy for the treatment of ST-segment elevation myocardial infarction? *J Am Coll Cardiol* 2006; **47**(7):1339–45.

45. Afolabi BA, Novaro GM, Pinski SL, Fromkin KR, Bush HS. Use of the prehospital ECG improves door-to-balloon times in ST

segment elevation myocardial infarction irrespective of time of day or day of week. *Emerg Med J* 2007; **24**(8):588–91.

46. Swor R, Hegerberg S, Hugh-McNally A, Goldstein M, McEachin CC. Prehospital 12-lead ECG: efficacy or effectiveness? *Prehosp Emerg Care* 2006; **10**(3):374–7.

47. Bata I, Armstrong PW, Westerhout CM et al. for the WEST Study Group. Time from first medical contact to reperfusion in ST Elevation Myocardial Infarction: a WEST sub-study. *Can J Cardiol* 2009; in press.

48. Larson DM, Menssen KM, Sharkey SW *et al* "False-positive" cardiac catheterization laboratory activation among patients with suspected ST-segment elevation myocardial infarction. *JAMA* 2007; **298**(23):2754–60.

49. Boersma E, Maas AC, Deckers JW, Simoons ML. Early thrombolytic treatment in acute myocardial infarction: reappraisal of the golden hour. *Lancet* 1996; **348**(9030):771–5.

50. Morrison LJ, Verbeek PR, McDonald AC, Sawadsky BV, Cook DJ. Mortality and prehospital thrombolysis for acute myocardial infarction: A meta-analysis. *JAMA* 2000; **283**(20):2686–92.

51. Bonnefoy E, Lapostolle F, Leizorovicz A *et al* Primary angioplasty versus prehospital fibrinolysis in acute myocardial infarction: a randomised study. *Lancet* 2002; **360**(9336):825–9.

52. Wallentin L, Goldstein P, Armstrong PW *et al* Efficacy and safety of tenecteplase in combination with the low-molecular-weight heparin enoxaparin or unfractionated heparin in the prehospital setting: the Assessment of the Safety and Efficacy of a New Thrombolytic Regimen (ASSENT)-3 PLUS randomized trial in acute myocardial infarction. *Circulation* 2003; **108**(2): 135–42.

53. Welsh RC, Goldstein P, Adgey J *et al* Variations in prehospital fibrinolysis process of care: insights from the Assessment of the Safety and Efficacy of a New Thrombolytic 3 Plus international acute myocardial infarction prehospital care survey. *Eur J Emerg Med* 2004; **11**(3):134–40.

54. Welsh RC, Chang W, Goldstein P *et al* Time to treatment and the impact of a physician on prehospital management of acute ST elevation myocardial infarction: insights from the ASSENT-3 PLUS trial. *Heart* 2005; **91**(11):1400–6.

55. Clawson JJ, Martin RL, Cady GA, Maio RF. The wake-effect – emergency vehicle-related collisions. *Prehosp Disaster Med* 1997; **12**(4):274–7.

56. Custalow CB, Gravitz CS. Emergency medical vehicle collisions and potential for preventive intervention. *Prehosp Emerg Care* 2004; **8**(2):175–84.

57. Gershlick AH, Stephens-Lloyd A, Hughes S *et al* Rescue angioplasty after failed thrombolytic therapy for acute myocardial infarction. *N Engl J Med* 2005; **353**(26):2758–68.

58. Armstrong PW. A comparison of pharmacologic therapy with/without timely coronary intervention vs. primary percutaneous intervention early after ST elevation myocardial infarction: the WEST (Which Early ST elevation myocardial infarction Therapy) study. *Eur Heart J* 2006; **27**(13):1530–8.

59. Buller CE, Welsh RC, Westerhout CM *et al* Guideline adjudicated fibrinolytic failure: incidence, findings, and management in a contemporary clinical trial. *Am Heart J* 2008; **155**(1):121–7.

60. Henry TD, Sharkey SW, Burke MN *et al* A regional system to provide timely access to percutaneous coronary intervention for

ST elevation myocardial infarction. *Circulation* 2007; **116**(7): 721–8.

61. Ting HH, Rihal CS, Gersh BJ *et al* Regional systems of care to optimize timeliness of reperfusion therapy for ST elevation myocardial infarction: the Mayo Clinic STEMI Protocol. *Circulation* 2007; **116**(7):729–36.

62. Smalling RW, Giesler GM, Julapalli VR *et al* Prehospital reduced-dose fibrinolysis coupled with urgent percutaneous coronary intervention reduces time to reperfusion and improves angiographic perfusion score compared with prehospital fibrinolysis alone or primary percutaneous coronary intervention: results of the PATCAR Pilot Trial. *J Am Coll Cardiol* 2007; **50**(16):1612–14.

63. ASSENT-4 PCI Investigators. Primary versus tenecteplase-facilitated percutaneous coronary intervention in patients with ST-segment elevation acute myocardial infarction (ASSENT-4 PCI): randomised trial. *Lancet* 2006; **367**(9510):569–78.

64. Ellis SG, Armstrong P, Betriu A *et al* Facilitated percutaneous coronary intervention versus primary percutaneous coronary intervention: design and rationale of the Facilitated Intervention with Enhanced Reperfusion Speed to Stop Events (FINESSE) trial. *Am Heart J* 2004; **147**(4):E16.

65. Welsh RC, Armstrong PW. It's a matter of time: contemporary prehospital management of acute ST elevation myocardial infarction. *Heart* 2005; **91**(12):1524–6.

66. Kainth A, Hewitt A, Sowden A *et al* Systematic review of interventions to reduce delay in patients with suspected heart attack. *Emerg Med J* 2004; **21**(4):506–8.

31 Reperfusion therapies for ST segment elevation myocardial infarction

Joseph B Muhlestein and Jeffrey L Anderson

Cardiovascular Department, Intermountain Medical Center, Murray, UT, USA

Introduction

The primary pathophysiology of acute ST segment elevation myocardial infarction (STEMI) is the total occlusion of a coronary artery, usually through thrombosis of a ruptured or eroded atherosclerotic plaque, with a subsequent lack of blood flow to the myocardium. This then results in a time-dependent "wave-front" of myocardial necrosis beginning at the subendocardium and moving towards the epicardial surface.[1] Although in a dog model that has very minimal collateral coronary circulation, the progression to complete transmural necrosis usually takes less than 3 hours, in humans the time may vary anywhere from 2 hours to 12 hours depending on the degree of available collateral coronary circulation, the degree of ischemic preconditioning and whether the thrombotic coronary occlusion is permanent or intermittent. The minimization of the total amount of myocardial necrosis during STEMI has been associated with improved long-term clinical outcomes. Although some evidence exists that myocardial salvage may be accomplished by a variety of pharmacologic maneuvers designed to reduce the oxygen demands of the heart, by far the most effective approach has been to produce reperfusion of the occluded artery as fast as possible, by either fibrinolytic therapy or mechanical means. Multiple studies have validated the "need for speed" approach to this effort and justified the mantra that "time is myocardium."

The benefits of therapy depend on the rate and extent to which myocardial reperfusion is effectively achieved.[2–4] Reperfusion is scored by the Thrombolysis In Myocardial Infarction (TIMI) visual[2] or frame-counts[5] methods supplemented, recently, by a TIMI myocardial perfusion (TMP) score.[6] Restoration of TIMI grade 3 (normal) epicardial flow is associated with lower mortality rates than TIMI grades 0–2 (3.7% vs 7.0%). Among those with TIMI 3 flow, lower mortality is associated with TMP grade 3 (0.7%) than with TMP grades 2 (2.9%) or 0–1 (5.4%). The factors differentiating epicardial and myocardial reperfusion are incompletely understood. Platelet and platelet–leukocyte aggregates, distal thrombus embolization and secreted vasoactive and thrombogenic factors have received recent attention, and a variety of targeted therapies, adjunctive to either fibrinolytic or mechanical reperfusion therapy and designed to further improve myocardial perfusion, are being actively studied.[7,8] However, despite the promise shown by multiple agents in the experimental situation, the results of clinical trials have been extremely disappointing and no trial to date has achieved its primary endpoint.[9]

Historic perspective

Although both fibrinolytic and mechanical approaches to coronary reperfusion therapy are presently used, depending on the clinical circumstances, from a historic perspective, fibrinolytic therapy was first developed and validated. In 1933, Tillet and Garner published their discovery of a streptococcal fibrinolysin.[10,11] Clinical application of streptokinase (SK) to AMI was first reported in 1958.[12] From then until 1979, at least 17 studies were published, but AMI pathophysiology was not well understood and results were inconclusive and poorly accepted.[13,14] With the establishment of the thrombotic nature of coronary occlusion[15] several groups demonstrated the feasibility of clinical fibrinolysis to achieve early reperfusion under angiographic monitoring (~75% success with intracoronary (IC) SK) in the period 1976–83.[16–19]

Randomized studies in AMI followed. Anderson *et al* reported in 1983[20] a benefit of early (<4h) IC SK on clinical, enzymatic, and imaging endpoints. Later therapy (at >6 hours) relieved ischemic pain but did not benefit regional myocardial function in another study.[21] The potential for

Evidence-Based Cardiology, 3rd edition. Edited by S. Yusuf, J.A. Cairns, A.J. Camm, E.L. Fallen, and B.J. Gersh. © 2010 Blackwell Publishing, ISBN: 978-1-4051-5925-8.

mortality benefit of IC SK was suggested by subsequent Western Washington and Dutch studies in a few hundred patients.[22–24] The logistic difficulties with intracoronary administration stimulated the re-evaluation of IV SK (Schröder *et al*[25]). By the mid-1980s, favorable comparisons with IC SK[26–28] and a larger outcomes study of IV SK (ISAM)[29] established the intravenous route for subsequent clinical trials.

Although intravenous fibrinolytic therapy is certainly superior to placebo in patients who present early with STEMI, there remain a number of problems associated with this approach. First, many patients have significant contra-indications to the use of fibrinolytic agents.[30] Second, even with the newer fibrinolytic agents, a small but significant risk of intracranial hemorrhage remains and results in death or disability, especially in the very old patients.[31] Third, fibrinolytics establish normal TIMI grade 3 flow in only 50–60% of the patients.[32,33] Only a third of treated patients have complete resolution of ST segment elevation, and only about 50% have >70% resolution of ST segment elevation 24–36 hours after fibrinolytic administration – a marker of lower mortality.[34] Since there are no absolutely reliable clinical signs or symptoms that indicate success of fibrinolytic therapy, it is difficult to evaluate whether the infarct artery is open with the treatment in an individual patient. Even in those patients with successful fibrinolysis, many go on to have reocclusion and reinfarction due to the ongoing vulnerability of the underlying atherosclerotic plaque.[35,36]

Mechanical reperfusion has the potential to overcome many of these limitations.[37] Direct (or primary) PCI, intervention on the infarct artery without prior fibrinolysis, can be done in many patients with contraindications to fibrinolytic therapy. The overall risk of intracranial bleeding is significantly lower with direct PCI.[38] With the strategy of direct PCI, there is an opportunity to evaluate the overall coronary anatomy, ventricular function, and intracardiac pressures essentially at the time of admission and possibly detect anatomic features or mechanical complications that would require earlier treatment with surgery. Another benefit of direct PCI is the availability of highly trained cardiac catheterization laboratory staff if circulatory resuscitation is needed. Additionally, there is a potential to significantly improve the proportion of patients who receive reperfusion with TIMI 3 flow. Early observational studies evaluating the potential of primary PCI were very promising.[39] This led to the performance of a number of randomized trials of fibrinolysis versus mechanical reperfusion therapy in STEMI, most of which demonstrated a significant superiority of primary PCI, especially among patients in which it was logistically feasible to accomplish reperfusion within 90 minutes of presentation (**Class I, Level A**).[40] As will be discussed in more detail later in this chapter, when all things are equal primary PCI is better than fibrinolytics.

Over the past decade, the results of multiple studies have led us to the present state in which, depending on a variety of circumstances, either fibrinolysis or mechanical reperfusion may be the treatment strategy of choice. This chapter will address in detail the evidence behind both approaches and provide guidelines to assist in choosing which form of reperfusion therapy to use when dealing with an individual patient. Potential adjunctive therapies to be used with each approach will be addressed in other chapters.

Fibrinolytic agents

General mechanisms of action and pharmacologic properties

Fibrinolysis is mediated by plasmin, a non-specific serine protease that degrades clot-associated fibrin and fibrinogen, disrupting a forming thrombus and facilitating reperfusion. The fibrinolytic (or "thrombolytic") agents are all plasminogen activators, directly or indirectly converting the proenzyme plasminogen to plasmin by cleaving the arginine 560- valine 561 bond (Fig. 31.1). Plasmin degrades several proteins, including fibrin, fibrinogen, prothrombin, and factors V and VII. The fibrinolytic agents differ in several properties, as summarized in the text and Table 31.1.

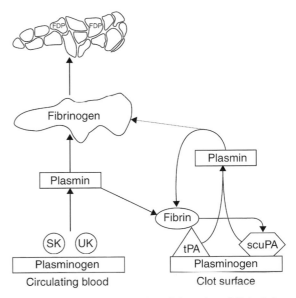

Figure 31.1 Schematic representation of the action of fibrinolytic enzymes. Streptokinase (SK) and urokinase (UK) work predominantly on circulating plasminogen, whereas tissue type plasminogen activator (tPA) and single chain urokinase-type plasminogen activator (scuPA) are relatively clot selective. (Modified with permission from Topol EJ. Clinical use of streptokinase and urokinase to treat acute myocardial infarction. *Heart Lung* 1987;**16**:760.)

Table 31.1 Comparison of fibrinolytic agents approved by the US FDA for intravenous use

	SK (streptokinase)	tPA (alteplase)	rPA (reteplase)	TNK (tenecteplase)
Dose	1.5 million units (MU) in 30–60 min	100 mg in 90 min[a]	10 U + 10 U, 30 min apart	30–50 mg over 5 seconds[b]
Circulating half-life (min)	≅20	≅6	≅18	≅20
Antigenic	Yes	No	No	No
Allergic reactions	Yes	No	No	No
Systemic fibrinogen depletion	Severe	Mild–moderate	Moderate	Minimal
Intracerebral hemorrhage	≅0.4%	≅0.7%	≅0.8%	≅0.7%
Patency (TIMI-2/3) rate, 90 min[c]	≅51%	≅73–84%	≅83%	≅77–88%
Lives saved per 100 treated	≅3[c]	≅4[d]	≅4	≅4
Cost per dose (approx US dollars)	290	2750	2750	2750

[a] Accelerated tPA given as follows: 15 mg bolus, then 0.75 mg/kg over 30 min (maximum 50 mg), then 0.50 mg/kg over 60 min (maximum 35 mg).
[b] TNK is dosed by weight (supplied in 5 mg/mL vials): 60 kg = 6 mL; 61–70 kg = 7 mL; 71–80 kg = 8 mL; 81–90 kg = 9 mL; 90 kg = 10 mL.
[c] Based on Granger et al[49] and Bode et al.[89]
[d] Based on the finding from the GUSTO trial[42] that tPA saves 1 more additional life per 100 treated than does SK.

Approved fibrinolytic agents

Streptokinase

Streptokinase (SK) is a 415-amino acid bacterial protein sharing homology with serine proteases.[41,42] Upon injection, SK forms a 1:1 stoichiometric complex with plasminogen or plasmin, activating a catalytic site that cleaves plasminogen to plasmin. The half-life of the SK complex is about 23 minutes. SK is antigenic, has little fibrin specificity, and causes substantial systemic lytic effects in clinical doses. Least expensive of fibrinolytics and still widely used globally, SK is administered by short-term (1 h) infusions.

Urokinase

Urokinase (UK) is a native, 2-polypeptide protein derived from human urine or renal cell cultures.[43] UK directly converts plasminogen to plasmin. It is non-antigenic and is cleared from the circulation predominantly by the liver with a half-life of 16 minutes. Clinically used doses produce moderately extensive systemic fibrinolysis. Its principal use in North America has been for intra-arterial (including intracoronary) fibrinolysis. It has not been approved for and currently is not available for IV use in acute myocardial infarction (AMI).

Tissue-type plasminogen activator (tPA)

Tissue-type plasminogen activator (tPA), a 526-amino acid single polypeptide chain, is the major intrinsic (physiologic) plasminogen activator.[44] The marketed form (alteplase) is manufactured by recombinant DNA technology (rtPA). tPA is converted by plasmin to a double-chain form with equivalent fibrinolytic activity.[45] tPA has greater activity in the locale of the thrombus and causes less systemic plasminemia, fibrinogenolysis, and proteolysis than SK. tPA is non-antigenic, is inhibited by a circulating plasminogen activator inhibitor (PAI-I), and is rapidly cleared (half-life about 5 minutes). This short half-life has necessitated bolus/infusion regimens (over 1–3 hours); bolus-only tPA regimens have been tested but abandoned in favor of longer-acting mutant forms of tPA.

Reteplase

Reteplase (rPA) was the first variant (mutant) of tPA to be developed and marketed.[46] It is a non-glycosylated, single chain deletion variant consisting only of the kringle 2 and proteinase (plasmin cleavage site) domains of human tPA. Fibrin specificity is lower and half-life longer (14–18 minutes) than tPA, allowing more convenient, double-bolus administration.

Tenecteplase

Tenecteplase (TNK-tPA) is a triple-site substitution variant of tPA: at amino acid 103, threonine (T) is replaced by asparagine, adding a glycosylation site; at site 117, asparagine (N) is replaced by glutamine, removing a glycosylation site; at a third site, four amino acids (lysine (K), histidine, arginine and arginine) are replaced by four alanines.[47] The first two changes decrease clearance rate (half-life 20 minutes), allowing for single bolus dosing. The third change confers greater fibrin specificity and resistance to PAI-1.

Efficacy of intravenous fibrinolytic therapy

Effects on coronary arterial patency

Because myocardial reperfusion is the postulated mechanism of benefit of fibrinolysis for MI, many angiographic studies have been undertaken to assess patency profiles of the infarct-related coronary artery after fibrinolylic therapy.[48] Granger *et al* summarized 14124 angiographic observations from 58 studies.[49] Because the extent of myocardial salvage is time dependent, early (0–90 min) patency has generally formed the primary endpoint in these studies. Without fibrinolytic therapy, spontaneous perfusion early after STEMI occurs in only 15% and 21% at 60 and 90 minutes after study entry, respectively, remains unchanged at 1 day, then gradually increases to about 60% by 3 weeks. All fibrinolytic regimens improve early patency rates. At 60 and 90 minutes, streptokinase had the lowest rates (48%, 51%), standard (3-hour) tPA infusions intermediate rates (about 60%, 70%), and accelerated (90-minute) tPA infusions the highest rates (74%, 84%). However, patency rates at >3 hours were similar for all regimens, and reocclusion rates were higher after tPA than non-fibrin specific (systemically active) agents (13% vs 8%) (IP = 0.002). The GUSTO angiographic study[50] embedded within a larger comparative mortality study,[42] directly demonstrated that early but not late patency rates accurately predict mortality differences among AMI therapies, providing direct support for the open artery hypothesis of fibrinolytic benefit.

Effect on mortality

By the late 1980s, accumulating clinical trials data provided support for a survival benefit of IV fibrinolysis.[51–53] The most important survival trials, comparing fibrinolysis to placebo or standard non-fibrinolytic care, are summarized below.

Gruppo Italiano per lo Studio della Streptochinasi nell' Infarto Miocardico (GISSI) This study[54] was the first "definitive" mortality trial. Eleven thousand eight hundred and six AMI patients with ST elevation were randomized to receive 1.5 million units (MU) of IV SK over 1 hour or standard therapy. Aspirin was not routinely given. In-hospital mortality was 10.7% in the SK group and 13.0% in the control group, a 17.6% risk reduction (P = 0.0002; relative risk (RR); 0.81). Survival differences remained at 1–2 years.[55] Benefit was time dependent and particularly large for treatment within 1 hour of symptom onset (47% mortality reduction, RR 0.49) but was not significant after 6 hours.

Second International Study of Infarct Survival (ISIS-2) This study[56] randomized 17187 patients with suspected AMI within 24 hours to IV SK (1.5 MU), aspirin (1 62.5 mg), both or neither (placebos) in a 2 × 2 factorial design. The 35-day vascular mortality rate (13.2% for the double placebo group) was reduced 23% by aspirin alone, 25% by SK alone, and 42% by combined aspirin and SK (all P < 0.00001). When both were given early (within 4 hours of symptom onset), a 53% odds reduction was achieved.

Anglo-Scandinavian Study of Early Thrombolysis (ASSET) This study[57] evaluated tPA (alteplase) with heparin versus heparin alone within a randomized, double blind, placebo-controlled design. ASSET enrolled 5013 patients within 5 hours of suspected AMI. Therapies were IV tPA (100 mg over 3 hours) plus heparin (5000U N bolus, then 1000 U/h), or placebo plus heparin. The 30-day mortality was lower in the tPA than the placebo group (7.2% vs 9.8%, P = 0.0011). Hemorrhagic risk was acceptable.

Fibrinolytic Therapy Trialists' (FTT) Collaborative Group This group[58] pooled data from nine controlled trials that randomized 1000 or more patients with suspected AMI. The database consisted of 58600 patients of whom 6177 (10.7%) died, 564 (1.0%) had strokes, and 436 had major non-cerebral bleeds. The 45000 patients who presented with ST elevation or bundle branch block (BBB) had an absolute mortality reduction of 30 per 1000 for treatment within the first 6 hours, 20 per 1000 for hours 7–12, and a statistically uncertain reduction of 13 per 1000 beyond 12 hours. These data led to the national guidelines (**Class I, Level A**) that all STEMI patients should undergo rapid evaluation for reperfusion therapy and have a reperfusion strategy implemented promptly after contact with the medical system.[59]

Subgroup analyses by presenting electrocardiogram (ECG) (Fig. 31.2) showed mortality reductions for those with ST elevation (21%, P < 0.00001) and bundle branch block (BBB) (25%) P < 0.01. Benefit was greater for those with anterior (37 lives saved per 1000 treated) compared with inferior (8 per 1000) or other (27 per 1000) AMI sites. The absolute benefit was greater in those with greater risk – for example, BBB (49 lives saved per 1000 treated) and anterior ST elevation (37 per 1000). Those with normal ECGs or with ST depression alone showed no benefit and adverse trends (7 and 14 more deaths per 1000, respectively).

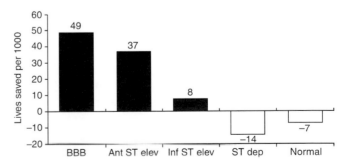

Figure 31.2 The effect of fibrinolytic therapy on mortality (lives saved per 1000 treated) in various patient subsets classified according to admission ECG. Patients presenting with bundle branch block and anterior ST segment elevations derived most benefit from fibrinolytic therapy. Patients with inferior ST segment elevation derived much less benefit, while those with ST depression or normal ECG did not benefit. (Based on data from FTT Collaborative Group.[57])

The FTT suggested that proportional mortality reduction was little influenced by systolic blood pressure or heart rate. Benefits also were confirmed for other high-risk groups, including those with prior MI and diabetes.

Benefits of very early (<1 hour) therapy

The magnitude of mortality reductions in FTT was dependent on time to therapy from symptom onset. For those with ST elevation or BBB, the absolute benefit was 39 (at 0–1 h), 30 (>1–3 h), 27 (>3–6 h), 21 (>6–12 h), and 7 (>12–24 h) lives saved per 1000 treated (Fig. 31.3).

Others also studied the benefits of therapy within 1 hour.[60] Boersma et al[61] reappraised very early therapy based on a larger database (50 246 patients, derived from all randomized trials of >100 patients). The absolute mortality reduction for treatment within 1 hour of symptom onset was 65 per 1000. The delay/benefit relation (Fig. 31.4) was non-linear. Other studies have demonstrated that if fibrinolytic therapy is given within 70 minutes of symptom onset, the mortality rate of STEMI can be as low as 1.4%[62] and in certain circumstances, very early therapy can even

result in aborted myocardial infarction.[63] This information has led to a push to provide fibrinolytic therapy in the prehospital setting. The ACC/AHA guidelines have given an indication (**Class IIa, Level A**) for the establishment of a prehospital fibrinolysis protocol in (1) settings in which physicians are present in the ambulance or (2) well-organized EMS systems with full-time paramedics who have 12-lead ECGs in the field with transmission capability, paramedic initial and ongoing training in ECG interpretation and STEMI treatment, on-line medical command, a medical director with training/experience in STEMI management, and an ongoing continuous quality improvement program.

Benefit of delayed (>6 hour) therapy

In contrast to earlier therapy, the benefit of fibrinolysis after 6 hours is less certain. The Late Assessment of Thrombolytic Efficacy (LATE) study[64] enrolled 5711 patients with evidence of AMI between 6 and 24 hours from symptom onset and randomized them to tPA (100 mg over 3 h) or placebo. A 26% relative mortality reduction (8.9% vs 11.9%, $P = 0.02$) was observed for those treated within 12 hours. The 12–24 hour subgroup showed a non-significant trend to benefit (8.7% vs 9.2% mortality rate). The South American EMERAS collaborative group[65] treated 4534 patients with IV SK or placebo within 24 hours after onset of suspected AMI and found a non-significant trend towards a mortality benefit between hours 7 and 12 (SK 11.7%, placebo 13.2%). Along with other late treatment trials,[58] these have provided the rationale for recommending fibrinolysis for hours 7–12 after the onset of AMI in patients with persistent symptoms and ECG changes.[66]

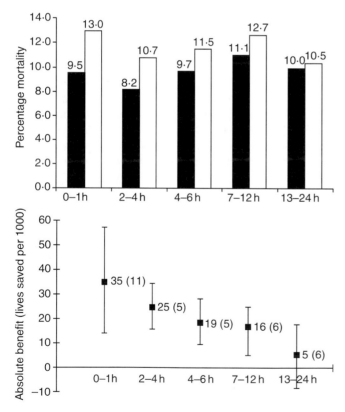

Figure 31.3 The effect of fibrinolytic therapy on mortality in various patient subsets classified according to duration of symptoms before treatment: (above) mortality in each subgroup of fibrinolytic treated (black bars) versus placebo-treated (white bars) patients; (below) absolute benefit (lives saved per 1000 treated, standard deviation in parentheses) with confidence intervals. (Based on data from FTT Collaborative Group.[57])

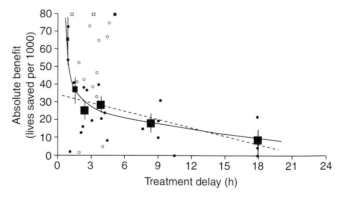

Figure 31.4 Absolute 35-day mortality reduction versus treatment delay: small closed dots, information from trials included in FTT analysis; open dots, information from additional trials; small squares, data beyond scale of X/Y cross. The linear (34.7–1.6X) and non-linear (19.4–0.6X + 29.3X⁻¹) closed regression lines are fitted within these data, weighted by the inverse of the variance of the absolute benefit at each data point. The black squares denote the average effects in six time-to-treatment groups (areas of squares inversely proportional to the variance of absolute benefits described). (Reproduced with permission from Antman et al[59].)

Risks of fibrinolytic therapy

Bleeding

Bleeding is the primary risk of fibrinolytic therapy. Intracranial (or intracerebral) hemorrhage (ICH) is the most important bleeding risk, occurring in about 0.5–1.0%, with substantial risk of fatality (44–75%) or disability.[67–71] Non-cerebral but not cerebral bleeding risk has benefited by increased fibrin selectivity. The absolute and relative contraindications to fibrinolytic therapy are summarized in Table 31.2.[59]

The risk of ICH varies with patient characteristics, the fibrinolytic agent, and adjunctive antithrombotic therapy. Simoons et al[70] identified four independent predictors of increased ICH risk: age >65 years (odds ratio (OR) 2.2; 95% confidence interval (CI) 1.4–3.51), weight <70 kg (OR 2.1; 95% CI 1.3–3.2), hypertension on admission (OR 2.0; 95% CI 1.2–3.2), and use of tPA (alteplase) (OR 1.6; 95% CI 1.0–2.5) versus SK. The GUSTO-1 group[71] identified seven

Table 31.2 Contraindications and cautions for fibrinolysis in STEMI*

Absolute contraindications

Any prior ICH

Known structural cerebral vascular lesion (e.g. arteriovenous malformation)

Known malignant intracranial neoplasm (primary or metastatic)

Ischemic stroke within 3 months EXCEPT acute ischemic stroke within 3 hours

Suspected aortic dissection

Active bleeding or bleeding diathesis (excluding menses)

Significant closed-head or facial trauma within 3 months

Relative contraindications

History of chronic, severe, poorly controlled hypertension

Severe uncontrolled hypertension on presentation (SBP greater than 180 mmHg or DBP greater than 110 mmHg)

History of prior ischemic stroke greater than 3 months, dementia, or known intracranial pathology not covered in contraindications

Traumatic or prolonged (greater than 10 minutes) CPR or major surgery (less than 3 weeks)

Recent (within 2–4 weeks) internal bleeding

Non-compressible vascular punctures

For streptokinase: prior exposure (more than 5 days ago) or prior allergic reaction

Pregnancy

Active peptic ulcer

Current use of anticoagulants: the higher the INR, the higher the risk of bleeding

ICH, intracranial hemorrhage; SBP, systolic blood pressure; DBP, diastolic blood pressure; CPR, cardiopulmonary resuscitation; INR, international normalized ratio; MI, myocardial infarction.

*Viewed as advisory for clinical decision making and may not be all-inclusive or definitive.

predictors of ICH: advanced age, lower weight, history of cerebrovascular disease, history of hypertension, higher systolic or diastolic pressure on presentation, and randomization to tPA (vs SK). In contrast, the incidence of non-cerebral bleeding is higher with SK.[72]

The safety of bolus compared with infusion administration of fibrinolysis for ICH was questioned by a meta-analysis of several different agents.[73] However, problems with the meta-analysis have been raised[74,75] and large, well-controlled trials of the two bolus agents in general use, RPA[76] and TNK-PA,[77] have not shown excess ICH rates compared with front-loaded rt-PA.

The critical importance of dose and adjunctive therapies to ICH risk is now realized. Excessive ICH was observed with tPA doses >100 mg.[48] Excessive adjunctive therapy (for example, heparin, hirudin, glycoprotein IIb/IIIa receptor inhibition) with fibrinolytics also has resulted in unacceptable rates of bleeding including ICH.[78–80] In the GUSTO-I trial, the risk of ICH increased with aPTT levels beyond 70 seconds.[81] Three concurrent trials[77,78,79] were stopped prematurely and reconfigured because of excessive hemorrhage. With lower doses of antithrombins, hemorrhage rates subsequently decreased. Recommendations for adjuvant heparin therapy have been adjusted downward to 60 U/kg bolus (maximum 4000 units) and 12 units/kg/h (maximum 1000 units), adjusted after 3 hours to maintain aPTT at 50–70 seconds for 48 hours.[66]

Previously, prolonged cardiopulmonary resuscitation (CPR) has been considered a contraindication to fibrinolytic therapy. However, Bottiger et al observed 90 patients with AMI who had out-of-hospital cardiac arrest.[82] Patients treated with heparin and tPA more frequently had return of spontaneous circulation (68% vs 44%, $P < 0.03$), admission to the ICU ($P < 0.01$), and survival to discharge (15% ~ 8%). Bleeding complications were not problematic.

Allergy, hypotension, and fever

Streptokinase is antigenic and may be allergenic although serious anaphylaxis or bronchoconstriction is rare (<0.2–0.5%).[56] In ISIS-3[69] any allergic-type reaction was reported after SK in 3.6% and tPA in 0.8%; only 0.3% and 0.1%, respectively, required treatment. Angioneurotic and periorbital edema, hypersensitivity vasculitis, serum sickness or renal failure due to interstitial nephritis, and purpuric rashes have been rarely reported, especially after repeat administration.[41,56,69] SK may acutely release bradykinin, a vasodilator. The incidence of clinical hypotension after SK (11.8%) was greater than after tPA (7.1 %);[69] only half of episodes required treatment.

Fever occurs in 5–30% of SK-treated patients. Delayed-type hypersensitivity may provoke fever and may respond to acetaminophen. The role of fibrinolytics in reports of splenic rupture, aortic dissection, and cholesterol embolization is uncertain.

Reinfarction

Although reperfusion may be effected by fibrinolytic therapy, repeat thrombosis and its associated reinfarction is a known, potentially devastating risk after fibrinolytic therapy. In a combined analysis of several fibrinolytic trials including more than 20 000 subjects, Gibson et al[83] reported that the frequency of symptomatic recurrent MI during the index hospitalization was 4.2%, and was associated with an increased 30-day mortality (16.4% vs 6.2%, $P = 0.001$).

Comparative fibrinolytic trials

After establishing the general utility of fibrinolysis in STE-AMI, clinical trials focused on comparisons with new drug regimens. The GISSI-2/International Study Group trial[84,85] randomized 20 891 patients with STEM1 <6h to tPA (alteplase, 100 mg/3 h) or SK (1.5 MU/L h) and to subcutaneous (SC) heparin (12 500 U twice daily) beginning 12 hours later, or no heparin. Aspirin and atenolol were given as standard therapies. In-hospital mortality was SK 8.5% and tPA 8.9% ($P = $ NS). ICH rates were 0.5% and 0.8% respectively; other major bleeds were most frequent with SK plus heparin. At 35 days, death or severe left ventricular dysfunction did not differ by fibrinolytic. Delayed, SC heparin added little benefit (RR 0.95; 95% CI 0.86–1.04).

The third ISIS study (ISIS-3)[69] randomized 41 299 patients with suspected AMI <24h old to receive SK (1.5 MU/L h), tPA (duteplase 0.6 MU/kg/4 h) or the streptokinase analog anisoylated plasminogen streptokinase activator complex (APSAC) (30 U/3 min) and to SC heparin (12 500 U, 4 hours after beginning thrombolytics and bid) or no heparin. Aspirin (162 mg/day) was given to all patients. The median time to treatment was 4 hours; 88% presented within 6 hours and had ST elevation. Mortality rates at 35 days were: SK 10.6%, APSAC 10.5%, and tPA 10.3% overall, and 10.0%, 9.9%, and 9.6%, respectively, in those with clear indications ($P = $ NS). Similar outcomes also were observed

after 6 months. SC heparin tended to improve 1-week mortality (7.4% vs 7.9%, $P = 0.06$) at the expense of increased bleeding, but mortality rates at 35 days were similar (10.3% vs 10.6%, $P = $ NS).

In comparing fibrinolytic regimens, GISSI-2 and ISIS-3 were limited by the suboptimal use of heparin for short-acting fibrin-selective tPA (SC dosing after a delay of 4–12 hours); treatment was relatively late (mean times >4 hours) and did not require ST elevation (ISIS-3), and tPA was not front-loaded.[86–88]

These concerns led to the proposal that tPA might be most effective if given in an accelerated dosing regimen and in combination with IV heparin. Table 31.3 summarizes the results of studies comparing various treatment strategies with accelerated dose tPA. The Global Use of Streptokinase and tPA for Occluded Coronary Arteries (GUSTO) study[42] randomized 41 021 patients with STEMI <6 h to:

- SK 1.5 MU/L h with SC heparin 12 500 U every 12 h starting 4 h after SK
- SK 1.5 MU/L h with IV heparin, 5000 U bolus then 1000 U/h, titrating aPTT to 60–85 seconds
- front-loaded tPA (15 mg bolus, 0.75 mg/kg (maximum 50 mg) over 30 minutes, then 0.50 mg/kg (maximum 35 mg) over 60 minutes, for a maximum of 100 mg over 90 minutes) and IV heparin as per the SK regimen
- a combination of tPA 1.0 mg/kg and SK 1.0 MU, administered concurrently over 60 minutes, plus IV heparin.

The primary endpoint, 30-day mortality, was lowest with accelerated tPA with IV heparin (6.3%), representing a 14% risk reduction ($P = 0.001$) compared to the two SK strategies (7.3%), which did not differ. Combined tPA and SK gave an intermediate outcome. The risk of hemorrhagic stroke was higher with tPA (0.7%) than SK (0.5%), but the combined endpoint of death or disabling stroke favored tPA (6.9% vs 7.8%, $P = 0.006$). Implications of GUSTO for selection of fibrinolytic regimens have been debated.

Table 31.3 Clinical endpoints in comparative trials of various agents with accelerated tPA

Endpoints	GUSTO-I		ASSENT-II		GUSTO-III		In-TIME-II		
	SK	tPA	SK + tPA	tPA	TNK	tPA	rPA	tPA	nPA
30-day death (%)	7.3	6.3*	7.0	6.2	6.2	7.2	7.5	6.6	6.8
Reinfarction (%)	3.7	4.0	4.0	3.8	4.1	4.2	4.2	5.5	5.0
Any stroke (%)	1.3	1.6	1.7	1.7	1.8	1.8	1.6	1.5	1.9
Hemorrhagic (%)	0.5	0.7*	0.9	0.9	0.9	0.9	0.9	0.6*	1.1*
Major bleed (%)	6.0	5.4*	6.1	5.9*	4.7*	1.2	1.0	0.6	0.5

*$P < 0.001$ for comparisons.

Comparative trials with bolus fibrinolytics

Reteplase

INJECT (International Joint Efficacy Comparison of Thrombolytics)[46] compared reteplase (rPA) and SK in a 6010-patient double-blind, randomized trial. Mortality rates at 35 days were rPA 9.0% and SK 9.5% (0.5% absolute reduction; 95% CI 1.9–0.96). On this basis "equivalence" (non-inferiority) of rPA to standard, SK therapy, was established and rPA approved. Reteplase was next favorably compared to tPA in an angiographic study, leading to a large mortality study. In RAPID 2 (Reteplase vs Alteplase Patency Investigation During acute myocardial infarction),[89] 90-minute TIM1 grade 2 or 3 patency rates among 324 patients were 83% vs 73% (rPA vs tPA, $P = 0.03$), with TIMI-3 flow rates of 60% vs 45%, $P = 0.01$. On this basis, a comparative mortality trial, GUSTO-3,[75] was undertaken and randomized 15059 patients 2:1 to rPA (two 10mg IV injections 30 minutes apart) or accelerated tPA (alteplase). A postulated advantage for rPA was not demonstrated (30-day mortality: rPA 7.5%, tPA 7.2%).

Tenecteplase

Tenecteplase (TNK-tPA), a fibrin-selective, single-bolus fibrinolytic, was evaluated in the TIMI-10 dose-finding trials.[90–91] In Phase II studies, a clear dose–response was observed both for coronary patency and hemorrhage (including ICH for the 50mg dose). With limitation and weight adjustment of TNK-tPA dose and reduction and earlier down-titration of heparin dosing, satisfactory bleeding rates and comparable TIMI-3 patency rates were demonstrated at 90 minutes compared to accelerated rt-PA.[92] The double-blind Phase III Assessment of the Safety and Efficacy of a New Thrombolytic-2 (ASSENT-2) mortality equivalence trial[77] compared weight-adjusted TNK (as a 30–50mg bolus over 5–10 seconds) and accelerated rt-PA. All patients received aspirin and heparin. Thirty-day mortality rates were virtually identical for TNK-tPA (6.18%) and rt-PA (6.15%) and met statistical criteria for equivalence. ICH rates also were identical (at 0.93% and 0.94%, respectively). However, major non-cerebral bleeding was lower with the more fibrin-selective TNK (4.66% vs 5.94%, $P < 0.0002$) as was need for blood transfusion (4.25% vs 5.49%, $P < 0.0002$). A lower mortality rate with TNK-tPA was observed among patients presenting 4 hours after symptom onset (7.0% vs 9.2%), which may be due to either greater activity of the more fibrin-specific TNK-tPA against older, fibrin-rich clots or chance.

Thus, none of the newer fibrinolytic regimens has surpassed accelerated tPA. However, the ease of administration of TNK-tPA, together with its reduced transfusion requirements, has led to its general acceptance and favored status in national guidelines.[59] Lower rates of dosing errors with bolus fibrinolytics such as TNK-tPA also may contribute to superior clinical outcomes.[93]

Fibrinolysis in the elderly

The appropriate use of fibrinolytics in the elderly continues to be debated. In an analysis of over 37000 Medicare patients with AMI age 65 or older who were eligible for fibrinolytic therapy,[94] 38% received fibrinolytic therapy and 4.2% received primary angioplasty. After multivariate adjustments, fibrinolytic therapy was not associated with improved 30-day survival (OR 1.01; 95% CI 0.94–1.09), whereas primary angioplasty was (OR 0.79; 95% CI 0.66–0.94). However, at 1 year, both fibrinolytic therapy (OR 0.84; 95% CI 0.79–0.89) and primary angioplasty (OR 0.71; 95% CI 0.61–0.83) were associated with lower mortality rates. Another Medicare analysis[95] suggested that fibrinolytic therapy might even be harmful in those over 75 years. In contrast, a large Swedish registry found a 12% risk reduction in the composite endpoint of cerebral bleeding and 1-year mortality.[96] Similarly, the Fibrinolytic Therapy Trialists' overview of randomized trials data in patients over 75 years reported 35-day mortality to be reduced (trend) from 29.4% to 26.0% with fibrinolytic therapy.[97] Analyses restricted to elderly patients with clear indications for fibrinolytic therapy suggested similar or greater absolute benefit from fibrinolytic therapy than in younger patients. Fibrinolytic regimens should be chosen to minimize the risk of ICH, which increases in the elderly. Weight-adjusting treatment regimens and avoidance of excessive heparin and other adjunctive antithrombotics (for example, Gp IIb/IIIa inhibitors) are important. When safety concerns predominate, SK, which carries a lower risk of ICH, or primary angioplasty should be considered as preferred reperfusion strategies in the elderly.

Fibrinolysis after early presentation

Time from onset of symptoms to fibrinolytic therapy is an important predictor of MI size and patient outcome.[98] The efficacy of fibrinolytic agents in lysing thrombus diminishes with the passage of time.[99] Fibrinolytic therapy administered within the first 2 hours (especially the first hour) can occasionally abort MI and dramatically reduces mortality.[100,101] This has lead the recent ACC/AHA guidelines to recommend that if there might be any delay in getting a patient to the catheterization laboratory who has presented with STEMI within 2 hours of symptom onset, then fibrinolysis might be the preferred therapy.[66] Additionally, the National Heart Attack Alert Working Group[102] recommends that emergency departments strive to achieve a 30-minute door-to-needle time to minimize treatment delays. Finally, prehospital fibrinolysis reduces treatment delays by up to 1 hour and reduces mortality by 17%.[103]

Primary angioplasty

Primary percutaneous coronary intervention (PCI) has been very successful in accomplishing mechanical reperfusion of the coronary artery in patients presenting with STEMI.[104] In the 1980s, the results of primary coronary angioplasty were reported from several single-center experiences.[105–108] These observational studies showed a patency rate of 87% to 95%, an in-hospital mortality rate of between 1.5% and 9%, and an increase in left ventricular ejection fraction from admission to discharge. Although these were not randomized, controlled studies, the results were better than those of fibrinolytic therapy. O'Keefe and co-workers reported 1000 consecutive patients undergoing primary coronary angioplasty at the Mid America Heart Institute.[109] The recanalization rate in infarct-related arteries was 94% and the mortality rate 7.8%. The independent risk factors for in-hospital mortality were cardiogenic shock, failure of reperfusion, age over 70 years, a left ventricular ejection fraction of 40% or less, and anterior myocardial infarction. The results encouraged further studies to test the superiority of primary coronary angioplasty.

Studies comparing primary PCI to fibrinolytic therapy

After the preliminary feasibility trials, a number of small randomized controlled trials compared various regimens of fibrinolytic therapy with balloon angioplasty. These studies were small in size compared to the studies of fibrinolytics versus placebo, and the results may not be generalizable. Also, the studies were limited in that third-generation fibrinolytics such as tenecteplase and reteplase along with modern regimens of heparin were not used; nor did they include the use of stents and glycoprotein IIb/IIIa receptor inhibitors in those patients treated by direct PCI. However, overall, the early randomized trials tended to favor direct balloon angioplasty over fibrinolysis in certain settings.

The PAMI (Primary Angioplasty in Myocardial Infarction) trial,[110,111] one of the first randomized studies, enrolled 395 patients with AMI seen within 12 hours of onset of chest pain. Patients were assigned randomly to undergo primary PTCA or receive intravenous t-PA infusion (100 mg over 3 hours). The trial demonstrated that primary PTCA reduced the composite outcome of in-hospital death, non-fatal reinfarction, recurrent ischemia or intracranial hemorrhage (OR 0.40; 95% CI 0.16–0.89) and also that of hospital days. At 2 years after reperfusion, patients treated with primary PTCA had a lower incidence of the composite of death, repeat myocardial infarction, repeat PTCA, recurrent ischemia, and hospital readmissions than patients who had t-PA.[112] Zijlstra et al[113] also reported significant

mortality benefit for direct angioplasty (OR 0.25; 95% CI 0.04–0.99).

Since these preliminary studies, a large number of other randomized clinical trials comparing primary PCI with fibrinolytic therapy have been performed. In a meta-analysis of 23 randomized STEMI trials comparing primary PCI with fibrinolytic therapy[114] (Fig. 31.5), there were significant reductions in short-term (4–6 weeks) and long-term (6–8 months) mortality, non-fatal MI, and stroke. Furthermore, when stratified according to the type of fibrinolytic agent, benefits of primary PCI were similar regardless of whether or not medical reperfusion was fibrin specific. Additionally, the analysis of the five trials involving patient transfer for primary PCI found similar treatment benefits, despite a mean treatment delay of 39 minutes with PCI.

The greatest absolute benefit of primary PCI occurs among patients at highest risk, as reported in several randomized trials. The Should We Emergently Revascularize Occluded Coronaries for Cardiogenic Shock (SHOCK) Trial[115] randomized 302 patients with cardiogenic shock to emergency revascularization versus medical stabilization, and demonstrated a significant improvement in mortality at at 6 months (50% versus 63% respectively, $P = 0.03$).

The importance of door-to-balloon time

Shorter door-to-balloon times have been shown in multiple analyses to be associated with lower mortality,[116] but this principle must be tied to the other critical time variable of symptom onset to presentation for medical care. Indeed "symptom onset-to-balloon" time may be a more critical time factor. For example, the Zwolle study group[117] analyzed data on 1791 patients who underwent primary PCI from 1994 to 2001. In their analysis, no relationship was found between door-to-balloon time and mortality. Instead, symptom onset-to-balloon time was significantly associated with angiographically favorable outcomes and 1-year mortality. Using multivariate analysis, a symptom onset-to-balloon time of more than 4 hours was identified as an independent predictor of 1-year mortality. But regardless of the time of symptom onset to patient presentation, the longer the door-to-balloon time, the longer the symptom onset-to-balloon time will also be. Because door-to-balloon time is something physicians have direct control over, it still remains a very important factor. To emphasize that point, a large cohort study of 29 222 STEMI patients treated with PCI within 6 hours of presentation at 395 hospitals that participated in the National Registry of Myocardial Infarction (NRMI)-3 and -4 from 1999 to 2002[118] showed that longer door-to-balloon time was associated with increased in-hospital mortality (mortality rate of 3.0%, 4.2%, 5.7%, and 7.4% for door-to-balloon times of 90

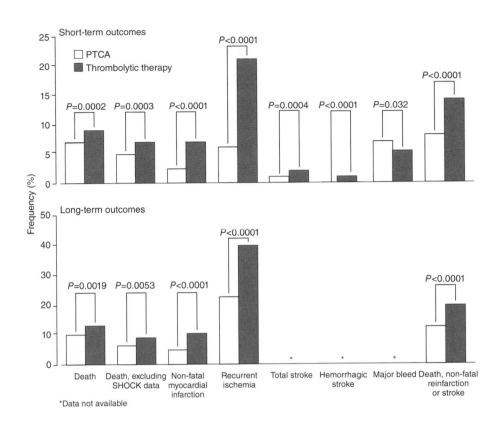

Figure 31.5 Short-term and long-term clinical outcomes in individuals treated with primary PTCA or thrombolytic therapy.

*Data not available

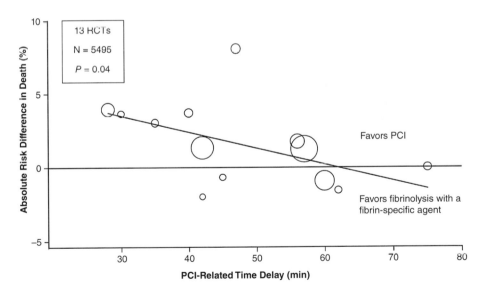

Figure 31.6 PCI versus lysis with fibrin-specific agents: is timing (almost) everything? RCT, randomized controlled trial; N, number of patients; PCI, percutaneous coronary intervention. (Modified from Nallamothu and Bates. *Am J Cardiol* 2003;**92**.824–6. Copyright 2003, with permission from Excerpta Medica, Inc.)

minutes or less, 91–120 minutes, 121–150 minutes, and more than 150 minutes, respectively; *P* for trend <0.01).

As the time delay for performing PCI increases, the mortality benefit for primary PCI over fibrinolysis decreases. When a STEMI patient presents to a center without interventional cardiology facilities, fibrinolytic therapy can generally be provided sooner than primary PCI.[119] Compared with a fibrin-specific lytic agent, a PCI strategy may not reduce mortality when a delay greater than 60 minutes is anticipated versus immediate administration of a lytic (Fig. 31.6).[120] This information has led to the National Guideline (**Class I, Level A**) stating that STEMI patients presenting to a facility without the capability for expert, prompt intervention with primary PCI within 90 minutes of first medical contact should undergo fibrinolysis unless contraindicated.[66] The balance of risk/benefit between the transfer of patients for PCI and more immediate treatment with fibrinolytic therapy remains uncertain. The DANAMI-2 trial

STEP 1: Assess Time and Risk
- Time since onset of symptoms
- Risk of STEMI
- Risk of fibrinolysis
- Time required for transport to a skilled PCI lab

STEP 2: Determine if Fibrinolysis or an Invasive Strategy is Preferred
If presentation is less than 3 hours and there is no delay to an invasive strategy, there is no preference for either strategy

Fibrinolysis is generally preferred if	**An Invasive Strategy is generally preferred if**

Early Presentation (less than or equal to 3 hours from symptom onset and delay to invasive strategy) (see below)
 	
Invasive Strategy is not an option
  Catheterization lab occupied/not available
  Vascular access difficulties
  Lack of access to a skilled PCI lab †‡
 	
Delay to Invasive Strategy
  Prolonged transport
  (Door-to-Balloon) – (Door-to-Needle) is greater than 1 hour *§
  Medical Contact-to-Balloon or Door-to-Balloon is greater than 90 minutes
	Skilled PCI lab available with surgical backup †‡
	  Medical Contact-to-Balloon or Door-to-Balloon is less than 90 minutes
	  (Door-to-Balloon) – (Door-to-Needle) is less than 1 hour *
	
	High Risk from STEMI
	  Cardiogenic shock
	  Killip class is greater than or equal to 3
	
	Contraindications to fibrinolysis including increased risk of bleeding and ICH
	
	Late Presentation
	  The symptom onset was greater than 3 hours ago
	
	Diagnosis of STEMI is in doubt

Figure 31.7 ACC/AHA 2004 guidelines for the assessement of reperfusion options for patients presenting with STEMI. STEMI = ST-elevation myocardial infarction; PCI = percutaneous coronary intervention; ICH = intracranial hemorrhage. *Applies to fibrin-specific agents. †Operator experience greater than a total of 75 Primary PCI cases/year. ‡Team experience greater than a total of 36 Primary PCI cases/year. §This calculation implies that the estimated delay to the implementation of the invasive strategy is greater than one hour versus initiation of fibrinolytic therapy immediately with a fibrin-specific agent.

(DANish trial in Acute Myocardial Infarction), found that patients treated at facilities without interventional cardiology capabilities had better composite outcomes with transfer for PCI within 2 hours of presentation than with pharmacologic reperfusion treatment at the local hospital.[121] Whether these results could be replicated elsewhere is not known. ACC/AHA practice guidelines for management of STEMI have made specific recommendations regarding the choice of primary PCI versus fibrinolytic therapy (Fig. 31.7) (**Class I, Level A**).[59]

Important technical aspects related specifically to mechanical reperfusion in the setting of STEMI

Balloon angioplasty versus coronary stents
Balloon angioplasty was the primary mode of mechanical reperfusion in most of the early primary PCI studies. However, soon after coronary stents became available for routine PCI, potential advantages of coronary stent deployment over "plain old balloon angioplasty (POBA)" during primary PCI were postulated. Through the placement of a coronary stent, a larger lumen diameter could be obtained and maintained, spontaneous or procedure-related coro-

nary arterial dissections could be sealed and the long-term risk of restenosis could be reduced.[122] However, the concern remained whether the acute plaque rupture and resulting thrombosis associated with STEMI would increase the risk of stent thrombosis.

To test this question, stent implantation in the setting of STEMI has been studied in comparison to fibrinolytic therapy and balloon angioplasty alone with and without concomitant Gp IIb/IIIa inhibitor therapy. Schomig *et al*[123] randomized 140 AMI patients to receive either accelerated intravenous tPA or direct coronary stenting plus abciximab. The median size of the infarct as measured by Tc^{99m} sestamibi scan was smaller in the stent plus abciximab group compared to the tPA group (14.3% vs 19.4%, $P = 0.002$). The combined endpoint of death, reinfarction or stroke was also lower in the stent plus abciximab group (8.5% vs 23.3%, $P = 0.02$). Le May *et al*,[124] in a smaller study of 123 AMI patients, reported that compared to accelerated tPA, stenting reduced the combined endpoint of death, reinfarction, stroke or repeat target vessel revascularization in a 6-month follow-up (24.2% vs 55.7%, $P < 0.001$). The median length of hospital stay was significantly reduced in the stented patients (4 days vs 7 days, $P = 0.001$). Kastrati *et al*[125] compared the administration of alteplase plus abciximab with stenting plus abciximab in 162 AMI patients. Stenting was associated with greater myocardial salvage than alteplase (median 13.6% vs 8.0%, $P = 0.007$). Stenting therefore results in superior outcomes to fibrinolytic therapy if done in appropriate settings.

Primary stenting has been compared with primary angioplasty in several studies.[126,127] In meta-analysis there were no differences in mortality (3.0% vs 2.8%) or reinfarction (1.8% vs 2.1%) rates. However, major adverse cardiac events were reduced (OR 0.52, $P < 0.001$), driven by the reduction in subsequent target vessel revascularization with stenting (OR 0.43, $P < 0.001$).

Preliminary reports suggest that compared with conventional bare metal stents (BMS), drug-eluting stents (DES) are not associated with increased risk when used for primary PCI in patients with STEMI. In a study by Lemos *et al*,[128] postprocedure vessel patency, biomarker release, and the incidence of short-term adverse events were similar in patients receiving sirolimus (n = 186) or bare metal (n = 183) stents. Thirty-day event rates of death, reinfarction or revascularization were 7.5% versus 10.4%, respectively ($P = 0.4$). There are also a handful of noteworthy randomized clinical trials directly evaluating the efficacy of DES in AMI. These studies include the Paclitaxel Eluting Stent versus Conventional Stent in Myocardial Infarction with ST-segment Elevation (PASSION),[129] the Trial to Assess the Use of the Cypher Stent in Acute Myocardial Infarction Treated with Balloon Angioplasty (TYPHOON),[130] the Sirolimus Eluting Stent Versus Bare Metal Stent in Acute Myocardial Infarction (SESAMI),[131] and the Comparison of Angioplasty with Infusion of Tirofiban or Abciximab and with Implantation of Sirolimus Eluting or Uncoated Stents for Acute Myocardial Infarction (MULTISTRATEGY trial).[132] These trials are summarized in Table 31.4. Despite the many differences in trial design and primary study endpoints, these trial data generally support the safety of using DES in patients with AMI. It has been consistently observed that DES

significantly reduce restenosis without increasing the short-term risk of thrombosis, as compared with BMS implantation.[133,134] No national guidelines regarding the use of coronary stents during primary PCI have been given. However, based on results of the above studies, we offer the following guidelines: when performing primary PCI for patients presenting with STEMI, coronary stents, either BMS (**Class I, Level A**) or DES (Class I, Level B), should be used whenever technically feasible.

Intracoronary aspiration/thrombectomy devices

Significant clot burden may complicate acute STEMI management. Prospective clinical studies have shown that intracoronary thrombectomy and thrombus aspiration may improve TIMI-3 flow, hasten ST segment elevation resolution, and enhance myocardial tissue perfusion and reduce MI. The Thrombus Aspiration during Percutaneous Coronary Intervention in Acute Myocardial Infarction (TAPAS) trial[135,136] showed that patients with STEMI benefit from aspiration thrombectomy. In TAPAS, patients presenting with STEMI were randomized to initial aspiration thrombectomy versus standard PCI regardless of the presence or absence of angiographically visible thrombus. At 1-year follow-up, cardiac death was 3.6% (19 of 535 patients) in the thrombus aspiration group and 6.7% (36 of 536) in the conventional PCI group (hazard ratio (HR) 1.93; 95% CI 1.11–3.37; $P = 0.020$). One-year cardiac death or non-fatal reinfarction occurred in 5.6% (30 of 535) of patients in the thrombus aspiration group and 9.9% (53 of 536) of patients in the conventional PCI group (HR 1.81; 95% CI 1.16–2.84; $P = 0.009$). Rheolytic thrombectomy, which employs a more sophisticated mechanism, has a greater potential to successfully remove a larger thrombus burden compared to manual aspiration. However, in a clinical trial of 480 STEMI patients (including those without visible clot) randomly assigned to PCI alone or PCI with AngioJet™ (Possis, Minneapolis, MN) catheter thrombectomy, there was a greater

Table 31.4 Combined analysis of randomized control trials of drug-eluting stents in myocardial infarction

	Death			TLR/TVR			Stent thrombosis			Restenosis		
	DES	BMS	p	DES	BMS	p	DES	BMS	p	DES	BMS	p
TYPHOON* (n = 712)	1.9%	1.4%	0.55	5.6%	13.4%	0.0004	3.3%	3.6%	0.80	7%	20%	na
PASSION* (n = 605)	4%	6.3%	0.20	5.3%	7.6%	0.23	1%	1%	0.99	–	–	
SESAMI* (n = 307)	1.8%	4.3%	0.36	5.0%	13.1%	0.015	3.1%	3.7%	0.43	9%	21%	na
MULTISTRATEGY# (n = 745)	3%	4%	0.42	3.2%	10.2%	<0.001	0.8%	1.1%	0.71	–	–	

* 1-year follow-up, #8 months follow-up.
DES, drug-eluting stent; BMS, bare metal stent; TLR, target lesion revascularization; TVR, target vessel revascularization.

infarct size measured by sestamibi imaging at 14–28 days with thrombectomy compared to PCI alone (12.5% vs 9.8%).[137] We therefore propose the following guideline: when performing primary PCI for STEMI, aspiration thrombectomy prior to balloon inflation should be performed whenever possible (**Class I, Level B**).

Embolization protection devices

Embolization protection devices, including the Guard-Wire™ (Medtronic Inc, Minneapolis, MN) balloon occluding device and FilterWire™ (Boston Scientific, Natick, MA) filter basket device, were designed to enhance myocardial tissue perfusion by reducing distal embolization of athero-thrombotic debris. Although both devices have demonstrated the ability to improve outcomes in elective PCI of degenerated saphenous vein grafts,[138,139] no benefit has been found when applied to native vessels in the setting of STEMI. In the Drug Elution and Distal Protection in ST-Elevation Myocardial Infarction (DEDICATION) Trial,[140] 626 patients with STEMI and undergoing primary PCI were randomized to distal protection using the Filter-Wire™ or standard therapy. There was no significant difference in the occurrence of the primary endpoint of complete ($\geq$70%) ST segment resolution (76% vs 72%, $P = 0.29$), no difference in maximum troponin-T (4.8 μg/L and 5.0 μg/L, $P = 0.87$) or maximum creatine kinase-MB (185 μg/L and 184 μg/L, $P = 0.99$), and no difference in median left ventricular wall motion index (1.70 vs 1.70, $P = 0.35$). The rate of major adverse cardiac and cerebral events 1 month after PCI was 5.4% with distal protection and 3.2% with conventional treatment ($P = 0.17$).

Likewise, in the Enhanced Myocardial Efficacy and Recovery by Aspiration of Liberated Debris (EMERALD) trial,[141] 501 patients presenting with STEMI and undergoing primary PCI or rescue intervention after failed thrombolysis were randomized to receive PCI with a balloon occlusion and aspiration distal microcirculatory protection system versus angioplasty without distal protection. The co-primary endpoints were ST segment resolution (STR) measured 30 minutes after PCI and infarct size measured by technetium Tc 99m sestamibi imaging between days 5 and 14 and secondary endpoints included major adverse cardiac events. Complete STR was achieved in a similar proportion reperfused with or without distal protection (63.3% (152/240) vs 61.9% (148/239), $P = 0.78$), and left ventricular infarct size was similar in both groups (median 12.0% (n = 229) vs 9.5% (n = 208), respectively; $P = 0.15$). Major adverse cardiac events at 6 months also occurred with similar frequency in the distal protection and control groups (10.0% vs 11.0%, respectively; $P = 0.66$). Based on these randomized trials we offer the following guideline: when performing primary PCI for STEMI, use of distal protection devices during balloon inflation is not generally recommended (**Class III, Level A**).

Although the explanation for the failure of these studies is unclear, smaller thrombus burden in native coronary arteries, premature embolization due to crossing the infarct-related stenotic lesion with the device, delayed reperfusion due to the occlusive nature of the device, and difficulty in protecting vulnerable side branches are thought to be several possibilities.

The use of bypass surgery in the setting of STEMI

With the advent of stents for acute vessel closures, the percentage of patients requiring emergency bypass surgery for acute myocardial infarction has fallen below 1% in contemporary randomized studies of direct PCI.[37,128] However, earlier studies of direct PC1 and observational registries reported this rate as 4–6%.[115,116,142] Bypass surgery may be required owing to anatomic considerations, such as left main disease or coronary disease not suitable for immediate PCI, or mechanical complications from the MI such as acute severe mitral regurgitation, ventricular septal defect or a failed PCI. Observational studies report that stable patients with acute MI can undergo bypass surgery with good results, but the complexity of performing cardiac surgery in patients with acute MI and potentially other manifestations like failed PCI or cardiogenic shock is definitely greater. Randomized studies comparing surgery to medical therapy or PC1 in this situation are lacking.

When bypass surgery was the only available therapy for acute coronary reperfusion in the 1970s, there were some studies that reported surprisingly good results. DeWood et al[143] reported on their experience with 187 patients treated with early coronary bypass surgery. In this observational study, all patients under 65 years of age who presented with ST segment elevation underwent cardiac catheterization. After exclusion of 28 patients (co-morbidity, diffuse or no coronary disease), 187 patients were treated with bypass surgery and 200 were treated medically. Although treatment was not randomly assigned, the groups were well balanced in terms of age, prior history, and presenting signs and symptoms. Hospital and long-term mortality was lower in the bypass patients (5.8% vs 11.5%, $P = 0.08$ in hospital; 11.7% vs 20.5%, $P < 0.03$ at 56 months). In surgical patients placed on cardiopulmonary bypass within 6 hours of symptoms, hospital mortality was 2%. Similar results have been reported in 261 patients treated with acute bypass surgery at the Iowa Heart Center (hospital mortality 5.7%).[144]

These findings, however, are limited by the fact that the comparisons between surgical and medical therapy were not randomized. Patients were excluded from the surgical cohort due to coronary anatomy, co-morbidity or shock. Thus, these excellent results are probably not generalizable to the larger population of acute infarct patients.

In the PAMI-2 study of AMI patients treated with direct angioplasty, 10.9% underwent cardiac surgery before hospital discharge, 57% of whom underwent the surgery urgently.[145] The in-hospital mortality was 6.4% in those who underwent surgery urgently versus 2.0% in the elective surgery group. The mortality associated with bypass surgery after AMI increases with the instability of the patient. Lee et al[116] reported on 316 patients undergoing bypass surgery after AMI, among whom the mortality was 1.2% in stable patients and 26% in patients with cardiogenic shock. Hochman et al[147] reported the results of a randomized study comparing medical therapy versus revascularization therapy in 304 patients with acute MI and cardiogenic shock. In the revascularization group 64% were treated with angioplasty and 36% with surgery. At 30 days the mortality was 46.7% in the revascularization group versus 56% in the medical therapy group ($P = 0.11$) but at 6 months the mortality was significantly lower in the revascularization group (50.3% vs 63.1%, $P = 0.027$). There was no difference in mortality between the angioplasty group (45.3%) and the surgery group (42%). Although patients have a high mortality when they present with AMI and cardiogenic shock, a revascularization strategy may improve the outcome in selected patients.

As a subgroup, patients ≥75 years of age had higher mortality with the revascularization strategy (RR 1.41; 95% CI 0.97–2.03) than medical therapy. Therefore, it is unclear at this time whether elderly patients in cardiogenic shock should undergo revascularization therapy in the setting of an acute MI.

The 2004 American College of Cardiology/American Heart Association practice guidelines for the treatment of AMI[59] recommend that acute bypass surgery should be undertaken in the following circumstances:

- failed PCI with persistent pain or hemodynamic instability in patients with coronary anatomy suitable for surgery
- persistent or recurrent ischemia refractory to medical therapy in patients who have coronary anatomy suitable for surgery, have a significant area of myocardium at risk, and are not candidates for PCI or fibrinolytic therapy
- at the time of surgical repair of postinfarction ventricular septal defect or mitral valve insufficiency
- cardiogenic shock in patients less than 75 years old with ST elevation or LBBB or posterior MI who develop shock within 36 hours of STEMI, have severe multi-vessel or left main disease, and are suitable for revascularization that can be performed within 18 hours of shock, unless further support is futile because of the patient's wishes or contra-indications/unsuitability for further invasive care
- life-threatening ventricular arrhythmias in the presence of greater than or equal to 50% left main stenosis and/or triple-vessel disease (**Class IIa, Level B**).

They also report that emergency CABG can be useful as the primary reperfusion strategy in patients who have suit-able anatomy and who are not candidates for fibrinolysis or PCI and who are in the early stages (6–12 hours) of an evolving STEMI, especially if severe multivessel or left main disease is present. Also emergency CABG can be effective in selected patients 75 years or older with ST elevation, LBBB or posterior MI who develop shock within 36 hours of STEMI, have severe triple-vessel or left main disease, and are suitable for revascularization that can be performed within 18 hours of shock (**Class IIa, Level B**).

Conclusion

Acute ST segment elevation myocardial infarction remains one of the most dramatic cardiovascular complications of the modern world. STEMI is generally initiated by the rupture of a coronary arterial atherosclerotic plaque, the end result of which is a total thrombotic occlusion of the vessel. The most important initial management of STEMI is the timely and effective reperfusion of the acutely occluded coronary artery. This may be accomplished either by pharmacologic means, using fibrinolytic agents, or by mechanical means, using PCI or CABG. The most appropriate method of reperfusion depends on the baseline characteristics of the patient, the specific details of the STEMI presentation and the availability of timely PCI. In general, when timely PCI is available within a door-to-balloon time of 90 minutes, it is the preferred method of reperfusion. In most other circumstances, fibrinolysis still remains a viable option for therapy.

References

1. Reimer KA, Lowe JE, Rasmussen MM, Jennings RB. The wavefront phenomenon of ischemic cell death. 1. Myocardial infarct size vs duration of coronary occlusion in dogs. *Circulation* 1977;**56**:786–94.
2. Chesebro JH, Knatterua B, Roberts R et al. Thrombolysis in Myocardial Infarction (TIMI) Trial, Phase I: a comparison between intravenous tissue plasminogen activator and intravenous streptokinase. Clinical findings through hospital discharge. *Circulation* 1987;**76**:142–54.
3. Anderson JL, Karagounis LA, Califf RM. Meta-analysis of five reported studies on the relation of early coronary patency grades with mortality and outcomes after acute myocardial infarction. *Am J Cardiol* 1996;**78**:1–8.
4. Ito II, Okamura A, Iwakura K et al. Myocardial perfusion patterns related to thrombolysis in myocardial infarction perfusion grades after coronary angioplasty in patients with acute anterior myocardial wall myocardial infarction. *Circulation* 1996;**93**:1993–9.
5. Gibson CM, Murphy SA, Rizzo MJ et al. Relationship between TIMI frame count and clinical outcomes after thrombolytic administration. Thrombolysis in Myocardial Infarction (TIMI) Study Group. *Circulation* 1999;**99**:1945–50.

6. Gibson CM, Cannon CP, Murphy SA *et al.* Relationship of TIMI myocardial perfusion grade to mortality after administration of thrombolytic drugs. *Circulation* 2000;**99**:1945–50.

7. Topel EJ. Toward a new frontier in myocardial reperfusion therapy: emerging platelet preeminence. *Circulation* 1998;**97**:211–18.

8. Svilaas T, Vlaar PJ, van der Horst IC *et al.* Thrombus aspiration during primary percutaneous coronary intervention. *N Engl J Med* 2008;**358**(6):557–67.

9. Dirksen MT, Laarman GJ, Simoons ML, Duncker DJ. Reperfusion injury in humans: a review of clinical trials on reperfusion injury inhibitory strategies. *Cardiovasc Res* 2007;**74**(3):343–55.

10. Tillet WS, Garner RL. The fibrinolytic activity of hemolytic streptococci. *J Exp Med* 1933;**58**:485–502.

11. Sherry S. The origin of thrombolytic therapy. *J Am Coll Cardiol* 1989;**14**:1085–92.

12. Fletcher AP, Alkjaersig N, Smyrniotis FE *et al.* Treatment of patients suffering from early acute myocardial infarction with massive and prolonged streptokinase therapy. *Trans Assoc Am Phys* 1958;**71**:287–97.

13. European Cooperative Study Group for Streptokinase Treatment in Acute Myocardial Infarction. Streptokinase in acute myocardial infarction. *N Engl J Med* 1979;**301**:797–802.

14. Sharma GV, Cella G, Parisi AF, Sasahara AA. Thrombolytic therapy. *N Engl J Med* 1982;**306**:1268–76.

15. DeWood MA, Spores J, Notske R *et al.* Prevalence of total coronary occlusion during the early hours of transmural myocardial infarction. *N Engl J Med* 1980;**303**:897–902.

16. Chazov El, Matveeva LS, Mazaev AV *et al.* Intracoronary administration of fibrinolysin in acute myocardial infarction (in Russian). *Ter Arkh* 1976;**48**:8–19.

17. Rentrop P, Blanke H, Karsch KR, Kaiser H, Kostering H, Leitz K. Selective intracoronary thrombolysis in acute myocardial infarction and unstable angina pectoris. *Circulation* 1981;**63**:307–17.

18. Rentrop KP, Blanke H, Karsch KR *et al.* Acute myocardial infarction: intracoronary application of nitroglycerin and streptokinase. *Clin Cardiol* 1979;**2**:354–63.

19. Ganz W, Ninomiya K, Hashida J *et al.* Intracoronary thrombolysis in acute myocardial infarction: experimental background and clinical experience. *Am Heart J* 1981;**102**:1145–9.

20. Anderson JL, Marshall HW, Bray BE *et al.* A randomized trial of intracoronary streptokinase in the treatment of acute myocardial infarction. *N Engl J Med* 1983;**308**:1312–18.

21. Khaja F, Walton JA Jr, Brymer JF *et al.* Intracoronary fibrinolytic therapy in acute myocardial infarction. Report of a prospective randomized trial. *N Engl J Med* 1983;**308**:1305–11.

22. Kennedy JW, Ritchie JL, Davis KB, Fritz JK. Western Washington randomized trial of intracoronary streptokinase in acute myocardial infarction. *N Engl J Med* 1983;**309**(24):1477–82.

23. Kennedy JW, Ritchie JL, Davis KB, Stadius ML, Maynard C, Fritz JK. The Western Washington randomized trial of intracoronary streptokinase in acute myocardial infarction. A 12-month follow-up report. *N Engl J Med* 1985;**312**:1073–8.

24. Simoons ML, Serruys PW, Brand M, Bar F, de Zwaan C, Res J *et al.* Improved survival after early thrombolysis in acute myocardial infarction. A randomized trial by the Interuniversity Cardiology Institute in the Netherlands. *Lancet* 1985;**2**:578–72.

25. Schröder R, Biamino G, von Leitner ER *et al.* Intravenous short-term infusion of streptokinase in acute myocardial infarction. *Circulation* 1983;**67**:536–48.

26. Rogers WJ, Mantle JA, Hood WP Jr *et al.* Prospective randomized trial of intravenous and intracoronary streptokinase in patients with acute myocardial infarction. *Circulation* 1983;**68**:1051–61.

27. Anderson JL, Marshall HW, Askins JC *et al.* A randomized trial of intravenous and intracoronary streptokinase in patients with acute myocardial infarction. *Circulation* 1984;**70**:606–18.

28. Alderman EL, Jutzy KR, Berte LE *et al.* Randomized comparison of intravenous versus intracoronary streptokinase for myocardial infarction. *Am J Cardiol* 1984;**54**:14–19.

29. ISAM Study Group. A prospective trial of intravenous streptokinase in acute myocardial infarction (I.S.A.M.). Mortality, morbidity, and infarct size at 21 days. *N Engl J Med* 1986;**314**:1465–71.

30. Cannon CP, Bahit MC, Haugland JM *et al.* Underutilization of evidence-based medications in acute ST elevation myocardial infarction. Results of the Thrombolysis in Myocardial Infarction (TIMI) 9 Registry. *Crit Pathways Cardiol* 2002;**1**:44.

31. Simoons ML, Maggioni AP, Knatterud G *et al.* Individual risk assessment for intracranial haemorrhage during thrombolytic therapy. *Lancet* 1993;**342**:1523–8.

32. GUSTO Angiographic Investigators. The effects of tissue plasminogen activator, streptokinase, or both on coronary artery patency, ventricular function, and survival after acute myocardial infarction. *N Engl J Med* 1993;**329**:1615–22.

33. TIMI Study Group. The Thrombolysis in Myocardial Infarction (TIMI) Trial, Phase 1 findings. *N Engl J Med* 1985;**312**:932–7.

34. Fu Y, Goodman S, Chang WC, Ven De Werf F, Granger CB, Armstrong PW. Time to treatment influences the impact of ST-segment resolution on one year prognosis: insights from the assessment of the saftery and efficacy of a new thrombolytic agent (ASSENT-2) trial. *Circulation* 2001;**104**:2653–9.

35. Hudson MP, Granger CB, Topol EJ *et al.* Early reinfarction after fibrinolysis: experience from the global utilization of streptokinase and tissue plasminogen activator (alteplase) for occluded coronary arteries (GUSTO-I) and global use of strategies to open occluded arteries (GUSTO-III) trials. *Circulation* 2001;**104**:1229–35.

36. Gibson CM, Cannon CP, Piana RN *et al.* Angiographic predictors of reocclusion after thrombolysis: results from the Thrombolysis in Myocardial Infarction (TIMI) 4 trial. *J Am Coll Cardiol* 1995;**25**:582–9.

37. Grines CL, Cox DA, Stone GW *et al.* Coronary angioplasty with or without stent implantation for acute myocardial infarction. *N Engl J Med* 1999;**341**:1949–56.

38. Reperfusion Therapy Consensus Group. Selection of reperfusion therapy for individual patients with evolving myocardial infarction. *Eur Heart J* 1997;**18**:1371–81.

39. O'Neill W, Timmis GC, Bourdillon PD *et al.* A prospective randomized clinical trial of intracoronary streptokinase versus coronary angioplasty for acute myocardial infarction. *N Engl J Med* 1986;**314**:812–18.

40. Weaver WD, Simes RJ, Betriu A *et al.* Comparison of primary coronary angioplasty and intravenous thrombolytic therapy for acute myocardial infarction: a quantitative review. *JAMA* 1997;**278**(23):2093–8.

41. Anderson JL, Smith BR. Streptokinase in acute myocardial infarction. In: Anderson JL, ed. Modern Management of Acute Myocardial Infarction in the Community Hospital. New York: Marcel Dekker, 1991.

42. GUSTO Investigators. An international randomized trial comparing four thrombolytic strategies for acute myocardial infarction. *N Engl J Med* 1993;**329**:673–82.

43. Rutherford RB, Comerota AJ. Urokinase. In: Messerli FH, ed. Cardiovascular Drug Therapy, 2nd edn. Philadelphia: WB Saunders, 1990.

44. Tifenbrunn AJ. Tissue-type plaminogen activator. In: Messerli FH, ed. Cardiovascular Drug Therapy, 2nd edn. Philadelphia: WB Saunders, 1990.

45. Rijken DC, Hoylaerts M, Collen D. Fibrinolytic properties of one-chain and two-chain human extrinsic (tissue-type) plaminogen activator. *J Biol Chem* 1982;**257**:2920–5.

46. International Joint Efficacy Comparison of Thrombolytics. Randomized, double-blind comparison of reteplase double bolus administration with streptokinase in acute myocardial infarction (INJECT): trial to investigate equivalence. *Lancet* 1995;**346**: 329–36.

47. Keyt BA, Paoni NF, Refino CJ *et al.* A faster-acting and more potent form of tissue plasminogen activator. *Proc Natl Acad Sci USA* 1994;**91**:3670–4.

48. Chesebro JH, Knatterud G, Roberts R *et al.* Thrombolysis in Myocardial Infarction (TIMI) Trial, Phase I: a comparison between intravenous tissue plasminogen activator and intravenous streptokinase. Clinical findings through hospital discharge. *Circulation* 1987;**76**:142–54.

49. Granger CB, White HD, Bates ER, Ohman EM, Califf RM. A pooled analysis of coronary arterial patency and left ventricular function after intravenous Thrombolysis for acute myocardial infarction. *Am J Cardiol* 1994;**74**:1220–8.

50. GUSTO Angiographic Investigators.The effects of tissue plasminogen activator, streptokinase, or both on coronary-artery patency, ventricular function, and survival after acute myocardial infarction. *N Engl J Med* 1993;**329**:1615–22.

51. Yusuf S, Collins R, Peto R *et al.* Intravenous and intracoronary fibrinolytic therapy in acute myocardial infarction: overview of results on mortality, re-infarction and side-effects from 33 randomized controlled trials. *Eur Heart J* 1985;**6**:556–85.

52. Yusuf S, Wittes J, Friedman L. Overview of results of randomized clinical trials in heart disease. I. Treatments following myocardial infarction. *JAMA* 1988;**260**:2088–93.

53. Yusuf S, Sleight P, Held P, McMahon S. Routine medical management of acute myocardial infarction. Lessons from overviews of recent randomized controlled trials. *Circulation* 1990; **82**:II 117–34.

54. Gruppo Italiano per lo Studio della Streptochinasi nell'Infarto Miocardico (GISSI). Effectiveness of intravenous thrombolytic treatment in acute myocardial infarction. *Lancet* 1986;**1**:397–402.

55. Gruppo Italiano per lo Studio della Streptochinasi nell'Infarto Miocardico (GISSI). Long-term effects of intravenous thrombolysis in acute myocardial infarction: final report of the GISSI study. *Lancet* 1987;**2**:871–4.

56. ISIS-2 (Second International Study of Infarct Survival) Collaborative Group. Randomized trial of intravenous streptokinase, oral aspirin, both, or neither among 17,187 cases of suspected acute myocardial infarction: ISIS-2. *Lancet* 1988;**2**:349–60.

57. Wilcox RG, von der Lippe G, Olsson CG, Jensen G, Skene AM, Hampton JR. Trial of tissue plasminogen activator for mortality reduction in acute myocardial infarction. Anglo-Scandinavian Study of Early Thrombolysis (ASSET). *Lancet* 1988;**2**:525–30.

58. Fibrinolytic Therapy Trialists' (FTT) Collaborative Group. Indications for fibrinolytic therapy in suspected acute myocardial infarction: collaborative overview of early mortality and major morbidity results from all randomized trials of more than 1000 patients. *Lancet* 1994;**343**:311–22.

59. Antman EM, Anbe DT, Armstrong PW *et al.* ACC/AHA guidelines for the management of patients with ST-elevation myocardial infarction. A report of the American College of Cardiology/American Heart Association Task Force on Practice Guidelines (Committee to Revise the 1999 Guidelines for the Management of patients with acute myocardial infarction). *J Am Coll Cardiol* 2004;**44**(3):E1-E211.

60. Gersh BJ, Anderson JL. Thrombolysis and myocardial salvage. Results of clinical trials and the animal paradigm – paradoxic or predictable? *Circulation* 1993;**88**:296–306.

61. Boersma E, Maas AC, Deckers JW, Simoons ML. Early thrombolytic treatment in acute myocardial infarction: reappraisal of the golden hour. *Lancet* 1996;**348**:771–5.

62. Weaver WD, Cerqueria M, Hallstrom AP *et al*, for the MITI Project Group. Early treatment with thrombolytic therapy: results from the myocardial infarction, triage and intervention pre-hospital trial. *JAMA* 1993;**270**:1211–16.

63. Taher T, Fu Y, Wagner GS *et al.* Aborted myocardial infarction in patients with ST-segment elevation: insights from the Assessment of the Safety and Efficacy of a New Thrombolytic Regimen-3 Trial Electrocardiographic Substudy. *J Am Coll Cardiol* 2004;**44**(1):38–43.

64. LATE Study Group. Late Assessment of Thrombolytic Efficacy (LATE) study with alteplase 6–24 hours after onset of acute myocardial infarction. *Lancet* 1993;**342**:759–66.

65. EMERAS (Estudio Multicentrico Estreptoquinasa Republicas de America del Sud) Collaborative Group.Randomized trial of late thrombolysis in patients with suspected acute myocardial infarction. *Lancet* 1993;**342**:767–72.

66. Antman EM, Hand M, Armstrong PW *et al.* 2007 Focused Update of the ACC/AHA 2004 Guidelines for the Management of Patients With ST-Elevation Myocardial Infarction: a report of the American College of Cardiology/American Heart Association Task Force on Practice Guidelines: developed in collaboration With the Canadian Cardiovascular Society endorsed by the American Academy of Family Physicians: 2007 Writing Group to Review New Evidence and Update the ACC/AHA 2004 Guidelines for the Management of Patients With ST-Elevation Myocardial Infarction, Writing on Behalf of the 2004 Writing Committee. *Circulation* 2008;**117**(2):296–329.

67. Anderson JL, Karagounis L, Allen A, Bradford MJ, Menlove RL, Pryor TA. Older age and elevated blood pressure are risk factors for intracerebral hemorrhage after thrombolysis. *Am J Cardiol* 1991;**68**:166–70.

68. Maggioni AP, Franzosi MG, Santoro E, White H, Van de Werf E, Tognoni G. The risk of stroke in patients with acute myocardial infarction after thrombolytic and antithrombotic treatment. Gruppo Italiano per lo Studio della Soprawivenza nell'Infarto Miocardico I1 (GISSI-2), and The International Study Group. *N Engl J Med* 1992;**327**:1–6.

69. ISIS-3 (Third International Study of Infarct Survival) Collaborative Group. ISIS-3: a randomized comparison of streptokinase vs tissue plasminogen activator vs anistreplase and of aspirin plus heparin vs aspirin alone among 41,299 cases of suspected acute myocardial infarction. *Lancet* 1992;**339**:753–70.

70. Simoons ML, Maggioni AP, Knatterud G *et al*. Individual risk assessment for intracranial haemorrhage during thrombolytic therapy. *Lancet* 1993;**342**:1523–8.

71. Gore Jim, Granger CB, Simoons ML *et al*. Stroke after thrombolysis. Mortality and functional outcomes in the GUSTO-1 trial. Global use of strategies to open occluded arteries. *Circulation* 1995;**92**:2811–18.

72. Berkowitz SD, Granger CB, Pieper KS *et al*. Incidence and predictors of bleeding after contemporary thrombolytic therapy for myocardial infarction. The Global Utilization of Streptokinase and Tissue Plasminogen activator for Occluded coronary arteries (GUSTO) I Investigators. *Circulation* 1997;**95**:2508–16.

73. Mehta SR, Eikelboom JW, Yusuf S. Risk of intracranial haemorrhage with bolus versus infusion thrombolytic therpy: a meta-analysis. *Lancet* 2000;**356**:449–54.

74. Armstrong PW, Granger C, Van de Werf E. Bolus fibrinolysis: risk, benefit, and opportunities. *Circulation* 2001;**103**:1171–3.

75. Anderson JL. Bolus thrombolytic treatment is associated a an increased risk of intracranial hemorrhage in patients with ST segment elevation infarction. A commentary. *Evidence-based Cardiovasc Med* 2000;**4**:110–11.

76. Global Use of Strategies to Open Occluded Coronary Arteries (GUSTO III) Investigators. A comparison of reteplase with alteplase for acute myocardial infarction. *N Engl J Med* 1997;**337**:1118–23.

77. Assessment of the Safety and Efficacy of a New Thrombolytic Investigators. Single-bolus tenecteplase compared with front-loaded alteplase in acute myocardial infarction: the ASSENT-2 double-blind Randomized Trial. *Lancet* 1999;**354**:716–22.

78. Global Use of Strategies to Open Occluded Coronary Arteries (GUSTO) IIa Investigators. Randomized trial of intravenous heparin versus recombinant hirudin for acute coronary syndromes. *Circulation* 1994;**90**:1631–7.

79. Antman EM. Hirudin in acute myocardial infarction. Safety report from the Thrombolysis and Thrombin Inhibition in Myocardial Infarction (TIMI) 9A Trial. *Circulation* 1994;**90**:1624–30.

80. Neuhaus KL, von Essen R, Tebbe U *et al*. Safety observations from the pilot phase of the randomized r-Hirudin Improvement of Thrombolysis (HITIII) study. A study of the Arbeitsgemeinschaft Leitender Kardiologischer Kranken-hausarzte (ALKK). *Circulation* 1994;**90**:1638–42.

81. Granger CB, Hirsch J, Califf RM *et al*. Activated partial thromboplastin time and outcome after thrombolytic therapy for acute myocardial infarction: results from the GUSTO-I trial. *Circulation* 1996;**93**:870–8.

82. Bottiger BW, Bode C, Kern S *et al*. Efficacy and safety of thrombolytic therapy after initially unsuccessful cardiopulmonary resuscitation: a prospective clinical trial. *Lancet* 2001;**357**:1583–5.

83. Gibson CM, Karha J, Murphy SA *et al*, for the TIMI Study Group. Early and long-term clinical outcomes associated with reinfarction following fibrinolytic administration in the Thrombolysis in Myocardial Infarction trials. *J Am Coll Cardiol* 2003;**42**:7–16.

84. Gruppo Italiano Per lo Studio della Sopravvivenza nell'Infarto Miocardico. GISSI-2: a factorial randomized trial of alteplase versus streptokinase and heparin versus no heparin among 12,490 patients with acute myocardial infarction. *Lancet* 1990;**336**:65–71.

85. International Study Group. In-hospital mortality and clinical course of 20891 patients with suspected acute myocardial infarction randomized between alteplase and streptokinase with or without heparin. *Lancet* 1990;**336**:71–5.

86. de Bono DP, Simoons ML, Tijssen J *et al*. Effect of early intravenous heparin on coronary patency, infarct size, and bleeding complications after alteplase thrombolysis: results of a randomised double blind European Cooperative Study Group trial. *Br Heart J* 1992;**67**:122–8.

87. Hsia J, Hamilton WP, Kleiman N, Roberts R, Chaitman BR, Ross AM. A comparison between heparin and low-dose aspirin as adjunctive therapy with tissue plasminogen activator for acute myocardial infarction. Heparin-Aspirin Reperfusion Trial (HART) Investigators. *N Engl J Med* 1990;**323**:1433–7.

88. Anderson JL, Karagounis LA. Does intravenous heparin or time-to-treatment/reperfusion explain differences between GUSTO and ISIS-3 results? *Am J Cardiol* 1994;**74**:1057–60.

89. Bode C, Smalling RW, Berg G *et al*. Randomized comparison of coronary thrombolysis achieved with double-bolus reteplase (recombinant plasminogen activator) and front-loaded, accelerated alteplase (recombinant tissue plasminogen activator) in patients with acute myocardial infarction. The RAPID II Investigators. *Circulation* 1996;**94**:891–8.

90. Cannon CP, McCabe CH, Gibson CM *et al*. TNK-tissue plasminogen activator in acute myocardial infarction. Results of the Thrombolysis in Myocardial Infarction (TIMI) 10A doseranging trial. *Circulation* 1997;**95**:351–6.

91. Cannon CP, Gibson CM, McCabe CH *et al*. TNK-tissue plasminogen activator compared with front-loaded alteplase in acute myocardial infarction: results of the TIMI 10B trial. Thrombolysis in Myocardial Infarction (TIMI) 10B Investigators. *Circulation* 1998;**98**:2805–14.

92. Van de Werf F, Cannon CP, Luyten A *et al*. Safety assessment of single-bolus administration of TNK tissue-plasminogen activator in acute myocardial infarction: the ASSENT-1 trial. The ASSENT-1 Investigators. *Am Heart J* 1999;**137**:786–91.

93. Cannon CP. Thrombolysis medication errors: benefits of bolus thrombolytic agents. *Am J Cardiol* 2000;**85**:17C–22C.

94. Berger AK, Radford MJ, Wang Y, Krumholz HM. Thrombolytic therapy in older patients. *J Am Coll Cardiol* 2000;**36**:366–74.

95. Thiemann DR, Coresh J, Schulman SP, Gerstenblith G, Oetgen WJ, Powe NR. Lack of benefit for intravenous thrombolysis in patients with myocardial infarction who are older than 75 years. *Circulation* 2000;**101**:2239–46.

96. Stenestrand U, Wallentin L. Fibrinolytic therapy in patients 75 years and older with ST-segment-elevation myocardial infarction: one-year follow-up of a large prospective cohort. *Arch Intern Med* 2003;**163**(8):965–71.

97. Fibrinolytic Therapy Trialists' (FTT) Collaborative Group. Indications for fibrinolytic therapy in suspected acute myocardial infarction: collaborative overview of early mortality and major morbidity results from all randomized trials of more than 1000 patients. *Lancet* 1994;**343**:311–22.

98. Boersma E, Maas AC, Deckers JW, Simoons ML. Early thrombolytic treatment in acute myocardial infarction: reappraisal of the golden hour. *Lancet* 1996;**348**:771–5.

99. Zeymer U, Tebbe U, Essen R, Haarmann W, Neuhaus KL, for the ALKK-Study Group. Influence of time to treatment on early infarct-related artery patency after different thrombolytic regimens. *Am Heart J* 1999;**137**:34–8.

100. Fibrinolytic Therapy Trialists' (FTT) Collaborative Group. Indications for fibrinolytic therapy in suspected acute myocardial infarction: collaborative overview of early mortality and major morbidity results from all randomised trials of more than 1000 patients. *Lancet* 1994;**343**:311–22.

101. Weaver WD, Cerqueira M, Hallstrom AP et al. Prehospital-initiated vs hospital-initiated thrombolytic therapy: the Myocardial Infarction Triage and Intervention trial. *JAMA* 1993;**270**: 1211–16.

102. National Heart Attack Alert Program Coordinating Committee, 60 Minutes to Treatment Working Group. Emergency department: rapid identification and treatment of patients with acute myocardial infarction. *Ann Emerg Med* 1994;**23**:311–29.

103. Morrison LJ, Verbeek PR, McDonald AC, Sawadsky BV, Cook DJ. Mortality and prehospital thrombolysis for acute myocardial infarction: a meta-analysis. *JAMA* 2000;**283**:2686–92.

104. Singh KP, Harrington RA. Primary percutaneous coronary intervention in acute myocardial infarction. *Med Clin N Am* 2007;**91**:639–55.

105. Hartzier GO, Rutherford BD, McConahay DR et al. Percutaneous transluminal coronary angioplasty with and without thrombolytic therapy for treatment of acute myocardial infarction. *Am Heart J* 1983;**106**:965–73.

106. Kimura T, Nosaka H, Ueno K, Nobuyoshi M. Role of coronary angioplasty in acute myocardial infarction. *Circulation* 1986;**74**(suppl II):22.

107. Rothbaum DA, Linnemeier TJ, Landin RJ et al. Emergency percutaneous transluminal coronary angioplasty in acute percutaneous transluminal coronary angioplasty in acute myocardial infarction: a 3 year experience. *J Am Coll Cardiol* 1987;**10**:264–72.

108. Miller PF, Brodie BR, Weintraub RA et al. Emergency coronary angioplasty for acute myocardial infarction. Results from a community hospital. *Arch Intern Med* 1987;**147**:1565–70.

109. O'Keefe JH, Bailey WL, Rutherford BD, Hartzler GO. Primary angioplasty for acute myocardial infarction in 1000 consecutive patients. Results in an unselected population and high-risk subgroups. *Am J Cardiol* 1993;**72**:107G–115G.

110. Grines CL Browne KF, Marco J et al. A comparison of immediate angioplasty with thrombolytic therapy for acute myocardial infarction. The Primary Angioplasty in Myocardial Infarction Study Group. *N Engl J Med* 1993;**328**:673–9.

111. Stone GW, Crines CL, Brwone KF et al. Predictors of in-hospital and 6-month outcome after acute myocardial infarction in the reperfusion era: the Primary Angioplasty in Myocardial Infarction (PAMI) trial. *J Am Coll Cardiol* 1995;**25**:370–7.

112. Nunn CM, O'Neill WW, Rothbaum D et al. Long-term outcome after primary angioplasty: report from the primary angioplasty in myocardial infarction (PAMI-I) trial. *J Am Coll Cardiol* 1999;**33**:640–6.

113. Zijlstra F, de Boer MJ, Hoornje JC et al. A comparison of immediate coronary angioplasty with intravenous streptokinase in acute myocardial infarction. *N Engl J Med* 1993;**328**:680–4.

114. Keeley EC, Boura JA, Grines CJ. Primary angioplasty versus intravenous thrombolytic therapy for acute myocardial infarction: a quantitative review of 23 randomized trials. *Lancet* 2003;**361**:13–20.

115. Hochman JS, Sleeper LA, White HD et al, for the Should We Emergently Revascularize Occluded Coronaries for Cardiogenic Shock (SHOCK) Investigators. One-year survival following early revascularization for cardiogenic shock. *JAMA* 2001;**285**:190–2.

116. Cannon CP, Gibson CM, Lambrew CT et al. Relationship of symptom-onset-to-balloon time and door-to-balloon time with mortality in patients undergoing angioplasty for acute myocardial infarction. *JAMA* 2000;**283**(22):2941–7.

117. De Luca G, Suryapranata H, Zijlstra F et al, for the ZWOLLE Myocardial Infarction Study Group. Symptom-onset-to-balloon time and mortality in patients with acute myocardial infarction treated by primary angioplasty. *J Am Coll Cardiol* 2003;**42**(6):991–7.

118. McNamara RL, Wang Y, Herrin J et al, for the NRMI Investigators. Effect of door-to-balloon time on mortality in patients with ST-segment elevation myocardial infarction. *J Am Coll Cardiol* 2006;**47**(11):2180–6.

119. Cannon CP, Antman EM, Walls R, Braunwald E. Time as an adjunctive agent to thrombolytic therapy. *J Thromb Thrombolysis* 1994;**1**:27–34.

120. Nallamothu BK, Bates ER. Percutaneous coronary intervention versus fibrinolytic therapy in acute myocardial infarction: is timing (almost) everything? *Am J Cardiol* 2003;**92**:824–6.

121. Andersen HR, Nielsen TT, Rasmussen K et al, for the DANAMI 2 Investigators. A comparison of coronary angioplasty with fibrinolytic therapy in acute myocardial infarction. *N Engl J Med* 2003;**349**:733–42.

122. Fischman DL, Leon MB, Baim DS et al. A randomized comparison of coronary-stent placement and balloon angioplasty in the treatment of coronary artery disease. Stent Restenosis Study Investigators. *N Engl J Med* 1994;**331**(8):496–501.

123. Schomig A, Kastrati A, Dirschinger J et al. Coronary stenting plus platelet glycoprotein IIb/IIIa blockade compared with tissue plasminogen activator in acute myocardial infarction. *N Engl J Med* 2000;**343**:385–91.

124. Le May MR, Labinaz M, Davies RF et al. Stenting versus thrombolysis in acute myocardial infarction trial (STAT). *J Am Coll Cardiol* 2001;**37**:985–91.

125. Kastrati A, Mehilli J, Dirshinger J et al. Myocardial salvage after coronary stenting plus abciximab versus fibrinolysis plus abciximab in patients with acute myocardial infarction: a randomized trial. *Lancet* 2002;**359**:920–5.

126. Zhu MM, Feit A, Chadow H, Alam M, Kwan T, Clark LT. Primary stent implantation compared with primary balloon angioplasty for acute myocardial infarction: a meta-analysis of randomized clinical trials. *Am J Cardiol* 2001;**88**:297–301.

127. Stone GW, Grines CL, Cox DA et al, for the Controlled Abciximab and Device Investigation to Lower Late Angioplasty Complications (CADILLAC) Investigators. Comparison of angioplasty with stenting, with or without abciximab, in acute myocardial infarction. *N Engl J Med* 2002;**346**:957–66.

128. Lemos PA, Saia F, Hofma SH et al. Short- and long-term clinical benefit of sirolimus-eluting stents compared to conventional

bare stents for patients with acute myocardial infarction. *J Am Coll Cardiol* 2004;**43**:704–8.

129. Laarman GJ, Suttorp MJ, Dirksen MT *et al.* Paclitaxel-eluting versus uncoated stents in primary percutaneous coronary intervention. *N Engl J Med* 2006;**355**:1105–13.

130. Spaulding C, Henry P, Teiger E *et al.* TYPHOON Investigators. Sirolimus-eluting versus uncoated stents in acute myocardial infarction. *N Engl J Med* 2006;**355**(11):1093–104.

131. Menichelli M, Parma A, Pucci E *et al.* Randomized trial of sirolimus-eluting stent versus bare-metal stent in acute myocardial infarction (SESAMI). *J Am Coll Cardiol* 2007;**49**(19):1924–30.

132. Valgimigli M, Percoco G, Ferrari R *et al.* Comparison of angioplasty with infusion of tirofiban or abciximab and with implantation of sirolimus-eluting or uncoated stents for acute myocardial infarction: the MULTISTRATEGY randomized trial. *JAMA* 2008;**299**(15):1788–99.

133. Kastrati A, Dibra A, Spaulding C *et al.* Meta-analysis of randomized controlled trials on drug-eluting stents vs. bare-metal stents in patients with acute myocardial infarction. *Eur Heart J* 2007;**28**(22):2706–13.

134. Stone GW, Lausky AJ, Pocock SJ *et al.* Paclitaxel-eluting stents versus bare-metal stents in acute myocardial infarction. *N Engl J Med* 2009;**360**:1946–59.

135. Svilaas T, Vlaar PJ, van der Horst IC *et al.* Thrombus aspiration during primary percutaneous coronary intervention. *N Engl J Med* 2008;**358**:557–67.

136. Vlaar PJ, Svilaas T, van der Horst IC *et al.* Cardiac death and reinfarction after 1 year in the Thrombus Aspiration during Percutaneous coronary intervention in Acute myocardial infarction Study (TAPAS): a 1-year follow-up study. *Lancet* 2008;**371**(9628):1915–20.

137. Ali A, Cox D, Dib N *et al.* Rheolytic thrombectomy with percutaneous coronary intervention for infarct size reduction in acute myocardial infarction: 30-day results from multicenter randomized study. *J Am Coll Cardiol* 2006; **48**:244–52.

138. Baim DS, Wahr D, George B *et al.* Randomized trial of a distal embolic protection device during percutaneous intervention of saphenous vein aorto-coronary bypass grafts. *Circulation* 2002;**105**:13–18.

139. Stone GW, Rogers C, Hermiller J *et al,* for the FilterWire EX Randomized Evaluation (FIRE) Investigators. Randomized comparison of distal protection with a filter-based catheter and a balloon occlusion and aspiration system during percutaneous intervention of diseased saphenous vein aorto-coronary bypass grafts. *Circulation* 2003;**108**:548–53.

140. Kelbaek H, Terkelsen CJ, Helqvist S *et al.* Randomized comparison of distal protection versus conventional treatment in primary percutaneous coronary intervention: the drug elution and distal protection in ST-elevation myocardial infarction (DEDICATION) trial. *J Am Coll Cardiol* 2008;**51**(9):899–905.

141. Stone GW, Webb J, Cox DA *et al,* for the Enhanced Myocardial Efficacy and Recovery by Aspiration of Liberated Debris (EMERALD) Investigators. Distal microcirculatory protection during percutaneous coronary intervention in acute st-segment elevation myocardial infarction: a randomized controlled trial. *JAMA* 2005;**293**:1063–72.

142. Grassman ED, Johnson SA, Krone RJ. Predictors of success and major complications for primary percutaneous transluminal coronary angioplasty in acute myocardial infarction. An analysis of the 1990 to 1994 Society fo Cardiac Angiography and Interventions registries. *J Am Coll Cardiol* 1997;**30**: 201–8.

143. DeWood MA, Spores J, Notske RN *et al.* Medical and surgical management of acute myocardial infarction. *Am J Cardiol* 1979;**44**:1356–64.

144. Phillips SJ, Zeff RH, Skinner JR *et al.* Reperfusion protocol and results in 738 patients with evolving myocardial infarction. *Ann Thorac Surg* 1986;**41**:119–25.

145. Stone GW, Brodie BR, Griffin JJ *et al.* Role of cardiac surgery in the hospital phase management of patients treated with primary angioplasty for acute myocardial infarction. *Am J Cardiol* 2000;**85**:1292–6.

146. Lee JH, Murrell HK, Strony J *et al.* Risk analysis of coronary bypass surgery after acute myocardial infarction. *Surgery* 1997;**122**:675–80.

147. Hochman JS, Sleeper LA, Webb JG *et al.* Early revascularization in acute myocardial infarction complicated by cardiogenic shock. *N Engl J Med* 1999;**341**:625–34.

32 Antithrombotic therapies for patients with ST segment elevation myocardial infarction

Andrew J Lucking and Keith A A Fox
University of Edinburgh, Edinburgh, Scotland, UK

Introduction

Acute coronary syndromes (ACS) are caused by rupture or erosion of an atherosclerotic plaque leading to exposure of plaque contents and constituents of the vessel wall to flowing blood.[1] Driven primarily by the aggregation and adhesion of platelets to collagen and von Willebrand factor (vWF), subsequent thrombin generation promotes thrombus formation that may ultimately result in total or partial vessel occlusion. The principal aim of initial management in patients presenting with ST segment elevation myocardial infarction (STEMI) is to restore normal flow in the infarct-related artery as soon as possible.[2,3] This has been shown to preserve left ventricular function[4] and improve survival rate.[5] Reperfusion may be achieved mechanically using percutaneous coronary intervention (PCI) or pharmacologically with a fibrinolytic agent. Given that thrombus formation and dissolution is a dynamic process, adjunctive antithrombotic therapy is important in both establishing and maintaining patency of the infarct-related vessel. In addition, antithrombotic agents help prevent complications of STEMI including deep vein thrombosis, pulmonary embolism and left ventricular thrombus. For the increasing number of patients treated with primary PCI, iatrogenic vessel injury and stent insertion can promote further local thrombosis and may result in acute vessel closure.[6,7] The beneficial role of antithrombotic therapies, particularly antiplatelet agents, in reducing these events is well established.[8–11] For those treated with a fibrinolytic agent, antithrombotic therapies are also important. Whilst fibrin-specific agents promote local clot lysis in the infarct-related vessel, they may result in a systemic prothrombotic state through enhanced thrombin generation[12] and platelet activation.[13]

Evidence-Based Cardiology, 3rd edition. Edited by S. Yusuf, J.A. Cairns, A.J. Camm, E.L. Fallen, and B.J. Gersh. © 2010 Blackwell Publishing, ISBN: 978-1-4051-5925-8.

Although the development of antithrombotic agents has focused primarily on reducing thrombotic and ischemic complications, the importance of safety as well as efficacy of novel agents and regimens is increasingly recognized. Antithrombotic therapy is associated with an increased risk of bleeding and accompanying adverse outcomes, including death. The relationship between antithrombotic therapy, bleeding and ischemic events is complex. Whilst the adverse effects of fatal and intracranial hemorrhage may be clear, bleeding may also result in the premature cessation of antithrombotic therapy or necessitate blood transfusion which are themselves associated with an increased incidence of ischemic complications.

This chapter will examine evidence for antithrombotic use in patients with acute STEMI. Where possible, in order to enhance clinical relevance, discussion will be presented according to reperfusion strategy: those who have undergone primary PCI; those who have received fibrinolytic therapy; and those who have received no specific reperfusion therapy.

Antiplatelet agents

The role of platelets in STEMI

Platelets are central to the pathophysiology of arterial thrombosis (Fig. 32.1). Following rupture or erosion of an atherosclerotic plaque, platelet adhesion, activation and aggregation occur sequentially, culminating in formation of a platelet-rich thrombus. Platelet adhesion is mediated by the interaction of platelet surface receptors with exposed subendothelial proteins including vWF and collagen. Subsequent activation involves a conformational change in platelet shape from smooth discoid to spiculated, vastly increasing the surface area available for thrombin generation. Following conformational change, degranulation and secretion of prothrombotic and inflammatory mediators propagate and amplify the thrombotic process. The final

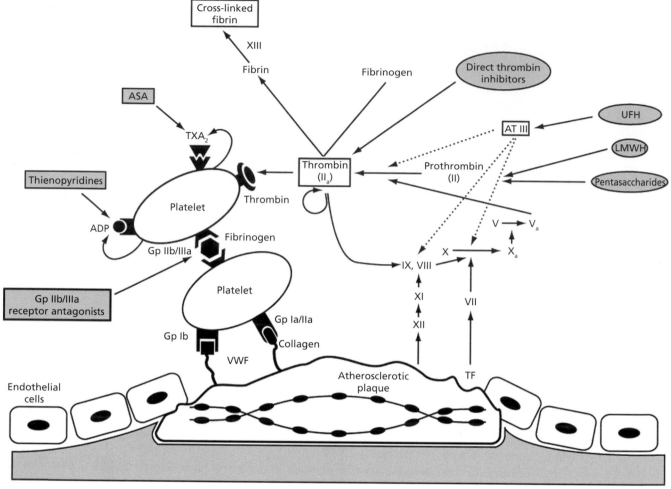

Figure 32.1 Schematic diagram showing the mechanisms responsible for thrombus formation at the site of a ruptured atherosclerotic plaque and the site of action of antithrombotic agents. ADP, adenosine diphosphate; ASA, acetylsalicyclic acid; AT III, antithrombin III; GP, glycoprotein receptor; LMWH, low molecular weight heparins; TF, tissue factor; TxA₂, thromboxane A₂; UFH, unfractionated heparin; VWF, von Willebrand factor.

step, platelet aggregation, involves glycoprotein IIb/IIIa receptor-mediated cross-linking of platelets via fibrinogen bridges.

Aspirin

Aspirin (acetylsalicylic acid, ASA) was the first antiplatelet therapy to be described and remains the principal agent used in the secondary prevention of all forms of cardiovascular disease. It exerts its antiplatelet effect by irreversibly inhibiting platelet cyclo-oxygenase 1. This results in decreased production of the platelet agonist and potent local vasoconstrictor, thromboxane A2.

The benefit of ASA in the context of acute myocardial infarction (MI) was established in the Second International Study of Infarct Survival (ISIS-2).[14] This 2 × 2 double-blind trial randomized patients (n = 17 187) to ASA (162.5 mg daily for one month), streptokinase (SK, 1.5 million IU over

one hour), both or neither. Aspirin reduced cardiovascular mortality at one month by 23% compared with placebo (9.4% versus 11.8%, relative risk reduction (RR) 23%, $P < 0.00001$). The benefit was maintained over at least 10 years of follow-up.[15] Aspirin also reduced rates of reinfarction (odds ratio (OR) 0.51) and stroke (OR 0.49) compared with placebo without a significant increase in major bleeding or stroke.

A 1992 meta-analysis suggested that ASA (loading dose 162–325 mg, maintenance dose 75–162 mg/day) reduces the incidence of vascular events (cardiovascular death, MI and stroke) following STEMI by almost a third (relative RR 30%).[16] Recent studies support earlier observations that compared to larger doses given long term, those in the range of 75–162 mg/day deliver efficacious antiplatelet activity[17] but with improved side-effect and safety profiles.[18]

Aspirin should be administered immediately to all patients with STEMI at a dose of 162–325 mg and continued indefinitely at a maintenance dose of 75–162 mg/day. The only exception is true aspirin allergy (**Class I, Level A**).

Thienopyridines

Thienopyridines exert their antiplatelet effect by irreversibly inhibiting the binding of adenosine diphosphate (ADP) to the platelet P2Y12 receptor. As their mechanism of action is distinct from that of ASA, the effect of dual therapy is additive. Clopidogrel is currently the most widely used thienopyridine, being as efficacious as ticlopidine but possessing a more benign safety profile.[19] Trials in patients with unstable angina (UA), non-STEMI[18] and more latterly STEMI have established it as a key component of contemporary integrated management protocols for all patients presenting with ACS. Despite clear benefits, it has a number of important limitations including a delayed onset of action,[20] a prolonged effect following cessation of therapy and interindividual variation in antiplatelet effect[21,22] that has been associated with an increased risk of ischemic events in poor responders.[21,23] These limitations have prompted the development of novel agents, including prasugrel, capable of more rapid, consistent and efficacious inhibition of ADP-induced platelet aggregation than clopidogrel.

Thienopyridines in patients receiving fibrinolytic therapy

The use of clopidogrel in combination with a fibrinolytic agent was investigated in the CLARITY-TIMI-28 (Clopidogrel as Adjunctive Reperfusion Therapy (Thrombolysis In Myocardial Infarction)) trial.[24] This study randomized patients (n = 3491) with STEMI to either clopidogrel (300 mg loading dose, followed by 75 mg/day) or placebo in addition to ASA and a standard thrombolytic regime. The initial clopidogrel dose was administered concurrently or within 10 minutes of fibrinolysis. All patients had coronary angiography performed prior to discharge. The primary endpoint (a composite of an occluded infarct-related artery at angiography or death/MI prior to angiography) occurred in 15.0% of those in the clopidogrel group compared with 21.7% of those receiving placebo (relative RR 31%, $P < 0.001$). At 30 days, clopidogrel reduced the odds of cardiovascular death, reinfarction or need for urgent revascularization by 20% compared with placebo (14.1% versus 11.6%, $P = 0.03$). The overall reduction in clinical events was similar to that in patients with UA and NSTEMI treated with clopidogrel.[25] Encouragingly, there was no increase in TIMI major or minor bleeding. A subsequent analysis of patients who underwent coronary artery bypass grafting during the index admission found no increase in bleeding from randomization to the end of follow-up or from the time of surgery to the end of follow-up, including patients in whom clopidogrel was continued until within five days of surgery.[26]

The COMMIT/CCS-2 (Clopidogrel and Metoprolol in Myocardial Infarction Trial/Second Chinese Cardiac) Study also investigated the role of clopidogrel in a substantial cohort of patients with STEMI managed in non-interventional settings (n = 45852).[27] Patients were randomized to clopidogrel 75 mg/day or placebo for up to four weeks (mean 15 days) in addition to ASA. In contrast to the CLARITY-TIMI-28 trial, no loading dose of clopidogrel was administered, patients >75 years old were not excluded and the delay between symptom onset and fibrinolysis was longer (just under three hours in CLARITY-TIMI-28 compared with over 10 hours in COMMIT/CCS-2). In addition, only 55% received fibrinolysis (all with urokinase, a non-fibrin specific agent), whereas in CLARITY-TIMI-28 all patients received fibrinolysis (approximately two-thirds with a fibrin-specific agent and the remainder with SK). Despite the absence of a loading dose in COMMIT/CCS-2, there was a lower incidence of death, reinfarction or stroke during the index admission (9.3% versus 10.1% in the placebo group, relative RR 9%, $P < 0.002$). Rates of major bleeding were low and similar in those treated with clopidogrel and placebo (0.58% versus 0.55%, $P = 0.59$).

Despite differences in the design of the two studies, the results of CLARITY-TIMI-28 and COMMIT-CCS-2 demonstrate that addition of clopidogrel to standard therapy including ASA and fibrinolysis is safe and reduces the incidence of major vascular events and mortality.

Clopidogrel 75 mg/day should be administered to all patients with STEMI undergoing fibrinolytic therapy (**Class I, Level A**) and continued for at least 14 days (**Class I, Level B**).

For patients less than 75 years of age, it is reasonable to administer a loading dose of clopidogrel 300 mg (**Class IIa, Level B**).

Thienopyridines in patients undergoing primary PCI

Three trials, CREDO (Clopidogrel for the Reduction of Events During Observation),[20] the PCI arm of the CURE (Clopidogrel in Unstable Angina to Prevent Recurrent Events) trial (PCI-CURE)[25] and PCI-CLARITY, a substudy of the CLARITY-TIMI-28 trial, have considerably strengthened the evidence for early administration of clopidogrel alongside ASA in patients undergoing PCI in a wide range of clinical settings.

The PCI-CLARITY (Clopidogrel as Adjunctive Reperfusion Therapy) trial was a prospective subgroup analysis of patients (n = 1863) from the CLARITY-TIMI-28 study who underwent PCI following mandated angiography[28] (PCI was performed between two and eight days following admission and *not* as the primary reperfusion strategy). As discussed above, a 300 mg loading dose of clopidogrel or placebo was administered at the time of fibrinolysis, in addition to standard therapy (ASA, fibrinolytic and unfractionated heparin (UFH) as appropriate). In contrast to other clopidogrel trials, patients in the control group also received clopidogrel (loading dose of 300–600 mg) after the diagnostic catheterization. All patients were given clopidogrel 75 mg/day for 30 days after the procedure. Thus, the trial compared pretreatment with clopidogrel with delayed administration at the time of PCI. In the pretreatment group, there was a 46% reduction in the odds of death, MI or stroke at 30 days compared with the delayed treatment group (3.6% versus 6.2%, P = 0.008). In addition, a 38% reduction in MI or stoke was observed prior to PCI (P = 0.028). The authors also performed a meta-analysis including data from CREDO (patients undergoing elective PCI) and PCI-CURE (patients with non-ST elevation acute coronary syndrome undergoing PCI) demonstrating a significant and consistent benefit of dual antiplatelet therapy initiated as early as possible prior to PCI.

Despite the size and consistency of data supporting the use of clopidogrel in the context of PCI, there have been no published studies specifically investigating its use in patients with STEMI undergoing primary PCI.

Limited data pertaining to the use of prasugrel in patients with STEMI undergoing PCI are available from the Trial to Assess Improvement in Therapeutic Outcomes by Optimizing Platelet Inhibition with Prasugrel–Thrombolysis in Myocardial Infarction (TRITON–TIMI) 38.[29] Moderate- to high-risk patients (n = 13 608) with ACS (with and without ST segment elevation) who were scheduled for PCI were randomized to either clopidogrel (300 mg loading dose followed by 75 mg daily) or prasugrel (60 mg loading dose followed by 10 mg daily) in addition to ASA and followed for a mean of 14.5 months. A quarter of the study population had STEMI (n = 3534) although the proportion of this subgroup that underwent primary compared to delayed PCI was not specified. In the overall study population, prasugrel reduced cardiovascular death, MI and stroke (9.9% with prasugrel versus 12.1% with clopidogrel, P < 0.001) and resulted in a marked reduction in stent thrombosis (2.4% versus 1.1% with clopidogrel, P < 0.001). Whilst all-cause mortality, MI, stroke and TIMI major bleeding (taken as a marker of overall clinical benefit) were reduced in the prasugrel group (12.2% versus 13.9% with clopidogrel, P < 0.004) there was an excess of TIMI major bleeding (2.4% versus 1.8%, P = 0.03) and fatal bleeding (0.4% versus 0.1%, P = 0.002). The balance of risk appeared to be in favor of prasugrel during the first few hours and days when it reduced ischemic events with little adverse effect on bleeding. Following this initial period, however, its ability to reduce ischemic events was limited and associated in the longer term with an excess of major bleeding compared to clopidogrel. It should be noted that study drugs were administered following angiography, and therefore prasugrel was effectively being compared with placebo for the first few hours following randomization as

conversion of clopidogrel to its active metabolite takes a number of hours.

Whilst the results from TRITON-TIMI-38 suggest that greater inhibition of platelet function can reduce ischemic events, there is an associated increase in major bleeding. Although a limited subgroup analysis has been performed to assess bleeding risk, further analysis of the existing data as well as forthcoming trials will be necessary to define more precisely the patient subgroups in whom most benefit is obtained as well as the optimal timing, duration and dose in patients with ACS including patients with STEMI.

Glycoprotein IIb/IIIa receptor antagonists

The glycoprotein (Gp) IIb/IIIa receptor antagonists inhibit the Gp IIb/IIIa integrin, found exclusively on platelets and megakaryocytes. The interaction of the receptor with its primary ligand, fibrinogen, is considered the final common pathway of platelet aggregation and blockade results in inhibition of aggregation irrespective of the initial agonist. There are close to 100 agonists known to stimulate platelet aggregation. Given the central role of platelets in arterial thrombosis and the fact that ASA and clopidogrel inhibit only the thromboxane A2 and ADP pathways respectively, the Gp IIb/IIIa receptor antagonists represent an attractive potential therapy in patients with STEMI.

There are three Gp IIb/IIIa receptor antagonists currently licensed for use. Abciximab is a chimeric (murine–human) monoclonal antibody directed against the IIb/IIIa receptor whereas tirofiban and eptifibatide are both small-molecule non-competitive IIb/IIIa inhibitors.

Gp IIb/IIIa receptor antagonists in patients receiving fibrinolytic therapy

The combination of a Gp IIb/IIIa receptor antagonist with a fibrinolytic agent (in full and reduced dose) has been evaluated extensively in efforts to improve the outcome from pharmacologic reperfusion.

Gp IIb/IIIa receptor antagonists and full-dose fibrinolytics The relatively small Combined Accelerated t-PA and Platelet Glycoprotein Integrin Receptor Blockade with Integrillin in Acute Myocardial Infarction (IMPACT-AMI) study randomized patients (n = 180) to alteplase and either placebo or one of six doses of eptifibatide (in addition to ASA and UFH).[30] The highest dose of eptifibatide (180 μg/kg bolus followed by an infusion at a rate of 0.75 μg/kg/min) achieved higher rates of TIMI 3 flow at 90 minutes compared with placebo (66% versus 39%, P = 0.007). The accompanying major bleeding rates were 3.9% and 5.4% respectively. A further pilot study (n = 181) investigated the efficacy of three doses of eptifibatide (180 μg/kg bolus followed by an infusion at a rate of 0.75, 1.33 or 2 μg/kg/min) compared with placebo in combination with full-dose

SK.[31] There appeared to be an increase in the rate of TIMI 3 flow at 90 minutes with eptifibatide (44% for the combined eptifibatide groups versus 31% in the placebo group, $P = 0.07$). However, rates of bleeding were higher in those treated with the highest dose of eptifibatide compared with the two lower doses and placebo (17% versus 11% versus 0% respectively, $P = 0.007$).

In summary, these small angiographic pilot studies suggested that whilst the addition of Gp IIb/IIIa receptor antagonists to full-dose fibrinolytics was effective at increasing target vessel patency, there appeared to be an excess in bleeding.

Gp IIb/IIIa receptor antagonists and reduced-dose fibrinolytics

Angiographic studies The TIMI-14 trial investigated abciximab use in combination with SK or alteplase.[32] Patients (n = 888) were randomized to one of four treatment groups: alteplase only (100 mg); abciximab only (0.25 mg/kg bolus followed by a 12 h infusion of 0.125 µg/kg/min); abciximab with 20–65 mg of alteplase; or abciximab with 0.5–1.5 million IU of SK. The highest rate of TIMI-3 flow was seen with abciximab in combination with 50 mg of alteplase (77% at 90 minutes versus 62% in the alteplase-only group, $P = 0.02$). Overall, there was no significant difference in major bleeding between these two groups (7% versus 6% respectively, $P = ns$). However, high bleeding rates led to discontinuation of treatment arms where abciximab was used in combination with SK.

The SPEED (Strategies for Patency Enhancement in the Emergency Department) trial randomized patients (n = 323) to either abciximab only (0.25 mg/kg bolus followed by a 12 h infusion of 0.125 µg/kg/min), reteplase only (two 10 mg boluses) or both (reteplase being given as a double bolus of 2.5–15 mg).[33] The rate of TIMI-3 flow with abciximab in combination with two 5 mg boluses of reteplase was 54% at 90 minutes. This compared with a rate of 47% in those given full-dose reteplase only. The rate of major bleeding was numerically higher with combination therapy compared with reteplase alone (9.8% versus 3.7%, $P = 0.11$).

In the INTRO-AMI (Integrellin and Low-Dose Thrombolytics in Acute Myocardial Infarction) study, eptifibatide was administered as a single (180 µg/kg) or double bolus (180 then 90 µg/kg or 180 then 180 µg/kg separated by 90 minutes), followed by an infusion of 1.33 or 2.00 µg/kg/min for 72 h in combination with 25 or 50 mg of alteplase.[34] The rate of TIMI-3 flow at 60 minutes was higher in those who received 50 mg of alteplase with eptifibatide 180 followed by 90 µg/kg bolus and a 1.33 µg/kg/min infusion compared to those receiving full-dose alteplase alone (56% versus 40%, $P = 0.04$). Rates of major bleeding and intracranial hemorrhage were again numerically higher in the group who received combination therapy (11% versus 6% and 3% versus 2% respectively; $P = ns$ for both).

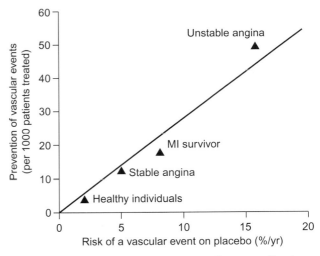

Figure 32.2 Clinical outcomes in the ASSENT-3,[46] GUSTO-V,[47] and HERO-2[48] trials: (a) mortality; (b) reinfarction.

Studies with clinical endpoints Following the potentially encouraging results seen in the angiographic pilot studies, randomized trials with clinical endpoints have investigated the potential of combining a Gp IIb/IIIa receptor antagonist with a fibrinolytic agent (Fig. 32.2).

The ASSENT-3 (Assessment of the Safety and Efficacy of a New Thrombolytic Regimen) trial randomized patients (n = 6095) within six hours of onset of STEMI to one of three treatment arms: full-dose tenecteplase and enoxaparin, half-dose tenecteplase and UFH plus abciximab or full-dose tenecteplase and UFH (control group). Compared with the control group, patients in the abciximab group had a significant reduction in the primary combined endpoint of death, reinfarction or refractory ischemia at 30 days (11.1% versus 15.4%, $P < 0.0001$), although there was no difference in mortality rates. Major bleeding (excluding intracranial hemorrhage) was increased (4.3% versus 2.2%, $P < 0.005$) and in those over 75 years old there was an approximately threefold increase (13.3% versus 4.1% respectively, $P = 0.0002$).

The GUSTO-V (Global Use of Strategies to Open Occluded Arteries) trial randomized patients (n = 16 588) with STEMI presenting within six hours of onset to either full-dose (two 10 U bolus doses) or half-dose reteplase (two 5 U bolus doses) plus full-dose abciximab.[35] Although there was a reduction in the reinfarction rate at 30 days with combination therapy (7.4% versus 8.8% with reteplase alone, $P < 0.001$), overall mortality was similar (5.9% for reteplase alone versus 5.6% for reteplase plus abciximab, $P = 0.43$) and remained so at one year (8.4% in both groups).[36] In addition, there were again concerns over increased bleeding in those treated with combination therapy, with an increase in moderate to severe bleeding (excluding intracranial hemorrhage, 4.6% versus 2.3%; $P < 0.001$) and a trend towards an increase in intracranial hemorrhage in those over 75 years old (2.1% versus 1.1%; $P = 0.07$).

The recently presented Facilitated Intervention with Enhanced Reperfusion to Stop Events (FINESSE) trial has helped to shed some light on the role of combining abciximab with a fibrinolytic agent. However, it is important to note that the trial was principally designed to evaluate whether facilitated PCI (with upstream delivery of abciximab with or without reteplase) was superior to primary PCI (with in-lab abciximab). Patients (n = 2452) with an estimated time to the catheterization laboratory of between one and four hours were randomized in a 1:1:1 fashion to upfront abciximab-facilitated primary PCI, half-dose reteplase/abciximab-facilitated PCI, or primary PCI with in-lab abciximab. Consistent with a recent meta-analysis,[37] the principal finding was that facilitated PCI provided no benefit and was associated with increased bleeding compared with standard primary PCI. There was no difference in the primary endpoint in the abciximab-only group compared to the combination group (9.8% versus 10.7% respectively, P = ns) but there was an increased incidence of TIMI major or minor bleeding (10.1% versus 14.5%, P = 0.008).

The use of abciximab in conjunction with half-dose reteplase or tenecteplase should be avoided in STEMI patients aged greater than 75 years due to an increased risk of intracranial hemorrhage (**Class III, Level B**).

Gp IIb/IIIa receptor antagonists in patients undergoing primary PCI

Primary PCI achieves TIMI-3 flow in the infarct-related artery in approximately 90% of patients. However, despite restoration of normal epicardial flow, flow within the downstream microvasculature and hence to the ischemic myocardium often remains impaired (the so-called "no reflow" phenomenon).[38–40] This may be a key determinant of long-term outcome as diminished microvascular flow is associated with increased cardiovascular complications and mortality.[40,41]

The role of Gp IIb/IIIa receptor antagonists in the setting of primary PCI has been evaluated in conjunction with ASA and UFH use. All trials referred to in the discussion below have evaluated the complementary role of Gp IIb/IIIa receptor antagonists in this context, unless otherwise stated.

Abciximab Abciximab is the most widely studied Gp IIb/IIIa receptor antagonist. It has consistently been shown to increase rates of TIMI-3 flow in the infarct-related vessel, in a time-dependent manner (Fig. 32.3).

The RAPPORT (ReoPro® and Primary PTCA Organization and Randomized Trial) study was the first substantive study to investigate the effect of abciximab on a clinical endpoint following primary PCI (n = 409).[42] It should be

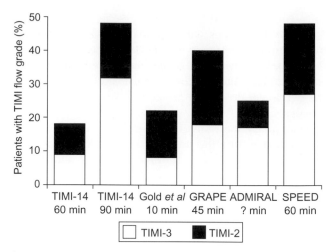

Figure 32.3 TIMI-2 and -3 flow rates in patients with acute MI treated with abciximab prior to angiography in the TIMI-14,[32] Gold et al,[95] GRAPE,[96] ADMIRAL,[43] and SPEED[33] trials. The time intervals between administration of the abciximab bolus and angiography are shown. GRAPE, glycoprotein recepter antagonist patency evaluation.

noted that stent use in this study was restricted to "bail-out" use only (i.e. abrupt vessel closure or dissection). The trial demonstrated a reduction in the 30-day rate of death, reinfarction or target vessel revascularization (TVR) in the abciximab group compared to placebo (11.2% versus 5.8%, P = 0.03).

The ADMIRAL (Abciximab before Direct Angioplasty and Stenting in Myocardial Infarction Regarding Acute and Long-Term Follow-up) study evaluated the effect of abciximab in patients (n = 300) with STEMI prior to primary PCI.[43] A 41% reduction in the primary endpoint of death, reinfarction and TVR was observed at 30 days in the abciximab group (6.0% versus 14.6% in placebo group, P = 0.01), with a similar reduction at six months (7.4% versus 15.9%, P = 0.02). The investigators attributed the better outcome to higher levels of TIMI 3 flow in the target vessel before (16.8% versus 5.4%, P = 0.01) and after (95.1% versus 86.7%, P = 0.04) PCI. The association between postprocedural TIMI 3 flow and a lower incidence of major adverse cardiac event (MACE) at 30 days has also been observed in other studies.

The larger CADILLAC (Controlled Abciximab and Device Investigation to Lower Late Angioplasty Complications) trial randomized patients (n = 2082) with STEMI using a 2 × 2 factorial design to either abciximab or placebo, and either angioplasty or stenting.[44] Patients were also given ASA, UFH and either clopidogrel or ticlopidine prior to going to the catheterization laboratory. The principal finding was a halving in the incidence of the composite endpoint (death, MI, stroke or TVR) at six months with stent insertion compared to angioplasty (20.0% versus 10.2%, P < 0.001). There was only a small additional benefit with abciximab (11.5% after stenting alone versus 10.2% after stenting plus abciximab, P = ns) although this may have been confounded by broad inclusion criteria and recruitment of a low-risk population coupled with relatively late administration of abciximab.

A meta-analysis of abciximab use in patients with STEMI undergoing primary PCI (n = 3266) demonstrated a reduction in the composite endpoint of death, reinfarction and need for TVR at 30 days (absolute RR 3.6%, relative RR 46%) and six months (absolute RR 3.2%, relative RR 20%).[45] A further meta-analysis of 11 trials (n = 27115) also demonstrated a reduction in short (30-day) and long-term (6–12 months) mortality (absolute RR 1% and 1.8% respectively; relative RR 29% for both) with abciximab use in the context of primary PCI.[46] Neither demonstrated an increased incidence of intracranial hemorrhage although the latter analysis indicated an increase in the rate of major bleeding (absolute risk increase 1.2%, relative risk increase 68%, $P < 0.001$).

With regard to when best to administer a GP IIb/IIIa receptor antagonist in patients undergoing primary PCI, a meta-analysis of six small studies had suggested a greater prevalence of TIMI 2 or 3 flow in the infarct-related artery prior to PCI with early administration (41.7% versus 29.8%, $P < 0.001$).[47] However, the FINESSE study (n = 2452) demonstrated no benefit of upstream (prior to catheter laboratory) administration of abciximab (or indeed upstream abciximb in combination with half-dose reteplase) compared to in-catheter laboratory administration.[48]

Tirofiban and eptifibatide Whilst tirofiban and eptifibatide share a common mechanism of action with abciximab, there have been no substantive trials with clinical endpoints to assess their role in primary PCI, although small placebo-controlled studies suggest an increase in TIMI 2 or 3 flow in the infarct-related artery following early administration of tirofiban[49] and eptifibatide[50,51] respectively. The EVA-AMI trial, presented at the American Heart Association 2007 Scientific Sessions, randomized STEMI patients (n = 400) undergoing primary PCI to abciximab or eptifibatide. There were no significant differences in the primary endpoint (the rate of ST segment resolution 60 minutes following PCI) or the incidence of ischemic or bleeding events during the index admission. Similar results supporting the non-inferiority of tirofiban compared to abciximab were observed in the MULTISTRATEGY trial (n = 745).[52]

Patients with STEMI undergoing primary PCI should be treated with abciximab (**Class I, Level A**) as soon as possible prior to the procedure (**Class I, Level B**).

As an alternative, patients undergoing primary PCI may be treated with tirofiban or eptifibatide (**Class IIb, Level B**).

It should be emphasized that virtually all studies to date investigating the role of Gp IIb/IIIa receptor antagonists in STEMI patients undergoing primary PCI have been conducted prior to the routine administration of clopidogrel. Interestingly, in the CADILLAC study, which failed to show a significant benefit of abciximab, patients *were* pretreated with a thienopyridine in addition to ASA. Whilst the study's broad entry criteria and subsequent recruitment of a relatively low-risk population may explain the lack of benefit with abciximab, it is possible that the routine administration of a thienopyridine diminished the relative efficacy of abciximab. The ON-TIME 2 study, showed a reduction in ST segment elevation at 60 minutes post-PCI (the primary endpoint) with tirofiban (initial 25 μg/kg bolus) compared with placebo.[53] Patients in this study were also pretreated with ASA and clopidogrel (600 mg) and although not powered for clinical endpoints, there were encouraging trends in MACE at 30 days.

Taken in conjunction with the results from the HORIZONS AMI trial, discussed below, it is clear that further studies are required to clarify the role of Gp IIb/IIIa receptor antagonists in STEMI patients pretreated with ASA and clopidogrel who are undergoing primary PCI.

Anticoagulant therapy

The coagulation cascade as a therapeutic target

Activation of the coagulation cascade plays an important role in thrombus formation during acute MI (see Fig. 32.1). Tissue factor, principally produced by monocytes within the plaque, binds to factor VII and initiates the extrinsic arm of the coagulation cascade, resulting in factor Xa generation. Factor Xa converts prothrombin to thrombin (factor IIa), the key enzyme responsible for the conversion of fibrinogen to its active form, fibrin. Multiple positive feedback mechanisms exist to enhance further production of factor Xa as well as promoting platelet activation and aggregation.

Under normal circumstances, the coagulation cascade is restrained by a number of mechanisms including the serine protease inhibitor antithrombin III (AT III). AT III binds to many of the activated coagulation factors, including thrombin and factor Xa, forming stable complexes that are no longer capable of proteolysis. The interaction between AT III and key coagulation factors is substantially enhanced by a number of endothelial cell proteoglycans. This catalytic function is reproduced by heparins.

Unfractionated heparin

Unfractionated heparin is the prototypical clinical anticoagulant. Despite important limitations (Table 32.1) it remains the most commonly used anticoagulant in clinical practice. It consists of a heterogenous mix of heparin mol-

Table 32.1 Clinical limitations of unfractionated heparin

Limitation	Clinical consequence
Non-specific binding to plasma proteins	Variability in anticoagulant effect
Cannot inactivate fibrin-bound thrombin	Reduced efficacy
Inhibited by platelet factor 4 and fibrin monomers	Leads to heparin resistance
Potential formation of antibodies against heparin	Can result in heparin-induced thrombocytopenia and thrombosis syndrome
Interaction with other drugs commonly used in the context of PCI	Variability in anticoagulant effect
Activates platelets	Potential for enhancing platelet aggregation

PCI, percutaneous coronary intervention.

Table 32.2 Benefits and risks associated with adjunctive delayed subcutaneous heparin in patients receiving streptokinase in the ISIS-3[22] and GISSI-2[21] studies

	Events per 1000 patients treated		
	ISIS-3	GISSI-2	Combined
Benefit			
Reduction in mortality	2.8	1.0	2.2[a]
Reduction in non-fatal MI	1.8	1.9	1.8
Risk			
Transfusions	2.6	4.5	3.2
Non-fatal strokes	0.5	0.6	0.6[b]

[a] Figures do not sum up because of rounding.
[b] Half of the patients had fully recovered by the time of discharge.

ecules, ranging in size from 5 to 35 kDa. It acts as an indirect inhibitor of factors IIa (thrombin) and Xa, exerting its effect by potentiating the action of AT III. Thrombin is the factor most sensitive to the effects of UFH, but requires "bridging" to the AT III/heparin complex by a heparin chain containing at least 18 saccharide units.

Unfractionated heparin in patients receiving fibrinolysis

Administration of fibrinolytic therapy results in a systemic prothrombotic state due to release of plasmin which activates platelets via the thrombin receptor[54] and triggers thrombin generation via activation of factor V.[55] The extent of thrombin activity induced by each agent appears to be directly related to the extent of free plasmin activity,[12] explaining why SK induces a more marked prothrombotic effect than the fibrin-specific agents alteplase, reteplase, and tenecteplase.[12] Exposure of clot-bound thrombin acts as a nidus for further thrombus formation and provides the rationale for the use of adjunctive anticoagulant therapy in patients treated with a fibrinolytic agent.

Angiographic studies A number of clinical trials have investigated the effect of UFH on vessel patency following fibrinolytic therapy.[5,56–60] Results are varied and interpretation is difficult owing to differences in use of ASA, fibrinolytic agent and regimen used and the timing of angiography. Overall, UFH does not appear to improve early (60–90 minute) infarct-related artery patency.[60] Although there may be some benefit at later time-points, no benefit was

seen when ASA was administered at a dose >100 mg which is now established clinical practice.

Clinical studies The Grupo Italiano per lo Studio della Sopravvivenza nell'Infarcto Miocardico (GISSI-2)[61] and the Third International Study of Infarct Survival (ISIS-3)[62] trials compared subcutaneous (SC) UFH with placebo as an adjunct to fibrinolysis in patients receiving SK, anistreplase and alteplase in addition to ASA (Table 32.2). In GISSI-2, patients (n = 20,891) were randomized to UFH or placebo 12 hours following administration of SK or alteplase. Unfractionated heparin was found to reduce mortality from 6.0% to 5.4% (relative RR 10%, $P < 0.05$). In ISIS-3 (n = 41 299), there was a trend towards a reduction in mortality with adjunctive UFH (7.4% versus 7.9% in the control group, $P = 0.06$). This may represent a benefit of four/five fewer deaths per 1000 during the treatment period, although due to substantial crossover of patients between treatment groups, it has been estimated that benefit was actually closer to seven lives per 1000 saved with UFH. At 30 days, although a similar trend remained, it was no longer statistically significant. Analysis of combined data from GISSI-2 and ISIS-3 suggested that in patients treated with SC UFH compared with control, there were two fewer deaths and two fewer non-fatal reinfarctions per 1000 patients, at the expense of three more transfusions and 0.6 more strokes (see Table 32.2).[63]

There is a paucity of data comparing the use of intravenous (IV) UFH in patients receiving fibrinolysis. Although four randomized controlled trials have addressed the issue and found no significant differences in mortality and rein-

Table 32.3 Effect of adjunctive intravenous heparin in patients treated with aspirin and fibrinolytic therapy

	Death (%)		Re-infarction (%)		Bleeding (%)	
	Control	Heparin	Control	Heparin	Control	Heparin
ISIS-2 Pilot (n = 626)[25]	6	8	5	1	1	0
ECSG (n = 1296)[18]	3	2	10	10	NA	NA
OSIRIS (n = 256)[26]	11	9	1	2	4	6
DUCCS (n = 250)[27]	9	12	4	9	8	15

DUCCS, Duke University Clinical Cardiology Study; ECSG, European Cooperative Study Group; NA, not available; OSIRIS, Optimization Study of Infarct Reperfusion Investigated by ST Monitoring.

farction, all lacked the statistical power to appropriately evaluate these clinical outcomes (Table 32.3).[56,57,64]

A meta-analysis of patients (n = 68000) treated with various UFH regimens (93% of whom received fibrinolytic therapy) demonstrated a modest reduction in mortality (8.6% versus 9.1% in control group, relative RR 5.5%, P = 0.03) and reinfarction (3.0% versus 3.3%, relative RR 9%, P – 0.04) at 35 days. Major bleeding was higher in those receiving UFH (1.0% versus 0.7% in control group, P = 0.001).[65]

In summary, the balance between risk and benefit is not straightforward. Benefits appear modest and are at the expense of major bleeds including intracranial hemorrhage.

Unfractionated heparin in patients undergoing primary PCI

UFH has been used since the advent of PCI, principally to avoid thrombus formation at the site of balloon injury, at vascular access points and within guide catheters. Various advances have led to a steady reduction in the amount of intraprocedural UFH used, including the widespread use of stents, high-pressure stent deployment and co-administration of increasingly potent antiplatelet therapies. There are no large-scale data to guide the use of UFH in PCI and thus it remains relatively empiric. The data that do exist have been acquired in small-scale studies and principally in patients undergoing elective procedures. A meta-analysis of six randomized controlled trials suggested optimal benefit with an initial bolus of 70–100 U/kg aiming for an activated clotting time (ACT) of 350–375 s. In patients treated with a Gp IIb/IIIa receptor antagonist, this should be reduced to 50–70 U/kg, aiming for an ACT of 200 s.[66]

UFH is a useful anticoagulant in patients with STEMI undergoing primary PCI. Dose should be adjusted for weight and when used in conjunction with a Gp IIb/IIIa receptor antagonist (**Class I, Level C**).

Unfractionated heparin in patients not receiving reperfusion therapy

Data from 21 trials (n – 5459) performed prior to the introduction of fibrinolytic therapy or the widespread use of ASA, beta-blockers or angiotensin-converting enzyme inhibitors demonstrated a reduction in venous thromboembolic events, stroke, reinfarction and death with the use of UFH compared to placebo.[63,64] Overall, a relative reduction in mortality of 25% (95% confidence interval (CI) 10–37%) was observed although there were 10 ± 4 additional episodes of major bleeding per 1000 patients treated. Overall, however, there are no substantive randomized data to guide the use of UFH in patients managed using current recommended regimens.

Low molecular weight heparin

Low molecular weight heparins (LMWHs) are derived from UFH by chemical and enzymatic depolymerization, resulting in preparations containing shorter heparin fragments (mean molecular weight of 4–5 kDa). In a similar way to UFH, LMWHs enhance the action of AT III but as the mean length of the heparin fragments is less, they have a reduced ability to bridge AT III to thrombin. As such bridging is not necessary to inhibit factor Xa, LMWHs exert their effect predominantly through inhibition of factor Xa. They possess a number of potential advantages over UFH (Table 32.4), including a more predictable level of anticoagulation eliminating the need for mandatory

Table 32.4 Comparison of unfractionated heparin, low molecular weight heparin, bivalirudin and fondaparinux

	UFH	LMWH	Bivalirudin	Fondaparinux
Mechanism of action	Potentiates AT III – principal effect is indirect inhibition of thrombin	Potentiates AT III – principal effect is indirect inhibition of factor Xa – some indirect inhibition of thrombin	Direct thrombin inhibitor	Potentiates action of AT III – results in specific indirect inhibition of factor Xa
Inhibition of fibrin-bound thrombin	No	No	Yes	No
Non-specific binding	Yes – to plasma proteins and cells	Yes – to plasma proteins and cells	No	No
Activation of platelets	Yes	Minimal	No – inhibits thrombin-mediated platelet activation	No
Pharmacokinetics	Non-linear	Non-linear (less so than UFH)	Linear	Linear
Risk of HIT	Yes	Yes (less than UFH)	No	No
Monitoring	Mandatory using ACT or aPTT	Not usually necessary; anti-Xa levels can be monitored	Not usually necessary; ACT or aPTT can be monitored	Not usually necessary; anti-Xa levels can be monitored
Reversal with protamine	Yes	Partial	No	No

ACT, activated clotting time; aPTT, activated partial prothromboplastin time; AT III, antithrombin III; LMWH, low molecular weight heparins; UFH, unfractionated heparin.

laboratory monitoring, a reduction in the incidence of thrombocytopenia, less platelet activation and an easier route of administration.

Low molecular weight heparin in patients receiving fibrinolysis

The use of LMWH with fibrinolytic therapy has been evaluated in a number of trials. Together, results suggest a modest advantage of LMWH over UFH that appears to be due to enhanced late patency of the infarct-related vessel and an associated reduction in reinfarction rate.

Dalteparin The Fragmin in Acute Myocardial Infarction (FRAMI) study[67] randomized patients (n = 776) to either dalteparin (150IU/kg twice daily) or placebo following fibrinolysis with SK. The only significant difference in clinical endpoints was an increase in major hemorrhage in those treated with dalteparin (2.9% versus 0.3% in control group, $P = 0.006$). The Biochemical Markers in Acute Coronary Syndromes (BIOMACS)-II study[68] also evaluated the use of adjunctive dalteparin (100IU/kg initially followed by 120IU/kg at 12 hours) in patients (n = 101) following SK. There was a trend towards increased rates of TIMI 3 flow at 20–28 hours (68% versus 51% in placebo group, $P = 0.10$) and a reduction in the incidence of recurrent ischemia (recorded on continuous electrocardiography)

from 38% to 16% ($P = 0.037$). There were no differences in major bleeding or clinical events.

In the Assessment of the Safety and Efficacy of a New Thrombolytic Agent (ASSENT)-PLUS trial,[69] patients (n = 439) were given alteplase and randomized to either adjunctive dalteparin (120IU/kg twice daily) for 4–7 days or IV UFH for 48 hours. Those treated with dalteparin had higher rates of infarct-related vessel patency between days 4 and 7 (86.6% versus 75.6%, $P = 0.003$). There was also a trend towards higher rates of TIMI 3 flow (69.3% versus 62.5%, $P = 0.16$). Although there were fewer reinfarctions at day seven in the dalteparin group (1.4% versus 5.4%, $P = 0.01$), there was no difference in the rate of reinfarction (6.5% versus 7.0%, P = ns) or the composite of death and reinfarction at 30 days.

Reviparin The Clinical Trial of Reviparin and Metabolic Modulation in Acute Myocardial Infarction Treatment Evaluation (CREATE),[70] performed in India and China, randomized STEMI patients (n = 15570) to weight-adjusted reviparin or placebo for seven days. Use of concomitant therapies was high (ASA in 97%, clopidogrel in 55%, beta-blockers in 66%, ACE inhibitors in 72%, and lipid-lowering agents in 66%). Fibrinolytic therapy, principally with non-fibrin specific agents, was the method of reperfusion in 73% of patients. The primary endpoint of death, MI or stroke was reduced in those treated with reviparin compared to placebo at seven days (9.6% versus 11.0%, $P = 0.0049$) and 30 days (11.8% versus 13.6%, $P = 0.0014$). Isolated mortality rates at seven and 30 days were also significantly reduced with reviparin. An excess in life-threatening bleeds not included in the primary endpoint was observed in those treated with reviparin (0.2% versus 0.1% with placebo, $P = 0.07$). Although its relevance to contemporary practice in the developed world is questionable (given that a greater proportion of patients are treated with primary PCI and fibrin-specific agents are more commonly used), the trial remains the only one to demonstrate a reduction in mortality with a LMWH.

Enoxaparin In the Acute Myocardial Infarction-Streptokinase (AMI-SK) trial (n = 496),[71] higher rates of vessel patency (87.6% versus 71.7%, $P < 0.001$) and TIMI 3 flow (70.3% versus 57.8%, $P = 0.01$) were observed at eight days in those treated with enoxaparin.

In the Heparin and Aspirin Reperfusion Therapy (HART)-II trial (n = 400),[72] rates of TIMI 2 or 3 flow at 90 minutes and rates of reocclusion at 5–7 days were similar in patients randomized to either UFH or enoxaparin for a minimum of three days following fibrinolysis with alteplase. There were no significant differences in rates of major bleeding in either study.

In the ASSENT-3 trial, patients (n = 6095) were randomized to full-dose tenecteplase with weight-adjusted UFH for at least 48 hours, full-dose tenecteplase with enoxaparin for seven days or reduced-dose tenecteplase with abciximab and UFH. The composite of death, reinfarction or refractory ischemia was significantly lower in those treated with enoxaparin than UFH (11.4%, RR 0.74, 95% CI 0.63–0.87, $P = 0.0002$). This advantage was driven primarily by a reduction in the rate of reinfarction. However, there was an increased incidence of bleeding complications in those treated with enoxaparin compared to UFH (Table 32.5).

The Enoxaparin and Thrombolysis Reperfusion for Acute Myocardial Infarction Treatment (ExTRACT-TIMI) 25 trial[73] randomized patients (n = 20 506) with STEMI undergoing fibrinolysis to receive either enoxaparin (30 mg IV bolus followed by 1 mg/kg throughout the index hospitalization) or UFH (60 U bolus followed by 12 U/kg/h for 48 hours). Importantly, therefore, the treatment groups varied not only in the antithrombin agent given but also in the duration of treatment. In addition, the dosing regimen was reduced in patients ≥75 years and/or with a creatinine clearance ≤30 mL/min. The primary endpoint of death or reinfarction at 30 days occurred in 12.0% of patients treated with UFH and 9.9% of those treated with enoxaparin (17% relative RR, $P < 0.001$). Non-fatal reinfarction occurred in

Table 32.5 Bleeding and stroke rates in the ASSENT-3,[46] GUSTO-V[47] and HERO-2[48] trials

	ASSENT-3			GUSTO-V		HERO-2	
	Tenecteplase + UF heparin	Tenecteplase + enoxaparin	Half-dose tenecteplase + UF Heparin + abciximab	Full-dose reteplase	Half-dose reteplase + abciximab	Streptokinase + UF heparin	Streptokinase + bivalirudin
Bleeding							
Severe (%)	2.16	3.04	4.31[a]	0.51	1.08[b]	0.47	0.68
Moderate (%)	–	–	–	1.79	3.47[b]	1.05	1.39[c]
Minor (%)	18.7	22.6	35.3[b]	11.4	20.01[b]	9.0	12.8[b]
Transfusions (%)	2.31	3.43[d]	4.16[b]	3.98	5.71[b]	1.11	1.39
Strokes							
All strokes (%)	1.52	1.62	1.49	0.88	0.97	0.90	1.24
Non-fatal disabling stroke	–	–	–	0.3	0.2	0.3	0.2
Intracranial (%) hemorrhages	0.93	0.88	0.94	0.59	0.62	0.39	0.55

[a] $P = 0.003$.
[b] $P < 0.0001$.
[c] $P = 0.05$.
[d] $P = 0.03$.
LMW, low molecular weight; UF, unfractionated

4.5% of the patients receiving UFH and 3.0% of those receiving enoxaparin (relative RR 33%, $P < 0.001$); 7.5% of patients given UFH died versus 6.9% of those given enoxaparin (relative RR 8%, $P = 0.11$). TIMI major bleeding was increased in the enoxaparin group compared to those receiving UFH (2.1% versus 1.4%, relative risk 1.53, $P < 0.001$) whilst rates of intracranial hemorrhage were similar (0.8% versus 0.7% respectively, $P = 0.14$). The composite of death, reinfarction or intracranial hemorrhage (a measure of overall clinical benefit) occurred in 12.2% of patients given UFH and 10.1% of those given enoxaparin (relative RR 17%, $P < 0.001$). In a prespecified analysis to look at concomitant clopidogrel use, the rate of TIMI major bleeding with enoxaparin compared with UFH was numerically but not statistically significantly higher in patients treated with clopidogrel (2.7% versus 1.0%) versus those who were not (2.1% versus 1.2%) ($P_{interaction} = 0.61$).[74] Overall clinical benefit remained in favor of enoxaparin over UFH, either with clopidogrel (absolute RR 2.4%, 95% CI 0.5–5.3%) or without (absolute RR 1.7%, 95% CI 0.5–3.0%) ($P_{interaction} = 0.61$). A further prespecified subgroup analysis assessed the effect of impaired renal function. This was possible due to relatively broad entry criteria resulting in the recruitment of patients with a wide spectrum of renal function. In line with data from previous trials and registry data, impaired renal function was a powerful independent predictor of adverse outcome including bleeding irrespective of treatment group.[75] Each successive 30 mL/min decline in creatinine clearance (CrCl) increased the risk of major or minor bleeding by approximately 50%. For patients with well-preserved renal function (CrCl >90 mL/min), the incidence of major bleeding was not significantly different between treatment groups. However, excess bleeding was observed in those with CrCl <30 mL/min treated with enoxaparin despite a halving of the maintenance dose. This raises the possibility that dose adjustment of enoxaparin may be required in patients with even moderate renal dysfunction (for example, CrCl 30–90 mL/min) to achieve a reduction in ischemic events while mitigating the risk of bleeding. Until alternative dosing regimens are developed, it also suggests that enoxaparin should not be administered to patients with CrCl <30 mL/min. More broadly, the analysis emphasises the high-risk nature of ACS patients with impaired renal function and suggests that dose reduction for enoxaparin and UFH in this patient subgroup should be investigated further.

The results of the ExTRACT-TIMI-25 trial are broadly in keeping with the results of meta-analyses of enoxaparin use in STEMI patients treated with fibrinolysis that indicate a reduction in reinfarction and recurrent ischemia, no improvement in overall mortality and an increase in major bleeding, especially in elderly patients and those with renal impairment.[76,77]

LMWHs are a useful alternative to UFH in STEMI in conjunction with fibrinolytic therapy and should be administered throughout the index hospitalization (up to eight days) (**Class I, Level A**).

Low molecular weight heparin in patients treated with primary PCI

The majority of data concerning safety and efficacy of LMWHs in the catheterization laboratory comes from studies in patients undergoing elective procedures or in patients with ACS managed with an early invasive strategy. Broadly, these data suggest that enoxaparin is a useful alternative to UFH when used as the primary anticoagulant in elective procedures.[78] In ACS patients managed using a contemporary antithrombotic regimen incorporating enoxaparin, it appears efficacious to perform PCI without additional anticoagulation although there is a small but significant increased risk of bleeding which is particularly relevant in the elderly and in those with renal impairment.[79,80] There are limited data regarding the safety and efficacy of LMWHs during PCI in the context of patients with STEMI.

Reviparin In the CREATE trial, 949 patients underwent primary PCI as their reperfusion strategy, although details of whether additional UFH was used periprocedurally are not provided and this cohort represented just 6.1% of the overall population. There was a trend towards a reduction in the primary endpoint of death, MI or stroke at seven days with reviparin compared to placebo (5.8% versus 7.3%, hazard ratio (HR) 0.79, 95% CI 0.48–1.31).

Enoxaparin In the ExTRACT-TIMI-25 trial, patients in the enoxaparin treatment group who subsequently underwent PCI following initial treatment with fibrinolysis (not primary PCI) without the use of additional UFH (n = 4676) had a lower incidence of the primary endpoint of death and reinfarction at 30 days compared to those in the UFH group (10.7% versus 13.8%, relative RR 23%, $P < 0.001$).[81] There were no differences in major bleeding (1.4% vs 1.6% respectively, $P = ns$).

In the Which Early ST Elevation Myocardial Infarction Therapy (WEST) study, patients with STEMI were randomized to fibrinolysis, protocol-specified rescue PCI and/or early angiography within 24h or primary PCI. Patients undergoing primary PCI (n = 33) were given ASA and clopidogrel at first contact and most received abciximab on arrival at the catheterization laboratory. Enoxaparin was administered at first contact (1 mg/kg SC). A supplemental dose (0.3–0.5 mg/kg IV) at the time of primary PCI was allowed in the original protocol and subsequently strongly encouraged following thrombotic complications in three of 36 patients during the early phase of the study enrolment. Use of UFH was precluded. Factor Xa levels were measured at the time of sheath insertion (prior to additional IV enoxaparin) and also at the end of the procedure. Initial anti-Xa levels 56 min (median, interquartile range 47–77) after SC enoxaparin were below the recommended therapeutic level of 0.5 U/mL in 85% of patients. Following PCI, at 126 min (118–185) after SC enoxaparin, in those without supplemental IV dosing (8/33) the second anti-Xa level was 0.44 U/mL (0.29–0.53); six of the eight patients remained <0.5 U/mL. With additional IV enoxaparin (25/33) the second anti-Xa level was 0.96 U/mL (0.82–1.16) 97 min (82–109) after SC enoxaparin; all patients had therapeutic levels of anti-Xa. This open-label study provides limited data on the role of enoxaparin in patients undergoing primary PCI but suggests that whilst a single SC enoxaparin dose fails to achieve adequate anticoagulation in the majority of STEMI patients, a regimen combining initial additional IV enoxaparin may provide effective early antithrombotic therapy in those undergoing primary PCI.

LMWHs are a reasonable alternative to UFH in patients with STEMI undergoing primary PCI (**Class IIb, Level B**).

Direct thrombin inhibitors

In contrast to UFH and LMWH, direct thrombin inhibitors (DTIs) bind to the substrate recognition and/or catalytic site of thrombin, resulting in its direct inhibition without the involvement of AT III. Due to their relatively small size, they are able to bind and inactivate fibrin-bound as well as free thrombin. They do not interact appreciably with plasma proteins or other drugs and are not inhibited by platelet factor IV and so display linear dose–response kinetics, resulting in predictable levels of anticoagulation. Additionally, in contrast to UFH, they do not activate platelets (see Table 32.4).[82]

Direct thrombin inhibitors in patients receiving fibrinolysis

Hirudin Hirudin is the prototypical DTI. It is a naturally occurring polypeptide found in the saliva of the leech. Clinically, it is used in a recombinant form – lepirudin.

The TIMI-5 trial randomized patients to either UFH or escalating doses of hirudin prior to fibrinolysis with alteplase. There was no significant difference in TIMI 3 flow at 90 minutes (57% in UFH group versus 65% in the hirudin group, *P* = ns) but there was a trend towards a reduced rate of reocclusion at 18–36 hours in those receiving hirudin (1.6% versus 6.7%, *P* = 0.07) and a lower combined rate of death or reinfarction (6.8% versus 16.7%). Based on this pilot study, the TIMI-9B and GUSTO-IIb trials evaluated the effect of hirudin given after the start of fibrinolysis on reinfarction and mortality. When the data from these two studies were combined, there was no reduction in mortality but the incidence of reinfarction was reduced by 14% (*P* = 0.024).

The Hirudin for the Improvement of Thrombolysis (HIT)-4 study randomized patients to UFH or hirudin (0.2 mg/kg IV bolus followed by 0.5 mg/kg SC twice daily)

in addition to SK. There was no effect on the combined endpoint of death/reinfarction/stroke/rescue angioplasty/refractory angina at 30 days (22.7% with hirudin versus 24.3% with UFH, *P* = ns). Rates of intracranial hemorrhage and major bleeding (3.3% versus 3.5%) were similar in both treatment groups.

Bivalirudin Bivalirudin is a synthetic, 20 amino acid peptide analog of the carboxy-terminal end of hirudin. It binds bivalently to thrombin and, once bound, is slowly cleaved by thrombin with resulting recovery of thrombin activity. It is cleared from plasma by a combination of proteolytic degradation and renal excretion. Its principal advantage over hirudin is a reduced incidence of bleeding complications, probably related to a shorter plasma half-life (approximately 25 minutes compared with 2–3 hours for hirudin).

In the Hirulog and Early Reperfusion or Occlusion (HERO)-1 trial, patients (n = 412) were given UFH, low-dose bivalirudin (0.125 mg/kg bolus followed by a 0.25 mg/kg/h infusion for 12 h, then 0.125 mg/kg/h) or high-dose bivalirudin (0.25 mg/kg bolus followed by a 0.5 mg/kg/h infusion for 12 h, then 0.25 mg/kg/h). TIMI 3 flow at 90–120 minutes was higher following bivalirudin than UFH (48% with high-dose bivalirudin, 46% with low-dose bivalirudin and 35% with UFH, *P* = 0.024).

The larger HERO-2 trial randomized patients (n = 17 073) to receive a bolus and 48 h infusion of bivalirudin or UFH immediately prior to SK. At 30 days, mortality was similar (10.8% in bivalirudin group versus 10.9% in UFH group, OR 0.96, 95% CI 0.90–1.09). After adjustments for gender differences between the two groups and for factors identified in the GUSTO risk model, the mortality estimate was 10.5% in the bivalirudin group and 10.9% in the UFH group (OR 0.96, 95% CI 0.86–1.07). Rates of reinfarction at 96 hours (adjudicated by an independent blinded committee) were less in the bivalirudin group (1.6% versus 2.3% in UFH group, OR 0.70, 95% CI 0.56–0.88, *P* = 0.001). Similarly, the combined rate of death and investigator-reported reinfarction was lower in the bivalirudin group (12.9% versus 14.2%, OR 0.90, 95% CI 0.82–0.99, *P* = 0.023). Whilst rates of intracranial bleeding and severe bleeding were low and similar in both treatment groups, moderate and minor bleeding were more common with bivalirudin than UFH (see Table 32.5). In a *post hoc* analysis, the rates of the composite endpoint of death/reinfarction/non-fatal disabling stroke were 12.7% in the bivalirudin versus 13.8% in the UFH group (*P* = 0.049) (see Fig. 32.3).

Univalent direct thrombin inhibitors The univalent DTIs include argatroban, inogatran, efegatran and D-Phe-Pro-Arg-CH$_2$Cl. Phase I studies have demonstrated their ability to enhance fibrinolytic therapy.

The Antithrombin-Argatroban in Acute Myocardial Infarction (ARGAMI-2) study randomized patients (n = 1001) to UFH or argatroban (120 μg bolus followed by a 4 μg/kg/min infusion for 72 h) in addition to fibrinolysis with SK or alteplase. A third treatment arm consisting of half-dose argatroban was terminated prematurely due to lack of efficacy. Mortality at 30 days was similar (5.5% in the argatroban group versus 5.7% in UFH group, P = ns). There was a trend towards less bleeding in patients who had received argatroban but no other difference in clinical event rates.

Meta-analysis of direct thrombin inhibitor trials

The Direct Thrombin Inhibitor Trialists' Collaborative Group performed a meta-analysis of 11 randomized controlled studies (n = 35 970) in which DTIs (hirudin, bivalirudin, argatroban, efegatran or inogatran) were compared with UFH in patients with ST segment elevation or non-ST segment elevation ACS.[83] There was no difference in mortality in those given DTIs compared with UFH immediately at the cessation of therapy (1.9% versus 2.0%; OR 0.97; 95% CI 0.83–1.13; P = 0.69), at seven days (2.2% versus 2.3%; OR 1.00; 95% CI 0.87–1.16; P = 0.95), at 30 days (3.6% versus 3.7%; OR 1.01; 95% CI 0.9–1.12; P = 0.90) or at six months (OR 1.00; 95% CI 0.91–1.09; P = 0.92). However, there was a reduction in the incidence of reinfarction compared with UFH at the cessation of therapy (2.8% versus 3.5%; OR 0.80; 95% CI 0.71–0.90; P < 0.001), seven days (3.2% versus 3.9%; OR 0.91; 95% CI 0.72–0.91; P < 0.001) and at 30 days (4.7% versus 5.3%; OR 0.87; 95% CI 0.79–0.95; P = 0.004). The combined incidence of death/MI was also reduced compared with UFH at cessation of therapy (4.3% versus 5.1%; OR 0.85; 95% CI 0.77–0.94; P = 0.001), at seven days (5.0% versus 5.8%; OR 0.88; 95% CI 0.80–0.96; P = 0.006) and at 30 days (7.4% versus 8.2%; OR 0.91; 95% CI 0.84–0.99; P = 0.02).

Five trials from this meta-analysis involved patients with STEMI. When combined with data from HERO-2 (Fig. 32.4), the results indicate that whilst DTIs have no effect on mortality alone, they do reduce the combined risk of death/reinfarction by 5% at 30 days compared with UFH. This is due primarily to a 20% reduction in the rate of reinfarction.

Bivalirudin is a useful alternative to UFH in STEMI in conjunction with fibrinolytic therapy (**Class I, Level B**).

Direct thrombin inhibitors in patients undergoing primary PCI

There are data from small studies to suggest that hirudin and argatroban may be safe and efficacious during PCI. The role of bivalirudin in patients undergoing elective procedures has been extensively studied and the recent Acute Catheterization and Urgent Intervention Triage Strategy (ACUITY) trial,[84] despite a number of limitations, has suggested that its use in ACS is safe and efficacious, including patients who are invasively managed with PCI.

The HORIZONS AMI trial[85] is the only substantive trial to investigate the role of a DTI in STEMI patients undergoing primary PCI. Patients (n = 3600) were randomized to UFH plus a glycoprotein IIb/IIIa receptor antagonist abciximab or eptifibatide) or bivalirudin monotherapy (plus glycoprotein IIb/IIIa receptor antagonist for large thrombus or refractory no flow only – used in only 7.2% of patients in the bivalirudin group). There was a reduction in overall clinical events (a composite of major bleeding and major adverse cardiovascular events) in the bivalirudin group at 30 days compared to the UFH and glycoprotein IIb/IIIa receptor antagonist group (12.1% versus 9.2% respectively, P = 0.006). Major bleeding alone at 30 days was also substantially reduced (8.3% versus 4.9%, P < 0.0001) and there was a significant reduction in cardiac death at 30 days (2.9% versus 1.8%, P = 0.035). The initial data demonstrate an excess in adverse events with bivalirudin only within the first 24 hours, probably related to an excess incidence of early stent thrombosis (1.3% versus 0.3% with UFH and glycoprotein IIb/IIIa receptor antagonist). However, the subsequent reduction in events seen in those treated with bivalirudin results in an overall benefit in favor of bivalirudin at 30 days, likely to be driven by a reduction in bleeding complications.

Bivalirudin is a reasonable alternative to the combination of UFH and a glycoprotein IIb/IIIa receptor antagonist in patients with STEMI undergoing primary PCI (**Class IIa, Level B**).

Factor Xa inhibitors

Fondaparinux is a synthetic inhibitor of factor Xa containing a key pentasaccharide moiety with structural similarity to the AT III binding site of UFH and LMWHs. It binds selectively to AT III, resulting in rapid and selective inhibition of factor Xa. It has a plasma half-life of around 15 hours and displays linear pharmacokinetics, obviating the need for routine monitoring (see Table 33.4).[86] Its role in the prevention and treatment of venous thromboembolic disease is well established.[86–88]

Factor Xa inhibitors in patients receiving fibrinolysis

The Synthetic Pentasaccharide as an Adjunct to Fibrinolysis in ST-Elevation Acute Myocardial Infarction (PENTALYSE) study compared fondaparinux with UFH in patients (n = 316) with STEMI.[89] All patients were given ASA and alteplase. Patients were randomized to receive UFH or one of three weight-adjusted doses of fondaparinux (4–6 mg, 6–10 mg or 10–12 mg) once daily for 5–7 days. The incidence of TIMI 3 flow at 90 minutes was similar in all groups (68% with UFH versus 64% in all fondaparinux groups). There was a trend towards a reduction in the rate of reocclusion at day 6 (0.9% versus 7.0% with UFH, P = 0.065) but rates of reinfarction at 30 days were similar (3.8% with fondaparinux versus 3.6% with UFH, P = 1.00). One patient who received fondaparinux (4 mg) suffered an

(a)

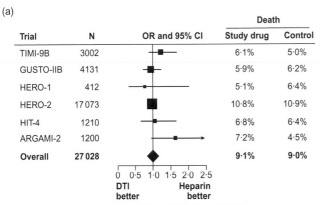

Trial	N	OR and 95% CI	Death Study drug	Control
TIMI-9B	3002		6·1%	5·0%
GUSTO-IIB	4131		5·9%	6·2%
HERO-1	412		5·1%	6·4%
HERO-2	17 073		10·8%	10·9%
HIT-4	1210		6·8%	6·4%
ARGAMI-2	1200		7·2%	4·5%
Overall	27 028		9·1%	9·0%

0 0·5 1·0 1·5 2·0 2·5
DTI better — Heparin better

Adjusted summary OR and 95% CI, P = 0·6806
Test for homogeneity of ORs: χ² = 5·8857, df = 4, P = 0·3175

(b)

Trial	N	OR and 95% CI	Re-infarction Study drug	Control
TIMI-9B	3002		4·3%	5·0%
GUSTO-IIB	4131		5·0%	6·0%
HERO-1	412		5·1%	8·6%
HERO-2	17 073		3·5%	4·5%
HIT-4	1210		4·5%	4·9%
ARGAMI-2	1200		2·9%	2·8%
Overall	27 028		3·9%	4·8%

0 0·5 1·0 1·5 2·0 2·5
DTI better — Heparin better

Adjusted summary OR and 95% CI, P = 0·0002
Test for homogeneity of ORs: χ² = 1·7769, df = 4, P = 0·8791

(c)

Trial	N	OR and 95% CI	Death/re-infarction Study drug	Control
TIMI-9B	3002		9·7%	9·3%
GUSTO-IIB	4131		9·9%	11·3%
HERO-1	412		9·9%	15·0%
HERO-2	17 073		13·0%	13·6%
HIT-4	1210		10·4%	10·9%
ARGAMI-2	1200		9·8%	6·5%
Overall	27 028		11·8%	12·4%

0 0·5 1·0 1·5 2·0 2·5
DTI better — Heparin better

Adjusted summary OR and 95% CI, P = 0·1756
Test for homogeneity of ORs: χ² = 8·4714, df = 4, P = 0·1321

(d)

Trial	N	OR and 95% CI	Stroke Study drug	Control
TIMI-9B	3002		1·1%	2·1%
GUSTO-IIB	4131		1·3%	0·8%
HERO-1	412		1·1%	1·4%
HERO-2	17 073		1·2%	1·0%
HIT-4	1210		1·0%	1·0%
ARGAMI-2	1200		0·4%	0·4%
Overall	27 028		1·2%	1·0%

0 0·5 1·0 1·5 2·0 2·5
DTI better — Heparin better

Adjusted summary OR and 95% CI, P = 0·2545
Test for homogeneity of ORs: χ² = 9·8726, df = 4, P = 0·0789

(e)

Trial	N	OR and 95% CI	Intracranial hemorrhage Study drug	Control
TIMI-9B	3002		0·4%	0·7%
GUSTO-IIB	4131		0·5%	0·4%
HERO-1	412		0·4%	0·0%
HERO-2	17 073		0·6%	0·4%
HIT-4	1210		0·2%	0·3%
ARGAMI-2	1200		0·0%	0·4%
Overall	27 028		0·5%	0·4%

0 0·5 1·0 1·5 2·0 2·5
DTI better — Heparin better

Adjusted summary OR and 95% CI, P = 0·3908
Test for homogeneity of ORs: χ² = 7·674, df = 4, P = 0.1751

(f)

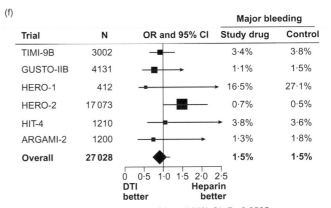

Trial	N	OR and 95% CI	Major bleeding Study drug	Control
TIMI-9B	3002		3·4%	3·8%
GUSTO-IIB	4131		1·1%	1·5%
HERO-1	412		16·5%	27·1%
HERO-2	17 073		0·7%	0·5%
HIT-4	1210		3·8%	3·6%
ARGAMI-2	1200		1·3%	1·8%
Overall	27 028		1·5%	1·5%

0 0·5 1·0 1·5 2·0 2·5
DTI better — Heparin better

Adjusted summary OR and 95% CI, P = 0·3535
Test for homogeneity of ORs: χ² = 11·11, df = 4, P = 0·0492

Figure 32.4 Thirty-day event rates in patients with ST-elevation MI, randomized to receive direct thrombin inhibitors (DTI) or unfractionated heparin in the HERO-1,[67] HERO-2,[48] TIMI-9B,[38] GUSTO-11B,[39] HIT-4,[65] and ARGAMI-2[73] trials: (a) death; (b) reinfarction; (c) death/reinfarction; (d) stroke; (e) intracranial hemorrhage; (f) major bleeding. HIT; hirudin for improvement of thrombolysis.

intracranial hemorrhage. Transfusion rates were 3.3% in those receiving fondaparinux versus 7.1% in those who received UFH (P = 0.21).

Data regarding the use of fondaparinux in patients with ACS have been gathered in the recent OASIS (Organization to Assess Strategies in Acute Ischemic Syndromes) trials. Whilst OASIS-5 compared the use of fondaparinux with enoxaparin in patients with ACS with or without ST elevation,[90] the OASIS-6 trial (n = 12 092) compared the use of fondaparinux to usual care (placebo in those in whom

UFH was not indicated or UFH for up to 48 hours followed by placebo for up to eight days) in patients with STEMI.[91] The first dose of fondaparinux (2.5 mg) was administered IV, followed by daily SC injections for up to eight days. There were no differences in the effects of fondaparinux between groups treated with UFH/placebo or placebo alone. Over the entire study population, fondaparinux reduced the primary endpoint of death or reinfarction at 30 days compared to treatment with placebo or UFH (9.7% versus 11.2%, relative RR 14%; $P = 0.008$). The benefit persisted at the study end (13.4% versus 14.8%, relative RR 9%; $P = 0.008$). In the subgroup who received thrombolytic therapy and were randomized to either fondaparinux or UFH (n = 2666) there was a reduction in death or reinfarction (relative RR 23%, $P = 0.003$) in those treated with fondaparinux although this was a modest sized subgroup analysis and should be interpreted with caution. Rates of bleeding were similar between groups (1.0% in the fondaparinux group versus 1.3% in the UFH/placebo group, $P = 0.13$).

Whilst parallels exist between OASIS-6 and the ExTRACT-TIMI-25 trial (discussed earlier), differences in inclusion criteria, study design and length of anticoagulant therapy preclude direct comparison. However, taken together with the results from OASIS-5, these studies provide strong evidence that a strategy of 48 hours of anticoagulation may be insufficient following MI. The premature cessation of anticoagulant therapy may result in reocclusion of the infarct-related artery and expose patients to an increased risk of recurrent infarction.

Fondaparinux is a useful alternative to UFH in STEMI patients who have received fibrinolytic therapy (**Class I, Level B**).

Factor Xa inhibitors in patients undergoing primary PCI

The OASIS-6 trial included patients with STEMI who underwent primary PCI (n = 3789). Whilst data from the study population as a whole demonstrated a benefit of fondaparinux over UFH or placebo on the primary endpoint of death and recurrent MI, this benefit was not seen in patients undergoing primary PCI. In addition, there was a higher rate of guiding catheter thrombosis and more coronary complications (abrupt coronary artery closure, new angiographic thrombus, catheter thrombus, no reflow, dissection or perforation) with fondaparinux.

Fondaparinux should not be used as the sole anticoagulant in patients with STEMI undergoing primary PCI (**Class III, Level B**).

Factor Xa inhibitors in patients not receiving reperfusion therapy

Compared to other contemporary trials involving patients with ACS, the OASIS-6 trial was unusual in that it included

patients with STEMI who did not receive reperfusion therapy (n = 2867). This subgroup formed almost a quarter of the overall cohort. Fondaparinux reduced the incidence of the primary endpoint (death or recurrent MI at 30 days) compared to UFH or placebo (relative RR 19%, $P = 0.04$).

Patients who do not receive reperfusion therapy should be treated throughout the index hospitalization (up to eight days) with fondaparinux in preference to UFH (**Class I, Level B**).

Conclusion

Antithrombotic therapy is a key component in the integrated management of patients presenting with STEMI. Optimal antithrombotic therapy requires antiplatelet and anticoagulant agents as well as consideration of the balance between efficacy and bleeding risk in each patient. The evaluation of novel agents and combination therapies continues at a phenomenal rate. All patients should be treated with ASA and a thienopyridine (currently clopidogrel) as soon as possible following diagnosis. The choice of anticoagulant therapy, in part, is dictated by the method of reperfusion undertaken. Whilst UFH is efficacious and remains widely used, evidence from recent large-scale trials favors the use of newer agents. Following fibrinolytic therapy, both fondaparinux and LMWHs improve clinical outcomes compared with UFH, although bleeding risk is increased with enoxaparin, especially in the elderly and those with renal impairment. Direct thrombin inhibitors appear to be a reasonable alternative to UFH, and preferred in settings of thrombocytopenia or prior heparin-induced thrombocytopenia. Whilst the use of a Gp IIb/IIIa receptor antagonist in conjunction with half-dose fibrinolytic may be considered in younger patients with a low risk of bleeding, it should be avoided in patients over 75 years of age given the increased risk of major bleeding, including intracranial hemorrhage.

In patients undergoing primary PCI, UFH has traditionally been administered based primarily on theoretical grounds and the experience of experts. There is evidence that the addition of a Gp IIb/IIIa receptor antagonist improves outcomes. Concern exists that fondaparinux and perhaps enoxaparin may not provide adequate periprocedural anticoagulation for patients undergoing PCI. There is now evidence from a single, moderately sized trial that bivalirudin is more efficacious than the combination of UFH plus a Gp IIb/IIIa receptor antagonist, removing the need for routine Gp IIb/IIIa receptor antagonist use. Further studies will be required to clarify whether this is applicable across the entire risk spectrum of STEMI patients.

For patients who have not undergone specific reperfusion therapy UFH appears to confer a modest benefit.

Compared to UFH, fondaparinux is efficacious, easy to administer and associated with a low incidence of bleeding. In order to further clarify the role of these newer agents, direct head-to-head trials of enoxaparin, fondaparinux and bivalirudin in STEMI patients undergoing primary PCI and fibrinolytic therapy are required. In addition, the role of novel antiplatelets[92,93] and inhibitors of tissue factor[94] remain to be defined.

Finally, bleeding complications in patients with ACS remain relatively common and may be as important to long-term outcome as ischemic events. Recent large studies have confirmed the importance of bleeding to overall outcome and helped identify patient subgroups at increased risk of bleeding. Given the strict inclusion criteria for most clinical trials, the risk of bleeding in the "real world" is likely to be higher. Central to the clinical decision-making process must be balancing the added antithrombotic effects of potent combination therapies against the accompanying increased risk of bleeding, especially in specific high-risk patient subgroups.

References

1. Zaman AG, Helft G, Worthley SG, Badimon JJ. The role of plaque rupture and thrombosis in coronary artery disease. *Atherosclerosis* 2000;**149**(2):251–66.

2. Thrombolysis in Myocardial Infarction (TIMI) Trial. Phase I findings. TIMI Study Group. *N Engl J Med* 1985;**312**(14): 932–6.

3. Simes RJ, Topol EJ, Holmes DR Jr *et al.* Link between the angiographic substudy and mortality outcomes in a large randomized trial of myocardial reperfusion. Importance of early and complete infarct artery reperfusion. GUSTO-I Investigators. *Circulation* 1995;**91**(7):1923–8.

4. White HD, Norris RM, Brown MA *et al.* Effect of intravenous streptokinase on left ventricular function and early survival after acute myocardial infarction. *N Engl J Med* 1987;**317**(14):850–5.

5. GUSTO Angiographic Investigators. The effects of tissue plasminogen activator, streptokinase, or both on coronary-artery patency, ventricular function, and survival after acute myocardial infarction. *N Engl J Med* 1993;**329**(22):1615–22.

6. Schuhlen H, Kastrati A, Pache J, Dirschinger J, Schomig A. Incidence of thrombotic occlusion and major adverse cardiac events between two and four weeks after coronary stent placement: analysis of 5,678 patients with a four-week ticlopidine regimen. *J Am Coll Cardiol* 2001;**37**(8):2066–73.

7. Wilson SH, Rihal CS, Bell MR, Velianou JL, Holmes DR Jr, Berger PB. Timing of coronary stent thrombosis in patients treated with ticlopidine and aspirin. *Am J Cardiol* 1999;**83**(7): 1006–11.

8. Barnathan ES, Schwartz JS, Taylor L *et al.* Aspirin and dipyridamole in the prevention of acute coronary thrombosis complicating coronary angioplasty. *Circulation* 1987;**76**(1):125–34.

9. Popma JJ, Ohman EM, Weitz J, Lincoff AM, Harrington RA, Berger P. Antithrombotic therapy in patients undergoing percutaneous coronary intervention. *Chest* 2001;**119**(1 suppl): 321S–336S.

10. Schwartz L, Bourassa MG, Lesperance J *et al.* Aspirin and dipyridamole in the prevention of restenosis after percutaneous transluminal coronary angioplasty. *N Engl J Med* 1988;**318**(26): 1714–19.

11. Kong DF, Califf RM, Miller DP *et al.* Clinical outcomes of therapeutic agents that block the platelet glycoprotein IIb/IIIa integrin in ischemic heart disease. *Circulation* 1998;**98**(25):2829–35.

12. Eisenberg PR. Role of heparin in coronary thrombolysis. *Chest* 1992;**101**(4 suppl):131S–139S.

13. Gurbel PA, Serebruany VL, Shustov AR *et al.* Effects of reteplase and alteplase on platelet aggregation and major receptor expression during the first 24 hours of acute myocardial infarction treatment. GUSTO-III Investigators. Global Use of Strategies to Open Occluded Coronary Arteries. *J Am Coll Cardiol* 1998;**31**(7):1466–73.

14. ISIS-2 (Second International Study of Infarct Survival) Collaborative Group. Randomized trial of intravenous streptokinase, oral aspirin, both, or neither among 17,187 cases of suspected acute myocardial infarction: ISIS-2. *Lancet* 1988;**2**(8607): 349–60.

15. Baigent C, Collins R, Appleby P, Parish S, Sleight P, Peto R. ISIS-2: 10 year survival among patients with suspected acute myocardial infarction in randomized comparison of intravenous streptokinase, oral aspirin, both, or neither. The ISIS-2 (Second International Study of Infarct Survival) Collaborative Group. *BMJ* 1998;**316**(7141):1337–43.

16. Roux S, Christeller S, Ludin E. Effects of aspirin on coronary reocclusion and recurrent ischemia after thrombolysis: a meta-analysis. *J Am Coll Cardiol* 1992;**19**(3):671–7.

17. Antithrombotic Trialists' Collaboration. Collaborative meta-analysis of randomized trials of antiplatelet therapy for prevention of death, myocardial infarction, and stroke in high risk patients. *BMJ* 2002;**324**(7329):71–86.

18. Peters RJ, Mehta SR, Fox KA *et al.* Effects of aspirin dose when used alone or in combination with clopidogrel in patients with acute coronary syndromes: observations from the Clopidogrel in Unstable angina to prevent Recurrent Events (CURE) study. *Circulation* 2003;**108**(14):1682–7.

19. Bhatt DL, Bertrand ME, Berger PB *et al.* Meta-analysis of randomized and registry comparisons of ticlopidine with clopidogrel after stenting. *J Am Coll Cardiol* 2002;**39**(1):9–14.

20. Steinhubl SR, Berger PB, Mann JT 3rd *et al.* Early and sustained dual oral antiplatelet therapy following percutaneous coronary intervention: a randomized controlled trial. *JAMA* 2002;**288**(19): 2411–20.

21. Serebruany VL, Steinhubl SR, Berger PB, Malinin AI, Bhatt DL, Topol EJ. Variability in platelet responsiveness to clopidogrel among 544 individuals. *J Am Coll Cardiol* 2005;**45**(2): 246–51.

22. Gurbel PA, Bliden KP. Durability of platelet inhibition by clopidogrel. *Am J Cardiol* 2003;**91**(9):1123–5.

23. Wang TH, Bhatt DL, Topol EJ. Aspirin and clopidogrel resistance: an emerging clinical entity. *Eur Heart J* 2006;**27**(6): 647–54.

24. Sabatine MS, Cannon CP, Gibson CM *et al.* Addition of clopidogrel to aspirin and fibrinolytic therapy for myocardial infarction with ST-segment elevation. *N Engl J Med* 2005;**352**(12):1179–89.

25. Mehta SR, Yusuf S, Peters RJ *et al.* Effects of pretreatment with clopidogrel and aspirin followed by long-term therapy in patients undergoing percutaneous coronary intervention: the PCI-CURE study. *Lancet* 2001;**358**(9281):527–33.

26. McLean DS, Sabatine MS, Guo W, McCabe CH, Cannon CP. Benefits and risks of clopidogrel pretreatment before coronary artery bypass grafting in patients with ST-elevation myocardial infarction treated with fibrinolytics in CLARITY-TIMI 28. *J Thromb Thrombolysis* 2007;**24**(2):85–91.

27. Chen ZM, Jiang LX, Chen YP *et al.* Addition of clopidogrel to aspirin in 45,852 patients with acute myocardial infarction: randomized placebo-controlled trial. *Lancet* 2005;**366**(9497): 1607–21.

28. Sabatine MS, Cannon CP, Gibson CM *et al.* Effect of clopidogrel pretreatment before percutaneous coronary intervention in patients with ST-elevation myocardial infarction treated with fibrinolytics: the PCI-CLARITY study. *JAMA* 2005;**294**(10): 1224–32.

29. Wiviott SD, Braunwald E, McCabe CH *et al.* Prasugrel versus clopidogrel in patients with acute coronary syndromes. *N Engl J Med* 2007;**357**(20):2001–15.

30. Ohman EM, Kleiman NS, Gacioch G *et al.* Combined accelerated tissue-plasminogen activator and platelet glycoprotein IIb/IIIa integrin receptor blockade with Integrilin in acute myocardial infarction. Results of a randomized, placebo-controlled, dose-ranging trial. IMPACT-AMI Investigators. *Circulation* 1997; **95**(4):846–54.

31. Ronner E, van Kesteren HA, Zijnen P *et al.* Safety and efficacy of eptifibatide vs placebo in patients receiving thrombolytic therapy with streptokinase for acute myocardial infarction; a phase II dose escalation, randomized, double-blind study. *Eur Heart J* 2000;**21**(18):1530–6.

32. Antman EM, Giugliano RP, Gibson CM *et al.* Abciximab facilitates the rate and extent of thrombolysis: results of the thrombolysis in myocardial infarction (TIMI) 14 trial. The TIMI 14 Investigators. *Circulation* 1999;**99**(21):2720–32.

33. Herrmann HC, Moliterno DJ, Ohman EM *et al.* Facilitation of early percutaneous coronary intervention after reteplase with or without abciximab in acute myocardial infarction: results from the SPEED (GUSTO-4 Pilot) Trial. *J Am Coll Cardiol* 2000; **36**(5):1489–96.

34. Brener SJ, Zeymer U, Adgey AA *et al.* Eptifibatide and low-dose tissue plasminogen activator in acute myocardial infarction: the integrilin and low-dose thrombolysis in acute myocardial infarction (INTRO AMI) trial. *J Am Coll Cardiol* 2002; **39**(3):377–86.

35. Topol EJ. Reperfusion therapy for acute myocardial infarction with fibrinolytic therapy or combination reduced fibrinolytic therapy and platelet glycoprotein IIb/IIIa inhibition: the GUSTO V randomized trial. *Lancet* 2001;**357**(9272):1905–14.

36. Lincoff AM, Califf RM, Van de Werf F *et al.* Mortality at 1 year with combination platelet glycoprotein IIb/IIIa inhibition and reduced-dose fibrinolytic therapy vs conventional fibrinolytic therapy for acute myocardial infarction: GUSTO V randomized trial. *JAMA* 2002;**288**(17):2130–5.

37. Keeley EC, Boura JA, Grines CL. Comparison of primary and facilitated percutaneous coronary interventions for ST-elevation myocardial infarction: quantitative review of randomized trials. *Lancet* 2006;**367**(9510):579–88.

38. Ito H, Maruyama A, Iwakura K *et al.* Clinical implications of the 'no reflow' phenomenon. A predictor of complications and left ventricular remodeling in reperfused anterior wall myocardial infarction. *Circulation* 1996;**93**(2):223–8.

39. Wu KC, Zerhouni EA, Judd RM *et al.* Prognostic significance of microvascular obstruction by magnetic resonance imaging in patients with acute myocardial infarction. *Circulation* 1998;**97**(8):765–72.

40. van 't Hof AW, Liem A, Suryapranata H, Hoorntje JC, de Boer MJ, Zijlstra F. Angiographic assessment of myocardial reperfusion in patients treated with primary angioplasty for acute myocardial infarction: myocardial blush grade. Zwolle Myocardial Infarction Study Group. *Circulation* 1998;**97**(23):2302–6.

41. Gibson CM, Cannon CP, Murphy SA *et al.* Relationship of TIMI myocardial perfusion grade to mortality after administration of thrombolytic drugs. *Circulation* 2000;**101**(2):125–30.

42. Brener SJ, Barr LA, Burchenal JE *et al.* Randomized, placebo-controlled trial of platelet glycoprotein IIb/IIIa blockade with primary angioplasty for acute myocardial infarction. ReoPro and Primary PTCA Organization and Randomized Trial (RAPPORT) Investigators. *Circulation* 1998;**98**(8):734–41.

43. Montalescot G, Barragan P, Wittenberg O *et al.* Platelet glycoprotein IIb/IIIa inhibition with coronary stenting for acute myocardial infarction. *N Engl J Med* 2001;**344**(25):1895–903.

44. Stone GW, Grines CL, Cox DA *et al.* Comparison of angioplasty with stenting, with or without abciximab, in acute myocardial infarction. *N Engl J Med* 2002;**346**(13):957–66.

45. Kandzari DE, Hasselblad V, Tcheng JE *et al.* Improved clinical outcomes with abciximab therapy in acute myocardial infarction: a systematic overview of randomized clinical trials. *Am Heart J* 2004;**147**(3):457–62.

46. De Luca G, Suryapranata H, Stone GW *et al.* Abciximab as adjunctive therapy to reperfusion in acute ST-segment elevation myocardial infarction: a meta-analysis of randomized trials. *JAMA* 2005;**293**(14):1759–65.

47. Montalescot G, Borentain M, Payot L, Collet JP, Thomas D. Early vs late administration of glycoprotein IIb/IIIa inhibitors in primary percutaneous coronary intervention of acute ST-segment elevation myocardial infarction: a meta-analysis. *JAMA* 2004;**292**(3):362–6.

48. Ellis SG, Tendera M, de Belder MA, *et al.* Facilitated PCI in patients with ST-elevation myocardial infarction. *N Engl J Med* 2008;**358**(21):2205–17.

49. Lee DP, Herity NA, Hiatt BL *et al.* Adjunctive platelet glycoprotein IIb/IIIa receptor inhibition with tirofiban before primary angioplasty improves angiographic outcomes: results of the TIrofiban Given in the Emergency Room before Primary Angioplasty (TIGER-PA) pilot trial. *Circulation* 2003;**107**(11): 1497–501.

50. Zeymer U, Zahn R, Schiele R *et al.* Early eptifibatide improves TIMI 3 patency before primary percutaneous coronary intervention for acute ST elevation myocardial infarction: results of the randomized integrilin in acute myocardial infarction (INTAMI) pilot trial. *Eur Heart J* 2005;**26**(19):1971–7.

51. Cutlip DE, Cove CJ, Irons D *et al.* Emergency room administration of eptifibatide before primary angioplasty for ST elevation acute myocardial infarction and its effect on baseline coronary flow and procedure outcomes. *Am J Cardiol* 2001;**88**(1):**A6**, 62–4.

52. Valgimigli M, Campo G, Percoco G et al. Comparison of angioplasty with infusion of tirofiban or abciximab and with implantation of sirolimus-eluting or uncoated stents for acute myocardial infarction: the MULTISTRATEGY randomized trial. *JAMA* 2008;**299**(15):1788–99.

53. Van't Hof AW, Ten Berg J, Heestermans T, et al. Prehospital initiation of tirofiban in patients with ST-elevation myocardial infarction undergoing primary angioplasty (On-TIME 2): a multicentre, double-blind, randomised controlled trial. *Lancet* 2008;**372**:537–46.

54. Eisenberg PR, Miletich JP. Induction of marked thrombin activity by pharmacologic concentrations of plasminogen activators in nonanticoagulated whole blood. *Thromb Res* 1989;**55**(5):635–43.

55. Lee CD, Mann KG. Activation/inactivation of human factor V by plasmin. *Blood* 1989;**73**(1):185–90.

56. O'Connor CM, Meese R, Carney R et al. A randomized trial of intravenous heparin in conjunction with anistreplase (anisoylated plasminogen streptokinase activator complex) in acute myocardial infarction: the Duke University Clinical Cardiology Study (DUCCS) 1. *J Am Coll Cardiol* 1994;**23**(1):11–18.

57. de Bono DP, Simoons ML, Tijssen J et al. Effect of early intravenous heparin on coronary patency, infarct size, and bleeding complications after alteplase thrombolysis: results of a randomized double blind European Cooperative Study Group trial. *Br Heart J* 1992;**67**(2):122–8.

58. Bleich SD, Nichols TC, Schumacher RR, Cooke DH, Tate DA, Teichman SL. Effect of heparin on coronary arterial patency after thrombolysis with tissue plasminogen activator in acute myocardial infarction. *Am J Cardiol* 1990;**66**(20):1412–17.

59. Hsia J, Hamilton WP, Kleiman N, Roberts R, Chaitman BR, Ross AM. A comparison between heparin and low-dose aspirin as adjunctive therapy with tissue plasminogen activator for acute myocardial infarction. Heparin-Aspirin Reperfusion Trial (HART) Investigators. *N Engl J Med* 1990;**323**(21):1433–7.

60. Topol EJ, George BS, Kereiakes DJ et al. A randomized controlled trial of intravenous tissue plasminogen activator and early intravenous heparin in acute myocardial infarction. *Circulation* 1989;**79**(2):281–6.

61. Gruppo Italiano per lo Studio della Sopravvivenza nell'Infarto Miocardico. GISSI-2: a factorial randomized trial of alteplase versus streptokinase and heparin versus no heparin among 12,490 patients with acute myocardial infarction. *Lancet* 1990; **336**(8707):65–71.

62. ISIS-3 (Third International Study of Infarct Survival) Collaborative Group. ISIS-3: a randomized comparison of streptokinase vs tissue plasminogen activator vs anistreplase and of aspirin plus heparin vs aspirin alone among 41,299 cases of suspected acute myocardial infarction. *Lancet* 1992;**339**(8796):753–70.

63. Collins R, Peto R, Baigent C, Sleight P. Aspirin, heparin, and fibrinolytic therapy in suspected acute myocardial infarction. *N Engl J Med* 1997;**336**(12):847–60.

64. ISIS (International Studies of Infarct Survival) Pilot Study. Randomized factorial trial of high-dose intravenous streptokinase, of oral aspirin and of intravenous heparin in acute myocardial infarction. *Eur Heart J* 1987;**8**(6):634–42.

65. Collins R, MacMahon S, Flather M et al. Clinical effects of anticoagulant therapy in suspected acute myocardial infarction: systematic overview of randomized trials. *BMJ* 1996;**313**(7058): 652–9.

66. Vainer J, Fleisch M, Gunnes P et al. Low-dose heparin for routine coronary angioplasty and stenting. *Am J Cardiol* 1996;**78**(8):964–6.

67. Kontny F, Dale J, Abildgaard U, Pedersen TR. Randomized trial of low molecular weight heparin (dalteparin) in prevention of left ventricular thrombus formation and arterial embolism after acute anterior myocardial infarction: the Fragmin in Acute Myocardial Infarction (FRAMI) Study. *J Am Coll Cardiol* 1997;**30**(4): 962–9.

68. Frostfeldt G, Ahlberg G, Gustafsson G et al. Low molecular weight heparin (dalteparin) as adjuvant treatment of thrombolysis in acute myocardial infarction – a pilot study: biochemical markers in acute coronary syndromes (BIOMACS II). *J Am Coll Cardiol* 1999;**33**(3):627–33.

69. Wallentin L, Dellborg DM, Lindahl B, Nilsson T, Pehrsson K, Swahn E. The low-molecular-weight heparin dalteparin as adjuvant therapy in acute myocardial infarction: the ASSENT PLUS study. *Clin Cardiol* 2001;24(3 suppl):I12–14.

70. Yusuf S, Mehta SR, Xie C et al. Effects of reviparin, a low-molecular-weight heparin, on mortality, reinfarction, and strokes in patients with acute myocardial infarction presenting with ST-segment elevation. *JAMA* 2005;**293**(4):427–35.

71. Simoons M, Krzeminska-Pakula M, Alonso A et al. Improved reperfusion and clinical outcome with enoxaparin as an adjunct to streptokinase thrombolysis in acute myocardial infarction. The AMI-SK study. *Eur Heart J* 2002;**23**(16):1282–90.

72. Ross AM, Molhoek P, Lundergan C et al. Randomized comparison of enoxaparin, a low-molecular-weight heparin, with unfractionated heparin adjunctive to recombinant tissue plasminogen activator thrombolysis and aspirin: second trial of Heparin and Aspirin Reperfusion Therapy (HART II). *Circulation* 2001;**104**(6):648–52.

73. Antman EM, Morrow DA, McCabe CH et al. Enoxaparin versus unfractionated heparin with fibrinolysis for ST-elevation myocardial infarction. *N Engl J Med* 2006;**354**(14):1477–88.

74. Sabatine MS, Morrow DA, Dalby A et al. Efficacy and safety of enoxaparin versus unfractionated heparin in patients with ST-segment elevation myocardial infarction also treated with clopidogrel. *J Am Coll Cardiol* 2007;**49**(23):2256–63.

75. Fox KA, Antman EM, Montalescot G et al. The impact of renal dysfunction on outcomes in the ExTRACT-TIMI 25 trial. *J Am Coll Cardiol* 2007;**49**(23):2249–55.

76. Theroux P, Welsh RC. Meta-analysis of randomized trials comparing enoxaparin versus unfractionated heparin as adjunctive therapy to fibrinolysis in ST-elevation acute myocardial infarction. *Am J Cardiol* 2003;**91**(7):860–4.

77. Murphy SA, Gibson CM, Morrow DA et al. Efficacy and safety of the low-molecular weight heparin enoxaparin compared with unfractionated heparin across the acute coronary syndrome spectrum: a meta-analysis. *Eur Heart J* 2007;**28**(12):2077–86.

78. Borentain M, Montalescot G, Bouzamondo A, Choussat R, Hulot JS, Lechat P. Low-molecular-weight heparin vs. unfractionated heparin in percutaneous coronary intervention: a combined analysis. *Catheter Cardiovasc Interv* 2005;**65**(2):212–21.

79. Wong GC, Giugliano RP, Antman EM. Use of low-molecular-weight heparins in the management of acute coronary artery syndromes and percutaneous coronary intervention. *JAMA* 2003;**289**(3):331–42.

80. Ferguson JJ, Califf RM, Antman EM et al. Enoxaparin vs unfractionated heparin in high-risk patients with non-ST-segment

elevation acute coronary syndromes managed with an intended early invasive strategy: primary results of the SYNERGY randomized trial. *JAMA* 2004;**292**(1):45–54.

81. Gibson CM, Murphy SA, Montalescot G *et al.* Percutaneous coronary intervention in patients receiving enoxaparin or unfractionated heparin after fibrinolytic therapy for ST-segment elevation myocardial infarction in the ExTRACT-TIMI 25 trial. *J Am Coll Cardiol* 2007;**49**(23):2238–46.

82. Aggarwal A, Sobel BE, Schneider DJ. Decreased platelet reactivity in blood anticoagulated with bivalirudin or enoxaparin compared with unfractionated heparin: implications for coronary intervention. *J Thromb Thrombolysis* 2002;**13**(3):161–5.

83. Direct Thrombin Inhibitor Trialists' Collaborative Group. Direct thrombin inhibitors in acute coronary syndromes: principal results of a meta-analysis based on individual patients' data. *Lancet* 2002;**359**(9303):294–302.

84. Stone GW, McLaurin BT, Cox DA *et al.* Bivalirudin for patients with acute coronary syndromes. *N Engl J Med* 2006;**355**(21): 2203–16.

85. Stone GW, Witzenbichler B, Guagliumi G *et al.* Bivalirudin during primary PCI in acute myocardial infarction. *N Engl J Med* 2008;**358**(21):2218–30.

86. Lewis BE, Wallis DE, Leya F, Hursting MJ, Kelton JG. Argatroban anticoagulation in patients with heparin-induced thrombocytopenia. *Arch Intern Med* 2003;**163**(15):1849–56.

87. Jang IK, Lewis BE, Matthai WH Jr, Kleiman NS. Argatroban anticoagulation in conjunction with glycoprotein IIb/IIIa inhibition in patients undergoing percutaneous coronary intervention: an open-label, nonrandomized pilot study. *J Thromb Thrombolysis* 2004;**18**(1):31–7.

88. Weitz JI, Hirsh J. New anticoagulant drugs. *Chest* 2001;**119** (1 suppl):95S–107S.

89. Coussement PK, Bassand JP, Convens C *et al.* A synthetic factor-Xa inhibitor (ORG31540/SR9017A) as an adjunct to fibrinolysis in acute myocardial infarction. The PENTALYSE study. *Eur Heart J* 2001;**22**(18):1716–24.

90. Yusuf S, Mehta SR, Chrolavicius S *et al.* Comparison of fondaparinux and enoxaparin in acute coronary syndromes. *N Engl J Med* 2006;**354**(14):1464–76.

91. Yusuf S, Mehta SR, Chrolavicius S *et al.* Effects of fondaparinux on mortality and reinfarction in patients with acute ST-segment elevation myocardial infarction: the OASIS-6 randomized trial. *JAMA* 2006;**295**(13):1519–30.

92. Greenbaum AB, Grines CL, Bittl JA *et al.* Initial experience with an intravenous P2Y12 platelet receptor antagonist in patients undergoing percutaneous coronary intervention: results from a 2-part, phase II, multicenter, randomized, placebo- and active-controlled trial. *Am Heart J* 2006;**151**(3):e681–689, e610.

93. Lefer AM, Campbell B, Scalia R, Lefer DJ. Synergism between platelets and neutrophils in provoking cardiac dysfunction after ischemia and reperfusion: role of selectins. *Circulation* 1998;**98**(13):1322–8.

94. Ott I, Malcouvier V, Schomig A, Neumann FJ. Proteolysis of tissue factor pathway inhibitor-1 by thrombolysis in acute myocardial infarction. *Circulation* 2002;**105**(3):279–81.

95. Gold HK, Garabedian HD, Dinsmore RE *et al.* Restoration of coronary flow in myocardial infarction by intravenous chimeric 7E3 antibody without exogenous plasminogen activators: observations in humans and animal. *Circulation* 1997;**95**:1755–9.

96. van den Merkhof LFM, Zijlstra F, Olsson H *et al.* Abciximab in the treatment of acute myocardial infarction eligible for primary percutaneous transluminal coronary angioplasty: Glycoprotein Receptor Antagonist Patency Evaluation (GRAPE) pilot study. *J Am Coll Cardiol* 1999;**33**:1528–32.

33 Complications after myocardial infarction

Peter L Thompson
University of Western Australia, Perth, Western Australia

Introduction

Despite major changes in treatment and prevention, myocardial infarction (MI) remains a common and lethal condition. The World Health Organization estimates that 7.6 million people died from cardiovascular disease in 2005, representing 30% of all global deaths,[1] and the global burden of coronary heart disease is projected to rise from around 47 million disability-adjusted life years (DALYs) in 1990 to 82 million DALYs in 2020.[2] The new definition of acute myocardial infarction, which has been expanded to include patients with clinical and electrocardiographic features of myocardial ischemia and an elevation of troponin outside the 99th percentile of the upper limit of the reference limit, will substantially increase the numbers of people who are diagnosed with acute myocardial infarction.[3] Reinfarction after myocardial infarction is a common complication, and mechanical complications include acute and chronic heart failure, cardiogenic shock, ventricular aneurysm, right ventricular infarction and failure, mitral regurgitation due to papillary muscle dysfunction or rupture, rupture of the interventricular septum and rupture of the free wall of the left ventricle. Electrical complications include ventricular fibrillation, ventricular tachycardia, atrial fibrillation, and atrioventricular block. Psychosocial and socioeconomic consequences are common and frequently neglected complications of myocardial infarction. Other chapters in this book cover the topics of left ventricular dysfunction and heart failure (Chapter 47), ventricular arrhythmias (Chapter 40), bradyarrhythmias (Chapter 41) and atrial fibrillation (Chapters 35–38).

The major complications of MI, such as left ventricular (LV) dysfunction, heart failure or ventricular and atrial arrhythmias, lend themselves to study with controlled clinical trials. However, for many of the acute complications of MI, clinical trials have not been performed, and clinical decision making must rely on evidence from other sources including uncontrolled trials, observational studies and inference from pathophysiologic data. The evidence base for managing the complications of MI will be discussed under the headings of clinical features and prognosis, and management.

Reinfarction, extension and expansion of infarction

The terminology of reinfarction can be confusing: the term *reinfarction* is used when there is new myocardial necrosis, *infarct extension* when an area of infarction extends to involve adjacent ischemic tissue[4] and *infarct expansion* when the infarcted tissue expands and contributes to hemodynamic deterioration. Infarct expansion does not require revascularization, but is treated by measures to control left ventricular dysfunction (see below). Reinfarction in patients with either non-ST segment elevation myocardial infarction (NSTEMI)[5] or ST elevation MI (STEMI)[6] may represent an extension of the initial necrosis or a new episode of infarction. The new universal definition of myocardial infarction recommends a diagnosis of reinfarction based on typical clinical features with a troponin elevation of >20% above earlier levels.[3] The evidence that the risk of reinfarction in NSTEMI is lessened by early angiography and revascularization is now strong. In a meta-analysis of seven trials with 8375 patients, all-cause mortality at one month was reduced by 25% at two years (relative risk (RR) 0.75, 95% confidence interval (CI) 0.63–0.90, $P = 0.001$) and the incidence of non-fatal myocardial infarction was reduced by 17% (RR 0.83, 95% CI 0.72–0.96, $P = 0.012$) in the early invasive group compared with the conservative group.[7] In STEMI treated with fibrinolysis, reinfarction can occur in 4–8% of patients. The reinfarction rate is significantly lower when primary percutaneous coronary intervention (PCI) is the initial treatment.[8]

Evidence-Based Cardiology, 3rd edition. Edited by S. Yusuf, J.A. Cairns, A.J. Camm, E.L. Fallen, and B.J. Gersh. © 2010 Blackwell Publishing, ISBN: 978-1-4051-5925-8.

Coronary reperfusion with fibrinolysis or PCI is strongly recommended and reduces the risk of reinfarction in STEMI (**Class I, Level A**).

In STEMI, PCI achieves better rates of reperfusion and is preferable to the use of fibrinolysis when available (**Class I, Level A**).

The risk of reinfarction in NSTEMI is reduced with early invasive investigation and revascularization where appropriate (**Class I, Level A**).

Left ventricular dysfunction and pulmonary congestion

Clinical features and prognosis

Pathophysiology

Adverse remodeling of the ventricle can occur immediately after coronary occlusion[9] and continues over the ensuing months and years, leading to an increase in end-diastolic and end-systolic volumes, an increase in the sphericity of the ventricle, and systolic bulging and thinning of the infarct zone, without necessarily any extension of the infarcted zone.[10] Results from autopsy studies suggested that MIs that involved greater than 40% of the left ventricle were usually fatal.[11] However, a more recent prospective study conducted in the reperfusion era showed that out of 16 patients with infarcts involving >40% of the myocardial mass and followed for 13 months, only one had persistent heart failure and subsequently died.[12] Extensive damage can occur as a consequence of one large infarction or multiple smaller ones. NSTEMI may also cause left ventricular dysfunction if there has been prior cumulative myocardial damage.[13]

Prognostic markers based on left ventricular dysfunction

The extent of LV dysfunction is a strong predictor of short- and long-term prognosis after MI. The Killip and Kimball[14] classification stratifies MI patients from low to very high risk based upon clinical signs of heart failure. It remains a reasonably accurate predictor of short-term survival. In patients undergoing primary percutaneous transluminal coronary angioplasty (PTCA), the in-hospital mortality was 2.4%, 7%, and 19% for Killip class I, II, and III respectively and six-month mortality was 4%, 10%, and 28% for class I, II, and III, respectively.[15] The Forrester classification, comprising four categories defined according to the presence or absence of pulmonary congestion and peripheral hypoperfusion, requires measurement of the pulmonary artery pressure using a balloon flotation catheter.[16] In postinfarction patients,[17] abnormal hemodynamic variables determined from right heart catheterization correlate strongly with a higher mortality even after adjusting for other prognostic variables. However, insertion of balloon

flotation catheters, while safe in experienced hands, has a recognized risk of adverse events, including ventricular tachyarrhythmias and pulmonary hemorrhage or infarction.[18] Meta-analyses of trials using pulmonary artery catheterization have failed to show any benefit on outcomes,[19] while increasing length of hospital stay.[20] Recent guidelines recommend the use of balloon flotation catheters only in severe or progressive congestive heart failure (CHF) or pulmonary edema, cardiogenic shock or progressive hypotension or suspected mechanical complications of acute infarction, i.e. ventricular septal defect (VSD), papillary muscle rupture or pericardial tamponade.[6]

Late (>30 days) postinfarction mortality was 3% in patients with an ejection fraction (EF) above 0.40, 12% when the EF was between 0.20 and 0.40, and 47% when it was below 0.20.[21] The presence of clinical signs of left ventricular failure is a strong indicator of a poor long-term prognosis but in most patients, more detailed assessment is necessary and the use of echocardiography or radionuclide assessment may provide information that cannot be obtained clinically.[22] Approximately two-thirds of patients with an ejection fraction low enough to indicate a poor long-term prognosis, e.g. <0.40, have no radiologic evidence of left ventricular failure.[23] The information obtained from assessing left ventricular function by echocardiography, radionuclide imaging or cardiac catheterization has been found to be of equivalent value in predicting one-year prognosis[24] and the choice of modality for assessment of left ventricular function depends on local availability and expertise. The left ventricular chamber volume has long been established as an important marker of long-term prognosis after myocardial infarction,[25] and the prevention of adverse remodeling by early coronary reperfusion is an important therapeutic aim in current treatment of myocardial infarction.[26] However, despite successful restoration of epicardial blood flow, left ventricular remodeling is still seen in a substantial number of patients, probably as a result of microvascular dysfunction in the coronary vessels.[27] Various methods of documenting this phenomenon have included measurements of the extent of recovery of ST segment elevation,[28] the myocardial blush grade on coronary angiography,[29] an index of microcirculatory resistance measured at angiography,[30] cardiac magnetic resonance imaging (MRI)[31] and myocardial contrast echocardiography.[32] The latter technique has been shown in a multicenter study to be superior to measurements of ST segment resolution and myocardial blush grade in predicting adverse remodeling.[32] Simple bedside scores based on readily available clinical data can also accurately stratify the risks of death and ischemic events in STEMI patients, as shown in large clinical trials such as the GUSTO,[33] GISSI[34] and TIMI trials,[35] in NSTEMI, as shown in the TIMI trials,[36] and in non-STE acute coronary syndromes as shown in the Global Registry of Acute Coronary Events (GRACE).[37]

Measurements of left ventricular function and diastolic volume predict short- and long-term prognosis after STEMI (**Level A**).

Clinical markers of prognosis can be used for risk stratification after STEMI and NSTEMI with a high degree of accuracy (**Level A**).

Biochemical markers

Biochemical markers of necrosis provide an index of the extent of left ventricular infarction, which in turn is correlated with the extent of left ventricular dysfunction. Creatine kinase was shown in the pre-reperfusion era to predict short- and long-term prognosis[38] but the introduction of reperfusion into routine clinical practice has reduced the utility of creatine kinase (CK) or CK-MB to reflect the extent of left ventricular dysfunction because of early, direct release of the myocardial enzymes into the plasma during reperfusion and high, early peaking of the serum levels. The use of newer markers such as troponins is now widespread. Both troponin-I[39] and troponin-T[40] correlate well with prognosis, and 96-hour troponin levels correlate well with infarct size.[41] B-type natriuretic peptide[42] and high sensitivity C-reactive protein[43] also correlate with cardiac failure and predict long-term prognosis after acute MI (AMI). A multimarker approach to using these biomarkers has been suggested, as patients with more than three abnormal biomarker levels have a worse prognosis than those with normal levels of biomarkers (hazard ratio (HR) 3.8 after correction for standard prognostic factors).[44]

Ninety-six hour troponin levels provide a quantitative index of the extent of infarction (**Level B**).

Management

Reperfusion therapy

While the role of early coronary reperfusion in improving outcomes has been well established, the relationship between improvements in left ventricular function and prognosis after reperfusion therapy has been surprisingly difficult to demonstrate. Although some of the early studies demonstrated clear benefits on left ventricular function from coronary thrombolysis,[45,46] the evidence since then has been conflicting, with some groups showing a worse left ventricular function despite an improved prognosis. In a meta-analysis of 10 studies enrolling 4088 patients treated with thrombolytic therapy versus control, only a modest improvement in left ventricular function was demonstrated after thrombolytic therapy.[47] By four days, mean LV ejection fraction was 53% versus 47% (thrombolytic versus control therapy, $P < 0.01$); by 10–28 days it was 54.1% and 51.5%, respectively. The reason for the discrepancy in the marked improvement in survival and the limited benefit on left ventricular function is not clear but is at least in part due to the fact that more patients not receiving fibrinolytic therapy die before LV function can be assessed post MI. Patients who have had coronary reperfusion after MI may have myocardium that is stunned[48] or even hibernating,[49] phenomena that may affect the assessment of ventricular function, and the preinfarction left ventricular function obviously impacts on the LV function during and after myocardial infarction. Stunned myocardium has been successfully reperfused but has not regained its normal contractile function, but has the potential to recover without any further reperfusion or revascularization. A study of 352 patients with anterior MI found that out of the 252 patients with abnormal LV function on day 1, 22% had complete and 36% had partial recovery of function by day 90.[50] Hibernating myocardium is underperfused and non-contractile because of persisting ischemia, but is not infarcted and may gradually improve its function with revascularization. The degree of success in achieving coronary patency with thrombolysis is an obvious confounding factor.[51] A detailed analysis correcting for these confounding factors concluded that left ventricular function is improved by successful coronary reperfusion.[52]

Overall, reperfusion therapy results in a modest improvement in systolic LV function (**Level B**).

Hemodynamic therapy

Improvements in hemodynamic status after myocardial infarction have not translated into better outcomes. For example, furosemide has been shown to reduce elevated LV filling pressures without adversely affecting cardiac output[53] but there is no evidence of improvement in outcomes with diuretic therapy in AMI. Nitrates have been shown to improve the hemodynamic status and adverse remodeling post AMI[54] but large clinical trials have not shown improved prognosis.[55,56] The calcium-sensitizing agent levosimendan has been evaluated in post-MI patients with cardiac failure and showed only a non-statistically significant trend towards improved outcome.[57] Infusion of the B-type natriuretic peptide nesiritide for acutely decompensated heart failure, including some patients with acute myocardial infarction, was initially reported to be safer than inotropic agents[58] but a meta-analysis of all trials showed an apparent adverse effect on outcomes.[59] In contrast, aldosterone antagonists have been shown to be beneficial in post-MI patients with left ventricular dysfunction and pulmonary congestion. The Randomized Aldactone Evaluation Study (RALES) studied patients with New York Heart Association class III–IV heart failure, many with remote myocardial infarction. Spironolactone treatment compared with placebo was associated with an 11% absolute risk reduction and 30% relative risk reduction in all-cause mortality over 24 months of follow-up.[60] The Eplerenone Post-Acute Myocardial Infarction Heart Failure Efficacy and Survival Study (EPHESUS) demonstrated that in post-MI patients with an ejection fraction <0.40 and heart failure or diabetes that compared with placebo, eplerenone significantly reduced overall mortality, cardiovascular mortality, and cardiac hospitalizations.[61]

Diuretics and nitrates can be used for relief of pulmonary congestion in acute MI, but there is no clinical trial evidence of benefit on outcomes (**Class I, Level B**).

Aldosterone antagonists (spironolactone and eplerenone) are indicated in post-MI patients with left ventricular dysfunction or pulmonary congestion (**Class I, Level A**).

Levosimendan may be considered as an alternative treatment in patients with severe cardiac failure following MI (**Class IIa, Level B**).

Nesiritide should not be used in patients with pulmonary congestion complicating myocardial infarction because of concerns about its safety profile (**Class III, Level A**).

ACE inhibitors for post-MI patients with left ventricular dysfunction

The beneficial effects of angiotensin-converting enzyme (ACE) inhibitors in the treatment of patients with left ventricular dysfunction complicating myocardial infarction have been striking. Eight large randomized, placebo-controlled trials have assessed the effect of an ACE inhibitor on mortality after MI. ACE inhibitors unequivocally reduce mortality overall, and the benefit appears to be greatest among patients with depressed LV function, overt heart failure or anterior infarction.[62–69]

In a meta-analysis of data from all the randomized trials involving more than 1000 patients in whom ACE inhibitor treatment was started within 36 hours of onset of myocardial infarction, there were results available on 98 496 patients from four eligible trials.[70] Among patients allocated to ACE inhibitors there was a 7% (95% CI 2–11%; $2P < 0.004$) proportional reduction in early mortality, an absolute reduction of five (SD, 2) deaths per 1000 patients. The absolute benefit was greatest in those patients with evidence of left ventricular dysfunction (i.e. Killip class 2–3, heart rate > = 100 bpm at entry) and in anterior MI. ACE inhibitor therapy also reduced the incidence of non-fatal manifestations of left ventricular dysfunction. During longer-term follow-up of patients enrolled in randomized controlled trials, ACE inhibitors have also been shown to be effective. In three long-term follow-up trials involving 5966 postinfarction patients, mortality was significantly lower with ACE inhibitors than with placebo (odds ratio (OR) 0.74, 95% CI 0.66–0.83).[71] Despite concerns that aspirin may blunt the effect of ACE inhibitors,[72] a detailed analysis of six long-term trials showed no adverse interaction between aspirin and ACE inhibitors.[73] The optimum timing of initiation of ACE inhibitor therapy has been studied in only a small number of direct comparative trials. In a direct comparison of early versus delayed administration, 352 patients with acute anterior myocardial infarction were randomized to early (1–14 days) or late (14–19 days) post-MI treatment with the ACE inhibitor ramipril and were followed by echocardiography. Those receiving early treatment had a greater improvement in ejection fraction, suggesting that such patients should be commenced on ACE inhibitor therapy early in their course of infarction.[74]

In considering treatment for left ventricular dysfunction, the hemodynamic benefits need to be balanced against the possible adverse effect. In the only ACE inhibitor trial that did not show a mortality benefit, CONSENSUS-II, treatment was begun early with an intravenous ACE inhibitor.[62]

All patients with post-MI LV dysfunction should be administered ACE inhibitors (**Class I, Level A**).

ACE inhibitors for post-MI patients without left ventricular dysfunction

Whether low-risk postinfarction patients without LV dysfunction derive benefit from ACE inhibitors is still controversial. The clear-cut benefits demonstrated in the HOPE[75] trial of ramipril in high-risk patients with coronary artery disease and the EUROPA trial of perindopril in post-AMI patients without left ventricular dysfunction[76] were not supported by the PEACE trial of trandolopril in lower risk patients.[77] A subsequent meta-analysis of the three trials supported the use of ACE inhibitors in the absence of LV dysfunction[78] and the totality of the evidence was examined in a meta-analysis of six trials including 16 772 patients randomized to ACE inhibitors and 16 728 patients randomized to placebo, which concluded that the benefits were favorable though modest,[79] consistent with the conclusion that the absolute benefit is proportional to the risk, with those at lowest risk benefiting least.[5]

ACE inhibitors are indicated for post-MI patients even in the absence of left ventricular dysfunction, but are more beneficial in patients at higher risk (**Class IIa, Level A**).

Cardiogenic shock

Clinical features and prognosis

Cardiogenic shock is a syndrome characterized by hypotension and peripheral hypoperfusion, usually accompanied by high LV filling pressures. The common clinical manifestations of these hemodynamic derangements include mental obtundation or confusion, cold and clammy skin, and oliguria or anuria. Cardiogenic shock is the most common cause of in-hospital mortality after MI.[80] When cardiogenic shock is not secondary to a correctable cause, such as arrhythmia, bradycardia, hypovolemia or a mechanical defect, short-term mortality is 80% or higher, depending upon the strictness of the definition. Despite the major improvements in treatment in the past two decades, the in-hospital mortality in a recent international registry for patients with cardiogenic shock treated with modern therapy in the late 1990s was 66%.[81] Old age, diabetes, previous infarction and extensive infarction as assessed either by enzymatic or electrocardiographic criteria are factors commonly associated with cardiogenic shock. Among patients receiving fibrinolytic therapy, the risk of cardiogenic shock increased by 47% with each decade increase in age.[82] Patients who survive to 30 days after cardiogenic shock have an excellent late survival, almost as good as patients without shock.[83]

Management

Inotropic drugs have been subjected to detailed study and widespread use in cardiogenic shock, but no benefit on mortality has been demonstrated.[84]

Newer drugs such as levosimendan may improve myocardial efficiency by their calcium-sensitizing effect, but levosimendan also has vasodilating properties, which make it unsuitable for patients in cardiogenic shock with significant hypotension.[85] Nesiritide has been shown to improve pulmonary capillary wedge pressure in patients with decompensated heart failure[86] but was subsequently shown to increase mortality.[87]

Intra-aortic balloon pumping has been used to stabilize patients with cardiogenic shock. Clear-cut benefits on hemodynamic status and coronary blood flow have been shown, but benefits on survival have not; in-hospital mortality remained at 83% despite the use of balloon pumping in a co-operative clinical trial.[88] Nevertheless, intra-aortic balloon pumping has a clear place in stabilizing the unstable cardiogenic shock patient for more definitive treatment such as coronary angioplasty or bypass surgery,[89] as has been demonstrated to improve coronary patency in a randomized trial in the setting of rescue angioplasty.[90] Newer methods of circulatory support have shown highly encouraging results[91,92] but benefits on survival remain to be established.

Fibrinolysis

Although the outcome of cardiogenic shock has been shown to be dependent on the patency of the infarct-related artery, clinical trials of fibrinolytic therapy have not shown a benefit in patients with established cardiogenic shock.[93] Alternative antithrombotic strategies may improve outcomes, but data are limited to observational studies.[94]

Fibrinolysis could be considered for the patient with cardiogenic shock if access to PCI is not readily available (**Class IIb, Level B**).

Percutaneous coronary intervention or CABG

Observational studies on the use of PCI in cardiogenic shock suggest that an aggressive approach with early revascularization reduces the mortality of patients with cardiogenic shock after MI,[95] and a registry report has suggested that an aggressive approach with reperfusion therapy and intra-aortic balloon pulsation treatment of patients in cardiogenic shock due to predominant LV failure is associated with lower in-hospital mortality rates than standard medical therapy.[96] In a controlled clinical trial of an aggressive approach involving early catheterization with revascularization and intra-aortic balloon pumping, in cardiogenic shock patients (the SHOCK trial),[97] 87% of patients in the invasive arm underwent revascularization (surgical or percutaneous). There was a clear trend at 30 days towards reduced mortality in the invasive group compared with the medical therapy group (46.7% vs 56.0%); however, this difference did not reach statistical significance. There was an early hazard in the first five days after assignment to the invasive approach, which was likely associated with procedure-related complications. However, after the first five days there was a statistically significant survival benefit in favor of the revascularization group, which persisted at one year, when survival in the early revascularization group was 46.7% compared with 33.6% in those treated with early medical stabilization (RR for death 0.7, 95% CI 0.54–0.95).[98]

Evidence from clinical trials and registries supports invasive intervention in patients with cardiogenic shock post MI. These patients should undergo urgent coronary angiography with a view to coronary angioplasty or, in selected patients, coronary bypass surgery (**Class I, Level A**).

Right ventricular infarction and failure

Clinical features and prognosis

Right ventricular (RV) infarction typically occurs in association with inferior or posterior MI, as a consequence of total occlusion of the right coronary artery proximal to its marginal branches[99] or of the proximal circumflex in patients with a dominant left coronary system. RV infarction was present in 54% of patients with inferior MI in one series, although clinical manifestations are usually evident in only 10–15%.[100] Right ventricular involvement in inferior infarction has been reported to increase the mortality by fivefold. A meta-analysis of six studies including 1198 patients confirmed that RV myocardial involvement was associated with an increased risk of death (OR 3.2, 95% CI 2.4–4.1), shock (OR 3.2, 95% CI 2.4–3.5), and arrhythmic complications.[101] Patients in the SHOCK trial registry with cardiogenic shock due to RV infarction had the same serious prognosis (hospital mortality in excess of 50%) as patients with shock due to predominant LV infarction.[102] Early reperfusion may improve the prognosis: in patients who have primary PCI for treatment of their cardiogenic shock, those with right ventricular infarction fared better than patients with cardiogenic shock due to left ventricular infarction.[103,104]

The clinical features of RV infarction complicating inferior MI include hypotension, an elevated jugular venous pressure and clear lung fields. Jugular venous distension on inspiration (Kussmaul's sign) has been reported to be a sensitive and specific sign of RV infarction.[105] The hemodynamic features of RV infarction may disappear with volume depletion or may emerge only after volume loading, making the clinical diagnosis elusive in some cases.

ST segment elevation in a right precordial lead (V_{4R}) has been reported to have a sensitivity of 70% and a specificity of nearly 100% for the diagnosis of RV infarction when the electrocardiogram is recorded within the first hours after the onset of symptoms. Echocardiography commonly reveals wall motion abnormalities of the right ventricle and interventricular septum. Bowing of the interatrial septum toward the left atrium indicates that the right atrial pressure exceeds the left atrial pressure,[106] and bowing of the interventricular septum into the right ventricle, compounding the dysfunction of the right ventricle,[107] both indicate a poor prognosis. Detection of a low RV EF and a segmental wall motion abnormality by radionuclide right ventriculography had a sensitivity of 92% and a specificity of 82% for identifying hemodynamically significant RV infarction in one study.[105] Assessment of RV function can help assess long-term prognosis, with patients with right ventricular ejection fraction having a risk of death four times that of patients with normal RV function.[108]

Patients with RV infarction complicating inferior MI have three times the risk of death of patients without RV infarction (**Level A**).

Patients with cardiogenic shock due to RV infarction have the same poor prognosis (>50% hospital mortality) as patients with LV infarction (**Level A**).

Management

Volume loading can normalize blood pressure and increase cardiac output.[109] Earlier studies of RV infarction demonstrated a marked response to volume loading.[110] Many of these patients were volume depleted secondary to aggressive diuresis in response to a raised venous pressure.

Volume loading can achieve hemodynamic improvement but has not been shown to improve outcomes (**Class I, Level B**).

Inotropic agents are often used in the treatment of right ventricular infarction when volume loading fails to improve cardiac output, but the effect of this on prognosis is unclear. The maintenance of atrioventricular synchrony is often critical to the maintenance of a satisfactory cardiac output; atrioventricular pacing has been shown to improve hemodynamics.[111] Successful reperfusion with fibrinolysis[112] or PCI[113] appears to reduce the incidence of RV infarction and

is associated with dramatic recovery of right ventricular function and reduced mortality. In contrast, unsuccessful right coronary artery reperfusion was associated with a high mortality.[114]

Reperfusion therapy in right ventricular infarction has not been studied in randomized trials but appears to be effective (**Level B**).

Left ventricular aneurysm

Clinical features and prognosis

Left ventricular aneurysms develop most commonly after large transmural anterior MIs, although in 5–15% of cases the site is inferior or posterior.[115] The diagnosis of aneurysm is less frequent in the reperfusion era, although documented trends have not been published. The coronary anatomy is an important determinant of the development of left ventricular aneurysm. Total occlusion of the left anterior descending artery in association with poor collateral blood supply is a significant determinant of aneurysm formation in anterior MI. Multivessel disease with either good collateral circulation or a patent left anterior descending artery is uncommonly associated with the development of left ventricular aneurysm.[116] Coronary patency also determines the likelihood of developing aneurysm.[117] A ventricular aneurysm can often be palpated as a dyskinetic region adjacent to the apical impulse. A third heart sound and signs of heart failure may also be detected. A non-specific marker of an aneurysm is ST segment elevation that persists weeks after the acute phase of infarction. Echocardiography can delineate LV aneurysms as well as left ventriculography and has a higher sensitivity in the detection of thrombus.[118] A left ventricular aneurysm may cause no problems, but may be associated with heart failure because the left ventricle functions at a mechanical disadvantage. Ventricular tachycardia late after infarction is commonly associated with an aneurysm, but its incidence may be reduced in patients receiving thrombolysis. In a non-randomized study of patients who developed a ventricular aneurysm after myocardial infarction, inducible ventricular tachycardia was less likely in patients who had received fibrinolytic therapy than those who had not (8% vs 88%; $P = 0.0008$) and there was a reduced incidence of sudden death on subsequent follow-up (0% vs 50%; $P = 0.002$).[119] A ventricular aneurysm also provides a nidus for the development of an intracavitary thrombus. The risk of a clinical embolic event, based on four observational studies, is approximately 5%[120] and is greatest within the first few weeks post infarction.

Management

Surgical removal of a left ventricular aneurysm is indicated in patients with heart failure that is difficult to control medically, in patients with recurrent ventricular tachycardia not controlled by other means, and in patients with embolic episodes in spite of adequate anticoagulation.[121] The earlier technique of linear excision of the aneurysm was associated with a high mortality, and has been supplanted by geometric reconstruction surgery in which the aneurysm is excluded from the left ventricular cavity, first described by Vincent Dor.[122] An overview of the reported results of the newer approach suggested substantially better outcomes,[123] but recent RCT revealed no benefit.[123a]

Surgical treatment of post-MI left ventricular aneurysms can help in the control of intractable cardiac failure (**Class IIB, Level C**).

A pseudoaneurysm is a rare complication of MI that develops when a myocardial rupture is sealed off by surrounding adherent pericardium. The aneurysmal sac may progressively enlarge but maintains a narrow neck, in contrast to a true ventricular aneurysm. In a series of 290 patients with LV pseudoaneurysms, congestive heart failure, chest pain and dyspnea were the most frequently reported symptoms, but >10% of patients were asymptomatic.[124] Physical examination revealed a murmur in 70% of patients. Almost all patients had electrocardiographic abnormalities, but only 20% of patients had ST segment elevation. Radiographic findings were frequently nonspecific but a mass was detected in more than one half of patients. Differentiation of left ventricular pseudoaneurysms from true aneurysms may be difficult, and can be enhanced with echocardiography[125] or magnetic resonance imaging.[126] Regardless of treatment, patients with LV pseudoaneurysms have a high mortality rate, but especially those who are managed non-surgically.[127] Surgical repair can be achieved, albeit with a high mortality.[128]

Surgery should be considered in all patients with LV pseudoaneurysms (**Class IIB, Level B**).

Free wall rupture

Clinical features and prognosis

Rupture of the free wall of the left ventricle is an almost uniformly fatal complication of MI that now probably accounts for 10–20% of in-hospital deaths.[129] In the GISSI trial, cardiac rupture was the cause of 19% of the deaths among patients aged 60 years or younger and 86% of deaths among those more than 70 years old.[130] Rupture occurs most frequently in elderly women.[131] Anterior infarctions, hypertension on admission and marked or persistent ST elevation are also risk factors for rupture.[132] The usual presentation is sudden collapse, associated electrical-mechanical dissociation, and failure to respond to cardiopulmonary resuscitation, although in some patients

ventricular rupture is subacute, allowing time for antemortem diagnosis.[133] This clinical entity is probably under-recognized and may be amenable to surgical repair. Premonitory symptoms of chest discomfort, a sense of impending doom and intermittent bradycardia signal impending myocardial rupture in many cases[134] and, if recognized, can lead to life-saving surgery[135] although, in one report[136] of 81 consecutive patients presenting with acute hypotension with electrical–mechanical dissociation, 19 survived with medical management alone. Urgent echocardiography is invaluable in the assessment of a patient who develops the above clinical features.[137]

Overall, reperfusion reduces the frequency of rupture[138] but a meta-analysis of 58 cases of rupture involving 1638 patients from four trials showed that the odds ratio (treated/control) of cardiac rupture was directly correlated with time to treatment ($P = 0.01$); late administration of fibrinolytic therapy may increase the risk of cardiac rupture.[139]

Management

Urgent surgical repair is mandatory for acute rupture[140] (**Class I, Level B**).

Pericarditis

Clinical features and prognosis

Pericarditis occurs in approximately 25% of patients with Q-wave infarctions and 9% of patients with non-Q wave infarctions;[141] it usually occurs within the first week.[142] A pericardial friction rub may be present but is not found in half of patients with typical symptoms and is not required for diagnosis or treatment. On the other hand, the only evidence of pericarditis in many patients is a transient pericardial rub, with no symptoms. Pericarditis following myocardial infarction is associated with a higher risk of death in the year post infarction, possibly due to the associated large effusion.[141]

Management

High-dose aspirin and non-steroidal anti-inflammatory drugs (NSAIDs) are recommended to treat the symptoms of postinfarction pericarditis, although no randomized studies have been done to document their efficacy. Prolonged administration of NSAIDs should be avoided. A serial echocardiographic study of patients with postinfarction pericarditis showed that patients treated with indomethacin or ibuprofen showed a greater tendency for infarct expansion, but it was not clear if the infarct expansion was due to the NSAIDs or to the selection for treatment of those with larger infarctions.[143] There is evidence that the adverse effects of the COX-2 inhibitors may affect endothelial function and enhance thrombosis by inhibiting the production of prostacyclin.[144] Recent reports indicate that the risks may be as high with all NSAIDs.[145,146] Until more observations become available, limited use of COX-2 inhibitors and NSAIDs in acute coronary syndromes is a sensible precaution.

A single dose or short-term treatment with a non-steroidal agent may be very effective for postinfarction pericarditis, but long-term therapy should be avoided (**Class IIb, Level B**).

Pericardial effusion and tamponade

A pericardial effusion can be detected by echocardiography in one-quarter of patients with acute Q-wave MI.[147] This finding correlates with the presence of heart failure and a poor prognosis. Cardiac tamponade is a rare complication of fibrinolytic therapy for acute MI, being reported in four of 392 consecutively treated patients in one series.[148] A large effusion and persistent pericarditis may be a sign of subacute rupture and should initiate consideration of surgical repair.

Dressler's syndrome

A form of postinfarction pericarditis, occurring 2–11 weeks after the acute event, was described in 1956 by Dressler.[149] The full syndrome includes prolonged or recurrent pleuritic chest pain, a pericardial friction rub, fever, pulmonary infiltrates or a small pulmonary effusion, and an increased sedimentation rate. There has been a striking reduction in the incidence of this postinfarction complication since the introduction of reperfusion into clinical practice.[150]

Non-steroidal anti-inflammatory drugs may be required for control of Dressler's syndrome, but there are no randomized trials to confirm their efficacy (**Class IIb, Level B**).

Cardiac thromboembolism

Clinical features and prognosis

The overall risk of stroke after MI estimated from published community-based studies is 11.1 ischemic strokes during hospitalization per 1000 MI, 12.2 at 30 days and 21.4 at one year.[151] In patients with large anterior STEMIs, left ventricular thrombi develop in up to 40%.[152] If left untreated, up to 15% of thrombi will dislodge and result in a symptomatic embolic event[153] This risk is higher in patients with large anterior infarctions[154,155] and patients with atrial fibrillation.[156] Emboli are more common within the first few months after infarction than later, and with large, irregular shaped thrombi, particularly those with frond-like appendages.[157]

When thrombus is visualized by echocardiography, the risk ratio for embolization is 5.45 (95% CI 3.0–9.8) according to a meta-analysis.[158] In NSTEMI, stroke is relatively uncommon but carries a high mortality. In a pooled analysis from six trials (n = 31 402) which included patients randomized to Gp IIb/IIIa inhibitors, there were 228 (0.7%) strokes: 155 (0.5%) non-hemorrhagic, 20 (0.06%) hemorrhagic, and 53 without computed tomography (CT) confirmation.[159] Older age, prior stroke and elevated heart rate were the strongest predictors of 30-day all-cause stroke. The risk of dying after a post-STEMI stroke is approximately 40%[160] and 25% after a NSTEMI stroke.[161] Fibrinolytic therapy is associated with an excess of stroke of four extra strokes on day one compared with placebo.[162] This risk is reduced if angioplasty is used instead of fibrinolytic therapy. In a meta-analysis comparing the effects of angioplasty with fibrinolysis, angioplasty was associated with a significant reduction in total stroke (0.7% vs 2.0%; $P = 0.007$) primarily due to a reduction in hemorrhagic stroke (0.1% vs 1.1%; $P < 0.001$).[163] In a Cochrane meta-analysis, the use of PCI compared with fibrinolysis significantly decreased the frequency of strokes of any cause by 66% (95% CI 28–84%) and no significant difference was observed for the incidence of major bleeding (RR 1.18, 95% CI 0.73–1.90) but the confidence intervals were large.[164]

PCI results in a lower risk of post-MI stroke compared with fibrinolysis (**Level B**).

Management

Anticoagulation with heparin followed by warfarin for six months has been shown to reduce the incidence of thromboembolism in patients with documented intracavitary thrombus (OR 0.14, 95% CI 0.04–0.52).[165] Meta-analysis of trials of anticoagulant therapy to prevent thrombus formation confirmed a benefit (OR 0.32, 95% CI 0.20–0.52) but no effect for antiplatelet drugs.[165] In a meta-analysis of all trials involving heparin administration in over 70 000 patients with acute myocardial infarction,[166] in the *absence* of aspirin, anticoagulant therapy reduced the risk of stroke to 1.1% from 2.1% (2P = 0.01), equivalent to 10 (95% CI 4) fewer strokes per 1000 (2P = 0.01). In the *presence* of aspirin, however, heparin was associated with a small non-significant excess of stroke and a definite excess of three major bleeds per 1000 (2P < 0.0001). An algorithm proposed by the STEMI guideline of the AHA and ACC of 2004 recommends the use of aspirin and warfarin for proven cardiogenic emboli, and aggressive investigation for other causes of stroke if there is no proof of a cardiac source of embolism.[6]

In post-MI patients, anticoagulation with aspirin and warfarin is recommended for proven cardiogenic emboli (**Class IIB, Level B**).

Acute mitral regurgitation

Clinical features and prognosis

Mitral regurgitation (MR) complicating acute myocardial infarction is usually due to dysfunction of the papillary muscles.[167] The milder form of mitral regurgitation is a relatively common complication of myocardial infarction, found in 19% of postinfarction patients who undergo left ventriculography[168] and 39% of those who undergo Doppler echocardiography.[169] Mitral regurgitation is an independent predictor of cardiovascular mortality in postinfarction patients; in patients studied with Doppler echocardiography, the hazard ratio for one-year mortality after adjustment for other prognostic variables was 2.31 (95% CI 1.03–5.20) for mild MR and 2.85 (95% CI 0.95–8.51) for moderate or severe MR.[170] The most severe form of mitral regurgitation results from complete rupture of the head of a papillary muscle and usually leads quickly to severe heart failure or cardiogenic shock. In the SHOCK trial registry, cardiogenic shock was associated with severe mitral regurgitation in 98 of 1190 patients.[171] The mitral regurgitation patients were more likely to be female and to have non-STEMI at the time of presentation, and to have inferior or posterior rather than anterior infarction.

Early diagnosis of mitral regurgitation complicating MI is important because mitral valve surgery can be life saving. Usually the diagnosis is evident clinically with a loud pansystolic murmur, maximal at the apex, and radiation to the axilla; however, if LV function is severely impaired or if left atrial pressure is very high, the murmur may be of low intensity or entirely absent. Echocardiographic examination is invaluable in confirming the diagnosis.[172] However, in some cases transthoracic echocardiography is nondiagnostic and transoesophageal echocardiography is required to assess the extent of the regurgitation. The presence of cardiogenic shock or severe failure with preserved LV function usually indicates that an important mechanical complication is present, and further investigation should be urgently pursued. If the mitral regurgitation is acute in its onset, the left atrium may not be greatly enlarged, and the pulmonary capillary wedge pressure tracing should exhibit large v waves. Large v waves are neither highly sensitive nor highly specific for severe chronic mitral regurgitation[173] but the correlation between giant v waves and severe acute mitral regurgitation is stronger.[174]

Management

Urgent mitral valve repair for severe post.infarction mitral regurgitation can give excellent long-term results[175] There is evidence from the SHOCK trial registry that transfer to a center skilled in mitral valve surgery for early operation

may be helpful.[171] The perioperative mortality associated with mitral valve surgery for postinfarction papillary muscle rupture is high, 27% in one series, but two-thirds of the survivors were still alive at seven years.[176] Patients with a low preoperative EF had the highest short-term and long-term mortality. Early reperfusion[177] has been shown to reduce the frequency of mitral regurgitation after myocardial infarction.[178] There have been reports of striking improvement in mitral regurgitation after emergency coronary angioplasty in patients with acute myocardial infarction.[179]

Urgent mitral valve repair is recommended for severe post-MI mitral regurgitation (**Class IIB, Level B**).

Ventricular septal rupture

Clinical features and prognosis

Rupture of the interventricular septum occurs in approximately 2% of patients with acute myocardial infarction.[180] The pathology of septal rupture is determined by the location of the associated myocardial infarction and has implications for surgical repair. Septal rupture complicating anterior infarction is usually apical and involves one direct perforation; septal rupture complicating inferior infarction often involves the posterior or basal septum with complex, serpiginous defects.[181] In the SHOCK trial registry of cardiogenic shock patients,[182] ventricular septal rupture occurred a median of 16h after infarction. The patients tended to be older ($P = 0.053$), were more often female ($P = 0.002$) and less often had previous infarction ($P < 0.001$), diabetes mellitus ($P = 0.015$) or smoking history ($P = 0.033$). The in-hospital mortality was higher in the shock patients with septal rupture (87% vs 61%, $P < 0.001$). Even when most patients undergo surgical repair, in-hospital or 30-day mortality remains high: 43–59%.[183,184] Early diagnosis may offer some hope of early repair. Most patients with septal rupture develop signs of acute right- and left-sided heart failure and a loud pansystolic murmur at the left sternal border. This may be difficult to distinguish from the murmur of acute mitral regurgitation. The murmur may be unimpressive or even absent when cardiac contractility is depressed. A large proportion of patients have a systolic thrill at the left sternal border. Echocardiography with Doppler color flow mapping is very sensitive and specific in the diagnosis of this condition; this technique also localizes the defect accurately and provides important prognostic information.[185]

Management

Early closure is now recognized to yield better results than attempting to wait for days or weeks until the conditions for surgery improve. Although early surgical intervention may increase operative mortality, overall mortality is reduced. In the SHOCK trial register, surgical repair was performed in 31 patients with rupture, of whom six (19%) survived. Of the 24 patients managed medically, only one survived.[182] Technical advances in repair have led to better outcomes, but mortality remains high.[186] Transcatheter closure has been described and in a report from a national register, there was success in deploying a device across the VSD in 16 of 18 patients. The 30-day mortality was 28%.[187,188]

Early surgical closure of post-MI septal rupture is recommended but there are no clinical trials to guide therapy (**Class IIB, Level C**).

Transcatheter closure is a feasible alternative to surgical closure of post-MI septal rupture (**Class IIB, Level C**).

Ventricular fibrillation and sustained ventricular tachycardia

Clinical features and prognosis

Sustained monomorphic ventricular tachycardia is not common in the early postinfarction period but the GISSI-3 database showed it is a marker of adverse prognosis, and a strong independent predictor of six-week mortality (HR 6.13, 95%CI 4.56–8.25).[189] Ventricular fibrillation (VF) occurring in the absence of cardiogenic shock, severe heart failure or hypotension (primary VF) has a good short-term prognosis[190] although one major study of primary VF showed higher hospital mortality.[191] Patients surviving early in-hospital VF complicating myocardial infarction experience no adverse effect on long-term survival following hospital discharge.[192] The frequency of VF has declined over the past 20 years, as noted by Antman and co-workers, who demonstrated from the randomized trials of prevention of ventricular fibrillation that the frequency in the 1970s was 5–10%, dropping through the 1980s to less than 2%.[193,194] The reasons for this may include admission of lower risk patients to coronary care units, wider use of beta-blocking drugs and more effective treatment of ventricular dysfunction and electrolyte imbalances in the coronary care unit. The prognosis of ventricular fibrillation depends on the associated clinical state. VF occurring in the presence of hemodynamic compromise has a high hospital mortality of 80%.[195]

Management

Meta-analyses of the clinical trials have shown that prophylactic lignocaine was effective in reducing the frequency of ventricular fibrillation, but paradoxically did not improve mortality and was associated with a possible adverse effect.[196,197] For this reason the use of intravenous lignocaine as prophylaxis against ventricular fibrillation has been virtually abandoned.

Intravenous beta-blockers have been shown to reduce mortality, particularly in high-risk patients, with an apparent benefit in reduction of ventricular fibrillation[198,199] (**Class IIB, Level B**).

Low serum potassium is associated with a higher risk of VF[200] especially in patients on diuretic therapy prior to their infarction.[201] The use of intravenous magnesium may reduce the risk of ventricular fibrillation but no benefit on outcome has been demonstrated. Clinical trials have demonstrated a benefit in selected patients.[202]

Postinfarction ventricular premature beats and non-sustained ventricular tachycardia

Clinical features and prognosis

While frequent ventricular premature beats (more than 10 per hour) in the postinfarction patient are an independent risk factor for subsequent mortality (both total mortality and sudden death), the significance of non-sustained ventricular tachycardia in this setting is controversial.[203] The suppression of these ventricular arrhythmias has consistently failed to improve survival.

Management

Antiarrhythmic drugs

Trials of prophylactic antiarrhythmic therapy have provided no support for this practice, which has been widespread in the past. A meta-analysis of 138 randomized trials of prophylactic antiarrhythmic drug therapy involving 98 000 postinfarction patients, reported by Teo *et al* in 1993,[204] showed that the mortality of patients randomized to receive class I agents was increased (OR 1.14, 95% CI 1.01–1.28, $P = 0.03$). Clinical trials have shown some support for the use of the predominantly class III drug amiodarone. Two randomized clinical trials, each with more than 1000 postinfarction patients with either frequent or repetitive ventricular extrasystoles (CAMIAT)[205] or an EF of 0.40 or less (EMIAT),[206] have compared amiodarone to placebo. EMIAT reported no difference in mortality between treatment groups but CAMIAT reported a decrease in the primary endpoint, a composite of resuscitated ventricular fibrillation or arrhythmic death (3.3% vs 6.0%, RR 48%, 95% CI 4–72%), and a trend toward decreased all-cause mortality. A subsequent analysis indicated that a beneficial interaction between amiodarone and beta-adrenergic blocker drugs may have contributed to the benefit of amiodarone in these trials.[207] A limitation of amiodarone therapy is the high incidence of serious adverse effects seen with long-term therapy. The clinical trial evidence that is now available does not appear to be strong enough to recommend amiodarone therapy to MI survivors with asymptomatic ventricular extrasystoles or a depressed EF. However, patients with symptomatic ventricular tachycardia as a long-term complication of MI often benefit from amiodarone therapy.

Implantable defibrillator

The implanted defibrillator reduced total mortality over 27 months in MADIT, a small randomized clinical trial in a specific high-risk subgroup of postinfarction patients.[208] Eligible patients had an EF of 0.35 or less, a documented episode of unsustained ventricular tachycardia, and inducible, nonsuppressible ventricular tachyarrhythmia during electrophysiologic study. The risk ratio for total mortality was 0.46 (95% CI 0.26–0.82). The MADIT II trial of 1200 post-MI patients with impaired left ventricular function was terminated early after observing a 30% reduction in mortality in patients randomized to receive an implantable defibrillator device compared to those receiving conventional treatment.[209] There is no evidence that early implantation of an implanted cardiac defibrillator (ICD) will improve prognosis.[210] The evidence supports a policy of implantation of an ICD in patients with LV dysfunction due to prior MI who are at least 40 days post MI, have an LVEF less than or equal to 30–40%, are NYHA functional class II or III, are receiving chronic optimal medical therapy, and who have reasonable expectation of survival with a good functional status for more than one year.[211]

The AVID (Amiodarone Versus Implantable Defibrillators) study included a group of patients with ventricular fibrillation or ventricular tachycardia associated with a low EF or hemodynamic compromise.[212] The effect of an implanted cardiac defibrillator was compared to therapy with amiodarone or sotalol, the treatment decision guided by Holter or electrophysiologic study. There was a statistically significant benefit of defibrillator therapy compared to drug therapy. Similar results have been reported in two smaller randomized trials: the Canadian Implantable Defibrillator Study[213] and the Cardiac Arrest Study Hamburg.[214] In a subgroup analysis of the AVID database, patients with better-preserved left ventricular function with ejection fractions in the range of 35–40%, cardioverter-defibrillator therapy had no advantage over drug therapy.[215] In a meta-analysis of the defibrillator secondary prevention trials (AVID, CASH and SIDS), there was a 28% reduction in the relative risk of death in favor of defibrillator therapy over amiodarone therapy.[216]

Overall, the evidence indicates that class I antiarrhythmic drugs should not be used to treat ventricular extrasystoles or unsustained ventricular tachycardia post infarction (**Class III, Level B**).

Amiodarone may be effective in some high-risk patients, but has a risk of side effects with long-term use (**Class IIb, Level B**).

Beta-blockers reduce total mortality and the incidence of reinfarction by one-quarter in postinfarction patients, and should be commenced early (**Class I, Level A**).

Patients with LV dysfunction due to MI and are at least 40 days post MI, have an LVEF less than or equal to 30–40%, are NYHA functional class II or III, are receiving chronic optimal medical therapy, and who have reasonable expectation of survival with a good functional status for more than one year should receive an ICD (**Class I, Level A**).

Atrial fibrillation

Clinical features and prognosis

Atrial fibrillation is a relatively common complication of myocardial infarction. In patients with MI treated with thrombolytic therapy in the GUSTO 1 trial, atrial fibrillation was present on admission in 2.5% and developed during hospitalization in an additional 7.9% of cases.[217] Patients with atrial fibrillation more often had underlying three-vessel disease and an incompletely patent infarct-related artery. In-hospital stroke developed more often (3.1%) in patients with atrial fibrillation compared to those without (1.3%) ($P = 0.0001$). Atrial fibrillation was more likely to complicate the in-hospital course of older patients with larger infarctions, worse Killip class and higher heart rates. The unadjusted mortality was higher at 30 days (14.3% vs 6.2%, $P = 0.0001$) and at one year (21.5% vs 8.6%, $P = 0.0001$) in patients with atrial fibrillation. The adjusted 30-day mortality ratio was 1.3 (95% CI 1.2–1.4). In a study from the GISSI trial, the incidence of in-hospital atrial fibrillation or flutter was 7.8%, and was associated with a worse prognosis.[218] After adjustment for other prognostic factors, atrial fibrillation remained an independent predictor of increased in-hospital mortality (adjusted RR 1.98, 95% CI 1.67–2.34). Four years after acute myocardial infarction, the negative influence of atrial fibrillation persisted (RR 1.78, 95% CI 1.60–1.99).

The onset of atrial fibrillation is usually after the first hospital day, and the usual underlying causes are heart failure, pericarditis and atrial ischemia, with heart failure being by far the most common.[219] In a study based on 106 780 US Medicare beneficiaries ≥65 years of age, patients were categorized on the basis of the presence of AF, and those with AF were further subdivided by timing of AF (present on arrival versus developing during hospitalization).[220] Of the AF patients, 11 510 presented with AF and 12 055 developed AF during hospitalization. Patients developing AF during hospitalization had a worse prognosis than patients who presented with AF. In another study, detailed analysis of the prognosis of AF in AMI showed that AF was an independent predictor of cardiac death when it developed within 24 hours (OR 2.5, 95% CI 1.2–5.0, $P = 0.0012$) and later (OR 3.7, 95% CI 1.8–7.5, $P = 0.0005$), but not when AF preceded the onset of AMI.[221]

Atrial fibrillation complicating acute myocardial infarction increases the incidence of mortality and stroke (**Level A**).

Management

Heart rate slowing is usually achieved with intravenous beta-blockers.[6] Amiodarone has been shown to be more effective than digoxin in achieving reversion to sinus rhythm.[222] In a prospective but not randomized study, the combination of amiodarone and digoxin was superior to amiodarone alone in restoring sinus rhythm faster, maintaining sinus rhythm longer, and allowing the use of a lower cumulative amount of amiodarone.[223] Studies comparing the effect of different treatment regimens on postinfarction atrial fibrillation have not addressed their effect on major outcomes.

Heart block and conduction disturbances

Clinical features and prognosis

Complete atrioventricular block occurred in 7.7% of patients with inferior MI in one large series.[224] In one series the in-hospital mortality rate was significantly higher (24.2% vs 6.3%, $P < 0.001$), but at hospital discharge the survivors had similar clinical characteristics to patients without complete atrioventricular block, and a similar mortality rate during the next year.[225] In a study of elderly patients who had suffered an acute MI, heart block was associated with increased in-hospital mortality but had no effect on prognosis at one year among hospital survivors.[226] There is some evidence that the widespread adoption of reperfusion therapy may have reduced the incidence of this complication of MI.[227] However, even in the "reperfusion era", among patients with inferior MI treated with fibrinolytic therapy, the development of complete atrioventricular block is associated with a relative risk of 4.5 for 21-day mortality.[228]

Management

In patients with inferior infarction, pacing is indicated if there is persistent high-grade atrioventricular block and hemodynamic instability.[229] In anterior infarction, the prognostic significance of atrioventricular block is even greater than for inferior MI. Patients with anterior MI and complete atrioventricular block had a 63% in-hospital mortality rate, compared with a 19% mortality rate in those without complete heart block.[224]

Transvenous pacing is required urgently for complete atrioventricular block complicating anterior infarction (**Class IIb, Level B**).

When right bundle branch block and left anterior hemiblock develop within the first few hours of infarction, prophylactic pacing may be considered but this practice remains controversial. If the patient survives, this type of heart block usually regresses, but there is a risk of complete heart block causing death after hospital discharge.[230] A small randomized trial showed no benefit of prophylactic placement of a permanent pacemaker.[231] The development of left or right bundle branch block, as a complication of MI is a marker of a larger infarct size and a higher mortality after hospital discharge[232] but is not an indication for prophylactic pacing. A randomized trial of pacing for bundle branch block complicating MI showed no advantage.[233] Left anterior hemiblock denotes neither a larger infarct size nor a worse prognosis.[234]

There is no clear indication for prophylactic pacing in post-MI conduction disturbance (**Class III, Level A**).

Psychosocial complications

Clinical features and prognosis

An estimated 20–50% of postinfarction patients have high levels of psychosocial stress, including anxiety, depression, denial, hostility, and social isolation.[235] A major depressive disorder may occur in as many as 15–20% of patients hospitalized with myocardial infarction[236] and depression has been shown to have a significantly adverse effect on outcome.[237] A meta-analysis of 16 cohorts involving 6367 MI patients showed that post-MI depression was significantly associated with an increased risk of all-cause mortality (OR 2.38, 95% CI 1.76–3.22, $P < 0.00001$) and cardiac mortality (OR 2.59, 95% CI 1.77–3.77, $P < 0.00001$).[238] The effects of depression are compounded by lifestyle factors, including isolation, which themselves have been shown to have an adverse effect.[239] Poor adherence to postinfarction therapies has been shown to be a possible mechanism for the adverse outcome of depressed postinfarction patients.[240]

Management

Cardiac rehabilitation programs provide psychologic and social support to patients after MI, in addition to education about risk factors and their modification. Randomized clinical trials of formal exercise programs post infarction have shown benefits on quality of life, but have not yielded definitive results individually on prognosis. In an overview that included 36 trials involving 4554 patients, after an average follow-up of three years, the OR was 0.80 for total mortality (95% CI 0.66–0.96), although the rate of non-fatal reinfarction was not reduced.[241] An overview of randomized trials of disease management programs in patients with known coronary disease (including myocardial infarction) showed improvements in processes of care, quality of life and functional status and admissions to hospital (RR 0.84, 95% CI 0.76–0.94), but no reductions in all-cause mortality (RR 0.91, 95% CI 0.79–1.04)) or recurrent myocardial infarction (RR 0.94, 95% CI 0.80–1.10).[242]

The effect of a specific nursing intervention designed to improve the psychologic and social status of postinfarction patients was assessed in the Montreal Heart Attack Readjustment Trial (M-HART). The 1376 patients were randomized to usual care or to a treatment plan consisting of nurse visits and telephone calls to patients exhibiting high levels of psychologic stress. The intervention had no effect on mortality in men, and was associated with an increased mortality in women that was of borderline statistical significance ($P = 0.069$).[243] The use of psychosocial intervention was compared to usual care in a study of 2481 post-MI patients who were depressed and with a low level of social support.[244] The intervention included cognitive behavioral therapy and pharmacotherapy for non-responders with severe depression. There was no significant difference between the two groups with regard to the primary endpoint of death and MI over a period of 48 months. A clinical trial of sertraline showed benefits on mood without any adverse effects on left ventricular function, QT interval or major cardiovascular outcomes.[245] Overall, while trials of psychosocial interventions have yielded inconsistent results with regard to hard cardiovascular endpoints such as death and MI, there is some evidence that these interventions improve functional status and quality of life.

Cardiac rehabilitation and support programs may improve quality of life but have not been shown to improve major cardiovascular outcomes (**Level B**).

If postinfarction depression is severe enough to require treatment, sertraline may be effective without adverse cardiac effects (**Class II, Level B**).

References

1. http://www.who.int/cardiovascular_diseases/en/index.html.
2. http://www.who.int/cardiovascular_diseases/en/cvd_atlas_13_coronaryHD.pdf.
3. Thygesen K, Alpert JS, White HD on behalf of the Joint ESC/ACCF/AHA/WHF Task Force for the Redefinition of Myocardial Infarction. Universal definition of myocardial infarction. *Circulation* 2007;**116**(22):2634–53.
4. Weisman HF, Healy B. Myocardial infarct expansion, infarct extension, and reinfarction: pathophysiologic concepts. *Prog Cardiovasc Dis* 1987;**30**:73–110.
5. Anderson JL, Adams CD, Antman EM *et al.* ACC/AHA 2007 guidelines for the management of patients with unstable angina/non-ST-elevation myocardial infarction: a report of the American College of Cardiology/American Heart Association Task Force on Practice Guidelines. *Circulation* 2007;**116**: e148–304.
6. Antman EM, Anbe DT, Armstrong PW *et al.* ACC/AHA guidelines for the management of patients with ST-elevation myocardial infarction: a report of the American College of Cardiology/American Heart Association Task Force on Practice Guidelines (Committee to Revise the 1999 Guidelines for the Management of Patients with Acute Myocardial Infarction). *Circulation* 2004;**110**:e82–292.
7. Bavry AA, Kumbhani DJ, Rassi AN, Bhatt DL, Askari AT. Benefit of early invasive therapy in acute coronary syndromes: a meta-analysis of contemporary randomized clinical trials. *J Am Coll Cardiol* 2006;**48**:1319–25.
8. Boden WE, Eagle K, Granger CB. Reperfusion strategies in acute ST-segment elevation myocardial infarction: a comprehensive review of contemporary management options. *J Am Coll Cardiol* 2007;**50**:917–29.
9. Braunwald E, Rutherford JD. Reversible ischemic left ventricular dysfunction: evidence for the "hibernating myocardium". *J Am Coll Cardiol* 1986;**8**:1467–70.
10. Pfeffer MA, Braunwald E. Ventricular remodeling after myocardial infarction. Experimental observations and clinical implications. *Circulation* 1990;**81**:1161–72.
11. Page DL, Caulfield JB, Kastor JA, DeSanctis RW, Saunders CA. Myocardial changes associated with cardiogenic shock. *N Engl J Med* 1971;**285**:133–7.
12. McCallister BD Jr, Christian TF, Gersh BJ, Gibbon RJ. Prognosis of myocardial infarctions involving more than 40% of the left ventricle after acute reperfusion therapy. *Circulation* 1993;**88**(4pt1):1470–5.
13. Fisher JP, Picard MH, Mikan JS *et al.* Quantitation of myocardial dysfunction in ischemic heart disease by echocardiographic endocardial surface mapping: correlation with hemodynamic status. *Am Heart J* 1995;**129**:1114–21.
14. Killip T, Kimball JT. Treatment of myocardial infarction in a coronary care unit: a two-year experience with 250 patients. *Am J Cardiol* 1967;**20**:457–64.
15. DeGeare VS, Boura JA, Grines LL, O'Neill WW, Grines CL. Predictive value of the Killip classification in patients undergoing primary percutaneous coronary intervention for acute myocardial infarction. *Am J Cardiol* 2001;**87**:1035–8.
16. Forrester JS, Diamond G, Chatterjee K, Swan HJC. Medical therapy of acute myocardial infarction by application of hemodynamic subsets. *N Engl J Med* 1976;**295**:1356–62,1404–14.
17. Zion MM, Balkin J, Rosenmann D *et al.* Use of pulmonary artery catheters in patients with acute myocardial infarction: analysis of experience in 5841 patients in the SPRINT Registry. *Chest* 1990;**98**:1331–5.
18. Ryan TJ, Antman EM, Brooks NH *et al.* 1999 update: ACC/AHA guidelines for the management of patients with acute myocardial infarction: executive summary and recommendations: a report of the American College of Cardiology/American Heart Association Task Force on Practice Guidelines (Committee on Management of Acute Myocardial Infarction). *Circulation* 1999;**100**:1016–30.
19. Shah MR, Hasselblad V, Stevenson LW *et al.* Impact of the pulmonary artery catheter in critically ill patients: meta-analysis of randomized clinical trials. *JAMA* 2005;**294**:1664–70.

20. Harvey S, Young D, Brampton W, Cooper A, Doig GS, Sibbald W, Rowan K. Pulmonary artery catheters for adult patients in intensive care. *Cochrane Database of Systematic Reviews* 2006, Issue 3. Art. No.: CD003408. DOI: 10.1002/14651858.CD003408.pub2.

21. Multicenter Postinfarction Research Group. Risk stratification and survival after myocardial infarction. *N Engl J Med* 1983 ;309:331–6.

22. Villanueva FS, Sabia PJ, Afrookteh A, Pollock SG, Hwang LJ, Kaul S. Value and limitations of current methods of evaluating patients presenting to the emergency room with cardiac-related symptoms for determining long-term prognosis. *Am J Cardiol* 1992;69:746–50.

23. Gottlieb S, Moss AJ, McDermott M, Eberly S. Interrelation of left ventricular ejection fraction, pulmonary congestion and outcome in acute myocardial infarction. *Am J Cardiol* 1992; 69:977–84.

24. Candell-Riera J, Permanyer-Miralda G, Castell J et al. Uncomplicated first myocardial infarction: strategy for comprehensive prognostic studies. *J Am Coll Cardiol* 1991;18:1207–19.

25. White HD, Norris RM, Brown MA, Brandt PW, Whitlock RM, Wild CJ. Left ventricular end-systolic volume as the major determinant of survival after recovery from myocardial infarction. *Circulation* 1987;76:44–51.

26. de Boer MJ, Suryapranata H, Hoorntje JC et al. Limitation of infarct size and preservation of left ventricular function after primary coronary angioplasty compared with intravenous streptokinase in acute myocardial infarction. *Circulation* 1994; 90:753–61.

27. Bolognese L, Carrabba N, Parodi G et al. Impact of microvascular dysfunction on left ventricular remodeling and long-term clinical outcome after primary coronary angioplasty for acute myocardial infarction. *Circulation* 2004;109:1121–6.

28. Sorajja P, Gersh BJ, Costantini C et al. Combined prognostic utility of ST-segment recovery and myocardial blush after primary percutaneous coronary intervention in acute myocardial infarction. *Eur Heart J* 2005;26:667–74.

29. Gibson CM, Cannon CP, Murphy SA et al. Relationship of TIMI myocardial perfusion grade to mortality after administration of thrombolytic drugs. *Circulation* 2000;101:125–30.

30. Fearon WF, Shah M, Ng M et al. Predictive value of the index of microcirculatory resistance in patients with ST-segment elevation myocardial infarction. *J Am Coll Cardiol* 2008;51:560–5.

31. Appelbaum E, Kirtane AJ, Clark A et al. Association of TIMI Myocardial Perfusion Grade and ST-segment resolution with cardiovascular magnetic resonance measures of microvascular obstruction and infarct size following ST-segment elevation myocardial infarction. *J Thromb Thrombolysis*. 2008 Feb 2. [Epub ahead of print]

32. Galiuto L, Garramone B, Scarà A et al, for AMICI Investigators. The extent of microvascular damage during myocardial contrast echocardiography is superior to other known indexes of post-infarct reperfusion in predicting left ventricular remodeling: results of the multicenter AMICI study. *J Am Coll Cardiol* 2008;51:552–9.

33. Califf RM, Pieper KS, Lee KL et al. Prediction of 1-year survival after thrombolysis for acute myocardial infarction in the global utilization of streptokinase and TPA for occluded coronary arteries trial. *Circulation* 2000;101:2231–8.

34. Marchioli R, Avanzini F, Barzi F et al, for GISSI-Prevenzione Investigators. Assessment of absolute risk of death after myocardial infarction by use of multiple-risk-factor assessment equations; GISSI-Prevenzione mortality risk chart. *Eur Heart J* 2001;22:2085–103.

35. Morrow DA, Antman EM, Charlesworth A et al. TIMI risk score for ST-elevation myocardial infarction: a convenient, bedside, clinical score for risk assessment at presentation: an intravenous nPA for treatment of infarcting myocardium early II trial sub study. *Circulation* 2000;102:2031–7.

36. Antman EM, Cohen M, Bernink PJ et al. The TIMI risk score for unstable angina/non-ST elevation MI: a method for prognostication and therapeutic decision-making. *JAMA* 2000;284: 835–42.

37. Eagle KA, Lim MJ, Dabbous OH et al, for GRACE Investigators. A validated prediction model for all forms of acute coronary syndrome: estimating the risk of 6-month post discharge death in an international registry. *JAMA* 2004;291:2727–33.

38. Thompson PL, Fletcher EE, Katavatis V. Enzymatic indices of myocardial necrosis: influence on short-and long-term prognosis after myocardial infarction. *Circulation* 1979;59:113–19.

39. Antman, EM, Tanasijevic, MJ, Thompson, B et al. Cardiac-specific troponin I levels to predict the risk of mortality in patients with acute coronary syndromes. *N Engl J Med* 1996; 335:1342–9.

40. Ohman, EM, Armstrong, PW, White, HD et al. Risk stratification with a point-of-care cardiac troponin T test in acute myocardial infarction. GUSTO III Investigators. Global Use of Strategies to Open Occluded Coronary Arteries. *Am J Cardiol* 1999;84:1281–6.

41. Steen H, Giannitsis E, Futterer S, Merten C, Juenger C, Katus HA. Cardiac troponin T at 96 hours after acute myocardial infarction correlates with infarct size and cardiac function. *J Am Coll Cardiol* 2006;48:2192–4.

42. Omland T, Persson A, Ng L et al. N-terminal pro-B-type natriuretic peptide and long-term mortality in acute coronary syndromes. *Circulation* 2002;106:2913–18.

43. Suleiman M, Aronson D, Reisner SA et al. Admission C-reactive protein levels and 30-day mortality in patients with acute myocardial infarction. *Am J Med* 2003;115:695–701.

44. Tello-Montoliu A, Marín F, Roldán V et al. A multimarker risk stratification approach to non-ST elevation acute coronary syndrome: implications of troponin T, CRP, NT pro-BNP and fibrin D-dimer levels. *J Intern Med* 2007;262:651–8.

45. White HD, Norris RM, Brown MA et al. Effect of intravenous streptokinase on left ventricular function and early survival after acute myocardial infarction. *N Engl J Med* 1987;317: 850–5.

46. National Heart Foundation of Australia Coronary Thrombolysis Group. Coronary thrombolysis and myocardial salvage by tissue plasminogen activator given up to 4 hours after onset of myocardial infarction. *Lancet* 1988;1: 203–7.

47. Granger CB, White HD, Bates ER, Ohman EM, Califf RM. A pooled analysis of coronary arterial patency and left ventricular function after intravenous thrombolysis for acute myocardial infarction. *Am J Cardiol* 1994;74(12):1220–8.

48. Bolli R. Myocardial 'stunning' in man. *Circulation* 1992;86: 1671–91.

49. Braunwald E, Rutherford JD. Reversible ischemic left ventricular dysfunction: evidence for the "hibernating myocardium". *J Am Coll Cardiol* 1986;**8**:1467–70.

50. Solomon SD, Glynn RJ, Greaves S *et al.* Recovery of ventricular function after myocardial infarction in the reperfusion era: the healing and early afterload reducing therapy study. *Ann Intern Med* 2001;**134**(6):451–8.

51. Marroquin OC, Lamas GA. Beneficial effects of an open artery on left ventricular remodelling after myocardial infarction. *Prog Cardiovasc Dis* 2000;**42**(6):471–83.

52. Lundergan CF, Ross AM, McCarthy WF *et al.* Predictors of left ventricular function after acute myocardial infarction: effects of time to treatment, patency, and body mass index: the GUSTO-I angiographic experience. *Am Heart J* 2001;**142**: 43–50.

53. Dikshit K, Vyden JK, Forrester JS *et al.* Renal and extrarenal hemodynamic effects of furosemide in congestive heart failure after myocardial infarction. *N Engl J Med* 1973;**288**:1087–90.

54. Jugdutt BI. Effect of nitrates on myocardial remodelling after acute myocardial infarction. *Am J Cardiol* 1996;**77**:17C–23C.

55. Gruppo Italiano per lo Studio della Sopravvivenza nell'infarto Miocardico. GISSI-3: effects of lisinopril and transdermal glyceryl trinitrate singly and together on 6-week mortality and ventricular function after acute myocardial infarction. *Lancet* 1994;**343**:1115–22.

56. ISIS-4 (Fourth International Study of Infarct Survival) Collaborative Group. ISIS-4: a randomised factorial trial assessing early oral captopril, oral mononitrate, and intravenous magnesium sulphate in 58,050 patients with suspected acute myocardial infarction. *Lancet* 1995;**345**:669–85.

57. Moiseyev VS, Poder P, Andrejevs N *et al*, for RUSSLAN Study Investigators. Safety and efficacy of a novel calcium sensitizer, levosimendan, in patients with left ventricular failure due to an acute myocardial infarction. A randomized, placebo-controlled, double blind study (RUSSLAN). *Eur Heart J* 2002;**23**:1422–32.

58. Silver M, Horton D, Ghali J, Elkayam U. Effect of nesiritide versus dobutamine on short-term outcomes in the treatment of patients with acutely decompensated heart failure. *J Am Coll Cardiol* 2002;**39**:798–803.

59. Sackner-Bernstein JD, Kowalski M, Fox M, Aaronson K. Short-term risk of death after treatment with nesiritide for decompensated heart failure: a pooled analysis of randomized controlled trials. *JAMA* 2005;**293**:1900–5.

60. Pitt B, Zannad F, Remme WJ *et al*, for the Randomized Aldactone Evaluation Study Investigators. The effect of spironolactone on morbidity and mortality in patients with severe heart failure. *N Engl J Med* 1999;**341**:709–17.

61. Pitt B, Remme W, Zannad F *et al*, for the Eplerenone Post-Acute Myocardial Infarction Heart Failure Efficacy and Survival Study Investigators. Eplerenone, a selective aldosterone blocker, in patients with left ventricular dysfunction after myocardial infarction. *N Engl J Med* 2003;**348**:1309–21.

62. Swedberg K, Held P, Kjekshus J *et al.* Effects of the early administration of enalapril on mortality in patients with acute myocardial infarction. *N Engl J Med* 1992;**327**:678–84.

63. Pfeffer MA, Braunwald E, Moye LA *et al.* Effect of captopril on mortality and morbidity in patients with left ventricular dysfunction after myocardial infarction. Results of the Survival and Ventricular Enlargement Trial. *N Engl J Med* 1992;**327**:669–77.

64. Gruppo Italiano per lo Studio della Sopravvivenza nell'Infarto Miocardico. GISSI-3: effects of lisinopril and transdermal glyceryl trinitrate singly and together on 6-week mortality and ventricular function after acute myocardial infarction. *Lancet* 1994;**343**:1115–22.

65. Acute Infarction Ramipril Efficacy (AIRE) Study Investigators. Effect of ramipril on mortality and morbidity of survivors of acute myocardial infarction with clinical evidence of heart failure. *Lancet* 1993;**342**:821–8.

66. Ambrosioni E, Borghi C, Magnani B. The effect of angiotensin-converting-enzyme inhibitor zofenopril on mortality and morbidity after anterior myocardial infarction. *N Engl J Med* 1995;**332**:80–5.

67. ISIS-IV Collaborative Group. A randomized factorial trial assessing early oral captopril, oral mononitrate and intravenous magnesium sulphate in 58050 patients with suspected acute myocardial infarction. *Lancet* 1995;**345**:669–85.

68. Kober L, Torp-Pedersen C, Carlsen JE *et al.* A clinical trial of the angiotensin-converting-enzyme inhibitor trandolapril in patients with left ventricular dysfunction after myocardial infarction. *N Engl J Med* 1995;**333**:1670–6.

69. Chinese Cardiac Study Collaborative Group. Oral captopril vs. placebo among 13634 patients with suspected acute myocardial infarction: interim report from the Chinese Cardiac Study (CCS–1). *Lancet* 1995;**345**:686–7.

70. ACE Inhibitor Myocardial Infarction Collaborative Group. Indications for ACE inhibitors in the early treatment of acute myocardial infarction: systematic overview of individual data from 100,000 patients in randomized trials. *Circulation* 1998;**97**:2202–12.

71. Flather MD, Yusuf S, Kober L *et al.* Long-term ACE-inhibitor therapy in patients with heart failure or left-ventricular dysfunction: a systematic overview of data from individual patients. ACE-Inhibitor Myocardial Infarction Collaborative Group. *Lancet* 2000;**355**:1575–81.

72. Peterson JG, Topol EJ, Sapp SK, Young JB, Lincoff AM, Lauer MS. Evaluation of the effects of aspirin combined with angiotensin-converting enzyme inhibitors in patients with coronary artery disease. *Am J Med* 2000;**109**:371–7.

73. Teo KK, Yusuf S, Pfeffer M *et al*, ACE Inhibitors Collaborative Group. Effects of long-term treatment with angiotensin-converting-enzyme inhibitors in the presence or absence of aspirin: a systematic review. *Lancet* 2002;**360**:1037–43.

74. Pfeffer MA, Greaves SC, Arnold JM *et al.* Early versus delayed angiotensin-converting enzyme inhibition therapy in acute myocardial infarction. The Healing and Early Afterload Reducing Therapy Trial. *Circulation* 1997;**95**:2643–51.

75. Yusuf S, Sleight P, Pogue J *et al*, Heart Outcomes Prevention Evaluation Study Investigators. Effects of an angiotensin-converting-enzyme inhibitor, ramipril, on cardiovascular events in high-risk patients (published correction appears in *N Engl J Med* 2000;342:748) *N Engl J Med* 2000;**342**:145–53.

76. Fox KM. European Trial on Reduction of Cardiac Events with Perindopril in Stable Coronary Artery Disease Investigators. Efficacy of perindopril in reduction of cardiovascular events among patients with stable coronary artery disease:

randomised, double-blind, placebo-controlled, multicentre trial (the EUROPA study). *Lancet* 2003;**362**:782–8.

77. Braunwald E, Domanski MJ, Fowler SE *et al.* Angiotensin-converting-enzyme inhibition in stable coronary artery disease. *N Engl J Med* 2004;**351**:2058–68.

78. Dagenais GR, Pogue J, Fox K, Simoons ML, Yusuf S. Angiotensin-converting-enzyme inhibitors in stable vascular disease without left ventricular systolic dysfunction or heart failure: a combined analysis of three trials. *Lancet* 2006;**368**:581–8.

79. Al-Mallah MH, Tleyjeh IM, Abdel-Latif AA, Weaver WD. Angiotensin-converting enzyme inhibitors in coronary artery disease and preserved left ventricular systolic function: a systematic review and meta-analysis of randomized controlled trials. *J Am Coll Cardiol* 2006;**47**:1576–83.

80. Goldberg RJ, Gore JM, Alpert JS *et al.* Cardiogenic shock after acute myocardial infarction. Incidence and mortality from a community wide perspective, 1975–1988. *N Engl J Med* 1991;**325**:1117–22.

81. Hochman JS, Boland J, Sleeper LA *et al.* Current spectrum of cardiogenic shock and effect of early revascularization on mortality. Results of an international registry. *Circulation* 1995;**91**:873–81.

82. Hasdai D, Califf RM, Thompson TD *et al.* Predictors of cardiogenic shock after thrombolytic therapy for acute myocardial infarction. *J Am Coll Cardiol* 2000;**35**:136–43.

83. Singh M, White J, Hasdai D *et al.* Long-term outcome and its predictors among patients with ST-segment elevation myocardial infarction complicated by shock: insights from the GUSTO-I trial. *J Am Coll Cardiol* 2007;**50**:1752–8.

84. Richard C, Ricome JL, Rimailho A, Bottineau G, Auzepy P. Combined hemodynamic effects of dopamine and dobutamine in cardiogenic shock. *Circulation* 1983;**67**:620–6.

85. De Luca L, Colucci WS, Nieminen MS, Massie BM, Gheorghiade M. Evidence-based use of levosimendan in different clinical settings. *Eur Heart J* 2006;**27**:1908–20.

86. Colucci WS, Elkayam U, Horton DP *et al.* Intravenous nesiritide, a natriuretic peptide, in the treatment of decompensated congestive heart failure. *N Engl J Med* 2000;**343**:246–53.

87. Sackner-Bernstein JD, Kowalski M, Fox M, Aaronson K. Short-term risk of death after treatment with nesiritide for decompensated heart failure. *JAMA* 2005;**293**:1900–5.

88. Scheidt S, Wilner G, Mueller H *et al.* Intra-aortic balloon counterpulsation in cardiogenic shock. Report of a co-operative clinical trial. *N Engl J Med* 1973;**288**:979–84.

89. Bengtson JR, Kaplan AJ, Pieper KS *et al.* Prognosis in cardiogenic shock after acute myocardial infarction in the interventional era. *J Am Coll Cardiol* 1992;**20**:1482–9.

90. Ohman EM, George BS, White CJ *et al*, the Randomized IABP Study Group. Use of aortic counterpulsation to improve sustained coronary artery patency during acute myocardial infarction: results of a randomized trial. *Circulation* 1994;**90**:792–9.

91. Park SJ, Nguyen DQ, Bank AJ, Ormaza S, Bolman RM 3rd. Left ventricular assist device bridge therapy for acute myocardial infarction. *Ann Thorac Surg* 2000;**69**:1146–51.

92. Thiele H, Lauer B, Hambrecht R, Boudriot E, Cohen HA, Schuler G. Reversal of cardiogenic shock by percutaneous left atrial-to-femoral arterial bypass assistance. *Circulation* 2001;**104**:2917–22.

93. Bates ER, Topol EJ. Limitations of thrombolytic therapy for acute myocardial infarction complicated by congestive heart failure and cardiogenic shock. *J Am Coll Cardiol* 1991;**18**:1077–84.

94. Hasdai D, Harrington RA, Hochman JS *et al.* Platelet glycoprotein IIb/IIIa blockade and outcome of cardiogenic shock complicating acute coronary syndromes without persistent ST-segment elevation. *J Am Coll Cardiol* 2000;**36**:685–92.

95. Berger PB, Holmes DR, Stebbins AL *et al*, for the GUSTO-1 Investigators. Impact of an aggressive invasive catheterization and revascularization strategy on mortality in patients with cardiogenic shock in the Global Utilization of Streptokinase and Tissue Plasminogen Activator for Occluded Coronary Arteries (GUSTO-1) Trial. *Circulation* 1997;**96**:122–7.

96. Sanborn TA, Sleeper LA, Bates ER *et al.* Impact of thrombolysis, intra-aortic balloon pump counterpulsation, and their combination in cardiogenic shock complicating acute myocardial infarction: a report from the SHOCK Trial Registry. Should we emergently revascularize occluded coronaries for cardiogenic shock? *J Am Coll Cardiol* 2000;**36**(3 suppl A):1123–9.

97. Hochman JS, Sleeper LA, Webb JG *et al.* Early revascularization in acute myocardial infarction complicated by cardiogenic shock. SHOCK Investigators. Should we emergently revascularize occluded coronaries for cardiogenic shock? *N Engl J Med* 1999;**341**:625–34.

98. Hochman JS, Sleeper LA, White HD *et al.* One-year survival following early revascularization for cardiogenic shock. *JAMA* 2001;**28**:190–2.

99. Kinch JW, Ryan TJ. Right ventricular infarction. *N Engl J Med* 1993;**330**:1211–17.

100. Zehender M, Kasper W, Kauder E *et al.* Eligibility for and benefit of thrombolytic therapy in inferior myocardial infarction: focus on the prognostic importance of right ventricular infarction. *J Am Coll Cardiol* 1994;**24**:362–9.

101. Mehta SR, Eikelboom JW, Natarajan MK, Diaz R, Yi C, Gibbons RJ, Yusuf S. Impact of right ventricular involvement on mortality and morbidity in patients with inferior myocardial infarction. *J Am Coll Cardiol* 2001;**37**:37–43.

102. Jacobs AK, Leopold JA, Bates E *et al.* Cardiogenic shock caused by right ventricular infarction: a report from the SHOCK registry. *J Am Coll Cardiol* 2003;**41**(8):1273–9.

103. Brodie BR, Stuckey TD, Hansen C, Bradshaw BH, Downey WE, Pulsipher MW. Comparison of late survival in patients with cardiogenic shock due to right ventricular infarction versus left ventricular pump failure following primary percutaneous coronary intervention for ST-elevation acute myocardial infarction. *Am J Cardiol* 2007;**99**:431–5.

104. Bowers TR, O'Neill WW, Grines C, Pica MC, Safian RD, Goldstein JA. Effect of reperfusion on biventricular function and survival after right ventricular infarction. *N Engl J Med* 1998;**338**:933–40.

105. Dell'Italia LJ, Starling MR, Crawford MH *et al.* Right ventricular infarction: identification by hemodynamic measurements before and after volume loading and correlation with noninvasive techniques. *J Am Coll Cardiol* 1984;**4**:931–9.

106. López-Sendón J, López de Sá E, Roldán I *et al.* Inversion of the normal interatrial septum convexity in acute myocardial infarction: incidence, clinical relevance and prognostic significance. *J Am Coll Cardiol* 1990;**15**:801–5.

107. Goldstein JA, Barzilai B, Rosamond TL, Eisenberg PR, Jaffe AS. Determinants of hemodynamic compromise with severe right ventricular infarction. *Circulation* 1990;**82**:359–68.

108. Larose E, Ganz P, Reynolds HG *et al.* Right ventricular dysfunction assessed by cardiovascular magnetic resonance imaging predicts poor prognosis late after myocardial infarction. *J Am Coll Cardiol* 2007;**49**:855–62.

109. Goldstein JA, Vlahakes GJ, Verrier ED *et al.* Volume loading improves low cardiac output in experimental myocardial infarction. *J Am Coll Cardiol* 1993;**2**:270–8.

110. Lloyd EA, Gersh BJ, Kennelly BM. Hemodynamic spectrum of "dominant" right ventricular infarction in 19 patients. *Am J Cardiol* 1981;**48**(6):1016–22.

111. Love JC, Haffajee CI, Gore JM, Alpert JS. Reversibility of hypotension and shock by atrial or atrioventricular sequential pacing in patients with right ventricular infarction. *Am Heart J* 1984;**108**:5–13.

112. Berger PB, Ruocco NA, Ryan TJ *et al.* Frequency and significance of right ventricular dysfunction during inferior wall left ventricular myocardial infarction treated with thrombolytic therapy (results from the Thrombolysis in Myocardial Infarction [TIMI] II trial). *Am J Cardiol* 1993;**71**:1148–52.

113. Bowers TR, O'Neill WW, Grines C, Pica MC, Safian RD, Goldstein JA. Effect of reperfusion on biventricular function and survival after right ventricular infarction. *N Engl J Med* 1998;**338**:933–40.

114. Schuler G, Hofmann M, Schwarz F *et al.* Effect of successful thrombolytic therapy on right ventricular function in acute inferior wall myocardial infarction. *Am J Cardiol* 1984;**54**:951–7.

115. Ba'albaki HA, Clements SD. Left ventricular aneurysm: a review. *Clin Cardiol* 1989;**12**:5 13.

116. Forman MB, Collins HW, Kopelman HA *et al.* Determinants of left ventricular aneurysm formation after anterior myocardial infarction: a clinical and angiographic study. *J Am Coll Cardiol* 1986;**8**:1256–62.

117. Popovic AD, Neskovic AN, Babic R *et al.* Independent impact of thrombolytic therapy and vessel patency on left ventricular dilation after myocardial infarction. Serial echocardiographic follow-up. *Circulation* 1994;**90**:800–7.

118. Sechtem U, Theissen P, Heindel W *et al.* Diagnosis of left ventricular thrombi by magnetic resonance imaging and comparison with angiocardiography, computed tomography and echocardiography. *Am J Cardiol* 1989;**64**:1195–9.

119. Sager PT, Perlmutter RA, Rosenfeld LE, McPherson CA, Wackers FJ, Batsford WP. Electrophysiologic effects of thrombolytic therapy in patients with a transmuralanterior myocardial infarction complicated by left ventricular aneurysm formation. *J Am Coll Cardiol* 1988;**12**:19–24.

120. Ba'albaki HA, Clements SD. Left ventricular aneurysm: a review. *Clin Cardiol* 1989;**12**:5–13.

121. Cohen M, Packer M, Gorlin R. Indications for left ventricular aneurysmectomy. *Circulation* 1983;**67**:717–22.

122. Dor V. Left ventricular reconstruction for ischemic cardiomyopathy. *J Card Surg* 2002;**17**:180–7.

123. Parolari A, Naliato M, Loardi C *et al.* Surgery of left ventricular aneurysm: a meta-analysis of early outcomes following different reconstruction techniques. *Ann Thorac Surg* 2007;**83**:2009–16.

123a. Jones RH, Velazquez EJ, Mickler RE *et al.* Coronary bypass surgery with or without surgical ventricular reconstruction. *N Engl J Med* 2009;**360**:1705–17.

124. Roberts WC, Morrow AG. Pseudoaneurysm of the left ventricle: an unusual sequel of myocardial infarction and rupture of the heart. *Am J Med* 1967;**43**:639–54.

125. Brown SL, Gropler RJ, Harris KM. Distinguishing left ventricular aneurysm from pseudoaneurysm: a review of the literature. *Chest* 1997;**111**:1403–9.

126. Konen E, Merchant N, Gutierrez C *et al.* True versus false left ventricular aneurysm: differentiation with MR imaging – initial experience. *Radiology* 2005;**236**:65–70.

127. Frances C, Romero A, Grady D. Left ventricular pseudoaneurysm. *J Am Coll Cardiol* 1998;**32**:557–61.

128. Eren E, Bozbuga N, Toker ME *et al.* Surgical treatment of postinfarction left ventricular pseudoaneurysm: a two-decade experience. *Tex Heart Inst J* 2007;**34**:47–51.

129. Reddy SG, Roberts WC. Frequency of rupture of the left ventricular free wall or ventricular septum among necroscopy cases of fatal acute myocardial infarction since introduction of coronary care units. *Am J Cardiol* 1989;**63**:906–11.

130. Maggioni AP, Maseri A, Fresco C *et al.* Age-related increase in mortality among patients with first myocardial infarctions treated with thrombolysis. The Investigators of the Gruppo Italiano per lo Studio della Sopravvivenza nell'Infarto Miocardico (GISSI-2). *N Engl J Med* 1993;**329**:1442–8.

131. Shapira I, Isakov A, Burke M, Almog C. Cardiac rupture in patients with acute myocardial infarction. *Chest* 1987;**92**:219–23.

132. Figueras J, Curos A, Cortadellas J, Sans M, Soler-Soler J. Relevance of electrocardiographic findings, heart failure, and infarct site in assessing risk and timing of left ventricular free wall rupture during acute myocardial infarction. *Am J Cardiol* 1995;**76**:543–7.

133. López-Sendón J, Gonzalez A, López de Sá E *et al.* Diagnosis of sub acute left ventricular wall rupture after acute myocardial infarction: sensitivity and specificity of clinical, hemodynamic and echocardiographic criteria. *J Am Coll Cardiol* 1992;**19**:1145–53.

134. Oliva PB, Hammill SC, Edwards WD. Cardiac rupture: a clinically predictable complication of acute myocardial infarction: a report of 70 cases with clinical-pathological correlations. *J Am Coll Cardiol* 1993;**22**:720–6.

135. Bashour T, Kabbani SS, Ellertson DG, Crew J, Hanna ES. Surgical salvage of heart rupture: report of two cases and review of the literature. *Ann Thorac Surg* 1983;**36**:209–13.

136. Figueras J, Cortadellas J, Evangelista A, Soler-Soler J. Medical management of selected patients with left ventricular free wall rupture during acute myocardial infarction. *J Am Coll Cardiol* 1997;**29**:512–18.

137. Purcaro A, Costantini C, Ciampani N *et al.* Diagnostic criteria and management of subacute ventricular free wall rupture complicating acute myocardial infarction. *Am J Cardiol* 1997;**80**:397–405.

138. Pollak H, Nobis H, Miczoch J Frequency of left ventricularfree wall rupture complicating acute myocardial infarction since the advent of thrombolysis. *Am J Cardiol* 1994;**74**:184–6.

139. Honan MB, Harrell FE Jr, Reimer KA *et al.* Cardiac rupture, mortality and the timing of thrombolytic therapy: a meta-analysis. *J Am Coll Cardiol* 1990;**16**:359–67.

140. McMullan MH, Maples MD, Kilgore TL, Hindman SH. Surgical experience with left ventricular free wall rupture. *Ann Thorac Surg* 2001;**71**:1894–8.

141. Tofler GH, Muller JE, Stone PH *et al.* Pericarditis in acute myocardial infarction: characterization and clinical significance. *Am Heart J* 1989;**117**:86–92.

142. Oliva PB, Hammill SC, Talano JV. Effect of definition on incidence of postinfarction pericarditis. Is it time to redefine postinfarction pericarditis? *Circulation* 1994;**90**:1537–41.

143. Jugdutt BI, Basualdo CA. Myocardial infarct expansion during indomethacin or ibuprofen therapy for symptomatic post infarction pericarditis. Influence of other pharmacologic agents during early remodelling. *Can J Cardiol* 1989;**5**:211–21.

144. Funk CD, FitzGerald GA. COX-2 inhibitors and cardiovascular risk. *J Cardiovasc Pharmacol* 2007;**50**:470–9.

145. Hippisley-Cox J, Coupland C. Risk of myocardial infarction in patients taking cyclo-oxygenase-2 inhibitors or conventional non-steroidal anti-inflammatory drugs: population based nested case-control analysis. *BMJ* 2005;**330**:1366.

146. Hennekens CH, Borzak S. Cyclooxygenase-2 inhibitors and most traditional nonsteroidal anti-inflammatory drugs cause similar moderately increased risks of cardiovascular disease. *J Cardiovasc Pharmacol Ther* 2008;**13**:41–50.

147. Sugiura T, Iwasaka T, Takayama Y *et al.* Factors associated with pericardial effusion in acute Q wave myocardial infarction. *Circulation* 1990;**81**:477–81.

148. Renkin J, De Bruyne B, Benit E *et al.* Cardiac tamponade early after thrombolysis for acute myocardial infarction: a rare but not reported hemorrhagic complication. *J Am Coll Cardiol* 1991;**17**:280–5.

149. Dressler W. A post-myocardial-infarction syndrome: preliminary report of a complication resembling idiopathic, recurrent, benign pericarditis. *JAMA* 1956;**160**:1379–83.

150. Shahar A, Hod H, Barabash GM, Kaplinsky E, Motro M. Disappearance of a syndrome: Dressler's syndrome in the era of thrombolysis. *Cardiology* 1994;**85**:255–8.

151. Witt BJ, Ballman KV, Brown RD Jr, Meverden RA, Jacobsen SJ, Roger VL. The incidence of stroke after myocardial infarction: a meta-analysis. *Am J Med* 2006;**119**:354.

152. Nihoyannopoulos P, Smith GC, Maseri A, Foale RA. The natural history of left ventricular thrombus in myocardial infarction: a rationale in support of masterly inactivity. *J Am Coll Cardiol* 1989;**14**:903–11.

153. Keren A, Goldberg S, Gottlieb S *et al.* Natural history of left ventricular thrombi: their appearance and resolution in the post-hospital period of acute myocardial infarction. *J Am Coll Cardiol* 1990;**15**:790–800.

154. Thompson PL, Robinson JS. Stroke after acute myocardial infarction: relation to infarct size. *BMJ* 1978;**2**:457.

155. Konrad MS, Coffey CE, Coffey KS *et al.* Myocardial infarction and stroke. *Neurology* 1984;**34**:1403–9.

156. Tanne D, Goldbourt U, Zion M *et al*, for the SPRINT Study Group. Frequency and prognosis of stroke/TIA among 4808 survivors of acute myocardial infarction. *Stroke* 1993;**24**:1490–5.

157. Keeley EC, Hillis LD. Left ventricular mural thrombus after acute myocardial infarction. *Clin Cardiol* 1996;**19**:83–6.

158. Vaitkus PT, Barnathan ES. Embolic potential, prevention and management of mural thrombus complicating anterior myocardial infarction: a meta-analysis. *J Am Coll Cardiol* 1993;**22**: 1004–9.

159. Westerhout CM, Hernández AV, Steyerberg EW *et al.* Predictors of stroke within 30 days in patients with non-ST-segment elevation acute coronary syndromes. *Eur Heart J* 2006;**27**: 2956–61.

160. Tanne D, Gottlieb S, Hod H *et al*, for the Secondary Prevention Reinfarction Israeli Nifedipine Trial (SPRINT) and Israeli Thrombolytic Survey Groups. Incidence and mortality from early stroke associated with acute myocardial infarction in the prethrombolytic and thrombolytic eras. *J Am Coll Cardiol* 1997;**30**:1484–90.

161. Westerhout CM, Hernández AV, Steyerberg EW *et al.* Predictors of stroke within 30 days in patients with non-ST-segment elevationacute coronary syndromes. *Eur Heart J* 2006;**27**: 2956–61.

162. Fibrinolytic Therapy Trialists' (FTT) Collaborative Group. Indications for fibrinolytic therapy in suspected acute myocardial infarction: collaborative overview of early mortality and major morbidity results from all randomised trials of more than 1000 patients. *Lancet* 1994;**343**:311–22.

163. Weaver WD, Simes RJ, Betriu A *et al.* Comparison of primary coronary angioplasty and intravenous thrombolytic therapy for acute myocardial infarction: a quantitative review. *JAMA* 1997;**278**:2093–8.

164. Cucherat M, Tremeau GG. Primary angioplasty versus intravenous thrombolysis for acute myocardial infarction. *Cochrane Database of Systematic Reviews* 2003, Issue 3. Art. No.: CD001560. DOI: 10.1002/14651858.CD001560.pub2.

165. Vaitkus PT, Berlin JA, Schwartz JS, Barnathan ES. Stroke complicating acute myocardial infarction: a meta-analysis of risk modification by anticoagulation and thrombolytic therapy. *Arch Intern Med* 1992;**152**:2020–4.

166. Collins R, MacMahon S, Flather M *et al.* Clinical effects of anticoagulant therapy in suspected acute myocardial infarction: systematic overview of randomised trials. *BMJ* 1996;**313**:652–9.

167. Izumi S, Miyatake K, Beppu S *et al.* Mechanism of mitral regurgitation in patients with myocardial infarction: a study using real-time two-dimensional Doppler flow imaging and echocardiography. *Circulation* 1987;**76**:777–85.

168. Lamas GA, Mitchell GF, Flaker GC *et al.* Clinical significance of mitral regurgitation after acute myocardial infarction. *Circulation* 1997;**96**:827–33.

169. Barzilai B, Gessler C, Pérez JE, Schaab C, Jaffe AS. Significance of Doppler-detected mitral regurgitation in acute myocardial infarction. *Am J Cardiol* 1988;**61**:220–3.

170. Feinberg MS, Schwammenthal E, Shlizerman L *et al.* Prognostic significance of mild mitral regurgitation by color Doppler echocardiography in acute myocardial infarction. *Am J Cardiol* 2000;**86**:903–7.

171. Thompson CR, Buller CE, Sleeper LA *et al.* Cardiogenic shock due to acute severe mitral regurgitation complicating acute myocardial infarction: a report from the SHOCK Trial Registry. Should we emergently revascularize occluded coronaries in cardiogenic shock? *J Am Coll Cardiol* 2000;**36**(3 suppl A):1104–9.

172. Patel AR, Mochizuki Y, Yao J, Pandian NG. Mitral regurgitation: comprehensive assessment by echocardiography. *Echocardiography* 2000;**17**:275–83.

173. Fuchs RM, Heuser RR, Yin FCP, Brinker JA. Limitations of pulmonary wedge v waves in diagnosing mitral regurgitation. *Am J Cardiol* 1982;**49**:849–54.

174. Baxley W, Kennedy JW, Field B, Dodge HT. Hemodynamics in ruptured chordae tendinae and chronic rheumatic mitral regurgitation. *Circulation* 1973;**48**:1288–94.

175. Birnbaum Y, Chamoun AJ, Conti VR, Uretsky BF. Mitral regurgitation following acute myocardial infarction. *Coron Artery Dis* 2002;**13**:337–44.

176. Kishon Y, Oh JK, Schaff HV et al. Mitral valve operation in postinfarction rupture of a papillary muscle: immediate results and long-term follow-up of 22 patients. *Mayo Clin Proc* 1992;**67**:1023–30.

177. Leor J, Feinberg MS, Vered Z et al. Effect of thrombolytic therapy on the evolution of significant mitral regurgitation in patients with a first inferior myocardial infarction. *J Am Coll Cardiol* 1993;**21**:1661–6.

178. Kinn JW, O'Neill WW, Benzuly KH, Jones DE, Grines CL. Primary angioplasty reduces risk of myocardial rupture compared to thrombolysis for acute myocardial infarction. *Cathet Cardiovasc Diagn* 1997;**42**:151–7.

179. Shawl FA, Forman MB, Punja S, Goldbaum TS. Emergent coronary angioplasty in the treatment of acute ischemic mitral regurgitation: long-term results in five cases. *J Am Coll Cardiol* 1989;**14**:986–91.

180. Moore CA, Nygaard TW, Kaiser DL, Cooper AA, Gibson RS. Postinfarction ventricular septal rupture: the importance of location of infarction and right ventricular function in determining survival. *Circulation* 1986;**74**:45–55.

181. Edwards BS, Edwards WD, Edwards JE. Ventricular septal rupture complicating acute myocardial infarction: identification of simple and complex types in 53 autopsied hearts. *Am J Cardiol* 1984;**54**:1201–5.

182. Menon V, Webb JG, Hillis LD et al. Outcome and profile of ventricular septal rupture with cardiogenic shock after myocardial infarction: a report from the SHOCK Trial Registry. Should we emergently revascularize occluded coronaries in cardiogenic shock? *J Am Coll Cardiol* 2000;**36**(3 suppl A):1110–16.

183. Lemery R, Smith HC, Giuliani ER, Gersh BJ. Prognosis in rupture of the ventricular septum after acute myocardial infarction and role of early surgical intervention. *Am J Cardiol* 1992;**70**:147–51.

184. Hill JD, Stiles QR. Acute ischemic ventricular septal defect. *Circulation* 1989;**79**(suppl I):I-112–I-115.

185. Helmcke F, Mahan EF, Nanda NC et al. Two-dimensional echocardiography and Doppler color flow mapping in the diagnosis and prognosis of ventricular septal rupture. *Circulation* 1990;**81**:1775–83.

186. Alvarez JM, Brady PW, Ross AM. Technical improvements in the repair of acute post infarction ventricular septal rupture. *J Cardiovasc Surg* 1992;**3**:198.

187. Holzer R, Balzer D, Amin Z et al. Transcatheter closure of postinfarction ventricular septal defects using the new Amplatzer muscular VSD occluder: results of a U.S. Registry. *Catheter Cardiovasc Interv* 2004;**61**(2):196–201.

188. Landzberg MJ, Lock JE. Transcatheter management of ventricular septal rupture after myocardial infarction. *Semin Thorac Cardiovasc Surg* 1998;**10**:128–32.

189. Volpi A, Cavalli A, Turato R, Barlera S, Santoro E, Negri E. Incidence and short-term prognosis of late sustained ventricular tachycardia after myocardial infarction: results of the Gruppo Italiano per lo Studio della Sopravvivenza nell'Infarcto Miocardio (GISSI-3) Data Base. *Am Heart J* 2001;**142**(1):87–92.

190. Tofler GH, Stone PH, Muller JE et al, for the MILIS Study Group. Prognosis after cardiac arrest due to ventricular tachycardia or ventricular fibrillation associated with acute myocardial infarction. *Am J Cardiol* 1987;**60**:755–61.

191. Volpi A, Maggioni A, Franzosi MG, Pampallona S, Mauri F, Tognoni G. In hospital prognosis of patients with acute myocardial infarction complicated by primary ventricular fibrillation. *N Engl J Med* 1987;**317**:257–61.

192. Volpi A, Cavalli A, Franzosi MG et al, the GISSI Investigators. One-year prognosis of primary ventricular fibrillation complicating acute myocardial infarction. *Am J Cardiol* 1989;**63**:1174–8.

193. Antman EM, Berlin JA. Declining incidence of ventricular fibrillation in myocardial infarction. Implications for the prophylactic use of lidocaine. *Circulation* 1992;**86**(3):764–73.

194. Henkel DM, Witt BJ, Gersh BJ et al. Ventricular arrhythmias after acute myocardial infarction: a 20-year community study. *Am Heart J* 2006;**151**:806–12.

195. Bigger JT, Dresdale RJ, Heissenbutter RH, Weld FM, Wit AL. Ventricular arrhythmias in ischemic heart disease: mechanism, prevalence, significance and management. *Prog Cardiovasc Dis* 1977;**19**:255–300.

196. MacMahon S, Collins R, Peto R, Koster RW, Yusuf S. Effects of prophylactic lignocaine in suspected acute myocardial infarction. An overview of results from the randomized, controlled trials. *JAMA* 1988;**260**:1910–16.

197. Da Silva RA, Hennekens CH, Lown B, Cascells W. Lignocaine prophylaxis in acute myocardial infarction: an evaluation of the randomised trials. *Lancet* 1981;**2**:855–8.

198. Norris RM, Barnaby PF, Brown MA et al. Prevention of ventricular fibrillation during acute myocardial infarction with intravenous propranolol. *Lancet* 1984;**2**:883–6.

199. Hjalmarson A, Herlitz J, Holmberg S et al. The Göteborg metoprolol trial: effects on mortality and morbidity in acute myocardial infarction. *Circulation* 1983;**67**:I26–32.

200. Nordrehaug JE, Lippe GVD. Hypokalaemia and ventricular fibrillation in acute myocardial infarction. *Br Heart J* 1983;**50**:525–9.

201. Stewart DE, Ikram H, Espiner EA, Nicholls MG. Arrhythmogenic potential of diuretic induced hypokalaemia in patients with mild hypertension and ischaemic heart disease. *Br Heart J* 1985;**54**:290–7.

202. Li J, Zhang Q, Zhang M, Egger M. Intravenous magnesium for acute myocardial infarction. *Cochrane Database of Systematic Reviews* 2007, Issue 2. Art. No.: CD002755. DOI: 10.1002/14651858.CD002755.pub2.

203. Maggioni AP, Zuanetti G, Franzosi MG et al. Prevalence and prognostic significance of ventricular arrhythmias after myocardial infarction in the fibrinolytic era. GISSI–2 results. *Circulation* 1993;**87**:312–22.

204. Teo K, Yusuf S, Furberg CD. Effects of prophylactic antiarrhythmic drug therapy in acute myocardial infarction: an

overview of results from randomized controlled trials. *JAMA* 1993;**270**:1589–95.

205. Cairns JA, Connolly SJ, Roberts R, Gent M. Randomised trial of outcome after myocardial infarction in patients with frequent or repetitive ventricular premature depolarisations: Canadian Amiodarone Myocardial Infarction Arrhythmia Trial (CAMIAT). *Lancet* 1997;**349**:675–82.

206. Julian DG, Camm AJ, Frangin G *et al.* Randomised trial of the effect of amiodarone on mortality in patients with left-ventricular dysfunction after recent myocardial infarction: European Myocardial Infarction Amiodarone Trial (EMIAT). *Lancet* 1997;**349**:667–74.

207. Boutitie F, Boissel JP, Connolly SJ *et al.* Amiodarone interaction with beta-blockers: analysis of the merged EMIAT (European Myocardial Infarct Amiodarone Trial) and CAMIAT (Canadian Amiodarone Myocardial Infarction Trial) databases. *Circulation* 1999;**99**:2268–75.

208. Moss AJ, Hall J, Cannom DS *et al.* Improved survival with an implanted defibrillator in patients with coronary disease at high risk for ventricular arrhythmia. Multicenter Automatic Defibrillation Implantation Trial (MADIT). *N Engl J Med* 1996;**335**:1933–40.

209. Moss AJ, Zareba W, Hall WJ *et al.* Prophylactic implantation of a defibrillator in patients with myocardial infarction and reduced ejection fraction. *N Engl J Med* 2002;**346**:877–83.

210. Wilber DJ, Zareba W, Hall WJ *et al.* Time dependence of mortality risk and defibrillator benefit after myocardial infarction. *Circulation* 2004;**109**:1082–4.

211. ACC/AHA/ESC. 2006 guidelines for management of patients with ventricular arrhythmias and the prevention of sudden cardiac death: a report of the American College of Cardiology/American Heart Association Task Force and the European Society of Cardiology Committee for Practice Guidelines (Writing Committee to Develop Guidelines for Management of Patients With Ventricular Arrhythmias and the Prevention of Sudden Cardiac Death). *J Am Coll Cardiol* 2006;**48**:e247–346.

212. Antiarrhythmics versus Implantable Defibrillators (AVID) Investigators. A comparison of antiarrhythmic-drug therapy with implantable defibrillators in patients resuscitated from near-fatal ventricular arrhythmias. *N Engl J Med* 1997;**337**:1576–83.

213. Connolly SJ, Gent M, Roberts RS *et al.* Canadian Implantable Defibrillator Study (CIDS): a randomized trial of the implantable cardioverter defibrillator against amiodarone. *Circulation* 2000;**101**:1287–302.

214. Kuck KH, Cappato R, Siebels J, Ruppel R. Randomized comparison of antiarrhythmic drug therapy with implantable defibrillators in patients resuscitated from cardiac arrest: the Cardiac Arrest Study Hamburg (CASH). *Circulation* 2000;**102**:748–54.

215. Domanski MJ, Sakseena S, Epstein AE *et al.* Relative effectiveness of the implantable cardioverter-defibrillator and antiarrhythmic drugs in patients with varying degrees of left ventricular dysfunction who have survived malignant ventricular arrhythmias. *J Am Coll Cardiol* 1999;**34**:1090–5.

216. Connolly SJ, Hallstrom AP, Cappato R *et al.* Meta-analysis of the implantable cardioverter defibrillator secondary prevention trials. AVID, CASH and CIDS studies; Antiarrythmics vs. Implantable Defibrillator Study, Cardiac Arrest Study Hamberg, Canadian Implantable Defibrillator Study. *Eur Heart J* 2000;**21**(24):2071–8.

217. Crenshaw BS, Ward SR, Granger CB *et al*, for the GUSTO-1 Trial Investigators. Atrial fibrillation in the setting of acute myocardial infarction: the GUSTO-1 experience. *J Am Coll Cardiol* 1997;**30**:406–13.

218. Pizzetti F, Turazza FM, Franzosi MG *et al*, GISSI-3 Investigators. Incidence and prognostic significance of atrial fibrillation in acute myocardial infarction: the GISSI-3 data. *Heart* 2001;**86**:527–32.

219. Sugiura T, Iwasaka T, Takahashi N *et al.* Factors associated with atrial fibrillation in Q wave anterior myocardial infarction. *Am Heart J* 1991;**121**:1409–12.

220. Rathore SS, Berger AK, Weinfurt KP *et al.* Acute myocardial infarction complicated by atrial fibrillation in the elderly: prevalence and outcomes *Circulation* 2000;**101**:969–74.

221. Sakata K, Kurihara H, Iwamori K *et al.* Clinical and prognostic significance of atrial fibrillation in acute myocardial infarction. *Am J Cardiol* 1997;**80**:1522–7.

222. Cowan JC, Gardiner P, Reid DS, Newell DJ, Campbell RW. A comparison of amiodarone and digoxin in the treatment of atrial fibrillation complicating suspected acute myocardial infarction. *J Cardiovasc Pharmacol* 1986;**8**:252–6.

223. Kontoyannis DA, Anastasiou-Nana MI, Kontoyannis SA, Zaga AK, Nanas JN. Intravenous amiodarone decreases the duration of atrial fibrillation associated with acute myocardial infarction. *Cardiovasc Drugs Ther* 2001;**15**:155–60.

224. Goldberg RJ, Zevallos JC, Yarzebski J *et al.* Prognosis of acute myocardial infarction complicated by complete heart block (the Worcester Heart Attack Study). *Am J Cardiol* 1992;**69**:1135–41.

225. Nicod P, Gilpin E, Dittrich H *et al.* Long-term outcome in patients with inferior myocardial infarction and complete atrioventricular block. *J Am Coll Cardiol* 1988;**12**:589–94.

226. Rathore SS, Gersh BJ, Berger PB, Oetgen WJ, Schulman KA, Solomon AJ. Acute myocardial infarction complicated by heart block in the elderly: prevalence and outcomes. *Am Heart J* 2001;**141**(1):47–54.

227. Harpaz D, Behar S, Gottlieb S, Boyko V, Kishon Y, Eldar M. Complete atrioventricular block complicating acute myocardial infarction in the thrombolytic era. SPRINT Study Group and the Israeli Thrombolytic Survey Group. Secondary Prevention Reinfarction Israeli Nifedipine Trial. *J Am Coll Cardiol* 1999;**34**:1721–8.

228. Berger PB, Ruocco NA Jr, Ryan TJ, Frederick MM, Jacobs AK, Faxon DP. Incidence and prognostic implications of heart block complicating inferior myocardial infarction treated with thrombolytic therapy: results from TIMI II. *J Am Coll Cardiol* 1992;**20**:533–40.

229. Ritter WS, Atkins JM, Blomqvist CG, Mullins CB. Permanent pacing in patients with transient trifascicular block during acute myocardial infarction. *Am J Cardiol* 1976;**38**:205–8.

230. Atkins JM, Leshin SJ, Blomqvist G, Mullins CB. Ventricular conduction blocks and sudden death in acute myocardial infarction. Potential indications for pacing. *N Engl J Med* 1973;**288**:281–4.

231. Grigg L, Kertes P, Hunt D, Goble A, Pitt A, Boxall J, Hale G. The role of permanent pacing after anterior myocardial infarction complicated by transient complete atrioventricular block. *Aust N Z J Med* 1988;**18**:685–8.

232. Ricou F, Nicod P, Gilpin E, Henning H, Ross J. Influence of right bundle branch block on short- and longterm survival after acute anterior myocardial infarction. *J Am Coll Cardiol* 1991;**17**:858–63.

233. Watson RD, Glover DR, Page AJ *et al.* The Birmingham Trial of permanent pacing in patients with intraventricular conduction disorders after acute myocardial infarction. *Am Heart J* 1984;**108**:496–501.

234. Bosch X, Theroux P, Roy D, Moise A, Waters DD. Coronary angiographic significance of left anterior fascicular block. *J Am Coll Cardiol* 1985;**5**:9 15.

235. Balady G, Fletcher BJ, Froelicher ES *et al.* Cardiac rehabilitation programs. A statement for healthcare professionals from the American Heart Association. *Circulation* 1994;**90**:1602–10.

236. Frasure-Smith N, Lesperance F, Talajic M. Depression following myocardial infarction. *JAMA* 1993;**270**:1819–25.

237. Carney RM, Blumenthal JA, Catellier D *et al.* Depression as a risk factor for mortality after acute myocardial infarction. *Am J Cardiol* 2003;**92**:1277–81.

238. van Melle JP, de Jonge P, Spijkerman TA *et al.* Prognostic association of depression following myocardial infarction with mortality and cardiovascular events: a meta-analysis. *Psychosom Med* 2004;**66**:814–22.

239. Ruberman W, Weinblatt E, Goldberg JD *et al.* Psychosocial influences on mortality after myocardial infarction. *N Engl J Med* 1984;**311**:552–9.

240. Ziegelstein RC, Fauerbach JA, Stevens SS *et al.* Patients with depression are less likely to follow recommendations to reduce cardiac risk during recovery from a myocardial infarction. *Arch Intern Med* 2000;**160**:1818–23.

241. O'Connor GT, Buring JE, Yusuf S *et al.* An overview of randomized trials of rehabilitation with exercise after myocardial infarction. *Circulation* 1989;**80**:234–44.

242. McAlister FA, Lawson FM, Teo KK, Armstrong PW. Randomised trials of secondary prevention programmes in coronary heart disease: systematic review. *BMJ* 2001;**323**: 957–62.

243. Frasure-Smith N, Lesperance F, Prince RH *et al.* Randomised trial of home-based psychosocial nursing intervention for patients recovering from myocardial infarction. *Lancet* 1997;**350**:473–9.

244. Berkman LF, Blumenthal J, Burg M *et al*, Enhancing Recovery in Coronary Heart Disease Patients Investigators (ENRICHD). Effects of treating depression and low perceived social support on clinical events after myocardial infarction: the Enhancing Recovery in Coronary Heart Disease Patients (ENRICHD) Randomized Trial. *JAMA* 2003;**289**:3106–16.

245. Glassman AH, O'Connor CM, Califf RM *et al.* Sertraline Antidepressant Heart Attack Randomized Trial (SADHEART) Group. Sertraline treatment of major depression in patients with acute MI or unstable angina. *JAMA* 2002;**288**:701–9.

An integrated approach to the management of patients after the early phase of ST segment elevation myocardial infarction

Pedro L Sánchez and Francisco Fernández-Avilés

Hospital General Universitario Gregorio Marañón, Madrid, Spain

Introduction

Regardless of the initial and immediate reperfusion management of patients with ST segment elevation acute myocardial infarction (STEMI), the main objective of the management of STEMI patients after the early phase should be to avoid early ischemic complications and long-term cardiac death. Thus, the therapeutic approach to prevention of these events depends upon the identification of those patients who are at the greatest risk of coronary instability and non-arrhythmic or arrhythmic death and the effectiveness of the available preventive measures and therapy. In addition, we also provide an overview of secondary prevention applicable not only to STEMI but also to the complete spectrum of the acute coronary syndrome. Mechanical or acute electrical complications are covered in Chapter 33. The evidence base for managing patients with STEMI and no clinical instability is discussed under the heading of risk stratification and management.

Invasive evaluation after the early phase of STEMI

Invasive evaluation is considered both after fibrinolytic therapy and in patients who did not undergo primary percutaneous coronary intervention (PCI) to minimize short-term ischemic complications. Furthermore, complete revascularization should also be considered in STEMI patients who undergo primary PCI of the culprit artery but with other severe stenosis. Cardiac catheterization and revascularization should always be considered in patients with recurrent ischemic chest discomfort or with poor left ventricular function.[1–3]

Evidence-Based Cardiology, 3rd edition. Edited by S. Yusuf, J.A. Cairns, A.J. Camm, E.L. Fallen, and B.J. Gersh. © 2010 Blackwell Publishing, ISBN: 978-1-4051-5925-8.

Ischemia-driven PCI after fibrinolysis

The DANAMI-1 trial[4] was the first and only prospective randomized study comparing an invasive strategy (PCI or coronary bypass surgery) with a conservative strategy in 1008 patients with a first STEMI and predischarge inducible myocardial ischemia after fibrinolysis. The primary combined endpoint (mortality, reinfarction, and admission with unstable angina) was significantly reduced even after long-term follow-up. Thus, patients who have received treatment with fibrinolysis and have inducible ischemia before discharge should undergo coronary angiography and be revascularized as appropriate.

Routine invasive evaluation and PCI early after fibrinolysis

Theoretically, in STEMI patients successfully reperfused with thrombolytics, routine mechanical repair of the infarct-related artery could eliminate residual stenosis, thus reducing reocclusion and related events. In the late 1980s studies of systematic cardiac catheterization and percutaneous procedures in STEMI patients with prior fibrinolytic therapy yielded disappointing results.[5–7] However, current interventional practice, including the use of stents, thienopyridines, and IIb/IIIa inhibitors, has led to studies that support the role of early routine angioplasty in the management of STEMI patients treated with fibrinolysis.

Six randomized studies (a total of 1835 patients) support routine coronary angiography and, if applicable, PCI shortly after fibrinolysis (SIAM III,[8] GRACIA-1,[9] CAPITAL-AMI,[10] the Leipzig Prehospital Fibrinolysis Study,[11] WEST[12] and CARESS-in-AMI.[12a] In the present era of stents and glycoprotein IIb/IIIa inhibitors, early elective stenting following fibrinolysis is feasible and safe. Moreover, it permits rapid patient risk stratification, substantially reduces hospitalization, improves left ventricular outcome, prevents reocclusion and, consequently, reduces the incidence of adverse coronary events at one year. Early routine PCI is defined as a planned early percutaneous repair of the culprit artery in patients with STEMI who have been successfully reperfused with fibrinolytics. It should be distinguished from facilitated and rescue PCI,[3] both examined elsewhere in this book as reperfusion strategies in STEMI.

Completeness of revascularization for multivessel coronary artery disease after primary PCI

Multivessel coronary disease is present in approximately 50% of patients with STEMI. Both the American College of Cardiology/American Heart Association (ACC/AHA) guidelines[1,13] and the European Society of Cardiology (ESC) guidelines[2,3] recommend that, in patients with multivessel disease, primary PCI should be directed only at the infarct-related artery, with no clear statement about PCI of non-culprit lesions. One exception may be a patient with severe multivessel disease and persistent shock after PCI of the infarct-related vessel, for whom same-procedure revascularization (or bypass surgery) may be considered to reduce the ischemic burden. However, PCI of non-culprit vessels simultaneously or soon after primary PCI in stabilized patients has seldom been studied in randomized controlled trials, and observational studies provide contradictory findings.

Two observational studies reported that multivessel PCI, although feasible, was associated with a higher incidence of major adverse cardiovascular events (MACE) than infarct-related artery revascularization.[14,15] Other observational studies have shown the opposite, with significantly improved clinical outcomes when complementary multivessel disease revascularization is performed,[16–18] even simultaneously.[17]

Two randomized trials (PRIMA,[19] HELP AMI[20]) evaluating the impact of complete revascularization in patients with STEMI also failed to give an answer. Although the hypothesis that complete and simultaneous revascularization could improve ejection fraction was supported by the PRIMA study, in HELP AMI (69 patients), the one-year incidence of repeat revascularization was similar between patients randomized to culprit lesion treatment only or to complete multivessel revascularization. Therefore, there is no evidence to recommend complete revascularization for multivessel coronary disease after primary PCI.

Invasive evaluation and PCI for patients initially not undergoing primary reperfusion

Patients often seek medical attention too late and either do not receive reperfusion therapy or reperfusion therapy fails to successfully recanalize the artery. Thus, it was suggested that achieving coronary patency in either of these situations might have a beneficial effect by preventing adverse left ventricular remodeling, improving left ventricular function,[21–23] increasing electrical stability, and providing collateral vessels to other coronary beds for protection against future events (the open artery hypothesis).

Two contemporary trials have recently re-evaluated this hypothesis: OAT (Occluded Artery Trial)[24] and TOSCA (Total Occlusion Study of Canada-2).[25] In the OAT,[24,26] 2166 stable high-risk (ejection fraction of <50% or proximal occlusion) patients with an occluded infarct artery 3–28 days after myocardial infarction (20% of whom received fibrinolytic therapy for the index event) were randomized to medical therapy or PCI. Exclusion criteria included NYHA class III or IV heart failure, rest angina, serum creatinine greater than 2.5 mg/dL, left main or three-vessel disease, clinical instability, or severe inducible ischemia on stress testing if the infarct zone was not akinetic or dyskinetic. PCI did not reduce the occurrence of death, reinfarction, or heart failure. Furthermore, there was a trend toward excess reinfarction during four years of follow-up in the invasive group compared with the medical therapy group.

In the TOSCA-2 trial,[25] 381 patients with an occluded native infarct-related artery (IRA) 3–28 days after myocardial infarction were randomized to PCI with stenting or optimal medical therapy alone. At one year, although patency of the infarct-related artery was significantly higher in the PCI group (83% vs 25%), left ventricular ejection fraction did not differ between the groups. These studies demonstrate that elective PCI of an occluded infarct-related artery 3–28 days after myocardial infarction in stable patients has no incremental benefit beyond optimal medical therapy in preserving ventricular function and preventing cardiovascular events.

Preventing cardiac remodeling

Although the mortality of patients with STEMI has decreased in recent years because of faster and more frequent administration of reperfusion treatment, some patients still experience poor clinical outcomes, which are closely linked to infarct size and onset of heart failure, among other factors. One of the main risks faced by patients with extensive infarctions who survive the hospitalization phase is the development of progressive ventricular dilation and dysfunction in the following months. Determinants of ventricular remodeling include large infarct size, anterior location, lack of patency of the infarct artery, use of thrombolytic agents, and lack of negative T-wave resolution. Although this left ventricular remodeling process could have a compensatory purpose, it often occurs in association with the development or worsening of heart failure and leads to greater mortality. In fact, heart failure is the main cause of cardiac mortality after the acute phase of STEMI;[27,28] therefore, treatments aimed at avoiding or reversing remodeling have been recognized as a goal of therapy and include pharmacologic interventions, stem cell transplantation, and mechanical interventions.

Pharmacologic therapy

Several trials have established that angiotensin-converting enzyme (ACE) inhibition, started in the early phase of STEMI with captopril, enalapril, ramipril, trandolapril, fosinopril or zofenopril, reduces adverse cardiac remodeling and mortality after STEMI.[29–36] The benefit is greater in high-risk patients such as those with depressed ejection fraction (SAVE,[29] TRACE[31]), those who develop heart failure after myocardial infarction (AIRE[30]), and those with anterior myocardial infarction (SMILE,[33] FAMIS[34]), although it can be extended to all STEMI patients (ISIS-4[35] and GISSI-3[36]).

Several meta-analyses of ACE inhibitors have confirmed their beneficial effects in patients with STEMI regardless of whether administration is early (within 48 hours of infarction) or late (>48 hours to 16 days).[32,37–39] The administration of an ACE inhibitor is associated with a significant reduction in mortality (50 lives saved per 1000 patients treated in high-risk patients and five lives saved in low-risk patients), a significant reduction in heart failure (absolute reduction of 3.5%), and significant reduction in the incidence of reinfarction (absolute reduction of 2.4%).

Angiotensin II receptor blockers have also been tested in patients with STEMI. Initial studies (OPTIMAAL[40] and VALIANT[41]) found that the angiotensin II receptor blockers losartan and valsartan, respectively, were not superior to captopril in high-risk patients after STEMI. Furthermore, the VALIANT study did not show any additional benefit with the combination of valsartan and captopril. Thus, angiotensin II receptor blockers should not be administered in addition to an ACE inhibitor immediately after myocardial infarction, although they are recommended as a substitute in patients who cannot tolerate ACE inhibitors.

Atrial natriuretic peptide has also been examined as a pharmacologic approach to preventing adverse remodeling early after STEMI. Atrial natriuretic peptide suppresses the renin-angiotensin-aldosterone system and endothelin-1, which stimulate left ventricular remodeling. Compared to nitroglycerin, atrial natriuretic peptide improved left ventricular ejection fraction and prevented left ventricular hypertrophy.[42] However, recent concerns about the possible adverse effects of infusing B-type natriuretic peptides have discouraged further studies.[43]

In addition to their antiarrhythmic properties, beta-blockers have beneficial effects on left ventricular remodeling after acute myocardial infarction and are associated with an improvement in left ventricular ejection fraction (LVEF), reduction in volume indexes, and incremental frac-

tional shortening. They should be given early after STEMI, and are more effective when combined with ACE inhibitors and as continued therapy.[44–46]

Stem cell therapy

The evidence that stem cells may reconstitute necrotic myocardium and improve cardiac function in animals[47] has led to clinical studies that initially examined the feasibility and safety of this therapy and later evaluated its efficacy in reversing adverse cardiac remodeling.[48] Pharmacologic mobilization of bone marrow stem cells with growth factors and catheter-based percutaneous intracoronary infusion of bone marrow-derived cells are the only methods that have been used to date for stem cell administration in patients with recent myocardial infarction.

Six Phase II randomized trials have evaluated the intracoronary administration of mononuclear bone marrow stem cells in patients with STEMI early after revascularization of the culprit artery; three studies failed to demonstrate a beneficial effect on improvement of ejection fraction,[49–51] and three showed an initial mid-term benefit.[52–54] The REPAIR-AMI trial,[53] also designed as a double-blind study, including 204 patients from 17 European centers, is the largest study performed to date. It showed a significant increase in the LVEF ($5.5 \pm 0.7\%$ versus $3.0 \pm 0.7\%$; $P = 0.014$) between stem cell recipients and patients who received placebo. Technical differences in the characteristics or handling of the infused stem cells might explain the different outcomes observed between trials.[55] A meta-analysis of 10 studies (Phase I and II) of intracoronary stem cell therapy involving 698 patients with recent acute myocardial infarction (within 14 days of the event) showed that stem cell therapy was associated with a significant increase in LVEF (3.0%), reduction in infarct size (−5.6%), reduction in end-systolic volume (−7.4 mL), and a trend toward reduced end-diastolic volume (−4.6 mL).[56] Intracoronary stem cell therapy was also associated with a significant reduction in recurrent AMI ($P = 0.04$) and with trends toward reduced death, rehospitalization for heart failure, and repeat revascularization. Thus, intracoronary stem cell therapy following PCI for STEMI appears to provide benefits for cardiac function and remodeling.

More conflicting results are observed in patients with acute myocardial infarction receiving granulocyte colony-stimulating factor (G-CSF). Although initial randomized studies showed a significant benefit in left ventricular remodeling,[57] four further studies did not find any differences in the left ventricular function among patients treated with the factor or placebo.[58–61] The divergent results may have been due to the absence of homing signals, timing of drug administration (in the study which showed a benefit, G-CSF was administered immediately after myocardial infarction, while in others administration was delayed for

3–5 days after revascularization), subpopulations of stem cells that were mobilized but not effective, and poorly defined study objectives. A meta-analysis including seven studies (Phase I and II) of G-CSF mobilized stem cells involving 318 patients with recent acute myocardial infarction (within 14 days of the event) showed that mobilization was associated with a significant increase in LVEF (2.9%) during follow-up, similar to that observed with intracoronary delivery of bone marrow-derived stem cells.

Mechanical interventions

Ventricular remodeling has been attributed to the segmental loss of viable myocardium due to myocardial infarction, which results in a redistribution of cardiac workload, with increased regional stress in the susceptible infarct and peri-infarct zones. Therefore, a reduction in wall stress early after an MI may help attenuate remodeling. Such a reduction in wall stress can be achieved by appropriate cardiac resynchronization therapy with biventricular pacing. The first reports on the feasibility and safety of this approach early after STEMI have recently been published.[62]

Preventing arrhythmic complications

All STEMI patients are at increased risk of sudden cardiac death, most often due to ventricular arrhythmias and especially in the first months after the episode of infarction.[63] Thus, identification of patients at risk is essential. Determinants of arrhythmic complications include reduced LVEF,[63–69] ventricular premature beats and non-sustained ventricular tachycardia,[64,65,70–72] late potentials,[73–75] QRS duration,[76] reduced heart variability,[77–81] and T-wave alternans.[75,82] Which risk factor to select and in which context is difficult to determine due to the limited amount of data directly comparing multiple risk factors. The most important initial parameter is probably LVEF, as most studies determining whether or not a patient who has had a myocardial infarction will require an implantable cardioverter defibrillator for primary prevention are based upon this parameter.[83–88]

Apart from LVEF, major scientific societies do not strongly recommend a routine non-invasive assessment of the risk of ventricular arrhythmias (including signal-averaged ECG, 24-hour ambulatory monitoring, heart rate variability, evoked potentials, or T-wave alternans) in patients recovering from STEMI.[1,2] Thus, the therapeutic approach to prevention of arrhythmic death depends upon the identification of high-risk patients and the implementation of proven therapeutic and preventive measures. Several large-scale studies have demonstrated that treatment with beta-blockers, ACE inhibitors, aldosterone antagonists, and statins results in reduction of all-cause mortality but also

of sudden cardiac death. In addition to optimal pharmacologic therapy, implantable cardioverter defibrillators (ICD) further decrease the risk of arrhythmic death.

Pharmacologic therapy

Beta-blockers

Several trials and meta-analyses from the pre-reperfusion era demonstrated that beta-blockers reduce mortality and reinfarction in patients recovering from acute myocardial infarction.[89,90] In the era of reperfusion therapy, convincing randomized data have shown that beta-blocker therapy improves survival during the acute phase of myocardial infarction. The CAPRICORN trial randomized 1959 patients with a LVEF of 40% or less to carvedilol or placebo 3–21 days after myocardial infarction.[91] There was a significant reduction in all-cause mortality from 15% to 12%. Furthermore, sustained ventricular tachyarrhythmic events were reduced by more than 70%,[92] confirming that treatment with beta-blockers (in addition to fibrinolysis or primary angioplasty, aspirin, and ACE inhibitors) reduces all-cause mortality and arrhythmic death.

ACE inhibitors

As pointed out previously, ACE inhibitors are one of the mainstay treatments for myocardial infarction and have been shown to improve survival. The best available data on the effect of ACE inhibitors on preventing sudden cardiac death come from a review of 15 randomized trials of ACE inhibitors which included 15104 patients.[93] Overall mortality was reduced by 17%, with a significant reduction of 20% for sudden cardiac death. This beneficial effect on sudden cardiac death of reducing ventricular remodeling has been recently confirmed in patients with non-STEMI without clinical heart failure or overt left ventricular systolic dysfunction enrolled in the HOPE trial.[94]

Aldosterone antagonists

Two trials (RALES[95] and EPHESUS[96]) of aldosterone antagonists found significant reductions of all-cause mortality and sudden cardiac death. The RALES trial evaluated the effect of spironolactone in patients with congestive heart failure, half of whom had a history of ischemic disease. The risk for sudden cardiac death was reduced by 29%. In the EPHESUS trial, eplerenone administered 3–14 days after myocardial infarction reduced the risk of sudden cardiac death by 21%.

Statins

There is no information available from randomized trials to indicate a benefit of statins for prevention of arrhythmia in patients with STEMI. However, two observational studies in patients with ICD noted a potential benefit of statins in preventing ventricular arrhythmias.[97,98]

Implantable cardioverter-defibrillator for primary prevention after the early phase of STEMI

The incidence of ventricular arrhythmias is higher during the first hours of an infarction, declines after the event, but remains elevated indefinitely in high-risk patients. The best approach to the selection of myocardial infarction patients to receive ICD therapy for primary prevention of sudden death has been explored in randomized trials in patients with left ventricular dysfunction and chronic myocardial infarction (MADIT 1,[83] MADIT 2,[85] CABG-Patch,[87] MUSTT,[84] and SCD-Heft[88]) and in patients with left ventricular dysfunction early after the infarction event (DINAMIT[86]).

Prophylactic use of an ICD has been shown to prolong life in patients with chronic myocardial infarction or ischemia and reduced left ventricular function[83–85,88] (see Chapter 40). However, as these studies have enrolled few patients with a recent myocardial infarction, the value of early ICD therapy is still uncertain. The DINAMIT trial is the only prospective randomized study comparing the role of prophylactic ICD compared with placebo in patients experiencing acute myocardial infarction within the preceding 6–40 days (average time from myocardial infarction to randomization was 18 days).[86] Inclusion criteria included LVEF ≤35% and reduced heart rate variability or elevated resting heart rate. The ICD group had a larger reduction (>50%) than the control group in risk of death due to arrhythmia; however, this effect was offset by a similarly large increase in the risk of death from non-arrhythmic causes. The unexpected increase in mortality from causes other than arrhythmia may have been due to subsequent heart failure, of which ventricular arrhythmias were a harbinger. Consequently, prophylactic ICD therapy is not currently recommended less than 40 days after myocardial infarction. In addition, a recent substudy of MADIT 2 demonstrated no survival benefit for patients in whom the time interval from the index infarction to ICD implantation was less than 18 months, creating uncertainty about the benefit of prophylactic ICD therapy early after myocardial infarction in patients with left ventricular dysfunction.[99]

Secondary prevention

After the initial phase, patients with STEMI carry a high risk of recurrence of ischemic events. Therefore, active secondary prevention is an essential element of long-term management.[100–102] A detailed review of all the measures available for secondary prevention is beyond the remit of this chapter; therefore, emphasis will be placed on the most important.

Discharge

Low-risk STEMI patients (age ≤70 years, LVEF >45%, one- or two-vessel disease, successful PCI, no persistent arrhythmias, early reperfusion from clinical onset) can be safely discharged on day 3 after STEMI.[103,104] Wide application of this management strategy may result in substantial cost savings.

Lifestyle

Although smoking cessation is difficult to achieve in the long term, observational studies show that the mortality rate of those who quit smoking in the following years is less than half that of those who continue to smoke.[105] This is, therefore, potentially one of the most effective of all secondary prevention measures. Active counseling with programs in which specially trained nurses maintain contact with patients over several months,[106] in addition to adjuvant therapy with nicotine replacement, bupropion and varenicline are necessary.[100–102] Physical activity is strongly encouraged. Regular, moderate, daily aerobic activity is preferred.[100–102] A healthy diet based on low salt intake and reduced intake of saturated fats is essential. Regular intake of fruit and vegetables should be encouraged. Moderate alcohol consumption may be beneficial.

Weight reduction

Obesity, particularly central or abdominal obesity, is often associated with other risk factors for cardiovascular disease (hypertension, dyslipidemia and insulin resistance). The theoretic goal is to achieve a body mass index (BMI) <25 kg/m² or a waist circumference <102 cm (40 inches) in men and <89 cm (35 inches) in women.[102] Although these are the long-term goals, an initial weight loss of 10% from baseline is a first step. Further weight reduction can be attempted if the initial 10% weight loss is successfully achieved and maintained. A multimodality approach including diet, increased physical activity, and possible pharmacologic therapy is recommended.

Blood pressure control

The goal for blood pressure is <140/<90 mmHg in almost all patients, including those with cardiovascular disease alone.[107] A lower goal (<130/<80 mmHg) is recommended only in patients with diabetes and/or chronic renal failure. Lifestyle interventions, particularly physical activity, weight loss, and pharmacotherapy are essential to achieve blood pressure control.

Management of diabetes

Glycemic balance abnormalities should be actively sought in every patient with acute coronary syndrome. In postmyocardial infarction diabetics, the 2006 ACC/AHA guidelines recommended an HbA1c goal of <7%, and ideally ≤6.5%.[102] Among patients with type 2 diabetes, aggressive management of lipids (LDL <70 mg/dL (1.8 mmol/L), HDL >40 mg/dL (1.1 mmol/L)), triglycerides <150 mg/dL (1.7 mmol/L)), and blood pressure (<130/<80 mmHg) appear to be at least as important as glycemic control. Lifestyle measures, in addition to weight loss in obese patients, and adapted pharmacotherapy are of great importance. In patients with impaired fasting glucose level or impaired glucose tolerance, no specific hypoglycemic treatment has been recommended except for lifestyle changes.

Interventions on lipid profile

Interventions on low-density lipoprotein cholesterol (LDL-c), high-density lipoprotein cholesterol (HDL-c), and triglycerides are an important component of the long-term management of STEMI. Most of the evidence has been obtained in the field of LDL-c reduction, which is best achieved with statins or a combination of statins and other lipid-lowering agents.

The use of statins, irrespective of cholesterol levels, has been addressed in the 4S,[108] CARE,[109] LIPID,[110] and HPS[111] trials, which compared statin therapy to placebo across a wide range of LDL-c. The concept that lower is better was tested in the PROVE IT,[112] IDEAL,[113] TNT,[114] and Phase A to Z trials,[115] which randomly assigned patients to more or less intense statin therapy. The last four trials showed greater clinical improvement with a more intense regimen and demonstrated a reduction in the incidence of stroke.

The ATP III guidelines recommended that the LDL-c goal should be less than 100 mg/dL (2.6 mmol/L) in all patients with myocardial infarction.[116] This goal is also recommended by the American guidelines for secondary prevention.[102] The modified ATP guidelines published in 2004,[117] and the American[118] and European[119] guidelines on the management of non-ST elevation acute coronary syndrome recommend an optional LDL goal of less than 70 mg/dL (1.8 mmol/L) for high-risk patients. Statins are therefore recommended for all STEMI patients irrespective of cholesterol levels and should be initiated early after admission to achieve LDL levels <100 mg/dL (2.6 mmol/L).

Antiplatelet agents and anticoagulants

Long-term aspirin therapy reduces the risk of reinfarction, stroke, and vascular death in STEMI patients by approximately 25%.[120] American and European guidelines[3,102] recommend indefinite daily oral aspirin therapy of 75–162 mg. Clopidogrel should be administered to all patients for whom aspirin is contraindicated. According to recently published recommendations for NSTEMI,[119] after PCI revascularization, clopidogrel (75 mg) must be continued for at least one month and ideally one year if a bare metal stent has been used or at least 12 months in the case of drug-eluting stents.

Although there is evidence of clinical benefit from warfarin plus aspirin compared with aspirin alone,[1] the applicability of this evidence to current practice is unclear, in part because most patients with STEMI are treated with dual antiplatelet therapy (aspirin and clopidogrel), and in part due to unproven applicability to current practice.[121] Thus warfarin should be considered for long-term use in patients with STEMI and persistent or paroxysmal atrial fibrillation, for at least three months in patients with left ventricular thrombus observed on an imaging study, and ideally indefinitely and at a lower dose in patients with left ventricular dysfunction and extensive regional wall motion abnormalities.[1]

Beta-blockers

Beta-blockers should be initiated in all STEMI patients and maintained indefinitely in the case of reduced left ventricular function, with or without symptoms of heart failure.[102] In other patients, beta-blockers may be useful, but evidence of their long-term benefit is not fully established. Low doses are generally recommended initially in patients with heart failure to minimize the risk of an acute worsening of cardiac function.

ACE inhibitors and angiotensin-II receptor blockers

ACE inhibitors and angiotensin receptor blockers decrease cardiovascular mortality and prevent cardiac adverse remodeling after myocardial infarction. For patients with reduced left ventricular function, an oral ACE inhibitor should be started on the first day after admission, in the absence of contraindications. For other patients, treatment should be initiated during hospitalization.

Influenza vaccination

Individuals with established cardiovascular disease and those at high risk are susceptible to the complications of influenza infection. Two randomized controlled trials have demonstrated a reduction in cardiovascular events as a result of influenza vaccination in this patient population.[122,123] The 2006 ACC/AHA guidelines recommended annual influenza vaccination using the inactivated preparation for all persons with atherosclerotic cardiovascular disease.[124]

Rehabilitation and return to physical activity

Two systematic reviews of exercise-based rehabilitation trials concluded that rehabilitation programs reduced mortality after infarction by 20–25%.[125,126] A Cochrane review of 8440 patients with coronary heart disease showed a 31% reduction in mortality.[127] However, these results must be viewed with caution as the studies were undertaken before the widespread use of aspirin, beta-blockers, and ACE inhibitors in postinfarction patients. After STEMI, patients should probably undergo an ECG-guided exercise test or an equivalent non-invasive test for ischemia within 4–7 weeks after discharge following the recommendations of NSTEMI patients.[119] However, applicability to current practice appears difficult. This approach could also help when giving patients advice on the level of physical activity including leisure, work, and sexual activity.

Evidence-based integrated approach to management of patients after the early phase of STEMI

Management of patients after the early phase of STEMI attempts to avoid early ischemic complications and late cardiac death (principally due to heart failure and arrhythmias).

Invasive evaluation after the early phase of STEMI

- Patients with recurrent ischemic chest discomfort or with left ventricular dysfunction should undergo coronary angiography and PCI or CABG as dictated by coronary anatomy (**Class I, Level B**).
- Patients who have received successful treatment with fibrinolysis should undergo routine coronary angiography and, if applicable, PCI after fibrinolysis (**Class I, Level A**).
- Patients who have received treatment with fibrinolysis and have inducible ischemia before discharge should be referred to coronary angiography and revascularized (**Class I, Level B**).
- Elective angiography and PCI of an occluded infarct artery 3–28 days after myocardial infarction should not be performed in stable patients (**Class III, Level B**).

Preventing cardiac remodeling

- ACE inhibitors should be prescribed following STEMI, because of confirmed beneficial effects on avoiding cardiac remodeling and mortality, whether they are begun early (within 48 hours of infarction) or later (more than 48 hours to 16 days) (**Class I, Level A**).
- Angiotensin II receptor blockers should not be combined with an ACE inhibitor in the immediate postinfarction setting. They are recommended in patients who cannot tolerate ACE inhibitors (**Class I, Level A**).
- Beta-blockers, especially when combined with ACE inhibitors, should be administered after acute myocardial infarction because of their beneficial effects on left ventricular remodeling and recurrent coronary events (**Class I, Level A**).
- Intracoronary stem cell therapy following PCI and mobilization of stem cells with G-CSF appears to provide benefits on cardiac function and remodeling (**Level B**).

Preventing arrhythmic complications

- Pharmacologic treatment with beta-blockers (**Class I, Level A**), ACE inhibitors (**Class I, Level A**), aldosterone antagonists (**Class I, Level A**), and statins (**Class I, Level B**) should be implemented to reduce the probability of sudden cardiac death.
- Prophylactic ICD therapy in patients with STEMI and severe left ventricular dysfunction is recommended but not less than 40 days after myocardial infarction (**Class I, Level A**).

Secondary prevention

- Lifestyle modification, smoking cessation (**Class I, Level B**), weight reduction (**Class I, Level B**), and physical activity (**Class I, Level B**) are recommended.
- Lipid-lowering diet (**Class I, Level B**) and statins (**Class I, Level A**) are recommended.
- Aspirin is recommended for all patients without contraindications (**Class I, Level A**). Clopidogrel in addition of aspirin is recommended in patients who have undergone coronary stenting (duration at least one month for bare metal stents and 12 months for drug-eluting stents) (**Class I, Level A**).
- Warfarin is recommended for patients with STEMI and persistent or paroxysmal atrial fibrillation (**Class I, Level A**), for patients with STEMI and left ventricular thrombus (**Class I, Level C**) and, ideally, indefinitely and at a lower dose in patients with left ventricular dysfunction and extensive regional wall motion abnormalities (Class IIa, Level A).
- Beta-blockers (**Class IIa, Level B**) and ACE inhibitors are recommended for all patients with STEMI (**Class IIa, Level B**).
- Annual influenza vaccination is recommended for all patients with STEMI (**Class I, Level B**).

References

1. Antman EM, Anbe DT, Armstrong PW *et al.* ACC/AHA guidelines for the management of patients with ST-elevation myocardial infarction – executive summary: a report of the American College of Cardiology/American Heart Association Task Force on Practice Guidelines (Writing Committee to Revise the 1999 Guidelines for the Management of Patients With Acute Myocardial Infarction). *Circulation* 2004;**110**:588–36.

atic review and meta-analysis of controlled clinical trials. *J Am Coll Cardiol* 2007;**50**:1761–7.

57. Ince H, Petzsch M, Kleine HD *et al.* Prevention of left ventricular remodeling with granulocyte colony-stimulating factor after acute myocardial infarction: final 1-year results of the Front-Integrated Revascularization and Stem Cell Liberation in Evolving Acute Myocardial Infarction by Granulocyte Colony-Stimulating Factor (FIRSTLINE-AMI) Trial. *Circulation* 2005;**112**:I73–80.

58. Ripa RS, Jorgensen E, Wang Y *et al.* Stem cell mobilization induced by subcutaneous granulocyte-colony stimulating factor to improve cardiac regeneration after acute ST-elevation myocardial infarction: result of the double-blind, randomized, placebo-controlled stem cells in myocardial infarction (STEMMI) trial. *Circulation* 2006;**113**:1983–92.

59. Zohlnhofer D, Ott I, Mehilli J *et al.* Stem cell mobilization by granulocyte colony-stimulating factor in patients with acute myocardial infarction: a randomized controlled trial. *JAMA* 2006;**295**:1003–10.

60. Engelmann MG, Theiss HD, Hennig-Theiss C *et al.* Autologous bone marrow stem cell mobilization induced by granulocyte colony-stimulating factor after subacute ST-segment elevation myocardial infarction undergoing late revascularization: final results from the G-CSF-STEMI (Granulocyte Colony-Stimulating Factor ST-Segment Elevation Myocardial Infarction) trial. *J Am Coll Cardiol* 2006;**48**:1712–21.

61. Ellis SG, Penn MS, Bolwell B *et al.* Granulocyte colony stimulating factor in patients with large acute myocardial infarction: results of a pilot dose-escalation randomized trial. *Am Heart J* 2006;**152**:(1051) e9–14.

62. Chung ES, Menon SG, Weiss R *et al.* Feasibility of biventricular pacing in patients with recent myocardial infarction: impact on ventricular remodeling. *Congest Heart Fail* 2007;**13**:9–15.

63. Marchioli R, Barzi F, Bomba E *et al.* Early protection against sudden death by n-3 polyunsaturated fatty acids after myocardial infarction: time-course analysis of the results of the Gruppo Italiano per lo Studio della Sopravvivenza nell'Infarto Miocardico (GISSI)-Prevenzione. *Circulation* 2002;**105**:1897–903.

64. No authors listed. Risk stratification and survival after myocardial infarction. *N Engl J Med* 1983;**309**:331–6.

65. Mukharji J, Rude RE, Poole WK *et al.* Risk factors for sudden death after acute myocardial infarction: two-year follow-up. *Am J Cardiol* 1984;**54**:31–6.

66. Zaret BL, Wackers FJ, Terrin ML *et al.* Value of radionuclide rest and exercise left ventricular ejection fraction in assessing survival of patients after thrombolytic therapy for acute myocardial infarction: results of Thrombolysis in Myocardial Infarction (TIMI) phase II study. The TIMI Study Group. *J Am Coll Cardiol* 1995;**26**:73–9.

67. Burns RJ, Gibbons RJ, Yi Q *et al.* The relationships of left ventricular ejection fraction, end-systolic volume index and infarct size to six-month mortality after hospital discharge following myocardial infarction treated by thrombolysis. *J Am Coll Cardiol* 2002;**39**:30–6.

68. Torp-Pedersen C, Kober L. Effect of ACE inhibitor trandolapril on life expectancy of patients with reduced left-ventricular function after acute myocardial infarction. TRACE Study Group. Trandolapril Cardiac Evaluation. *Lancet* 1999;**354**:9–12.

69. Solomon SD, Zelenkofske S, McMurray JJ *et al.* Sudden death in patients with myocardial infarction and left ventricular dysfunction, heart failure, or both. *N Engl J Med* 2005;**352**:2581–8.

70. Maggioni AP, Zuanetti G, Franzosi MG *et al.* Prevalence and prognostic significance of ventricular arrhythmias after acute myocardial infarction in the fibrinolytic era. GISSI-2 results. *Circulation* 1993;**87**:312–22.

71. Volpi A, De Vita C, Franzosi MG *et al.* Determinants of 6-month mortality in survivors of myocardial infarction after thrombolysis. Results of the GISSI-2 data base. The Ad hoc Working Group of the Gruppo Italiano per lo Studio della Sopravvivenza nell'Infarto Miocardico (GISSI)-2 Data Base. *Circulation* 1993;**88**:416–29.

72. Ruberman W, Weinblatt E, Goldberg JD, Frank CW, Chaudhary BS, Shapiro S. Ventricular premature complexes and sudden death after myocardial infarction. *Circulation* 1981;**64**:297–305.

73. Denes P, el-Sherif N, Katz R *et al.* Prognostic significance of signal-averaged electrocardiogram after thrombolytic therapy and/or angioplasty during acute myocardial infarction (CAST substudy). Cardiac Arrhythmia Suppression Trial (CAST) SAECG Substudy Investigators. *Am J Cardiol* 1994;**74**:216–20.

74. Zimmermann M, Sentici A, Adamec R, Metzger J, Mermillod B, Rutishauser W. Long-term prognostic significance of ventricular late potentials after a first acute myocardial infarction. *Am Heart J* 1997;**134**:1019–28.

75. Ikeda T, Sakata T, Takami M *et al.* Combined assessment of T-wave alternans and late potentials used to predict arrhythmic events after myocardial infarction. A prospective study. *J Am Coll Cardiol* 2000;**35**:722–30.

76. Savard P, Rouleau JL, Ferguson J *et al.* Risk stratification after myocardial infarction using signal-averaged electrocardiographic criteria adjusted for sex, age, and myocardial infarction location. *Circulation* 1997;**96**:202–13.

77. Farrell TG, Bashir Y, Cripps T *et al.* Risk stratification for arrhythmic events in postinfarction patients based on heart rate variability, ambulatory electrocardiographic variables and the signal-averaged electrocardiogram. *J Am Coll Cardiol* 1991;**18**:687–97.

78. Kleiger RE, Miller JP, Bigger JT Jr, Moss AJ. Decreased heart rate variability and its association with increased mortality after acute myocardial infarction. *Am J Cardiol* 1987;**59**:256–62.

79. Cripps TR, Malik M, Farrell TG, Camm AJ. Prognostic value of reduced heart rate variability after myocardial infarction: clinical evaluation of a new analysis method. *Br Heart J* 1991;**65**:14–9.

80. Malik M, Camm AJ, Janse MJ, Julian DG, Frangin GA, Schwartz PJ. Depressed heart rate variability identifies postinfarction patients who might benefit from prophylactic treatment with amiodarone: a substudy of EMIAT (The European Myocardial Infarct Amiodarone Trial). *J Am Coll Cardiol* 2000;**35**:1263–75.

81. Singh N, Mironov D, Armstrong PW, Ross AM, Langer A. Heart rate variability assessment early after acute myocardial infarction. Pathophysiological and prognostic correlates. GUSTO ECG Substudy Investigators. Global Utilization of Streptokinase and TPA for Occluded Arteries. *Circulation* 1996;**93**:1388–95.

82. Rosenbaum DS, Jackson LE, Smith JM, Garan H, Ruskin JN, Cohen RJ. Electrical alternans and vulnerability to ventricular arrhythmias. *N Engl J Med* 1994;**330**:235–41.

83. Moss AJ, Hall WJ, Cannom DS *et al.* Improved survival with an implanted defibrillator in patients with coronary disease at high risk for ventricular arrhythmia. Multicenter Automatic Defibrillator Implantation Trial Investigators. *N Engl J Med* 1996;**335**:1933–40.

84. Buxton AE, Lee KL, Fisher JD, Josephson ME, Prystowsky EN, Hafley G. A randomized study of the prevention of sudden death in patients with coronary artery disease. Multicenter Unsustained Tachycardia Trial Investigators. *N Engl J Med* 1999;**341**:1882–90.

85. Moss AJ, Zareba W, Hall WJ *et al.* Prophylactic implantation of a defibrillator in patients with myocardial infarction and reduced ejection fraction. *N Engl J Med* 2002;**346**:877–83.

86. Hohnloser SH, Kuck KH, Dorian P *et al.* Prophylactic use of an implantable cardioverter-defibrillator after acute myocardial infarction. *N Engl J Med* 2004;**351**:2481–8.

87. Bigger JT Jr. Prophylactic use of implanted cardiac defibrillators in patients at high risk for ventricular arrhythmias after coronary-artery bypass graft surgery. Coronary Artery Bypass Graft (CABG) Patch Trial Investigators. *N Engl J Med* 1997;**337**:1569–75.

88. Bardy GH, Lee KL, Mark DB *et al.* Amiodarone or an implantable cardioverter-defibrillator for congestive heart failure. *N Engl J Med* 2005;**352**:225–37.

89. Gottlieb SS, McCarter RJ, Vogel RA. Effect of beta-blockade on mortality among high-risk and low-risk patients after myocardial infarction. *N Engl J Med* 1998;**339**:489–97.

90. Beta-Blocker Pooling Project (BBPP). Subgroup findings from randomized trials in post infarction patients. The Beta-Blocker Pooling Project Research Group. *Eur Heart J* 1988;**9**:8–16.

91. Dargie HJ. Effect of carvedilol on outcome after myocardial infarction in patients with left-ventricular dysfunction: the CAPRICORN randomised trial. *Lancet* 2001;**357**:1385–90.

92. McMurray J, Kober L, Robertson M *et al.* Antiarrhythmic effect of carvedilol after acute myocardial infarction: results of the Carvedilol Post-Infarct Survival Control in Left Ventricular Dysfunction (CAPRICORN) trial. *J Am Coll Cardiol* 2005;**45**:525–30.

93. Domanski MJ, Exner DV, Borkowf CB, Geller NL, Rosenberg Y, Pfeffer MA. Effect of angiotensin converting enzyme inhibition on sudden cardiac death in patients following acute myocardial infarction. A meta-analysis of randomized clinical trials. *J Am Coll Cardiol* 1999;**33**:598–604.

94. Teo KK, Mitchell LB, Pogue J, Bosch J, Dagenais G, Yusuf S. Effect of ramipril in reducing sudden deaths and nonfatal cardiac arrests in high-risk individuals without heart failure or left ventricular dysfunction. *Circulation* 2004;**110**:1413–17.

95. Pitt B, Zannad F, Remme WJ *et al.* The effect of spironolactone on morbidity and mortality in patients with severe heart failure. Randomized Aldactone Evaluation Study Investigators. *N Engl J Med* 1999;**341**:709–17.

96. Pitt B, Remme W, Zannad F *et al.* Eplerenone, a selective aldosterone blocker, in patients with left ventricular dysfunction after myocardial infarction. *N Engl J Med* 2003;**348**:1309–21.

97. Hohnloser SH. Prevention of recurrent life-threatening arrhythmias: will lipid-lowering therapy make a difference? *J Am Coll Cardiol* 2000;**36**:773–5.

98. Chiu JH, Abdelhadi RH, Chung MK *et al.* Effect of statin therapy on risk of ventricular arrhythmia among patients with coronary artery disease and an implantable cardioverter-defibrillator. *Am J Cardiol* 2005;**95**:490–1.

99. Wilber DJ, Zareba W, Hall WJ *et al.* Time dependence of mortality risk and defibrillator benefit after myocardial infarction. *Circulation* 2004;**109**:1082–4.

100. Smith SC Jr, Blair SN, Bonow RO *et al.* AHA/ACC Guidelines for Preventing Heart Attack and Death in Patients With Atherosclerotic Cardiovascular Disease: 2001 update. A statement for healthcare professionals from the American Heart Association and the American College of Cardiology. *J Am Coll Cardiol* 2001;**38**:1581–3.

101. De Backer G, Ambrosioni E, Borch-Johnsen K *et al.* European guidelines on cardiovascular disease prevention in clinical practice. Third Joint Task Force of European and Other Societies on Cardiovascular Disease Prevention in Clinical Practice. *Eur Heart J* 2003;**24**:1601–10.

102. Smith SC Jr, Allen J, Blair SN *et al.* AHA/ACC guidelines for secondary prevention for patients with coronary and other atherosclerotic vascular disease: 2006 update: endorsed by the National Heart, Lung, and Blood Institute. *Circulation* 2006;**113**:2363–72.

103. Grines CL, Marsalese DL, Brodie B *et al.* Safety and cost-effectiveness of early discharge after primary angioplasty in low risk patients with acute myocardial infarction. PAMI-II Investigators. Primary Angioplasty in Myocardial Infarction. *J Am Coll Cardiol* 1998;**31**:967–72.

104. De Luca G, Suryapranata H, van 't Hof AW *et al.* Prognostic assessment of patients with acute myocardial infarction treated with primary angioplasty: implications for early discharge. *Circulation* 2004;**109**:2737–43.

105. Aberg A, Bergstrand R, Johansson S *et al.* Cessation of smoking after myocardial infarction. Effects on mortality after 10 years. *Br Heart J* 1983;**49**:416–22.

106. Taylor CB, Houston-Miller N, Killen JD, DeBusk RF. Smoking cessation after acute myocardial infarction: effects of a nurse-managed intervention. *Ann Intern Med* 1990;**113**:118–23.

107. Chobanian AV, Bakris GL, Black HR *et al.* The Seventh Report of the Joint National Committee on Prevention, Detection, Evaluation, and Treatment of High Blood Pressure: the JNC 7 report. *JAMA* 2003;**289**:2560–72.

108. No authors listed. Randomised trial of cholesterol lowering in 4444 patients with coronary heart disease: the Scandinavian Simvastatin Survival Study (4S). *Lancet* 1994;**344**:1383–9.

109. Sacks FM, Pfeffer MA, Moye LA *et al.* The effect of pravastatin on coronary events after myocardial infarction in patients with average cholesterol levels. Cholesterol and Recurrent Events Trial investigators. *N Engl J Med* 1996;**335**:1001–9.

110. Tonkin AM, Colquhoun D, Emberson J *et al.* Effects of pravastatin in 3260 patients with unstable angina: results from the LIPID study. *Lancet* 2000;**356**:1871–5.

111. MRC/BHF. Heart Protection Study of cholesterol lowering with simvastatin in 20,536 high-risk individuals: a randomised placebo-controlled trial. *Lancet* 2002;**360**:7–22.

112. Cannon CP, Braunwald E, McCabe CH *et al.* Intensive versus moderate lipid lowering with statins after acute coronary syndromes. *N Engl J Med* 2004;**350**:1495–504.

113. Pedersen TR, Faergeman O, Kastelein JJ *et al.* High-dose atorvastatin vs usual-dose simvastatin for secondary prevention

after myocardial infarction: the IDEAL study: a randomized controlled trial. *JAMA* 2005;**294**:2437–45.

114. LaRosa JC, Grundy SM, Waters DD *et al*. Intensive lipid lowering with atorvastatin in patients with stable coronary disease. *N Engl J Med* 2005;**352**:1425–35.

115. de Lemos JA, Blazing MA, Wiviott SD *et al*. Early intensive vs a delayed conservative simvastatin strategy in patients with acute coronary syndromes: phase Z of the A to Z trial. *JAMA* 2004;**292**:1307–16.

116. Third Report of the National Cholesterol Education Program (NCEP) Expert Panel on Detection, Evaluation, and Treatment of High Blood Cholesterol in Adults (Adult Treatment Panel III) final report. *Circulation* 2002;**106**:3143–421.

117. Grundy SM, Cleeman JI, Merz CN *et al*. Implications of recent clinical trials for the National Cholesterol Education Program Adult Treatment Panel III guidelines. *Circulation* 2004;**110**:227–39.

118. Anderson JL, Adams CD, Antman EM *et al*. ACC/AHA 2007 guidelines for the management of patients with unstable angina/non-ST-Elevation myocardial infarction: a report of the American College of Cardiology/American Heart Association Task Force on Practice Guidelines (Writing Committee to Revise the 2002 Guidelines for the Management of Patients With Unstable Angina/Non-ST-Elevation Myocardial Infarction) developed in collaboration with the American College of Emergency Physicians, the Society for Cardiovascular Angiography and Interventions, and the Society of Thoracic Surgeons endorsed by the American Association of Cardiovascular and Pulmonary Rehabilitation and the Society for Academic Emergency Medicine. *J Am Coll Cardiol* 2007;**50**:e1–e157.

119. Bassand JP, Hamm CW, Ardissino D *et al*. Guidelines for the diagnosis and treatment of non-ST-segment elevation acute coronary syndromes. *Eur Heart J* 2007;**28**:1598–660.

120. Antithrombotic Trialists' Collaboration. Collaborative meta-analysis of randomised trials of antiplatelet therapy for prevention of death, myocardial infarction, and stroke in high risk patients. *BMJ* 2002;**324**:71–86.

121. Husted SE, Ziegler BK, Kher A. Long-term anticoagulant therapy in patients with coronary artery disease. *Eur Heart J* 2006;**27**:913–19.

122. Gurfinkel EP, Leon de la Fuente R, Mendiz O, Mautner B. Flu vaccination in acute coronary syndromes and planned percutaneous coronary interventions (FLUVACS) Study. *Eur Heart J* 2004;**25**:25–31.

123. Ciszewski A, Bilinska ZT, Brydak LB *et al*. Influenza vaccination in secondary prevention from coronary ischaemic events in coronary artery disease: FLUCAD study. *Eur Heart J* 2008;**29**(11):1350–8.

124. Davis MM, Taubert K, Benin AL *et al*. Influenza vaccination as secondary prevention for cardiovascular disease: a science advisory from the American Heart Association/American College of Cardiology. *J Am Coll Cardiol* 2006;**48**:1498–502.

125. O'Connor GT, Buring JE, Yusuf S *et al*. An overview of randomized trials of rehabilitation with exercise after myocardial infarction. *Circulation* 1989;**80**:234–44.

126. Oldridge NB, Guyatt GH, Fischer ME, Rimm AA. Cardiac rehabilitation after myocardial infarction. Combined experience of randomized clinical trials. *JAMA* 1988;**260**:945–50.

127. Jolliffe J, Rees K, Taylor RRS, Thompson DR, Oldridge N, Ebrahim S. Exercise-based rehabilitation for coronary heart disease. *Cochrane Database of Systematic Reviews* 2001, Issue 1. Art. No.: CD001800. DOI: 10.1002/14651858.CD001800.

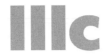

Arrhythmias

A John Camm and John A Cairns, Editors

35 Atrial fibrillation: rhythm and rate control therapies

Irina Savelieva,[1] Albert L Waldo[2] and A John Camm[1]

[1]Department of Cardiology, Division of Cardiac and Vascular Science, St George's University of London, London, UK

[2]Department of Medicine, Cardiovascular Medicine, Case Western Reserve University School of Medicine, and University Hospitals Case Medical Center, Cleveland, OH, USA

Introduction

The Framingham Study in the US and the Rotterdam Study in Europe have estimated lifetime risk for development of atrial fibrillation (AF) to be 1 in 4 for men and women 40 years of age and older.[1,2] Projected data from two population-based studies in the US predict a 2.5 to 3-fold increase in the number of patients with AF by 2050.[3,4] The high lifetime risk for AF and increased longevity underscore the important public health burden posed by this arrhythmia across the world. Because AF has multiple etiologies and a broad variety of presentations it demands a range of therapeutic responses. The primary pathologies underlying or promoting the occurrence of AF vary more than for any other cardiac arrhythmia, ranging from autonomic imbalance through organic heart disease to metabolic disorders, such as diabetes mellitus, metabolic syndrome, and hyperthyroidism. A rational approach to management of the individual case depends on careful assessment of the temporal pattern of the arrhythmia, associated cardiovascular disease, and any particular features suggesting the advisability or risks of any particular treatment regimen. The nature of AF and of individual patient factors change over time, requiring a flexible approach to long-term management.

AF usually tends to recur and may follow a predictable pattern. Paroxysmal AF generally progresses to persistent and/or permanent over time. In the Canadian Registry of AF (CARAF) 8–9% of patients with new-onset paroxysmal AF developed a sustained arrhythmia by the end of the first year; about 25% were in permanent AF by 5 years.[5] Rates appear to be higher for those with a persistent variety, with 35–40% developing the permanent arrhythmia by the end of the first year since diagnosis.[6,7] Between two-thirds and three-quarters of patients had documented recurrence of AF within 5 years, despite continuous antiarrhythmic drug therapy.[5] However, even these projections may represent conservative estimates because of undiscovered silent arrhythmias.[8] Progression of AF relates to progression of the underlying disease and to continuous structural remodeling of the atria, including changes associated with ageing (e.g. fatty metamorphosis, myocyte degeneration, and fibrosis). As the arrhythmia becomes more sustained, restoration and maintenance of sinus rhythm become more challenging.

Principles of therapy

The fundamental principles of therapy for AF include primary prevention (i.e. treating the conditions that are commonly associated with the development of the arrhythmia); cardioversion of first-onset or recurrent AF which fails to self-terminate; secondary prevention (i.e. specific antiarrhythmic drugs or catheter ablation to suppress recurrence of paroxysmal or persistent AF once the arrhythmia has occurred); control of ventricular rates during recurrent or permanent AF; and anticoagulation to prevent thromboembolism. Treatment of underlying heart disease, such as hypertension and heart failure may *per se* deter the occurrence of new AF by alleviating and/or delaying remodeling of the atria (primary prevention). Although secondary prevention usually implies the use of specific antiarrhythmic agents to prevent recurrent AF, continuous treatment of underlying heart disease (e.g. stringent blood pressure control in hypertension) is likely to contribute to the reduction of recurrence and also to delay the progression to permanent AF. Treatment of the underlying heart disease to prevent AF is often referred as "upstream" therapy.[9] There is evidence that beta-blockers, which have very modest antiarrhythmic properties, and traditionally

Evidence-Based Cardiology, 3rd edition. Edited by S. Yusuf, J.A. Cairns, A.J. Camm, E.L. Fallen, and B.J. Gersh. © 2010 Blackwell Publishing, ISBN: 978-1-4051-5925-8.

non-antiarrhythmic drugs, such as angiotensin-converting enzyme inhibitors, angiotensin receptor blockers, and statins, may have the antiarrhythmic potential, additional to any treatment effect on the underlying disease. This is discussed in Chapter 36.

Non-pharmacologic rhythm control therapy with catheter-based pulmonary vein isolation and left atrial ablation can be used to treat some forms of AF. However, the eventual impact of catheter-based techniques, particularly for long-term rhythm control and in patients with significant underlying heart disease, is not yet known.[10] Drug therapy remains, therefore, the mainstream for management of AF. Rate control is the primary treatment strategy in permanent AF and it is also relevant to all forms of the arrhythmia.

Studies of rate and rhythm control strategies

Two prime treatment strategies are rhythm control and rate control. Intuitively, rhythm control is a more attractive treatment strategy as sinus rhythm offers physiologic control of heart rate and regularity, normal atrial activation and contraction, the correct sequence of atrioventricular activation, and normal valve function. It might be an ideal approach for both stroke prevention and symptom alleviation. Nevertheless, during the 1980s and 1990s, the potential downside of available antiarrhythmic drug therapy became clear. A series of studies showed that under certain conditions, antiarrhythmic drugs could become proarrhythmic and, thereby, potentially lethal.[11,12] And for amiodarone, although proarrhythmia uniquely was an infrequent clinical problem, pulmonary fibrosis, a potentially lethal adverse effect, could develop.[13]

The difficulties in rhythm control management, principally the high AF recurrence rate, and the concern for serious adverse effects associated with antiarrhythmic drug therapy finally led to rate versus rhythm control studies. The major studies were the Atrial Fibrillation Follow up Investigation of Rhythm Management (AFFIRM) trial[14], the RAte Control versus Electrical Cardioversion (RACE) trial[15] and, most recently, the Atrial Fibrillation Congestive Heart Failure (AF CHF) trial[16] (Table 35.1). There were also a series of pilot studies performed, including the Pharmacological Intervention in Atrial Fibrillation (PIAF),[17] Strategies of Treatment of Atrial Fibrillation (STAF),[18] and How to Treat Chronic Atrial Fibrillation (HOT CAFÉ),[19] among others. They all directly and prospectively compared the effect of rhythm control treatment strategies versus rate control strategies on patient outcomes. It should be emphasized that it is likely none of these studies would have been performed if an antiarrhythmic drug or drugs were available which suppressed AF with >90% efficacy and an acceptable adverse effect profile.

AFFIRM

AFFIRM was a randomized clinical trial that compared two treatment strategies for AF in 4060 patients with paroxysmal or persistent AF and one or more risk factors (age ≥65, hypertension, diabetes, poor left ventricular function, congestive heart failure, or a prior stroke or transient ischemic attack) associated with a high risk of stroke and death, with at least 6 hours of AF in the last 6 months (with one episode in the previous 12 weeks).[14] The primary endpoint was all-cause mortality. A combined secondary endpoint consisted of death, disabling stroke or anoxic encephalopathy, major bleed or cardiac arrest. Quality of life and functional capacity were also assessed in a subset of patients. Throughout the study, the prevalence of sinus rhythm was high in the rhythm control arm, although it declined with time (82.4% at 1 year, 73.3% at 3 years, and 62.6% at 5 years). The prevalence of sinus rhythm in the rate control arm was higher than anticipated (42.9% at 1 year, 38.5% at 3 years, and 34.6% at 5 years).

A total of 356 patients in the rhythm control arm and 306 patients in the rate control arm died during this study. Overall survival at 1, 3, and 5 years was 96%, 87%, and 76% in the rhythm control arm, and 96%, 89%, and 79% in the rate control arm (Fig. 35.1).[14] Although there was no significant difference between the two groups ($P = 0.08$), a trend towards better survival in the rate control arm appeared after the first 1½ years. The secondary combined endpoint (death, disabling stroke or anoxic encephalopathy, major bleed or cardiac arrest) was not significantly different between the arms ($P = 0.33$) (Fig. 35.2).[20] No major differences were noted in functional status or quality of life.

A total of 77 ischemic strokes occurred in the rate control arm compared with 80 in the rhythm control arm ($P = 0.79$).[14] Most strokes in both arms occurred in patients who were either not taking warfarin or who had an INR <2.0. In the rhythm control arm, 22% of strokes occurred in patients whose INR was <2, and more than one-half (57%) occurred in patients not taking warfarin. Thus, 79% of patients in the

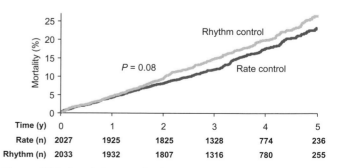

Figure 35.1 Cumulative mortality from any cause in the rate control and rhythm control arms of the AFFIRM study. Time zero is the day of randomization. Data have been truncated at 5 years. (From Wyse *et al.*[14], with permission.)

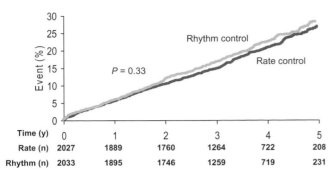

Figure 35.2 Cumulative events for the secondary endpoint of death, disabling stroke or anoxic encephalopathy, major bleed or cardiac arrest in the AFFIRM trial. Time zero is the day of randomization. Data have been truncated at 5 years. (From Waldo[20], with permission.)

rhythm control arm who had a stroke either were not taking warfarin or the INR was subtherapeutic. These stroke outcomes probably should not be surprising in patients with stroke risk factors because of the likely recurrence of AF in a large percentage of patients and the fact that there is an important incidence of asymptomatic AF.

RACE

RACE was a multicenter, randomized trial in 522 patients.[15] It tested the hypothesis that rate control is not inferior to the maintenance of sinus rhythm for the treatment of persistent AF. The primary endpoint was a composite of cardiovascular death, hospital admission for heart failure, thromboembolic complications, severe bleeding, pacemaker implantation, and severe adverse effects of therapy. Rate control was achieved by keeping the ventricular response rates <100 beats per minute with control of symptoms. Rhythm control consisted of serial use of antiarrhythmic drug therapy and electrical cardioversion, if required, to maintain sinus rhythm.

At 3-year follow-up, only 40% of rhythm control patients and 10% of rate control patients were in sinus rhythm. In this trial, 17.2% of patients achieved the primary endpoint in the rate control arm, versus 22.6% of patients in the rhythm control arm (absolute difference 5.4%; 90% confidence interval (CI) −11% to 0.4%). Therefore, the RACE trial demonstrated that rate control met the criteria for non-inferiority to rhythm control, indicating that rate control is an acceptable primary treatment option for patients with AF.

PIAF

The PIAF pilot study[17] compared rate control using diltiazem with rhythm control using amiodarone. Other atrioventricular node blocking drugs could be used if diltiazem failed to control the ventricular rate. The trial enrolled 252 patients with persistent AF. The primary endpoint was improvement in AF-related symptoms. At follow-up, 56%

of patients in the rhythm control arm and 10% of patients in the rate control arm were in sinus rhythm ($P < 0.001$). At 1 year, a similar proportion of patients in both groups reported improved symptoms (76 patients in the rate control arm vs 70 patients in the rhythm control arm, $P = 0.317$). Amiodarone restored sinus rhythm in 23% of patients. The distance walked in 6 minutes was greater in the rhythm control arm, but quality of life measures did not differ. Hospital admission rates were higher in the rhythm control arm (87/127 (69%) vs 30/125 (24%), $P = 0.001$), and adverse drug effects caused more frequent therapy changes in this arm as well (31 (25%) vs 17 (14%), $P = 0.036$). Overall, although the two groups in the PIAF study had similar clinical results, exercise tolerance was better with rhythm control. However, this advantage in favor of rhythm control was offset by more frequent hospital admissions.

STAF

In this pilot study, 200 patients with persistent AF were randomized to rate control or rhythm control, and followed for a mean of 19.6 ± 8.9 months.[18] There was no difference between the two strategies for the primary combined endpoint of death, cardiopulmonary resuscitation, stroke or transient ischemic attack, and systemic embolism. Hospitalization was significantly more frequent in the rhythm control arm, explained by the need to perform multiple cardioversions and to change antiarrhythmic drug therapy. In short, the data showed similar outcomes in both arms, supporting the concept that rate control is a legitimate primary treatment option. Moreover, the study suggested there was no benefit in attempting rhythm control in patients at high risk for recurrence of AF. A limitation of this study was that two-thirds of the patients had AF for more than 6 months at the time of entry into the study, and only 23% of the patients in the rhythm control arm were in sinus rhythm after 36 months of follow-up.

HOT CAFÉ

The HOT CAFÉ study was a randomized, multicenter, prospective trial in 205 patients with a clinically overt, persistent first episode of AF.[19] The primary endpoint was a composite of death from any cause, thromboembolic complications (especially disabling ischemic stroke), and intracranial or other major hemorrhage. Secondary endpoints included rate control, sinus rhythm maintenance, and discontinuation of therapy, especially if due to a potential proarrhythmic effect, hemorrhage, hospitalization, new or worsening congestive heart failure, or change in exercise tolerance. Patients were followed for a mean of 1.7 ± 0.4 years (maximum follow-up, 2.5 years). Antiarrhythmic drugs used included disopyramide, propafenone, sotalol, and amiodarone. At the end of the study, 63.5% of patients in the rhythm control arm remained in sinus rhythm.

Table 35.1 Studies of rate versus rhythm control in atrial fibrillation

Study	PIAF	STAF	HOT CAFÉ	RACE
No. of patients	252	200	205	522
Follow-up, years	1	1.6	1.7	2.3
Primary endpoint	Symptom improvement	Composite of ACM, cardiovascular events, CPR, TE	Composite of ACM, TE, bleeding	Composite of CVD, hospitalizations for CHF, TE, bleeding, pacemaker, AAD adverse effects
Difference in primary endpoint	Symptom improved in 70 RhyC vs 76 RC patients ($P = 0.317$)	5.54%/yr vs 6.09%/yr RhyC vs RC ($P = 0.99$)	No difference (OR, 10.98; 95% CI, 0.28–22.3; $P > 0.71$)	22.6% vs 17.2% RhyC vs RC (HR, 0.73; 90% CI, 0.53–1.01; $P = 0.11$)
Mortality	N/A	2.5%/year vs 4.9%/year RhyC vs RC	3 (2.9%) vs 1 (1%) RhyC vs RC	6.8% vs 7% (n.s.)
Thromboembolic event	N/A	3.1%/year vs 0.6%/year RhyC vs RC	3 (2.9%) vs 1 (1%) RhyC vs RC	Trend towards more TE in RhyC 7.9% vs 5.5% RhyC vs RC
Heart failure	N/A	Improved: 16 vs 26; worsened: 39 vs 29 RhyC vs RC patients ($P = 0.18$)	No difference	4.5% vs 3.5% RhyC vs RC
Hospitalizations	69% vs 24% RhyC vs RC ($P = 0.001$)*	54% vs 26% RhyC vs RC ($P < 0.01$)	74% vs 12% RhyC vs RC ($P < 0.001$); excluding DCC, 1.03 vs 0.05 per patient RhyC vs RC	More in RhyC*
Quality of life	No difference, but better functional capacity in RhyC	No difference	Not assessed, but better functional capacity in RhyC	No difference
Other findings	Better exercise tolerance but more AAD adverse effects in RhyC (25% vs 14%; $P = 0.036$)	18 out of total 19 primary endpoint events occurred during AF	Better exercise tolerance ($P < 0.001$), smaller LA and LV sizes, better LV systolic function in RhyC	On-treatment analysis: more CHF in RC; Echo substudy: smaller LA and LV sizes, better LV systolic function in RhyC

AAD, antiarrhythmic drugs; ACM, all-cause mortality; AF, atrial fibrillation; AF CHF, Atrial Fibrillation and Congestive Heart Failure; AFFIRM, Atrial Fibrillation Follow-up Investigation of Rhythm Management; CHF, congestive heart failure; CI, confidence intervals; CPR, cardiopulmonary resuscitation; CRRAFT, Control of Rate versus Rhythm in rheumatic study in rheumatic Atrial Fibrillation Trial; CVD, cardiovascular death; HOT CAFÉ, HOw to Treat Chronic Atrial Fibrillation; HR, hazard ratio; J-RHYTHM, Japanese Rhythm management trial for atrial fibrillation; LA, left atrium; LV, left ventricle; OR, odds ratio; PAF, Paroxysmal Atrial Fibrillation 2; PIAF, Pharmacological Intervention in Atrial Fibrillation; RACE, Rate Control versus Electrical Cardioversion; RC, rate control; RhyC, rhythm control; SE, systemic embolism; STAF, Strategies of Treatment of Atrial Fibrillation; TE, thromboembolic event; TIA, transient ischemic attack. *, including cardioversion; †, reported as an adverse event

Although it was not reported, it is likely that very few, if any, patients in the rate control arm were in sinus rhythm because patients had to be in AF for at least 7 days at entry into the study. There were no significant differences in the primary endpoint between rate and rhythm control patients (odds ratio (OR) 1.98; 95% CI 0.28–22.3; $P > 0.71$), nor were there significant differences in secondary endpoints, except that the incidence of hospital admissions was much lower in the rate control than the rhythm control arm (12% vs 74%, respectively; $P < 0.001$).

AFFIRM	AF-CHF	J-RHYTHM	CRRAFT	PAF 2
4060	1376	823	144 (rheumatic AF, 73% had valvular intervention)	137 (after atrioventricular node ablation and pacing)
3.5 All-cause mortality	3.1 Cardiovascular mortality	1.6 Composite of ACM, stroke, SE, major bleeding, CHF hospitalization, adverse effects	1 Improvement in exercise tolerance, functional class, and quality of life	1.3 Prevention of permanent AF
23.8% vs 21.3% RhyC vs RC (HR, 1.15; 95% CI, 0.99–1.34; $P = 0.08$)	27% vs 25% RhyC vs RC (HR, 1.06; 95% CI, 0.86–1.3; $P = 0.59$)	15.3% vs 22% RhyC vs RC ($P = 0.0128$)	Significant improvement in all outcomes with RhyC	Permanent AF: 21% vs 37% RhyC vs RC (OR, 0.43; 95% CI, 0.18–0.98; $P = 0.027$)
As above	32% vs 33% RhyC vs RC ($P = 0.68$)	4 (1%) vs 3 (0.7%) RhyC vs RC	0 vs 5 events RhyC vs RC ($P = 0.023$)	N/A
Stroke: 7.1% vs 5.5% RhyC vs RC ($P = 0.79$) SE: 0.4% vs 0.5% RhyC vs RC ($P = 0.62$)	3% vs 4% RhyC vs RC ($P = 0.32$)	2.39% vs 2.97% RhyC vs RC	1 TIA in RhyC vs 0 events in RC	3 (4%) vs 1 (1%) RhyC vs RC ($P = 0.30$)
2.7% vs 2.1% RhyC vs RC ($P = 0.58$)	28% vs 31% RhyC vs RC ($P = 0.17$)	0.5% vs 1.5% RhyC vs RC	CHF functional class improved: 60% vs 17.5% RhyC vs RC; worsened: 4.4% vs 10% ($P = 0.0014$)	22% vs 10% RhyC vs RC ($P = 0.05$)
80% vs 73% RhyC vs RC ($P < 0.001$)	During the first year 46% vs 39% RhyC vs RC ($P = 0.0063$)	N/A	8.9% vs 15% RhyC vs RC ($P = 0.51$)	For CHF, 18% vs 7% RhyC vs RC ($P = 0.05$)
No difference, but trend towards better functional capacity in RhyC	Not yet available	Symptom frequency was lower with RhyC ($P = 0.0027$)	Improved by ≥ 1 score: 86.7% vs 50% RhyC vs RC ($P = 0.033$)	No difference
On-treatment analysis: maintenance of sinus rhythm was associated with lower mortality (HR, 0.53; 95% CI, 0.39–0.72; $P < 0.0001$)	On-treatment analysis: no survival benefit from maintenance of sinus rhythm (HR, 1.11; 95% CI, 0.78–1.58; $P = 0.568$)	Symptoms or adverse effects leading to crossover occurred in 11% RhyC vs 16.6% RC patients ($P = 0.0142$)	N/A	N/A

Meta-analysis of these studies has demonstrated no significant excess or reduced mortality with either strategy but hinted at a trend towards better survival when rate control was the primary treatment approach (OR 0.87; 95% CI 0.74–1.02; $P = 0.09$).[21]

Following these publications, there has been a general movement away from rhythm control in patients who are able to tolerate the arrhythmia when the ventricular rate is adequately controlled. The major limitation of the studies which compared two strategies was inability to achieve a clear difference with respect to rhythm and rate status in the two arms as a significant proportion of patients in the rhythm control arm failed to maintain sinus rhythm and many patients in the rate control arm were in sinus rhythm at the end of the study. A subsequent, retrospective, on-treatment analysis of time-dependent covariates on outcome in the AFFIRM trial has shown that the presence of sinus rhythm conferred a considerable reduction of 47% in the risk of death irrespective of the treatment strategy.[22] However, antiarrhythmic drug use was associated with a 42% increase in the risk of death. This has been interpreted as showing that when sinus rhythm is included as a separate factor, the sinus rhythm variable expresses the beneficial effect and the antiarrhythmic drug variable expresses the detrimental effects. Thus, use of antiarrhythmic drugs is associated with increased mortality. However, when sinus rhythm was removed as a separate factor from the analysis, antiarrhythmic drugs were not associated with mortality, presumably because the beneficial antiarrhythmic effects of antiarrhythmic drugs offset their adverse effects. In short, it suggested that in patients with AF, if one could achieve sinus rhythm safely and effectively, sinus rhythm would confer a favorable outcome.

AF CHF

Retrospective studies in patients with left ventricular dysfunction and AF previously showed that there is as high as a twofold increased mortality compared with patients in sinus rhythm.[23,24] These and similar observations triggered a large randomized, open-label trial, AF CHF. The AF CHF investigators compared rate and rhythm control strategies specifically in 1376 patients with an ejection fraction of 35% or less and NYHA II–IV heart failure who were followed for a mean of 37 months.[15] For patients randomized to the rhythm control arm, aggressive therapy to prevent AF and maintain sinus rhythm was recommended. Amiodarone was the drug of choice for AF suppression and sinus rhythm maintenance, but sotalol and dofetilide were used in selected cases. For patients randomized to the rate control arm, beta-blockers with digitalis were used to achieve the target heart rate of <80 beats per minute at rest and <110 beats per minute during a 6-minute walk test. Atrioventricular node ablation and pacemaker therapy were recommended for patients who were otherwise unable to meet rate control targets.

The study showed no benefit of rhythm control on top of optimal medical therapy with regard to the primary endpoint (cardiovascular mortality) as well as prespecified secondary endpoints including total mortality, worsening heart failure, stroke, and hospitalization. Cardiovascular death occurred in 182 (26.7%) of the patients in the rhythm control group compared with 175 (25.2%) in the rate control arm (hazard ratio (HR) 1.058, 95% CI 0.86–1.30; $P = 0.59$) (Fig. 35.3).[15] During the course of the study, 21% of patients crossed over from rhythm to rate control, primarily because of the inability to maintain sinus rhythm, but 10% crossed from the rate control arm to rhythm control, primarily because of worsening heart failure. Similar to the AFFIRM trial, the AF CHF trial conducted a retrospective on-treatment analysis of outcomes and showed that AF does not predict cardiovascular or all-cause mortality once the severity of clinical symptoms and mitral regurgitation is known.[24a] These results further indicate that rate control is a legitimate primary treatment option for patients with heart failure.

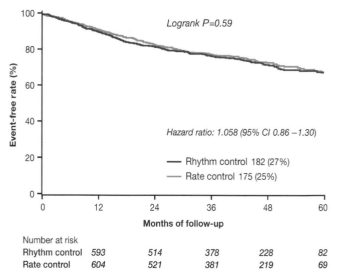

Figure 35.3 Kaplan–Meier estimates of death from cardiovascular causes (primary outcome) in the AF CHF study. AF CHF, Atrial Fibrillation in Congestive Heart Failure. (From Roy *et al*[16], with permission.)

The results of the AF CHF trial likely reflect the considerable improvement in the management of heart failure as well as the management of stroke prevention in patients with AF. In the years since the publication of the retrospective studies which identified a twofold increase in mortality in patients with AF and heart failure compared to patients with sinus rhythm and heart failure, therapy with beta-blockers, afterload reducers, statins, and aldosterone antagonists has considerably improved outcome. We learn once again from the AF CHF trial that because of new, improved and better applied therapies which produce better outcomes, historic controls are often an invalid comparator. A contemporary comparator will reflect the changes, usually the improvements, in patient care that occur over time, which, in turn, will change (usually improve) patient outcomes.

Importantly, the results of rate versus rhythm control studies highlighted the limitations of current therapies to achieve and maintain sinus rhythm. Long-term maintenance of sinus rhythm has proven difficult to achieve in patients with persistent AF, and the method is time-consuming and expensive due to the costs of the antiarrhythmic drugs and the increased need for hospitalization. Thus, the unmet need for safer and more effective antiarrhythmic agents to reverse this trend is clear.

Pharmacologic cardioversion for atrial fibrillation

Pharmacologic cardioversion is considered to be most effective if initiated within 7 days after the onset of the arrhythmia in which case restoration of sinus rhythm can be achieved in nearly 70% of patients, but the success rate decreases significantly as AF persists beyond this limit. The likelihood of spontaneous conversion varies greatly, but is mainly determined by the nature of the arrhythmia (paroxysmal or persistent), the duration of the index episode, the overall duration of AF, the number of recurrences, and the severity of underlying heart disease.[25] Systematic analysis of placebo-controlled studies of pharmacologic cardioversion for AF has shown that among patients with AF of less than 24 hours, 66% spontaneously converted to sinus rhythm compared with only 17% of those with the arrhythmia of longer duration (OR 1.8).[26]

The choice of an antiarrhythmic drug for cardioversion of AF depends on the underlying heart disease.[5] Class IC antiarrhythmic agents (propafenone and flecainide), sotalol, and ibutilide are recommended for cardioversion of AF in patients with moderate structural heart disease or hypertension without left ventricular hypertrophy and are contraindicated in patients with a history of heart failure, myocardial infarction with left ventricular dysfunction, and significant left ventricular hypertrophy (>1.4 cm). Amiodarone and dofetilide can be used in patients presenting with symptoms of heart failure and known advanced heart disease. Propafenone, flecainide and sotalol are less effective for cardioversion with increased duration of the arrhythmia, and in such patients the choice of drugs is limited to dofetilide, ibutilide and amiodarone. Intravenous formulations of antiarrhythmic drugs are typically used for cardioversion, particularly when the AF is of short duration; however, oral forms of propafenone, flecainide, sotalol and amiodarone are available and may be used in loading doses. Although oral quinidine and oral or intravenous procainamide (class IA antiarrhythmic agents) are available in some countries, there has been a significant decrease in their use worldwide. Antiarrhythmic drugs recommended by the ACC/AHA/ESC guidelines are listed in Table 35.2.

Propafenone and flecainide

In placebo-controlled, randomized studies, intravenous propafenone and flecainide were effective in cardioversion of recent (usually 1–72 h)-onset AF, with conversion rates as high as 80–90% within an hour after the start of infusion.[27–29] The advantage of propafenone and flecainide is the possibility of oral administration for cardioversion of AF; the conversion rates are comparable to those achieved with intravenous formulations, although the effect is usually delayed.[30–36] In a meta-analysis of 1843 patients from 27 studies, intravenous or oral propafenone demonstrated a placebo-subtracted efficacy of 31.5% at 4 hours and 32.9% at 8 hours.[30] Thus, after administration of a loading single oral dose of propafenone (usually 450–600 mg) or flecainide (usually 200–300 mg), sinus rhythm

was restored in, respectively, 51–59% at 3 hours and 72–78% at 8 hours, compared with respective conversion rates of 18% and 39% on placebo.[31] Across the studies, the success rates ranged from 56% to 83% for propafenone and from 57% to 68% for flecainide. The conversion times ranged from 110 ± 59 to 287 ± 352 minutes and 110 ± 82 to 190 ± 147 minutes for propafenone and flecainide, respectively.[32–34] Both drugs have been given a **Class I** recommendation for cardioversion of recent-onset (less than 7 days) AF in patients without significant structural heart disease (**Level A**). The drugs are considered relatively ineffective for termination of AF of longer duration (**Class IIb, Level B**).

"Pill in the pocket" approach

The high efficacies of oral propafenone and flecainide in cardioversion of AF have formed the basis for the use of these drugs for termination of the arrhythmia outside the hospital setting. In patients with no or minimal structural heart disease and relatively infrequent (perhaps less than 12 per year) paroxysms of AF of distinct onset which, although symptomatic, do not cause significant hemodynamic compromise (e.g. hypotension), a loading single dose of either drug has proven safe and effective for expedient cardioversion to sinus rhythm.[37] In a key feasibility study, a selected cohort of 210 patients who had been successfully treated in hospital with either oral flecainide or propafenone for paroxysmal AF were given a supply of the relevant drug and asked to take a single oral dose within 5 minutes of noticing palpitations. In comparison with their own historic control data, as a result of the "pill in the pocket" strategy, the number of visits to emergency departments fell to 4.9 a month (from 45.6 visits a month during the previous period, $P < 0.001$), despite the same frequency of arrhythmia episodes.[38]

However, the experience with this strategy is limited, neither propafenone nor flecainide is licensed for patients to use for self-treating single attacks, and it is mandatory that the efficacy and safety of this strategy are first tested in hospital. It is unknown how valuable the "pill in the pocket" approach will be in the long term because AF tends to progress to sustained over time. Long-term anticoagulation will be needed in high-risk individuals. It is generally recommended that patients should not be taking a prophylactic antiarrhythmic drug. There is always the danger of development of atrial flutter with 1:1 atrioventricular conduction due to slowing of the atrial rate, associated with dangerous widening of the QRS complex (due to the enhanced (use-dependent) sodium channel blocking effect) and rarely left ventricular dysfunction secondary to the negative inotropic effect. Atrial flutter was reported in 2.5–20% of patients who received oral loading doses of propafenone or flecainide for conversion of AF (5–7% on average), and 2–14% of patients developed hypotension.[34] Therefore, concomitant administration of an atrioventricular node-blocking agent (a beta-blocker, verapamil or

Table 35.2 Antiarrhythmic drugs for pharmacologic cardioversion of atrial fibrillation

Drug	Route	Dose	AF ≤7 days		AF >7 days		Potential adverse effects
			Class	LOE	Class	LOE	
Flecainide	Oral or intravenous	Loading dose 200–300 mg or 1.5–3.0 mg/kg over 10–20 min	I	A	IIb	B	Rapidly conducted atrial flutter; ventricular proarrhythmia in patients with myocardial ischemia; possible deterioration of ventricular function in the presence of organic heart disease
Propafenone	Oral or intravenous	Loading dose 450–600 mg or 1.5–2.0 mg/kg over 10–20 min	I	A	IIb	B	
Ibutilide	Intravenous	1 mg over 10 min; repeat 1 mg if necessary	IIa	A	IIa	A	QT prolongation; torsades de pointes; hypotension
Sotalol	Intravenous	80 mg initial dose; then 160–320 mg in divided doses	III	A	III	B	QT prolongation; torsades de pointes; bradycardia; hypotension
	Oral	80 mg initial dose; then 160–320 mg in divided doses	IIb	B	III	B	
Dofetilide	Oral	125–500 mg twice daily*	I	A	I	I	QT prolongation; torsades de pointes; contraindicated if creatinine clearance < 20 mL/min
Amiodarone	Oral or intravenous	Inpatient: 1200–1800 mg daily in divided doses until 10 g total; then 200–400 mg daily Outpatient: 600–800 mg daily until 10 g total; then 200–400 mg daily 5–7 mg/kg over 30–60 min intravenously; then 1200–1800 mg daily oral until 10 g total; then 200–400 mg daily	IIa	A	IIa	A	Hypotension; bradycardia; QT prolongation; torsades de pointes (risk <1%); phlebitis (intravenous) gastrointestinal upset; constipation (oral); multiorgan toxicity in the long term
Quinidine†	Oral	750–1500 mg in divided doses over 6–12 hours + rate-slowing drug (e.g. verapamil)	IIb	B	IIb	B	QT prolongation; torsades de pointes; QRS widening; rapid atrial flutter; hypotension; gastrointestinal upset
Procainamide†	Intravenous	1000 mg over 30 min (33 mg/min) followed by 2 mg/min infusion	IIb	B	IIb	C	QRS widening; torsades de pointes; rapid atrial flutter

AF, atrial fibrillation; LOE, level of evidence;

* dose depends on creatinine clearance: >60 mL/min – 500 mg; 40–60 mL/min – 250 mg; 20–40 mL/min – 125 mg twice daily; contraindicated if creatinine clearance <20 mL/min;

† limited use or withdrawn agents.

diltiazem) is warranted. Transient atrioventricular block, QRS widening, and left bundle branch block occurred in approximately 2–8%. Class IC drugs usually are ineffective for conversion of atrial flutter. They slow conduction within the re-entrant circuit and prolong the atrial flutter cycle length, but rarely interrupt the circuit and there is greater risk of 1:1 atrioventricular conduction. The efficacy rates have been reported to be as low as 13–40%.[39]

Sotalol

Intravenous sotalol generally is ineffective for acute cardioversion of AF of any duration (**Class III, Level A**). The conversion rate in one study was 11–13% with sotalol vs 14% on placebo in the double-blind phase and 30% in the open-label phase.[40] In a direct comparison study with ibutilide in 308 patients with AF or flutter of 3 hours to 45 days, sotalol 1.5 mg/kg (n = 103) restored sinus rhythm in only 11% of patients with AF and 19% of patients with flutter and was significantly inferior to ibutilide.[41] Even among patients with very recent onset AF (<48 hours), only 12% converted to sinus rhythm at 3 hours with oral sotalol 80–160 mg and a further 12% converted to sinus rhythm at 8 hours after receiving a cumulative dose of 160–240 mg.[42] In this study, the conversion rates for sotalol were significantly lower than for oral quinidine in combination with digoxin (36% and 71% at 3 and 8 hours, respectively). In the Sotalol Amiodarone Atrial Fibrillation Efficacy Trial (SAFE-T), 24.2% of patients with persistent AF treated with sotalol converted to sinus rhythm within 28 days, compared with 27.1% on amiodarone and only 0.8% on placebo.[43] Sotalol may offer a modest benefit of facilitating spontaneous conversion to sinus rhythm and, in addition, can ensure ventricular rate control in patients awaiting electrical cardioversion (**Class IIb, Level B**).

The antifibrillatory effect of sotalol is limited by reverse use dependency of its effect on atrial refractoriness: sotalol prolongs the atrial effective refractory period at normal and slow atrial rates, but not during rapid AF. The adverse effects of sotalol include hypotension, bradycardia, QT interval prolongation and associated ventricular proarrhythmia (torsades de pointes). Bradycardia and hypotension were the most common with intravenous sotalol, with an incidence of 6.5% and 3.7%, respectively.[43] Polymorphic ventricular tachycardia or torsades de pointes was reported in 1% of men and 4.1% of women who received sotalol for ventricular tachyarrhythmias.[44] The risk of proarrhythmia is increased in the presence of left ventricular hypertrophy because of increased duration and inhomogeneity of repolarization in the hypertrophied myocardium, increased transmural dispersion of repolarization, disruption of gap junction coupling, and a greater likelihood of ischemia and fibrosis. Sotalol levels are also increased in renal failure and torsades de pointes is more likely under these conditions.

Ibutilide

In randomized, placebo-controlled studies and direct comparisons with procainamide and sotalol, the class III drug ibutilide has proven more effective for cardioversion of atrial flutter than AF.[41,45–47] The overall conversion rates for atrial flutter were reported to be almost twofold higher than for AF (56–70% vs 31–44%).[41,46] In direct comparison studies, ibutilide 2 mg cardioverted 70% of atrial flutter compared with only 19% on sotalol[41] and 14% on procainamide.[47] Higher doses of ibutilide administered as a single bolus of 2 mg or two successive infusions of 1 mg are usually required for termination of AF. Thus, in the Ibutilide/Sotalol Comparator Study, patients with AF were twice as likely to convert to sinus rhythm after receiving a 2 mg infusion than those who received a 1 mg infusion (44% vs 20%).[41] The antiarrhythmic effect of ibutilide decreased if the arrhythmia had persisted for more than 7 days – from 71% to 57% for atrial flutter and from 46% to 18% for AF. Nevertheless, ibutilide is recommended for cardioversion of AF (**Class IIa, Level A**).

Unlike sotalol and procainamide (a class IA agent), ibutilide does not produce significant hypotension but like many of the class III antiarrhythmic drugs, it may cause QT interval prolongation and ventricular proarrhythmia. In the ibutilide trials, the incidence of polymorphic ventricular tachycardia or torsades de pointes requiring electrical cardioversion was 0.5–1.7% and the incidence of self-terminating polymorphic ventricular tachycardia was 2.6–6.7%.[48] There are insufficient data to support the use of ibutilide in patients with significant structural heart disease as many controlled studies of ibutilide have only enrolled patients with mild or moderate underlying heart disease. Ibutilide 2 mg administered intravenously on top of long-term therapy with oral amiodarone in patients referred for electrical cardioversion terminated AF in 39% of patients and flutter in 54%.[49] The QT interval was significantly prolonged, but there was only one case of non-sustained polymorphic tachycardia.

Dofetilide

In small (less than 100 patients) randomized, double-blind, placebo-controlled studies, dofetilide administered intravenously at 8 µg/kg restored sinus rhythm in about one-third of patients presenting with atrial flutter or AF compared with 0–3.3% on placebo.[50,51] As with ibutilide, the conversion rates were significantly higher for atrial flutter than for AF (54–64% vs 14.5–24%).[50,51] In a double-blind, dose-ranging, pharmacokinetic study, dofetilide 8 µg/kg was confirmed as the most effective dose with an acceptable rate of adverse events: 39% of patients in the dofetilide group converted to sinus rhythm compared with 6% in the placebo group.[52] In line with the conversion rates observed with other antiarrhythmic agents, the likelihood of pharmacologic conversion on dofetilide decreased as the duration of AF increased: the drug was effective in 67% of patients with arrhythmia onset within 24 hours of treatment, 36% of patients with AF of 1–7 days, and 24% of patients with AF of more than 7 days.

Two medium-size prospective studies, SAFIRE-D (Symptomatic Atrial Fibrillation Investigative Research on Dofetilide) and EMERALD (European and Australian Multicenter Evaluative Research on Dofetilide), reported a modest 30% cardioversion rate of persistent AF with high-dose (1000 µg daily) oral dofetilide compared with 1.2% of spontaneous conversion on placebo[53] and 5% on sotalol.[54] In the pooled analysis from the DIAMOND (Danish Investigations of Arrhythmia and Mortality ON Dofetilide) studies in patients with symptomatic heart failure and an ejection fraction ≤35% (DIAMOND-CHF) or myocardial infarction with left ventricular dysfunction (DIAMOND-MI), oral dofetilide had a neutral effect on mortality and also demonstrated a greater rate of conversion to sinus rhythm (44% vs 14%).[24]

Oral dofetilide is considered safe and relatively effective for pharmacologic cardioversion of AF including arrhythmia duration of more than 7 days (**Class I, Level A**). Intravenous dofetilide is rarely used for pharmacologic cardioversion. However, dofetilide has been reported to prolong the QT interval and cause torsades de pointes. This effect is dose related. Therefore, it is mandatory that dofetilide be initiated in hospital and that patients should be monitored for 3 days. In addition, the dose of dofetilide requires adjustment to creatinine clearance.

Amiodarone

Amiodarone is currently assigned a **Class IIa, Level A** indication for cardioversion of AF of any duration. Meta-analysis of 13 randomized controlled studies in 1174 patients has shown that IV amiodarone was 44% more effective in converting AF compared with placebo, but its antiarrhythmic effect was delayed by 24 hours.[55] At 8 hours, the probability of restoration of sinus rhythm was 65% higher with flecainide or propafenone than with amiodarone. In a double-blind direct comparison with dofetilide, amiodarone cardioverted only 4% of patients with AF compared with 35% on dofetilide and 4% on placebo.[56] In one study, amiodarone administered intravenously as a bolus of 300 mg for 1 hour followed by infusion of 20 mg/kg for 24 hours and oral treatment for 4 weeks cardioverted 80% of AF.[57] However, spontaneous conversion rates in this study were also high (40%). Amiodarone given at a high single loading oral dose of 30 mg/kg (approx. 2.4 g) was less effective than oral propafenone 600 mg at 4 hours (16% vs 37%) and comparable with propafenone at 24 hours (56% vs 47%), but the median time to conversion to

sinus rhythm was significantly shorter with propafenone than amiodarone (2.4 vs 6.9 hours).[58]

Intravenous amiodarone has a modest effect on atrial refractoriness and therefore is moderately effective in terminating the arrhythmia in the emergency setting, but unlike class IC agents, amiodarone does not have any negative inotropic effect, controls the ventricular rate, and is associated with a low incidence of torsades de pointes. All this makes it safe to use in patients with advanced structural heart disease. Amiodarone prolongs the QT interval but, unlike pure class III agents, exhibits a low arrhythmogenic potential (less than 1%).[59] The most common effects of intravenous amiodarone are hypotension and relative bradycardia. There is limited experience with the use of intravenous amiodarone for termination of AF in critically ill patients.[60]

The mortality and morbidity study CHF-STAT (Congestive Heart Failure Survival Trial of Antiarrhythmic Therapy) in 667 patients with a mean ejection fraction of 25% has shown that long-term treatment with oral amiodarone 400 mg daily for the first year and 300 mg daily for the remainder of the 4.5-year trial had a neutral effect on survival but was associated with greater rates of conversion to sinus rhythm compared with placebo (31% vs 7.7%).[61] The SAFE-T study randomized 665 patients with persistent AF (74–80% less than 1 year) to therapy with amiodarone, sotalol or placebo for 28 days prior to carrying out electrical cardioversion.[43] The amiodarone regimen for this period was 800 mg for the first 2 weeks and 600 mg for the next 2 weeks. Of 267 patients who received amiodarone, 27.1% converted to sinus rhythm compared with 0.8% out of 137 in the placebo group. In a study of 95 patients with a mean AF of almost 2 years, amiodarone prescribed 600 mg daily for 4 weeks restored sinus rhythm in 34% of patients compared with 0% in the placebo group.[62]

Procainamide, quinidine, and disopyramide

The class IA drug procainamide has been shown to facilitate conversion of AF of less than 48 hours, but its efficacy is limited in AF of longer duration.[47,63–65] The conversion rates with procainamide administered intravenously at a dose 1000–1200 mg over 30 minutes ranged from 21% to 70%. In direct comparison studies, the efficacy of procainamide was comparable to that of propafenone (69.5% vs 48.7%)[64] and flecainide (65% vs 92%).[65] In a randomized, single-blind, placebo-controlled study in 362 patients with AF of less than 48 hours, the conversion rates with IV procainamide, propafenone, and amiodarone were 68.5%, 80.2%, and 89.1%, respectively.[66] Propafenone produced the most rapid effect, with a median time to conversion of 1h, followed by procainamide (3h) and amiodarone (9h). The non-target effects of procainamide are vasodilation and hypotension due to the alpha-adrenergic properties, anticholinergic action, atrioventricular node blockade, worsening heart failure, and lupus erythematosus. The drug is no longer used routinely for cardioversion of AF (**Class IIb, Level B**).

Quinidine given orally in a cumulative dose of up to 1200–2400 mg over 24 hours has been shown to cardiovert 60–80% of recent-onset AF; it is more effective than sotalol[67] and in some studies it was as effective as intravenous amiodarone.[68] The effect usually occurs within 12 hours of treatment. Quinidine poses increased risk of torsades de pointes which is observed at a rate of 6%; it widens the QRS complex, causes gastrointestinal side effects in a significant proportion of patients, and is contraindicated in individuals with structural heart disease. The poor safety profile of quinidine has led to a decrease in its use for acute cardioversion of AF (**Class IIb, Level B**).

There is limited evidence for the efficacy of intravenous disopyramide for acute pharmacologic cardioversion in patients with AF. In one study, disopyramide administered as a bolus of 2 mg/kg over 5 minutes restored sinus rhythm in 10 of 14 (71%) patients with self-limiting lone AF and 3 of 7 (43%) patients with atrial flutter.[69] There are concerns, however, that the adverse effects such as proarrhythmia, hypotension, asystole, and non-target effects resulting from anticholinergic activity of disopyramide may offset its modest antiarrhythmic potential (**Class IIb, Level B**).[5]

Other agents

One-quarter to one-half of patients with AF have low serum magnesium levels.[70] The electrophysiologic effects of magnesium include prolongation of the atrial and atrioventricular node refractory periods which are essential determinants of ventricular rates and maintenance of AF. Meta-analysis of eight studies in 476 patients showed that magnesium sulfate, administered intravenously at an initial dose of 1200–5000 mg over 1–30 minutes (in some studies followed by a second dose or continuous infusion for 2–6 hours), was superior to placebo or the active comparator in cardioverting AF with an odds ratio of 1.6 (95% CI 1.07–2.39).[70] Time to conversion was 3.8–14.9 hours and the most common side effects were sensations of warmth and flushing. In addition to its antifibrillatory action, magnesium produced effective ventricular rate control. There was no correlation between serum magnesium levels and the response. However, magnesium is not routinely used for pharmacologic cardioversion of AF (**Class IIb, Level B**), but it may potentiate the effect of other antiarrhythmic agents, e.g. in patients with refractory AF.

Digitalis, beta-blockers, and calcium antagonists usually are ineffective for acute conversion of AF (**Class III**).[27,71,72] The DAAF (Digitalis in Acute Atrial Fibrillation) study has shown no difference in cardioversion rates at 16 hours between intravenous digoxin and placebo (51% vs 46%).[73] Moreover, the drug has been shown to have a profibrillatory effect due to its cholinergic effects which may cause a non-uniform reduction in conduction velocity and effective refractory periods of the atria, and to delay the reversal of remodeling after restoration of sinus rhythm.[74] Digoxin is not indicated for pharmacologic cardioversion of AF (**Class III, Level A**). Short-acting intravenous beta-blockers (e.g. esmolol) and non-dihydropyridine calcium antagonists (verapamil and diltiazem) are more commonly used for rate control than for restoration of sinus rhythm.

Antiarrhythmic drugs and electrical cardioversion

Antiarrhythmic drugs can be used to facilitate electrical cardioversion and to prevent immediate or early recurrence of AF (**Class IIa, Level B**). Synergistic action of antiarrhythmic drugs may be due to prolongation of atrial refractoriness, conversion of AF to a more organized atrial rhythm (e.g. flutter) which may be cardioverted with less energy, the suppression of atrial premature beats that may re-initiate AF, and prevention of atrial remodeling. The disadvantages are increased risk of ventricular proarrhythmia and bradycardia.

Pretreatment with ibutilide lowered the energy requirement by approximately 30% and improved the success rate of cardioversion, including those who previously had failed electrical cardioversion.[75] Flecainide administered intravenously increased the likelihood of converting to sinus rhythm by 16% and significantly reduced the energy requirement.[76] Intravenous sotalol was synergistic with internal electrical cardioversion by preventing reinitiation of AF. Sotalol suppressed atrial premature beats and prolonged the coupling interval of atrial premature beats, thus reducing risk of early recurrence.[77] Higher success rates of electrical cardioversion for persistent AF were reported in patients pretreated with oral amiodarone compared with diltiazem (88% vs 56%).[78] The results with calcium antagonists were controversial. Thus, in the VEPARAF (VErapamil Plus Antiarrhythmic drugs Reduce Atrial Fibrillation) trial, adjunctive treatment with verapamil reduced the AF recurrence rate from 35% to 20%.[79] In the VERDICT (Verapamil versus Digoxin Cardioversion Trial), only 47% of patients in the verapamil-treated group and 53% of those in the digoxin-treated group remained free from recurrence of the arrhythmia during the first month after cardioversion.[80]

New agents for pharmacologic cardioversion

Vernakalant

Vernakalant is a new arrhythmic drug agent with an affinity for ion channels specifically involved in the repolarization processes in atrial tissue, in particular, the ultrarapid potassium repolarization current I_{Kur}. Although I_{Kur} current is the main target of vernakalant, its mechanism of action involves blockade of several ion channels such as I_{to}, and I_{Na}, but there is little impact on major currents responsible for ventricular repolarization, such as I_{Kr} and I_{Ks} currents. The intravenous formulation of vernakalant is under regulatory body review for pharmacologic cardioversion of AF.

The efficacy of vernakalant was investigated in one dose-finding study, three medium-size randomized clinical studies, and a phase IV open-label study (Table 35.3).[81-84] In the randomized, double-blind, placebo-controlled Atrial arrhythmia Conversion Trials (ACT I and II), vernakalant was significantly more effective than placebo in converting AF of less than 7 days (51.7% and 51.2% compared with 4% and 3.6%, respectively, $P < 0.001$).[82,83] Vernakalant was administered as a 10-minute infusion of 3 mg/kg and if AF

persisted after 15 minutes, a second infusion of 2 mg/kg was given. The median time to conversion was 8–11 minutes and the majority of patients (75–82%) converted after the first dose. The highest efficacy was observed for AF of up to 72 hours (70–80%). The results were reproduced in the open-label ACT IV study in which vernakalant restored sinus rhythm in 50.9% within 14 minutes after the start of treatment. Vernakalant was significantly less effective in converting AF of more than 7 days and did not convert atrial flutter.

The drug was well tolerated, with no significant QT prolongation or drug-related torsades de pointes. However, in the ACT I study, the QTc values after infusion were greater in the vernakalant group than in the placebo group, and 24% of patients in the vernakalant group had QTc >500 ms as opposed to 15% in the placebo group, but no torsades de pointes was reported during the first 24 hours after

Table 35.3 Summary of clinical studies of vernakalant in atrial fibrillation

Study	Number of patients	Patient characteristics	Dose of vernakalant	Placebo controlled	Primary endpoint	Outcome vs placebo/control
CRAFT	56	AF 3–72 h	IV 0.5 mg/kg +1 mg/kg or IV 2 mg/kg + 3 mg/kg	Yes	Conversion to SR during infusion or within 30 minutes after the last infusion	Converted to SR: 61% vs 5%, $P < 0.001$; patients in SR at 30 minutes 56% vs 5%, $P = 0.016$; only higher dose was effective
ACT I	336	AF 3 h–45 days (3 h–7 days, n = 220; 8–45 days, n = 116)	IV 3 mg/kg + 2 mg/kg	Yes	Conversion to SR within 90 minutes of drug initiation in AF 3 h–7 days	Converted to SR: 51.7% vs 4%, $P < 0.001$
ACT II	150	AF 3–72 h between 24 h and 7 days after cardiac surgery	IV 3 mg/kg + 2 mg/kg	Yes	Conversion to SR within 90 minutes of drug initiation in AF 3 h–7 days	Converted to SR: 47% vs 14%, $P < 0.001$
ACT III	262	AF 3 h–45 days (3 h–7 days, n = 170; 8–45 days, n = 69)	IV 3 mg/kg + 2 mg/kg	Yes	Conversion to SR within 90 minutes of drug initiation in AF 3 h–7 days	Converted to SR: 51.2% vs 3.6%, $P < 0.001$
ACT IV	167	AF 3 h–45 days (3 h–7 days, n = 170; 8–45 days, n = 69)	IV 3 mg/kg + 2 mg/kg	No	Conversion to SR within 90 minutes of drug initiation in AF 3 h–7 days	Converted to SR: 50.9%
Prevention, phase IIa	159	After pharmacologic (vernakalant) or electrical cardioversion for persistent AF	Oral 300 or 600 mg bid	Yes	SR at 1 month	Maintained SR at 1 month: 61% (each group) vs 43% on placebo, $P = 0.028$
Prevention, phase IIb	446	Persistent AF after pharmacologic (vernakalant) or electrical cardioversion	Oral 150, 300 or 500 mg bid	Yes	SR at 3 months	Maintained SR at 3 months on 500 mg bid: 51% vs 37% on placebo, $P < 0.05$; lower doses reduced AF rates, but not significant vs placebo

ACT, Atrial arrhythmia Conversion Trial; AF, atrial fibrillation; CRAFT, Controlled Randomized Atrial Fibrillation Trial; IV, intravenous; SR, sinus rhythm. Reproduced with permission from Savelieva et al.[84]

infusion.[82] The most common (>5%) side effects of vernakalant were dysgeusia, sneezing, and nausea.

Prevention of atrial fibrillation

Prophylactic antiarrhythmic drug therapy generally is not recommended after a first episode of AF, either self-terminating or after pharmacologic or electrical cardioversion.[5] However, this approach can be appropriate in a small proportion of patients as paroxysmal AF tends to become persistent or permanent. After cardioversion, approximately 25–50% patients will have recurrence of AF within the first 1–2 months (early recurrence).[85] Thereafter, the recurrence rate is about 10% per year (late recurrence). Prophylactic antiarrhythmic drug therapy is recommended for the vast majority of patients with paroxysmal AF when paroxysms occur frequently and are associated with significant symptoms or lead to worsening left ventricular function, and for patients with persistent AF when the likelihood of maintenance of sinus rhythm is uncertain, especially in the presence of risk factors for recurrence such as left atrial enlargement, evidence for depressed atrial function, left ventricular dysfunction, underlying cardiovascular pathology, long duration of the arrhythmia, advanced age, and female gender) (**Class I, Level A**).

The choice of antiarrhythmic drug for prevention of AF is dictated by the presence and nature of underlying heart disease (Fig. 35.4).

A systematic review of 44 studies in 11 322 patients has shown that antiarrhythmic drugs significantly reduced AF recurrence after cardioversion; the number of patients needed to treat to prevent a recurrence ranged from two to nine depending on the agent used.[86] Antiarrhythmic drugs may also render AF less symptomatic, less frequent, and less sustained or may promote conversion to sinus rhythm. The majority of large, high-quality studies were conducted in patients with persistent AF, i.e. AF requiring electrical or pharmacologic therapy to terminate. This was probably because the recurrence of a persistent episode is more "predictable," is likely to occur during the first year, and is easier to recognize and document, especially when the time to first symptomatic recurrence is used as an endpoint. Hence, the results of many trials of the efficacy of antiarrhythmic drugs for the prevention of recurrences of persistent AF were extrapolated on the patient populations with a paroxysmal (self-terminating) arrhythmia.

Beta-blockers

Beta-blockers generally are modestly effective in preventing AF (**Class IIb, Level B**) and are mainly used for rate control. An exception is AF caused by thyrotoxicosis or, rarely, lone adrenergically mediated AF when beta-blockers may be a first-line therapy (**Class I**).[87,88] In anecdotal reports beta-blockers were superior to placebo or were as effective as sotalol for prevention of persistent AF.[89,90] In a medium-size (n = 394), double-blind, placebo-controlled study, treatment with metoprolol 100 mg daily was associated with a modest reduction in arrhythmia recurrence at 3 months after electrical cardioversion from 60% in the placebo arm to 48% in the metoprolol arm.[89] Patients who received metoprolol had slower ventricular rates during the recurrence of AF and were probably less symptomatic. In another study, 58% of

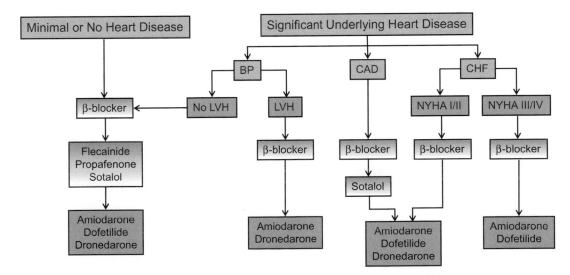

Figure 35.4 Selection of antiarrhythmic drugs for prevention of atrial fibrillation.

patients treated with bisoprolol 5mg daily and 59% of patients treated with sotalol 160mg daily maintained sinus rhythm at 1 year after cardioversion.[90]

Some beta-blockers such as carvedilol may be more potent antiarrhythmics because of their direct effects on cardiac ion channels beyond their antiadrenergic action. In addition, carvedilol has antioxidant activity and may protect the atrial myocardium from oxidative injury caused by fast atrial rates and ischemia. In direct comparisons, carvedilol demonstrated no benefit over bisoprolol, although a higher proportion of patients treated with carvedilol completed the 1-year study in sinus rhythm (68% v 54%)[91] although this trend was not significant and the number of patients was small (n = 90). Beta-blockers may, however, prevent AF associated with congestive heart failure: a meta-analysis of seven studies in 11952 patients has shown that therapy with beta-blockers, on background therapy with ACE inhibitors and diuretics, was associated with a statistically significant reduction in the incidence of new-onset AF from 39 to 28 per 1000 patient-years (a 27% reduction in relative risk) during mean follow-up of 1.35 years (**Class I, Level A**).[92]

Quinidine

Quinidine has been used for treatment of AF since the discovery of its antiarrhythmic properties in early 1920s. In a meta-analysis of six randomized controlled trials in 808 patients, published in 1990, the proportions of patients remaining in sinus rhythm at 3, 6, and 12 months were 69%, 58%, and 50% in the quinidine group compared with 45%, 33%, and 25% in the control group.[93] In a 2006 analysis which included two recent large-scale studies of quinidine, PAFAC (Prevention of Atrial Fibrillation After Cardioversion) and SOPAT (Suppression Of Paroxysmal Atrial Tachyarrhythmias), quinidine reduced the incidence of recurrent AF by 49%.[86] The antiarrhythmic effect of quinidine was offset by high all-cause mortality and sudden death in the quinidine-treated patients compared with controls (2.9% vs 0.8%; OR 2.98).[93] The foremost safety issue for quinidine is its propensity to cause ventricular proarrhythmia including torsades de pointes, even at low or subtherapeutic doses. In earlier studies, the incidence of quinidine-induced ventricular proarrhythmias was reported to be 15%.[12]

Following the reports of increased mortality associated with quinidine and the development of newer antiarrhythmic drugs which are better tolerated, the use of quinidine has significantly decreased worldwide. However, the PAFAC[94] and SOPAT[95] trials showed no adverse effect on mortality, probably because in these studies, quinidine was used at lower doses (320–480mg as opposed to 1000–1800 g daily in the previous trials[93]), in combination with verapamil, and in patients with less significant structural heart disease. The number of patients with previous myocardial infarction (2.9–5%) and coronary artery disease (17–21%) was low.

In the PAFAC (848 patients with persistent AF) and SOPAT studies (1012 patients with similar clinical characteristics), which both employed daily transtelephonic ECG monitoring for arrhythmia detection, quinidine was superior to placebo and was as effective as sotalol in maintenance of sinus rhythm after cardioversion. The overall efficacy of antiarrhythmic drug therapy was modest: at 1 year, only about 30–35% of patients had no AF recurrence (including asymptomatic episodes detected during daily transtelephonic ECG transmissions) compared with 20–23% in the placebo arm. As for the safety concerns, there were five reports of ventricular tachycardia of more than 10 beats in patients treated with quinidine, four in the PAFAC study and one in the SOPAT study, but no torsades de pointes, which did occur in the sotalol arm of the PAFAC study. Nevertheless, the modest efficacy of quinidine and concerns about its safety have led to the withdrawal of quinidine from the list of drugs available for treatment of AF (**Class III, Level A**).

Disopyramide

Disopyramide is rarely used for treatment of AF because of its negative inotropic effect, the torsadogenic potential, and poor tolerance due to antimuscarinic properties. However, the use of disopyramide is advocated in patients with lone, vagally mediated AF (**Class IIa, Level B**). Although it was commonly prescribed for ventricular arrhythmias, data on the efficacy of disopyramide in AF are sparse. In a randomized, double-blind placebo-controlled study of 90 patients, disopyramide maintained sinus rhythm in 70% of patients at 1 month and 54% of patients at 1 year after cardioversion; the corresponding values for placebo were 39% and 30%, respectively.[96] In a small, double-blind study of 56 patients, disopyramide 250mg tid was not significantly different from propafenone 300mg tid in maintaining sinus rhythm at 6 months after cardioversion (67% vs 55%) but was associated with a significantly higher withdrawal rate due to adverse events, including two cases of heart failure and fast ventricular rates during AF in one patient.[97]

Propafenone and flecainide

Propafenone and flecainide are recommended as first-line therapy (**Class I, Level A**) for AF in patients without significant structural heart disease, i.e. patients without congestive heart failure, left ventricular dysfunction, hypertrophy, previous myocardial infarction or coronary artery disease. Both propafenone and flecainide reduced the recurrence rate by two-thirds, with no advantage of one drug over the other.[86] A number of randomized, controlled studies addressed the long-term efficacy of class IC antiarrhythmic drugs in AF.[98–104] In the Propafenone Atrial Fibrillation Trial (PAFT) of 102 patients, the likelihood of maintenance of sinus rhythm at 6 months after cardioversion was 67% with low-dose propafenone (450 mg) compared with 35% on placebo, with no increase in drug-related side effects (10% on propafenone vs 14% on placebo).[99] The UK PSVT (Paroxysmal Supraventricular Tachycardia) study evaluated the safety and efficacy of propafenone, 600 mg and 900 mg daily, and showed that both regimens were effective but a dose of 900 mg was associated with a less favorable adverse events profile.[100] In a meta-analysis of propafenone, the incidence of recurrent AF was 55.4% (51.3–59.7%) at 6 months and 56.8% (52.3–61.3%) at 1 year.[101] All-cause mortality associated with propafenone was 0.3%.

The efficacy of a sustained-release (SR) propafenone formulation which allows twice-daily dosing has been studied in the North American Recurrence of Atrial Fibrillation Trial (RAFT)[103] and its European equivalent, ERAFT.[104] Both studies have shown that propafenone SR is superior to placebo in prolonging time to first symptomatic recurrence of paroxysmal AF in patients with minor structural heart disease. In the RAFT study, which included 523 patients with onset of AF within 1–1.5 years prior to enrolment, time to AF recurrence was prolonged from 41 days on placebo to 112, 291, and >300 days on propafenone SR 225, 325, and 425 mg twice daily. Sixty-five percent of patients treated with the highest dose of 425 mg twice daily were free of symptomatic AF at the end of follow-up compared with only 20% in the placebo group, although the adverse effect rate was higher than with low-dose regimens.[103] The ERAFT study randomized 293 patients with paroxysmal AF of longer duration (approximately 5 years) and more frequent paroxysms to propafenone SR 325 mg or 425 mg twice daily or placebo. The time to the first recurrence of the arrhythmia was shorter than in the RAFT study, but still was prolonged from 5 days on placebo to 19 and 24 days on lower and high-dose propafenone.[104]

Several placebo-controlled and comparator trials of another class IC antiarrhythmic drug, flecainide, including the Flecainide Multicenter Atrial Fibrillation Study, have consistently reported a 70–80% likelihood of maintaining sinus rhythm after 1 year with an acceptable risk–benefit relationship.[105–108] In direct comparisons, flecainide and propafenone prevented AF in 77% and 75% patients, respectively.[106] In 239 patients, the antiarrhythmic effect of flecainide at a maximum dose of 300 mg daily was comparable to that of quinidine given at a maximum dose of 1500 mg daily, but 30% in the quinidine group withdrew from the 1-year study because of the side effects compared with 18% in the flecainide group.[107] In the Flecainide Atrial Fibrillation study in 123 patients with paroxysmal AF or flutter, flecainide demonstrated a linear dose–response, with only

7.7% and 9.4% of patients remaining free from the arrhythmia on the lowest doses (25 mg and 50 mg twice daily, respectively) compared with 39.4% of patients who received a standard therapeutic dose of 100 mg twice daily.[108]

Other class IC drugs

Drugs with class IC mode of action other than flecainide and propafenone are available in some countries, e.g. pilsicainide is available in Japan; cibenzoline is used in Japan and France. Pilsicainide is modestly effective in cardioversion of recent-onset AF (45% vs 8.6% on placebo) but is ineffective in AF of longer duration.[109] The drug showed no superiority over other members of its class in maintaining sinus rhythm in the long term and exhibited a similar adverse event profile to other class IC agents. In direct comparisons with cibenzoline which, in addition to sodium channels, also blocks potassium repolarization currents (I_{Kr} and I_{Ks}) and the acetylcholine-activated potassium current (I_{KAch}), the efficacy of pilsicainide was 8–59% at 6 months and 3–41% at 1 year.[110] The corresponding values for cibenzoline were 29–59% at 6 months and 16–50% at 1 year.

Sotalol

Selected randomized trials of the efficacy of class III antiarrhythmic drugs for conversion of AF and maintenance of sinus rhythm are summarized in Table 35.4. Several randomized, placebo-controlled and comparator studies have reported that sotalol is an effective and safe prophylactic antiarrhythmic drug for AF in the absence of heart failure, myocardial infarction or hypertension with significant left ventricular hypertrophy (**Class I, Level A**) (Table 35.4, Fig. 35.5).[111–113] Because of its beta-blocking effect, sotalol offers the additional benefit of ventricular rate slowing during recurrences. In the d,l-Sotalol Atrial Fibrillation/Flutter dose efficacy study of 253 patients, sotalol significantly prolonged the median time to first symptomatic recurrence of the arrhythmia documented by transtelephonic monitoring from 27 days on placebo to 106, 229, and 175 days (for 80, 120, and 160 mg twice-daily regimens, respectively).[111] In this study, sotalol 120 mg twice daily was found to be both safe and effective compared with lower and higher dose regimens. In direct comparisons, sotalol was as effective as propafenone (73% vs 63%)[112] and quinidine (74% vs 68%)[113] or quinidine plus verapamil (50% in each group)[95] in maintaining sinus rhythm after 1 year. Sotalol 160 mg twice daily was superior to an investigational class III antiarrhythmic agent azimilide in 658 patients with persistent AF.[114] Sotalol prolonged the median time to recurrence of sustained AF after electrical cardioversion to 28 days compared with 14 days for azimilide and 12 days for placebo. In a meta-analysis of nine randomized controlled studies in 1538 patients, sotalol reduced the recurrence rate by 47%.[86]

Table 35.4 Selected studies of class III antiarrhythmic drugs for conversion and/or maintenance of sinus rhythm in patients with atrial fibrillation

Study	Drug	No of patients	Follow-up
Ibutilide Repeat Dose Study[46]	Ibutilide 1.5 mg or 2 mg IV vs placebo	266; 50% AFL	24 hours
Randomized study of Ibutilide[47] vs Procainamide[40]	Ibutilide 1–2 mg IV vs procainamide 1.2 g IV	127; 33% AFL	24 hours
Ibutilide/Sotalol Comparator Study (ISCS)[41]	Ibutilide 1 mg or 2 mg IV vs d,l-sotalol 1.5 mg/kg IV	319; 18.5% AFL	72 hours
d,l-Sotalol Atrial Fibrillation/ Flutter Study Group[111]	d,l-Sotalol 160, 240, 320 mg	253; 20% AFL	1 year
SOCESP[113]	Sotalol 160–320 mg vs quinidine 600–800 mg	121	6 months
Bellandi[112]	Sotalol 240 mg vs propafenone 450–900 mg vs placebo	300	1 year
PAFAC[94]	Sotalol 320 mg vs quinidine + verapamil 320/160 mg vs placebo	848	1 year
SOPAT[95]	Sotalol 320 mg vs quinidine + verapamil 480/240 mg, 320/160 mg vs placebo	1012	1 year
CTAF[115]	Amiodarone 200 mg vs sotalol 160–320 mg or propafenone 450–600 mg	403	1.3 year
CHF-STAT[50,61]	Amiodarone 800 mg for 2 weeks; 400 mg for 50 weeks; maintenance dose 300 mg vs placebo	667; 103 with AF at baseline	4.5 years
SAFE-T[43]	Amiodarone 300 mg for the 1st year, 200 mg thereafter vs sotalol 320 mg vs placebo	665	4.5 years
DDAFFS[51]	Dofetilide 8 μg/kg IV vs placebo	96; 18% AFL	24 hours
DIAMOND-AF[24]	Dofetilide 500 μg vs placebo	506	1.5 years
SAFIRE-D[53]	Dofetilide 250, 500, 1000 μg vs placebo	225	1 year
EMERALD[54]	Dofetilide 250, 500, 1000 μg vs sotalol 160 mg vs placebo	671	Phase 1: 72 h; Phase 2: 2 years

AF, atrial fibrillation; AFL, atrial flutter; CHF-STAT, Congestive Heart Failure Survival Trial of Antiarrhythmic Therapy; CTAF, Canadian Trial of Atrial Fibrillation; DDAFS, Danish Dofetilide in Atrial Fibrillation and Flutter Study; DIAMOND-AF, Danish Investigations of Arrhythmia and Mortality ON Dofetilide; EMERALD, European and Australian Multicenter Evaluative Research on Dofetilide; PAFAC, Prevention of Atrial Fibrillation After Cardioversion; SAFE-T, Sotalol Amiodarone Atrial Fibrillation Efficacy Trial; SAFIRE-D, Symptomatic Atrial Fibrillation Investigative Research on Dofetilide; SOCESP, Cardiology Society of São Paulo Investigators; SOPAT, Suppression Of Paroxysmal Atrial Tachyarrhythmias.

Conversion rate	Maintenance of sinus rhythm	Torsade de pointes
47% converted on ibutilide vs 2% on placebo ($P < 0.0001$); 63% AFL vs 31% AF ($P < 0.0001$)	N/A	8.3% on ibutilide; 1.7% required electrical cardioversion
58.3% converted on ibutilide vs 18.3% on procainamide ($P < 0.0001$)	N/A	0.8% on ibutilide
AFL: 76% converted on ibutilide vs 14% on placebo ($P = 0.001$)		
AF: 51% converted on ibutilide vs 21% on placebo ($P = 0.005$)		
AFL: 70% converted on ibutilide 1.5 mg vs 56% on ibutilide 1 mg vs 19% on sotalol ($P < 0.05$ vs sotalol)	N/A	0.9% on ibutilide 2 mg; 0.5% required electrical cardioversion; none on sotalol
AF: 44% converted on ibutilide 1.5 mg vs 20% on ibutilide 1 mg vs 11% on sotalol ($P < 0.05$ for ibutilide 1.5 mg vs sotalol)		
N/A	Free from AF: 30%, 40%, 45% on sotalol 160, 240, 320 mg vs 28% on placebo	None
	Time to 1st AF recurrence: 106, 229, 175 days on sotalol 160 ($P = 0.111$), 240 ($P = 0.001$), 320 mg ($P = 0.012$) vs 27 days on placebo	
N/A	74% on sotalol vs 68% on quinidine ($P = 0.43$)	5% on sotalol vs 2% on quinidine
	Time to 1st AF recurrence 69 vs 10 days ($P < 0.05$); AF ≤72 h: 93% in sinus rhythm on sotalol vs 64% on quinidine ($P = 0.01$); AF > 72 h: 33% in sinus rhythm relapsed on sotalol vs 68% on quinidine ($P < 0.05$)	
N/A	73% in sinus rhythm on sotalol vs 63% on propafenone vs 35% on placebo ($P = 0.001$)	4% on sotalol; 2% required cardioversion
N/A	33% in sinus rhythm on sotalol vs 35% on quinidine and 17% on placebo	2.3% on sotalol; ventricular tachycardia 0.5% on sotalol vs 1.1% on quinidine
N/A	~50% in sinus rhythm on sotalol and quinidine vs 38% on placebo	Ventricular tachycardia 0.4% on quinidine high dose
	Time to 1st AF recurrence: 146 days on sotalol ($P = 0.0007$) vs 149 (low dose; $P = 0.0006$) and 150 (high dose; $P = 0.0061$) on quinidine vs 106 on placebo	
N/A	65% in sinus rhythm on amiodarone vs 37% on sotalol or propafenone ($P < 0.001$)	1 (1%) on propafenone
31.3% on amiodarone vs 7.7% on placebo ($P = 0.002$)	New-onset AF: 4% on amiodarone vs 8% on placebo ($P = 0.005$)	Not stated
27.1% converted on amiodarone, 24.2% on sotalol vs 0.8% on placebo ($P < 0.001$ for both drugs)	63% in sinus rhythm on amiodarone vs 49% on sotalol vs 18% on placebo ($P < 0.001$)	1 (0.4%) on sotalol
	Time to 1st AF recurrence: 487 days on amiodarone, 74 days on sotalol vs 6 days on placebo ($P < 0.001$ for both drugs)	
30.3% converted on dofetilide vs 3.3% on placebo ($P < 0.006$)	N/A	3% on dofetilide
44% on dofetilide vs 14% on placebo ($P < 0.001$)	79% in sinus rhythm on dofetilide vs 46% on placebo ($P < 0.001$)	3.3% on dofetilide
6.1% ($P = 0.015$), 9.8% ($P = 0.015$), 19.9% ($P < 0.001$) on dofetilide 250, 500, 100 µg vs 1.2% on placebo	40%, 37%, 58% on dofetilide vs 25% on placebo	0.8% on dofetilide 1 (0.4%) proarrhythmic death
6%, 11%, 29% on dofetilide vs 5% on sotalol at 72 hours	66% in sinus rhythm on dofetilide 1000 µg vs 21% on placebo at 1 year	3 (0.45%) torsades de pointes 1 (0.15%) sudden death

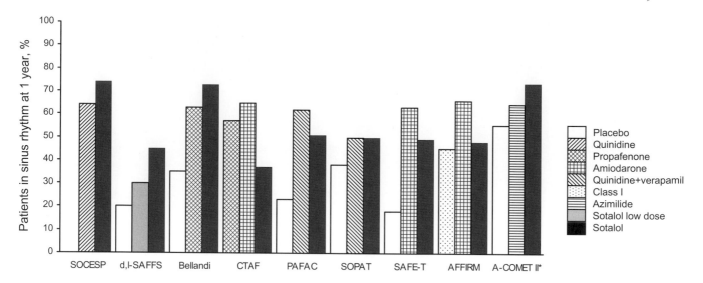

Figure 35.5 Efficacy of sotalol in comparison with other antiarrhythmic drugs for maintenance of sunus rhythm in patients with atrial fibrillation. A-COMET II, Azimilide CardiOversion MaintEnance Trial II; AFFIRM, Atrial Fibrillation Follow-up Investigation of Rhythm Management; CTAF, Canadian Trial of Atrial Fibrillation; d,l-SAFFS, d,l-Sotalol Atrial Fibrillation/Flutter Study; PAFAC, Prevention of Atrial Fibrillation After Cardioversion; SOCESP, Cardiology Society of São Paulo Investigators; SOPAT, Suppression Of Paroxysmal Atrial Tachyarrhythmias; * at 6 months.

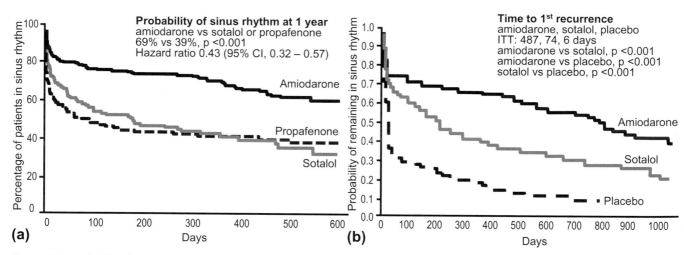

Figure 35.6 Probability of remaining free from recurrent atrial fibrillation with amiodarone and sotalol in the Canadian Trial of Atrial Fibrillation (CTAF) (a) and in the Sotalol Amiodarone Atrial Fibrillation Efficacy Trial (SAFE-T) (b). ITT, intention to treat. (Modified from references Singh et al.[43] and Roy et al.[115], with permission.)

However, subsequent studies reported limited efficacy of sotalol compared with amiodarone and the combination of quinidine and verapamil.[43,94,115] In the Canadian Trial of Atrial Fibrillation (CTAF), sotalol was significantly inferior to amiodarone for the long-term maintenance of sinus rhythm (Fig. 35.6).[115] The PAFAC study demonstrated a 50% recurrence rate with sotalol during 1 year of daily transtelephonic ECG monitoring compared with 38% on the combination of quinidine and verapamil.[94] In the

SAFE-T study, sotalol 160 mg twice daily was superior to placebo, but less effective than amiodarone in prevention of AF recurrence after pharmacologic or electrical cardioversion (the median time to a recurrence was 6 days on placebo, 74 days on sotalol, and 487 days on amiodarone).[43] At 2 years, approximately 30% of patients treated with sotalol remained in sinus rhythm compared with 60% of patients on amiodarone and 10% of patients on placebo. However, a prespecified subgroup analysis revealed that

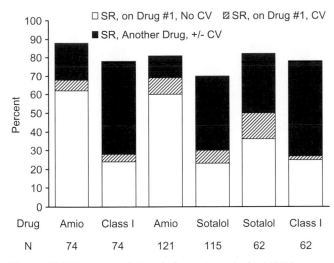

Figure 35.7 Prevalence of sinus rhythm at 1 year in the AFFIRM substudy.[116] Patients are included only if they were randomized 1 year or more before the termination of the substudy. Amio, amiodarone; CV, cardioversion; SR, sinus rhythm.

this difference was driven by the superiority of amiodarone and a relative inefficacy of sotalol in patients without ischemic heart disease, whereas both drugs were equally modestly effective in patients with ischemic heart disease: the proportion of patients in sinus rhythm at 2 years was approximately 40% in the amiodarone group and 35% in the sotalol group. The efficacy of sotalol was similar to that of class I antiarrhythmic drugs and inferior to that of amiodarone in the AFFIRM substudy (48%, 45%, and 66%, respectively) (Fig. 35.7).[116]

Hypotension and bradycardia were the most common cardiovascular adverse effects of sotalol with an incidence of 6–10%, while ventricular proarrhythmias associated with prolongation of the QT interval were reported in 1–4% of patients and were dose related.[112,113] In A-COMET II (Azimilide CardiOversion MaintEnance Trial-II), eight (3.5%) out of 223 patients treated with sotalol 320 mg daily withdrew from the study because of a significant QT interval prolongation compared with two (0.9%) of 224 patients in the placebo group.[114] In the SAFE-T trial, only one patient (0.4%) in the sotalol group had an episode of torsades.[43]

Dofetilide

Unlike class IC agents and sotalol, dofetilide is safe to use in patients with previous myocardial infarction and/or congestive heart failure (**Class I, Level A**). In the DIAMOND AF substudy of DIAMOND-CHF and DIAMOND-MI trials, 506 patients with AF at baseline were more likely to remain in sinus rhythm on treatment with

dofetilide 500 µg twice daily compared with placebo (79% vs 42%).[24] Dofetilide had no effect on mortality in patients in whom AF persisted during the study, but restoration and maintenance of sinus rhythm were associated with a 56% reduction in death. In the DIAMOND-CHF (n = 1518) and DIAMOND MI (n = 1510) studies, patients treated with dofetilide had a lower incidence of new-onset AF than those on placebo (1.23% vs 3.78%)[117,118]; this effect was more pronounced in patients with NYHA class III and IV heart failure enrolled in DIAMOND-CHF (1.98% vs 6.55%).[117]

In the dose-ranging SAFIRE-D study of 325 patients with persistent AF or flutter for 2–26 weeks, dofetilide exhibited a dose-related effect: 40%, 37%, and 58% patients receiving 250, 500, and 1000 µg of dofetilide, respectively, were in sinus rhythm after 1 year compared with 25% in the placebo group.[53] The median time to relapse was 31, 179, and more than 365 days for dofetilide groups and 27 days for placebo. Dofetilide was almost twice as effective for the long-term prevention of atrial flutter than of AF (73% vs 40%).

The major safety concern about dofetilide is its torsadogenic potential which is dose related. For instance, the incidence of torsades de pointes with dofetilide ranges from almost "zero" at doses below 250 µg bid to 10% or greater at doses higher than 500 µg bid.[12] In the randomized controlled studies, the incidence of torsades de pointes varied between 0.6% and 3.3%, with more than three-quarters of episodes occurring during the first 3–4 days of drug initiation. Dofetilide is excreted predominantly via the kidneys and its dose should be adjusted for creatinine clearance (see Table 35.2); the drug should not be prescribed in patients with significantly impaired renal function (creatinine clearance less than 20), hypokalemia, hypomagnesemia or a QT interval of longer than 500 ms. If the QT interval is prolonged to >500 ms or by >15% versus baseline, the dose should be reduced.

Azimilide

Although initial reports on azimilide were encouraging,[119] the recent A-STAR (Supraventricular TachyArrhythmia Reduction) and A-COMET II trials, in patients with persistent AF, have failed to show any antiarrhythmic benefit of azimilide.[114,120] The ALIVE (AzimiLide PostInfarct SurviVal Evaluation) trial of 3717 patients with a recent myocardial infarction and left ventricular dysfunction has shown a neutral effect of azimilide on all-cause mortality, including in patients with a significantly reduced ejection fraction.[121] Fewer patients who started the trial in sinus rhythm developed AF on azimilide and there was a trend to higher pharmacologic conversion rates in the azimilide arm than in the placebo arm (26.8% vs 10.8%); (P = 0.076).[122] The marginal efficacy and unacceptably high rates of torsade de pointes proarrhythmia prevent the use of azimilide for treatment of AF.

Amiodarone

The potential of amiodarone to maintain sinus rhythm in patients with AF and a relative cardiac safety in patients with significant structural heart disease has been repeatedly shown in observational and prospective, randomized, controlled studies. The CTAF trial randomized 403 patients with mixed paroxysmal and persistent AF to amiodarone 10 mg/kg for 2 weeks, followed by 300 mg per day for 4 weeks and a maintenance dose of 200 mg and either sotalol 160–320 mg per day (depending on gender, body mass, and creatinine clearance) or propafenone 450–600 mg (depending on age and body weight).[115] The incidence of recurrent AF lasting more than 10 minutes was reduced by 57% in the amiodarone group compared with the sotalol or propafenone group (31% vs 61%) (see Fig. 35.6). Data from the CHF-STAT substudy showed that patients who received amiodarone at a maintenance dose of 300 mg per day converted to sinus rhythm more frequently (31.3% vs 7.7% on placebo), had fewer recurrences, and were half as likely to develop new AF compared with placebo.[61]

Despite prolonging cardiac repolarization, amiodarone has a low torsadogenic potential.[12] For instance, a literature review reported that the incidence of torsades de pointes was only 0.7% in 2878 patients treated with amiodarone in 17 uncontrolled studies, while no proarrhythmic effects were described among 1464 patients treated in seven controlled studies.[59] The residual risk of torsades de pointes with amiodarone occurs chiefly in patients with other risk factors, such as bradycardia or hypokalemia. The reason for the low propensity of amiodarone to cause torsades de pointes is not clear, but is presumably related to its complex mode of action which involves class I, II and IV effects alongside its class III properties. It has also been suggested that amiodarone does not increase the heterogeneity of refractoriness in the myocardial layers and does not increase transmural dispersion of repolarization.[123]

Given its neutral effect on all-cause mortality, amiodarone should be considered a drug of choice for management of AF in patients with congestive heart failure, hypertrophic cardiomyopathy and hypertension with significant left ventricular hypertrophy (**Class I, Level A**). However, although several studies besides the CHF-STAT have reported on the relative safety of amiodarone,[124,125] recent subgroup analyses from the Sudden Cardiac Death in Heart Failure Trial (SCD-HeFT) suggested that amiodarone was associated with excess mortality in patients with NYHA III heart failure.[126]

Amiodarone may cause multiple non-target effects, which range from transient and relatively trivial (e.g. gastrointestinal disturbances) to partially preventable (e.g. skin toxicity) and medically correctable (e.g. underactive thyroid) to serious such as pulmonary toxicity, liver damage, hyperthyroidism, bradycardia, significant or irreversible neurologic symptoms (e.g. peripheral neuropathy), and visual disturbances (e.g. optic neuritis). The adverse effects of amiodarone seem to occur less frequently at low doses (100–200 mg daily) than with higher maintenance doses (300–400 mg daily), but idiosyncratic reactions can arise. Amiodarone is not therefore recommended as first-line therapy in patients with little or no structural heart disease for whom therapy with class IC drugs or sotalol is more appropriate.

Dronedarone

Dronedarone is an investigational agent with multiple electrophysiologic effects which are similar to those of amiodarone, but it is devoid of iodine atoms and is believed to have a better side-effect profile with significantly less reporting of pulmonary fibrosis, ocular adverse effects, and skin photosensitivity. Dronedarone does not significantly prolong the QT interval and, like amiodarone, probably has a low potential for causing torsades de pointes.

The antiarrhythmic potential of dronedarone and the effects on mortality and morbidity have been studied in a dose-finding study, two high-quality, medium-size efficacy and safety trials, and a recently completed large-scale survival trial (Table 35.5).[127–129] The efficacy of dronedarone in preventing AF recurrences after electrical cardioversion was clearly demonstrated in a dose-ranging study where 400 mg bid proved to be the most effective dose.[127] The EURIDIS (EURopean trial In atrial fibrillation or flutter patients receiving Dronedarone for the maintenance of Sinus rhythm) and its American-Australian-African equivalent ADONIS have shown that dronedarone 400 mg twice daily (n = 828) was superior to placebo (n = 409) in prevention of recurrent AF and was also effective in controling ventricular rates.[128] In the European trial, the median time to the recurrence of arrhythmia (the primary endpoint) was 41 days in the placebo group and 96 days in the dronedarone group ($P = 0.01$). In the American-Australian-African counterpart, the corresponding time was 59 and 158 days ($P = 0.002$). Figure 35.8 shows the probability of recurrent AF on dronedarone and placebo based in the pooled EURIDIS and ADONIS studies.

The efficacy and safety of dronedarone were directly compared to that of amiodarone in the DIONYSOS (Efficacy and Safety of Dronedarone versus Amiodarone for the Maintenance of Sinus Rhythm in Patients with Atrial Fibrillation) study in 504 patients with persistent AF who underwent electrical cardioversion (data on file). The primary

Table 35.5 Summary of clinical studies of dronedarone in atrial fibrillation

Study	Number of patients	Patient characteristics	Dose of dronedarone	Placebo controlled	Primary endpoint	Follow-up, months	Outcome
DAFNE	199	Post cardioversion	400 mg bid 600 mg bid 800 mg bid	Yes	Time to first AF recurrence	6	Dronedarone 400 mg bid significantly prolonged median time to first AF recurrence v placebo: 60 vs 5.3 days. Relative risk reduction, 55%; (95% CI, 28–72% $P = 0.001$)
EURIDIS	615	Persistent or paroxysmal AF	400 mg bid	Yes	Time to first AF recurrence	12	Median time to first AF recurrence was 41 days on dronedarone v 96 days on placebo, $P = 0.01$
ADONIS	630	Persistent or paroxysmal AF	400 mg bid	Yes	Time to first AF recurrence	12	Median time to first AF recurrence was 59 days on dronedarone vs 158 days on placebo, $P = 0.002$
EURIDIS and ADONIS pooled	1237	Persistent or paroxysmal AF	400 mg bid	Yes, n = 409	All-cause mortality and hospitalizations *post hoc* analysis	12	Reduced on dronedarone vs placebo: 22.8% vs 30.9% (HR, 0.73; 95% CI, 0.57–0.93; $P = 0.01$)
ERATO	630	Permanent AF with ventricular rates >80 bpm on rate controlling therapy	400 mg bid	Yes	Mean 24-hour ventricular rate at 2 weeks	1	Ventricular rates were 12 bpm lower on dronedarone v placebo; $P < 0.0001$
ANDROMEDA	617	Congestive heart failure; EF <0.35; 38% had a history of AF; 25% in AF at randomization	400 mg bid	Yes	All-cause mortality and hospitalization for heart failure	Median, 2	Stopped early because of increased mortality in the dronedarone arm: 8% vs 3.8% on placebo (HR, 2.3; 95% CI, 1.07–4.25; $P = 0.03$) Primary endpoint: 17.1% on dronedarone vs 12.6% on placebo (HR, 1.38; 95% CI, 0.92–2.09; $P = 0.12$)
ATHENA	4628	Paroxysmal or persistent AF with risk factors	400 mg bid	Yes	All-cause mortality and hospitalizations for cardiac causes	21	Dronedarone reduced the primary endpoint vs placebo by 24% ($P < 0.001$)
DIONYSOS	504	Persistent AF	400 mg bid	No, amiodarone is used as an active comparator	AF recurrence and premature drug discontinuation for side effects or lack of efficacy	7	Primary endpoint events on dronedarone vs amiodarone: 184 (73.9%) vs 141 (55.3%); p < 0.01 AF recurrence: 36.5% vs 24.3% Drug discontinuation: 26 (10.4%) vs 34 (13.3%)

ACE, angiotensin-converting enzyme; ADONIS, American-Australian-African trial with DronedarONe In atrial fibrillation or flutter for the maintenance of Sinus rhythm; AF, atrial fibrillation; ANDROMEDA, ANtiarrhythmic trial with DROnedarone in Moderate to severe heart failure Evaluating morbidity DecreAse; ATHENA, A placebo-controlled, double-blind, parallel arm Trial to assess the efficacy of dronedarone 400 mg bid for the prevention of cardiovascular Hospitalization or death from any cause in patiENts with Atrial fibrillation/atrial flutter; bpm, beats per minute; DAFNE, Dronedarone Atrial FibrillatioN study after Electrical cardioversion; DIONYSOS, Efficacy and Safety of Dronedarone vs Amiodarone for the Maintenance of Sinus Rhythm in patients with Atrial Fibrillation; EF, ejection fraction; ERATO, Efficacy and Safety of Dronedarone for the Control of Ventricular Rate; EURIDIS, EURopean trial In atrial fibrillation or flutter patients receiving Dronedarone for the maintenance of Sinus rhythm.
Reproduced from: Savelieva et al.[84]

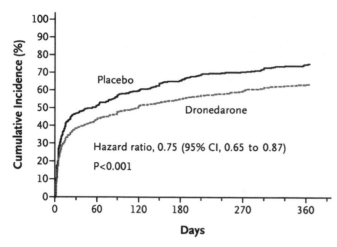

Figure 35.8 EURIDIS and ADONIS pooled analysis. Times to first recurrence of atrial fibrillation or flutter. ADONIS, American-Australian-African trial In atrial fibrillation or flutter patients receiving DronedarONe for the maIntenance of Sinus rhythm; EURIDIS, EURopean trial in a trial fibrillation or flutter patients receiving dronedarone for the maintenance of sinus rhythm. (Modified from Singh *et al.*[128], with permission.)

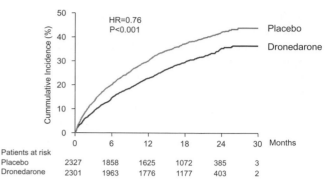

Figure 35.9 Time to first cardiovascular hospitalization or death in the ATHENA trial. ATHENA = A placebo controlled, double blind Trial to assess the efficacy of dronedarone for the prevention of cardiovascular Hospitalization or death from any cause in patiENts with Atrial fibrillation and flutter. Reproduced from Hohnloser *et al.*[129], with permission.

endpoint was recurrence of AF or premature drug discontinuation secondary to adverse effects or lack of efficacy. After a mean follow-up of 7 months, 36.5% patients in the dronedarone group and 24.3% patients in the amiodarone group had a recurrence of AF. Dronedarone was better tolerated, with fewer episodes of thyroid dysfunction (2 vs 15), neurological side effects (3 vs 17), and bradycardia (8 vs 22) compared with amiodarone. However, gastrointestinal disorders (diarrhea, vomiting, nausea) were more common with dronedarone than amiodarone (32 vs 13).

The *post hoc* analysis of the EURIDIS and ADONIS studies showed that patients treated with dronedarone had a 27% reduction in relative risk of hospitalization for cardiovascular causes and death (22.8% vs 30.9% on placebo).[128] Subsequently, a further Phase III randomized controlled study (ATHENA: A placebo controlled, double blind Trial to assess the efficacy of dronedarone for the prevention of cardiovascular Hospitalization or death from any cause in patiENts with Atrial fibrillation and flutter) has been undertaken in 4628 high-risk patients.[129] Dronedarone prolonged time to first cardiovascular hospitalization or death from any cause (the composite primary endpoint) by 24% (*P* < 0.001) compared with placebo (Fig. 35.9). This effect was driven by the reduction in cardiovascular hospitalizations (25%), particularly hospitalizations for AF (37%) and acute coronary syndromes (30%). All-cause mortality was similar in the dronedarone and placebo groups (5% and 6%, respectively); however, dronedarone significantly reduced deaths from cardiovascular causes (2.7% vs 3.9%; *P* = 0.03).

The ANDROMEDA (ANtiarrhythmic trial with DROnedarone in Moderate to severe heart failure Evaluating morbidity DecreAse) study was initiated to explore the effects of dronedarone on all-cause death and hospitalizations for heart failure in patients with NYHA class III or IV heart failure. The trial was stopped prematurely after 627 patients out of the 1000 planned were enrolled, because an interim safety analysis revealed an excess of deaths in the dronedarone arm compared with placebo (8% vs 13.8%; HR 2.13; 95% CI 1.07–4.25; *P* = 0.03).[130] The adverse outcome of ANDROMEDA appears largely explained by an increase in creatinine in the dronedarone-treated patients being misinterpreted as progressive renal failure (it was due to its effect on renal tubular excretion), prompting inappropriate discontinuation of otherwise life-saving treatment with angiotensin-converting enzyme inhibitors or angiotensin receptor-blocking drugs. Consequently, excess mortality related to dronedarone was secondary to heart failure. The risk of death was the greatest in patients with severely depressed ventricular function and there were more hospitalizations for heart failure in the dronedarone arm. In the subsequent analysis of a small proportion (n = 200) of patients with class III heart failure enrolled in the ATHENA trial, therapy with dronedarone was, in fact, associated with a lower likelihood of hospitalizations or death from cardiovascular cause as well as lower all-cause mortality compared with placebo.[130a]

Investigational antiarrhythmic agents

A raft of other amiodarone analogs is currently at various stages of development.[84] Celivarone (SSR149744C) has been studied in a Phase II dose-ranging study, MAIA (MAintenance of sinus rhythm In patients with recent

Atrial fibrillation or flutter) in 673 patients who were randomized to one of four doses (50, 100, 200 or 300 mg once daily) or placebo. As with dronedarone, the higher doses of celivarone tended to be less effective than the lower doses. The lowest incidence of the recurrence at 90 days was 52.1% in the celivarone 50 mg compared with 67.1% in the placebo group. No proarrhythmia or thyroid dysfunction was reported in this short-term study. The results of the double-blind placebo-controlled CORYFREE (COntrolled Dose Ranging studY of the eFficacy and safEty of SSR149744c 300 or 600 mg for the Conversion of Atrial Fibrillation/flutter) trial are expected. There is ongoing research into the development of an amiodarone derivative with modified bonds within the molecule allowing rapid hydrolization by esterases, resulting in a more rapid action, a shorter half-life and possibly a better risk–benefit ratio. Another amiodarone derivative, budiodarone (ATI-2042) which shares its mixed ion channel effects but has a different metabolic pathway, a shorter half-life, and low propensity to tissue accumulation, has recently proven to reduce AF burden by up to 75.5% over 12 weeks of treatment in 110 patients with paroxysmal AF (reported at the Heart Rhythm Society Late Breaking Trials Session in 2009).

An oral formulation of vernakalant has been investigated in two medium-size Phase II studies (Table 35.3).[84] In a double-blind, placebo-controlled study (n = 446), patients treated with vernakalant 600 mg twice daily were more likely to maintain sinus rhythm at 3 months after pharmacologic or electrical cardioversion compared with placebo (51% vs 37%).

There were no reports of torsade de pointes or drug-related deaths. There is evidence that an antianginal drug, ranolazine, may also produce an antiarrhythmic effect due to multiple channel blockade, particularly late sodium current blockade. Phase III studies of ranolazine in AF are presently planned.

Where to initiate antiarrhythmic drug therapy

The issue of the proper site for initiation of antiarrhythmic drug therapy for AF revolves around considerations of risk and practicality. In-hospital initiation under monitored conditions conveys benefits of accurate assessment of the efficacy and prompt recognition of adverse effects, such as bradycardia, conduction abnormalities, excessive QT interval prolongation, proarrhythmia, and intolerance or idiosyncrasy. Patients in AF in whom sinus node function or the QT interval duration during sinus rhythm are unknown and patients at anticipated high risk of developing adverse effects should not be prescribed antiarrhythmic drugs outside the hospital setting that are known to aggravate their condition. For some antiarrhythmic agents, e.g. dofetilide, there is formal mandate for in-hospital initiation.

In the absence of proarrhythmic concerns and formal labeling, convenience and cost effectiveness favor out-of-hospital initiation, e.g. oral propafenone and flecainide in patients with lone AF or AF associated with hypertension without significant left ventricular hypertrophy. The same approach is valid for amiodarone, given its long elimination half-life period and low probability of developing torsades de pointes. Dronedarone has proven a safe and well tolerated agent with an added benefit of ventricular rate control and can, therefore, be initiated on an outpatient basis. An ECG control or transtelephonic ECG monitoring should be arranged to provide surveillance of heart rate, PR and QT interval durations, QRS width, and assessment of the efficacy of treatment.

Antiarrhythmic drug use after left atrial ablation

After left atrial ablation-based therapies, the incidence of AF or atrial tachycardia has been reported to be 45% during the first 3 months despite antiarrhythmic drugs.[131] [131]. The arrhythmia recurrence is more common in patients with persistent AF, older individuals, and in patients with structural heart disease. In many cases, early recurrence of AF after ablation is transient and is thought to be secondary to inflammation after radiofrequency injury, nerve ending damage and resulting imbalance of the cardiac autonomic nervous system, and a delayed effect of ablation associated with "maturation" of lesions. Early AF often subsides after 3 months (the blanking period) upon the resolution of inflammation and restoration of autonomic regulation, without the need for reablation. Therefore antiarrhythmic drug therapy to suppress early recurrence of AF is commonly employed for the first 1–3 months after ablation or if the arrhythmia recurs after discontinuation of the antiarrhythmic drug. These are usually the same agents that have been previously ineffective, but may now be efficacious because of a synergistic effect with ablation (an example of so-called "hybrid" therapy). Amiodarone has been reported to be most commonly prescribed because of its antifibrillatory as well as atrioventricular conduction slowing properties. The use of antiarrhythmic drugs increases the probability of maintaining sinus rhythm by about 20–30% as suggested by the worldwide surveys on catheter ablation for AF conducted in 1995–2002 and 2003–2006.[132,132a]

The synergistic effect of antiarrhythmic drugs (mainly propafenone, flecainide, and sotalol) has recently been demonstrated in the 5A (AntiArrhythmics After Ablation of Atrial fibrillation) study in 110 patients randomized to receive antiarrhythmic drugs or no therapy for at least 6 weeks after ablation (presented at the Annual Sessions of the Heart Rhythm Society in 2008). The composite endpoint was the occurrence of atrial arrhythmias lasting more than 24 hours or symptomatic arrhythmias, need for cardioversion or hospitalization for atrial arrhythmias, and intolerance of antiarrhythmic drugs. About one-quarter of patients had reablation. The recruitment for the study was terminated early because of significantly fewer events in the drug-treated group compared with patients who received no drug therapy. However, because of a short minimum follow-up period of 6 weeks that falls within the blanking period, the study has failed to show whether antiarrhythmic drug therapy can offer any benefit beyond the blanking period when the majority of patients would receive an antiarrhythmic drug anyway according to the current practice.

About 10% of patients, however, develop regular fast atrial tachycardias which are either focal or re-entrant (atypical atrial flutter), are refractory to antiarrhythmic drugs, and often require additional ablation. The incidence of late (more than 1 year) recurrence of AF after ablation is currently at 5–10%, but it is likely to be higher when long-term follow-up data become available and the procedure is more widely used.[131]

Pharmacologic rate control

Acute rate control

Beta-blockers and calcium antagonists

Randomized controlled studies have shown that intravenous verapamil, diltiazem, and beta-blockers (usually esmolol) can accomplish rapid control of the ventricular response rate (**Class I, Level B/C**) (Table 35.6).[133–139] The decrease in the ventricular rate (approximately 20–30%),

time to the maximum effect (20–30 minutes), the conversion rate (12–25%), and the adverse reactions (usually hypotension and bradycardia, although left ventricular dysfunction and high-degree heart block may occur) have been reported to be the same with both beta-blockers and calcium antagonists. Beta-blockers are preferable in patients with a history of myocardial infarction or if thyrotoxicosis is suspected as a cause of the arrhythmia, whereas verapamil and diltiazem are preferred in patients with chronic obstructive airways disease.[139] The majority of patients (70–75%) responded to the first bolus of diltiazem and verapamil with heart rate reductions to below 100 bpm.[137,138] In patients with pre-excitation syndrome and AF, agents which slow atrioventricular conduction can cause the impulse to travel in the anterograde direction via the accessory pathway rather than via the atrioventricular node. Because the accessory pathway, unlike the atrioventricular node, is capable of conducting very rapidly at a 1:1 ratio, this may lead to AF with extremely fast ventricular rates that may degenerate into ventricular fibrillation.

Digoxin

Intravenous digoxin is no longer the treatment of choice when rapid rate control is essential because of its delayed onset of the therapeutic effect (more than 60 minutes). In a direct comparison with diltiazem, the peak effect of digoxin was not observed until 3 hours, whereas diltiazem significantly decreased the ventricular rate within 5 minutes.[136] Some reported no significant effect or lack of persistent rate control with digoxin in patients with continuous AF and symptomatic bradyarrhythmias or pauses when AF converted to sinus rhythm.[140] However, because of its positive inotropic action, digoxin can be used in patients with poor

Table 35.6 Drugs for acute rate control in atrial fibrillation

Drug	Route of administration	Dose	Onset	Recommendation (Class)	Level of evidence
Esmolol	Intravenous	0.5 mg/kg over 1 min followed by 0.05–0.2 mg/kg/min infusion	5 min	I	C*
Metoprolol	Intravenous	2.5–5 mg over 2 min followed by repeat doses if necessary	5 min	I	C*
Propranolol	Intravenous	0.15 mg/kg	5 min	I	C*
Diltiazem	Intravenous	0.25 mg/kg over 2 min followed by 5–15 mg/h infusion	2–7 min	I	B
Verapamil	Intravenous	0.075–0.15 mg/kg over 2 min	3–5 min	I	B
Digoxin	Intravenous	0.25 mg each 2 h, max 1.5 mg	2 h	IIb†	B
Amiodarone	Intravenous	As for cardioversion‡	6–8 h	IIb‡	C
Sotalol	Intravenous	1–1.5 mg/kg over 5–10 min	15–30 min	III	B

* For all beta-blockers;
† a Class I indication in patients with poor ventricular function and moderately fast ventricular rates, level of evidence B;
‡ Class IIa indication in patients with poor ventricular function and moderately fast ventricular rates, level of evidence C.

ventricular function and moderately fast ventricular rates (**Class I, Level B**). One important advantage of digoxin is its ability to convert atrial flutter to AF and, thereby, make ventricular rate control easier to accomplish. However, this approach is rarely practical in the emergency setting.

Amiodarone

Amiodarone suppresses atrioventricular conduction by inhibiting the L-type calcium current ($I_{Ca,L}$), (the major determinant of the action potential of the atrioventricular nodal cells), and producing a sympatholytic effect. Amiodarone also has mild beta-blocking properties. There is anecdotal evidence that intravenous amiodarone may be effective in ventricular rate control when other agents have no effect on ventricular response or are contraindicated. Intravenous infusion of amiodarone was associated with a decrease in ventricular rates by 37 beats per minute and an increase in systolic blood pressure by 24 mmHg in 38 patients with hemodynamically unstable AF refractory to electrical cardioversion and intravenous agents, such as esmolol, diltiazem, digoxin, and procainamide.[60] The atrioventricular blocking effect of amiodarone is complemented by its antifibrillatory action. The disadvantages of IV amiodarone are slow onset of action and increased risk of phlebitis. Although amiodarone is not routinely used for acute rate control, it is given a **Class IIa, Level C** recommendation in patients with AF *and* congestive heart failure and, unlike digoxin, has the potential to restore sinus rhythm.

Sotalol

Sotalol usually is ineffective in cardioverting AF, but can slow down the ventricular rate due to its beta-blocking properties.[43] In 140 patients with recent-onset AF, intravenous infusions of either sotalol 1.5 mg/kg over 10 minutes or amiodarone 10 mg/kg in 30 minutes helped to facilitate rate control compared with IV digoxin, but the overall conversion rate within 12 hours was modest with either agent.[141] The potential negative inotropic effect of sotalol precludes its use for rate control in patients with left ventricular dysfunction and the proarrhythmic (torsadogenic) potential of sotalol due to QT interval prolongation reduces its value as a rate-controling agent (**Class III, Level B**).

Clonidine, adenosine, and magnesium

There is limited evidence on the use of clonidine and magnesium for ventricular rate control. The rationale for the use of clonidine in AF is its central sympatholytic activity of directly blocking alpha-2 adrenoreceptors in the lower brainstem region and its ability to stimulate parasympathetic outflow, resulting in prolongation of the refractoriness of the atrioventricular node. In 40 hemodynamically stable patients with new-onset (less than 24 hours) rapid AF, clonidine, given orally at a dose of 0.1 mg and repeated at 2-hour intervals if rate control was not achieved, reduced ventricular rates by 44 beats per minute over a 6-hour follow-up. This effect was comparable to that of verapamil and digoxin, both administered intravenously (the mean heart rate reduction was 52 and 42 beats per minute, respectively).[142] Clonidine was associated with a greater reduction of systolic blood pressure compared with verapamil.

In a meta-analysis of trials in 303 patients and a rapid ventricular rate, intravenous magnesium effectively reduced the ventricular rate to below 90–100 within 5–15 minutes of infusion (OR 1.96; 95% CI 1.24–3.08).[70] Magnesium had a synergistic effect on the atrioventricular node when given with digoxin or diltiazem[139] and also produced an antifibrillatory effect. The overall response rate, including rate control and conversion to sinus rhythm, was significantly higher in patients who received the magnesium infusion compared with placebo or an active comparator (86% v 56%; OR 4.61; 95% CI 2.67–7.96).[70]

Adenosine, in its present formulation, is not suitable for rate control (**Class III, Level A**) because of its extremely short half-life, lack of the antifibrillatory effect, and the potential to induce AF, particularly in the presence of an accessory pathway. The incidence of AF after a central venous intravenous adenosine infusion for supraventricular tachycardia is about 10–15%.[143]

New agents for acute rate control

Several adenosine derivatives with a high specificity for adenosine A1 receptors, tecadenoson, selodenoson, and capadenoson, are currently under investigation. The high affinity for A1 receptors enables effective rate control without reducing the blood pressure or causing bronchospasm as a result of stimulating A2 receptors. Tecadenoson has an immediate onset of action in about 30 seconds and has a half-life of approximately 30 minutes and may prove to be a potent and safe drug for urgent rate control and possibly even cardioversion of AF. Selodenoson has an even longer half-life of 150 minutes and is available in an oral formulation. Tecadenoson has been mainly studied for cardioversion of supraventricular tachycardias.[144] Undesirable symptoms commonly reported with adenosine, such as flushing, dyspnea, and chest pain, occurred less frequently. Tecadenoson shortens atrial action potential duration and may therefore induce AF. However, in contrast to adenosine, the effect on atrial refractoriness is smaller than the blocking effect on the atrioventricular node, and risk of AF is therefore expected to be low. In the Phase III TEMPEST (Trial to Evaluate the Management of Paroxysmal supraventricular tachycardia during Electrophysiologic Study with Tecadenoson), AF as an adverse event was reported in 2% of patients.[144] Selodenoson demonstrated a statistically and clinically significant decrease in ventricular rate compared with placebo in a small double-blind Phase II trial.[145] Final results are pending from three other Phase II studies in patients with spontaneous AF with uncontrolled ventricular rates.

Rate control in paroxysmal and persistent atrial fibrillation

Beta-blockers and calcium antagonists

Rate control is an essential constituent of management of AF and is pertinent to all types of the arrhythmia. In paroxysmal and persistent AF, rate control is important during the recurrence or prior to electrical cardioversion. Non-dihydropyridine calcium antagonists and beta-blockers are drugs of choice (**Class I, Level B/C**). They are also commonly prescribed in combination with the class IC agents propafenone and flecainide to prevent fast ventricular rates due to 1:1 atrioventricular conduction when recurrent AF evolves to flutter.

Digoxin

Digoxin should be avoided if the arrhythmia is self-terminating or electrical cardioversion is planned and rhythm control is pursued. This is because digoxin abbreviates the atrial action potential by several mechanisms, including increased intracellular calcium, augmentation of the transient outward potassium I_{to} current, and a vagotonic effect which can be proarrhythmic in the atria.[146] Thus digoxin can promote the recurrence or perpetuation of atrial fibrillation and offset the effect of antiarrhythmic agents. In a randomized, double-blind, placebo-controlled, crossover study in 43 patients with frequent symptomatic paroxysms of atrial fibrillation, the median time to the occurrence of two episodes of the arrhythmia documented by patient-activated monitors was prolonged from 13.5 days in the placebo group to 18.7 days in the digoxin group during 2-month follow-up.[147] However, no significant difference was detected between digoxin and placebo in terms of the number and duration of atrial fibrillation episodes. It is likely that digoxin used as monotherapy reduced the frequency of symptomatic atrial fibrillation by lowering the ventricular rate response and increasing the regularity. The heart rate during symptomatic episodes was reduced by approximately 15 beats per minute.

Sotalol and amiodarone

Some antiarrhythmic drugs, such as sotalol, amiodarone, and dronedarone, slow atrioventricular conduction and thus offer an additional benefit of ventricular rate control during recurrences of AF. Although much of the evidence for the rate-controling effects of antiarrhythmic drugs comes from studies in permanent AF, antiarrhythmic drugs are not commonly employed for long-term rate control and therefore will be discussed in this section.

Sotalol has been relatively well studied for rate control.[148–150] In the randomized, double-blind, parallel, placebo-controlled Sotalol Atrial Fibrillation Study in 60 patients, the combination of digoxin and dl-sotalol, at either 80 or 160 mg/day, resulted in a statistically signifi-

cant reduction in heart rate at rest and with exercise during both exercise testing and ambulatory monitoring.[148] In patients with AF of more than 1 month, sotalol and metoprolol on the background of digoxin were equally effective in reducing the resting heart rate, but sotalol surpassed metoprolol during exercise.[150] Although there were no reports of torsades de pointes, sotalol significantly prolonged the QT interval both at rest and during exercise. In the CHF-STAT study, amiodarone reduced the mean and maximal ventricular rates by 16–20% and 14–22%, respectively.[61] However, sotalol and amiodarone are not routinely employed for long-term rate control, e.g. in permanent or accepted AF, because of proarrhythmic and non-target side effects (**Class IIb, Level B/C**).

Dronedarone

In the EURIDIS and ADONIS studies, dronedarone was not only effective in suppressing recurrent AF, but also reduced the ventricular rate response during the recurrence of the arrhythmia by 12–15 beats per minute compared with placebo.[128] Similar reductions in ventricular rates were achieved in the ATHENA trial including patients who progressed to permanent AF. The ability of the drug to control ventricular rates was prospectively assessed in the ERATO (Efficacy and Safety of Dronedarone for the Control of Ventricular Rate) study of 174 patients with AF with a resting heart rate of more than 80 beats per minute despite standard therapy with beta-blockers, calcium antagonists, and digitalis.[151] At 2 weeks, dronedarone lowered the mean 24-hour ventricular rate (the primary endpoint) by 12 beats per minute and limited the peak heart rate during a maximal symptom-limited exercise test by 24 beats per minute compared with placebo without affecting the overall exercise capacity.

Rate control in permanent atrial fibrillation

Elements of rate control

Several questions remain to be answered about rate control therapy in AF. These include how best to measure successful therapy and what is the optimal heart rate. Current guidelines define adequate rate control as maintenance of the ventricular rate response between 60 and 80 at rest and 90 and 115 during moderate exercise.[5] Few systematic studies have explored the effect of rate-slowing drugs on chronotropic competence in AF or defined upper limits of the appropriate ventricular rate response during exercise.[152,153] Measuring the systolic velocity integral of aortic blood flow with Doppler ultrasound to assess the effect of different ventricular rates on cardiac output in 60 patients with AF, Rawles demonstrated that rates of up to 90 maintain good cardiac output at rest, while during exercise, ventricular rates of 90–140 might be necessary in order to maintain equivalent cardiac outputs to patients in sinus rhythm.[153] However, no controlled clinical trials have validated these values with regard to their effects on morbidity or mortality.

Atrial contraction contributes 20–40% of the total stroke volume. Loss of atrial contraction may cause a marked decrease in cardiac output, especially in patients with impaired diastolic filling, hypertension, and left ventricular hypertrophy. Hence, although rapid ventricular rates can be detrimental, they should not be too low either. Pharmacologic ventricular rate control can have other problems, such as being associated with periods of bradycardia (usually sinus) alternating with tachycardia (usually AF) in the same patient.[154] This often requires placement of a pacemaker to prevent bradycardia and permit adequate drug therapy to control ventricular rates. It also sometimes leads to atrioventricular node ablation by radiofrequency ablation with placement of a permanent pacemaker system to control ventricular rate optimally.

Adequate rate control probably encompasses more than the mere prevention of fast ventricular rates. The effect of excessively irregular rhythm is rarely acknowledged in practice as an important constituent of effective rate control, despite some evidence that the rhythm irregularity *per se* may contribute to ventricular dysfunction.[155] Randomized studies comparing atrioventricular node ablation and atrioventricular node modification in AF provided indirect evidence that not only rate control but also regularization of the rhythm were essential for improving cardiac performance.[156]

Methods of assessment of rate control

Ventricular rate control at rest does not always translate into effective control during exercise. Few data exist that define the most robust method of assessment of rate control and explore whether different methods can provide comparable information or whether the combination of two or theoretically more tests may provide better results. In a small study in patients with permanent AF, ventricular rates assessed after 5 minutes of rest, after a 50-yard walk and after 1 minute of stair stepping exercise correlated with ventricular rates derived from 24-hour Holter recordings.[157] Thus, the heart rate at rest was slower than the mean heart rate obtained from the Holter recording, on average, by 20 beats per minute, but when combined with the heart rate after a 50-yard walk, the resulting heart rate was similar to the mean rate on Holter. The heart rate after 1 minute of stair stepping was similar to the maximum ventricular rates during Holter monitoring. Ambulatory 24-hour ECG monitoring is considered sufficient for assessment of rate control in elderly and sedentary individuals, whereas in younger individuals, an exercise stress test may be necessary.[5] The AFFIRM trial[14] used those criteria in establishing clinical ventricular rate control, but the RACE trial[15] took a more lenient approach, accepting simply a ventricular rate less than 100 beats per minute. The mean heart rate across all follow-up visits for patients in AF was lower in AFFIRM.[158] Event-free survival for the occurrence of the primary endpoint did not differ (64% in AFFIRM vs 66% in RACE). Patients with mean ventricular rates during AF within the AFFIRM (≤80 beats per minute) or RACE (<100 beats per minute) criteria had a better outcome than patients with ventricular rates ≥100 beats per minute (HR 0.69 and 0.58, respectively for ≤80 and <100 compared with ≥100 beats per minute). Perhaps the closeness to 80 beats per minute of the mean ventricular rates in these studies tells the story best. A RACE II study was instigated to assess whether maintaining strict rate control, i.e. mean resting heart rate less than 80 beats per minute and heart rate during mild exercise less than 110 beats per minute, can offer any additional benefit to standard practice.[159]

Drugs for rate control

Digoxin, beta-blockers, verapamil, and diltiazem, are commonly employed (Table 35.7).[5] Digoxin is effective in controling ventricular rates at rest by prolongation of atrioventricular node conduction and refractoriness through vagal stimulation, by direct effects on the atrioventricular node, and by increasing the amount of concealed conduction in the atrioventricular node due to the increased rate at which atria discharge (**Class I, Level B**). However, the effect of digoxin is negated during exercise when most vagal tone is lost and atrioventricular conduction is further enhanced by the increased sympathetic tone.[160] Therefore, digoxin as monotherapy can be effective in older, sedentary patients, but a combination with beta-blockers or calcium antagonists is often necessary to achieve rate control in the majority of patients.

Non-dihydropyridine calcium antagonists and beta-blockers are effective as primary pharmacologic therapy for rate control (**Class I, Level B/C**); however, multiple adjustments of drug type and dosage and a combination of two agents may be needed to achieve the desired effect.[160–164] For example, in the AFFIRM trial, only 58% of patients in the rate control group achieved adequate rate control with the first drug or combination; drug switches occurred in 37% of the patients and drug combinations were commonly used.[164] Overall, adequate rate control was ascertained in 80% of patients at 5 years (most frequently on a beta-blocker with or without digoxin), but these patients were followed carefully to assess rate control at each follow-up visit and frequent drug switches were allowed. Digoxin alone was effective in only 58% of patients.

Atrial fibrillation after cardiac surgery

Prevalence and risk factors

Pooled data from the control arms of 40 randomized clinical trials and three large observational studies have shown

Table 35.7 Drugs for long-term rate control in atrial fibrillation

Drug	Dose	Class of recommendation	Level of evidence	Potential adverse effects
Digoxin	Loading dose: 250 μg every 2 hours; up to 1500 μg; maintenance dose 125–250 μg daily	I	B	Bradycardia; atrioventricular block; atrial arrhythmias; ventricular tachycardia
Diltiazem	120–360 mg daily	I	B	Hypotension; atrioventricular block; heart failure
Verapamil	120–360 mg daily	I	B	Hypotension; atrioventricular block; heart failure
Atenolol	50–100 mg daily	I	C*	Hypotension; bradycardia; heart failure; deterioration of chronic obstructive pulmonary disease or asthma
Metoprolol	50–200 mg daily	I	C*	
Propranolol	80–240 mg daily	I	C*	
Bisoprolol	5–10 mg daily	I	C*	
Carvedilol	25–100 mg daily	I	C*	
Sotalol	80–320 mg	IIb[†]	C	Bradycardia; QT prolongation; torsades de pointes (risk <1%); photosensitivity; pulmonary toxicity; polyneuropathy; hepatic toxicity; thyroid dysfunction; gastrointestinal disturbances
Amiodarone	800 mg daily for 1 week, then 600 mg daily for 1 week, then 400 mg daily for 406 weeks; maintenance dose 200 mg daily	IIb[†]	C	Bradycardia; QT prolongation; torsades de pointes (risk <1%); photosensitivity; pulmonary toxicity; polyneuropathy; hepatic toxicity; thyroid dysfunction; gastrointestinal disturbances

* For all beta-blockers;
[†] useful during recurrence of atrial fibrillation.

that, in the absence of prophylactic antiarrhythmic drug therapy, AF may occur in about 30% of patients after isolated coronary artery bypass grafting, 40% of patients after valve surgery, and 50% of patients after combined coronary artery and valvular surgery.[165] Postoperative AF occurs predominantly during the first 4 days and is associated with increased morbidity and mortality, largely due to stroke and circulatory failure, and longer hospital stay. More than 90% patients present with a paroxysmal or first-onset form of the arrhythmia. Atrial flutter and atrial tachycardias, including multifocal atrial tachycardia, are also common.

Clinical factors that convey a higher risk for the development of postoperative atrial tachyarrhythmias include advanced age, male sex, a previous history of AF, hypertension, congestive heart failure, valvular heart disease, chronic obstructive pulmonary disease, chronic renal failure, previous cardiac surgery, left atrial enlargement, inadequate cardioprotection and hypothermia, right coronary artery grafting, and a longer bypass time.[166] The incidence of postoperative atrial tachyarrhythmias may be lower with minimally invasive techniques, especially for valvular surgery.[167] The pathophysiology of AF after cardiac surgery relates primarily to sterile pericarditis that accompanies the surgery. This results in perioperative changes in atrial electrophysiology, including increased dispersion of atrial refractoriness, decreased atrial conduction velocity, and changes in atrial transmembrane potential.

Rate versus rhythm control

The rhythm control strategy, including electrical or pharmacologic restoration of sinus rhythm with subsequent prophylactic antiarrhythmic therapy, should be considered in hemodynamically unstable or highly symptomatic patients with postoperative AF. If AF is well tolerated, rate control may be sufficient as AF after isolated coronary bypass surgery is often self-limiting and there is a high likelihood of spontaneous conversion to sinus rhythm, usually within 6 weeks. Although digoxin and non-dihydropyridine calcium antagonists (verapamil, diltiazem) are effective in slowing atrioventricular conduction, beta-blockers should be considered the first-line choice because of their beneficial effects on the hyperadrenergic postoperative state. In comparator studies, diltiazem produced a more rapid rate-slowing effect than digoxin (median times to a 20% or more decrease in ventricular rates were 2 minutes and more than 3.5 hours, respectively).[168] At 2 and 6 hours, the proportion of patients who achieved adequate rate control was significantly higher in the diltiazem-treated group compared with the digoxin-treated group (75% vs 35% and 85% vs 45%, respectively). Digoxin in combination with either beta-blockers or a non-dihydropyridine calcium antagonist will often provide effective therapy in otherwise difficult cases.

Pharmacologic prevention of postoperative AF

Beta-blockers

The best evidence for efficacy in prevention of postoperative AF has been accumulated for beta-blockers, sotalol, and amiodarone (Fig. 35.10).[165] Two earlier meta-analyses of randomized controlled studies have shown that treatment with beta-blockers may reduce the incidence of AF by approximately 50%.[169,170] In a meta-analysis of 27 trials in 3840 patients, therapy with beta-blockers reduced risk of postoperative AF by 61%; there was also a trend towards shorter length of stay.[165] In the large Beta-blocker Length Of Stay (BLOS) study in 1000 patients, 85% of whom had isolated coronary artery bypass grafting, therapy with metoprolol 100–150 mg per day initiated immediately after surgery was associated with a small but statistically significant reduction in the incidence of AF compared with placebo, but had no effect on the length of hospital stay.[171] Current guidelines give a **Class I, Level A** recommendation for beta-blockers for prevention of AF after heart surgery. The downside of beta-blockers is that they may increase risk of bradycardia (5–10%) and risk of longer ventilation (1–2%). In a retrospective analysis, carvedilol was reported to be superior to other beta-blockers, predominantly metoprolol or atenolol, with respect to efficacy and safety.[172] Temporary cardiac pacing using temporary epicardial wire electrodes placed at the time of surgery in most patients should permit use of beta-blockers in the face of bradycardia.

Sotalol

In eight randomized controlled studies in 1294 patients, sotalol has been reported to reduce the incidence of postoperative AF by 65% compared with placebo, but it had no impact on length of hospital stay, strokes or mortality.[165] Sotalol may be more effective in the prevention of AF than beta-blockers because of its potential incremental benefit due to its class III antiarrhythmic property.[173] However, the use of sotalol risks bradycardia and torsades de pointes, especially in patients with electrolyte disturbances. In direct comparisons, both sotalol and amiodarone were effective and safe in reducing postoperative AF in patients undergoing isolated coronary artery bypass surgery (25% vs 17%), but sotalol was significantly inferior to amiodarone in patients who had aortic valve replacement alone or in combination with coronary surgery (82% vs 7%).[174] When the results of several studies were pooled, there were no differences between the two drugs with respect to the incidence of AF, length of stay, and adverse events.[175] Sotalol was designated **Class IIb, Level B** for prevention of postoperative AF.

Amiodarone

There is compelling evidence from randomized, controlled studies and meta-analyses that treatment with amiodarone may reduce the incidence and duration of postoperative AF, and also control the ventricular rate (**Class IIa, Level A**).[176–183] The Amiodarone Reduction in Coronary Heart (ARCH) study of 300 patients who had undergone coronary bypass surgery has shown a significant reduction in the incidence of postoperative AF with IV amiodarone compared with placebo (35% vs 47%).[181] In the Prevention of Arrhythmias that Begin Early After Revascularization (PAPABEAR) trial of 601 patients undergoing isolated coronary artery bypass surgery, treatment with amiodarone 10 mg/kg per day starting 7 days before surgery was associated with a significant decrease in the incidence of postoperative AF compared with placebo (30% vs 16%), reflecting a 52% reduction in relative risk.[182] The number of patients needed to be treated in order to prevent one episode of the arrhythmia was 7.5. However, there was no difference between amiodarone and placebo groups with respect to complications or length of hospital stay.

A meta-analysis of 19 studies which enrolled 3295 patients, among whom 1639 had received amiodarone and 1656 were in the control group, has shown that therapy with amiodarone halved the incidence of postoperative AF.[165] In addition, amiodarone reduced the occurrence of ventricular tachyarrhythmias by 61% and strokes by 47%. In contrast with other therapies, treatment with amiodarone was associated with a statistically significant shorter

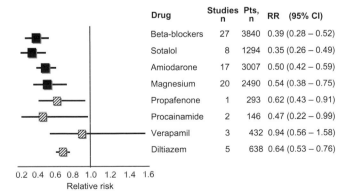

Drug	Studies n	Pts, n	RR (95% CI)
Beta-blockers	27	3840	0.39 (0.28 – 0.52)
Sotalol	8	1294	0.35 (0.26 – 0.49)
Amiodarone	17	3007	0.50 (0.42 – 0.59)
Magnesium	20	2490	0.54 (0.38 – 0.75)
Propafenone	1	293	0.62 (0.43 – 0.91)
Procainamide	2	146	0.47 (0.22 – 0.99)
Verapamil	3	432	0.94 (0.56 – 1.58)
Diltiazem	5	638	0.64 (0.53 – 0.76)

0.2 0.4 0.6 0.8 1.0 1.2 1.4 1.6
Relative risk

Figure 35.10 Meta-analysis of pharmacologic prevention of atrial fibrillation after heart surgery. Hatched boxes indicate agents that have not been rigorously tested. (Data from Mitchell *et al*[165].)

length of hospital stay, although the difference from the control group was small (0.6 days), resulting in cost savings of marginal statistical significance (data on costs were available in six studies). Adverse events such as hypotension and bradycardia necessitating inotropic and chronotropic support or pacing may limit the routine use of amiodarone to prevent postoperative AF.

Other agents

Ibutilide and dofetilide have proven to be effective for pharmacologic cardioversion of atrial tachyarrhythmias after cardiac surgery. In 302 patients, 101 of whom presented with atrial flutter, ibutilide restored sinus rhythm in 57% compared with 15% on placebo.[184] Conversion rates at all doses were higher for atrial flutter than for AF (78% vs 44%). In 133 patients undergoing isolated coronary artery bypass grafting or combined with valvular surgery, therapy with dofetilide at doses adjusted according to glomerular filtration rates and started on the day of operation resulted in a modest decrease in the incidence of AF compared with placebo (36% vs 18%).[185] Although there were no cases of torsades de pointes in this study, the QT-prolonging effect and the proarrhythmic potential of dofetilide and ibutilide are of significant concern and the drugs are not routinely used in the early postoperative period.

Magnesium sulfate has been reported to reduce the incidence and number of episodes of AF by 46% in a pooled analysis of 20 studies in 2490 patients.[186] The effect was comparable to that of beta-blockers, sotalol, and amiodarone and no adverse events were reported. The favorable effects of magnesium may relate to restoration of electrolyte balance after surgery. Alternatively, the stimulating effects of magnesium on the sodium/potassium pump may act beneficially by inducing a calcium channel-blocking effect. However, magnesium is not commonly employed as a primary agent for prevention or treatment of AF and is usually adjunctive to beta-blockers or antiarrhythmic drugs.

Class I antiarrhythmic drugs have been shown to be moderately effective in prevention of atrial tachyarrhythmias after cardiac surgery. The results from the Clinical Outcomes from the Prevention of Post-operative Arrhythmia (COPPA) II study in 293 patients who had undergone coronary bypass have shown that treatment with propafenone 675 mg daily reduced the incidence of postoperative AF by 38% compared with placebo, but did not change length of stay.[187] Propafenone administered intravenously at a dose of 2 mg/kg produced a more rapid effect on restoration of sinus rhythm compared with intravenous procainamide given at a dose of 20 mg/kg to maximum of 1000 mg (59% vs 18% at 15 minutes) but there was no significant difference in the conversion rates at 1 hour (76% vs 61%).[188] The proarrhythmic potential and the negative inotropic effect of propafenone in patients prone to ischemia or patients with previous myocardial infarction limit the use of propafenone early after heart surgery. Procainamide was associated with a significantly higher incidence of hypotension than propafenone (27% vs 7%) which was clinically relevant and required discontinuation of the drug in 9% of cases. Procainamide does not appear to be significantly more effective than placebo in the prevention of AF and there are concerns about its negative inotropic effect in patients with depressed ventricular function.[189]

Several randomized controlled studies have suggested the beneficial role of agents with anti-inflammatory properties, such as statins, or specific anti-inflammatory drugs such as corticosteroids; these therapies are discussed in detail in Chapter 36.

Conclusion

It is important to emphasize that the rate versus rhythm control trials provide good evidence to help guide therapy. They consistently demonstrate that rate control is a legitimate primary therapeutic option. Importantly, the results of these trials should not be interpreted to mean that a rate control strategy is better than a rhythm control strategy. The strategy of choice must be decided on a patient-by-patient basis. Thus, considering presently available therapy of AF, the first decision to be made with each patient is which strategy to pursue: rate control or rhythm control. Rational antiarrhythmic treatment of AF starts with classification of AF into one of its subtypes: recent onset, paroxysmal, persistent or permanent. Only then can the goal of treatment be identified: to restore sinus rhythm with the option of prophylactic drug treatment or to accept AF as the dominant rhythm.

Antiarrhythmic treatment is further guided by the duration of the arrhythmia, the tendency for recurrence after conversion, and the potential side effects of drugs. At some stage during treatment, rate control is useful in all three subtypes of AF but especially in the permanent form. Pharmacologic cardioversion can be accomplished with intravenous or oral antiarrhythmic drugs, but it is most effective in recent-onset AF. In persistent AF of longer duration, restoration of sinus rhythm is accomplished by electrical cardioversion and antiarrhythmic drugs are employed for prevention of recurrence. Most patients cannot be cured of AF: almost all will experience recurrence of the arrhythmia sooner or later after the first attack despite drug treatment. Therefore, the primary goal of treatment is to reduce morbidity (and possibly mortality) rather than simply to suppress the arrhythmia.

In the last several decades the proarrhythmic effect of antiarrhythmic drugs has been widely recognized. In addition, negative inotropic and extracardiac side effects further limit the use of traditional antiarrhythmic agents. Furthermore, there have been surprisingly few trials designed to demonstrate their efficacy in reducing mortality, significant morbidity or healthcare costs. There has recently been a significant effort by the pharmaceutical industry to develop new agents for the management of patients with AF and it now seems likely that several of these agents will be approved and will become available for the control of AF and flutter.

References

1. Lloyd-Jones DM, Wang TJ, Leip EP, Larson MG, Levy D et al. Lifetime risk for development of atrial fibrillation: the Framingham Heart Study. *Circulation* 2004;**110**:1042–6.

2. Heeringa J, van der Kuip DA, Hofman A, Kors JA, van Herpen G, Stricker BH et al. Prevalence, incidence and lifetime risk of atrial fibrillation: the Rotterdam study. *Eur Heart J* 2006;**27**:949–53.

3. Go AS, Hylek EM, Phillips KA, Chang Y, Henault LE, Selby JV, Singer DE. Prevalence of diagnosed atrial fibrillation in adults: national implications for rhythm management and stroke prevention: the AnTicoagulation and Risk Factors in Atrial Fibrillation (ATRIA) Study. *JAMA* 2001;**285**:2370–5.

4. Miyasaka Y, Barnes ME, Gersh BJ, Cha SS, Bailey KR, Abhayaratna WP et al. Secular trends in incidence of atrial fibrillation in Olmsted County, Minnesota, 1980 to 2000, and implications on the projections for future prevalence. *Circulation* 2006;**114**:119–25.

5. Kerr CR, Humphries KH, Talajic M, Klein GJ, Connolly SJ, Green M et al. Progression to chronic atrial fibrillation after the initial diagnosis of paroxysmal atrial fibrillation: results from the Canadian Registry of Atrial Fibrillation. *Am Heart J* 2005;**149**:489–96.

6. Lehto M, Kahla R. Persistent atrial fibrillation: a population based study of patients with their first cardioversion. *Int J Cardiol* 2003;**92**:145–50.

7. Levy S, Maarek M, Coumel P et al, on behalf of the College of French Cardiologists. Characterization of different subsets of atrial fibrillation in general practice in France: the ALFA Study. *Circulation* 1999;**99**:3028–35.

8. Savelieva I, Camm AJ. Clinical relevance of silent atrial fibrillation: prevalence, prognosis, quality of life, and management. *J Interv Card Electrophysiol* 2000;**4**:369–82.

9. Savelieva I, Camm AJ. Atrial fibrillation and heart failure: natural history and pharmacological treatment. *Europace* 2004;**5** (suppl 1):S5–19.

10. Savelieva I, Camm AJ. Update on atrial fibrillation: Part II. *Clin Cardiol* 2008;**31**:102–8.

11. Coplen SE, Antman EM, Berlin JA, Hewitt P, Chalmers TC. Efficacy and safety of quinidine therapy for maintenance of sinus rhythm after cardioversion. A meta-analysis of randomized control trials. *Circulation* 1990;**82**:1106–16.

12. Camm AJ. Safety considerations in the pharmacological management of atrial fibrillation. *Int J Cardiol* 2008;**127**:299–306.

13. Jafar-Fesharaki M, Scheinman MM. Adverse effects of amiodarone. *Pacing Clin Electrophysiol* 1998;**21**:108–20.

14. Wyse DG, Waldo AL, DiMarco JP, Domanski MJ, Rosenberg Y, Schron EB et al. A comparison of rate control and rhythm control in patients with atrial fibrillation. *N Engl J Med* 2002;**347**:1825–33.

15. Van Gelder IC, Hagens VE, Bosker HA, Kingma JH, Kamp O, Kingma T et al, for the RAte Control versus Electrical cardioversion for persistent atrial fibrillation study group. A comparison of rate control and rhythm control in patients with recurrent persistent atrial fibrillation. *N Engl J Med* 2002;**347**: 1834–40.

16. Roy D, Talajic M, Nattel S, Wyse DG, Dorian P, Lee KL et al, for the Atrial Fibrillation and Congestive Heart Failure Investigators. Rhythm control versus rate control for atrial fibrillation and heart failure. *N Engl J Med* 2008;**358**:2667–77.

17. Hohnloser SH, Kuck KH, Lilienthal J. Rhythm or rate control in atrial fibrillation – pharmacological intervention in atrial fibrillation (PIAF): a randomised trial. *Lancet* 2002;**356**: 1789–94.

18. Carlsson J, Miketic S, Windeler J, Coneo A, Haun S, Mills S, Walter S, Tebbe U. Randomized trial of rate-control versus rhythm-control in persistent atrial fibrillation. The Strategies of Treatment of Atrial Fibrillation Study. *J Am Coll Cardiol* 2003;**41**:1690–6.

19. Opolski G, Torbicki A, Kosior DA, Szulc M, Wozakowska-Kaplon B, Kolodziej P, Achremczyk P. Rate control vs rhythm control in patients with nonvalvular persistent atrial fibrillation: the results of the Polish How To Treat Chronic Atrial Fibrillation Study. *Chest* 2004;**126**:476–86.

20. Waldo AL. Lessons learned from the AFFIRM trial – treatment of patients with atrial fibrillation at risk for stroke. *ACC Curr J Rev* 2004;**13**:68–72.

21. De Denus S, Sanoski CA, Carlsson J, Opolski G, Spinler SA. Rate vs rhythm control in patients with atrial fibrillation: a meta-analysis. *Arch Intern Med* 2005;**165**:258–62.

22. Corley SD, Epstein AE, DiMarco JP et al, for the AFFIRM Investigators. Relationships between sinus rhythm, treatment, and survival in the Atrial Fibrillation Follow-Up Investigation of Rhythm Management (AFFIRM) Study. *Circulation* 2004;**109**:1509–13.

23. Dries DL, Exner DV, Gersh BJ, Domanski MJ, Waclawiw MA, Stevenson LV. Atrial fibrillation is associated with an increased risk for mortality and heart failure progression in patients with asymptomatic and symptomatic left ventricular systolic dysfunction: A retrospective analysis of the SOLVD trials. Studies Of Left Ventricular Dysfunction. *J Am Coll Cardiol* 1998;**32**:695–703.

24. Pedersen OD, Bagger H, Keller N, Marchant B, Kober L, Torp-Pedersen C, for the Danish Investigation of Arrhythmia and Mortality ON Dofetilide Study Group. Efficacy of dofetilide in the treatment of atrial fibrillation-flutter in patients with reduced left ventricular function. A Danish Investigations of Arrhythmia and Mortality ON Dofetilide (DIAMOND) Substudy. *Circulation* 1001;**104**:292–6.

24a. Talajic M, Khairy P, Levesque S, Connolly S, Dorian P, Hohnloser SH et al. Maintenance of sinus rhythm is not associated with improved survival in patients with atrial fibrillation and heart failure. *Circulation* 2008; Abstract supplement: Abstract 4095.

25. Danias PG, Caulfield TA, Weigner MJ, Silverman DI, Manning WJ. Likelihood of spontaneous conversion of atrial fibrillation to sinus rhythm. *J Am Coll Cardiol* 1998;**31**:588–92.

26. Slavik RS, Tisdale JE, Borzak S. Pharmacologic conversion of atrial fibrillation: a systematic review of available evidence. *Prog Cardiovasc Dis* 2001;**44**:121–52.

27. Fresco C, Proclemer A, on behalf of the PAFIT-2 Investigators. Management of recent onset atrial fibrillation. *Eur Heart J* 1996;**17**(suppl C):C41–7.

28. Bianconi L, Mennuni M, and PAFIT-3 Investigators. Comparison between propafenone and digoxin administered intravenously to patients with acute atrial fibrillation. *Am J Cardiol* 1998;**82**:584–8.

29. Boriani G, Biffi M, Capucci A, Broffoni T, Rubino I, Della Casa S et al. Oral propafenone to convert recent-onset atrial fibrillation in patients with and without underlying heart disease: a randomized, controlled trial. *Ann Intern Med* 1997;**126**:621–5.

30. Reimold SC, Maisel WH, Antman EM. Propafenone for the treatment of supraventricular tachycardia and atrial fibrillation: a meta-analysis. *Am J Cardiol* 1998;**82**:66N–71N.

31. Capucci A, Boriani G, Botto GL, Lenzi T, Rubino I, Falcone C et al. Conversion of recent-onset atrial fibrillation to sinus rhythm by a single oral loading dose of propafenone or flecainide. *Am J Cardiol* 1994;**74**:503–5.

32. Azpitarte J, Alvarez M, Baun O, García R, Moreno E, Martín F et al. Value of single oral loading dose of propafenone in converting recent-onset atrial fibrillation: results of a randomized double-blind, controlled study. *Eur Heart J* 1997;**18**:1649–54.

33. Alp NJ, Bell JA, Shahi M. Randomised double blind trial of oral versus intravenous flecainide for the cardioversion of acute atrial fibrillation. *Heart* 2000;**84**:37–40.

34. Deneer VH, Borgh MB, Kingma JH, Lie-A-Huen L, Brouwers JR. Oral antiarrhythmic drugs in converting recent onset atrial fibrillation. *Pharm World Sci* 2004;**26**:66–78.

35. Khan IA. Single oral loading dose of propafenone for pharmacological cardioversion of recent-onset atrial fibrillation. *J Am Coll Cardiol* 2001;**37**:542–7.

36. Khan IA. Oral loading single dose flecainide for pharmacological cardioversion of recent-onset atrial fibrillation. *Int J Cardiol* 2003;**87**:121–8.

37. Camm AJ, Savelieva I. Some patients with paroxysmal atrial fibrillation should carry flecainide or propafenone to self treat. *BMJ* 2007;**334**:637.

38. Alboni P, Botto GL, Baldi N, Luzi M, Russo V, Gianfranchi L et al. Outpatient treatment of recent-onset atrial fibrillation with the "pill-in-the-pocket" approach. *N Engl J Med* 2004;**351**:2384–91.

39. Crijns HJGH, van Gelder IC, Kingma JH, Dunselman PH, Gosselink AT, Lie KI. Atrial flutter can be terminated by a class III antiarrhythmic drug, but not by a class IC drug. *Eur Heart J* 1995;**15**:1403–8.

40. Sung RJ, Tan HL, Karagounis L et al, for the Sotalol Multicenter Study Group. Intravenous sotalol for termination of supraventricular tachycardia and atrial fibrillation and flutter: a multicenter, randomized, double-blind, placebo-controlled study. *Am Heart J* 1995;**129**:739–48.

41. Vos MA, Golitsyn SR, Stangl K et al, for the Ibutilide/Sotalol Comparator Study Group. Superiority of ibutilide (a new class III agent) over d,l-sotalol in converting atrial flutter and atrial fibrillation. *Heart* 1998;**79**:568–75.

42. Halinen MO, Huttunen M, Paakkinen S, Tarssanen L. Comparison of sotalol with digoxin-quinidine for conversion of acute atrial fibrillation to sinus rhythm (the Sotalol-Digoxin-Quinidine Trial). *Am J Cardiol* 1995;**76**:495–8.

43. Singh BN, Singh SN, Reda DJ et al, for the Sotalol Amiodarone Atrial Fibrillation Efficacy Trial (SAFE-T) Investigators. Amiodarone versus sotalol for atrial fibrillation. *N Engl J Med* 2005;**352**:1861–72.

44. Lehmann MH, Hardy S, Archibald D, Quart B, MacNeil DJ. Sex difference in risk of torsades de pointes with d,l-sotalol. *Circulation* 1996;**94**:2534–41.

45. Ellenbogen KA, Stambler BS, Woof MA, Wood MA, VanderLugt JT. Efficacy of intravenous ibutilide for rapid termination of atrial fibrillation and atrial flutter: a dose-response study. *J Am Coll Cardiol* 1996;**28**:130–6.

46. Stambler BS, Wood MA, Ellenbogen KA, Perry KT, Wakefield LK, VanderLugt JT and the Ibutilide Repeat Dose Investigators. Efficacy and safety of repeated intravenous doses of ibutilide for rapid conversion of atrial flutter or fibrillation. *Circulation* 1996;**94**:1613–21.

47. Volgman AS, Carberry PA, Stambler B, Lewis WR, Dunn GH, Perry KT et al. Conversion efficacy and safety of intravenous ibutilide compared with intravenous procainamide in patients with atrial flutter or fibrillation. *J Am Coll Cardiol* 1998;**31**:1414–9.

48. Kowey PR, Vanderlught JT, Luderer JR. Safety and risk/benefit analysis of ibutilide for acute conversion of atrial fibrillation/flutter. *Am J Cardiol* 1996;**78**:46A–52A.

49. Glatter K, Yang Y, Cjatterjee K, Modin G, Cheng J, Kayser S, Scheinman MM. Chemical cardioversion of atrial fibrillation or flutter with ibutilide in patients receiving amiodarone therapy. *Circulation* 2001;**103**:253–7.

50. Falk RH, Pollak A, Singh SN, Friedrich T. Intravenous dofetilide, a class III antiarrhythmic agent, for the termination of sustained atrial fibrillation or flutter. Intravenous Dofetilide Investigators. *J Am Coll Cardiol* 1997;**29**:385–90.

51. Nørgaard BL, Wachtell K, Christensen PD, Madsen B, Johansen JB, Christiansen EH et al. Efficacy and safety of intravenously administered dofetilide in acute termination of atrial fibrillation and flutter: a multicenter, randomized, double blind, placebo-controlled study. *Am Heart J* 1999;**137**:1062–9.

52. Lindeboom JE, Kingma JH, Crijns HJ, Dunselman PH. Efficacy and safety of intravenous dofetilide for rapid termination of atrial fibrillation and atrial flutter. *Am J Cardiol* 2000;**85**:1031–3.

53. Singh S, Zoble RG, Yellen L et al, for the Dofetilide Atrial Fibrillation Investigators. Efficacy and safety of oral dofetilide in converting to and maintaining sinus rhythm in patients with chronic atrial fibrillation or atrial flutter: the Symptomatic Atrial Fibrillation Investigative Research on Dofetilide (SAFIRE-D) Study. *Circulation* 2000;**102**:2385–90.

54. Greenbaum RA. European and Australian Multicenter Evaluative Research on Atrial Fibrillation Dofetilide (EMERALD). *Circulation* 1999;**99**:2486–91.

55. Chevalier P, Durand-Dubief A, Burri H, Cucherat M, Kirkorian G, Touboul P. Amiodarone versus placebo and classic drugs for cardioversion of recent-onset atrial fibrillation: a meta-analysis. *J Am Coll Cardiol* 2003;**41**:255–62.

56. Bianconi L, Castro A, Dinelli M, Alboni P, Pappalardo A, Richiardi E, Santini M. Comparison of intravenously administered dofetilide versus amiodarone in the acute termination of atrial fibrillation and flutter. A multicentre, randomized, double-blind, placebo-controlled study. *Eur Heart J* 2000;**21**:1265–73.

57. Vardas PE, Kochiadakis GE, Igoumenidis NE, Tsatsakis AM, Simantirakis EN, Chlouverakis GI. Amiodarone as a first-choice drug for restoring sinus rhythm in patients with atrial fibrillation: a randomized, controlled study. *Chest* 2000;**117**:1538–45.

58. Blanc J, Voinov C, Maarek M, on behalf of the Parsifal Study Group. Comparison of oral loading dose of propafenone and amiodarone for converting recent-onset atrial fibrillation. *Am J Cardiol* 1999;**84**:1029–32.

59. Hohnloser SH, Klingenheben T, Singh BN. Amiodarone-associated proarrhythmic effects. A review with special reference to torsade de pointes tachycardia. *Ann Intern Med* 1994;**121**:529–35.

60. Clemo HF, Wood MA, Gilligan DM, Ellenbogen KA. Intravenous amiodarone for acute heart rate control in the critically ill patient with atrial tachyarrhythmias. *Am J Cardiol* 1998;**81**:594–8.

61. Deedwania PC, Singh BN, Ellenbogen K, Fisher S, Fletcher R, Singh SN, for the Department of Veterans Affairs CHF-STAT Investigators. Spontaneous conversion and maintenance of sinus rhythm by amiodarone in patients with heart failure and atrial fibrillation: observations from the Veterans Affairs Congestive Heart Failure Survival Trial of Antiarrhythmic Therapy (CHF-STAT). *Circulation* 1998;**98**:2574–9.

62. Galperín J, Elizari MV, Chiale PA *et al*, for the GEFCA Investigators-GEMA Group. Efficacy of amiodarone for the termination of chronic atrial fibrillation and maintenance of normal sinus rhythm: a prospective, multicenter, randomized, controlled, double blind trial. *J Cardiovasc Pharmacol Ther* 2001;**6**:341–50.

63. Kochiadakis GE, Igoumenidis NE, Solomou MC, Parthenakis FI, Christakis-Hampsas MG, Chlouverakis GI *et al*. Conversion of atrial fibrillation to sinus rhythm using acute intravenous procainamide infusion. *Cardiovasc Drugs Ther* 1998;**12**:75–81.

64. Mattioli AV, Lucchi GR, Vivoli D, Mattioli G. Propafenone versus procainamide for conversion of atrial fibrillation to sinus rhythm. *Clin Cardiol* 1998;**21**:763–6.

65. Madrid AH, Moro C, Marin-Huerta E, Mestre JL, Novo L, Costa A. Comparison of flecainide and procainamide in cardioversion of atrial fibrillation. *Eur Heart J* 1993;**14**:1127–31.

66. Kochiadakis GE, Igoumenidis NE, Hamilos ME, Marketou ME, Chlouverakis GI, Vardas PE. A comparative study of the efficacy and safety of procainamide versus propafenone versus amiodarone for the conversion of recent-onset atrial fibrillation. *Am J Cardiol* 2007;**99**:1721–5.

67. Hohnloser SH, Van de Loo A, Baedeker F. Efficacy and proarrhythmic hazards of pharmacologic cardioversion of atrial fibrillation: prospective comparison of sotalol versus quinidine. *J Am Coll Cardiol* 1995;**26**:852–8.

68. Kerin NZ, Faitel K, Naini M. The efficacy of intravenous amiodarone for the conversion of chronic atrial fibrillation: amiodarone vs quinidine for conversion of atrial fibrillation. *Arch Intern Med* 1996;**156**:49–53.

69. Camm J, Ward D, Spurrell RA. The effect of intravenous disopyramide phosphate on recurrent paroxysmal tachycardias. *Br J Clin Pharmacol* 1979;**8**:441–9.

70. Onalan O, Crystal E, Daoulah A, Lau C, Crystal A, Lashevsky I. Meta-analysis of magnesium therapy for the acute management of rapid atrial fibrillation. *Am J Cardiol* 2007;**99**:1726–32.

71. Falk RH, Knowlton AA, Bernard SA, Gotlieb NE, Battinelli NJ. Digoxin for converting recent-onset atrial fibrillation to sinus rhythm. *Ann Intern Med* 1987;**106**:503–6.

72. Noc M, Stajer D, Horvat M. Intravenous amiodarone versus verapamil for acute conversion of paroxysmal atrial fibrillation to sinus rhythm. *Am J Cardiol* 1990;**65**:679–80.

73. Digitalis in Acute Atrial Fibrillation (DAAF) Trial Group. Results of a randomized, placebo-controlled multicentre trial in 239 patients. *Eur Heart J* 1997;**18**:649–54.

74. Tieleman RG, Blaauw Y, Van Gelder IC, De Langen CD, de Kam PJ, Grandjean JG *et al*. Digoxin delays recovery from tachycardia-induced electrical remodeling of the atria. *Circulation* 1999;**100**:1836–42.

75. Oral H, Souza JJ, Michand GF, Knight BP, Goyal R, Strickberger SA, Morady F. Facilitating transthoracic cardioversion of atrial fibrillation with ibutilide pretreatment. *N Engl J Med* 1999;**340**:1849–54.

76. Boriani J, Biffi M, Capucci A, Bronzetti G, Ayers GM, Zannoli R *et al*. Favorable effects of flecainide in transvenous internal cardioversion of atrial fibrillation. *J Am Coll Cardiol* 1999;**33**:333–41.

77. Tse HF, Lau CP, Ayers GM. Incidence and modes of onset of early reinitiation of atrial fibrillation after successful internal cardioversion, and its prevention by intravenous sotalol. *Heart* 1999;**82**:319–24.

78. Capucci A, Villani GQ, Aschieri D, Rosi A, Piepoli MF. Oral amiodarone increases the efficacy of direct-current cardioversion in restoration of sinus rhythm in patients with chronic atrial fibrillation. *Eur Heart J* 2000;**21**:66–73.

79. De Simone A, De Pasquale M, De Matteis C, Canciello M, Manzo M, Sabino L *et al*. Verapamil plus antiarrhythmic drugs reduce atrial fibrillation recurrences after an electrical cardioversion (VEPARAF Study). *Eur Heart J* 2003;**24**:1425–9.

80. Van Noord T, Van Gelder IC, Tieleman RG, Bosker HA, Tuinenburg AE, Volkers C *et al*. VERDICT: the Verapamil versus Digoxin Cardioversion Trial: a randomized study on the role of calcium lowering for maintenance of sinus rhythm after cardioversion of persistent atrial fibrillation. *J Cardiovasc Electrophysiol* 2001;**12**:766–9.

81. Roy D, Rowe BH, Stiell IG *et al*, for the CRAFT Investigators. A randomized, controlled trial of RSD1235, a novel antiarrhythmic agent, in the treatment of recent onset atrial fibrillation. *J Am Coll Cardiol* 2004;**44**:2355–61.

82. Roy D, Pratt CM, Torp-Pedersen C *et al*, for the Atrial Arrhythmia Conversion Trial Investigators. Vernakalant hydrochloride for rapid conversion of atrial fibrillation: a phase 3, randomized, placebo-controlled trial. *Circulation* 2008;**117**:1518–25.

83. Roy D, Pratt C, Juul-Møller S *et al*, for the ACT III Investigators. Efficacy and tolerance of RSD1235 in the treatment of atrial fibrillation or atrial flutter: results of a phase III, randomized, placebo-controlled, multicenter trial. *J Am Coll Cardiol* 2006;**47**(suppl A):10A.

84. Savelieva I, Camm J. Anti arrhythmic drug therapy for atrial fibrillation: current anti arrhythmic drugs, investigational agents, and innovative approaches. *Europace* 2008;**10**:647–65.

85. Van Gelder IC, Crijns HJGM, Van Gilst WH, Verwer R, Lie KI. Prediction of uneventful cardioversion and maintenance of sinus rhythm from direct-current electrical cardioversion of chronic atrial fibrillation and flutter. *Am J Cardiol* 1991;**68**:41–6.

86. Lafuente-Lafuente C, Mouly S, Longas-Tejero MA, Mahe I, Bergmann JF. Antiarrhythmic drugs for maintaining sinus rhythm after cardioversion of atrial fibrillation: a systematic review of randomized controlled trials. *Arch Intern Med* 2006;**166**:719–28.

87. Geffner DL, Hershman JM. Beta-adrenergic blockade for the treatment of hyperthyroidism. *Am J Med* 1992;**93**:61–8.

88. Coumel P. Autonomic influences in atrial tachyarrhythmias. *J Cardiovasc Electrophysiol* 1996;**7**:999–1007.

89. Kühlkamp V, Schirdewan A, Stangl K, Homberg M, Ploch M, Beck OA. Use of metoprolol CR/XL to maintain sinus rhythm after conversion from persistent atrial fibrillation: a randomized, double-blind, placebo-controlled study. *J Am Coll Cardiol* 2000;**36**:139–46.

90. Plewan A, Lehmann G, Ndrepepa G, Schreieck J, Alt EU, Schömig A, Schmitt C. Maintenance of sinus rhythm after electrical cardioversion of persistent atrial fibrillation: sotalol vs bisoprolol. *Eur Heart J* 2001;**22**:1504–10.

91. Katritsis DG, Panagiotakos DB, Karvouni E, Giazitzoglou E, Korovesis S, Paxinos G *et al*. Comparison of effectiveness of carvedilol versus bisoprolol for maintenance of sinus rhythm after cardioversion of persistent atrial fibrillation. *Am J Cardiol* 2003;**92**:1116–19.

92. Nasr IA, Bouzamondo A, Hulot JS, Dubourg O, Le Heuzey JY, Lechat P. Prevention of atrial fibrillation onset by beta-blocker treatment in heart failure: a meta-analysis. *Eur Heart J* 2007;**28**:457–62.

93. Coplen SE, Antman EM, Berlin JA, Hewitt P, Chalmers TC. Efficacy and safety of quinidine therapy for maintenance of sinus rhythm after cardioversion. A meta-analysis of randomized control trials. *Circulation* 1990;**82**:1106–16.

94. Fetsch T, Bauer P, Engberding R *et al*, for the Prevention of Atrial Fibrillation after Cardioversion Investigators. Prevention of atrial fibrillation after cardioversion: results of the PAFAC trial. *Eur Heart J* 2004;**25**:1385–94.

95. Patten M, Maas R, Bauer P *et al*, for the SOPAT Investigators. Suppression of paroxysmal atrial tachyarrhythmias – results of the SOPAT trial. *Eur Heart J* 2004;**25**:1395–404.

96. Karlson BW, Torstensson I, Abjörn C, Jansson SO, Peterson LE. Disopyramide in the maintenance of sinus rhythm after electroconversion of atrial fibrillation. A placebo-controlled one-year follow-up study. *Eur Heart J* 1988;**9**:284–90.

97. Crijns HJ, Gosselink AT, Lie KI. Propafenone versus disopyramide for maintenance of sinus rhythm after electrical cardioversion of chronic atrial fibrillation: a randomized, double-blind study. PRODIS Study Group. *Cardiovasc Drugs Ther* 1996;**10**:145–52.

98. Pritchett ELC, McCarthy EA, Wilkinson WE. Propafenone treatment of symptomatic paroxysmal supraventricular arrhythmias: a randomized, placebo-controlled, crossover trial in patients tolerating oral therapy. *Ann Intern Med* 1991;**114**:539–44.

99. Stroobandt R, Stiels B, Hoebrechts R, on behalf of the Propafenone Atrial Fibrillation Trial Investigators. Propafenone for conversion and prophylaxis of atrial fibrillation. *Am J Cardiol* 1997;**79**:418–23.

100. UK Propafenone PSVT Study Group. A randomized, placebo-controlled trial of propafenone in the prophylaxis of paroxysmal supraventricular tachycardia and paroxysmal atrial fibrillation. *Circulation* 1995;**92**:2550–7.

101. Reimold SC, Maisel WH, Antman EM. Propafenone for the treatment of supraventricular tachycardia and atrial fibrillation: a meta-analysis. *Am J Cardiol* 1998;**82**:66N–71N.

102. Dogan A, Ergene O, Nazli C, Kinay O, Altinbas A, Ucarci Y *et al*. Efficacy of propafenone for maintaining sinus rhythm in patients with recent onset or persistent atrial fibrillation after conversion: a randomized, placebo-controlled study. *Acta Cardiol* 2004;**59**:255–61.

103. Pritchett EL, Page RL, Carlson M *et al*, for the Rythmol Atrial Fibrillation Trial (RAFT) Investigators. Efficacy and safety of sustained-release propafenone (propafenone SR) for patients with atrial fibrillation. *Am J Cardiol* 2003;**92**:941–6.

104. Meinertz T, Lip GYH, Lombardi F *et al*, for the ERAFT Investigators. Efficacy and safety of propafenone sustained release in the prophylaxis of symptomatic paroxysmal atrial fibrillation (The European Rythmol/Rytmonorm Atrial Fibrillation Trial [ERAFT] Study). *Am J Cardiol* 2002;**90**:1300–6.

105. Pietersen AH, Hellemann H, for the Danish-Norwegian Flecainide Multicenter Atrial Fibrillation Study Group. Usefulness of flecainide for prevention of paroxysmal atrial fibrillation and flutter. *Am J Cardiol* 1991;**67**:713–7.

106. Chimienti M, Cullen MT Jr, Casadei G. Safety of long-term flecainide and propafenone in the management of patients with symptomatic paroxysmal atrial fibrillation: report from the Flecainide And Propafenone Italian Study Investigators. *Am J Cardiol* 1996;**77**:60A–75A.

107. Naccarelli GV, Dorian P, Hohnloser S, Coumel P, for the Flecainide Multicenter Atrial Fibrillation Study Group. Prospective comparison of flecainide versus quinidine for the treatment of paroxysmal atrial fibrillation/flutter. *Am J Cardiol* 1996;**77**:53A–9A.

108. Atarashi H, Ogawa S, Inoue H, Hamada C, for the Flecainide Atrial Fibrillation Investigators. Dose-response effect of flecainide in patients with symptomatic paroxysmal atrial fibrillation and/or flutter monitored with trans-telephonic electrocardiography: a multicenter, placebo-controlled, double-blind trial. *Circ J* 2007;**71**:294–300.

109. Okishige K, Fukunami M, Kumagai K *et al*, for the Pilsicainide Suppression Trial for Persistent Atrial Fibrillation II Investigators. Pharmacological conversion of persistent atrial fibrillation into sinus rhythm with oral pilsicainide: pilsicainide suppression trial for persistent atrial fibrillation II. *Circ J* 2006;**70**:657–61.

110. Komatsu T, Sato Y, Tachibana H, Nakamura M, Horiuchi D, Okumura K. Randomized crossover study of the long-term effects of pilsicainide and cibenzoline in preventing recurrence of symptomatic paroxysmal atrial fibrillation: influence of the duration of arrhythmia before therapy. *Circ J* 2006;**70**:667–72.

111. Benditt DG, Williams JH, Jin J *et al*, for the d,l-Sotalol Atrial Fibrillation/Flutter Study Group. Maintenance of sinus rhythm with oral d,l-sotalol therapy in patients with symptomatic atrial fibrillation and/or atrial flutter. *Am J Cardiol* 1999;**84**:270–7.

112. Bellandi F, Simonetti I, Leoncini M, Frascarelli F, Giovannini T, Maioli M, Dabizzi RP. Long-term efficacy and safety of propafenone and sotalol for the maintenance of sinus rhythm after conversion of recurrent symptomatic atrial fibrillation. *Am J Cardiol* 2001;**88**:640–5.

113. De Paola AAV, Veloso HH, for the SOCESP Investigators. Efficacy and safety of sotalol versus quinidine for the maintenance

of sinus rhythm after conversion of atrial fibrillation. *Am J Cardiol* 1999;**84**:1033–7.

114. Lombardi F, Borggrefe M, Ruzyllo W, Lüderitz B, for the A-COMET-II Investigators. Azimilide vs. placebo and sotalol for persistent atrial fibrillation: the A-COMET-II (Azimilide-CardiOversion MaintEnance Trial-II) trial. *Eur Heart J* 2006;**27**:2224–31.

115. Roy D, Talajic M, Dorian P *et al*, for the Canadian Trial of Atrial Fibrillation Investigators. Amiodarone to prevent recurrence of atrial fibrillation. *N Engl J Med* 2000;**342**:913–20.

116. AFFIRM First Antiarrhythmic Drug Substudy Investigators. Maintenance of sinus rhythm in patients with atrial fibrillation: an AFFIRM Substudy of First Antiarrhythmic Drug. *J Am Coll Cardiol* 2003;**42**:20–9.

117. Torp-Pedersen C, Møller M, Bloch-Thomsen PE *et al*, for the Danish Investigations of Arrhythmia and Mortality on Dofetilide Study Group. Dofetilide in patients with congestive heart failure and left ventricular dysfunction. *N Engl J Med* 1999;**341**:857–65.

118. Køber L, Bloch Thomsen PE, Møller M *et al*, for the Danish Investigations of Arrhythmia and Mortality on Dofetilide (DIAMOND) Study Group. Effect of dofetilide in patients with recent myocardial infarction and left-ventricular dysfunction: a randomised trial. *Lancet* 2000;**356**:2052–8.

119. Pritchett EL, Page RL, Connolly SJ, Marcello SR, Schnell DJ, Wilkinson WE. Antiarrhythmic effects of azimilide in atrial fibrillation: efficacy and dose-response. *J Am Coll Cardiol* 2000;**36**:794–802.

120. Kerr CR, Connolly SJ, Kowey P *et al*, for the A-STAR Investigators. Efficacy of azimilide for the maintenance of sinus rhythm in patients with paroxysmal atrial fibrillation in the presence and absence of structural heart disease. *Am J Cardiol* 2006;**98**:215–18.

121. Camm AJ, Pratt CM, Schwartz PJ *et al*, for the AzimiLide post Infarct surVival Evaluation (ALIVE) Investigators. Mortality in patients with recent myocardial infarction: a randomized, placebo-controlled trial of azimilide using heart rate variability for risk stratification. *Circulation* 2004;**109**:990–6.

122. Pratt CM, Singh SN, Al-Khalidi HR *et al*, for the ALIVE Investigators. The efficacy of azimilide in the treatment of atrial fibrillation in the presence of left ventricular systolic dysfunction: Results from the Azimilide Postinfarct Survival Evaluation (ALIVE) trial. *J Am Coll Cardiol* 2004;**43**:1211–16.

123. Sicouri S, Moro S, Litovsky S, Elizari MV, Antzelevitch C. Chronic amiodarone reduces transmural dispersion of repolarization in the canine heart. *J Cardiovasc Electrophysiol* 1997;**8**:1269–79.

124. Boutitie F, Boissel JP, Connolly SJ, Camm AJ, Cairns JA, Julian DG *et al*. Amiodarone interaction with beta-blockers: analysis of the merged EMIAT (European Myocardial Infarct Amiodarone Trial) and CAMIAT (Canadian Amiodarone Myocardial Infarction Trial) databases. The EMIAT and CAMIAT Investigators. *Circulation* 1999;**99**:2268–75.

125. Doval HC, Nul DR, Grancelli HO, Perrone SV, Bortman GR, Curiel R. Randomised trial of low-dose amiodarone in severe congestive heart failure. Grupo de Estudio de la Sobrevida en la Insuficiencia Cardiaca en Argentina (GESICA). *Lancet* 1994;**344**:493–8.

126. Bardy GH, Lee KL, Mark DB *et al*, for the Sudden Cardiac Death in Heart Failure Trial (SCD-HeFT) Investigators. Amiodarone or an implantable cardioverter-defibrillator for congestive heart failure. *N Engl J Med* 2005;**352**:225–37.

127. Touboul P, Brugada J, Capucci A, Crijns HJ, Edvardsson N, Hohnloser SH. Dronedarone for prevention of atrial fibrillation: a dose-ranging study. *Eur Heart J* 2003;**24**:1481–7.

128. Singh BN, Connolly SJ, Crijns HJ *et al*, for the EURIDIS and ADONIS Investigators. Dronedarone for maintenance of sinus rhythm in atrial fibrillation or flutter. *N Engl J Med* 2007;**357**:987–99.

129. Hohnloser SH, Crijns HJ, van Eickels M, Gaudin C, Page RL, Torp-Pedersen C, Connolly SJ; ATHENA Investigators. *Effect of dronedarone on cardiovascular events in atrial fibrillation. N Engl J Med* 2009;**360**:668–78.

129a. Page RL, Connolly SJ, Crijns HJ, van Eickels M, Gaudin C, Torp-Petersen C, Hohnloser SH. Rhythm- and rate-controlling effects of dronedarone in patients with atrial fibrillation: insights from the ATHENA trial. *Circulation* 2008; Abstract Supplement: Abstract 4097.

130. Køber L, Torp-Pedersen C, McMurray JJ *et al*, for the Dronedarone Study Group. Increased mortality after dronedarone therapy for severe heart failure. *N Engl J Med* 2008;**358**:2678–87.

130a. Hohnloser SH, Connolly SJ, Crijns HJ, Gaudin C, van Eickels M, Page RL, Torp-Pedersen C. Effects of dronedarone on clinical outcomes in patients with atrial fibrillation and congestive heart failure: insights from ATHENA. Heart Rhythm Society Late Breaking Trials Session II, 2009.

131. Calkins H, Brugada J, Packer DL *et al*, for the Heart Rhythm Society; European Heart Rhythm Association; European Cardiac Arrhythmia Society; American College of Cardiology, American Heart Association; Society of Thoracic Surgeons. HRS/EHRA/ECAS expert consensus statement on catheter and surgical ablation of atrial fibrillation: recommendations for personnel, policy, procedures and follow-up. A report of the Heart Rhythm Society (HRS) Task Force on Catheter and Surgical Ablation of Atrial Fibrillation developed in partnership with the European Heart Rhythm Association (EHRA) and the European Cardiac Arrhythmia Society (ECAS); in collaboration with the American College of Cardiology (ACC), American Heart Association (AHA), and the Society of Thoracic Surgeons (STS). Endorsed and approved by the governing bodies of the American College of Cardiology, the American Heart Association, the European Cardiac Arrhythmia Society, the European Heart Rhythm Association, the Society of Thoracic Surgeons, and the Heart Rhythm Society. *Europace* 2007;**9**:335–79.

132. Cappato R, Calkins H, Chen SA, Davies W, Iesaka Y, Kalman J *et al*. Worldwide survey on the methods, efficacy, and safety of catheter ablation for human atrial fibrillation. *Circulation* 2005;**111**:1100–5.

132a. Cappato R, Calkins H, Chen SA, Davies W, Iesaka Y, Kalman J, Kim YH, Klein G, Natale A, Packer D, Skanes A. *Prevalence and causes of fatal outcome in catheter ablation of atrial fibrillation. J Am Coll Cardiol* 2009;**53**:1798–803.

133. Waxman HL, Myerburg RJ, Appel R, Sung RJ. Verapamil for control of ventricular rate in paroxysmal supraventricular tachycardia and atrial fibrillation or flutter: a double-blind randomized cross-over study. *Ann Intern Med* 1981;**94**:1–6.

134. Ellenbogen KA, Dias VC, Plumb VJ, Heywood JT, Mirvis DM. A placebo-controlled trial of continuous intravenous diltiazem

infusion for 24-hour rate control during atrial fibrillation and atrial flutter: a multicenter study. *J Am Coll Cardiol* 1991;**185**:891–7.

135. Byrd RC, Sung RJ, Marks J, Parmley WW. Safety and efficacy of esmolol (ASL-8052: an ultrashort-acting beta-adrenergic blocking agent) for control of ventricular rate in supraventricular tachycardias. *J Am Coll Cardiol* 1984;**3**:394–9.

136. Schreck DM, Rivera AR, Tricarico VJ. Emergency management of atrial fibrillation and flutter: intravenous diltiazem versus intravenous digoxin. *Ann Emerg Med* 1997;**29**:135–40.

137. Gonzalez R, Scheinman MM. Treatment of supraventricular arrhythmias with intravenous and oral verapamil. *Chest* 1981;**80**:465–70.

138. Salerno DM, Dias VC, Kleiger RE, Tschida VH, Sung RJ, Sami M, Giorgi LV. Efficacy and safety of intravenous diltiazem for treatment of atrial fibrillation and atrial flutter. The Diltiazem-Atrial Fibrillation/Flutter Study Group. *Am J Cardiol* 1989;**63**:1046–51.

139. Khan IA, Nair CK, Singh N, Gowda RM, Nair RC. Acute ventricular rate control in atrial fibrillation and atrial flutter. *Int J Cardiol* 2004;**97**:7–13.

140. Jordaens L, Trouerbach J, Calle P, Tavernier R, Derycke E, Vertongen P et al. Conversion of atrial fibrillation to sinus rhythm and rate control by digoxin in comparison to placebo. *Eur Heart J* 1997;**18**:643–8.

141. Thomas SP, Guy D, Wallace E, Crampton R, Kijvanit P, Eipper V, Ross DL, Cooper MJ. Rapid loading of sotalol or amiodarone for management of recent onset symptomatic atrial fibrillation: a randomized, digoxin-controlled trial. *Am Heart J* 2004;**147**:e3.

142. Simpson CS, Ghali WA, Sanfilippo AJ, Moritz S, Abdollah H. Clinical assessment of clonidine in the treatment of new-onset rapid atrial fibrillation: a prospective, randomized clinical trial. *Am Heart J* 2001;**142**:e3.

143. Strickberger SA, Man KC, Daoud EG, Goyal R, Brinkman K, Knight BP et al. Adenosine-induced atrial arrhythmia: a prospective analysis. *Ann Intern Med* 1997;**127**:417–22.

144. Ellenbogen KA, O'Neill G, Prystowsky EN et al, for the TEMPEST Study Group. Trial to evaluate the management of paroxysmal supraventricular tachycardia during an electrophysiology study with tecadenoson. *Circulation* 2005;**111**:3202–8.

145. Cheng J, Beard J, on behalf of the DTI0009 Study Group. DTI0009, a novel selective A1 agonist, suppresses AV nodal conduction without hypotensive effect. *Circulation* 2002;**106**(suppl II):II–545.

146. Sticherling C, Oral H, Horrocks J, Chough SP, Baker RL, Kim MH et al. Effects of digoxin on acute, atrial fibrillation-induced changes in atrial refractoriness. *Circulation* 2000;**102**:2503–8.

147. Murgatroyd FD, Gibson SM, Baiyan X et al, for the Controlled Randomized Atrial Fibrillation Trial (CRAFT) Investigators. Double-blind placebo-controlled trial of digoxin in symptomatic paroxysmal atrial fibrillation. *Circulation* 1999;**99**:2765–70.

148. Brodsky M, Saini R, Bellinger R, Zoble R, Weiss R, Powers L. Comparative effects of the combination of digoxin and dl-sotalol therapy versus digoxin monotherapy for control of ventricular response in chronic atrial fibrillation: dl-Sotalol Atrial Fibrillation Study Group. *Am Heart J* 1994;**127**:572–7.

149. Singh S, Saini RK, DiMarco J, Kluger J, Gold R, Chen YW. Efficacy and safety of sotalol in digitalized patients with chronic atrial fibrillation. The Sotalol Study Group. *Am J Cardiol* 1991;**68**:1227–30.

150. Kochiadakis GE, Kanoupakis EM, Kalebubas MD, Igoumenidis NE, Vardakis KE, Mavrakis HE, Vardas PE. Sotalol vs metoprolol for ventricular rate control in patients with chronic atrial fibrillation who have undergone digitalization: a single-blinded crossover study. *Europace* 2001;**3**:73–9.

151. Davy JM, Herold M, Hoglund C et al, for the ERATO Study Investigators. Dronedarone for the control of ventricular rate in permanent atrial fibrillation: the Efficacy and safety of dRonedArone for the cOntrol of ventricular rate during atrial fibrillation (ERATO) study. *Am Heart J* 2008;**156**:527.

152. Lewis RV, Irvine N, McDevitt DG. Relationships between heart rate, exercise tolerance and cardiac output in atrial fibrillation: the effects of treatment with digoxin, verapamil and diltiazem. *Eur Heart J* 1988;**9**:777–81.

153. Rawles JM. What is meant by a "controlled" ventricular rate in atrial fibrillation? *Br Heart J* 1990;**63**:157–61.

154. Waldo AL. A perspective on rate control in the treatment of atrial fibrillation. *Clin Cardiol* 2004;**27**:121–4.

155. Daoud EG, Weiss R, Bahu M, Knight BP, Bogun F, Goyal R et al. Effect of an irregular ventricular rhythm on cardiac output. *Am J Cardiol* 1996;**78**:1433–6.

156. Twidale N, McDonald T, Nave K, Seal A. Comparison of the effects of AV nodal ablation versus AV nodal modification in patients with congestive heart failure and uncontrolled atrial fibrillation. *Pacing Clin Electrophysiol* 1998;**21**:641–51.

157. Wasmer K, Oral H, Sticherling C, Clough S, Baker R, Tada H et al. Assessment of ventricular rate in patients with chronic atrial fibrillation. *J Am Coll Cardiol* 2001;**37**:93A.

158. Van Gelder IC, Wyse DG, Chandler ML et al, for the RACE and AFFIRM Investigators. Does intensity of rate-control influence outcome in atrial fibrillation? An analysis of pooled data from the RACE and AFFIRM studies. *Europace* 2006;**8**:935–42.

159. Van Gelder IC, Van Veldhuisen DJ, Crijns HJ, Tuininga YS, Tijssen JG, Alings AM et al. RAte Control Efficacy in permanent atrial fibrillation: a comparison between lenient versus strict rate control in patients with and without heart failure. Background, aims, and design of RACE II. *Am Heart J* 2006;**152**:420–6.

160. David D, Segni ED, Klein HO, Kaplinsky E. Inefficacy of digitalis in the control of heart rate in patients with chronic atrial fibrillation: beneficial effect of an added beta adrenergic blocking agent. *Am J Cardiol* 1979;**44**:1378–82.

161. Farshi R, Kistner D, Sarma JS, Longmate JA, Singh BN. Ventricular rate control in chronic atrial fibrillation during daily activity and programmed exercise: a crossover open-label study of five drug regimens. *J Am Coll Cardiol* 1999;**33**:304–10.

162. Corbelli R, Masterson M, Wilkoff BL. Chronotropic response to exercise in patients with atrial fibrillation. *Pacing Clin Electrophysiol* 1990;**13**:179–87.

163. Khand AU, Rankin AC, Martin W, Taylor J, Gemmell I, Cleland JG. Carvedilol alone or in combination with digoxin for the management of atrial fibrillation in patients with heart failure? *J Am Coll Cardiol* 2003;**42**:1944–51.

164. Olshansky B, Rosenfeld LE, Warner AL et al, for the AFFIRM Investigators. The Atrial Fibrillation Follow-up Investigation of Rhythm Management (AFFIRM) study: approaches to control rate in atrial fibrillation. *J Am Coll Cardiol* 2004;**43**:1201–8.

165. Mitchell LB. Prophylactic therapy to prevent atrial arrythmia after cardiac surgery. *Curr Opin Cardiol* 2007;**22**:18–24.

166. Mathew JP, Fontes ML, Tudor IC *et al*, for the Investigators of the Ischemia Research and Education Foundation; Multicenter Study of Perioperative Ischemia Research Group. A multicenter risk index for atrial fibrillation after cardiac surgery. *JAMA* 2004;**291**:1720–9.

167. Scherer M, Sirat AS, Dogan S, Aybek T, Moritz A, Wimmer-Greinecker G. Does totally endoscopic access for off-pump cardiac surgery influence the incidence of postoperative atrial fibrillation in coronary artery bypass grafting? A preliminary report. *Cardiovasc Eng* 2006;**6**:118–21.

168. Tisdale JE, Padhi ID, Goldberg AD, Silverman NA, Webb CR, Higgins RS *et al*. A randomized, double blind comparison of intravenous diltiazem and digoxin for atrial fibrillation after coronary bypass surgery. *Am Heart J* 1998;**135**:739–47.

169. Kowey PR, Taylor JE, Rials SJ, Marinchak RA. Meta-analysis of the effectiveness of prophylactic drug therapy in preventing supraventricular arrhythmia early after coronary artery bypass grafting. *Am J Cardiol* 1992;**69**:963–5.

170. Andrews TC, Reimold SC, Berlin JA, Antman EM. Prevention of supraventricular arrhythmias after coronary artery bypass surgery. A meta-analysis of randomized trials. *Circulation* 1991;**84**(suppl III):III-236–III-244.

171. Connolly SJ, Cybulsky I, Lamy A, Roberts RS, O'Brien B, Carroll S *et al*. Beta-Blocker Length Of Stay (BLOS) study. Double-blind, placebo-controlled, randomized trial of prophylactic metoprolol for reduction of hospital length of stay after heart surgery: the beta-Blocker Length Of Stay (BLOS) study. *Am Heart J* 2003;**145**:226–32.

172. Merritt JC, Niebauer M, Tarakji K, Hammer D, Mills RM. Comparison of effectiveness of carvedilol versus metoprolol or atenolol for atrial fibrillation appearing after coronary artery bypass grafting or cardiac valve operation. *Am J Cardiol* 2003;**92**:735–6.

173. Parikka H, Toivonen L, Heikkila L, Virtanen K, Järvinen A. Comparison of sotalol and metoprolol in the prevention of atrial fibrillation after coronary artery bypass surgery. *J Cardiovasc Pharm* 1998;**31**:67–73.

174. Mooss AN, Wurdeman RL, Sugimoto JT, Packard KA, Hilleman DE, Lenz TL *et al*. Amiodarone versus sotalol for the treatment of atrial fibrillation after open heart surgery: the Reduction in Postoperative Cardiovascular Arrhythmic Events (REDUCE) trial. *Am Heart J* 2004;**148**:641–8.

175. Wurdeman RL, Mooss AN, Mohiuddin SM, Lenz TL. Amiodarone vs. sotalol as prophylaxis against atrial fibrillation/flutter after heart surgery: a meta-analysis. *Chest* 2002;**121**:1203–10.

176. Daoud EG, Strickberger SA, Man KC, Goyal R, Deeb GM, Bolling SF *et al*. Preoperative amiodarone as prophylaxis against atrial fibrillation after heart surgery. *N Engl J Med* 1997;**337**:1785–91.

177. Redle JD, Khurama S, Marzan R, McCullough PA, Stewart JR, Westveer DC *et al*. Prophylactic oral amiodarone compared with placebo for prevention of atrial fibrillation after coronary artery bypass surgery. *Am Heart J* 1999;**138**:144–50.

178. Giri S, White CM, Dunn AB, Felton K, Freeman-Bosco L, Reddy P *et al*. Oral amiodarone for prevention of atrial fibrillation after open heart surgery, the Atrial Fibrillation Suppression Trial (AFIST): a randomised placebo-controlled trial. *Lancet* 2001;**357**:830–6.

179. White CM, Caron MF, Kalus JS, Rose H, Song J, Reddy P *et al*. Atrial Fibrillation Suppression Trial II. Intravenous plus oral amiodarone, atrial septal pacing, or both strategies to prevent post-cardiothoracic surgery atrial fibrillation: the Atrial Fibrillation Suppression Trial II (AFIST II). *Circulation* 2003;**108**(suppl 1):II200–6.

180. Crystal E, Garfinkle MS, Connolly S, Ginger T, Sleik K, Yusuf S. Interventions for preventing post-operative atrial fibrillation in patients undergoing heart surgery. *Cochrane Database of Systematic Reviews* 2004, Issue 4. Art. No.: CD003611. DOI: 10.1002/14651858.CD003611.pub2.

181. Guarnieri T, Nolan S, Gottlieb SO, Dudek A, Lowry DR. Intravenous amiodarone for the prevention of atrial fibrillation after open heart surgery: the Amiodarone Reduction in Coronary Heart (ARCH) Trial. *J Am Coll Cardiol* 1999;**34**:343–7.

182. Mitchell LB, Exner DV, Wyse DG, Connolly CJ, Prystai GD, Bayes AJ *et al*. Prophylactic Oral Amiodarone for the Prevention of Arrhythmias that Begin Early After Revascularization, Valve Replacement, or Repair: PAPABEAR: a randomized controlled trial. *JAMA* 2005;**294**:3093–100.

183. Bagshaw SM, Galbraith PD, Mitchell LB, Sauve R, Exner DV, Ghali WA. Prophylactic amiodarone for prevention of atrial fibrillation after cardiac surgery: a meta-analysis. *Ann Thorac Surg* 2006;**82**:1927–37.

184. VanderLugt JT, Mattioni T, Denker S *et al*, for the Ibutilide Investigators. Efficacy and safety of ibutilide fumarate for the conversion of atrial arrhythmias after cardiac surgery. *Circulation* 1999;**100**:369–75.

185. Serafimovski N, Burke P, Khawaja O, Sekulic M, Machado C. Usefulness of dofetilide for the prevention of atrial tachyarrhythmias (atrial fibrillation or flutter) after coronary artery bypass grafting. *Am J Cardiol* 2008;**101**:1574–9.

186. Miller S, Crystal E, Garfinkle M, Lau C, Lashevsky I, Connolly SJ. Effects of magnesium on atrial fibrillation after cardiac surgery: a meta-analysis. *Heart* 2005;**91**:618–23.

187. Kowey PR, Yannicelli D, Amsterdam E, COPPA-II Investigators. Effectiveness of oral propafenone for the prevention of atrial fibrillation after coronary artery bypass grafting. *Am J Cardiol* 2004;**94**:663–5.

188. Geelen P, O'Hara GE, Roy N, Talajic M, Roy D, Plante S, Turgeon J. Comparison of propafenone versus procainamide for the acute treatment of atrial fibrillation after cardiac surgery. *Am J Cardiol* 1999;**84**:345–7.

189. Gold MR, O'Gara PT, Buckley MJ, DeSanctis RW. Efficacy and safety of procainamide in preventing arrhythmias after coronary artery bypass surgery. *Am J Cardiol* 1996;**78**:975–9.

36 Atrial fibrillation: upstream therapies

Antonios Kourliouros, Irina Savelieva, Marjan Jahangiri and A John Camm
St George's University of London, London, UK

Introduction

Atrial fibrillation (AF) has been described as an "epidemic" due to its rising prevalence in our aging population. AF is a leading cause of thromboembolism and is also asscociated with impaired quality of life and increased overall mortality. Available treatment strategies consist of heart rate control, rhythm control and prevention of thromboembolism. Antiarrhythmic agents still form the mainstay of pharmacologic therapy for AF. However, despite their proven efficacy in symptom control and prevention of hemodynamic complications, they do not offer a definitive treatment. Comprehensive understanding of the mechanisms leading to AF is paramount for the development of targeted and potentially curative treatments.

Current evidence suggests that the pathogenesis of AF is multifactorial. Observations at the level of atrial cardiomyocytes and interstitium reveal cellular degeneration with hypertrophy and extracellular matrix protein proliferation leading to fibrosis. It has been described that interstitial fibrosis predisposes to tissue anisotropy by creating areas with different conduction properties, which can either block or initiate a conduction wavelet and lead to re-entry circuits and AF. Although this structural remodeling can generate an inflammatory response, inflammation may also play a direct role in the development of atrial fibrosis and act as a trigger for the development of AF in the presence of a susceptible anatomic substrate. Finally, the ionic current changes and action potential abnormalities associated with the development of AF are also accountable for the self-perpetuation of the arrhythmia.

Upstream management of AF refers to therapies that target the responsible substrate and aim to prevent the development of the arrhythmia in the first place or delay its occurrence and domestication. Experimental and clinical data have highlighted the potential effect of angiotensin-converting enzyme inhibitors (ACEI), angiotensin receptor blockers (ARB), statins, n-3 polyunsaturated fatty acids (PUFA) and corticosteroids on the prevention of AF. The proposed mechanisms by which these agents exhibit their protective effect are shown in Table 36.1.

Angiotensin-converting enzyme inhibitors and angiotensin receptor blockers for the prevention of atrial fibrillation

In a meta-analysis of 12 published randomized controlled trials (RCT) evaluating the effect of ACEIs/ARBs on new or recurrent AF, the difference in the underlying cardiovascular pathology of the studied populations led to significant variability in outcomes.[1] Although ACEIs/ARBs conferred a statistically significant risk reduction of 28% in AF, this effect was more pronounced in high-risk heart failure patients (44% relative risk reduction), and absent in the hypertension subgroup analysis. This finding was consistent even when the meta-analysis was revisited by another group, which included data from patients with cardiovascular disease but preserved left ventricular ejection fraction (LVEF), receiving ramipril or placebo.[2] In another meta-analysis,[3] additional to their marked benefit in patients with heart failure, ACEIs/ARBs were also found to be effective in the prevention of AF in patients with hypertension and following myocardial infarction (23% and 11% risk reduction, respectively). Finally, Anand and colleagues, having identified 9 RCTs with new onset AF (and not recurrent) as a reported outcome, demonstrated that ACEIs were more efficacious in primary AF prevention than ARBs.[4] Overall, most of the studies examined did not specify AF as a primary endpoint and AF outcomes were analysed *post hoc*, which may have led to multiple testing errors. This evidence-based assessment of the efficacy of ACEIs/ARBs in AF prevention focuses on patient groups with similar underlying cardiovascular pathology.

Evidence-Based Cardiology, 3rd edition. Edited by S. Yusuf, J.A. Cairns, A.J. Camm, E.L. Fallen, and B.J. Gersh. © 2010 Blackwell Publishing, ISBN: 978-1-4051-5925-8.

Table 36.1 Upstream therapies for prevention of atrial fibrillation

Drugs	Mode of action	Evidence base
ACEIs and ARBs	Targeting underlying heart disease (e.g. hypertension, heart failure) and unloading the atria Preventing structural remodeling: antifibrotic, antiapoptotic, and anti-inflammatory effects Antioxidant effects via PPAR-dependent pathways Direct electrophysiologic effects on ion channels (e.g. inhibition of I_{Kur}, I_{to}) Preventing gap junctional remodeling Modulating the autonomous nervous system: antisympathetic activity Modulating thrombogenesis (e.g. antiplatelet effects, P-selectin inhibition)	Good experimental data Retrospective analyses of large RCTs Small prospective studies Three meta-analyses Ongoing RCTs
Statins	Reducing cardiovascular events and the development of underlying heart disease Preventing substrate formation: anti-inflammatory and antioxidant effects Protecting the atrial mycardium during ischemia via increased eNOS activity Preventing matrix remodeling via inhibition of MMPs Preventing electrical remodeling by reducing downregulation of the I_{Ca} Modulating thrombogenesis (e.g. improved rheology, antiplatelet effects, fibrinogen reduction)	Experimental data Retrospective analyses of RCTs and observational studies Prospective study in electrical cardioversion Prospective studies in CABG Three meta-analyses Ongoing RCTs
Corticosteroids	Anti-inflammatory effects	Indirect evidence based on CRP reduction Small prospective studies Prospective studies in CABG and aortic valve surgery
PUFA	Preventing stretch-induced electrical remodeling Direct electrophysiologic effects on ion channels (inhibition of I_{Na}, I_{Ca}) Reducing proarrhythmic eicosanoids in the myocardium Anti-inflammatory and antioxidant effects Preventing matrix remodeling via MMP-dependent mechanism	Experimental data Clinical experience: preventing ventricular fibrillation Analyses from the population-based studies Prospective study in CABG and after cardioversion Ongoing RCTs

ACEIs and ARBs for the prevention of AF in patients with heart failure

The beneficial effects of ACEI/ARB therapy in patients with heart failure are well established. Their potential antiarrhythmic effect was initially examined in a cohort of 30 patients with congestive heart failure (CHF) and persistent AF who were randomized to lisinopril 10 mg or placebo and treated with electrical cardioversion.[5] Despite the higher rate of maintenance of sinus rhythm (SR) in the lisinopril group, the AF risk reduction was not statistically significant in this small group of patients.

The first study to demonstrate a statistically significant reduction in AF due to ACEI treatment was the TRAndolapril Cardiac Evaluation (TRACE) trial.[6] Patients admitted to hospital with acute MI and documented LVEF ≤36% were randomized to trandolapril (up to 4 mg/day) or placebo. During the follow-up period of 2–4 years, the incidence of AF was 5.3% in the plecebo group and 2.8% in the treatment group, yielding a 55% risk reduction in AF due

to trandolapril. Although the antiarrhythmic effect of trandolapril remained consistent after adjustment for progressive LVEF decline in the placebo group, it is likely that AF reduction may just reflect the distinct attenuation of LV remodeling following MI due to ACE inhibition. The results of the SOLVD (Studies Of Left Ventricular Dysfunction) trial, which examined the effect of ACE inhibition on AF in patients with LV dysfunction, supported the beneficial role of enalapril.[7] With an absolute risk reduction of 18%, enalapril use was strongly associated with maintenance of SR during the 2.9 years of follow-up. Once again, it is likely that the efficacious management of underlying cardiac disease might have been responsible for this reduction in AF rather than any potential direct antiarrhythmic effect of enalapril.

In 4395 patients with documented heart failure who were randomized to valsartan or placebo in the context of the Val-HeFT study,[8] new-onset AF occurred in 5.1% of those on valsartan versus 7.95% receiving placebo (odds ratio (OR) 0.63, 95% confidence interval (CI) 0.49–0.81).

Table 36.2 Clinical studies of ACEIs and ARBs for the prevention of atrial fibrillation

Study, date	n	Baseline rhythm	Underlying disease	Design	Drug	Groups	Add. Intervent	Endpoint	Mean follow-up	Risk reduction
Van de Berg,[5] 1995	30	Persistent AF	Congestive heart failure	Double-blind RCT	Lisinopril	Lisinopril vs placebo	DCCV	AF recurrence	84 days	No effect
CAPPP,[10] 1999	10985	Sinus rhythm & AF	Primary hypertension	Open-label RCT (AF secondary outcome)	Captopril	Captopril vs conventional antihypertensives	–	AF occurrence	6.1 years	No effect of captopril on AF prevention
STOP-H2,[11] 1999	6614	Sinus rhythm & AF	Primary hypertension	Open-label RCT (AF secondary outcome)	Enalapril or lisinopril	ACEIs vs calcium antagonists vs conventional antihypertensives	–	AF occurrence	5 years	No effect of ACEIs on AF prevention
TRACE,[6] 1999	1577	Sinus rhythm	Post-MI, LV dysfunction	Double-blind RCT with retrospective analysis	Trandolapril	Trandolapril vs placebo	–	AF occurrence	2–4 years	55%
Madrid,[18] 2002	154	Persistent AF	Any, 21% lone AF	Open-label RCT	Irbesartan	Irb+amio vs amio	DCCV	Time to 1st recurrence	254 days	65%
Ueng,[19] 2003	145	Persistent AF	Any, 20% lone AF	Open-label RCT	Enalapril	Enalapril+amio vs amio	DCCV	Time to 1st recurrence	270 days	69%
SOLVD,[7] 2003	374	Sinus rhythm	LV dysfunction	Double-blind RCT with retrospective analysis	Enalapril	Enalapril vs placebo	–	AF occurrence	2.9 years	78%
Madrid,[20] 2004	90	Persistent AF	None, lone AF	Open-label RCT	Irbesartan	Amio vs amio+irb 150 mg vs amio+irb 300 mg	DCCV	Time to 1st recurrence	220 days	53% reduction by amio+irb 300mg
LIFE,[13] 2005	8851	Sinus rhythm	HTN, LV hypertrophy	Double-blind RCT with retrospective analysis	Losartan	Losartan-based vs atenolol-based therapy	–	New-onset AF	4.8 years	33%
Val-HeFT,[8] 2005	4395	Sinus rhythm	Congestive heart failure	Double-blind RCT with retrospective analysis	Valsartan	Valsartan vs placebo	–	AF occurrence	23 months	37%
CHARM,[9] 2006	6379	Sinus rhythm	Congestive heart failure	Double-blind RCT (AF prespecified)	Candesartan	Candesartan vs placebo	–	Time to new AF	37.7 months	20%
HOPE,[2] 2007	8335	Sinus rhythm	CAD + other cardiovascular risk factor	Double-blind RCT with retrospective analysis	Ramipril	Ramipril vs placebo	–	AF occurrence	4.5 years	No effect
CAPRAF,[21] 2007	171	Persistent AF	Any, 48% lone AF	Double-blind RCT (AF secondary outcome)	Candesartan	Candesartan vs. placebo	DCCV	AF recurrence	6 months	No effect
VALUE,[14] 2008	13760	Sinus rhythm	HTN, other cardiovascular risk factors	Double-blind RCT (AF secondary outcome)	Valsartan	Valsartan-based vs. amlodipine-based therapy	–	AF occurrence	4.2 years	16% (unadjusted)
TRANSCEND,[15] 2008	5926	Sinus rhythm	Coronary, peripheral vascular or cerebrovascular disease	Double-blind RCT (AF secondary outcome)	Telmisartan	Telmisartn vs. placebo	–	AF occurrence	56 months	No effect
ONTARGET,[16] 2008	25620	Sinus rhythm	Coronary, peripheral vascular or cerebrovascular disease	Double-blind RCT (AF secondary outcome)	Telmisartan	Telmisartan vs telmisartin + ramipril vs. ramipril	–	AF occurrence	56 months	No effect
GISSI-AF,[22] 2009	1442	≥2 episodes of AF or successful DCCV	Cardiovascular disease, lone AF (12%)	Double-blind RCT	Valsartan	Valsartan vs. placebo	±DCCV	Time to first recurrence and proportion of patients with ≥1 recurrence	12 months	No effect

This risk reduction in AF due to valsartan was not influenced by concomitant treatment with other ACE inhibitors (93% of cases). In addition, AF occurrence was associated with a 40% increase in overall mortality. Despite the efficacy of valsartan in the prevention of AF, its capacity to reduce mortality was not proven, probably due to the relatively low rate of AF in this study population. In the CHARM study,[9] the effect of candesartan on new-onset AF was a prespecified secondary outcome in the cohort of 6379 patients with symptomatic heart failure and absence of the arrhythmia. The reduction in AF caused by candesartan (target dose 32 mg/d) versus placebo (5.55% vs 6.74%), remained significant following adjustment for prespecified co-variates that are known to influence overall prognosis and AF development (OR 0.80, 95% CI 0.65–0.99). The design of this study allowed for the analysis of subgroups with CHF but preserved LVEF (in contrast to the SOLVD and Val-HeFT studies), and CHF with or without concomitant ACEI treatment. Although no significant heterogeneity was observed in subgroup analysis, the beneficial effect of candesartan was more pronounced in patients with reduced LVEF, irrespective of ACEI treatment (adjusted OR 0.77, 95% CI 0.59–0.99).

The available data from these large-scale studies are highly suggestive of the preventive role of ACEIs/ARBs in avoiding new or recurrent AF in patients with heart failure. Although this association was often either a *post hoc* finding or a secondary endpoint, the size of the studies and the consistency of their results provide satisfactory evidence on the efficacy of ACEIs/ARBs in this setting. Therefore, the use of ACEIs/ARBs for the prevention of AF in patients with CHF is recommended (**Class I, Level A**).

ACEIs and ARBs for the prevention of AF in patients with hypertension and/or coronary artery disease

The efficacy of ACEIs/ARBs for the treatment of primary hypertension is recognized. Large studies, which aimed to identify whether their antihypertensive capacity is associated with a reduction in overall cardiovascular mortality and morbidity, included AF occurrence in their secondary endpoints. More specifically, the Captopril Prevention Project (CAPPP) was a multicenter randomized trial evaluating the effect of captopril (50–100 mg) versus conventional antihypertensive treatment with beta-blockers and/or diuretics, on fatal and non-fatal myocardial infarction and stroke and other cardiovascular deaths.[10] Cardiovascular mortality was lower in the captopril group, albeit not statistically significant. No difference was observed upon analyses of secondary outcomes with the inclusion of new AF, between the two groups. These findings were in line with its contemporary, the Swedish Trial in Old Patients with Hypertension-2 (STOP-H2) study,[11] which compared

the efficacy of conventional antihypertensives (diuretics, beta-blockers), ACEIs (enalapril 10 mg, lisinopril 10 mg) and calcium antagonists (felodipine 2.5 mg, isradipine 2.5 mg) on cardiovascular morbidity and mortality in patients aged 70–84 years. All three therapies were similarly effective against these primary outcomes, and no superiority of ACEIs was observed in the prevention of AF when compared to conventional antihypertensives. However, in another multicenter trial (LIFE),[12] patients with hypertension and documented LV hypertrophy benefited from losartan-based treatments, which significantly reduced new-onset AF when compared to atenolol-based treatment (OR 0.67, 95% CI 0.55–0.83). The enhanced regression of LV hypertrophy caused by losartan, as evaluated on the echocardiographic substudy within LIFE,[13] may have led to reduced atrial overload and dilation, and therefore a reduction in AF. New-onset AF was a prespecified outcome within the VALUE trial.[14] Valsartan-based antihypertensive treatment led to a reduction in AF occurrence when compared to amlodipine in patients with hypertension and other cardiovascular risk factors. In contrast, two contemporary RCTs evaluating the role of telmisartan versus placebo,[15] and telmisartan with or without ramipril,[16] did not show any preventative effect on AF occurrence in patients with coronary, peripheral or cerebrovascular disease.

In conclusion, due to the limited number of studies, their design and significant heterogeneity, the efficacy of ACEIs/ARBs in the prevention of AF in hypertensive patients with cardiovascular risk factors, although plausible, requires further evaluation (**Class IIa, Level B**).

ACEIs and ARBs for secondary prevention of AF

The efficacy of amiodarone in the maintenance of sinus rhythm in patients with persistent AF is well documented.[17] The addition of irbesartan (150–300 mg/d) to amiodarone (400 mg) therapy before electrical cardioversion for persistent AF led to a 65% reduction in the risk of AF recurrence over a two-month follow-up.[18] This open-label randomized trial was the first to describe the possible association of ARBs and maintenance of sinus rhythm. However, it was limited by the fact that the irbesartan treatment group was more likely to receive beta-blockade, which is known to be protective for AF, and that asymptomatic recurrences that terminated spontaneously could not have been effectively captured. In a similar study evaluating the effect of enalapril on AF recurrence following electrical cardioversion and amiodarone, a 69% risk reduction was observed in patients on combined enalapril and amiodarone treatment at four weeks.[19] Finally, Madrid and colleagues[20] examined the effect of increasing doses of irbesartan in addition to amiodarone treatment on AF recurrence after electrical cardioversion in patients with "lone" persistent AF. Maintenance of SR was higher in the irbesartan 300 mg plus amiodarone group (77%), when compared to the irbesartan 150 mg plus amiodarone group (65%) and to amiodarone alone (52%). The risk reduction conferred by high-dose irbesartan was 53% after appropriate adjustments at the two-month follow-up.

Although a combination therapy of amiodarone with ACEIs/ARBs appears superior to amiodarone alone, the efficacy of monotherapy with ACEIs/ARBs was not tested in any of those trials. In addition, their open-label design and the lack of placebo group may have influenced the accuracy of their outcomes. In an attempt to overcome these important limitations, Tveit and colleagues designed a double-blind placebo-controlled trial examining the effect of the ARB candesartan on AF recurrence following successful electrical cardioversion in patients not receiving adjunct antiarrhythmics.[21] Six-week pretreatment with candesartan (16 mg) followed by a 6-month therapy after electrical cardioversion did not influence AF recurrence rates when compared with placebo. Similarly, the more recent GISSI-AF study, which examined the role of valsartan (vs. placebo) in AF prevention in patients with documented symptomatic AF and/or successful electrical cardioversion, did not demonstrate any effect attributed to valsartan treatment.[22] The main outcome measures were time to first AF recurrence and proportion of patients with more than one AF episodes during the first year; the treatment arm received valsartan gradually adjusted to 320 mg daily, in addition to established antiarrhythmic regimens. Despite the relatively short follow-up and the underrepresentation of patients with heart failure (8%), the negative results from this study encourage the scepticism regarding the efficacy of ARBs in secondary AF prevention.

Therefore, the beneficial effect of ACEIs/ARBs in secondary prevention is not yet established and will need to be validated further (**Class IIb, Level B**). Ongoing trials aim to create a clearer picture on the antiarrhythmic potential of ACEIs/ARBs. ACTIVE I is a partial factorial placebo-controlled, double blind trial evaluating the capacity of irbesartan (titrated to 300 mg/day) to prevent AF recurrence in patients with paroxysmal or persistent AF, which is a prespecified secondary outcome.[23] The Angiotensin II antagonist in paroxysmal atrial fibrillation (ANTIPAF) trial focuses on the effect of olmesartan (40 mg/day) on reduction of episodes of paroxysmal AF as a primary endpoint, and assesses both symptomatic and asymptomatic paroxysms with the use of transtelephonic ECG monitoring.[24]

Statins for the prevention and treatment of atrial fibrillation

Several studies have suggested the possible prophylactic effect of statins on new-onset AF and on AF recurrence following successful electrical or chemical cardioversion.

A systematic review and meta-analysis evaluating the efficacy of statins on AF prevention demonstrated variability in outcomes between observational studies and RCTs.[25] Interestingly, the antiarrhythmic effect of statins was less pronounced in RCTs and did not reach statistical significance, whereas observational studies yielded a 23% relative risk reduction in patients on statins, which was statistically significant (OR 0.77, 95% CI 0.70–0.85) and associated with no apparent heterogeneity. Many reasons may account for this discrepancy, such as the potentially underpowered AF detection in a large RCT, longer mean follow-up of observational studies and variability in methods of AF detection. It is also evident that the patient populations, presence and type of AF at baseline, type of intervention performed, and primary outcome of interest differed between studies. Another meta-analysis focusing only on RCTs demonstrated that statin use was associated with a significant decrease in the incidence or recurrence of AF (OR 0.39, 95% CI 0.10–0.85). However, the variability in clinical settings and significant heterogeneity between studies is, once again, supportive but not confirmatory of the overall beneficial effect of statins on AF.[26] This is why our evidence-based analysis examines the effect of statins on patients according to their baseline heart rhythm, underlying cardiovascular pathology and type of intervention performed.

Statins for the prevention of AF in patients with coronary artery disease

The first association of statin use with prevention of AF in patients with chronic coronary artery disease (CAD) was shown by Young-Xu and colleagues in an observational longitudinal study with a five-year follow-up.[27] Patients receiving statins had a 9% incidence of new-onset AF compared with 15% in patients not on statins. Following adjustment for potential confounders, the risk reduction in AF remained statistically significant (OR 0.37, 95% CI 0.18–0.76). This effect was independent of changes in baseline and follow-up cholesterol levels, indicating that the potential antiarrhythmic effect of statins extends beyond their lipid-lowering capacity.

High-dose statin use and its possible impact on AF in patients with acute coronary syndrome (ACS) was examined *post hoc* within the Myocardial Ischemia Reduction with Aggressive Cholesterol Lowering (MIRACL) study.[28] Atorvastatin 80 mg or placebo was administered to patients with ACS within four days of admission to hospital and for a period of 16 weeks. The incidence of new-onset AF (1.6% and 1.8%, respectively) in patients without the arrhythmia prior to randomization and the rate of freedom from recurrence in patients with known AF, were not influenced by intensive statin treatment. However, the short duration of follow-up (16 weeks) with limited ECG record-

Table 36.3 Clinical studies of statins for the prevention of atrial fibrillation

Study, date	Design	N	Setting	Statin type	Mean follow-up	Risk reduction
Dotani,[46] 2000	Retrospective	323	CABG	Any brand	1 year	77%
Siu,[38] 2003	Retrospective	62	Lone persistent AF following DCCV	Simvastatin (20 ± 13 mg) Atorvastatin (10 ± 3 mg)	44 months	69%
Young-Xu,[27] 2003	Observational	449	Stable CAD	Any brand	5 years	63%
Colivicchi,[39] 2004	Observational	851	Persistent AF, HTN and electrical or chemical cardioversion	Atorvastatin (12 ± 4 mg) Simvastatin (20 ± 7 mg)	1 year	25%
Merckx,[30] 2004	Observational	667	LA dilation, LVH	Any brand	6.5 years	67%
MIRACL,[28] 2004	Prospective randomized, placebo controlled	3086	ACS	Atorvastatin 80 mg	16 weeks	No effect
Tveit,[40] 2004	Prospective randomized, open label	114	AF >48 hours, DCCV	Pravastatin 40 mg	6 weeks	No effect
Amar,[47] 2005	Observational	131	Major non-cardiac thoracic surgery	Any brand	7–9 days post-op	74%
Ozaydin,[41] 2006	Prospective randomized, open label	48	Persistent AF, DCCV	Atorvastatin 10 mg	3 months	81%
Amit,[35] 2005	Retrospective	264	Post pacemaker	Any brand	359 days	No effect
Marin,[48] 2006	Prospective, observational	234	CABG	Any brand	1 month	48%
ARMYDA,[49] 2006	Prospective randomized, double blind, placebo controlled	200	Cardiac surgery	Atorvastatin 40 mg vs placebo	1 month	61%
SCD-HeFT,[34] 2006	Prospective randomized, placebo controlled	2521	Heart failure, LVEF ≤35%	Any brand	45.5 months	28%
ADVANCENT[SM,33] 2006	Retrospective, registry	25268	LVEF ≤40%	Any brand + other lipid-lowering agents	–	31%
García-Ferrández,[42] 2006	Prospective randomized	54	Persistent AF, DCCV	Atorvastatin 80 mg	3 months	No effect
Richter,[44] 2007	Retrospective	234	Paroxysmal or persistent AF, RF ablation	Any brand	12.7 months	No effect
Al Chekakie,[45] 2007	Retrospective	177	Paroxysmal or persistent AF, RF ablation	Any brand	13.8 months	No effect
Tsai,[36] 2007	Prospective randomized, open label	106	Post pacemaker	Atorvastatin 20 mg	1 year	67%
Ramani,[29] 2007	Retrospective, registry	1526	ACS	Any brand	–	43%
Ozaydin,[51] 2007	Observational	326	CABG	Any brand	1 week post-op	53%
Mariscalc,[52] 2007	Observational	405	CABG	Any brand	Hospital stay	42%
Kourliourcs,[53] 2008	Observational	623	Cardiac surgery	Any brand	Hospital stay	44%
Lertsburapa,[54] 2008	Observational	555	Cardiac surgery	Any brand	1 month	40%
Song,[50] 2008	Prospective randomised, open-label	124	Off-pump CABG	Atorvastatin 20 mg	1 month	66%
Gillis,[37] 2008	Observational	185	Post pacemaker	Any brand	1 year	67%
Almroth,[43] 2009	Prospective randomised, double-blind, placebo-controlled	234	Persistent AF, DCCV	Atorvastatin 80 mg	1 month	No effect
Pellegrini,[31] 2009	Post hoc analysis of randomised, placebo-controlled trial	2673	CAD	Any brand	4.1 years	55%

ings may be responsible for the very low incidence of new-onset AF, which potentially renders this analysis underpowered. In a retrospective study,[29] 1526 patients admitted to hospital with suspected ACS and no history of arrhythmia were evaluated by the development of new AF and statin use. A risk reduction of 43% was present in statin users following adjustment for potential confounders (OR 0.57, 95% CI 0.39–0.83).

Echocardiographic risk factors for the development of AF, such as left ventricular hypertrophy (LVH) (wall thickness ≥10 mm) and left atrial dilation (≥40 mm) were evaluated in another study by Merckx and colleagues.[30] In this cohort analysis of patients with the above echocardiographic features and CAD, but no evidence of LV failure, statin use was found to be protective for the development of future AF, especially with advanced age. Finally, in a post hoc analysis of the Heart and Estrogen/Progestin Replacement Study (HERS), including women with prior coronary disease, statins were associated with 65% lower odds of AF at baseline and with a 55% risk reduction in new-onset AF during follow-up.[31]

The efficacy of statins in reducing morbidity and coronary mortality in anginal and/or postinfarction patients is recognized and their use is therefore recommended. The possible additional effect of statins on AF prevention further supports the recommendation in this group of patients (**Class IIa, Level B**).

Statins for the prevention of AF in patients with heart failure

Congestive heart failure and AF often co-exist. The prevalence of AF in the CHF population varies from 13% to 27%. The Framingham Heart Study confirmed that new-onset AF against the background of CHF significantly increases mortality (hazard ratio (HR) 2.7, 95% CI 1.9–3.7).[32] The efficacy of statins in the prevention of AF in CHF patients has been examined in patients with LV dysfunction (LVEF ≤40%) on the ADVANCENT[SM] registry.[33] The significant reduction in prevalence of AF in patients on statins was even more pronounced than that achieved from ACEIs/ARBs, and was independent of their lipid-lowering properties. This observation is in line with the findings from the Sudden Cardiac Death Heart Failure Trial (SCD-HeFT), in which statins were as efficacious as amiodarone in the prevention of atrial arrhythmias in patients with symptomatic heart failure and LVEF ≤35%.[34] However, this group included cases of atrial flutter in addition to AF, and therefore, the absolute effect of statin use on AF is not clearly specified. Overall, although statins may have a place in CHF, their potential antiarrhythmic effect is less well established in this setting and requires further investigation (**Class IIb, Level B**).

Statins for the prevention of AF in patients with permanent pacemakers

It is recognized that the incidence of supraventricular arrhythmias and AF in particular is increased in patients with conduction abnormalities and presence of permanent pacemakers. In an observational study of 264 patients with pacemakers implanted predominantly for atrioventricular block and sinus bradycardia, Amit and colleagues[35] demonstrated no impact of statin treatment on the incidence of AF. However, the heterogeneity between the groups, with patients on statins being more likely to suffer from CAD, hypertension and previous AF, was one of the main limitations of the study. A randomized open-label trial assessing the effect of atorvastatin 20 mg on paroxysmal AF or atrial high rate episodes (AHE) in patients with pacemakers demonstrated the protective effect of atorvastatin on the arrhythmia, with a 67% risk reduction in new PAF/AHEs in a one-year period.[36] Similarly, in an observational cohort study of patients with history of paroxysmal AF who underwent pacemaker implantation (>90% sinus node disease), statin use was associated with a 67% relative risk reduction in AF recurrence.[37] Overall, the available clinical evidence is still limited before any strong recommendations for statin use can be made in this setting (**Class IIb, Level B**).

Statins in patients with AF following cardioversion

The first study to evaluate the effect of statin treatment on AF recurrence following successful external electrical cardioversion (DCCV) was reported by Siu and colleagues.[38] Sixty-two patients with persistent-lone AF were retrospectively evaluated for a mean of 44 months after DCCV. AF recurrence was 40% in the statin group versus 84% in the no statin group at two years, leading to a significant reduction in AF (relative risk 0.31, 95% CI 0.103–0.905). In an observational study by Colivicchi and colleagues,[39] patients with persistent AF against a background of essential hypertension who underwent successful chemical or electrical cardioversion were examined for the development of recurrent AF for one year. Due to the non-randomized nature of the study, a propensity model was constructed and following appropriate adjustments, atorvastatin and simvastatin use was associated with a significant reduction in AF recurrence (HR 0.75, 95% CI 0.63–0.89). Four randomized trials, with primary endpoint being AF recurrence following successful DCCV, yielded controversial results. In an open-label study of 114 patients with AF >48 hours who were scheduled for DCCV, the statin group received pravastatin 40 mg for three weeks before and six weeks after the procedure.[40] Pravastatin did not confer any benefit on the immediate success of cardioversion or AF recurrence. However, in another randomized controlled trial, atorvastatin 10 mg administered 48 hours before and for three months following DCCV, in addition to standard antiarrhythmic therapy, led to a significant reduction in AF recurrence.[41] In a similar cohort of patients, intensive atorvastatin treatment (80 mg) had no effect on recurrent AF.[42] The only double-blind placebo-controlled trial to examine the role of statins in sinus rhythm maintenance following successful electrical cardioversion showed a small (and not statistically significant) benefit in patients receiving intensive atorvastatin treatment who were not on routine antiarrhythmic therapy.[43] In conclusion, in view of certain methodological issues and conflicting results among studies, the indicated use of statins is less well established for sinus rhythm maintenance following electrical cardioversion (**Class IIb, Level B**).

Statins in AF patients following catheter ablation

In recent years, catheter ablation for the treatment of AF has become a commonly performed procedure mainly indicated for the presence of symptomatic AF refractory or intolerant to at least one class I or III antiarrhythmic medication. However, rates of AF recurrence vary considerably according to the duration of AF, presence of structural abnormalities, use of antiarrhythmic medications, and type of procedure performed. Two contemporary retrospective studies assessing catheter ablation outcomes did not show any significant reduction in AF recurrence due to statin use, with or without ACEIs/ARBs.[44,45] Differences in baseline characteristics, treatment and duration of AF are some of the inherent limitations of such studies (**Class III, Level C**).

Statins for the prevention of AF in patients undergoing cardiac surgery

The rate of AF following cardiac surgery ranges from 10% to 50%, with a peak incidence on the second and third postoperative days. The exact etiology of postoperative AF remains unknown but pre-existing structural remodeling under the influence of the augmented inflammatory response due to cardiopulmonary bypass, myocardial ischemia and cardiotomy may be contributing factors.

The first evidence of the possible preventive effect of statins on arrhythmias following cardiac surgery came from a study by Dotani and colleagues.[46] Patients on statins had a significantly lower incidence of post-CABG "new arrhythmias" requiring treatment (OR 0.23, 95% CI 0.08–0.65, $P = 0.006$). While statins were also found to be beneficial in AF prevention following non-cardiac thoracic surgery,[47] the first prospective study to associate statin use with a reduction in AF following CABG surgery was

reported by Marin and colleagues.[48] In their cohort of 234 consecutive patients, history of AF and non-use of statins were independent risk factors for the postoperative arrhythmia. ARMYDA-3 (Atorvastatin for Reduction of Myocardial Dysrhythmia After cardiac surgery) is the only double-blind, placebo-controlled randomized trial to assess the effect of statins on postoperative AF.[49] Two hundred patients were randomized to atorvastatin 40 mg or placebo for seven days before cardiac surgery until discharge. Postoperative AF occurred in 57% of the control group compared with 35% of patients on atorvastatin (OR 0.39, 95% CI 0.18–0.85, $P = 0.017$). Although not statistically significant, the placebo group included more patients who received combined coronary and valve surgery, whereas beta-blocker use was also less prevalent. Since then, additional studies have supported the beneficial effect of statins on AF after CABG,[50–52] with the addition of a possible dose-dependent effect.[53,54] A meta-analysis evaluating adverse postoperative outcomes according to preoperative statin treatment, demonstrated a significant 33% relative risk reduction in postoperative AF.[55] Therefore, statin use is recommended in patients undergoing cardiac surgery for the prevention of postoperative AF (**Class I, Level A**).

N-3 polyunsaturated fatty acids for the prevention of atrial fibrillation

The role of nutritional factors in the development of AF has recently been suggested following observations of reduced risk of fatal arrhythmias in populations with high fish consumption.[56] The n-3 polyunsaturated fatty acids (PUFA) eicosapentaenoic acid (EPA) and docosahexaenoic acid (DHA), the active ingredients in fish oil, were found to be protective against fatal arrhythmias in clinical and experimental studies.[57,58] The effect of PUFAs on AF was examined in a population-based cohort study of 4815 individuals ≥65 years, within the Cardiovascular Health Study (CHS).[59] Individuals consuming tuna or other fish ≥5 times per week had a significantly lower incidence of AF (19 per 1000 person-years), when compared to those who consumed fish <1 time per month (33 per 1000 person-years). Although the higher fish consumption group exhibited a more favorable cardiovascular risk profile, multivariate adjustment for possible confounders confirmed the significant risk reduction in new AF (HR 0.65, 95% CI 0.51–0.87, $P = 0.001$). These beneficial effects were attributable to tuna/other broiled or baked fish and not to fried fish or fish sandwich, the frequent consumption of which was positively associated with the development of AF. Aside from the possible confounding of other lifestyle determinants and increased cardiovascular risk factors, this finding may also be explained by the fact that frying increases the content of n-6 fatty acids, *trans* fatty acids and oxidation

Table 36.4 Clinical studies on PUFAs for the prevention of atrial fibrillation

Study, year	n	Design	Groups	Mean age (years)	Mean follow-up	AF incidence	Risk reduction
Cardiovascular Health Study,[59] 2004	4815	Prospective cohort study	Quartiles according to baked/broiled fish consumption (<1/mo, 1–3/mo, 1–4/wk, ≥5/wk)	72.8	12 years	20%	35% between highest and lowest quartile
Danish Diet, Cancer and Health Study,[60] 2005	47949	Prospective cohort study	Quintiles according to average daily PUFA intake from fish (0.16g, 0.36g, 0.52g, 0.74g, 1.29g)	56	5.7 years	1%	No effect
Calo,[64] 2005	160	Randomized, open label	PUFAs 2g/day vs control for ≥5 days before CABG until hospital discharge	65.6	28 days	15% PUFA, 33% controls	68%
Phycisians' Health Study,[61] 2006	17679	Prospective cohort study	Quintiles according to dietary fish intake (<1/mo, 1–3/mo, 1–2/wk, 2–5/wk, ≥5/wk)	Unknown	15 years	7%	Increased AF risk in highest vs lowest quintile
Rotterdam Study,[62] 2006	5184	Prospective cohort study	Tertiles of EPA + DHA daily intake (≤43mg, 43–144mg, ≥144mg)	67.4	6.4 years	6%	No effect
Erdogan,[65] 2007	108	Randomized, placebo-controlled trial	PUFA vs placebo for 4wks before and 1 year after DCCV for persistent AF	66.5	1 year	80% recurrence	No effect
Women's Health Initiative,[63] 2008	46704	Cohort analysis	Quartiles according to estimated dietary fish and omega-3 intake	Unknown	6 years	0.8%	No effect

Table 36.5 Clinical studies on corticosteroids for the prevention of atrial fibrillation

Study, year	Design	N	Setting	Drug	Follow-up	Risk reduction
Yared,[68] 2000	Randomized, double-blind, placebo-controlled trial, *post hoc* analysis	235	Cardiac surgery, any	DEX 0.6mg/kg IV after induction of anesthesia	Hospital discharge	DEX reduced post-op AF from 32% to 19%
Halvorsen,[69] 2003	Randomized, double-blind, placebo-controlled trial	300	CABG	DEX 4mg IV after induction and same dose morning after surgery	Hospital discharge	No effect
Dernellis,[75] 2004	Randomized, placebo-controlled trial	104	Persistent AF after chemical ± electrical cardioversion	Methylprednisolone 16mg for 4 weeks tapered to 4mg for 4 months (+ propafenone 450 mg/day to all patients)	23.6 months	9.6% recurrent AF in steroid group vs 50% in placebo
Huerta,[77] 2005	Population-based cohort study	5710	Asthma and/or COPD	Respiratory drugs, including oral and inhaled steroids	–	2.7 times increased risk of AF with oral steroids
Rubens,[70] 2005	Prospective randomized	68	Cardiac surgery	CPB control, SMA-CPB, SMA-CPB-MPSS, MPSS alone	Hospital discharge	AF reduction from 38% without MPSS to 12% with MPSS
Prasongsukarn,[71] 2005	Randomized, double-blind, placebo-controlled trial	88	CABG	Methylprednisolone 1 g IV before CPB followed by DEX 4mg IV/6h for first 24h post-op	Hospital discharge	50%
Rotterdam Study,[76] 2006	Population-based cohort study	385	New-onset AF	Any oral or parenteral steroids administered 1 month before AF diagnosis	–	Increased AF in steroid users
Yared,[72] 2007	Randomized, double-blind, placebo-controlled trial	78	CABG + valve surgery	DEX 0.6mg/kg IV after induction of anesthesia	Hospital discharge	No effect
Halonen,[73] 2007	Randomized, double-blind, placebo-controlled trial	241	CABG and/or AVR	Hydrocortisone 100mg, 1 dose pre-op, then 1 dose/8h for 3 days post-op	Hospital discharge	46%

products, which are associated with adverse cardiac outcomes.

The Danish Diet, Cancer, and Health Study was a large cohort analysis of 47 949 individuals, assessing, amongst others, the effect of n-3 fatty acids on AF.[60] With a mean follow-up of 5.7 years and a cohort of patients with no history of cardiac disease, increased consumption of fish oil did not influence the incidence of AF. The authors suggest that apart from other methodologic issues that may have affected outcomes such as additional intake of fish oil capsules, patients on the top quintile of fish oil consumption were likely to be older and suffer from hypertension, factors which are known to be associated with AF. Moreover, findings from the Physicians' Health Study of 17 679 men during a 15-year follow-up demonstrated that high estimated omega-3 fatty acid consumption is positively associated with AF (OR 1.37, 95% CI 0.90–2.28) and that there is a statistically significant trend for AF occurrence with increasing fish consumption.[61] In another prospective population-based study (The Rotterdam Study),[62] no effect on AF was observed between patients on the highest and the lowest tertiles according to fish intake (relative risk 1.25, 95% CI 0.95–1.67). Similarly, estimated dietary omega-3 fatty acid intake did not influence the development of AF during follow-up in a cohort analysis of Women's Health Initiative Study.[63]

Many factors may be responsible for the variability in outcomes seen in these population-based studies. Differences in mean age (72.8 years in CHS, 67.4 in Rotterdam and 56 in Danish studies) could explain the lower incidence of observed AF in the "no benefit" studies (20% CHS vs 6% in Rotterdam and 1% in Danish studies), as well as dietary changes and new cardiac conditions during follow-up, which may have contributed to inconsistent results.

The possible prophylactic effect of PUFAs on AF occurrence following CABG was examined in an open-label randomized study of 160 patients.[64] PUFAs (850–882 mg EPA and DHA in a 1:2 ratio) were administered for a minimum of five days before surgery until discharge. Patient characteristics and perioperative variables were not significantly different between treatment and control groups. The incidence of postoperative AF was reduced in patients on PUFAs (15.2%), compared to controls (33.3%) (OR 0.35, 95% CI 0.16–0.76) and, along with age, PUFA use remained an independent predictor for postoperative AF (OR 0.32, 95% CI 0.10–0.98, P = 0.013). In addition, the treatment group had a significantly shorter length of hospital stay (7.3 ± 2.1 days vs 8.2 ± 2.6 days).

A recent randomized placebo-controlled study of 108 patients with persistent AF, who underwent successful electrical cardioversion, did not demonstrate differences in AF recurrence between those on PUFAs and the placebo group.[65]

The antiarrhythmic effects of PUFAs on AF are not confirmed since large epidemiologic studies yielded controversial results. The two randomized trials on the effect of PUFAs on postoperative AF and AF recurrence following successful electrical cardioversion were also inconsistent.

These findings may indicate a differential effect according to underlying medical conditions, cardiovascular risk factors and types of intervention performed. Further controlled studies are necessary to delineate the possible antiarrhythmic effect of PUFAs on AF (**Class IIb, Level B**).

Corticosteroids for the prevention of atrial fibrillation

The first evidence to associate AF with inflammation was reported in 1997, when Frustaci and colleagues demonstrated histologic changes consistent with myocarditis in atrial tissue of patients with lone AF.[66] The increased rate of AF following cardiac surgery highlights the role of inflammation in the development of the arrhythmia.

Elevated plasma C-reactive protein (CRP) levels have been associated with an increased risk of cardiovascular events and its predictive value has been validated in various prospective epidemiologic studies.[67] Corticosteroids exhibit a potent anti-inflammatory capacity and their role in AF prevention has been examined mainly within the context of cardiothoracic surgery.[68–73] A recent meta-analysis of clinical trials assessing the efficacy of corticosteroids on postoperative AF demonstrated a 45% reduction in the arrhythmia with an associated statistically significant reduction in length of hospital stay by 1.6 days.[74] With insignificant heterogeneity between studies or publication bias, this meta-analysis also suggests that only intermediate doses confer a statistically significant protective effect. Finally, the odds of postoperative pneumonia, urinary tract infections and gastrointestinal bleeding were increased, albeit not significantly, whereas overall mortality was decreased.

In patients with persistent AF, the use of low-dose glucocorticoid treatment in addition to prophylactic propafenone was associated with a significant reduction in the rate of recurrence after chemical or electrical cardioversion.[75] Patients who received 16 mg methylprednisolone for four weeks tapered to 4 mg for four months had a 9.6% incidence of recurrent AF compared with 50% of the placebo group without any severe side effects. Methylprednisolone significantly reduced CRP by 80% in the first month. Follow-up CRP levels were also correlated significantly with the risk of recurrent AF. This preventive capacity of corticosteroids in AF was not validated in a later nested-cohort analysis within the Rotterdam Study.[76] In contrast, the risk of new-onset AF was significantly increased with corticosteroid use (OR 3.75, 95% CI 2.38–5.87) and, moreover, this effect was more pronounced with high-dose steroids, independent of their indication, suggesting a potential direct arrhythmogenic effect of steroids. Due to the nature of this study, a possible diagnosis bias, with patients using steroids receiving more ECGs and rendering AF diagnosis more likely, cannot be eliminated. In addition, the case population consisted of older people with hypertension, heart failure and previous MI, and despite appropriate adjustment with multivariate regression, a selection bias may also be present. However, the observation that steroids may lack any antiarrhythmic effect, but that they may induce AF instead, was further supported by another nested-cohort study from the UK General Practice Research Database.[77] Upon comparison of the case group, with documented arrhythmia and asthma and/or chronic obstructive pulmonary disease, to controls with the same respiratory conditions, oral steroids, especially short-term use, were associated with an increased risk of AF (OR 2.7, 95% CI 1.9–3.8).

The impact of corticosteroids in the prevention of AF remains controversial. Although intermediate-dose steroids appear to confer a relative reduction in AF post cardiac surgery (**Class IIa, Level B**), high-dose steroids may be arrhythmogenic in this setting as well as in the background of asthma and COPD. More trials are required to establish the efficacy of corticosteroids in AF and, more importantly, to delineate their safety if used for arrhythmia prevention alone.

Conclusion

Atrial fibrillation is an important health problem due to the associated risk of stroke, all-cause mortality and its rising prevalence in our aging population. The objective of available treatment modalities for AF is to reduce morbidity (and possibly mortality) through restoration of sinus rhythm, heart rate control when rhythm conversion is not feasible, and prevention of thromboembolism. However, most patients with a first-detected episode of AF, symptomatic or not, will experience recurrence and possibly domestication of the arrhythmia despite treatment. It is evident that available antiarrhythmic regimens, although potentially efficacious in symptom control and prevention of hemodynamic complications, do not offer a definitive treatment or cure.

Upstream therapies refer to pharmacologic agents that target and modulate the substrate responsible for the development and perpetuation of AF. The use of angiotensin-converting enzyme inhibitors, angiotensin receptor blockers, statins, n-3 polyunsaturated fatty acids and corticosteroids in the context of AF prevention, which is beyond their recommended conventional indications, has delivered promising results. Although their efficacy is dependent on the nature of underlying cardiovascular pathology, type and chronicity of AF, and other therapeutic interventions performed, most studies concur in the beneficial impact of upstream therapies in AF prevention.

Experimental data suggest that this effect is predominantly achieved by amelioration of atrial structural changes and inflammatory response associated with the arrhythmia, as well as modulating risk factors for cardiovascular disease, which eventually lead to AF. Further evaluation of upstream therapies through well-defined clinical trials and experimental studies will provide additional evidence for their use as adjuncts to antiarrhythmic treatments or as stand-alone therapy for the prevention of AF.

References

1. Healey JS, Baranchuk A, Crystal E et al. Prevention of atrial fibrillation with angiotensin-converting enzyme inhibitors and angiotensin receptor blockers: a meta-analysis. *J Am Coll Cardiol* 2005;**45**:1832–9.
2. Salehian O, Healey J, Stambler B et al. Impact of ramipril on the incidence of atrial fibrillation: results of the Heart Outcomes Prevention Evaluation study. *Am Heart J* 2007;**154**:448–53.
3. Jibrini MB, Molnar J, Arora R. Prevention of atrial fibrillation by way of abrogation of the renin-angiotensin system: a systematic review and meta-analysis. *Am J Ther* 2008;**15**:36–43.
4. Anand K, Moos AN, Hee TT, Mohiuddin SM. Meta-analysis: inhibition of renin-angiotensin system prevents new-onset atrial fibrillation. *Am Heart J* 2006;**152**:217–22.
5. Van Den Berg MP, Crijns HJ, Van Veldhuisen DJ, Griep N, De Kam PJ, Lie KI. Effects of lisinopril in patients with heart failure and chronic atrial fibrillation. *J Card Fail* 1995;**1**:355–63.
6. Pedersen OD, Bagger H, Kober L, Torp-Pedersen C. Trandolapril reduces the incidence of atrial fibrillation after acute myocardial infarction in patients with left ventricular dysfunction. *Circulation* 1999;**100**:376–80.
7. Vermes E, Tardif JC, Bourassa MG et al. Enalapril decreases the incidence of atrial fibrillation in patients with left ventricular dysfunction: insight from the Studies Of Left Ventricular Dysfunction (SOLVD) trials. *Circulation* 2003;**107**:2926–31.
8. Maggioni AP, Latini R, Carson PE et al. Valsartan reduces the incidence of atrial fibrillation in patients with heart failure: results from the Valsartan Heart Failure Trial (Val-HeFT). *Am Heart J* 2005;**149**:548–57.
9. Ducharme A, Swedberg K, Pfeffer MA et al. Prevention of atrial fibrillation in patients with symptomatic chronic heart failure by candesartan in the Candesartan in Heart failure: Assessment of Reduction in Mortality and morbidity (CHARM) program. *Am Heart J* 2006;**152**:86–92.
10. Hansson L, Lindholm LH, Niskanen L et al. Effect of angiotensin-converting-enzyme inhibition compared with conventional therapy on cardiovascular morbidity and mortality in hypertension: the Captopril Prevention Project (CAPPP) randomized trial. *Lancet* 1999;**353**:611–16.
11. Hansson L, Lindholm LH, Ekbom T et al. Randomized trial of old and new antihypertensive drugs in elderly patients: cardiovascular mortality and morbidity the Swedish Trial in Old Patients with Hypertension-2 study. *Lancet* 1999;**354**:1751–6.
12. Wachtell K, Lehto M, Gerdts E et al. Angiotensin II receptor blockade reduces new-onset atrial fibrillation and subsequent stroke compared to atenolol: the Losartan Intervention For End

Point Reduction in Hypertension (LIFE) study. *J Am Coll Cardiol* 2005;**45**:712–19.

13. Devereux RB, Dahlof B, Gerdts E *et al.* Regression of hypertensive left ventricular hypertrophy by losartan compared with atenolol: the Losartan Intervention for Endpoint Reduction in Hypertension (LIFE) trial. *Circulation* 2004;**110**:1456–62.

14. Schmieder RE, Kjeldsen SE, Julius S, McInnes GT, Zanchetti A, Hua TA. Reduced incidence of new-onset atrial fibrillation with angiotensin II receptor blockade: the VALUE trial. *J Hypertens* 2008;**26**:403–11.

15. Yusuf S, Teo K, Anderson C, Pogue J, Dyal L, Copland I *et al.* Effects of the angiotensin-receptor blocker telmisartan on cardiovascular events in high-risk patients intolerant to angiotensin-converting enzyme inhibitors: a randomised controlled trial. *Lancet* 2008;**372**:1174–83.

16. Yusuf S, Teo KK, Pogue J, Dyal L, Copland I, Schumacher H *et al.* Telmisartan, ramipril, or both in patients at high risk for vascular events. *N Engl J Med* 2008;**358**:1547–59.

17. Roy D, Talajic M, Dorian P *et al.* Amiodarone to prevent recurrence of atrial fibrillation. Canadian Trial of Atrial Fibrillation Investigators. *N Engl J Med* 2000;**342**:913–20.

18. Madrid AH, Bueno MG, Rebollo JM *et al.* Use of irbesartan to maintain sinus rhythm in patients with long-lasting persistent atrial fibrillation: a prospective and randomized study. *Circulation* 2002;**106**:331–6.

19. Ueng KC, Tsai TP, Yu WC *et al.* Use of enalapril to facilitate sinus rhythm maintenance after external cardioversion of longstanding persistent atrial fibrillation. Results of a prospective and controlled study. *Eur Heart J* 2003;**24**:2090–8.

20. Madrid AH, Marin IM, Cervantes CE *et al.* Prevention of recurrences in patients with lone atrial fibrillation. The dose-dependent effect of angiotensin II receptor blockers. *J Renin Angiotensin Aldosterone Syst* 2004;**5**:114–20.

21. Tveit A, Grundvold I, Olufsen M, Seljeflot I, Abdelnoor M, Arnesen H *et al.* Candesartan in the prevention of relapsing atrial fibrillation. *Int J Cardiol* 2007;**120**:85–91.

22. Disertori M, Latini R, Maggioni AP *et al.* Rationale and design of the GISSI-Atrial Fibrillation Trial: a randomized, prospective, multicentre study on the use of valsartan, an angiotensin II AT1-receptor blocker, in the prevention of atrial fibrillation recurrence. *J Cardiovasc Med (Hagerstown)* 2006;**7**:29–38.

23. Connolly S, Yusuf S, Budaj A *et al.* Rationale and design of ACTIVE: the atrial fibrillation clopidogrel trial with irbesartan for prevention of vascular events. *Am Heart J* 2006;**151**:1187–93.

24. Goette A, Breithardt G, Fetsch T *et al.* Angiotensin II antagonist in paroxysmal atrial fibrillation (ANTIPAF) trial: rationale and study design. *Clin Drug Investig* 2007;**27**:697–705.

25. Liu T, Li L, Korantzopoulos P, Liu E, Li G. Statin use and development of atrial fibrillation: a systematic review and meta-analysis of randomized clinical trials and observational studies. *Int J Cardiol* 2008;**126**(2):160–70.

26. Fauchier L, Pierre B, de Labriolle A, Grimard C, Zannad N, Babuty D. Antiarrhythmic effect of statin therapy and atrial fibrillation a meta-analysis of randomized controlled trials. *J Am Coll Cardiol* 2008;**51**:828–35.

27. Young-Xu Y, Jabbour S, Goldberg R, Blatt CM, Graboys T, Bilchik B, Ravid S. Usefulness of statin drugs in protecting against atrial fibrillation in patients with coronary artery disease. *Am J Cardiol* 2003;**92**:1379–83.

28. Schwartz GG, Olsson AG, Chaitman B, Goldberg J, Szarek M, Sasiela WJ. Effect of intensive statin treatment on the occurrence of atrial fibrillation after acute coronary syndrome: an analysis of the MIRACL trial. *Circulation* 2004;**110**(suppl III):740.

29. Ramani G, Zahid M, Good CB, Macioce A, Sonel AF. Comparison of frequency of new-onset atrial fibrillation or flutter in patients on statins versus not on statins presenting with suspected acute coronary syndrome. *Am J Cardiol* 2007;**100**:404–5.

30. Merckx KL, Tieleman RG, Folkeringa RJ *et al.* Use of statins is associated with reduced incidence of atrial fibrillation in patients with left ventricular hypertrophy and left atrial dilatation. *Heart Rhythm* 2004;**1**(suppl):S105.

31. Pellegrini CN, Vittinghoff E, Lin F, Hulley SB, Marcus GM. Statin use is associated with lower risk of atrial fibrillation in women with coronary disease: the HERS trial. *Heart* 2009;**95**:704–8.

32. Wang TJ, Larson MG, Levy D *et al.* Temporal relations of atrial fibrillation and congestive heart failure and their joint influence on mortality: the Framingham Heart Study. *Circulation* 2003;**107**:2920–5.

33. Hanna IR, Heeke B, Bush H *et al.* Lipid-lowering drug use is associated with reduced prevalence of atrial fibrillation in patients with left ventricular systolic dysfunction. *Heart Rhythm* 2006;**3**:881–6.

34. Dickinson MG, Hellkamp AS, Ip JH *et al.* Statin therapy was associated with reduced atrial fibrillation and flutter in heart failure patients in SCD-HEFT. *Heart Rhythm* 2006;**3**(suppl): S49.

35. Amit G, Katz A, Bar-On S, Gilutz H, Wagshal A, Ilia R, Henkin Y. Association of statin therapy and the risk of atrial fibrillation in patients with a permanent pacemaker. *Clin Cardiol* 2006;**29**:249–52.

36. Tsai CT, Wang YC, Lai LP, Lin JL. Atorvastatin prevents atrial fibrillation in patients with implantation of a pacemaker: a prospective randomized trial. *Heart Rhythm* 2007;**4**(suppl):S119.

37. Gillis AM, Morck M, Exner DV, Soo A, Rose MS, Sheldon RS *et al.* Beneficial effects of statin therapy for prevention of atrial fibrillation following DDDR pacemaker implantation. *Eur Heart J* 2008;**29**:1873–80.

38. Siu CW, Lau CP, Tse HF. Prevention of atrial fibrillation recurrence by statin therapy in patients with lone atrial fibrillation after successful cardioversion. *Am J Cardiol* 2003;**92**:1343–5.

39. Colivicchi F, Ammirati F, Santini M. Effects of statin therapy on the recurrence of persistent atrial fibrillation in patients with essential hypertension: A propensity score-adjusted analysis. *Heart Rhythm* 2004;**1**(suppl):S168.

40. Tveit A, Grundtvig M, Gundersen T *et al.* Analysis of pravastatin to prevent recurrence of atrial fibrillation after electrical cardioversion. *Am J Cardiol* 2004;**93**:780–2.

41. Ozaydin M, Varol E, Aslan SM *et al.* Effect of atorvastatin on the recurrence rates of atrial fibrillation after electrical cardioversion. *Am J Cardiol* 2006;**97**:1490–3.

42. Garcia-Fernandez A, Marin F, Mainar L, Roldan V, Martinez JG. Effect of statins on preventing recurrence of atrial fibrillation after electrical cardioversion. *Am J Cardiol* 2006;**98**:1299–300.

43. Almroth H, Hoglund N, Boman K, Englund A, Jensen S, Kjellman B *et al.* Atorvastatin and persistent atrial fibrillation following cardioversion: a randomized placebo-controlled multicentre study. *Eur Heart J* 2009;**30**:827–33.

44. Richter B, Derntl M, Marx M, Lercher P, Gossinger HD. Therapy with angiotensin-converting enzyme inhibitors, angiotensin II receptor blockers, and statins: no effect on ablation outcome after ablation of atrial fibrillation. *Am Heart J* 2007;**153**:113–19.

45. Al Chekakie MO, Akar JG, Wang F *et al.* The effects of statins and renin-angiotensin system blockers on atrial fibrillation recurrence following antral pulmonary vein isolation. *J Cardiovasc Electrophysiol* 2007;**18**:942–6.

46. Dotani MI, Elnicki DM, Jain AC, Gibson CM. Effect of preoperative statin therapy and cardiac outcomes after coronary artery bypass grafting. *Am J Cardiol* 2000;**86**:1128–30, A6.

47. Amar D, Zhang H, Heerdt PM, Park B, Fleisher M, Thaler HT. Statin use is associated with a reduction in atrial fibrillation after noncardiac thoracic surgery independent of C-reactive protein. *Chest* 2005;**128**:3421–7.

48. Marin F, Pascual DA, Roldan V *et al.* Statins and postoperative risk of atrial fibrillation following coronary artery bypass grafting. *Am J Cardiol* 2006;**97**:55–60.

49. Patti G, Chello M, Candura D *et al.* Randomized trial of atorvastatin for reduction of postoperative atrial fibrillation in patients undergoing cardiac surgery: results of the ARMYDA-3 (Atorvastatin for Reduction of MYocardial Dysrhythmia After cardiac surgery) study. *Circulation* 2006;**114**:1455–61.

50. Song YB, On YK, Kim JH, Shin DH, Kim JS, Sung J *et al.* The effects of atorvastatin on the occurrence of postoperative atrial fibrillation after off-pump coronary artery bypass grafting surgery. *Am Heart J* 2008;**156**:373 e9–16.

51. Ozaydin M, Dogan A, Varol E *et al.* Statin use before by-pass surgery decreases the incidence and shortens the duration of postoperative atrial fibrillation. *Cardiology* 2007;**107**:117–21.

52. Mariscalco G, Lorusso R, Klersy C *et al.* Observational study on the beneficial effect of preoperative statins in reducing atrial fibrillation after coronary surgery. *Ann Thorac Surg* 2007;**84**:1158–64.

53. Kourliouros A, De Souza A, Roberts N *et al.* Dose-related effect of statins on atrial fibrillation after cardiac surgery. *Ann Thorac Surg* 2008;**85**:1515–20.

54. Lertsburapa K, White CM, Kluger J, Faheem O, Hammond J, Coleman CI. Preoperative statins for the prevention of atrial fibrillation after cardiothoracic surgery. *J Thorac Cardiovasc Surg* 2008;**135**:405–11.

55. Liakopoulos OJ, Choi YH, Haldenwang PL, Strauch J, Wittwer T, Dorge H *et al.* Impact of preoperative statin therapy on adverse postoperative outcomes in patients undergoing cardiac surgery: a meta-analysis of over 30,000 patients. *Eur Heart J* 2008;**29**:1548–59.

56. Albert CM, Hennekens CH, O'Donnell CJ *et al.* Fish consumption and risk of sudden cardiac death. *JAMA* 1998;**279**:23–8.

57. Leaf A, Albert CM, Josephson M *et al.* Prevention of fatal arrhythmias in high-risk subjects by fish oil n-3 fatty acid intake. *Circulation* 2005;**112**:2762–8.

58. Jahangiri A, Leifert WR, Patten GS, McMurchie EJ. Termination of asynchronous contractile activity in rat atrial myocytes by n-3 polyunsaturated fatty acids. *Mol Cell Biochem* 2000;**206**:33–41.

59. Mozaffarian D, Psaty BM, Rimm EB *et al.* Fish intake and risk of incident atrial fibrillation. *Circulation* 2004;**110**:368–73.

60. Frost L, Vestergaard P. n-3 Fatty acids consumed from fish and risk of atrial fibrillation or flutter: the Danish Diet, Cancer, and Health Study. *Am J Clin Nutr* 2005;**81**:50–4.

61. Aizer A, Gaziano JM, Manson JE, Buring JE, Albert CM. Relationship between fish consumption and the development of atrial fibrillation in men. *Heart Rhythm* 2006;**3**(suppl 1):S5.

62. Brouwer IA, Heeringa J, Geleijnse JM, Zock PL, Witteman JC. Intake of very long-chain n-3 fatty acids from fish and incidence of atrial fibrillation. The Rotterdam Study. *Am Heart J* 2006;**151**:857–62.

63. Berry J, Passman R, Prineas RJ, van Horn L, Tinker L, Wu L *et al.* Fish and omega-3 fatty acid intake and incident atrial fibrillation: the women's health initiative. *Heart Rhythm* 2008;**5**(Suppl):S22.

64. Calo L, Bianconi L, Colivicchi F *et al.* N-3 Fatty acids for the prevention of atrial fibrillation after coronary artery bypass surgery: a randomized, controlled trial. *J Am Coll Cardiol* 2005;**45**:1723–8.

65. Erdogan A, Bayer M, Kollath D *et al.* Omega AF study: polyunsaturated fatty acids (PUFA) for prevention of atrial fibrillation relapse after successful external cardioversion. *Heart Rhythm* 2007;**4**(suppl 1):S185–6.

66. Frustaci A, Chimenti C, Bellocci F, Morgante E, Russo MA, Maseri A. Histological substrate of atrial biopsies in patients with lone atrial fibrillation. *Circulation* 1997;**96**:1180–4.

67. Ridker PM. Clinical application of C-reactive protein for cardiovascular disease detection and prevention. *Circulation* 2003;**107**:363–9.

68. Yared JP, Starr NJ, Torres FK *et al.* Effects of single dose, postinduction dexamethasone on recovery after cardiac surgery. *Ann Thorac Surg* 2000;**69**:1420–4.

69. Halvorsen P, Raeder J, White PF *et al.* The effect of dexamethasone on side effects after coronary revascularization procedures. *Anesth Analg* 2003;**96**:1578–83.

70. Rubens FD, Nathan H, Labow R *et al.* Effects of methylprednisolone and a biocompatible copolymer circuit on blood activation during cardiopulmonary bypass. *Ann Thorac Surg* 2005;**79**:655–65.

71. Prasongsukarn K, Abel JG, Jamieson WR *et al.* The effects of steroids on the occurrence of postoperative atrial fibrillation after coronary artery bypass grafting surgery: a prospective randomized trial. *J Thorac Cardiovasc Surg* 2005;**130**:93–8.

72. Yared JP, Bakri MH, Erzurum SC *et al.* Effect of dexamethasone on atrial fibrillation after cardiac surgery: prospective, randomized, double-blind, placebo-controlled trial. *J Cardiothorac Vasc Anesth* 2007;**21**:68–75.

73. Halonen J, Halonen P, Jarvinen O *et al.* Corticosteroids for the prevention of atrial fibrillation after cardiac surgery: a randomized controlled trial. *JAMA* 2007;**297**:1562–7.

74. Baker WL, White CM, Kluger J, Denowitz A, Konecny CP, Coleman CI. Effect of perioperative corticosteroid use on the incidence of postcardiothoracic surgery atrial fibrillation and length of stay. *Heart Rhythm* 2007;**4**:461–8.

75. Dernellis J, Panaretou M. Relationship between C-reactive protein concentrations during glucocorticoid therapy and recurrent atrial fibrillation. *Eur Heart J* 2004;**25**:1100–7.

76. van der Hooft CS, Heeringa J, Brusselle GG *et al.* Corticosteroids and the risk of atrial fibrillation. *Arch Intern Med* 2006;**166**:1016–20.

77. Huerta C, Lanes SF, Garcia Rodriguez LA. Respiratory medications and the risk of cardiac arrhythmias. *Epidemiology* 2005;**16**:360–6.

37 Atrial fibrillation: antithrombotic therapy

John A Cairns[1] and Stuart Connolly[2]
[1] University of British Columbia, Vancouver, Canada
[2] McMaster University, Hamilton, Ontario, Canada

Definitions, incidence and natural history

Stroke and non-central nervous system (CNS) embolism have long been known to be important complications of atrial fibrillation (AF). In several case series, 50–70% of embolic strokes were found to result in either death or severe neurologic deficit.[1] The Framingham Study[2,3] documented an annual 4.5% incidence of stroke among individuals with rheumatic AF, although those with AF in the absence of other disease and whose age is under 60 years (so-called "lone atrial fibrillation") have an extremely low risk of stroke.[4,5] The terms "non-rheumatic atrial fibrillation" and "non-valvular atrial fibrillation" (NVAF) are not entirely synonymous, although they are often used interchangeably. Non-valvular atrial fibrillation has become the preferred term for patients with AF in the absence of mitral valve disease, a prosthetic valve or mitral valve repair.[6] Paroxysmal AF is defined as an episode lasting up to seven days, whereas persistent AF is defined as a duration beyond seven days. Both paroxysmal and persistent AF are designated as recurrent AF if they resolve spontaneously or in response to treatment and then recur. Persistent AF is defined as permanent if cardioversion fails or AF lasts for more than one year and cardioversion has not been attempted.

Data from the placebo groups of five landmark randomized clinical trials among patients with non-valvular AF[7–12] found a mean 4.5% annual incidence of stroke (range 3–7%) and a mean 5.0% annual incidence of stroke plus other systemic emboli (range 3–7.4%); over half the strokes resulted in death or permanent disability.[13] Patients were selected for entry into these trials according to a variety of criteria, including the absence of contraindications to warfarin and in some instances to aspirin, willingness to participate in a clinical trial and the echocardiographic exclusion of rheumatic valvular disease. Although generalizations to a wider population must be made cautiously, the observed rates of stroke and other systemic embolism are similar to those reported in earlier cohorts and likely are representative of those in the general population.

Antithrombotic management

Oral anticoagulant therapy

Prior to 1990, anticoagulation was usually prescribed for AF patients who had mitral stenosis, a prosthetic heart valve, prior arterial embolism or who were to undergo electrical cardioversion. Anticoagulation was generally not prescribed long-term for patients with non-rheumatic AF. In the late 1980s, the observations of the Framingham Study, together with evidence for the efficacy and increased safety of regimens of lower-dose warfarin, prompted the initiation of five randomized controlled trials of warfarin versus control or placebo for the primary prevention of thromboembolism among patients with non-rheumatic (non-valvular) AF (Table 37.1).[13] The trials enrolled patients with AF detected on a routine or screening electrocardiogram, whose mean age was 69 years. AFASAK[10] and SPINAF[9] excluded patients with intermittent AF, whereas the proportion of intermittent AF in CAFA[8] was 7%, in BAATAF[7] 16% and in SPAF[12] 34%. Previous stroke or transient ischemic attack was infrequent. Treatment allocation was randomized in all trials; the international normalized ratio (INR) ranges varied from a lower limit of 1.4 to an upper limit of 4.5. There was a double-blind comparison of warfarin to placebo in CAFA and SPINAF, and an open-label comparison in BAATAF. AFASAK compared warfarin, aspirin and aspirin placebo. SPAF allocated patients as being warfarin eligible (group 1) or warfarin ineligible (group 2). Group 1 patients were randomized to open-label warfarin, aspirin 325 mg/day or aspirin placebo; group 2 patients were randomized to aspirin or aspirin placebo.

Evidence-Based Cardiology, 3rd edition. Edited by S. Yusuf, J.A. Cairns, A.J. Camm, E.L. Fallen, and B.J. Gersh. © 2010 Blackwell Publishing, ISBN: 978-1-4051-5925-8.

Table 37.1 Non-rheumatic atrial fibrillation: designs of randomized trials

Trial	Sample size	Warfarin	INR	Aspirin
BAATAF[7]	420	Open	1.5–2.7*	
CAFA[8]	383	Blind	2.0–3.0	
SPINAF[9]	536	Blind	1.4–2.8*	
AFASAK[10,11]	1007	Open	2.8–4.2	75 mg/day
SPAF[12]	1330	Open	2.0–4.5*	325 mg/day

AFASAK, Copenhagen Atrial Fibrillation Aspirin Anticoagulation; BAATAF, Boston Area Anticoagulation Trial for Atrial Fibrillation; CAFA, Canadian Atrial Fibrillation Anticoagulation; INR, international normalized ratio; SPAF, Stroke Prevention in Atrial Fibrillation; SPINAF, Stroke Prevention in Non-rheumatic Atrial Fibrillation

*INRs estimated by investigators from prothrombin time ratios.

Four of the trials[7,9,10,12] were stopped early by their Data and Safety Monitoring Boards (DSMB) because interim analyses were strongly positive, whereas the fifth[8] was stopped early because of the strongly positive results from two other trials. The primary outcomes varied somewhat among the trials. However, it is possible to determine the rates of ischemic stroke and major bleeding (intracranial, transfusion of two or more units, hospitalization) from each trial, to make comparisons and to pool the results. The Atrial Fibrillation Investigators overview[13] was a collaborative prospective meta-analysis which provides reliable summary data based on individual patient information. The overall risk of ischemic stroke of 4.5% per year (identical to that documented in the Framingham Study) was reduced to 1.4% per year with warfarin, a relative risk reduction (RRR) of 68% (95% confidence interval (CI) 50–79%) and an absolute reduction of 31 strokes for every 1000 patients treated ($P < 0.001$). A major concern with warfarin is hemorrhage, which was carefully documented in each trial. The rate of major hemorrhage with warfarin was 1.3% per year versus 1% per year in controls, an increase of three major hemorrhages per 1000 patients treated, including an excess of intracranial hemorrhage of two per year for every 1000 patients treated. A more recent meta-analysis[14] of these five trials calculated a RRR of 66% for ischemic stroke, and 61% for ischemic stroke or intracranial hemorrhage. This overview calculated a significant 31% RRR of all-cause mortality. Hence, the overall picture is one of major benefit from warfarin, with only a modest and statistically insignificant increase in the risk of major extracranial hemorrhage and cerebral hemorrhage (**Level A**).

The European Atrial Fibrillation Trial (EAFT) compared oral anticoagulants, aspirin and placebo in patients with non-rheumatic AF who had experienced a transient ischemic attack (TIA) or stroke within the preceding three months.[15] The annual risk of recurrence was 12% among the placebo patients, dramatically higher than the 4.5% annual risk in the overall population of patients with non-rheumatic AF. The relative risk reduction by anticoagulants was 66% ($P < 0.001$), virtually identical to that calculated in the overview of the five major randomized controlled trials, but the absolute reduction of strokes was much greater (84 per year per 1000 patients) because of the high baseline risk of stroke in this population. Major extracranial bleeding was more frequent on anticoagulants versus placebo (excess of 21 per year per 1000), but this adverse event was far outweighed by the reduction of major or moderately disabling strokes by anticoagulants (**Level A**).

A recent meta-anlysis[16] of primary and secondary prevention trials has assessed the outcome of all stroke (ischemic plus hemorrhagic), providing a more clinically meaningful summary than the outcome of ischemic stroke only. The relative risk reduction was 64% overall, about 60% in primary prevention trials (absolute risk reduction [ARR] was 27/1000 patients/year) (Table 37.2) and about 68% for secondary prevention (ARR 84/1000 patients/year). There was an excess of major extracranial bleeding of 3/1000 patients/year with adjusted dose oral anticoagulation versus control.

Aspirin therapy

Comparisons of aspirin and placebo resulted in a somewhat less impressive risk reduction for stroke of about 16% (NS) in AFASAK,[10] 44% ($P = 0.02$) in SPAF[12] and 17% (NS) in the European Atrial Fibrillation Trial (EAFT)[15] (Table 37.3). A recently updated meta-analysis[16] which included the Low Dose Aspirin, Stroke and Atrial Fibrillation pilot study (LASAF),[17] the Japan Atrial Fibrillation Stroke Trial,[18] atrial fibrillation patients from the European Stroke Prevention Study 2 (ESPS-2)[19] and the United Kingdom TIA Study (UK-TIA)[20] found a statistically significant 22% RRR (95% CI 2–39%) of all strokes (ischemic plus hemorrhagic) in five trials of aspirin versus placebo, and a 19% RRR (95% CI 1–35%) when two trials of aspirin versus no treatment were included. The ARR was 0.8%/year in primary prevention trials and 2.5%/year in secondary prevention trials. Hence, aspirin can be expected to reduce the risk of ischemic stroke and all strokes, with an ARR of about one half that of warfarin and with a somewhat lower risk of major extracranial bleeding of 0.2%/year versus 0.3%/year (**Level A**).

Aspirin versus oral anticoagulants

Direct comparisons of oral anticoagulants and aspirin have been undertaken in nine trials[16,21] (Table 37.4). AFASAK[10] included 671 patients who were randomized to warfarin (INR 2.8–4.2) or aspirin 75 mg/day. SPAF-II[22] studied 715 patients aged 75 years or less and 385 patients aged over 75 years, with each group randomly allocated to either

Table 37.2 Non-rheumatic atrial fibrillation: outcomes of primary prevention randomized trials of warfarin*

| Trial | All stroke (ischemic plus hemorrhagic) | | | | Major extracranial bleed** Absolute risk increase events/1000 pt/yr |
	Control events/1000 pt/yr	Warfarin events/1000 pt/yr	Relative risk reduction (%)	Absolute risk reduction events/1000 pt/yr	
BAATAF[7]	30	6	78	24	
CAFA[8]	37	25	33	12	
SPINAF[9]	48	14	70	33	
AFASAK[10,11]	48	22	54	26	
SPAF[12]	78	38	60	47	
Overview[13]	45	18	60	27	3

*Data from Hart et al[16]
**Major bleed defined as a bleeding event requiring 2 U of blood or requiring hospital admission.

Table 37.3 Non-rheumatic atrial fibrillation: outcomes of primary and secondary prevention randomized trials of aspirin

| Trial | All strokes (ischemic and hemorrhagic) | | | |
	Control events/ 1000 pt/yr	Aspirin events/ 1000 pt/yr	Relative risk reduction % (95% CI)	Absolute risk reduction events/1000 pt/yr
Trials of aspirin vs placebo				
AFASAK[10]	48	39	17	9
SPAF[12]	60	35	44	25
EAFT[15]	122	103	11	19
ESPS-2[19]	207	138	29	69
UK-TIA[20]	67	58 (300 mg/day)	17	9
	67	60 (1200 mg/day)	14	7
Overview of 5 aspirin-placebo trials[16]	88	69	22 (2 to 39)	19 primary prevention 25 secondary prevention
Trials of aspirin vs no treatment				
LASAF[17]	22	27 (125 mg/day)	−17	−5
	6	22 (125 mg/2 days)	67	16
JAST[18]	20	22	−10	−2
Overview of 7 aspirin trials[16]	63	52	19 (−1 to 35)	8 primary prevention 25 secondary prevention

*Data from Hart et al[16]

warfarin (INR 2.0–4.5) or aspirin (325 mg/day). EAFT[15] randomized 455 anticoagulation-eligible patients with recent TIA or minor ischemic stroke to oral anticoagulant (INR 2.5–4.0) or aspirin (300 mg/day). AFASAK-2[23] randomized 339 patients into a primary prevention trial which compared warfarin (INR 2–3) to aspirin (300 mg/day). PATAF[24] randomized 272 patients into a primary prevention trial which compared warfarin (INR 2.5–3.5) to aspirin (150 mg/day). A meta-analysis[16] and an update[21] found a statistically significant 39% (95% CI 19–53) RRR of all strokes (ischemic plus hemorrhagic) with anticoagulants, equivalent to an ARR of about 9 events/1000 patients/year for primary prevention and 70 events/1000 patients/year

for secondary prevention (**Level A**). Major extracranial hemorrhage occurred with an excess of about 2/1000/year on warfarin.[16]

In SPAF II warfarin was superior to aspirin for reducing ischemic stroke, but the risk of intracranial hemorrhage was increased with warfarin, particularly in patients >75 years of age. When patients of all ages were considered, there was an ARR of 0.8%/year ($P = $ NS) in ischemic stroke or systemic embolus with warfarin, but when all strokes were compared, the ARR was only 0.3%/year ($P = $ NS). The relatively high rates of intracranial bleeding may be attributable to the use of prothrombin time monitoring, the high INR range chosen and the very elderly population. If the

Table 37.4 Non-rheumatic atrial fibrillation: outcomes of primary and secondary randomized trials of adjusted dose anticoagulation vs aspirin*

Trial	All strokes (ischemic and hemorrhagic)			
	Anticoagulation events/1000 pt/yr	Aspirin events/1000 pt/yr	Relative risk reduction % (95% CI)	Absolute risk reduction events/1000 pt/yr
AFASAK[10]	22	39	45	17
SPAF-II[22]				
Age ≤75	17	19	10	2
Age ≥75	50	55	10	5
EAFT[15]	39	109	67	70
AFASAK-2[23]	31	25	−23	−6
PATAF[24]	7	10	20	3
Vemmos et al	0	40	100	400
Chinese ATAFS	17	29	43	12
WASPO	0	0	not calculated	not calculated
BAFTA[25]	26	49	47	23
Overview[21]	25	41	39	9 primary prevention
			(19 to 53)	70 secondary prevention

* Data from Hart et al[16,21]

SPAF II results were to be excluded from the meta-analysis, the RRR of all strokes (ischemic and hemorrhagic) with anticoagulation would be greater than 39%.

The Birmingham Atrial Fibrillation Treatment of the Aged (BAFTA) Trial[25] was a randomized, open-label study of warfarin (INR 2.0–3.0) versus aspirin (75 mg/day) which is particularly relevant to several areas of uncertainty in current practice, because the patients were aged 75 years and greater (mean 81.5 years). They were recruited from and managed within general practices in England and Wales and the primary outcome included fatal or disabling stroke (ischemic and hemorrhagic), intracranial hemorrhage, and clinically significant arterial embolism. Warfarin reduced the annual risk of the primary outcome from 3.8% to 1.8%, a RRR of 52% (P = 0.003), and an ARR of 2% per year. The annual risk of extracranial hemorrhage was 1.4% (warfarin) versus 1.6% (aspirin). It should be noted that 40% of patients were on warfarin prior to study entry and that the study subjects represented only an estimated 10% of those with AF in the geographic region. Nevertheless, the results provide powerful evidence for the relative efficacy and safety of warfarin over aspirin for the treatment of NVAF in carefully selected elderly patients in real-life clinical practice settings.

Adjusted Dose Anticoagulation compared to warfarin/aspirin combinations, low or fixed dose anticoagulation, and to alternative antiplatelet regimens

The SPAF III trial[26] was undertaken in an attempt to reduce the rates of major hemorrhage with warfarin,

while improving on the stroke prevention achievable by aspirin alone. Patients at high risk of embolic stroke (at least one of impaired LV function, systolic hypertension, prior thromboembolism, or female gender plus age over 75 years) were randomly allocated warfarin 1–3 mg/day plus aspirin 325 mg/day or warfarin (INR 2–3). The trial was discontinued early after a mean follow-up of 1.2 years, because the rate of the composite primary outcome of ischemic stroke or systemic embolus was significantly higher in those given combination therapy than in those given adjusted-dose warfarin (7.9% vs 1.9% per year, P < 0.0001). Rates of disabling stroke and of the composite of ischemic stroke, systemic embolus or vascular death were also significantly and markedly increased. The rates of major bleeding were similar in the two treatment groups.

AFASAK 2[22] was designed to compare regimens of aspirin 300 mg/day, fixed-dose warfarin (1.25 mg/day) plus aspirin 300 mg/day and fixed-dose warfarin 1.25 mg/day to warfarin (INR 2.0–3.0). The trial was stopped early when the results of SPAF III became available. Adjusted-dose warfarin was superior to each of the three comparison regimens at this point. It is clear that in high-risk patients, regimens of low fixed-dose warfarin in combination with aspirin do not provide adequate protection against thromboembolism (**Level A**).

Three trials (AFASAK 2,[22] MWNAF[27] and PATAF[23]) compared low or fixed doses of warfarin with standard warfarin (INR 2.0–3.0 or 2.5–3.5) but none showed a benefit. A meta-analysis[24] calculated a statistically insignificant 38% RRR for all strokes with the adjusted-dose warfarin (**Level A**).

The SIFA study[28] compared the antiplatelet agent indobufen to warfarin (INR 2.0–3.5), randomizing 916 patients with recent ischemic stroke or TIA. During a one-year follow-up, the RRR by warfarin was 21% (95% CI 54–60%) (**Level A**).

The FFAACS[29] study compared the oral anticoagulant fluindione (INR 2.0–2.6) to fluindione plus aspirin 100 mg/day in high-risk patients with AF, but was stopped early because of excess hemorrhage in the combination group. The NAS-PAEF study[30] randomized 495 high-risk AF patients to acencoumarol (INR 2.0–3.0) or acencoumarol (INR 1.4–2.4) plus the cyclo-oxygenase inhibitor triflusal (600 mg/day). There were 714 lower risk patients randomized to acencoumarol (INR 2.0–3.0), triflusal or triflusal plus acencoumarol (INR 1.25–2.0). The achieved INRs differed less than was intended between the acencoumarol alone group (mean INR 2.5) and the combination therapy groups (mean INRs 1.93 and 2.17 in the low- and high-risk strata, respectively). The hazard ratio (HR) of the combination versus acencoumarol alone for the outcome of ischemic stroke or systemic embolus was 0.44 in both groups. When severe bleeding was combined with the primary outcome of vascular death, TIA or non-fatal stroke, there was an ARR of 2.3%/year ($P < 0.05$) with the combination in the intermediate risk group and an ARR of 1.74%/year ($P = NS$) in the high-risk group (**Level B**). These results suggest that it may yet be possible to find a regimen of antiplatelet agent and lower dose anticoagulant, but the appropriate INR range is likely to be only marginally less than the standard 2.0–3.0.

The ACTIVE program comprised three separate interrelated trials, including ACTIVE-W,[31] which used a non-inferiority design to compare the combination of clopidogrel (75 mg/day) plus aspirin (recommended at 75–100 mg/day) to anticoagulation (INR 2.0–3.0), among patients with AF who were eligible and willing to take anticoagulation. The trial was stopped early (only 27% of expected events had occurred) at the recommendation of the DSMB, because of an extremely low likelihood of eventually concluding non-inferiority of the clopidogrel/aspirin combination. Among the 6706 patients enrolled and followed for a median of 1.28 years, the risk ratio with the combination for the composite outcome of stroke, non-CNS embolus, myocardial infarction and vascular death was 1.44 (95% CI 1.18–1.76, $P = 0.0003$), and for all stroke was 1.72 (95% CI 1.24–4.37, $P = 0.002$) (**Level A**). Somewhat surprisingly, the risk ratio for major bleeding was 1.10 (95% CI 0.83–1.45) with the combination.

The ACTIVE-A trial[31a] compared the combination of clopidogrel (75 mg/day) plus aspirin to aspirin alone among 7554 patients with AF at increased risk of stroke and for whom vitamin K antagonist therapy was unsuitable. After a mean 3.6 years the risk of major vascular events was reduced by the combination (RR 0.89; 95%

CI 0.81, 0.98; $P = 0.01$). However, major bleeding was increased (2.0% vs 1.3%/year, RR 1.57; 95% CI 1.29, 1.92; $P < 0.001$).

Other anticoagulants

Warfarin and other vitamin K antagonists are very effective in reducing the incidence of stroke and systemic embolus. However, the narrow therapeutic margin and the interactions with many other drugs and foods necessitate frequent monitoring and patient diligence. There is a substantial risk of major hemorrhage, particularly in elderly patients. Ximelagatran is an oral direct thrombin inhibitor, with predictable and stable pharmacokinetics and relatively low potential for interactions with other drugs and with foods. Coagulation monitoring and dose adjustments are not required. This agent was evaluated in two large trials employing non-inferiority designs.[32,33] In both, it was concluded that ximelagatran was non-inferior (i.e. not unacceptably inferior) to warfarin.

SPORTIF III[32] randomized 3410 patients with AF and one or more stroke risk factors to open-label warfarin (INR 2.0–3.0) or ximelagatran (36 mg bid). During a mean 17.4-month follow-up, the incidence of the primary outcome (all stroke or systemic embolus) by intention to treat was reduced to 1.6%/year with ximelagatran from 2.3%/year with warfarin (ARR 0.7%/year, 95% CI –0.1–1.4 %, $P = 0.10$ and RRR 29%, 95% CI –6.5–52%). The incidence of major bleeding was similar in the two groups, but the total of minor or major bleeding was less frequent with ximelagatran (25.8%/year vs 29.8%/year, RRR 14%, 95% CI 4–22%, $P = 0.007$). The authors concluded that ximelagatran was "at least as effective" as warfarin for the prevention of stroke and systemic embolism.

SPORTIF V[33] compared ximelagatran to warfarin among 3922 patients in a study of almost identical design, except that it was double blind. During a mean follow-up of 20 months, the incidence of the primary outcome was 1.6%/year with ximelagatran and 1.2%/year with warfarin (ARR –0.45%/year, 95% CI –1.0–0.13%/year, but $P < 0.001$ for the predefined non-inferiority margin). The incidence of major bleeding was similar in the two groups, whereas major or minor bleeding was less frequent with ximelagatran (37% vs 47%/year, 95% CI –14% to –6.0%/year, $P < 0.001$). The authors concluded that "ximelagatran was non-inferior to well-controlled warfarin".

Both studies found an excess of patients with elevations of alanine transaminase (ALT) to greater than three times the upper limit of normal, usually within the first six months (6.0% vs 1% in SPORTIF III and 6.0% vs 0.8% in SPORTIF V). Furthermore, the claim of non-inferiority was based on the choice of non-inferiority margins that were excessive.[34] The commonly accepted approach is to estimate the efficacy of the currently accepted therapy (in this case warfarin vs placebo) from a meta-analysis and then to choose a non-inferiority margin which would represent preservation of at least 50% of the benefit of the accepted therapy compared to placebo. If the non-inferiority margin had been chosen according to the FDA recommendations, SPORTIF III would still have reached a conclusion of non-inferiority, but SPORTIF V would not, nor would a meta-analysis of the two studies. The FDA did not approve the new agent, having concluded that the more convenient dose and monitoring regimens and less total bleeding did not outweigh their concerns about hepatic toxicity and the appropriateness of the chosen non-inferiority margins (**Level B**).

Dabigatran is another oral direct thrombin inhibitor which is being compared to warfarin (INR 2-3) among patients with AF with at least one additional risk factor for stoke in the RE-LY trial. Enrollment is complete (18 113 patients) and results are expected in 2009.

There are several available oral, direct acting Factor Xa inhibitor drugs which have proven effective and safe in studies of deep venous thrombosis and offer promise in the setting of AF. In the AVERROES trial, apixaban (5 mg bid) is being compared to aspirin (81–324 mg daily) among patients with AF at more than very low risk of stroke in whom vitamin K antagonist therapy is unsuitable. The expected enrollment is 5600 patients with completion in 2010. In the ARISTOTLE trial, apixaban (5 mg bid) is being compared to warfarin (INR 2.5) among patients with AF at somewhat higher risk of stroke. The expected enrollment is 15 000 patients with completion in 2010. In the ROCKET AF trial, rivaroxaban (20 mg/day) is being compared to warfarin (INR 2.5) among patients with AF at risk of stroke and suitable for warfarin therapy. The expected enrollment is 14 000 patients with completion in 2010. In the ENGAGE AF TIMI 48 trial, DU-176b (high and low dose regimens) is being compared to warfarin among patients with AF at risk of stroke and suitable for warfarin therapy. The expected enrollment is 16 500 patients with completion in 2011.

Risk stratification (stroke or systemic embolus)

Rigorous and current data for stroke risk come from analyses of the placebo patients in large clinical trials of antithrombotic therapy. The Atrial Fibrillation Investigators overview[13] calculated the annual risk of stroke to be 4.5% among the total group of control patients in the five major primary prevention randomized trials of anticoagulation. The statistically significant multivariate predictors of stroke were previous stroke or TIA, increasing age, history of hypertension, and diabetes. Annual stroke risk ranged from 0 (112 patients <60 years age) to 1.3% (patients <80 years age with no other risk factors), to 11.7% (patients with prior stroke or TIA). A recent systematic review[35] examined the evidence identifying independent risk factors for stroke as reported in seven studies (including the AFI overview[13]) selected according to rigorously defined criteria. The absolute annual risk of stroke varied 20-fold among patients grouped by various risk factors. Independent risk factors for stroke (Table 37.5) were the same as those previously identified[13]: stroke/TIA (RR 2.5), age (RR 1.5/decade), history of hypertension (RR 2.0) and diabetes mellitus (RR 1.7). Female sex was an independent risk factor in three of six cohorts, but coronary artery disease and clinical congestive heart failure were not found to be independent risk factors in any of the studies which met the inclusion criteria. Congestive heart failure and reduced ejection fraction have been identified as univariant risk factors[13,36,37] and are included in current risk classification schemes.[6,38] The review emphasized a variety of shortcomings of the studies, including inconsistencies in definitions of some of the risk factors, the use of antiplatelet therapies, and the stroke outcomes (ischemic strokes only, all strokes, strokes plus other systemic emboli and strokes plus TIAs) (**Level A**).

The data from the Atrial Fibrillation Investigators overview[13] and the SPAF group[35] were combined to create the

Table 37.5 Risk factors for stroke in patients with non-vascular atrial fibrillation*

Risk factor	Multivariate RR (%)	95% CI (%)	Prevalence of risk factor in patient cohorts (% and range)	Observed range of absolute stroke rate/year with only this risk factor (%)
Stroke/TIA	2.5	1.8–3.5	7 (0–14)	6–9
Age	1.5/decade	1.3–1.7	Mean age range 62–79 yrs	1.5–3.0 for age >75 yr.
History of hypertension	2.0	1.6–2.5	48 (42–53)	1.5–3.0
Diabetes mellitus	1.7	1.4–2.0	15 (14–18)	2.0–3.5

*Data from Stroke Risk in Atrial Fibrillation Working Group[35]
RR, relative risk; CI, confidence interval

CHADS$_2$ index[38] which assigns 1 point each for congestive heart failure, hypertension, age 75 years or older and diabetes mellitus and 2 points for a history of stroke or TIA. The scheme was validated and compared to the other two schemes among 1733 Medicare beneficiaries aged 65–95 years, who had been discharged from hospital with non-rheumatic AF and not prescribed warfarin. The CHADS$_2$ index was the most accurate predictor of stroke, with the annual stroke rate increasing by about 1.5% for each 1-point increase in CHADS$_2$ score (from 1.9 with a score of 0 to 18.2% with a score of 6). This scheme was also evaluated in comparison to several others among 2580 patients receiving aspirin in six prospective trials.[39] The CHADS$_2$ index identified increments in stroke risk similar to those identified in the prior validation, and was better at discriminating medium- and high-risk patients than the other schema. The CHADS$_2$ index has become the favored choice for determining risk of stroke and guiding choice of antithrombotic therapy.[6]

Several cohort studies[1] have demonstrated a more consistent lower annual stroke risk in patients with paroxysmal (transient) AF than in those with persistent (chronic or sustained) AF. On the other hand, the SPAF trial found similar annual rates of ischemic stroke in patients with "recurrent" (3.2%) and "chronic" (3.3%) AF,[40] and a meta-analysis of the control groups in five large trials showed no difference.[13] Current practice guidelines do not differentiate between paroxysmal and persistent AF (**Class I, Level A**). However, it is possible that the risk of stroke is less in patients whose episodes of AF are brief (<1 day) and self-terminating.[41]

The short-term risk of stroke appears to be higher in patients with recent-onset atrial fibrillation than in those with atrial fibrillation for more than 1–2 years.[42,43] In the European Atrial Fibrillation Trial,[15] among patients with prior stroke, the annual recurrence rate was 12% without treatment. Several case series reported recurrence rates of 0.1–1.3%/day during the first two weeks following a cardioembolic stroke.[44] The high rate of recurrence, although not observed in every study, suggested that there is some urgency in initiating anticoagulation following the occurrence of embolic stroke in patients with AF. The International Stroke Trial Collaborative Group addressed this concern with a large randomized trial of 18 451 patients with ischemic stroke who were randomized within 24 hours of onset to SC unfractionated heparin (5000 IU bid or 12 500 IU bid), aspirin 300 mg/day, both or neither and maintained for 14 days or until prior hospital discharge.[44] CT scan was performed to exclude intracranial hemorrhage when possible and was mandatory in comatose patients. Among the 3169 patients with AF, both doses of heparin were significantly more effective for the prevention of recurrent stroke of ischemic or unknown type. However, both heparin regimens resulted in significantly more symp-

tomatic intracranial hemorrhage, and there was no significant difference among the regimens in the rate of the composite outcome of recurrent stroke or symptomatic intracranial hemorrhage, nor of all-cause mortality. Patients with AF had a higher mortality than patients without AF (16.9% vs 7.5%), probably due to greater mean age and larger cerebral infarcts. The rate of recurrence within 14 days, of stroke of ischemic or unknown type, was 3.9% among patients with AF, considerably lower than reported in earlier studies, but still higher than in patients without AF in this study. The results indicate that heparin is not indicated in the acute management of embolic stroke among patients with AF (**Level A**). Based upon their study and a combined analysis with the Chinese Acute Stroke Trial,[45] the authors recommend that AF patients who experience ischemic stroke should be given aspirin 300 mg/day with conversion to warfarin (INR 2.0–3.0) after 14 days[44] (**Class IIa, Level A**). When stroke occurs in AF patients receiving warfarin, subsequent management should be guided by the INR measured at the time of onset of the stroke. If the INR was below the conventional therapeutic range it is probably sufficient to reinstitute warfarin with meticulous attention to maintaining INR in the range of 2.0–3.0. If the INR was in the therapeutic range, it is reasonable to raise the intensity of warfarin to an INR range of 2.5–3.5 (**Class IIb, Level C**).

The risk of stroke in patients with thyrotoxic AF is substantial, although the mechanism and the relative role of congestive heart failure are uncertain. The risk of stroke is also substantial among patients with hypertrophic cardiomyopathy and AF. These risks have not been rigorously evaluated, and antithrombotic therapies for patients with AF and thyrotoxicosis or hypertrophic cardiomyopathy should be based upon the presence of validated stroke risk factors[46] (**Class I, Level C**).

Risk of hemorrhage

The efficacy of warfarin for the prevention of ischemic stroke must be balanced against the risk of major hemorrhage, particularly cerebral hemorrhage, which is usually fatal. The risk of major hemorrhage is increased by the intensity of anticoagulation, advanced age, and hypertension.[47,48] It is likely to be higher in clinical practice than in the rigorous setting of a clinical trial. The 3.1% absolute reduction of ischemic stroke observed in the initial five randomized controlled trials was accompanied by an absolute excess risk of major hemorrhage of only 0.3%. The INR ranges chosen varied from a low of 1.4 to a high of 4.5. In SPAF II[21] the greater efficacy of warfarin over aspirin for the prevention of ischemic stroke was outweighed by excess cerebral hemorrhage in patients over age 75 years (mean 80 years), likely related to the chosen INR of 2.0–4.5.

The HEMORR$_2$HAGES scheme was developed from three previously published prediction rules and all four approaches were then evaluated in a population of elderly patients with AF.[49] The scheme allotted points for hepatic or renal disease, ethanol abuse, malignancy, age >75 years, reduced platelets, prior bleed, hypertension, anemia, excessive falls or neuropsychiatric disease and prior stroke. The scheme provided good discrimination among patients with an annual risk of hospitalization for hemorrhage which ranged from 1.9% to 12.3% (**Level C**).

Recent practice guidelines[6,46] stress the importance of appropriate antithrombotic therapy for AF, and yet practice surveys indicate that rates of compliance range from rather low[50–54] to reasonably high.[55] Hylek et al[56] point out that randomized trials and most observational cohorts underestimate the risks of major hemorrhage because they include few patients over 80 years of age, and infrequently include patients in the initial phase of warfarin therapy when the risk of major hemorrhage is highest. They enrolled 472 patients age ≥65 years (153 ≥80 years), with ECG-verified AF, who were new to warfarin and whose care was established at the study institution and whose warfarin was managed by the on-site anticoagulation clinic. The patients were enrolled on the first day of warfarin and followed for one year between 2001 and 2003 (complete follow-up in 100%). A total of 90% of patients ≥80 years of age had a CHADS$_2$ score ≥2, and of the patients ≥80 years, 95.3% had at least an intermediate risk of major hemorrhage. Anticoagulation control was very good, with 56% of person time within the INR range of 2.0–3.0, 29% below 2.0, 11% within 3.0–<4.0, and only 2% ≥4.0. Even within this optimized setting, the rate of major hemorrhage was 7.2 per 100 patient-years (intracranial hemorrhage was 2.5 per 100 patient-years). The incidence of major hemorrhage was 13.08% for patients ≥80 years versus 4.75% for those <80 years. The risk during the first 90 days of therapy was three times that of the remainder of the year. The risk of major hemorrhage was increased 20 times among patients with an INR >4.0. Most of the intracranial bleeds occurred in patients ≥75 years of age. The rate of major hemorrhage was higher in patients with higher CHADS$_2$ scores.

In contrast, the BAFTA study[25] found that in patients aged >75 years, warfarin was more efficacious than aspirin in preventing all strokes (ischemic plus hemorrhagic) and did not cause more extracranial hemorrhage (1.4%/year with warfarin vs 1.6%/year with aspirin). The lower bleeding risk may be attributable to more restrictive patient selection for a clinical trial than for the Hylek survey and the fact that 40% of them had been taking warfarin safely prior to entering the trial.

These observations point to the challenges in choosing the optimal antithrombotic therapy for very elderly patients to ensure a favorable risk–benefit ratio.[57] For those with no stroke risk factors other than age ≥75 years, it is reasonable to consider aspirin in preference to warfarin.[6] Nevertheless, ischemic stroke with its dire consequences is relatively frequent, and the competing risk of intracranial hemorrhage with warfarin may be acceptable. If warfarin is to be used, great care must be taken to rigorously maintain the selected therapeutic INR with frequent monitoring in the first three months and more often than the "standard" monthly interval subsequently (**Class I, Level C**).

For most patients who are candidates for warfarin, an INR range of 2.0–3.0 with a target of 2.5 appears optimal.[6,46] In a large cohort of patients the risk of ischemic stroke, severity of stroke and mortality rose sharply when INR fell to 1.5–1.9, but the risk of intracranial hemorrhage did not rise until INR values exceeded 3.9.[58] A recent meta-analysis[59] of studies which assigned hemorrhagic and thromboembolic events in patients taking anticoagulants to discrete INR ranges found that 44% of hemorrhages occurred when INRs were above the therapeutic range, 48% of thromboembolic events took place when below it and that the mean proportion of events that occurred when the patient's INR was outside the therapeutic range was higher in the studies of shorter follow-up. Patients with a previous TIA or minor stroke may benefit from a somewhat higher INR of 2.0–3.9 with a target of 3.0.[6,60] Patients at higher risk of cerebral hemorrhage, particularly those over the age of 75, may benefit from a somewhat lower INR range of 1.6–2.5 with a target of 2.0,[6] although protection against ischemic stroke drops off sharply when INRs fall below this target (**Class IIa, Level C**).

Rate versus rhythm control

Management strategies for AF have generally been focused on rhythm control (attempting to establish and sustain normal sinus rhythm by the use of various proven pharmacologic agents and appropriate electrical cardioversion) or rate control (attempting to maintain resting and exercise heart rates below optimal levels, without specific attempts to establish or maintain sinus rhythm). An overview[61,62] of the five trials which compared the strategies of rhythm with rate control in AF found a mortality of 13.0% with rate control versus 14.6% with rhythm control (OR 0.87, $P = 0.09$). The rates of ischemic stroke and major hemorrhage were similar. The AFFIRM trial,[63] by far the largest, randomized 4060 patients of mean age 69.7 years and found a trend toward lower survival in the rhythm control group, which also had significantly more hospitalizations and adverse drug effects. Anticoagulation (INR 2.0–3.0) was mandated in the rate control group (85% maintained warfarin) and strongly encouraged in the rhythm control group, but could be stopped at the physician's discretion if sustained sinus rhythm was achieved (70% maintained warfarin). Ischemic stroke occurred at an annual rate of about 1% in each group, and in most instances the patient was either off warfarin or the INR was <2.0. The authors concluded that continuous anticoagulation is warranted in all patients with AF and one or more risk factors for stroke, whether or not sinus rhythm appears to be restored and maintained, and this approach is recommended by consensus groups[6,46] (**Class I, Level A**).

Choice of antithrombotic therapy

Table 37.6 is derived from the practice guidelines of the AHA/ACC/ESC consensus process[6] and incorporates concepts of varying risks of thromboembolism with age and other risk factors, and embodies concepts of varying hemorrhagic risk with increasing age. The schema differs somewhat from that developed by the ACCP consensus process[46] which recommends aspirin in a dose of 325 mg/day, definite warfarin for patients ≥75 years even with no other risk factors, not differentiating between moderate- and high-risk factors, and not considering weak or less validated risk factors. The Atrial Fibrillation Working Group has recently published a comparison of 12 risk stratification schemes.[64] They conclude that additional research is required to "identify and strengthen a single scheme around which standard recommendations could be developed".

For the present, tables such as Table 37.6 can provide broad guidance to the clinician in decisionmaking about antithrombotic therapy for AF. However, experienced clinical judgment is required to decide optimal therapy depending on the competing risks (ischemic stroke/other systemic embolus versus cerebral and other major hemorrhage); anticoagulant monitoring (quality and availability of monitoring and the willingness/ability of the patient to maintain a safe regimen); and individual patient preferences (perspectives on the competing risks of ischemic stroke and major hemorrhage and the inconvenience and complexity of warfarin therapy). Eventually, pharmacogenomic algorithms may allow more rapid and safe determinations of initial warfarin dosage, particularly among

Table 37.6 Choice of antithrombotic therapies for patients with non-rheumatic atrial fibrillation (based on AHA/ACC/ESC Guidelines 2006[6])

Clinical risk factors*	Age (years)		
	<65	65–74	≥75
No	Aspirin (81–325 mg/day) (**Class I, Level A**)	Aspirin (81–325 mg/day) (**Class I, Level A**) or Warfarin (INR 2.0–3.0, target 2.5) (**Class I, Level A**)	Aspirin (81–325 mg/day) (**Class I, Level A**) or Warfarin (INR 2.0–3.0, target 2.5) (**Class I, Level A**) Consider INR 1.6–2.5, target 2.0 (**Class IIb, Level C**)
	Consider no antithrombotic therapy (**Class IIb, Level C**) Consider warfarin (INR 2.0–3.0, target 2.5) for females or coronary artery disease (**Class IIa, Level B**)		
1 moderate risk factor# in addition to age ≥75 yr	Aspirin (75–325 mg/day) or Warfarin (INR 2.0–3.0, target 2.5) (**Class IIa, Level B**)	Aspirin (75–325 mg/day) or Warfarin (INR 2.0–3.0, target 2.5) (**Class IIa, Level B**)	Warfarin (INR 2.0–3.0, target 2.5) (**Class I, Level A**) Consider INR 1.6–2.5, target 2.0 (**Class IIb, Level C**)
Any high risk factor* or >1 moderate risk factor	Warfarin (INR 2.0–3.0, target 2.5) (**Class I, Level A**)	Warfarin (INR 2.0–3.0, target 2.5) (**Class I, Level A**)	Warfarin (INR 2.0–3.0, target 2.5) (**Class I, Level A**) Consider INR 1.6–2.5, target 2.0 (**Class IIb, Level C**)

Hypertension, heart failure or LVEF ≤ 35%, diabetes mellitus.

* Previous stroke, TIA or embolism; mitral stenosis; prosthetic heart valve.

patients whose warfarin requirements are particularly low or high.[64a]

Cardioversion

Although the randomized trials have shown no improvement in major outcomes including thromboembolism with a rhythm control strategy versus rate control, individual patients may gain symptomatic benefit and even long-term freedom from AF following electrical or pharmacologic cardioversion. The strongest predictor of initial and persistent success with cardioversion is short duration of the atrial fibrillation before cardioversion. In general, it may be expected that atrial fibrillation occurring in conjunction with surgery, viral illness, alcohol or other pharmacologic excess, or in association with thyrotoxicosis or pulmonary embolus, has a high likelihood of reversion with persistence of sinus rhythm if there has been resolution of the precipitating cause. Successful and sustained reversion to sinus rhythm is associated with relatively young age and freedom from underlying heart disease. Some patients have intolerable symptoms and poor exercise tolerance during AF and may prefer attempted rhythm control to rate control. The rate of initial success in restoring sinus rhythm is high but in the contemporary AFFIRM trial, vigorous efforts to establish and sustain sinus rhythm resulted in prevalences of 82.5%, 73.3% and 62.6% at one, three and five years, respectively.[63]

Although no study has rigorously documented the incidence of systemic embolism following electrical, pharmacologic or spontaneous cardioversion, it is widely believed that in many patients cardioversion acutely increases the risk of stroke. This perception forms the rationale for anticoagulation of patients prior to cardioversion. The best available study used a prospective cohort design to detect a reduction of postcardioversion systemic embolism from 5.3% to 0.8% among anticoagulated patients.[65] It is generally believed that a newly formed thrombus will become organized and adherent to the left atrial wall within two weeks of formation. Transesophageal echocardiography (TEE) reveals that in the majority of patients thrombus resolves, rather than simply becoming firmly adherent to the wall of the left atrium or left atrial appendage.[66] Accordingly, anticoagulation is usually recommended for about three weeks before cardioversion[6,46] (**Class I, Level C**). A study that pooled data from 32 studies found that 98% of thromboembolic events occurred within 10 days of cardioversion of atrial fibrillation or flutter.[67] However, evidence exists that even after successful electroversion, atrial contraction may not normalize for some weeks,[68,69] and therefore maintenance of anticoagulation for about four weeks following cardioversion seems prudent[6,46] (**Class I, Level C**). There is a lack of evidence that the incidence of thromboembolism is less with pharmacologic than with electrical cardioversion, and accordingly anticoagulant management should not differ[6] (**Class I, Level C**). New-onset atrial fibrillation is generally not thought to warrant anticoagulation if cardioversion is undertaken within 48 hours of its onset.[6,46] If cardioversion is unsuccessful or if AF has been recurrent, anticoagulation may be commenced subsequently.

Emergency cardioversion may be required because of ischemia or hemodynamic compromise in some situations, and should not be delayed even if the AF has been present for more than 48 hours and the patient is not already anticoagulated. In such a situation, concomitant heparinization may offer some benefit (**Class I, Level C**).

The potential role of TEE for the detection of atrial thrombi and the simplification and shortening of the anticoagulation regimen in association with cardioversion was studied in a consecutive series of 230 patients.[70] Atrial thrombi were detected in 15%. Of 196 patients without thrombi, 95% were successfully cardioverted without prolonged anticoagulation, and none had a clinical thromboembolic event. However, a subsequent study[71] and a meta-analysis of several clinical studies[72] indicate that the absence of thrombi on TEE does not mean that a period of four weeks of anticoagulation following cardioversion may be safely omitted (**Class I, Level C**).

The Assessment of Cardioversion Utilizing Echocardiography (ACUTE) pilot study[73] was followed by a multicenter randomized prospective of trial of 1222 patients with atrial fibrillation of more than two days' duration.[74] All patients were anticoagulated and assigned to therapy guided by the findings on TEE or to conventional therapy. If TEE showed no thrombus, the patient underwent cardioversion and continued on anticoagulant therapy for four weeks. If thrombus was detected, warfarin was given for three weeks, TEE was repeated and, if the thrombus had resolved, cardioversion was performed and warfarin continued for four weeks. If thrombus was still detected after three weeks of anticoagulation, no cardioversion was attempted but warfarin was continued for four weeks further. The patients randomized to no TEE received warfarin for three weeks and then underwent cardioversion followed by a further four weeks of warfarin. At eight weeks after the assignment of management strategy, there was no significant difference between the two therapeutic groups (TEE vs no TEE) in the rate of embolic events or the prevalence of sinus rhythm. The TEE strategy resulted in fewer total hemorrhagic events, most of them minor. Right or left heart thrombi were identified in 13.8% of patients who underwent TEE. Of those patients with thrombi detected, 88.2% had a thrombus in the left atrial appendage. Patients may be anticoagulated and screened by TEE and cardioversion performed immediately if no thrombus is detected, and then receive at least four further weeks of anticoagulation.

If thrombus is detected, patients should undergo at least three weeks of anticoagulation prior to cardioversion, followed by a further four weeks of anticoagulation. Among those patients with atrial thrombi detected, the value of repeat TEE after the initial three weeks of anticoagulation is uncertain. In centers where TEE is readily available and the interpretations reliable, a TEE-guided management strategy may safely shorten the time to cardioversion by comparison with standard anticoagulant regimens (**Class I, Level A**). The cost-effectiveness of such an approach depends very much on local and national patterns of practice and cost structures.

Left atrial radiofrequency ablation is increasingly used to treat AF, raising questions about the role of warfarin in such patients. In general, the procedure should be conducted with the patient off warfarin and the INR in the normal range. Warfarin should then be restarted with INR 2.0–3.0 for at least the next several months, and continued indefinitely in patients with a CHADS$_2$ of 3 or more,[41] with consideration given to discontinuing warfarin in young patients with very low CHADS$_2$ scores and who are free of even asymptomatic AF after several months (**Class IIb, Level B**).

Atrial flutter

There is a widespread perception that the risk of stroke is less with atrial flutter than with atrial fibrillation. A retrospective analysis of a large database of elderly hospitalized patients confirmed this perception, calculating a stroke risk ratio of 1.4 with atrial flutter and 1.6 with AF.[75] By eight years of follow-up more than half the patients with atrial flutter had developed AF, and these patients were more likely to experience a stroke. The development of AF was more likely among patients with congestive heart failure, rheumatic heart disease, hypertension and diabetes mellitus. Although there are no rigorous prospective data on the incidence of stroke among patients with atrial flutter, nor randomized trials of the value of anticoagulation, it is generally recommended that patients with atrial flutter be risk stratified and treated in the same manner as patients with AF[6,46] (**Class I, Level C**).

Retrospective studies of patients with atrial flutter undergoing cardioversion suggest that the risk of thromboembolism is less than that for patients with AF, but nevertheless clinically important.[76] Case series note a very low incidence of thromboemboli when patients with atrial flutter are adequately anticoagulated prior to cardioversion.[77] It is generally recommended that patients with atrial flutter who are to be cardioverted receive an anticoagulant regimen identical to that for patients with AF[6,46] (**Class I, Level C**).

Atrial fibrillation and coronary artery disease

There are extensive data available on the efficacy of warfarin at various intensities, combinations of warfarin and aspirin, aspirin alone and clopidogrel among survivors of acute myocardial infraction (AMI).[78,79] Practice guidelines favor the use of aspirin 75–162 mg/day, and the substitution of clopidogrel 75 mg/day or warfarin (INR 2.5–3.5) for patients allergic to aspirin.[78,79] However, when AF is present following AMI, warfarin therapy is usually required for stroke prophylaxis. An INR range of 2.5–3.5 may be appropriate for the first few months post AMI, followed by the standard range of 2.0–3.0 long term.[6,46,78] Aspirin should generally not be given concurrently (**Class I, Level B**). A prospective cohort study based on Swedish coronary care unit admissions of patients discharged with AF following AMI found that oral anticoagulants were given to only 30% of such patients, and yet this therapy was associated with a 7% reduction of one-year mortality after adjustment for confounding variables[80] (**Level C**).

For patients undergoing percutaneous coronary intervention (PCI), maintenance aspirin is supplemented by clopidogrel which is begun prior to PCI and maintained for several months subsequently, the duration being longer for drug-eluting than bare metal stents.[78,79,81] AF patients who are receiving warfarin monotherapy, and who undergo PCI, may have the warfarin interrupted for 48 hours prior to PCI and reinstituted as soon as possible after the procedure, with the substitution of aspirin (75–81 mg/day) during the period off warfarin. Clopidogrel should be administered according to the same approaches as for patients without AF[46,78,79,81] (**Class I, Level C**). In patients at particularly high risk of stent thrombosis, triple therapy with warfarin, clopidogrel and aspirin may be appropriate[78,81] (**Class IIb, Level C**). The risk of bleeding is increased when warfarin is given in conjunction with aspirin and/or clopidogrel, and careful monitoring with INR 2.0–2.5 is recommended (**Class I, Level C**).

Interruption of warfarin therapy in relation to surgical procedures

Warfarin should generally be discontinued prior to surgical or diagnostic procedures which have a risk of bleeding. Given that the risk of stroke among patients with AF ranges from <1% to >20%/year, it is generally recommended that warfarin may be safely discontinued for up to a week (four days prior to and three days after surgery) in most patients with AF[82] (**Class IIa, Level C**). For those at particularly high risk of stroke (mechanical valve prosthesis or recent stroke), IV unfractionated heparin or SC

LMWH may be given preoperatively. It is likely that most potentially hemorrhagic dental procedures, if undertaken with appropriate surgical skill and the use of hemostatic mouthwash, can be done without discontinuing warfarin, provided the preoperative INR is under 3.0[83] (**Class IIa, Level B**).

Conclusion and recommendations

Patients with persistent or paroxysmal atrial fibrillation should generally receive chronic antithrombotic therapy with warfarin or aspirin regardless of whether a strategy of rate control or rhythm control has been selected (see Table 38.6) (**Class I, Level A**). Antithrombotic therapy should generally be sustained indefinitely, unless a clearly reversible cause of atrial fibrillation (e.g. pulmonary embolism, thyrotoxicosis, viral infection, perioperative, alcohol excess) has resolved and sinus rhythm has resumed (**Class I, Level C**).

Major risk factors for thromboembolism include the presence of mitral stenosis, a prosthetic heart and a history of prior stroke, TIA or non-CNS systemic embolism; moderate risk factors include age ≥ 75 year, history of hypertension, heart failure or moderate to severe LV dysfunction and diabetes mellitus. Warfarin is more effective than aspirin in preventing thromboemboli, but carries a higher risk of hemorrhage. The choice of agent is governed by the perceived balance between the risk of thromboembolism and the risk of hemorrhage in each individual patient and should include appropriate consideration of patient preferences (**Class I, Level A**).

Among patients with persistent or paroxysmal AF, age is an important determinant of the risk of thromboembolism even in the absence of other moderate or major risk factors. When the patient is <65 years and is free of any moderate or major risk factors for thromboembolic events (CHADS$_2$ = 0), the risk of thromboembolism is very low and aspirin therapy is preferable to warfarin (**Class I, Level A**). Consideration should be given even to no antithrombotic therapy (**Class IIb, Level C**). In the age range 65–74 years (CHADS$_2$ = 0), the risk of thromboembolism is increased and either aspirin or warfarin may be indicated. Patient preferences and risk factors for hemorrhage should influence the choice (**Class IIa, Level A**). When the patient is aged ≥ 75 years the risk of thromboembolism is further increased, even in the absence of other risk factors (CHADS$_2$ = 1). However, the risk of major hemorrhage, and particularly intracranial hemorrhage, also rises. Either aspirin or warfarin may be appropriate (**Class I, Level A**). If warfarin is to be used, consideration should be given to a reduced intensity of anticoagulation (INR 1.6–2.5, target 2.0), recognizing that maintaining an adequate intensity of anticoagulation with a target of 2.0 is difficult and requires frequent monitoring (**Class IIb, Level C**).

Patients aged 74 or less with one moderate risk factor for thromboembolism (CHADS$_2$ = 1) should receive either aspirin or warfarin. Risks of thromboembolism and hemorrhage as well as patient preferences should influence the choice (**Class I, Level A**).

Patients with more than one moderate risk factor or one major risk factor for thromboembolism (CHADS$_2 \geq 2$) should receive warfarin (**Class I, Level A**).

Patients with AF who experience an episode of thromboembolism with an INR below the therapeutic range should continue on oral anticoagulation with more meticulous monitoring and dose adherence. If the episode occurs at an INR in the therapeutic range, consideration should be given to maintaining a higher range (INR 2.5–3.5), with intensive monitoring to avoid any levels over 4.0 (**Class IIb, Level C**).

Patients undergoing cardioversion (electrical or pharmacologic) for AF of uncertain or known duration of 48 hours or longer should generally receive oral anticoagulation for about three weeks prior to the procedure and for at least four weeks afterwards (**Class I, Level C**). Patients with more than one episode of AF or who are at high risk of thromboembolism should have oral anticoagulation continued indefinitely even if sinus rhythm persists at four weeks (**Class I, Level C**). If cardioversion is required on an urgent basis because of hemodynamic instability in patients with AF of uncertain or greater than 48 hours duration, cardioversion should not be delayed. Concomitant anticoagulation should be established using IV unfractionated heparin (activated partial thromboplastin time (APTT) 1.5–2.0 times reference control) and maintained until oral anticoagulation can be achieved and sustained for at least four weeks (**Class I, Level C**).

New-onset AF does not require anticoagulation if cardioversion is undertaken within 48 hours of its onset.[6,46] If cardioversion is unsuccessful or if AF has been recurrent, anticoagulation may be commenced subsequently (**Class I, Level C**).

In appropriate centers TEE-guided management can offer a safe, cost-effective and convenient alternative to standard anticoagulant regimens. If AF is of uncertain or known duration of 48 hours or longer, TEE may be performed. If there is no LA thrombus, IV heparin may be commenced, cardioversion undertaken, and oral anticoagulation maintained for at least four weeks. (An alternative would be to administer oral anticoagulation initially for at least five days and then to perform TEE.) If thrombus is detected on TEE, anticoagulation should be continued for a total of three weeks, followed by cardioversion and sustained oral anticoagulation for at least four weeks further (**Class I, Level B**).

Patients undergoing LA radiofrequency ablation should have warfarin stopped and INR in the normal range. Warfarin should then be restarted and maintained indefinitely for patients with a CHADS$_2$ score of 3 or less, with consideration given to discontinuing warfarin in young patients with very low CHADS$_2$ scores and who are free of even asymptomatic AF after several months (**Class IIb, Level B**).

The antithrombotic management of patients with atrial flutter should be generally be similar to that for patients with AF (**Class I, Level C**).

Patients with AF following myocardial infarction should receive warfarin (INR 2.5–3.5 for the first few months and 2.0–3.0 long term) and aspirin should generally not be given concurrently (**Class IIb, Level C**).

AF patients who are to undergo PCI should have the warfarin interrupted for 48 hours prior to PCI and reinstituted as soon as possible after the procedure, with the substitution of aspirin (75–81 mg/day) during the period off warfarin. Clopidogrel should be administered according to the same approaches as for patients without AF, with triple therapy reserved for patients at particularly high risk of stent thrombosis. The INR should be kept in the range 2.0–2.5 in such patients[46,78,79,81] (**Class IIb, Level C**).

In patients about to undergo surgical or diagnostic procedures that carry a risk of bleeding, if the INR is 2.0–3.0, oral anticoagulation may be safely discontinued for up to four days before and three days after the procedure. With expert management, most potentially hemorrhagic dental procedures do not require cessation of anticoagulation if the INR is 2.0–3.0 (**Class IIa, Level B**).

References

1. Cairns JA, Connolly SJ. Nonrheumatic atrial fibrillation: risk of stroke and role of antithrombotic therapy. *Circulation* 1991;**84**: 469–81.

2. Kannel WB, Abbot RD, Savage DD *et al.* Epidemiologic features of chronic atrial fibrillation: the Framingham Study. *N Engl J Med* 1982;**306**:1018–22.

3. Wolf PA, Dawber TR, Thomas E Jr *et al.* Epidemiologic assessment of chronic atrial fibrillation and risk of stroke: the Framingham Study. *Neurology* 1978;**28**:973–7.

4. Brand FN, Abbott RD, Kannel WB *et al.* Characteristics and prognosis of lone atrial fibrillation: 30-year follow-up in the Framingham Study. *JAMA* 1985;**254**:3449–53.

5. Kopecky SL, Gersh BJ, McGoon MD *et al.* The natural history of lone atrial fibrillation: a population-based study over three decades. *N Engl J Med* 1987;**317**:669–74.

6. Fuster V, Rydén LE, Cannon AS *et al.* ACC/AHA/ESC guidelines for the management of patients with atrial fibrillation: A report of the American College of Cardiology/American Heart Association Task Force on Practice Guidelines and the European Society of Cardiology Committee for Practice Guidelines. *Circulation* 2006;**114**:257–354.

7. Boston Area Anticoagulation Trial of Atrial Fibrillation Investigators. The effect of low-dose warfarin on the risk of stroke in patients with nonrheumatic atrial fibrillation. *N Engl J Med* 1990;**323**:1505–11.

8. Connolly SJ, Laupacis A, Gent M *et al*, for the CAFA Study Coinvestigators. Canadian Atrial Fibrillation Anticoagulation (CAFA) Study. *J Am Coll Cardiol* 1991;**18**:349–55.

9. Ezekowitz MD, Bridgers SL, James KE *et al.* Warfarin in the prevention of stroke associated with nonrheumatic atrial fibrillation. *N Engl J Med* 1992;**327**:406–12.

10. Petersen P, Boysen G, Godtfredsen J *et al.* Placebo-controlled, randomised trial of warfarin and aspirin for prevention of thromboembolic complications in chronic atrial fibrillation: the Copenhagen AFASAK study. *Lancet* 1989;**i**:175–9.

11. Petersen P, Boysen G. Letter to Editor. *N Engl J Med* 1990;**323**: 482.

12. Stroke Prevention in Atrial Fibrillation Investigators. Stroke prevention in atrial fibrillation study: final results. *Circulation* 1991;**84**:527–39.

13. Atrial Fibrillation Investigators. Risk factors for stroke and efficiency of antithrombotic therapy in atrial fibrillation analysis of pooled later from five randomized controlled trials. *Arch Intern Med* 1994;**154**:1449–57.

14. Aguilar MI, Hart R. Oral anticoagulants for preventing stroke in patients with non-valvular atrial fibrillation and no previous history of stroke or transient ischemic attacks. *Cochrane Database of Systematic Reviews* 2005, Issue 3. Art. No.: CD001927. DOI: 10.1002/14651858.CD001927.pub2.

15. EAFT (European Atrial Fibrillation Trial) Study Group. Secondary prevention in non-rheumatic atrial fibrillation after transient ischemic attack or minor stroke. *Lancet* 1993;**342**: 1255–62.

16. Hart RG, Pearce LA, Aguilare MI. Meta-analysis: antithrombotic therapy to prevent stroke in patients who have non-valvular atrial fibrillation. *Ann Intern Med* 2007;**146**:857–67

17. Posada IS, Barriales V, for the LASAF Pilot Study Group. Alternate-day dosing of aspirin in atrial fibrillation. *Am Heart J* 1999;**138**:137–43.

18. Japan Arial Fibrillation Stoke Trial Group. Low-dose aspirin for prevention of stroke in low-risk patients with atrial fibrillation: Japan Arial Fibrillation Stroke Trial. *Stroke* 2006;**37**:447–51.

19. Diener HC, Cunha L, Forbes C, Sivenius J, Smets P, Lowenthal A. European Stroke Prevention Study 2. Dipyridamole and acetylsalicylic acid in the secondary prevention of stroke. *J Neurol Sci* 1996;**143**:1–13.

20. Benavente O, Hart R, Koudstaal P, Laupacis A, McBride R. Antiplatelet therapy for preventing stroke in patients with non-valvular atrial fibrillation and no previous history of stroke or transient ischemic attacks. In: Warlow C, Van Gijn J, Sandercock P, eds. Stroke Module of the Cochrane Database of Systematic Reviews. Oxford: The Cochrane Collaboration, 1999. CD-ROM available from BMJ Publishing Group (London).

21. Hart RG, Pearce LA, Aguilar MI. Adjusted-dose warfarin versus aspirin for preventing stroke in patients with atrial fibrillation. *Ann Intern Med* 2007;**147**:590–92.

22. Stroke Prevention in Atrial Fibrillation Investigators. Warfarin versus aspirin for prevention of thromboembolism in atrial fibrillation. Stroke Prevention in Atrial Fibrillation II Study. *Lancet* 1994;**343**.687–91.

23. Gullov AL, Koefoed BG, Petersen P *et al.* Fixed minidose warfarin and aspirin alone and in combination vs. adjusted-dose warfarin for stroke prevention in atrial fibrillation. Second Copenhagen Atrial Fibrillation, Aspirin, and Anticoagulation Study. *Arch Intern Med* 1998;**158**:1513–21.

24. Hellemons BS, Langenberg M, Lodder J *et al.* Primary prevention of arterial thromboembolism in non-rheumatic atrial fibrillation in primary care: randomized controlled trial comparing two intensities of coumarin with aspirin. *BMJ* 1999;**319**:958–64.

25. Mant J, Hobbs R, Roalfe A *et al.* Warfarin versus aspirin for stroke prevention in an elderly community population with atrial fibrillation (the Birmingham Atrial Fibrillation Treatment of the Aged Study, BAFTA): and randomized controlled trial. *Lancet* 2007;**370**:493–503.

26. Stroke Prevention in Atrial Fibrillation Investigators. Adjusted-dose warfarin versus low-intensity, fixed-dose warfarin plus aspirin for high-risk patients with atrial fibrillation: the Stroke Prevention in Atrial Fibrillation III randomized clinical trial. *Lancet* 1996;**348**:633–8.

27. Pengo V, Zasso A, Barbero F *et al.* Effectiveness of fixed minidose warfarin in the prevention of thromboembolism and vascular death in nonrheumatic atrial fibrillation. *Am J Cardiol* 1998;**82**:433–37.

28. Morocutti C, Amabile G, Fattapposta F *et al.* Indobufen versus warfarin in the secondary prevention of major vascular events in nonrheumatic atrial fibrillation. SIFS (Studio Italiano Fibrillazione Ariale) Investigators. *Stroke* 1997;**28**:1015–21.

29. Lechat P, Lardoux H, Mallet A *et al.* Anticoagulant (fluindione)-aspirin combination in patients with high-risk atrial fibrillation. A randomized trial (Fluindione, Fibrillation Auriculaire, Aspirin et Contraste Spontane; FFAACS). *Cerebrovasc Dis* 2001;**12**:245–52.

30. Perez-Gomez F, Alegria E, Berjon J *et al.* Comparative effects of antiplatelet, anticoagulant, or combined therapy in patients with valvular and nonvalular atrial fibrillation. A randomized multicenter study. *J Am Coll Cardiol* 2004;**44**:1557–66.

31. ACTIVE Writing Group on behalf of the ACTIVE Investigators. Connolly S, Pogue J, Hart R *et al.* Clopidogrel plus aspirin versus oral anticoagulation for atrial fibrillation in the Atrial fibrillation Clopidogrel Trial with Irbesartan for prevention of Vascular Events (ACTIVE W): a randomized controlled trial. *Lancet* 2006;**367**:1903–12.

31a. The ACTIVE Investigators. Effect of clopidogrel added to aspirin in patients with atrial fibrillation. *N Engl J Med* 2009;**360**:2066–78.

32. Executive Steering Committee on behalf of the SPORTIF III Investigators. Stroke prevention with the oral direct thrombin inhibitor ximelagatran compared with warfarin for the prevention of thromboembolism in patients with non-valvular atrial fibrillation (SPORTIF III); a randomized trial. *Lancet* 2003;**362**:1691–8.

33. SPORTIF Executive Steering Committee for the SPORTIF V Investigators. Ximelagatran vs. warfarin for stroke prevention in patients with non-valvular atrial fibrillation. A randomized trial. *JAMA* 2005;**293**:690–8.

34. Kaul S, Diamond GA, Weintraub WS. Trials and tribulations of non-inferiority. The ximelagatran experience. *J Am Coll Cardiol* 2005;**46**:1986–95.

35. Stroke Risk in Atrial Fibrillation Working Group. Independent predictors of stroke in patients with atrial fibrillation. A systematic review. *Neurology* 2007;**69**:546–54.

36. Stroke Prevention in Atrial Fibrillation Investigation. Prevention of thromboembolism in atrial fibrillation: I Clinical features of patients at risk. *Ann Intern Med* 1992;**116**:1–5.

37. Stroke Prevention in Atrial Fibrillation Investigation. Prevention of thromboembolism in atrial fibrillation: II Echocardiographic features of patients at risk. *Ann Intern Med* 1992;**116**:6–12.

38. Gage BF, Waterman AD, Shannon, Boechler M, Rich MW, Radford MJ. Validation of clinical classification schemes for predicting stroke. Results from the National Registry of Atrial Fibrillation. *JAMA* 2001;**285**:2864–70.

39. Gage BF, van Walraven C, Pearce L *et al.* Selecting patients with atrial fibrillation for anticoagulation. Stroke risk stratification in patients taking aspirin. *Circulation* 2004;**110**:2287–92.

40. Hart RG, Pearce LA, Rothbart RM *et al*, for the Stroke Prevention in Atrial Fibrillation Investigators. Stroke with intermittent atrial fibrillation: incidence and predictors during aspirin therapy. *J Am Coll Cardiol* 2000;**35**:183–7.

41. Wyse DG. Anticoagulation in atrial fibrillation: a contemporary viewpoint. *Heart Rhythm* 2007;**4**:S34–S-39.

42. Petersen P, Godtfredsen J. Embolic complications in paroxysmal atrial fibrillation. *Stroke* 1986;**17**:622–6.

43. Wolf PA, Kannel WB, McGee DL *et al.* Duration of atrial fibrillation and eminence of stroke: the Framingham Study. *Stroke* 1983;**14**:664–7.

44. Saxena R, Lewis S, Berge E *et al*, for the International Stroke Trial Collaborative Group. Risk of early death and recurrent stroke and effect of heparin in 3169 patients with acute ischemic stroke and atrial fibrillation in the International Stroke Trial. *Stroke* 2001;**32**:2333–7.

45. Chen ZM, Sandercock P, Pan HC *et al.* Indications for early aspirin use in acute ischemic stroke: a combined analysis of 40 000 randomized patients from the Chinese Acute Stroke Trial and the International Stroke Trial: indications for early aspirin. *Stroke* 2000;**31**:1240–9.

46. Singer DE, Albers GW, Dalen JE, Go AS, Halperin J, Manning WJ. Antithrombotic therapy in atrial fibrillation. *Chest* 2004;**126**:429S-456S.

47. Hylek EM, Singer DE. Risk factors for intracranial hemorrhage in patients taking warfarin. *Ann Intern Med* 1994;**120**:897–902.

48. Fihu SD, Callahan CM, Martin DC *et al.* The risk for and severity of bleeding complications in elderly patients treated with warfarin. *Ann Intern Med* 1996;**124**:970–9.

49. Gage BF, Yan Y, Milligan PE *et al.* Clinical classification schemes for predicting hemorrhage: results from the National Registry of Atrial Fibrillation (NRAF). *Am Heart J* 2006;**151**: 713–19.

50. Waldo AL, Becker RC, Tapson VF, Colgan KJ. Hospitalized patients with atrial fibrillation and a high risk of stroke are not being provided with adequate anticoagulation. *J Am Coll Cardiol* 2005;**46**:1729–36.

51. Rowan SB, Bailey DN, Bublitz CE, Anderson RJ. Trends in anticoagulation for atrial fibrillation in the U.S.: an analysis of the national ambulatory medical care survey database. *J Am Coll Cardiol* 2007;**49**:1561–5.

52. Glazer NL, Dublin S, Smith NL *et al.* Newly detected atrial fibrillation and compliance with antithrombotic guidelines. *Arch Intern Med* 2007;**167**:246–52.

53. Simpson SR, Wilson C, Hannaford PC, Williams D. Evidence for age and sex differences in the secondary prevention of stroke in Scottish primary care. *Stroke* 2005;**36**:1771–5.

54. Hylek EM, D'Antonio J, Evans-Molina C, Shea C, Henault LE, Regan S. Translating the results of randomized trials into clinical

practice: the challenge of warfarin candidacy among hospitalized elderly patients with atrial fibrillation. *Stroke* 2006;**37**: 1075–80.

55. Nieuwlaat R, Capucci A, Lip GYH *et al.* Antithrombotic treatment in real-life atrial fibrillation patients: a report from the Euro Heart Survey on Atrial Fibrillation. *Eur Heart J* 2006;**27**: 3018–26.

56. Hylek EM, Evans-Molina C, Shea C, Henault LE, Regan S. Major hemorrhage and tolerability of warfarin in the first year of therapy among elderly patients with atrial fibrillation. *Circulation* 2007;**115**:2689–96.

57. Wyse DG. Bleeding while starting anticoagulation for thromboembolism prophylaxis in elderly patients with atrial fibrillation. *Circulation* 2007;**115**:2684–86.

58. Hylek EM, Go AS, Chang Y *et al.* Effect of intensity of oral anticoagulation on stroke severity and mortality in atrial fibrillation. *N Engl J Med* 2003;**349**:1019–26.

59. Oake N, Fergusson DA, Forster AJ, van Walraven C. Frequency of adverse events in patients with poor anticoagulation: a meta-analysis. *Can Med Assoc J* 2007;**176**:1589–94.

60. European Atrial Fibrillation Trial Study Group. Optimal oral anticoagulant therapy in patients with nonrheumatic atrial fibrillation and recent cerebral ischemia. *N Engl J Med* 1995;**333**:5–10.

61. Pelargonio G, Prystowsky EN. Rate versus rhythm control in the management of patients with atrial fibrillation. *Nature Clin Prac* 2005;**2**:514–21.

62. de Denus S, Sanoski CA, Carlsson J, Opolski G, Spinler SA. Rate vs. rhythm control in patients with atrial fibrillation: a meta-analysis. *Arch Intern Med* 2005;**165**:258–62.

63. Wyse DG, Waldo AL, DiMarco JP *et al.* A comparison of rate control and rhythm control in patients with atrial fibrillation. *N Engl J Med* 2002;**347**:1825–33.

64. Stroke Risk in Atrial Fibrillation Working Group. Comparison of 12 risk stratification schemes to predict stroke in patients with non-valvular atrial fibrillation. *Stroke* 2008;**39**:1901–10.

64a. The International Warfarin Pharmacogenetics Consortium. Estimation of the warfarin dose with clinical and pharmacogenetic data. *N Engl J Med* 2009;**360**:753–64.

65. Bjerkelund CJ, Orning OM. The efficacy of anticoagulant therapy in preventing embolism related to DC electrical conversion of atrial fibrillation. *Am J Cardiol* 1969;**23**:208.

66. Collins LJ, Silverman DI, Douglas PS, Manning WJ. Cardioversion of nonrheumatic atrial fibrillation: reduced thromboembolic complications with 4 weeks of precardioversion anticoagulation are related to atrial thrombus resolution. *Circulation* 1995;**92**:160–3.

67. Berger M, Schweitzer P. Timing of thromboembolic events after electrical cardioversion of atrial fibrillation or flutter: a retrospective analysis. *Am J Cardiol* 1998;**82**:1545–7, A8.

68. Manning WJ, Leeman DE, Gotch PJ *et al.* Pulsed Doppler evaluation of atrial mechanical function after electrical cardioversion of atrial fibrillation. *J Am Coll Cardiol* 1989;**13**:617–23.

69. Padraig GO, Puleo PR, Bolli R *et al.* Return of atrial mechanical function following electrical cardioversion of atrial dysrhythmias. *Am Heart J* 1990;**120**:353–9.

70. Manning WJ, Silverman DI, Keightly CS *et al.* Transesophageal echocardiographically facilitated early cardioversion from atrial fibrillation using short-term anticoagulation – final results of a prospective 4.5 year study. *J Am Coll Cardiol* 1995;**25**: 1354–61.

71. Black IW, Falkin D, Sagar KB *et al.* Exclusion of atrial thrombus by transesophageal echocardiography does not preclude embolism after cardioversion of atrial fibrillation: a multicenter study. *Circulation* 1994;**89**:2509–13.

72. Moreyra E, Finkelhor RS, Debul RD. Limitations of transesophageal echocardiography in the risk assessment of patients before nonanticoagulated cardioversion from atrial fibrillation and flutter: an analysis of pooled trials. *Am Heart J* 1995; **129**:71–5.

73. Klein AL, Grimm RA, Black IW *et al.* Cardioversion guided by transesophageal echocardiography: the ACUTE Pilot Study. *Ann Intern Med* 1997;**126**:200–9.

74. Klein AL, Grimm RA, Murray RD *et al.* Use of transesophageal echocardiography to guide cardioversion in patients with atrial fibrillation. *N Engl J Med* 2001;**344**:1411–20.

75. Biblo LA, Yuan Z, Quan KJ, Mackall JA, Rimm AA. Risk of stroke in patients with atrial flutter. *Am J Cardiol* 2001;**87**:346–9.

76. Gallagher MM, Hennessy BJ, Edvardsson N *et al.* Embolic complications of direct current cardioversion of atrial arrhythmias: association with low intensity of anticoagulation at the time of cardioversion. *J Am Coll Cardiol* 2002;**40**:926–33.

77. Elhendy A, Gentile F, Khandheria BK *et al.* Thromboembolic complications after electrical cardioversion in patients with atrial flutter. *Am J Med* 2001;**111**:433–8.

78. Antman EM, Hand M, Armstrong PW *et al.* 2007 focused update of the ACC/AHA 2004 guidelines for the management of patients with ST-elevation myocardial infarction. *Circulation* 2008;**117**;296–329.

79. Harrington RA, Becker RC, Ezekowitz M *et al.* Antithrombotic therapy for coronary artery disease. *Chest* 2004;**126**:513S-548S.

80. Stenestrand U, Lindback JL, Wallentin L, for the RIKS-HIA Registry. Anticoagulation therapy in atrial fibrillation in combination with acute myocardial infarction influences long-term outcome. A prospective cohort study for the Register of Information and Knowledge about Swedish Heart Intensive Care Admissions. *Circulation* 2005;**112**:3225–31.

81. King SB, Smith SC, Hirshfeld JW *et al.* 2007 focused update of the ACC/AHA/SCAI 2005 guideline update for percutaneous coronary intervention. *Circulation* 2008;**117**:261–95.

82. Kearon C, Hirsh J. Management of anticoagulation before and after elective surgery. *N Engl J Med* 1997;**336**:1506–11.

83. Patatanian E, Fugate SE. Hemostatic mouthwashes in anticoagulated patients undergoing dental extraction. *Ann Pharmacother* 2006;**40**:2205–10.

38 Ablation therapy for atrial fibrillation

Conor D Barrett,[1] Chi Keong Ching,[2] Luigi Di Biase,[3] Claude S Elayi,[4]
David J Burkhardt,[3] Rodney Horton[3] and Andrea Natale[3]

[1] Cardiac Arrhythmia Service, Massachusetts General Hospital Heart Center, Boston, MA, USA
[2] Department of Cardiology, National Heart Centre Singapore, Singapore
[3] Texas Cardiac Arrhythmia Institute, St David's Medical Center, Austin, TX, USA
[4] Division of Cardiovascular Medicine, Gill Heart Institute, University of Kentucky, Lexington, KY, USA

Introduction

The past decade has witnessed major advances in the treatment of atrial fibrillation (AF). Following the seminal observations of Haissaguerre et al[1] who recognized the importance of the role of ectopic beats from the pulmonary veins (PVs) in the initiation of AF, percutaneous catheter ablation has evolved as a curative therapy and has been effective in maintaining sinus rhythm in patients with paroxysmal AF. The purpose of this chapter is to discuss the role of ablative therapy and those trials which compare ablation to pharmacologic therapy or to the "ablate and pace" strategy. Because of its necessarily invasive nature, a description is also given of reported complications and studies which have applied strategies to quantify and prevent them.

Advantages of rhythm control

The main advantage in maintaining sinus rhythm is the relief of symptoms. A significant number of patients with AF complain of palpitations, dizziness, fatigue or dyspnea. Contributory factors include lack of atrial contraction, a rapid ventricular rate, an irregular ventricular rhythm and a reduced cardiac output. In patients with poor ventricular rate control in atrial fibrillation, symptoms of congestive heart failure may result from tachycardia-mediated cardiomyopathy.

In patients with valvular disease (for example, mitral stenosis) or those with a less compliant left ventricle (for example, those with left ventricular hypertrophy), the absence of co-ordinated atrial mechanical activity may result in a reduction in ventricular preload and a consequent reduction in cardiac output. The more rapid heart rates further impair ventricular filling by shortening diastolic filling time. Even in patients with controlled ventricular rates, irregular R-R intervals are associated with a 15% reduction in cardiac output.[2] Effective rhythm control thus aims to restore normal atrial function, increase ventricular preload and slow the ventricular rate, thereby enhancing cardiac output. These improvements in hemodynamics lead to increased exercise tolerance.[3] Other benefits of the maintenance of sinus rhythm include avoidance of tachycardia-induced cardiomyopathy,[4] a possible reduction of embolic risk and a potential decrease in mortality.

A few large clinical trials have been published comparing treatment strategies for AF. In particular, the AF Follow-up Investigation of Rhythm Management (AFFIRM),[5] Rate Control versus Electrical cardioversion for AF (RACE)[6] and Strategies for Treatment of AF (STAF)[7] trials compared rate control and rhythm control approaches using antiarrhythmic drugs (AADs). For a full discussion of these trials see Chapter 35. Adopting an intention-to-treat analysis, these trials concluded that there was no mortality difference between the two approaches. Hence, for the type of patients enrolled, a rate control approach may be adequate treatment for AF when compared with a rhythm control strategy with AADs.

However, it would be incorrect to extrapolate that sinus rhythm offers no benefit over AF. The aforementioned trials were not comparisons of sinus rhythm with AF. They compared a rate control strategy to a pharmacologic rhythm control strategy with AADs which was only poorly effective. When the data in the AFFIRM trial were analyzed according to the patient's actual rhythm, the benefit of sinus rhythm over AF became apparent. In a subgroup analysis by Scott et al, the presence of sinus rhythm was one of the most powerful independent predictors of survival, along with the use of warfarin, even after adjustment for all other relevant clinical variables.[8] Patients in sinus rhythm were almost half as likely to die compared with those with AF (adjusted hazard ratio 0.53; 99% confidence interval (CI) 0.39–0.72; $P < 0.0001$). This benefit was offset

Evidence-Based Cardiology, 3rd edition. Edited by S. Yusuf, J.A. Cairns, A.J. Camm, E.L. Fallen, and B.J. Gersh. © 2010 Blackwell Publishing, ISBN: 978-1-4051-5925-8.

apparently by the use of AAD therapy, which may have increased the risk of death. Of note, these trials largely excluded highly symptomatic patients who might benefit most from sinus rhythm.

Inadequacy of non-ablative rhythm control

The failure of AFFIRM, RACE or STAF trials to show any difference between rate and rhythm control strategies is perhaps a testament to the ineffectiveness of the rhythm control strategies that were used. The main modalities for non-ablative rhythm control are AADs and device-based therapy. Meta-analysis of randomized trials looking at the efficacy of AADs showed that up to 32% of the placebo arm patients were in sinus rhythm, compared to 55% of the patients who were assigned to receive ADD therapy.[9]

Evidently, AADs do not reliably cure AF but serve to reduce the burden of AF in some patients. Even in patients who were able to maintain sinus rhythm while on AADs, debilitating side effects were not uncommon in the published trials. Of the AADs, amiodarone had the highest success rate in maintaining sinus rhythm. However, the side-effect profile of amiodarone led to its discontinuation in up to 30% of patients due to intolerable skin discoloration, pulmonary fibrosis, thyroid dysfunction, neurologic or ophthalmic disorders.[10]

Device-based therapy has demonstrated poor efficacy for the treatment of AF. Antitachycardia devices can deliver burst atrial pacing and may convert atrial tachycardia or atrial flutter to sinus rhythm but such rapid pacing usually fails to terminate AF.[11] Atrial defibrillators can terminate AF with a high success rate.[12] However, repeated shocks lead to patient discomfort, making this option intolerable for the majority of patients. Dual site and overdrive atrial pacing,[13] which were expected to be beneficial, have failed to demonstrate consistent reduction in AF burden or improvement in AF symptoms.

Another option for patients who have AF with ventricular rates that are uncontrolled despite maximum tolerated AV nodal blocking agents is the so-called "ablate and pace strategy." The PABA-CHF trial (Pulmonary vein antrum isolation vs AV Node ABlation with Bi-ventricular pacing for Atrial Fibrillation in Congestive Heart Failure), which is currently in press, compared such a strategy to pulmonary vein isolation. This trial is discussed below in the section on randomized controlled trials.

Catheter ablation of atrial fibrillation

Pulmonary vein isolation (PVI), or radiofrequency (RF) ablation for AF directly eliminates or isolates the initiating factors for AF and offers the possibility of a "cure" without subjecting the patient to the side effects of AADs. It is well established that the pulmonary veins play a major role in triggering and maintaining AF. Haissaguerre et al[1,14] demonstrated that up to 94% of patients had triggers in one or more pulmonary vein (PV). Sites outside the pulmonary veins may trigger AF in 6–10% of patients.[15,16]

AF has also been reported to be maintained by micro re-entrant circuits ("rotors") that exhibit high frequency and periodic activity, from which spiral wavefronts of activation radiate into the surrounding atrial tissue.[17] Of interest, the dominant rotors in AF are localized primarily in the pulmonary vein-left atrium (PV-LA) region.[18] Vagal inputs may also be important in both triggering and maintaining AF; many of these inputs are clustered close to the PV-LA junction.[19]

The primary goal of radiofrequency catheter ablation for AF is to electrically disconnect the PVs from the rest of the atrium by ablating around the atrial aspect of the veins. Most centers worldwide, regardless of further adjunctive ablation strategies, recognize that PVI is of the foremost importance in AF ablation. The inhomogeneity of left atrial and LA antral anatomy poses significant challenges in PV isolation. The PV is a "funnel-shaped" structure with a large proximal end, known as the antrum. The antrum of each PV blends into the posterior wall of the LA. In order to maximize success and minimize the complication of PV stenosis it is advisable for ablation to be performed around the entire antrum at the posterior left atrial wall.

Most centers performing AF ablation are ablating at the PV antrum and not at the true PV ostium, thus minimizing the risk of PV stenosis. Different centers may refer to ablation at the antrum by various names such as LA catheter ablation, circumferential PV antrum isolation or extraostial isolation. The lesion sets produced by these various approaches are very similar. A typical PV isolation RF ablation lesion set is shown in Plate 38.1.

Randomized controlled trials of catheter ablation for atrial fibrillation

There are five published randomized controlled trials comparing RF ablation with pharmacologic treatment. The sixth published randomized controlled trial compared ablation with no other treatment after patients had undergone prior treatment with amiodarone and direct current (DC) cardioversion. These six published trials are summarized in Table 38.1. Another trial was presented in 2006 but is not yet published. One further trial (in press) compared outcomes in patients with refractory AF who underwent ablation with those who underwent an "ablate and BiV-pace" procedure. At least four further multicenter, randomized trials are in the recruitment stages: AATAC-HF (Ablation v Amiodarone for Treatment of Atrial Fibrillation in patients with Congestive Heart Failure and an implanted ICD/CRTD), CASTLE-AF (Catheter Ablation versus STandard conventional treatment in heart failure patients with Left ventricular dysfunction and Atrial Fibrillation), RAAFT-2 (first line Radiofrequency Ablation versus Antiarrhythmic drugs for Atrial Fibrillation Treatment) and CABANA (Catheter ABlation versus ANtiarrhythmic drug therapy for Atrial Fibrillation – pilot trial).

In a study published in 2003, Krittayaphong et al[20] reported on 30 patients with long-standing AF who did not respond satisfactorily to drug treatment. These patients were randomized to treatment with amiodarone (n = 15) or RF ablation (n = 15) and were followed up for 1 year. In the ablation arm, the patients underwent PVI and further ablation in the right atrium. The study reported that freedom from AF was better in the RF ablation group (78.6%) as compared to the amiodarone group (40%) (P = 0.018). There was also a difference in favor of the RF ablation group in terms of subjective measurements of symptoms relating to AF and quality of life. Amiodarone was not observed to have a significant effect on symptoms of AF or quality of life in this study. In the RF ablation group, one patient suffered a stroke. Amiodarone was associated with adverse effects in 47% of patients, necessitating discontinuation in one patient. The authors concluded that RF ablation was an effective alternative treatment in patients with long-standing AF refractory to medical therapy.

Wazni et al[21] studied 70 patients (RAAFT pilot study), 67 with paroxysmal and three with persistent AF. None of the included patients had previously been treated for AF; therefore each patient's allotted treatment was the first-line treatment for that individual. Patients were randomized to receive either PVI using RF ablation (n = 33) or antiarrhythmic drug treatment (n = 37), with a 1-year follow-up. At the end of 1-year follow-up, 63% of patients who received antiarrhythmic drugs had at least one recurrence of symptomatic AF compared with 13% of patients who received PVI (P < 0.001). There were significantly decreased hospitalization rates and improved quality of life measurements in the PVI group. In the antiarrhythmic drug group, the mean number of AF episodes decreased from 12 to six, after initiating therapy. In the ablation group there was one asymptomatic PV stenosis and no severe PV stenosis. There was no thromboembolic event in either group. There was a higher rate of documented bradycardia in the AAD group, occurring in 9% of patients. Overall, the authors concluded that PVI may be a feasible first-line approach for treating patients with symptomatic AF. This is the only published trial to date comparing outcomes in patients who were AAD naïve at the time of recruitment.

Stabile et al[22] (CACAF, Catheter Ablation for the Cure of Atrial Fibrillation study) studied 137 patients with both paroxysmal and persistent AF in whom treatment with

AAD had already been unsuccessful. Patients were randomized to continue their current drug regimen (n = 69) or to continue medications and additionally undergo RF ablation (n = 68). RF ablation involved PVI, ablation of the cavotricuspid isthmus and ablation from the left inferior pulmonary vein to the mitral valve (mitral isthmus). The follow-up period was 13 months, including a 1-month blanking period. The primary endpoint of the study was the absence of any documented recurrence of atrial arrhythmia lasting >30 s in the 1-year follow-up period, following the blanking period. After completion of follow-up, 91% of patients in the non-ablation group had at least one recurrence compared to 44% (P < 0.001) of patients in the ablation group. Of the recurrences in the ablation group, four patients developed an atrial flutter and 26 had recurrence of atrial fibrillation. The success observed in the ablation group must, of course, be viewed in terms of observed complications. In the ablation group there was a major complication rate of 4.4%. Complications were due to a stroke in one patient, a pericardial effusion requiring pericardiocentesis in one patient and transient diaphragmatic paralysis in one further patient. No pulmonary vein stenosis was reported. In the AAD group one patient suffered sudden death, one patient had a transient ischemic attack and two died from cancer. Comparing the median per patient number of hospitalizations in the 1 year of follow-up between the two groups, no statistically significant difference was observed between the ablation and control groups. It was concluded that ablation therapy combined with antiarrhythmic drug therapy is superior to antiarrhythmic drug therapy alone in preventing atrial arrhythmia recurrences in patients with paroxysmal or persistent AF in whom antiarrhythmic drug therapy had already failed.

Pappone et al[23] (APAF, Ablation for Paroxysmal Atrial Fibrillation trial) randomized 198 patients with paroxysmal AF who had previously failed AAD therapy. The patients included in this study had a longer history of paroxysmal AF with a mean of 6 ± 5 years. These patients were randomized to circumferential PV ablation (n = 99) or to medical treatment (n = 99) with the maximum tolerated dose of amiodarone, flecainide or sotalol, either as single drug or in combination. Analysis was performed according to the intention-to-treat principle. Of note, 42 of 99 patients who were randomized to drug treatment crossed over and received catheter ablation, which was permitted under the study protocol after 3 months of therapy. All patients received warfarin and were followed for 12 months. In the RF ablation group, a repeat ablation was performed in 9% of patients; this was for atrial tachycardia (3%) and AF (6%). At the completion of follow-up, 86% of patients in the RF ablation group and 22% in the AAD group who did not require a second AAD were free from recurrent AF or atrial tachycardia (P < 0.001). Amiodarone was, overall, administered to 61 patients in the group, either alone or in combination with flecainide. Based on intention-to-treat analysis, after 1 year of follow-up, 93% of the RF ablation group and 35% of the AAD group were free of all atrial tachyarrhythmias ($P < 0.01$). However, there was a high rate of crossover from the AAD arm to the RF ablation arm, with 42% of patients crossing over to the RF ablation arm. One transient ischemic attack and one pericardial effusion occurred in the RF ablation group. Side effects leading to drug withdrawal were observed in 23 patients in the AAD group; they included thyroid dysfunction (seven patients receiving amiodarone), 1:1 atrial flutter or a wide complex tachycardia (three patients receiving flecainide), and sexual dysfunction (11 patients receiving sotalol). The authors concluded that RF ablation was more successful than AADs for prevention of paroxysmal AF, with an observed low complication rate in the RF ablation group.

Oral et al[24] reported on 146 patients with persistent AF who were randomized to either RF ablation or medical management. The study was designed such that all patients, regardless of randomized group, received amiodarone for the initial 6 weeks after recruitment. Patients assigned to RF ablation then underwent PVI and had amiodarone continued for a further 3 months following ablation. Patients in the control group, who did not convert to SR on amiodarone therapy, underwent up to two direct current cardioversions in the first 3 months and continued amiodarone for 3 months following cardioversion. Those who reverted to AF after this time in the control group were permitted to resume therapy with amiodarone or cross over to RF ablation. Analysis was by the intention-to-treat principle. There were 77 patients included in the RF ablation arm and 69 in the control arm. A second ablation procedure was performed in 32% of patients in the RF group because of recurrence of AF (26%) or emergence of an atypical atrial flutter (6%) following the initial RF ablation procedure. By the intention-to-treat analysis at the end of 1-year follow-up, 74% of patients in the RF ablation group and 58% of those in the non-ablation group were free of atrial tachyarrhythmias in the absence of AAD therapy. There was, however, a very high crossover rate observed. Of the 69 patients in the non-ablation group, 77% (53 patients) crossed over to undergo RF ablation for recurrent AF within 1 year. Of those in the control group who were not on AAD therapy or did not undergo RF ablation at the end of 1 year, only 4% were in sinus rhythm. The authors reported no observed procedure- or AAD-related complications, with the exception of the 6% of patients who developed atrial flutter following RF ablation. The authors concluded that RF ablation offers a good strategy for maintenance of sinus rhythm for the majority of patients with symptomatic persistent AF, independent of long-term AAD use.

The results of these six trials were pooled in a recent meta-analysis,[25] giving a total of 578 randomized patients. This analysis has to be viewed with the knowledge that there was heterogeneity in patients included, AF patterns and treatment strategies among the different published trials. Nonetheless, it was observed that compared to presence or absence of AAD therapy, RF ablation was more effective in preventing AF recurrence. Following 1-year follow-up, AF was present in 72 of the 291 patients (25%) who underwent RF ablation. This compared to 193 of 287 patients (67%) in those who were not assigned to undergo RF ablation. It is noteworthy that RF ablation was the better treatment in all six studies, whether they included patients with paroxysmal, persistent or "permanent" atrial fibrillation. Also, RF ablation resulted in better rates of sinus rhythm at 1 year in those patients who had previously failed AAD and in those who had not undergone prior treatment with AAD therapy.

Another trial, the Ablation versus AntiArrhythmic drugs for Atrial fibrillation [A4] trial, was presented in 2006.[26] This multicenter, international trial randomized 59 patients to AAD therapy and 53 patients to RF ablation, after having failed treatment with at least one class I or class III AAD. All patients had symptomatic paroxysmal AF of at least 6 months' duration. Follow-up entailed ambulatory ECG monitoring at 2, 3, 6 and 12 months, as well as monitoring for patient symptoms. The primary endpoint of this study was recurrence of AF of a duration greater than 3 minutes, after a 3-month blanking period from initiation of AAD therapy or ablation. After 3 months, crossover was permitted and in fact 37 patients in the AAD arm crossed over to the RF arm by the end of the study. Repeat ablation and multiple AAD trials were permitted in the first 3 months. Patients randomized to the ablation arm underwent a mean of 1.8 ablations. At the completion of the study, after 1 year of follow-up, 75% of patients in the RF ablation group and 7% of patients in the AAD therapy group were free of atrial arrhythmia. The best outcomes in the AAD group were observed in those patients who received amiodarone for the first time, with 25% being free of AF at 1 year. This still was inferior to the observed results in the RF ablation group. Complications referable to RF ablation included cardiac tamponade (n = 2), pulmonary vein stenosis (n = 1), and groin hematomas (n = 2). In patients treated with AADs, one patient developed hyperthyroidism and one died unrelated to therapy, due to cancer. This trial, in similarity to the published trials, supported the use of RF ablation for patients with symptomatic AF over the use of AADs.

Another strategy (the "ablate and pace" strategy) has been used in patients with symptomatic AF in whom it has not been possible to control ventricular rates. The procedure involves ablation of the AV junction and implantation of a pacemaker, thus avoiding rapid ventricular rates in atrial fibrillation. This historically has involved implantation of a right ventricular pacemaker lead with or without (for patients with "permanent" atrial fibrillation) implantation of an atrial lead. Such patients, following successful AV junction ablation, will become pacemaker dependent with chronic right ventricular pacing. This can have a deleterious effect; in patients in SR this has been shown to increase the likelihood of hospitalization for heart failure and death.[27]

The OPSITE trial (Optimal Pacing SITE) examined the role of RV, LV and BiV pacing in patients who had undergone AV junction ablation for permanent AF after failure of drug treatment.[28] The primary endpoints were exercise capacity and quality of life. Compared to RV pacing, this study demonstrated no significant improvement with LV-only pacing and a modest improvement with BiV pacing.

Subsequent to this, the PAVE trial (left ventricular-based cardiac stimulation Post AV nodal Ablation Evaluation) was published by Doshi et al.[29] This was a prospective, randomized, multicenter, patient-blinded trial comparing RV pacing with BiV pacing in patients who had undergone AV junction ablation for persistent AF which was refractory to medical management. The primary endpoints were change in quality of life, change in the 6-minute walk test and change in LV ejection fraction (LVEF) at the end of 6 months' follow-up. At the end of the study there was no significant difference in quality of life, but there were modest but significant differences in LVEF and 6-minute walk distance. The largest benefit in terms of change in the 6-minute walk distance was observed in patients who had pre-existing LVEF <45% or NYHA class II–III symptoms as compared to those with normal LVEF or NYHA class I symptoms.

Following publication of these trials, the question arose as to whether RF ablation for AF (PVI) would prove superior to the best available "ablate and pace" strategy in patients with pre-existing heart failure and LV systolic dysfunction. The PABA-CHF trial was a prospective, international multicenter study which included patients with systolic heart failure (LVEF ≤ 40% and NYHA class II–III) and symptomatic AF which had proven to be drug unresponsive. Patients with both paroxysmal and persistent AF were included and were then randomized to undergo either PVI or AV junction ablation with biventricular pacing (AVJA-BiV). Patients in the PVI group who were still in AF at 3 months underwent a further RF ablation procedure. Patients were followed up over 6 months with clinical measurements, echocardiograms and monitoring for both symptomatic and asymptomatic episodes of AF recurrence. The primary endpoint was a composite of LVEF, 6-minute walk distance and the Minnesota Living with Heart Failure (MLWHF) score at 6 months.[30]

Of the 81 patients included, 41 underwent PVI (49% paroxysmal), 40 underwent AVJA-BiV (54% paroxysmal) and follow-up data were available on all. The trial reached its primary composite endpoint favoring the PVI group as compared to the AVJA-BiV group. There were improvements favoring the PVI group in the prespecified composites at 6 months, including the MLWHF score (61 v 79, $P < 0.0001$), longer 6-minute walk distances (340 v 297 m, $P = 0.0002$) and higher LVEF (35% v 28%, $P = 0.0001$). After 6 months of follow-up of patients who had undergone PVI, 88% were free of AF while maintained on AADs and 71% were free of AF without AAD therapy. Other relative measures of improvement in the PVI group, as compared to the AVJA-BiV group, included improvement in LA size (4.5 v 4.9 cm, $P = 0.003$) and less progression of AF severity (0% v 32%, $P < 0.0001$). There were no major complications or mortalities in either group. In the RF ablation group, there were three groin hematomas, one pericardial effusion, two asymptomatic mild PV stenoses and one incidence of pulmonary edema. In the AVJA-BiV group there were two cases of generator pocket hematoma, one pneumothorax, two LV lead dislodgments and two cases of high LV lead capture thresholds at follow-up. The authors concluded that, in patients with heart failure and depressed LVEF who have atrial fibrillation, treatment with PVI as compared to AVJA-BiV resulted in improvements in quality of life (as measured by the MLWHF tool), 6-minute walk test, LVEF and LA dimensions. This was achieved without the inherent pacemaker dependence which follows AV junction ablation. The PABA-CHF study adds support to the use of PVI for systolic heart failure patients with drug-refractory AF.

Non-randomized trials of atrial fibrillation ablation in patient subgroups

Apart from the PABA-CHF trial, there are no randomized trials in the cardiomyopathy subpopulations of patients with AF. However, there are some published data which do offer some insight and are at least hypothesis generating. In patients with congestive heart failure, studies have been published which suggest that PVI has a positive effect on LVEF, with an improvement from $42 \pm 9\%$ to $56 \pm 8\%$ observed in one study.[31] Tondo et al also noted significant improvement in LVEF (from $33 \pm 2\%$ to $47 \pm 3\%$) following RF ablation for AF.[32] Significant improvements in quality of life measures were observed in another study as reported by Chen et al.[33] A non-significant improvement in LVEF was observed in this study. Hsu et al first reported significant improvements in LVEF (of $21 \pm 13\%$), symptoms, quality of life measures and exercise capacity in patients with congestive heart failure and documented depressed LV systolic function.[34] Similar findings have also been reported in a smaller study[35] (Table 38.1).

Another well-recognized group of patients who are susceptible to the development of AF are those with hypertrophic cardiomyopathy (HCM). Medical treatment of AF in

Table 38.1 Randomized controlled trials of ablation

Trial	AF type	Prior AAD treatment	Number of patients	RF ablation patients	Control patients	Control	Follow-up (months)	AF free RFA (%)	AF free control (%)	P value
Krittayaphong et al[20]	Persistent	Yes	30	15	15	AAD	12	78.6	40	0.018
Wazni et al[21]*	Paroxysmal	No	70	33	37	AAD	12	87	13	<0.001
Stabile et al[22]**	All	Yes	137	68	69	AAD	13	55.9	8.7	<0.001
Pappone et al[23]	Paroxysmal	Yes	198	99	99	AAD	12	93	35	<0.01
Oral et al[24]***	Persistent	Yes	146	77	69	AAD/none	12	74	58	0.05
Jais et al[26]****	Paroxysmal	Yes	112	53	59	AAD	12	75	7	<0.001

* There were 63 patients with paroxysmal AF and 3 with persistent AF.

** Patients in the RF group also continued AAD treatment throughout the study.

*** Crossover to RF from the control arm was permitted after 3 months. There was a high rate of crossover; 77% of patients crossed over by the end of the study. The tabulated results are an intention-to-treat analysis. In the control arm, 3 (4%) patients were in SR in the absence of AAD therapy or RF ablation.

**** Crossover to RF from the control arm was permitted after 3 months.

AF, atrial fibrillation; AAD, antiarrhythmic drug (see text for details); RF, radiofrequency.

this population can be quite difficult. Again, no randomized data are available in this subpopulation but results of two studies suggest a promising role for catheter ablation in this group of patients. It is not surprising that the reported success rates are not as high as those reported in patients without HCM. In one series of 27 patients with HCM undergoing RF ablation for AF, a success rate of 70% was observed, seven of the patients having required a second ablation procedure.[36] Another study, in 33 patients, observed a success rate of 62% in returning patients to SR following RF ablation in patients with AF and HCM.[37]

All of these studies have several limitations including the small sample size, the enrollment of selected groups of patients, being performed either in a single center or in institutions with highly experienced operators. In addition, many of the consecutive series originated from centers with exceptional experience and the observed success and complication rates might not reflect what could be achieved in less specialized institutions.

Complications of catheter ablation of atrial fibrillation

Extensive ablation within the atria coupled with instrumentation with various catheters in the setting of aggressive anticoagulation during RF ablation sets the stage for potential complications. Nonetheless, overall complication rates are relatively low. A variety of these complications have been reported. While the majority occurred during or within 48 hours of the procedure, some are known to have an insidious course with a relatively late presentation. This section reviews the published literature on these complications so that they can be prevented or diagnosed accurately and treated appropriately if they do occur.

Cerebrovascular events

The incidence of thromboembolism in AF ablation ranges from 0.5% to 2.8%.[38] A worldwide survey reported cerebral thromboembolism in 67 patients (20 strokes and 47 transient ischemic attacks) out of 7154 patients who underwent left atrial instrumentation for ablation of AF.[39] Prevention remains the best strategy for reducing thromboembolic events during AF ablation. Continuation of warfarin in its therapeutic range throughout the periprocedural period has recently proved to be a safe alternative to bridging with enoxaparin or heparin, which have been demonstrated to increase the risk of procedure-related bleeding.[40]

PV stenosis

The incidence of PV stenosis, defined as >70% narrowing, was reported to occur in 3.4% of patients in one series.[41] The pathogenesis of PV stenosis is probably due to initial ablation too close to the true PV ostium, which precipitates a healing reaction culminating in proliferation of the elastic lamina/intima. The incidence of PV stenosis has decreased as a result of PV isolation at the antrum, which is a considerable distance from the true PV ostia. With this technique in one study, the incidence of PV stenosis was found to be 0.9% (16 out of 1780 patients).[42] The clinical presentation of these patients was variable and included no symptoms, mild dyspnea to severe dyspnea with hemoptysis, fever, and pleuritic chest pain. An algorithm was devised to calculate the cumulative stenosis index (CSI) which is the sum of percentage stenosis of the ipsilateral veins divided by the total number of ipsilateral veins. The study concluded that patients with a CSI ≥75% and a relative lung perfusion of ≤25% have the greatest risk of severe symptoms and lung diseases. In these patients, early and, when required, repeated PV intervention (with venoplasty and/or stenting) should be considered for improvement of pulmonary blood flow and prevention of associated lung disease.

Esophageal injury and fistula

The posterior wall of the LA is adjacent to the esophagus. RF ablation procedures may substantially elevate the temperature at the LA–esophageal interface and may be observed within the esophageal lumen.[43] Atrio-esophageal fistulas may then result from thermal injury leading to tissue necrosis and fistula formation between the posterior LA and esophagus. A report of three patients with this complication after percutaneous RF ablation in experienced centers was published in 2004 [44,45]

Via an anonymous volunteer reporting method, a series of nine patients who had this complication was later reported.[46] A variety of clinical presentations occurred within 2 weeks of the ablation procedures, including neurologic findings consistent with multiple embolic strokes (with intravascular gas on CT), endocarditis, chest pain associated with ST segment elevation, and gastrointestinal bleeding. All nine patients developed septic shock and died; autopsy confirmed the presence of atrio-esophageal fistula.

Although the incidence of atrio-esophageal fistula is rare, it is almost always fatal. Recently, a case of successful temporary esophageal stenting to seal off an esophageal perforation following LA catheter ablation was reported.[47]

Continuous monitoring of esophageal temperature may be an option to enhance safety during posterior LA wall ablation. Alternative strategies in avoiding esophageal injury during AF ablation include empirically decreasing the power delivered and duration of lesions when ablating on the posterior LA wall, pre-procedure ingestion of Gastrograffin dye, tagging the esophagus on a three-dimensional electroanatomic mapping system and merging a three-dimensional recreated image of the esophagus with an electroanatomic map of the LA.

Organized atrial tachyarrhythmias

Organized left atrial tachyarrhythmia (OLAT) following segmental or wide area circumferential PVI and LA circumferential ablation with additional linear ablation has been variably reported as ranging from 2.5% to 27%. The mechanism of these OLATs has been described as macro re-entry, micro re-entry and "focal." The macro re-entry OLATs are most often due to re-entry mediated by gaps in linear ablation lines. Such a gap functions as a slowly conducting isthmus in the re-entry circuit, commonly located at the LA roof, posterior wall or mitral isthmus.

These macro re-entry OLATs are often symptomatic, necessitating a repeat ablation. On the other hand, focal OLATs typically originate from PV ostial or antral regions that have partially recovered conduction to the LA. Of note, centers that adopt a strategy of wide area circumferential PV ablation and linear LA ablations[48,49] appear to experience an increased prevalence of OLATs. This demonstrates that the inability to create contiguous linear lesions and/or recovery of partial conduction along such lesions can be proarrhythmic. An example of an OLAT (later shown to be due to macro re-entry) and the electroanatomic map are shown in Figure 38.1 and Plates 38.2 and 38.3.

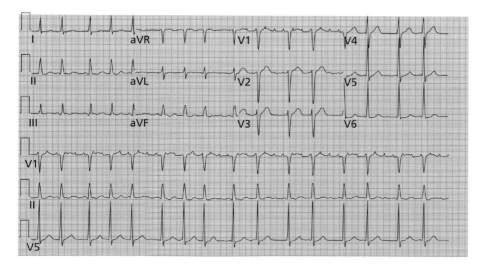

Figure 38.1 Atypical flutter in a patient following previous RF ablation for atrial fibrillation. A 12-lead ECG of a patient who was highly symptomatic of an atypical atrial flutter which occurred months following a PVI procedure.

Phrenic nerve injury

During RF ablation for AF, phrenic nerve (PN) injury may occur when isolating the superior vena cava (SVC) from the right atrium or the right superior pulmonary vein from the left atrium. A series of 17 patients who sustained PN injury following catheter ablation or AF, inappropriate sinus tachycardia or ventricular tachycardia with a variety of energy sources including RF ablation (13 patients), cryo-ablation (one patient), ultrasound balloon ablation (two patients) and laser balloon ablation (one patient) has been reported.[50] All patients recovered within a median time of 6 months.

Needless to say, the most effective way to prevent PNI is to deliver RF energy away from the PN. Too close a proximity to the PN can be demonstrated by high-output pacing at the proposed region of ablation where PN capture occurs. Ablation at these regions is not advisable. Preabla-tion pacing at the level of the PV antrum (as far as feasible from the PV ostia) or the SVC–RA junction when perform-ing isolation of these veins for AF could represent a poten-tial strategy to minimize the risk of PN injury. A novel method of protecting the PN during epicardial catheter ablation, by using a balloon catheter in the pericardial space to mechanically separate the left PN from the abla-tion catheter, has been recently reported.[51] Early recogni-tion of transient PN injury by fluoroscopy during RF ablation may result in fewer cases of persistent injury.

Other complications

Other complications include air embolism, cardiac tam-ponade, mitral valve damage and rare instances of acute pyloric spasm and gastric hypomotility observed following posterior LA lesions.[52] In summary, the short-term safety with newer ablation techniques has improved, but serious and potentially life-threatening complications persist.

Conclusion

Ablation of atrial fibrillation is appropriate in symptomatic patients who have failed medical therapy (**Class I, Level A**).

Ablation of atrial fibrillation should be considered in patients with congestive heart failure who are unrespon-sive to AAD (**Class I, Level B**). The benefits of ablation of atrial fibrillation in congestive heart failure have been dem-onstrated by one randomized trial and several consecutive series.

Ablation of atrial fibrillation may be considered for first-line therapy in patients with recurrent atrial fibrillation (**Class IIb, Level B**).

Several larger ongoing trials are comparing AAD therapy with ablation for AF (AATAC-HF, CASTLE-AF, RAAFT-2

and CABANA trials). These studies will be important in deciding whether catheter ablation for AF can be adopted as a reasonable first-line strategy compared to the current strategy of initiating AAD, thus negating the inherent dangers associated with long-term AAD therapy. If the results of these trials concur with the pilot RAAFT study, ablation as first-line therapy may then become a Class I recommendation.

References

1. Haissaguerre M, Jais P, Shah DC, Takahashi A, Hocini M, Quiniou G et al. Spontaneous initiation of atrial fibrillation by ectopic beats originating in the pulmonary veins. *N Engl J Med* 1998;**339**:659–66.
2. Daoud EG, Weiss R, Bahu M, Knight BP, Bogun F, Goyal R et al. Effect of an irregular ventricular rhythm on cardiac output. *Am J Cardiol* 1996;**78**:1433–6
3. Gosselink AT, Bijlsma EB, Landsman ML, Crijns HJ, Lie KI. Long-term effect of cardioversion on peak oxygen consumption in chronic atrial fibrillation. A 2-year follow-up. *Eur Heart J* 1994;**15**:1368–72.
4. Grogan M, Smith HC, Gersh BJ, Wood DL. Left ventricular dys-function due to atrial fibrillation in patients initially believed to have idiopathic dilated cardiomyopathy. *Am J Cardiol* 1992;**15**:1570–3.
5. Wyse DG, Waldo AL, DiMarco JP et al, for the Atrial Fibrillation Follow-up Investigation of Rhythm Management (AFFIRM) Investigators. A comparison of rate control and rhythm control in patients with atrial fibrillation. *N Engl J Med* 2002;**347**:1825–33.
6. Hagens VE, Vermeulen KM, TenVergert EM et al, for the RACE study group. Rate control is more cost-effective than rhythm control for patients with persistent atrial fibrillation –results from the RAte Control versus Electrical cardioversion (RACE) study. *Eur Heart J* 2004;**25**:1542–9.
7. Carlsson J, Miketic S, Windeler J et al, for the STAF Investigators. Randomized trial of rate-control versus rhythm-control in per-sistent atrial fibrillation: the Strategies of Treatment of Atrial Fibrillation (STAF) study. *J Am Coll Cardiol* 2003;**41**:1690–6.
8. Corley SD, Epstein AE, DiMarco JP et al, for the AFFIRM Inves-tigators. Relationships between sinus rhythm, treatment, and survival in the Atrial Fibrillation Follow-Up Investigation of Rhythm Management (AFFIRM) Study. *Circulation* 2004;**109**:1509–13.
9. Nichol G, McAlister F, Pham B, Laupacis A, Shea B, Green M et al. Meta-analysis of randomised controlled trials of the effective-ness of antiarrhythmic agents at promoting sinus rhythm in patients with atrial fibrillation. *Heart* 2002;**87**:535–43.
10. Chun SH, Sager PT, Stevenson WG, Nademanee K, Middlekauff HR, Singh BN. Long-term efficacy of amiodarone for the main-tenance of normal sinus rhythm in patients with refractory atrial fibrillation or flutter. *Am J Cardiol* 1995;**76**:47–50.
11. Mitchell AR, Spurrell PA, Cheatle L, Sulke N. Effect of atrial antitachycardia pacing treatments in patients with an atrial defi-brillator: randomised study comparing subthreshold and nominal pacing outputs. *Heart* 2002;**87**:433–7.

12. Packer DL, Asirvatham S, Munger TM. Progress in nonpharmacologic therapy of atrial fibrillation. *J Cardiovasc Electrophysiol* 2003;**14**(12 suppl):S296–309.

13. Lau CP, Tse HF, Yu CM *et al*, for the New Indication for Preventive Pacing in Atrial Fibrillation (NIPP-AF) Investigators. Dual-site atrial pacing for atrial fibrillation in patients without bradycardia. *Am J Cardiol* 2001;**88**:371–5.

14. Haïssaguerre M, Jaïs P, Shah DC, Garrigue S, Takahashi A, Lavergne T *et al*. Electrophysiological end point for catheter ablation of atrial fibrillation initiated from multiple pulmonary venous foci. *Circulation* 2000;**101**:1409–17.

15. Finta B, Haines DE. Catheter ablation therapy for atrial fibrillation. *Cardiol Clin* 2004;**22**:127–45, ix.

16. Arruda M, Mlcochova H, Prasad SK, Kilicaslan F, Saliba W, Patel D *et al*. Electrical isolation of the superior vena cava: an adjunctive strategy to pulmonary vein antrum isolation improving the outcome of AF ablation. *J Cardiovasc Electrophysiol* 2007;**18**:1261–6.

17. Jalife J. Rotors and spiral waves in atrial fibrillation. *J Cardiovasc Electrophysiol* 2003;**14**: 776–80.

18. Arora R, Verheule S, Scott L, Navarrete A, Katari V, Wilson E *et al*. Arrhythmogenic substrate of the pulmonary veins assessed by high-resolution optical mapping. *Circulation* 2003;**107**: 1816–21.

19. Pappone C, Santinelli V, Manguso F, Vicedomini G, Gugliotta F, Augello G *et al*. Pulmonary vein denervation enhances long-term benefit after circumferential ablation for paroxysmal atrial fibrillation. *Circulation* 2004;**109**:327–34.

20. Krittayaphong R, Raungrattanaamporn O, Bhuripanyo K, Sriratanasathavorn C, Pooranawattanakul S, Punlee K, Kangkagate C. A randomized clinical trial of the efficacy of radiofrequency catheter ablation and amiodarone in the treatment of symptomatic atrial fibrillation. *J Med Assoc Thai* 2003;**86**(suppl 1):S8–16.

21. Wazni OM, Marrouche NF, Martin DO, Verma A, Bhargava M, Saliba W *et al*. Radiofrequency ablation vs antiarrhythmic drugs as first-line treatment of symptomatic atrial fibrillation: a randomized trial. *JAMA* 2005;**293**:2634–40.

22. Stabile G, Bertaglia E, Senatore G, De Simone A, Zoppo F, Donnici G *et al*. Catheter ablation treatment in patients with drug-refractory atrial fibrillation: a prospective, multi-centre, randomized, controlled study (Catheter Ablation For The Cure Of Atrial Fibrillation Study). *Eur Heart J* 2006;**27**:216–21.

23. Pappone C, Augello G, Sala S, Gugliotta F, Vicedomini G, Gulletta S *et al*. A randomized trial of circumferential pulmonary vein ablation versus antiarrhythmic drug therapy in paroxysmal atrial fibrillation: the APAF Study. *J Am Coll Cardiol* 2006;**48**: 2340–7.

24. Oral H, Pappone C, Chugh A, Good E, Bogun F, Pelosi F Jr *et al*. Circumferential pulmonary-vein ablation for chronic atrial fibrillation. *N Engl J Med* 2006;**354**:934–41.

25. Gjesdal K, Vist GE, Bugge E, Rossvoll O, Johansen M, Norderhaug I, Ohm OJ. Curative ablation for atrial fibrillation: a systematic review. *Scand Cardiovasc J* 2008;**42**:3–8.

26. Jais P, Cauchemez B, Macle L, Daoud E, Khairy P, Subbiah R *et al*. Catheter ablation versus antiarrhythmic drugs for atrial fibrillation: the A4 Study. *Circulation* 2008;**118**:2498–505.

27. Wilkoff BL, Cook JR, Epstein AE *et al*, for the Dual Chamber and VVI Implantable Defibrillator Trial Investigators. Dual-chamber pacing or ventricular backup pacing in patients with an implantable defibrillator: the Dual Chamber and VVI Implantable Defibrillator (DAVID) Trial. *JAMA* 2002;**288**:3115–23.

28. Brignole M, Gammage M, Puggioni E *et al*, for the Optimal Pacing SITE (OPSITE) Study Investigators. Comparative assessment of right, left, and biventricular pacing in patients with permanent atrial fibrillation. *Eur Heart J* 2005;**26**:712–22.

29. Doshi RN, Daoud EG, Fellows C *et al*, for the PAVE Study Group. Left ventricular-based cardiac stimulation post AV nodal ablation evaluation (the PAVE study). *J Cardiovasc Electrophysiol* 2005;**16**:1160–5.

30. Khan MN, Jais P, Cummings J, Di Biase L, Sanders P, Martin DO *et al*. Pulmonary vein antrum isolation vs. AV node ablation with bi-ventricular pacing for atrial fibrillation. *N Engl J Med* 2008;**359**(17):1778–85.

31. Gentlesk PJ, Sauer WH, Gerstenfeld EP, Lin D, Dixit S, Zado E *et al*. Reversal of left ventricular dysfunction following ablation of atrial fibrillation. *J Cardiovasc Electrophysiol* 2007;**18**:9–14.

32. Tondo C, Mantica M, Russo G, Avella A, De Luca L, Pappalardo A *et al*. Pulmonary vein vestibule ablation for the control of atrial fibrillation in patients with impaired left ventricular function. *Pacing Clin Electrophysiol* 2006;**29**:962–70.

33. Chen MS, Marrouche NF, Khaykin Y, Gillinov AM, Wazni O, Martin DO *et al*. Pulmonary vein isolation for the treatment of atrial fibrillation in patients with impaired systolic function. *J Am Coll Cardiol* 2004;**43**:1004–9.

34. Hsu LF, Jaïs P, Sanders P, Garrigue S, Hocini M, Sacher F *et al*. Catheter ablation for atrial fibrillation in congestive heart failure. *N Engl J Med* 2004;**351**:2373–83.

35. Efremidis M, Sideris A, Xydonas S, Letsas KP, Alexanian IP, Manolatos D *et al*. Ablation of atrial fibrillation in patients with heart failure: reversal of atrial and ventricular remodelling. *Hellenic J Cardiol* 2008;**49**:19–25.

36. Kilicaslan F, Verma A, Saad E, Themistoclakis S, Bonso A, Raviele A *et al*. Efficacy of catheter ablation of atrial fibrillation in patients with hypertrophic obstructive cardiomyopathy. *Heart Rhythm* 2006;**3**:275–80.

37. Bunch TJ, Munger TM, Friedman PA, Asirvatham SJ, Brady PA, Cha YM *et al*. Substrate and procedural predictors of outcomes after catheter ablation for atrial fibrillation in patients with hypertrophic cardiomyopathy. *J Cardiovasc Electrophysiol* 2008;**19**: 1009–14.

38. Iesaka Y. Complications of catheter ablation of atrial fibrillation: cause, prevention and management. *J Cardiovasc Electrophysiol* 2006;**17**:S50–5.

39. Cappato R, Calkins H, Chen SA, Davies W, Iesaka Y, Kalman J *et al*. Worldwide survey on the methods, efficacy, and safety of catheter ablation for human atrial fibrillation. *Circulation* 2005;**111**:1100–5.

40. Wazni OM, Beheiry S, Fahmy T, Barrett C, Hao S, Patel D *et al*. Atrial fibrillation ablation in patients with therapeutic international normalized ratio: comparison of strategies of anticoagulation management in the periprocedural period. *Circulation* 2007;**116**:2531–4.

41. Saad EB, Rossillo A, Saad CP, Martin DO, Bhargava M, Erciyes D *et al*. Pulmonary vein stenosis after radiofrequency ablation of atrial fibrillation: functional characterization, evolution, and influence of the ablation strategy. *Circulation* 2003;**108**:3102–7.

42. Di Biase L, Fahmy TS, Wazni OM, Bai R, Patel D, Lakkireddy D et al. Pulmonary vein total occlusion following catheter ablation for atrial fibrillation: clinical implications after long-term follow-up. *J Am Coll Cardiol* 2006;**48**:2493–9.

43. Cummings JE, Barrett CD, Litwak KN, Di Biase L, Chowdhury P, Oh S et al. Esophageal luminal temperature measurement underestimates esophageal tissue temperature during radiofrequency ablation within the canine left atrium: comparison between 8 mm tip and open irrigation catheters. *J Cardiovasc Electrophysiol* 2008;**19**:641–4.

44. Scanavacca MI, D'ávila A, Parga J, Sosa E. Left atrial-esophageal fistula following radiofrequency catheter ablation of atrial fibrillation. *J Cardiovasc Electrophysiol* 2004;**15**:960–2.

45. Pappone C, Oral H, Santinelli V, Vicedomini G, Lang CC, Manguso F et al. Atrio-esophageal fistula as a complication of percutaneous transcatheter ablation of atrial fibrillation. *Circulation* 2004;**109**:2724–6.

46. Cummings JE, Schweikert RA, Saliba WI, Burkhardt JD, Kilikaslan F, Saad E, Natale A. Brief communication: atrial-esophageal fistulas after radiofrequency ablation. *Ann Intern Med* 2006;**144**:572–4.

47. Bunch TJ, Nelson J, Foley T, Allison S, Crandall BG, Osborn JS et al. Temporary esophageal stenting allows healing of esophageal perforations following atrial fibrillation ablation procedures. *J Cardiovasc Electrophysiol* 2006;**17**:435–9.

48. Mesas CE, Pappone C, Lang CC, Gugliotta F, Tomita T, Vicedomini G et al. Left atrial tachycardia after circumferential pulmonary vein ablation for atrial fibrillation: electroanatomic characterization and treatment. *J Am Coll Cardiol* 2004;**44**:1071–9.

49. Pappone C, Manguso F, Vicedomini G, Gugliotta F, Santinelli O, Ferro A et al. Prevention of iatrogenic atrial tachycardia after ablation of atrial fibrillation: a prospective randomized study comparing circumferential pulmonary vein ablation with a modified approach. *Circulation* 2004;**110**:3036–42.

50. Bai R, Patel D, Di Biase L, Fahmy TS, Kozeluhova M, Prasad S et al. Phrenic nerve injury after catheter ablation: should we worry about this complication? *J Cardiovasc Electrophysiol* 2006;**17**:944–8.

51. Buch E, Vaseghi M, Cesario DA, Shivkumar K. A novel method for preventing phrenic nerve injury during catheter ablation. *Heart Rhythm* 2007;**4**:95–8.

52. Shah D, Dumonceau JM, Burri H, Sunthorn H, Schroft A, Gentil-Baron P et al. Acute pyloric spasm and gastric hypomotility: an extracardiac adverse effect of percutaneous radiofrequency ablation for atrial fibrillation. *J Am Coll Cardiol* 2005;**46**:327–30.

39 Supraventricular tachycardia

Erica D Penny-Peterson and Gerald V Naccarelli

Penn State University College of Medicine, Hershey, PA, USA

Introduction

Supraventricular arrhythmias encompass tachycardias that require atrial or atrioventricular (AV) nodal tissue for initiation and maintenance (Box 39.1). The duration of symptoms may be paroxysmal or incessant. Origins include atrial musculature, AV nodal tissue, sinus node and pulmonary veins.[1-4] There are several forms which can be categorized as AV node dependent or AV node independent (Box 39.2).

Paroxysmal supraventricular tachycardia (PSVT) is generally a narrow complex tachycardia that excludes atrial flutter, atrial fibrillation and multifocal atrial tachycardia. Its incidence is 35 per 100 000 persons and higher in females.[1,2] PSVTs associated with cardiovascular disease typically occur in older males and often originate in atrial tissue.[5] More than 50% of these patients also have associated atrial fibrillation.[6]

Typical symptoms from PSVT include palpitations, light-headedness, and chest pain. Overt syncope is rare.[1,7] However, some patients are minimally symptomatic. PSVTs are prognostically benign rhythms and often well tolerated. Hemodynamic compromise is uncommon but is more likely to occur in patients with significant structural heart disease. Incessant forms of PSVT can cause a tachycardia-mediated cardiomyopathy. Tachycardia-mediated cardiomyopathy can be reversed by either preventing the arrhythmia or control of the ventricular response either by pharmacologic or ablative treatments. Several studies have documented an improvement in left ventricular ejection fraction after catheter ablation in patients who had PSVT with rapid rates.[8,9]

SVT mechanisms include re-entry, automaticity, and triggered activity.[4,10] Automaticity is a disorder of impulse initiation. It occurs when the sinus node impulse is blocked or slowed. This allows ectopic pacemakers located in the atria, coronary sinus, pulmonary veins or AV junction to reach threshold and overdrive the sinus node. Impulse formation may also occur when the sinus node is exposed to excessive adrenergic stimulation or reduced vagal input, resulting in inappropriate sinus tachycardia.[11]

Rarely, SVTs may be secondary to triggered activity.[10] Triggered activity is a disorder of impulse conduction, mainly repolarization, in which the previous action potential or summation of action potentials creates depolarizing oscillations in the membrane potential. Early afterdepolarizations (EAD) occur during phase 2 or phase 3 of the action potential. Late or delayed afterdepolarizations (DAD) occur during phase 4 of the action potential. These afterdepolarizations are capable of reaching the membrane potential threshold and initiating a new action potential. An example of a triggered arrhythmia is non-paroxysmal atrial tachycardia with block secondary to digitalis toxicity.[12] Steinbeck *et al* demonstrated an increase in rate secondary to a shift of the dominant pacemaker cells to a group of cells near the sinoatrial border in rabbit atrial preparations exposed to ouabain, suggesting that these triggered foci are not in the SA node but in the perisinus atrium.[13] DAD is associated with calcium overload.

Re-entry is the most common mechanism for SVT.[1,2,4,10,14] Sixty percent of re-entry is AV nodal, 30% is atrioventricular re-entry, 10% is atrial or sinoatrial re-entry tachycardia. If the tachycardia is secondary to re-entry, initiation and termination of the tachycardia are reproducible with programmed electrical stimulation.[10]

History and physical examination are important and can give clues to mechanism and type of arrhythmia. If there is a gradual increase in rate with initiation or decrease with termination, automaticity is likely. Abrupt initiation and termination favor re-entry. An irregular rhythm may be more suggestive of atrial fibrillation, atrial flutter or multifocal atrial tachycardia.

A 12-lead ECG is helpful in the evaluation of PSVT. The morphology and relationship between P waves and the

Evidence-Based Cardiology, 3rd edition. Edited by S. Yusuf, J.A. Cairns, A.J. Camm, E.L. Fallen, and B.J. Gersh. © 2010 Blackwell Publishing, ISBN: 978-1-4051-5925-8.

BOX 39.1 Nomenclature

Sinus tachycardia	STACH
Atrioventricular nodal re-entrant tachycardia	AVNRT
Atrioventricular re-entrant tachycardia	AVRT
Atrial tachycardia	ATACH
Inappropriate sinus tachycardia	IAST
Sinoatrial reentrant tachycardia	SANRT
Non-paroxysmal junctional tachycardia	NPJT
Junctional ectopic tachycardia	JET
Atrial fibrillation	AF
Atrial flutter	AFL
Multifocal atrial tachycardia	MAT

BOX 39.2 Classification of supraventricular tachycardias

AV node independent
- Sinus tachycardia
- Inappropriate sinus tachycardia
- Sinus node re-entrant tachycardia
- Atrial tachycardia
- Atrial flutter
- Atrial fibrillation
- Multifocal atrial tachycardia
- Junctional ectopic tachycardia

AV node dependent
- Slow-fast AVNRT
- Fast-slow AVNRT
- Orthodromic AVRT (WPW)
- Antidromic AVRT (WPW) – pre-existed
- PJRT (slow conducting CBT)

QRS (PR or RP) are helpful in making a more specific diagnosis and allow the diagnosis of atrioventricular nodal re-entrant tachycardia (AVNRT) or atrioventricular re-entrant tachycardia (AVRT) in 80–85% of cases.[15] Once the rhythm has been terminated, the tachycardia should be compared to a resting 12-lead electrocardiogram. However, 20% of ECG interpretations may incorrectly characterize PSVT. Therefore, a 12-lead ECG should not be the sole diagnostic test to determine mechanism.[16]

Vagal maneuvers such as Valsalva, the diving reflex, breath holding, and carotid sinus massage can be helpful in terminating tachycardia or in revealing clues to the etiology of the arrhythmia (**Class I, Level B**).[1,16] Intravenous adenosine can also be used to aid in the diagnosis. AVNRT and AVRT are excluded if tachycardia persists with block in the AV node. If the tachycardia is not terminated by vagal maneuvers and IV adenosine, the most likely etiology is an AV node-independent tachycardia. Intravenous AV node blocking agents, such as IV verapamil or diltiazem, may be attempted if adenosine fails to help therapeutically and/or clarify the mechanistic diagnosis.

An echocardiogram may be useful if there is a suspicion of structural heart disease. Findings are useful in determining if patients can be treated with class IC agents or help in defining anatomy and/or congenital defects in patients prior to an ablation procedure.[1,7] Thyroid function and electrolytes should be evaluated. Electrophysiology study is helpful in patients in whom the mechanism and etiology cannot be determined with the above information and also in those patients with a history of tachycardia but no documented tachycardia on 12-lead ECG or Holter monitor. Patients with continued symptoms despite AV nodal blocking agents and those who desire to maintain normal rhythm with an antiarrhythmic agent are appropriate to refer for an electrophysiology study. Patients with hemodynamically unstable SVT, patients who do not wish to take medications but are interested in invasive catheter ablation, patients with evidence of pre-excitation, and those with a wide complex tachycardia requiring differentiation of SVT from VT are also candidates for an electrophysiology study.[1–3]

Acute management of SVT focuses on termination or conversion of SVT to sinus rhythm or control of ventricular rate. Intravenous L-type calcium channel antagonists have proven efficacious for acute management of narrow complex hemodynamically stable SVT[1,17–20] (**Class I, Level A**). Verapamil and diltiazem are calcium channel antagonists which slow or depress the effects of sinus node and AVN function by inhibiting membrane transport of calcium. Sung *et al* studied the conversion rate of SVT to sinus rhythm in 20 patients with re-entrant SVT randomized to verapamil or placebo. Fifteen of 19 patients converted to sinus versus 1/16 patients with placebo.[18] Waxman *et al* confirmed in a double-blind randomized trial that IV low- and high-dose verapamil were superior to placebo in slowing the ventricular rate and converting PSVT to sinus rhythm.[19] The IV Diltiazem Study Group determined that the conversion rate by IV diltiazem (0.05 mg/kg) was 84%. The limitation of diltiazem and verapamil therapy is hypotension.[20]

Adenosine is an alpha-1 receptor inhibitor in cardiac muscle cells. It prevents the influx of calcium into the cell and thus depresses conduction of the SA node and AVN.[21] It has been proven through double-blind randomized placebo-controlled trials to be as efficacious and safe as verapamil.[22,23] Glatter *et al* evaluated 229 patients with SVT during an electrophysiology study and determined that the rate of conversion to sinus rhythm with adenosine was 85% for AVRT and 86% for AVNRT.[22] This is comparable to the conversion rate with verapamil.[20] DiMarco *et al* evaluated the efficacy and safety of adenosine in two prospective, randomized trials. Results of this study determined that the rate of adverse events/side effects was 36%, were typically mild and lasted less than 1 minute. Also, when compared to verapamil, time to termination was much faster, occurring in 30 seconds.[23] Adenosine is an effective treatment for the acute termination of narrow complex SVT (**Class I, Level A**).[1] However, recurrence rate of SVT after adenosine was found to be 57% within 5 minutes of adenosine.[24]

There are no large randomized double-blinded placebo-controlled trials evaluating the efficacy and safety of selective beta-1 adrenergic blockers, digoxin or amiodarone (**Class IIb, Level C**).[1] Evidence is based on small clinical trials, expert opinion and clinical experience. Intravenous esmolol and metoprolol were proven to decrease ventricular rate by 15% in patients with SVT.[25,26] Patients were also able to be switched to oral digoxin, propranolol, verapamil, metoprolol and quinidine successfully without losing therapeutic effect.[25] Short-term intravenous amiodarone has a high rate of conversion of SVT to sinus rhythm with low risk of toxicity.[27,28] Vietti-Ramus et al demonstrated that high-dose IV amiodarone had an 88% conversion rate and 100% conversion if atrial flutter and atrial fibrillation were excluded. Time to conversion was between 30 minutes and up to 20 hours.[27] Given safer and better options as noted above, intravenous amiodarone for acute symptoms of SVT is a **Class IIb, Level C** recommendation.[1]

The goals of long-term management of PSVT are arrhythmia suppression or significant decrease in frequency and duration of symptomatic episodes. If PSVT recurrence rates are high, long-term management with an antiarrhythmic or catheter-based ablation should be considered. Flecainide is a class IC antiarrhythmic that is proven efficacious and safe in the treatment of PSVT (**Class IIa, Level B**). Henthorn et al performed a double-blind placebo-controlled trial evaluating time to first recurrence in 34 patients with PSVT.[29] The time to first recurrence in the flecainide group was 55 days compared to 11 days with placebo. Freedom from symptoms during 60 days was 70% of the flecainide group and 15% of the placebo group. Anderson et al performed a similar double-blind placebo-controlled trial evaluating chronic therapy with flecainide to increase the time to recurrent SVT.[30] Of patients on flecainide, 82% were symptom free versus 24% on placebo. There were no proarrhythmic events or deaths during treatment with flecainide. In a multicenter trial evaluating the safety and efficacy of oral flecainide (100–200 mg bid), 87% of patients improved symptomatically.[31] Minor subjective side effects such as headache, dizziness and abnormal vision occurred but these were rarely severe enough to necessitate discontinuation of flecainide.

Propafenone, a class IC agent with beta-adrenergic blocker properties, has also been proven efficacious and safe in the long-term management of PSVT[1,32] (**Class IIa, Level B**). A 6-month randomized placebo-controlled trial evaluating recurrence rates after treatment with 300 mg tid, 300 mg bid, and 150 mg bid of propafenone compared with placebo revealed that the recurrence rate in the propafe-

none group was one-fifth of that seen in the placebo group.[33] In the UK Propafenone PSVT Study Group, 100 patients with PSVT, paroxysmal atrial fibrillation or atrial flutter were evaluated comparing propafenone 300 mg bid or tid and placebo. This therapy was proven efficacious and safe for the prophylaxis of recurrent PSVT. Patients who could tolerate higher doses of propafenone had a trend towards fewer episodes compared to when treated with lower doses.[34]

Multiple class III antiarrhythmics have been evaluated in the long-term treatment of PSVT. A multicenter randomized, double-blind placebo-controlled trial has been performed with sotalol to evaluate its efficacy and safety (**Class IIa, Level C**). Recurrent SVT was less frequent in the sotalol group versus placebo. There were no adverse events of cardiac death, heart failure or proarrhythmia in patients receiving either 160 mg or 80 mg bid.[35]

Amiodarone was assessed in 121 patients with atrial tachyarrhythmias refractory to digoxin, beta-blockers, and other antiarrhythmics over 27 months and 81% did not have recurrent episodes.[36] Amiodarone was discontinued in 6% because of adverse side effects.[36] Therefore, amiodarone can be used as long-term management of PSVT for pharmacologic control but is generally not used due to long-term end-organ toxicity (**Class IIa, Level C**).

The efficacy of dofetilide was compared to propafenone and placebo in 122 patients over 6 months. The endpoints were episode-free periods and reduction in the frequency of symptomatic PSVT, assessed using diaries and event recorders. Episode-free rates were 50% in the dofetilide group, 54% in the propafenone group and 6% in the placebo group.[37] The results of this study confirmed that dofetilide, a class III antiarrhythmic agent, was as efficacious as propafenone in preventing recurrence and in decreasing frequency of PSVT (**Class IIa, Level C**). Although an effective alternative, the use of dofetilide is usually limited to the treatment of AF/atrial flutter due to its proarrhythmia potential (**Class IIa, Level C**).

The pill-in-the-pocket method has been evaluated in the management of PSVT that occurs infrequently.[38] This approach can effectively terminate SVT and reduce hospitalizations and cost of care. Alboni et al evaluated the conversion rate within 2 hours and the safety profile of a single oral dose of flecainide, diltiazem and propranolol, and placebo in 33 patients with inducible SVT during electrophysiology studies.[39] The conversion rate was 52% for placebo, 61% with flecainide and 94% with combination diltiazem and propranolol.[39] Patients were discharged on the most effective medication for conversion based on results of electrophysiology study. At 1 year, the rate of emergency room consultation decreased from 100% at baseline to 9%. Adverse events included hypotension, bradycardia and an episode of syncope.[39]

Catheter ablation for the treatment of PSVT is a first-line acceptable alternative to pharmacologic therapy in very symptomatic patients or in patients with high-risk professions seeking a definitive cure (**Class I, Level B**).[1,40] Cure rates for AVNRT and AVRT are greater than 95% with low risks of heart block, tamponade, and vascular complications.[7] Catheter ablation improves quality of life and reduces healthcare costs in symptomatic patients compared to pharmacologic management.[40]

Sinus tachycardia

Sinus tachycardia is usually a response to physiologic stimulus such as fever, infection, anemia, exercise, hypotension or pain and is corrected by treating the underlying etiology. Acute myocardial infarction is an indication to treat sinus tachycardia with medications (e.g. beta-blockers). Sinus tachycardia in this setting is consistent with higher 30-day mortality and poor outcomes.[41,42]

Inappropriate sinus tachycardia

Inappropriate or non-physiologic sinus tachycardia is a tachycardia out of proportion to metabolic demands.[1,4] The exact mechanism has not been well defined. It is hypothesized that there is abnormal automaticity, enhanced automaticity or an abnormal response to autonomic tone.[43,44] The prognosis is usually benign unless the tachycardia is rapid and incessant such that a tachycardia-mediated cardiomyopathy is induced. There are no randomized trials of treatment of inappropriate sinus tachycardia. Treatment is empiric and if the tachycardia is due to excessive sympathetic tone, beta-blockers may be helpful and are considered first-line treatment (**Class I, Level C**). Calcium antagonists have a more limited role (**Class IIa, Level C**).[45] If vagal suppression is the underlying etiology, heart rate control may be more difficult. Catheter ablation or modification of the sinus node has been performed but long-term success is limited and based only on several small studies (**Class IIb, Level C**).[46,47] Although heart rate is slower with modification, symptoms do not improve consistently. Common complications of sinus node ablation include the need for permanent pacemaker, phrenic nerve damage and trauma to the superior vena cava leading to superior vena cava syndrome.

Sinus node re-entry

Mapping during tachycardia demonstrates superior to inferior and right to left activation,[47,48] similar to normal sinus rhythm. Sinus node reentrant tachycardia terminates abruptly with vagal maneuvers and adenosine unlike physiologic and inappropriate sinus tachycardia. There are no randomized, double-blind placebo-controlled trials for the therapy of sinus node reentrant tachycardia. Patients are generally managed with beta-blockers or calcium channel antagonists (**Class I, Level C**). Catheter ablation can be used in patients with persistent symptoms despite medication, but complications such as phrenic nerve damage and intra-atrial block limit the use of this technique (**Class IIb, Level C**).[3,48,49]

Atrial tachycardia

In 2001 the Joint Expert Group from the Working Group on Arrhythmias of European Society of Cardiology and North American Society of Pacing and Electrophysiology classified atrial tachycardias according to mechanism and anatomy.[50] Focal and intra-atrial tachycardias have been described. Associated clinical scenarios in which atrial tachycardia may be sustained include acute myocardial infarction, infection, electrolyte abnormalities, hypoxia, and cardiac stimulants such as theophylline and cocaine.[1,4,51] Formerly, it was generally accepted that the mechanism of focal atrial tachycardia was enhanced automaticity, but three mechanisms are currently recognized (enhanced automaticity, triggered activity, and micro re-entry) and can be difficult to discriminate clinically. There is variable response to Valsalva maneuvers and adenosine.[11,52–54] In a study performed by Engelstein et al, adenosine was used to distinguish different mechanisms of atrial tachycardia during electrophysiologic study. There was no effect on intra-atrial re-entrant or macro re-entrant atrial tachycardias.[53] Triggered activity may respond to adenosine due to its ability to shorten the action potential and reduce the time available for early afterdepolarizations.[53] In automatic atrial tachycardias varying degrees of heart block may develop in response to adenosine. P-wave morphology may assist in locating the focus and planning of catheter ablation. Kristler et al developed an algorithm determining location of focal atrial tachycardias based on P-wave morphology.[55,56]

Acute treatment focuses on control of ventricular rate and management of symptoms. Atrial tachycardia is rarely terminated with adenosine (**Class IIa, Level C**).[52–54] Direct current cardioversion seldom terminates automatic focal atrial tachycardia but may terminate atrial tachycardia resulting from micro re-entry or triggered activity.[1,4] It is used in hemodynamically unstable atrial tachycardia (**Class I, Level B**). Clinical trials evaluating the efficacy and safety of pharmacologic agents in the acute treatment of atrial tachycardia are lacking. Guidelines are based on clinical experience. Intravenous verapamil (**Class IIa, Level C**) and beta-blockers (**Class I, Level C**) may be beneficial in cases where slow conduction is a critical component of the re-entry circuit or to control the ventricular rate through slowing of the AV node without affecting the atrial rate.[57] Intravenous amiodarone may also be an alternative for rate control acutely, especially in patients with left ventricular dysfunction (**Class IIa, Level C**). Digoxin is typically not used acutely due to its delayed onset of action (**Class III, Level C**).

Long-term management is based on symptoms and prevention of tachycardia-induced cardiomyopathy.[58] Beta-blockers or non-dihydropyridine calcium channel antagonists may be beneficial for rate control (**Class I, Level C**).[19,25,26] Class IA, class IC, and class III agents may be used for suppression (**Class IIa, Level C**).[1,59,60] Flecainide achieves complete suppression in 56%, reduced symptoms or frequency in 8% and no response 36% of patients with either atrial tachycardia or atrial fibrillation.[59]

Catheter ablation may be attempted for recurrent symptoms or failed pharmacologic treatment (**Class I, Level B**).[61] The success rate is approximately 86% with an 8% recurrence. Complications are related to the origin of the tachycardia and the site of ablation.[1,2,61] Cardiac perforation can occur, ablating both right- and left-sided focal atrial tachycardias. Heart block is possible near areas of the septum and coronary sinus ostium.

Paroxysmal atrial tachycardia with AV block or variable conduction is classified as a focal tachycardia. Its mechanism is generally accepted as being triggered activity with characteristics similar to enhanced automaticity.[3,4] Paroxysmal atrial tachycardia is associated with acute pulmonary disease and digoxin toxicity.[3] Efforts at rhythm control with antiarrhythmics have been suboptimal. Treatment involves treating the underlying pathologic disease state, discontinuing digoxin and in rare instances giving digoxin antibody (Digibind).[1,62,63]

Intra-atrial re-entrant tachycardia, also known as re-entrant atrial tachycardia, is a macro re-entrant arrhythmia. It may be extremely difficult to differentiate between intra-atrial and focal atrial tachycardia without electrophysiologic techniques. Intra-atrial re-entrant tachycardia is the mechanism of 6% of atrial tachycardias referred to electrophysiology studies.[64] It is generally associated with structural heart disease and congenital heart disease with atrial surgical scars. The response to vagal maneuvers is approximately less than 25% due to reduced autonomic innervation of atrial tissue compared to the sinus and AV node.[16] The treatment is empiric based on case reports or small studies. Class IC agents may be attempted if the patient has no known structural heart disease. Amiodarone is an acceptable alternative because of its efficacy but is limited by its side-effect profile with long-term use. Calcium channel antagonists and beta-blockers (**Class I, Level C**) are useful for rate control but rarely resolve symptoms except in combination with a membrane-active antiarrhythmic.[1,3,4] Drug resistance, adverse effects of drugs and persistent symptoms are indications for catheter ablation

(**Class I, Level B**). There is a high recurrence rate with catheter ablation. Collins *et al* studied congenital heart disease patients with atrial arrhythmias and acute success rates with catheter ablation.[65]

Multifocal atrial tachycardia

Multifocal atrial tachycardia is described as an atrial tachycardia with variable PR intervals and at least three distinct P-wave morphologies.[3,66] The mechanism is thought to be either triggered activity or abnormal automaticity. Multifocal atrial tachycardia is seen in less than 1% of PSVT.[66] It is associated with chronically and severely ill patients. Disease states that are common to this arrhythmia are pulmonary disease, cardiac disease, and sepsis. More than 60% will have associated pulmonary disease which can be exacerbated by theophylline and beta-adrenergic agonists used in these patients.[67,68] Associated arrhythmias include atrial flutter, atrial fibrillation and atrial tachycardias.[69] The overall prognosis of a patient with multifocal atrial tachycardia is poor, with mortality rates of up to 30–60%.[69] Interestingly, death is usually not secondary to the arrhythmia but due to the underlying disease. Therapy is aimed at treating the underlying disease state.[1,66] However, ventricular rates of 150 and rarely over 200 may require treatment if causing significant symptoms or hemodynamic instability. Pharmacologic therapy is aimed at decreasing the ventricular rate with AV nodal blocking agents. Membrane-active antiarrhythmics and cardioversion tend to be less effective and recurrence of multifocal atrial tachycardia is common. Digoxin is not of proven efficacy and may increase the risk of paroxysmal atrial tachycardia with variable conduction because of digoxin toxicity.[69] Given the high rate of chronic obstructive lung disease, verapamil and diltiazem in a continuous intravenous infusion are commonly used to control ventricular rates.[70,71] The use of verapamil or diltiazem is limited by the occurrence of hypotension. Beta-blockers can also be used if tolerated.[72] Magnesium supplementation has also been studied.[73] Drug-resistant patients may be referred for radiofrequency ablation of the AV junction.[74,75] This is not curative but does decrease the ventricular response. Given the limited options, the best choice is treatment of the underlying disease state and control of ventricular rates as needed.[1,66]

Atrial flutter

Atrial flutter is a macro re-entrant atrial tachycardia typically associated with organic heart disease.[1] It is more common in males and the elderly, can co-exist with atrial fibrillation and is common after cardiac surgery.[1,6,50] Long-term sequelae may include tachycardia-mediated cardiomyopathy and thromboembolic events.[76]

In 2001 the Working Group on Arrhythmias of the European Society of Cardiology and North American Society of Pacing and Electrophysiology attempted to develop a standardized classification.[50] Typical atrial flutter is a macro re-entrant tachycardia circulating around the tricuspid annulus with an area of slow conduction in the cavotricuspid region. Therefore, these atrial flutters were designated as cavotricuspid-dependent atrial flutter and all others were designated as cavotricuspid-independent atrial flutter.[50] Vagal maneuvers or adenosine may be helpful to slow ventricular conduction through the AV node to reveal the flutter waves and exclude other forms of paroxysmal supraventricular tachycardias[1,16] (**Class I, Level C**).

Acute treatment is based on symptoms and hemodynamics of the patient.[1,76] If there is hemodynamic instability, emergency cardioversion is performed (**Class I, Level C**). Cardioversion in hemodynamically stable patients can be accomplished with direct current cardioversion with 50–100J biphasic (**Class I, Level C**) or with ibutilide 1 mg over 10 minutes (**Class IIa, Level A**). Ibutilide has an acceptable rate of conversion to sinus rhythm of approximately 50–60%.[1,77–81] Stambler et al performed a multicenter randomized placebo-controlled trial evaluating the efficacy and safety of ibutilide in the conversion of atrial fibrillation and atrial flutter to sinus rhythm in 266 patients. The rate of conversion of atrial flutter was 63% and dosing regimens of ibutilide (1 mg × 2 or 1 mg and 0.5 mg) did not affect the efficacy.[77] Trials comparing ibutilide to other class III or class IC agents have proven it to be superior in pharmacologic conversion of atrial flutter to sinus rhythm.[79–81] Non-sustained polymorphic ventricular tachycardia and torsades de pointes requiring cardioversion may occur up to 4 hours post infusion with a reported incidence of 0.9–8.3% in clinical trials[77–81]; therefore, ibutilide must be given in a monitored setting. Intravenous magnesium prior to infusion of ibutilide, ruling out hypokalemia and avoiding use in patients with prolonged QT intervals may prevent polymorphic VT/torsades de pointes. Intravenous class IC antiarrhythmic agents are not highly effective at the acute conversion of atrial flutter to sinus rhythm[82] (**Class IIb, Level A**).

In postsurgical patients with an epicardial wire, pacing the atrium at a cycle length 10 ms less than the tachycardia cycle length may terminate atrial flutter or convert the flutter to atrial fibrillation. Prospective, randomized clinical trials have demonstrated that transesophageal atrial pacing is as efficacious as direct current cardioversion for atrial flutter.[83] In the asymptomatic patient, rate control is the goal and can be achieved with AV nodal blocking agents.[84–88] IV diltiazem (**Class I, Level C**) and IV digoxin (**Class IIb, Level C**) were compared in a prospective, randomized open-label trial in the emergency room and diltiazem was superior in controling ventricular rates.[84] A similar randomized, double-blind trial was performed in post coronary bypass patients. Diltiazem controlled rates more rapidly than digoxin but overall rate control after 12–24 hours was similar.[85] Rate control may be difficult and warrant conversion to sinus rhythm.

If a patient has symptomatic atrial flutter, long-term treatment is focused on maintaining sinus rhythm, maintaining control of ventricular rates or curing the patient with catheter-based ablation. For symptomatic patients it is important to convert to sinus with direct current cardioversion, an antiarrhythmic agent or both.[1,76,89] A 3-year study demonstrated that only 42% of patients maintained sinus rhythm after direct cardioversion without an antiarrhythmic.[89] Predictors of failure to convert to sinus rhythm include severe left atrial dilation, dilated cardiomyopathy and chronic atrial flutter of prolonged duration. Pharmacologic control with antiarrhythmic drugs is reasonable and if there is no evidence of coronary artery disease or cardiomyopathy, class IC agents may be used.[29–34] It is important to give an AV nodal blocking agent with these antiarrhythmic drugs due to the risk of 1:1 conduction and sudden cardiac death.

The risk of thromboembolic events is comparable or slightly lower than with atrial fibrillation.[89–92] Post cardioversion the risk is approximately 1%.[89] In patients with atrial flutter and risk factors for stroke or who require cardioversion of atrial flutter of more than 48 hours duration, therapeutic anticoagulation with warfarin is warranted, as with atrial fibrillation.

Catheter ablation techniques to cure atrial flutter are highly effective and have low complication rates. Success rates acutely are 95–100% with chronic success rates of 85–95%.[1,93] This is now an acceptable first-line therapy for atrial flutter.[93–96] The Loire-Ardeche-Drome-Isere-Puy-de-Dome (LADIP) trial demonstrated that long-term success in suppressing atrial flutter was greater in first-time patients with atrial flutter ablation (**Class I, Level B**) versus patients treated with cardioversion and oral amiodarone (**Class IIb, Level C**). Rates of subsequent atrial fibrillation were not significantly different between the two groups.[94] Another prospective randomized trial comparing ablation versus pharmacologic rhythm control as first-line therapy proved that ablation of atrial flutter improved quality of life, reduced recurrent atrial flutter rates, reduced future hospitalizations, and reduced the incidence of atrial fibrillation in follow-up.[96]

However, most studies have demonstrated that atrial flutter ablations have no impact on the incidence of atrial fibrillation.[94,97] In patients receiving antiarrhythmic drugs for atrial fibrillation with subsequent drug-induced atrial flutter, treatment with atrial flutter ablation and continuing pharmacologic control of atrial fibrillation is efficacious and safe.[98,99] Despite the claim of long-term success, approximately 60% of patients will be diagnosed with atrial fibrillation within a 5-year period.[95,97] The risk of the procedure is low but complete heart block, perforation with tamponade, coronary artery damage, and thromboembolic events may occur.[1,93] Patients who cannot be converted to sinus rhythm or who fail anatomic ablation may be referred for palliative ablation of the AV junction.

AV nodal re-entrant tachycardia

AV nodal re-entrant tachycardia (AVNRT) is the most common form of PSVT in adults, accounting for more than 50% of cases.[1–4,10] It is more common in females. There are rare cases in young children and infants. On physical exam, neck pulsations may be evident from simultaneous contraction of the atria and ventricles.[2,100]

The anatomy of the AV junction is important to understand the mechanism of AVNRT. The AV node has right and left posterior extensions. It is hypothesized that there are atrial inputs superiorly, posteriorly and from the left atrium.[101] The superior inputs are near the apex of the triangle of Koch and the posterior or inferior inputs are near the coronary sinus ostium.[101] One hypothesis is that the transitional cells or atrial inputs involve the slow and fast pathways. The fast pathway is located superiorly and posteriorly to the apex of the triangle of Koch. The slow pathway is made of multiple strands anteriorly and inferior to the coronary sinus ostium[102] and there may be multiple slow pathways present in a single individual.[103] The fast pathway has faster conduction and a longer effective refractory period compared to the slow pathway and is more responsive to adrenergic stimuli, such as catecholamines and isoproterenol. Slow-fast AVNRT is the most common form,[3–4,102] present in 75% of cases. The atypical fast-slow variant occurs in about 5–10% of cases. A slow-slow variant occurs in about 5–10% of cases.[3–4,102]

Normal conduction through the AV node is via a single AV nodal pathway. However, dual AV nodal pathways are commonly noted in patients during electrophysiologic testing.[104,105] Although dual AV nodal pathways are common, only a small percentage will support clinical tachycardia.

Acute treatment is determined by how well the arrhythmia is tolerated.[1–3] If there is hemodynamic instability, direct current cardioversion is favored. Termination may occur with intravenous adenosine 6 mg or 12 mg.[21–24] The rate of termination of AVNRT after intravenous adenosine is approximately 86–95% (**Class I, Level A**), and adenosine is as effective as verapamil based on various clinical trials.[21–24,106] Vagal maneuvers may also be beneficial[16] (**Class I, Level B**). AV nodal blocking agents, such as beta-blockers and calcium channel antagonists and digoxin, slow antegrade pathway conduction (**Class IIa, Level C**).[17–20,25–28,107]

Curative measures versus suppression of recurrent arrhythmia through ablation or pharmacologic therapy are long-term therapy goals. Class IC agents typically affect the retrograde fast pathway and are one of the most effective pharmacologic options[20–34] (**Class IIb, Level B**). In the Flecainide Supraventricular Tachycardia Study Group, the number of symptom-free patients after chronic oral flecainide therapy increased from 24% to 82%.[30] Sotalol (**Class IIa, Level B**) and amiodarone (**Class IIb, Level C**) may have beneficial effects on both antegrade and retrograde parts of the circuit.[35,107]

In patients with recurrent episodes despite pharmacologic therapy, those not willing to take medications or patients in high-risk professions, such as commercial pilots, radiofrequency catheter ablation is a reasonable option[1,108] (**Class I, Level B**). The target is the slow pathway anterior and posterior to the CS ostium and tricuspid annulus. The target is found via an anatomic approach, characteristic electrograms or a combination of the two.[108] The anatomic approach places the ablation catheter anterior and inferior to the CS ostium near the tricuspid annulus. Endpoints include elimination of slow pathway or dual AV nodal physiology and of inducible AVRNT. The success rate is approximately 95% with low recurrence rates.[1,93,108] Complications include complete heart block requiring a permanent pacemaker in approximately 1%.[93,109]

In patients with only one documented episode or very infrequent episodes, it is reasonable to advise vagal maneuvers, pill-in-the-pocket therapy, rate control options, catheter ablation or no treatment. All of the above in this setting are considered Class I, Level C recommendations.[1]

Automatic junctional tachycardia

Automatic junctional tachycardias (AJTs) occur secondary to increased automaticity within the AV junction.[1,3,4,110] Electrophysiology studies in selected patients have demonstrated increased response to exercise and isoproterenol and decreased response to propranolol. This suggests a catecholamine-sensitive or dependent junctional focus.[111,112] There are no randomized, placebo-controlled trials for the treatment of AJT. Treatment is based on clinical experience and small case series, mainly in infants and children. Most will respond to beta-blockers (**Class IIa, Level C**) but may require class IC agents or amiodarone (**Class IIa, Level C**) in addition to AV nodal agents.[113] Ablation of the junctional focus or His bundle is reserved for incessant, drug-resistant forms and treatment recommendations are based on case reports[114–116] (**Class IIa, Level C**).

Non-paroxysmal junctional tachycardia occurs in the presence of structural heart disease. Examples include myocardial infarction, myocarditis, post surgery, and digoxin toxicity in the setting of atrial fibrillation.[117,118]

Treatment is typically not indicated. Resolution occurs with correction of underlying pathology (**Class I, Level C**).[119] Beta-blockers may be useful in some settings (**Class IIa, Level C**).[1]

Atrioventricular reciprocating tachycardia

Atrioventricular reciprocating tachycardias are re-entrant arrhythmias that involve an accessory pathway in one limb of the circuit. The prevalence of manifest pre-excitation is 0.15–0.25% in the population and of those studied in the electrophysiologic laboratory, up to 13% will have multiple pathways.[1,120] There tends to be a male predominance. Typically, structural heart disease is absent. However, 5–10% of patients with Epstein's anomaly will have Wolff–Parkinson–White syndrome with right-sided accessory pathways predominating. There have been case reports of familial occurrence of accessory pathways without and in association with dilated cardiomyopathy.[121,122]

The prognosis depends on the electrophysiologic properties of the accessory pathway.[1,122–124] Localization of the accessory pathway may be predicted based on the vector of the delta wave on ECG.[125]

Arrhythmias associated with accessory pathways or Wolff–Parkinson–White (WPW) syndrome include orthodromic AV reciprocating tachycardia, antidromic reciprocating tachycardia, atrial flutter and atrial fibrillation, and permanent junctional reciprocating tachycardia. Orthodromic AV reciprocating tachycardia is the most common paroxysmal supraventricular tachycardia in WPW syndrome.[1,3] It is a macro re-entrant tachycardia that uses the AVN as the antegrade limb and the accessory pathway as the retrograde limb. There are some patients with no ECG evidence of pre-excitation who have orthodromic tachycardia with retrograde conduction over an accessory pathway; 20–30% of patients with accessory pathways have such concealed bypass tracts.[1,3,126] Diagnosis is determined during electrophysiologic studies. Most concealed pathways are left sided.

The permanent form of junctional reciprocating tachycardia involves an accessory pathway with slow conduction and decremental properties. Typically, there is no evidence of pre-excitation during sinus rhythm and the concealed pathway participates in orthodromic tachycardia in the retrograde direction. It is typically seen in children and young adults and may become incessant and result in tachycardia-mediated cardiomyopathy.[126] The most common location of the pathway is posteroseptal near the ostium of the coronary sinus.

Antidromic tachycardia is a macro re-entrant tachycardia which occurs in 5–10% of patients with WPW syndrome.[1,3] This circuit uses the pathway as the antegrade limb, resulting in a wide QRS complex during tachycardia. Atrial fibrillation and atrial flutter may occur in 20–30% of patients with pathways that conduct antegrade.[1,3] Accessory pathway conduction is sodium channel dependent, often resulting in short refractory periods and fast conduction; thus antegrade pathways may conduct 1:1 with atrial flutter at rates 300 bpm and faster with atrial fibrillation with a risk of ventricular fibrillation and sudden death under these conditions. The risk of sudden death is increased by the presence of a short refractory period of the antegrade pathway (<250 ms), multiple accessory pathways, and a shortest pre-excited R-R during atrial fibrillation of <220 ms.[127]

Treatment of accessory pathways is guided by symptoms or associated arrhythmias such as atrial fibrillation. Symptomatic patients are best treated with catheter ablation (**Class I, Level B**).[1] Asymptomatic patients or patients with WPW pattern are generally low risk for sudden death. Observation is usually the best option (**Class I, Level C**).[1,123,124]

Acute treatment of orthodromic SVT may be accomplished with vagal maneuvers (**Class I, Level B**), adenosine (**Class I, Level A**), diltiazem (**Class I, Level B**), verapamil (**Class I, Level A**), and intravenous beta-blockers (**Class I, Level B**) and amiodarone (**Class I, Level B**).[16–28] If there is hemodynamic compromise, direct current cardioversion is favored (**Class IIa, Level C**). The target of pharmacologic therapy is the weak limb of the circuit, usually the AV node. Adenosine has limited value in determining the mechanism of AVRNT versus AVRT in a narrow QRS tachycardia (**Class I, Level A**). Adenosine has a short duration of action, does not cause hypotension and has been proven to be as effective and safe as verapamil[23] (**Class I, Level A**). Procainamide is a class IA antiarrhythmic which slows conduction of both atrial and ventricular tissue and increases the effective refractory period of the accessory pathway, atrium and ventricle. It has been proven efficacious in treatment of orthodromic tachycardia.[128] Antidromic tachycardia or pre-excited atrial fibrillation presents with a wide QRS due to antegrade conduction via the accessory pathway. Treatment is best managed with cardioversion if there is hemodynamic instability. If the patient is hemodynamically stable the safest pharmacologic agent to terminate tachycardia or slow the ventricular response is procainamide[128] but this is not generally available nowadays. AV node blockers slow conduction of the AV node and may lead to unopposed conduction of the accessory pathway. This could result in ventricular fibrillation, especially in the setting of atrial fibrillation.[129–132] Therefore, these agents must be avoided in WPW patients with atrial fibrillation (**Class III Level B**).

Catheter ablation is preferred as a definitive cure in long-term management of symptomatic patients (**Class I, Level B**). Patients who decline an invasive approach who have low-risk pathways for sudden death may be treated with class IC, IA or class III antiarrhythmics or AV nodal agents for rate control except digoxin and verapamil (**Class III, Level C**). There are no randomized, placebo-controlled trials to demonstrate the efficacy and safety of antiarrhythmic agents in this patient population. Most recommendations are based on small case series and expert opinion. Class IC agents have been proven to be efficacious and safe[133–135] (**Class IIa, Level C**). Vassiliadis et al determined that 40% of patients with WPW syndrome responded to an initial dose of oral propafenone, and 60% responded after an increase in dose without developing significant adverse reactions or proarrhythmic events.[133] In an open-label uncontrolled trial with oral flecainide, Cockrell et al studied 63 symptomatic patients with tachycardias involving accessory pathways during electrophysiology study.[135] Prevention or slowed inducible AVRT was demonstrated in 70%. Adverse reaction to flecainide occurred in hospitalized but not in discharged patients.[135] It is reasonable to use oral class IC antiarrhythmics for the prevention of AVRT. It may be reasonable to initiate this in a monitored setting and ensure the patient does not have structural heart disease.

Class III agents prolong the refractory period of the atria, ventricles and accessory pathway (both retrograde and antegrade).[136–138] Sotalol has been shown to be effective and safe during electrophysiology studies[136] (**Class IIa, Level C**). The success of intravenous and oral sotalol during electrophysiology study was predictive of long-term success of oral sotalol in preventing recurrent SVT.[136] There are multiple studies demonstrating that amiodarone is a reasonable option in orthodromic, antidromic and prevention of pre-excited atrial fibrillation.[137,138]

Class IA agents were the first antiarrhythmics to be used in WPW but were replaced by safer class IC agents. The use of class IA agents is limited by multiple side effects (e.g. gastrointestinal and anticholinergic effects). In patients with pre-excited atrial fibrillation, disopyramide slows the ventricular response by prolongation of the refractory period of the accessory pathway.[139]

Catheter-based ablation is a first-line therapy for symptomatic patients and patients with documented atrial fibrillation.[1,140] Ablation may be offered to patients who have high-risk professions or those who have failed medications (**Class I, Level B**). Approximately 50% of accessory pathways are located in the left lateral AV groove, 30% are posteroseptal, 20% are right free wall, and <5% are anteroseptal. The curative ablation site is at the earliest atrial electrogram or ventricular electrogram and the site of the accessory potential.[140] Difficult ablations may occur secondary to catheter instability, especially on the right, oblique pathways (the atrial insertion and ventricular insertion are not parallel). The success rate is approximately 90–95% with low recurrence, <5% with left-sided pathways and higher with right-sided pathways.[93,140] Pos-

teroseptal and anteroseptal pathway ablations have a slightly lower success rates with a risk of AV block in the paraseptal area. Some ablations may need to be performed within the CS due to an epicardial location.

References

1. ACC/AHA/ESC. Guidelines for the management of patients with supraventricular arrhythmias. Executive Summary: A report of the American College of Cardiology/American Heart Association Task Force on practice guidelines and the European Society of Cardiology Committee for Practice Guidelines *Circulation* 2003;**108**:1871–909.
2. Etienne Delacretaz MD. Supraventricular tachycardia. *N Engl J Med* 2006;**354**:1039–51.
3. Ganz L, Friedman PL. Supraventricular tachycardia. *N Engl J Med* 1995;**332**:162–73.
4. Wellens H. 25 years of insights into mechanisms of supraventricular arrhythmias. *PACE* 2003;**26**:1916–21.
5. LA Orejarena, Vidaillet H Jr, DeStefano F *et al*. Paroxysmal supraventricular tachycardia in the general population. *J Am Coll Cardiol* 1998;**31**:150–7.
6. Granada J, Uribe W, Chyou PH *et al*. Incidence and predictors of atrial flutter in the general population. *J Am Coll Cardiol* 2000;**36**:2242–6.
7. Ferguson JD, DiMarco JP. Contemporary management of paroxysmal supraventricular tachycardia. *Circulation* 2003;**107**(8):1096–9.
8. Nerheim P, Birger-Botkin S, Piracha L, Olshansky B. Heart failure and sudden death in patients with tachycardia-induced cardiomyopathy and recurrent tachycardia. *Circulation* 2004;**110**:247–52.
9. Luchsinger JA, Steinberg JS. Resolution of cardiomyopathy after ablation of atrial flutter. *J Am Coll Cardiol* 1998;**32**(1):205–10.
10. Zipes DP. Mechanisms of clinical arrhythmias. *PACE* 2003;**26**:1778–92.
11. Chen SA, Chiang CE, Yang CJ *et al*. Sustained atrial tachycardia in adult patients. Electrophysiological characteristics, pharmacological response, possible mechanisms, and effects of radiofrequency ablation. *Circulation* 1994;**90**(3):1262–78.
12. Rosen MR. Cellular electrophysiology of digitalis toxicity. *J Am Coll Cardiol.* 1985;**5**(5 suppl A):22A–33A.
13. Steinbeck G, Bonke FI, Allessie MA, Lammers WJ. The effect of ouabain on the isolated sinus node preparation of the rabbit studied with microelectrodes. *Circ Res* 1980;**46**(3):406–14.
14. Akhtar M, Jazayeri MR, Sra J *et al*. Atrioventricular nodal reentry. Clinical, electrophysiological, and therapeutic considerations. *Circulation* 1993;**88**:282–95.
15. Stevenson WG, Sager PT, Friedman PL. Entrainment techniques for mapping atrial and ventricular tachycardias. *J Cardiovasc Electrophysiol* 1995;**6**(3):201–16.
16. Waxman MB, Wald RW, Sharma AD *et al*. Vagal techniques for termination of paroxysmal supraventricular tachycardia. *Am J Cardiol* 1980;**46**:655–64.
17. Singh BN, Nademanee K, Baky SH. Calcium antagonists. Clinical use in the treatment of arrhythmias. *Drugs* 1983;**25**:125–53.

18. Sung RJ, Elser B, McAllister RG Jr. Intravenous verapamil for termination of re-entrant supraventricular tachycardias: Intracardiac studies correlated with plasma verapamil concentrations. *Ann Intern Med* 1980;**93**:682–9.

19. Waxman HL, Myerburg RJ, Appel R, Sung RJ. Verapamil for control of ventricular rate in paroxysmal supraventricular tachycardia and atrial fibrillation or flutter: a double-blind randomized cross-over study. *Ann Intern Med* 1981;**94**:1–6.

20. Dougherty AH, Jackman WM, Naccarelli GV, Friday KJ, Dias VC. Acute conversion of paroxysmal supraventricular tachycardia with intravenous diltiazem. IV Diltiazem Study Group. *Am J Cardiol* 1992;**70**:587–92.

21. DiMarco JP, Sellers TD, Lerman BB *et al.* Diagnostic and therapeutic use of adenosine in patients with supraventricular tachyarrhthmias. *J Am Coll Cardiol* 1985;**6**:417–25.

22. Glatter KA, Cheng J, Dorostkar P *et al.* Electrophysiologic effects of adenosine in patients with supraventricular tachycardia. *Circulation* 1999;**99**:1034–40.

23. DiMarco JP, Miles WH, Akhtar M *et al.* Adenosine for paroxysmal supraventricular tachycardia: Dose ranging and comparison with Verapamil: Assessment in placebo-controlled, multicenter trials. The Adenosine for PSVT Study Group. *Ann Intern Med* 1990;**113**:104–10.

24. Cairns CB, Niemann JT. Intravenous adenosine in the emergency department management of paroxysmal supraventricular tachycardia. *Ann Emerg Med* 1991;**20**:717–21.

25. Das G, Tshida V, Gray R *et al.* Efficacy of esmolol in the treatment and transfer of patients with supraventricular tachyarrhythmias to alternate oral antiarrhythmic agents. *J Clin Pharmacol* 1988;**28**:746–50.

26. Amsterdam EA, Kulcyski J, Ridgeway MG. Efficacy of cardioselective beta-adrenergic blockade with intravenously administered metoprolol in the treatment of supraventricular tachyarrhythmias. *J Clin Pharmacol* 1991;**31**:714–18.

27. Vietti-Ramus G, Veglio F, Marchisio U *et al.* Efficacy and safety of short intravenous amiodarone in supraventricular tachyarrhythmias. *Int J Cardiol* 1992;**35**:77–85.

28. Holt P, Crick JC, Davies DW, Curry P. Intravenous amiodarone in the acute termination of supraventricular arrhythmias. *Int J Cardiol* 1985;**8**:67–79.

29. Henthorn RW, Waldo AL, Anderson JL *et al.* Flecainide acetate prevents recurrence of symptomatic paroxysmal supraventricular tachycardia. The Flecainide Supraventricular Tachycardia Study Group. *Circulation* 1991;**83**:119–25.

30. Anderson JL, Platt ML, Guarnieri T *et al.* Flecainide acetate for paroxysmal supraventricular tachyarrhythmias. The Flecainide Supraventricular Tachycardia Study Group. *Am J Cardiol* 1994;**74**:578–84.

31. Hopson JR, Buxton AE, Rinkenberger RL *et al.* Safety and utility of flecainide acetate in the routine care of patients with supraventricular tachyarrhthmias: results of a multicenter trial. The Flecainide Supraventricular Tachycardia Study Group. *Am J Cardiol* 1996;**77**:72A-82A.

32. Coumel P, Leclercq JF, Assayag P. European experience with the antiarrhythmic efficacy of propafenone for supraventricular and ventricular arrhythmias. *Am J Cardiol* 1984;**54**:60–6.

33. Pritchett EL, McCarthy EA, Wilkinson WE. Propafenone treatment of symptomatic paroxysmal supraventricular arrhythmias. A randomized placebo-controlled, crossover trial in patients tolerating oral therapy. *Ann Intern Med* 1991;**114**: 539–44.

34. UK Propafenone PSVT Study Group. A randomized, placebo-controlled trial of propafenone in the prophylaxis of paroxysmal supraventricular tachycardia and paroxysmal atrial fibrillation. *Circulation* 1995;**92**:2550–7.

35. Wanless RS, Anderson K, Joy M, Joseph SP. Multicenter comparative study of the efficacy and safety of sotalol in the prophylactic treatment of patients with paroxysmal supraventricular tachyarrhythmias. *Am Heart J* 1997;**133**:441–6.

36. Graboys TB, Podrid PJ, Lown B. Efficacy of amiodarone for refractory supraventricular tachyarrhythmias. *Am Heart J* 1983;**106**:870–6.

37. Tendera M, Wnuk-Wojnar A, Kulakowski P *et al.* Efficacy and safety of dofetilide in the prevention of symptomatic episodes of paroxysmal supraventricular tachycardia: A 6-month double-blind comparison with propafenone and placebo. *Am Heart J* 2001;**142**:93–8.

38. Margolis B, DeSilva RA, Lown B. Pill in the pocket (SVT) episodic drug treatment in the management of paroxysmal arrhythmias. *Am JM Cardiol* 1980;**45**:621–6.

39. Alboni P, Tomasic C, Menozzi C, Bottoni N. Efficacy and safety of out of hospital self-administered single-dose oral drug treatment in the management of infrequent well tolerated paroxysmal supraventricular tachycardia. *J Am Coll Cardiol* 2001;**37**:548–53.

40. Goldberg AS, Bathina MN, Mickelsen S *et al.* Long-term outcomes on quality-of-life and health care cost in patients with supraventricular tachycardia (radiofrequency catheter ablation versus medical therapy). *Ann Intern Med* 2000;**133**:864–76.

41. DeSanctis RW, Block P, Hutter AM Jr. Tachyarrhythmias in myocardial infarction. *Circulation* 1972;**45**:681–702.

42. Crimm A, Severance HW Jr, Coffey K *et al.* Prognostic significance of isolated sinus tachycardia during first three days of acute myocardial infarction. *Am J Med* 1984;**76**:983–8.

43. Bauernfeind RA, Amat-Y-Leon F, Dhingra RC, Kehoe R. Chronic nonparoxysmal sinus tachycardia in otherwise healthy persons. *Ann Intern Med* 1979;**91**:702–10.

44. Morillo CA, Klein GJ, Thakur RK *et al.* Mechanism of 'inappropriate' sinus tachycardia. Role of sympathovagal balance. *Circulation* 1994;**90**:873–7.

45. Brady, PA, Low PA, Shen WK. Inappropriate sinus tachycardia, postural orthostatic tachycardia syndrome, and overlapping syndromes. *Pacing Clin Electrophysiol* 2005;**28**:1112–21.

46. Callans DJ, Ren JF, Schwartzman D, Gottlieb CD. Narrowing of the superior vena cava-right atrium junction during radiofrequency catheter ablation for inappropriate sinus tachycardia: analysis with intracardiac echocardiography. *J Am Coll Cardiol* 1999;**33**:1667–70.

47. Krahn AD, Yee R, Klein GJ, Morillo C. Inappropriate sinus tachycardia: evaluation and therapy. *J Cardiovasc Electrophysiol* 1995;**6**:1124–8.

48. Gomes JA, Mehta D, Langan MN. Sinus node re-entrant tachycardia. *PACE* 1995;**18**:1045–57.

49. Sanders WE, Sorrentino RA, Greenfield RA, Shenasa H, Hamer ME, Wharton JM. Catheter ablation of sinoatrial node re-entrant tachycardia. *J Am Coll Cardiol* 1994;**23**:926–34.

50. ACC/AHA/ESC. 2006 Guidelines for the management of patients with atrial fibrillation: A report of the American College of Cardiology/American Heart Association Task Force

on Practice Guidelines and the European Society of Cardiology Committee for Practice Guidelines. *J Am Coll Cardiol* 2006;**48**:e149–e246.

51. Haines DE, DiMarco JP. Sustained intraatrial re-entrant tachycardia: clinical, electrocardiographic and electrophysiologic characteristics and long-term follow-up. *J Am Coll Cardiol* 1990;**15**:1345–54.

52. Kall JG, Dopp D, Olshansky B *et al*. Adenosine-sensitive atrial tachycardia. *PACE* 1995;**18**:300–6.

53. Engelstein ED, Lippman N, Stin KM, Lerman BB. Mechanism-specific effects of adenosine on atrial tachycardia. *Circulation* 1994;**89**:2645–54.

54. Markowitz S, Stein K, Mittal S, Slotwinder D. Differential effects of adenosine on focal and macro-re-entrant atrial tachycardia. *J Cardiovacs Electrophysiol* 1999;**10**:489–502.

55. Kister PM, Roberts-Thomson KC, Haqqani HM, Fynn SP. P-wave morphology in focal atrial tachycardia: development of an algorithm to predict the anatomic site of origin. *J Am Coll Cardiol* 2006;**48**:1010–17.

56. De Groot NM, Schalij MJ. Fragmented, long-duration, low-amplitude electrograms characterize the origin of focal atrial tachycardia. *J Cardiovasc Electrophysiol* 2006;**17**:1086–92.

57. Stock JP. Beta adrenergic blocking drugs in the clinical management of cardiac arrhythmias. *Am J Cardiol* 1966;**18**:444–9.

58. Jeong YH, Choi KJ, Song JM, Hwang ES. Diagnostic approach and treatment strategy in tachycardia-induced cardiomyopathy. *Clin Cardiol* 2008;**31**:172–8.

59. Berns E, Rinkenberger RL, Jeang MK, Dougherty AH. Efficacy and safety of flecainide acetate for atrial tachycardia or fibrillation. *Am J Cardiol* 1987;**59**:1337–41.

60. Kunze KP, Kuck KH, Schluter M, Bleifeld W. Effect of encainide and flecainide on chronic ectopic atrial tachycardia. *J Am Coll Cardiol* 1986;**7**:1121–6.

61. Higa S, Tai CT, Lin YJ, Liu TY. Focal atrial tachycardia: new insight from noncontact mapping and catheter ablation. *Circulation* 2004;**109**:84–91.

62. Rose MR, Glassman E, Spencer FC. Arrhythmias following cardiac surgery: relation to serum digoxin levels. *Am Heart J* 1975;**89**:288–94.

63. Antman EM, Wenger TL, Butler VP Jr, Haber E. Treatment of 150 cases of life-threatening digitalis intoxication with digoxin-specific Fab antibody fragments. Final report of a multicenter study. *Circulation* 1990;**81**:1744–52.

64. Josephson ME. *Clinical Cardiac Electrophysiology: Techniques and Interpretations*, 2nd edn. Philadelphia: Lea and Febiger, 1993.

65. Collins KK, Love BA, Walsh EP, Saul JP. Location of acutely successful radiofrequency catheter ablation of intraatrial re-entrant tachycardia in patients with congenital heart disease. *Am J Cardiol* 2004;**86**:969–74.

66. Kastor JA. Multifocal atrial tachycardia. *N Engl J Med* 1990;**322**:1713–7.

67. Levine JH, Michael JR, Guarnieri T. Multifocal atrial tachycardia: a toxic effect of theophylline. *Lancet* 1985;**5**:12–14.

68. Marchlinski FE, Miller JM. Atrial arrhythmias exacerbated by theophylline. Response to verapamil and evidence for triggered activity in man. *Chest* 1985;**88**:931–4.

69. Wang K, Goldfarb BL, Gobel FL, Richman HG. Multifocal atrial tachycardia. *Arch Intern Med* 1977;**137**:161–4.

70. Hazard PB, Burnett CR. Verapamil in multifocal atrial tachycardia. Hemodynamic and respiratory changes. *Chest* 1987;**91**:68–70.

71. Salerno DM, Anderson B, Sharkey PJ, Iber C. *Ann Intern Med* 1987;**107**:623–8.

72. Arsura EL, Soar M, Lefkin AS, Scher DL. Metoprolol in the treatment of multifocal atrial tachycardia. *Crit Care Med* 1987;**15**:591–4.

73. Iseri LT, Fairshter RD, Hardemann JL, Brodsky MA. Magnesium and potassium therapy in multifocal atrial tachycardia. *Am Heart J* 1985;**110**:789–94.

74. Tucker KJ, Law J, Rodriques MJ. Treatment of refractory recurrent multifocal atrial tachycardia with atrioventricular junction ablation and permanent pacing. *J Invasive Cardiol* 1995;**7**:207–12.

75. Ueng KC, Lee SH, Wu DJ, Lin CS. Radiofrequency catheter modification of atrioventricular junction in patients with COPD and medically refractory multifocal atrial tachycardia. *Chest* 2000;**117**:52–9.

76. Wellens H. Contemporary management of atrial flutter. *Circulation* 2002;**106**:649–52.

77. Stambler BS, Wood MA, Ellengogen KA, Perry KT. Efficacy and safety of repeated intravenous doses of ibutilide for rapid conversion of atrial flutter or fibrillation. *Circulation* 1996;**94**:1613–21.

78. Ellenbogen KA, Stambler BS, Wood MA, Sager PT. Efficacy of intravenous ibutilide for rapid termination of atrial fibrillation and atrial flutter: a dose-response study. *J Am Coll Cardiol* 1996;**28**:130–6.

79. Volgman AS, Carberry PA, Stambler BS, Lewis WR. Conversion efficacy and safety of intravenous ibutilide compared with intravenous procainamide in patients with atrial flutter or fibrillation. *J Am Coll Cardiol* 1998;**31**:1414–19.

80. Stambler BS, Wood MA, Ellenbogen KA. Antiarrhythmic actions of intravenous ibutilide compared with procainamide during human atrial flutter and fibrillation: electrophysiological determinants of enhanced conversion efficacy. *Circulation* 1997;**96**:4298–306.

81. Ibutilide/Sotalol Comparator Study Group. Superiority of ibutilide over DL-sotalol in converting atrial flutter and atrial fibrillation. *Heart* 1998;**79**:568–75.

82. Suttorp MJ, Kingma JH, Jessurun ER, Lie-A-Huen L. The value of class IC antiarrhythmic drugs for acute conversion of paroxysmal atrial fibrillation or flutter to sinus rhythm. *J Am Coll Cardiol* 1990;**16**:1722–7.

83. Tucker KJ, Wilson C. A comparison of transesophageal atrial pacing and direct current cardioversion for termination of atrial flutter: a prospective, randomized clinical trial. *Br Heart J* 1993;**69**:530.

84. Schreck DM, Rivera AR, Tricarico VJ. Emergency management of atrial fibrillation and flutter: Intravenous diltiazem versus intravenous digoxin. *Ann Emerg Med* 1997;**29**:135–40.

85. Tisdale JE, Padhi ID, Goldberg AD, Silverman NA. A randomized, double-blind comparison of intravenous diltiazem and digoxin for atrial fibrillation after coronary bypass surgery. *Am Heart J* 135;**5**:739–47.

86. Ellenbogen KA, Dias VC, Plumb VJ, Heywood JT. A placebo-controlled trial of continuous intravenous diltiazem infusion for 24-hour heart rate control during atrial fibrillation and atrial flutter: a multicenter study. *J Am Coll Cardiol* 1991;**18**:891–7.

87. Goldenberg IF, Lewis WR, Dias VC, Heywood JT. Intravenous diltiazem for the treatment of patients with atrial fibrillation or flutter and moderate to severe congestive heart failure. *Am J Cardiol* 1995;**15**:638–9.

88. Mooss AN, Wurdeman RL, Mohiuddin SM, Reyes AP. Esmolol versus diltiazem in the treatment of postoperative atrial fibrillation/atrial flutter after open heart surgery. *Am Heart J* 2000;**140**:176.

89. Crijns HJ, Van Gelder IC, Tieleman RG, Brugemann J. Long-term outcome of electrical cardioversion in patients with chronic atrial flutter. *Heart* 1997;**77**:56–61.

90. Lanzarotti CJ, Olshansky B. Thromboembolism in chronic atrial flutter: is the risk underestimated? *J Am Coll Cardiol* 1997;**30**:1506–11.

91. Biblo LA, Yuan Z, Quan KJ, Mackall JA. Risk of stroke in patients with atrial flutter. *Am J Cardiol* 2001;**87**:346–9.

92. Hallagan SC, Gersh BJ, Brown RD Jr, Rosales AG. The natural history of lone atrial flutter. *Ann Intern Med* 2004;**140**:265–8.

93. Scheinman MM, Huang S. The 1998 NASPE prospective catheter ablation registry. *Pacing Clin Electrophysiol* 2000;**23**: 1020–8.

94. Da Costa A, Thevenin J, Roche F, Romeyer-Bouchard C. Results form LADIP trial on atrial flutter, a multicenter prospective randomized study comparing amiodarone and radiofrequency ablation after first episode of symptomatic atrial flutter. *Circulation* 2006;**114**:1676–81.

95. Tai CT, Chen SA, Chiang CE, Lee SH. Long-term outcome of radiofrequency catheter ablation for typical atrial flutter: risk prediction of recurrent arrhythmias. *J Cardiovasc Electrophysiol* 1998;**9**:115–21.

96. Natale A, Newby K, Pisano E, Leonelli F. Prospective randomized comparison of antiarrhythmic versus first-line radiofrequency ablation in patients with atrial flutter. *J Am Coll Cardiol* 2000;**35**:1898–904.

97. Luria DM, Hodge DO, Monahan KH, Haroldson JM. Effect of radiofrequency ablation of atrial flutter on the natural history of subsequent atrial arrhythmias. *J Cardiovasc Electrophysiol* 2008;**10**:435–9.

98. Reithmann C, Hoffmann E, Spitzlberger G, Dorwarth U. Catheter ablation of atrial flutter due to amiodarone therapy for paroxysmal atrial fibrillation. *Eur Heart J* 2000;**21**:565–72.

99. Huang DT, Monahan KM, Zimetbaum P, Papageorgiou P. Hybrid pharmacologic and ablative therapy: a novel and effective approach for the management of atrial fibrillation. *J Cardiovasc Electrophysiol* 1998;**9**:462–9.

100. Gursoy S, Steurer G, Brugada J, Andries E, Brugada P. The hemodynamic mechanism of pounding in the neck in atrioventricular nodal re-entrant tachycardia. *N Engl J Med* 1992;**327**:772–4.

101. Gonzalez MD, Contreras LJ, Cardona F, Klugewicz CJ. Demonstration of a Left atrial input to the atrioventricular node in humans. *Circulation* 2002;**106**:2930–4.

102. Heidbuchel H, Jackman WM. Characterization of subforms of AV nodal re-entrant tachycardia. *Europace* 2004;**6**:316–29.

103. Tai CT, Chen SA, Chiang CE, Lee SH. Multiple antegrade atrioventricular node pathways in patients with atrioventricular node re-entrant tachycardia. *J Am Coll Cardiol* 1996;**28**:725–31.

104. Denes P, Wu D, Dhingra RC, Chuquimia R, Rosen KM. Demonstration of dual A-V nodal pathways in patients with paroxysmal supraventricular tachycardia. *Circulation* 1973;**48**: 549–55.

105. Mazgalev T, Tchou P. Atrioventricular nodal conduction gap and dual pathway electrophysiology. *Circulation* 1995;**92**:2705–14.

106. Rankin AC, Brooks R, Ruskin JN, McGovern BA. Adenosine and the treatment of supraventricular tachycardia. *Am J Med* 1992;**92**:655–64.

107. Gambhir DS, Bhargava M, Nair M, Arora R. comparison of electrophysiologic effects and efficacy of single-dose intravenous and long-term oral amiodarone therapy in patients with AV nodal re-entrant tachycardia. *Indian Heart J* 1996;**48**:133–7.

108. Nakagawa H, Jackman WM. Catheter ablation of paroxysmal supraventricular tachycardia. *Circulation* 2007;**116**:2465–78.

109. Hintringer F, Hartikaninen J, Davies DW, Heald SC. Prediction of atrioventricular block during radiofrequency ablation of the slow pathway of the atrioventricular node. *Circulation* 1995;**92**:3490–6.

110. Srivathsan K, Gami AS, Barrett R, Monahan K. Differentiating atrioventricular nodal re-entrant tachycardia from junctional tachycardia: novel application of delta H-A interval. *J cardiovasc Electrophysiol* 2008;**19**:1–6.

111. Kumagai K, Yamato H, Yamanouchi Y, Matsuo K. Automatic junctional tachycardia in an adult. *Clin cardiol* 1990;**13**:813–16.

112. Ruder MA, Davis JC, Eldar M, Abott M. Clinical and electrophysiologic characterization of automatic junctional tachycardia in adults. *Circulation* 1986;**73**:930–7.

113. Villain E, Vetter VL, Garcia JM, Herre J. Evolving concepts in the management of congenital junctional ectopic tachycardia. A multicenter study. *Circulation* 1990;**81**:1713–14.

114. Ehlert FA, Goldberger JJ, Deal BJ, Benson DW. Successful radiofrequency energy ablation of automatic junctional tachycardia preserving normal atrioventricular nodal conduction. *Pacing Clin Electrophysiol* 1993;**16**:54–61.

115. Handan M, Van Hare GF, Fisher W. Selective catheter ablation of the tachycardia focus in patients with nonre-entrant junctional tachycardia. *Am J Cardiol* 1996;**78**:1292–7.

116. Scheinman MM, Gonzalez RP, Cooper MW. Clinical and electrophysiologic features and role of catheter ablation techniques in adult patients with automatic atrioventricular junctional tachycardia. *Am J Cardiol* 1994;**74**:565–72.

117. Storstein O, Hansteen V, Hatle L. Studies on digitalis: XIII: a prospective study of 649 patients on maintenance treatment with digitoxin. *Am Heart J* 1977;**93**:434–43.

118. Knoebel SB, Rasmussen S, Lovelace DE, Anderson GJ. Nonparoxysmal junction tachycardia in acute myocardial infarction: computer-assisted detection. *Am J Cardiol* 1975;**35**:825–30.

119. Palileo EV, Bauernfeind RA, Swiryn SP, Wyndham CR. Chronic nonparoxysmal junctional tachycardia. *Chest* 1981;**80**:106–8.

120. Munger TM, Packer DL, Hammill SC, Feldman BJ. A population study of the natural history of Wolff-Parkinson-White syndrome in Olmsted County, Minnesota, 1953 to 1989. *Circulation* 1993;**87**:866–73.

121. Light PE. Familial Wolff-Parkinson-White syndrome: a disease of glycogen storage or ion channel dysfunction? *J Cardiovasc Electrophysiol* 2006;**17**(S1):58–61.

122. Scheinman MM. History of Wolff-Parkinson-White syndrome. *Pacing Clin Electrophysiol* 2005;**28**:152–6.

123. Pappone C, Santinelli V, Rosanio S, Vicedomini G. Usefulness of invasive electrophysiologic testing to stratify the risk of arrhythmic events in asymptomatic patients with Wolff-Parkinson-White pattern. Results from a large prospective long-term follow-up study. *J Am Coll Cardiol* 2003;**41**:239–44.

124. Wellens HJ. Should catheter ablation be performed in asymptomatic patients with Wolff-Parkinson-White syndrome? When to perform catheter ablation in asymptomatic patients with a Wolff-Parkinson-White syndrome electrocardiogram. *Circulation* 2005;**112**:2201–7.

125. Fitzpatrick AP, Gonzales RP, Lesh MD, Modin GW. New algorithm for the localization of accessory atrioventricular connections using a baseline electrocardiogram. *J Am Coll Cardiol* 1994;**23**:107–16.

126. Dorostkar PC, Silka MJ, Morady F, Dick M 2nd. Clinical course of persistent junctional reciprocating tachycardia. *J Am Coll Cardiol* 1999;**33**:366–75.

127. Wellens HJ, Bar FW, Dassen WR, Brugada P. Effect of drugs in the Wolff-Parkinson-White syndrome. Importance of initial length of effective refractory period of the accessory pathway. *Am J Cardiol* 1980;**46**:665–9.

128. Mandel WJ, Laks MM, Obayashi K, Hayakawa H. The Wolff-Parkinson-White syndrome: pharmacologic effects of procainamide. *Am Heart J* 1975;**90**:744–54.

129. Sellers TD Jr, Bashore TM, Gallagher JJ. Digitalis in the pre-excitation syndrome. Analysis during atrial fibrillation. *Circulation* 1977;**56**:260–7.

130. Garratt C, Antoniou A, Ward D, Camm AJ. Misuse of verapamil in pre-excited atrial fibrillation. *Lancet* 1989;**1**: 367–9.

131. Gulamhusein S, Ko P, Carruthers SG, Klein GJ. Acceleration of the ventricular response during atrial fibrillation in Wolff-Parkinson-White syndrome after verapamil. *Circulation* 1982;**65**:348–54.

132. McGovern B, Garan H, Ruskin JN. Precipitation of cardiac arrest by verapamil in patients with Wolff-Parkinson-White syndrome. *Ann Intern Med* 1986;**104**:791–4.

133. Vassiliadis I, Papoutsakis P, Kallikazaros I, Stefanadis C. Propafenone in the prevention of non-ventricular arrhythmias associated with Wolff-Parkinson-White syndrome. *Int J Cardiol* 1990;**27**:63–70.

134. Kim SS, Lal R, Ruffy R. Treatment of paroxysmal re-entrant supraventricular tachycardia with flecainide acetate. *Am J Cardiol* 1986;**58**:80–5.

135. Cockrell JL, Scheinman MM, Titus C, Helmy I. Safety and efficacy of oral flecainide therapy in patients with atrioventricular re-entrant tachycardia. *Ann Intern Med* 1991;**114**:189–94.

136. Kunze KP, Schluter M, Kuck KH. Sotalol in patients with Wolff-Parkinson-White syndrome. *Circulation* 1987;**75**:1050–7.

137. Feld GK, Nademanee K, Stevenson W, Weiss J. clinical and electrophysiologic effects of amiodarone in patients with atrial fibrillation complicating the Wolff-Parkinson-White syndrome. *Am Heart J* 1988;**115**:102–7.

138. Wellens HJ, Lie KI, Bar FW, Wesdorp JC. Effect of amiodarone in the Wolff-Parkinson-White syndrome. *Am J Cardiol* 1976;**38**:189–94.

139. Kerr CR, Prystowsky EN, Smith WM, Cook L. Electrophysiologic effects of disopyramide phosphate in patients with Wolff-Parkinson-White syndrome. *Circulation* 1982;**65**:869–78.

140. Jackman WM, Wang XZ, Friday KJ, Roman CA. Catheter ablation of accessory atrioventricular pathways (Wolff-Parkinson-White Syndrome) by radiofrequency current. *N Engl J Med* 1991;**324**:1605–11.

40 Prevention and treatment of life-threatening ventricular arrhythmia and sudden death

Carlos A Morillo[1] and Adrian Baranchuk[2]

[1] Hamilton Health Sciences, McMaster University, Hamilton, Ontario, Canada
[2] Kingston General Hospital, Queen's University, Kingston, Ontario, Canada

Introduction

Sudden cardiac death (SCD) remains a major public health problem; however, in the last two decades a series of well-conducted randomized clinical trials have provided solid evidence that has lead to significant changes in guidelines and recommendations.[1] The incidence of SCD varies among reports. In Canada it has been estimated that 40 000 deaths annually are due to cardiovascular disease; 50% of these deaths are sudden.[2] In the United States the annual incidence of SCD is 450,000.[3,4] The global European incidence of sudden death is difficult to calculate, however, the Maastricht study reported an annual incidence of out-of-hospital sudden death of 1 in 1000 inhabitants, which is quite similar to the North American estimates.[5,6] One of the limitations in determining the true estimate of SCD is the lack of uniform criteria to define and classify the mode of death. Most studies define SCD as death occurring within an hour of initiating symptoms.

Risk stratification

Identifying subjects at risk of SCD has proven to be a complex task. Over the past two decades several methods of risk stratification have been developed and evaluated. Different methods have been used in clinical trials of antiarrhythmic agents to select a population at high risk of SCD. The most simple and widely used markers include the degree of reduction in left ventricular ejection fraction (LVEF), and functional class as assessed by the New York Heart Association (NYHA) classification. Direct assessment of ventricular ectopy derived from the 24-hour ambulatory ECG recording and susceptibility to induced

Evidence-Based Cardiology, 3rd edition. Edited by S. Yusuf, J.A. Cairns, A.J. Camm, E.L. Fallen, and B.J. Gersh. © 2010 Blackwell Publishing, ISBN: 978-1-4051-5925-8.

ventricular arrhythmias by programmed electrical stimulation have also been reported.[6] Methods that identify potential triggers such as signal-averaged ECG and more recently T-wave alternans or modulators of autonomic function like heart rate variability, baroreflex sensitivity and turbulence have all been assessed individually or in combination, with disappointing results.[7] To date, LVEF reduction with a threshold around <35% continues to be the easiest and most powerful predictor of both total mortality and SCD.

Although the most prevalent cause of SCD is coronary artery disease, it is important to highlight that non-ischemic dilated cardiomyopathy with depressed LVEF and congenital cardiomyopathies and channelopathies with preserved LVEF have a significant incidence of SCD as primary manifestation.

Suppression of ventricular arrhythmias and sudden cardiac death

Ventricular ectopy is considered an electrical trigger of sustained ventricular arrhythmias and potentially SCD. Several trials evaluated the role of ventricular arrhythmia suppression and its effect on cardiac mortality in patients with coronary artery disease.

The International Mexiletine and Placebo Antiarrhythmic Coronary Trial (IMPACT)[8] included 630 patients with recent myocardial infarction who were randomly assigned to treatment with mexiletine or placebo. After an average follow up of nine months, the mortality on mexiletine was 7.6% and on placebo was 48% (P = NS). The Cardiac Arrhythmic Suppression Trial (CAST)[9] enrolled 1727 patients with recent onset of myocardial infarction and with asymptomatic, or mildly symptomatic, ventricular arrhythmia (≥6 ventricular premature ventricular complexes per hour), potentially suppressible by a class I antiarrhythmic drug (encainide, flecainide or moricizine), who were randomized to the active antiarrhythmic drug or placebo and followed for arrhythmic death. The trial was halted early because of an increased incidence of arrhythmic cardiac death and non-fatal cardiac arrests in patients treated with encainide and flecainide (4.5% vs 1.2%, risk ratio (RR) 3.6, 95% confidence interval (CI) 1.7–8.5). In a meta-analysis of the results of 138 trials of antiarrhythmic prophylactic therapy in patients after myocardial infarction,[10] there were 660 deaths among 11 712 patients allocated to receive class I agents and 571 deaths among 11 517 corresponding control patients (51 trials: odds ratio (OR) 1.14; 95% CI 1.01–1.28; $P = 0.03$). Based on this evidence, class I antiarrhythmic agents have been abandoned for the reduction of the the risk of SCD in patients with ischemic cardiomyopathy and non-sustained ventricular arrhythmia.

Class III antiarrhythmic agents were tested in a series of randomized studies. The two largest trials using amiodarone are the Canadian Amiodarone Myocardial Infarction Arrhythmia Trial (CAMIAT)[11] and the European Myocardial Infarction Amiodarone Trial (EMIAT).[12] Both showed a reduction in arrhythmic death but no significant reduction in overall death. Meta-analysis of data from all 13 randomized controlled trials of amiodarone (89% of patients, after myocardial infarction) showed a significant reduction in total mortality (OR 0.87, 95% CI 0.78–0.99) and a significant reduction in arrhythmic death (OR 0.71, 95% CI 0.59–0.85).[13,14]

Analysis of the interaction between the treatment and baseline factors suggested an important positive relationship between beta-blocker use and amiodarone effect,[15] such that patients on beta-blockers received a significantly greater benefit from amiodarone than those not on beta-blockers. More recently, the association of amiodarone and beta-blockers has been demonstrated to markedly reduce the incidence of appropriate ICD therapy. In the Optimal Pharmacological Therapy in Cardioverter Defibrillator Patients (OPTIC) trial,[16] amiodarone plus beta-blocker significantly reduced the risk of appropriate ICD shocks compared with beta-blocker alone (HR 0.27; 95% CI 0.14–0.52; $P < 0.001$) or sotalol (HR 0.43; 95% CI 0.22–0.85; $P = 0.02$).

D-Sotalol, a pure class III agent, was evaluated for prevention of SCD in a placebo-controlled trial of 3121 patients with recent myocardial infarction and LVEF <40%, or symptomatic heart failure with a remote myocardial infarction (Survival with Oral d-sotalol, SWORD trial).[17] Among 1549 patients assigned to d-sotalol there were 78 deaths (5.0%) compared to 48 (3.1%) among the 1572 patients assigned to placebo (RR 1.65, 95% CI 1.15–2.36). Presumed arrhythmic deaths (RR 1.77, 95% CI 1.15–2.74) accounted for the excess mortality in the d-sotalol group. This proarrhythmic fatal effect of d-sotalol was greater in patients with a left ventricular ejection fraction of 31–40% than in those with lower ejection fractions (RR 4.0 vs 1.2, $P = 0.007$). In a multicenter double-blind randomized study, Julian *et al* reported the effect of sotalol 320 mg once daily compared

with placebo in patients surviving an AMI.[18] Treatment was started 5–14 days after infarction in 1456 patients (60% being randomized to sotalol and 40% to placebo). Patients were followed for 12 months. The mortality rate was 7.3% (64 patients) in the sotalol group and 8.9% (52 patients) in the placebo group. The mortality was 18% lower in the sotalol than in the placebo group, but this difference was not statistically significant.

Another pure class III compound, dofetilide, was tested in patients with symptomatic heart failure. In the Danish Investigations of Arrhythmia and Mortality on Dofetilide (DIAMOND), 1518 patients were randomized to dofetilide or placebo.[19,20] The study treatment was initiated in hospital and included three days of cardiac monitoring and dose adjustment. During a median follow-up of 18 months, 311 patients in the dofetilide group (41%) and 317 patients in the placebo group (42%) died (OR 0.95; 95% CI 0.81–1.11). Treatment with dofetilide significantly reduced the risk of hospitalization for worsening congestive heart failure (CHF), rate of conversion and risk of recurrence of atrial fibrillation. There were 25 cases of torsades de pointes in the dofetilide group (3.3%), compared to none in the placebo group. Dofetilide has also been tested in a randomized trial of 1510 patients with severe LVEF ≤35% after recent myocardial infarction (DIAMOND MI trial).[21] The primary endpoint was all-cause mortality. No significant difference was found between the dofetilide and placebo groups in overall mortality (31% vs 32%). The cardiac mortality (26% vs 28%) and arrhythmic mortality (17% vs 18%) were also similar. There were seven cases of torsades de pointes ventricular tachycardia, all in the dofetilide group. In the Azimilide Postinfarct Survival Evaluation (ALIVE) trial the effect of azimilide, another pure class III agent, was evaluated in 3717 patients with recent myocardial infarction, with LVEF <35% and with low heart rate variability. Azimilide had no effect on mortality (HR 1.0).[22]

Other studies have tested antiarrhythmic agents in patients with sustained ventricular arrhythmias. The endpoints were arrhythmic death, recurrence of sustained ventricular arrhythmia or reinducibility of ventricular tachycardia during programmed electrical stimulation. Steinbeck *et al*[23] conducted a prospective randomized trial in 170 patients to investigate whether electrophysiologic study (EPS)-guided antiarrhythmic therapy improved the long-term outcome of patients with spontaneous and inducible sustained ventricular arrhythmia compared with metoprolol therapy not guided by EPS. In 55 patients ventricular tachycardia was not inducible during the baseline EPS, thereby precluding further serial drug testing. These patients were treated with metoprolol. The two-year incidence of the composite outcome was the same for EPS-guided therapy compared to metoprolol (46% vs 48%).

The Electrophysiological Study Versus Electrocardiographic Monitoring (ESVEM) study[24,25] included patients with inducible ventricular tachycardia and any of the following: (i) history of cardiac arrest, (ii) sustained ventricular tachycardia or (iii) syncope. They were randomly assigned to undergo serial testing to determine efficacy of antiarrhythmic drugs either by performing EPS or by 24-hour ambulatory ECG monitoring. Patients (n = 486) received long-term treatment with the first antiarrhythmic drug that was determined to be effective on the basis of either repeated EPS or 24-hour Holter. The ESVEM study concluded that therapies guided by EPS or Holter monitoring were comparable. The secondary outcome, related to the efficacy of individual antiarrhythmic drugs, concluded that sotalol was more effective than the class I drugs tested. The actuarial probability of a recurrence of arrhythmia after a drug was deemed efficacious by either strategy was significantly lower for patients treated with sotalol than for patients treated with other antiarrhythmic agents (RR 0.43; 95% CI 0.29–0.62). Sotalol significantly reduced the risk of all-cause mortality (RR 0.50; 95% CI 0.30–0.80), cardiac mortality (0.50; $P = 0.02$) and arrhythmic death (0.50; $P = 0.04$).

In the Cardiac Arrest in Seattle: Conventional versus Amiodarone Drug Evaluation (CASCADE) study, antiarrhythmic drug therapy was evaluated in survivors of out-of-hospital ventricular fibrillation (VF).[26] Amiodarone without EPS or Holter guidance was compared to class I antiarrhythmic agents (quinidine, procainamide, their combination, or flecainide), selected by serial EPS or Holter monitoring. Most of the 228 randomized patients had coronary artery disease with a prior myocardial infarction, and the mean LVEF was 35 ± 10%. During a mean follow-up of six years, amiodarone improved survival compared to class I agents (53% vs 40%, $P = 0.007$).

The Sudden Cardiac Death in Heart Failure Trial (SCD-HeFT) randomly assigned 2521 patients with NYHA class II or III CHF and a LVEF of 35% or less to conventional therapy for CHF plus placebo (847 patients), conventional therapy plus amiodarone (845 patients), or conventional therapy plus a conservatively programmed, shock-only, single-lead ICD (829 patients).[27] Placebo and amiodarone were administered in a double-blind fashion. The primary endpoint was death from any cause. Mortality was 29% in the placebo group and 28% in the amiodarone group. As compared with placebo, amiodarone was associated with a similar risk of death (HR1.06; 97.5% CI 0.86–1.30; $P = 0.53$).

Beta-blockers and prevention of sudden cardiac death

Beta-blockers are the agent most frequently studied in postmyocardial infarction patients for the prevention of death, with more than 12 large trials reported. A meta-analysis of the beta-blocker trials, reported in 1985, showed a significant reduction in mortality during treatment after myocardial infarction.[28] This meta-analysis also indicated a highly significant 30% reduction in sudden cardiac death with beta-blockers. The risk of non-sudden death was also decreased by 12%, but this difference was not significant. Recent beta-blocker trials in CHF patients also show a reduction in both overall deaths and SCD.[29-32] Beta-blockers are effective against arrhythmic death (20–30% reduction) and non-arrhythmic deaths, and reduce overall mortality significantly. Beta-blocker therapy is indicated in all patients at high risk for SCD.

In summary, antiarrhythmic drugs have been extensively evaluated in randomized trials as prophylactic agents against death, but little tested against recurrence of arrhythmia. Class I antiarrhythmic drugs are harmful and are proscribed in patients with ischemic heart disease and reduced LVEF. Amiodarone has a moderate effect against SCD and a neutral effect on other deaths, therefore its overall effect on total mortality is modest. Pure class III agents are at best neutral and, in the case of d-sotalol, actually harmful. Pure class III antiarrhythmic agents clearly do not reduce mortality or SCD when used prophylactically in high-risk patients. The different results of d-sotalol, dofetilide and azimilide trials are probably due to differences in the design of the studies and differences in risk of torsades de pointes between the agents.

Recommendations

- Beta-blockers are indicated in patients with myocardial infarction or congestive heart failure for the prevention of death (**Class I, Level A**).
- Amiodarone, usually in combination with beta-blockers, can be useful for patients with LV dysfunction due to prior MI and symptoms due to VT unresponsive to beta-blockers (**Class IIa, Level B**).
- Sotalol is reasonable therapy to reduce symptoms resulting from ventricular tachyarrhythmia (VT) for patients with LV dysfunction due to prior MI unresponsive to beta-blockers. Amiodarone or sotalol is reasonable adjunctive therapies for patients with implantable cardioverter-defibrillators (ICD) to improve symptoms due to frequent episodes of sustained VT or VF in patients with LV dysfunction due to prior MI.
- Amiodarone is reasonable therapy to reduce symptoms due to recurrent hemodynamically stable VT for patients with LV dysfunction due to prior MI who cannot or refuse to have an ICD implanted (**Class IIb, Level C**).
- Amiodarone may be reasonable therapy for patients with LV dysfunction due to prior MI with an ICD indication, who cannot or refuse to have an ICD implanted (**Class IIb, Level C**).
- Class Ic antiarrhythmics should be avoided in patients with coronary artery disease or LV dysfunction (**Class III, Level A**).

Upstream therapy and prevention of sudden cardiac death

The effect of angiotensin-converting enzyme (ACE) inhibitors on the risk of SCD following myocardial infarction has been demonstrated in randomized trials.[33–35] A recent meta-analysis incorporated data from 15 trials that included 15 104 patients having 900 SCD.[35] ACE inhibitor therapy resulted in a significant reduction in total mortality (OR 0.83, 95% CI 0.71–0.97), cardiovascular death (OR 0.82, 95% CI 0.69–0.97) and SCD (OR 0.80, 95% CI 0.70–0.92). Also, the meta-analysis suggested that a reduction in SCD risk with ACE inhibitors was an important component of overall survival benefit, the magnitude of effect on SCD being the same as on overall mortality.

Interestingly, in the Heart Outcome Prevention Evaluation (HOPE) Study[36] involving cardiovascular patients without a significant decrease in left ventricular function (LVEF >40%), the ACE inhibitor ramipril significantly decreased the incidence of cardiac arrest (RR 0.62, 95% CI 0.41–0.94). The mechanism by which ACE inhibitors reduce SCD is poorly understood. In addition to attenuation of remodeling, thereby reducing the substrate for ventricular tachyarrhythmia, they provide significant neurohumoral modulation and protection from future ischemic events.

Angiotensin receptor blockers (ARB) are potentially antiarrhythmic; this effect can be explained by blockade of the angiotensin II receptor type I leading to inhibition of the proarrhythmic effects of angiotensin II.[37] Several trials of different angiotensin receptor blockers have demonstrated equivalent effects to those of ACE inhibitors on cardiac and overall mortality. However, with the exception of the CHARM trials, the addition of an ARB to an ACE inhibitor has not yielded any added benefits.[38] In summary, ARBs should be used as alternative therapy in patients intolerant to ACE inhibitors.

In the Randomized Aldactone Evaluation Study (RALES),[39] aldactone was evaluated in patients having NYHA III–IV. After a mean follow-up of 24 months, the incidence of SCD was significantly decreased (RR 0.71, 95% CI 0.54–0.95). The magnitude of this effect was similar to the effect on total mortality (RR 0.70, 95% CI 0.68–0.72). In the EPHESUS trial patients with an acute myocardial infarction complicated by symptomatic LV dysfunction were randomized to standard therapy versus standard therapy plus eplerenone.[40] Eplerenone significantly reduced all-cause mortality, cardiovascular death and the risk of cardiovascular death or hospitalization. Interestingly SCD was also significantly reduced (RR 0.79, 95% CI 0.64–0.97). Either spironolactone or eplerenone is recommended as adjunctive therapy in patients with heart failure with LV dysfunction and NYHA class III–IV.

The role of n-3 polyunsaturated fatty acids for the prevention of SCD has been assessed in a number of randomized trials. The Diet And Reinfarction Trial randomized 2033 men with recent myocardial infarction and reported a significant reduction in both cardiac and total mortality (RR 0.71, 95% CI 0.54–0.93).[41] In a larger study, the GISSI-Prevenzione Trial,[42] treatment with n-3 polyunsaturated fatty acids in 11 324 postmyocardial infarction patients significantly decreased the incidence of SCD (RR 0.74, 95% CI 0.58–0.93), also significantly decreasing total cardiac mortality and coronary mortality by a similar extent (RR 0.78 and 0.80, respectively, both significant). A recent systematic review of 48 RCTs (36 913 participants) and 41 cohort studies did not document a clear effect of omega 3 fats on total mortality, combined cardiovascular events or cancer.[43] The pooled estimate of this meta-analysis showed no strong evidence of reduced risk of total mortality (relative risk 0.87, 95% CI 0.73–1.03) or combined cardiovascular events (0.95, 0.82–1.12) in participants taking additional omega 3 fats. When data from the subgroup of studies of long-chain omega 3 fats were analyzed separately, total mortality (0.86, 0.70–1.04; 138 events) and cardiovascular events (0.93, 0.79–1.11) were not clearly reduced. Neither RCTs nor cohort studies suggested increased risk of cancer with a higher intake of omega 3 (trials: 1.07, 0.88–1.30; cohort studies: 1.02, 0.87–1.19), but clinically important harm could not be excluded.

In summary, the effects of fish oils on SCD and cardiovascular morbidity and mortality remain debated. The protective effect of fish oils may be limited to patients with a previous myocardial infarction. Current guidelines recommend that patients with documented coronary artery disease consume approximately 1 g of EPA+ DHA per day, preferably from oily fish although supplements can also be considered.[44]

Thus, accumulated evidence supports the wide use of upstream interventions in appropriate patients.

Recommendations

- ACE inhibitors and, in ACE-intolerant patients, ARBs are indicated in patients with myocardial infarction or congestive heart failure for the prevention of death (**Class I, Level A**).
- Polyunsaturated fatty acids (1 g of EPA+ DHA per day) are recommended in patients with known cardiovascular disease for the prevention of cardiovascular outcomes (**Class IIa, Level B**).

Implantable cardioverter-defibrillators for prevention of sudden cardiac death

Several studies have assessed the effectiveness of ICDs for the prevention of SCD in high-risk populations. The primary risk stratifier is a LVEF ≤35%. In some instances the presence of non-sustained VT or the induction of VT during programmed electrical stimulation have been used as inclusion criteria. These trials may be classified according to the underlying anatomic substrate:
• Coronary artery disease and depressed LVEF: MADIT,[45] CABG-Patch,[46] MUSTT,[47] MADIT II,[48] DINAMIT[49]
• Dilated non-ischemic cardiomyopathy (DCM) and depressed LVEF: CAT,[50] AMIOVIRT,[51] DEFINITE[52]
• LVEF <35% independent of the etiology of the underlying cardiomyopathy: SCD-HeFT.[27]

Primary prevention of SCD in ischemic cardiomyopathy

The rationale for the CABG-Patch trial was developed at a time when a thoracotomy was required for implantation of an ICD. Thus patients scheduled for CABG and with LVEF ≤35% were further stratified for risk of arrhythmic death by signal-averaged ECG.[46] There were 900 high-risk patients randomized to receive an ICD or not at the time of CABG. Antiarrhythmic drug use was similar between the two groups. There were 52 patients randomized to ICD who either never received a device or who had it removed. There were 198 deaths (102 in the ICD group and 96 in the control group) for an overall mortality rate of 21.8% during an average follow-up of 32 ± 16 months. The hazard ratio was 1.07 (95% CI 0.81–1.42), indicating no benefit from the ICD in this patient population. Secondary analysis showed that the ICD did reduce arrhythmic death; this potential benefit was offset by an unexplained increase in non-arrhythmic deaths.

The Multicenter Automatic Defibrillator Implantation Trial (MADIT)[45] included patients with LVEF <35% and recent myocardial infarction who were screened with programmed ventricular stimulation. Patients with inducible VT or VF were enrolled in the study if inducibility of VT could not be suppressed by procainamide. There were 196 patients randomized to receive either an ICD or "conventional" therapy. The choice of conventional therapy was at the discretion of the investigator. Amiodarone and beta-blockers, the only drugs proven effective against VT and VF, were used predominantly but sporadically (in 45% and 5%, respectively, of "conventional" patients at last contact). The trial was terminated prematurely when about 75% of planned enrollment had occurred, because of marked benefit derived from ICD treatment (HR 0.46; 95% CI 0.26–0.82; P = 0.009). When the specific causes of death were examined, the ICD not only reduced arrhythmic death, but also appeared to reduce non-arrhythmic cardiac death, and deaths of unknown cause, which is unexplained and biologically implausible.

The Multicenter Unsustained Tachycardia Trial (MUSTT)[47] was a randomized trial of electrophysiologically guided antiarrhythmic therapy in patients with coronary artery disease, LVEF ≤0.40 and asymptomatic, non-sustained ventricular tachycardia. Seven hundred and four patients who satisfied these criteria, and in whom sustained VT was induced by programmed stimulation, were randomly assigned to receive either antiarrhythmic drug tailored by electrophysiologic testing, including drugs and ICDs (if drugs failed to suppress inducibility), or no antiarrhythmic therapy. The primary endpoint of cardiac arrest or death from arrhythmia was reached in 25% of those receiving electrophysiologically guided therapy, and in 32% of those assigned to no antiarrhythmic therapy (relative risk 0.73, 95% CI 0.53–0.99). Five-year total mortality was 42% in patients receiving EPS-guided therapy, versus 48% in controls (RR 0.80, 95% CI 0.64–1.01). In a non-randomized analysis the primary endpoint was less frequent among patients who received ICDs compared to patients discharged without an ICD (relative risk 0.24; 95% CI 0.13–0.45; P < 0.001). In contrast, the primary endpoint was similar among those receiving antiarrhythmic therapy compared to those on no therapy.

The second Multicenter Automatic Defibrillator Implantation Trial (MADIT II)[48] included patients with LVEF ≤30% but *without* evidence of sustained VT/VF and excluded those with recent (<1 month) myocardial infarction, coronary artery bypass graft (CABG) or percutaneous transluminal coronary angioplasty (PTCA) (<2 months). There were 1232 patients randomly assigned to receive an ICD (742 patients) or conventional medical therapy (490 patients). During an average follow-up of 20 months, the mortality rates were 19.8% in the conventional therapy group and 14.2% in the defibrillator group (HR 0.69, 95% CI 0.51–0.93). MADIT II was a landmark trial expanding ICD indications to patients with severe LVEF impairment due to ischemic cardiomyopathy but with no evidence of sustained ventricular arrhythmia.

Identifying those subjects with coronary artery disease (CAD) and severe LV dysfunction who will derive the greatest benefit from prophylactic ICD therapy remains a challenge. Several MADIT II subgroup studies have been reported including survival in elderly patients, QRS duration, and clinical risk factors, and time after MI.[53-57] An important question is whether ICD therapy maintains its efficacy in elderly subjects, addressed by Huang *et al* in a MADIT II substudy.[54] Among 1232 patients enrolled with prior infarct and LVEF ≤0.30, 204 were ≥75 years old and of those, 121 underwent ICD implant.

The hazard ratio for mortality in patients ≥75 years assigned to ICD compared with those in conventional therapy was 0.56 (95% CI 0.29–1.08; P = 0.08) after a mean follow-up of 17.2 months. Comparatively, the hazard ratio in patients <75 years assigned to ICD was 0.63 (0.45–0.88; P = 0.01) after 20.8 months. The ICD was associated with an equivalent reduction of mortality in elderly and younger patients. Dhar et al evaluated the prognostic significance of prolonged QRS relative to arrhythmic outcomes in medically and ICD-treated patients enrolled in MADIT II.[55] In the medically treated arm, prolonged QRS was a significant independent predictor of SCD (HR 2.12; 95% CI 1.20–3.76; P = 0.01). However, in the ICD-treated arm, prolonged QRS did not predict SCD or rapid VT/VF (HR 0.77; 95% CI 0.47–1.24; P = 0.28). The difference in the prognostic effect of prolonged QRS in these two groups was significant (P < 0.01). These results suggest that in MADIT II patients, prolonged QRS does not predict SCD/VT/VF in ICD-treated patients but does predict SCD in medically treated patients. This underscores the non-equivalence of VT/VF and SCD and the need for caution in inferring risk of SCD when using non-randomized databases that include only patients with ICDs.

Clinical risk factors may be useful to identify subjects who would benefit from a prophylactic ICD implant. Goldenberg et al developed a simple clinical risk score (NYHA class >II, age >70 years, BUN >26 mg/dl, QRS duration >0.12 s, and atrial fibrillation) using a proportional-hazards regression analysis for the end point of all-cause mortality in patients allocated to the conventional therapy arm of MADIT II.[56] A prespecified subgroup of very high-risk (VHR) patients (BUN ≥50 mg/dL and/or serum creatinine ≥2.5 mg/dL) was excluded. The benefit of the ICD was then assessed within risk score categories and separately in VHR patients. Crude mortality rates in the conventional group were 8% and 28% in patients with 0 and ≥1 risk factors, respectively, and 43% in VHR patients. ICD therapy was associated with a 49% reduction in the risk of death (P < 0.001) among patients with ≥1 risk factors (n = 786), whereas no ICD benefit was identified in patients with 0 risk factors (n = 345; HR 0.96; P = 0.91) and in VHR patients (n = 60; HR 1.00; P > 0.99). Patients that derive the greatest benefit from a prophylactic ICD are at intermediate risk, in contrast, low-risk and VHR patients have attenuated efficacy with an ICD.

One of the most important questions that clinicians pose when having to determine whether an asymptomatic patient with CAD and a LVEF ≤30% will benefit from ICD therapy is the time from most recent MI, evaluated by Wilber et al in a substudy of the MADIT II trial.[57] Mortality rates (deaths per 100 person-years of follow-up) in both treatment groups were analyzed by time from MI divided into quartiles (<18, 18–59, 60–119, and > = 120 months). In conventional care patients, these rates increased as time

from MI increased (7.8%, 8.4%, 11.6%, 14.0%; P = 0.03). Mortality rates in ICD patients were consistently lower in each quartile and showed minimal increases over time (7.2%, 4.9%, 8.2%, 9.0%; P = 0.19). Covariate-adjusted hazard ratios for risk of death associated with ICD therapy were 0.97 (95% CI 0.51–1.81; P = 0.92) for recent MI (<18 months) and 0.55 (95% CI 0.39–0.78; P = 0.001) for remote MI (> = 18 months). These investigators concluded that the survival benefit associated with ICDs appears to be greater for remote MI and remains substantial for up to 15 years after MI.

In summary, the efficacy of prophylactic ICD therapy based on the MADIT II criteria seems to be maintained in elderly patients, particularly in those without significant co-morbidities. QRS duration does not appear to be of use to further stratify patients that will benefit and some clinical risk factors such as impaired renal function, NYHA class, age >70 and atrial fibrillation may be helpful to identify patients at intermediate risk of dying, and who derive the greatest benefit from ICD therapy. Nonetheless none of these findings has been transferred into current guidelines and larger trials and prolonged follow-up are needed.

The most appropriate timing for the insertion of an ICD after an acute myocardial infarction (AMI) had not been specifically addressed in previous clinical trials. The Defibrillator in Acute Myocardial Infarction Trial (DINAMIT)[49] was a randomized trial that compared ICD versus no ICD in a group of patients recruited during the period immediately following an acute myocardial infarction (6–40 days). Inclusion criteria were LVEF <35% and depressed heart rate variability defined as standard deviation of the N–N interval (SDNN) ≤70 ms. There was no difference in the primary outcome of overall mortality between the two groups (95% CI 0.76–1.55; P = 0.66) (follow-up 30 ± 13 months). However, there was a reduction in arrhythmic deaths that was offset by an increase in non-arrhythmic deaths in the ICD group. The conclusion of the DINAMIT study reinforces the need to delay the decision to implant an ICD by at least six weeks in patients with a recent myocardial infarction. Reassessment of LVEF at the end of this waiting time is required in order to confirm the severity of LV dysfunction. This trial also highlights the presence of competing risks in the early post-AMI phase that may offset the benefits of the ICD.

Primary prevention of SCD in non-ischemic dilated cardiomyopathy (DCM)

Non-ischemic dilated cardiomyopathy is a term that encompasses a variety of etiologies that may lead to the final outcome of dilated cardiomyopathy. This should be noted when interpreting the various different clinical trials reported to date. In the Cardiomyopathy Trial (CAT)[50] patients with recent onset of DCM and LVEF ≤30% were randomly assigned to ICD vs no ICD. The primary end-point was all-cause mortality at one year of follow-up. The trial was terminated after the inclusion of 104 patients (50 ICD, 54 control) because the all-cause mortality rate at one year did not reach the expected 30% in the control group. Mean follow-up was 22.8 ± 4.3 months; no SCD occurred during the first or second year. Cumulative survival was not significantly different between the two groups (93% and 80% in the control group versus 92% and 86% in the ICD group after two and four years, respectively). The lack of benefit for the ICD group could be explained by the uncertain evolution of a recently diagnosed DCM with some patients having spontaneous recovery of LVEF to near normal values.

The Amiodarone Versus Implantable Cardioverter-defibrillator Randomized Trial (AMIOVIRT)[51] randomized 103 patients with DCM, LVEF <35% and asymptomatic non-sustained ventricular tachycardia to receive either amiodarone or an ICD. The primary endpoint was total mortality; secondary endpoints included arrhythmia-free survival, quality of life, and costs. The study was stopped when the prospective stopping rule for futility was reached. The percentages of patients surviving at one year (90% vs 96%) and three years (88% vs. 87%) in the amiodarone and ICD groups, respectively, were not statistically different ($P = 0.8$). Quality of life was also similar with each therapy ($P = NS$). Amiodarone showed a trend towards improved arrhythmia-free survival ($P = 0.1$) and lower costs during the first year of therapy ($8879 v. $22 039, $P = 0.1$).

In the Defibrillators in Non-Ischemic Cardiomyopathy Treatment Evaluation (DEFINITE)[52] study, 458 patients with DCM, LVEF <36% and premature ventricular complexes or non-sustained VT were randomized to receive standard medical therapy alone versus standard medical therapy plus a single-chamber ICD. Standard medical therapy included ACE inhibitors (86%) and beta-blockers (85%); mean LVEF was 21%. During a mean follow-up of 29 ± 14.4 months, there were 68 deaths: 28 in the ICD group and 40 in the standard therapy group (HR 0.65; 95% CI 0.40–1.06; $P = 0.08$). The mortality rate at two years was 14.1% in the standard therapy group and 7.9% in the ICD group. There were 17 sudden deaths from arrhythmia: three in the ICD group and 14 in the standard therapy group (HR 0.20; 95% CI 0.06–0.71; $P = 0.006$). The conclusion was that the addition of an ICD to standard treatment that should include an ACE inhibitor plus a beta-blocker significantly reduces SCD but has minimal impact in reducing overall mortality.

Primary prevention of SCD in patients with dilated cardiomyopathy

The Sudden Cardiac Death in Heart Failure Trial (SCD-HeFT)[27] was the largest trial including DCM patients. It

randomly assigned 2521 patients with NYHA class II or III heart failure and a LVEF ≤35% to conventional therapy for heart failure plus placebo conventional therapy plus amiodarone, or conventional therapy plus a conservatively programmed, shock-only, single-lead ICD. The primary endpoint was death from any cause. Median LVEF was 25%, 70% were in heart failure NYHA class II and 30% were in class III. The cause of heart failure was ischemic in 52% and non-ischemic in 48%. During a median follow-up of 45.5 months, there were 244 deaths (29%) in the placebo group, 240 (28%) in the amiodarone group, and 182 (22%) in the ICD group. The risk of death on amiodarone was similar to that on placebo (HR 1.06; 97.5% CI 0.86–1.30; $P = 0.53$) while ICD therapy was associated with a decreased risk of death (HR 0.77; 97.5% CI 0.62–0.96; $P = 0.007$) and an absolute decrease in mortality of 7.2 percentage points after five years in the overall population, independent of whether the cause of heart failure was ischemic or non-ischemic (Fig. 40.1). Of note, ICD therapy had a 46% relative risk reduction in mortality in patients with NYHA class II (HR 0.54; 97.5% CI 0.40–0.74) (Fig. 41.3). In contrast, patients with NYHA class III had no benefit from ICD therapy (HR 1.16; 97.5% CI 0.8–1.61). There is no obvious biologic reason for this unexpected result, but it is possible that patients with more advanced heart failure die from pump failure, and resynchronization therapy or heart transplant may be the therapies of choice. These findings should be interpreted with caution since other trials such as MADIT II have not reproduced these findings. Current guidelines recommend prophylactic ICD therapy in patients with both NYHA Class II and III.

ICD for secondary prevention of SCD

All the secondary prevention trials comparing amiodarone versus ICD in patients surviving VT/VF were extensively described in the previous edition of this book.[58] The three largest of these were the Canadian Implantable Defibrillator Study (CIDS),[59] the Antiarrhythmic versus Implantable Defibrillator (AVID)[60] and the Cardiac Arrest Study Hamburg (CASH).[61] CASH enrolled patients with prior VF, whereas CIDS and AVID study enrolled both patients with prior VF as well as patients with hemodynamically unstable VT. CIDS also enrolled patients with decreased LV function, syncope and inducible VT.

A meta-analysis including the three trials[62] showed a significant reduction in death from any cause with the ICD, with a summary HR (ICD vs amiodarone) of 0.72 (95% CI 0.60–0.87; $P = 0.0006$). For the outcome of arrhythmic death the HR was 0.50 (95% CI 0.37–0.67; $P < 0.0001$). Survival was extended by a mean of 4.4 months by the ICD over a follow-up period of six years. Patients with LVEF ≤35% derived significantly more benefit from ICD therapy than those with better LV function (HR 1.2, 95% CI 0.86–1.76 in

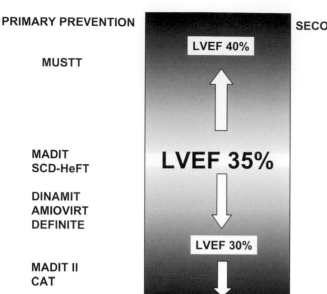

PRIMARY PREVENTION

MUSTT

MADIT
SCD-HeFT

DINAMIT
AMIOVIRT
DEFINITE

MADIT II
CAT

LVEF 40%

LVEF 35%

LVEF 30%

SECONDARY PREVENTION

CIDS
AVID
CASH

Figure 40.1 Clinical trials evaluating the role of ICD in both primary and secondary indications. LVEF <35% is the threshold suggested by most primary prevention trials. Graded color towards an LVEF of 40% suggests that the benefit of ICD is less marked than in patients with more severe deterioration of LVEF.

patients with LVEF >35% vs HR 0.66, 95% CI in patients with LVEF ≤35%, $P_{interaction}$ = 0.011). The point estimates of ICD benefit from the three studies were consistent with each other ($P_{heterogeneity}$ = 0.306).

Among patients presenting with life-threatening sustained VT or VF the balance of evidence now favors ICD therapy over amiodarone, particularly in those with impaired LV function (<35%). In light of the modest prolongation of life conferred by the ICD and its high cost, where resources are limited, efforts should be directed towards identifying patients in higher-risk groups and considering amiodarone as a reasonable alternative.

Antiarrhythmic drugs as adjunctive ICD therapy

ICDs and antiarrhythmic drugs should not be considered as exclusive alternatives.[63] In fact, a significant proportion of ICD patients receive concomitant antiarrhythmic therapy to help control supraventricular tachyarrhythmia, recurrent ventricular arrhythmia and frequent appropriate and inappropriate ICD shocks. Indeed, the ICD does not prevent VT/VF, only its fatal consequences.

In the OPTIC[16] study, 412 patients with an ICD were randomized to receive blinded amiodarone + beta-blocker vs sotalol alone vs beta-blocker alone for one year. The primary outcome was ICD shock for any reason; they occurred in 12 patients (10.3%) assigned to amiodarone plus beta-blocker, 26 (24.3%) assigned to sotalol, and 41 (38.5%) assigned to beta-blocker alone. A reduction in the risk of shock was observed with use of either amiodarone plus beta-blocker or sotalol versus beta-blocker alone (HR 0.44; 95% CI 0.28–0.68; P < 0.001). Amiodarone plus beta-

blocker significantly reduced the risk of shock compared with beta-blocker alone (HR 0.27; 95% CI 0.14–0.52; P < 0.001) and with sotalol (HR 0.43; 95% CI 0.22–0.85; P = 0.02). The rates of study drug discontinuation at one year were 18.2% for amiodarone, 23.5% for sotalol, and 5.3% for beta-blocker alone. Adverse pulmonary and thyroid events and symptomatic bradycardia were more common among patients randomized to amiodarone. Amiodarone should be initiated in ICD patients presenting with frequent shocks both appropriate and inappropriate; sotalol is not as effective but is an acceptable alternative. ICD therapy whether appropriate or inappropriate leads to serious discomfort and anxiety in patients with ICDs. The OPTIC trial provides strong evidence that both sotalol and amiodarone are highly effective in preventing shocks and should be initiated once either inappropriate or appropriate shocks are documented.

The Shock Inhibition Evaluation with Azimilide (SHIELD) trial randomized 633 ICD recipients in a double-blind, placebo-controlled study to evaluate the effect of daily doses of 75 or 125 mg of azimilide on recurrent symptomatic ventricular tachyarrhythmias and ICD therapies.[64] The total of all-cause shocks plus symptomatic ventricular tachycardia (VT) terminated by antitachycardia pacing (ATP) was significantly reduced by azimilide, with relative risk reductions of 57% (HR 0.43, 95% CI 0.26–0.69, P = 0.0006) at the 75 mg dose and 47% (HR 0.53, 95% CI 0.34–0.83, P = 0.0053) at the 125 mg dose. The reductions in all-cause shocks with both doses of azimilide did not achieve statistical significance. The incidence of all appropriate ICD therapies (shocks or ATP-terminated VT) was reduced significantly among patients taking 75 mg azimil-

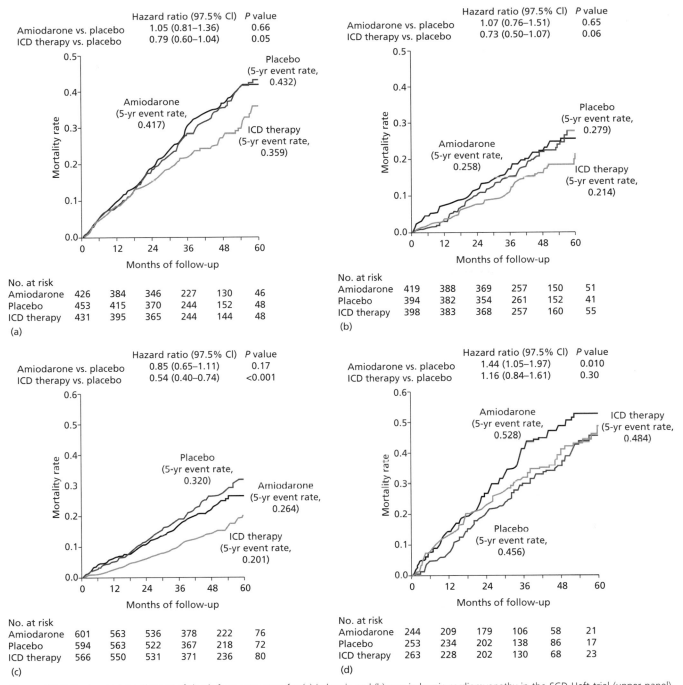

Figure 40.2 Kaplan–Meier estimates of death from any cause for (a) ischemic and (b) non ischemic cardiomyopathy in the SCD-Heft trial (upper panel). Kaplan–Meier estimates of death from any cause in NYHA Class II (c) and III patients (d). (From Bardy et al[27]).

ide (HR 0.52, 95% CI 0.30–0.89, $P = 0.017$) and those taking 125 mg of azimilide (HR 0.38, 95% CI 0.22–0.65, $P = 0.0004$). Azimilide significantly reduced the recurrence of VT or ventricular fibrillation terminated by shocks or ATP in ICD patients, thereby reducing the burden of symptomatic ventricular tachyarrhythmias.

Three randomized clinical trials have assessed the effect of omega 3 fatty acids in patients with an ICD and previous VT/VF.[65–67] Raitt and collaborators randomized 200 patients with an ICD and a recent episode of sustained VT or VF, in a double-blind, placebo-controlled trial, to receive fish oil 1.8 g/d, 72% omega 3 PUFAs, or placebo; they were

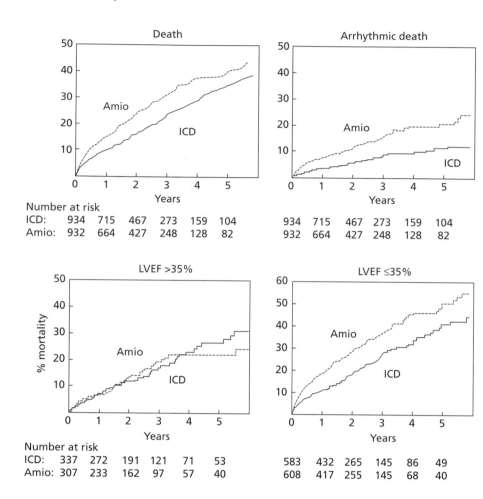

Figure 40.3 Meta-analysis of clinical trials evaluating the role of ICD therapy for secondary prevention of SCD. The upper panel shows the cumulative risk of fatal events for the amiodarone and ICD treatment arms and the lower panel shows the cumulative risk for death according to LVEF ≤35% or ≥35%. (From Conolly et al[62]).

followed up for a median of 718 days (range 20–828 days).[65] Time to first episode of ICD treatment for VT/VF was the primary outcome. Patients randomized to receive fish oil had ICD therapy for VT/VF at six, 12, and 24 months, 46% (5%), 51% (5%), and 65% (5%) compared with 36% (5%), 41% (5%), and 59% (5%) for patients randomized to receive placebo (*P* = 0.19). Recurrent VT/VF events were more common in patients randomized to receive fish oil (*P* < 0.001). These investigators concluded that fish oil supplementation did not reduce the risk of VT/VF and may be proarrhythmic in some patients.

Leaf *et al* randomized 402 patients with ICDs to double-blind treatment with either fish oil or an olive oil daily supplement for 12 months.[66] The primary endpoint was a composite of time to first ICD event for VT/VF or death from any cause. Treatment with the fish oil supplement showed a trend toward a prolonged time to the first ICD event or death from any cause (risk reduction of 28%; *P* = 0.057). In patients "on treatment" for at least 11 months, the antiarrhythmic benefit of fish oil was improved for those with confirmed events (risk reduction of 38%; *P* = 0.034). The authors interpreted these findings as evidence that for individuals at high risk of fatal ventricular

arrhythmias, regular daily ingestion of fish oil fatty acids may significantly reduce potentially fatal ventricular arrhythmias.

The Study on Omega-3 Fatty acids and ventricular Arrhythmia (SOFA) was a randomized, parallel, placebo-controlled, double-blind trial that recruited 546 patients with ICDs and prior documented VT/VF.[67] Patients were randomly assigned to receive 2 g/d of fish oil (n = 273) or placebo (n = 273) for a median period of 356 days. The primary outcome was a composite of appropriate ICD intervention for VT/VF or all-cause death. The primary endpoint occurred in 81 (30%) patients taking fish oil vs 90 (33%) patients taking placebo (HR 0.86; 95% CI 0.64–1.16; *P* = 0.33). This study did not indicate evidence of benefit or harm of omega 3 PUFAs in patients with an ICD and prior VT/VF. A recent meta-analysis pooled the data from the described trials that included a total of 573 patients who received fish oil and 575 patients who received a control; at one year there was no overall effect of fish oil on the relative risk of ICD discharge.[68] Significant heterogeneity was observed between trials and this meta-analysis was unable to show any significant effect on the relative risk of ICD therapy.

In summary, adjunctive therapy for the prevention of recurrent shocks has clinical relevance primarily by improving quality of life by preventing both appropriate and inappropriate shocks and potentially prolonging device longevity. Amiodarone and sotalol have both shown significant reductions in device therapy and are recommended for patients with recurrent shocks. Azimilide has shown some promising results but there has been no head-to-head comparison with amiodarone or sotalol. There is currently no strong evidence that supports the routine use of fish oils for the reduction of ICD therapies.

Prevention of less common cardiomyopathies and channelopathies

Several less common disorders may manifest with SCD as primary clinical presentation and include a heterogeneous group of cardiomyopathies such as hypertrophic cardiomyopathy (HCM), arrhythmogenic right ventricular dysplasia/cardiomyopathy (ARVD/C) and Chagas' disease. Channelopathies such as the Brugada syndrome, long QT syndrome and catecholaminergic polymorphic VT are among the most frequent genetic disorders. Some of these conditions have a very low prevalence and there are no data from randomized clinical trials. Nonetheless, SCD is a relatively frequent and devastating clinical presentation that affects young people and their siblings.[69,70] The level of evidence for all these disorders is C, and larger studies assessing the role of primary prevention are needed.[6,71]

Hypertrophic cardiomyopathy

HCM is a relatively common cardiac disorder (adult prevalence about 1:500) in which SCD is a devastating component, which may occur at any age but particularly in young, often asymptomatic patients. Risk factors for SCD have been derived from observational studies and international registries. Major risk factors include prior cardiac arrest; family history of SCD, syncope or spontaneous sustained or non-sustained VT, LV thickness >30 mm and an abnormal blood pressure response to exercise.[6,71] The implant of an ICD for secondary prevention of SCD is widely accepted based on small observational studies and expert opinion.[71]

The prophylactic use of an ICD is also appropriate in those individuals with any of the aforementioned risk factors. It remains unclear which risk factor has the highest predictive accuracy and *a single* risk factor may be a sufficient indication for an ICD for primary prophylaxis. Maron *et al*[72] recently reported data from a multicenter registry that included 506 patients with HCM with an ICD implanted for either primary or secondary prophylaxis. The mean follow-up was 3.7 ± 2.8 years. The primary outcome was appropriate shocks delivered by the ICD.

ICD therapy appropriately terminated ventricular tachycardia/fibrillation in 103 patients (20%). Intervention rates were 10.6% per year for secondary prevention after cardiac arrest (five-year cumulative probability, 39% (SD, 5%)), and 3.6% per year for primary prevention (five-year probability, 17% (SD, 2%)). Time to first appropriate discharge was up to 10 years, with a 27% probability of receiving therapy five years or more after implantation. For primary prevention, 35% of patients with appropriate ICD interventions had undergone implantation for only a single risk factor; likelihood of appropriate discharge was similar in patients with one, two, three or more risk markers (3.83, 2.65, and 4.82 per 100 person-years, respectively; $P = 0.77$). An important proportion of ICD discharges occurred in primary prevention patients who had undergone implantation for a single risk factor. In summary, patients with HCM and a secondary prevention indication have a 10.6% yearly rate of appropriate shocks in contrast to patients with a primary indication who have a 3.6% yearly rate of appropriate shocks independent of the risk factors previously mentioned.

Arrhythmogenic right ventricular cardiomyopathy (ARVC)

ARVC may manifest as SCD in younger patients and selected subjects may be at higher risk for SCD. There is some evidence identifying high-risk subgroups derived from observational studies and it is reasonable to recommend the use of an ICD in these patients.[73] Risk factors that identify patients that may be at risk of life-threatening arrhythmias include induction of VT during electrophysiologic testing, detection of non-sustained VT on ambulatory ECG monitoring, male gender, severe RV dilation and extensive RV involvement.[74] Presentation at an age <5 years, LV involvement, prior cardiac arrest and unexplained syncope may also serve as markers of increased risk for SCD.[6,75] However it is important to realize that these risk factors have not been validated in large prospective series. There is a wide variation in presentation and course of ARVC patients; however, patients presenting with syncope, sustained VT or SCD appear to be a higher-risk group.

The role of ICD therapy for primary prevention of SCD in patients with ARVC is unclear and no data from randomized clinical trials are available. The decision to implant an ICD for primary prophylaxis in patients with ARVC may be prompted by the presence of one or more of the following markers: family history of SCD or ARVC, syncope, extensive RV involvement, and LV involvement.[6]

Chagas' cardiomyopathy

Chagas' disease is an endemic parasitic disease that affects more than 100 million people in Latin America. Recent migration patterns have made North America and Europe also vulnerable and several cases have been reported in the last years.[76–78] Dilated cardiomyopathy, progressive heart failure, conduction disorders and life-threatening arrhythmias are common clinical presentations.[78] SCD is the principal cause of death in Chagas' disease, accounting for about 55–65% of deaths affecting individuals during their most productive years, leading to an estimated SCD incidence of 24 per 1000 patient-years.[78] There is a lack of controlled trials in the prevention or treatment of SCD associated with Chagas' disease.

The Chagas Cardiomyopathy Bisoprolol Intervention Study (CHARITY)[79] is an ongoing randomized trial conducted in Colombia, testing bisoprolol vs placebo in a population with Chagas' disease and symptomatic heart failure. SCD is one of the secondary outcomes. The Benznidazole Evaluation For Interrupting Trypanosomiasis (BENEFIT) trial is a large randomized double-blind trial that is testing the hypothesis whether treatment with the anti-trypanosomal agent benznidazol reduces both PCR serology and clinical outcomes that include SCD, ventricular tachycardia, overall mortality and cardiac mortality.[80]

Current data from registries and small observational trials suggest that the ICD has a similar beneficial effect in patients with Chagas' cardiomyopathy compared to other non-ischemic dilated cardiomyopaties.[81,82] Of note, progression of LV dysfunction and heart failure is more aggressive in patients with Chagas' cardiomyopathy and may affect the overall benefit of ICD therapy in this population. Further studies will be needed to clarify the role of ICD therapy in the prevention of SCD.

Brugada syndrome

The diagnosis of Brugada syndrome is based on characteristic 12-lead ECG manifestations that include J point segment elevation in leads V1–V3 and right bundle branch block pattern that may be intermittent.[83] The disease is transmitted in an autosomal dominant pattern with more than 90% of cases being male. The genetic alteration has been localized to the cardiac sodium channel gene (SCN5A).[84]

Identifying asymptomatic subjects that are at increased risk of SCD is of clinical importance but remains a controversial topic. There are no data indicating that family history predicts SCD in patients with Brugada syndrome. Similarly there is no evidence that asymptomatic subjects with no family history are at low risk. Patients with a spontaneous characteristic ECG pattern compared to ECG changes elicited by pharmacologic challenge appear to have a worse prognosis.[85] Furthermore, patients with a spontaneous characteristic ECG pattern and syncope have a sixfold higher risk of SCD compared with patients without syncope and spontaneous ECG changes.[85]

Some investigators promote the use of EPS to identify patients with asymptomatic Brugada syndrome at high risk of SCD.[6,83] This practice remains highly controversial as other investigators have reported a low accuracy for EPS to predict SCD.[83–85] In summary, it appears reasonable to offer an ICD in patients who have survived a cardiac arrest and present with polymorphic VT or syncope together with spontaneous characteristic Brugada ECG pattern. Primary prevention with an ICD in asymptomatic patients with the Brugada syndrome is based on individual patient selection.[6,86]

Long QT syndrome

The long QT syndrome is frequently associated with SCD. Long-term therapy with beta-blockers, permanent pacing or left cervicothoracic ganglionic sympathectomy have been reported to reduce cardiac events.[6,87,88] A number of clinical markers have been suggested as risk stratifiers for SCD. History of syncope, family history of SCD, cardiac arrest, torsades de pointes and type of long QT (LQTS 2–3) have been suggested by some investigators as markers of SCD.[87] ICD is recommended for patients who have a recurrence of syncope or VF while receiving beta-blockers. Primary prevention with an ICD may be indicated in patients felt to be at very high risk and those unable to receive beta-blockers. Genetic analysis may in the future aid in identifying patients at higher risk of SCD and may justify implanting an ICD for primary prevention.[6,88]

Catecholaminergic polymorphic VT

Cathecholaminergic polymorphic VT (CPVT) is an inherited disease characterized by life-threatening arrhythmias (usually triggered by emotion or exercise). The mortality rate in untreated individuals is 30–50% by age 40.[89] Non-sustained or sustained bidirectional VT is a frequent clinical presentation, usually triggered by exercise. Irregular polymorphic VT or VF can also be seen in these patients. Beta-blockers are the therapy of choice. If syncope recurs on appropriate beta-blocker therapy an ICD is indicated.[6,89,90]

Application of current evidence in under-represented populations

Translating evidence derived from clinical trials may be challenging in specific under-represented populations. In most clinical trials testing the ICD, patients over 75 years of age have been under-represented and the benefits of ICD therapy in this subgroup remain debatable. A recent study combined individual data from the CIDS, AVID and CASH studies and divided the population into those aged ≥75 and

<75 years.[91] Overall, 1866 patients were included in this analysis; 252 patients were aged ≥75 years old (13.5%). LVEF was similar in both groups (32.6 ± 13.7 vs 33.8 ± 14.9%, $P = 0.20$) as was baseline NYHA class III or IV (12.3 vs 11.8%, $P = 0.38$). Older patients were less likely to have VF as their presenting arrhythmia (39 vs 53%, $P = 0.0001$). Over a mean follow-up of 2.3 years, older patients were more likely to die from both non-arrhythmic (8.74% per year vs 3.96% per year, $P = 0.001$) and arrhythmic death (6.73% per year vs 3.84% per year, $P = 0.03$). The ICD significantly reduced all-cause and arrhythmic death in patients aged <75 years (all-cause death HR 0.69, 95% CI 0.56–0.85, $P < 0.0001$; arrhythmic death HR 0.44, 95% CI 0.32–0.62, $P < 0.0001$), but not in patients aged ≥75 years old (all-cause death HR 1.06, 95% CI 0.69–1.64, $P = 0.79$; arrhythmic death HR 0.90, 95% CI 0.42–1.95, $P = 0.79$).

Evidence from observational studies suggests that elderly patients with multiple co-morbidities may derive less benefit from ICD therapy, possibly due to competing risks that dilute the effects of ICD therapy. End-stage renal failure has been identified as a potential co-morbidity that reduces the benefit of ICD.[92,93] ICD therapy should not be withheld based on age alone; however, careful consideration of the risk of non-arrhythmic death among elderly patients and patients with multiple co-morbidities, especially end-stage renal disease, should be taken into account when considering ICD implantation.

Cardiac resynchronization therapy and ICD for SCD prevention

Whether ICD therapy alone or combined with cardiac resynchronization therapy in appropriate heart failure candidates has an impact on SCD remains a matter of debate. The Comparison Of Medical therapy, Pacing, And defibrillatION in heart failure (COMPANION)[94] trial included 1520 patients with advanced heart failure (NYHA class III–IV) due to ischemic or non-ischemic cardiomyopathy

---

BOX 40.1 Recommendations for ICD therapy

Primary prevention

Class I
- Patients with ischemic heart disease with or without mild to moderate symptoms and LVEF <35%, due to prior MI who are at least 40 days post MI (measured at least one month post MI and three months post coronary revascularization procedure) and are in NYHA class II or III (**Level A**)
- Patients with LVEF <30%, due to prior MI who are at least 40 days post-MI (measured at least one month post MI and three months post coronary revascularization procedure) and are in NYHA class I (**Level A**)
- Patients with non-ischemic cardiomyopathy LVEF <35%, and NYHA functional class II–III (**Level B**)
- Patients with familial or inherited conditions such as, but not limited to, long QT syndrome, hypertrophic cardiomyopathy, Brugada syndrome or ARVD and at a high risk for life-threatening ventricular tachyarrhythmias (**Level C**)
- Patients with non-sustained VT due to prior MI who are at least 40 days post MI (measured at least one month post MI and three months post coronary revascularization procedure) LVEF <40% and inducible VF or sustained VT at electrophysiologic study (**Level B**)

Class IIa
- Patients with non-ischemic cardiomyopathy with unexplained syncope and, LVEF <30% (**Level C**)
- Patients with sustained VT with normal or near normal LVEF (**Level C**)
- Patients with HCM who have one or more risk factors for SCD (**Level C**)

- Patients with ARVD/C who have one or more risk factors for SCD (**Level C**)
- Patients with long QT syndrome with syncope and/or VT while receiving beta-blockers (**Level C**)
- Patients with Brugada syndrome with unexplained syncope or documented VT that has not resulted in cardiac arrest (**Level C**)
- Patients with catecholaminergic polymorphic VT who present with syncope/documented sustained VT while receiving beta-blockers (**Level C**)
- Patients with Chagas' cardiomyopathy and LVEF <35% and NYHA II or III (**Level C**)

Secondary prevention

Class I
- Patients with aborted cardiac arrest due to VF/VT not due to a transient or reversible cause (**Level A**)
- Spontaneous sustained VT in association with structural heart disease (**Level B**)
- Syncope of undetermined origin with clinically relevant, hemodynamically significant sustained VT or VF induced at electrophysiology study (**Level B**)
- Spontaneous sustained VT in patients who do not have structural heart disease that is not amenable to other treatments (**Level B**)

Class IIa
- Patients with unexplained syncope non-ischemic dilated cardiomyopathy and LVEF <35% (**Level C**)
- Patients in hospital with sustained VT awaiting for cardiac transplantation (**Level C**)

and a QRS interval of at least 120 msec who were randomly assigned to optimal pharmacologic therapy alone or in combination with cardiac resynchronization therapy (CRT) with either a pacemaker or a pacemaker/defibrillator. The primary composite endpoint was the time to death or hospitalization for any cause. Mean LVEF was 22% and all the patients had a QRS duration >150 ms. The total annual mortality in the control group was 19% and the addition of ICD to biventricular pacing reduced the relative risk by 36% (HR 0.64, 95% CI 0.48–0.86). This benefit was maintained independent of type of cardiomyopathy.

The CArdiac REsynchronization Heart Failure (CARE-HF)[95] study randomized 813 patients with advanced heart failure (NYHA class III–IV), QRS prolongation (>120 msec) and LVEF <35% who were followed for a mean of 29.4 months. The primary endpoint (time to death from any cause or an unplanned hospitalization for a major cardiovascular event) was significantly reduced in the CRT compared to medical therapy group (HR 0.63; 95% CI 0.51–0.77; $P < 0.001$). Death was also significantly reduced in the CRT compared to medical therapy group (HR 0.64; 95% CI 0.48–0.85; $P < 0.002$). The extended CARE-HF follow-up also observed a significant reduction in SCD (HR 0.54, 95% CI 0.35–0.84, $P = 0.005$).[96] Thus it is reasonable to recommend CRT + ICD when there is an overlapping indication (advanced heart failure, EF <35%, QRS duration >120 msec).

References

1. Baranchuk A, Morillo CA. Guidelines for the prevention of sudden cardiac death: filling the gap. In: Gulizia M (ed) *Emerging Pathologies in Cardiology*. Milan: Springer, 2005; 223–30.
2. Tang AS, Ross H, Simpson CS et al. Canadian Cardiovascular Society/Canadian Heart Rhythm Society. Position Paper on Implantable Cardioverter Defibrillator (ICD) Use in Canada. *Can J Cardiol* 2005;**21**(suppl A):11A–18A.
3. Josephson M, Wellens HJJ. Implantable defibrillators and sudden cardiac death. *Circulation* 2004;**109**:2685–91.
4. American Heart Association. *2002 Heart and Stroke Statistical Update*. Dallas, TX: American Heart Association, 2001.
5. Vreede-Swagemakers JJM, Gorgels APM, Dubois-Arbouw WI et al. Out-of-hospital cardiac arrest in the 1900s: a population-based study in the Maastricht area on incidence, characteristics and survival. *J Am Coll Cardiol* 1997;**30**:1500–5.
6. Epstein AE, DiMarco JP, Ellenbogen KA et al. ACC/AHA/HRS 2008 guidelines for device-based therapy for cardiac rhythm abnormalities. *J Am Coll Cardiol* 2008;**51**:e1–62.
7. Albert CM, Ruskin JN. Risk stratifiers for sudden cardiac death (SCD) in the community: primary prevention of SCD. *Cardiovasc Res* 2001;**50**:186–96.
8. International Mexiletine and Placebo Antiarrhythmic Coronary Trial. I. Report on arrhythmia and other findings. Impact Research Group. *J Am Coll Cardiol* 1984;**4**:1148–63.
9. Cardiac Arrhythmia Suppression Trial (CAST) Investigators. Preliminary report: effect of encainide and flecainide on mortality in a randomized trial of arrhythmia suppression after myocardial infarction. *N Engl J Med* 1989;**321**:406–12.
10. Teo KK, Yusuf S, Furberg CD. Effects of prophylactic antiarrhythmic drug therapy in acute myocardial infarction. An overview of results from randomized controlled trials. *JAMA* 1993;**270**:1589–95.
11. Cairns JA, Connolly SJ, Roberts R, Gent M. Randomised trial of outcome after myocardial infarction in patients with frequent or repetitive ventricular premature depolarisations: CAMIAT. Canadian Amiodarone Myocardial Infarction Arrhythmia Trial Investigators. *Lancet* 1997;**349**:675–82.
12. Julian DG, Camm AJ, Frangin G et al. Randomised trial of effect of amiodarone on mortality in patients with left-ventricular dysfunction after recent myocardial infarction: EMIAT. European Myocardial Infarct Amiodarone Trial Investigators. *Lancet* 1997;**349**:667–74.
13. Amiodarone Trials Meta-Analysis Investigators. Effect of prophylactic amiodarone on mortality after acute myocardial infarction and in congestive heart failure: meta-analysis of individual data from 6500 patients in randomised trials. *Lancet* 1997;**350**:1417–24.
14. Connolly SJ. Evidence-based analysis of amiodarone efficacy and safety. *Circulation* 1999;**100**:2025–34.
15. Boutitie F, Boissel JP, Connolly SJ et al. Amiodarone interaction with beta-blockers: analysis of the merged EMIAT (European Myocardial Infarct Amiodarone Trial) and CAMIAT (Canadian Amiodarone Myocardial Infarction Trial) databases. The EMIAT and CAMIAT Investigators. *Circulation* 1999;**99**:2268–75.
16. Connolly SJ, Dorian P, Roberts RS et al. Comparison of beta-blockers, amiodarone plus beta-blockers, or sotalol for prevention of shocks from implantable cardioverter defibrillators: the OPTIC Study: a randomized trial. *JAMA* 2006;**295**:165–71.
17. Waldo AL, Camm AJ, deRuyter H et al. Effect of d-sotalol on mortality in patients with left ventricular dysfunction after recent and remote myocardial infarction. The SWORD Investigators. Survival With Oral d-Sotalol. *Lancet* 1996;**348**:7–12.
18. Julian DG, Prescott RJ, Jackson FS, Szekely P. Controlled trial of sotalol for one year after myocardial infarction. *Lancet* 1982;**22**;1:1142–7.
19. Torp-Pedersen C, Moller M, Bloch-Thomsen PE et al. Dofetilide in patients with congestive heart failure and left ventricular dysfunction. Danish Investigations of Arrhythmia and Mortality on Dofetilide Study Group. *N Engl J Med* 1999;**341**:857–65.
20. Torp-Pedersen C, Moller M, Bloch-Thomsen PE et al. Dofetilide in patients with congestive heart failure and left ventricular dysfunction. *N Engl J Med* 1999;**341**:857–65.
21. Kober L, Bloch Thomsen PE, Moller M et al. Effect of dofetilide in patients with recent myocardial infarction and left-ventricular dysfunction: a randomised trial. *Lancet* 2000; **356**:2052–8.
22. Camm AJ, Pratt CM, Schwartz PJ et al. Mortality in patients after a recent myocardial infarction: a randomized, placebo-controlled trial of azimilide using heart rate variability for risk stratification. *Circulation* 2004;**8**(109):990–6.
23. Steinbeck G, Andresen D, Bach P et al. A comparison of electrophysiologically guided antiarrhythmic drug therapy with beta-blocker therapy in patients with symptomatic, sustained ventricular tachyarrhythmias. *N Engl J Med* 1992;**327**:987–92.
24. Mason JW. A comparison of seven antiarrhythmic drugs in patients with ventricular tachyarrhythmias. Electrophysiologic

Study versus Electrocardiographic Monitoring Investigators. *N Engl J Med* 1993;**329**:452–8.

25. Mason JW. A comparison of electrophysiologic testing with Holter monitoring to predict antiarrhythmic-drug efficacy for ventricular tachyarrhythmias. Electrophysiologic Study versus Electrocardiographic Monitoring Investigators. *N Engl J Med* 1993;**329**:445–51.

26. Greene HL. The CASCADE Study: randomized antiarrhythmic drug therapy in survivors of cardiac arrest in Seattle. CASCADE Investigators. *Am J Cardiol* 1993;**72**:70F–4F.

27. Bardy GH, Lee KL, Mark DB *et al.* Amiodarone or an implantable cardioverter-defibrillator for congestive heart failure. *N Engl J Med* 2005;**352**:225–37.

28. Yusuf S, Peto R, Lewis J, Collins R, Sleight P. Beta blockade during and after myocardial infarction: an overview of the randomized trials. *Prog Cardiovasc Dis* 1985;**27**:335–71.

29. Carson P. Beta-blocker therapy in heart failure. *Cardiol Clin* 2001;**19**:267–78, vi.

30. Cardiac Insufficiency Bisoprolol Study II (CIBIS-II): a randomised trial. *Lancet* 1999;**353**:9–13.

31. Metoprolol CR/XL Randomised Intervention Trial in Congestive Heart Failure (MERIT-HF). Effect of metoprolol CR/XL in chronic heart failure. *Lancet* 1999;**353**:2001–7.

32. Cohn JN, Johnson G, Ziesche S *et al.* A comparison of enalapril with hydralazine-isosorbide dinitrate in the treatment of chronic congestive heart failure. *N Engl J Med* 1991;**325**:303–10.

33. Kober L, Torp-Pedersen C, Carlsen JE *et al.* A clinical trial of the angiotensin-converting-enzyme inhibitor trandolapril in patients with left ventricular dysfunction after myocardial infarction. Trandolapril Cardiac Evaluation (TRACE) Study Group. *N Engl J Med* 1995;**333**:1670–6.

34. Cleland JG, Erhardt L, Murray G, Hall AS, Ball SG. Effect of ramipril on morbidity and mode of death among survivors of acute myocardial infarction with clinical evidence of heart failure. A report from the AIRE Study Investigators. *Eur Heart J* 1997;**18**:41–51.

35. Domanski MJ, Exner DV, Borkowf CB, Geller NL, Rosenberg Y, Pfeffer MA. Effect of angiotensin converting enzyme inhibition on sudden cardiac death in patients following acute myocardial infarction. A meta-analysis of randomized clinical trials. *J Am Coll Cardiol* 1999;**33**:598–604.

36. Yusuf S, Sleight P, Pogue J, Bosch J, Davies R, Dagenais G. Effects of an angiotensin-converting-enzyme inhibitor, ramipril, on cardiovascular events in high-risk patients. The Heart Outcomes Prevention Evaluation Study Investigators. *N Engl J Med* 2000;**342**:145–53.

37. Boriani G, Valzania C, Diemberger I *et al.* Potential of non-antiarrhythmic drugs to provide an innovative upstream approach to the pharmacological prevention of sudden cardiac death. *Expert Opin Investig Drugs* 2007;**16**:605–23.

38. Arshad A, Mandava A, Kamath G, Musat D. Sudden cardiac death and the role of medical therapy. *Prog Cardiovasc Dis* 2008;**50**:420–38.

39. Pitt B, Zannad F, Remme WJ *et al.* The effect of spironolactone on morbidity and mortality in patients with severe heart failure. Randomized Aldactone Evaluation Study Investigators. *N Engl J Med* 1999;**341**:709–17.

40. Pitt B, Remme WJ, Zannad F *et al.* Eplerenone, a selective aldosterone blocker, in patients with left ventricular dysfunction after myocardial infarction. *N Engl J Med* 2003;**348**:1309–21.

41. Burr ML, Fehily AM, Gilbert JF *et al.* Effects of changes in fat, fish and fiber intakes on death and myocardial infarction: Diet and Reinfarction Trial (DART). *Lancet* 1989;**2**:757–61.

42. Gruppo Italiano per lo Studio della Sopravvivenza nell'Infarto Miocardico. Dietary supplementation with *n*-3 polyunsaturated fatty acids and vitamin E after myocardial infarction: results of the GISSI-Prevenzione trial. *Lancet* 1999;**354**:447–55.

43. Hooper L, Thompson RL, Harrison RA *et al.* Risks and benefits of omega 3 fats for mortality, cardiovascular disease, and cancer: systematic review. *BMJ* 2006;**332**:752–60.

44. Kris-Etherton P, Harris WS, Appel LJ. Fish consumption, fish oil, omega-3 fatty acids and cardiovascular disease. *Circulation* 2002;**106**:2747–57.

45. Moss AJ, Hall WJ, Cannom DS *et al.* Multicenter Automatic Defibrillator Implantation Trial Investigators. Improved survival with an implanted defibrillator in patients with coronary disease at high risk for ventricular arrhythmia. *N Engl J Med* 1996;**335**:1933–40.

46. Bigger JT Jr. Prophylactic use of implanted cardiac defibrillators in patients at high risk for ventricular arrhythmias after coronary-artery bypass graft surgery. Coronary Artery Bypass Graft (CABG) Patch Trial Investigators. *N Engl J Med* 1997; **337**:1569–75.

47. Multicenter Unsustained Tachycardia Trial Investigators. A randomized study of the prevention of sudden death in patients with coronary artery disease. *N Engl J Med* 1999;**341**:1882–90.

48. Moss AJ, Zareba W, Hall WJ *et al.* Prophylactic implantation of a defibrillator in patients with myocardial infarction and reduced ejection fraction. *N Engl J Med* 2002;**346**:877–83.

49. Hohnloser SH, Kuck KH, Dorian P *et al.* Prophylactic use of an implantable cardioverter-defibrillator after acute myocardial infarction. DINAMIT investigators. *N Engl J Med* 2004;**351**: 2481–8.

50. Bansch D, Antz M, Boczor S *et al.* Primary prevention of sudden cardiac death in idiopathic dilated cardiomyopathy: the Cardiomyopathy trial (CAT). *Circulation* 2002;**105**:1453–8.

51. Strickberger SA, Hummel JD, Bartlett TG *et al.* Amiodarone versus implantable cardioverter-defibrillator: randomized trial in patients with nonischemic dilated cardiomyopathy and asymptomatic nonsustained ventricular tachycardia-AMIO-VIRT. *J Am Coll Cardiol* 2003;**41**:1707–12.

52. Kadish A, Dyer A, Daubert JP *et al.* Prophylactic defibrillator implantation in patients with nonischemic dilated cardiomyopathy. *N Engl J Med* 2004;**350**:2151–8.

53. Moss AJ. MADIT-II: substudies and their implications. *Card Electrophysiol Rev.* 2003;**7**:430–3.

54. Huang DT, Sesselberg HW, McNitt S *et al.* MADIT-II Research Group. Improved survival associated with prophylactic implantable defibrillators in elderly patients with prior myocardial infarction and depressed ventricular function: a MADIT-II substudy. *J Cardiovasc Electrophysiol* 2007;**18**:833–8.

55. Dhar R, Alsheikh-Ali AA, Estes NA 3rd *et al.* Association of prolonged QRS duration with ventricular tachyarrhythmias and sudden cardiac death in the Multicenter Automatic Defibrillator Implantation Trial II (MADIT-II). *Heart Rhythm* 2008;**5**:807–13.

56. Goldenberg I, Vyas AK, Hall WJ *et al,* MADIT II Investigators. Risk stratification for primary implantation of a cardioverter-defibrillator in patients with ischemic left ventricular dysfunction. *J Am Coll Cardiol* 2008;**51**:288–96.

57. Wilber DJ, Zareba W, Hall WJ et al. Time dependence of mortality risk and defibrillator benefit after myocardial infarction. Circulation 2004;109(9):1082–4.

58. Crystal E, Connolly SJ, Dorian P. Prevention and treatment of life-threatening ventricular arrhythmia and sudden death. In: Yusuf S, Cairns J, Camm J, Fallen E, Gersh B (eds) Evidence-based Cardiology, 2nd edn. Oxford: Blackwell, 2002; 577–86.

59. Connolly SJ, Gent M, Roberts RS et al. Canadian Implantable Defibrillator Study (CIDS): a randomized trial of the implantable cardioverter defibrillator against amiodarone. Circulation 2000;101:1297–302.

60. Antiarrhythmics versus Implantable Defibrillators (AVID) Investigators. A comparison of antiarrhythmic-drug therapy with implantable defibrillators in patients resuscitated from near-fatal ventricular arrhythmias. N Engl J Med 1997;337: 1576–83.

61. Kuck KH, Cappato R, Siebels J, Ruppel R. Randomized comparison of antiarrhythmic drug therapy with implantable defibrillators in patients resuscitated from cardiac arrest: the Cardiac Arrest Study Hamburg (CASH). Circulation 2000;102:748–54.

62. Connolly SJ, Hallstrom AP, Cappato R et al. Meta-analysis of the implantable cardioverter defibrillator secondary prevention trials. AVID, CASH and CIDS studies. Antiarrhythmics vs Implantable Defibrillator study. Cardiac Arrest Study Hamburg. Canadian Implantable Defibrillator Study. Eur Heart J 2000;21:2071–8.

63. Dorian P. Combination ICD and drug treatments – best options. Resuscitation 2000;45:S3–6.

64. Dorian P, Borggrefe M, Al-Khalidi HR et al. SHock Inhibition Evaluation with azimiLiDe (SHIELD) Investigators. Placebo-controlled, randomized clinical trial of azimilide for prevention of ventricular tachyarrhythmias in patients with an implantable cardioverter defibrillator. Circulation 2004;110:3646–54.

65. Raitt MH, Connor WE, Morris C et al. Fish oil supplementation and risk of ventricular tachycardia and ventricular fibrillation in patients with implantable defibrillators: a randomized controlled trial. JAMA 2005;293:2884–91.

66. Leaf A, Albert CM, Josephson M et al. Fatty Acid Antiarrhythmia Trial Investigators. Prevention of fatal arrhythmias in high-risk subjects by fish oil n-3 fatty acid intake. Circulation 2005;112(18):2762–8.

67. Brouwer IA, Zock PL, Camm AJ et al, SOFA Study Group. Effect of fish oil on ventricular tachyarrhythmia and death in patients with implantable cardioverter defibrillators: the Study on Omega-3 Fatty Acids and Ventricular Arrhythmia (SOFA) randomized trial. JAMA 2006;295:2613–9.

68. Jenkins DJ, Josse AR, Beyene J et al. Fish-oil supplementation in patients with implantable cardioverter defibrillators: a meta-analysis. CMAJ 2008;178:157–64.

69. Gregoratos G, Abrams J, Epstein AE et al. ACC/AHA/NASPE 2002 guideline update for implantation of cardiac pacemakers and antiarrhythmia devices: summary article. Circulation 2002;106:2145–61.

70. Priori SG, Aliot E, Blømstrom-Lundqvist C et al. Task force on sudden death, European Society of Cardiology. Summary of recommendations. Europace 2002;4:3–18.

71. Priori SG, Aliot E, Blømstrom-Lundqvist C et al. Update of the guidelines on sudden cardiac death of the European society of cardiology. Eur Heart J 2003;24:13–15.

72. Maron BJ, Spirito P, Shen WK et al. Implantable cardioverter-defibrillators and prevention of sudden cardiac death in hypertrophic cardiomyopathy. JAMA 2007;298:405–12.

73. Link MS, Wang PJ, Haugh CJ et al. Arrhythmogenic right ventricular dysplasia: clinical results with implantable cardioverter defibrillators. J Interv Card Electrophysiol 1997;1:41–8.

74. Dalal D, Nasir K, Bomma C et al. Arrhythmogenic right ventricular dysplasia: a United States experience. Circulation 2005;112: 3823–32.

75. Piccini JP, Dalal D, Roguin A et al. Predictors of appropriate implantable defibrillator therapies in patients with arrhythmogenic right ventricular dysplasia. Heart Rhythm 2005;2:1188–94.

76. Baranchuk A, Rosas F, Morillo CA. Enfermedad de Chagas en países desarrollados: mito o realidad? (Chagas' disease in developed countries: myth or reality?) In: Rosas F, Vanegas D, Cabrales M (eds) Enfermedad de Chagas. Bogotá, Colombia: Sociedad Colombiana de Cardiología, Sociedad Española de Cardiologia, 2007: 217–19.

77. Bern C, Montgomery SP, Herwaldt BL et al. Evaluation and treatment of Chagas' disease in the United States: a systematic review. JAMA 2007;298:2171–81.

78. Rassi A Jr, Rassi A, Little WC et al. Development and validation of a risk score for predicting death in Chagas' heart disease. N Engl J Med 2006;355:799–808.

79. Quiros FR, Morillo CA, Casas JP et al. CHARITY: Chagas Cardiomyopathy Bisoprolol Intervention Study. A randomized double-blind placebo force-titration controlled study with bisoprolol in patients with chronic heart failure secondary to Chagas cardiomyopathy [NCT00323973]. Trials 2006;9;7–21.

80. Marin-Neto JA, Rassi A Jr, Morillo CA et al. Rationale and design of a randomized placebo-controlled trial assessing the effects of etiologic treatment in Chagas' cardiomyopathy: the Benznidazole Evaluation for Interrupting Trypanosomiasis (BENEFIT). Am Heart J 2008;156:37–43.

81. Dubner S, Valero E, Pesce R et al. A Latin American registry of implantable cardioverter defibrillators: the ICD-LABOR study. Ann Noninvas Electrocardiol 2005;10:420–8.

82. Cardinalli-Neto A, Bestetti RB, Cordeiro JA et al. Predictors of all-cause mortality for patients with chronic Chagas' heart disease receiving implantable cardioverter defibrillator therapy. J Cardiovasc Electrophysiol 2007;18:1236–40.

83. Brugada J, Brugada R, Brugada P. Right bundle-brunch block and ST-segment elevation in leads V1 through V3: a marker for sudden death in patients without demonstrable structural heart disease. Circulation 1998;97:457–60.

84. Priori SG, Napolitano C, Gasparini M et al. Clinical and genetic heterogeneity of right bundle branch block and ST-segment elevation syndrome: a prospective evaluation of 52 families. Circulation 2000;102:2509–15.

85. Sacher F, Probst V, Iesaka Y et al. Outcome after implantation of a cardioverter-defibrillator in patients with Brugada syndrome: a multicenter study. Circulation 2006;114:2317–24.

86. Sarkozy A, Boussy T, Kourgiannides G et al. Long-term follow-up of primary prophylactic implantable cardioverter-defibrillator therapy in Brugada syndrome. Europace 2007; 28:334–44.

87. Priori SG, Schwartz PJ, Napolitano C et al. Risk stratification in the long-QT syndrome. N Engl J Med 2003;348:1866–74.

88. Zareba W, Moss AJ, Daubert JP *et al.* Implantable cardioverter defibrillator in high-risk long QT syndrome patients. *J Cardiovasc Electrophysiol* 2003;**14**:337–41.

89. Liu N, Colombi B, Raytcheva-Buono EV *et al.* Catecholaminergic polymorphic ventricular tachycardia. *Herz* 2007;**32**:212–17.

90. Sumitomo N, Harada K, Nagashima M *et al.* Catecholaminergic polymorphic ventricular tachycardia: electrocardiographic characteristics and optimal therapeutic strategies to prevent sudden death. *Heart* 2003;**89**:66–70.

91. Healey JS, Hallstrom AP, Kuck KH *et al.* Role of the implantable defibrillator among elderly patients with a history of life-threatening ventricular arrhythmias. *Eur Heart J* 2007;**28**:1746–9.

92. Herzog C, Schuling L, Weihandl M *et al.* Survival of dialysis patients after cardiac arrest and the impact of implantable cardioverter defibrillators. *Kidney* 2005;**68**:818–82.

93. Robin J, Weinberg W, Tiogson J *et al.* Renal dialysis as a risk factor for appropriate therapies and mortality in implantable cardioverter-defibrillator recipients. *Heart Rhythm* 2006;**3**:1196–201.

94. Bristow MR, Saxon LA, Boehmer J *et al.* Cardiac-resynchronization therapy with or without an implantable defibrillator in advanced chronic heart failure. *N Engl J Med* 2004;**350**:2140–50.

95. Cleland JGF, Daubert JC, Erdmann E *et al.* The Effect of cardiac resynchronization on morbidity and mortality in heart failure. *N Engl J Med* 2005;**352**:1539–49.

96. Cleland JGF, Daubert JC, Erdmann E *et al.* Longer-term effect of cardiac resynchronization therapy on mortality in heart failure. The Cardiac Resynchronization-Heart Failure (CARE-HF) trial extension phase. *Eur Heart J* 2006;**27**:1928–32.

Pacemaker therapy, including cardiac resynchronization therapy

William D Toff[1] and A John Camm[2]

[1]Department of Cardiovascular Sciences, University of Leicester, Leicester, UK
[2]Cardiac and Vascular Sciences, St George's University of London, London, UK

Introduction and historical perspective

The development and implementation of the first fully implantable cardiac pacemaker in 1958 transformed the outlook for patients with symptomatic bradycardia and Stokes–Adams attacks.[1] Since then, technologic advances and innovation over five decades have enabled the development of increasingly sophisticated pacing systems, better able to simulate the normal cardiac activation sequence, and a wide variety of different pacing modes is now available.

Initially, pacemakers were only implanted for atrioventricular (AV) block, but their use was soon extended to the management of symptomatic bradycardia associated with sinus node disease. In recent years, improved understanding of pathophysiologic mechanisms has prompted the assessment of pacemaker therapy in other conditions such as neurocardiogenic syncope, hypertrophic cardiomyopathy and paroxysmal atrial fibrillation. Most recently, the development of cardiac resynchronization therapy using biventricular pacing has emerged as an important treatment for selected patients with heart failure. With the emergence of new indications for pacing and the availability of a vast array of different pacing modes and techniques, an evidence-based approach to the practice of cardiac pacing has become increasingly important.

Goals of cardiac pacing

The fundamental aims of cardiac pacing are to relieve symptoms, to improve the quality of life and, in some instances, to prolong survival. The achievement of these aims is mediated by improvements in hemodynamic func-

Evidence-Based Cardiology, 3rd edition. Edited by S. Yusuf, J.A. Cairns, A.J. Camm, E.L. Fallen, and B.J. Gersh. © 2010 Blackwell Publishing, ISBN: 978-1-4051-5925-8.

tion and functional capacity, reduction in cardiovascular morbidity, and prevention of sudden death. Any consideration of the utility and optimal mode of pacing must have regard to all of these factors. It is important to note that hemodynamic differences between alternative pacing modes do not always translate into significant differences in clinical outcomes and comprehensive assessment in randomized clinical trials is therefore essential. It is also important to bear in mind that inappropriate pacing or complications from pacing may result in new or worse symptoms and increased cardiovascular morbidity. This is perhaps best exemplified by the pacemaker syndrome.[2]

Current pacing practice

The most recent world survey of cardiac pacing reported that there were over 540 000 new pacemaker implants in the 43 contributing countries in 2005[3] and the number of new implants is continuing to rise.[3–5] There is considerable national and regional variation in the implant rate. In the USA in 2005, there were approximately 752 new implants per million population. In Europe, figures ranged from 101 per million (Russia) to 789 per million (Belgium).[3] These variations may partly reflect differences in the age distribution and morbidity of the relevant populations but availability of resources and variations in standards of medical care and attitudes to pacing may also be relevant. There has also been some suggestion, in the past, of inappropriate and excessive pacemaker implantation.[6]

In an effort to define appropriate pacing practice, a joint task force subcommittee of the American College of Cardiology (ACC) and the American Heart Association (AHA) has published guidelines for permanent pacemaker implantation, most recently in 2008 (Table 41.1).[7] Similar guidelines have also been published in Europe by a task force of the European Society of Cardiology (ESC), in collaboration with the European Heart Rhythm Association.[8]

Table 41.1 ACC/AHA/HRS guidelines: indications for permanent cardiac pacing[7]

Condition	Class I	Class IIa	Class IIb	Class III
Acquired AV block in adults				
First-degree		First- or second-degree AV block with symptoms similar to those of pacemaker syndrome or hemodynamic compromise (B)	First- or second-degree AV block, with or without symptoms, associated with neuromuscular diseases such as myotonic muscular dystrophy, Erb dystrophy or peroneal muscular atrophy (B)	Asymptomatic first-degree AV block (B)
Second-degree	Second-degree AV block with associated symptomatic bradycardia regardless of site or type of block (B)	See above	See above	Asymptomatic type I second-degree block at the supra-His (AV node) level or not known to be intra- or infra-Hisian (C)
	Asymptomatic type II second-degree AV block with a wide QRS, including isolated RBBB (B)	Asymptomatic type II second-degree AV block with a narrow QRS (B)		
	Second-degree AV block during exercise in the absence of myocardial ischemia (C)	Asymptomatic second-degree block at intra- or infra-His levels found at EPS (B)		
Third-degree (CHB)	CHB and advanced second-degree AV block at any anatomic level associated with any of the following: • Bradycardia with symptoms (including heart failure) or ventricular arrhythmia presumed due to AV block (C) • Arrhythmias and other conditions requiring drug therapy that results in symptomatic bradycardia (C) • Sinus rhythm, with documented asystole ≥3 s, an escape rate <40/min or an infranodal escape rhythm in awake, symptom-free patients (C) • AF and bradycardia with one or more pauses ≥5 s in awake, symptom-free patients (C) • Prior catheter ablation of the AV junction (C) • Postoperative AV block that is not expected to resolve after cardiac surgery (C)	Persistent third-degree AV block with an escape rate >40/min in asymptomatic adults without cardiomegaly (C)	AV block in the setting of drug use and/or toxicity when block is expected to recur even after the drug is withdrawn (B)	AV block that is expected to resolve and is unlikely to recur (for example, drug toxicity, Lyme disease, transient increased vagal tone or during hypoxia in sleep apnea syndrome without symptoms) (B)

Continued on p. 638

Table 41.1 *Continued*

Condition	Class I	Class IIa	Class IIb	Class III
	• Neuromuscular diseases, such as myotonic muscular dystrophy, Kearns–Sayre syndrome, Erb dystrophy or peroneal muscular atrophy with or without symptoms (B) Asymptomatic persistent third-degree AV block at any anatomic site with mean awake ventricular rates ≥40/min if cardiomegaly or LV dysfunction is present or block is infranodal (B) Third-degree AV block during exercise in the absence of myocardial ischemia (C)			
Chronic bifascicular or trifascicular block	Associated with advanced second-degree AV block or intermittent CHB (B)	Syncope not demonstrated to be due to AV block when other likely causes have been excluded, specifically VT (B)	Neuromuscular diseases such as myotonic muscular dystrophy, Erb dystrophy or peroneal muscular atrophy with bifascicular or any fascicular block, with or without symptoms (C)	Fascicular block without AV block or symptoms (B)
	Associated with type II second-degree AV block (B)	Incidental finding at EPS of markedly prolonged HV interval (≥100 ms) in asymptomatic patients (B)		Fascicular block with first-degree AV block without symptoms (B)
	Alternating bundle branch block (C)	Incidental finding at EPS of pacing-induced infra-His block that is not physiological (B)		
AV block after the acute phase of myocardial infarction (MI)	Persistent second-degree AV block in the His–Purkinje system with alternating bundle branch block or third-degree AV block within or below the His–Purkinje system after ST elevation MI (B)	None	Persistent second- or third-degree AV block at the AV node level, even in the absence of symptoms (B)	Transient AV block in the absence of intraventricular conduction defects (B)
	Transient advanced second- or third-degree infranodal AV block and associated bundle branch block. If the site of block is uncertain, an EPS may be necessary (B)			Transient AV block in the presence of isolated left anterior fascicular block (B)
	Persistent and symptomatic second- or third-degree AV block (C)			New bundle branch block or fascicular block in the absence of AV block (B) Persistent asymptomatic first-degree AV block in the presence of bundle branch block or fascicular block (B)

Table 41.1 *Continued*

Condition	Class I	Class IIa	Class IIb	Class III
Sinus node dysfunction (SND)	SND with documented symptomatic bradycardia, including frequent sinus pauses that produce symptoms (C)	SND with heart rate <40/min when a clear association between significant symptoms consistent with bradycardia and the actual presence of bradycardia has not been documented (C)	Minimally symptomatic patients with chronic heart rates <40/min whilst awake (C)	SND in asymptomatic patients (C)
	Symptomatic chronotropic incompetence (C)	Syncope of unexplained origin when clinically significant abnormalities of sinus node function are discovered or provoked at EPS (C)		SND in patients in whom the symptoms suggestive of bradycardia have been clearly documented to occur in the absence of bradycardia (C)
	Symptomatic sinus bradycardia that results from required drug therapy for medical conditions (C)			SND with symptomatic bradycardia due to nonessential drug therapy (C)
Hypersensitive carotid sinus syndrome and neurocardiogenic syncope	Recurrent syncope caused by spontaneously occurring carotid sinus stimulation and carotid sinus pressure that induces ventricular asystole of >3 s (C)	Syncope without clear, provocative events and with a hypersensitive cardio-inhibitory response >3 s (C)	Significantly symptomatic neurocardiogenic syncope associated with bradycardia documented spontaneously or at the time of tilt-table testing (B)	Hypersensitive cardio-inhibitory response to carotid sinus stimulation without symptoms or with vague symptoms (C)
				Situational vasovagal syncope in which avoidance behavior is effective and preferred (C)
Pacing to prevent tachycardia	Sustained pause-dependent VT, with or without QT prolongation (C)	High-risk patients with congenital long-QT syndrome (C)	Prevention of symptomatic, drug-refractory, recurrent AF in patients with co-existing sinus node disease (B)	Frequent or complex ventricular ectopic activity without sustained VT in the absence of the long-QT syndrome (C)
				Torsades de pointes VT due to reversible causes (A)
				Prevention of AF in patients without any other indication for pacemaker implantation (B)
Pacing with devices that automatically detect and pace to terminate tachycardia	None	Symptomatic recurrent SVT that is reproducibly terminated by pacing when catheter ablation and/or drugs fail to control the arrhythmia or produce intolerable side effects (C)	None	Presence of an accessory pathway that has the capacity for rapid anterograde conduction (C)

Continued on p. 640

Table 41.1 *Continued*

Condition	Class I	Class IIa	Class IIb	Class III
Hypertrophic cardiomyopathy (HCM)	SND or AV block in patients with hypertrophic cardiomyopathy as described above (C)	None	Medically refractory, symptomatic patients with HCM and significant resting or provoked LV outflow tract obstruction (A). (A dual-chamber ICD should be considered when risk factors for sudden death are present)	Asymptomatic or medically controlled patients (C) Symptomatic patients without evidence of LV outflow obstruction (C)
Cardiac resynchronization therapy (CRT) in patients with severe systolic heart failure	For patients who have LV EF ≤35%, QRS duration ≥120 ms and sinus rhythm, CRT with or without ICD is indicated for the treatment of NYHA class III or ambulatory class IV heart failure symptoms with optimal medical therapy (A)	For patients who have LV EF ≤35%, QRS duration ≥120 ms and atrial fibrillation, CRT with or without an ICD is reasonable for the treatment of NYHA class III or ambulatory class IV heart failure symptoms on optimal medical therapy (B) For patients with LV EF ≤35% with NYHA class III or ambulatory class IV symptoms who are receiving optimal medical therapy and who have frequent dependence on ventricular pacing, CRT is reasonable (C)	For patients with LV EF ≤35% with NYHA class I or II symptoms who are receiving optimal medical therapy and who are undergoing implantation of a permanent pacemaker and/or ICD with anticipated frequent ventricular pacing, CRT may be considered (C)	CRT is not indicated for asymptomatic patients with reduced LV EF in the absence of other indications for pacing (B) CRT Is not indicated for patients whose functional status and life expectancy are limited predominantly by chronic non-cardiac conditions (C)
After cardiac transplantation	Persistent inappropriate or symptomatic bradycardia not expected to resolve and other Class I indications for permanent pacing (C)	None	Prolonged or recurrent relative bradycardia, which limits rehabilitation or discharge after postoperative recovery from cardiac transplantation (C) Syncope after cardiac transplantation even when bradyarrhythmia has not been documented (C)	None

Table 41.1 *Continued*

Condition	Class I	Class IIa	Class IIb	Class III
Children, adolescents and patients with congenital heart disease	Advanced second- or third-degree AV block associated with symptomatic bradycardia, ventricular dysfunction or low cardiac output (C)	Congenital heart disease and sinus bradycardia for the prevention of recurrent episodes of intra-atrial re-entrant tachycardia; SND may be intrinsic or secondary to antiarrhythmic treatment (C)	Transient postoperative third-degree AV block that reverts to sinus rhythm with residual bifascicular block (C)	Transient postoperative AV block with return of normal AV conduction in the otherwise asymptomatic patient (B)
	Sinus node dysfunction with correlation of symptoms during age-inappropriate bradycardia (B)	Congenital third-degree AV block beyond the first year of life with an average heart rate <50/min, abrupt pauses in ventricular rate that are 2 or 3 times the basic cycle length, or associated with symptoms due to chronotropic incompetence (B)	Congenital third-degree AV block in asymptomatic children or adolescents with an acceptable rate, a narrow QRS complex, and normal ventricular function (B)	Asymptomatic bifascicular block with or without first-degree AV block after surgery for congenital heart disease in the absence of prior transient complete AV block (C)
	Postoperative advanced second- or third-degree AV block that is not expected to resolve or that persists at least 7 days after cardiac surgery (B)	Sinus bradycardia with complex congenital heart disease with a resting heart rate <40/min or pauses in ventricular rate >3 s (C)	Asymptomatic sinus bradycardia after biventricular repair of congenital heart disease with a resting heart rate <40/min or pauses in ventricular rate >3 s (C)	Asymptomatic type I second-degree AV block (C)
	Congenital third-degree AV block with a wide QRS escape rhythm, complex ventricular ectopy, or ventricular dysfunction (B)	Congenital heart disease an impaired hemodynamics due to sinus bradycardia or loss of AV synchrony (C)		Asymptomatic sinus bradycardia with the longest R–R interval <3 s and the minimum rate >40/min (C)
	Congenital third-degree AV block in the infant with a ventricular rate <55/min or with congenital heart disease and a ventricular rate <70/min (C)	Unexplained syncope in the patient with prior congenital heart surgery complicated by transient complete heart block with residual fascicular block after a careful evaluation to exclude other causes of syncope (B)		

CHB, complete heart block; CHF, congestive heart failure; EPS, electrophysiology study; VT, ventricular tachycardia; RBBB, right bundle branch block.

The grade of evidence supporting each recommendation is indicated in parentheses:

(A) data derived from multiple randomized clinical trials involving a large number of individuals

(B) data derived from a limited number of trials involving comparatively small numbers of patients or from well-designed data analyses of non-randomized studies or observational data registries

(C) recommendation based on consensus opinion of experts.

Class I – conditions for which there is evidence and/or general agreement that pacing is beneficial, useful and effective.

Class II – conditions for which there is conflicting evidence and/or a divergence of opinion about the usefulness/efficacy of pacing.

Class III – conditions for which there is evidence and/or general agreement that pacing is not useful/effective and in some cases may be harmful.

Class II is subdivided into Class IIa – weight of evidence/opinion is in favor of usefulness/efficacy and Class IIb – usefulness/efficacy is less well established by evidence/opinion.

Based on Epstein *et al.*[7]

Conventional indications for pacing

The principal indication for cardiac pacing is to relieve or prevent symptoms associated with bradycardia. In high-grade AV block, however, there is evidence that survival may also be improved by pacing, even in the absence of symptoms, and pacing should be considered on prognostic grounds alone.

Where significant symptoms are clearly associated with documented bradycardia, the requirement for pacing will rarely be in doubt. In other contexts, the cause of symptoms may be unclear and it is important to note that the most common symptoms are non-specific and prevalent in the elderly population, even in the absence of bradycardia.

The most common causes of bradycardia requiring pacing are impaired impulse formation, as in sinus node disease, or a disturbance of cardiac conduction, as in AV block. These conditions account for the vast majority of primary pacemaker implants.[3] The remainder includes patients paced for a variety of conditions, including carotid sinus syndrome, cardio-inhibitory forms of neurocardiogenic syncope and others.

Atrioventricular block

First-degree atrioventricular block

Isolated prolongation of the PR interval may be a normal variant in healthy young subjects.[9] In older subjects, it is more often associated with underlying pathology, such as conducting system fibrosis or coronary artery disease, but it does not usually give rise to symptoms and pacing is not generally indicated.

Occasionally, symptoms may arise if the PR interval is markedly prolonged. Atrial systole may then closely follow delayed ventricular systole from the previous cycle, resulting in a comparable hemodynamic disturbance to that seen in the pacemaker syndrome[10,11] and a favorable response to dual-chamber pacing has been reported.[12] Symptomatic first-degree AV block with a demonstrable improvement during temporary dual-chamber pacing may reasonably be considered at least a **Class IIa**[13] and perhaps even a Class I[14] indication for pacing (**Level B**).

Second-degree atrioventricular block

When second-degree AV block of any type is associated with clearly attributable symptoms, pacing is indicated. In the absence of symptoms, the situation is more complex. Prognosis is thought to relate to the site of block, proximal block at the level of the AV node being more benign than distal block in the His–Purkinje system.[15] The ECG classification into Mobitz type I (Wenckebach), Mobitz type II or advanced (2:1, 3:1 or 4:1) second-degree AV block is purely descriptive and the site of block cannot always be inferred although electrophysiologic studies have shown that type I block is most commonly proximal whereas type II block is almost always distal.[16] In the past, type I second-degree AV block has often been regarded as benign but evidence from the Devon Heart Block and Bradycardia Survey (a non-randomized, observational study) suggests that in unpaced patients aged 45 years or over, even amongst those without attributable symptoms, there is an increased incidence of adverse outcomes (symptomatic bradycardia, higher degree AV block or impaired survival) compared to the general population and that pacing is associated with improved survival.[17,18] Guidelines differ in their conclusions but published opinion suggests that pacing should be considered in asymptomatic type I second-degree AV block, particularly in older patients with structural heart disease[19,20] (**Class IIa, Level C**). In young subjects, however, asymptomatic type I second-degree AV block occurring during sleep or associated with athletic training is more likely to reflect high resting vagal tone and pacing is unnecessary.[21,22] In type II second-degree AV block, progression to complete AV block is common, particularly when the QRS complex is wide,[15] and pacing is indicated even in the absence of symptoms (**Class I, Level C**).

Complete atrioventricular block

In symptomatic complete AV block, pacing usually, although not invariably, improves the symptoms and should always be considered. Irrespective of symptoms, however, untreated acquired complete heart block is associated with significantly impaired survival. Overall mortality may exceed 50% at 1 year, the outlook being worse in older patients (>80 years) and those with associated non-rheumatic structural heart disease.[23] Male sex and a history of syncope have also been associated with a worse outlook in some studies[24] but there is conflicting evidence regarding syncope.[25] Transient AV block carries a more favorable prognosis, with a 1-year mortality of 36%, compared with 70% in patients with permanent AV block,[23] but a significant proportion of patients (38–39% over median follow-up of 36–54 months) progress to permanent AV block and become pacemaker dependent when paced.[26]

Observational studies of outcome in paced patients during the early days of cardiac pacing suggested that pacing in complete AV block could improve survival to approach that of a similar age- and sex-matched group.[24] Mortality was higher in those with a history of myocardial infarction but not influenced by pre-pacing QRS duration or morphology, ventricular rate (dichotomized about 40/min) or whether AV block was intermittent or constant.[27] In a more recent study of patients aged ≥65 years, paced for symptomatic, high-grade AV block, overall survival was less than expected for an age- and sex-matched cohort.[28] However, in patients aged <80 years without structural heart disease, survival was normal. Congestive heart failure, chronic obstructive pulmonary disease, age, syncope, insulin-dependent diabetes and male gender emerged as independent predictors of increased mortality. There have been no prospective randomized trials to assess the impact of pacing in high-grade AV block but the prevalence of symptoms, the high mortality without pacing, the strength of the data from observational studies, and the absence of any alternative therapy suggest that such a trial is neither ethical nor necessary. The vast majority of patients with complete AV block should be paced, whether or not they have symptoms (**Class I, Level C**)

Congenital complete atrioventricular block

In patients surviving to adulthood, the prognosis of congenital complete AV block has previously been regarded as benign, based largely on retrospective studies of a small series of patients.[29] More recent data concerning long-term follow-up (7–30 years) of 102 patients with isolated congenital complete AV block, who survived without symptoms to the age of 15 years, suggests a less favorable outlook.[30] Stokes–Adams attacks occurred in 27 patients, of whom eight died (six during the first attack) and six others required cardiac resuscitation. All survivors received pacemakers. A further eight patients had repeated fainting spells requiring pacing and 27 others were paced for other reasons (fatigue, effort dyspnea, dizziness, ectopics during exercise, mitral regurgitation or slow ventricular rates). Of 40 patients followed for 30 years, only four remained asymptomatic without pacing. The only significant predictor of risk was QTc prolongation, which was seen in seven patients, all of whom had Stokes–Adams attacks and three of whom died. In contrast to previous studies, low ventricular rates, widened QRS complexes, poor chronotropic response to exercise and ectopics were not predictive of future Stokes–Adams attacks or death. These data support the authors' recommendation of prophylactic pacing in adolescents and adults with congenital complete AV block, even without symptoms, notwithstanding the fact that a number of questions remain unanswered (**Class IIa, Level C**).[31]

Fascicular block

In asymptomatic subjects with unifascicular block (right bundle branch block, left anterior hemiblock or left posterior hemiblock), the risk of progression to high-grade AV block is remote[32] and pacing is not indicated (**Class III, Level C**). In asymptomatic bifascicular block (left bundle branch block or right bundle branch block with left anterior or posterior hemiblock), the risk of progression to high-grade AV block is in the region of 2% per annum. Prognosis

is principally determined by the presence or absence of underlying structural heart disease and prophylactic pacing is not routinely indicated (**Class III, Level B**).[33] Progression to high-grade AV block is more commonly seen in patients with a history of syncope but should not be presumed to be the cause without further assessment. If high-grade AV block is documented, pacing is mandatory (**Class I, Level B**). When the cause of syncope remains unclear, an electrophysiology study may help identify patients likely to benefit from pacemaker implantation. A prolonged HV interval >100 ms and His–Purkinje block during atrial pacing have high specificity for prediction of subsequent progression to high-grade AV block.[34,35] Less marked HV prolongation (>70 ms) is more common but its significance is uncertain.[36] Sensitivity for disclosure of latent high-grade AV block may be markedly enhanced by the use of intravenous disopyramide during the study but this is not advised in patients with impaired left ventricular (LV) function.[37] The electrophysiology study may also be of value to identify inducible ventricular tachycardia,[38] which argues against the empiric use of permanent pacing in this context. However, in patients with bifascicular block and a history of syncope for which no other cause is apparent despite thorough evaluation, including an electrophysiology study, empiric pacing may be the most expeditious course. This strategy is principally justified for relief of symptoms as pacing does not appear to influence mortality or the incidence of sudden death in this context (**Class IIa, Level B**).[33]

Atrioventricular and bundle branch block after myocardial infarction

Transient conduction disturbance is a relatively common complication of acute myocardial infarction. Long-term prognosis is principally determined by the extent of myocardial injury. When AV block complicates inferior myocardial infarction, it typically resolves within a few days and rarely persists beyond 2 or 3 weeks. In anterior infarction, however, AV block may reflect extensive septal necrosis and the prognosis is poor despite pacing.[39] Patients with high-grade AV block persisting for more than 3 weeks after myocardial infarction should be considered for permanent pacing (**Class I, Level C**).

The occurrence of an intraventricular conduction disturbance (apart from isolated left anterior hemiblock) in patients with acute myocardial infarction identifies a group with poor short-term and long-term prognosis and an increased risk of sudden death.[40] The poor prognosis in this group, however, is mainly attributable to a high incidence of malignant ventricular arrhythmia, pump failure, and electromechanical dissociation, rather than progressive conduction disturbance. A prospective study of 50 patients randomized to pacing or control groups and followed for 5 years showed no significant difference in survival.[41]

However, evidence from a retrospective multicenter study of patients with bundle branch block complicating myocardial infarction indicates that transient high-degree AV block during the acute phase is associated with a high incidence of recurrent AV block and sudden death that may be reduced by pacemaker implantation.[42,43] The risk appears to be particularly high in patients with block involving the right bundle and at least one fascicle of the left bundle (**Class I, Level B**).[43,44]

Sinoatrial disease

Sinoatrial disease encompasses a wide spectrum of arrhythmia including sinus bradycardia, sinus arrest, sino-atrial block, sick sinus syndrome, the tachycardia–bradycardia syndrome and chronotropic incompetence (failure to reach at least 80% of the maximum predicted heart rate at peak exertion).[45] The prognosis in sinoatrial disease is generally good unless myocardial ischemia, heart failure or systemic embolism is present.[46] Permanent pacing is indicated for the relief of symptoms that are due to bradycardia.

The efficacy of pacing in sick sinus syndrome has been assessed in a randomized trial.[47] One hundred and seven patients with symptomatic sick sinus syndrome were randomized to receive no treatment, oral theophylline or permanent dual chamber adaptive rate (DDDR) pacing. Patients were excluded in very severe cases, defined as symptomatic resting sinus rate <30/min, sinus pauses >3s or heart failure refractory to treatment with angiotensin-converting enzyme (ACE) inhibitors and diuretics. During a mean follow-up period of 19 months, both pacing and theophylline were associated with a lower incidence of heart failure compared with no treatment (3%, 3% and 17% respectively) but only pacing was associated with a significantly lower incidence of syncope (6%, 17% and 23% respectively). Pacing remains the treatment of choice for patients with symptomatic sick sinus syndrome (**Class I, Level B/C**). In the absence of long-term follow-up data to confirm efficacy and safety, theophylline or other pharmacologic means of chronotropic support cannot be recommended.

Pacing does not appear to improve survival in sinoatrial disease[48] and it is not generally indicated in asymptomatic patients (**Class III, Level C**). Such patients, however, should be followed closely to assess progression. Athletically trained subjects may have sinus rates as low as 30/min during sleep with pauses of almost 3s.[49] These findings usually reflect high vagal tone and do not require pacing in the absence of symptoms. If lower rates or longer pauses are observed during sleep or if similar findings occur during the day, particularly if there is evidence of progression with time, prophylactic pacing may be justified on empiric grounds although there are no supportive data (**Class IIb, Level C**).

Mode selection in AV block and sinus node disease

In AV block, the essential requirement is that the ventricle be paced. When sinus rhythm and chronotropic competence are preserved, dual-chamber pacing with atrial tracking will ensure the maintenance of AV synchrony and physiologic rate adaptation. When sinus rhythm is absent or when chronotropic incompetence is present, an extrinsic sensor may be used to provide rate adaptation with either ventricular or dual-chamber pacing, as appropriate. In isolated sinoatrial disease, rate support can be achieved by single-chamber pacing in the atrium or ventricle, or by dual-chamber pacing.

Both dual-chamber pacing and adaptive rate single-chamber pacing have been shown to offer benefits in terms of improved hemodynamics, increased treadmill exercise tolerance and reduced symptoms when compared with single rate ventricular pacing in small randomized cross-over studies.[50–58] The mean patient age in most of these studies was younger than the typical paced population although similar benefits have also been reported in patients aged 75 years or over.[59] Nonetheless, the long-term clinical benefit of physiologic pacing in the elderly has been questioned.[60] Small-scale quality of life studies have yielded conflicting results although physiologic pacing, with preservation of AV synchrony and rate adaptation, does appear to offer advantages in terms of symptoms and there is considerable evidence of patient preference for physiologic modes.[61] Single-chamber ventricular pacing is associated with an increased risk of pacemaker syndrome, which has been estimated to occur in between 7% and 20% of patients.[2] It has, however, been suggested that a subclinical form may be present in many apparently asymptomatic patients.[62] Data from retrospective studies suggest that ventricular pacing is associated with an increased risk of atrial fibrillation (AF), heart failure, and thromboembolism.[46,63] and with increased mortality in some patient groups.[64–66]

The Danish trial reported by Anderson and colleagues, was the first prospective randomized trial of pacemaker mode selection.[67] In this study, 225 patients with sick sinus syndrome were randomized to either single-chamber atrial (AAI) or single-chamber ventricular (VVI) pacing and followed for a mean of 3.3 years. Neither the incidence of AF or stroke nor survival differed significantly between the two groups, although the incidence of a combined end-point of stroke plus peripheral embolism was significantly lower in the atrial paced group. Extended follow-up of the same group of patients was reported after a mean of 5.5 years.[68] The previously identified benefits of atrial pacing were enhanced, with a significantly lower incidence of AF, thromboembolism and heart failure in the atrial paced group. All-cause mortality and mortality due to cardiovascular causes were also significantly lower in the atrial paced group. Only four of 110 patients in the atrial paced group developed second- or third-degree AV block, requiring pacemaker upgrade (0.6% per annum).[69]

The Pacemaker Selection in the Elderly (PASE) study randomized 407 patients, aged 65 or older (mean age 76 years), to ventricular or dual-chamber pacing.[70] All patients received DDDR pacing systems and mode randomization was achieved by programming of the pacemaker. The group included 175 patients with sinus node disease, 201 patients with AV block and 31 patients with other diagnoses. The study was powered to assess differences in health-related quality of life. As would be expected, there was marked improvement in quality of life (SF-36) after pacemaker implantation but there were no significant differences between groups in relation to pacing mode. It is noteworthy that 26% of the patients randomized to ventricular pacing crossed over to dual-chamber pacing because of symptoms attributed to pacemaker syndrome. Whilst potentially significant in itself, the high crossover rate confounds interpretation of the data, particularly in respect of clinical outcomes. In a multivariate analysis, a decrease in systolic blood pressure to <110 mmHg during ventricular pacing at the time of pacemaker implantation ($P = 0.001$), use of beta-blockers at the time of randomization ($P = 0.01$) and non-ischemic cardiomyopathy ($P = 0.04$) were the only variables that predicted crossover.[71]

The Canadian Trial of Physiologic Pacing (CTOPP), the largest reported to date, included 2568 patients aged 18 years or older (mean age 73 years), with either AV block (60%) or sinus node disease (40%), who were randomized to receive either a ventricular (VVIR) or a physiologic pacemaker.[72–74] In the physiologic arm, investigators selected either an atrial (AAIR) or a dual-chamber (DDDR) system. Adaptive rate pacing was used in both groups if chronotropic incompetence was evident and in patients with complete AV block randomized to receive ventricular pacing. Over a mean follow-up of 3 years there was no significant difference in the primary outcome of cardiovascular death or stroke (VVIR 5.5% per annum vs physiologic 4.9% per annum; relative risk reduction 9.4%; 95% confidence interval (CI) −10.5 to 25.7; $P = 0.33$). Neither was there any significant difference in all-cause mortality or in hospital admission for heart failure. There was, however, a significant, albeit modest reduction in AF (defined as an episode lasting more than 15 minutes) associated with physiologic pacing (VVIR 6.6% per annum vs physiologic 5.3% per annum; relative risk reduction 18.0%; 95% CI −0.3 to 32.6; $P = 0.05$), which became evident after about 2 years. Perioperative complications were more common with physiologic pacing (VVIR 3.8% vs physiologic 9.0%; $P < 0.001$) mainly in relation to the pacing lead(s). There was a trend suggesting that younger patients (<74 years) might have a reduced risk of stroke or cardiovascular death with physiologic pacing.

Subgroup analysis of the CTOPP data suggests that the benefits of physiologic pacing may be influenced by pacemaker dependency.[75] This was assessed in 87% of the enrolled patients by recording the unpaced heart rate at the first follow-up visit (2–8 months post implant). In patients with unpaced heart rates ≤60/min, the incidence of cardiovascular death or stroke was lower with physiologic pacing (VVIR 6.4% per annum vs physiologic 4.1% per annum; relative risk reduction 35.5%; 95% CI 12 to 53). By contrast, the treatment effect of physiologic pacing was slightly negative in patients with unpaced heart rates >60/min (VVIR 4.1% per annum vs physiologic 4.3% per annum; relative risk reduction −1.9%; 95% CI −50 to 31). The difference in treatment effect between the two groups was of only borderline significance ($P = 0.058$).

Quality of life improved with pacing but there were no significant differences according to pacing mode irrespective of pacemaker dependency.[76] A limited economic analysis in a subset of 472 patients showed that physiologic pacing was not cost-effective according to generally accepted standards unless used selectively in patients likely to be pacemaker dependent.[77]

The CTOPP investigators subsequently reported the results of extended follow-up after a mean of 6.4 years. The previously observed difference in the rate of AF persisted, with a relative risk reduction in the physiologic group of 20.1% (95% CI 5.4 to 32.5; $P = 0.009$) but there was no significant difference in the rate of cardiovascular death or stroke.[78]

The Mode Selection Trial (MOST) assessed the benefits of adaptive rate, dual-chamber pacing compared with adaptive rate, single-chamber, ventricular pacing in 2110 patients aged ≥21 years, with sinus node dysfunction.[79] A DDDR pacing system was implanted in all patients and the pacing mode was randomized to VVIR or DDDR. After a median follow-up of 33.1 months, there was no difference in the incidence of the primary endpoint, death or non-fatal stroke, between the groups (VVIR 23.0% vs DDDR 21.5%; $P = 0.48$).[80] However, dual-chamber pacing was associated with a lower incidence of AF (hazard ratio (HR) 0.79; 95% CI 0.66 to 0.94; $P = 0.008$). Heart failure scores were also significantly improved but this did not result in a lower incidence of hospitalization for heart failure in the primary unadjusted analysis (VVIR 12.3%; DDDR 10.3%; HR 0.82; 95% CI 0.63 to 1.06; $P = 0.13$). Quality of life was substantially improved by pacing with a small but significant advantage for the dual-chamber mode in three of the eight subscales of the SF-36.[81] Crossover from VVIR to DDDR mode occurred in 374 patients but 61 patients subsequently switched back, resulting in a crossover rate at final follow-up of 31.4%. Almost half of the crossovers were attributed to pacemaker syndrome. The high crossover rate in PASE and MOST, where a mode change only required reprogramming of the device, contrasts with the low rates in CTOPP (2.7% at 3 years) and UKPACE (3.1% at 3 years), in which replacement of the pacing system would have been required. Although the high crossover rate in MOST complicates interpretation of the data, an analysis based on treatment received showed that it had no impact on the primary endpoint or other key clinical outcomes.[82] An economic analysis suggested that dual-chamber pacing in this patient group is cost-effective at conventionally accepted levels both within the 4-year time horizon of the trial and projected over the lifetime of the patients.[83]

The United Kingdom Pacing and Cardiovascular Events (UKPACE) trial enrolled patients aged ≥70 years with high-grade AV block. Prior to the trial, national registry data showed evidence of ageism in clinical practice, with elderly patients being much less likely to receive dual-chamber pacemakers than those who were younger.[84] In the trial, 2021 patients were randomly assigned to receive either single-chamber or dual-chamber pacemakers and followed for a minimum of 3 years. In the single-chamber arm, assignment to VVI or VVIR was also randomized. After median follow-up of 4.6 years, there was no significant difference in the primary outcome of all-cause mortality (VVIR 7.2% per annum vs DDDR 7.4% per annum; HR 0.96; 95% CI 0.83 to 1.11; $P = 0.33$). Median follow-up for other events was 3 years and showed no significant difference in the rates of AF, heart failure or a composite of stroke, transient ischemic attack (TIA) or other thromboembolism.[85] When VVI and VVIR pacing were compared separately with dual-chamber pacing, there was a significantly higher rate of stroke, TIA or other thromboembolism with VVI pacing than with DDD (2.5% per annum vs 1.7%; $P = 0.04$) but there were no other significant differences. Complications related to the implantation procedure were more common in the dual-chamber group than in the single-chamber group (7.8% vs 3.5%; $P < 0.001$), as were complications before hospital discharge (10.4% vs 6.1%; $P < 0.001$). Preliminary analysis of quality of life showed improvement with pacing but no significant difference according to randomized pacing mode. Suspected pacemaker syndrome occurred in only 2.7% of those receiving single-chamber pacing[86] and crossover from single- to dual-chamber pacing in 3.1%.[85]

The Danish Multicenter Randomized Study on Atrial Inhibited versus Dual-Chamber Pacing in Sick Sinus Syndrome (DANPACE) aims to examine the relative merits of single-lead atrial pacing (AAIR) and dual-chamber pacing (DDDR) in patients aged ≥18 years with sick sinus syndrome (including tachycardia-bradycardia syndrome) and normal AV conduction.[87] The primary outcome measure is all-cause mortality. Secondary outcomes include cardiovascular mortality, AF, thromboembolism, quality of life and

cost–benefit. Recruitment of 1415 patients (reduced from an original target of 1900) was completed in June 2008 and follow-up will be concluded in 2009.

A prior pilot study randomized 177 patients with sick sinus syndrome and normal AV conduction to single-chamber atrial pacing (AAIR), or dual-chamber pacing (DDDR) with either a short AV delay or a fixed long AV delay. During a mean follow-up of 2.9 years, echocardiography showed no significant changes in left atrial or ventricular diameter or in LV fractional shortening in the atrial pacing group. However, left atrial diameter increased in both of the dual-chamber groups and LV fractional shortening decreased in the dual-chamber group with short AV delay.[88] The incidence of AF was significantly lower in the atrial pacing group (7.4%) than in the dual-chamber groups with short (12.3%) or long (17.5%) AV delay, the benefit being most evident in patients with brady-tachy syndrome.[89]

The benefits of physiologic pacing have been addressed in four other trials for which only limited data are available. An Italian study reported on 210 patients with high-grade AV block (100 patients) or sick sinus syndrome (110 patients) with no prior AF, randomly assigned to ventricular (VVI or VVIR) or atrial-based (AAI, DDD, DDDR or VDD) pacing.[90] The incidence of chronic AF was lower with atrial-based than with ventricular pacing, particularly in those with sick sinus syndrome. The Pacemaker Atrial Tachycardia (PAC-A-TACH) trial assessed the effect of pacing mode on atrial tachyarrhythmia recurrence in 198 patients with the tachycardia-bradycardia syndrome.[91] All patients received dual-chamber, adaptive rate pacemakers programmed to either VVIR or DDDR pacing. After a median of 23.7 months follow-up, 44% of patients crossed over from VVIR to DDD (due to pacemaker syndrome in 28% and atrial tachyarrhythmia in 13%) and 9% crossed over from DDDR to VVIR (due to recurrent atrial tachyarrhythmia in 7% and atrial lead problems in 2%). Intention-to-treat analysis showed no significant difference in atrial tachyarrhythmia recurrence rates at 1 year (VVIR 43%; DDDR 48%; $P = 0.09$). Mortality, a secondary outcome, was significantly higher in the VVIR group and the trial was stopped after follow-up of approximately 2 years in all patients. Cumulative mortality was 21% in the VVIR group and 5% in the DDDR group ($P < 0.001$). Pacing mode (risk ratio 4.3; 95% CI 1.6 to 11.4; $P = 0.004$) and prior history of myocardial infarction (risk ratio 3.1; 95% CI 1.4 to 6.7; $P = 0.006$) were identified as independent predictors of mortality.[92] The Systematic Trial of Pacing to Prevent Atrial Fibrillation (STOP-AF) randomly assigned 227 patients with sick sinus syndrome, all implanted with a DDDR pacing system, to either atrial-based (AAI or DDD) or ventricular pacing.[93,94] The results have not yet been presented or published. Finally, the ongoing Pacing the Octagenarian Plus (POPP) trial is comparing the effect of single-chamber

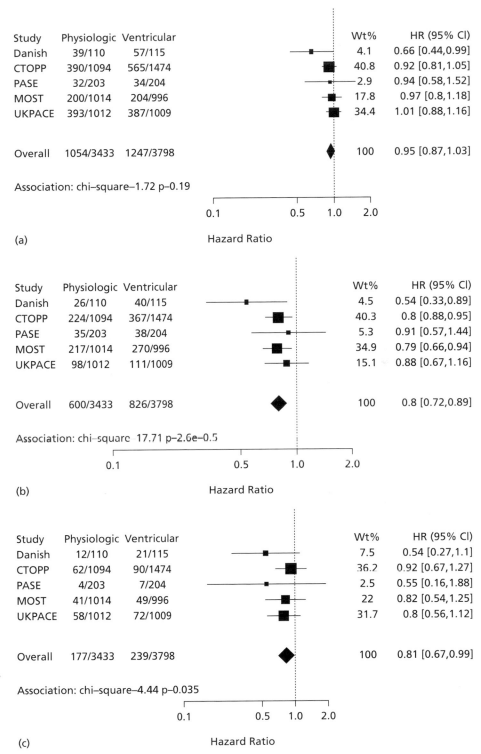

Figure 41.1 Effect of pacing mode, expressed as the HR and 95% CI. An HR <1.0 is shown to the left of the center line and favors atrial-based pacing. CIs that cross 1.0 signify a statistically non-significant effect. (a) All-cause mortality. (b) Incidence of atrial fibrillation. (c) Incidence of stroke (Reproduced with permission from Healey et al.[96])

(VVIR) and dual-chamber (DDDR) pacing on hospitalization for cardiovascular causes, functional capacity and quality of life in the very elderly.[95]

A prospectively planned meta-analysis of patient-level data from five of the trials (the Danish Trial, PASE, CTOPP, MOST and UKPACE) demonstrated a reduction in AF with atrial-based pacing (HR 0.80; 95% CI 0.72 to 0.89; P = 0.00003) and in stroke (HR 0.81; 95% CI 0.67 to 0.99; P = 0.035).[96] There was no significant reduction in mortality or heart failure and no convincing evidence that any patient subgroup derived special benefit from atrial-based pacing. The key findings are shown in Figure 41.1.

Two systematic reviews have comprehensively assessed the various parallel group and crossover randomized controlled trials comparing single-chamber ventricular pacing and dual-chamber pacing.[97,98] The aggregated data indicate an overall advantage for dual-chamber pacing, related to the lower incidence of AF and the reduction in pacemaker syndrome. These benefits must be weighed against the increased implant complications and cost. The overall estimate of cost-effectiveness of dual-chamber pacing varied between around UK £9000 and around UK £30000 per quality-adjusted life-year, according to the assumptions made about the incidence and severity of pacemaker syndrome.[98]

A new paradigm for physiologic pacing

The results of the various prospective randomized trials suggest that the clinical benefits of physiologic or dual-chamber pacing may previously have been overestimated. Pacemaker recipients are often elderly with multiple co-morbidities and a high mortality from non-cardiovascular causes. Against this background, it may be unrealistic to expect a marked effect of pacing mode on quality of life, clinical events and mortality, all of which may be more influenced by other factors. A further explanation for the limited clinical benefits of physiologic pacing might be that the conventional placement of the ventricular lead at the right ventricular apex causes interventricular and intraventricular dyssynchrony that could offset the hemodynamic advantage of preserved AV synchrony. It has long been recognized that eccentric ventricular stimulation results in impaired LV performance.[99] Pacing at the right ventricular apex produces an activation sequence similar to that of left bundle branch block, the acquired form of which is associated with an adverse prognosis particularly in patients with heart failure.[32,100,101] Whilst this may partly reflect advanced underlying disease, there is some evidence that the conduction disturbance is an independent marker of adverse outcomes.[101] Paradoxically, the problem may be accentuated by dual-chamber pacing. In an analysis of patients in the MOST study with normal baseline QRS duration, the cumulative percentage of ventricular beats that were paced was greater with dual-chamber than with single-chamber pacing and a higher cumulative percentage of ventricular pacing was associated with an increased risk of heart failure hospitalization and AF with either pacing mode.[102] Further data suggesting a deleterious effect of right ventricular apical pacing have emerged from studies of pacing strategies in implantable cardioverter defibrillator (ICD) recipients. In the Dual-chamber and VVI Implantable Defibrillator (DAVID) trial, 506 patients with an ICD capable of dual-chamber adaptive rate pacing were randomly assigned to back-up ventricular pacing at 40/min

or dual-chamber adaptive rate pacing at 70/min. All patients had ejection fraction ≤40% but no indication for cardiac pacing. Over 1 year, the incidence of the composite endpoint of death or hospitalization for heart failure was significantly increased in the dual-chamber paced group (HR 1.61; 95% CI 1.06 to 2.44).[103] Similarly, in a subgroup analysis of the Multicenter Automatic Defibrillator Implantation Trial (MADIT) II, which tested the benefit of a prophylactic ICD (single- or dual-chamber with back-up pacing) in patients with prior myocardial infarction and LV ejection fraction ≤30%, patients who were predominantly paced had an increased incidence of new or worsening heart failure.[104]

Recognition of the potential importance of dyssynchrony from right ventricular pacing has prompted a re-evaluation of what constitutes "physiologic" pacing and a new paradigm is emerging.[105,106] The key considerations are that, in addition to preserving AV synchrony, the selected therapy should minimize unnecessary ventricular pacing and minimize intraventricular and interventricular dyssynchrony when ventricular pacing is required.

Minimizing ventricular pacing

In patients with sinus node disease and normal AV conduction, single-chamber atrial pacing permits ventricular activation via the intrinsic conduction system, with complete avoidance of ventricular pacing. Although the subsequent development of AV conduction disturbance is infrequent (circa 1.7% per annum),[107] many physicians prefer to implant a dual-chamber system to insure against the risk. It is, however, noteworthy that the Danish study was the only randomized trial to use single-lead atrial pacing as the sole physiologic comparator and showed the greatest clinical benefits from physiologic pacing, including a reduction in mortality. The DANPACE trial will provide further information about the relative merits of the two approaches in due course.

If a ventricular lead is placed prophylactically or due to the presence of intermittent AV conduction disturbance, there are several programming options to minimize ventricular pacing although none will truly emulate normal physiology. Fixed, long AV delays are only partially effective in reducing ventricular pacing and may compromise upper-rate behavior and predispose to pacemaker-mediated tachycardia.[108] Other options include the use of the DDIR mode, which provides back-up pacing in the ventricle without tracking the atrial rhythm, and algorithms that permit automatic extension of the AV interval (AV search hysteresis) to favor intrinsic ventricular activation.[109,110] A number of manufacturers have recently introduced dual-chamber devices with new algorithms that combine functional AAIR pacing with ventricular monitoring and back-up DDDR pacing, when required.

These algorithms have been shown to be effective in reducing the cumulative percentage of ventricular pacing.[111,112] The recently reported Search AV Extension and Managed Ventricular Pacing for Promoting Atrioventricular Conduction (SAVE PACe) trial showed a lower incidence of AF with the use of AV search hysteresis and minimal ventricular pacing algorithms than with conventional dual-chamber pacing in patients with sinus node disease and normal AV conduction after a mean follow-up of 1.7 years (HR 0.6; 95% CI 0.41 to 0.88; $P = 0.009$).[113] The programming in the conventional dual-chamber arm of the study resulted in a particularly high frequency of ventricular pacing (median 99%), which may have amplified the apparent benefit of the new algorithms but the study nonetheless added to the evidence suggesting benefit from the avoidance of unnecessary ventricular pacing. Attention has been drawn to a potential disadvantage of the algorithms, which may permit or induce very long PR intervals, resulting in potentially significant AV desynchronization in some patients.[114] Further trials are in progress to assess the clinical utility of these new approaches.[115–117]

An additional consideration when programming devices to minimize ventricular pacing is the use of adaptive rate pacing using extrinsic sensors to determine the pacing rate. The Advanced Elements of Pacing Trial (ADEPT) demonstrated, perhaps surprisingly, that rate modulation using current dual-chamber pacemaker technology does not provide measurable improvements in either quality of life or exercise capacity in patients with a blunted heart rate response to exercise.[118] Although there was no difference in the prespecified composite clinical endpoint, rate modulation was associated with a higher frequency of hospitalization for heart failure. It may be that the advantages of restoring chronotropic competence are attenuated by the deleterious effects of increased ventricular pacing. The findings suggest that sensor-driven adaptive rate pacing should be avoided in the absence of chronotropic incompetence and that cautious programming is advisable when it is used.

Minimizing ventricular dyssynchrony

In patients who have permanent AV block and in those who are likely to require more than occasional ventricular pacing, the intraventricular and interventricular dyssynchrony associated with pacing at the right ventricular apex may be attenuated by the use of alternative or multiple pacing sites in the right ventricle, or biventricular pacing.

Alternative and multisite pacing
Numerous small and relatively short-term studies have shown improved hemodynamic function using pacing sites in the right ventricular outflow tract but results have been inconsistent, probably reflecting differences in patient selection, lead positioning and duration of follow-up.[119–121] The septal aspect of the outflow tract appears to be the optimal site[122] but the precise location for maximum hemodynamic advantage may vary between patients. The attainment of a suitable lead position requires sound knowledge of the anatomy, aided by radiologic and electrocardiographic confirmation of optimal lead placement.[123] Another approach that has been investigated is the use of direct His bundle or para-Hisian pacing, which would be expected to achieve the most physiologic ventricular activation pattern in patients with intact distal conduction.[124–126] The technique has been shown to be feasible and to improve hemodynamic and functional outcomes compared with pacing at the right ventricular apex but accurate lead placement is technically challenging and its role remains uncertain. Bifocal right ventricular pacing, with leads at the apex and in the outflow tract, has also been assessed, predominantly in patients with heart failure and conventional indications for cardiac resynchronization therapy.[127–129] Improved hemodynamic and functional outcomes have been demonstrated in the short and medium term and the technique may have a role in this setting for patients in whom transvenous placement of the LV lead is unsuccessful and surgical placement of an epicardial lead is not an option.[129]

Biventricular pacing
Recognition that the dyssynchrony associated with pacing at the right ventricular apex is analogous to that induced by left bundle branch block has prompted consideration of biventricular pacing in patients with a bradycardic indication for pacing, NYHA class III or IV heart failure and impaired LV function. Patients requiring pacing for bradycardia were generally excluded from the trials of biventricular pacing in heart failure but extrapolation of their results suggests that it may be an attractive therapeutic option in this setting. It might also be of prophylactic benefit, even in those without heart failure or impaired LV function at the time of implant. The utility of biventricular pacing in patients paced for bradycardia was first demonstrated in observational studies in which patients with class III and IV heart failure, previously implanted with a right ventricular pacing system, were upgraded to a biventricular pacing system. The procedure was shown to be feasible and to result in improved NYHA class, ejection fraction and symptoms or quality of life after 3–6 months' follow-up.[130,131] In a pilot, randomized, crossover trial in patients with advanced heart failure, requiring replacement of conventional pacing systems, biventricular pacing was associated with improved hemodynamics, NYHA functional class, 6-minute walk distance and quality of life.[132]

The first randomized trial to assess biventricular pacing as a primary strategy in patients requiring anti-bradycardia pacing was the Post AV Nodal Ablation Evaluation (PAVE) trial, which compared right ventricular apical pacing and biventricular pacing in 184 patients, with or without heart failure or LV impairment, who were undergoing AV node ablation for AF.[133] After 6 months follow-up, biventricular pacing was associated with a greater improvement in 6-minute walk distance and ejection fraction was preserved, contrasting with a small fall with right ventricular apical pacing. A subsequent smaller 3-month crossover study in severely symptomatic patients with permanent AF, uncontrolled heart rate or heart failure undergoing AV node ablation showed only modest or no benefit from biventricular or LV pacing compared with right ventricular apical pacing, possibly due to the short follow-up.[134] More recently, the Homburg Biventricular Pacing Evaluation (HOBIPACE) compared biventricular pacing with conventional right ventricular pacing in 30 patients with AV block requiring pacing, LV dilation ($\geq 60\,mm$) and reduced ejection fraction ($\leq 45\%$) in a 3-month crossover design.[135] Biventricular pacing was superior with regard to LV function, quality of life and exercise capacity, the benefit being similar for patients in sinus rhythm and in AF.

Biventricular pacing has subsequently been compared with conventional dual-chamber pacing in a randomized parallel group study of 50 patients, unselected with regard to baseline ejection fraction, being paced for high-grade AV block.[136] After 12 months follow-up, ejection fraction was preserved, N-terminal pro-BNP fell and NYHA class improved in the biventricular paced group, whereas ejection fraction decreased and N-terminal pro-BNP and NYHA class were unchanged in the dual-chamber paced group.

Further trials are ongoing to assess the benefits of biventricular pacing as an alternative to conventional pacing in patients with impaired LV function and mild to moderate heart failure (the Biventricular versus Right Ventricular Pacing in Patients with AV Block (BLOCK-HF) trial),[137] without advanced heart failure (the Preventing Ventricular Dysfunction in Pacemaker Patients Without Advanced Heart Failure (PREVENT-HF) study),[138] with preserved LV function (the Pacing to Avoid Cardiac Enlargement (PACE) trial),[139] and unselected with regard to ejection fraction or heart failure at enrolment (the Biventricular Pacing for Atrioventricular Block to Prevent Cardiac Desynchronization (BioPace) study).[140]

Comment and recommendations

The available data suggest that dual-chamber pacing confers a modest advantage over single-chamber ventricular pacing due to the reduced risk of AF, the avoidance of pacemaker syndrome and a possible small benefit in quality of life. Interpretation of the data regarding pacemaker syndrome is complicated by the divergent estimates of mode intolerance between trials in which the mode randomization was achieved by software programming (PASE, PAC-A-TACH and MOST) and those in which it was achieved by hardware selection (the Danish study, CTOPP and UKPACE). Each design has strengths and weaknesses but software randomization trials are more vulnerable to the effect of investigator bias.[141] In the software randomization trials, crossover rates ranged from 26% to 44%, whereas in the hardware randomization trials, they did not exceed 5%. The true incidence of mode intolerance is most likely between the two extremes. Notwithstanding these uncertainties, dual-chamber pacing is the recommended mode for the majority of patients with sinus node disease or AV block, except in the presence of permanent AF (**Class I/IIa, Level A**). In patients with isolated sinus node disease and no evident abnormality of AV conduction on ECG or at implant, single-chamber atrial pacing remains an attractive option and provides the most physiologic pattern of ventricular activation.[142] Retrospective analysis of pooled data from 28 studies suggests that the risk of subsequent AV block, is low (0.6% per annum)[143] and this is supported by data from the Danish study.[69] Many physicians will nevertheless prefer to implant a dual-chamber system with features and programming tailored to provide functional AAIR pacing with minimal unnecessary ventricular activation.[144] The choice of pacing mode should take account of individual patient factors and in elderly patients with high-degree AV block, single-chamber ventricular pacing (VVIR) is a reasonable option. Adaptive rate pacing should be provided if there is evidence of chronotropic incompetence but unnecessarily aggressive programming of rate response should be avoided. In patients who are likely to require frequent ventricular pacing, alternative pacing sites, such as the septal aspect of the right ventricular outflow tract, may confer an advantage by minimizing dyssynchrony but further data are required before this approach can be recommended for routine practice. Ongoing trials will clarify the role of biventricular pacing in patients requiring pacing for bradycardia. It is, however, a reasonable option to consider, on an individual basis, in patients with NYHA class III or IV heart failure, a low ejection fraction ($\leq 35\%$) and a high anticipated requirement for ventricular pacing (**Class IIa, Level B**). Consideration should also be given to implanting a combined device in patients with a conventional indication for an ICD.

New indications for pacing

Neurocardiogenic syncope

Neurocardiogenic syncope describes the clinical syndromes of syncope resulting from inappropriate autonomic responses, manifested as abnormalities in the control of peripheral vascular resistance and heart rate.[145] It is thought to account for the largest proportion of faints in clinical practice. The most common forms are carotid sinus syndrome and vasovagal syncope but other related syndromes include cough, deglutition, and micturition syncope. A systematic approach to evaluate patients with syncope is essential and comprehensive guidelines have recently been published.[146,147] Carotid sinus massage[148,149] and tilt-table testing[150] are useful diagnostic tools in carotid sinus syndrome and vasovagal syncope respectively, enabling abnormal reflex responses to be categorized as cardio-inhibitory (asystole >3s, bradycardia or AV block), vasodepressor (fall in systolic blood pressure >50mmHg) or mixed. This has invited assessment of the utility of cardiac pacing which might be expected to benefit patients with predominantly cardio-inhibitory or mixed responses.

Carotid sinus syndrome

Early reports of pacing in carotid sinus syndrome confirmed its efficacy in some patients but persistent symptoms were seen in those with a significant vasodepressor response or hypotension during ventricular pacing.[151] The latter was improved by AV sequential pacing and it was suggested that this was the appropriate mode in patients with mixed responses. Attention has been drawn to the variable natural history of the condition, which may remit spontaneously, and the importance of a control group when evaluating therapy has been emphasized.[152] A prospective randomized trial of pacing in patients with severe carotid sinus syndrome randomized 60 patients to pacing (VVI in 18 and DDD in 14 patients) or no therapy (28 patients).[153] During a mean follow-up of 36 months, syncope recurred in 16 (57%) of the non-paced group and only three (9%) of the paced group; 19 patients (68%) in the non-paced group were eventually paced because of the severity of symptoms. Pacing is now the treatment of choice in all but the mildest forms of carotid sinus syndrome. Recent evidence suggests that carotid sinus syndrome is underdiagnosed and that comprehensive assessment of patients presenting with syncope, dizziness or falls may identify a significant number of otherwise unrecognized patients who may benefit from pacing.[154]

In the Syncope And Falls in the Elderly – Pacing And Carotid sinus Evaluation (SAFE PACE) trial, 24264 patients with falls or syncope were identified from a total of 71299 emergency room attendees aged ≥50 years during a 29-month period.[155] Patients with evident extrinsic or medical explanations for falling and those with cognitive impairment were excluded, leaving a residuum of 3384 non-accidental fallers. Of these, 1624 consented to and underwent carotid sinus massage, yielding 257 patients with cardio-inhibitory or mixed carotid sinus hypersensitivity, of whom 175 (mean age 73 years) were randomized to pacing or no

pacing and followed for 1 year, to test the hypothesis that dual-chamber pacing, with a rate drop response algorithm, might reduce the frequency of further falls. Paced patients were significantly less likely to fall (odds ratio 0.42; 95% CI 0.23 to 0.75) and syncope and injurious events were less frequent. A larger, multicenter, randomized controlled trial, SAFE PACE 2,[156] was subsequently undertaken to further evaluate these findings in a wider cultural setting and to clarify the relationship between symptoms and arrhythmia by the use of an implantable loop recorder in the non-paced patients. No data from this trial are currently available. However, a small crossover trial, comparing pacing (DDD with rate drop response) and no pacing (ODO mode) for 6 months each in 34 patients with recurrent unexplained falls and carotid sinus hypersensitivity has recently been reported.[156a] This failed to confirm the benefit from pacing that was observed in SAFE PACE but there was a high attrition rate, with only 25 patients completing both phases, and the study was consequently underpowered and inconclusive.

Comment and recommendations

Recurrent syncope caused by spontaneously occurring carotid sinus stimulation with a cardio-inhibitory response to carotid sinus massage (asystole >3s) is a **Class I, Level C** indication for pacing. Recurrent syncope without clear provocative events and with a cardio-inhibitory response to carotid sinus massage is a **Class IIa, Level C** indication for pacing. European guidelines also require that the asystolic response to carotid sinus massage be accompanied by syncope or presyncope. The role of pacing in patients with a history of recurrent falls (without clear evidence of syncope) and cardio-inhibitory carotid sinus hypersensitivity is uncertain and should be considered on an individualized basis (**Class IIb, Level B**).

Vasovagal syndrome

Pacing has also been evaluated in the so-called "malignant" form of vasovagal syndrome, characterized by recurrent syncope with only brief or absent prodromal symptoms. Evidence from several studies using temporary pacing during tilt testing indicates that pacing rarely prevents vasovagal syncope, reflecting the fact that hypotension precedes the onset of bradycardia in most patients. However, dual-chamber pacing does attenuate the evolution of the final and most extreme degrees of hypotension and may thereby prolong the symptomatic presyncopal period in selected patients with a documented cardio-inhibitory component.[157] A retrospective review of 37 patients receiving predominantly dual-chamber implanted pacemakers, followed for a mean of 50.2 months, reported symptomatic improvement in 89% with 62% remaining free of syncope and 27% completely asymptomatic. The collective syncopal burden was reduced from 136 to 11 episodes per year.[158]

The North American Vasovagal Pacemaker Study (VPS)[159] randomized patients with a history of frequent syncope (≥6 lifetime episodes) and a cardio-inhibitory response on tilt testing to receive either no pacing or DDI pacing with a pacemaker incorporating a specialized rate drop-sensing algorithm designed to detect the characteristic pattern of onset of bradycardia that is seen in vasovagal syndrome. The fall in heart rate is typically more marked than occurs with natural diurnal fluctuation yet less precipitous than that seen at the onset of complete AV block or asystole. On detection of a characteristic rate drop, pacing commences with a high initial intervention rate that gradually decreases.[160] It had been intended to enroll 284 patients, but the study was stopped after enrolment of only 54 patients due to substantial benefit in the paced group. During follow-up, syncope recurred in 22% of patients who were paced compared with 70% of those who were not (relative risk reduction 85.4%; 95% CI 59.7 to 94.7; $P = 0.000022$). There was no significant effect on presyncope (reported by 63% of paced patients and 74% of non-paced patients).

The Vasovagal International Study (VASIS) Group subsequently reported a multicenter European trial of similar design.[161] Forty-two patients with at least three syncopal episodes in the preceding 2 years and a cardio-inhibitory response to tilt testing were randomized to DDI pacing with rate hysteresis (n = 19) or no pacing (n = 23). Syncope recurred in only one (5%) of the paced patients but in 14 (61%) of the unpaced patients ($P = 0.0006$). The median time to first syncope in the unpaced group was 5 months.

The Syncope Diagnosis and Treatment (SYDIT) study compared the relative efficacy of dual-chamber pacing with a rate drop-sensing algorithm and pharmacologic therapy with atenolol.[162] Patients were eligible if they had at least three syncopal episodes in the preceding 2 years and a positive response to tilt testing (syncope with relative bradycardia). The study was terminated after 93 patients had been enrolled, as an interim analysis showed a significant effect in favor of pacing. Syncope recurred in only 4.3% of the paced group (after a median of 390 days) compared with 25.5% of the pharmacologically treated group (after a median of 135 days) (odds ratio 0.133; 95% CI 0.028 to 0.632; $P = 0.004$).

Less encouraging results have since been reported from two double-blind, placebo-controlled trials. In the second Vasovagal Pacemaker Study (VPS II),[163] the inclusion criteria were similar to those of the first VPS but in contrast to that study, VASIS and SYDIT, all patients received a pacemaker and were randomized to DDD pacing with a rate drop response algorithm (n = 48) or no pacing (ODO mode; n = 52). Over 6 months follow-up, syncope recurred in 33% of the paced group, compared with 42% of the non-paced group. The relative risk reduction in time to syncope with DDD pacing was 30% but this was not significant (95% CI −33% to 63%; $P = 0.14$).

In the Vasovagal Syncope and Pacing (SYNPACE) trial,[164] 29 patients with severe recurrent vasovagal syncope, reproduced on tilt-testing, all received a pacemaker which was randomly assigned to be programmed on (DDD pacing with rate drop response; n = 16) or off (inactive OOO mode; n = 13). During a median follow-up of 715 days, there was no significant improvement in syncope recurrence (50% of the paced group and 38% of the non-paced group) or in time to first syncope.

The difference in outcomes between the blinded and unblinded trials suggests a significant placebo or "expectation of benefit" effect from pacemaker implantation. This is supported by the results of a meta-analysis including data from nine randomized trials of pacing for vasovagal syncope.[165] The analysis showed that permanent pacing reduced the risk of recurrent syncope in the unblinded trials (odds ratio 0.09; 95% CI 0.04 to 0.22) but not in the double-blind trials (odds ratio 0.83; 95% CI 0.41 to 1.70). The accumulated data do not support the use of pacing as first-line therapy for vasovagal syncope. However, attention has been drawn to the limitations of the trials, all of which were relatively small, with even the largest (VPS II) being limited in power to rule out a modest benefit from pacing.[166,167] There was also variation in the enrolment criteria, including the requirement for a positive (cardio-inhibitory) tilt test. Pacing would only be expected to benefit patients in whom syncopal episodes were wholly or predominantly mediated by bradycardia or asystole. The utility of tilt testing to identify such patients is limited by poor reproducibility and a lack of correlation between the responses to tilt testing and the mechanism of spontaneous syncope.[146,168] The use of an implantable loop recorder to document the cardiac rhythm during spontaneous syncope and guide further therapy has shown promise and is being further evaluated in a randomized trial.[169,170]

Comment and recommendations

Pacing should not be considered as first-line therapy for the majority of patients with vasovagal syncope. The initial focus should be on conservative measures, such as education, reassurance and physical maneuvers, which may be particularly useful when there are prodromal symptoms.[146] Pacing may, however, be considered in patients with severe recurrent syncope refractory to other measures, in whom profound bradycardia or asystole is documented during tilt testing or spontaneous episodes. The uncertain benefits and the associated risks of pacing should be discussed with the patient (**Class IIa, Level B**).

Hypertrophic cardiomyopathy

The ability of pacing at the right ventricular apex to reduce the LV outflow tract (LVOT) gradient in patients with hypertrophic cardiomyopathy has been recognized for over 30 years.[171] The benefits are thought to be due to eccentric activation of the septum, which may increase the LVOT diameter and decrease systolic anterior movement of the mitral valve during systole. Initial clinical studies showed encouraging short- and medium-term results, with decreased symptoms and improved exercise capacity associated with reductions of LVOT gradient in the region of 60%.[172–175] Favorable LV remodeling has also been observed after prolonged pacing.[176–178] Three prospective randomized crossover trials subsequently confirmed the ability of pacing to reduce the LVOT gradient. There was variable improvement in symptoms with evidence of a significant placebo effect but no significant change in exercise tolerance.[179–184] One study suggested an increased benefit from pacing in patients aged 65 years or over.[184]

Comment and recommendations

The role of dual-chamber pacing in the management of patients with hypertrophic obstructive cardiomyopathy remains controversial. The accumulated data suggest that pacing cannot be considered as primary or routine treatment but it may benefit some patients with symptoms refractory to drug therapy, significant outflow obstruction and contraindications for septal ablation or surgery (**Class IIb, Level A**). The acute hemodynamic response to pacing is not a reliable predictor of symptomatic or functional improvement and temporary pacing studies are thus of little value in patient selection.[175,176,184] Complete heart block is a recognized complication of both transcoronary alcohol septal ablation and surgical septal myectomy, for which permanent pacing may be required (**Class I, Level C**).[185,186] In patients at high risk of sudden death, an ICD may also be indicated.

Atrial fibrillation

The limited success of drug therapy in suppressing paroxysmal AF has prompted the assessment of various pacing strategies, even in patients with no other indication for pacemaker implantation. Possible mechanisms by which pacing might suppress AF in this context include reduction of bradycardia, overdrive suppression of atrial premature beats, elimination of compensatory pauses and reduction in inter- or intra-atrial conduction delay and dispersion of refractoriness that might otherwise favor re-entry. Atrial rate support has been shown to be of benefit in a small series of selected patients with the vagally mediated, pause-dependent form of AF, although concomitant drug therapy may still be required.[187] In a broader context, the use of atrial-based pacing,[188,189] atrial overdrive[190–193] and a variety of AF suppression algorithms[194–199] has been assessed in patients with and without conventional indications for pacing. Results have been inconsistent but generally disappointing. A possible confounder in some of the

studies is the potentially deleterious effect of inappropriate ventricular pacing, which may be increased by the use of atrial overdrive pacing algorithms and predispose to both tachycardia-related cardiomyopathy and the development of AF. The combination of atrial overdrive suppression algorithms with techniques to minimize ventricular pacing might attenuate these effects and this is currently being assessed.[115] Other techniques that have been assessed include biatrial pacing in patients with inter- or intra-atrial conduction delay,[200–204] and dual-site[205–209] or alternative site pacing (on the interatrial septum or at the coronary sinus os)[210–215]. Once again, results have been inconsistent with no clear evidence of clinical benefit.

Comment and recommendations

The use of pacing as a primary antiarrhythmic strategy in the management of AF is not justified by the available data. Interpretation of the data is confounded by variability in the pattern and frequency of arrhythmia, the clinical characteristics of the patients, and the endpoints and outcome measures between the studies, many of which have been small and underpowered. In patients with conventional indications for pacing, the use of a device with preventive algorithms may be justified in selected cases. These pacing modalities may be most effective when used as hybrid therapy with antiarrhythmic drugs. Indeed, it may be that much of the benefit in some of the studies is attributable to the facilitation of increased antiarrhythmic drug therapy by pacing. Pacing is not indicated for the prevention of AF in patients without other indications for pacemaker implantation (**Class III, Level B**).

Long QT syndrome

Patients with the long QT syndrome are at high risk of syncope and sudden death, usually due to polymorphic ventricular tachycardia. There are compelling data from observational studies[216–218] and from the International Long QT Syndrome Registry[219,220] indicating that cardiac pacing, with concomitant beta-blockade, may reduce the rate of recurrent syncope and sudden death. The benefit of pacing is thought to be due to the prevention of bradycardia and pauses, together with rate-related shortening of the QT interval. Unfortunately, for pacing to be effective, relatively high rates (>80/min) may be required[221] with the attendant disadvantage of reduced battery life and the potential risk of tachycardia-induced cardiomyopathy.[222]

Careful attention to pacemaker programming is essential.[223] Features that allow slowing of the heart rate below the programmed lower rate limit, such as hysteresis and sleep functions, and algorithms that may favor the occurrence of pauses should be disabled. Specific rate-smoothing algorithms that are capable of preventing postextrasystolic pauses may be useful.[224] There is indirect experimental and clinical evidence to suggest that pacing might be of particular value in patients with the LQT3 genotype,[225–227] which is particularly associated with increased dispersion of repolarization during bradycardia and with arrhythmia occurring during sleep,[228] but it should not be inferred that other genotypes will not benefit from pacing. Further data are required to clarify the extent to which therapy in the long QT syndrome can be guided by genotype. Pacing should be considered as an adjuvant to beta-blockade in all patients with long QT syndrome and symptomatic bradycardia or high-grade AV block, and whenever there is evidence of pause-dependent malignant arrhythmias (**Class I, Level C**). In high-risk patients, an ICD may also be indicated.

Postcardiac transplantation

Bradycardia, usually due to transient sinus node dysfunction or AV block, may occur in almost two-thirds of patients in the first few weeks following orthotopic cardiac transplantation.[229] Recovery from transient AV block usually occurs within 16 days but transient sinus node dysfunction may persist for several weeks and the optimum time for consideration of permanent pacemaker implantation is uncertain.[230] In some cases, temporary treatment with oral theophylline may avert the need for permanent pacing.[231] The proportion of transplant recipients receiving permanent pacing for persistent bradycardia ranges from 2.8% to 29% in different centers.[232] The variation may reflect differences in the incidence of bradycardia and the criteria for permanent pacing although differences in surgical technique may also be relevant.[233] In paced transplant recipients, bradycardia often resolves and pacemaker usage decreases during the first few months.[234] Deferring consideration of permanent pacing until 3 weeks after transplantation may mean that some patients with transient sinus node dysfunction are spared unnecessary pacemaker implantation. Deferral is also associated with a commensurate increase in pacemaker usage in those paced. However, even with this strategy, less than half of those using their pacemakers at 3 months continue to do so at 6 months and there are no clear predictive factors to guide patient selection.[235]

Following heterotopic cardiac transplantation, the donor and recipient hearts beat independently of one another, the denervated donor heart typically beating at a faster rate. Competitive contraction of the two hearts may be deleterious and LV function in the recipient heart is improved when the two hearts beat out of phase. Acute studies have shown that paced linkage of the two hearts to produce consistent counterpulsation may result in significant functional improvement.[236] This technique has been evaluated in a chronic study using permanent dual-chamber pacemakers with the atrial channel connected to the donor atrium and the "ventricular" channel connected to the recipient atrium.[237] Paced linkage was associated with significant improvements in symptoms, general health, energy, levels of activity and maximum cardiac output in the donor heart.

Sleep apnea

Sleep apnea with hypersomnolence is estimated to affect 2–4% of middle-aged adults, although asymptomatic forms may be more frequent.[238] The condition is associated with an increased risk of hypertension and cardiovascular disease, including bradyarrhythmia.[239] It has been noted that treatment of the condition in patients with asymptomatic bradycardia occurring only during sleep may reduce the need for pacemaker implantation, provided that advanced disease of the sinus node or AV conducting system has been excluded.[240] Conversely, there have been reports of improvements in sleep-disordered breathing following pacemaker implantation in patients with sinus node dysfunction and AV block.[241]

Following similar observations in patients receiving atrial overdrive pacing for the suppression of atrial tachyarrhythmia, the efficacy of atrial overdrive was assessed in a randomized crossover trial.[242] A group of 15 patients with sinus node disease and sleep apnea, identified on screening, showed improved apnea and hypopnea indices during atrial overdrive pacing, compared with intrinsic rhythm. The mechanism of benefit is unclear but might relate to increased sympathetic activity during pacing. Surprisingly, both obstructive and central forms of sleep apnea were improved, suggesting a central mechanism affecting both respiratory rhythm and pharyngeal motor neurone activity.[243] However, subsequent studies failed to show significant benefit from atrial overdrive pacing in patients with obstructive sleep apnea with[244–247] or without[248–250] a bradycardia-related indication for pacing. A distinguishing feature of the earlier positive study, which might account for the discrepant findings, was that more than half of the patients had central sleep apnea and all had a significant number of central events. Improvements in apnea-hypopnea index and sleep quality have also been demonstrated after cardiac resynchronization therapy but only in those who responded to resynchronization, suggesting that the benefits are mediated by improved heart failure status rather than a specific effect of pacing.[251]

Neither pacing nor cardiac resynchronization therapy is currently indicated in patients without conventional indications for device therapy (**Class III, Level A**). In patients with sleep apnea who have an implanted device, atrial overdrive pacing and cardiac resynchronization therapy may improve symptoms but other specific therapies such as continuous positive airway pressure are more effective and may also be required (**Class IIb, Level A**).

Cardiac resynchronization therapy

Background

In the early 1990s, the use of dual-chamber pacing in patients with heart failure but no bradyarrhythmic indication for pacing was extensively explored. This was initially prompted by the suggestion that dual-chamber pacing with a short AV delay might improve cardiac function in dilated cardiomyopathy by improving the relationship between atrial and ventricular systole, thereby decreasing presystolic, mitral and tricuspid regurgitation and increasing ventricular filling time.[252] Initial hemodynamic and clinical studies yielded encouraging results[253,254] but others failed to show any significant benefit.[255,256] It might have been anticipated that patients with a prolonged PR interval and increased QRS duration would be most likely to benefit and this was confirmed in hemodynamic and short-term clinical studies.[257–259] Intraventricular conduction delay may be present in up to 40% of patients with severe heart failure.[260] This results in asynchronous contraction of the left and right ventricles, which may adversely affect hemodynamic function. Cardiac resynchronization therapy (CRT) aims to reverse these changes by using biventricular pacing to resynchronize left and right ventricular activation and by ensuring AV synchrony with an optimal AV delay if sinus rhythm is preserved. Biatrial synchronization may also be used in the presence of interatrial conduction delay.

The potential hemodynamic benefit of biventricular pacing was first demonstrated in an acute study in humans in 1983[261] but it was not until 1994 that the clinical application of the technique was reported in a patient with severe drug-refractory congestive heart failure.[262] Early case reports documented short-term clinical and hemodynamic improvement in patients with class III and IV heart failure using three- or four-chamber atrio-biventricular pacing.[262–264] Acute hemodynamic studies demonstrated decreased pulmonary capillary wedge pressure and increased peak LV dP/dt, systolic blood pressure and cardiac index during biventricular pacing.[264–268] Similar or greater improvements in some parameters were also reported with LV pacing alone.[265–268] The early studies of biventricular pacing used an epicardial pacing lead, implanted by limited thoracotomy or thoracoscopy, to pace the left ventricle, with a standard endocardial lead in the right ventricle. This approach has been superseded by the development of a technique for pacing the left ventricle by means of a lead introduced transvenously via the coronary sinus, with the tip located in one of the posterior or lateral cardiac veins overlying the LV free wall.[269] A coronary sinus angiogram is often used to create an anatomic map to guide placement of the specialized leads that have been developed for this type of pacing.[270]

Encouraging preliminary data regarding the clinical utility of CRT were reported from two non-randomized studies: InSync[271,272] and the French pilot study.[273] Several randomized trials have subsequently been completed in Europe and the USA to further assess the efficacy of CRT in ischemic and non-ischemic dilated cardiomyopathy. These include a number of short-term crossover and parallel group studies assessing the impact of CRT on symptoms, functional capacity and ventricular remodeling, and two larger studies designed to assess the impact on morbidity and mortality.

Randomized trials

The first Pacing Therapy in Congestive Heart Failure (PATH-CHF) trial was a single-blind randomized crossover trial, designed to evaluate the short- and long-term effects of univentricular and biventricular pacing in patients with NYHA class III or IV heart failure despite optimal medical therapy.[274,275] Patients were required to have a QRS duration ≥120 ms and a PR interval ≥150 ms. Two dual-chamber pacemakers were implanted, one with endocardial leads in the right atrium and ventricle, the other with an endocardial lead in the right atrium and a lead attached to the epicardial surface of the left ventricle via a limited thoracotomy. During the acute phase of the study, right and left univentricular pacing were compared with biventricular pacing, at preselected AV delays, using a randomized crossover design. Overall, biventricular and LV pacing had similar hemodynamic effects and increased LV dP/dt and pulse pressure more than right ventricular pacing. Pacing site had a greater influence on hemodynamics than the AV delay. During the chronic phase of the study, 41 patients were randomized to either atrio-biventricular pacing or the best atrio-univentricular mode (determined during the acute phase) for a 4-week period. This was followed by a 4-week wash-out phase without pacing and a further 4 weeks in the alternative mode. Compared with baseline, active pacing showed significant benefits in terms of peak oxygen consumption and 6-minute walk distance, with similar benefits in the univentricular and biventricular modes. Quality of life and NYHA functional class improved during the first pacing period but there was evidence of a placebo or carry-over effect, in that improvements were not eliminated during the subsequent wash-out period. There was, however, a further significant improvement during the second active pacing period, suggesting a genuine treatment effect. On completion of the crossover phase, patients were assigned to their best pacing mode and followed for 1 year. During that time, the number of days spent in hospital for heart failure was significantly lower than in the year before implantation.

The PATH-CHF II trial assessed the effects of atrial-synchronized left univentricular pacing. This was a randomized crossover study, in which 86 patients with NYHA class II–IV heart failure were stratified according to QRS duration (120 ms to 150 ms v >150 ms) and outcomes were compared after 3-month periods of either LV or inactive pacing.[276] The long QRS group showed increased exercise tolerance and improved quality of life with active pacing, whereas the short QRS group showed no improvement in either outcome.

The Multi-Site Stimulation in Cardiomyopathy (MUSTIC) trial assessed the efficacy of transvenous biventricular pacing using a randomized blinded crossover design to compare outcomes after 12 weeks each of active and inactive pacing.[277] Patients had severe but stable heart failure due to idiopathic or ischemic LV systolic dysfunction (NYHA class III) despite optimal medical therapy, ejection fraction <35%, LV end-diastolic diameter (EDD) >60 mm, QRS duration >150 ms and no conventional indication for pacing. Sixty-seven patients in sinus rhythm were enrolled, of whom nine were withdrawn before randomization and 10 failed to complete the two crossover periods. In the 48 patients who completed the study, the 6-minute walk distance improved by 23% ($P < 0.001$) after 3 months of biventricular pacing. Quality of life scores improved by 32% ($P < 0.001$) and peak oxygen uptake by 8% ($P < 0.03$). Hospitalizations were decreased by two-thirds ($P < 0.05$). Active pacing was preferred by 85% of the patients ($P < 0.001$). At the end of the crossover phase, patients were programmed to their preferred mode; the clinical benefits were maintained at 1-year reassessment.[278,279]

The MUSTIC study had a separate limb for patients in AF, which enrolled 64 patients in NYHA class III with LV systolic dysfunction, chronic AF, a slow ventricular rate requiring pacing, and a broad paced QRS (≥200 ms).[280] There was a high drop-out rate and only 37 patients were successfully implanted and completed both crossover phases. An intention-to-treat analysis showed no benefit from CRT on exercise capacity or quality of life compared with right univentricular pacing. However, an analysis excluding patients in whom delivery of effective therapy was unsuccessful due to a low percentage of ventricular pacing, showed modest but statistically significant improvements. Eighty-five percent of patients preferred biventricular pacing and hospitalizations were less frequent during the CRT phase.

The Multicenter InSync Randomized Clinical Evaluation (MIRACLE) was a double-blind, parallel-group, randomized trial to assess the benefit of CRT in patients with NYHA class III or IV heart failure, on optimal and stable medical therapy, with ejection fraction ≤35%, LV EDD ≥55 mm and QRS duration ≥130 ms.[281] After baseline evaluation and successful implantation of a transvenous CRT pacing system, 453 patients were randomly assigned to receive active CRT or a control group with no pacing and followed for 6 months. In the CRT group, there were 12 deaths. In the control group, 16 patients died, two received a transplant and five missed the 6-month visit. One patient in each group withdrew due to device-related complications. Amongst those who completed the study, patients assigned to CRT had significant improvements in 6-minute walk distance, quality of life, NYHA class, peak oxygen consumption, and a composite heart failure score and there were fewer hospitalizations for heart failure. Echocardiography showed evidence of reverse LV remodeling, improved systolic and diastolic function, and decreased mitral regurgitation in the CRT group.[282]

MIRACLE ICD was a study of similar design in which 369 patients with an indication for an ICD received an ICD with CRT capability (CRT-D) and were randomly assigned to CRT on or CRT off.[283] After 6 months follow-up, CRT was associated with improved quality of life, functional status, treadmill time and peak oxygen uptake, although there was no difference in the change in 6-minute walk distance (a co-primary endpoint). In contrast to the earlier study in patients without an ICD indication, there were no significant differences in changes in LV size or function, overall heart failure status or rates of hospitalization. The MIRACLE ICD investigators also enrolled 222 patients with NYHA class II heart failure into a parallel study reported separately as MIRACLE ICD II.[284] Of the 191 successfully implanted patients, 186 were randomly assigned to CRT on or off. After 6 months follow-up, there was no significant improvement in exercise capacity but there were significant improvements in LV size and function, and a composite assessment of clinical status.

The CONTAK CD study assessed the safety and efficacy of CRT combined with an ICD in patients with NYHA class II–IV heart failure, ejection fraction ≤35%, QRS duration ≥120 ms and a conventional indication for an ICD.[285] The study began with a 3-month crossover design (n = 248) but later changed to a 6-month parallel group study (n = 333). The primary endpoint was also changed from peak oxygen consumption to a heart failure composite. The initial implants had an epicardial LV lead (11% of cases) but a transvenous lead was used subsequently (89% of cases). Of 581 enrolled patients, 501 were successfully implanted and 490 were randomly assigned to CRT on or CRT off. Three-month follow-up data from the crossover study were combined with 6-month data from the parallel study. CRT was associated with a non-significant 15% reduction in heart failure progression. There was a significant increase in peak oxygen consumption but only non-significant changes in NYHA class and quality of life, except for the subgroup in NYHA class III or IV, in which all functional status outcomes improved. CRT was associated with decreased LV dimensions and increased ejection fraction. Interpretation of the data is complicated by the change in study design and the power of the study was diminished by a lower than anticipated event rate, possibly due to improved medical therapy during the course of the study, and the short fol-low-up in the crossover phase.

The Comparison of Medical Therapy, Pacing and Defibrilla-tion in Heart Failure (COMPANION) trial included 1520 patients with class III or IV heart failure due to ischemic or non-ischemic cardiomyopathy, ejection fraction ≤35%, QRS width ≥120ms and sinus rhythm, who were randomly assigned in a 1:2:2 ratio to optimal pharmacologic therapy alone or with the addition of a CRT pacing system (CRT-P) or a CRT pacing system with defibrillation capability (CRT-D).[286] The primary endpoint was death or hospitalization from any cause. As compared with optimal pharmacologic therapy, CRT-P reduced the primary endpoint (HR 0.81; 95% CI 0.69 to 0.96; *P* = 0.014) and all-cause mortality (HR 0.76; 95% CI 0.58 to 1.01; *P* = 0.06). CRT-D (HR 0.64; 95% CI 0.48 to 0.86; *P* = 0.003). CRT was associated with early and sustained improvements in NYHA class, 6-minute walk distance, and quality of life.[286,287]

The Cardiac Resynchronization-Heart Failure (CARE-HF) trial enrolled 813 patients with class III or IV heart failure due to LV systolic dysfunction, ejection fraction ≤35% and QRS >120ms, who were randomly assigned to receive optimal medical therapy with or without CRT.[288] Echocar-diographic evidence of dyssynchrony was also required in patients with QRS between 120ms and 149ms. Patients with atrial arrhythmias were excluded. The primary end-point was a composite of death from any cause or unplanned hospitalization for a major cardiovascular event. After mean follow-up of 29.4 months, the incidence of the primary endpoint was significantly lower in the group receiving CRT (HR 0.63; 95% CI 0.51 to 0.77; *P* < 0.001). There was also a significant reduction in all-cause mortality (HR 0.64; 95% CI 0.48 to 0.85; *P* < 0.002) accompanied by significant improvements in symptoms, ejection fraction, NYHA class and quality of life. Echocardiography at 3 months and 18 months showed evidence of reverse remodeling with a lower end-systolic volume index and decreased mitral regurgitation. N-terminal pro-brain natriuretic peptide was also reduced. Extended follow-up for a further 8 months showed reduced mortality (HR 0.60; 95% CI 0.47 to 0.77; *P* < 0.0001), sudden death (HR 0.54; 95% CI 0.35 to 0.84; *P* = 0.005) and death due to heart failure (HR 0.55; 95% CI 0.37 to 0.82; *P* = 0.003).[289] In secondary analyses, no baseline characteristics or markers of response at 3 months emerged as useful predictors of the effect of CRT on mortality.[290,291]

The accumulated data from the various trials of CRT have been summarized in several systematic reviews and meta-analyses.[292–297] The aggregated data suggest that in patients with class III or IV heart failure due to LV systolic dysfunction with prolonged QRS duration, CRT reduces all-cause mortality and major cardiovascular morbidity, and improves quality of life (Fig. 41.2). Overall implant success rates are estimated at 93% (95% CI 92.2 to 93.7%) with a periprocedural complication rate of 4.3% (95% CI

3.6 to 5.1%), peri-implant mortality of 0.3% (95% CI 0.1 to 0.6%) and no other significant safety concerns.[295] Using currently accepted implant criteria, it is estimated that 1–3% of patients discharged alive after hospital admission for heart failure and 15–20% of patients attending special-ized heart failure clinics may be candidates for CRT.[298] Economic analyses based on outcome data from the ran-domized trials suggest that CRT is a cost-effective thera-peutic option using currently accepted thresholds in Europe and the USA.[294,299–301]

Unresolved issues in CRT

Notwithstanding the strong evidence base for CRT in patients meeting the enrolment criteria for the various ran-domized trials, there are several areas of clinical practice in which the available data are inconclusive.

Atrial fibrillation

The benefits of CRT depend on the effective delivery of biventricular pacing. In the presence of AF, which is a common occurrence in advanced heart failure, spontane-ous ventricular activation by intrinsic conduction through an intact AV node may result in a marked reduction in the percentage of biventricular paced beats. Long-term clinical outcome data on the effectiveness of CRT in AF are limited, as both the COMPANION and CARE HF trials included only patients with sinus rhythm. Some data are available from the MUSTIC-AF study[280] and several observational studies[302–308] which suggest that CRT may be beneficial, provided adequate biventricular pacing is achieved. Data from a European registry including 162 patients with per-manent AF and 511 in sinus rhythm suggest that CRT in patients with AF results in similar improvements in ven-tricular function and functional capacity to those observed in patients with sinus rhythm but only after AV node abla-tion, which was performed when biventricular pacing occurred ≤85% of the time.[304] Comparable benefits were not seen in the group of patients who continued with pharma-cologic rate control, even though biventricular pacing was achieved for over 85% of the time. Further data from an extension of the same registry, including 243 patients with permanent AF and 1042 in sinus rhythm, showed similar mortality in both groups after a median follow-up of 34 months.[307] In the patients with AF, survival was signifi-cantly improved in those who underwent ablation and CRT compared with those who received CRT alone. There were imbalances in some important baseline characteristics between the groups and these findings require verification in a prospective randomized trial. It might be supposed that reversal of structural changes in the atria and ventri-cles following CRT might favor spontaneous cardioversion and retention of sinus rhythm but observational data do not support that hypothesis.[303] Similarly, in patients in

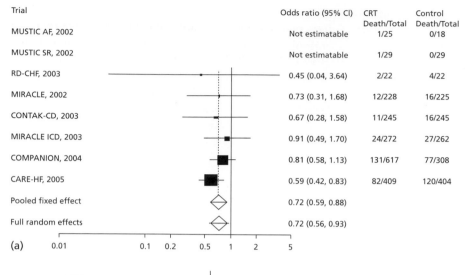

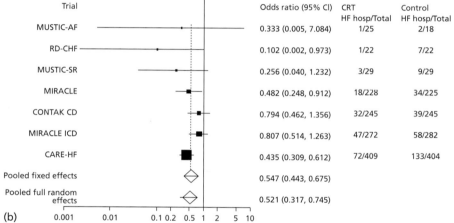

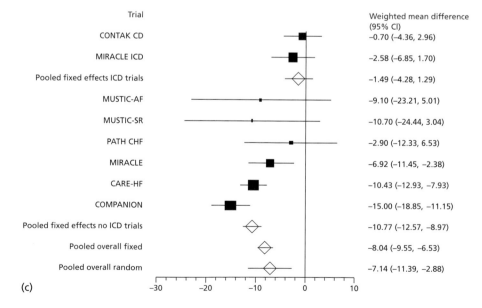

Figure 41.2 Effect of CRT on (a) mortality, (b) hospitalization for heart failure, (c) quality of life assessed by Minnesota Living with Heart Failure Questionnaire. All data from randomized trials. (Reproduced with permission from Freemantle et al.[292])

sinus rhythm, CRT does not appear to influence the incidence of AF.[309]

Non-responders to CRT

A significant minority of patients fulfilling the criteria for CRT fail to benefit fully or at all from the therapy. The response to CRT may be characterized in terms of symptomatic or functional benefit, morbidity, mortality or cardiac remodeling and hemodynamic improvement but there is no universally agreed definition of what constitutes therapeutic success. Rates of non-response of 20–30% are often quoted but even higher rates have been reported, particularly in studies using objective parameters of LV remodeling.[310] The difference may partly reflect the well-recognized placebo effect of device implantation. Reasons for non-response include variability in the pattern and reversibility of intraventricular dyssynchrony,[311] suboptimal position of the LV lead[312] and factors related to the myocardial substrate, such as extensive scar tissue or transmural scar tissue at the LV pacing site in ischemic patients.[313] A wide variety of echocardiographic markers of dyssynchrony have been assessed for their ability to predict the response to CRT but no ideal approach has been found.[314,315] In the recently published Predictors of Response to CRT (PROSPECT) study, a wide range of conventional echocardiographic and tissue Doppler-based methods was evaluated but no single measure was found to improve patient selection for CRT beyond current guidelines.[316] It remains to be seen whether newer echocardiographic techniques that have shown some promise, such as speckle tracking[317] and three-dimensional imaging,[318] or cardiac magnetic resonance[319] will prove more successful.

Optimal positioning of the LV lead may be limited by the coronary venous anatomy. This is most often characterized by performing a coronary sinus venogram at the time of the CRT implant but non-invasive imaging by computed tomography has been shown to be feasible and may in the future enable anatomic limitations to be identified in advance.[320] The use of targeted lead placement using echocardiographic guidance has been evaluated in a randomized trial (the Investigating Non-Response to Cardiac Resynchronization: Evaluation of Methods to Eliminate Non-Response & Target Appropriate Lead Location (INCREMENTAL) study). Preliminary results have been presented and suggest that this approach may increase the responder rate in patients with ischemic cardiomyopathy.[321] In non-responders, repositioning of a suboptimally located LV lead should be considered. Surgical placement of an epicardial lead may facilitate targeted therapy when a satisfactory lead position cannot be achieved transvenously.[322] The available surgical options include direct lead placement via a small left thoracotomy, video-assisted thoracoscopy or robotic surgery.[323] A recent innovation that may improve the response to CRT is the addition of a third

ventricular lead in either the right or left ventricle to achieve multisite pacing.[324–326] Encouraging initial results have been reported from small studies but further evaluation is required to determine the utility of this approach in non-responders and as primary therapy.

After implantation of a CRT device, individualized adjustment of the programmed AV and interventricular delay may improve the effectiveness of cardiac resynchronization.[327,328] Further complexity is added by the observation that the optimal settings may vary during exercise and over time during follow-up.[329,330] Techniques used to determine the optimal response include echocardiography, impedance cardiography, acoustic cardiography, surface or intracardiac electrocardiography and non-invasive hemodynamic monitoring.[331–333] The optimal method and the long-term impact of optimization on clinical outcomes have not yet been determined. Clinical trials are ongoing to assess the utility of the various approaches both at the time of the initial implant and during follow-up.

CRT in patients with narrow QRS complexes

The finding that LV dyssynchrony is present in up to 43% of heart failure patients with narrow QRS complexes (<120 ms)[334] has prompted the evaluation of CRT in this setting. Small observational studies showed improvements in symptoms, NYHA class, 6-minute walk distance and ejection fraction, with echocardiographic evidence of reverse remodeling after 3–6 months follow-up. The changes were similar to those observed in CRT recipients with broad QRS complexes.[335–337] The results of two randomized studies, however, were disappointing.

In the Resynchronization Therapy in Normal QRS (RethinQ) trial, 172 patients with standard indications for an ICD, NYHA class III heart failure, ejection fraction ≤35%, QRS duration <130 ms and echocardiographic evidence of mechanical dyssynchrony were implanted with an ICD with CRT capability and randomly assigned to CRT on or off.[338] After 6 months follow-up, there were no significant differences between the groups in a primary endpoint based on peak oxygen uptake during cardiopulmonary exercise testing, except in a prespecified subgroup with QRS duration ≥120 ms. NYHA class was improved in the CRT group compared with the controls but there were no significant differences in quality of life, 6-minute walk distance, echocardiographic measures or heart failure events requiring intravenous therapy. The Evaluation of Screening Techniques in Electrically-Normal, Mechanically-Dyssynchronous Heart Failure Patients Receiving Cardiac Resynchronization Therapy (ESTEEM-CRT) trial was an unblinded single-arm feasibility study, in which 68 patients with NYHA class III heart failure, ejection fraction ≤35%, QRS duration <120 ms and echocardiographic evidence of mechanical dyssynchrony were implanted with an ICD with CRT capability and assessed 1 month post-implant and again after 6 months.[339] Patients' symptoms improved but there were no changes in exercise performance or echocardiographic measures. The symptomatic improvement was attributed to bias from the unblinded assessment or a placebo effect.

It is unclear whether these negative findings reflect ineffectiveness of CRT in patients with a narrow QRS complex, the influence of confounding factors compromising the response in relatively small short-term studies or the limitations of our current understanding and the available tools for assessing dyssynchrony, as demonstrated in the PROSPECT study. Some limited encouragement may be offered by the DESIRE study, which attempted to identify CRT responders on the basis of simple echocardiographic indices of dyssynchrony, regardless of QRS width, in a group of 64 patients with class III or IV heart failure, ejection fraction $\leq$40%, LV EDD $\geq$27 mm/m^2 and QRS <150 ms.[340] Patients were assigned to one of two groups after enrolment according to the presence or absence of dyssynchrony on a baseline echocardiogram. After 6 months follow-up, 55% of the patients showed clinical improvement, including 70% of those with dyssynchrony and 42% of those without ($P < 0.04$). Baseline QRS did not predict response to CRT. Unfortunately, the design of the study rendered it susceptible to a possible placebo effect and assessment bias, and the modest sensitivity and specificity of the echocardiographic measures of dyssynchrony inevitably limit their clinical utility. Further insights may come from the ongoing Echocardiography Guided Cardiac Resynchronization Therapy (Echo-CRT) trial, which is examining the effect of CRT on mortality and hospitalization for heart failure in ICD recipients with advanced heart failure, ejection fraction $\leq$35%, ventricular dyssynchrony on echocardiography and QRS duration <130 ms.[341] At present, CRT is not recommended in patients with a narrow QRS.

CRT in patients with class I or II heart failure

The favorable effects of CRT in patients with advanced heart failure invite speculation that patients with less severe symptoms might also benefit and that earlier intervention might prevent disease progression. Some support for this hypothesis comes from the MIRACLE ICD II trial,[284] which assessed the efficacy of CRT in 186 ICD recipients with NYHA class II heart failure, and similarly from the findings in the subset of 263 patients with class I or II heart failure in the CONTAK CD study.[285] Both studies showed evidence of reverse remodeling after CRT although there was no improvement in exercise capacity or quality of life. Reverse remodeling and improved ejection fraction after CRT were also demonstrated in an observational study of 50 patients with NYHA class II heart failure, the changes being similar to those observed in a parallel group in NYHA class III or IV.[342] Further evidence was provided by a subgroup analysis of data from the CARE-HF trial, which

showed beneficial effects on morbidity and mortality even in a group of 175 patients whose symptoms improved to NYHA class I or II after enrolment but prior to randomization and delivery of CRT.[343]

More recently, the REsynchronization reVErses Remodeling in Systolic Left vEntricular Dysfunction (REVERSE) trial assessed whether CRT could attenuate progression of heart failure and reverse LV remodeling in patients with mild or resolved symptoms (NYHA class I or II) and LV dysfunction.[344] Patients were enrolled in Europe and North America with QRS duration $\geq$120 ms, ejection fraction $\leq$40% and LV EDD $\geq$55 mm. A total of 610 patients were successfully implanted with a CRT device, with ICD capability if indicated, and randomly assigned to CRT on or off. After 1 year, CRT had no significant impact on the primary endpoint, a composite reflecting clinical status.[345] There was, however, evidence of reverse remodeling, with decreased LV end-systolic and end-diastolic volumes and increased ejection fraction. Time to first hospitalization for heart failure was increased in the CRT group but there was no difference in quality of life or 6-minute walk distance. Two-year follow-up of the 262 European patients has recently been reported.[346] Worsening of the clinical composite score was less frequent with CRT active than in the control group (19% vs 34%; $P = 0.01$). Echocardiographic improvements were sustained but again there was no difference in quality of life or functional status, possibly due to the mild initial symptoms. The study suggests that CRT may modify disease progression in patients with mild symptoms but firm conclusions must await the results of two larger ongoing trials comparing CRT-D with ICD alone in patients in NYHA class I and II (MADIT-CRT)[347] or class II (The Resynchronization/ Defibrillation for Ambulatory Heart Failure Trial – RAFT).[348] These trials are powered for composite primary endpoints including mortality and heart failure events or hospitalization.

Incremental benefit of combined CRT and ICD therapy

There is substantial overlap between the current indications for CRT and those for a primary prevention ICD, as defined by MADIT II[349] and the Sudden Cardiac Death in Heart Failure Trial (SCD-HeFT).[350] In patients with indications for both devices, the implantation of a combined CRT-D system is a logical option although it cannot be assumed that the mortality benefit of combined therapy will be greater than that of either device alone. The only trial to have randomly assigned patients to receive CRT-P or CRT-D was COMPANION,[286] which was not designed to make a direct comparison of the two options. The finding that the reduction in all-cause mortality with CRT-D was significant whereas that with CRT-P was not must be interpreted with caution, as the follow-up was relatively short with a median of only 14 months. It is important also to note that both COMPANION and CARE-HF[288] excluded patients with a conventional indication (at that time) for an ICD. A degree of complexity is added by the fact that improvement in NYHA class after initiation of CRT may move the patient into or out of a category for which ICD efficacy has been demonstrated. The incremental benefit of CRT-D is further called into question by the finding in the CARE-HF trial that CRT-P reduced not only death due to heart failure but also sudden death, and by observational data suggesting a reduction in susceptibility to ventricular arrhythmia after upgrading from ICD therapy to CRT-D.[351] A provocative and concerning finding in COMPANION was that the need for ICD therapy in CRT-treated patients was associated with more advanced disease and predicted a number of major adverse outcomes, including risk of subsequent sudden death.[352] It is also noteworthy that a subgroup analysis in SCD-HeFT showed the benefits of ICD therapy to be limited to patients in NYHA class II, with no clear advantage to those in class III who comprise the main group for which CRT is currently indicated.[350] The incremental benefit of CRT-D over CRT-P is currently uncertain[297,353] and a matter of ongoing debate.[354,355] Economic analysis suggests that CRT-D is unlikely to be a cost-effective option compared with CRT-P in the treatment of patients with class III and IV heart failure due to LV dysfunction but it is more likely to be so in younger patients (<60 years) or those with a high risk of sudden death (>7% per annum).[356] A trial directly comparing CRT-P and CRT-D would be of considerable value. Meanwhile, the decision as to whether or not to offer CRT-D rather than CRT-P to individual patients with indications for both CRT and an ICD must be made on an individual basis.

Comment and recommendations

There is considerable evidence that CRT, with or without an ICD, can improve a wide range of hemodynamic and clinical outcomes, including mortality, in patients who have NYHA class III or IV heart failure despite optimal medical therapy, with LV ejection fraction ≤35%, increased QRS duration (≥120 ms) and sinus rhythm (**Class I, Level A**). Patients in atrial fibrillation may also benefit, provided a sufficiently high proportion of biventricular paced beats can be achieved by AV node ablation or otherwise, although further studies are required in this area (**Class IIa, Level B**). Further data are also required to clarify the role of CRT in patients with mild or moderate symptoms. CRT cannot be recommended for patients with narrow QRS complexes (**Class III, Level A**).

Future perspectives

The role of pacemaker therapy in the treatment of symptomatic bradycardia is now firmly established. Some ques-

tions remain regarding mode selection, particularly regarding the role of single-chamber atrial pacing in patients with isolated sinus node disease, and the optimal location of the atrial and ventricular leads. Further technologic developments will bring new device algorithms to minimize ventricular pacing, new tools to facilitate selective site pacing, and pacing systems that are compatible with magnetic resonance imaging.[357] Future clinical trials are likely to enhance our understanding of the role of pacing in indications other than sinus node disease and AV block and to clarify the potential role of CRT in patients with conventional indications for pacing and in those with less advanced disease. Techniques for achieving cardiac resynchronization are likely to improve, as are methods to predict those who will respond. In the longer term, there is the promise of exciting new developments that may transform the way in which pacemaker therapy is delivered. The use of cardiac stimulation mediated by ultrasound energy, as an alternative to implanted leads, has recently been reported.[358] Biologic therapies are evolving and there is hope that a biologic pacemaker, achieved using gene therapy or stem cell technology, might ultimately become a clinical reality.[359] A key message from the first 50 years of cardiac pacing is that new technologies and innovations in pacemaker therapy must be critically evaluated in well-designed clinical trials to achieve a proper understanding of their clinical utility and to facilitate their further evolution.

References

1. Elmqvist R, Senning A. An implantable pacemaker for the heart. In: Smyth CN, ed. *Medical Electronics* (Proceedings of the Second International Conference on Medical Electronics, Paris, 1959). London: Iliffe, 1960: 253–4.
2. Travill CM, Sutton R. Pacemaker syndrome: an iatrogenic condition. *Br Heart J* 1992;**68**:163–6.
3. Mond HG, Irwin M, Ector H, Proclemer A. The World Survey of Cardiac Pacing and Cardioverter-Defibrillators: Calendar Year 2005. *PACE* 2008;**31**:1202–12.
4. Ector H, Vardas P, on behalf of the European Heart Rhythm Association, European Society of Cardiology. Current use of pacemakers, implantable cardioverter defibrillators, and resynchronization devices: data from the registry of the European Heart Rhythm Association. *Eur Heart J* 2007;**9**(suppl I):144–9.
5. Network Devices Survey Group. Heart Rhythm Devices: UK National Survey 2007 (version 1.1). London: Department of Health; 2009. http://www.devicesurvey.com (accessed 10 June 2009).
6. Greenspan AM, Kay HR, Berger BC et al. Incidence of unwarranted implantation of permanent cardiac pacemakers in a large medical population. *N Engl J Med* 1988;**318**:158–63.
7. Epstein AE, DiMarco JP, Ellenbogen KA et al. ACC/AHA/HRS 2008 guidelines for device-based therapy of cardiac rhythm abnormalities: a report of the American College of Cardiology/American Heart Association Task Force on Practice Guidelines

(Writing Committee to revise the ACC/AHA/NASPE 2002 guideline for implantation of cardiac pacemakers and antiarrhythmia devices): developed in collaboration with the American Association for Thoracic Surgery and Society of Thoracic Surgeons. *Circulation* 2008;**117**:e350–408.

8. Vardas PE, Auricchio A, Blanc JJ *et al.* Guidelines for cardiac pacing and cardiac resynchronization therapy. The Task Force for Cardiac Pacing and Cardiac Resynchronization Therapy of the European Society of Cardiology. Developed in collaboration with the European Heart Rhythm Association. *Europace* 2007;**9**:959–98.

9. Bexton RS, Camm AJ. First degree atrioventricular block. *Eur Heart J* 1984;**5**(suppl A):107–9.

10. Chirife R, Ortega DE, Salazar AL. "Pacemaker syndrome" without a pacemaker. Deleterious effects of first-degree AV block. *RBM* 1990;**12**(3):22.

11. Zornosa JP, Crossley GH, Haisty WK Jr *et al.* Pseudo-pacemaker syndrome: a complication of radiofrequency ablation of the AV junction. *PACE* 1992;**15**:590.

12. Mabo P, Varin C, Vauthier M *et al.* Deleterious hemodynamic consequences of isolated long PR intervals: correction by DDD pacing. *Eur Heart J* 1992;**13**(suppl):225.

13. Barold SS. Indications for permanent cardiac pacing in first-degree AV block: class I, II, or III? *PACE* 1996;**19**:747–51.

14. Wharton JM, Ellenbogen KA. Atrioventricular conduction system disease. In: Ellenbogen KA, Kay GN, Wilkoff BL, eds. Clinical Cardiac Pacing. Philadelphia: WB Saunders, 1995.

15. Dhingra RC, Denes P, Wu D *et al.* The significance of second degree atrioventricular block and bundle branch block. *Circulation* 1974;**49**:638–46.

16. Puech P, Grolleau R, Guimond C. Incidence of different types of AV-block and their localisation by His bundle recordings. In: Wellens HJJ, Lie KI, Janse MJ, eds. *The Conduction System of the Heart: Structure, Function and Clinical Implications.* Philadelphia: Lea and Febiger, 1976.

17. Shaw DB, Kekwick CA, Veale D, Gowers J, Whistance T. Survival in second degree atrioventricular block. *Br Heart J* 1985;**53**:587–93.

18. Shaw DB, Gowers JI, Kekwick CA, New KHJ, Whistance AWT. Is Mobitz type I atrioventricular block benign in adults? *Heart* 2004;**90**:169–74.

19. Campbell RWF. Chronic Mobitz type I second degree atrioventricular block: has its importance been underestimated? *Br Heart J* 1985;**53**:585–6.

20. Connelly DT, Steinhaus DM. Mobitz type I atrioventricular block: an indication for permanent pacing? *PACE* 1996;**19**:261–4.

21. Grossman M. Second degree heart block with Wenckebach phenomenon: its occurrence over a period of several years in a young healthy adult. *Am Heart J* 1958;**56**:607–10.

22. Meytes I, Kaplinsky E, Yahini JH, Hanne-Papara N, Neufeld HN. Wenckebach A-V block: a frequent feature following heavy physical training. *Am Heart J* 1975;**90**:426–30.

23. Johansson BW. Complete heart block. A clinical hemodynamic and pharmacological study in patients with and without an artificial pacemaker. *Acta Med Scand* 1966;**180**(suppl 451):1–127.

24. Edhag O, Swahn Å. Prognosis of patients with complete heart block or arrhythmic syncope who were not treated with artificial pacemakers. *Acta Med Scand* 1976;**200**:457–63.

25. Rosenqvist M, Nordlander R. Survival in patients with permanent pacemakers. *Cardiol Clin* 1992;**10**:691–703.

26. Rosenqvist M, Edhag KO. Pacemaker dependence in transient high grade atrioventricular block. *PACE* 1984;**7**:63–70.

27. Ginks W, Leatham A, Siddons H. Prognosis of patients paced for chronic atrioventricular block. *Br Heart J* 1979;**41**:633–6.

28. Shen WK, Hammill SC, Hayes DL *et al.* Long-term survival after pacemaker implantation for heart block in patients ≥65 years. *Am J Cardiol* 1984;**74**:560–4.

29. Campbell M, Emanuel R. Six cases of congenital heart block followed for 34–40 years. *Br Heart J* 1966;**59**:587–90.

30. Michaëlsson M, Jonzon A, Riesenfeld T. Isolated congenital complete atrioventricular block in adult life. *Circulation* 1995;**92**:442–9.

31. Friedman RA. Congenital AV block. Pace me now or pace me later? *Circulation* 1995;**92**:283–5.

32. Rowlands DJ. Left and right bundle branch block, left anterior and left posterior hemiblock. *Eur Heart J* 1984;**5**(suppl A):99–105.

33. McAnulty JH, Rahimtoola SH, Murphy E *et al.* Natural history of "high-risk" bundle branch block. Final report of a prospective study. *N Engl J Med* 1982;**307**:137–43.

34. Scheinman MM, Peters RW, Sauvé MJ *et al.* Value of the H-Q interval in patients with bundle branch block and the role of prophylactic permanent pacing. *Am J Cardiol* 1982;**50**:1316–22.

35. Dhingra RC, Wyndham C, Bauernfeind RA *et al.* Significance of block distal to His bundle induced by atrial pacing in patients with chronic bifascicular block. *Circulation* 1979;**60**:1455–64.

36. Ward DE, Camm AJ. Atrioventricular conduction delays and block. In: Ward DE, Camm AJ, eds. *Clinical Electrophysiology of the Heart.* London: Edward Arnold, 1987.

37. Englund A, Bergfeldt L, Rosenqvist M. Disopyramide stress test: a sensitive and specific tool for predicting impending high degree atrioventricular block in patients with bifascicular block. *Br Heart J* 1995;**74**:650–5.

38. Click RL, Gersch BJ, Sugrue DD *et al.* Role of electrophysiologic testing in patients with symptomatic bundle branch block. *Am J Cardiol* 1987;**59**:817–23.

39. Ginks WR, Sutton R, Oh W, Leatham A. Long-term prognosis after acute anterior infarction with atrioventricular block. *Br Heart J* 1977;**39**:186–9.

40. Col JJ, Weinberg SL. The incidence and mortality of intraventricular conduction defects in acute myocardial infarction. *Am J Cardiol* 1972;**29**:344–50.

41. Watson RDS, Glover DR, Page AJF *et al.* The Birmingham trial of permanent pacing in patients with intraventricular conduction disorders after acute myocardial infarction. *Am Heart J* 1984;**108**:496–501.

42. Hindman MC, Wagner GS, JaRo M *et al.* The clinical significance of bundle branch block complicating acute myocardial infarction. 1. Clinical characteristics, hospital mortality and one-year follow up. *Circulation* 1978;**58**:679–88.

43. Hindman MC, Wagner GS, JaRo M *et al.* The clinical significance of bundle branch block complicating acute myocardial infarction. 2. Indications for temporary and permanent pacemaker insertion. *Circulation* 1978;**58**:689–99.

44. Ritter WS, Atkins J, Blomqvist CG, Mullins CB. Permanent pacing in patients with transient trifascicular block during acute myocardial infarction. *Am J Cardiol* 1976;**38**:205–8.

45. Katritsis D, Camm AJ. Chronotropic incompetence: a proposal for definition and diagnosis. *Br Heart J* 1993;**70**:400–2.

46. Sutton R, Kenny RA. The natural history of sick sinus syndrome. *PACE* 1986;**9**:1110–14.

47. Alboni P, Menozzi C, Brignole M *et al.* Effects of permanent pacemaker and oral theophylline in sick sinus syndrome. The THEOPACE study: a randomized controlled trial. *Circulation* 1997;**96**:260–6.

48. Shaw DB, Holman RR, Gowers JI. Survival in sino atrial disorder (sick-sinus syndrome). *BMJ* 1980;**280**:139–41.

49. Talan DA, Bauernfeind RA, Ashley WW, Kanakis C Jr, Rosen KM. Twenty-four hour continuous ECG recordings in long-distance runners. *Chest* 1982;**82**:19–24.

50. Kruse I, Arnman K, Conradson T-B, Rydén L. A comparison of the acute and long-term hemodynamic effects of ventricular inhibited and atrial synchronous ventricular inhibited pacing. *Circulation* 1982;**65**:846–55.

51. Perrins EJ, Morley CA, Chan SL, Sutton R. Randomized controlled trial of physiological and ventricular pacing. *Br Heart J* 1983;**50**:112–17.

52. Boon NA, Frew AJ, Johnston JA, Cobbe SM. A comparison of symptoms and intra-arterial ambulatory blood pressure during long term dual-chamber atrioventricular synchronous (DDD) and ventricular demand (VVI) pacing. *Br Heart J* 1987;**58**:34–9.

53. Benditt DG, Mianulli M, Fetter J *et al.* Single-chamber cardiac pacing with activity-initiated chronotropic response: evaluation by cardiopulmonary exercise testing. *Circulation* 1987;**75**:184–91.

54. Lipkin DP, Buller N, Frenneaux M, *et al.* Randomized crossover trial of rate responsive Activitrax and conventional fixed rate ventricular pacing. *Br Heart J* 1987;**58**:613–16.

55. Smedgård P, Kristensson B-E, Kruse I, Rydén L. Rate-responsive pacing by means of activity sensing versus single rate ventricular pacing: a double-blind cross-over study. *PACE* 1987;**10**:902–15.

56. Rediker DE, Eagle KA, Homma S, Gillam LD, Harthorne JW. Clinical and hemodynamic comparison of VVI versus DDD pacing in patients with DDD pacemakers. *Am J Cardiol* 1988;**61**:323–9.

57. Mitsuoka T, Kenny RA, Au Yeung T *et al.* Benefits of dual-chamber pacing in sick sinus syndrome. *Br Heart J* 1988;**60**:338–47.

58. Hummel J, Barr E, Hanich R *et al.* DDDR pacing is better tolerated than VVIR in patients with sinus node disease. *PACE* 1990;**13**:504.

59. Hargreaves MR, Channon KM, Cripps TR, Gardner M, Ormerod OJM. Comparison of dual-chamber and ventricular rate responsive pacing in patients over 75 with complete heart block. *Br Heart J* 1995;**74**:397–402.

60. Petch M. Who needs dual-chamber pacing? *BMJ* 1993;**307**:215–16.

61. Linde C. How to evaluate quality-of-life in pacemaker patients: problems and pitfalls. *PACE* 1996;**19**:391–7.

62. Sulke N, Dritsas A, Bostock J *et al.* "Subclinical" pacemaker syndrome: a randomized study of symptom free patients with ventricular demand (VVI) pacemakers upgraded to dual-chamber devices. *Br Heart J* 1992;**67**:57–64.

63. Camm AJ, Katritsis D. Pacing for sick sinus syndrome – a risky business? *PACE* 1990;**13**:695–9.

64. Alpert MA, Curtis JJ, Sanfelippo JF *et al.* Comparative survival after permanent ventricular and dual-chamber pacing for patients with chronic high degree atrioventricular block with and without pre-existent congestive heart failure. *J Am Coll Cardiol* 1986;**7**:925–32.

65. Linde-Edelstam C, Gullberg B, Norlander R, *et al.* Longevity in patients with high degree atrioventricular block paced in the atrial synchronous or the fixed rate ventricular inhibited mode. *PACE* 1992;**15**:304–13.

66. Rosenqvist M, Brandt J, Schuller H. Long-term pacing in sinus node disease: effects of stimulation mode on cardiovascular morbidity and mortality. *Am Heart J* 1988;**116**:16–22.

67. Andersen HR, Thuesen L, Bagger JP, Vesterlund T, Thomsen PE. Prospective randomized trial of atrial versus ventricular pacing in sick-sinus syndrome. *Lancet* 1994;**344**:1523–8.

68. Andersen HR, Nielsen JC, Thomsen PEB *et al.* Long-term follow up of patients from a randomized trial of atrial versus ventricular pacing for sick sinus syndrome. *Lancet* 1997;**350**:1210–16.

69. Andersen HR, Nielsen JC, Bloch Thomsen PE *et al.* Atrioventricular conduction during long-term follow up of patients with sick sinus syndrome. *Circulation* 1998;**98**:1315–21.

70. Lamas GA, Orav EJ, Stambler BS *et al.* Quality of life and clinical outcomes in elderly patients treated with ventricular pacing as compared with dual-chamber pacing. *N Engl J Med* 1998;**338**:1097–104.

71. Ellenbogen KA, Stambler BS, Orav EJ *et al.* Clinical characteristics of patients intolerant to VVIR pacing. *Am J Cardiol* 2000;**86**:59–63.

72. Connolly SJ, Kerr CR, Gent M *et al.* Effects of physiologic pacing versus ventricular pacing on the risk of stroke and death due to cardiovascular causes. *N Engl J Med* 2000;**342**:1385–91.

73. Skanes AC, Krahn AD, Yee R *et al.* Progression to chronic atrial fibrillation after pacing: the Canadian Trial of Physiologic Pacing. *J Am Coll Cardiol* 2001;**38**:167–72.

74. Baranchuk A, Healey JS, Thorpe KE *et al.* The effect of atrial-based pacing on exercise capacity as measured by the 6-minute walk test: a substudy of the Canadian Trial of Physiological Pacing (CTOPP). *Heart Rhythm* 2007;**4**:1024–8.

75. Tang ASL, Roberts RS, Kerr C *et al.* Relationship between pacemaker dependency and the effect of pacing mode on cardiovascular outcomes. *Circulation* 2001;**103**:3081–5.

76. Newman D, Lau C, Tang ASL *et al.* Effect of pacing mode on health-related quality of life in the Canadian Trial of Physiologic Pacing. *Am Heart J* 2003;**145**:430–7.

77. O'Brien BJ, Blackhouse G, Goeree R *et al.* Cost-effectiveness of physiologic pacing: results of the Canadian Health Economic Assessment of Physiologic Pacing. *Heart Rhythm* 2005;**2**:270–5.

78. Kerr CR, Connolly SJ, Abdollah H *et al.* Canadian Trial of Physiological Pacing: effects of physiological pacing during long-term follow-up. *Circulation* 2004;**109**:357–62.

79. Lamas GA, Lee K, Sweeney M *et al.* The Mode Selection Trial (MOST) in sinus node dysfunction: design, rationale, and baseline characteristics of the first 1000 patients. *Am Heart J* 2000;**140**:541–51.

80. Lamas GA, Lee KL, Sweeney MO *et al.* Ventricular pacing or dual-chamber pacing for sinus-node dysfunction. *N Engl J Med* 2002;**346**:1854–62.

81. Fleischmann KE, Orav EJ, Lamas GA *et al.* Pacemaker implantation and quality of life in the Mode Selection Trial (MOST). *Heart Rhythm* 2006;**3**:653–9.

82. Hellkamp AS, Lee KL, Sweeney MO, Link MS, Lamas GA, for the MOST Investigators. Treatment crossovers did not affect randomized treatment comparisons in the Mode Selection Trial (MOST). *J Am Coll Cardiol* 2006;**47**:2260–6.

83. Rinfret S, Cohen DJ, Lamas GA *et al.* Cost-effectiveness of dual-chamber pacing compared with ventricular pacing for sinus node dysfunction. *Circulation* 2005;**111**:165–72.

84. Toff WD, Skehan JD, de Bono DP, Camm AJ. The United Kingdom Pacing and Cardiovascular Events (UKPACE) trial. *Heart* 1997;**78**:221–3.

85. Toff WD, Camm AJ, Skehan JD, for the United Kingdom Pacing and Cardiovascular Events (UKPACE) Trial Investigators. Single-chamber versus dual-chamber pacing for high-grade atrioventricular block. *N Engl J Med* 2005;**353**:145–55.

86. Toff WD, Camm AJ, Skehan JD, for the UKPACE Investigators. Low incidence of pacemaker syndrome in elderly patients paced for high-grade atrioventricular block. *Heart Rhythm* 2004;**1**(suppl I):383.

87. Andersen HR, Svendsen JH, for the DANPACE Investigators. The Danish Multicenter Randomized Study on Atrial Inhibited versus Dual-Chamber Pacing in Sick Sinus Syndrome (The DANPACE Study). Purpose and design of the study. *Heart Drug* 2001;**1**:67–70.

88. Nielsen JC, Kristensen L, Andersen HR *et al.* A randomized comparison of atrial and dual-chamber pacing in 177 consecutive patients with sick sinus syndrome: echocardiographic and clinical outcome. *J Am Coll Cardiol* 2003;**42**:614–23.

89. Kristensen L, Nielsen JC, Mortensen PT, Pedersen OL, Pedersen AK, Andersen HR. Incidence of atrial fibrillation and thromboembolism in a randomised trial of atrial versus dual-chamber pacing in 177 patients with sick sinus syndrome. *Heart* 2004;**90**:661–6.

90. Mattioli AV, Vivoli D, Mattioli G. Influence of pacing modalities on the incidence of atrial fibrillation in patients without prior atrial fibrillation. A prospective study. *Eur Heart J* 1998,**19**:282–6.

91. Wharton JM, Sorrentino RA, Campbell P *et al.* Effect of pacing modality on atrial tachyarrhythmia recurrence in the tachycardia-bradycardia syndrome: preliminary results of the Pacemaker Atrial Tachycardia Trial. *Circulation* 1998; **98**(suppl I):I–494.

92. Wharton JM, Sorrentino RA, Criger D *et al.* Predictors of death in VVI-R and DDD-R paced patients with the tachycardia-bradycardia syndrome. *J Am Coll Cardiol* 1999; **33**(suppl A):153A.

93. Charles RG, McComb JM. Systematic trial of pacing to prevent atrial fibrillation (STOP-AF). *Heart* 1997;**78**:224–5.

94. Charles RG. Personal communication.

95. University of Calgary, Calgary Health Trust. Pacing the Octogenarian Plus Population (POPP): a comparison of physiologic versus ventricular pacing in those who are 80 years of age and older. Available from: http://www.clinicaltrials.gov/ct2/show/record/NCT00116987 NLM Identifier: NCT00116987.

96. Healey JS, Toff WD, Lamas GA *et al.* Cardiovascular outcomes with atrial-based pacing compared with ventricular pacing: meta-analysis of randomized trials, using individual patient data. *Circulation* 2006;**114**:11–17.

97. Dretzke J, Toff WD, Lip GYH, Raftery J, Fry-Smith A, Taylor RRS. Dual chamber versus single chamber ventricular pacemakers for sick sinus syndrome and atrioventricular block. *Cochrane Database of Systematic Reviews* 2004, Issue 2. Art. No.: CD003710. DOI: 10.1002/14651858.CD003710.pub2.

98. Castelnuovo E, Stein K, Pitt M, Garside R, Payne E. The effectiveness and cost-effectiveness of dual-chamber pacemakers compared with single-chamber pacemakers for bradycardia due to atrioventricular block or sick sinus syndrome: systematic review and economic evaluation. *Health Technology Assessment* 2005;**9**:No. 43.

99. Wiggers CJ. The muscular reactions of the mammalian ventricles to artificial surface stimuli. *Am J Physiol* 1925;**73**:346–78.

100. Francia P, Balla C, Paneni F, Volpe M. Left bundle-branch block – pathophysiology, prognosis, and clinical management. *Clin Cardiol* 2007;**30**:110–15.

101. Baldasseroni S, Opasich C, Gorini M *et al.* Left bundle-branch block is associated with increased 1-year sudden and total mortality rate in 5517 outpatients with congestive heart failure: a report from the Italian network on congestive heart failure. *Am Heart J* 2002;**143**:398–405.

102. Sweeney MO, Hellkamp AS, Ellenbogen KA *et al.* Adverse effect of ventricular pacing on heart failure and atrial fibrillation among patients with normal baseline QRS duration in a clinical trial of pacemaker therapy for sinus node dysfunction. *Circulation* 2003;**107**:2932–7.

103. Wilkoff BL, Cook JR, Epstein AE *et al*, for the Dual-chamber and VVI Implantable Defibrillator Trial Investigators. Dual-chamber pacing or ventricular backup pacing in patients with an implantable defibrillator: the Dual-chamber and VVI Implantable Defibrillator (DAVID) Trial. *JAMA* 2002;**288**:3115–23.

104. Steinberg JS, Fischer A, Wang P *et al.* The clinical implications of cumulative right ventricular pacing in the multicenter automatic defibrillator trial II. *J Cardiovasc Electrophysiol* 2005;**16**:359–65.

105. Gillis AM. Redefining physiologic pacing: lessons learned from recent clinical trials. *Heart Rhythm* 2006;**3**:1367–72.

106. Sweeney MO, Prinzen FW. A new paradigm for physiologic ventricular pacing. *J Am Coll Cardiol* 2006;**47**:282–8.

107. Kristensen L, Nielsen JC, Pedersen AK, Mortensen PT, Andersen HR. AV block and changes in pacing mode during long-term follow-up of 399 consecutive patients with sick sinus syndrome treated with an AAI/AAIR pacemaker. *PACE* 2001;**24**:358–65.

108. Nielsen JC, Pedersen AK, Mortensen PT, Andersen HR. Programming a fixed long atrioventricular delay is not effective in preventing ventricular pacing in patients with sick sinus syndrome. *Europace* 1999;**1**:113–20.

109. Stierle U, Krüger D, Vincent AM *et al.* An optimized AV delay algorithm for patients with intermittent atrioventricular conduction. *PACE* 1998;**21**:1035–43.

110. Melzer C, Sowelam S, Sheldon TJ *et al.* Reduction of right ventricular pacing in patients with sinus node dysfunction using an enhanced search AV algorithm. *PACE* 2005;**28**:521–7.

111. Gillis AM, Pürerfellner H, Israel CW *et al.* Reducing unnecessary right ventricular pacing with the managed ventricular

pacing mode in patients with sinus node disease and AV block. *PACE* 2006;**29**:697–705.

112. Pioger G, Leny G, Nitzsché R, Ripart A. AAIsafeR limits ventricular pacing in unselected patients. *PACE* 2007;**30**(suppl 1):S66–70.

113. Sweeney MO, Bank AJ, Nsah E *et al.* Minimizing ventricular pacing to reduce atrial fibrillation in sinus-node disease. *N Engl J Med* 2007;**357**:1000–8.

114. Sweeney MO, Ellenbogen KA, Tang ASL, Johnson J, Belk P, Sheldon T. Severe atrioventricular decoupling, uncoupling, and ventriculoatrial coupling during enhanced atrial pacing: incidence, mechanisms, and implications for minimizing right ventricular pacing in ICD patients. *J Cardiovasc Electrophysiol* 2008;**19**:1175–80.

115. Funck RC, Boriani G, Manolis AS *et al.* The MINERVA study design and rationale: a controlled randomized trial to assess the clinical benefit of minimizing ventricular pacing in pacemaker patients with atrial tachyarrhythmias. *Am Heart J* 2008;**156**:445–51.

116. Quesada A, Botto G, Erdogan A *et al.* Managed ventricular pacing vs. conventional dual-chamber pacing for elective replacements: the PreFER MVP study: clinical background, rationale, and design. *Europace* 2008;**10**:321–6.

117. Medtronic-Vitatron, Vitatron GmbH. *A randomized, prospective multicenter study to determine the incidence of atrial fibrillation and heart failure in correlation to stimulation modes of pacemakers (Mode Evaluation in Sick Sinus Syndrome Trial – MODEST).* Available from: http://www.clinicaltrials.gov/ct2/show/NCT00161551 NLM Identifier: NCT00161551.

118. Lamas GA, Knight JD, Sweeney MO *et al.* Impact of rate-modulated pacing on quality of life and exercise capacity – evidence from the Advanced Elements of Pacing Randomized Controlled Trial (ADEPT). *Heart Rhythm* 2007;**4**:1125–32.

119. de Cock CC, Giudici MC, Twisk JW. Comparison of the haemodynamic effects of right ventricular outflow-tract pacing with right ventricular apex pacing: a quantitative review. *Europace* 2003;**5**:275–8.

120. Gammage MD, Marsh AM. Randomized trials for selective site pacing: do we know where we are going? *PACE* 2004;**27**:878–82.

121. Manolis AS. The deleterious consequences of right ventricular apical pacing: time to seek alternative site pacing. *PACE* 2006;**29**:298–315.

122. Hillock RJ, Stevenson IH, Mond HG. The right ventricular outflow tract: a comparative study of septal, anterior wall, and free wall pacing. *PACE* 2007;**30**:942–7.

123. Mond HG, Hillock RJ, Stevenson IH, McGavigan AD. The right ventricular outflow tract: the road to septal pacing. *PACE* 2007;**30**:482–91.

124. Deshmukh PM, Romanyshyn M. Direct His-bundle pacing: present and future. *PACE* 2004;**27**:862–70.

125. Zanon F, Baracca E, Aggio S *et al.* A feasible approach for direct his-bundle pacing using a new steerable catheter to facilitate precise lead placement. *J Cardiovasc Electrophysiol* 2006;**17**:29–33.

126. Occhetta E, Bortnik M, Magnani A *et al.* Prevention of ventricular desynchronization by permanent para-Hisian pacing after atrioventricular node ablation in chronic atrial fibrillation: a crossover, blinded, randomized study versus

apical right ventricular pacing. *J Am Coll Cardiol* 2006;**47**:1938–45.

127. Vlay SC. Alternate site biventricular pacing: Bi-V in the RV – is there a role? *PACE* 2004;**27**:567–9.

128. Res JC, Bokern MJ, de Cock CC *et al.* The BRIGHT study: bifocal right ventricular resynchronization therapy: a randomized study. *Europace* 2007;**9**:857–61.

129. Barold SS, Audoglio R, Ravazzi PA, Diotallevi P. Is bifocal right ventricular pacing a viable form of cardiac resynchronization? *PACE* 2008;**31**:789–94.

130. Leon AR, Greenberg JM, Kanuru N *et al.* Cardiac resynchronization in patients with congestive heart failure and chronic atrial fibrillation: effect of upgrading to biventricular pacing after chronic right ventricular pacing. *J Am Coll Cardiol* 2002;**39**:1258–63.

131. Baker CM, Christopher TJ, Smith PF, Langberg JJ, Delurgio DB, Leon AR. Addition of a left ventricular lead to conventional pacing systems in patients with congestive heart failure: feasibility, safety, and early results in 60 consecutive patients. *PACE* 2002;**25**:1166–71.

132. Leclercq C, Cazeau S, Lellouche D *et al.* Upgrading from single-chamber right ventricular to biventricular pacing in permanently paced patients with worsening heart failure: The RD-CHF Study. *PACE* 2007;**30**(suppl 1):S23–30.

133. Doshi RN, Daoud EG, Fellows C *et al.* Left ventricular-based cardiac stimulation post AV nodal ablation evaluation (the PAVE study). *J Cardiovasc Electrophysiol* 2005;**16**:1160–5.

134. Brignole M, Gammage M, Puggioni E *et al.* Comparative assessment of right, left, and biventricular pacing in patients with permanent atrial fibrillation. *Eur Heart J* 2005;**26**:712–22.

135. Kindermann M, Hennen B, Jung J, Geisel J, Böhm M, Fröhlig G. Biventricular versus conventional right ventricular stimulation for patients with standard pacing indication and left ventricular dysfunction: the Homburg Biventricular Pacing Evaluation (HOBIPACE). *J Am Coll Cardiol* 2006;**47**:1927–37.

136. Albertsen AE, Nielsen JC, Poulsen SH *et al.* Biventricular pacing preserves left ventricular performance in patients with high-grade atrio-ventricular block: a randomized comparison with DDD(R) pacing in 50 consecutive patients. *Europace* 2008;**10**:314–20.

137. Curtis AB, Adamson PB, Chung E, Sutton MS, Tang F, Worley S. Biventricular versus right ventricular pacing in patients with AV block (BLOCK HF): clinical study design and rationale. *J Cardiovasc Electrophysiol* 2007;**18**:965–71.

138. de Teresa E, Gómez-Doblas JJ, Lamas G *et al.* Preventing ventricular dysfunction in pacemaker patients without advanced heart failure: rationale and design of the PREVENT-HF study. *Europace* 2007;**9**:442–6.

139. Fung JW, Chan JY, Omar R *et al.* The Pacing to Avoid Cardiac Enlargement (PACE) trial: clinical background, rationale, design, and implementation. *J Cardiovasc Electrophysiol* 2007;**18**:735–9.

140. Funck RC, Blanc JJ, Mueller HH *et al.* Biventricular stimulation to prevent cardiac desynchronization: rationale, design, and endpoints of the 'Biventricular Pacing for Atrioventricular Block to Prevent Cardiac Desynchronization (BioPace)' study. *Europace* 2006;**8**:629–35.

141. Gribbin GM, McComb JM. Pacemaker trials: software or hardware randomization? *PACE* 1998; **21**:1503–7.

142. Santini M, Ricci R. Is AAI or AAIR still a viable mode of pacing? *PACE* 2001;**24**:276–81.

143. Rosenqvist M, Obel IWP. Atrial pacing and the risk for AV block: is there a time for change in attitude? *PACE* 1989;**12**:97–101.

144. Barold SS. Permanent single-chamber atrial pacing is obsolete. *PACE* 2001;**24**:271–5.

145. Quan KJ, Carlson MD, Thames MD. Mechanisms of heart rate and arterial blood pressure control: implications for the pathophysiology of neurocardiogenic syncope. *PACE* 1997; **20**:764–74.

146. Brignole M, Alboni P, Benditt DG *et al.* Guidelines on management (diagnosis and treatment) of syncope – update 2004. *Europace* 2004;**6**:467–537.

147. Strickberger SA, Benson DW, Biaggioni I *et al.* AHA/ACCF Scientific Statement on the evaluation of syncope: from the American Heart Association Councils on Clinical Cardiology, Cardiovascular Nursing, Cardiovascular Disease in the Young, and Stroke, and the Quality of Care and Outcomes Research Interdisciplinary Working Group; and the American College of Cardiology Foundation: in collaboration with the Heart Rhythm Society: endorsed by the American Autonomic Society. *Circulation* 2006;**113**:316–27.

148. Morley CA, Sutton R. Carotid sinus syncope. *Int J Cardiol* 1984;**6**:287–93.

149. Brignole M, Menozzi C. Methods other than tilt testing for diagnosing neurocardiogenic (neurally mediated) syncope. *PACE* 1997;**20**:795–800.

150. Kenny RA, Ingram A, Bayliss J, Sutton R. Head-up tilt: a useful test for investigating unexplained syncope. *Lancet* 1986;**i**:1352–5.

151. Morley CA, Perrins EJ, Grant P *et al.* Carotid sinus syncope treated by pacing. Analysis of persistent symptoms and role of atrioventricular sequential pacing. *Br Heart J* 1982;**47**:411–18.

152. Sugrue DD, Gersh BJ, Holmes DR, Wood DL, Osborn MJ, Hammill SC. Symptomatic "isolated" carotid sinus hypersensitivity: natural history and results of treatment with anticholinergic drugs or pacemaker. *J Am Coll Cardiol* 1986;**7**:158–62.

153. Brignole M, Menozzi C, Lolli G, Bottoni N, Gaggioli G. Long-term outcome of paced and nonpaced patients with severe carotid sinus syndrome. *Am J Cardiol* 1992;**69**:1039–43.

154. Dey AB, Bexton RS, Tynan MM, Charles RG, Kenny RA. The impact of a dedicated "syncope and falls" clinic on pacing practice in Northeastern England. *PACE* 1997;**20**:815–17.

155. Kenny RAM, Richardson DA, Steen N, Bexton RS, Shaw FE, Bond J. Carotid sinus syndrome: a modifiable risk factor for nonaccidental falls in older adults (SAFE PACE). *J Am Coll Cardiol* 2001;**38**:1491–6.

156. Kenny RA for the SAFE PACE 2 study group. SAFE PACE 2: Syncope And Falls in the Elderly – Pacing And Carotid Sinus Evaluation. *Europace* 1999;**1**:69–72.

156a. Parry SW, Steen N, Bexton RS, Tynan M, Kenny RA. Pacing in elderly recurrent fallers with carotid sinus hypersensitivity (PERF-CSH): a randomised, double-blind, placebo controlled crossover trial. *Heart* 2009;**95**:405–9.

157. Petersen MEV, Sutton R. Cardiac pacing for vasovagal syncope: a reasonable therapeutic option? *PACE* 1997;**20**:824–6.

158. Petersen MEV, Chamberlain-Webber R, Fitzpatrick AP *et al.* Permanent pacing for cardioinhibitory malignant vasovagal syndrome. *Br Heart J* 1994;**71**:274–81.

159. Connolly SJ, Sheldon R, Roberts RS, Gent M on behalf of the Vasovagal Pacemaker Study Investigators. The North American Vasovagal Pacemaker Study (VPS). A randomized trial of permanent cardiac pacing for the prevention of vasovagal syncope. *J Am Coll Cardiol* 1999;**33**:16–20.

160. Sutton R, Petersen MEV. First steps towards a pacing algorithm for vasovagal syncope. *PACE* 1997;**20**:827–8.

161. Sutton R, Brignole M, Menozzi C *et al.* Dual-chamber pacing in the treatment of neurally mediated tilt-positive cardioinhibitory syncope. Pacemaker versus no therapy: a multicenter randomized study. *Circulation* 2000;**102**:294–9.

162. Ammirati F, Colivicchi F, Santini M, for the Syncope Diagnosis and Treatment Study Investigators. Permanent cardiac pacing versus medical treatment for the prevention of recurrent vasovagal syncope. A multicenter, randomized, controlled trial. *Circulation* 2001;**104**:52–7.

163. Connolly SJ, Sheldon R, Thorpe KE *et al.* Pacemaker therapy for prevention of syncope in patients with recurrent severe vasovagal syncope: Second Vasovagal Pacemaker Study (VPS II): a randomized trial. *JAMA* 2003;**289**:2224–9.

164. Raviele A, Giada F, Menozzi C *et al.* A randomized, double-blind, placebo-controlled study of permanent cardiac pacing for the treatment of recurrent tilt-induced vasovagal syncope. The vasovagal syncope and pacing trial (Synpace). *Eur Heart J* 2004;**25**:1741–8.

165. Sud S, Massel D, Klein GJ *et al.* The expectation effect and cardiac pacing for refractory vasovagal syncope. *Am J Med* 2007;**120**:54–62.

166. Trim GM, Krahn AD, Klein GJ, Skanes AC, Yee R. Pacing for vasovagal syncope after the second vasovagal pacemaker study: a matter of judgement. *Cardiac Electrophysiol Rev* 2003;**7**:416–20.

167. Brignole M, Sutton R. Pacing for neurally mediated syncope: is placebo powerless? *Europace* 2007;**9**:31–3.

168. Brignole M, Sutton R, Menozzi C *et al.* Lack of correlation between the responses to tilt testing and adenosine triphosphate test and the mechanism of spontaneous neurally mediated syncope. *Eur Heart J* 2006;**27**:2232–9.

169. Brignole M, Sutton R, Menozzi C *et al.* Early application of an implantable loop recorder allows effective specific therapy in patients with recurrent suspected neurally mediated syncope. *Eur Heart J* 2006;**27**:1085–92.

170. Brignole M. International study on syncope of uncertain aetiology 3 (ISSUE 3): pacemaker therapy for patients with asystolic neurally-mediated syncope: rationale and study design. *Europace* 2007;**9**:25–30.

171. Bourdarias JP, Lockhart A, Ourbak P, *et al.* Hemodynamique des cardiomyopathies obstructives. *Arch Mal Coeur* 1964;**57**:737–8.

172. McDonald K, McWilliams E, O'Keefe B *et al.* Functional assessment of patients treated with permanent dual-chamber pacing as a primary treatment for hypertrophic cardiomyopathy. *Eur Heart J* 1988;**9**:893–8.

173. Fananapazir L, Cannon RO, Tripodi D, Panza JA. Impact of dual-chamber permanent pacing in patients with obstructive hypertrophic cardiomyopathy with symptoms refractory to verapamil and beta-adrenergic blocker therapy. *Circulation* 1992;**85**:2149–61.

174. Jeanrenaud X, Goy JJ, Kappenberger L. Effects of dual-chamber pacing in hypertrophic obstructive cardiomyopathy. *Lancet* 1992;**339**:1318–23.

175. Slade AKB, Sadoul N, Shapiro L *et al*. DDD pacing in hypertrophic cardiomyopathy: a multicentre clinical experience. *Heart* 1996;**75**:44–9.

176. Daubert JC. Pacing and hypertrophic cardiomyopathy. *PACE* 1996;**19**:1141–2.

177. Fananapazir L, Epstein ND, Curiel RV, Panza JA, Tripodi D, McAreavey D. Long-term results of dual-chamber (DDD) pacing in obstructive hypertrophic cardiomyopathy: evidence for progressive symptomatic and hemodynamic improvement and reduction of left ventricular hypertrophy. *Circulation* 1994;**90**:2731–42.

178. Pavin D, Gras D, De Place C, Leclercq C, Mabo P, Daubert C. Long-term effect of DDD pacing in patients with hypertrophic obstructive cardiomyopathy: is there a left ventricular remodelling? *PACE* 1996;**19**:680.

179. Nishimura RA, Trusty JM, Hayes DL *et al*. Dual-chamber pacing for hypertrophic cardiomyopathy: a randomized, double-blind, crossover trial. *J Am Coll Cardiol* 1997;**29**:435–41.

180. Kappenberger L, Linde C, Daubert C *et al*. Pacing in hypertrophic obstructive cardiomyopathy. A randomized crossover study. *Eur Heart J* 1997;**18**:1249–56.

181. Linde C, Gadler F, Kappenberger L, Ryden L, for the PIC Study Group. Placebo effect of pacemaker implantation in obstructive hypertrophic cardiomyopathy. *Am J Cardiol* 1999;**83**:903–7.

182. Kappenberger LJ, Linde C, Jeanrenaud X *et al*. Clinical progress after randomized on/off pacemaker treatment for hypertrophic obstructive cardiomyopathy. *Europace* 1999;**1**:77–84.

183. Gadler F, Linde C, Daubert C *et al*. Significant improvement of quality of life following atrioventricular synchronous pacing in patients with hypertrophic obstructive cardiomyopathy. Data from 1 year of follow up. *Eur Heart J* 1999;**20**: 1044–50.

184. Maron BJ, Nishimura RA, McKenna WJ, Rakowski H, Josephson ME, Kieval RS. Assessment of permanent dual-chamber pacing as a treatment for drug-refractory symptomatic patients with obstructive hypertrophic cardiomyopathy: a randomized, double-blind, crossover study (M-PATHY). *Circulation* 1999;**99**: 2927–33.

185. Lawrenz T, Lieder F, Bartelsmeier M *et al*. Predictors of complete heart block after transcoronary ablation of septal hypertrophy: results of a prospective electrophysiological investigation in 172 patients with hypertrophic obstructive cardiomyopathy. *J Am Coll Cardiol* 2007;**49**:2356–63.

186. Smedira NG, Lytle BW, Lever HM *et al*. Current effectiveness and risks of isolated septal myectomy for hypertrophic obstructive cardiomyopathy. *Ann Thorac Surg* 2008;**85**:127–33.

187. Coumel P, Friocourt P, Mugica J, Attuel P, Leclerq JF. Long term prevention of vagal atrial arrhythmias by atrial pacing at 90/min: experience with 6 cases. *PACE* 1983;**6**:552–60.

188. Gillis AM, Wyse DG, Connolly S *et al*. Atrial pacing periablation for prevention of paroxysmal atrial fibrillation. *Circulation* 1999;**99**:2553–8.

189. Gillis AM, Connolly SJ, Lacombe P *et al*. Randomized crossover comparison of DDDR versus VDD pacing after atrioventricular junction ablation for prevention of atrial fibrillation. *Circulation* 2000;**102**:736–41.

190. Ward KJ, Willett JE, Bucknall C, Gill JS, Kamalvand K. Atrial arrhythmia suppression by atrial overdrive pacing: pacemaker Holter assessment. *Europace* 2001;**3**:108–14.

191. Levy T, Walker S, Rex S, Paul V. Does atrial overdrive pacing prevent paroxysmal atrial fibrillation in paced patients? *Int J Cardiol* 2000;**75**:91–7.

192. Garrigue S, Barold SS, Cazeau S *et al*. Prevention of atrial arrhythmias during DDD pacing by atrial overdrive. *PACE* 1998;**21**:1751–9.

193. Wiberg S, Lönnerholm S, Jensen SM, Blomström P, Ringqvist I, Blomström-Lundqvist C. Effect of right atrial overdrive pacing in the prevention of symptomatic paroxysmal atrial fibrillation: a multicenter randomized study, the PAF-PACE study. *PACE* 2003;**26**:1841–8.

194. Silberbauer J, Sulke N. The role of pacing in rhythm control and management of atrial fibrillation. *J Interv Card Electrophysiol* 2007;**18**:159–86.

195. Carlson MD, Ip J, Messenger J *et al*. A new pacemaker algorithm for the treatment of atrial fibrillation: results of the Atrial Dynamic Overdrive Pacing Trial (ADOPT). *J Am Coll Cardiol* 2003;**42**:627–33.

196. Gold M, Hoffmann E. The impact of atrial prevention pacing on AF burden: primary results of the study for atrial fibrillation reduction (SAFARI). *Europace* 2006;**8**(S1):222–3.

197. Blanc JJ, De Roy L, Mansourati J *et al*. Atrial pacing for prevention of atrial fibrillation: assessment of simultaneously implemented algorithms. *Europace* 2004;**6**:371–9.

198. Camm AJ, Sulke N, Edvardsson N *et al*. Conventional and dedicated atrial overdrive pacing for the prevention of paroxysmal atrial fibrillation: the AFTherapy study. *Europace* 2007;**9**:1110–18.

199. Sulke N, Silberbauer J, Boodhoo L *et al*. The use of atrial overdrive and ventricular rate stabilization pacing algorithms for the prevention and treatment of paroxysmal atrial fibrillation: the Pacemaker Atrial Fibrillation Suppression (PAFS) study. *Europace* 2007;**9**:790–7.

200. Daubert C, Mabo P, Berder V. Arrhythmia prevention by permanent atrial resynchronization in advanced interatrial block. *Eur Heart J* 1990;**11**:237.

201. Daubert C, Mabo P, Berder V *et al*. Permanent dual atrium pacing in major interatrial conduction block: a four years experience. *PACE* 1993;**16**:885.

202. Mabo P, Daubert JC, Bouhour A, for the SYNBIAPACE Study Group. Biatrial synchronous pacing for atrial arrhythmia prevention: the SYNBIAPACE study. *PACE* 1999;**22**:755.

203. Mirza I, James S, Holt P. Biatrial pacing for paroxysmal atrial fibrillation: a randomized prospective study into the suppression of paroxysmal atrial fibrillation using biatrial pacing. *J Am Coll Cardiol* 2002;**40**:457–63.

204. Crystal E, Connolly SJ, Sleik K, Ginger TJ, Yusuf S. Interventions on prevention of postoperative atrial fibrillation in patients undergoing heart surgery: a meta-analysis. *Circulation* 2002;**106**:75–80.

205. Saksena S, Prakash A, Hill M *et al*. Prevention of recurrent atrial fibrillation with chronic dual-site right atrial pacing. *J Am Coll Cardiol* 1996;**28**:687–94.

206. Delfaut P, Saksena S, Prakash A, Krol RB. Long-term outcome of patients with drug refractory atrial flutter and fibrillation after single- and dual-site right atrial pacing for arrhythmia prevention. *J Am Coll Cardiol* 1998; **32**:1900–8.

207. Saksena S, Prakash A, Ziegler P *et al*. Improved suppression of recurrent atrial fibrillation with dual-site right atrial pacing

and antiarrhythmic drug therapy. *J Am Coll Cardiol* 2002;**40**:1140–50.

208. Lau CP, Tse HF, Yu CM *et al*. Dual-site atrial pacing for atrial fibrillation in patients without bradycardia. *Am J Cardiol* 2001;**88**:371–5.

209. Bennett DH. Comparison of the acute effects of pacing the atrial septum, right atrial appendage, coronary sinus os, and the latter two sites simultaneously on the duration of atrial activation. *Heart* 2000;**84**:193–6.

210. Baillin SJ, Adler S, Giudici M. Prevention of chronic atrial fibrillation by pacing in the region of Bachmann's bundle: results of a multicenter randomized trial. *J Cardiovasc Electrophysiol* 2001;**12**:912–17.

211. Padeletti L, Pieragnoli P, Ciapetti C *et al*. Randomized crossover comparison of right atrial appendage pacing versus interatrial septum pacing for prevention of paroxysmal atrial fibrillation in patients with sinus bradycardia. *Am Heart J* 2001;**142**:1047–55.

212. Padeletti L, Pürerfellner H, Adler SW *et al*. Combined efficacy of atrial septal lead placement and atrial pacing algorithms for prevention of paroxysmal atrial tachyarrhythmia. *J Cardiovasc Electrophysiol* 2003;**14**:1189–95.

213. Hermida JS, Kubala M, Lescure FX *et al*. Atrial septal pacing to prevent atrial fibrillation in patients with sinus node dysfunction: results of a randomized controlled study. *Am Heart J* 2004;**148**:312–17.

214. Hakacova N, Velimirovic D, Margitfalvi P, Hatala R, Buckingham TA. Septal atrial pacing for the prevention of atrial fibrillation. *Europace* 2007;**9**:1124–8.

215. de Voogt W, van Hemel N, de Vusser P *et al*. No evidence of automatic atrial overdrive pacing efficacy on reduction of paroxysmal atrial fibrillation. *Europace* 2007;**9**:798–804.

216. Moss AJ, Liu JE, Gottlieb S *et al*. Efficacy of permanent pacing in the long QT syndrome. *Circulation* 1991;**84**:1524–9.

217. Eldar M, Griffin JC, Van Hare GF *et al*. Combined use of beta-adrenergic blocking agents and long-term cardiac pacing for patients with the long QT syndrome. *J Am Coll Cardiol* 1992;**20**:830–7.

218. Dorostkar PC, Eldar M, Belhassen B, Scheinman MM. Long-term follow-up of patients with long-QT syndrome treated with beta-blockers and continuous pacing. *Circulation* 1999;**100**:2431–6.

219. Schwartz PJ. The Long QT Syndrome. New York: Futura, 1997.

220. Zareba W, Priori SG, Moss AJ *et al*. Permanent pacing in the long QT syndrome patients. *PACE* 1997;**20**:1097.

221. Viskin S, Alla SR, Baron HV *et al*. Mode of onset of torsade de pointes in congenital long QT syndrome. *J Am Coll Cardiol* 1996;**28**:1262–8.

222. Klein H, Levi A, Kaplinsky E, DiSegni E, David D. Congenital long-QT syndrome: deleterious effect of long-term high-rate ventricular pacing and definitive treatment by cardiac transplantation. *Am Heart J* 1996;**132**:1079–81.

223. Viskin S. Cardiac pacing in the long QT syndrome: review of available data and practical recommendations. *J Cardiovasc Electrophysiol* 2000;**11**: 593–600.

224. Viskin S, Fish R, Roth A, Copperman Y. Prevention of torsade de pointes in the congenital long QT syndrome: use of a pause prevention pacing algorithm. *Heart* 1998;**79**:417–19.

225. Priori SG, Napolitano C, Cantù F, Brown AM, Schwartz PJ. Differential response to Na⁺ channel blockade, β-adrenergic

226. Schwartz PJ, Priori SG, Locati EH *et al*. Long QT syndrome patients with mutations of the SCN5A and HERG genes have differential responses to Na⁺ channel blockade and to increases in heart rate. *Circulation* 1995;**92**:3381–6.

227. Shimizu W, Antzelevitch C. Sodium channel block with mexiletine is effective in reducing dispersion of repolarization and preventing torsade des pointes in LQT2 and LQT3 models of the long-QT syndrome. *Circulation* 1997;**96**:2038–47.

228. Schwartz PJ, Priori SG, Spazzolini C *et al*. Genotype-phenotype correlation in the long-QT syndrome: gene-specific triggers for life-threatening arrhythmias. *Circulation* 2001;**103**:89–95.

229. Jacquet L, Ziady G, Stein K *et al*. Cardiac rhythm disturbances early after orthotopic heart transplantation: prevalence and importance of the observed abnormalities. *J Am Coll Cardiol* 1990;**16**:832–7.

230. Holt ND, Tynan MM, Scott CD, Parry G, Dark JH, McComb JM. Permanent pacemaker use after cardiac transplantation: completing the audit cycle. *Heart* 1996;**76**:435–8.

231. Bertolet BD, Eagle DA, Conti JB, Mills RM, Belardinelli L. Bradycardia after heart transplantation: reversal with theophylline. *J Am Coll Cardiol* 1996;**28**:396–9.

232. Holt ND, McComb JM. Cardiac transplantation and pacemakers: when and what to implant. *Card Electrophysiol Rev* 2002;**6**:140–51.

233. DiBiase A, Tse TM, Schnittger I, Wexler L, Stinson EB, Valantine HA. Frequency and mechanism of bradycardia in cardiac transplant recipients and need for pacemakers. *Am J Coll Cardiol* 1991;**67**:1385–9.

234. Heinz G, Kratochwill C, Schmid S *et al*. Sinus node dysfunction after orthotopic heart transplantation: the Vienna experience 1987–1993. *PACE* 1994;**17**:2057–63.

235. Scott CD, Omar I, McComb JM, Dark JH, Bexton RS. Long-term pacing in heart transplant recipients is usually unnecessary. *PACE* 1991;**14**:1792–6.

236. Morris-Thurgood J, Cowell R, Paul V *et al*. Hemodynamic and metabolic effects of paced linkage following heterotopic cardiac transplantation. *Circulation* 1994;**90**:2342–7.

237. Morris-Thurgood J, Paul VE, Dyke C *et al*. Chronic linkage after heterotopic heart transplantation. *Transplant Proc* 1997;**29**: 580.

238. Young T, Palta M, Dempsey J, Skatrud J, Weber S, Badr S. The occurrence of sleep-disordered breathing among middle-aged adults. *N Engl J Med* 1993;**328**:1230–5.

239. Stegman SS, Burroughs JM, Henthorn RW. Asymptomatic bradyarrhythmias as a marker for sleep apnea: appropriate recognition and treatment may reduce the need for pacemaker therapy. *PACE* 1996;**19**:899–904.

240. Grimm W, Koehler U, Fus E *et al*. Outcome of patients with sleep apnea-associated severe bradyarrhythmias after continuous positive airway pressure therapy. *Am J Cardiol* 2000;**86**:688–92.

241. Kato I, Shiomi T, Sasanabe R *et al*. Effects of physiological cardiac pacing on sleep-disordered breathing in patients with chronic bradydysrhythmias. *Psychiatry Clin Neurosci* 2001;**55**:257–8.

242. Garrigue S, Bordier P, Jaïs P *et al*. Benefit of atrial pacing in sleep apnea syndrome. *N Engl J Med* 2002;**346**:404–12.

243. Gottlieb DJ. Cardiac pacing – a novel therapy for sleep apnea? *N Engl J Med* 2002:**346**:444–5.

244. Pépin JL, Defaye P, Garrigue S, Poezevara Y, Lévy P. Overdrive atrial pacing does not improve obstructive sleep apnoea syndrome. *Eur Respir J* 2005;**25**:343–7.

245. Simantirakis EN, Schiza SE, Chrysostomakis SI et al. Atrial overdrive pacing for the obstructive sleep apnea-hypopnea syndrome. *N Engl J Med* 2005;**353**:2568–77.

246. Lüthje L, Unterberg-Buchwald C, Dajani D, Vollmann D, Hasenfuss G, Andreas S. Atrial overdrive pacing in patients with sleep apnea with implanted pacemaker. *Am J Respir Crit Care Med* 2005;**172**:118–22.

247. Shalaby AA, Atwood CW, Hansen C et al. Analysis of interaction of acute atrial overdrive pacing with sleep-related breathing disorder. *Am J Cardiol* 2007;**99**:573–8.

248. Unterberg C, Lüthje L, Szych J, Vollmann D, Hasenfuss G, Andreas S. Atrial overdrive pacing compared to CPAP in patients with obstructive sleep apnoea syndrome. *Eur Heart J* 2005;**26**:2568–75.

249. Krahn AD, Yee R, Erickson MK et al. Physiologic pacing in patients with obstructive sleep apnea: a prospective, randomized crossover trial. *J Am Coll Cardiol* 2006;**47**:379–83.

250. Sharafkhaneh A, Sharafkhaneh H, Bredikus A, Guilleminault C, Bozkurt B, Hirshkowitz M. Effect of atrial overdrive pacing on obstructive sleep apnea in patients with systolic heart failure. *Sleep Med* 2007;**8**:31–6.

251. Simantirakis EN, Schiza SE, Siafakas NS, Vardas PE. Sleep-disordered breathing in heart failure and the effect of cardiac resynchronization therapy. *Europace* 2008;**10**:1029–33.

252. Brecker SJD, Xiao HB, Sparrow J, Gibson D. Effects of dual-chamber pacing with short atrioventricular delay in dilated cardiomyopathy. *Lancet* 1992;**340**:1308–12.

253. Hochleitner M, Hörtnagl H, Fridrich L, Gschnitzer F. Long-term efficacy of physiologic dual-chamber pacing in the treatment of end-stage idiopathic dilated cardiomyopathy. *Am J Cardiol* 1992;**70**:1320–5.

254. Auricchio A, Sommariva L, Salo RW, Scafuri A, Chiariello L. Improvement of cardiac function in patients with severe congestive heart failure and coronary artery disease by dual-chamber pacing with shortened AV delay. *PACE* 1993;**16**:2034–43.

255. Linde C, Gadler F, Edner M et al. Results of atrioventricular synchronous pacing with optimized delay in patients with severe congestive heart failure. *Am J Cardiol* 1995;**75**:919–23.

256. Gold MR, Feliciano Z, Gottlieb SS, Fisher ML. Dual-chamber pacing with a short atrioventricular delay in congestive heart failure: a randomized study. *J Am Coll Cardiol* 1995;**26**:967–73.

257. Nishimura RA, Hayes DL, Holmes DR Jr, Tajik AJ. Mechanism of hemodynamic improvement by dual-chamber pacing for severe left ventricular dysfunction: an acute Doppler and catheterisation hemodynamic study. *J Am Coll Cardiol* 1995;**25**:281 8.

258. Paul V, Cowell R, Morris-Thurgood J et al. First-degree heart block in heart failure: is this a class I indication for dual-chamber pacing? *PACE* 1995;**18**:906.

259. Brecker SJD, Gibson DG. What is the role of pacing in dilated cardiomyopathy? *Eur Heart J* 1996;**17**:819–24.

260. Wilensky RL, Yudelman P, Cohen AI et al. Serial electrocardiographic changes in idiopathic dilated cardiomyopathy confirmed at necropsy. *Am J Cardiol* 1988;**62**:276–83.

261. de Teresa E, Chamorro JL, Pulpon LA et al. An even more physiological pacing. Changing the sequence of ventricular activation. In: Steinbech K, Glogar D, Laszkovics A et al, eds. *Cardiac Pacing.* Proceedings of the VIIth World Symposium on Cardiac Pacing. Darmstadt, Germany: Steinkopff Verlag, 1983:395–400.

262. Cazeau S, Ritter P, Bakdach S et al. Four chamber pacing in dilated cardiomyopathy. *PACE* 1994;**17**:1974–9.

263. Bakker PF, Meijburg H, de Jonge N et al. Beneficial effects of biventricular pacing in congestive heart failure. *PACE* 1994;**17**:820.

264. Cazeau S, Ritter P, Lazarus A et al. Multi-site pacing for end-stage heart failure. *PACE* 1996;**19**:1748–57.

265. Blanc JJ, Etienne Y, Gilard M et al. Evaluation of different ventricular pacing sites in patients with severe heart failure. *Circulation* 1997;**96**:3273–7.

266. Leclercq C, Cazeau S, Le Breton H et al. Acute hemodynamic effects of biventricular DDD pacing in patients with end-stage heart failure. *J Am Coll Cardiol* 1998;**32**:1825–31.

267. Auricchio A, Stellbrink C, Block M et al. Effect of pacing chamber and atrioventricular delay on acute systolic function of paced patients with congestive heart failure. *Circulation* 1999;**99**:2993–3001.

268. Kass DA, Chen C-H, Curry C et al. Improved left ventricular mechanics from acute VDD pacing in patients with dilated cardiomyopathy and ventricular conduction delay. *Circulation* 1999;**99**:1567–73.

269. Daubert JC, Ritter P, Le Breton H et al. Permanent left ventricular pacing with transvenous leads inserted into the coronary veins. *PACE* 1998;**21**:239–45.

270. Walker S, Levy T, Rex S, Brant S, Paul V. Initial United Kingdom experience with the use of permanent, biventricular pacemakers. Implantation procedure and technical considerations. *Europace* 2000;**2**:233–9.

271. Gras D, Mabo P, Tang T et al. Multisite pacing as a supplemental treatment of congestive heart failure: preliminary results of the Medtronic Inc. InSync study. *PACE* 1998;**21**:2249–55.

272. Gras D, Ritter P, Lazarus A et al. Long-term outcome of advanced heart failure patients with cardiac resynchronisation therapy. *PACE* 2000;**23**:658.

273. Leclercq C, Cazeau S, Ritter P et al. A pilot experience with permanent biventricular pacing to treat advanced heart failure. *Am Heart J* 2000;**140**:862–70.

274. Auricchio A, Stellbrink C, Block M et al. Effect of pacing chamber and atrioventricular delay on acute systolic function of paced patients with congestive heart failure. *Circulation* 1999;**99**:2993–3001.

275. Auricchio A, Stellbrink C, Sack S et al. Long-term clinical effect of hemodynamically optimized cardiac resynchronization therapy in patients with heart failure and ventricular conduction delay. *J Am Coll Cardiol* 2002;**39**:2026–33.

276. Auricchio A, Stellbrink C, Butter C et al. Clinical efficacy of cardiac resynchronization therapy using left ventricular pacing in heart failure patients stratified by severity of ventricular conduction delay. *J Am Coll Cardiol* 2003;**42**:2109–16.

277. Cazeau S, Leclercq C, Lavergne T et al. Effects of multisite biventricular pacing in patients with heart failure and intraventricular conduction delay. *N Engl J Med* 2001;**344**:873–80.

278. Linde C, Leclercq C, Rex S et al. Long-term benefits of biventricular pacing in congestive heart failure: results from the

MUltisite STimulation in cardiomyopathy (MUSTIC) study. *J Am Coll Cardiol* 2002;**40**:111–18.

279. Linde C, Braunschweig F, Gadler F, Bailleul C, Daubert JC. Long-term improvements in quality of life by biventricular pacing in patients with chronic heart failure: results from the Multisite Stimulation in Cardiomyopathy study (MUSTIC). *Am J Cardiol* 2003;**91**:1090–5.

280. Leclercq C, Walker S, Linde C *et al*. Comparative effects of permanent biventricular and right-univentricular pacing in heart failure patients with chronic atrial fibrillation. *Eur Heart J* 2002;**23**:1780–7.

281. Abraham WT, Fisher WG, Smith AL *et al*. Multicenter InSync Randomized Clinical Evaluation. Cardiac resynchronization in chronic heart failure. *N Engl J Med* 2002;**346**:1845–53.

282. St John Sutton MG, Plappert T, Abraham WT *et al*. Effect of cardiac resynchronization therapy on left ventricular size and function in chronic heart failure. *Circulation* 2003;**107**:1985–90.

283. Young JB, Abraham WT, Smith AL *et al*. Combined cardiac resynchronization and implantable cardioversion defibrillation in advanced chronic heart failure: the MIRACLE ICD Trial. *JAMA* 2003;**289**:2685–94.

284. Abraham WT, Young JB, León AR *et al*. Effects of cardiac resynchronization on disease progression in patients with left ventricular systolic dysfunction, an indication for an implantable cardioverter-defibrillator, and mildly symptomatic chronic heart failure. *Circulation* 2004;**110**:2864–8.

285. Higgins SL, Hummel JD, Niazi IK *et al*. Cardiac resynchronization therapy for the treatment of heart failure in patients with intraventricular conduction delay and malignant ventricular tachyarrhythmias. *J Am Coll Cardiol* 2003;**42**:1454–9.

286. Bristow MR, Saxon LA, Boehmer J *et al*. Cardiac-resynchronization therapy with or without an implantable defibrillator in advanced chronic heart failure. *N Engl J Med* 2004;**350**:2140–50.

287. De Marco T, Wolfel E, Feldman AM *et al*. Impact of cardiac resynchronization therapy on exercise performance, functional capacity, and quality of life in systolic heart failure with QRS prolongation: COMPANION trial sub-study. *J Card Fail* 2008;**14**:9–18.

288. Cleland JG, Daubert JC, Erdmann E *et al*. The effect of cardiac resynchronization on morbidity and mortality in heart failure. *N Engl J Med* 2005;**352**:1539–49.

289. Cleland JG, Daubert JC, Erdmann E *et al*. Longer-term effects of cardiac resynchronization therapy on mortality in heart failure [the CArdiac REsynchronization-Heart Failure (CARE-HF) trial extension phase]. *Eur Heart J* 2006;**27**:1928–32.

290. Richardson M, Freemantle N, Calvert MJ, Cleland JG, Tavazzi L, for the CARE-HF Study Steering Committee and Investigators. Predictors and treatment response with cardiac resynchronization therapy in patients with heart failure characterized by dyssynchrony: a pre-defined analysis from the CARE-HF trial. *Eur Heart J* 2007;**28**:1827–34.

291. Cleland J, Freemantle N, Ghio S *et al*. Predicting the long-term effects of cardiac resynchronization therapy on mortality from baseline variables and the early response a report from the CARE-HF (Cardiac Resynchronization in Heart Failure) Trial. *J Am Coll Cardiol* 2008;**52**:438–45.

292. Freemantle N, Tharmanathan P, Calvert MJ, Abraham WT, Ghosh J, Cleland JG. Cardiac resynchronisation for patients with heart failure due to left ventricular systolic dysfunction – a systematic review and meta-analysis. *Eur J Heart Fail* 2006;**8**:433–40.

293. Rivero-Ayerza M, Theuns DA, Garcia-Garcia HM, Boersma E, Simoons M, Jordaens LJ. Effects of cardiac resynchronization therapy on overall mortality and mode of death: a meta-analysis of randomized controlled trials. *Eur Heart J* 2006;**27**:2682–8.

294. Fox M, Mealing S, Anderson R *et al*. The clinical effectiveness and cost-effectiveness of cardiac resynchronisation (biventricular pacing) for heart failure: systematic review and economic model. *Health Technol Assess* 2007;**11**(47):iii–iv, ix–248.

295. McAlister FA, Ezekowitz J, Hooton N *et al*. Cardiac resynchronization therapy for patients with left ventricular systolic dysfunction: a systematic review. *JAMA* 2007;**297**:2502–14.

296. McAlister FA, Ezekowitz J, Dryden DM *et al*. Cardiac resynchronization therapy and implantable cardiac defibrillators in left ventricular systolic dysfunction. *Evid Rep Technol Assess (Full Rep)* 2007;**152**:1–199.

297. Lam SK, Owen A. Combined resynchronisation and implantable defibrillator therapy in left ventricular dysfunction: Bayesian network meta-analysis of randomised controlled trials. *BMJ* 2007;**335**(7626):925.

298. McAlister FA, Tu JV, Newman A *et al*. How many patients with heart failure are eligible for cardiac resynchronization? Insights from two prospective cohorts. *Eur Heart J* 2006;**27**:323–9.

299. Feldman AM, de Lissovoy G, Bristow MR *et al*. Cost effectiveness of cardiac resynchronization therapy in the Comparison of Medical Therapy, Pacing, and Defibrillation in Heart Failure (COMPANION) trial. *J Am Coll Cardiol* 2005;**46**:2311–21.

300. Calvert MJ, Freemantle N, Yao G *et al*. Cost-effectiveness of cardiac resynchronization therapy: results from the CARE-HF trial. *Eur Heart J* 2005;**26**:2681–8.

301. Yao G, Freemantle N, Calvert MJ, Bryan S, Daubert JC, Cleland JG. The long-term cost-effectiveness of cardiac resynchronization therapy with or without an implantable cardioverter-defibrillator. *Eur Heart J* 2007;**28**:42–51.

302. Molhoek SG, Bax JJ, Bleeker GB *et al*. Comparison of response to cardiac resynchronization therapy in patients with sinus rhythm versus chronic atrial fibrillation. *Am J Cardiol* 2004;**94**:1506–9.

303. Kiès P, Leclercq C, Bleeker GB *et al*. Cardiac resynchronisation therapy in chronic atrial fibrillation: impact on left atrial size and reversal to sinus rhythm. *Heart* 2006;**92**:490–4.

304. Gasparini M, Auricchio A, Regoli F *et al*. Four-year efficacy of cardiac resynchronization therapy on exercise tolerance and disease progression: the importance of performing atrioventricular junction ablation in patients with atrial fibrillation. *J Am Coll Cardiol* 2006;**48**:734–43.

305. Delnoy PP, Ottervanger JP, Luttikhuis HO *et al*. Comparison of usefulness of cardiac resynchronization therapy in patients with atrial fibrillation and heart failure versus patients with sinus rhythm and heart failure. *Am J Cardiol* 2007;**99**:1252–7.

306. Khadjooi K, Foley PW, Chalil S *et al*. Long-term effects of cardiac resynchronisation therapy in patients with atrial fibrillation. *Heart* 2008;**94**:879–83.

307. Gasparini M, Auricchio A, Metra M *et al*. Long-term survival in patients undergoing cardiac resynchronization therapy: the importance of performing atrio-ventricular junction ablation in

patients with permanent atrial fibrillation. *Eur Heart J* 2008;**29**: 1644–52.

308. Tolosana JM, Hernandez Madrid A, Brugada J et al. Comparison of benefits and mortality in cardiac resynchronization therapy in patients with atrial fibrillation versus patients in sinus rhythm (Results of the Spanish Atrial Fibrillation and Resynchronization [SPARE] Study). *Am J Cardiol* 2008;**102**: 444–9.

309. Hoppe UC, Casares JM, Eiskjaer H et al. Effect of cardiac resynchronization on the incidence of atrial fibrillation in patients with severe heart failure. *Circulation* 2006;**114**:18–25.

310. Birnie DH, Tang AS. The problem of non-response to cardiac resynchronization therapy. *Curr Opin Cardiol* 2006;**21**: 20–6.

311. Breithardt OA, Stellbrink C, Kramer AP et al. Echocardiographic quantification of left ventricular asynchrony predicts an acute hemodynamic benefit of cardiac resynchronization therapy. *J Am Coll Cardiol* 2002;**40**:536–45.

312. Butter C, Auricchio A, Stellbrink C et al. Effect of resynchronization therapy stimulation site on the systolic function of heart failure patients. *Circulation* 2001;**104**:3026–9.

313. Ypenburg C, Schalij MJ, Bleeker GB et al. Impact of viability and scar tissue on response to cardiac resynchronization therapy in ischaemic heart failure patients. *Eur Heart J* 2007; **28**:33–41.

314. Bax JJ, Abraham T, Barold SS et al. Cardiac resynchronization therapy: Part 1 – issues before device implantation. *J Am Coll Cardiol* 2005;**46**:2153–67.

315. Gorcsan J 3rd, Abraham T, Agler DA et al. Echocardiography for cardiac resynchronization therapy: recommendations for performance and reporting – a report from the American Society of Echocardiography Dyssynchrony Writing Group endorsed by the Heart Rhythm Society. *J Am Soc Echocardiog* 2008;**21**:191–213.

316. Chung ES, Leon AR, Tavazzi L et al. Results of the Predictors of Response to CRT (PROSPECT) trial. *Circulation* 2008;**117**: 2608–16.

317. Suffoletto MS, Dohi K, Cannesson M, Saba S, Gorcsan J 3rd. Novel speckle-tracking radial strain from routine black-and-white echocardiographic images to quantify dyssynchrony and predict response to cardiac resynchronization therapy. *Circulation* 2006;**113**:960–8.

318. Kapetanakis S, Kearney MT, Siva A, Gall N, Cooklin M, Monaghan MJ. Real-time three-dimensional echocardiography: a novel technique to quantify global left ventricular mechanical dyssynchrony. *Circulation* 2005;**112**:992–1000.

319. Helm RH, Lardo AC. Cardiac magnetic resonance assessment of mechanical dyssynchrony. *Curr Opin Cardiol* 2008;**23**:440–6.

320. Van de Veire NR, Marsan NA, Schuijf JD et al. Noninvasive imaging of cardiac venous anatomy with 64-slice multi-slice computed tomography and noninvasive assessment of left ventricular dyssynchrony by 3-dimensional tissue synchronization imaging in patients with heart failure scheduled for cardiac resynchronization therapy. *Am J Cardiol* 2008;**101**: 1023–9.

321. Exner DV. *A Randomized comparison of targeted versus usual left ventricular lead placement*. The INCREMENTAL Study. Presented at the Heart Rhythm Society, 29th Annual Scientific Sessions, San Francisco, California, USA, 15 May 2008.

322. Doll N, Piorkowski C, Czesla M et al. Epicardial versus transvenous left ventricular lead placement in patients receiving cardiac resynchronization therapy: results from a randomized prospective study. *Thorac Cardiovasc Surg* 2008;**56**:256–61.

323. Mair H, Jansens JL, Lattouf OM, Reichart B, Dabritz S. Epicardial lead implantation techniques for biventricular pacing via left lateral mini-thoracotomy, video-assisted thoracoscopy, and robotic approach. *Heart Surg Forum* 2003;**6**:412–17.

324. Alonso C, Goscinska K, Ritter P, Jauvert G, Lazarus A, Cazeau S. Upgrading from biventricular to triple-ventricular pacing guided by echocardiography: a pilot study. *Heart Rhythm* 2005;**2**(suppl):S325.

325. Leclercq C, Gadler F, Kranig W et al. A randomized comparison of triple-site versus dual-site ventricular stimulation in patients with congestive heart failure. *J Am Coll Cardiol* 2008;**51**: 1455–62.

326. Lenarczyk R, Kowalski O, Kukulski T et al. Mid-term outcomes of triple-site vs. conventional cardiac resynchronization therapy: A preliminary study. *Int J Cardiol* 2009;**133**:87–94.

327. Bax JJ, Abraham T, Barold SS et al. Cardiac resynchronization therapy: Part 2 – issues during and after device implantation and unresolved questions. *J Am Coll Cardiol* 2005;**46**:2168–82.

328. Hasan A, Abraham WT. Optimization of cardiac resynchronization therapy after implantation. *Curr Treat Options Cardiovasc Med* 2008;**10**:319–28.

329. Valzania C, Biffi M, Martignani C et al. Cardiac resynchronization therapy: variations in echo-guided optimized atrioventricular and interventricular delays during follow-up. *Echocardiography* 2007;**24**:933–9.

330. Valzania C, Eriksson MJ, Boriani G, Gadler F. Cardiac resynchronization therapy during rest and exercise: comparison of two optimization methods. *Europace* 2008;**10**:1161–9.

331. Zuber M, Toggweiler S, Roos M, Kobza R, Jamshidi P, Erne P. Comparison of different approaches for optimization of atrioventricular and interventricular delay in biventricular pacing. *Europace* 2008;**10**:367–73.

332. Gold MR, Niazi I, Giudici M et al. A prospective comparison of AV delay programming methods for hemodynamic optimization during cardiac resynchronization therapy. *J Cardiovasc Electrophysiol* 2007;**18**:490–6.

333. Whinnett ZI, Davies JE, Nott G et al. Efficiency, reproducibility and agreement of five different hemodynamic measures for optimization of cardiac resynchronization therapy. *Int J Cardiol* 2008;**129**:216–26.

334. Yu CM, Lin H, Zhang Q, Sanderson JE. High prevalence of left ventricular systolic and diastolic asynchrony in patients with congestive heart failure and normal QRS duration. *Heart* 2003;**89**:54–60.

335. Achilli A, Sassara M, Ficili S et al. Long-term effectiveness of cardiac resynchronization therapy in patients with refractory heart failure and "narrow" QRS. *J Am Coll Cardiol* 2003;**42**: 2117–24.

336. Bleeker GB, Holman ER, Steendijk P et al. Cardiac resynchronization therapy in patients with a narrow QRS complex. *J Am Coll Cardiol* 2006;**48**.2243–50.

337. Yu CM, Chan YS, Zhang Q et al. Benefits of cardiac resynchronization therapy for heart failure patients with narrow QRS complexes and coexisting systolic asynchrony by echocardiography. *J Am Coll Cardiol* 2006;**48**:2251–7.

338. Beshai JF, Grimm RA, Nagueh SF *et al.* Cardiac-resynchronization therapy in heart failure with narrow QRS complexes. *N Engl J Med* 2007;**357**:2461–71.

339. Leon AR, Niazi I, Herrman K *et al.* Chronic evaluation of CRT in narrow QRS patients with mechanical dyssynchrony from a multicenter study: ESTEEM-CRT. *Heart Rhythm* 2008;**5**(suppl 5):S23–S24.

340. Cazeau SJ, Daubert JC, Tavazzi L, Frohlig G, Paul V. Responders to cardiac resynchronization therapy with narrow or intermediate QRS complexes identified by simple echocardiographic indices of dyssynchrony: the DESIRE study. *Eur J Heart Fail* 2008;**10**:273–80.

341. Biotronik Inc. Echocardiography Guided Cardiac Resynchronization Therapy (EchoCRT). Available from: http://www.clinicaltrials.gov/ct2/show/record/NCT00683696 NLM Identifier: NCT00683696.

342. Bleeker GB, Schalij MJ, Holman ER, Steendijk P, van der Wall EE, Bax JJ. Cardiac resynchronization therapy in patients with systolic left ventricular dysfunction and symptoms of mild heart failure secondary to ischemic or nonischemic cardiomyopathy. *Am J Cardiol* 2006;**98**:230–5.

343. Cleland JG, Freemantle N, Daubert JC, Toff WD, Leisch F, Tavazzi L. Long-term effect of cardiac resynchronisation in patients reporting mild symptoms of heart failure: a report from the CARE-HF study. *Heart* 2008;**94**:278–83.

344. Linde C, Gold M, Abraham WT, Daubert JC, for the REVERSE Study Group. Rationale and design of a randomized controlled trial to assess the safety and efficacy of cardiac resynchronization therapy in patients with asymptomatic left ventricular dysfunction with previous symptoms or mild heart failure – the REsynchronization reVErses Remodeling in Systolic left vEntricular dysfunction (REVERSE) study. *Am Heart J* 2006;**151**:288–94.

345. Linde C, Abraham WT, Gold MR *et al.* Randomized trial of cardiac resynchronization in mildly symptomatic heart failure patients and in asymptomatic patients with left ventricular dysfunction and previous heart failure symptoms. *J Am Coll Cardiol* 2008;**52**:1834–43.

346. Daubert JC. 24-month results from the European cohort of the REsynchronization reVErses Remodeling in Systolic left vEntricular dysfunction trial. Presented at the American College of Cardiology, 58th Annual Scientific Sessions, Orlando, Florida, USA, 31 March 2009.

347. Moss AJ, Brown MW, Cannom DS *et al.* Multicenter automatic defibrillator implantation trial-cardiac resynchronization therapy (MADIT-CRT): design and clinical protocol. *Ann Noninvasive Electrocardiol* 2005;**10**(4 suppl):34–43.

348. Tang AS, Wells GA, Arnold M *et al.* Resynchronization/defibrillation for ambulatory heart failure trial: rationale and trial design. *Curr Opin Cardiol* 2008;**24**:1–8.

349. Moss AJ, Zareba W, Hall WJ *et al.* Prophylactic implantation of a defibrillator in patients with myocardial infarction and reduced ejection fraction. *N Engl J Med* 2002;**346**:877–83.

350. Bardy GH, Lee KL, Mark DB *et al.* Amiodarone or an implantable cardioverter-defibrillator for congestive heart failure. *N Engl J Med* 2005;**352**:225–37.

351. Ermis C, Seutter R, Zhu AX *et al.* Impact of upgrade to cardiac resynchronization therapy on ventricular arrhythmia frequency in patients with implantable cardioverter-defibrillators. *J Am Coll Cardiol* 2005;**46**:2258–63.

352. Saxon LA, Bristow MR, Boehmer J *et al.* Predictors of sudden cardiac death and appropriate shock in the Comparison of Medical Therapy, Pacing, and Defibrillation in Heart Failure (COMPANION) Trial. *Circulation* 2006;**114**:2766–72.

353. McAlister FA, Ezekowitz J, Dryden DM *et al.* Cardiac resynchronization therapy and implantable cardiac defibrillators in left ventricular systolic dysfunction. Evid Rep Technol Assess *No.152.* AHRQ Publication No. 07-E009. Rockville, MD: Agency for Healthcare Research and Quality, 2007.

354. Ellenbogen KA, Wood MA, Klein HU. Why should we care about CARE-HF? *J Am Coll Cardiol* 2005;**46**:2199–203.

355. Daubert JC, Leclercq C, Mabo P. There is plenty of room for cardiac resynchronization therapy devices without back-up defibrillators in the electrical treatment of heart failure. *J Am Coll Cardiol* 2005;**46**:2204–7.

356. Bond M, Mealing S, Anderson R, Dean J, Stein K, Taylor RS. Is combined resynchronisation and implantable defibrillator therapy a cost-effective option for left ventricular dysfunction? *Int J Cardiol* 2008 Aug 12 (epub ahead of print).

357. Roguin A, Schwitter J, Vahlhaus C *et al.* Magnetic resonance imaging in individuals with cardiovascular implantable electronic devices. *Europace* 2008;**10**:336–46.

358. Lee KL, Lau CP, Tse HF *et al.* First human demonstration of cardiac stimulation with transcutaneous ultrasound energy delivery: implications for wireless pacing with implantable devices. *J Am Coll Cardol* 2007;**50**:877–83.

359. Rosen MR, Brink PR, Cohen IS, Robinson RB. Cardiac pacing: from biological to electronic … to biological? *Circ Arrhythmia Electrophysiol* 2008;**1**:54–61.

42 Syncope

David G Benditt, Fei Lu and Scott Sakaguchi

Cardiac Arrhythmia Center, University of Minnesota Medical School, Minneapolis, MN, USA

Introduction

Syncope is a symptom in which transient loss of consciousness (TLOC) occurs as a consequence of a spontaneously self-limited period of cerebral hypoperfusion.[1-3] A wide range of conditions may be responsible for triggering syncope; in many instances the faint is relatively benign (e.g. vasovagal faint) but others (e.g. certain cardiac arrhythmias) may have more serious implications. In any case, whether the underlying problem is "innocent" or potentially life-threatening, syncope may lead to physical injury, accidents that put others at risk, and economic loss. Consequently, the management goals are to identify the specific causes(s) of the symptoms, and thereafter develop a treatment plan designed to prevent recurrences.[1]

This chapter provides a brief summary of the major causes of syncope, including nomenclature concerns, but focuses principally on clinical management (diagnosis and treatment), particularly changing treatment concepts for neurally mediated reflex syncope and orthostatic syncope. Whenever possible, the recommendations provided here are adapted from the European Society of Cardiology Syncope Task Force guidelines.[1] However, that was not always possible. In such cases, we have either elected not to provide a "level" of recommendation or, when it seemed reasonable, to indicate by means of an asterisk (*) that the recommendation is based on the authors' opinion.

Nomenclature

"Syncope" must be distinguished from the many other forms of transient loss of consciousness (TLOC) or "TLOC/syncope mimics" (Fig. 42.1). Unfortunately, physicians remain uncertain regarding this distinction. Despite the efforts of some,[1-4] the confusion continues to be exacerbated by imprecise writing in the medical literature.[5-7] For example, the recent scientific statement from the American College of Cardiology Foundation (ACCF) and the American Heart Association (AHA) confuses the definition of "true syncope" with the broader concept of TLOC.[5] Similar imprecise characterization of syncope may be found in a widely cited report from the Framingham Study[6] and in a relatively recent clinical review article in the *British Medical Journal*.[7] Inaccurate advice from seemingly authoritative sources unnecessarily confounds the "syncope" evaluation and results in the undertaking of expensive but low-yield tests such as electroencephalograms (EEGs) and imaging studies of the head. In an effort to clarify matters, several groups have attempted to both address the vagaries of terminology[1-4] and develop more cost-effective ways to evaluate syncope patients.[1,8-14]

Incidence, natural history, and prognosis

Frequency in the population

Syncope has been variably reported to account for approximately 1–3 % of emergency department (ED) visits (the 1% is the more recent estimate) and 1–6% of general hospital admissions in the United States.[15-17] In numerical terms, the National Hospital Ambulatory Medical Care Survey of 2006 in the United States noted that primary diagnoses of "syncope and collapse" (ICD-9; 780.2) had increased from approximately 887 000 ED visits in 2001 to greater than 1 125 000 ED visits in 2006. On the other hand, "syncope and collapse" listed among all US hospital discharge diagnoses in the 2006 National Hospital Discharge Survey remained relatively constant over this same time period: 405 000 in 2001 and 411 000 in 2006. This suggests, perhaps, that ED physicians are becoming less hesitant to have such patients evaluated on an outpatient basis.

Evidence-Based Cardiology, 3rd edition. Edited by S. Yusuf, J.A. Cairns, A.J. Camm, E.L. Fallen, and B.J. Gersh. © 2010 Blackwell Publishing, ISBN: 978-1-4051-5925-8.

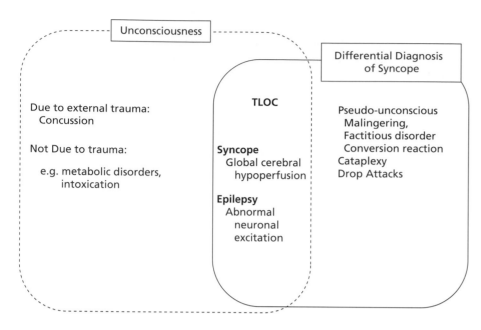

Figure 42.1 Schematic illustrating the relationship of "syncope" to other conditions that cause real or apparent transient loss of consciousness (TLOC). Syncope is characterized by causing TLOC as a result of a self-limited inadequacy of cerebral perfusion.

In part, variations among published reports examining epidemiologic aspects of "syncope" may relate to the terminology issues alluded to above. In any event, as pointed out by Sheldon and Serletis,[18] conventional clinical epidemiologic terms such as "prevalence" (the proportion of people with the disease) and "incidence" (the proportion of people acquiring the disease in a sampling interval) are not readily applicable to the problem of understanding the epidemiology of "syncope". For instance, these authors argue quite insightfully that syncope prevalence must approach zero since at any point in time very few people are unconscious. Similarly, since syncope is a transient symptom that vanishes, its true "incidence" is difficult to assess. Sheldon and Serletis[18] suggest more meaningful indices such as cumulative proportion, cumulative event rate or cumulative incidence.

Given the limitations noted above, it is possible to obtain from the literature a rough sense of the "burden" of syncope in various population subsets. Thus, the Framingham Study (in which biennial examinations were carried out over a 26-year period in 5209 free-living individuals) reported occurrence of at least one syncope event in approximately 3% of men and 3.5% of women in a relatively broad-based free-living population sample.[19] The first syncope occurred at an average age of 52 years (range 17–78 years) for men and 50 years (range 13–87 years) for women. Further, while syncope occurred at virtually all ages, syncope burden tended to increase with advancing age from 8/1000 person-exams in the 35–44 year old age group to approximately 40/1000 person-exams in the ≥75 year age group.

In more selected populations, syncope has been estimated to occur in 15% of children <18 years of age, 25% of the young military population, and in up to 23% of a nursing home population >70 years of age.[15,16,18–24] However,

with respect to the elderly patient, the reported frequency may well be an underestimate since up to 20% of these individuals are believed to be forgetful for such episodes (i.e. retrograde amnesia).

Two reports provide the most up-to-date assessment of syncope burden among free-living persons. Ganzeboom et al[22] surveyed medical students in The Netherlands and found that 39% had fainted at least once by about age 25 (women 47% versus men 24%). A Canadian report indicated that the likelihood of at least one faint was 37% by age 60, and almost all first spells occurred by age 40.[24] Combined, these studies suggest that 40% of people faint at least once in their lives.

Recurrence rates

Among patients who have experienced syncope, it has been estimated that syncope recurrences occur in about 30%.[19,22,24] About one-third of patients have recurrences of syncope by 3 years of follow-up, with most recurrences occurring within the first 2 years. Predictors of recurrence of syncope include:
- age <45 years
- a psychiatric diagnosis, and
- a long history of prior syncope recurrences; in particular, patients with more than six syncope spells and a positive tilt-table test (i.e. suggestive that syncope is of neurally mediated reflex origin) have a high risk of syncope recurrence (>50% over 2 years).

Mortality

The presence and severity of co-existing structural heart disease are the most important predictors of mortality risk in syncope patients. Thus, among individuals with cardiac syncope (i.e. primary cardiac arrhythmia, an ischemic episode or severe valvular heart disease), the 1-year mortality is high (ranging between 18% and 33%) compared to that for patients with either non-cardiac (including "vasovagal") causes of syncope (0–12%) or unexplained syncope. The risk of death differences are even more striking when considering "sudden cardiac death" events: the 1-year incidence of sudden death is approximately 24% in patients with a cardiac cause versus about 3% in the other two groups.[6,19]

Although patients with cardiac syncope have higher mortality rates compared with those of non-cardiac or unknown causes, cardiac syncope patients do not as a rule appear to exhibit a higher mortality when compared with matched controls having similar degrees of heart disease.[25–29] There are, however, some important exceptions to this rule. These include severe aortic stenosis (average survival without valve replacement of 2 years), hypertrophic cardiomyopathy in which syncope at diagnosis is a predictor of increased sudden death risk, and possibly patients with heart failure and severe left ventricular dysfunction.[29] The mortality risk associated with syncope in the setting of one of the channelopathies (e.g. Brugada syndrome, long QT syndrome (LQTS)) or in the presence of arrhythmogenic right ventricular dysplasia (ARVD) may reasonably be considered to fall into this exception as well, if the syncope is known to be due to ventricular tachyarrhythmias.

A number of subgroups of syncope patients can be identified who have an excellent prognosis. These include young healthy individuals without heart disease and normal electrocardiogram (ECG), individuals with the most common forms of neurally mediated reflex syndromes (i.e. vasovagal faint, most situational faints) and syncope of unknown cause (5% first-year mortality). Patients with carotid sinus syndrome (CSS) may be expected to have a more worrisome prognosis given the close association of CSS with underlying atherosclerotic cardiovascular disease. However, syncope may result in injury. Major morbidity such as fractures and motor vehicle accidents are reported in 6% of patients, and minor injury such as laceration and bruises in 29%. Recurrent syncope is associated with fractures and soft tissue injury in approximately 12% of patients.

Prognostic issues remaining to be resolved

Failing to distinguish the additional risks associated with recurrent syncope from the risks accompanying any underlying co-morbidity (especially heart disease) is a common error. The result is that physicians may overlook the need to address syncope risk directly as they focus on the treatment of the underlying heart disease (or occasionally vice versa).

For instance, implantable cardioverter-defibrillator (ICD) therapy is often recommended in patients with syncope and left ventricular ejection fraction (LVEF) <30%. Clearly, an ICD may well be indicated, but it would be indicated even in the absence of syncope. On the other hand, while the ICD may prevent sudden death, it takes time to detect an arrhythmia and initiate treatment; consequently, it may not protect the patient from injury due to recurrent syncope (even if the syncope is due to ventricular tachyarrhythmias). Further assessment of the patient is needed.

The impact of syncope has been a particular concern in "channelopathy" patients, specifically in LQTS or Brugada pattern.[30–33] With regard to LQTS, in one large prospective observational trial in >800 patients,[30] cardiovascular endpoints including apparent syncope, cardiac arrest and sudden death occurred in 23% of patients. Syncope was associated with a fivefold increased risk of cardiac arrest or sudden death, but it was not a sensitive predictor of death risk. Similarly, in patients with the so-called Brugada pattern on ECG who have a history of syncope, the observation has been made that syncope is not a sensitive predictor of or risk factor for sudden death. In a multicenter study, 40% of 220 Brugada patients implanted with an ICD had a history of syncope, but the patients with syncope were not at a higher risk of appropriate ICD discharge than those who had been asymptomatic.[31] Similarly, in a large meta-analysis encompassing 1140 patients (262 of them (23%) with a history of syncope), the patients with syncope had the same risk of ventricular tachyarrhythmias as those who had been without syncope, and a significantly lower risk than those presenting with documented cardiac arrest.[33]

Pathophysiology

The syncope victim is usually in the upright position at the onset of the attack. Syncope in the supine position should raise the possibility of marked bradycardia or very rapid tachyarrhythmias. Supine syncope due to neural reflex hypotension has also been reported, but is believed to be uncommon.

The relationship of upright posture to increased susceptibility to transient cerebral hypoperfusion is readily understandable since in humans, upright posture substantially reduces the safety factor for cerebral perfusion. Upon arising from being seated or supine, approximately 500–1000 mL of blood moves relatively rapidly from the central circulation to the venous system below the diaphragm. Physiologic adaptive countermeasures, including peripheral vaso- and venoconstriction, enhanced muscle pump activity, thoracic respiratory pump action, and moderate tachycardia, automatically come into play to prevent an otherwise inevitable drop in cerebral blood flow. Additionally, the "autoregulatory" nature of the cerebrovascular circulation helps to maintain flow despite fluctuation of perfusion pressure. Thus, the healthy well-hydrated human is usually able to cope quite effectively with even very abrupt positional change. On the other hand, despite built-in compensatory mechanisms, many individuals (even those in good health) may experience transient symptomatic hypotension when moving quickly from the supine or seated to upright posture. In the vast majority, this scenario is typically abrupt in onset, occurs promptly after posture change (i.e. "immediate" hypotension), is brief in duration, and is manifest only as a temporary loss of vision (so-called "gray-out").[34] The immediate hypotensive event is rarely a cause for concern. However, of a more serious nature, in some patients frank syncope may occur after movement to upright posture (so-called postural or "orthostatic" faints). In these cases, the faint is usually somewhat delayed after the postural change, suggesting that the mechanism is more than just the "immediate" hypotensive response.[35] In some of these patients there appears to be a more complete failure of physiologic adaptation mechanisms, due to diseases of the autonomic nervous system. In the majority of cases, however, more commonly encountered conditions are the cause, including:

- drug therapy (e.g. diuretics, vasodilators)
- generalized frailty in a chronically ill individual
- dehydration
- recent exposure to extended periods of bedrest or gravitation-reduced environment.

Quite often, hypotension leading to syncope is the result of neurally mediated reflex disturbances of blood pressure control (e.g. vasovagal faint, situational faints, carotid sinus syndrome, etc.). Vasovagal and situational faints (e.g. post-micturition syncope) are among the most frequent causes of syncope in all age groups, and are the most common of the so-called neurally mediated reflex syncope syndrome (Box 42.1). In some of these cases the predominant outcome of inappropriate neural reflex activity is parasympathetic-induced bradycardia or asystole (so-called cardio-inhibitory syncope). In others, symptomatic hypotension is due primarily to inappropriate vasodilation (i.e. vasodepressor syncope). In most cases, however, both phenomena contribute.[1,36,37]

Primary cardiac arrhythmias are a less frequent cause of syncope in the general population than are the conditions noted above. Nonetheless, when at fault (usually in individuals with structural heart disease) they are important to identify since they may have a worrisome prognosis, and they can usually be treated effectively whether by drugs, ablation or implantable devices.

Paroxysmal supraventricular and ventricular tachycardias (SVT, VT), intermittent atrioventricular (AV) block or sinus node pauses are among the most common primary cardiac arrhythmias associated with syncope. However, the basis for syncope in the setting of these arrhythmias may be complex. By way of example, an abrupt blood pressure decrease starting immediately after tachyarrhythmia onset occurs even in patients with normal hearts. Certainly, the rapid heart rate plays an important role in this phenomenon. However, other factors may contribute. Sudden atrial distension and vigorous atrial contraction against closed AV valves (in tachycardias with AV dissociation) may cause not only a reduced forward flow but also a neurally mediated reflex vasodilation that may undermine the effectiveness of adaptive vaso- and venoconstrictive mechanisms. Further, in elderly or infirm patients, muscle pump and respiratory pump activity may be compromised, thereby increasing the chance that perfusion pressure may fall below the autoregulation capability of the cerebrovascular bed.

In patients with cardiac disease such as hypertrophic cardiomyopathy (HCM) or aortic stenosis, both SVT and VT may cause cardiac syncope. However, neurally mediated reflex hypotension may also contribute; the triggers are believed to come from the heart itself, presumably via excessive stretch on ventricular and atrial mechanoreceptors.

Diagnosis

The European Society Task Force on Syncope guidelines,[1] the American College of Cardiology Task Force report on tilt-table testing,[38] the American Academy of Emergency Medicine practice guidelines[39] and the ACC/AHA Scientific Statement on Syncope[5] provide recommendations regarding the appropriate strategy for diagnosis and treatment of syncope (Fig. 42.2), including risk-stratification advice regarding the need for hospitalization. For the most part these recommendations have been primarily "expert" consensus-based documents. However, recently several observational studies and randomized clinical trials have begun to contribute to our better understanding of how syncope management practices might be improved.

Classification of the causes of syncope

Box 42.1 provides a classification of the principal causes of syncope likely to be encountered in general internal medicine or family practice. However, it should be borne in mind that a single diagnosis may not be sufficient; more than one cause may contribute to the clinical picture (especially in the older patient).

Neurally mediated reflex syncope

The vasovagal (or "common") and situational faints occur in virtually all age groups, and may be triggered by any of a variety of factors, including prolonged standing (particu-

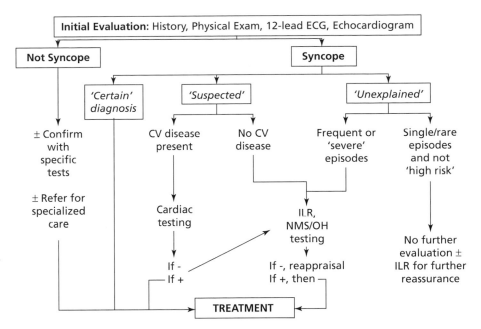

Figure 42.2 Algorithm, modified from that proposed by the European Society of Cardiology Syncope Task Force guidelines,[1] depicting an approach to the clinical evaluation of syncope. As discussed in the text, a careful initial evaluation by an experienced clinician can often provide a "certain" diagnosis of the cause of syncope. In such cases, no further evaluation is needed, and treatment as needed may begin. However, in many instances the outcome of the initial assessment is only a "suspected" diagnosis or even an "unexplained" cause. In such cases, further selective testing is needed. An appropriate pathway is indicated here. See text for details. ILR, implantable or insertable loop recorder; NMS, neurally mediated reflex syncope; OH, orthostatic hypotension; TLOC, transient loss of consciousness.

BOX 42.1 Syncope and syncope mimics: a classification

Syncope
- Neurally mediated reflex syncope
  - Vasovagal faint
  - Carotid sinus syncope
  - Situational faints (e.g. cough syncope, post micturition, defecation, etc.)
  - Pain triggered
- Orthostatic syncope
  - Chronic blood/plasma loss (e.g. hemorrhage, diarrhea)
  - Primary autonomic failure syndromes (e.g. pure autonomic failure, multiple system atrophy, Parkinson's disease with autonomic failure)
  - Secondary autonomic failure syndromes (neuropathies: diabetic, alcohol, amyloid)
  - Drugs (vasodilators, diuretics)
- Primary cardiac arrhythmias
  - Sinus node dysfunction (including bradycardia/tachycardia syndrome)
  - AV conduction system disease
  - Paroxysmal supraventricular and ventricular tachycardias
  - Channelopathies (LQTS, Brugada, etc.)
  - Implanted device (pacemaker, ICD) malfunction

- Structural cardiovascular or cardiopulmonary disease
  - Severe aortic stenosis
  - Acute myocardial infarction/ischemia
  - Cardiac valvular disease/ischemia infarction
  - Atrial myxoma, ball-valve thrombus
  - Obstructive cardiomyopathy
  - Pericardial disease/tamponade
  - Prosthetic valve malfunction
  - Pulmonary embolus
  - Pulmonary hypertension
  - Subclavian steal syndrome
- Cerebrovascular
  - Vascular steal syndromes
  - Acute hypoxemia
  - Migraine

Syncope mimics – disorders resembling syncope
- Seizures
- Psychogenic "syncope" (conversion reaction)
- Hyperventilation (hypocapnia)
- Intoxications
- Accidental falls (usually in elderly/infirm persons)

---

larly in warm, emotionally charged environments), unpleasant sights, and pain. The diagnosis is most often suspected from the medical history; however, the history is not always definitive, especially in the elderly.[40] In such cases, the accounts of eye-witnesses become crucial and tilt-table testing (**Class IIa, Level C**) and use of implantable loop recorders (**Class I, Level B**) become important diagnostic tests.[1,41–45] The ATP test, although controversial

(**Class IIb*, Level C**), may also prove helpful to the clinician, especially in the older patient in whom pacemaker therapy is a consideration.[46–49]

Carotid sinus syndrome is one form of neurally mediated reflex syncope that tends to occur in older male patients, probably related to higher predilection to atherosclerotic cardiovascular disease in that population. Published experience suggests that CSS may be a more important cause of non-accidental "falls" or "spells" in older individuals than had previously been appreciated.[50] The condition is suspected by careful history taking, but its presence is confirmed when symptoms are reproduced during carotid sinus massage (best undertaken with the patient in the upright position secured on a tilt-table), particularly if there is concomitant induction of an asystolic pause, paroxysmal AV block, and/or a marked drop in systemic arterial pressure (**Class I, Level B**). In the absence of symptom reproduction, a pause of ≥5 seconds is often considered sufficient to support the diagnosis (assuming other etiologies of syncope have been excluded). An implantable loop recorder (ILR) may also prove helpful in suggesting the diagnosis of CSS, but limitations include absence of direct correlation of syncope with carotid stimulation, and the possibility of "missing" a major vasodepressor hypotension episode since it is not yet possible to monitor systemic pressure with these devices.

Orthostatic (postural) syncope

Frank syncope induced by moving from supine or seated to upright posture is an important problem in elderly or less physically fit individuals, or patients who are volume depleted. Iatrogenic factors such as excessive diuresis or aggressive prescription of antihypertensive drugs may be important contributors. Inadequate fluid intake, especially by older persons who have diminished thirst drive or who purposely avoid fluids due to genitourinary system issues, is another important contributor. Less often, primary forms of autonomic nervous system dysfunction are the underlying predisposing cause, including pure autonomic failure, multiple system atrophy, and Parkinson's disease.[51–53]

In most clinical practices overt primary autonomic dysfunction is relatively rare. Nevertheless, becoming familiar with its presentations may be of value in determining the cause of orthostatic symptoms in some patients, and perhaps better understanding symptoms in a much larger group of patients who have less well-defined disorders, such as postural orthostatic tachycardia syndrome (POTS). Furthermore, as the features of autonomic dysfunction become more widely appreciated, subtly affected patients will be identified more often. For instance, Low et al[54] reviewed an experience in 155 patients referred for assessment of suspected orthostatic hypotension. Findings in this referral population revealed that among the most severely affected symptomatic patients (n = 90, mean age 64 years), pure autonomic failure accounted for 33%, multisystem atrophy for 26%, and autonomic/diabetic neuropathy for 31%. Finally, secondary autonomic dysfunction due to neuropathies associated with chronic diseases (e.g. diabetes mellitus), toxic agents (e.g. alcohol) or infections (e.g. Guillain–Barré syndrome) are relatively common in medical practice, and may also cause syncope in association with orthostatic hypotension.

Primary cardiac arrhythmias

Primary cardiac arrhythmias (i.e. those rhythm disturbances arising as a result of cardiac conduction system disturbances, anomalous electrical connections, myocardial disease or "channelopathies") are less frequent causes of syncope than either the neurally mediated or orthostatic triggers, but they are of importance due to their more worrying prognostic implications. In general terms, the arrhythmias most often associated with syncope or near-syncope are the bradyarrhythmias accompanying sinus node dysfunction or AV block, and the tachyarrhythmias of ventricular origin. Only a very brief overview is provided here as these conditions are discussed in detail elsewhere in this volume.

Sinus node dysfunction Sinus node dysfunction (SND) comprises various sinus node and/or atrial arrhythmias that may result in persistent or intermittent periods of inappropriate slow (sinus bradycardia, sinus pauses, sinoatrial exit block) or, on the other hand, excessively fast heart beating (most often atrial fibrillation or atrial flutter), or both manifestations at different times in the same individual.[55,56] SND may be considered to be "intrinsic" or "extrinsic". Intrinsic SND is closely associated with structural disturbances in the atria (e.g. fibrosis, chamber enlargement) resulting from aging, disease or prior cardiac surgery. Extrinsic SND may be due to autonomic nervous system influences, cardioactive drugs, and/or metabolic disturbances.[57–59] In terms of syncope, bradyarrhythmias associated with SND appear to be the more important culprits than tachyarrhythmias.[56]

Disturbances of atrioventricular conduction Disturbances of AV conduction range from relatively innocent abnormalities (e.g. first-degree AV block) to complete conduction failure (third-degree AV block).[60–62] As a rule, however, it is the more severe forms of acquired AV block (that is, Mobitz type II block, "high-grade" and complete AV block) that are most closely associated with syncope. In contrast to acquired forms of AV block, congenital complete AV block was for a long time considered to be relatively benign. However, it is now known that syncope is more common and mortality greater in congenital AV block patients than had previously been suspected.[60]

Whether syncope occurs in patients with various forms of bundle branch block or fascicular conduction system disease depends both on the risk of developing high-grade or complete AV block and on the risk of occurrence of ventricular tachyarrhythmias.[62] Diagnostic electrophysiologic testing may be useful in such cases.

Ventricular tachyarrhythmias Ventricular tachyarrhythmias (VT) have been reported to be responsible for syncope in up to 20% of patients referred for electrophysiologic assessment. Risk factors favoring VT as a cause of syncope include underlying structural heart disease, underlying conduction system disease, congenital or drug-induced LQTS or other so-called "channelopathies". The latter conditions present special risks of both syncope and sudden death.[63-68] Syncope in channelopathy patients may be due to any cause (including vasovagal faints), but the specific and most critical risk is syncope due to polymorphic VT, including torsades de pointes. The mere presence of a "history of syncope" is not sufficient reason to implicate a VT as the cause and consequently, while ICD therapy in such a situation (i.e. no evidence of a VT) is recommended by guidelines (**Class IIb, Level B**), there continues to be room for debate.[68] In any case, the assumption that VT is the cause of syncope should not be taken lightly even if an ICD has been placed. An ICD may prevent premature death, but may act too late to prevent syncope (or, as alluded to already, may not even be relevant to the cause of syncope in a particular individual).[25,28,29]

Supraventricular tachyarrhythmias Supraventricular tachycardias are relatively infrequent causes of syncope.[1,69,70] Tachycardia rate, the volume status and posture of the patient at time of onset of the arrhythmia, the presence of associated structural cardiopulmonary disease, the integrity of reflex peripheral vascular compensation, and the promptness with which normal cardiac activity resumes after termination of the tachycardia are key factors determining whether hypotension of sufficient severity to cause syncope occurs.[70]

Structural cardiovascular or cardiopulmonary disease

Structural cardiac or cardiopulmonary disease is often present in syncope patients, particularly those in older age groups. However, in these cases it is usually arrhythmias associated with structural disease, rather than the abnormal structure itself, that are more often the cause of symptoms. In terms of syncope directly attributable to structural disease, the most common is that which occurs in conjunction with acute myocardial ischemia or infarction, pulmonary embolism and pulmonary hypertension. The basis of syncope in these conditions is multifactorial, including both the hemodynamic impact of the specific lesion as well as neurally mediated reflex effects.

Syncope may also occur and be a presenting feature in conditions in which there is fixed or dynamic obstruction to left ventricular outflow (e.g. aortic stenosis, hypertrophic obstructive cardiomyopathy (HOCM)). In such cases symptoms are often provoked by physical exertion, but may also develop if an otherwise benign arrhythmia should occur (e.g. atrial fibrillation). The basis for the faint is in part inadequate blood flow due to the mechanical obstruction. However, especially in the case of valvular aortic ste-

nosis, ventricular mechanoreceptor-mediated bradycardia and vasodilation is thought to be an important contributor. In obstructive cardiomyopathy, neural reflex mechanisms may also play a role in causing syncope, but atrial tachyarrhythmias (particularly atrial fibrillation) or ventricular tachycardia (even at relatively modest rates) can also trigger hypotension.[71-74]

Cerebrovascular, neurologic, and psychiatric disturbances

Cerebrovascular disease and neurologic disturbances are rarely the cause of true syncope.[1] However, these conditions may result in a clinical picture that can be mistaken for syncope even by experienced practitioners. For example, temporal lobe epilepsy may closely mimic (or induce) neurally mediated reflex bradycardia and hypotension. In such cases, neurologic consultation becomes essential.

Fixed cerebrovascular disease is almost never responsible for syncope due to the redundancy of the cerebral circulation (multiple vessels accessing the circle of Willis).[75] Consequently, searching for carotid artery disease in syncope patients by Doppler studies or angiography is rarely useful. On the other hand, global cerebrovascular spasm (possibly as part of a migraine syndrome) could trigger syncope. However, as well as can be determined, the frequency with which this mechanism occurs is vanishingly small; most faints in "migraineurs" are of vasovagal origin.[75]

Psychiatric conditions do not cause syncope, but may result in syncope mimics. Thus, conversion reactions may be responsible for symptoms that are difficult to distinguish from loss of consciousness events. Similarly, anxiety attacks may be associated with severe hyperventilation resulting in hypocapnia and transient alkalosis that cause "syncope-like" symptoms. Considerable effort (including multiple consultations to various specialists) is often expended before a pseudo-syncope diagnosis is comfortably established. When these conditions are suspected, psychiatric consultation is needed.

Strategy for the diagnostic evaluation

Structure of the syncope evaluation

The ultimate goal of the diagnostic evaluation is to establish a sufficiently strong correlation between symptoms and detected abnormalities to permit both an assessment of prognosis and initiation of an appropriate treatment plan. Care must be taken to avoid assuming that the mere presence of an abnormality provides a basis for the patient's symptoms.

A careful history and physical examination form the basis for the initial assessment of the syncope patient (see Fig. 42.2). Alone, these first steps provide a diagnosis in a substantial proportion of patients, especially in younger individuals in whom vasovagal faints predominate and the history is clear-cut. However, in many other cases even an experienced history-taker cannot be certain of the diagnosis, and further testing is needed. In this regard, the front-line physician must determine whether such testing requires hospitalization or if outpatient evaluation is safe (i.e. minimal chance of mortality or syncope recurrence with either injury or necessitating hospitalization within the next few weeks to months). Thus, patients who may be safely evaluated outside hospital include those "low-risk" individuals who exhibit any of the following features: absence of evident structural heart disease and a normal ECG, history of recurrent syncope over many years or suspicion that the presentation is that of a "syncope mimic" (e.g. psychogenic pseudo-syncope). Unfortunately, however, apart from these very low-risk patients, it is difficult to "risk stratify" moderate- to high-risk TLOC/syncope patients.[76,77]

Although, as noted earlier, ED practice patterns in the US may be changing, hospital admission for syncope management remains very frequent despite the fact that in many instances outpatient assessment would be just as safe and far less expensive. Potentially, greater availability of "syncope management units" (SMU), "rapid access black-out clinics" (best illustrated by that in Manchester, UK) or "TLOC/syncope clinics" may reduce inappropriate hospital admissions.

Medical history taking The first step in the assessment of the patient with presumed syncope is to obtain a detailed medical history of the events, including interviewing bystanders and relatives.[1,40,78–82] Throughout the history taking, it is important to bear in mind that co-morbidities may contribute to syncope susceptibility. Consequently, it is essential to pay attention to other disease conditions that may be present.

Unfortunately, the utility of history taking is limited by the practitioner's clinical experience. Consequently, the availability of a more structured history-taking instrument may prove helpful. Several reports have provided insight into this aspect of the clinical care pathway.[40,80]

In the most recent of the structured history-taking approaches, a quantitative method was applied by the Calgary Syncope Symptom Study in assessing whether vasovagal syncope could be distinguished from epilepsy and if vasovagal syncope could be distinguished from other causes of syncope.[80] With regard to the syncope versus seizures question, the findings in 539 patients in whom the cause of loss of consciousness was known (various types of epilepsy, vasovagal syncope, and cardiac arrhythmias) were assessed. A point score to differentiate syncope from seizures was derived, and proved to have a sensitivity of 94% and a specificity of 94%. Historical aspects suggestive of seizure activity included preceding emotional stress, "déjà vu" sensation, unusual posturing or motor activity during an event, confusion upon awakening or tongue injury. Conversely, syncope was favored by separate episodes of pre-syncope, diaphoresis or an event precipitated by prolonged standing or sitting.

In terms of the second issue, the causes of syncope were known in 323 patients. The point score correctly classified 90% of patients, diagnosing vasovagal syncope with 89% sensitivity and 91% specificity.[80] Factors favoring vasovagal syncope included pre-syncope or syncope with orthostatic stress, pain or medical settings, and a prodrome of warmth or diaphoresis. Elements suggesting causes other than vasovagal syncope included a history of cardiac conduction system disease, supraventricular tachycardia, diabetes or findings such as cyanosis during syncope or having a first syncope at age >35 years.

The medical history is not equally valuable in all age groups. Del Rosso *et al*[81] found that the medical history was only one-fifth (5% v 25%) as effective for defining a cause of syncope in individuals >65 years compared to younger patients. Further, recollection of prodromal symptoms was also less in older versus younger individuals. Consequently, the evaluation of the elderly "fainter" inevitably will require greater reliance on ancillary tests.

Physical examination Physical findings that suggest a basis for syncope include:
• orthostatic hypotension: the frequency of orthostatic fainting is low in young patients; it has been reported to account for 30% of faints in patients >75 years of age[82]
• abnormal response to carotid sinus massage (CSM): this is unusual in younger fainters, but becomes an important condition as individuals age. CSM is usually recommended as part of the syncope evaluation in all syncope patients >55 years of age. A CSM-induced pause >3 seconds duration is considered abnormal and, while not definitive, raises the possibility of carotid sinus syndrome as a cause of symptoms
• upper extremity differences in blood pressure/pulse suggesting subclavian steal or aortic dissection
• pathologic cardiac murmurs (e.g. aortic stenosis, HCM) or vascular bruits
• evidence of pulmonary hypertension (often supported by echocardiographic findings).
The 12-lead ECG is part of the initial evaluation, although it only infrequently (<5% of cases) identifies a specific cause of syncope. However, 12-lead ECG findings such as a Q-wave, left ventricular hypertrophy, a prolonged QT interval, Brugada syndrome pattern or ventricular pre-excitation pattern may suggest the presence of organic heart disease or electrophysiologic abnormality, that helps to direct further testing. Similarly, echocardiography is increasingly considered to be an element of the initial evaluation (especially in North America), although its use may

be best reserved for instances when the status of underlying cardiac disease is unclear based on history or prior studies. For the most part, the value of the echocardiogram is in assessing left ventricular function and occasionally evaluating the severity of suspected structural abnormalities such as aortic or mitral valvular stenosis, or pulmonary hypertension.

If the initial evaluation (history, physical examination, 12-lead ECG, and echocardiogram) provides a "definite" diagnosis, no further testing is needed and if warranted, treatment may be started. However, the initial evaluation is often only suggestive of a basis for loss of consciousness or is non-diagnostic. In such cases the investigation must be continued, but can be directed more effectively based on the "initial evaluation" findings (see Fig. 42.2).

Additional testing As a rule, if structural heart disease is deemed absent by initial evaluation and there is no history of "palpitations", then neurally mediated reflex syncope or orthostatic hypotension is by far the most likely cause of syncope. In this setting, tilt-table testing in conjunction with related assessment of autonomic nervous system function (e.g. carotid sinus massage, response to cough, etc.) is the most useful diagnostic approach. However, it may be reasonably argued that an ILR might be an even more cost-effective strategy at this stage.[41–44]

If abnormal cardiac findings were identified on the initial evaluation, then the next step should be determining their functional significance by hemodynamic and/or angiographic assessment. In addition, since cardiac arrhythmias are a common cause of syncope in patients with structural cardiac disease, assessing the patient's susceptibility to tachy- and bradyarrhythmias becomes a priority. The strategy for this latter step will depend on an estimate of the immediate mortality risk. In low-risk settings, non-invasive techniques (for example, ambulatory ECG) or ILRs may be reasonable (see below). On the other hand, if the risk is assessed to be higher (e.g. low LVEF, clinically relevant valvular heart disease), then invasive electrophysiologic testing is warranted. Such testing may be helpful even in patients with low LVEF and criteria for ICD therapy, for reasons explained earlier. Tilt-table testing would follow if the diagnosis remains in doubt.[1] Only infrequently should specialized neurologic studies be ordered early in the evaluation (for example, if the history was suggestive of a seizure disorder rather than syncope).[1,83,84]

Electrocardiographic (ECG) recordings Documenting the cardiac rhythm (and, if possible, the corresponding arterial blood pressure) during a spontaneous episode is perhaps the single most valuable observation in the evaluation of syncope. However, most syncope patients have a symptom frequency (i.e. interval between events) measured in weeks

or months, but not days. Consequently, syncope–ECG correlation is rarely achieved with 24-hour or 48-hour Holter monitoring (yield is variably reported as 6% and 20%, but may in fact be much less). Longer term ambulatory ECG recording is usually needed.

Both wearable and implantable long-term (weeks to months) ECG monitor systems are available. Unfortunately, conventional event recorders often have limited diagnostic utility in syncope if the patient has to apply the recorder to the chest just prior to or immediately following the period of unconsciousness. In the absence of a very prolonged premonitory warning period or the presence of a very astute bystander, such use is often impossible. To circumvent these latter limitations, a continuously attached event recorder system using wireless telemetry (so-called mobile cardiac outpatient telemetry, MCOT) has recently been introduced. These devices not only permit the recording of transient events, but also offer the ability for critical data to be transmitted without need for patient interaction. In a recent report, MCOT (Cardionet Inc, San Diego, CA) provided a significantly higher diagnostic yield when compared with a conventional patient-activated external looping event monitor (LOOP) in a 17-center prospective clinical trial with patients randomized to either LOOP or MCOT for up to 30 days.[85] A total of 266 patients who completed the monitoring period were analyzed. A diagnosis was made in 88% of MCOT subjects compared with 75% of LOOP subjects ($P = 0.008$). Currently, MCOT is only available in the USA.[85,86]

Implantable loop recorders (ILRs) such as the Reveal® family (Medtronic Inc, Minneapolis, MN) and Confirm® (St Jude Medical Inc, St Paul, MN) have become important tools for capturing transient arrhythmias.[41–45,87,88] On the downside, although remote downloading of stored data is now available (e.g. Carelink®, Medtronic Inc), these ILRs still require manual interaction by the patient or other individual in order to initiate transmission. A newer generation ILR (Sleuth®, Transoma Inc, St Paul, MN) overcomes this latter limitation by providing wireless download capability that operates without need for human interaction.

ILRs have been the subject of several important studies that illustrate their value in the diagnosis of the causes of syncope. In the ISSUE 2 diagnosis study,[45] 343 patients with suspected reflex syncope underwent tilt-table testing (positive in 164, 48%). In addition, 180 patients underwent an adenosine triphosphate (ATP) test (positive in 53, 29%). All patients also had an ILR placed. Syncope was documented by the ILR in 106 (26%) patients at a median of 3 months follow-up. An asystolic pause was more frequently found during spontaneous syncope than during tilt-testing (45% v 21%, $P = 0.02$), although there was a trend for those with an asystolic response on tilt-test also to have an asystolic response during spontaneous syncope (75% v 37%, $P = 0.1$). Patients with positive ATP test responses showed syncope recurrence rates and apparent mechanism of syncope similar to those with negative ATP tests.

In the Eastbourne Syncope Assessment (EaSyAS) trial,[88] 201 patients (median age 74) with recurrent unexplained syncope were randomized to receive an ILR or conventional diagnostic strategy. During follow-up (median duration, 17 months), an ECG diagnosis was obtained in 42 (43%) ILR patients compared to eight (6%) patients in the conventional diagnosis group (hazard ratio (HR) 6.53, 95% confidence interval (CI) 3.73–11.4, P < 0.001).

Exercise testing is usually of limited utility in assessing the basis of syncope unless the medical history indicates that the events are clearly related to physical exertion. Thus, when selectively employed, exercise testing may permit detection of rate-dependent AV block, exercise-induced tachyarrhythmias or the exercise-associated variant of neurally mediated syncope.[89,90] Finally, although the signal-averaged ECG (SAECG) cannot provide direct evidence for the cause of syncope, such testing may be helpful in patients with ischemic heart disease if "normal"; a normal SAECG tends to exclude susceptibility to ventricular tachyarrhythmias.[91–94] Similarly, a negative T-wave alternans (TWA) test tends to reduce the likelihood of a life-threatening tachyarrhythmia being the cause of the patients' symptoms.[95,96]

In summary, the basis of infrequent but recurring syncope episodes is unlikely to be established by either conventional 24- or 48-hour ambulatory ECG recording, or by conventional external "event" recorders. The longer monitoring capabilities of MCOT systems provide some distinct advantages. Nevertheless, even MCOT may be difficult for patients to tolerate for more than 2–3 weeks. Consequently, in such a setting, consideration should be given to utilizing an ILR. ILRs have proved to be cost-effective, with the majority of ILR patients providing symptom–ECG correlation within a year of device placement.

Imaging techniques Echocardiography is the most widely employed imaging technique in the syncope evaluation, but it rarely provides a definitive basis for symptoms. Nonetheless, the echocardiogram is invaluable in many syncope evaluations given the importance of identifying underlying structural heart disease in these patients. Further, in some cases the echocardiogram may provide direct clues to the cause if, for example, HOCM, severe valvular aortic stenosis, intracardiac tumor (e.g. myxoma) or anomalous origin of one of the coronary arteries is detected.

Head-up tilt-table testing and electrophysiologic testing To date, the head-up tilt-table test is the only diagnostic tool to have been subjected to sufficient clinical scrutiny to assess its effectiveness in the diagnostic evaluation of vasovagal syncope. The evidence supporting its utility in this setting is sufficiently convincing, and both the ESC Syncope Task Force and an ACC "expert" task force have provided recommendations regarding indications for and methodology of appropriate use of the tilt-table laboratory[1,38] (**Class II, Level B**). Such testing, especially when undertaken in the absence of drugs, appears to discriminate well between symptomatic patients and asymptomatic control subjects; this remains true even when nitroglycerin (so-called "Italian protocol") or isoproterenol is used. Tilt-table testing at 60, 70, and 80 degrees exhibited specificities of 92%, 92%, and 80% respectively with low-dose isoproterenol provocation.[97] On the other hand, equally strong evidence indicates that head-up tilt is not useful to predict treatment effectiveness (**Class III, Level B**). The ISSUE study clearly demonstrated that the physiologic observations on the tilt-table do not reliably correspond to those obtained when spontaneous faints are recorded.[44,45,98] Thus, tilt-table tests may demonstrate susceptibility to vasovagal faints, but do not provide insight into whether the spontaneous events are cardio-inhibitory, vasodepressor or "mixed" in nature. On the other hand, recordings made by ILRs during spontaneous faints are highly reproducible and therefore predictive of mechanism of subsequent events.[99]

Although there are no large randomized studies, there is reasonably strong evidence to indicate that electrophysiologic testing (EPS) is most likely to be diagnostic in individuals with underlying structural heart disease[100–104] (**Class II, Level B**). For example, in a review by Camm and Lau,[69] testing was clearly more successful in patients with structural cardiac disease (71%) than in patients without (36%). However, care must be taken in interpreting EPS findings in syncope patients. Fujimura et al[105] found that among 21 syncope patients with known symptomatic sinus pauses or AV block, EPS only correctly identified 3/8 of the former (sensitivity 37.5%) and 2/13 of the latter patients (sensitivity 15.4%). On the other hand, although firm evidence is lacking, the induction of sustained re-entry supraventricular or ventricular tachycardia in a syncope patient is highly likely to be significant. These arrhythmias are rarely inconsequential bystanders.

The combination of tilt-table testing and invasive EPS has been evaluated in syncope patients, but the reports are few, date from the pre-ILR era (i.e. a true "gold standard" was not available to confirm findings), and were not controlled. By way of example, Sra et al[104] reported EPS results in conjunction with head-up tilt testing in 86 consecutive patients referred for evaluation of unexplained syncope. EPS was abnormal in 29 (34%) of patients, with the majority of these (21 patients) exhibiting inducible sustained monomorphic VT. Among the remaining patients, head-up tilt testing proved positive in 34 (40%) cases, while 23 patients (26%) remained undiagnosed. In general, patients exhibiting positive electrophysiologic findings were older, more frequently male, and had lower LVEFs and more structural heart disease than patients with positive head-up tilt tests or patients in whom no diagnosis was determined. Using a similar approach, Fitzpatrick *et al*[106] analyzed findings in 322 syncope patients. Conventional EPS provided a basis for syncope in 229 of 322 cases (71%), with 93 patients having a normal study. Among the patients with abnormal EPS findings, AV conduction disease was diagnosed in 34%, sinus node dysfunction in 21%, CSS in 10%, and an inducible sustained tachyarrhythmia in 6%. In the 93 patients with normal EPS, tilt-table testing was undertaken in 71 cases, and resulted in syncope consistent with a vasovagal faint, in 53/71 (75%) of this subset.

Neurologic studies Conventional neurologic laboratory studies (EEG, head CT and MRI) have a low diagnostic yield in unselected syncope patients. For instance, among the 433 syncope evaluations reviewed by Kapoor,[107] the EEG proved helpful in only three cases. Consequently, these studies should be restricted to those situations in which other clinical observations suggest nervous system disease (see discussion earlier). On the other hand, given the importance of dysautonomic causes of syncope and related syndromes (i.e. orthostatic syncope, POTS, inappropriate sinus tachycarda),[108–111] tilt-table testing and other tests of autonomic function have an increasingly important role to play (see earlier discussion).

Syncope management units

The ineffectiveness of conventional approaches to evaluation of the suspected syncope patient is widely recognized, and has been highlighted by two major studies from Italy, OESIL and EGSYS.[9,112,113] Both illustrated the inefficiency of the standard approach. Further, in each case a follow-up study (OESIL-2, EGSYS-2) demonstrated that a more standardized guideline-based care pathway (such as could be provided in a structured multidisciplinary syncope management unit (SMU), as recommended by the ESC Syncope Task Force) significantly improved diagnostic yield and reduced hospital admissions, resource consumption, and overall costs.[114–116] Two different models of syncope facilities have been developed, one primarily centered within emergency departments (ED)[117] and the other within the cardiology or medicine department.[116]

The SMU operating primarily within an ED usually has risk stratification (i.e. identifying those individuals who can be sent for outpatient assessment versus those needing hospital admission) as its principal goal. In this regard, the prospective single-center SEEDS study[115] evaluated the hypothesis that a designated syncope unit in the ED improves diagnostic yield and reduces hospital admission for patients with syncope who were considered to be at intermediate risk for an adverse cardiovascular outcome. Patients were randomly allocated to one or other of two treatment arms: syncope unit evaluation or standard care.

The study enrolled 103 individuals, with 51 patients randomized to SMU care. Comparing SMU versus standard care patients, a presumptive diagnosis was established in 34 (67%) and five (10%) patients respectively, and hospital admission was required for 22 (43%) and 51 (98%) patients, respectively. The SMU care pathway reduced total patient-hospital days from 140 to 64. Thus, the SMU appeared to improve diagnostic yield and cost-effectiveness of care significantly.

In another ED-based study, a previously developed rule set (the so-called "San Francisco Syncope Rule") was applied.[116] This strategy combined the presence of any of the following observations to risk stratify patients: an abnormal ECG, symptoms of shortness of breath, a hematocrit <30%, systolic blood pressure <90 mmHg or a history of congestive heart failure. The rule was 98% sensitive and 56% specific to predict serious outcomes (defined as death, myocardial infarction, arrhythmia, pulmonary embolism, stroke, subarachnoid bleed, significant hemorrhage or any condition resulting in a return ED visit and hospitalization) in 791 patients referred to a teaching hospital. However, in one external validation cohort,[117] the San Francisco Syncope Rule had a lower sensitivity and specificity (89% and 42%).

The SMU model adopted in some Italian hospitals is a functional or "virtual" unit managed inside the department of cardiology. Where appropriate, patients are jointly managed with other specialists. The patients may be referred to the unit from any of several sites, including the ED, inpatient services or outpatient clinics.

In the context of the more structured approach to the syncope evaluation, EGSYS-2[9–11] provided a prospective, controlled, multicenter study designed to determine if a "standardized" method of care is superior to the usual care.[10] There were 929 patients in the usual care pathway and 745 patients in the standardized care group. At the end of the evaluation, the standardized care group had a 17% lower hospitalization rate (39% v 47%), 11% shorter in-hospital stay (7.2 ± 5.7 v 8.1 ± 5.9 days) and 26% fewer tests performed per patient (median 2.5 v 3.4). Additionally, standardized care patients had 75% fewer discharges with "unexplained syncope" (standardized 5% v usual care 20%). The mean cost per patient was 19% lower (€1127 v 1394), and the mean cost per diagnosis was 29% lower (€1240 v 1753) in the standardized care group.

SMUs of the type discussed here, while strongly advocated by the ESC Syncope Task Force,[1] are only infrequently found in either North America or Europe. In 2005, a survey of United States and Canadian medical centers revealed that only four of 28 reporting centers (4/28, 14%) had organized an SMU.[118] Of the centers with an SMU, the unit was described as a "physical space" in one case and as a "virtual unit" (i.e. not a defined physical entity) in the others.

Treatment

The effectiveness of syncope prevention varies, depending upon the specific diagnosis. Thus, susceptibility to syncope due to a well-documented, inducible, and ablatable SVT should be entirely eliminated (**Class I, Level B**). Similarly, although effectiveness of treatment is not likely to be as outstanding as the ablation example, the evidence supporting the utility of cardiac pacing in CSS and acquired AV block is substantial (**Class IIa, Level B**). On the other hand, evidence favoring the effectiveness of pharmacologic management in vasovagal syncope is much weaker (**Level C**, with the possible exception of midodrine – **Level B**).

Neurally mediated reflex syncope

The initial treatment of most patients with neurally mediated syncopal syndromes comprises reassurance and education. The education component must focus on avoidance of triggering events (e.g. hot crowded environments, dehydration, effects of cough, etc.), recognition of premonitory symptoms, and maneuvers to abort the episode (e.g. leg crossing, muscle tensing, supine posture).

Acute intervention by medical personnel is rarely possible in the case of the vasovagal fainter. However, affected individuals can be taught physical counter-maneuver techniques that may prove useful for aborting evolving episodes if there is enough warning. For instance, leg crossing with leg and thigh muscle tensing can abruptly increase blood pressure and potentially avert an imminent faint (**Class IIa, Level B**).[119] Arm tensing (tugging), squatting or lowering the head to a more dependent position are other useful maneuvers.

The multicenter, prospective, randomized Physical Counter-pressure Maneuver (PCM) trial[119] assessed the effectiveness of physical counter-pressure maneuvers (PCM) in 223 patients (38 ±15 years) with recurrent vasovagal syncope and recognizable warning symptoms: 117 patients were randomized to standardized conventional therapy alone and 106 patients received conventional therapy plus training in counter-pressure maneuvers (i.e. leg crossing, arm tensing). The median yearly syncope burden during follow-up was significantly lower in the group trained in PCM than in the control group ($P < 0.004$); overall, 51% of the patients with conventional treatment and 32% of the patients trained in PCM experienced a syncope recurrence ($P < 0.005$).

In the case of vasovagal syncope, when symptoms are recurrent or severe or threaten lifestyle or occupation, a prevention strategy is needed. In this context, and given a highly motivated patient with recurrent vasovagal symptoms, the prescription of progressively prolonged periods of enforced upright posture (so-called "tilt-training" or "standing training") or other physical maneuvers may be useful for reducing syncope susceptibility (**Class IIb***, **Level B**).[120,121] The goal of tilt-training (more accurately termed standing training) is to normalize neurovascular response to orthostatic stress[32]. Initially the "tilt-training" concept used repeated in-hospital exposure to postural stress by tilt-table tests until syncope was no longer inducible. However, this approach is impracticable. Currently, the method entails home "standingtraining" for progressively longer periods of time over 10–12 weeks. At the beginning, the recommended standing duration is 3–5 minutes twice daily; standing duration is then gradually lengthened every 3–4 days to as much as 30–40 minutes twice daily.

The value of tilt-training remains controversial. Nonrandomized studies suggest that it reduces susceptibility to recurrent vasovagal syncope if undertaken consistently.[120,121] However, compliance is a limitation and randomized observations have been less encouraging.[122,123] A randomized study using a hard clinical endpoint (i.e. syncope recurrence or syncope burden) is needed before we can derive any solid conclusion regarding efficacy of the tilt-training approach.

Despite the safety, portability, and inexpensive nature of most physical treatments for reducing susceptibility to vasovagal faints, their inconvenience is a problem. Consequently, many vasovagal fainters (and their doctors) still search for a pharmacologic approach. In this regard, so-called "volume expanders" (e.g. electrolyte-containing drinks, fludrocortisone, salt tablets) are safest. However, with rare exceptions,[124] their effectiveness is largely anecdotal (**Class IIb***, **Level B**). A controlled trial with fludrocortisone in adults is currently ongoing (the POST2 study).

Beta-adrenergic blocking drugs were among the first agents proposed for use in preventing vasovagal syncope. Early small studies suggested benefit but more recent observations, including the placebo-controlled, double-blind POST trial,[125] raise doubts (**Class IIb*, Level B+**).

Other agents that have been used in difficult-to-treat vasoavgal fainters include midodrine (a vasoconstrictor), disopyramide, and serotonin reuptake inhibitors. However, for any of these only a small experience currently exists.[126–134] Midodrine may be an exception in that several single-center studies, including a controlled trial in which instruction regarding maintenance of hydration served as a control, tend to support its effectiveness[132–134] (**Class IIa, Level B**).

Cardiac pacing is highly successful in CSS (**Class IIa, Level B**) when bradycardia has been documented[135] but is less effective in other forms of neurally mediated faints. In this regard, early trials provided strong supportive evidence of efficacy of cardiac pacing in vasovagal syncope.[136–138] However, in these studies the control group did not receive a pacemaker. More recent reports, in which pacemakers were placed in both the treatment and control groups, have tended to downplay the value of cardiac pacing in this setting.[139,140]

The value of establishing the specific characteristic of the neurally mediated faint for determining treatment strategy has recently been addressed in the ISSUE-2 study.[45] This trial used a strategy of early ILR use, with therapy delayed until documentation of syncope was obtained. In ISSUE-2, 53 patients received ILR-based specific therapy, mostly pacemaker therapy (n = 47), and 50 patients received counseling (education and reassurance). The 1-year recurrence rate in patients assigned to a specific therapy was 10% compared with 41% in the patients without specific therapy (80% relative risk reduction for patients, and 92% for burden). The 1-year recurrence rate in patients with pacemakers was 5%.

Orthostatic syncope

Reducing susceptibility to symptomatic orthostatic hypotension necessitates multiple strategies. Education focusing on predisposing factors such as abrupt posture change, dehydration or concomitant illness is important. Thereafter, whenever possible, non-essential offending medications (e.g. diuretics, vasodilators) should be eliminated.

Patients should also be taught about physical counter-maneuvers (see earlier) designed to ameliorate problems associated with upright posture. However, care must be taken to alert older or infirm patients to risks of falling when applying maneuvers such as leg crossing.[141] Thereafter, longer-term prevention may include "tilt-training".[120,121]

Other physical maneuvers designed to diminish displacement of central volume to the lower extremities during upright posture include use of anti-gravitational hose and/or abdominal binders, elevation of the head of the bed at night, and (currently in investigation) a portable breathing device that increases impedance during inspiration (ITD).[142,143] With regard to the latter, Melby *et al*[143] utilized the ITD in a short-term acute intervention study in normal controls and patients with a history of orthostatic hypotension. Both groups were studied after abrupt movement from a gravitationally neutral position to upright standing. Findings indicated that the reduced intrathoracic pressure associated with breathing through the ITD was accompanied by a lesser fall of systemic pressure upon assuming the upright posture. More recently, van Thijs *et al*[144] employed a similar approach and observed essentially the same potential benefit. A longer term controlled trial is needed.

In terms of pharmacologic treatment, increased dietary salt and/or use of salt-retaining steroids (i.e. principally fludrocortisone) is usually the first step (**Class IIb, Level C**), followed if needed by judicious dosing with the arterial and venous constrictor midodrine. Additional benefit has been reported with the use of agents such as erythropoietin in order to increase circulating blood volume. Unfortunately, however, often the older orthostatic hypotension patient is also susceptible to supine hypertension. This combination results in an obvious therapeutic dilemma requiring very careful individualized manipulation of the various treatment options.

Cardiac arrhythmias

Evidence supports cardiac pacemaker therapy in patients with syncope due to bradyarrhythmias (**Class I, Level B**).[145,146] In the case of paroxysmal supraventricular tachyarrhythmias (PSVT) with syncope, there is little in the way of long-term follow-up studies examining the efficacy of conventional antiarrhythmic drug treatment. However, transcatheter ablation has become a very safe and cost-effective treatment option.

In the case of syncope due to VT, the almost ubiquitous presence of underlying left ventricular dysfunction increases proarrhythmic risk associated with most antiarrhythmic drug therapy. In these cases, despite early consideration of class 3 agents (particularly amiodarone), there remains the difficulty of assuring effective prophylaxis; consequently, transcatheter ablation and ICDs are increasingly important considerations. Currently, ablation techniques are appropriate first choices in only a few forms of VT, specifically symptomatic patients with right ventricular outflow tract tachycardia and bundle branch re-entry tachycardia (**Class IIb, Level B**).

With regard to implantable devices for symptomatic VT, several prospective treatment trials provide evidence favoring ICD efficacy (**Class I, Level A**) compared to pharmacologic approaches, especially in the setting of diminished left ventricular function.[63,147–151] Although these studies did not directly target syncope patients, it is reasonable to extend the observations to those syncope patients in whom ventricular tachyarrhythmias and poor left ventricular function are identified.[152]

In the subset of patients in whom structural cardiovascular or cardiopulmonary disease is the cause of syncope, treatment is best directed at amelioration of the specific structural lesion. However, it may be impossible to eliminate the underlying problem adequately. For instance, modifying outflow gradients in HOCM is not readily achieved by pharmacologic or surgical therapies. Therefore, although controversial, cardiac pacing continues to be employed (often as an ICD) in individuals who have experienced syncope or who have a worrisome family history (**Class IIb, Level B**).[153–156]

Cost-effectiveness issues

Syncope occurs in all age groups and can be responsible for considerable morbidity and lifestyle disturbance.[1,9,12–14,157–159] Consequently, lost productivity, economic derangement, and loss of vocation are important considerations when assessing the manner in which syncope is to be evaluated and treated.[43,160–163] Currently, in contrast to earlier reports,[162,163] given availability of ILRs, better understanding of the limitations of previously used testing strategies, and evidence favoring the structured SMU approach to syncope management, there is the potential to markedly improve the frequency with which a specific diagnosis is obtained, thereby reducing the cost per specific diagnosis.

Conclusion

Syncope is a common medical problem with many potential causes and a tendency to recur. Assessment of each patient must be thorough, with particular attention paid to recognition and evaluation of structural cardiac and/or vascular disease. Box 42.2 summarizes the key steps that need to be addressed.

When structural cardiovascular disease is thought likely, hemodynamic and angiographic studies are often needed to address severity and direct appropriate treatment strategy. On the other hand, syncope in the absence of structural cardiovascular disease is more often either neurally medi-

ated reflex in origin or the result of orthostatic hypotension (often drug induced). In such cases, without the diagnosis being clear from the medical history and physical examination alone, autonomic function testing (particularly tilt-table testing) is warranted to confirm the diagnostic suspicion.

The treatment of syncope has been the subject of relatively few clinical trials and consequently treatment recommendations are based principally on "expert consensus". Given this important limitation, when structural cardiovascular disturbances or primary cardiac arrhythmias are the cause, appropriately directed therapy is likely to be highly effective. On the other hand, in neurally mediated reflex faints and orthostatic hypotension leading to syncope, documentation of pharmacologic treatment efficacy (with the possible exception of midodrine) is less convincing, and physical counter-maneuvers have become increasingly important; this is the case for both acute intervention (e.g. leg crossing and muscle tensing) and long-term benefits (i.e. tilt-training).

A small but increasing number of clinical observational reports and randomized placebo-controlled trials have recently improved our understanding of the TLOC/syncope complex. However, not every element of syncope/TLOC management can be subjected to such intense evaluation. The role of expert consensus opinion, both in day-to-day care as well as in practice guideline development, remains essential.

Acknowledgment

The authors would like to thank Wendy Markuson and Barry LS Detloff for assistance in preparation of the manuscript.

BOX 42.2 Key messages: the evaluation of the syncope patient

The goals
- establish a correlation between symptoms and detected abnormalities
- assess prognosis
- ascertain if evaluation requires hospitalization
- initiate appropriate treatment plan.

Key steps
- obtain detailed medical history (including bystanders/relatives)
- determine presence of underlying structural heart disease
- consider need for obtaining ECG/symptom correlation

Factors determining need for further tests
- evidence for structural cardiovascular disease
- certainty of the initial clinical impression,
- number and frequency of syncopal events
- occurrence of injury or accident
- family history of syncope or sudden death
- occupation, avocation

References

1. Brignole M, Alboni P, Benditt D et al. Guidelines on management (diagnosis and treatment) of syncope. Europace 2004;**6**:467–537.
2. van Thijs RD, Benditt DG, Mathias CJ, Schondorf R, Sutton R, Wieling W, van Dijk JG. Unconscious confusion – a literature search for definitions of syncope and related disorders. Clin Autonom Res 2004;**15**:35–9.
3. van Thijs RD, Wieling W, Kaufmann H, van Dijk JG. Defining and classifying syncope. Clin Autonom Res 2004;**14**(supp 1): 4–8.
4. Benditt DG on behalf of the Ad Hoc Syncope Consortium. The ACCF/AHA Scientific Statement on Syncope: a document in need of thoughtful revision. Europace **2006**;8:1017–21, Clin Autonom Res 2006;**18**:363–8.
5. Strickberger SA, Benson DW Jr, Biaggioni I et al. AHA/ACCF scientific statement on the evaluation of syncope. J Am Coll Cardiol **2006**;47:473–84, Circulation 2006;**113**:316–27.

6. Soteriades ES, Evans JC, Larson MG *et al.* Incidence and prognosis of syncope. *N Engl J Med* 2002;**347**:878–85.

7. Chen-Scarabelli C, Scarabelli TM. Neurocardiogenic syncope. *BMJ* 2004;**329**:336–41.

8. Benditt DG, Brignole M. Syncope: is a diagnosis a diagnosis? *J Am Coll Cardiol* 2003;**41**:791–4.

9. Brignole M, Menozzi C, Bartoletti A *et al.*, for the Evaluation of Guidelines in Syncope Study 2 (EGSYS-2) Group. A new management of syncope: prospective guideline-based evaluation of patients referred urgently to general hospitals. *Eur Heart J* 2006;**27**:76–82.

10. Brignole M, Menozzi C, Bartoletti A *et al.* A new management of syncope: prospective systematic guideline-based evaluation of patients referred urgently to general hospitals. *Eur Heart J* 2006;**27**:76–82.

11. Benditt DG. Syncope management guidelines at work: first steps towards assessing clinical utility. *Eur Heart J* 2006;**27**:7–9.

12. Kenny RA, O'Shea D, Walker HF. Impact of a dedicated syncope and falls facility for older adults on emergency beds. *Age Ageing* 2002;**31**:272–5.

13. Shen WK, Decker WW, Smars PA *et al.* Syncope evaluation in the emergency department study (SEEDS): a multidisciplinary approach to syncope management. *Circulation* 2004;**119**: 3636–45.

14. Bartoletti A, Brignole M, Proclemer A *et al.* How is syncope studied in the Italian hospitals? *Italian Heart J* 2004; **5**(suppl):472–9.

15. Gendelman HE, Linzer M, Gabelman M *et al.* Syncope in a general hospital population. *NY State J Med* 1983;**83**:116–65.

16. Wayne HH Syncope: physiological considerations and an analysis of the clinical characteristics in 510 patients. *Am J Med* 1961;**30**:418–38.

17. Blanc J-J, L'Her C, Touiza A *et al.* Prospective evaluation and outcome of patients admitted for syncope over a 1 year period. *Eur Heart J* 2002;**23**:815–20.

18. Sheldon RS, Serletis A. Epidemiological aspects of transient loss of consciousness/syncope. In: Benditt DG, Brignole M, Raviele A, Wieling W, eds. *Syncope and Transient Loss of Consciousness. A Multidisciplinary Approach.* Oxford: Blackwell Publishing, 2007 pp 8–14.

19. Savage DD, Corwin L, McGee DL *et al.* Epidemiologic features of isolated syncope: the Framingham Study. *Stroke* 1985;**16**:626–9.

20. Dermkesian G, Lamb LE. Syncope in a population of healthy young adults. *JAMA* 1958;**168**: 1200–7.

21. Driscoll DJ, Jacobsen SJ, Porter CJ, Wollan PC. Syncope in children and adolescents. *J Am Coll Cardiol* 1997;**29**:1039–45.

22. Ganzeboom KS, Colman N, Reitsma JB, Shen WK, Wieling W. Prevalence and triggers of syncope in medical students. *Am J Cardiol* 2003;**91**:1006–8.

23. Koshman ML, Ritchie D, for the Investigators of the Syncope Symptom Study and the Prevention of Syncope Trial. Age of first faint in patients with vasovagal syncope. *J Cardiovasc Electrophysiol* 2006;**17**(1):49–54.

24. Serletis A, Rose S, Sheldon AG, Sheldon RS. Vasovagal syncope in medical students and their first-degree relatives. *Eur Heart J* 2006;**27**(16):1965–70.

25. Pires LA, May LM, Ravi S *et al.* Comparison of event rates and survival in patients with unexplained syncope without documented ventricular tachyarrhythmias versus patients with documented sustained ventricular tachyarrhythmias both treated with implantable cardioverter-defibrillators. *Am J Cardiol* 2000;**85**(6):725–8.

26. Olshansky B, Hahn EA, Hartz VL *et al.* Clinical significance of syncope in the electrophysiologic study versus electrocardiographic monitoring (ESVEM) trial. The ESVEM Investigators. *Am Heart J* 1999;**137**(5):878–86.

27. Steinberg JS, Beckman K, Greene HL *et al.* Follow-up of patients with unexplained syncope and inducible ventricular tachyarrhythmias: analysis of the AVID registry and an AVID substudy. Antiarrhythmics Versus Implantable Defibrillators. *J Cardiovasc Electrophysiol* 2001;**12**(9):996–1001.

28. Knight BP, Goyal R, Pelosi F *et al.* Outcome of patients with nonischemic dilated cardiomyopathy and unexplained syncope treated with an implantable defibrillator. *J Am Coll Cardiol* 1999;**33**:1964–70.

29. Olshansky B, Poole JE, Johnson G *et al.* Syncope predicts the outcome of cardiomyopathy patients: analysis of the SCD-HeFT study. *J Am Coll Cardiol* 2008;**51**:1277–82.

30. Sauer A, Moss A, McNitt S *et al.* Long QT syndrome in adults. *J Am Coll Cardiol* 2007;**49**: 329–37.

31. Sacher F, Probst V, Iesaka Y *et al.* Outcome after implantation of a cardioverter-defibrillator in patients with Brugada syndrome. A multicenter study. *Circulation* 2006;**114**:2317–24.

32. Andrea Sarkozy A, Boussy T, Kourgiannides G *et al.* Long-term follow-up of primary prophylactic implantable cardioverter-defibrillator therapy in Brugada syndrome. *Eur Heart J* 2007;**28**(22):334–44.

33. Paul M, Schulze-Bahr E, Gerss J *et al.* Impact of programmed ventricular stimulation in patients with Brugada syndrome (abstract). A metanalysis of worldwide published data. *Eur Heart J* 2006;**27**:470.

34. Wieling W, Krediet CTP, Van Dijk N *et al.* Initial hypotension: review of a forgotten condition. *Clin Sci* 2007;**112**:157–65.

35. Gibbons CH, Freeman R. Delayed orthostatic hypotension. *Neurology* 2006;**67**:28–32.

36. Kenny RA, Bayliss J, Ingram A, Sutton R. Head up tilt: a useful test for investigating unexplained syncope. *Lancet* 1986;**1**: 1352–4.

37. Sutton R, Petersen M, Brignole M, Ravieli A, Menozzi C, Giani P. Proposed classification for tilt induced vasovagal syncope. *Eur J Cardiac Pacing Electrophysiol* 1992;**2**:180–3.

38. Benditt DG, Ferguson DW, Grubb BP *et al.* Tilt-table testing for assessing syncope. An American College of Cardiology expert consensus document. *J Am Coll Cardiol* 1996;**28**(1): 263–75.

39. Huff SJ, Decker WW, Quinn JV *et al*, for the American College of Emergency Physicians Clinical Policies Subcommittee. Clinical policy: critical issues in the evaluation and management of patients presenting with syncope. *Ann Emerg Med* 2007;**49**:431–44.

40. Alboni P, Brignole M, Menozzi C *et al.* The diagnostic value of history in patients with syncope with or without heart disease. *J Am Coll Cardiol* 2001;**37**:1921–8.

41. Krahn AD, Klein GJ, Yee R, Takle-Newhouse T, Norris C. Use of an extended monitoring strategy in patients with problematic syncope. Reveal Investigators. *Circulation* 1999;**26**(99): 406–10.

42. Krahn AD, Klein GJ, Yee R, Skanes AC. Randomized assessment of syncope trial: conventional diagnostic testing versus a prolonged monitoring strategy. *Circulation* 2001;3(104): 46–51.

43. Krahn AD, Klein GJ, Yee R, Hoch JS, Skanes AC. Cost implications of testing strategy in patients with syncope. Randomized Assessment of Syncope trial. *J Am Coll Cardiol* 2003;**42**: 495–501.

44. Brignole M, Sutton R, Menozzi C, Garcia-Civera R, Moya A, Wieling W *et al.* Early application of an implantable loop recorder allows a mechanism-based effective therapy in patients with recurrent suspected neurally mediated syncope. *Eur Heart J* 2006;**27**(6):1085–92.

45. Moya A, Brignole, M, Sutton R *et al.*, for the International Study on Syncope of Uncertain Etiology 2 (ISSUE 2) Group. Reproducibility of implantable loop recorder electrocardiographic findings in recurrent syncope and presyncope, and during asymptomatic periods, in patients with suspected neurally mediated reflex syncope. *Eur Heart J* 2007;**102**:1518–23.

46. Parry SW, Nath S, Bourke JP, Bexton RS, Kenny RA. Adenosine test in the diagnosis of unexplained syncope: marker of conducting tissue disease or neurally mediated syncope? *Eur Heart J* 2006;**27**:1396–400.

47. Flammang D, Pelleg A, Benditt DG. The adenosine triphosphate (ATP) test for evaluation of syncope of unknown origin. *J Cardiovasc Electrophysiol* 2005;**16**(12):1388–9.

48. Brignole M, Donateo P, Menozzi C. The diagnostic value of ATP testing in patients with unexplained syncope. *Europace* 2003;**5**: 425–8.

49. Brignole M, Sutton R, Menozzi C *et al.* Lack of correlation between the responses to tilt testing and adenosine triphosphate test and the mechanism of spontaneous neurally mediated syncope. *Eur Heart J* 2006;**27**:2232–9.

50. Kenny RAM, Richardson DA, Steen N *et al.* Carotid sinus syndrome: a modifiable risk factor for nonaccidental falls in older adults (SAFE PACE). *J Am Coll Cardiol* 2001;**38**:1491–6.

51. Mathias CJ. Autonomic diseases – clinical features and laboratory evaluation. *J Neurol Neurosurg Psychiatry* 2003;**74**; 31–41.

52. Mathias CJ. Autonomic diseases – management. *J Neurol Neurosurg Psychiatry* 2003;**74**;42–7.

53. Mathias CJ. Role of autonomic evaluation in the diagnosis and management of syncope. *Clin Autonom Res* 2004;**14**;S1, 45–54.

54. Low PA, Opfer-Gherking TL, McPhee BR *et al.* Prospective evaluation of clinical characteristics of orthostatic hypotension. *Mayo Clin Proc* 1995;**70**:617–22.

55. Kaplan BM, Langendorf R, Lev M, Pick A. Tachycardia-bradycardia syndrome (so-called "sick sinus syndrome"). *Am J Cardiol* 1973;**26**:497–508.

56. Rubenstein JJ, Schulman CL, Yurchak PM *et al.* Clinical spectrum of the sick sinus syndrome. *Circulation* 1972;**6**:5–13.

57. Ogawa H, Inoue T, Miwa S, Fujimoto T, Ohnishi Y, Fukuzaki H. Heart rate responses to autonomic drugs in sick sinus syndrome – correlation with syncope and electrophysiologic data. *Jap Circ J* 1991;**55**:15–23.

58. Linker NJ, Camm AJ. Drug effects on the sinus node. A clinical perspective. *Cardiovasc Drugs Ther* 1988;**2**:165–70.

59. Strickberger SA, Fish RD, Lamas GA *et al.* Comparison of effects of propranolol versus pindolol on sinus rate and pacing frequency in sick sinus syndrome. *Am J Cardiol* 1993;**71**:53–6.

60. Michaelsson M, Jonzon A, Riesenfeld T. Isolated congenital complete atrioventricular block in adult life. *Circulation* 1995;**92**:442–9.

61. Scheinman MM, Peters RW, Sauve MJ *et al.* Value of H-Q interval in patients with bundle branch block and the role of prophylactic permanent pacing. *Am J Cardiol* 1982;**50**:1316–22.

62. Da Costa A, Gulian JL, Romeyer-Bouchard C *et al.* Clinical predictors of cardiac events in patients with isolated syncope and negative electrophysiologic study. *Int J Cardiol* 2006;**109**: 28–33.

63. Buxton AE, Lee KL, Fisher JD, Josephson ME, Prystowsky EN, Hafley G. A randomized study of the prevention of sudden death in patients with coronary artery disease. Multicenter Unsustained Tachycardia Trial Investigators. *N Engl J Med* 1999;**341**:1882–90.

64. Moss AJ, Schwartz PJ, Crampton RS *et al.* The long QT syndrome: prospective longitudinal study of 328 families. *Circulation* 1991;**84**:1136–44.

65. Sauer A, Moss A, McNitt S *et al.* Long QT syndrome in adults. *J Am Coll Cardiol* 2007;**49**:329–37

66. Brugada P, Brugada J. Right bundle branch block, persistent ST-segment elevation and sudden cardiac death: a distinct clinical and electrocardiographic syndrome. A multicenter report. *J Am Coll Cardiol* 1992;**20**:1391–6.

67. Antzelevitch C, Brugada P, Borggrefe M *et al.* Brugada syndrome: report of the second consensus conference. *Circulation* 2005;**111**:659–70.

68. Rosso R, Glick A, Glickson M *et al*, for the Israeli Working Group on Cardiac Pacing and Electrophysiology. Outcome after implantation of cardioverter defibrillator in patients with Brugada syndrome: a multicenter Israeli study (ISRABRU). *Isr Med Assoc J* 2008;**10**:462–4.

69. Camm AJ, Lau CP. Syncope of undetermined origin: diagnosis and management. *Prog Cardiol* 1988;**1**:139–56.

70. Leitch JW, Klein GJ, Yee R *et al.* Syncope associated with supraventricular tachycardia: an expression of tachycardia or vasomotor response. *Circulation* 1992;**85**:1064–71.

71. Thaman R, Elliott PM, Shah JS *et al.* Reversal of inappropriate peripheral vascular responses in hypertrophic cardiomyopathy. *J Am Coll Cardiol* 2005;**46**:883–92.

72. Barletta G, Lazzeri C, Franchi F, Del Bene R, Michelucci A. Hypertrophic cardiomyopathy: electrical abnormalities detected by the extended-length ECG and their relation to syncope. *Int J Cardiol* 2004;**97**:43–8.

73. Fox WC, Lockette W. Unexpected syncope and death during intense physical training: evolving role of molecular genetics. *Aviat Space Environ Med* 2003;**74**:1223–30.

74. Manganelli F, Betocchi S, Ciampi Q *et al.* Comparison of hemodynamic adaptation to orthostatic stress in patients with hypertrophic cardiomyopathy with or without syncope and in vasovagal syncope. *Am J Cardiol* 2002;**89**:1405–10.

75. van Dijk JG. Cerebrovascular disorders as the primary cause of syncope. In: Benditt DG, Blanc J-J, Brignole M, Sutton R, eds. *The Evaluation and Treatment of Syncope*, 2nd edn. Oxford: Blackwell Publishing, 2005, pp 213–15.

76. Reed MJ, Newby DE, Coull AJ, Jacques KG, Prescott RJ, Gray AJ. The Risk stratification Of Syncope in the Emergency department (ROSE) pilot study: a comparison of existing syncope guidelines. *Emergency Med J* 2007;**24**:270–5.

77. Costantino G, Perego F, Dipaola F *et al*. Short- and long-term prognosis of syncope, risk factors, and role of hospital admission: results from the STePS (short-term prognosis of syncope) study. *J Am Coll Cardiol* 2008;**51**:276–83.

78. Calkins H, Shyr Y, Frumin H, Schork A, Morady F. The value of clinical history in the differentiation of syncope due to ventricular tachycardia, atrioventricular block and neurocardiogenic syncope. *Am J Med* 1995;**98**:365–73.

79. Linzer M, Yang EH, Estes III M *et al*. Diagnosing syncope. Part 1. Value of history, physical examination, and electrocardiography. *Ann Intern Med* 1997;**126**:989–99.

80. Sheldon R, Rose S, Connolly S *et al*. Diagnostic criteria for vasovagal syncope based on quantitative history. *Eur Heart J* 2006;**27**:344–50.

81. Del Rosso A, Alboni P, Brignole M, Menozzi C, Raviele A. Relation of clinical presentation of syncope to the age of patients. *Am J Cardiol* 2005;**96**:1431–5.

82. Ungar A, Mussi C, Del Rosso A *et al*, for the Italian Group for the Study of Syncope in the Elderly. Diagnosis and characteristics of syncope in older patients referred to geriatric departments. *J Am Geriatr Soc* 2006;**54**:1531–6.

83. Kapoor W. Evaluation and outcome of patients with syncope. *Medicine* 1990;**69**:160–75.

84. Grubb BP, Gerard G, Rousch K *et al*. Differentiation of convulsive syncope and epilepsy with head up tilt table testing. *Ann Intern Med* 1991;**115**:871–6.

85. Rothman SA, Laughlin JC, Seltzer J *et al*. The diagnosis of cardiac arrhythmias: a prospective multi-center randomized study comparing mobile cardiac outpatient telemetry versus standard loop event monitoring. *J Cardiovasc Electrophysiol* 2007;**18**:241–7.

86. Olson JA, Fouts AM, Padanilam BJ *et al*. Utility of mobile cardiac outpatient telemetry for the diagnosis of palpitations, presyncope, syncope, and the assessment of therapy efficacy. *J Cardiovasc Electrophysiol* 2007;**18**:1–5.

87. Deharo JC, Jego C, Lanteaume A *et al*. An implantable loop recorder study of highly symptomatic vasovagal patients: the heart rhythm observed during a spontaneous syncope is identical to the recurrent syncope but not correlated with the head-up tilt test or ATP test. *J Am Coll Cardiol* 2006;**47**:587–93.

88. Farwell DJ, Freemantle N, Sulke N. The clinical impact of implantable loop recorders in patients with syncope. *Eur Heart J* 2006;**27**:351–6.

89. Sakaguchi S, Shultz J, Remole C, Adler S, Lurie K, Benditt D. Syncope associated with exercise, a manifestation of neurally mediated syncope. *Am J Cardiol* 1995;**75**:476–81.

90. Calkins H, Seifert M, Morady F. Clinical presentation and long term follow-up of athletes with exercise-induced vasodepressor syncope. *Am Heart J* 1995;**129**:1159–64.

91. Kuchar DL, Thorburn CW, Sammel NL. Signal-averaged electrocardiogram for evaluation of recurrent syncope. *Am J Cardiol* 1986;**58**:949–53.

92. Folino AF, Bauce B, Frigo G, Nava A. Long-term follow-up of the signal-averaged ECG in arrhythmogenic right ventricular cardiomyopathy: correlation with arrhythmic events and echocardiographic findings. *Europace*. 2006;**8**:423–9.

93. Grimm W, Christ M, Bach J, Muller HH, Maisch B. Noninvasive arrhythmia risk stratification in idiopathic dilated cardiomyopathy: results of the Marburg Cardiomyopathy Study. *Circulation* 2003;**108**:2883–91.

94. Gomes JA, Cain ME, Buxton AE, Josephson ME, Lee KL, Hafley GE. Prediction of long-term outcomes by signal-averaged electrocardiography in patients with unsustained ventricular tachycardia, coronary artery disease, and left ventricular dysfunction. *Circulation* 2001;**104**:436–41.

95. Bloomfield DM, Bigger JT, Steinman RC *et al*. Microvolt T wave alternans and the risk of death or sustained ventricular arrhythmias in patients with left ventricular dysfunction. *J Am Coll Cardiol* 2006;**47**:456–63.

96. Chow T, Kereiakes DJ, Bartone C *et al*. Microvolt T wave alternans identifies patients with ischemic cardiomyopathy who benefit form implantable cardioverter defibrillator therapy. *J Am Coll Cardiol* 2006;**49**:50–8.

97. Natale A, Akhtar M, Jazayeri M *et al*. Provocation of hypotension during head-up tilt testing in subjects with no history of syncope or presyncope. *Circulation* 1995;**92**:54–8.

98. Moya A, Brignole M, Menozzi C *et al*, for the ISSUE Investigators. Mechanism of syncope in patients with isolated syncope and in patients with tilt-positive syncope. *Circulation* 2001;**104**:1261–7.

99. Moya A, Brignole M, Sutton R *et al*. Reproducibility of electrocardiographic findings in patients with suspected reflex neurally mediated syncope. *Am J Cardiol* 2008;**102**:1518–23.

100. Akhtar M, Shenasa M, Denker S, Gilbert CJ, Rizwi N. Role of cardiac electrophysiologic studies in patients with unexplained recurrent syncope. *PACE* 1983;**6**:192–201.

101. Morady F, Shen E, Schwartz A *et al*. Long-term follow-up of patients with recurrent unexplained syncope evaluated by electrophysiologic testing. *J Am Coll Cardiol* 1983;**2**: 1053–9.

102. Mittal S, Iwai S, Stein KM *et al*. Long-term outcome of patients with unexplained syncope treated with an electrophysiologic-guided approach in the implantable cardioverter-defibrillator era. *J Am Coll Cardiol* 1999;**34**:1082–9.

103. Mittal S, Hao SC, Iwai S *et al*. Significance of inducible ventricular fibrillation in patients with coronary artery disease and unexplained syncope. *J Am Coll Cardiol* 2001;**38**:371–6.

104. Sra JS, Anderson AJ, Sheikh SH *et al*. Unexplained syncope evaluated by electrophysiologic studies and head-up tilt testing. *Ann Intern Med* 1991;**114**:1013–19.

105. Fujimura O, Yee R, Klein GJ *et al*. The diagnostic sensitivity of electrophysiologic testing in patients with syncope caused by bradycardia. *N Engl J Med* 1989;**321**:1703–7.

106. Fitzpatrick A, Theodorakis G, Vardas P *et al*. The incidence of malignant vasovagal syndrome in patients with recurrent syncope. *Eur Heart J* 1991;**12**:389–94.

107. Kapoor W. Evaluation and outcome of patients with syncope. *Medicine* 1990;**69**:160–75.

108. Grubb BP. Neurocardiogenic syncope and related disorders of orthostatic intolerance. *Circulation* 2005;**111**(22):2997–3006.

109. Thieben MJ, Sandroni P, Sletten DM *et al*. Postural orthostatic tachycardia syndrome: the Mayo clinic experience. *Mayo Clin Proc* 2007;**82**:308–13.

110. Yusuf S, Camm AJ. The sinus tachycardias. *Nature Clin Pract Cardiovasc Med* 2005;**2**:44–52.

111. Chiale PA, Garro HA, Schmidberg J et al. Inappropriate sinus tachycardia may be related to an immunologic disorder involving cardiac beta-adrenergic receptors. *Heart Rhythm* 2006;**3**: 1182–6.

112. Ammirati F, Colivicchi F, Minardi G et al. The management of syncope in the hospital: the OESIL Study (Osservatorio Epidemiologico della Sincope nel Lazio). *G Ital Cardiol* 1999;**29** :533–9.

113. Desertori M, Brignole MM, Menozzi C et al. Management of patients with syncope referred urgently to general hospitals. *Europace* 2003;**5**:283–91.

114. Ammirati F, Colivicchi F, Santini M. Implementation of a simplified diagnostic algorithm in a multicentre prospective trial – the OESIL 2 Study (Osservatorio Epidemiologico della Sincope nel Lazio. *Eur Heart J* 2000;**21**:935–40.

115. Shen W, Decker W, Smars P et al. Syncope evaluation in the emergency department study (SEEDS). A multidisciplinary approach to syncope management. *Circulation* 2004;**110**: 3636–45.

116. Quinn J, McDermott D, Stiell I et al. Prospective validation of the San Francisco Syncope Rule to predict patients with serious outcomes. *Ann Emerg Med* 2006;**47**:448–54.

117. Sun BC, Mangione CM, Merchant G. External validation of the San Francisco Syncope Rule. *Ann Emerg Med* 2007;**49**:420–7.

118. Benditt DG, Lu F, Lurie KG, Sakaguchi S. Organization of syncope management units: the North American experience. In: Raviele A, ed. *Cardiac Arrhythmias*. Milan: Springer-Verlag Italia, 2005, pp 655–8.

119. van Dijk N, Quartieri F, Blanc JJ, Garcia-Civera R, Brignole M, Moya A, Wieling W. Effectiveness of physical counterpressure maneuvers in preventing vasovagal syncope. The Physical Counterpressure Manoeuvres Trial (PCM-Trial). *J Am Coll Cardiol* 2006;**48**:1652–7.

120. Ector H, Reybrouck T, Heidbuchel H, Gewillig M, Van de Werf F. Tilt training: a new treatment for recurrent neurocardiogenic syncope or severe orthostatic intolerance. *PACE* 1998;**21**: 193–6.

121. Reybrouck T, Ector H. Tilt training: a new challenge in the treatment of neurally mediated syncope. *Acta Cardiologica* 2006;**61**:183–9.

122. Kinay O, Yazici M, Nazli C et al. Tilt training for recurrent neurocardiogenic syncope: effectiveness, patient compliance, and scheduling the frequency of training sessions. *Jpn Heart J* 2004;**45**:833–43.

123. Gurevitz O, Barsheshet A, Bar-Lev D et al. Tilt training: does it have a role in preventing vasovagal syncope? *Pacing Clin Electrophysiol* 2007;**30**:1499–505.

124. Salim MA, Di Sessa TG. Effectiveness of fludrocortisone and salt in preventing syncope recurrence in children: a double-blind, placebo-controlled, randomized trial. *J Am Coll Cardiol* 2005;**45**:484–8.

125. Sheldon R, Connolly S, Rose S et al, for the POST Investigators. Prevention of Syncope Trial (POST): a randomized, placebo-controlled study of metoprolol in the prevention of vasovagal syncope. *Circulation* 2006;**113**:1164–70.

126. Fitzpatrick AP, Ahmed R, Williams S et al. A randomized trial of medical therapy in malignant vasovagal syndrome or neu-

rally mediated bradycardia/hypotension syndrome. *Eur J Cardiac Pacing Electrophysiol* 1991;**1**:191–202.

127. Brignole M, Menozzi C, Gianfranchi L et al. A controlled trial of acute and long-term medical therapy in tilt-induced neurally mediated syncope. *Am J Cardiol* 1992;**70**:339–42.

128. Morillo CA, Leitch JU, Yee R et al. A placebo-controlled trial of intravenous and oral disopyramide for prevention of neurally mediated syncope induced by head-up tilt. *J Am Coll Cardiol* 1993;**22**:1843–8.

129. Moya A, Permanyer-Miralda G, Sagrista-Sauleda J et al. Limitations of head-up tilt test for evaluating the efficacy of therapeutic interventions in patients with vasovagal syncope: results of a controlled study of etilefrine versus placebo. *J Am Coll Cardiol* 1995;**25**:65–9.

130. Jankovic J, Gilden JL, Hiner BC, Brown DC, Rubin M. Neurogenic orthostatic hypotension: a double-blind placebo-controlled study with midodrine. *Am J Med* 1993;**95**:38–48.

131. Sra J, Maglio C, Biehl M, Dhala A, Blanck Z, Deshpande S et al. Efficacy of midodrine hydrochloride in neurocardiogenic syncope refractory to standard therapy. *J Cardiovasc Electrophysiol* 1997;**8**:42–6.

132. Ward CR, Gray JC, Gilroy JJ, Kenny RA. Midodrine: a role in the management of neurocardiogenic syncope. *Heart* 1998;**79**:45–9.

133. Samniah N, Sakaguchi S, Lurie KG, Iskos D, Benditt DG. Efficacy and safety of midodrine hydrochloride in patients with refractory vasovagal syncope. *Am J Cardiol* 2001;**88**(1): 80–3.

134. Perez-Lugones A, Schweikert R, Pavia S, Sra J, Akhtar M, Jaeger F et al. Usefulness of midodrine in patients with severely symptomatic neurocardiogenic syncope: a randomized control study. *J Cardiovascul Electrophysiol* 2001;**12**(8):935–8.

135. Gregoratos G, Abrams J, Epstein AE et al. ACC/AHA/NASPE 2002 guideline update for implantation of cardiac pacemakers and antiarrhythmia devices: summary article. *Circulation* 2002;**106**:2145–61.

136. Connolly SJ, Sheldon R, Roberts RS, Gent M, for the Vasovagal Pacemaker Study Investigators. The North American Vasovagal Pacemaker Study (VPS): a randomized trial of permanent cardiac pacing for the prevention of vasovagal syncope. *J Am Coll Cardiol* 1999;**33**:16–20.

137. Sutton R, Brignole M, Menozzi C et al. Dual-chamber pacing is efficacious in treatment of neurally mediated tilt-positive cardioinhibitory syncope. Pacemaker versus no therapy: a multicentre randomized study. *Circulation* 2000;**102**: 294–9.

138. Ammirati F, Colivicchi F, Santini M et al. Permanent cardiac pacing versus medical treatment for the prevention of recurrent vasovagal syncope. A multicenter, randomised, controlled trial. *Circulation* 2001;**104**: 52–7.

139. Connolly SJ, Sheldon R, Thorpe KE et al for the VPS II Investigators. Pacemaker therapy for prevention of syncope in patients with recurrent severe vasovagal syncope: second Vasovagal Pacemaker Study (VPS II). *JAMA* 2003;**289**: 2224–9.

140. Raviele A, Giada F, Menozzi C et al. The Vasovagal Syncope and Pacing Trial (SYNPACE). A randomised, double-blind, placebo-controlled study of permanent pacing for treatment of recurrent tilt-induced vasovagal syncope. *Eur Heart J* 2004;**25**:1741–8.

141. Wieling W, Van Lieshout JJ, Van Leeuwen AM. Physical maneuvers that reduce postural hypotension in autonomic failure. *Clin Autonom Res* 1993;**3**:57–65.

142. Melby DP, Cytron JA, Benditt DG. New approaches to the treatment and prevention of neurally-medicated reflex (neurocardiogenic) syncope. *Curr Cardiol Rep* 2004;**6**:385–90.

143. Melby DP, Lu F, Sakaguchi S, Zook M, Benditt DG. Increased impedance to inspiration ameliorates hemodynamic changes associated with movement to upright posture in orthostatic hypotension: a randomized pilot study. *Heart Rhythm* 2007;**4**:128–35.

144. van Thijs RD, Wieling W, van den Aardweg JG, van Dijk JG. Respiratory countermaneuvers in autonomic failure. *Neurology* 2007;**69**:582–5.

145. Rosenqvist M, Brandt J, Schuller H. Long-term pacing in sick sinus node disease: effects of stimulation mode on cardiovascular morbidity and mortality. *Am Heart J* 1988;**116**:16–22.

146. Andersen HR, Thuesen L, Bagger JP *et al.* Prospective randomised trial of atrial versus ventricular pacing in sick-sinus syndrome. *Lancet* 1994;**344**:1523–8.

147. Zipes DP, Camm AJ, Borggrefe M *et al.* ACC/AHA/ESC 2006 guidelines for management of patients with ventricular arrhythmias and the prevention of sudden cardiac death. *Europace* 2006;**8**:746–837.

148. Moss AJ, Zareba W, Hall WJ *et al.* Prophylactiic implantation of a defibrillator in patients with myocardial infarction and reduced ejection fraction. *N Engl J Med* 2002;**346**:877–83.

149. Moss AJ, Hall WJ, Cannom DS, Daubert JP, Higgins SL, Klein H *et al.* Improved survival with an implanted defibrillator in patients with coronary disease at high risk for ventricular arrhythmia. *N Engl J Med* 1996;**335**:1933–40.

150. Antiarrhythmics versus Implantable Defibrillators (AVID) Investigators. A comparison of antiarrhythmic drug therapy with implantable defibrillators in patients resuscitated from near-fatal ventricular arrhythmias. *N Engl J Med* 1997;**337**:1576–83.

151. Bardy GH, Lee KL, Mark DB *et al* for Sudden Cardiac Death in Heart Failure Trial (SCD-HeFT) Investigators. Amiodarone or an implantable cardioverter-defibrillator for congestive heart failure *N Engl J Med* 2005;**352**:225–37.

152. Middelkauff HR, Stevenson WG, Stevenson LW, Saxon LA. Syncope in advanced heart failure: high risk of sudden death regardless of origin of syncope. *J Am Coll Cardiol* 1993;**21**: 110–16.

153. Fananapazir L, Epstein ND, Curiel RV *et al.* Long-term results of dual-chamber (DDD) pacing in obstructive cardiomyopathy. Evidence for progressive symptomatic and hemodynamic improvement and reduction of left ventricular hypertrophy. *Circulation* 1994;**90**:2731–42.

154. Kappenberger L, Linde C, Dauberet C *et al.* Pacing in hypertrophic obstructive cardiomyopathy. A randomized crossover trial. *Eur Heart J* 1997;**18**:1249–56.

155. Maron BJ, Cecchi F, McKenna WJ. Risk factors and stratification for sudden cardiac death in patients with hypertrophic cardiomyopathy. *Br Heart J* 1994;**72**(suppl):S13–18.

156. Maron BJ, Spirito P, Shen WK *et al.* Implantable cardioverter-defibrillators and prevention of sudden cardiac death in hypertrophic cardiomyopathy *JAMA* 2007;**298**:405–12.

157. van der Velde N, van den Meiracker AH, Pols HAP, Stricker BH, van der Cammen TJM. Withdrawal of fall-risk-increasing drugs in older persons: effect on tilt-table test outcomes. *J Am Geriatr Soc* 2007;**55**:734–9.

158. van Thijs RD, Kruit MC, van Buchem MA, Ferrari MD, Launer LJ, van Dijk JG. Syncope in migraine: the population-based CAMERA study. *Neurology* 2006;**66**:1034–7.

159. Grubb BP. Neurocardiogenic syncope and related disorders of orthostatic intolerance. *Circulation* 2005;**111**:2997–3006.

160. Kapoor W, Karpf M, Maher Y *et al.* Syncope of unknown origin: the need for a more cost-effective approach to its evaluation. *JAMA* 1982;**247**:2687–91.

161. Calkins H, Byrne M, El-Atassi R, Kalbfleisch S, Langberg JJ, Morady F. The economic burden of unrecognized vasodepressor syncope. *Am J Med* 1993;**95**:473–9.

162. Rockx MA, Hoch JS, Klein GJ, Yee R, Skanes AC, Gula LJ, Krahn AD. Is ambulatory monitoring for "community-acquired" syncope economically attractive? A cost-effectiveness analysis of a randomized trial of external loop recorders versus Holter monitoring. *Am Heart J* 2005;**150**:1065.

163. Steinberg LA, Knilans TK. Syncope in children: diagnostic tests have a high cost and low yield. *J Pediatr* 2005;**146**:355–8.

Cardiopulmonary resuscitation

Michael Colquhoun

School of Medicine, Cardiff University, Cardiff, Wales, UK

Introduction

Cardiac arrest may complicate any type of heart disease, but is particularly common in coronary heart disease; one half of all deaths caused by the condition present as sudden cardiac death.[1] Approximately 400 000–460 000 individuals in the USA[2] and 700 000 in Europe[3] experience sudden cardiac arrest each year, making the condition a major health problem (**Level C**).[2,3] Unexpected cardiac arrest also remains an important problem in hospital with an incidence of 0.174 ± 0.087 per bed per year reported in one recent large American multicenter cohort study.[4]

The modern era of resuscitation began with the development of defibrillators suitable for clinical use[5,6] and the demonstration of the effectiveness of expired air ventilation and closed chest compression that extended the time available for successful defibrillation.[7,8] The development of the portable defibrillator made resuscitation outside hospital a practical proposition. Particular credit goes to Pantridge in Belfast who recognized that hospital-based coronary care units would have limited impact on mortality in a condition where 60% of deaths occurred within one hour of the onset of symptoms.[9] He developed the first mobile coronary care unit in the world and the report of 10 patients admitted alive to hospital following defibrillation[10] acted as a stimulus to the development of similar strategies for managing cardiac arrest worldwide.

Establishing an evidence base for resuscitation practice

The development of effective resuscitation strategies led to a demand for standardized guidelines for clinical practice.

Evidence-Based Cardiology, 3rd edition. Edited by S. Yusuf, J.A. Cairns, A.J. Camm, E.L. Fallen, and B.J. Gersh. © 2010 Blackwell Publishing, ISBN: 978-1-4051-5925-8.

A commitment to foster an international evidence base for resuscitation practice and publish consistent guidelines for practice led to the foundation of the International Liaison Committee on Resuscitation (ILCOR). A regular five-year cycle of evidence review and publication of guidelines is now well established.[11–14]

The ILCOR methodology is based on a rigorous evaluation of *all* the available evidence relating to a specific topic using standardized worksheets,[15,16] which remain accessible at www.c2005.org.[17] In 2005, guidelines for practice were published with only minor differences between those of the European Resuscitation Council[18,20] and the American Heart Association.[19,21]

In this chapter, the basis for the practice of resuscitation of adult subjects is reviewed in the light of the evidence evaluation process described above. Common to nearly all resuscitation attempts is the application of basic life support to maintain breathing and a circulation until definitive treatment with defibrillation or other advanced techniques can be implemented. It is one of the few strategies proved to improve outcome from cardiac arrest and is the subject of the first section.

The remainder of the chapter is concerned with advanced life support topics. Defibrillation is considered in detail in the second section; it is the only definitive treatment for the majority of patients with cardiac arrest, and one of the few techniques with an unequivocal evidence base for its effectiveness. The third section is concerned with other advanced life support techniques that aim to maintain breathing and the circulation while treatment to restore the circulation is given.

Adult basic life support

Recognition of cardiac arrest

The prompt recognition of cardiac arrest is the key to starting resuscitation with the minimum of delay; recent studies have helped clarify the most accurate methods for diagnosing cardiac arrest. The traditional method of palpating the carotid pulse has now been shown to be unreliable[22,23] (**Level B**) although there is no convincing evidence that checking for movement, breathing or coughing is superior[24] (**Level C**). Agonal gasps are common after the onset of cardiac arrest and bystanders often report that such subjects are breathing when interrogated by ambulance call takers. This can result in CPR being withheld or delayed[25] (**Level C**). It is recommended therefore that rescuers should start CPR in an unresponsive (unconscious) victim who is not moving or breathing. Even if the victim is taking occasional gasps, cardiac arrest should be suspected and CPR started (**Class IIa**).

Airway and ventilation

Opening the airway

Several prospective studies using clinical or radiologic indicators of airway patency have shown that the head tilt–chin lift method is practicable, safe and effective[26–28] (**Level C**). This was confirmed in a case series[29] (**Level C**). It is recommended that rescuers should use this method to open the airway (**Class IIa**). No study has evaluated the use of routine finger sweeps to clear the airway in the absence of an obvious obstruction; finger sweeps should only be employed if a visible obstruction is present in the oropharynx (**Class IIb**).

Ventilation

Manikin studies[30] and one human study[31] showed that when no advanced airway (e.g. a tracheal tube) was present a tidal volume of 1 L produced significantly more gastric distension than 500 mL (**Level C**). In anethetized patients with no advanced airway in place, ventilation with 455 mL of room air was associated with acceptable although reduced oxygen saturation when compared with 719 mL. There was no difference in oxygen saturation between volumes of 624 mL and 719 mL[32] (**Level C**). Another study compared patients in cardiac arrest mechanically ventilated with oxygen at 12 L per minute. Smaller volumes of 500 mL were associated with a higher arterial PCO_2 and worse acidosis but no differences in PaO_2 than with volumes of 1 L[33] (**Level B**).

Small case series[34] and an animal study[35] showed that hyperventilation is associated with increased intrathoracic pressure, decreased coronary and cerebral perfusion and (in the animal study) decreased return of spontaneous circulation (ROSC). A case series of patients showed that ventilation rates of >10 min[−1] and inspiratory times of >1 s were associated with poor survival[37] (**Level C**). In summary, larger tidal volumes and higher ventilation rates may be detrimental while the adverse consequences of smaller volumes appear acceptable.

The recommended technique for mouth-to-mouth ventilation using exhaled air or bag-valve-mask ventilation using room air or oxygen is to give one breath within an inspiratory time of 1 s (**Class IIa**) sufficient to make the chest rise (**Class IIa**). After an advanced airway is in place (e.g. tracheal tube, Combitube™, laryngeal mask airway, etc.), the patient should be ventilated with supplementary oxygen sufficient to make the chest rise. In such patients the lungs should be ventilated at a rate of 8–10 ventilations min[−1] without pausing during chest compressions to deliver ventilations (**Class IIa**). There were insufficient data to recommend for or against the use of mechanical ventilators.

Chest compressions

The crucial importance of chest compressions has been increasingly recognized in recent years (for review of the subject see Chamberlain, Handley and Colquhoun).[36] Unfortunately there is increasing evidence that compressions are performed particularly badly in practice. In recent treatment recommendations, particular emphasis is placed on ways of increasing the number and quality of chest compressions during resuscitation attempts.

Hand position

There is insufficient evidence to recommend any one specific hand position when performing chest compressions in adults. Based on manikin studies in healthcare professionals demonstrating shorter pauses between ventilations and compressions[37] and improved performance[38] it is recommended that the hands should be placed 'in the centre of the chest' with the dominant hand in contact with the sternum (**Class IIa, Level C**).

Rate and depth

Studies in humans have given conflicting results; in one study a rate of 120 min[−1] provided improved hemodynamics over standard cardiopulmonary resuscitation (CPR)[39] (**Level C**). Studies that employed mechanical compression, however, have showed no improvement with rates of up to 140 min[−1] compared to 60 min[−1][40,41] (**Level C**). Observational studies show that hospital healthcare providers[42,43] and emergency medical services (EMS) personnel[44,45] give fewer compressions than currently recommended (**Level C**). These studies[43,44] also showed that compression depth is often inadequate.

In animal models of cardiac arrest, deeper compressions correlated with increased ROSC and 24-hour survival than standard compression depths[46–48] (**Level C**).

Decompression of the chest

In one animal study incomplete chest recoil was associated with increased intrathoracic pressure, decreased venous return and decreased coronary and cerebral perfusion.[49] There are no comparable human data. Lifting the hands slightly but completely off the chest between compressions allowed full recoil of the chest in a manikin study[50] (**Level C**). Observational studies in human CPR[35] and manikin studies[50] have shown that incomplete chest recoil is common during CPR (**Level C**).

Duty cycle

This term describes the time spent in compression as a proportion of the time between the start of one compression and the next. Coronary blood flow is determined in part by duty cycle (reduced when >50%) and the extent of chest relaxation at the end of each compression[51] (**Level C**). There is a lack of clinical evidence from human studies, but data from animal or mathematical models suggest a cycle of 20–50% is optimal[46,52–55] (**Level C**).

A duty cycle of 50% is much easier to achieve than cycles where compressions constitute a smaller percentage of the time,[56] an important practical issue for both performance and training (**Level C**).

Following analysis of this evidence, it is recommended that chest compressions should be performed with the hands placed in the center of the chest (**Class IIa**) at a rate of at least 100 min[-1] (**Class IIa**), compressing the sternum to a depth of at least 4–5 cm. Rescuers should allow complete recoil of the chest between compressions (**Class IIb**). It is reasonable to use a duty cycle of 50% (**Class IIb**). Rescuers should minimize interruption of chest compressions for checking the pulse, analyzing rhythm or performing other activities (**Class IIa**).

A manikin study showed that compression depth deteriorated within one minute, but rescuers only became aware of fatigue after five minutes[57] (**Level C**). In consequence, it is recommended that where feasible, rescuers should rotate the duties of compression regardless of whether they feel fatigued (**Class IIb**).

Compression ventilation sequence

Interrupting compressions Observational studies and secondary analysis of randomized trials have shown that interruption of chest compressions is commonplace[42,44,58] (**Level C**). Animal studies consistently show that interruptions in chest compression are associated with reduced ROSC, survival and postresuscitation myocardial dysfunction[59–61] (**Level C**). One retrospective study that employed ventricular fibrillation (VF) waveform analysis to predict the probability of defibrillation showed that interruptions in chest compression were associated with a reduced chance of conversion to another rhythm[62] (**Level C**).

On the basis of this evidence it is recommended that rescuers should minimize interruptions to chest compression (**Class IIa**).

Compression/ventilation ratio during CPR The number of compressions delivered per minute is determined by the compression rate, the compression/ventilation ratio and the time required to provide ventilation. Evidence from clinical studies shows that rescuers tend to ventilate too quickly and perform too few chest compressions when observed in actual resuscitation attempts. One observational study showed that paramedics perform ventilation at excessive rates in intubated patients and the same was found in a study of hospital responders both with and without an advanced airway in place[35,42,44] (**Level C**). A study of downloads from automated external defibrillators (AEDs) used by EMS personnel showed that chest compressions are frequently delivered at rates other than those recommended in guidelines. Adherence to recommended rates appeared to be associated with improved outcome[45] (**Level C**). A comparable study in trained lay responders in public access defibrillation (PAD) schemes showed widely differing rates of compression, often given too quickly, but pauses were also commonplace.[63] The compression/ventilation ratios employed also varied considerably. The AED algorithms (that require a "hands-off" period during rhythm analysis) were responsible for some of the pauses, but many were prolonged and unexplained. The outcome was that the number of compressions given was very much lower than recommended in guidelines (**Level C**).

Animal studies consistently show that hyperventilation is associated with lower coronary and cerebral perfusion and poorer survival while chest compressions given continuously or with minimal interruptions are associated with improved hemodynamics and improved survival[59,60,64–66] (**Level C**).

Various compression/ventilation ratios have been applied in animal models of cardiac arrest but without a consistent outcome on which to recommend any one particular ratio.[67–69] There are no adequate data from human studies. A mathematical analysis suggested that a ratio of 30/2 would provide the best blood flow and oxygen delivery[70] (**Level C**).

To optimize the number of compressions delivered, to reduce interruptions and simplify instruction (and skill retention), it is recommended that a single compression/ventilation ratio of 30/2 be used by the lone rescuer of infants, children and adults (**Class IIa**). Compressions should be delivered at a rate of at least 100 per minute (**Class IIa**).

Initial steps in the resuscitation sequence may include:
- opening the airway while assessing the patient
- giving 2–5 breaths while initiating resuscitation
- continuing resuscitation with a compression/ventilation ratio of 30/2.

Chest compression-only CPR

There have been no prospective human studies of compression-only CPR. A randomized prospective trial of compression-only CPR prior to EMS arrival in Seattle (a city with a very rapid EMS response time) showed a trend towards improved survival in those receiving compressions only, but the difference was not statistically significant[71] (**Level B**). Animal studies have shown compression-only CPR to be as effective as conventional CPR with ventilation in the first few minutes after the onset of cardiac arrest.[64–66] A compression/ventilation ratio of 30/2 maintained arterial oxygen saturation at two-thirds of normal whereas compressions only resulted in oxygen desaturation within two minutes.[69]

In observational studies of adult cardiac arrest treated by lay persons trained in standard CPR, survival with compression-only CPR was better than when victims received no CPR, but not as good as when victims received both compressions and ventilations[72,73] (**Level C**).

On the basis of this evidence, the recommendation is that rescuers should provide compression-only CPR if they are unwilling to perform airway and breathing maneuvers or if they are untrained and uncertain how to undertake CPR (**Class IIa**).

Advanced life support: defibrillation

Procedures before defibrillation

The precordial thump

There are no prospective studies of the precordial thump. Case series have reported VF or pulseless ventricular tachycardia (VT) converted to a perfusing rhythm following a precordial thump.[74–76] The likelihood of success was higher in VT[74–78] but decreased rapidly with time.[76] Observational studies also report that other arrhythmias including unstable supraventricular tachycardia (SVT) were terminated by a precordial thump[79,80] (**Level C**).

Observational studies show that an effective precordial thump is delivered by a closed fist from a height of 5–40 cm.[75,76,78] Adverse events include acceleration of the rate of VT, conversion of VT into VF, the production of complete heart block and asystole.[75,77,78,81–84] Current data do not allow these events to be reliably predicted (**Level C**).

The recommendation for practice is that one immediate precordial thump may be considered after a monitored arrest if a defibrillator is not immediately available (**Class Indeterminate**).

CPR before defibrillation

One study that employed a retrospective control group[85] (**Level C**) and one prospective study[86] (**Level B**) showed that 1.5–3 minutes of CPR before attempted defibrillation improved ROSC and survival in adults with out-of-hospital VF or VT when the response interval was ≥4–5 min. Another randomized trial reported that adults with VF or VT outside hospital did not benefit from 1.5 min of CPR[87] (**Level B**). Animal studies of VF of ≥5 min duration report that CPR before defibrillation (very often with concomitant adrenaline) improved survival rates[88–91] (**Level C**).

The ILCOR recommendation reflects this evidence: 1.5–3 min of CPR before attempted defibrillation may be considered in adults with out-of-hospital VF or VT where EMS response times are greater than 4–5 min (**Class IIb**). There was no evidence to support or refute the strategy in hospital.

Defibrillator electrode–patient interface

No studies have investigated the influence of electrode position on the outcome of human cardiac arrest. The subject has been investigated during conversion of stable atrial fibrillation or by the use of surrogate endpoints such as transthoracic impedance (TTI). Cardioversion of perfused myocardium in stable atrial fibrillation (AF) may not be the same as defibrillation of ischemic myocardium and caution is required when extrapolating from such studies. Many studies in AF have investigated the influence of electrode position and have lead to current recommendations. For references see [92] (**Level B or C**).

One human study documented higher success with larger electrodes[93]; 12.8 cm pads were superior to 8 cm (**Level B**). Several studies have confirmed lower TTI with increased electrode size (**Level B or C**). One animal study reported increased myocardial damage in dogs with smaller electrodes (4.3 cm compared with 8 or 12 cm)[94] (**Level C**).

The recommendation is that electrodes should be placed on the exposed chest in an anterolateral position (**Class IIa**). Acceptable alternatives are the anteroposterior and apex-posterior position (**Class IIa**). Placing the electrode on the female breast increased TTI[95] and in consequence the electrode should be placed underneath or lateral to the left breast (**Level C**).

Self-adhesive defibrillation pads versus paddles

One randomized trial[96] and two retrospective series[97,98] showed that the TTI was similar with both types of electrode (**Level B, C**). One randomized study showed similar effectiveness in converting AF[99] (**Level C**).

Self-adhesive pads are safe and effective and are an acceptable alternative to standard defibrillation paddles (**Class IIa**). There are important practical advantages with pads for routine monitoring and for perioperative or prehospital use.

Waveform analysis

Analysis of the VF waveform has the potential to improve the timing and effectiveness of countershocks. Evidence comes from retrospective analysis of human series and animal models (**Level C**). The technology is advancing rapidly but is not yet available in routine clinical practice.

Defibrillator shock waveform

A major advance in defibrillator technology in recent years has been the introduction of biphasic waveforms. Randomized clinical studies in human cardiac arrest[100–102] (**Level B**), reanalysis of the data in one study,[103] two observational studies[104,105] (**Level C**) and many animal studies show that biphasic waveforms using equal or lower energy levels are superior to or at least as effective as monophasic waveforms for terminating VF. A meta-analysis of seven randomized trials in patients in the electrophysiology laboratory[105] concluded that biphasic waveforms defibrillate with similar efficacy at lower energies than monophasic 200 J shocks, and greater efficacy than monophasic shocks of the same energy (**Level A**). No specific biphasic waveform has yet been demonstrated to be superior. One retrospective study[106] showed a higher hospital discharge rate with a monophasic truncated exponential (MTE) waveform compared to a biphasic truncated exponential (BTE) waveform. Survival was a secondary endpoint, however, and there were many confounding factors, not least the higher incidence of bystander CPR in the MTE group.

The recommendation for practice is that biphasic shocks are safe and effective for the termination of VF when compared with monophasic defibrillators (**Class IIa**).

First shock energy levels

Many clinical studies have compared initial biphasic shock energies of 100–200 J without clearly showing an advantage for either[100–102,104,106,107] (**Level B, C**). These studies also investigated subsequent energy levels ranging from 150 J to 300 J for VF refractory to the initial shock but without clearly demonstrating an optimal level. Other laboratory studies of stable patients evaluated termination of induced VF by energy levels of 115–200 J No clinical or laboratory study has convincingly shown greater benefit or harm from any currently used energy level. A hospital study compared first shock efficacy of monophasic damped sinusoidal (MDS) waveforms of low (100–240 J), intermediate (300–320 J) and high (400–440 J) without demonstrating a statistically significant benefit for any level.[108]

There is currently insufficient evidence to recommend a specific energy level for the first or subsequent biphasic shock. ILCOR recommend that with a biphasic defibrillator it is reasonable to use 150–200 J with a BTE waveform or 120 J with a rectilinear waveform (**Class IIa**). For a monophasic defibrillator an initial shock of 360 J is considered a reasonable option (**Class IIa**).

Second and subsequent shocks

Fixed versus escalating energy levels

Only one small human study compared fixed energy with escalating energies for subsequent shocks from a biphasic defibrillator. There was no clear benefit for either strategy[109] (**Level C**). No recommendation for either strategy could therefore be made.

One shock versus three shock sequence

No clinical or animal studies have compared a protocol that employs a single shock with one that employs three successive shocks before the resumption of chest compressions. Many studies have investigated the efficacy of first or subsequent shocks; success is defined as the termination of VF for ≥5s after the shock. This is an assessment made on the ECG, however, and does not necessarily indicate the return of the circulation.

The efficacy of the first shock given by a variety of waveforms and energy levels has been investigated in several trials of out-of-hospital VF.[92] A summary of the results is as follows.
• With a 200 J MDS waveform first shock success was 77–91%.
• With a 200 J MTE waveform, the rate was 54–63%.
• With a 150 J BTE waveform (four studies) and one using a 200 J BTE waveform, first shock success was 86–98%.
• With a 120 J rectilinear biphasic waveform first shock success rate was 85%.
Although the first shock success at converting the rhythm was relatively high, the average rate of ROSC with the first shock for all three waveforms was only 21% (range 13–23%).

Second and third shock success rate

Where the patient remained in VF after the first shock:
• with the MDS waveform with increasing energy levels (200 J to 200–300 J to 360 J), the combined success of the second and or third shocks was 68–72%
• with the MTE waveform with increasing energy levels (200 J to 200–360 J) the combined success of the second and/or third shocks was 27–60%
• with the fixed (non-escalating) 150 J BTE waveform, the combined success of the second and or third shocks was 50–90%.
The single study that used a rectilinear escalating waveform (120 J to 150–200 J reported combined success of second and/or third shocks of 85%.

In the absence of any evidence for a clearly superior strategy, ILCOR recommended that practice should concentrate on procedures that optimize the chances of successful defibrillation regardless of the precise energy, waveform or shock sequence. These priorities were to recognize the potential need for defibrillation as soon as possible, provide CPR until a defibrillator is available and minimize interruptions to chest compressions (**Class I**).

A one-shock strategy may improve outcome by reducing interruptions in chest compressions. A stacked sequence of three shocks can be optimized by the immediate resumption of effective chest compressions after each shock (irrespective of the rhythm) and by minimizing the "hands-off" periods for rhythm analysis or other procedures.

Advanced life support: other considerations

Airway and ventilation

Methods to secure and maintain the airway and the different strategies and devices used to provide ventilation during resuscitation attempts are evaluated in detail during the ILCOR evidence evaluation process. Detailed consideration of these topics is outside the scope of this chapter and the reader is referred to the original ILCOR documents.[110]

Drugs used in the management of cardiac arrest

Vasopressors

Despite the widespread use of vasopressors, principally adrenaline/epinephrine during resuscitation attempts, and several trials involving vasopressin, there is no placebo-controlled trial showing that the routine use of any vasopressor during human cardiac arrest increases survival to hospital discharge.

Vasopressin Despite promising preliminary data and numerous animal studies, two large randomized trials of cardiac arrest in humans did not show a benefit (in terms of ROSC or survival) for vasopressin 40 U (repeated in one trial) compared with adrenaline 1 mg (repeated) as the initial vasopressor whether in hospital[111] or out of hospital[112] (**Level A**). In one of the trials,[112] *post hoc* analysis suggested an improvement to hospital discharge for the subset of patients initially in asystole in patients receiving vasopressin compared to adrenaline, but neurologically intact survival was not different in the two groups. Subsequently, meta-analysis of five randomized trials[113] showed no statistically significant differences between vasopressin and adrenaline for ROSC, death within 24 hours or death before hospital discharge. Subgroup analysis based on presenting cardiac rhythm did not show any benefit in terms of death before hospital discharge (**Level A**).

Alpha-methyl noradrenaline When vasopressors like adrenaline that possesses both alpha- and beta-adrenergic effects are administered during cardiac arrest, the beta effects increase myocardial oxygen consumption with the risk of increased myocardial ischemia. Alpha-1 but not alpha-2 receptors have been identified in the ventricular myocardium, and it has been suggested that the selective alpha-2 agonist alpha-methyl noradrenaline may offer advantages by producing vasoconstriction (with attendant increase in coronary perfusion) while avoiding the positive inotropic and chronotropic effects of adrenaline. Animal work has been encouraging but no human study has been reported (**Level C**).[114,116]

Endothelin Several animal studies have demonstrated improved coronary or cerebral perfusion pressure with endothelin-1. This did not result in improved myocardial blood flow, however. No human trial has been reported.

Conclusions Despite the lack of placebo-controlled trials, adrenaline has been the standard vasopressor and remains the drug of choice. It is considered appropriate to administer a 1 mg dose of epinephrine IV/IO every 3–5 minutes during adult cardiac arrest (**Class IIb**). Current evidence does not support or refute the use of any other vasopressor or combination during human cardiac arrest. There is insufficient evidence to support the use of vasopressin either alone or in combination with adrenaline in any cardiac arrest rhythm (**Class III**).

Antiarrhythmic drugs

There is no evidence that the administration of any antiarrhythmic drug during resuscitation increases survival to hospital discharge.

Amiodarone

Two randomized clinical trials in adults have shown that the administration of of amiodarone by paramedics to adult patients in out-of-hospital cardiac arrest with shock-refractory VF/pulseless VT improved survival to hospital admission (but not to hospital discharge) when compared to placebo[117] or lidocaine[118] (**Level A**). Other lower level studies in humans or animals document a consistent improvement in the response to defibrillatory shocks in VF or VT.

Despite the lack of long-term outcome data, it is deemed reasonable to use amiodarone for VF/VT refractory to initial shocks (**Class IIb**).

Other drugs and fluids

There is no evidence that buffers, aminophylline, atropine, calcium or magnesium given routinely during human cardiac arrest increase survival to hospital discharge (**Class III**). There are reports that fibrinolytic agents may have a role when the arrest is caused by pulmonary embolism (**Class IIa**).

Aminophylline Ischemia is a potent stimulus for the release of adenosine which may slow the heart and possibly produce or maintain asystole. Methylxanthines like aminophylline block adenosine receptors and on this basis a role for the use of aminphylline in the management of bradyasystolic arrest has been proposed. In a small case series, 15 consecutive patients with cardiac arrest due to asystole or to non-perfusing bradyarrhythmias, who failed to respond to intravenous atropine and epinephrine, were treated with aminophylline (rapid intravenous injection of 250 mg). Establishment of a stable heart rhythm with sufficient blood pressure to allow discontinuation of closed-chest cardiac massage was achieved in 11 of 15 (73%) patients. All 11 patients were alive 60 minutes after resuscitation. One patient survived, without neurologic damage[119] (**Level C**). Subsequently, three randomized trials of its use were unable to show any increase in ROSC[120–122] but the numbers recruited into the trial were small. No trial has shown an effect on survival to hospital discharge. There is no evidence of harm following its use, but overall there is insufficient evidence to advocate a role for its routine use (**Class IIb, Level B**).

Atropine Five prospective but non-randomized studies in adults[123–127] and one retrospective case[128] series failed to show any consistent benefit following the use of atropine (**Level C**). The use of atropine has not been associated with harm, however, and there have been anecdotal reports of survival following its use in asystolic cardiac arrest. In the absence of agents with more evidence to support their use, atropine maintains a role in the management of asystole (**Class Indeterminate**). Atropine remains the first-line drug treatment for acute symptomatic bradycardia (**Class IIa**).

Buffers Sodium bicarbonate has been widely used in the past in the management of cardiac arrest. There are no randomized controlled trials to support its use and recent resuscitation guidelines have curtailed its unrestricted use. Retrospective reports of its uncontrolled use are largely inconclusive although one study reported that EMS systems that gave sodium bicarbonate earlier and more frequently had increased rates of ROSC, hospital discharge and better long-term neurologic survival[129] (**Level C**). Animal studies are also inconclusive. The drug has been used successfully to treat hypotension and arrhythmias complicating tricyclic overdosage, but only one report described the successful treatment of VF arrest[130] (**Level C**).

The routine use of sodium bicarbonate during cardiac arrest (especially outside hospital) or after ROSC is not recommended (**Class III**). It may be considered for life-threatening hyperkalemia or cardiac arrest associated with hyperkalemia, tricyclic overdosage or pre-existing metabolic acidosis (**Class IIb**).

Magnesium Randomized trials of magnesium in adult cardiac arrest[131–4] (**Level B**) and lower degrees of evidence including animal studies have not shown an increased rate of ROSC when magnesium was given during CPR. One small case series reported benefit in patients in shock-resistant and adrenaline/lidocaine-resistant VF.[135]

There are insufficient data to recommend or refute the use of magnesium in cardiac arrest. It should be given in hypomagnesemia and retains a place in the management of torsades de pointes (**Class IIa**).

Fibrinolytic drugs Up to 70% of patients with sudden cardiac arrest have underlying acute myocardial infarction or pulmonary embolism. Both conditions are potentially responsive to fibrinolytic therapy. Adult patients have been successfully resuscitated following the administration of fibrinolytic drugs after the initial failure of standard resuscitation procedures, particularly when the cause has been pulmonary embolism. One large clinical trial, however, failed to show a significant treatment effect when administered to patients with pulseless electrical activity (PEA) outside hospital.[136] Other small studies or case reports were inconclusive with regard to improving outcome, but did not report an increase in bleeding complications (**Level C**).

In the Thrombolysis in Cardiac Arrest (TROICA) trial 1050 patients suffering from witnessed out-of-hospital arrest of presumed cardiac origin were randomly assigned to tenecteplase (TNK) or placebo, plus standard therapy. Interim data analysis showed that the addition of TNK to standard CPR did not increase the 30-day survival rate (18.2% vs 20.2%, P = NS) nor the hospital admission rate (59.0% vs 59.5%, P = NS). The symptomatic intracranial hemorrhage (1% vs 0%) and major bleeding (8.9% vs 7.4%) rates were not significantly different between groups. This preliminary data analysis showed that the probability that the study would demonstrate overall superiority of tenecteplase over placebo was low and the recruitment was suspended[137] (**Level B**).

Thrombolysis should be considered in cardiac arrest caused by proven or suspected pulmonary embolism (**Class IIa**). The data do not support its routine use in other situations.

Techniques and devices to assist the circulation during cardiac arrest

Because CPR is often of poor quality and deteriorates with time, and because interruptions of chest compressions are common, a variety of approaches has been adopted to improve the quality of CPR by the use of prompt devices or by other techniques. A separate approach is to use mechanical methods to undertake chest compressions, thereby eliminating dependence on rescuers.

Transcutaneous pacing for asystole

Three randomized trials[138–140] have failed to demonstrate an improvement in the rate of hospital admission or survival to discharge when pacing was attempted in asystolic patients in the prehospital arena or the emergency department (**Level A**). Pacing is therefore not recommended for this group of patients (**Class III**). It retains its established role in the treatment of bradycardia (**Class I**).

CPR prompt devices

Unprompted CPR is often of poor quality and interruptions to chest compressions are frequent[42,44,45,63] (**Level C**). Studies in adults, children or experimental animals or with manikins have consistently shown improvement in end-tidal CO_2 or quality of CPR when feedback is provided to guide the rescuer[141–151] (**Level C**). Several such aids are now available either as stand-alone devices or incorporated into the AED or electrodes. Further studies are required to investigate the effect on patient outcomes resulting from the introduction of these devices into practice. In the meantime, it is considered that CPR prompt devices may be useful in both out-of-hospital and in-hospital settings (**Class IIb**).

Active compression decompression (ACD) CPR

ACD devices are designed to adhere to the chest (usually by a suction cup) so that after chest compression is complete, lifting the device actively expands the chest. This causes a greater reduction in intrathoracic pressure than would result from passive expansion and thereby increases venous return and cardiac output during subsequent chest compressions. Initial studies were promising, reporting improved survival[152–4] (**Level A, B**).

However, subsequent Cochrane meta-analysis of 10 trials (in 4062 patients) comparing ACD with standard CPR outside hospital did not show an improvement in either short-term survival or hospital discharge[155] (**Level A**). Similarly, analysis of two hospital-based trials (826 patients) comparing ACD with standard CPR after arrest in hospital did not show improvement in either short-term survival or hospital discharge[155] (**Level A**). At present there is insufficient evidence to recommend for or against the use of ACD.

Load-distributing band CPR

This chest compression device features a backboard and a band that is placed circumferentially around the chest. The band is constricted pneumatically to produce chest compression. Case control[156,157] and laboratory studies[158,159] with encouraging results prompted the conduct of two larger clinical studies of the device. One study, comparing results before and after the introduction of the device into an EMS system, reported improvements in ROSC, hospital admission and discharge rates[160] (**Level C**). The second study, a randomized multicenter trial, was stopped prematurely as patients in the device group showed worse neurologic outcomes and a trend toward worse survival than with manual CPR[161] (**Level A**). An accompanying editorial[162] tried to reconcile the apparently contradictory results. Further randomized trials of the device are planned and until more data are available, the device cannot be recommended for routine practice. At present it is recommended that properly trained personnel may use the device as an adjunct to CPR for patients with cardiac arrest in the out-of-hospital or in-hospital setting (**Class IIb**).

Mechanical (piston) CPR

Although this method of providing mechanical CPR has been around for several years, published evidence to support its use is scanty. Prospective randomized studies in humans have demonstrated improvement in surrogate outcomes like end-tidal CO_2 or mean arterial blood pressure when it has been employed both in and outside hospital.[163–6] The device has proved capable of performing chest compressions that adhere more closely to guidelines than manual compressions, particularly during the transport of patients. Reports of its effect on immediate resuscitation or ultimate survival when used in clinical practice are lacking. At present the recommendation is that mechanical piston CPR may be considered for patients in cardiac arrest in circumstances that make manual resuscitation difficult (**Class IIb**).

Lund University Cardiac Arrest System (LUCAS) CPR device

This is a gas-driven device that incorporates a suction cup to apply chest compressions and to achieve active decompression. Promising improvements in hemodynamics were reported in pigs when compared to manual CPR.[167,168] A small case series reported promising results[169] although outcome data were incomplete (**Level C**). The device has been used successfully during the transport of severely hypothermic patients to a center with cardiopulmonary bypass[170,171] and during prolonged resuscitation from PEA complicating anaphylaxis[172] (**Level C**).

A prospective randomized clinical trial comparing the device with manual CPR in out-of-hospital cardiac arrest reported no significant difference in ROSC, hospital admission or discharge[173] (**Level B**). The LUCAS device was applied late, however (18 min after arrest) and the trial highlighted the complexity of conducting such evaluation. Further trials are planned and will help establish the place of the device. Important injuries have been noted in a small number of patients in whom the device was used.[174]

Conclusion

The principles of evidence-based medicine are increasingly applied to the management of cardiac arrest. International collaboration to agree upon the scientific basis of practice is well established. The formulation of sound guidelines for practice is limited, however, by a lack of robust scientific evidence in many areas. There are additional problems with the conduct of clinical trials that might help this process: the population studied is heterogeneous, different treatment strategies are common, recording data is difficult under the circumstances and many confounding factors are usually present. The design and conduct of trials with sufficient statistical power to evaluate potentially small benefits present further challenges. The low levels of evidence often quoted in this chapter attest to these problems but by critically examining the evidence base in this way, areas of ignorance and potentially poor practice may readily be identified. That is a necessary stage toward obtaining better evidence and providing more effective management.

References

1. Myerburg RJ, Kessler KM, Castellanos A. Sudden cardiac death: epidemiology, transient risk and intervention assessment. *Ann Intern Med* 1993;**119**(12): 1187–97.

2. American Heart Association. *Heart Disease and Stroke Statistics – 2005 Update*. Dallas, TX: American Heart Association, 2005.

3. Sans S, Kesteloot H, Kromhout D. The burden of cardiovascular diseases mortality in Europe. Task Force of the European Society of Cardiology on cardiovascular mortality and morbidity. Statistics in Europe. *Eur Heart J* 1997;**18**:1231–48.

4. Peberdy MA, Kaye W, Ornato JP *et al.* Cardiopulmonary resuscitation in adults in the hospital: a report of 14,720 cardiac arrests from the National Registry of Cardiopulmonary Resuscitation. *Resuscitation* 2003;**58**:297–308.

5. Beck CS, Pritchard WH, Fell HS. Ventricular fibrillation of long duration abolished by electric shock. *JAMA* 1947;**135**: 985–6.

6. Zoll PM, Linenthal AJ, Gibson W *et al.* Termination of ventricular fibrillation in man by externally applied electric countershock. *N Engl J Med* 1956;**254**:727–32.

7. Safer P, Elam JO. Manual versus mouth to mouth methods of artificial respiration *Anesthesiology* 1958;**19**:111–12.

8. Kouwenhoven WB, Jude JR, Knickerbocker CG. Closed chest cardiac massage. *JAMA* 1960;**173**:1064–7.

9. McNeilly RH, Pemberton J Duration of last attack in 998 fatal cases of coronary artery disease and its relation to possible cardiac resuscitation. *BMJ* 1968;**iii**:139–42.

10. Pantridge JF, Geddes JS. A mobile intensive care unit in the management of myocardial infarction. *Lancet* 1967;**ii**:271–3.

11. Chamberlain DA, Cummins RO, Montgomery WH *et al.* International collaboration in resuscitation medicine. *Resuscitation* 2005;**67**:163–5.

12. Guidelines for cardiopulmonary resuscitation (CPR) and emergency cardiac care (ECC). *JAMA* 1992;**286**:2135–302.

13. International Liaison Committee on Resuscitation. The International Liaison Committee on Resuscitation (ILCOR) – past, present and future. *Resuscitation* 2005;**67**:157–61.

14. American Heart Association with the International Liaison Committee on Resuscitation. Guidelines 2000 for cardiopulmonary resuscitation and emergency cardiovascular care – an international consensus on science. *Resuscitation* 2000;**46**: 1–447.

15. Morley PT, Zaritsky A. The evidence evaluation process for the 2005 International Consensus Conference on cardiopulmonary Resuscitation and emergency cardiovascular care science with treatment recommendations. *Resuscitation* 2005;**67**:167–70.

16. International Liaison Committee on Resuscitation. 2005 international consensus on cardiopulmonary resuscitation and emergency cardiovascular care science with treatment recommendations. Part 1 Introduction. *Resuscitation* 2005;**67**: 181–6.

17. http://www.c2005.org/presenter.jhtml?identifier=3022512

18. International Liaison Committee on Resuscitation. 2005 International consensus on cardiopulmonary resuscitation and emergency cardiovascular care with treatment recommendations. *Resuscitation* 2005;**67**:157–341.

19. International Liaison Committee on Resuscitation. 2005 International consensus on cardiopulmonary resuscitation and emergency cardiovascular care science with treatment recommendations. *Circulation* 2005; 112: III-1–III-136.

20. European Resuscitation Council. Guidelines for resuscitation 2005. *Resuscitation* 2005;**67**(suppl 1):S1-S189.

21. American Heart Association. 2005 Guidelines for cardiopulmonary resuscitation and emergency cardiac care. *Circulation* 2005;**112**(suppl I):IV-1–IV-211.

22. Bahr J, Klinger H, Panzer W *et al.* Skills of lay people in checking the carotid pulse. *Resuscitation* 1997;**35**:23–6.

23. Eberle B, Dick W, Schneider T *et al.* Checking the carotid pulse check: diagnostic accuracy of first responders in patients with and without a pulse. *Resuscitation* 1996;**33**:107–16.

24. Ruppert M, Reith MW, Widmann JH *et al.* Checking for breathing: evaluation of the diagnostic capability of emergency medical services personnel, physicians, medical students and lay persons. *Ann Emerg Med* 1999;**34**:720–9.

25. Hauff SR, Rea TD, Culley LL *et al.* Factors impeding dispatcher-assisted telephone cardiopulmonary resuscitation. *Ann Emerg Med* 2003;**42**:731–7.

26. Guildner CW. Resuscitation: opening the airway. A comparative study of techniques for opening an airway obstructed by the tongue. *JACEP* 1976: **5**:588–90.

27. Greene DG, Elam JO, Dobkin AB, Studley CL. Cineflourographic study of hyperextension of the neck and upper airway patency. *JAMA* 1961;**176**:570–3.

28. Morikawa S, Safar P, Decarlo J. Influence of the head-jaw position upon upper airway patency. *Anesthesiology* 1961;**22**: 265–70.

29. Elam JO, Greene DG, Schneider MA *et al.* Head tilt method of oral resuscitation. *JAMA* 1960;**172**:812–15.

30. Zecha-Stallinger A, Wenzel V, Wagner-Bergner HG *et al.* A strategy to optimise the performance of the mouth to bag resuscitator using smaller tidal volumes: effects on lung and gastric

ventilation in a bench model of an unprotected airway. *Resuscitation* 2004;**61**:69–74.

31. Wenzel V, Keller C, Idris AH *et al.* Effects of smaller tidal volumes during basic life support ventilation in patients with respiratory arrest: good ventilation, less risk? *Resuscitation* 1999;**43**:25–9.

32. Dorges V, Ocker H, Hagelberg S *et al.* Optimisation of tidal volumes given with self-inflatable bags without additional oxygen. *Resuscitation* 2000;**43**:195–9.

33. Langhelle A, Sunde K, Wik L, Steen PA. Arterial blood-gases with 500- versus 1000-ml tidal volumes during out-of-hospital CPR. *Resuscitation* 2000;**45**:27–33.

34. Aufderheide TP, Lurie KG, Death by hyperventilation: a common and life-threatening problem during cardiopulmonary resuscitation. *Crit Care Med* 2004;**32**:S345-S351.

35. Aufderheide TP, Sigurdsson G, Pirrallo RG *et al.* Hyperventilation-induced hypotension during cardiopulmonary resuscitation. *Circulation* 2004;**109**:1960–5.

36. Chamberlain DA, Handley AJ, Colquhoun MC. Time for change (editorial). *Resuscitation* 2003;**58**:237–47.

37. Kundra P, Dey S, Ravishankar M. Role of dominant hand position during external cardiac compression. *Br J Anaesth* 2000;**84**:491–3.

38. Handley AJ. Teaching hand placement for chest compression – a simpler technique. *Resuscitation* 2002;**53**:29–36.

39. Swenson RD, Weaver WD, Niskanen RA *et al.* Hemodynamics in humans during conventional and experimental methods of cardiopulmonary resuscitation. *Circulation* 1988;**78**:630–9.

40. Ornato JP, Gonzalez ER, Garnett AR *et al.* Effect of cardiopulmonary resuscitation compression rate on end-tidal carbon dioxide concentration and arterial pressure in man. *Crit Care Med* 1988;**16**:241–5.

41. Milander MM, Hiscok PS, Sanders AB *et al.* Chest compression and ventilation rates during cardiopulmonary resuscitation: the effects of audible tone guidance. *Acad Emerg Med* 1995;**2**:708–13.

42. Abella BS, Alvarado JP, Myklebust H *et al.* Quality of cardiopulmonary resuscitation during in-hospital cardiac arrest. *JAMA* 2005;**293**:305–10.

43. Abella BS, Sandbo N, Vassilatos P *et al.* Chest compression rates during cardiopulmonary resuscitation are suboptimal: a prospective study during in-hospital cardiac arrest. *Circulation* 2005;**111**:428–34.

44. Wik L, Kramer-Johansen J, Myklebust H *et al.* Quality of cardiopulmonary resuscitation during out-of-hospital cardiac arrest. *JAMA* 2005;**293**:299–304.

45. Ko PC, Chen WJ, Lin CH, Ma MH, Lin FY. Evaluating the quality of prehospital cardiopulmonary resuscitation by reviewing automated external defibrillator records and survival for out-of-hospital witnessed arrests. *Resuscitation* 2005;**64**:163–9.

46. Kern KB, Carter AB, Showen RL *et al.* Twenty-four hour survival in a canine model of cardiac arrest comparing three methods of manual cardiopulmonary resuscitation. *J Am Coll Cardiol* 1986;**7**:859–67.

47. Babbs CF, Voorhees WD, Fitzgerald KR *et al.* Relationship of blood pressure and flow during CPR to chest compression amplitude: evidence for an effective compression threshold. *Ann Emerg Med* 1983;**12**:527–32.

48. Bellamy RF, DeGuzman LR, Pedersen DC. Coronary blood flow during cardiopulmonary resuscitation in swine. *Circulation* 1984;**69**:174–80.

49. Yannopoulos D, McKnite S, Aufderheide TP *et al.* Effects of incomplete chest wall decompression during cardiopulmonary resuscitation on coronary and cerebral perfusion pressures in a porcine model of cardiac arrest. *Resuscitation* 2005;**64**:363–72.

50. Aufderheide TP, Pirrallo RG, Yannopoulos D *et al.* Incomplete chest wall decompression: a clinical evaluation of CPR performance by EMS personnel and assessment of alternative manual chest compression–decompression techniques. *Resuscitation* 2005;**64**:353–62.

51. Wolfe JA, Maier GW, Newton JR Jr *et al.* Physiologic determinants of coronary blood flow during external cardiac massage. *J Thorac Cardiovasc Surg* 1988;**95**:523–32.

52. Feneley MP, Maier GW, Kern KB *et al.* Influence of compression rate on initial success of resuscitation and 24 hour survival after prolonged manual cardiopulmonary resuscitation in dogs. *Circulation* 1988;**77**:240–50.

53. Swart GL, Mateer JR, DeBehnke DJ *et al.* The effect of compression duration on hemodynamics during mechanical high-impulse CPR. *Acad Emerg Med* 1994;**1**:430–7.

54. Halperin HR, Tsitlik JE, Guerci AD *et al.* Determinants of blood flow to vital organs during cardiopulmonary resuscitation in dogs. *Circulation* 1986;**73**:539–50.

55. Talley DB, Ornato JP, Clarke AM. Computer-aided characterization and optimization of the Thumper compression waveform in closed-chest CPR. *Biomed Instrum Technol* 1990;**24**:283–8.

56. Handley AJ, Handley SA. Improving CPR performance using an audible feedback system suitable for incorporation into an automated external defibrillator. *Resuscitation* 2003;**57**:57–62.

57. Hightower D, Thomas SH, Stone CK, Dunn K, March JA. Decay in quality of closed-chest compressions over time. *Ann Emerg Med* 1995;**26**:300–3.

58. van Alem AP, Sanou BT, Koster RW. Interruption of cardiopulmonary resuscitation with the use of the automated external defibrillator in out-of-hospital cardiac arrest. *Ann Emerg Med* 2003;**42**:449–57.

59. Berg RA, Sanders AB, Kern KB *et al.* Adverse hemodynamic effects of interrupting chest compressions for rescue breathing during cardiopulmonary resuscitation for ventricular fibrillation cardiac arrest. *Circulation* 2001;**104**:2465–70.

60. Yu T, Weil MH, Tang W *et al.* Adverse outcomes of interrupted precordial compression during automated defibrillation. *Circulation* 2002;**106**:368–72.

61. Kern KB, Hilwig RW, Berg RA, Sanders AB, Ewy GA. Importance of continuous chest compressions during cardiopulmonary resuscitation: improved outcome during a simulated single lay-rescuer scenario. *Circulation* 2002;**105**:645–9.

62. Eftestol T, Sunde K, Steen PA. Effects of interrupting precordial compressions on the calculated probability of defibrillation success during out-of-hospital cardiac arrest. *Circulation* 2002;**105**:2270–3.

63. Whitfield R, Colquhoun M, Chamberlain DA, Newcombe R, Davies CS, Boyle R. The Department of Health National Defibrillator Programme: analysis of downloads from 250 deployments of public access defibrillators. *Resuscitation* 2005;**64**:269–77.

64. Berg RA, Hilwig RW, Kern KB, Ewy GA. "Bystander" chest compressions and assisted ventilation independently improve outcome from piglet asphyxial pulseless "cardiac arrest". *Circulation* 2000;**101**:1743–8.

65. Berg RA, Kern KB, Hilwig RW et al. Assisted ventilation does not improve outcome in a porcine model of single-rescuer bystander cardiopulmonary resuscitation. *Circulation* 1997;**95**: 1635–41.

66. Berg RA, Kern KB, Hilwig RW, Ewy GA. Assisted ventilation during 'bystander' CPR in a swine acute myocardial infarction model does not improve outcome. *Circulation* 1997;**96**:4364–71.

67. Sanders AB, Kern KB, Berg RA, Hilwig RW, Heidenrich J, Ewy GA. Survival and neurologic outcome after cardiopulmonary resuscitation with four different chest compression–ventilation ratios. *Ann Emerg Med* 2002;**40**:553–62.

68. Dorph E, Wik L, Stromme TA, Eriksen M, Steen PA. Quality of CPR with three different ventilation:compression ratios. *Resuscitation* 2003; **58**:193–201.

69. Dorph E, Wik L, Stromme TA, Eriksen M, Steen PA. Oxygen delivery and return of spontaneous circulation with ventilation:compression ratio 2:30 versus chest compressions only CPR in pigs. *Resuscitation* 2004;**60**:309–18.

70. Babbs CF, Kern KB. Optimum compression to ventilation ratios in CPR under realistic, practical conditions: a physiological and mathematical analysis. *Resuscitation* 2002;**54**:147–57.

71. Hallstrom A, Cobb L, Johnson E, Copass M. Cardiopulmonary resuscitation by chest compression alone or with mouth-to-mouth ventilation. *N Engl J Med* 2000;**342**:1546–53.

72. van Hoeyweghen RJ, Bossaert LL, Mullie A et al. Quality and efficiency of bystander CPR. Belgian Cerebral Resuscitation Study Group. *Resuscitation* 1993;**26**:47–52.

73. Waalewijn RA, Tijssen JG, Koster RW. Bystander initiated actions in out-of-hospital cardiopulmonary resuscitation: results from the Amsterdam Resuscitation Study (ARRESUST). *Resuscitation* 2001;**50**:273–9.

74. Befeler B. Mechanical stimulation of the heart; its therapeutic value in tachyarrhythmias. *Chest* 1978;**73**:832–8.

75. Volkmann H, Kühnert H, Paliege R et al. Terminierung von Kammertachykardien durch mechanische Herzstimulation mit Präkordialschlägen. (Termination of ventricular tachycardias by mechanical cardiac pacing by means of precordial thumps.) *Zeitschrift für Kardiologie* 1990;**79**:717–724.

76. Caldwell G, Millar G, Quinn E. Simple mechanical methods for cardioversion: defence of the precordial thump and cough version. *BMJ* 1985;**291**:627–30.

77. Morgera T, Baldi N, Chersevani D, Medugno G, Camerini F. Chest thump and ventricular tachycardia. *Pacing Clin Electrophysiol* 1979;**2**:69–75.

78. Rahner E, Zeh E. Die Regularisierung von Kammertachykardien durch präkordialen Faustschlag. (The regularization of ventricular tachycardias by precordial thumping.) *Medizinsche Welt* 1978;**29**:1659–63.

79. Cotoi S, Moldovan D, Carasca E. Precordial thump in the treatment of cardiac arrhythmias (electrophysiologic considerations). *Physiologie* 1980;**17**:285–8.

80. Cotoi S. Precordial thump and termination of cardiac reentrant tachyarrhythmias. *Am Heart J* 1981;**101**:675–7.

81. Gertsch M, Hottinger S, Hess T. Serial chest thumps for the treatment of ventricular tachycardia in patients with coronary artery disease. *Clin Cardiol* 1992;**15**:181–8.

82. Krijne R. Rate acceleration of ventricular tachycardia after a precordial chest thump. *Am J Cardiol* 1984;**53**:964–5.

83. Sclarovsky S, Kracoff OH, Agmon J. Acceleration of ventricular tachycardia induced by a chest thump. *Chest* 1981;**80**:596–9.

84. Yakaitis RW, Redding JS. Precordial thumping during cardiac resuscitation. *Crit Care Med* 1973;**1**:22–6.

85. Cobb LA, Fahrenbruch CE, Walsh TR et al. Influence of cardiopulmonary resuscitation prior to defibrillation in patients with out-of-hospital ventricular fibrillation. *JAMA* 1999;**281**: 1182–8.

86. Wik L, Hansen TB, Fylling F et al. Delaying defibrillation to give basic cardiopulmonary resuscitation to patients with out-of-hospital ventricular fibrillation: a randomized trial. *JAMA* 2003;**289**:1389–95.

87. Jacobs IG, Finn JC, Oxer HF, Jelinek GA. CPR before defibrillation in out-of-hospital cardiac arrest: a randomized trial. *Emerg Med Australas* 2005;**17**:39–45.

88. Berg RA, Hilwig RW, Kern KB, Ewy GA. Precountershock cardiopulmonary resuscitation improves ventricular fibrillation median frequency and myocardial readiness for successful defibrillation from prolonged ventricular fibrillation: a randomized, controlled swine study. *Ann Emerg Med* 2002;**40**: 563–70.

89. Berg RA, Hilwig RW, Ewy GA, Kern KB. Precountershock cardiopulmonary resuscitation improves initial response to defibrillation from prolonged ventricular fibrillation: a randomized, controlled swine study. *Crit Care Med* 2004;**32**:1352–7.

90. Kolarova J, Ayoub IM, Yi Z, Gazmuri RJ. Optimal timing for electrical defibrillation after prolonged untreated ventricular fibrillation. *Crit Care Med* 2003;**31**:2022–28.

91. Niemann JT, Cairns CB, Sharma J, Lewis RJ. Treatment of prolonged ventricular fibrillation: immediate countershock versus high-dose epinephrine and CPR preceding countershock. *Circulation* 1992;**85**:281–7.

92. International Liaison Committee on Resuscitation. 2005 International consensus on cardiopulmonary resuscitation and emergency cardiovascular care with treatment recommendations. Part 3 Defibrillation. *Resuscitation* 2005;**67**:203–11.

93. Thomas ED, Ewy GA, Dahl CF, Ewy MD. Effectiveness of direct current defibrillation: role of paddle electrode size. *Am Heart J* 1977;**93**:463–7.

94. Dahl CF, Ewy GA, Warner ED, Thomas ED. Myocardial necrosis from direct current countershock: effect of paddle electrode size and time interval between discharges. *Circulation* 1974;**50**: 956–61.

95. Pagan-Carlo LA, Spencer KT, Robertson CE et al. Transthoracic defibrillation: importance of avoiding electrode placement directly on the female breast. *J Am Coll Cardiol* 1996;**27**:449–52.

96. Deakin CD, McLaren RM, Petley GW et al. A comparison of transthoracic impedance using standard defibrillation paddles and self-adhesive defibrillation pads. *Resuscitation* 1998;**39**: 43–6.

97. Kerber RE, Martins JB, Kelly KJ et al. Self-adhesive preapplied electrode pads for defibrillation and cardioversion. *J Am Coll Cardiol* 1984;**3**:815–20.

98. Kerber RE, Martins JB, Ferguson DW *et al.* Experimental evaluation and initial clinical application of new self-adhesive defibrillation electrodes. *Int J Cardiol* 1985;**8**:57–66.

99. Kirchhof P, Monnig G, Wasmer K *et al.* A trial of self-adhesive patch electrodes and hand-held paddle electrodes for external cardioversion of atrial fibrillation (MOBIPAPA). *Eur Heart J* 2005;**26**:1292–7.

100. Morrison LJ, Dorian P, Long J *et al.* Out-of-hospital cardiac arrest rectilinear biphasic to monophasic damped sine defibrillation waveforms with advanced life support intervention trial (ORBIT). *Resuscitation* 2005;**66**:149–57.

101. van Alem AP, Chapman FW, Lank P *et al.* A prospective, randomised and blinded comparison of first shock success of monophasic and biphasic waveforms in out-of-hospital cardiac arrest. *Resuscitation* 2003;**58**:17–24.

102. Schneider T, Martens PR, Paschen H *et al.* Multicenter, randomized, controlled trial of 150-J biphasic shocks compared with 200- to 360-J monophasic shocks in the resuscitation of out-of-hospital cardiac arrest victims. Optimized Response to Cardiac Arrest (ORCA) Investigators. *Circulation* 2000;**102**:1780–7.

103. Martens PR, Russell JK, Wolcke B *et al.* Optimal Response to Cardiac Arrest study: defibrillation waveform effects. *Resuscitation* 2001;**49**:233–43.

104. Stothert JC, Hatcher TS, Gupton CL *et al.* Rectilinear biphasic waveform defibrillation of out-of-hospital cardiac arrest. *Prehosp Emerg Care* 2004;**8**:388–92.

105. Faddy SC, Powell J, Craig, JC. Biphasic and monophasic shocks for transthoracic defibrillation: a meta analysis of randomised controlled trials. *Resuscitation* 2003;**58**:9–16.

106. Carpenter J, Rea TD, Murray JA, Kudenchuk PJ, Eisenberg MS. Defibrillation waveform and post-shock rhythm in out-of-hospital ventricular fibrillation cardiac arrest. *Resuscitation* 2003;**59**:189–96.

107. White RD, Russell JK. Refibrillation, resuscitation and survival in out-of-hospital sudden cardiac arrest victims treated with biphasic automated external defibrillators. *Resuscitation* 2002;**55**:17–23.

108. Tang W, Weil MH, Sun S *et al.* The effects of biphasic and conventional monophasic defibrillation on postresuscitation myocardial function. *J Am Coll Cardiol* 1999;**34**:815–22.

109. Walsh SJ, McClelland AJ, Owens CG *et al.* Efficacy of distinct energy delivery protocols comparing two biphasic defibrillators for cardiac arrest. *Am J Cardiol* 2004;**94**:378–80.

110. International Liaison Committee on Resuscitation. 2005 International consensus on cardiopulmonary resuscitation and emergency cardiovascular care with treatment recommendations. Part 4 Advanced life support. *Resuscitation* 2005;**67**:214–17.

111. Stiell IG, Hebert PC, Wells GA *et al.* Vasopressin versus epinephrine for inhospital cardiac arrest: a randomised controlled trial. *Lancet* 2001;**358**:105–9.

112. Wenzel V, Krismer AC, Arntz HR *et al.* A comparison of vasopressin and epinephrine for out-of-hospital cardiopulmonary resuscitation. *N Engl J Med* 2004;**350**:105–13.

113. Aung K, Htay T. Vasopressin for cardiac arrest: a systematic review and meta-analysis. *Arch Intern Med* 2005;**165**:17–24.

114. Klouche K, Weil MH, Tang W *et al.* A selective alpha(2)-adrenergic agonist for cardiac resuscitation. *J Lab Clin Med* 2002;**140**:27–34.

115. Klouche K, Weil MH, Sun S *et al.* A comparison of alpha-methylnorepinephrine, vasopressin and epinephrine for cardiac resuscitation. *Resuscitation* 2003;**57**:93–100.

116. Sun S, Weil MH, Tang W *et al.* alpha-Methylnorepinephrine, a selective alpha2-adrenergic agonist for cardiac resuscitation. *J Am Coll Cardiol* 2001;**37**:951–6.

117. Kudenchuk PJ, Cobb LA, Copass MK *et al.* Amiodarone for resuscitation after out-of-hospital cardiac arrest due to ventricular fibrillation. *N Engl J Med* 1999;**341**:871–8.

118. Dorian P, Cass D, Schwartz B *et al.* Amiodarone as compared with lidocaine for shock-resistant ventricular fibrillation. *N Engl J Med* 2002;**346**:884–90.

119. Viskin S, Belhassen B, Roth R *et al.* Aminophylline for bradyasystolic cardiac arrest refractory to atropine and epinephrine. *Ann Intern Med* 1993;**118**:279–81.

120. Mader TJ, Gibson P. Adenosine receptor antagonism in refractory asystolic cardiac arrest: results of a human pilot study. *Resuscitation* 1997;**35**:3–7.

121. Mader TJ, Smithline HA, Gibson P. Aminophylline in undifferentiated out-of-hospital asystolic cardiac arrest. *Resuscitation* 1999;**41**:39–45.

122. Mader TJ, Smithline HA, Durkin L *et al.* A randomized controlled trial of intravenous aminophylline for atropine-resistant out-of-hospital asystolic cardiac arrest. *Acad Emerg Med* 2003;**10**:192–7.

123. Stiell IG, Wells GA, Field B *et al.* Advanced cardiac life support in out-of-hospital cardiac arrest. *N Engl J Med* 2004;**351**:647–56.

124. Stiell IG, Wells GA, Hebert PC *et al.* Association of drug therapy with survival in cardiac arrest: limited role of advanced cardiac life support drugs. *Acad Emerg Med* 1995;**2**:264–73.

125. Engdahl J, Bang A, Lindqvist J, Herlitz J. Can we define patients with no and those with some chance of survival when found in asystole out of hospital? *Am J Cardiol* 2000;**86**:610–14.

126. Engdahl J, Bang A, Lindqvist J, Herlitz J. Factors affecting short- and long-term prognosis among 1069 patients with out-of-hospital cardiac arrest and pulseless electrical activity. *Resuscitation* 2001;**51**:17–25.

127. Dumot JA, Burval DJ, Sprung J *et al.* Outcome of adult cardiopulmonary resuscitations at a tertiary referral center including results of "limited" resuscitations. *Arch Intern Med* 2001;**161**:1751–8.

128. Tortolani AJ, Risucci DA, Powell SR, Dixon R. In-hospital cardiopulmonary resuscitation during asystole. Therapeutic factors associated with 24-hour survival. *Chest* 1989;**96**:622–6.

129. Bar-Joseph G, Abramson NS, Kelsey SF *et al.* Improved resuscitation outcome in emergency medical systems with increased usage of sodium bicarbonate during cardiopulmonary resuscitation. *Acta Anaesthesiol Scand* 2005;**49**:6–15.

130. Sandeman DJ, Alahakoon TI, Bentley SC. Tricyclic poisoning – successful management of ventricular fibrillation following massive overdose of imipramine. *Anaesth Intensive Care* 1997;**25**:542–5.

131. Thel MC, Armstrong AL, McNulty SE *et al.* Randomised trial of magnesium in in-hospital cardiac arrest. Duke Internal Medicine Housestaff. *Lancet* 1997;**350**:1272–6.

132. Allegra J, Lavery R, Cody R *et al.* Magnesium sulfate in the treatment of refractory ventricular fibrillation in the prehospital setting. *Resuscitation* 2001;**49**:245–9.

133. Fatovich D, Prentice D, Dobb G. Magnesium in in-hospital cardiac arrest. *Lancet* 1998;**351**:446.

134. Hassan TB, Jagger C, Barnett DB. A randomised trial to investigate the efficacy of magnesium sulphate for refractory ventricular fibrillation. *Emerg Med J* 2002;**19**:57–62.

135. Baraka A, Ayoub C, Kawkabani N. Magnesium therapy for refractory ventricular fibrillation. *J Cardiothorac Vasc Anesth* 2000;**14**:196–9.

136. Abu-Laban RB, Christenson JM, Innes GD *et al.* Tissue plasminogen activator in cardiac arrest with pulseless electrical activity. *N Engl J Med* 2002;**346**:1522–8.

137. Böttiger BW, Arntz H-R, Chamberlain DA *et al.* for the TROICA Trial Investigators and the European Resuscitation Council Study Group. Thrombolysis during resuscitation for out-of-hospital cardiac arrest. *New Engl J Med* 2008;**359**:2651–62.

138. Hedges JR, Syverud SA, Dalsey WC *et al.* Prehospital trial of emergency transcutaneous cardiac pacing. *Circulation* 1987;**76**:1337–43.

139. Barthell E, Troiano P, Olson D *et al.* Prehospital external cardiac pacing: a prospective, controlled clinical trial. *Ann Emerg Med* 1988;**17**:1221–6.

140. Cummins RO, Graves JR, Larsen MP *et al.* Out-of-hospital transcutaneous pacing by emergency medical technicians in patients with asystolic cardiac arrest. *N Engl J Med* 1993;**328**:1377–82.

141. Kern KB, Sanders AB, Raife J *et al.* A study of chest compression rates during cardiopulmonary resuscitation in humans: the importance of rate-directed chest compressions. *Arch Intern Med* 1992;**152**:145–9.

142. Berg RA, Sanders AB, Milander M *et al.* Efficacy of audio-prompted rate guidance in improving resuscitator performance of cardiopulmonary resuscitation on children. *Acad Emerg Med* 1994;**1**:35–40.

143. Barsan WG, Levy RC. Experimental design for study of cardiopulmonary resuscitation in dogs. *Ann Emerg Med* 1981;**10**:135–7.

144. Milander MM, Hiscok PS, Sanders AB *et al.* Chest compression and ventilation rates during cardiopulmonary resuscitation: the effects of audible tone guidance. *Acad Emerg Med* 1995;**2**:708–13.

145. Chiang WC, Chen WJ, Chen SY *et al.* Better adherence to the guidelines during cardiopulmonary resuscitation through the provision of audio-prompts. *Resuscitation* 2005;**64**:297–301.

146. Boyle AJ, Wilson AM, Connelly K *et al.* Improvement in timing and effectiveness of external cardiac compressions with a new non-invasive device: the CPR-Ezy. *Resuscitation* 2002;**54**:63–7.

147. Wik L, Thowsen J, Steen PA. An automated voice advisory manikin system for training in basic life support without an instructor. A novel approach to CPR training. *Resuscitation* 2001;**50**:167–72.

148. Wik L, Myklebust H, Auestad BH, Steen PA. Retention of basic life support skills 6 months after training with an automated voice advisory manikin system without instructor involvement. *Resuscitation* 2002;**52**:273–9.

149. Elding C, Baskett P, Hughes A. The study of the effectiveness of chest compressions using the CPR-plus. *Resuscitation* 1998;**36**:169–73.

150. Thomas SH, Stone CK, Austin PE *et al.* Utilization of a pressure-sensing monitor to improve in-flight chest compressions. *Am J Emerg Med* 1995;**13**:155–7.

151. Handley AJ, Handley SA. Improving CPR performance using an audible feedback system suitable for incorporation into an automated external defibrillator. *Resuscitation* 2003;**57**:57–62.

152. Cohen TJ, Goldner BG, Maccaro PC *et al.* A comparison of active compression–decompression cardiopulmonary resuscitation with standard cardiopulmonary resuscitation for cardiac arrests occurring in the hospital. *N Engl J Med* 1993;**329**:1918–21.

153. Tucker KJ, Redberg RF, Schiller NB, Cohen TJ. Active compression–decompression resuscitation: analysis of transmitral flow and left ventricular volume by transesophageal echocardiography in humans. Cardiopulmonary Resuscitation Working Group. *J Am Coll Cardiol* 1993;**22**:1485–93.

154. Plaisance P, Lurie KG, Vicaut E *et al.* A comparison of standard cardiopulmonary resuscitation and active compression–decompression resuscitation for out-of-hospital cardiac arrest. French Active Compression–Decompression Cardiopulmonary Resuscitation Study Group. *N Engl J Med* 1999;**341**:569–75.

155. Lafuente-Lafuente C, Melero-Bascones M. Active chest compression-decompression for cardiopulmonary resuscitation. *Cochrane Database of Systematic Reviews* 2004, Issue 4. Art. No.: CD002751. DOI: 10.1002/14651858.CD002751.pub2.

156. Casner M, Anderson D, Isaacs SM. The impact of a new CPR assist device on the rate of return of spontaneous circulation in out of hospital cardiac arrest. *Prehosp Emerg Med* 2005;**9**:61–7.

157. Timerman S, Cardoso LF, Ramires JA, Halperin H. Improved hemodynamic performance with a novel chest compression device during treatment of in-hospital cardiac arrest. *Resuscitation* 2004;**61**:273–80.

158. Halperin H, Berger R, Chandra N *et al.* Cardiopulmonary resuscitation with a hydraulic-pneumatic band. *Crit Care Med* 2000; 28: N203-N206.

159. Halperin HR, Paradis N, Ornato JP *et al.* Cardiopulmonary resuscitation with a novel chest compression device in a porcine model of cardiac arrest: improved hemodynamics and mechanisms. *J Am Coll Cardiol* 2004;**44**:2214–20.

160. Ong MEH, Ornato JP, Edwards DP *et al.* Use of an automated, load-distributing band chest compression device for out-of-hospital cardiac arrest resuscitation. *JAMA* 2006;**295**:2629–37.

161. Hallstrom A, Rea TD, Sayre MR *et al.* Manual chest compression vs use of an automated chest compression device during resuscitation following out-of-hospital cardiac arrest: a randomized trial. *JAMA* 2006;**295**:2620–8.

162. Lewis RJ, Niemann JT. Manual vs device-assisted CPR: reconciling apparently contradictory results. *JAMA* 2006;**295**:2661–4.

163. Dickinson ET, Verdile VP, Schneider RM, Salluzzo RF. Effectiveness of mechanical versus manual chest compressions in out-of-hospital cardiac arrest resuscitation: a pilot study. *Am J Emerg Med* 1998;**16**:289–92.

164. McDonald JL. Systolic and mean arterial pressures during manual and mechanical CPR in humans. *Ann Emerg Med* 1982;**11**:292–5.

165. Ward KR, Menegazzi JJ, Zelenak RR *et al.* A comparison of chest compressions between mechanical and manual CPR by monitoring end-tidal PCO2 during human cardiac arrest. *Ann Emerg Med* 1993;**22**:669–74.

166. Sunde K, Wik L, Steen PA. Quality of mechanical, manual standard and active compression–decompression CPR on the arrest site and during transport in a manikin model. *Resuscitation* 1997;**34**:235–42.

167. Steen S, Liao Q, Pierre L, Paskevicius A, Sjoberg T. Evaluation of LUCAS, a new device for automatic mechanical compression and active decompression resuscitation. *Resuscitation* 2002;**55**: 285–99.

168. Rubertsson S, Karlsten R. Increased cortical cerebral blood flow with LUCAS; a new device for mechanical chest compressions compared to standard external compressions during experimental cardiopulmonary resuscitation. *Resuscitation* 2005;**65**:357–63.

169. Steen S, Sjöberg T, Olsson P, Young M. Treatment of out of hospital cardiac arrest with LUCAS, a new device for automatic mechanical compression and active decompression resuscitation. *Resuscitation* 2005;**67**:25–30.

170. Holmström P, Boyd J, Sorsa M, Kuisma M. A case of hypothermic cardiac arrest treated with an external chest compression device (LUCAS) during transport to re-warming. *Resuscitation* 2005;**67**:139–41.

171. Wik L, Kiil S. Use of an automatic mechanical chest compression device (LUCAS) as a bridge to establishing cardiopulmonary bypass for a patient with hypothermic cardiac arrest. *Resuscitation* 2005;**66**:391–4.

172. Vatsgar TT, Ingebrigtsen O, Fjose LO *et al.* Cardiac arrest and resuscitation with an automatic mechanical chest compression device (LUCAS) due to anaphylaxis of a woman receiving caesarean section because of pre-eclampsia. *Resuscitation* 2006;**68**:155–9.

173. Axelsson C, Nestin J, Svensson L *et al.* Clinical consequences of the introduction of mechanical chest compression in the EMS system for treatment of out-of-hospital cardiac arrest: a pilot study. *Resuscitation* 2006;**71**:47–55.

174. Englund E, Kongstad PC. Active compression-decompression CPR necessitates follow-up post mortem. *Resuscitation* 2006;**68**: 161–3.

44 Arrhythmias due to monogenic disorders

Dawood Darbar, Prince Kannankeril and Dan M L Roden

Departments of Medicine, Pediatrics, and Pharmacology, Vanderbilt University School of Medicine, Nashville, TN, USA

Introduction

Monogenic diseases are caused by single genetic defects, follow Mendelian inheritance, and are classified as autosomal dominant, autosomal recessive or X-linked. Over 5000 monogenic diseases have been identified, and more than 1000 genes responsible for these disorders are known. The prevalence of monogenic diseases ranges from 1 in 1000 individuals in the most common forms to 1 in 200 000 in the rarest. The identification and study of the genetic substrates of these diseases are important not only because they contribute to the development of diagnostic tests for affected individuals but also because they promote understanding of the function of different proteins in humans. Consequently, genetic testing is currently applied not only for diagnostic evaluation, but also as a research tool for the study of pathophysiology of inherited arrhythmia syndromes. In cardiology, there are two major clusters of monogenic disorders: the cardiomyopathies due to alterations in sarcomeric and in cytoskeletal proteins, and the arrhythmogenic diseases that are caused by mutations in ion channels and ion channel-controlling proteins, e.g. the congenital long QT syndromes (LQTS), the Brugada syndrome, catecholaminergic polymorphic ventricular tachycardia (CPVT), Andersen–Tawil syndrome, conduction system disease, and atrial fibrillation (AF).

What we have learned from the genetics of monogenic arrhythmia syndromes

The identification of genes responsible for the inherited arrhythmia syndromes has contributed greatly to our understanding of the substrate for arrhythmia develop-

Evidence-Based Cardiology, 3rd edition. Edited by S. Yusuf, J.A. Cairns, A.J. Camm, E.L. Fallen, and B.J. Gersh. © 2010 Blackwell Publishing, ISBN: 978-1-4051-5925-8.

ment. More importantly, it has provided practical information when managing affected patients with these disorders. The identification of a mutation allows us to suspect the diagnosis independent of the clinical features of the syndrome. When screening family members of a genotyped proband, an unexpectedly large number of carriers is identified among relatives initially considered unaffected based on clinical phenotyping. For example, up to 32% of carriers of LQTS-related mutations can have a normal QTc.[1] As silent carriers have a 50% probability of transmitting LQTS to their offspring and they are more likely to develop cardiac arrhythmias compared to an age-matched population,[2] knowing the genotype status of an individual has practical implications. In addition, silent carriers of a LQTS-related genetic defect still have a 20% risk of becoming symptomatic.[2] Thus, the most immediate contribution of genetic information to clinical practice is that of providing a novel and useful parameter for risk stratification that can be used alone or in combination with other clinical variables. Currently, only in the congenital LQTS do we have data on hundreds of genotyped patients with long clinical follow-up but emerging data for other diseases such as CPVT are becoming available. As progress is made in our understanding of the links between DNA defects and clinical phenotype, genotyping patients with inherited arrhythmia disorders is even more likely to contribute to the clinical management of patients.

Complexity beyond monogenic arrhythmia disorders

Since the initial discovery of mutations in *KCNQ1*, *KCNH2*, and *SCN5A* cardiac ion channel genes by Keating and colleagues over a decade ago,[3–5] hundreds of mutations have been identified in various ion channel subunits and in proteins important for the proper functioning of cardiac ion channels. Although it was initially assumed that all carriers of pathogenic mutations would manifest the corresponding phenotype, it soon became apparent that the clinical consequences of genetic defects are far more variable than expected. Some of this variability is related to incomplete penetrance and variable expressivity. The penetrance of a monogenic disease is defined as the percentage of individuals with a mutant allele who develop the phenotype of the related disease and it can vary from 10% to 100%. The expressivity of a disease is defined as the different phenotypical manifestations that can be observed among carriers of the same genetic defect. Consequently, the combination of variable penetrance and expressivity dictates that carriers of a DNA mutation may manifest either no clinical phenotype or phenotypes that are not the classic "textbook" type. Thus, genotyping patients affected by "simple" monogenic diseases is more complicated than initially envisioned.

Another important concept when considering monogenic diseases is genetic heterogeneity. Analogous to the genetics of inherited cardiomyopathies, in arrhythmia disorders the "same" phenotype is associated with multiple genetic defects. At present, nine genes are known to cause the phenotype of the congenital LQTS and explain 60–75% of the clinically diagnosed cases. Similarly, two genes have been associated with CPVT and they account for half of the patients with the phenotype.[6] Two genes are known to cause the Brugada syndrome, but several other genes are likely to be implicated because so far only 20% of clinical diagnoses result in positive results at genetic testing.[7] Perhaps an obvious question that stems from these considerations is whether we should refer to all genetic variants with the same name, such as LQTS. Should all individuals with the same ECG marker, e.g., prolonged QT interval, ST segment elevation in the right precordial leads, adrenergically driven polymorphic ventricular tachycardia (VT), be grouped under the same diagnosis, when we know that

each genetic variant has a distinguishing clinical phenotype? This may be more than semantics as there are emerging data that the genetic substrate is a major determinant of prognosis in patients harboring different genetic mutations.[2]

In the future we may consider each genetic variant as a separate disease based on the specific defect as this would avoid the difficulty of trying to fit the complex and overlapping phenotypes into clinical categories. This would not only simplify the categorization of overlapping syndromes but also the clinical profiles: Brugada syndrome with conduction defects, Brugada syndrome with atrial arrhythmias, conduction defects with sinus abnormalities, Brugada syndrome with prolonged QT interval, etc. All these conditions could be grouped in the category of sodium channel disease and its full spectrum of abnormalities. This is complicated even further as it is now established that mutations in one gene may lead not only to variable phenotypes within the same disease, but also to profoundly different diseases. The most emblematic example of this diversity is represented by mutations in the lamin A/C gene, which are known to cause at least eight phenotypes (allelic diseases) as different as dilated cardiomyopathy, Emery–Dreifuss muscular dystrophy, familial partial lipodystrophy, Charcot–Marie–Tooth disease, mandibuloacral dysplasia, Hutchinson–Gilford progeria, lipoatrophy with diabetes, and hepatic steatosis hypertrophic cardiomyopathy. In inherited arrhythmia disorders, three diseases have been associated with mutations of the cardiac sodium channel gene (LQTS, Brugada syndrome, and progressive conduction disturbances)[4,8] and three diseases (LQTS, short QT syndrome and familial AF) have been associated with mutations in the *KCNQ1* gene encoding for the alpha-subunit of the potassium channel conducting the slow component of the delayed rectifier (I_{Ks}).[5,9,10] It is therefore

Table 44.1 Atrial arrhythmias due to monogenic disorders

Phenotype	Rhythm	Inheritance	Locus	Ion channel /protein	Gene
AF	AF	AD	10q22–24	–	–
			11p15	I_{Ks}	KCNQ1
			6q14–16	–	–
			21q22	I_{Kr}	KCNE2
			17q23	I_{K1}	KCNJ2
			12p13	I_{Kur}	KCNA5
	AF	AR	5p13		
SND	Sinus bradycardia, AF	AD		HCN4	HCN4
Atrial standstill	SND, AF	AD	3q21	I_{Na}	SCN5A
WPW syndrome	AVRT	AD			PRKAG2
Progressive conduction disease	AVB	AD	19q13 3q21	I_{Na}	SCN5A

AD, autosomal dominant; AF, atrial fibrillation; AR, autosomal recessive; AVRT, atrioventricular re-entrant tachycardia; AVB, atrioventricular block; SND, sinus node dysfunction; WPW, Wolff–Parkinson–White.

obvious that the identification of a mutation in a given gene cannot establish the diagnosis of a single disease and the identification of a mutation in an individual with a known disease is not enough to predict the phenotype of that individual.

We will now discuss individual inherited monogenic arrhythmia disorders.

Atrial fibrillation

Atrial fibrillation (AF), the most common cardiac arrhythmia in clinical practice, affects approximately 2% of the United States population and results in substantial morbidity and mortality.[11] The increasing prevalence of AF parallels the increasing age of the general population.[12] AF is also the most common arrhythmia requiring drug therapy. The limited success of current interventions for AF is partially the result of heterogeneity of the underlying electrical substrate and incomplete understanding of fundamental mechanisms in disease pathogenesis. Although some of the risk factors associated with AF have been identified, relatively little is known about the underlying molecular events leading to the arrhythmia.[13] One approach to unraveling the molecular pathogenesis of AF is through the identification of genes responsible for familial forms of the disease. Evidence for the heritability of AF has come from several sources including the study of AF kindreds who exhibit the arrhythmia as a primary disease, the analysis of AF presenting in the setting of another familial cardiac disease, and the analysis of common population genetic variants, i.e. DNA polymorphisms, that may predispose to AF.

Monogenic forms of lone AF

Monogenic familial AF was first reported in 1943[14] and while it may be uncommon, there has been no attempt to determine the prevalence of familial AF. Heritability of AF is further suggested by two recent population-based studies demonstrating that AF in first-degree relatives was associated with an increased risk of developing AF.[12,15] One study showed that 5% of patients with AF and up to 15% of individuals with lone AF may have a familial form of the disease.[16,17]

A gene locus for AF was first reported in 1997, based on genetic mapping in three Spanish families.[18] However, the gene responsible for AF in these kindreds has not yet been identified, but resides within a relatively large chromosomal region spanning 14 centiMorgans (cM). In addition, three other loci on chromosomes 6q14–16,[19] 5p13[20] and 10p11-q21[21] have been reported, with no genes yet identified. In 2002, a novel AF locus on chromosome 5p15 was identified by genome-wide linkage analysis of a

four-generation kindred.[22] Importantly, this study established an abnormally prolonged P-wave (>155 ms) determined by signal-averaged ECG analysis as an "endophenotype" that improved statistical power of the linkage study in this family. Collectively, these reports support the idea that familial AF is a genetically heterogeneous disease much like many other inherited arrhythmia syndromes.[16]

Recently, the first genes for AF have been identified, providing a link between ion channelopathies and the arrhythmia. In a four-generation Chinese family in which LQTS and early-onset AF co-segregate, a mutation (S140G) in *KCNQ1* gene on chromosome 11p15.5 has been reported.[10] Functional analysis of the S140G mutant revealed a gain-of-function effect in KCNQ1/KCNE1 and KCNQ1/KCNE2 currents, which contrasts with the dominant negative or loss-of-function effects of *KCNQ1* mutations previously associated with LQTS. More recently, the same group established a link between *KCNE2* and AF by identification of a mutation in two families with AF.[23] The mutation R27C also caused a gain-of-function when co-expressed with *KCNQ1* but had no effect when expressed with *KCNH2*. Recently, a truncating mutation in *KCNA5* encoding a voltage-gated potassium channel ($K_V1.5$) underlying the ultra-rapid delayed rectifier current (I_{Kur}) was associated with familial AF.[24] These studies firmly establish the role of potassium channels in the pathogenesis of some forms of familial AF, but resequencing studies in large cohorts suggest that mutations in these channels are a rare cause of the arrhythmia.[25]

AF associated with other monogenic diseases

Studies of other cardiac monogenic disorders have also provided evidence for the genetic contribution to the etiology of AF. These include diseases such as hypertrophic cardiomyopathy, skeletal myopathies, familial amyloidosis, and atrial myopathies. It is likely that AF in these cases is related at least in part to non-specific structural changes in the atria caused by the underlying cardiac pathology, but AF is uniquely prominent in some kindreds with each of these conditions.[26] AF can also present in other ion channelopathies like congenital LQTS type 4,[27] Brugada syndrome[28] and short QT syndrome.[29] The high incidence of atrial arrhythmias in patients with short QT syndrome and gain of function mutations in I_{Ks}[30] point to an important role for shortening of the action potential in the development of AF. Sodium channel gene (*SCN5A*) defects have also been associated with a syndrome of early-onset dilated cardiomyopathy and AF.[31] Moreover, mutations in the gene for the nuclear membrane protein lamin A/C (*LMNA*) have pleiotropic non-cardiac and cardiac manifestations including dilated cardiomyopathy, AF, and conduction system disease.[32] Collectively, these studies attest to the heterogeneous nature of AF and strongly suggest that defects in many more genes remain to be identified.

AF associated with cardiac or systemic diseases

Most patients with AF have one or more identifiable risk factors, but many or even most patients with these same risk factors do not develop AF. Thus, it is likely that genetic determinants favor AF in some individuals with identifiable risk factors. Studies comparing cases of non-familial AF to age- and gender-matched controls (association studies) have provided insight into the genetic basis of "acquired" AF. One study evaluated a polymorphism in *KCNE1* and AF and identified an association with the 38G allele. While the 38G allele appears to reduce I_{Ks},[33] mice lacking *KCNE1* are prone to AF due to an unexpected increase in I_{Ks},[34] suggesting that the consequences of ion channel mutations are not always straightforward. In addition, common DNA polymorphisms in *GNB3*,[35] *KCNE5*,[36] and *SCN5A* have all been associated with AF.[37] Over the last several years increasing evidence has arisen that renin-angiotensin-aldosterone (RAAS) activation may be an important risk factor for the development of AF. Retrospective analyses suggest that angiotensin-converting enzyme (ACE) inhibitor therapy is associated with a lower incidence of AF and a placebo-controlled trial found a similar beneficial effect of adding the angiotensin receptor blocker (ARB) irbesartan to amiodarone.[38] Additionally, a case–control study of 250 Taiwanese subjects with AF and 250 controls identified polymorphisms in this pathway as risk factors for AF.[39] Added support for the role of RAAS activation in the pathophysiology of AF comes from a recent study which demonstrated a pharmacogenetic interaction between the ACE *I/D* polymorphism and efficacy of antiarrhythmic drug therapy in patients with lone AF.[40]

The above studies in aging patients with non-familial AF in the presence of underlying heart disease suggest some form of heritable contribution to the pathogenesis of the more common forms of AF. These data are promising and may help clarify why some people develop AF under specific circumstances while others may not.

Uncovering common genes for AF

A logical consequence of the availability of comprehensive genomic maps is the advent of high-density genome-wide searches for modest gene effects using large-scale testing of single nucleotide polymorphisms (SNPs). Such an approach has been suggested to tackle complex human diseases such as AF. Early proponents suggested the study of coding or promoting variants with potential functional significance. Collins *et al* subsequently proposed that non-coding or evenly spaced SNPs with high density could be used to track disease loci through linkage disequilibrium.[41] The availability of high-density mapping of marker SNPs and assessment of genomic structure, together with emerging information on functional pathways, have begun to provide powerful means of identifying genetic susceptibilities to AF. In the first genome-wide association study of AF, a novel locus on chromosome 4q25 has recently been identified which confers a 1.6–2.0 (95% confidence interval)-fold increased risk of the arrhythmia across multiple different populations.[42]

Atrial flutter

While there is significant overlap among the risk factors for AF and atrial flutter, in general these arrhythmias exhibit quite distinct biology and electrophysiology.[13] Atrial flutter is commonly associated with the later stages of a broad range of congenital heart disease (CHD). There is extensive heterogeneity particularly in the most profound structural disorders, but increasing evidence of a heritable component to many forms of CHD is accumulating. The association of CHD with atrial flutter has been attributed to abnormal atrial patterning, which may range from the extreme to the subtle, often with no other obvious manifestations. Interestingly, atrial flutter was found to be more strongly associated with the locus on chromosome 4q25 than AF, at least suggesting that there may be common factors underlying the clinical presentation of some forms of these two arrhythmias.[42] Given the intrinsic biases of genome-wide association studies, these links might be far downstream of the primary causation, but nevertheless may have substantial effects on a population basis.

Sinus nodal failure

Classic Mendelian genetics have revealed several distinctive mechanisms for sinus nodal disease. Mutations in the cardiac transcription factors Nkx 2.5 and Tbx 2.5 both cause defects in the differentiation and maintenance of specialized conduction tissues (particularly those of the AV node) and each causes subtle abnormalities of sinus impulse generation.[8,43–45] Similarly, several primary arrhythmic syndromes including some forms of the LQTS also result in perturbations of sinus rhythm.[46] While in many instances potential mechanisms have been framed in terms of effects on transmembrane ion currents, data from genetic models of *SCN5A* and AnkB disease suggest that subtle trophic effects on myocardial structures may also play a role.[47,48] Genetic models may also inform human studies at an earlier stage. Murine null alleles of the pacemaker channels *HCN2* and *HCN4* first directly implicated these channels in normal sinus rhythm, and subsequent human genetic

Table 44.2 Genetic arrhythmia syndromes associated with ventricular arrhythmias

Syndrome	Inheritance	Locus	Ion channel/protein	Gene
LQT syndrome (RW)	AD	11p15		
LQT1			I_{Ks}	KCNQ1
LQT2			I_{Kr}	KCNH2
LQT3			I_{Na}	SCN5A
LQT4			ankyrin B	ANK2
LQT5			I_{Ks}	KCNE1
LQT6			I_{Kr}	KCNE2
LQT7			I_{K1}	KCNJ2
LQT8			$I_{Ca\text{-}L}$	CACNA1C
LQT9			Caveolin-3	CAV3
LQT10			I_{Na}	SCN4B
LQT syndrome (JLN)	AR	11p15	I_{Ks}	KCNQ1
		21q22	I_{Kr}	KCNE1
Catecholaminergic polymorphic VT	AD	1q42		RYR2
	AR	1p13-p11		CASQ2
		7p14-p22		
Brugada syndrome	AD	3p21	I_{Na}	SCN5A
		3p22–25	I_{Na}	GPDL-1
Short QT syndrome	AD	21q22	I_{Kr}	KCNH2
		21q22	I_{Ks}	KCNQ1
		17q23	I_{K1}	KCNJ2
Arrhythmogenic RV Cardiomyopathy	AD	14q23–24		
ARVC1		1q42	Ryanodine receptor 2	RYR2
ARVC2		14q11-q12		
ARVC3		2q32		
ARVC4		3p23		
ARVC5		10p12-p14		
ARVC6		10q22		
ARVC7		6p28	Desmoplakin	DSP
ARVC8		12p11	Plakophilin-2	PKP2
ARVC9		18q12.1-q12.2	Desmoglein-2	DSG2
		18q12.1	Desmocollin-2	DSC2
Naxos disease	AR	17q21	Plakoglobin	JUP

JLN, Jervell–Lange-Nielsen; LQT, long QT; RV, right ventricular; RW, Romano–Ward; VT, ventricular tachycardia. See Table 44.1 for remaining abbreviations.

studies have identified mutations in the *HCN4* gene in sinoatrial disease.[49–52]

Other atrial arrhythmias

Virtually every known myocardial disease has been associated with some form of atrial arrhythmia. However, there are some rare associations which appear to be considerably more specific. A number of metabolic disorders, including mitochondrial diseases, glycogen or other storage disorders, are strongly associated with prominent evidence of AV conduction disease, often with overt ventricular preexcitation as well as frequent macro re-entrant and other atrial arrhythmias. For example, dominant mutations in the AMP-activated protein kinase gamma subunit (PRKAG2) have been shown to result in massive myocardial thickening, AV conduction system disease and ventricular preexcitation.[53] These families had previously been included under the rubric of hypertrophic cardiomyopathy on the basis of their inheritance patterns, adult-onset and echocardiographic features. AF and atrial flutter are common, but high-grade AV block is the dominant clinical arrhythmia in these kindreds. Clinical studies suggest that in many cases asymptomatic individuals are maximally pre-excited at rest, and therefore probably dependent on accessory AV connections from an early age.[54] These data defined a novel subset of "hypertrophic cardiomyopathy" illustrating the potential utility of molecular nosology for cardiac disease, but also offer some unique insights into the mechanisms of normal AV electrical development.[53]

Ventricular arrhythmias

Congenital long QT syndromes

The congenital LQTS are a group of genetic disorders that affect cardiac ion channels, characterized by prolongation of the QT interval, and risk for the life-threatening ventricular tachycardia torsades de pointes. Shortly after the autosomal recessive syndrome of congenital deafness, prolongation of the QT interval, and sudden death was described by Anton Jervell and Fred Lange-Nielsen in 1957,[55] Romano and Ward each independently described an "autosomal dominant" form without congenital deafness.[56,57] In the late 1990s the first five LQTS genes were identified, all of which encode ion channel subunits that underlie the cardiac action potential.[3–5,58] The most commonly affected genes, *KCNQ1* and *KCNH2* (underlying LQT1 and LQT2 respectively), encode proteins that form the alpha-subunits of two major repolarizing potassium currents, I_{Ks} and I_{Kr}. Two other LQTS genes encode for the corresponding beta-subunits (*KCNE1* and *KCNE2* underlying LQT5 and LQT6, respectively). The other major LQTS gene, *SCN5A* (underlying LQT3), encodes the alpha-subunit of the cardiac sodium channel. It is now accepted that patients with "Romano–Ward syndrome" carry a single mutation, while homozygous mutations (or compound heterozygotes) of *KCNQ1* or *KCNE1* cause Jervell–Lange-Nielsen (JLN) syndrome.[59,60] The extracardiac finding of congenital deafness requires the presence of two mutant alleles, and results from lack of functioning I_{Ks} in the inner ear.[61] JLN syndrome patients are also highly susceptible to arrhythmias; thus arrhythmia risk seems partly dependent on "gene dosage."[62] These five classic forms of congenital LQTS result from mutations which reduce outward currents (I_{Ks} or I_{Kr}) or enhance inward current (I_{Na}), thereby prolonging action potential duration and, in turn, prolonging the QT interval.

Additional ion channel mutations have been associated with rare arrhythmia syndromes (Andersen–Tawil syndrome, *KCNJ2*, and Timothy syndrome, *CACNA1C*) which may include QT prolongation, as well as significant extracardiac phenotypes.[63,64] Andersen–Tawil syndrome patients do not uniformly display prolonged QT intervals, and due to clinical features that differ from LQTS, this syndrome is better termed ATS1 rather than LQT7.[65] The previously termed LQT4 has been linked to mutations in *ANK2*, encoding the structural protein ankyrin-B, which when mutated results in altered localization and expression of ion channels.[27] Patients with *ANK2* mutations do not uniformly have prolonged QT intervals, and it has been suggested that LQT4 be renamed "sick sinus syndrome associated with bradycardia" or "ankyrin-B syndrome."[66]

The incidence of congenital LQTS has been estimated at 1 in 5000, and the incidence of JLN syndrome estimated as 1 in 500 congenitally deaf individuals. Without treatment, 13% of LQTS patients will suffer cardiac arrest or sudden death prior to 40 years of age; when syncopal events are included, 36% will have symptoms by age 40.[2] The JLN syndrome is more severe, with 90% experiencing syncope, cardiac arrest or sudden death by age 18, and mortality exceeding 25% even with therapy.[62] Important clinical differences among affected patients depending on the underlying affected gene have been observed – so-called genotype-phenotype correlation. As the majority (>90%) of genotyped LQTS patients have LQT1, LQT2 or LQT3,[67] most of the differences are observed among these genotypes and include different ECG T-wave patterns,[68] clinical course,[69] triggers of cardiac events,[70] response to sympathetic stimulation,[71,72] and effectiveness and limitations of beta-blocker therapy.[73]

Pharmacologic therapy for LQTS

Despite the genotype-specific aspects mentioned above, evidence-based therapeutic recommendations, for the most part, disregard the underlying genotype.[74] This is practical, as approximately one-third of patients with an unambiguous clinical diagnosis of LQTS do not have mutations in any of the known LQTS genes. Beta-blockers and lifestyle modifications, including restriction from vigorous exercise and avoidance of drugs which prolong the QT interval, are recommended for all patients with a clinical diagnosis of LQTS[73] (**Class I, Level B**). While there are no placebo-controlled clinical trials of beta-blockers in LQTS, the data from retrospective comparisons of cohorts with and without therapy, event rates before and after beta-blocker therapy, and data from the International Registry provide convincing evidence (60% reduction in risk for cardiac events, and LQTS-related death).[73,75,76] Aside from beta-blockers no pharmacologic intervention has been supported by enough data to warrant evidence-based recommendations. Sodium channel blockers seem a logical choice for patients with LQT3, and mexiletine has been shown to shorten the QT interval both in *in vitro* models of LQT3 and in a small cohort of LQT3 patients.[77,78] Concerns about the safety of flecainide were raised when intravenous flecainide elicited a Brugada syndrome phenotype in six out of 13 LQT3 patients.[79] However, in eight LQT3 patients with a specific *SCN5A* mutation, oral flecainide shortened the QT and was safely tolerated chronically.[80] Elevating serum potassium, both acutely[81] and chronically with oral potassium and spironolactone, shortens the QT interval in LQT2.[82] Despite these potentially beneficial effects on repolarization, a reduction in cardiac events has yet to be demonstrated with any drug other than beta-blockers.

Non-pharmacologic therapy for LQTS

Patients who have suffered a cardiac arrest should receive an implantable cardioverter-defibrillator (ICD), as 14% of those individuals will experience cardiac arrest or sudden death within 5 years, even with beta-blocker therapy[73] (**Class I, Level B**). Patients with recurrent syncope on beta-blocker therapy also should undergo ICD implantation, as 19% will have subsequent cardiac arrest, appropriate ICD shock or death[83,84] (**Class IIa, Level B**). Patients who do not meet the above criteria may be considered for prophylactic ICD implantation if they are in a category associated with a higher risk of cardiac arrest[74] (**Class IIb, Level B**). A combination of risk factors, including age, gender, genotype, history of syncope, and QT duration, contributes to an individual's risk.[2]

The largest LQTS study to date investigates predictors of life-threatening events during the high-risk period of adolescence (2772 patients between age 10 and 20 years).[85] In this group, male gender (between age 10 and 12), QTC ≥530, and recent syncope increased the risk for cardiac arrest or sudden death, while genotype was not predictive. In a recent large study of adults (812 patients >18 years), female gender, QTc ≥500, and interim syncope increases the risk of life-threatening events.[75] Genotype did not increase risk of cardiac arrest or sudden death, but LQT2 patients were at increased risk of any cardiac event. Previous studies suggested that patients with LQT2 or LQT3 had a higher risk of symptoms or death on beta-blockers compared to LQT1 patients.[2,70,73] The JLN syndrome would be considered a high-risk category, with 27% suffering cardiac arrest or sudden death on beta-blocker therapy, and 51% remaining or becoming symptomatic on therapy[63] (**Class IIb, Level B**). Timothy syndrome (LQT8), associated with syndactyly and multiorgan dysfunction, is perhaps the most severe form of LQTS, with 10 of the first 17 described children dead at an average age of 2.5 years.[64] Left cardiac sympathetic denervation (LCSD) may be considered for patients with LQTS and syncope or cardiac arrest despite beta-blocker therapy, those intolerant to beta-blockers or those with ICDs to reduce appropriate shocks (**Class IIb, Level B**). The published experience with LCSD is from 147 "high-risk" patients – 75% with cardiac events despite beta-blockers, nearly half with a history of cardiac arrest, and an average QTc of 543 ± 65 ms.[86] LCSD was highly effective in reducing the frequency and occurrence of syncope and cardiac arrest in this high-risk group, with a 91% reduction in cardiac events. The 5-year survival was 95%, and 65% were asymptomatic or had only a single episode of syncope during 7 years of follow-up. Protection was not complete, however, as 34% had cardiac arrest or sudden death after LCSD.

Short QT syndrome

Just as abnormally long QT intervals increase the risk of sudden death, it has been recognized since the 1990s that excessively short QT intervals are also associated with increased mortality.[87] In 2000, a new genetic arrhythmia syndrome was suggested when persistently short QT intervals were noted in a family with atrial fibrillation and in an unrelated patient who suffered sudden death.[88,89] Subsequently, two other families with short QT intervals, short atrial and ventricular effective refractory periods and inducible ventricular fibrillation (VF) at electrophysiology study were reported.[30] The ECG in these patients with "short QT syndrome" reveals not only a short QT interval, but an absence of the ST segment and abnormally tall T-waves in many. In short QT syndrome patients, identification of "gain-of-function" mutations in KCNH2, KCNQ1, and KCNJ2 followed only 4–5 years after the initial description of the syndrome.[29,90,91]

The true prevalence of short QT syndrome is unknown, but it appears to be exquisitely rare. In two separate population studies of 10–12 000 subjects, a QTc <320 was observed rarely (0–0.1%), and those with the shortest QT values did not have higher mortality than the rest of the population.[92,93] No ECGs with QTc <300 were observed in a hospital-based study of >100 000 patients.[94] The rarity of the syndrome, and the fact that it is relatively newly recognized, results in a small cohort of published cases (29 in the largest study).[95] The reported cases of short QT syndrome have absolute QT intervals between 210 and 320 ms, and corrected QT intervals between 250 and 340 ms, as well as a personal or family history of sudden death or aborted sudden death.[95,96] Cardiac arrest is the most frequent symptom (31%) and, unfortunately, is often the first clinical presentation. As with any new syndrome, the initially recognized cases are the most severe, therefore the high incidence of sudden death in these patients is not terribly surprising. The risk for VF in short QT syndrome may stem from an increased transmural dispersion of repolarization.[97] Other symptoms include presyncope, syncope, palpitations, and atrial fibrillation. Electrophysiology study may be useful to confirm the diagnosis, as short atrial and ventricular refractory periods accompany the syndrome; however, the predictive value of inducible VF is poor (only three of six patients with a history of VF had inducible VF at electrophysiology study).[95] Defibrillator therapy has been recommended for these patients, but is complicated by the potential for frequent inappropriate shocks due to oversensing of the high-amplitude T-waves in this disorder[98] (**Class IIa, Level C**). As more patients with short QT syndrome are identified, clinical heterogeneity will likely be uncovered and risk stratification may become possible. Multiple drugs, including flecainide, sotalol, ibutilide, and quinidine, have been tested in a few short QT syndrome patients.[99] Quinidine significantly prolonged the QT interval and ventricular refractory period, and prevented inducibility of VF. Interestingly, quinidine seems to prolong the QT to greater degrees in patients with *KCNH2* mutations.[95] At this time, there are no data on the efficacy of quinidine to reduce symptoms or clinical events, but the effects in patients and in *in vitro* models suggest that quinidine may be useful to reduce appropriate ICD shocks or in those who refuse an ICD[100] (**Class IIb, Level C**).

Catecholaminergic polymorphic ventricular tachycardia

Catecholaminergic polymorphic ventricular tachycardia (CPVT) is a genetic arrhythmia syndrome that may lead to syncope or sudden death in young children with normal hearts.[101] Linkage of CPVT to chromosome 1q42-q43[102] was followed by identification of mutations in the cardiac ryanodine receptor (RYR2).[103] Mutations in calsequestrin 2 (*CASQ2*) have also been identified in an autosomal recessive form of CPVT.[104,105] A third locus has been linked to chromosome 7p14-p22 in a family with autosomal recessive CPVT, but the gene has not yet been identified.[106] Abnormal calcium release from the SR seems to be a common mechanism underlying CPVT mutations. Experimental studies simulating adrenergic stimulation in the setting of abnormal calcium release reveal epicardial origin of ectopic beats increasing transmural dispersion of repolarization, providing the substrate for catecholaminergic VT. Furthermore, bidirectional VT results as a consequence of alternation in the origin of ectopic activity between endocardial and epicardial regions.[107]

The familial transmission, risk of physical or emotional stress, and benefits of beta-blocker therapy have been recognized since the early reports of CPVT.[101,108] Swimming-triggered events, previously thought to be specific for LQT1, have been associated with CPVT as well.[109] The incidence of CPVT is unknown, but it is likely underdiagnosed. A high index of suspicion is necessary, with exercise testing often required to make the diagnosis. In contrast to LQTS, the baseline ECG is normal, although resting sinus bradycardia has been noted.[110] Exercise induces a characteristic bidirectional VT, which may be asymptomatic; however, polymorphic VT and ventricular fibrillation may also occur.[111] Electrophysiology study with programmed ventricular stimulation usually does not provoke any arrhythmias. The disease is highly lethal, with a mortality rate in untreated individuals of 30–50% by age 40.[112] Beta-blockers are recommended for all patients with CPVT[74] (**Class I, Level C**). In one series, 98% of patients were symptom free for 2 years on beta-blockers[110] but a second study with longer follow-up (40–50 months) revealed arrhythmias in 18/39 CPVT patients on beta-blockers.[111] Defibrillator therapy is recommended for CPVT patients who have survived cardiac arrest (**Class I, Level C**) and for those with syncope or sustained VT on beta-blockers[74] (**Class IIa, Level C**).

Brugada syndrome

Brugada syndrome refers to a typical ECG pattern (ST elevation in the right precordial or, rarely, inferior leads) associated with a risk of ventricular arrhythmias and sudden death.[113] With improved recognition of the syndrome, it is now apparent that most, if not all cases of sudden unexplained nocturnal death syndrome (SUNDS)[114] and some sudden infant death syndrome (SIDS) cases are due to Brugada syndrome.[115,116]

The first Brugada syndrome gene to be identified was *SCN5A*, the same gene underlying LQT3.[9] Brugada syndrome *SCN5A* mutations result in reduced sodium current, as opposed to augmented late sodium current in LQT3. Experimental studies have revealed that loss of sodium current leaves the transient outward current (I_{to}) unopposed, resulting in the characteristic ECG as well as an increased risk for ventricular tachycardia and fibrillation.[117] Interestingly, fever has been reported to unmask the ECG findings and elicit storms of ventricular tachycardia in Brugada syndrome.[118,119] Correspondingly, some mutations have temperature-dependent functional consequences.[120] Only 20% of Brugada syndrome patients have *SCN5A* mutations, suggesting that other genes are also important. In one large Brugada syndrome family, a mutation in glycerol-3-phosphate dehydrogenase 1-like gene (*GPD1L*), which also affects sodium current, has been identified.[121] Additionally, mutations in *CACNA1C* have been identified in patients with Brugada syndrome and shorter than normal QT intervals.[122]

The electrocardiographic findings in Brugada syndrome are dynamic and may be concealed, but can be unmasked by sodium channel-blocking drugs such as flecainide, ajmaline or procainamide.[123] This makes determination of the true prevalence difficult. Large population studies from Japan estimate the prevalence at between 0.1% and 0.7%, but it is likely lower in North America and Europe.[124,125] The prevalence is lower among schoolchildren (0.02%), who may not yet manifest ECG changes.[126] The disease expression is significantly affected by gender as well, as 90% of diagnosed patients are male. An ICD is the only proven effective therapy and is recommended for patients with Brugada syndrome and a previous cardiac arrest as they are at the highest risk for a recurrence (69% at 54 months of follow-up)[74,127] (**Class I, Level B**). A single randomized controlled trial comparing an ICD to beta-blockers was performed in survivors of SUNDS, most of whom had Brugada syndrome. In total there were seven deaths (18%) in the beta-blocker group and no deaths in the ICD group but there were a total of 12 ICD patients who received ICD discharges due to recurrent ventricular fibrillation.[128] An ICD is also recommended for patients with a spontaneous Brugada-pattern ECG who have a history of syncope, as these patients have a recurrence rate of 19% at 26 months of follow-up[129] (**Class IIa, Level C**). Patients with no history of syncope, and who require drug challenge to elicit the Brugada ECG are at minimal risk, and may be clinically monitored (**Class IIa, Level C**). Although quinidine, likely by blocking I$_{to}$, has demonstrated some protective effects,[130,131] recommended use in Brugada syndrome is an adjunct to ICD or for the treatment of electrical storm[74] (**Class IIb, Level C**). The role of electrophysiology study for risk stratification is controversial, with differing results in separate large cohorts.[132–134] The negative predictive value in asymptomatic individuals appears high, while the positive predictive value is poor in all cohorts studied. At this time, an electrophysiology study may be considered in asymptomatic individuals with a spontaneous Brugada ECG, as they have an intermediate risk of sudden death[74] (**Class IIb, Level C**).

Hypertrophic cardiomyopathy

Hypertrophic cardiomyopathy (HCM) represents a genetically diverse group of disorders associated with a variety of cardiac arrhythmias. HCM typically displays an autosomal dominant pattern of inheritance, with most cases attributable to defects in various components of the cardiac sarcomere.[135] Mutations in PRKAG2 underlie a specific phenotype consisting of HCM, Wolff–Parkinson–White (WPW) syndrome, premature conduction disease, and the presence of glycogen vacuoles in myocytes.[136] Various arrhythmias are observed in HCM, including atrial fibrillation and flutter, ventricular tachycardia and ventricular fibrillation. HCM is covered in detail in Chapter 50; here we will limit our discussion to risk stratification and treatment of ventricular arrhythmias and sudden death.

It is important to recognize that treatment strategies for relief of left ventricular outflow obstruction and associated symptoms such as exercise intolerance and chest pain are independent of arrhythmia and SD management. The SD risk in HCM varies with age (2–4% per year in children, 1% per year in adults), and HCM is the leading cause of sudden death in young athletes in the United States.[137] Various major risk factors for sudden death have been identified, including prior cardiac arrest (ventricular fibrillation), spontaneous sustained ventricular tachycardia, family history of SD, history of syncope, septal thickness >3 cm, abnormal blood pressure response to exercise, and nonsustained ventricular tachycardia.[138] An ICD is indicated for patients with a history of sustained ventricular fibrillation or tachycardia, as these patients have a high rate of appropriate ICD discharge (11% per year)[74,139] (**Class I, Level C**). Additionally, an ICD is recommended for patients

with two or more major risk factors, and should be considered for patients with one major risk factor (**Class IIa, Level C**). Amiodarone has shown survival benefit in nonrandomized studies[140] but is likely inferior to ICD, and is therefore indicated only when an ICD is not feasible[74] (**Class IIa, Level C**). Patients with symptoms suggestive of arrhythmias such as palpitations or syncope or presenting with sustained supraventricular arrhythmias should undergo comprehensive invasive electrophysiology testing, as should patients with WPW on ECG. Electrophysiology testing for risk stratification is controversial, with one group presenting data suggesting poorer outcome in patients with inducible VT[141] (**Class IIb, Level C**). Many feel that the electrophysiology study adds little to noninvasive means of risk stratification.[142]

Arrhythmogenic right ventricular cardiomyopathy

Arrhythmogenic right ventricular cardiomyopathy (ARVC) is a genetic cardiomyopathy characterized by ventricular arrhythmias and structural abnormalities of the right ventricle, resulting from progressive fibrofatty infiltration of right ventricular myocardium.[143] It may be a relatively common cause of ventricular tachycardia in young patients with previously unrecognized heart disease, and accounts for up to 10% of unexpected sudden death,[144] though its prevalence may vary by geographic location.[145] The diagnosis of ARVC is based on clinical criteria including structural abnormalities, tissue characterization, abnormalities in depolarization or repolarization, arrhythmias, and family history.[146] These criteria are often subjective and may be too stringent, especially for family members of patients with known ARVC.[147] Familial occurrence of ARVC is well recognized, most commonly with autosomal dominant inheritance.

Genetic heterogeneity has been firmly established, and linkage analysis has identified nine distinct genetic loci. To date, five genes have been identified in autosomal-dominant ARVC: the cardiac ryanodine receptor (RYR2) in ARVC2,[148] desmoplakin (DSP) in ARVC8,[149] plakophilin-2 (PKP2) in ARVC9,[150] desmoglein-2 (DSG2)[151] and desmocollin-2 (DSC2).[152] ARVC2 is a rare and atypical form, with only mild structural abnormalities and a characteristic bidirectional VT very similar to CPVT. It is still unclear whether such patients fulfil the diagnostic criteria for ARVC. Mutations in the non-coding region of the transforming growth factor β3 have been identified in one kindred with ARVC1.[153] One form of ARVC, inherited in an autosomal-recessive fashion, is associated with wooly hair and palmoplantar keratoderma (Naxos disease) and caused by mutations in plakoglobin (JUP).[154] Five of the seven identified genes encode key components of the desmosome – protein complexes which provide structural and functional integrity to adjacent cells, suggesting that ARVC is a disease of the desmosome.

Management is problematic in patients with ARVC. Patients may simultaneously be at risk for lethal arrhythmias, yet experience frequent, short episodes of minimally symptomatic arrhythmias. The annual incidence of sudden death ranges from 0.08% to 9%, and ARVC is the top cause of SD in athletes in one Italian series.[155] Patients with ARVC who have a history of aborted sudden cardiac death or sustained ventricular tachycardia warrant placement of an ICD[74] (**Class I, Level B**). Otherwise, there is currently little information available to help decide which patients merit placement of a prophylactic ICD. Several clinical features have been proposed as markers of an increased risk of sudden death, including disease severity, history of syncope, family history of sudden death, and left ventricular involvement; an ICD can be considered in these patients[74] (**Class IIa, Level C**). Adjunctive medical or attempted ablation therapy is often necessary to limit the frequency discharges, especially for minimally symptomatic arrhythmias. Response to beta-blockers is variable, but sotalol or amiodarone can be effective for prevention of VT[74,156] (**Class IIa, Level C**). Catheter ablation may be used as adjunctive therapy, but remains unproven as long-term therapy in this condition (**Class IIb, Level C**). The role of electrophysiology testing is unclear at this time, but had excellent negative predictive value in one study among individuals with "probable ARVC" (three Task Force criteria), suggesting that low-risk individuals may be identified[157] (**Class IIb, Level C**).

Conclusion

In the last decade the identification of gene defects in a vast array of monogenic disorders has revolutionized our understanding of the basic mechanisms underlying numerous disease processes. Mutations in cardiac ion channels have been identified as the basis of a wide range of inherited arrhythmia syndromes, including congenital long and short QT syndromes, Brugada syndrome, Lenegre syndrome, Andersen–Tawil syndrome, and familial atrial fibrillation. More recently, it has been observed that not only transmembrane cardiac ion channels cause cardiac arrhythmias, but also intracellular channel and non-ion conduction proteins that may be pathophysiologically linked to inherited arrhythmias. The identification of genes underlying the inherited arrhythmia syndromes has greatly contributed to our understanding of the substrates for arrhythmia development but an unexpected complexity has emerged in the genotype/phenotype relationship. Phenotypic expression of a given mutation does not always appear to be uniform in patients, implying a contribution from environmental factors and/or presence of other genetic modifiers. The marked clinical heterogeneity associated with these inherited arrhythmia syndromes has led to the development of a multifactorial ("multiple hits") concept of arrhythmogenesis in which causal gene mutations have a major effect on disease that is further modified by factors such as age, gender, autonomic tone, and environmental triggers.

References

1. Priori SG, Napolitano C, Schwartz PJ. Low penetrance in the long-QT syndrome: clinical impact. *Circulation* 1999;**99**: 529–33.
2. Priori SG, Schwartz PJ, Napolitano C *et al.* Risk stratification in the long-QT syndrome. *N Engl J Med* 2003;**348**:1866–74.
3. Curran ME, Splawski I, Timothy KW, Vincent GM, Green ED, Keating MT. A molecular basis for cardiac arrhythmia: HERG mutations cause long QT syndrome. *Cell* 1995;**80**:795–803.
4. Wang Q, Shen J, Splawski I *et al.* SCN5A mutations associated with an inherited cardiac arrhythmia, long QT syndrome. *Cell* 1995;**80**:805–11.
5. Wang Q, Curran ME, Splawski I *et al.* Positional cloning of a novel potassium channel gene: KVLQT1 mutations cause cardiac arrhythmias. *Nat Genet* 1996;**12**:17–23.
6. Mohamed U, Napolitano C, Priori SG. Molecular and electrophysiological bases of catecholaminergic polymorphic ventricular tachycardia. *J Cardiovasc Electrophysiol* 2007;**18**:791–7.
7. Rossenbacker T, Priori SG. The Brugada syndrome. *Curr Opin Cardiol* 2007;**22**:163–70.
8. Schott JJ, Alshinawi C, Kyndt F *et al.* Cardiac conduction defects associate with mutations in SCN5A. *Nat Genet* 1999;**23**:20–1.
9. Chen Q, Kirsch GE, Zhang D *et al.* Genetic basis and molecular mechanism for idiopathic ventricular fibrillation. *Nature* 1998;**392**:293–6.
10. Chen YH, Xu SJ, Bendahhou S *et al.* KCNQ1 gain-of-function mutation in familial atrial fibrillation. *Science* 2003;**299**:251–4.
11. Feinberg WM, Blackshear JL, Laupacis A, Kronmal R, Hart RG. Prevalence, age distribution, and gender of patients with atrial fibrillation. Analysis and implications. *Arch Intern Med* 1995;**155**:469–73.
12. Fox CS, Parise H, D'Agostino RB Sr *et al.* Parental atrial fibrillation as a risk factor for atrial fibrillation in offspring. *JAMA* 2004;**291**:2851–5.
13. Levy S, Camm AJ, Saksena S *et al.* International consensus on nomenclature and classification of atrial fibrillation: a collaborative project of the Working Group on Arrhythmias and the Working Group of Cardiac Pacing of the European Society of Cardiology and the North American Society of Pacing and Electrophysiology. *J Cardiovasc Electrophysiol* 2003;**14**:443–5.
14. Wolff L. Familial auricular fibrillation. *N Engl J Med* 1943;**229**: 396–7.
15. Arnar DO, Thorvaldsson S, Manolio TA *et al.* Familial aggregation of atrial fibrillation in Iceland. *Eur Heart J* 2006;**27**:708–12.
16. Darbar D, Herron KJ, Ballew JD *et al.* Familial atrial fibrillation is a genetically heterogeneous disorder. *J Am Coll Cardiol* 2003;**41**:2185–92.

17. Ellinor PT, Yoerger DM, Ruskin JN, Macrae CA. Familial aggregation in lone atrial fibrillation. *Hum Genet* 2005;**118**:1–6.

18. Brugada R, Tapscott T, Czernuszewicz GZ *et al.* Identification of a genetic locus for familial atrial fibrillation. *N Engl J Med* 1997;**336**:905–11.

19. Ellinor PT, Shin JT, Moore RK, Yoerger DM, MacRae CA. Locus for atrial fibrillation maps to chromosome 6q14–16. *Circulation* 2003;**107**:2880–3.

20. Oberti C, Wang L, Li L *et al.* Genome-wide linkage scan identifies a novel genetic locus on chromosome 5p13 for neonatal atrial fibrillation associated with sudden death and variable cardiomyopathy. *Circulation* 2004;**110**:3753–9.

21. Volders PG, Zhu Q, Timmermans C *et al.* Mapping a novel locus for familial atrial fibrillation on chromosome 10p11-q21. *Heart Rhythm* 2007;**4**:469–75.

22. Darbar D, Jahangir A, Hammill SC, Gersh BJ. P wave signal-averaged electrocardiography to identify risk for atrial fibrillation. *Pacing Clin Electrophysiol* 2002;**25**:1447–53.

23. Yang Y, Xia M, Jin Q *et al.* Identification of a KCNE2 gain-of-function mutation in patients with familial atrial fibrillation. *Am J Hum Genet* 2004;**75**:899–905.

24. Olson TM, Alekseev AE, Liu XK *et al.* Kv1.5 channelopathy due to KCNA5 loss-of-function mutation causes human atrial fibrillation. *Hum Mol Genet* 2006;**15**:2185–91.

25. Ellinor PT, Petrov-Kondratov VI, Zakharova E *et al.* Potassium channel gene mutations rarely cause atrial fibrillation. *BMC Med Genet* 2006;**7**:70.

26. Gruver EJ, Fatkin D, Dodds GA *et al.* Familial hypertrophic cardiomyopathy and atrial fibrillation caused by Arg663His beta-cardiac myosin heavy chain mutation. *Am J Cardiol* 1999;**83**:13H–18H.

27. Mohler PJ, Schott JJ, Gramolini AO *et al.* Ankyrin-B mutation causes type 4 long-QT cardiac arrhythmia and sudden cardiac death. *Nature* 2003;**421**:634–9.

28. Morita H, Kusano-Fukushima K, Nagase S *et al.* Atrial fibrillation and atrial vulnerability in patients with Brugada syndrome. *J Am Coll Cardiol* 2002;**40**:1437–44.

29. Priori SG, Pandit SV, Rivolta I *et al.* A novel form of short QT syndrome (SQT3) is caused by a mutation in the KCNJ2 gene. *Circ Res* 2005;**96**:800–7.

30. Gaita F, Giustetto C, Bianchi F *et al.* Short QT syndrome: a familial cause of sudden death. *Circulation* 2003;**108**:965–70.

31. Olson TM, Michels VV, Ballew JD *et al.* Sodium channel mutations and susceptibility to heart failure and atrial fibrillation. *JAMA* 2005;**293**:447–54.

32. Fatkin D, MacRae C, Sasaki T *et al.* Missense mutations in the rod domain of the lamin A/C gene as causes of dilated cardiomyopathy and conduction-system disease. *N Engl J Med* 1999;**341**:1715–24.

33. Ehrlich JR, Zicha S, Coutu P, Hebert TE, Nattel S. Atrial fibrillation-associated minK38G/S polymorphism modulates delayed rectifier current and membrane localization. *Cardiovasc Res* 2005;**67**:520–8.

34. Temple J, Frias P, Rottman J *et al.* Atrial fibrillation in KCNE1-null mice. *Circ Res* 2005;**9**:9.

35. Schreieck J, Dostal S, von Beckerath N *et al.* C825T polymorphism of the G-protein beta3 subunit gene and atrial fibrillation: association of the TT genotype with a reduced risk for atrial fibrillation. *Am Heart J* 2004;**148**:545–50.

36. Ravn LS, Hofman-Bang J, Dixen U *et al.* Relation of 97T polymorphism in KCNE5 to risk of atrial fibrillation. *Am J Cardiol* 2005;**96**:405–7.

37. Chen LY, Ballew JD, Herron KJ, Rodeheffer RJ, Olson TM. A common polymorphism in SCN5A is associated with lone atrial fibrillation. *Clin Pharmacol Ther* 2007;**81**:35–41.

38. Madrid AH, Bueno MG, Rebollo JM *et al.* Use of irbesartan to maintain sinus rhythm in patients with long-lasting persistent atrial fibrillation: a prospective and randomized study. *Circulation* 2002;**106**:331–6.

39. Tsai CT, Lai LP, Lin JL *et al.* Renin-angiotensin system gene polymorphisms and atrial fibrillation. *Circulation* 2004;**109**:1640–6.

40. Darbar D, Motsinger AA, Ritchie MD, Gainer JV, Roden DM. Polymorphism modulates symptomatic response to antiarrhythmic drug therapy in patients with lone atrial fibrillation. *Heart Rhythm* 2007;**4**:743–9.

41. Collins FS, Guyer MS, Charkravarti A. Variations on a theme: cataloging human DNA sequence variation. *Science* 1997;**278**:1580–1.

42. Gudbjartsson DF, Arnar DO, Helgadottir A *et al.* Variants conferring risk of atrial fibrillation on chromosome 4q25. *Nature* 2007;**1**:1.

43. Basson CT, Huang T, Lin RC *et al.* Different TBX5 interactions in heart and limb defined by Holt-Oram syndrome mutations. *Proc Natl Acad Sci USA* 1999;**96**:2919–24.

44. Donofrio MT, Gullquist SD, Mehta ID, Moskowitz WB. Congenital complete heart block: fetal management protocol, review of the literature, and report of the smallest successful pacemaker implantation. *J Perinatol* 2004;**24**:112–17.

45. Kasahara H, Wakimoto H, Liu M *et al.* Progressive atrioventricular conduction defects and heart failure in mice expressing a mutant Csx/Nkx2.5 homeoprotein. *J Clin Invest* 2001;**108**:189–201.

46. Keating MT, Sanguinetti MC. Molecular and cellular mechanisms of cardiac arrhythmias. *Cell* 2001;**104**:569–80.

47. Papadatos GA, Wallerstein PM, Head CE *et al.* Slowed conduction and ventricular tachycardia after targeted disruption of the cardiac sodium channel gene Scn5a. *Proc Natl Acad Sci USA* 2002;**99**:6210–15.

48. Mohler PJ, Rivolta I, Napolitano C *et al.* Nav1.5 E1053K mutation causing Brugada syndrome blocks binding to ankyrin-G and expression of Nav1.5 on the surface of cardiomyocytes. *Proc Natl Acad Sci USA* 2004;**101**:17533–8.

49. Ludwig A, Budde T, Stieber J *et al.* Absence epilepsy and sinus dysrhythmia in mice lacking the pacemaker channel HCN2. *EMBO J* 2003;**22**:216–24.

50. Stieber J, Herrmann S, Feil S *et al.* The hyperpolarization-activated channel HCN4 is required for the generation of pacemaker action potentials in the embryonic heart. *Proc Natl Acad Sci USA* 2003;**100**:15235–40.

51. Milanesi R, Baruscotti M, Gnecchi-Ruscone T, DiFrancesco D. Familial sinus bradycardia associated with a mutation in the cardiac pacemaker channel. *N Engl J Med* 2006;**354**:151–7.

52. Nof E, Luria D, Brass D *et al.* Point mutation in the HCN4 cardiac ion channel pore affecting synthesis, trafficking, and functional expression is associated with familial asymptomatic sinus bradycardia. *Circulation* 2007;**116**:463–70.

53. Arad M, Benson DW, Perez-Atayde AR *et al*. Constitutively active AMP kinase mutations cause glycogen storage disease mimicking hypertrophic cardiomyopathy. *J Clin Invest* 2002;**109**:357–62.

54. Mehdirad AA, Fatkin D, DiMarco JP *et al*. Electrophysiologic characteristics of accessory atrioventricular connections in an inherited form of Wolff-Parkinson-White syndrome. *J Cardiovasc Electrophysiol* 1999;**10**:629–35.

55. Jervell A, Lange-Nielsen F. Congenital deaf-mutism, functional heart disease with prolongation of the Q-T interval and sudden death. *Am Heart J* 1957;**54**:59–68.

56. Romano C, Gemme G, Pongiglione R. Rare cardiac arrythmias of the pediatric age. Ii. Syncopal attacks due to paroxysmal ventricular fibrillation. *Clin Pediatr (Bologna)* 1963;**45**:656–83.

57. Ward OC. A new familial cardiac syndrome in children. *J Ir Med Assoc* 1964;**54**:103–6.

58. Splawski I, Tristani-Firouzi M, Lehmann MH, Sanguinetti MC, Keating MT. Mutations in the hminK gene cause long QT syndrome and suppress IKs function. *Nat Genet* 1997;**17**: 338–40.

59. Schulze-Bahr E, Wang Q, Wedekind H *et al*. KCNE1 mutations cause jervell and Lange-Nielsen syndrome. *Nat Genet* 1997; **17**:267–8.

60. Tyson J, Tranebjaerg L, Bellman S *et al*. IsK and KvLQT1: mutation in either of the two subunits of the slow component of the delayed rectifier potassium channel can cause Jervell and Lange-Nielsen syndrome. *Hum Mol Genet* 1997;**6**:2179–85.

61. Neyroud N, Tesson F, Denjoy I *et al*. A novel mutation in the potassium channel gene KVLQT1 causes the Jervell and Lange-Nielsen cardioauditory syndrome. *Nat Genet* 1997;**15**:186–9.

62. Schwartz PJ, Spazzolini C, Crotti L *et al*. The Jervell and Lange-Nielsen syndrome: natural history, molecular basis, and clinical outcome. *Circulation* 2006;**113**:783–90.

63. Plaster NM, Tawil R, Tristani-Firouzi M *et al*. Mutations in Kir2.1 cause the developmental and episodic electrical phenotypes of Andersen's syndrome. *Cell* 2001;**105**:511–19.

64. Splawski I, Timothy KW, Sharpe LM *et al*. Ca(V)1.2 calcium channel dysfunction causes a multisystem disorder including arrhythmia and autism. *Cell* 2004;**119**:19–31.

65. Zhang L, Benson DW, Tristani-Firouzi M *et al*. Electrocardiographic features in Andersen-Tawil syndrome patients with KCNJ2 mutations: characteristic T-U-wave patterns predict the KCNJ2 genotype. *Circulation* 2005;**111**:2720–6.

66. Mohler PJ, Le Scouarnec S, Denjoy I *et al*. Defining the cellular phenotype of "ankyrin-B syndrome" variants: human ANK2 variants associated with clinical phenotypes display a spectrum of activities in cardiomyocytes. *Circulation* 2007;**115**: 432–41.

67. Splawski I, Shen J, Timothy KW *et al*. Spectrum of mutations in long-QT syndrome genes. KVLQT1, HERG, SCN5A, KCNE1, and KCNE2. *Circulation* 2000;**102**:1178–85.

68. Moss AJ, Zareba W, Benhorin J *et al*. ECG T-wave patterns in genetically distinct forms of the hereditary long QT syndrome. *Circulation* 1995;**92**:2929–34.

69. Zareba W, Moss AJ, Schwartz PJ *et al*. Influence of genotype on the clinical course of the long-QT syndrome. International Long-QT Syndrome Registry Research Group. *N Engl J Med* 1998;**339**:960–5.

70. Schwartz PJ, Priori SG, Spazzolini C *et al*. Genotype-phenotype correlation in the long-QT syndrome: gene-specific triggers for life-threatening arrhythmias. *Circulation* 2001;**103**:89–95.

71. Shimizu W, Noda T, Takaki H *et al*. Diagnostic value of epinephrine test for genotyping LQT1, LQT2, and LQT3 forms of congenital long QT syndrome. *Heart Rhythm* 2004;**1**:276–83.

72. Noda T, Takaki H, Kurita T *et al*. Gene-specific response of dynamic ventricular repolarization to sympathetic stimulation in LQT1, LQT2 and LQT3 forms of congenital long QT syndrome. *Eur Heart J* 2002;**23**:975–83.

73. Moss AJ, Zareba W, Hall WJ *et al*. Effectiveness and limitations of beta-blocker therapy in congenital long-QT syndrome. *Circulation* 2000;**101**:616–23.

74. Zipes DP, Camm AJ, Borggrefe M *et al*. ACC/AHA/ESC 2006 Guidelines for Management of Patients With Ventricular Arrhythmias and the Prevention of Sudden Cardiac Death: a report of the American College of Cardiology/American Heart Association Task Force and the European Society of Cardiology Committee for Practice Guidelines. *Circulation* 2006;**114**: e385–484.

75. Sauer AJ, Moss AJ, McNitt S *et al*. Long QT syndrome in adults. *J Am Coll Cardiol* 2007;**49**:329–37.

76. Schwartz PJ. Management of long QT syndrome. *Nat Clin Pract Cardiovasc Med* 2005;**2**:346–51.

77. Shimizu W, Antzelevitch C. Sodium channel block with mexiletine is effective in reducing dispersion of repolarization and preventing torsade des pointes in LQT2 and LQT3 models of the long-QT syndrome. *Circulation* 1997;**96**:2038–47.

78. Schwartz PJ, Priori SG, Locati EH *et al*. Long QT syndrome patients with mutations of the SCN5A and HERG genes have differential responses to Na+ channel blockade and to increases in heart rate. Implications for gene-specific therapy. *Circulation* 1995;**92**:3381–6.

79. Priori SG, Napolitano C, Schwartz PJ, Bloise R, Crotti L, Ronchetti E. The elusive link between LQT3 and Brugada syndrome: the role of flecainide challenge. *Circulation* 2000;**102**: 945–7.

80. Benhorin J, Taub R, Goldmit M *et al*. Effects of flecainide in patients with new SCN5A mutation: mutation-specific therapy for long-QT syndrome? *Circulation* 2000;**101**:1698–706.

81. Compton SJ, Lux RL, Ramsey MR *et al*. Genetically defined therapy of inherited long-QT syndrome. Correction of abnormal repolarization by potassium. *Circulation* 1996;**94**:1018–22.

82. Etheridge SP, Compton SJ, Tristani-Firouzi M, Mason JW. A new oral therapy for long QT syndrome: long-term oral potassium improves repolarization in patients with HERG mutations. *J Am Coll Cardiol* 2003;**42**:1777–82.

83. Zareba W, Moss AJ, Daubert JP, Hall WJ, Robinson JL, Andrews M. Implantable cardioverter defibrillator in high-risk long QT syndrome patients. *J Cardiovasc Electrophysiol* 2003;**14**: 337–41.

84. Vincent GM. Risk assessment in long QT syndrome: the Achilles heel of appropriate treatment. *Heart Rhythm* 2005;**2**:505–6.

85. Hobbs JB, Peterson DR, Moss AJ *et al*. Risk of aborted cardiac arrest or sudden cardiac death during adolescence in the long-QT syndrome. *JAMA* 2006;**296**:1249–54.

86. Schwartz PJ, Priori SG, Cerrone M *et al*. Left cardiac sympathetic denervation in the management of high-risk

patients affected by the long-QT syndrome. *Circulation* 2004;**109**:1826–33.

87. Algra A, Tijssen JG, Roelandt JR, Pool J, Lubsen J. Heart rate variability from 24-hour electrocardiography and the 2-year risk for sudden death. *Circulation* 1993;**88**:180–5.

88. Gussak I, Brugada P, Brugada J *et al.* Idiopathic short QT interval: a new clinical syndrome? *Cardiology* 2000;**94**:99–102.

89. Hong K, Bjerregaard P, Gussak I, Brugada R. Short QT syndrome and atrial fibrillation caused by mutation in KCNH2. *J Cardiovasc Electrophysiol* 2005;**16**:394–6.

90. Brugada R, Hong K, Dumaine R *et al.* Sudden death associated with short-QT syndrome linked to mutations in HERG. *Circulation* 2004;**109**:30–5.

91. Bellocq C, van Ginneken AC, Bezzina CR *et al.* Mutation in the KCNQ1 gene leading to the short QT-interval syndrome. *Circulation* 2004;**109**:2394–7.

92. Gallagher MM, Magliano G, Yap YG *et al.* Distribution and prognostic significance of QT intervals in the lowest half centile in 12,012 apparently healthy persons. *Am J Cardiol* 2006;**98**:933–5.

93. Anttonen O, Junttila MJ, Rissanen H, Reunanen A, Viitasalo M, Huikuri HV. Prevalence and prognostic significance of short QT interval in a middle-aged Finnish population. *Circulation* 2007;**116**:714–20.

94. Reinig MG, Engel TR. The shortage of short QT intervals. *Chest* 2007;**132**:246–9.

95. Giustetto C, Di Monte F, Wolpert C *et al.* Short QT syndrome: clinical findings and diagnostic-therapeutic implications. *Eur Heart J* 2006;**27**:2440–7.

96. Schimpf R, Wolpert C, Gaita F, Giustetto C, Borggrefe M. Short QT syndrome. *Cardiovasc Res* 2005;**67**:357–66.

97. Extramiana F, Antzelevitch C. Amplified transmural dispersion of repolarization as the basis for arrhythmogenesis in a canine ventricular-wedge model of short-QT syndrome. *Circulation* 2004;**110**:3661–6.

98. Schimpf R, Wolpert C, Bianchi F *et al.* Congenital short QT syndrome and implantable cardioverter defibrillator treatment: inherent risk for inappropriate shock delivery. *J Cardiovasc Electrophysiol* 2003;**14**:1273–7.

99. Gaita F, Giustetto C, Bianchi F *et al.* Short QT syndrome: pharmacological treatment. *J Am Coll Cardiol* 2004;**43**:1494–9.

100. Milberg P, Tegelkamp R, Osada N *et al.* Reduction of dispersion of repolarization and prolongation of postrepolarization refractoriness explain the antiarrhythmic effects of quinidine in a model of short QT syndrome. *J Cardiovasc Electrophysiol* 2007;**18**:658–64.

101. Leenhardt A, Lucet V, Denjoy I, Grau F, Ngoc DD, Coumel P. Catecholaminergic polymorphic ventricular tachycardia in children. A 7-year follow-up of 21 patients. *Circulation* 1995;**91**:1512–19.

102. Swan H, Piippo K, Viitasalo M *et al.* Arrhythmic disorder mapped to chromosome 1q42-q43 causes malignant polymorphic ventricular tachycardia in structurally normal hearts. *J Am Coll Cardiol* 1999;**34**:2035–42.

103. Priori SG, Napolitano C, Tiso N *et al.* Mutations in the cardiac ryanodine receptor gene (hRyR2) underlie catecholaminergic polymorphic ventricular tachycardia. *Circulation* 2001;**103**:196–200.

104. Eldar M, Pras E, Lahat H. A missense mutation in the CASQ2 gene is associated with autosomal-recessive catecholamine-induced polymorphic ventricular tachycardia. *Trends Cardiovasc Med* 2003;**13**:148–51.

105. Postma AV, Denjoy I, Hoorntje TM *et al.* Absence of calsequestrin 2 causes severe forms of catecholaminergic polymorphic ventricular tachycardia. *Circ Res* 2002;**91**:e21–6.

106. Bhuiyan ZA, Hamdan MA, Shamsi ET *et al.* A novel early onset lethal form of catecholaminergic polymorphic ventricular tachycardia maps to chromosome 7p14-p22. *J Cardiovasc Electrophysiol* 2007;**30**:30.

107. Nam GB, Burashnikov A, Antzelevitch C. Cellular mechanisms underlying the development of catecholaminergic ventricular tachycardia. *Circulation* 2005;**111**:2727–33.

108. Coumel P. Catecholaminergic polymorphic ventricular tachyarrhythmias in children. *Card Electrophysiol Rev* 2002;**6**:93–5.

109. McPate MJ, Duncan RS, Milnes JT, Witchel HJ, Hancox JC. The N588K-HERG K+ channel mutation in the 'short QT syndrome': mechanism of gain-in-function determined at 37 degrees C. *Biochem Biophys Res Commun* 2005;**334**:441–9.

110. Postma AV, Denjoy I, Kamblock J *et al.* Catecholaminergic polymorphic ventricular tachycardia: RYR2 mutations, bradycardia, and follow up of the patients. *J Med Genet* 2005;**42**:863–70.

111. Priori SG, Napolitano C, Memmi M *et al.* Clinical and molecular characterization of patients with catecholaminergic polymorphic ventricular tachycardia. *Circulation* 2002;**106**:69–74.

112. Liu N, Colombi B, Raytcheva-Buono EV, Bloise R, Priori SG. Catecholaminergic polymorphic ventricular tachycardia. *Herz* 2007;**32**:212–17.

113. Brugada P, Brugada J. Right bundle branch block, persistent ST segment elevation and sudden cardiac death: a distinct clinical and electrocardiographic syndrome. A multicenter report. *J Am Coll Cardiol* 1992;**20**:1391–6.

114. Vatta M, Dumaine R, Varghese G *et al.* Genetic and biophysical basis of sudden unexplained nocturnal death syndrome (SUNDS), a disease allelic to Brugada syndrome. *Hum Mol Genet* 2002;**11**:337–45.

115. Priori SG, Napolitano C, Giordano U, Collisani G, Memmi M. Brugada syndrome and sudden cardiac death in children. *Lancet* 2000;**355**:808–9.

116. Todd SJ, Campbell MJ, Roden DM, Kannankeril PJ. Novel Brugada SCN5A mutation causing sudden death in children. *Heart Rhythm* 2005;**2**:540–3.

117. Yan GX, Antzelevitch C. Cellular basis for the Brugada syndrome and other mechanisms of arrhythmogenesis associated with ST-segment elevation. *Circulation* 1999;**100**:1660–6.

118. Saura D, Garcia-Alberola A, Carrillo P, Pascual D, Martinez-Sanchez J, Valdes M. Brugada-like electrocardiographic pattern induced by fever. *Pacing Clin Electrophysiol* 2002;**25**:856–9.

119. Dinckal MH, Davutoglu V, Akdemir I, Soydinc S, Kirilmaz A, Aksoy M. Incessant monomorphic ventricular tachycardia during febrile illness in a patient with Brugada syndrome: fatal electrical storm. *Europace* 2003;**5**:257–61.

120. Dumaine R, Towbin JA, Brugada P *et al.* Ionic mechanisms responsible for the electrocardiographic phenotype of the Brugada syndrome are temperature dependent. *Circ Res* 1999;**85**:803–9.

121. London B, Sanyal S, Michalec M, Pfahnl A, Shang L, Kerchner L. A mutation in the glycerol-3-phosphate dehydrogenase 1-like gene (GPD1L) causes Brugada syndrome. *Heart Rhythm* 2006;**3**(5, suppl 1):S32.

122. Antzelevitch C, Pollevick GD, Cordeiro JM *et al.* Loss-of-function mutations in the cardiac calcium channel underlie a new clinical entity characterized by ST-segment elevation, short QT intervals, and sudden cardiac death. *Circulation* 2007;**115**: 442–9.

123. Brugada R, Brugada J, Antzelevitch C *et al.* Sodium channel blockers identify risk for sudden death in patients with ST-segment elevation and right bundle branch block but structurally normal hearts. *Circulation* 2000;**101**:510–15.

124. Matsuo K, Akahoshi M, Nakashima E *et al.* The prevalence, incidence and prognostic value of the Brugada-type electrocardiogram: a population-based study of four decades. *J Am Coll Cardiol* 2001;**38**:765–70.

125. Miyasaka Y, Tsuji H, Yamada K *et al.* Prevalence and mortality of the Brugada-type electrocardiogram in one city in Japan. *J Am Coll Cardiol* 2001;**38**:771–4.

126. Oe H, Takagi M, Tanaka A *et al.* Prevalence and clinical course of the juveniles with Brugada-type ECG in Japanese population. *Pacing Clin Electrophysiol* 2005;**28**:549–54.

127. Brugada J, Brugada R, Antzelevitch C, Towbin J, Nademanee K, Brugada P. Long-term follow-up of individuals with the electrocardiographic pattern of right bundle-branch block and ST-segment elevation in precordial leads V1 to V3. *Circulation* 2002;**105**:73–8.

128. Nademanee K, Veerakul G, Mower M *et al.* Defibrillator Versus beta-Blockers for Unexplained Death in Thailand (DEBUT): a randomized clinical trial. *Circulation* 2003;**107**:2221–6.

129. Antzelevitch C, Brugada P, Borggrefe M *et al.* Brugada Syndrome. Report of the Second Consensus Conference. Endorsed by the Heart Rhythm Society and the European Heart Rhythm Association. *Circulation* 2005;**17**:17.

130. Hermida JS, Denjoy I, Clerc J *et al.* Hydroquinidine therapy in Brugada syndrome. *J Am Coll Cardiol* 2004;**43**:1853–60.

131. Belhassen B, Glick A, Viskin S. Efficacy of quinidine in high-risk patients with Brugada syndrome. *Circulation* 2004;**110**:1731–7.

132. Brugada J, Brugada R, Brugada P. Determinants of sudden cardiac death in individuals with the electrocardiographic pattern of Brugada syndrome and no previous cardiac arrest. *Circulation* 2003;**108**:3092–6.

133. Priori SG, Napolitano C, Gasparini M *et al.* Natural history of Brugada syndrome: insights for risk stratification and management. *Circulation* 2002;**105**:1342–7.

134. Eckardt L, Probst V, Smits JP *et al.* Long-term prognosis of individuals with right precordial ST-segment-elevation Brugada syndrome. *Circulation* 2005;**111**:257–63.

135. Lind JM, Chiu C, Semsarian C. Genetic basis of hypertrophic cardiomyopathy. *Expert Rev Cardiovasc Ther* 2006;**4**:927–34.

136. Gollob MH, Green MS, Tang AS *et al.* Identification of a gene responsible for familial Wolff-Parkinson-White syndrome. *N Engl J Med* 2001;**344**:1823–31.

137. Maron BJ, Shirani J, Poliac LC, Mathenge R, Roberts WC, Mueller FO. Sudden death in young competitive athletes. Clinical, demographic, and pathological profiles. *JAMA* 1996;**276**:199–204.

138. Maron BJ, McKenna WJ, Danielson GK *et al.* American College of Cardiology/European Society of Cardiology clinical expert consensus document on hypertrophic cardiomyopathy. *J Am Coll Cardiol* 2003;**42**:1687–713.

139. Maron BJ, Spirito P, Shen WK *et al.* Implantable cardioverter-defibrillators and prevention of sudden cardiac death in hypertrophic cardiomyopathy. *JAMA* 2007;**298**:405–12.

140. McKenna WJ, Oakley CM, Krikler DM, Goodwin JF. Improved survival with amiodarone in patients with hypertrophic cardiomyopathy and ventricular tachycardia. *Br Heart J* 1985;**53**: 412–16.

141. Fananapazir L, Tracy CM, Leon MB *et al.* Electrophysiologic abnormalities in patients with hypertrophic cardiomyopathy. A consecutive analysis in 155 patients. *Circulation* 1989;**80**: 1259–68.

142. Behr ER, Elliott P, McKenna WJ. Role of invasive EP testing in the evaluation and management of hypertrophic cardiomyopathy. *Card Electrophysiol Rev* 2002;**6**:482–6.

143. Calkins H. Arrhythmogenic right-ventricular dysplasia/cardiomyopathy. *Curr Opin Cardiol* 2006;**21**:55–63.

144. Tabib A, Loire R, Chalabreysse L *et al.* Circumstances of death and gross and microscopic observations in a series of 200 cases of sudden death associated with arrhythmogenic right ventricular cardiomyopathy and/or dysplasia. *Circulation* 2003;**108**: 3000–5.

145. Corrado D, Basso C, Thiene G. Sudden cardiac death in young people with apparently normal heart. *Cardiovasc Res* 2001;**50**: 399–408.

146. McKenna WJ, Thiene G, Nava A *et al.* Diagnosis of arrhythmogenic right ventricular dysplasia/cardiomyopathy. Task Force of the Working Group Myocardial and Pericardial Disease of the European Society of Cardiology and of the Scientific Council on Cardiomyopathies of the International Society and Federation of Cardiology. *Br Heart J* 1994;**71**:215–18.

147. Hamid MS, Norman M, Quraishi A *et al.* Prospective evaluation of relatives for familial arrhythmogenic right ventricular cardiomyopathy/dysplasia reveals a need to broaden diagnostic criteria. *J Am Coll Cardiol* 2002;**40**:1445–50.

148. Tiso N, Stephan DA, Nava A *et al.* Identification of mutations in the cardiac ryanodine receptor gene in families affected with arrhythmogenic right ventricular cardiomyopathy type 2 (ARVD2). *Hum Mol Genet* 2001;**10**:189–94.

149. Rampazzo A, Nava A, Malacrida S *et al.* Mutation in human desmoplakin domain binding to plakoglobin causes a dominant form of arrhythmogenic right ventricular cardiomyopathy. *Am J Hum Genet* 2002;**71**:1200–6.

150. Gerull B, Heuser A, Wichter T *et al.* Mutations in the desmosomal protein plakophilin-2 are common in arrhythmogenic right ventricular cardiomyopathy. *Nat Genet* 2004;**36**: 1162–4.

151. Pilichou K, Nava A, Basso C *et al.* Mutations in desmoglein-2 gene are associated with arrhythmogenic right ventricular cardiomyopathy. *Circulation* 2006;**113**:1171–9.

152. Heuser A, Plovie ER, Ellinor PT *et al.* Mutant desmocollin-2 causes arrhythmogenic right ventricular cardiomyopathy. *Am J Hum Genet* 2006;**79**:1081–8.

153. Beffagna G, Occhi G, Nava A *et al.* Regulatory mutations in transforming growth factor-beta3 gene cause arrhythmogenic

right ventricular cardiomyopathy type 1. *Cardiovasc Res* 2005;**65**:366–73.

154. McKoy G, Protonotarios N, Crosby A *et al.* Identification of a deletion in plakoglobin in arrhythmogenic right ventricular cardiomyopathy with palmoplantar keratoderma and woolly hair (Naxos disease). *Lancet* 2000;**355**:2119–24.

155. Furlanello F, Bertoldi A, Dallago M *et al.* Cardiac arrest and sudden death in competitive athletes with arrhythmogenic right ventricular dysplasia. *Pacing Clin Electrophysiol* 1998;**21**:331–5.

156. Wichter T, Paul TM, Eckardt L *et al.* Arrhythmogenic right ventricular cardiomyopathy. Antiarrhythmic drugs, catheter ablation, or ICD? *Herz* 2005;**30**:91–101.

157. Piccini JP, Dalal D, Roguin A *et al.* Predictors of appropriate implantable defibrillator therapies in patients with arrhythmogenic right ventricular dysplasia. *Heart Rhythm* 2005;**2**:1188–94.

45 Arrhythmogenic right ventricular cardiomyopathy

Deirdre Ward[1] and Perry M Elliott[2]
[1]Trinity College, Dublin, Ireland
[2]University College London, London, UK

Introduction

Arrhythmogenic right ventricular cardiomyopathy (ARVC) is a disorder characterized clinically by ventricular arrhythmia, heart failure and sudden death, and histologically by cardiomyocyte loss and replacement with fibrous or fibrofatty tissue. The estimated prevalence of ARVC is 1 in 5000 of the population. It is an important cause of sudden cardiac deaths in athletes and in people under 35 years. In many individuals, the disease is caused by mutations in genes that encode different components of the intercalated disc of cardiomyocytes. Clinically, ARVC is difficult to diagnose, usually requiring integration of data from family members, electrocardiography and a range of imaging techniques. Management of ARVC focuses on treatment of symptomatic arrhythmia, prevention of sudden cardiac death and, in the later stages of the disease, heart failure management.

History

In 1952 Dr Henry Uhl described a case of "almost total absence of the myocardium of the right ventricle" in an 8-month-old girl.[1] The case was characterized by complete heart block and right ventricular failure. At post mortem the myocardium of the left ventricle was normal and there was a sharp demarcation line between this and the very abnormal right ventricle in which there was virtually complete loss of the myocardium. There was no evidence of ischemic change or inflammation and the cause was assumed to be a maldevelopment or dysplastic process.

The first description of an ARVC was in 1978, when detailed electrocardiography readings of four French

patients with right ventricular dysplasia associated with arrhythmia were reported.[2] In the same journal there was a report of two French patients in their sixth decade of life presenting with recurrent ventricular tachycardia of left bundle branch bock (LBBB) morphology resistant to medical therapy. Clinical examination, angiography and ultimately post-mortem examination identified what was described as "the parchment right ventricle syndrome of the adult."[3]

A case series of 24 patients published 4 years later identified the characteristics of the typical patient with what is now called arrhythmogenic right ventricular cardiomyopathy. The mean age at presentation (in those who had symptoms) was 39 years, and the male/female ratio was 2.7:1. Almost 90% of the patients had T-wave inversion in the right precordial leads. Ventricular postexcitation waves (epsilon waves) were present in one-third of patients. All but one of the patients had spontaneously occurring ventricular tachycardia with a LBBB configuration. In those who underwent echocardiography, the ratio of right to left ventricular size was increased, and wall motion abnormality of the right ventricle was seen in the majority. One patient had a wall motion abnormality of the posterior wall of the left ventricle. Morphologic findings were confirmed in 13 patients during surgical intervention. The right ventricle was invariably enlarged and there were discrete areas of segmental dilation associated with dyskinetic wall motion and aneurysms. The authors reported the most common location of these right ventricular aneurysms to be the anterior surface of the right ventricular outflow tract, apex and inferior wall, and coined the term "the triangle of dysplasia." There was frequently an increase in subepicardial fat over these areas and depletion in the numbers of muscle fibers. The amount of fibrosis was variable. On microscopy some hypertrophy of the remaining myofibers was noted, and there was a varying degree of lymphocytic infiltration.[4] One of the patients came from a family reported 4 years earlier in a description of seven cases of familial ventricular tachycardia.[5]

Evidence-Based Cardiology, 3rd edition. Edited by S. Yusuf, J.A. Cairns, A.J. Camm, E.L. Fallen, and B.J. Gersh. © 2010 Blackwell Publishing, ISBN: 978-1-4051-5925-8.

The first gene mutation to be associated with ARVC was identified in patients with a recessive cardiocutaneous syndrome characterized by wooly hair, palmoplantar keratoderma and ARVC common on the Greek island of Naxos.[6] The locus for Naxos disease was mapped to chromosome 17 (17q21), and subsequently a deletion in the gene encoding plakoglobin was identified as the disease-causing mutation.[7,8] Plakoglobin is a constituent protein in both adherens and desmosomal cell–cell junctions. Subsequent evaluation of other related desmosomal genes in ARVC patients with more typical autosomal dominant disease has identified disease-causing mutations in a further four genes encoding other desmosomal proteins.

The structure of the right ventricle renders it inherently more difficult to image than the left ventricle, but improvements in imaging techniques over the past decade have broadened the clinical spectrum of the disease by identifying patients at an earlier, often asymptomatic stage. Cardiac magnetic resonance imaging in particular has demonstrated a high prevalence of left ventricular involvement in many patients, illustrating the heterogeneity in disease expression.[9–13]

Epidemiology

In most populations the prevalence of ARVC is unknown. An apparent cluster of disease is reported in the Veneto region of Italy, with a frequency of 1 per 5000, but it is unclear whether this is a true clustering or a reflection of local interest and expertise in the disease. Nevertheless, the limited information available suggests that ARVC is an important cause of premature sudden cardiac death. A retrospective review of a French post-mortem series identified ARVC as a likely cause of death in 10% of the population aged 1–65 years.[14] Prospective studies of an Italian cohort aged 12–35 years found evidence of ARVC in 12% of those who suffered a sudden cardiac death.[15] A population-based study from the USA identified pathologic changes of ARVC in 17% of sudden death victims under 40 years of age.[16] Other authors report that up to 25% of sudden deaths in athletes are due to ARVC.[17]

Pathology

In the early stages, abnormal pathologic findings are localized to the apical, inflow and infundibular areas of the right ventricle.[4] With disease progression, the left ventricle, particularly the posterolateral wall, is often involved, with relative sparing of the interventricular septum. In some cases, the pathologic abnormalities may be confined to the left ventricle.[18,19]

Macroscopic examination of the heart shows diffuse or focal thinning of the right ventricular wall, affecting the subepicardium more than the subendocardium, with aneurysm formation in up to 50% of cases.[18,20] Histologically, there is myocardial atrophy and fibro-fatty replacement. Islands or strands of surviving myocytes exhibit a combination of degenerative change with myocyte vacuolation, often associated with focal mononuclear inflammatory cell infiltrates.[21–24] In some cases, typical histologic findings may be present in the absence of any macroscopic features.[25] A second histologic pattern, characterized by transmural infiltration of adipose tissue without fibrous replacement or wall thinning, has been considered to be an earlier stage of the condition[22,26] but this can be a normal finding, particularly in older women.[20]

A number of studies have reported evidence of apoptosis in ARVC which is not found in normal controls, patients undergoing post-transplant surveillance or in patients with structurally normal hearts and VT arising from the RV outflow tract.[27–30] Apoptosis is more common in patients with a short (less than 6 months) clinical history and acute symptoms and signs.[27] Apoptosis is present to an equivalent degree in children and adults with ARVC.[28]

Endomyocardial biopsies from some ARVC patients have been found to contain enteroviral RNA with homology to Coxsackie virus type B. In one study similar proportions of patients with myocarditis or dilated cardiomyopathy were positive for viral RNA but none of the control patients with non-inflammatory cardiac disorders.[31] Other studies have failed to confirm these findings, which may reflect patient selection and differences between inherited and sporadic, non-familial forms of ARVC.[32–37]

Genetics

Systematic family studies have shown that ARVC is inherited in up to 50% of cases.[38] Numerous genetic loci have been identified (Table 45.1). The mode of transmission is usually autosomal dominant with variable penetrance, but autosomal recessive forms are well recognized and provided the first insights into the genetic basis of ARVC. In 1986, an autosomal recessive syndrome characterized by cardiomyopathy, wooly hair and palmoplantar keratoderma was described in families from the Greek island of Naxos.[6] The cardiac phenotype of this syndrome replicates the clinical and histopathologic characteristics of typical ARVC.[39] Subsequent molecular genetic investigations in families with Naxos disease revealed a homozygous mutation in the gene encoding plakoglobin, a member of the armadillo protein family found in adherens and desmosomal junctions between cardiomyocytes. Families with a similar cardiocutaneous phenotype are reported from other Mediterranean areas,[40–43] India[44] and South America.[45] The

Table 45.1 Genetic loci identified in association with ARVC

Subtype	Loci	Reference
ARVC 1	14q23–24	Rampazzo, 1994[53]
	Transforming growth factor β3 (?)	Beffagna, 2005[54]
ARVC 2	1q42–43	Rampazzo, 1995[107]
	Ryanodine 2 receptor	Tiso, 2001[52]
ARVC 3	14q12–22	Severini, 1996[108]
ARVC 4	2q32	Rampazzo, 1997[109]
ARVC 5	3p23	Ahmad, 1998[110]
ARVC 6	10q22.3	Melberg, 1999[111]
ARVC 7	10p12–14	Li, 2000[112]
ARVC 8	6p24	Rampazzo, 2002[113]
	Desmoplakin	
ARVC 9	12p11	Gerull, 2004[46]
	Plakophilin 2	
ARVC 10	18q12.1–12.2	Pilichou, 2006[94]
	Desmoglein 2	
ARVC 11	18q12.1	Syrris, 2006[114]
	Desmocollin 2	

cause in many of these families is an autosomal recessively inherited mutation in the gene encoding desmoplakin.

The intercalated discs are end-to-end connections between cardiomyocytes that maintain mechanical and electrical integrity between cells. They consist of three main components: the adherens junction, the desmosome, and gap junctions. Desmosomes are the secondary mechanical intercellular junctions, present in abundance in epithelial tissues and the myocardium. Plakoglobin links the intermediate filament network to the cytoplasmic tails of the cadherin proteins which extend into the intercellular space and have adhesive functions, although the precise mechanism by which they achieve this function is unknown. Desmoplakin is a protein of the plakin family of cytolinkers and is located deeper in the cytoplasmic plaque of the desmosome. It appears to be an obligate component of the desmosomal junction.[37]

The involvement of plakoglobin and desmoplakin genes in these recessive forms of ARVC led to the examination of these and other desmosomal protein genes in the more common dominant ARVC phenotype. Plakoglobin has only been associated with autosomal recessive ARVC to date. Desmoplakin, on the other hand, accounts for 16% of dominant ARVC cases. Genes implicated only in autosomal dominant disease include plakophilin 2 (PKP2) accounting for 25–43% of cases,[46–48] desmoglein (DSG2) (10% of cases), and desmocollin (DSC2).

The discovery that many cases of ARVC are "desmosomal" diseases has led to a simplistic theory of pathogenesis in which disruption of desmosomal integrity causes separation of myocardial cells under conditions of mechan-ical stress. Detached myocytes die and are replaced by fibro-fatty tissue. The predilection for the right ventricle can be explained by the relative thinness of the RV walls in comparison with the left ventricle; the tendency for lesions to develop in the "triangle of dysplasia" is explained by the fact that the RV inflow, apex and outflow are the regions of maximal mechanical stress.

While this theory may explain the ultrastructural changes associated with ARVC and, indeed, the apparently aggressive form of the disease in those who partake in endurance training,[49] it does not account for the disproportionate tendency to arrhythmia. Evaluation of a small number of patients with Naxos disease has shown that expression of connexin 43, a major gap junction protein, is markedly reduced in both the left and right ventricles, even at an early age of disease development. A reduction in the number and size of the gap junctions may result in an electrical coupling defect which increases the propensity to arrhythmia and may explain the occurrence of sudden death in patients without marked morphologic changes.[50]

Two non-desmosomal genes have been associated with ARVC. Mutations in the ryanodine receptor gene (RYR2) were reported in association with a localized form of ARVC, but mutations in this gene more typically cause catecholaminergic polymorphic VT (CPVT) and are no longer classified as a subtype of ARVC.[51,52] A mutation in the transforming growth factor beta 3 (TGFβ3) gene has also been described, but the mutation occurs in an intronic region of the gene and only one of the three originally described ARVC1 families has a TGFβ3 mutation. Functional studies have shown an alteration in the expression of the TGFβ3 gene resulting in increased fibrosis. Whether this represents true ARVC or not remains controversial.[53,54]

Natural history

The natural history of ARVC can be divided into four phases.[38] In phase one (the "concealed" phase) patients are asymptomatic with few if any morphologic abnormalities. In the absence of systematic post-mortem evaluation of the right ventricle, the diagnosis may be missed at this stage and so the incidence of sudden death in this phase may be underestimated. In the second (electrical) phase, symptoms of arrhythmia occur and morphologic structural and functional abnormalities are easier to identify. The third phase is marked by the classic right ventricular functional abnormalities that can progress to right ventricular failure with relatively preserved left ventricular function. The final or end-stage is associated with the development of biventricular systolic impairment. Although a useful disease paradigm, it is not inevitable that affected persons will progress through all phases as described. Moreover, multiple (mostly unknown) factors influence the clinical manifestations and natural history of the condition. It is generally thought that physical training and exercise both increase the risk of arrhythmic events in affected individuals and result in more aggressive disease progression.[17,49,55–57] Some patients demonstrate left ventricular involvement early in the disease, and may have predominant left ventricular disease.[58–60]

Clinical features

The first presentation of the disease is often sudden cardiac death in previously asymptomatic individuals, including young children and teenagers.[14,55,61,62] Occasionally, patients will have experienced syncope in the months preceding their death.[14,56,63] An imbalance of adrenergic activity has been suggested as a possible factor in the genesis of lethal ventricular arrhythmias; thus exposure to catecholamines (particularly during exercise) may increase the risk of sudden death.[64]

Patients usually present with symptoms between the second and fifth decades of life. Syncope, palpitations and chest pain are common, but family studies have shown that most affected individuals are asymptomatic, particularly in the early stages.[65,66] With disease progression, features of right and later biventricular failure may be present.

Diagnosis

Accurate diagnosis of ARVC is notoriously difficult at post mortem and in living patients. The gold standard for making the diagnosis is the demonstration of transmural fibro-fatty replacement of right ventricular myocardium. However, endomyocardial biopsy has a substantial false-negative rate caused by the patchy distribution of the disease and the fact that the interventricular septum, which is the site of choice for endomyocardial biopsy, is often relatively spared. In an attempt to address this difficulty, a task force of international experts was convened, under the auspices of the Scientific Council of the International Society and Federation of Cardiology (ISFC) and the European Society of Cardiology Working Group on Myocardial and Pericardial Diseases. The Task Force reviewed the evidence available at the time in order to agree a set of clinical diagnostic criteria. They grouped clinical criteria into six categories, and assigned either major or minor status to each criterion depending on the degree of specificity for the diagnosis. A cumulative scoring system was devised with agreed thresholds for making a clinical diagnosis. The presence of two major criteria from different categories, or one major and two minor, or four minor criteria, all from different categories, is considered diagnostic of ARVC[67] (Box 45.1).

BOX 45.1 Criteria for diagnosis of ARVC (adapted from McKenna *et al*[67])

1. **Family history**
Major
  - Familial disease confirmed at necropsy or surgery
Minor
  - Family history of premature sudden death (<35 years) due to suspected right ventricular cardiomyopathy
  - Family history of clinical diagnosis based on the present criteria
2. **Tissue characterization of walls**
Major
  - Fibro-fatty replacement of myocardium demonstrated on endomyocardial biopsy
3. **Global and/or regional dysfunction and structural alterations**
Major
  - Severe dilation and reduction in systolic function of RV with no (or only mild) impairment of LV
  - Localized RV aneurysms (akinetic or dyskinetic areas with diastolic bulging)
  - Severe segmental dilation of the RV
Minor
  - Mild global RV dilation and/or reduction in ejection fraction with normal LV
  - Mild segmental dilation of RV
  - Regional RV hypokinesia
4. **Depolarization/conduction abnormalities**
Major
  - Epsilon waves or localized prolongation of the QRS complex in V1–V3 (>110 ms)
Minor
  - Late potentials demonstrated on signal-averaged ECG
5. **Repolarization abnormalities**
Minor
  - Inverted T-waves in right precordial leads (V2 and V3)
  - (individuals >12 years of age; in the absence of right bundle branch block)
6. **Arrhythmias**
Minor
  - Sustained and non-sustained ventricular tachycardia with LBBB morphology (documented on ECG, Holter or exercise testing)
  - Frequent ventricular extrasystoles (>1000 over 24-hr Holter monitoring)

Imaging

Morphologic abnormalities of the right ventricle are challenging to identify *in vivo*, particularly when they are relatively subtle. At the time of publication of the Task Force criteria the most commonly used imaging modality was cine-angiography of the right ventricle. This has been largely replaced by transthoracic echo which, in addition to the detection of ARVC, has a major role in the exclusion of congenital heart disease such as partial anomalous venous drainage, Ebstein's anomaly and other causes of isolated right ventricular abnormalities.[68,69] The major challenge when using echo to assess the right ventricle is the chamber's complex three-dimensional structure. Together with the segmental nature of the disease, this means that structure and function should be assessed using multiple views.[70] The echocardiographic features of ARVC include: right ventricular dilation and hypokinesia; aneurysms; regional wall motion abnormalities, including dyskinesia of the inferobasal right ventricular segment; increased echogenicity of the moderator band; and right ventricular apical hypertrabeculation.[63,68,71–73] Tricuspid annular early diastolic velocities are reduced[70,74] but strain rate imaging has not yet been found to be a reliable diagnostic tool in ARVC. Three-dimensional echo may be a more accurate method of assessing right ventricular systolic function[75] but larger studies are needed to validate the technique.

Cardiac magnetic resonance imaging is generally considered to be the imaging modality of choice in ARVC, but unfamiliarity with normal right ventricular morphology and function has led to high interobserver error and poor reproducibility in some series.[76,77] The presence of intramyocardial fat deposition in the right ventricle must also be interpreted with caution, as fat in the right ventricle is present in a large proportion of "normal" individuals (up to 85%), and the frequency and severity increase with age, body weight and female gender.[20,23,78] Diagnostic accuracy can be improved by using standardized acquisition and analysis protocols. Using genetic status as the gold standard, a single-center experience has suggested that magnetic resonance imaging has a sensitivity of 96% and a specificity of 78%.[13]

In the current Task Force criteria, right ventricular abnormalities were only considered significant in the absence of significant left ventricular disease. However, gadolinium-enhanced cardiac MR imaging has reported evidence of LV involvement in 84% of patients.[79] It is likely that the next iteration of the Task Force guidelines will be modified to take into account the biventricular nature of disease in patients with ARVC.

ECG

The most frequent electrocardiographic marker of ARVC is the presence of precordial T-wave inversion. Studies have reported a very wide range in prevalence (19–94%),[80–83] with the lowest prevalence rates in evaluations of large families, reflecting incomplete penetrance, and the highest rates in case series of probands where selection bias may lead to an overestimation of the true prevalence of this disease marker.[66,82]

The presence of epsilon waves on the ECG (any electrical potential in V1–V3 occurring after the QRS complex where the Q–epsilon interval exceeds the QRS duration in V6 by more than 25 ms)[72] may be highly specific for a diagnosis of ARVC but they are found in only one-quarter to one-third of patients.[81,84] A modified method of lead placement may enhance detection of epsilon waves.[72]

Localized QRS prolongation (in excess of 110 ms) in the right precordial leads is considered a major criterion for ARVC. More recently, investigators have looked at QRS dispersion (the numeric difference in QRS duration between the right precordial leads and V6) which is a strong independent predictor of sudden death if the value is greater than 40 ms.[84]

Signal-averaged ECG

The presence of late potentials on signal-averaged ECG is consistent with ARVC, but they are also found frequently after myocardial ischemia. The prevalence in case series varies which may reflect a wide range of disease severity as late potentials have a positive correlation with the extent of ventricular fibrosis, reduced right ventricular systolic function and significant morphologic abnormalities on imaging.[85,86]

Ventricular arrhythmia

The occurrence of VT with left bundle branch morphology is a non-specific finding, but in the context of other diagnostic features, it is supportive of the diagnosis. In addition to ARVC, left bundle morphology VT occurs in myocardial ischemia, dilated cardiomyopathy and right ventricular outflow tract VT. The presence of ventricular ectopy above a threshold of 1000 ectopics in 24 hours should raise suspicion of ARVC in an appropriate clinical scenario, but merits minor status only as a result of low specificity.

Diagnosis in relatives

In the early years following the first description of the disease, ARVC was thought to be almost always sporadic. Case reports emerged subsequently describing families with clinical evidence of ARVC with wide variation in disease characteristics and severity between family members.[57,87–90] In a later series of seven families, over 50% of evaluated relatives were affected with a slight male predominance (63% of men and 53% of women affected), autosomal dominant transmission with incomplete penetrance and variable clinical expression.[91]

Systematic evaluation of relatives of 67 index cases found evidence of familial disease in 28% of cases using the Task Force criteria. A further 11% of families had non-diagnostic abnormalities on ECG, ambulatory ECG monitoring or echocardiography. The authors proposed a modification of the diagnostic criteria to be applied to first-degree relatives of an index case where ARVC is proven. In this scheme, the presence of late potentials on signal-averaged ECG or a single minor criterion on ECG, echocardiography or ambulatory monitoring should be considered diagnostic. The authors also proposed that, in the setting of a positive family history, a threshold of 200 ventricular ectopics over a 24-hour monitoring period is sufficiently sensitive to diagnose ARVC (Box 45.2).[92] These criteria have been tested in a small number of studies in genetically characterized families, where application of the Task Force criteria would identify 54–66% of gene carriers. Use of the proposed modified criteria increased this figure to between 70% and almost 100%.[59,93]

Genetic testing was not possible at the time of the Task Force review. DNA screening for desmosomal gene mutations identifies disease-causing mutations in over 40% of probands who have a clinical diagnosis of ARVC.[94] In the setting of familial disease, with 50% risk of mutation inheritance and variable age-related penetrance which mandates repeated clinical evaluation of all adult relatives, mutation analysis in the proband and predictive testing in relatives is probably cost-effective if a disease-causing mutation is identified. Co-existence of two distinct desmosomal gene mutations within families has been reported, although the frequency of this occurrence has not yet been clarified.[94] Screening of all desmosomal genes in all probands is therefore required, rather than concentrating on "hotspot" genes or exons. As with any inherited condition, the potential clinical, psychologic and financial implications of mutation identification in an asymptomatic individual mean that formal genetic counseling and informed consent are mandatory prior to gene testing.

Management

Patients with proven or suspected ARVC are discouraged from active sports participation or endurance training. Other simple measures include avoidance of stimulants and abstention from recreational drug usage, although there are no data to prove an association between either activity and sudden death.

Pharmacologic therapy is generally recommended in patients with well-tolerated VT or symptomatic ventricular ectopy. The only comparative study of pharmacologic agents in spontaneously occurring and inducible VT identified sotalol as the most efficacious agent[95] (**Class IIB, Level C**). In practice, both sotalol and amiodarone are widely used, although long-term side effects of amiodarone therapy in relatively young patients are a cause for concern. These agents may also be useful in patients with implantable cardioverter defibrillators (ICD) who have had recurrent therapies.

Before the advent of radiofrequency and cryoablation therapies, surgical disarticulation of the RV and surgical resection of segments of RV myocardium were advocated for the suppression of recurrent or incessant arrhythmia.[96,97] In the modern era, success rates of 60–90% for catheter ablation of re-entry circuits have been reported, although up to 60% of patients relapse, probably due to the development of new arrhythmic foci.[98] The number of lesions required for successful therapy may be up to 38 per patient, which is a cause for concern in patients with thinned and fibrosed RV myocardium.[99] Catheter ablation has a more accepted role in patients with ICDs who experience recurrent appropriate therapies (**Level C**).

Current joint ACC/AHA/ESC guidelines for ICD implantation are summarized in Box 45.3.[100] Much of the information on risk identification is provided by retrospective analysis of discharge rates from ICDs implanted for primary and secondary prophylaxis in patients with advanced disease. Data from three separate populations identify a prior cardiac arrest, a history of VT with hemodynamic compromise, major morphologic abnormalities of the right ventricle and left ventricular involvement as independent risk predictors. Programmed ventricular stimulation has also been advocated as a risk predictor, but results vary. In one study, electrophysiology testing had poor positive and negative predictive accuracy, was the only independent predictor of rapid (>240 beats/min) VT in another, and was predictive of appropriate ICD therapy in patients with a history of sustained ventricular arrhythmia in a third. None of the patients in these studies were genetically characterized.[101–104]

BOX 45.2 Proposed modification of Task Force criteria for the diagnosis of familial ARVC (adapted from Hamid *et al*[92])

Proven ARVC in a first-degree relative plus one of the following:

1. **Structural or functional abnormality of the right ventricle:**
   - Mild global RV dilation of the RV and/or reduction in ejection fraction with normal LV
   - Mild segmental dilation of the RV
   - Regional RV hypokinesia
2. **Arrhythmia:**
   - Ventricular tachycardia with LBBB morphology (documented on ECG, Holter monitoring or during exercise testing)
   - >200 ventricular extrasystoles over 24 hours (Holter monitor)
3. **ECG:**
   - T-wave inversion in the right precordial leads (V2 and V3)
4. **Signal-averaged ECG:**
   - Demonstration of late potentials

BOX 45.3 Indications for defibrillator implantation (ICD) in ARVC (adapted from ACC/AHA/ESC Guidelines[100])

Class I
Sustained VT/VF
+ already on optimal medical treatment
+ anticipated survival >1 year (with good functional status) (Level B)

Class IIa
Primary prophylaxis in any of the following:
• Extensive disease (including LV involvement)
• ≥1 affected family member experienced SCD*
• Unexplained syncope (where VT/VF have not been excluded)
+ already on optimal medical therapy
+ anticipated survival ≥1 year (with good functional status) (Level C)

Class IIb
VT inducible on EP studies (Level C)

*Presence of >1 premature sudden cardiac death in a family must be considered in relation to the number of persons at risk within that pedigree.

VT, ventricular tachycardia (>30 seconds duration, rate >120bpm); VF, ventricular fibrillation; LV, left ventricle; SCD, sudden cardiac death; EP, electrophysiologic.

One small study has identified QRS dispersion on standard ECG as a predictor of risk. ARVC patients in whom the difference between maximum and minimum QRS duration in any ECG leads was > 40ms had a higher risk of sudden death.[84] The presence of late potentials on signal-averaged ECG has not yet been found to identify a higher risk population. The use of three-dimensional voltage mapping during EP studies may become a useful tool for risk stratification. In one study, a borderline association between the occurrence of significant arrhythmia and reduced and fractionated voltage signals has been demonstrated. The location of these areas of altered signal intensity correlated well with endomyocardial biopsies.[105] Definite or probable indications for ICD implantation in ARVC are summarized in Box 45.3.

Patients with symptomatic arrhythmia may be managed differently in North America compared with European centers, with a lower threshold for device implantation in the former. Whether the common practice of ICD implantation in all those diagnosed clinically with ARVC can or will be extended to those with a genetic diagnosis in the future is uncertain. In addition to the usually encountered device complications at implant and revision, progressive fibrosis and wall thinning can make it difficult to achieve satisfactory lead position and may increase the risk of perforation.

The incidence of inappropriate device therapy in patients with ARVC ranges from 10% to 23%.[101,102,106] The use of cardiac resynchronization has not been evaluated specifically in ARVC. Cardiac transplantation may be necessary in patients with advanced heart failure, and occasionally for intractable arrhythmia.

Future directions

Research is ongoing to improve our ability to diagnose and risk stratify ARVC patients. Advanced imaging techniques, electrical mapping technologies and identification of new genes are likely to provide new insights. Stem cell therapy does not look promising, not least because cells that differentiate into contracting myocardial cells have not been able to generate gap junctions, which is already a fundamental problem in ARVC. Disease-modifying therapy may be a promising area for progress, particularly if we can gain better understanding of the various genetic, infective, environmental and lifestyle factors that currently influence disease penetrance and progression.

References

1. Uhl HS. A previously undescribed congenital malformation of the heart: almost total absence of the myocardium of the right ventricle. *Bull Johns Hopkins Hosp* 1952;**91**(3):197–209.
2. Frank R, Fontaine G, Vedel J, Mialet G, Sol C, Guiraudon G et al. [Electrocardiology of 4 cases of right ventricular dysplasia inducing arrhythmia]. *Arch Mal Coeur Vaiss* 1978;**71**(9):963–72.
3. Vedel J, Frank R, Fontaine G, Drobinski G, Guiraudon G, Brocheriou C et al. [Recurrent ventricular tachycardia and parchment right ventricle in the adult. Anatomical and clinical report of 2 cases]. *Arch Mal Coeur Vaiss* 1978;**71**(9):973–81.
4. Marcus FI, Fontaine GH, Guiraudon G, Frank R, Laurenceau JL, Malergue C et al. Right ventricular dysplasia: a report of 24 adult cases. *Circulation* 1982;**65**(2):384–98.
5. Waynberger M, Coutadon M, Peltier JM, Ducloux G, Jallut H, Slama R. [Familial ventricular tachycardia. Apropos of 7 cases]. *Nouv Presse Med* 1974;**3**(30):1857–60.
6. Protonotarios N, Tsatsopoulou A, Patsourakos P, Alexopoulos D, Gezerlis P, Simitsis S et al. Cardiac abnormalities in familial palmoplantar keratosis. *Br Heart J* 1986;**56**(4):321–6.
7. Coonar AS, Protonotarios N, Tsatsopoulou A, Needham EW, Houlston RS, Cliff S et al. Gene for arrhythmogenic right ventricular cardiomyopathy with diffuse nonepidermolytic palmoplantar keratoderma and woolly hair (Naxos disease) maps to 17q21. *Circulation* 1998;**97**(20):2049–58.
8. McKoy G, Protonotarios N, Crosby A, Tsatsopoulou A, Anastasakis A, Coonar A et al. Identification of a deletion in plakoglobin in arrhythmogenic right ventricular cardiomyopathy with palmoplantar keratoderma and woolly hair (Naxos disease). *Lancet* 2000;**355**(9221):2119–24.
9. Tandri H, Calkins H, Nasir K, Bomma C, Castillo E, Rutberg J et al. Magnetic resonance imaging findings in patients meeting

task force criteria for arrhythmogenic right ventricular dysplasia. *J Cardiovasc Electrophysiol* 2003;**14**(5):476–82.

10. Tandri H, Friedrich MG, Calkins H, Bluemke DA. MRI of arrhythmogenic right ventricular cardiomyopathy/dysplasia. *J Cardiovasc Magn Reson* 2004;**6**(2):557–63.

11. Tandri H, Saranathan M, Rodriguez ER, Martinez C, Bomma C, Nasir K *et al.* Noninvasive detection of myocardial fibrosis in arrhythmogenic right ventricular cardiomyopathy using delayed-enhancement magnetic resonance imaging. *J Am Coll Cardiol* 2005;**45**(1):98–103.

12. Keller DI, Osswald S, Bremerich J, Bongartz G, Cron TA, Hilti P *et al.* Arrhythmogenic right ventricular cardiomyopathy: diagnostic and prognostic value of the cardiac MRI in relation to arrhythmia-free survival. *Int J Cardiovasc Imaging* 2003;**19**(6): 537–43; discussion 45–7.

13. Sen-Chowdhry S, Prasad SK, Syrris P, Wage R, Ward D, Merrifield R *et al.* Cardiovascular magnetic resonance in arrhythmogenic right ventricular cardiomyopathy revisited: comparison with task force criteria and genotype. *J Am Coll Cardiol* 2006;**48**(10):2132–40.

14. Tabib A, Loire R, Chalabreysse L, Meyronnet D, Miras A, Malicier D *et al.* Circumstances of death and gross and microscopic observations in a series of 200 cases of sudden death associated with arrhythmogenic right ventricular cardiomyopathy and/or dysplasia. *Circulation* 2003;**108**(24):3000–5.

15. Corrado D, Basso C, Rizzoli G, Schiavon M, Thiene G. Does sports activity enhance the risk of sudden death in adolescents and young adults? *J Am Coll Cardiol* 2003;**42**(11):1959–63.

16. Shen WK, Edwards WD, Hammill SC, Bailey KR, Ballard DJ, Gersh BJ. Sudden unexpected nontraumatic death in 54 young adults: a 30-year population-based study. *Am J Cardiol* 1995;**76**(3):148–52.

17. Corrado D, Thiene G, Nava A, Rossi L, Pennelli N. Sudden death in young competitive athletes: clinicopathologic correlations in 22 cases. *Am J Med* 1990;**89**(5):588–96.

18. Hughes SE, McKenna WJ. New insights into the pathology of inherited cardiomyopathy. *Heart* 2005;**91**(2):257–64.

19. Gallo P, d'Amati G, Pelliccia F. Pathologic evidence of extensive left ventricular involvement in arrhythmogenic right ventricular cardiomyopathy. *Hum Pathol* 1992 Aug;**23**(8):948–52.

20. Tansey DK, Aly Z, Sheppard MN. Fat in the right ventricle of the normal heart. *Histopathology* 2005;**46**(1):98–104.

21. Fornes P, Ratel S, Lecomte D. Pathology of arrhythmogenic right ventricular cardiomyopathy/dysplasia – an autopsy study of 20 forensic cases. *J Forensic Sci* 1998;**43**(4):777–83.

22. Basso C, Thiene G, Corrado D, Angelini A, Nava A, Valente M. Arrhythmogenic right ventricular cardiomyopathy. Dysplasia, dystrophy, or myocarditis? *Circulation* 1996;**94**(5):983–91.

23. Burke AP, Farb A, Tashko G, Virmani R. Arrhythmogenic right ventricular cardiomyopathy and fatty replacement of the right ventricular myocardium: are they different diseases? *Circulation* 1998;**97**(16):1571–80.

24. d'Amati G, Leone O, di Gioia CR, Magelli C, Arpesella G, Grillo P *et al.* Arrhythmogenic right ventricular cardiomyopathy: clinicopathologic correlation based on a revised definition of pathologic patterns. *Hum Pathol* 2001;**32**(10):1078–86.

25. Burke AP, Robinson S, Radentz S, Smialek J, Virmani R. Sudden death in right ventricular dysplasia with minimal gross abnormalities. *J Forensic Sci* 1999;**44**(2):438–43.

26. Fontaine G, Fontaliran F, Zenati O, Guzman CE, Rigoulet J, Berthier JL *et al.* Fat in the heart. A feature unique to the human species? Observational reflections on an unsolved problem. *Acta Cardiol* 1999;**54**(4):189–94.

27. Valente M, Calabrese F, Thiene G, Angelini A, Basso C, Nava A *et al.* In vivo evidence of apoptosis in arrhythmogenic right ventricular cardiomyopathy. *Am J Pathol* 1998;**152**(2):479–84.

28. Nishikawa T, Ishiyama S, Nagata M, Sakomura Y, Nakazawa M, Momma K *et al.* Programmed cell death in the myocardium of arrhythmogenic right ventricular cardiomyopathy in children and adults. *Cardiovasc Pathol* 1999;**8**(4):185–9.

29. Nagata M, Hiroe M, Ishiyama S, Nishikawa T, Sakomura Y, Kasanuki H *et al.* Apoptotic cell death in arrhythmogenic right ventricular cardiomyopathy: a comparative study with idiopathic sustained ventricular tachycardia. *Jpn Heart J* 2000;**41**(6):733–41.

30. Yamaji K, Fujimoto S, Ikeda Y, Masuda K, Nakamura S, Saito Y *et al.* Apoptotic myocardial cell death in the setting of arrhythmogenic right ventricular cardiomyopathy. *Acta Cardiol* 2005;**60**(5):465–70.

31. Grumbach IM, Heim A, Vonhof S, Stille-Siegener M, Mall G, Gonska BD *et al.* Coxsackievirus genome in myocardium of patients with arrhythmogenic right ventricular dysplasia/ cardiomyopathy. *Cardiology* 1998;**89**(4):241–5.

32. Kearney DL, Towbin JA, Bricker JT, Radovancevic B, Frazier OH. Familial right ventricular dysplasia (cardiomyopathy). *Pediatr Pathol Lab Med* 1995;**15**(1):181–9.

33. Heim A, Grumbach I, Hake S, Muller G, Pring-Akerblom P, Mall G *et al.* Enterovirus heart disease of adults: a persistent, limited organ infection in the presence of neutralizing antibodies. *J Med Virol* 1997;**53**(3):196–204.

34. Heim A, Grumbach I, Stille-Siegener M, Figulla HR. Detection of enterovirus RNA in the myocardium of a patient with arrhythmogenic right ventricular cardiomyopathy by in situ hybridization. *Clin Infect Dis* 1997;**25**(6):1471–2.

35. Calabrese F, Angelini A, Thiene G, Basso C, Nava A, Valente M. No detection of enteroviral genome in the myocardium of patients with arrhythmogenic right ventricular cardiomyopathy. *J Clin Pathol* 2000;**53**(5):382–7.

36. Bowles NE, Ni J, Marcus F, Towbin JA. The detection of cardiotropic viruses in the myocardium of patients with arrhythmogenic right ventricular dysplasia/cardiomyopathy. *J Am Coll Cardiol* 2002;**39**(5):892–5.

37. Getsios S, Huen AC, Green KJ. Working out the strength and flexibility of desmosomes. *Nat Rev Mol Cell Biol* 2004;**5**(4): 271–81.

38. Corrado D, Fontaine G, Marcus FI, McKenna WJ, Nava A, Thiene G *et al.* Arrhythmogenic right ventricular dysplasia/ cardiomyopathy: need for an international registry. Study Group on Arrhythmogenic Right Ventricular Dysplasia/Cardiomyopathy of the Working Groups on Myocardial and Pericardial Disease and Arrhythmias of the European Society of Cardiology and of the Scientific Council on Cardiomyopathies of the World Heart Federation. *Circulation* 2000;**101**(11):E101–6.

39. Fontaine G, Fontaliran F, Frank R. Arrhythmogenic right ventricular cardiomyopathies: clinical forms and main differential diagnoses. *Circulation* 1998;**97**(16):1532–5.

40. Alcalai R, Metzger S, Rosenheck S, Meiner V, Chajek-Shaul T. A recessive mutation in desmoplakin causes arrhythmogenic

right ventricular dysplasia, skin disorder, and woolly hair. *J Am Coll Cardiol* 2003;**42**(2):319–27.

41. Djabali K, Martinez-Mir A, Horev L, Christiano AM, Zlotogorski A. Evidence for extensive locus heterogeneity in Naxos disease. *J Invest Dermatol* 2002;**118**(3):557–60.

42. Narin N, Akcakus M, Gunes T, Celiker A, Baykan A, Uzum K *et al*. Arrhythmogenic right ventricular cardiomyopathy (Naxos disease): report of a Turkish boy. *Pacing Clin Electrophysiol* 2003;**26**(12):2326–9.

43. Tosti A, Misciali C, Piraccini BA, Fanti PA, Barbareschi M, Ferretti RM. Woolly hair, palmoplantar keratoderma, and cardiac abnormalities: report of a family. *Arch Dermatol* 1994;**130**(4): 522–4.

44. Rao BH, Reddy IS, Chandra KS. Familial occurrence of a rare combination of dilated cardiomyopathy with palmoplantar keratoderma and curly hair. *Indian Heart J* 1996;**48**(2): 161–2.

45. Carvajal-Huerta L. Epidermolytic palmoplantar keratoderma with woolly hair and dilated cardiomyopathy. *J Am Acad Dermatol* 1998;**39**(3):418–21.

46. Gerull B, Heuser A, Wichter T, Paul M, Basson CT, McDermott DA *et al*. Mutations in the desmosomal protein plakophilin-2 are common in arrhythmogenic right ventricular cardiomyopathy. *Nat Genet* 2004;**36**(11):1162–4.

47. van Tintelen JP, Entius MM, Bhuiyan ZA, Jongbloed R, Wiesfeld AC, Wilde AA *et al*. Plakophilin-2 mutations are the major determinant of familial arrhythmogenic right ventricular dysplasia/cardiomyopathy. *Circulation* 2006;**113**(13):1650–8.

48. Dalal D, James C, Devanagondi R, Tichnell C, Tucker A, Prakasa K *et al*. Penetrance of mutations in plakophilin-2 among families with arrhythmogenic right ventricular dysplasia/cardiomyopathy. *J Am Coll Cardiol* 2006;**48**(7):1416–24.

49. Kirchhof P, Fabritz L, Zwiener M, Witt H, Schafers M, Zellerhoff S *et al*. Age- and training-dependent development of arrhythmogenic right ventricular cardiomyopathy in heterozygous plakoglobin-deficient mice. *Circulation* 2006;**114**(17): 1799–806.

50. Kaplan SR, Gard JJ, Protonotarios N, Tsatsopoulou A, Spiliopoulou C, Anastasakis A *et al*. Remodeling of myocyte gap junctions in arrhythmogenic right ventricular cardiomyopathy due to a deletion in plakoglobin (Naxos disease). *Heart Rhythm* 2004;**1**(1):3–11.

51. Bauce B, Nava A, Rampazzo A, Daliento L, Muriago M, Basso C *et al*. Familial effort polymorphic ventricular arrhythmias in arrhythmogenic right ventricular cardiomyopathy map to chromosome 1q42–43. *Am J Cardiol* 2000;**85**(5):573–9.

52. Tiso N, Stephan DA, Nava A, Bagattin A, Devaney JM, Stanchi F *et al*. Identification of mutations in the cardiac ryanodine receptor gene in families affected with arrhythmogenic right ventricular cardiomyopathy type 2 (ARVD2). *Hum Mol Genet* 2001;**10**(3):189–94.

53. Rampazzo A, Nava A, Danieli GA, Buja G, Daliento L, Fasoli G *et al*. The gene for arrhythmogenic right ventricular cardiomyopathy maps to chromosome 14q23-q24. *Hum Mol Genet* 1994;**3**(6):959–62.

54. Beffagna G, Occhi G, Nava A, Vitiello L, Ditadi A, Basso C *et al*. Regulatory mutations in transforming growth factor-beta3 gene cause arrhythmogenic right ventricular cardiomyopathy type 1. *Cardiovasc Res* 2005;**65**(2):366–73.

55. Thiene G, Nava A, Corrado D, Rossi L, Pennelli N. Right ventricular cardiomyopathy and sudden death in young people. *N Engl J Med* 1988;**318**(3):129–33.

56. Corrado D, Basso C, Thiene G, McKenna WJ, Davies MJ, Fontaliran F *et al*. Spectrum of clinicopathologic manifestations of arrhythmogenic right ventricular cardiomyopathy/dysplasia: a multicenter study. *J Am Coll Cardiol* 1997;**30**(6):1512–20.

57. Nava A, Thiene G, Canciani B, Scognamiglio R, Daliento L, Buja G *et al*. Familial occurrence of right ventricular dysplasia: a study involving nine families. *J Am Coll Cardiol* 1988;**12**(5): 1222–8.

58. Norman M, Simpson M, Mogensen J, Shaw A, Hughes S, Syrris P *et al*. Novel mutation in desmoplakin causes arrhythmogenic left ventricular cardiomyopathy. *Circulation* 2005;**112**(5): 636–42.

59. Bauce B, Basso C, Rampazzo A, Beffagna G, Daliento L, Frigo G *et al*. Clinical profile of four families with arrhythmogenic right ventricular cardiomyopathy caused by dominant desmoplakin mutations. *Eur Heart J* 2005;**26**(16):1666–75.

60. De Pasquale CG, Heddle WF. Left sided arrhythmogenic ventricular dysplasia in siblings. *Heart* 2001;**86**(2):128–30.

61. Corrado D, Basso C, Schiavon M, Thiene G. Screening for hypertrophic cardiomyopathy in young athletes. *N Engl J Med* 1998;**339**(6):364–9.

62. Pawel BR, de Chadarevian JP, Wolk JH, Donner RM, Vogel RL, Braverman P. Sudden death in childhood due to right ventricular dysplasia: report of two cases. *Pediatr Pathol* 1994;**14**(6): 987–95.

63. Daliento L, Turrini P, Nava A, Rizzoli G, Angelini A, Buja G *et al*. Arrhythmogenic right ventricular cardiomyopathy in young versus adult patients: similarities and differences. *J Am Coll Cardiol* 1995;**25**(3):655–64.

64. Wichter T, Schafers M, Rhodes CG, Borggrefe M, Lerch H, Lammertsma AA *et al*. Abnormalities of cardiac sympathetic innervation in arrhythmogenic right ventricular cardiomyopathy : quantitative assessment of presynaptic norepinephrine reuptake and postsynaptic beta-adrenergic receptor density with positron emission tomography. *Circulation* 2000;**101**(13):1552–8.

65. Hulot JS, Jouven X, Empana JP, Frank R, Fontaine G. Natural history and risk stratification of arrhythmogenic right ventricular dysplasia/cardiomyopathy. *Circulation* 2004;**110**(14): 1879–84.

66. Dalal D, Nasir K, Bomma C, Prakasa K, Tandri H, Piccini J *et al*. Arrhythmogenic right ventricular dysplasia: a United States experience. *Circulation* 2005;**112**(25):3823–32.

67. McKenna WJ, Thiene G, Nava A, Fontaliran F, Blomstrom-Lundqvist C, Fontaine G *et al*. Diagnosis of arrhythmogenic right ventricular dysplasia/cardiomyopathy. Task Force of the Working Group Myocardial and Pericardial Disease of the European Society of Cardiology and of the Scientific Council on Cardiomyopathies of the International Society and Federation of Cardiology. *Br Heart J* 1994;**71**(3):215–18.

68. Tome Esteban MT, Garcia-Pinilla JM, McKenna WJ. [Update in arrhythmogenic right ventricular cardiomyopathy: genetic, clinical presentation and risk stratification]. *Rev Esp Cardiol* 2004;**57**(8):757–67.

69. Alizad A, Seward JB. Echocardiographic features of genetic diseases: part 1. Cardiomyopathy. *J Am Soc Echocardiogr* 2000;**13**(1):73–86.

70. Lindstrom L, Wilkenshoff UM, Larsson H, Wranne B. Echocardiographic assessment of arrhythmogenic right ventricular cardiomyopathy. *Heart* 2001;**86**(1):31–8.

71. Atalay S, Imamoglu A, Gumus H, Gurdal M, Ozenci M. Value of the echocardiographic findings of arrhythmogenic right ventricular dysplasia with left ventricular involvement in a child. *Pediatr Cardiol* 1996;**17**(1):40–2.

72. Fontaine G, Fontaliran F, Hebert JL, Chemla D, Zenati O, Lecarpentier Y *et al.* Arrhythmogenic right ventricular dysplasia. *Annu Rev Med* 1999;**50**:17–35.

73. Yoerger DM, Marcus F, Sherrill D, Calkins H, Towbin JA, Zareba W *et al.* Echocardiographic findings in patients meeting task force criteria for arrhythmogenic right ventricular dysplasia: new insights from the multidisciplinary study of right ventricular dysplasia. *J Am Coll Cardiol* 2005;**45**(6):860–5.

74. Daubert C, Descaves C, Foulgoc JL, Bourdonnec C, Laurent M, Gouffault J. Critical analysis of cineangiographic criteria for diagnosis of arrhythmogenic right ventricular dysplasia. *Am Heart J* 1988;**115**(2):448–59.

75. Kjaergaard J, Hastrup Svendsen J, Sogaard P, Chen X, Bay Nielsen H, Kober L *et al.* Advanced quantitative echocardiography in arrhythmogenic right ventricular cardiomyopathy. *J Am Soc Echocardiogr* 2007;**20**(1):27–35.

76. Bomma C, Rutberg J, Tandri H, Nasir K, Roguin A, Tichnell C *et al.* Misdiagnosis of arrhythmogenic right ventricular dysplasia/cardiomyopathy. *J Cardiovasc Electrophysiol* 2004;**15**(3):300–6.

77. Bluemke DA, Krupinski EA, Ovitt T, Gear K, Unger E, Axel L *et al.* MR Imaging of arrhythmogenic right ventricular cardiomyopathy: morphologic findings and interobserver reliability. *Cardiology* 2003;**99**(3):153–62.

78. Basso C, Thiene G. Adipositas cordis, fatty infiltration of the right ventricle, and arrhythmogenic right ventricular cardiomyopathy. Just a matter of fat? *Cardiovasc Pathol* 2005;**14**(1):37–41.

79. Sen-Chowdhry S, Syrris P, Ward D, Asimaki A, Sevdalis E, McKenna WJ. Clinical and genetic characterization of families with arrhythmogenic right ventricular dysplasia/cardiomyopathy provides novel insights into patterns of disease expression. *Circulation* 2007;**115**(13):1710–20.

80. Fontaine G, Umemura J, Di Donna P, Tsezana R, Cannat JJ, Frank R. [Duration of QRS complexes in arrhythmogenic right ventricular dysplasia. A new non-invasive diagnostic marker]. *Ann Cardiol Angeiol (Paris)* 1993;**42**(8):399–405.

81. Peters S, Trummel M. Diagnosis of arrhythmogenic right ventricular dysplasia-cardiomyopathy: value of standard ECG revisited. *Ann Noninvasive Electrocardiol* 2003;**8**(3):238–45.

82. Nava A, Bauce B, Basso C, Muriago M, Rampazzo A, Villanova C *et al.* Clinical profile and long-term follow-up of 37 families with arrhythmogenic right ventricular cardiomyopathy. *J Am Coll Cardiol* 2000;**36**(7):2226–33.

83. Pinamonti B, Sinagra G, Salvi A, Di Lenarda A, Morgera T, Silvestri F *et al.* Left ventricular involvement in right ventricular dysplasia. *Am Heart J* 1992;**123**(3):711–24.

84. Turrini P, Corrado D, Basso C, Nava A, Bauce B, Thiene G. Dispersion of ventricular depolarization-repolarization: a noninvasive marker for risk stratification in arrhythmogenic right ventricular cardiomyopathy. *Circulation* 2001;**103**(25):3075–80.

85. Oselladore L, Nava A, Buja G, Turrini P, Daliento L, Livolsi B *et al.* Signal-averaged electrocardiography in familial form of arrhythmogenic right ventricular cardiomyopathy. *Am J Cardiol* 1995;**75**(15):1038–41.

86. Turrini P, Angelini A, Thiene G, Buja G, Daliento L, Rizzoli G *et al.* Late potentials and ventricular arrhythmias in arrhythmogenic right ventricular cardiomyopathy. *Am J Cardiol* 1999;**83**(8):1214–19.

87. Zanardi F, Occari G, Cavazzini L, Grandi E, Tomasi AM. [Familial arrhythmogenic dysplasia of the right ventricle. Observation of 3 cases]. *G Ital Cardiol (Rome)* 1986;**16**(1):4–14.

88. Nava A, Scognamiglio R, Thiene G, Canciani B, Daliento L, Buja G *et al.* A polymorphic form of familial arrhythmogenic right ventricular dysplasia. *Am J Cardiol* 1987;**59**(15):1405–9.

89. Nava A, Martini B, Thiene G, Buja GF, Canciani B, Scognamiglio R *et al.* [Arrhythmogenic right ventricular dysplasia. Study of a selected population]. *G Ital Cardiol (Rome)* 1988;**18**(1):2–9.

90. Hirooka Y, Urabe Y, Imaizumi T, Takeshita A, Tajimi T, Koyanagi S *et al.* The usefulness of equilibrium radionuclide ventriculography in the diagnosis of arrhythmogenic right ventricular dysplasia and a report of cases of a familial occurrence. *Jpn Circ J* 1988;**52**(6):511–17.

91. Nava A, Canciani B, Thiene G, Scognamiglio R, Buja G, Martini B *et al.* [Analysis of the mode of transmission of right ventricular dysplasia]. *Arch Mal CoeurVaiss* 1990;**83**(7):923–8.

92. Hamid MS, Norman M, Quraishi A, Firoozi S, Thaman R, Gimeno JR *et al.* Prospective evaluation of relatives for familial arrhythmogenic right ventricular cardiomyopathy/dysplasia reveals a need to broaden diagnostic criteria. *J Am Coll Cardiol* 2002;**40**(8):1445–50.

93. Syrris P, Ward D, Asimaki A, Sen-Chowdhry S, Ebrahim HY, Evans A *et al.* Clinical expression of plakophilin-2 mutations in familial arrhythmogenic right ventricular cardiomyopathy. *Circulation* 2006;**113**(3):356–64.

94. Pilichou K, Nava A, Basso C, Beffagna G, Bauce B, Lorenzon A *et al.* Mutations in desmoglein-2 gene are associated with arrhythmogenic right ventricular cardiomyopathy. *Circulation* 2006;**113**(9):1171–9.

95. Wichter T, Borggrefe M, Haverkamp W, Chen X, Breithardt G. Efficacy of antiarrhythmic drugs in patients with arrhythmogenic right ventricular disease. Results in patients with inducible and noninducible ventricular tachycardia. *Circulation* 1992;**86**(1):29–37.

96. Katsumoto K, Niibori T. [Surgical treatment of a case of arrhythmogenic right ventricular dysplasia with local myocardial resections]. *Nippon Kyobu Geka Gakkai Zasshi* 1989;**37**(9):1984–8.

97. Agarwal SC, Furniss SS, Forty J, Tynan M, Bourke JP. Pacing to restore right ventricular contraction after surgical disconnection for arrhythmia control in right ventricular cardiomyopathy. *Pacing Clin Electrophysiol* 2005;**28**(10):1122–6.

98. Corrado D, Basso C, Nava A, Thiene G. Arrhythmogenic right ventricular cardiomyopathy: current diagnostic and management strategies. *Cardiol Rev* 2001;**9**(5):259–65.

99. Verma A, Kilicaslan F, Schweikert RA, Tomassoni G, Rossillo A, Marrouche NF *et al.* Short- and long-term success of substrate-based mapping and ablation of ventricular tachycardia in arrhythmogenic right ventricular dysplasia. *Circulation* 2005;**111**(24):3209–16.

100. Zipes DP, Camm AJ, Borggrefe M, Buxton AE, Chaitman B, Fromer M *et al.* ACC/AHA/ESC 2006 guidelines for management of patients with ventricular arrhythmias and the prevention of sudden cardiac death: a report of the American College of Cardiology/American Heart Association Task Force and the European Society of Cardiology Committee for Practice Guidelines (Writing Committee to Develop guidelines for management of patients with ventricular arrhythmias and the prevention of sudden cardiac death) developed in collaboration with the European Heart Rhythm Association and the Heart Rhythm Society. *Europace* 2006;**8**(9):746–837.

101. Corrado D, Leoni L, Link MS, Della Bella P, Gaita F, Curnis A *et al.* Implantable cardioverter-defibrillator therapy for prevention of sudden death in patients with arrhythmogenic right ventricular cardiomyopathy/dysplasia. *Circulation* 2003;**108**(25):3084–91.

102. Wichter T, Paul M, Wollmann C, Acil T, Gerdes P, Ashraf O *et al.* Implantable cardioverter/defibrillator therapy in arrhythmogenic right ventricular cardiomyopathy: single-center experience of long-term follow-up and complications in 60 patients. *Circulation* 2004;**109**(12):1503–8.

103. Roguin A, Bomma CS, Nasir K, Tandri H, Tichnell C, James C *et al.* Implantable cardioverter-defibrillators in patients with arrhythmogenic right ventricular dysplasia/cardiomyopathy. *J Am Coll Cardiol* 2004;**43**(10):1843–52.

104. Piccini JP, Dalal D, Roguin A, Bomma C, Cheng A, Prakasa K *et al.* Predictors of appropriate implantable defibrillator therapies in patients with arrhythmogenic right ventricular dysplasia. *Heart Rhythm* 2005;**2**(11):1188–94.

105. Corrado D, Basso C, Leoni L, Tokajuk B, Bauce B, Frigo G *et al.* Three-dimensional electroanatomic voltage mapping increases accuracy of diagnosing arrhythmogenic right ventricular cardiomyopathy/dysplasia. *Circulation* 2005;**111**(23): 3042–50.

106. Hodgkinson KA, Parfrey PS, Bassett AS, Kupprion C, Drenckhahn J, Norman MW *et al.* The impact of implantable cardioverter-defibrillator therapy on survival in autosomal-dominant arrhythmogenic right ventricular cardiomyopathy (ARVD5). *J Am Coll Cardiol* 2005;**45**(3):400–8.

107. Rampazzo A, Nava A, Erne P, Eberhard M, Vian E, Slomp P *et al.* A new locus for arrhythmogenic right ventricular cardiomyopathy (ARVD2) maps to chromosome 1q42-q43. *Hum Mol Genet* 1995;**4**(11):2151–4.

108. Severini GM, Krajinovic M, Pinamonti B, Sinagra G, Fioretti P, Brunazzi MC *et al.* A new locus for arrhythmogenic right ventricular dysplasia on the long arm of chromosome 14. *Genomics* 1996;**31**(2):193–200.

109. Rampazzo A, Nava A, Miorin M, Fonderico P, Pope B, Tiso N *et al.* ARVD4, a new locus for arrhythmogenic right ventricular cardiomyopathy, maps to chromosome 2 long arm. *Genomics* 1997;**45**(2):259–63.

110. Ahmad F, Li D, Karibe A, Gonzalez O, Tapscott T, Hill R *et al.* Localization of a gene responsible for arrhythmogenic right ventricular dysplasia to chromosome 3p23. *Circulation* 1998;**98**(25):2791–5.

111. Melberg A, Oldfors A, Blomstrom-Lundqvist C, Stalberg E, Carlsson B, Larrson E *et al.* Autosomal dominant myofibrillar myopathy with arrhythmogenic right ventricular cardiomyopathy linked to chromosome 10q. *Ann Neurol* 1999;**46**(5): 684–92.

112. Li D, Ahmad F, Gardner MJ, Weilbaecher D, Hill R, Karibe A *et al.* The locus of a novel gene responsible for arrhythmogenic right-ventricular dysplasia characterized by early onset and high penetrance maps to chromosome 10p12-p14. *Am J Hum Genet* 2000;**66**(1):148–56.

113. Rampazzo A, Nava A, Malacrida S, Beffagna G, Bauce B, Rossi V *et al.* Mutation in human desmoplakin domain binding to plakoglobin causes a dominant form of arrhythmogenic right ventricular cardiomyopathy. *Am J Hum Genet* 2002;**71**(5): 1200–6.

114. Syrris P, Ward D, Evans A, Asimaki A, Gandjbakhch E, Sen-Chowdhry S *et al.* Arrhythmogenic right ventricular dysplasia/cardiomyopathy associated with mutations in the desmosomal gene desmocollin-2. *Am J Human Genet* 2006;**79**(5):978–84.

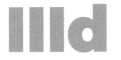

Specific cardiovascular disorders: left ventricular dysfunction

Salim Yusuf, Editor

46

Epidemiology and prevention of heart failure and management of asymptomatic left ventricular systolic dysfunction

J Paul Rocchiccioli and John J V McMurray
BHF Glasgow Cardiovascular Research Centre, University of Glasgow, Glasgow, Scotland, UK

Epidemiology of heart failure

Despite the considerable burden of heart failure (HF), its epidemiology is still poorly defined, especially in primary care.[1] A precise analysis of the epidemiology must take into account the difficulty in defining the syndrome itself, particularly in a predominantly elderly population in whom symptoms and signs are less specific. An ideal estimate of the true epidemiology would be based on surveys in random samples of the general population, using validated questionnaires and targeted physical examinations in conjunction with objective measures of left ventricular systolic dysfunction (LVSD) such as imaging and possibly supported by validated biomarkers. Broadly speaking, contemporary studies can be divided into those analyzing the prevalence and incidence of "symptomatic" HF (further divided into those with preserved and reduced LV ejection fraction [LVEF]) and those investigating the prevalence of LVSD (of which a significant proportion of patients will be asymptomatic).

Prevalence of symptomatic HF (Table 46.1)

Studies utilizing a range of designs suggest that the prevalence of HF is around 2–5% of the population of the developed world, increasing considerably with age. Whilst age-adjusted incidence has remained stable in the last two decades, prevalence may be increasing.[2] Furthermore, approximately half of all patients with symptomatic HF have preserved LVEF.[3] Prevalence varies widely from 0.4% to 19% in older age groups based on general practice (GP)

studies in the UK. The GP Research Database, involving 211 general practices in England and Wales (representing 2.6% of the national population), reported an overall prevalence (physician diagnosis) of 12.2/1000 in men and 15.8/1000 in women, increasing to 190/1000 in those over 85 years.[4] The substantial increase in prevalence with aging has been confirmed in additional UK primary care studies.[5,6]

Several population-based observational studies have been undertaken in North America and continental Europe (see Table 46.1). The prevalence of symptomatic HF in the USA is reported to be of the order of 2.2% and similarly increases considerably with age.[7,8] The European EPICA study of 5434 individuals attending general practices in Portugal reported that prevalence was 44.6/1000 in those >25 years and increased noticeably in the elderly.[9] These data are supported by contemporary data from across Northern and Southern Europe.[10–14] A significant proportion of patients with symptomatic HF have preserved LVEF. In the Olmsted County Study, 55% of symptomatic patients had preserved LVEF, an observation which is consistent with several other epidemiologic studies (Fig. 46.1).[3]

Prevalence of LVSD (Table 46.2)

A number of studies have used an objective measure of LVEF to estimate the population prevalence of LVSD. The Glasgow MONICA Study included 1640 subjects aged 25–74 who were assessed by questionnaire, electrocardiography and transthoracic echocardiography (TTE).[15] Prevalence of LVSD (LVEF <0.30) was 2.9% and increased with age. A cohort of 2267 subjects from the Rotterdam Study (which used a combination of clinical criteria and prescribing patterns to define HF) underwent echocardiography.[10] Prevalence of LVSD (defined by fractional shortening <25%) was 5.5% in men and 2.2% in women. Similar data come from the UK, USA and Australia.[7,16,17]

Evidence-Based Cardiology, 3rd edition. Edited by S. Yusuf, J.A. Cairns, A.J. Camm, E.L. Fallen, and B.J. Gersh. © 2010 Blackwell Publishing, ISBN: 978-1-4051-5925-8.

Table 46.1 Reported prevalence of symptomatic heart failure

Type of study	Location	No. patients	Mean age (yrs)	Overall prevalence (%)			Prevalence in older age groups
				Male	**Female**	**All**	
Surveys of treated patients							
General practice research database (1998)[4]	UK – national data	698 467	–	1.2	1.6	–	19 (>85y)
Mair *et al* (1996)[5]	UK – regional primary care	17 400	–	–	–	1.5	8.5 (>65y)
Clarke *et al* (1995)[6]	UK – regional primary care	993 872	–	–	–	0.8–1.6	4–6 (>70y)

							Proportion with preserved LVEF (%)		
							Male	**Female**	**All**
Population screening using echocardiography									
Olmsted County (2003)[7]	USA – regional data	2042	63	2.7	1.7	2.2	4.4 (>75y)	–	–	44
EPICA (2002)[9]	Portugal – regional data	5434	68	4.3	4.4	4.4	12.8 (70–79y) 16.7 (>85y)	20	55	40
Cardiovascular Health Study (2001)[8]	USA – national data	4842	74	–	–	8.8	14–18 (>85y)	42	67	55
Helsinki Ageing Study (1997)[11]	Finland – regional data	501	–	5.2	9.3	8.2	–	–	–	72
Asturias (2001)[12]	Spain – regional data	391	60	6.6	3.3	4.9	18 (>80y)	–	–	59
Västeras (2001)[13]	Sweden – regional data	433	75	4.0	9.5	6.7	–	–	–	46
Rotterdam Study (1999)[10]	Netherlands – regional data	1698	65	3.7	4.0	3.9	13.0 (>85y)	–	–	71
Poole (1999)[14]	UK – regional data	817	76	12.8	2.9	7.5	12.1 (>80y)	–	–	68

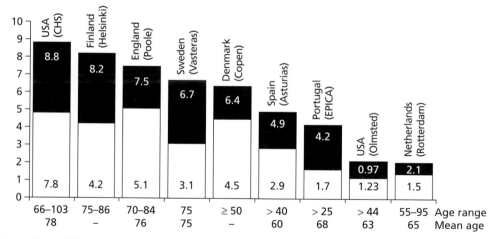

Figure 46.1 Prevalence of heart failure in cross-sectional, population-based and echocardiographic studies. Black bars show percentage prevalence; lower portion of bars shows the proportion of cases associated with preserved systolic function. LV, left ventricular. (Reproduced with permission from Hogg *et al.*[3])

Incidence of symptomatic HF (Table 46.3)

An estimate of the incidence of HF is more difficult to define, but there are considerable data, particularly from large population-based studies. In the Framingham Heart Study, at 34 years follow-up, incidence was approximately 2/1000 person-years in subjects aged 45–54, increasing to 40/1000 in men aged 85–94.[18] Similar rates are reported from the Olmsted County Study and UK and Finnish pop-

ulation studies.[4,19,20] In the UK, Cowie and colleagues reported incidence in referrals from primary care. They identified new cases from a population of 151 000 in London, through surveillance of hospital admissions and through referrals to a rapid-access HF clinic.[21] Diagnosis of HF was determined by a panel of cardiologists and supported by echocardiography. Incidence was 1.3/1000 overall for those ≥25 years. Incidence increased with age and was higher in men than women. Overall, only 29% of

Table 46.2 Reported population prevalence of LVSD

Study	Location	Type of study	Definition of LVSD	No. patients	Mean age	Overall prevalence (%)			Proportion in older age group (%)	Proportion with asymptomatic LVSD (%)
						Male	Female	Overall		
Glasgow MONICA[15]	Glasgow, UK	Cross-sectional survey	LVEF ≤ 30%	1640	50	2.9	4.0	2.9	6.4 men 4.9 women (65–74y)	48
Rochester Epidemiology Project[7]	Olmsted County, Minnesota, USA	Cross-sectional survey	LVEF ≤ 40%	2042	63	3.6	1.0	2.0	4.4 (>75y)	55
Rotterdam Study[10]	Rotterdam, Netherlands	Prospective cohort study	FS ≤ 25%	2267	66	5.5	2.2	3.7	10.3 (85–94y)	60
Canberra Study[17]	Canberra, Australia	Cross-sectional survey	LVEF ≤ 50%	1275	69	8.7	3.1	5.9	14.4 (>80y)	59
ECHOES[12]	West Midlands, UK	Cross-sectional survey	LVEF ≤ 40%	3960	61	3.0	0.7	1.8	3.6 (>75y)	50

LVEF, left ventricular ejection fraction; FS, fractional shortening.

Table 46.3 Reported population incidence of heart failure

Study	Location	Type of study	Year of study	No. patients	Age (years)	Overall incidence (per 1000 per year)			Proportion in older age group (per 1000 per year)
						Male	Female	Overall	
Framingham[18]	Framingham, USA	Prospective cohort study	1948–88	9504	70	NA	7.2	4.7	27 men 22 women (80–89y)
Rochester Epidemiology Project[19]	Olmsted County, Minnesota, USA	Cross-sectional survey	1981–1991	2042	All ages	2.8	3.4	2.4	60 both sexes (>79y)
Cowie et al[21]	Hillingdon, London, UK	Cross-sectional study (rapid-access HF clinic)	1995–6	151 000	>25	1.3	1.4	1.2	11.6 both sexes 16.8 men 9.6 women (>85y)
REACH Study[22]	Michigan, USA	Retrospective study of administrative databases	1989–99	29 686	All ages	NA	3.7	4.2	46 men 40 women (>85y)
General Practice Research Database[4]	England and Wales, UK	Retrospective cohort study using national data	1996	698 467	40–84	4.2	4.4	3.9	15–19 (75–79y)
Remes et al[20]	Four rural communities in Finland	Population-based surveillance study	1986–88	11 000	45–74	2.3–2.7	4.0	1.0	4.4–4.8 (64–74y)

patients referred had an adjudicated final diagnosis of HF, illustrating the difficulty of classification on the basis of clinical assessment alone.

The age-adjusted incidence of HF appears to be stable. In the Resource Utilization Among Congestive Heart Failure (REACH) Study, which was a retrospective study using administrative databases of outpatient visits and hospitalizations in Michigan, USA, the incidence of HF in 1999 was 3.7/1000 person-years in men and 4.2/1000 person-years in women of all ages with no changes between 1989 and 1999.[22] In a similar analysis of the Framingham Heart Study, incidence was examined in four periods: 1950–69, 1970–79, 1980–89 and 1990–99.[18] When compared with the rate for the period from 1950 to 1969, incidence remained virtually unchanged among men in the three subsequent periods but declined by 31–40% among women.

Incidence of HF with preserved ejection fraction

The body of evidence suggests that approximately 40–50% of patients have preserved EF (HF-PEF). An analysis of the Olmsted County Study identified 6076 patients with incident HF identified from the general population between 1987 and 2001 and suggested that about half had preserved EF (47%) whereas studies in patients hospitalized with HF suggest lower proportions (e.g. 31% in a study undertaken in Ontario, Canada).[23,24] The EuroHeart Failure Survey reported on the characteristics and outcome of 6806 patients admitted to 115 European hospitals with HF between March 2000 and May 2001.[25] Forty-six percent of patients had HF-PEF (LVEF ≥40%); these patients were more likely to be older, hypertensive and have a history of chronic atrial fibrillation, whereas coronary artery disease (CAD) was more prevalent in the systolic HF group ($P < 0.001$). The observed variations in the reported propor-

tion of HF-PEF in these studies are partly explained by the differing thresholds for differentiating HF-PEF from systolic HF and the proportion of patients undergoing quantitative assessment of LVEF. Nevertheless, these data indicate that a significant proportion of patients have HF-PEF.

HF morbidity: hospitalizations

Despite the limitations of administrative databases, there is evidence that age-adjusted hospitalization rates have significantly increased in the developed countries over the last two decades (Fig. 46.2), emphasizing the growing global nature of this problem.[1] In the USA and UK, HF is the most common cause of hospitalization in people aged ≥65 years.[26,27] In Scotland, the number of hospital admissions for HF increased by 16% in men and 12% in women between 1990 and 1996, with some apparent plateauing by 1993–94.[28] Similar data have been reported in The Netherlands.[29]

Men tend to be younger than women at index admission, but because of greater female longevity, overall admission numbers are roughly equal. The NHS Heart Failure Survey determined that 50% of patients with admissions for HF were male but that female patients were older (mean 80 v 75 years, $P < 0.001$).[30] Overall, the typical HF patient is getting older. In The Netherlands between 1985 and 1995, mean age rose from 71.2 to 72.9 years in men and from 75.0 to 77.7 years in women.[30] Elderly patients are more likely to have prolonged admissions, be managed by non-specialists, and be burdened by co-morbid conditions prolonging their admission.[31] An admission to hospital with HF is frequently prolonged and in many cases followed by readmission within a relatively short time, particularly amongst the very elderly. In England and Wales, mean length of stay is 7 (IQR [interquartile range] 4–14) and 8 (IQR 4–14) days

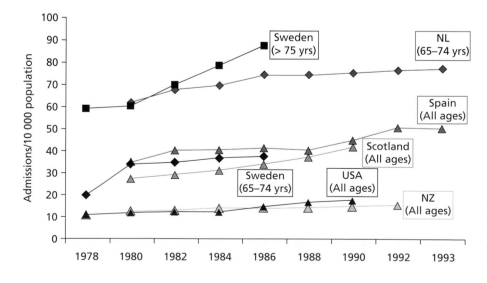

Figure 46.2 Comparison of heart failure admissions rates per annum (recorded hospital admission/10 000 population at risk) in Western developed countries, 1978–1993. (Adapted with permission from data in McMurray *et al*, Heart 2000;83:596–602.)

for men and women respectively.[31] Transfer to a non-specialist unit adds another 2 days. Readmission to hospital is both common and costly. In Scottish hospitals in 2002, the average 30-day readmission rate was 5.3% (lowest 3.3%, highest 7.3%) and may be even higher in the USA.[26,32]

HF mortality

HF prognosis remains poor despite considerable therapeutic advances. However, official statistics continue to specifically attribute only a small proportion of deaths to HF. This reflects a common policy of coding the cause of death as the underlying etiology (e.g. CAD) rather than as HF itself. Population level data suggest that HF-related mortality is comparable to that of cancer; in the Framingham Heart Study the 5-year mortality was as high as 75% in men.[33] Similarly, in a UK study, 1- and 5-year mortality following a first hospitalization was 43% and 73% respectively, with increasing relative risks with increasing age.[34] In Scotland between 1986 and 1995, crude mortality rates in incident HF were 19.9% at 30 days, 44.5% at 1 year and 76.5% at 5 years.[35] Median survival was 1.47 years in men and 1.39 years in women.

In the Rotterdam Study, survival rates from *prevalent* cases of HF were more favorable, with 1- and 5- year survival rates of 89% and 59% respectively.[36] This still, however, represents a threefold increase in the age- and gender-matched risk of death compared to the general population. However, prognosis appears to be improving. In 2000, MacIntyre *et al* demonstrated a fall in 30-day case fatality rates by 26% in men and 17% in women between 1986 and 1995.[35] Similar reductions were seen with longer term mortality. In the Framingham Study, 1- and 5-year mortality rates in men declined from 30% to 70% in 1950–69 and to 28% and 59% in 1990–99, with similar decreases in women.[33] In the Olmsted County Study, age-adjusted 5-year survival improved from 43% in 1979–84 to 52% in 1996–2000. Similar compeling reductions in mortality were identified in data from nearly 300 000 hospitalizations from the Swedish Hospital Registry between 1988 and 2000.[37] These improvements in outcome temporally correlate with the emergence of evidence-based therapies offering potential incremental benefits.

Prognosis of HF-PEF

With respect to hospitalization rates, in the Olmsted County Study, 24% of patients with HF-PEF were never hospitalized, 51% hospitalized once, and 25% hospitalized more than twice over a 5-year period.[38] Patients with systolic HF had significantly more hospitalizations (41% once and 49% more than twice over the same 5-year period). In hospital cohort studies, the reported rates of rehospitalization are similar between those with low and preserved EF. In the aforementioned Canadian EFFECT Study, there was no significant difference in either 30-day (4.5% v 4.9% for HF-PEF and systolic HF respectively, $P = 0.66$) or 1-year readmission rates (13.5% v 16.1% for HF-PEF and systolic HF respectively, $P = 0.09$) in patients who survived the index HF admission.[39]

Similarly, in the EuroHeart Failure Survey, rates of early (within 12 weeks) readmission were almost identical (and impressively high) between both groups (22% and 21% for HF-PEF and systolic HF respectively, $P = 0.47$), indicating that, regardless of LV EF, approximately one in five patients may experience an early (and costly) readmission to hospital.[25]

In terms of mortality, in the Framingham Study, patients with systolic HF had an annual mortality rate of 18.9% compared to 4.1% in age- and sex-matched controls with HF-PEF (over 6.2 years follow-up).[40] Median survival was 4.3 years in those with systolic HF and 7.1 years in those with HF-PEF. A contemporary insight into comparative prognosis comes from the Candesartan in Heart Failure Reduction in Mortality (CHARM) Study which enrolled 7601 patients with symptomatic HF (over 25% of whom had preserved LVEF). The CHARM investigators related baseline LVEF to outcome in 7599 patients with symptomatic HF (of whom 55% were receiving a beta-blocker) randomized to receive candesartan or placebo.[41] Over a median follow-up of 38 months, the hazard ratio (HR) for all-cause mortality increased by 39% for every 10% reduction in LVEF below 45% (HR 1.39; 95% confidence interval (CI) 1.32–1.46).

In contrast to the aforementioned population-based and clinical trial data, two contemporary hospital-based cohort studies suggest that there is little difference in outcome between these patient groups. In the Canadian EFFECT Study, both 30-day (7.1% v 5.3%, $P = 0.08$) and 1-year mortality (25.5% v 22.2%, $P = 0.07$) rates were broadly similar between systolic HF and HF-PEF respectively.[39] Similarly, 5-year survival rates were only marginally better in those with HF-PEF in the Olmsted County Study (HR 0.96, 95% CI 0.93–1.00, $P = 0.03$).[23] It is difficult to accurately explain the differences between these data and those observed in the CHARM population which may suggest the need for care in extrapolating clinical course from trials to the general population.

Epidemiology of HF in the developing world

Data describing the epidemiology of HF in the developing world are scarce and are somewhat limited to single-center hospital-based studies. This reflects the relative difficulty of conducting large-scale studies in communities with finite resources. Furthermore, studies often lack objective measures of LV function and accurate determinants of etiology principally because of inaccessibility to specialist tests. Whereas cardiovascular disease is the principal cause of death in the developed world, it represents only around a quarter of deaths in the developing nations. In contrast, whereas mortality rates have generally declined in the developed world, cardiovascular events are accelerating elsewhere (particularly Asia), in parallel with the emergence of industrialization, "Western" lifestyle and greater longevity.[42] This is often referred to as "epidemiologic transition". Current projections predict that in the next two decades, cardiovascular disease (and undoubtedly associated HF) will emerge as the dominant cause of death in these regions.

In the early 1980s a case series of 315 HF patients admitted to a regional hospital in Nigeria suggested that HF accounted for 7% of all admissions.[43] Almost half were deemed attributable to "cardiomyopathy" (in many cases undefined) and 10% due to rheumatic heart disease. There was also regional variation between Northern and Southern Nigeria, where hypertension accounted for 13% and 35% of cases respectively. Accurate analyses of the contribution of coronary disease were lacking. In contrast, in a small single-center case series undertaken in Kenya in 1999, HF accounted for only 3.3% of hospital admissions.[44] Rheumatic heart disease was attributed in 32% of cases followed by undefined cardiomyopathy in 25%. Only 2.2% of cases were attributed to coronary disease (the assumption made in the presence of ECG features of previous myocardial infarction).

The Heart of Soweto Study mapped the emergence of cardiovascular disease in a geographically stable impoverished population in South Africa.[45] A total of 1593 cases of newly diagnosed cardiovascular disease were identified during 2006. HF was the most common primary diagnosis (44%), of whom 53% had moderate-to-severe LVSD. Approximately one-third (35%) were attributed to cardiomyopathy, a further third (33%) to hypertension and only 9% to ischemic etiology and 8% to primary valvular disease (predominantly rheumatic heart disease). Nevertheless, 59% of all patients had modifiable cardiovascular risk factors, which could influence future risk and illustrates the changing epidemiology in this region.

Profound epidemiologic transitions have taken place in many parts of the Middle East, Central and Southern America and Asia with a resultant increase in the burden of cardiovascular disease. In Oman between 1992 and 1994, the prevalence of HF was 5.17/1000.[46] Ischemic heart disease was the most commonly attributed cause (51.7%) followed by hypertension (24.9%) and idiopathic cardiomyopathy (8.3%). Overall, only 15.7% of patients had HF-PEF (defined as LVEF ≥50%).

In Central and Southern America several case series indicate that the incidence of HF is higher (up to 9.4% of medical admissions in one Brazilian study) and often attributed to modifiable causes, particularly CAD (around

a third) and hypertension (around 20%).[47,48] The relative contribution of Chagas' disease varied between 4% and 20%. In Asian countries such as China, India and Malaysia, cardiovascular disease is now the leading cause of death and in a similar fashion to the West, CAD and hypertension have now replaced rheumatic valve disease as the dominant cause of HF which accounts for up to 6% of medical admissions.[49–51]

Epidemiology of asymptomatic left ventricular systolic dysfunction

Prevalence of asymptomatic left ventricular systolic dysfunction (ALVSD)

In a systematic review, Wang and colleagues identified 11 studies estimating the prevalence of ALVSD.[52] After adjustment for factors including the definition of LVSD, they suggested 3–6% as a reasonable estimate. Prevalence appears to be 2–8-fold greater in men than in women, and increases significantly with age. Therefore, the prevalence of ALVSD is at least twice that of symptomatic HF.

Prognosis of ALVSD

Randomized controlled trials provide the largest source of data on prognosis in ALVSD but are limited by their underrepresentation of the "average" patient. In the Survival and Ventricular Enlargement (SAVE) trial of post-myocardial infarction (MI) LVSD, 13% of patients developed overt HF during median follow-up of 37 months.[53] Similarly, during a median 3-year follow-up, 16% of the placebo-treated patients in the Study of Left Ventricular Dysfunction-Prevention (SOLVD-P) died, with 5% dying within the first year following randomization.[54] Nearly one-third progressed to overt HF and 5% died suddenly. Mortality and HF risk were associated with the degree of baseline systolic dysfunction (mean LVEF was 28%). Several population-based observational studies have confirmed that ALVSD is associated with an increased risk of cardiovascular mortality, all-cause mortality and non-fatal cardiovascular events, including the development of symptomatic HF.[55]

Etiology of heart failure

Heart failure is a classic illustration of the cardiovascular disease continuum, where multiple overlapping mechanisms are involved in disease progression and the disease progressively worsens, providing the opportunity to influence the process. The greatest opportunity for reducing the incidence and excessive mortality and morbidity of HF is through preventive strategies. The ACC/AHA staged approach recognizes that there are established risk factors and behaviors known to be associated with increased risk (Fig. 46.3). Interventions designed to interrupt these processes could slow or halt disease progression and are therefore potential preventive targets. Table 46.4 illustrates the common risk factors identified as preventive targets in the ACC/AHA and CCS guidelines.

LVSD progresses gradually, often beginning with an index myocardial injury (such as MI) which leads to a progressive loss of functioning myocytes. The loss of

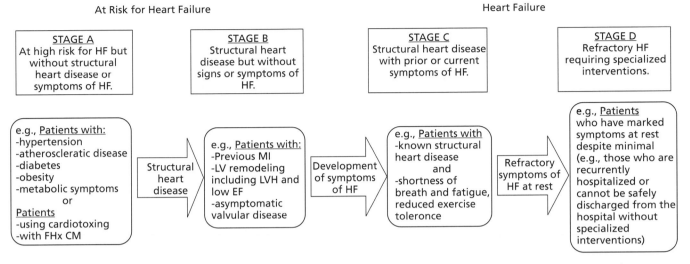

Figure 46.3 ACC/AHA guidelines for the evaluation of chronic HF: evolution of HF by stage. EF, ejection fraction; FHx CM, family history of cardiomyopathy; LVH, left ventricular hypertrophy. (Reproduced with permission from the American College of Cardiology Foundation.)

Table 46.4 Risk factors for the development of heart failure

ACC/AHA Stage A ("at risk")	ACC/AHA Stage B ("structural heart disease")
Hypertension*	Previous myocardial infarction
Atherosclerotic disease* (especially coronary artery disease)	LV remodeling
Diabetes mellitus*	Left ventricular hypertrophy
Hyperlipidemia*	Left ventricular systolic dysfunction (asymptomatic)
Smoking*	Asymptomatic valvular heart disease (especially mitral and aortic regurgitation)
Obesity	
Older age	
Male sex	
Physical inactivity	
Heavy alcohol use	
Valvular heart disease (especially rheumatic valve disease)	
Chronic arrhythmia	
Infection	
Chagas' disease	
HIV	
Enteroviruses (especially Coxsackie B)	
Thyroid dysfunction	
Drug induced	
Anthracyclines	
Cyclophsophamide	
Mitoxantrone	
Paclitaxel	
Trastuzumab	
Amphetamine abuse	
Cocaine abuse	

*Most important targets for prevention.

cardiac function occurs as a consequence of ventricular remodeling, a process by which ventricular shape, dimension and function are altered. Remodeling consists of a multitude of maladaptive pathophysiologic processes including myocyte hypertrophy, necrosis and apoptosis and myocardial interstitial fibrosis and is exacerbated by activation of neurohormonal and inflammatory pathways.[56] The remodeling process may persist despite any further discrete myocardial injury and is accelerated in the face of ongoing risk factors such as hypertension, diabetes mellitus, cigarette smoking and elevated cholesterol.

In the developed world, CAD, either alone or in combination with hypertension, appears to be the dominant cause of HF.[1,57] It is, however, difficult to definitively determine the primary etiology in a patient with multiple risk factors. Earlier studies which relied on non-invasive methods may have been unable to precisely determine the etiology (CAD in particular). In the Bromley Heart Failure Study, the percentage with unknown cause declined from 42% to 10% after cardiac catheterization and nuclear perfusion scanning.[57] Variations in the frequencies of causes of HF can also be explained by differences in the study population and in the methods used to allocate HF diagnosis and underlying precipitant.

Coronary artery disease and myocardial infarction

In the original Framingham cohort, monitored until 1965, hypertension appeared to be the most common cause of HF (in 30% of men and 20% of women, and as co-factor in a further 33% and 25% respectively). However, in subsequent years, CAD emerged as the dominant etiology (increasing from 22% in the 1950s to almost 70% in the 1970s).[58] Similarly, in the Glasgow MONICA Study, 95% of symptomatic individuals had evidence of CAD.[15] Those with symptomatic HF were also more likely to have a past history of MI and ongoing angina pectoris. In asymptomatic individuals, 71% had evidence of CAD. As such, preventive strategies for CAD are also likely to be effective in preventing HF.

There are surprisingly few data describing the epidemiology of HF following acute MI. This again reflects the heterogeneous characteristics of the population. Clinical trials may provide a comprehensive data source but are confounded by bias related to inclusion criteria. Multivariable analyses from the Argatroban in Acute Myocardial Infarction (ARGMI)-2 trial suggest that risk of post-MI HF increases with age, anterior and Q-wave infarcts and in those with prior history of MI.[59] Those with significant LVSD were also more likely to have symptomatic HF on presentation and have associated co-morbid conditions. The Worcester Heart Attack Study (MA, USA) has systematically evaluated the community incidence of MI and sub-

sequent HF in a stable population over a 26-year period (1975–2001).[60] Over this period the incidence of first MI decreased although the proportion of HF complicating MI rose from 40.1% in the mid 1970s, peaking in the early 1980s at 45.5%. Since then, there has been a gradual reduction in the proportion of HF, with a rate of 39.9% in 2001. Whilst the risk of death from HF declined in a parallel fashion, the adjusted odds ratio (OR) in the 2001 cohort was significantly higher (OR 1.37, 95% CI 1.13–1.64 compared with 1975–8). This has been confirmed by the most recent analyses, reflecting an MI population that is typically older and more often burdened by co-morbid conditions, particularly diabetes, and thus reflecting the evolution of the epidemiology of HF as a whole.

Hypertension

The measurable contribution of hypertension appears to have declined; Kannel and colleagues demonstrated a decline in the contribution of hypertension per decade through 1950–87 of approximately 5% in men and 30% in women.[61] This may reflect the parallel introduction of efficacious antihypertensives, as well as improved diagnostic discrimination in the assessment of suspected CAD (with the advent of coronary angiography). Nevertheless, whilst the risk of HF associated with hypertension is measurably smaller than that associated with CAD, hypertension contributes considerably to the epidemiology of HF as it occurs more frequently.[59] Additionally, ECG evidence of left ventricular hypertrophy in the presence of hypertension carries an approximate 15-fold increased risk of HF.[62]

Diabetes mellitus

Dysglycemia is directly implicated in HF pathophysiology with accumulating evidence that diabetes is associated with accelerated myocardial fibrosis, hypertrophy and progressive dysfunction.[63] Diabetes confers a twofold increased risk of HF, and this may be proportionately greater in younger individuals and in women.[64] Those most at risk are generally older, with higher baseline $HbA1_c$ and Body Mass Index (BMI), established diabetic microvascular complications, longer duration of disease and on insulin, and experiencing coronary disease.[65–67]

In an analysis of the Randomized Evaluation of Strategies for Left Ventricular Dysfunction (RESOLVD) Study, 27% of patients had documented diabetes, 8% had undiagnosed diabetes, and a further 9% had abnormal fasting glucose levels.[68] Further compeling evidence of the negative contribution of diabetes comes from the CHARM program. Diabetes emerged as one of the most powerful predictors of outcome, with an approximate doubling of risk of death or the composite outcome of cardiovascular death or HF hospitalization.[69] Recent evidence indicates that elevated fasting glucose alone is an independent predictor of future HF hospitalization, suggesting that impaired glucose tolerance and insulin resistance is prognostically significant even without overt diabetes.[70]

Obesity and cardiometabolic risk factors

Cardiometabolic risk factors include: abdominal adiposity, hypertriglyceridemia, high total cholesterol, low HDL cholesterol, hypertension and fasting hyperglycemia. The relationship between lipid abnormalities and atherosclerosis is well established. Similarly, both elevated triglycerides and high ration of total to high-density lipoprotein (HDL) cholesterol have been found to be associated with increased risk of HF.[71] In an analysis of the Framingham Heart Study, each incremental increase in BMI of $1\,kg/m^2$ was associated with a 5% and 7% increased risk of HF in men and women respectively, with 11% of cases of HF in men and 14% in women being directly attributed to obesity.[72] Similarly, the NHANES-I follow-up study suggested that obesity was associated with a 30% higher risk of incident HF.[62]

Tobacco smoking

Multivariable analyses from epidemiologic studies and clinical trial registries indicate that tobacco smoking is an independent risk factor for the future development of HF. A prior history of cigarette smoking was found in 42% of men and 24% of women who developed HF from the Framingham Study and approximately 17% of all incident cases could be attributed to cigarette smoking in the NHANES-I survey.[18,62] There is both a direct and independent relationship between smoking and the development of ALVSD as well as a dose–response relationship strongly supporting causality.[73]

Special circumstances

Valvular heart disease

Although the measurable contribution of valvular heart disease has decreased (secondary to the decreased incidence of rheumatic heart disease in the developed nations), patients with HF frequently have valvular abnormalities. In the Glasgow MONICA Study, 25% of patients with symptomatic LVSD had abnormalities on echocardiography which may contribute to morbidity.[15] Nevertheless, as discussed above, even in the developed world, atherosclerotic disease now dominates.

Other causes of cardiomyopathy

Long-term heavy alcohol consumption (>11 units per day) is a particularly important (and largely preventable) cause of dilated cardiomyopathy, especially in men in their late forties.[74] An ever increasing list of candidate drugs (both therapeutic and recreational) is implicated in HF etiology.[75]

Special attention should be given to individuals receiving anthracycline and immunotherapy-based cancer treatment. In survivors of childhood cancer, the relative risk of HF is 15.1 times greater than siblings and is greatest with previous anthracycline-based chemotherapy or thoracic irradiation. Trastuzumab is a monoclonal antibody directed against the HER-2 receptor (expressed in around 25% of breast cancers). Although very effective in the management of these cancers (which are often more aggressive) trastuzumab has been linked with an increased risk of cardiomyopathy (prevalence of up to 11% in some studies).[76] With broadening clinical indications for its use, we may see more reports of trastuzumab-related cardiotoxicity (particularly when used in combination with other cardiotoxic agents).

Recently, concern has been directed towards the thiazolidinediones (TZDs), insulin-sensitizing agents used in the management of type-2 diabetes, with both case report and clinical trial data suggesting an increased incidence of fluid retention and possibly decompensation of HF.[77]

In Latin America, Chagas' disease is an important and preventable cause of HF. Chagas' is caused by the protozoan parasite *Trypanosoma cruzi,* and transmitted through its principal vector, the triatomine bug, which is endemic in Latin America. Infection is closely linked to socio-economic status, with the impoverished and those in rural communities being most at risk. It is estimated that 25 million people worldwide are infected or at risk of Chagas', with seroprevalence rates as high as 40%.[78] These estimates may underestimate the true prevalence and the population at risk (which includes up to 500 000 immigrants in the USA). Dilated cardiomyopathy occurs in up to 30% of infected individuals between 10–20 years after initial infection and is associated with a typically worse prognosis than "idiopathic" cardiomyopathies.[79]

Renal disease

Renal impairment is strongly associated with the development of cardiovascular disease and death. End-stage renal disease is associated with a CVD risk 20–30 times that of the general population. In particular, microalbuminuria is a well-characterized risk factor for HF in diabetics, in whom the presence of elevated urine albumin excretion increases risk by 3–5-fold.[67] In the Heart Outcomes Prevention Evaluation (HOPE) trial, microalbuminuria was a predictor of HF and other cardiovascular events in both diabetics and non-diabetics.[80]

Preventive strategies

Preventive strategies include public health policy, the specific targeting of high-risk individuals and secondary prevention in those with established cardiovascular disease (ACC/AHA Stage A). Many patients have more than one risk factor; therefore, optimal treatment of all risk factors may produce benefits that are at least additive, if not synergistic. Interpretation of clinical trial data may be difficult. Whilst some treatment strategies may appear to be intuitively effective (e.g. reperfusion therapy following MI), direct evidence of reduction of HF risk may be lacking and therefore, assigning appropriate evidence recommendations may be difficult. Tables 46.5 and 46.6 summarize the best available clinical trial data directly supporting treatments for the prevention of HF and supporting evidence recommendations for these strategies.

Treatment of hypertension

Treatment of both systolic and diastolic hypertension is associated with a considerable reduction in the incidence of HF with several randomized controlled trials and meta-analyses demonstrating reductions of the order of 30–50% across the spectrum of disease severity and in all age groups (see Table 46.6).[81–85] Indeed, the elderly may have most to gain, with considerable reductions in cardiovascular events; particularly HF.[86] Is there a difference between antihypertensive agents or is adequate BP reduction enough? The most compeling data support the use of diuretics, inhibitors of the renin-angiotensin-aldosterone system (RAAS) and beta-blockers, whereas calcium channel blockers appear somewhat less effective and alpha-antagonists may be potentially detrimental.

The International Nifedipine GITS (INIGHT) Study compared long-acting nifedipine with the thiazide diuretic co-amilozide.[87] There was a significantly higher rate of HF amongst patients treated with nifedipine (0.8% v 0.3%, $P = 0.028$) although again there was no significant differ-

ence in other cardiovascular outcome measures. The Nordic Diltiazem trial (NORDIL) randomized patients to diltiazem or "conventional" beta-blocker or thiazide-based therapy.[88] Incidence of HF was approximately 20% higher in those treated with diltiazem (2.5/1000 per year v 2.1/1000 per year) although this difference was not statistically significant.

The Antihypertensive and Lipid-Lowering Treatment to Prevent Heart Attack Trial (ALLHAT) remains the largest randomized controlled antihypertensive trial conducted to date and allowed direct comparison of several regimens (see Table 46.6).[89] The doxazosin arm of the study was terminated early because of an increased incidence of cardiovascular events, particularly HF, relative to chlorthalidone (relative risk (RR) 2.04, 95% CI 1.79–2.32). This differential effect on HF was consistently observed amongst all subgroups. Previous smaller trials have suggested that alpha-antagonists increase plasma volume and plasma norepinephrine levels, adding biologic plausibility to the potential detrimental effects of doxazosin.[90] The remaining arms of the ALLHAT study included 33 357 patients assigned to chlorthalidone, lisinopril or amlodipine.[91] At 5 years, systolic BP was significantly lower in the chlorthalidone-treated group. The amlodipine group had a 35% higher risk of hospitalized and fatal HF compared with chlorthalidone (RR 1.35, 95% CI 1.21–1.50, $P < 0.001$) and a 23% higher risk compared with the lisinopril group (RR 1.23, 95% CI 1.09–1.38, $P < 0.01$). There was no significant difference between lisinopril and chlorthalidone.

These findings are supported by the Blood Pressure Lowering Treatment Trialists' Collaboration (BPLTCC) meta-analysis of 29 trials involving over 162 000 patients which demonstrated superiority of ACE inhibitor, beta-

Table 46.5 Evidence-based practice recommendations for the prevention of heart failure

Preventive strategy	ACC/AHA	HFSA*	Australian*	Canadian	ESC
Treatment of hypertension	I-A	I-A	I-A	I-A	I-A
Treatment of atherosclerosis and secondary prevention of coronary artery disease					
ACE inhibitor	I-A	I-A	I-B	I-A	I-B
Beta-blocker (post MI)	I-A	I-A	I-B	–	–
Lipid-lowering therapy	I-C	I-A¶	I-B	I-A	I-A¶
Optimizing treatment of diabetes					
Glycemic control	I-C	I-A¶	–	–	–
ACE inhibitors	IIa-A	I-A¶	–	–	I-A
Angiotensin receptor blockers (in patients with microalbuminuria)	IIa-C	I-A¶	–	–	I-A
Treatment of obesity	–	I-C	–	–	–
Smoking cessation	I-C	I-A	–	I-C	–

* "Is recommended" (HFSA) and "should be treated with "(Australian) are considered equivalent to Class I recommendation.

¶ Heart failure guidelines refer specifically to relevant national clinical practice guidelines for diabetes or secondary prevention of atherosclerosis which make the reported recommendations.

Table 46.6 Clinical trials providing evidence for prevention of heart failure

Study	Inclusion criteria	Intervention	HF event relative risk reduction
Antihypertensive agents			
STOP[82]	Hypertension – 70–84 y	Beta-blocker v placebo	53% (P = 0.031)
SHEP[83]	Isolated systolic hypertension –>60 y	Chlorthalidone 12.5 mg (plus atenolol 25 mg) v placebo	51% (P < 0.01)
Syst-Eur[84]	Isolated systolic hypertension –>60 y	Nitrenidipine 10–40 mg (plus enalapril 5–10 mg + hydrochlorothiazide 12.5–25 mg) v placebo	29% (P = 0.12)
ALLHAT[89,91]	Hypertension –>55 y	Chlorthalidone 12.5–25 mg v amlodipine 2.5–10 mg v lisinopril 10–40 mg v doxazosin 2–8 mg	See text
VALUE[94]	Hypertension –>50 y	Valsartan 80–160 mg v amlodipine 5–10 mg	37% (P = 0.004)
JIKEI[85]	Hypertension – 20–79 y	Valsartan 40–160 mg v + "conventional" treatment v "conventional" treatment alone	47% (P = 0.0293)
Secondary prevention of coronary artery disease			
HOPE[80]	Vascular disease or diabetes + risk factors	Ramipril 10 mg v placebo	23% (P < 0.01)
EUROPA[101]		Perindopril 8 mg v placebo	39% (P = 0.002)
PEACE[102]		Trandalopril 2–4 mg v placebo	25% (P = 0.02)
CURE[112]	Acute coronary syndromes	Clopidogrel 75 mg v placebo	18% (P = 0.03)
Optimizing diabetic care			
UKPDS[65]	Type 2 diabetes (T2DM)	Glycemic control	See text
RENAAL[97]	T2DM, hypertension, nephropathy	Losartan 50–100 mg v placebo	32% (P = 0.005)
IDNT[95]	T2DM, hypertension, nephropathy	Irbesartan 300 mg v amlodipine 10 mg v placebo	28% (P = 0.048)
Hyperlipidemia			
4S[104]	Stable coronary artery disease	Simvastatin 20–40 mg v placebo	21% (P < 0.015)
TNT[107]		Atorvastatin 10 mg v atorvastatin 80 mg	26% (P = 0.01)
CARE[105]		Pravastatin 40 mg v placebo	21% (P = 0.10)
VA-HIT[106]		Gemfibrozil 1200 mg v placebo	22% (P = 0.04)
PROVE-IT[108]	Acute coronary syndromes	Atorvastatin 80 mg v pravastatin 40 mg	45% (P = 0.008)

blocker or diuretic-based regimens over calcium channel blockers in reducing the risk of HF, despite almost identical BP reductions.[92] Indeed, for every outcome other than HF, the differences in the observed risk were directly related to degree of blood pressure reduction.

The newest class of antihypertensive drug showing efficacy in prevention of HF are the angiotensin receptor blockers (ARBs). This group has shown particular efficacy in reducing major cardiovascular events in diabetics with established nephropathy (and in many cases, associated hypertension). The Losartan Intervention for Endpoint reduction in hypertension (LIFE) study compared losartan and atenolol in 9193 patients with significant hypertension (BP 160–200/95–115 mmHg).[93] After mean follow-up of just under 5 years the primary composite endpoint of cardiovascular morbidity and death was lower in the losartan group (HR 0.87, 95% CI 0.77–0.98, P = 0.021) with a trend towards a reduction in HF admissions. The Valsartan Antihypertensive Long-term Use Evaluation (VALUE) trial ran-

domized 15 235 high-risk patients to a regimen based on the ARB valsartan or CCB amlodipine, with the addition of hydrochlorothiazide to each as necessary.[94] Primary outcome was time to first cardiac event (a composite which included hospitalization or death due to HF). Whilst there was no difference in the primary outcome between either group, in a subsequent analysis of the 46% receiving monotherapy, valsartan emerged as superior in reducing incident HF (HR 0.63, 95% CI 0.461–0.962. P = 0.004).

These studies illustrate the substantial benefits of antihypertensive therapy across a spectrum of hypertension severity, with even modest reductions in BP among patients with stage 1 and 2 hypertension producing tremendous benefits. Amongst diabetics and patients with established atherosclerosis, inhibitors of the RAAS have been particularly effective.[92,95–97] It is estimated that only 52% of Americans with established hypertension are receiving treatment, and only 23% are adequately controlled.[98] Similarly almost half of patients with previous MI have uncontrolled hypertension.[99] There is therefore, considerable room for improvement and prevention in such high-risk individuals. Optimal BP control in line with contemporary guidelines should be the primary goal, the choice of drugs guided by concomitant medical problems (e.g. CAD, diabetes or renal disease) (**Class I, Level A**).

Treatment of atherosclerosis and prevention of myocardial infarction

ACE inhibitors

ACE inhibitors play a pivotal role in the secondary prevention of MI and in patients with chronic stable atherosclerosis. The ACE Inhibitor Myocardial Infarction Collaborative Group undertook a systematic review of trials of ACE inhibition in the early (0–36 hours) phase of acute MI.[100] Data were available from four randomized controlled trials involving nearly 100 000 patients. Results were consistent, with a significant 7% relative risk reduction in 30-day mortality and a significant but small 1.4% absolute risk reduction in the incidence of non-fatal HF.

In patients with established cardiovascular disease, long-term treatment with an ACE inhibitor may decrease the risk of death and further major cardiovascular events, including HF, although studies have yielded variable results. The aforementioned HOPE trial randomized 9297 patients aged 55 years or older with diabetes mellitus or established vascular disease (but without evidence of HF) to receive ramipril or placebo.[80] Ramipril decreased the incidence of HF by 23% (OR 0.77, 95% CI 0.67–0.97, $P < 0.001$). This benefit appeared independent of blood pressure. Similar results were observed with perindopril in the EURopean trial On reduction of cardiac events with Perindopril in stable coronary Artery disease (EUROPA) Study.[101] Perindopril was associated with a significant 20% relative risk reduction in the primary endpoint (OR 0.8, 95% CI 0.09–0.29, $P = 0.0003$) with a 39% relative risk reduction in HF hospitalizations (OR 0.69, 95% CI 0.17–0.56, $P = 0.002$). In contrast to HOPE and EUROPA, the Prevention of Events with Angiotensin Converting Enzyme inhibition (PEACE) trial failed to show any incremental benefit of adding ACE inhibitor (trandolapril) to otherwise optimal therapy on the composite endpoint of cardiovascular death, MI or coronary revascularization.[102] There was, however, a significant reduction in the composite rate of death or hospitalization due to HF (OR 0.75, 95% CI 0.59–0.95, $P = 0.02$). To control for apparent differences in risk profiles, baseline therapies and follow-up between the different trials, two comprehensive meta-analyses have combined the findings of these and smaller studies and persuasively demonstrate a significant reduction in all-cause mortality, cardiovascular mortality and hospitalization for HF (OR 0.77, 95% CI 0.67–0.90, $P = 0.0007$).[96,103] As such, all patients with stable CAD should be considered for treatment with an ACE inhibitor (**Class I, Level A**).

Lipid-lowering therapy

The Scandinavian Simvastatin Survival Study (4S) randomized 4444 patients (mean age 60 years) with known CAD and serum cholesterol 5.5–8.0 mmol/L, and without clinical evidence of HF, to receive simvastatin (20 mg initially, increased to 40 mg if cholesterol remained >5.2 mmol/L) or placebo.[104] Primary endpoint was total mortality. After 5-years follow-up there was a significant 30% reduction in total mortality ($P < 0.0003$) with a 21% relative risk reduction in the incidence of HF ($P < 0.015$). The relative risk reduction for major coronary events was independent of baseline cholesterol and similar across all subgroups. Risk of HF was closely related to ischemic events, particularly MI and comorbid diabetes. The Cholesterol and Recurrent Events (CARE) trial randomized 1283 elderly patients aged 65–75 years (mean 69 years) with prior history of MI and total cholesterol <6.2 mmol/L to receive pravastatin 40 mg or placebo.[105] There was a significant reduction in the primary composite endpoint of non-fatal MI or CAD death (39% relative risk reduction, $P = 0.001$) and a trend towards reductions in incident HF (23% relative risk reduction, $P = 0.10$).

The Veterans' Affairs Co-operative Studies Program High-density Lipoprotein Cholesterol Intervention trial (VA-HIT) randomized 2531 male patients with established CAD, low HDL cholesterol and no more than moderately elevated LDL cholesterol to receive either the fibrate gemfibrozil 1200 mg or placebo.[106] Primary endpoint was non-fatal MI or death from CAD. After 5.1 years follow-up gemfibrozil was associated with a significant reduction in the primary endpoint and a 22% relative risk reduction in HF hospitalization (OR 0.78, 95% CI 0.62–0.98, $P = 0.04$).

In a meta-analysis of six recently conducted randomized controlled trials comparing intensive with moderate lipid-lowering therapy (with a statin) in patients with recent acute coronary syndrome (ACS) and stable CAD, intensive therapy showed greater efficacy in reducing total mortality, although this was restricted to patients with recent ACS.[107] Nevertheless, intensive therapy was associated with a significant reduction in risk of HF hospitalization in both patient groups (RR 0.63, 95% CI 0.46–0.86 and OR 0.77, 95% CI 0.64–0.092 respectively). These substantial reductions in heart failure admission rates may be independent of ischemic events. In the Pravastatin or Atorvastatin Evaluation and InfecTion (PROVE-IT) trial, 4162 patients with low baseline rates of HF were randomized to receive intensive (atorvastatin 80 mg) or moderate (pravastatin 40 mg) statin therapy following stabilization for a recent ACS.[108] Hospitalization rates for HF were significantly reduced in the intensive therapy group (HR 0.55, 95% CI 0.35–0.85, $P = 0.008$) and this benefit appeared independent of recurrent ischemic events. Consequently, lipid-lowering therapy (in accordance with local primary and secondary prevention guidelines) is strongly recommended in all patients with CAD to prevent HF (**Class I, Level A**).

Antiplatelets

Antiplatelet drugs, notably aspirin, have been shown to produce short-term benefits in preventing mortality and cardiovascular events after MI and in patients with cardiovascular disease.[109] Aspirin is universally accepted as first-line treatment of CAD. However, two prospective outcome trials, including patients with HF, have failed to demonstrate significant beneficial effects on mortality specifically related to HF.[110,111]

Clopidogrel exerts its antiplatelet effects through antagonism of adenosine diphosphate-induced platelet aggregation. Combination of clopidogrel with aspirin, which acts via the thromboxane-mediated aggregation pathway, may have an additive effect, producing incremental clinical benefits, particularly in high-risk patients. The Clopidogrel in Unstable Angina to Prevent Recurrent Events trial investigators randomized 12 562 patients who had presented within 24 hours of onset of ACS (excluding ST elevation MI) to receive aspirin and clopidogrel (loading dose of 300 mg followed by 75 mg daily) or placebo for 12 months.[112] Clopidogrel was associated with a significant 20% relative risk reduction in the primary composite outcome measure of death from cardiovascular causes, non-fatal MI or stroke (HR 0.80, 95% CI 0.72–0.90, $P < 0.001$). There was also a significant reduction in incidence of in-hospital HF (HR 0.82, 95% CI 0.69–0.98, $P = 0.03$). This was of a similar magnitude to the reduction in ischemic events, suggesting that through prevention of recurrent ischemia, intensive antiplatelet therapy can prevent heart failure following ACS (**Class IIa, Level B**).

Optimizing treatment of diabetes

Considering diabetes as an integral part of the cardiovascular risk continuum, strategies to prevent HF should largely focus on optimal treatment of hypertension, reducing ischemic events and optimizing diabetes care as a whole. It is difficult, however, to determine if improving glycemic control reduces heart failure incidence *per se*, largely due to a paucity of good data from large trials. In the UK Prospective Diabetes Study Group (UKPDS), every 1% reduction in HbA1$_c$ was associated with a 16% reduction in risk of incident HF (95% CI 3–26, $P = 0.016$).[65] Whilst several observational and interventional studies have demonstrated a linear relationship between percentage HbA1$_c$ and subsequent risk of HF, the converse, that aggressive reduction in HbA1$_c$ modifies risk of heart failure, remains largely unproven.[66,113] Nevertheless, glycemic control in patients with diabetes is recommended to reduce future heart failure risk (**Class I, Level A**).

Treatment of obesity

Effective weight reduction strategies have been shown to improve many of the adverse effects of obesity. Some small studies specifically investigating bariatric surgery in the management of morbid obesity have demonstrated measurable reductions in LV mass with tandem improvements in LV systolic and diastolic function.[114,115] Nevertheless, there is no firm evidence on which to base recommendations for weight loss targets as a preventive strategy for HF. Contemporary practice guidelines suggest a BMI of <30 as a clinical target (**Class I, Level C**).

Smoking cessation

There is considerable evidence that smoking cessation prevents subsequent cardiovascular events in those with established coronary disease.[116,117] Similarly, smoking cessation appears to have substantial benefits on decreasing morbidity and mortality in patients with established heart failure.[73] In the SOLVD study, non-smokers or former smokers showed improved outcome when compared with current smokers. These and other observational data suggest that smoking cessation may positively impact on HF outcome, particularly in those with established cardiovascular disease (**Class I, Level A**).

Others

In patients at risk of "cardiomyopathy", clinical vigilance and early treatment of asymptomatic LVSD is the key. Precipitating causes should be sought and corrected. Drug-induced LVSD may be responsible for only a small proportion but may be easily overlooked and relies on a thorough history and clinical awareness of potential culprits. In those receiving high-dose anthracycline chemotherapy regimens, a variety of cardioprotectant strategies have been attempted but without much success.[118] The most promising is the free radical scavenger dexrazoxane which may reduce the incidence and severity of cardiomyopathy associated with doxorubicin.[118]

In 2007 the WHO launched a "Global Network for Chagas' Elimination" with the primary goal of eliminating Chagas' disease by 2010. This complements national programs to control Chagas' such as the "Southern Cone Initiative" which, through a combination of housing improvements and insecticide spraying, have resulted in significant reductions in transmission.[119] The use of antiparasitic therapy (principally benzidazole) has been evaluated in several small randomized and non-randomized controlled trials. These studies have been evaluated by the Cochrane Collaboration which suggests potential for asymptomatic patients.[120] Large-scale randomized controlled trials are indicated, with one under way.[121]

The prevention of rheumatic heart disease relies on accurate diagnosis and effective administration of secondary prophylaxis. The WHO recommends a program based upon monthly injections of penicillin after a first episode of acute rheumatic fever, and continued until the third decade as an effective (and affordable) strategy to prevent rheumatic heart disease.[122] Despite this, many impoverished nations have no national secondary prophylaxis program. The prevention of these infectious causes of HF is perhaps more closely tied to national public health policy than specific therapeutic interventions.

Management of asymptomatic left ventricular systolic dysfunction

Neurohormonal activation is evident in ALVSD and therefore, therapeutic manipulation may provide clinical benefits. ALVSD is more often managed in primary care and by non-specialists, and therefore, may go unrecognized or untreated. Patients with ALVSD may also be reluctant to commit to a lifetime of medication in the absence of symptoms, especially when faced by side effects and prescription costs. Most of the existing evidence comes from studies in patients with CAD incidentally found to have ALVSD. There are only limited data for non-ischemic etiologies. Table 46.7 summarizes the evidence-based recommendations.

ACE inhibitors

The milestone trials in the treatment of ALVSD using ACE inhibitors are the SOLVD-P and the SAVE trials.[53,54] The SOLVD-P trial randomized 4228 asymptomatic or mildly symptomatic patients with LVEF ≤35%, primarily with CAD (83%), to receive enalapril or placebo. After median follow-up of 37 months, patients receiving enalapril showed a trend toward increased survival and a significant reduction in the risk of development of HF. Extended 12-year follow-up demonstrated a statistically significant 14%

reduction in mortality.[123] The SAVE trial randomized 2231 patients with ALVSD (LVEF ≤40%) following MI to receive placebo or captopril. Mean baseline LVEF was 31%. After median follow-up of 19 months there was a significant 22% relative risk reduction in HF hospitalization and a 36% relative risk reduction in death due to worsening HF.

Finally the Trandolapril Cardiac Evaluation (TRACE) study randomized 1749 patients with MI and LVEF <35% (31% of whom were asymptomatic) to trandolapril or placebo for up to 50 months.[124] Trandolapril produced a 22% relative risk reduction in total mortality and a 29% relative risk reduction in death due to worsening HF.

Taken together, these trials unequivocally support the use of ACE inhibitors in ALVSD, particularly in patients with CAD. Consequently, ACE inhibitors are indicated in all patients with ALVSD post MI (**Class I, Level A**) and in patients with ALVSD even if they have not experienced MI (**Class I, Level A**).

Beta blockers

Treatment with beta-blockers has been shown to provide significant incremental benefits in symptomatic patients treated with an ACE inhibitor. Moreover, beta-blockers have been demonstrated to induce reverse remodeling, reducing LV dimensions and increasing LVEF. In a *post hoc* analysis of the SOLVD-P trial, the benefit of adding beta-blockers to ACE inhibitors in ALVSD became apparent.[125] Those patients receiving both agents (25%) had significantly lower rates of mortality and hospitalization for HF. Similarly, a retrospective analysis of the SAVE trial found that the 35% of patients who were receiving both agents had a 30% lower risk of death and a 21% lower risk of progression to symptomatic HF that was independent of

Table 46.7 Evidence-based recommendations for the management of ALVSD

	ACC/AHA	HFSA*	Australian*	Canadian	ESC
ACE inhibitors	I-A	I-A	I-A	I-A (LVEF <35%) I-B (LVEF 45–40%)	I-A
Beta-blockers					
Prior MI	I-A	I-B	I-B	I-B	I-B
No prior MI	I-C	I-C	–	IIa-C	–
Angiotensin receptor blockers					
Prior MI (intolerant of ACE inhibitor)	I-B	I-C[†]	–	–	I-A[§]
No prior MI (intolerant of ACE inhibitor)	IIa-C	–	–	–	–
Implantable cardioverter defibrillator					
Prior MI (LVEF ≤30%)	IIa-B	–	–	–	IIa-B
No prior MI (LVEF ≤30%)	IIb-C	–	–	–	IIb-C

* "Is recommended" (HFSA) and "should be treated with" (Australian) are considered equivalent to Class I recommendation.
[†] No specific distinction made between prior MI and no prior MI.
[§] "In acute MI with signs of heart failure *or* LVSD".

captopril use.[126] The Australia-New Zealand Heart Failure trial randomized 415 patients with LVSD (LVEF <45%) due to CAD (30% of whom were asymptomatic) to carvedilol or placebo.[127] Most patients were concurrently treated with an ACE inhibitor (86%). After a median 19-month follow-up there was a 26% relative risk reduction in mortality or HF hospitalization with carvedilol. Carvedilol also produced significant improvements in LVEF.

The Carvedilol Post-Infarct Survival Control in LV Dysfunction (CAPRICORN) trial randomized 1959 patients with LVEF ≤40% (mean 33%) post MI to receive carvedilol or placebo.[128] Fifty-three percent of patients were asymptomatic and nearly all received ACE inhibitors (98%). Although there was no difference in the primary composite endpoint of all-cause mortality or cardiovascular hospital admission, there was a significant 23% relative risk reduction in all-cause mortality with carvedilol. In a subgroup analysis of the asymptomatic patients, carvedilol treatment produced a 31% relative risk reduction in all-cause mortality. In an echocardiographic substudy of the same study, carvedilol resulted in statistically significant reductions in LV volumes and superior improvements in LVEF indicating a reversal of LV remodeling.[129]

The more specific effects of ACE inhibitors and beta-blockers on LV remodeling were evaluated in the Carvedilol ACE Inhibitor Remodelling Mild CHF Evaluation (CARMEN) trial which assigned 572 patients with heart failure (LVEF ≤40%) to enalapril, carvedilol or combination of both;[130] 8% of patients were asymptomatic. Primary endpoint was change in LV end-systolic volume at 6 and 8 months. Carvedilol alone and the combination of both drugs appeared to be most efficacious. Patients who were treated with ACE inhibitor alone had no change in LV dimensions and a small, late increase in LVEF. The recently published Reversal of Ventricular Remodelling with Toprol-XL (REVERT) trial has extended these data, demonstrating that beta-blocker therapy can ameliorate LV remodeling.[131] When considering that initiation of a beta-blocker is better tolerated in asymptomatic or mildly symptomatic individuals, an early approach to combined beta-blocker and ACE inhibitor therapy in these patients seems most appropriate. Consequently, beta-blockers are indicated in all patients with ALVSD post MI (**Class I, Level B**) and in patients with ALVSD without history of MI (**Class I, Level C**).

Angiotensin receptor blockers (ARBs)

Clinical trial evidence supporting the use of ARBs in ALVSD is currently limited to the post-MI population. The Valsartan in Acute Myocardial Infarction (VALIANT) trial randomized 14 703 patients with LVSD (mean LVEF 35%) 0.5 to 10 days post MI to receive the ARB valsartan (target dose 160 mg bd) the ACE inhibitor captopril or a combination of both.[132] Twenty-eight percent had no symptoms of HF. After a median follow-up period of nearly 25 months, valsartan was as effective as captopril in reducing the primary endpoint of total mortality, even in asymptomatic patients. The combination of both drugs conferred no additional benefit, whilst increasing the risk of adverse events.

The Optimal Trial in Myocardial Infarction with the Angiotensin II Antagonist Losartan (OPTIMAAL) trial randomized 5477 patients 50 years of age or older with either clinical HF or echocardiographic evidence of LVSD post MI to receive the ARB losartan (at target dose 50 mg once daily) or captopril (at target dose 50 mg three times daily).[133] The primary endpoint was all-cause mortality. Approximately one-third of the study population were asymptomatic. There was a non-significant trend in mortality favoring captopril, although losartan was better tolerated. These results suggest that the efficacy of an ARB in post-MI LVSD either varies depending on agent used (valsartan being efficacious and losartan not) or by dosing. In the VALIANT trial, valsartan was more rapidly titrated and reported equivalent non-inferior reductions in events when compared with captopril. In contrast, the OPTIMAAL investigators observed a significantly higher early event rate in this high-risk population, suggesting that the dosing regimen of losartan may have been suboptimal.

Consequently, ARBs are indicated in patients with ALVSD post MI who are intolerant of ACE inhibitors (**Class I, Level B**) and may be beneficial in ALVSD in patients without a history of MI who are intolerant of ACE inhibitors (**Class IIa, Level C**).

Aldosterone antagonists (AA)

The Eplerenone Post-Acute Myocardial Infarction Heart Failure Efficacy and Survival Study (EPHESUS) randomized 6632 patients LVEF ≤40% and clinical or radiologic HF (or diabetes mellitus) after MI to receive the selective AA eplerenone 50 mg once daily or placebo (in addition to standard therapy).[54,134] There was a significant 15% relative risk reduction in all-cause mortality with further benefits in reducing hospital admissions. These benefits were achieved despite high baseline use of ACE inhibitors and beta-blockers, demonstrating the incremental advantage for these high-risk patients; 10% of patients were asymptomatic (all diabetics). In a recent cardiac magnetic resonance imaging study, eplerenone significantly reduced LV remodeling (assessed by LV systolic volume index) over a 6-month period compared with placebo in 100 patients with ALVSD post MI (RAP Weir, presentation at the American Heart Association Scientific Congress, Orlando, 2007). These patients were otherwise optimally treated in accordance with contemporary guidelines.

Consequently, the AA eplerenone should be considered in diabetic patients with ALVSD post MI although a level of recommendation cannot be made on the basis of the available evidence. Further adequately powered clinical endpoint studies are indicated to explore the broader application of aldosterone antagonists in ALVSD, particularly in such high-risk groups.

Implantable cardioverter-defibrillators (ICDs)

Despite advances in pharmacologic treatment, patients continue to experience significant mortality. In the SOLVD-P trial, 5% of patients suffered sudden cardiac death that was not preceded by worsening HF and in the Framingham population, 43% of patients with ALVSD died suddenly.[54,55] It is presumed that a significant proportion of these sudden deaths are arrhythmic in etiology. This has led to the investigation of ICDs as a preventive strategy in high-risk patients. Early studies targeted therapy to those considered most at risk on the basis of electrophysiologic testing, and confirmed a significant reduction in mortality. Subsequently, "primary prevention" devices have been proven to be efficacious in preventing sudden cardiac death in patients without electrophysiologic testing and in patients with both ischemic and non-ischemic LVSD. A considerable proportion of asymptomatic patients were included in the landmark studies.

The Multicenter Automatic Defibrillator Implantation Trial II (MADIT-II) randomized 1232 patients with past history of MI (at least 1 month) and LVEF ≤30% to receive conventional medical therapy or medical therapy plus ICD.[135] Median follow-up was 20 months. Approximately one-third of each group were asymptomatic. ICD was associated with a 31% relative risk reduction in death compared with medical therapy alone. Asymptomatic patients were conferred the same survival benefits as those with overt symptoms. The Defibrillators in Non-ischemic Cardiomyopathy Treatment Evaluation (DEFINITE) Study investigated the role of ICD in patients with non-ischemic cardiomyopathy.[136] Four hundred and fifty-eight patients (22% of whom were asymptomatic) with LVEF ≤36% were randomized to receive conventional medical therapy or medical therapy plus ICD. Device implantation produced a non-significant 35% relative risk reduction in total mortality ($P = 0.08$). In contrast to the MADIT-II population, only symptomatic NYHA III patients received mortality benefit.

Consequently, ICD implantation should be considered in patients with ALVSD and LVEF ≤30% post MI on optimal medical therapy and in whom a reasonable survival with good functional status of more than 1 year can be expected (**Class IIa, Level B**). Implantation may be considered in patients with non-ischemic cardiomyopathy with LVSD but this remains an area of debate (**Class IIb, Level C**).

Conclusion

Heart failure affects approximately 2–5% of the population and is associated with considerable morbidity and mortality. Whilst the age-adjusted incidence appears to have remained stable, prevalence is thought to be increasing, principally as a consequence of aging of the population and improved survival from CAD. The prevalence of ALVSD may be even greater, indicating that many patients go unrecognized and untreated. Therapies aimed at modifying the abnormal neurohormonal activation that is characteristic of LVSD have been proven to prevent progression of ALVSD to overt HF, particularly post MI.

Early identification of those at risk and modification of risk factors is critical to reduce the population burden. Future strategies may include the use of devices and novel therapeutic agents as well as screening for asymptomatic patients. Together with effective preventive measures, this may decelerate this growing epidemic.

References

1. Mosterd A, Hoes AW. Clinical epidemiology of heart failure. *Heart* 2007;**93**(9):1137–46.
2. Stewart S, MacIntyre K, Capewell S, McMurray JJ. Heart failure and the aging population: an increasing burden in the 21st century? *Heart* 2003;**89**(1):49–53.
3. Hogg K, Swedberg K, McMurray J. Heart failure with preserved left ventricular systolic function; epidemiology, clinical characteristics, and prognosis. *J Am Coll Cardiol* 2004;**43**(3): 317–27.
4. Office for National Statistics. Key Health Statistics from General Practice 1998. Office for National Statistics, London.
5. Mair FS, Crowley TS, Bundred PE. Prevalence, aetiology and management of heart failure in general practice. *Br J Gen Pract* 1996;**46**(403):77–9.
6. Clarke KW, Gray D, Hampton JR. How common is heart failure? Evidence from PACT (prescribing analysis and cost) data in Nottingham. *J Public Health Med* 1995;**17**(4): 459–64.
7. Redfield MM, Jacobsen SJ, Burnett JC Jr, Mahoney DW, Bailey KR, Rodeheffer RJ. Burden of systolic and diastolic ventricular dysfunction in the community: appreciating the scope of the heart failure epidemic. *JAMA* 2003;**289**(2):194–202.
8. Mittelmark MB, Psaty BM, Rautaharju PM, Fried LP, Borhani NO, Tracy RP *et al.* Prevalence of cardiovascular diseases among older adults. The Cardiovascular Health Study. *Am J Epidemiol* 1993;**137**(3):311–7.
9. Ceia F, Fonseca C, Mota T, Morais H, Matias F, de Sousa A *et al.* Prevalence of chronic heart failure in Southwestern Europe: the EPICA study. *Eur J Heart Fail* 2002;**4**(4):531–9.
10. Mosterd A, Hoes AW, de Bruyne MC, Deckers JW, Linker DT, Hofman A *et al.* Prevalence of heart failure and left ventricular dysfunction in the general population; The Rotterdam Study. *Eur Heart J* 1999;**20**(6):447–55.

11. Kupari M, Lindroos M, Iivanainen AM, Heikkila J, Tilvis R. Congestive heart failure in old age: prevalence, mechanisms and 4-year prognosis in the Helsinki Ageing Study. *J Intern Med* 1997;**241**(5):387–94.

12. Cortina A, Reguero J, Segovia E, Rodriguez Lambert JL, Cortina R *et al.* Prevalence of heart failure in Asturias (a region in the north of Spain). *Am J Cardiol* 2001;**87**(12):1417–19.

13. Hedberg P, Lonnberg I, Jonason T, Nilsson G, Pehrsson K, Ringqvist I. Left ventricular systolic dysfunction in 75-year-old men and women; a population-based study. *Eur Heart J* 2001 ;**22**(8):676–83.

14. Morgan S, Smith H, Simpson I, Liddiard GS, Raphael H, Pickering RM *et al.* Prevalence and clinical characteristics of left ventricular dysfunction among elderly patients in general practice setting: cross sectional survey. *BMJ* 1999;**318**(7180): 368–72.

15. McDonagh TA, Morrison CE, Lawrence A, Ford I, Tunstall-Pedoe H, McMurray JJ *et al.* Symptomatic and asymptomatic left-ventricular systolic dysfunction in an urban population. *Lancet* 1997;**350**(9081):829–33.

16. Davies M, Hobbs F, Davis R, Kenkre J, Roalfe AK, Hare R *et al.* Prevalence of left-ventricular systolic dysfunction and heart failure in the Echocardiographic Heart of England Screening study: a population based study. *Lancet* 2001;**358**(9280): 439–44.

17. Abhayaratna WP, Smith WT, Becker NG, Marwick TH, Jeffery IM, McGill DA. Prevalence of heart failure and systolic ventricular dysfunction in older Australians: the Canberra Heart Study. *Med J Aust* 2006;**184**(4):151–4.

18. Ho KK, Pinsky JL, Kannel WB, Levy D. The epidemiology of heart failure: the Framingham Study. *J Am Coll Cardiol* 1993;**22**(4 suppl A):6A–13A.

19. Senni M, Tribouilloy CM, Rodeheffer RJ, Jacobsen SJ, Evans JM, Bailey KR *et al.* Congestive heart failure in the community: trends in incidence and survival in a 10-year period. *Arch Intern Med* 1999;**159**(1):29–34.

20. Remes J, Reunanen A, Aromaa A, Pyorala K. Incidence of heart failure in eastern Finland: a population-based surveillance study. *Eur Heart J* 1992;**13**(5):588–93.

21. Cowie MR, Wood DA, Coats AJ, Thompson SG, Poole-Wilson PA, Suresh V *et al.* Incidence and aetiology of heart failure; a population-based study. *Eur Heart J* 1999;**20**(6):421–8.

22. McCullough PA, Philbin EF, Spertus JA, Kaatz S, Sandberg KR, Weaver WD. Confirmation of a heart failure epidemic: findings from the Resource Utilization Among Congestive Heart Failure (REACH) study. *J Am Coll Cardiol* 2002;**39**(1): 60–9.

23. Owan TE, Hodge DO, Herges RM, Jacobsen SJ, Roger VL, Redfield MM. Trends in prevalence and outcome of heart failure with preserved ejection fraction. *N Engl J Med* 2006;**355**(3): 251–9.

24. Sosin MD, Bhatia GS, Davis RC, Connolly DL, Lip GY. Heart failure: treatment and ethnic origin. *Lancet* 2003;**362**(9387): 919–20.

25. Lenzen MJ, Scholte op Reimer WJ, Boersma E, Vantrimpont PJ, Follath F, Swedberg K *et al.* Differences between patients with a preserved and a depressed left ventricular function: a report from the EuroHeart Failure Survey. *Eur Heart J* 2004;**25**(14): 1214–20.

26. Haldeman GA, Croft JB, Giles WH, Rashidee A. Hospitalization of patients with heart failure: National Hospital Discharge Survey, 1985 to 1995. *Am Heart J* 1999;**137**(2):352–60.

27. McMurray J, McDonagh T, Morrison CE, Dargie HJ. Trends in hospitalization for heart failure in Scotland 1980–1990. *Eur Heart J* 1993;**14**(9):1158–62.

28. Stewart S, MacIntyre K, MacLeod MM, Bailey AE, Capewell S, McMurray JJ. Trends in hospitalization for heart failure in Scotland, 1990–1996. An epidemic that has reached its peak? *Eur Heart J* 2001;**22**(3):209–17.

29. Mosterd A, Reitsma JB, Grobbee DE. Angiotensin converting enzyme inhibition and hospitalisation rates for heart failure in the Netherlands, 1980 to 1999: the end of an epidemic? *Heart* 2002;**87**(1):75–6.

30. Nicol ED, Fittall B, Roughton M, Cleland JG, Dargie H, Cowie MR. NHS heart failure survey: a survey of acute heart failure admissions in England, Wales and Northern Ireland. *Heart* 2008;**94**(2):172–7.

31. Jong P, Vowinckel E, Liu PP, Gong Y, Tu JV. Prognosis and determinants of survival in patients newly hospitalized for heart failure: a population-based study. *Arch Intern Med* 2002;**162**(15):1689–94.

32. Stewart S, Demers C, Murdoch DR, McIntyre K, MacLeod ME, Kendrick S *et al.* Substantial between-hospital variation in outcome following first emergency admission for heart failure. *Eur Heart J* 2002;**23**(8):650–7.

33. Levy D, Kenchaiah S, Larson MG, Benjamin EJ, Kupka MJ, Ho KK *et al.* Long-term trends in the incidence of and survival with heart failure. *N Engl J Med* 2002;**347**(18):1397–402.

34. Blackledge HM, Tomlinson J, Squire IB. Prognosis for patients newly admitted to hospital with heart failure: survival trends in 12 220 index admissions in Leicestershire 1993–2001. *Heart* 2003;**89**(6):615–20.

35. MacIntyre K, Capewell S, Stewart S, Chalmers JW, Boyd J, Finlayson A *et al.* Evidence of improving prognosis in heart failure: trends in case fatality in 66 547 patients hospitalized between 1986 and 1995. *Circulation* 2000;**102**(10):1126–31.

36. Mosterd A, Cost B, Hoes AW, de Bruijne MC, Deckers JW, Hofman A *et al.* The prognosis of heart failure in the general population: The Rotterdam Study. *Eur Heart J* 2001;**22**(15): 1318–27.

37. Schaufelberger M, Swedberg K, Koster M, Rosen M, Rosengren A. Decreasing one-year mortality and hospitalization rates for heart failure in Sweden; Data from the Swedish Hospital Discharge Registry 1988 to 2000. *Eur Heart J* 2004;**25**(4):300–7.

38. Senni M, Tribouilloy CM, Rodeheffer RJ, Jacobsen SJ, Evans JM, Bailey KR *et al.* Congestive heart failure in the community: a study of all incident cases in Olmsted County, Minnesota, in 1991. *Circulation* 1998;**98**(21):2282–9.

39. Bhatia RS, Tu JV, Lee DS, Austin PC, Fang J, Haouzi A *et al.* Outcome of heart failure with preserved ejection fraction in a population-based study. *N Engl J Med* 2006;**355**(3):260–9.

40. Vasan RS, Larson MG, Benjamin EJ, Evans JC, Reiss CK, Levy D. Congestive heart failure in subjects with normal versus reduced left ventricular ejection fraction: prevalence and mortality in a population-based cohort. *J Am Coll Cardiol* 1999;**33**(7):1948–55.

41. Solomon SD, Anavekar N, Skali H, McMurray JJ, Swedberg K, Yusuf S *et al.* Influence of ejection fraction on cardiovascular

outcomes in a broad spectrum of heart failure patients. *Circulation* 2005;**112**(24):3738–44.

42. Pearson TA. Cardiovascular disease in developing countries: myths, realities, and opportunities. *Cardiovasc Drugs Ther* 1999;**13**(2):95–104.

43. Antony KK. Pattern of cardiac failure in Northern Savanna Nigeria. *Trop Geogr Med* 1980;**32**(2):118–25.

44. Oyoo GO, Ogola EN. Clinical and sociodemographic aspects of congestive heart failure patients at Kenyatta National Hospital, Nairobi. *East Afr Med J* 1999;**76**(1):23–7.

45. Sliwa K, Wilkinson D, Hansen C, Ntyintyane L, Tibazarwa K, Becker A *et al.* Spectrum of heart disease and risk factors in a black urban population in South Africa (the Heart of Soweto Study): a cohort study. *Lancet* 2008;**371**(9616):915–22.

46. Agarwal AK, Venugopalan P, de Bono D. Prevalence and aetiology of heart failure in an Arab population. *Eur J Heart Fail* 2001;**3**(3):301–5.

47. Barretto AC, Nobre MR, Wajngarten M, Canesin MF, Ballas D, Serro-Azul JB. [Heart failure at a large tertiary hospital of Sao Paulo]. *Arq Bras Cardiol* 1998;**71**(1):15–20.

48. Diaz A, Ferrante D, Badra R, Morales I, Becerra A, Varini S *et al.* Seasonal variation and trends in heart failure morbidity and mortality in a South American community hospital. *Congest Heart Fail* 2007;**13**(5):263–6.

49. Yao C, Wu Z, Wu Y. The changing pattern of cardiovascular diseases in China. *World Health Stat Q* 1993;**46**(2):113–18.

50. Krishnaswami S, Joseph G, Richard J. Demands on tertiary care for cardiovascular diseases in India: analysis of data for 1960–89. *Bull WHO* 1991;**69**(3):325–30.

51. Chong AY, Rajaratnam R, Hussein NR, Lip GY. Heart failure in a multiethnic population in Kuala Lumpur, Malaysia. *Eur J Heart Fail* 2003;**5**(4):569–74.

52. Wang TJ, Levy D, Benjamin EJ, Vasan RS. The epidemiology of "asymptomatic" left ventricular systolic dysfunction: implications for screening. *Ann Intern Med* 2003;**138**(11):907–16.

53. Pfeffer MA, Braunwald E, Moye LA, Basta L, Brown EJ Jr, Cuddy TE *et al.* Effect of captopril on mortality and morbidity in patients with left ventricular dysfunction after myocardial infarction. Results of the Survival And Ventricular Enlargement trial. The SAVE Investigators. *N Engl J Med* 1992;**327**(10): 669–77.

54. SOLVD Investigators. Effect of enalapril on survival in patients with reduced left ventricular ejection fractions and congestive heart failure. The SOLVD Investigators. *N Engl J Med* 1991; **325**(5):293–302.

55. Wang TJ, Evans JC, Benjamin EJ, Levy D, LeRoy EC, Vasan RS. Natural history of asymptomatic left ventricular systolic dysfunction in the community. *Circulation* 2003;**108**(8):977–82.

56. Mann DL, Bristow MR. Mechanisms and models in heart failure: the biochemical model and beyond. *Circulation* 2005;**111**(21):2837–49.

57. Fox KF, Cowie MR, Wood DA, Coats AJ, Gibbs JS, Underwood SR *et al.* Coronary artery disease as the cause of incident heart failure in the population. *Eur Heart J* 2001;**22**(3):228–36.

58. Levy D, Larson MG, Vasan RS, Kannel WB, Ho KK. The progression from hypertension to congestive heart failure. *JAMA* 1996;**275**(20):1557–62.

59. Rott D, Behar S, Hod H, Feinberg MS, Boyko V, Mandelzweig L *et al.* Improved survival of patients with acute myocardial infarction with significant left ventricular dysfunction undergoing invasive coronary procedures. *Am Heart J* 2001;**141**(2): 267–76.

60. Botkin NF, Spencer FA, Goldberg RJ, Lessard D, Yarzebski J, Gore JM. Changing trends in the long-term prognosis of patients with acute myocardial infarction: a population-based perspective. *Am Heart J* 2006;**151**(1):199–205.

61. Kannel WB, Ho K, Thom T. Changing epidemiological features of cardiac failure. *Br Heart J* 1994;**72**(2 suppl):S3–S9.

62. He J, Ogden LG, Bazzano LA, Vupputuri S, Loria C, Whelton PK. Risk factors for congestive heart failure in US men and women: NHANES I epidemiologic follow-up study. *Arch Intern Med* 2001;**161**(7):996–1002.

63. Young ME, McNulty P, Taegtmeyer H. Adaptation and maladaptation of the heart in diabetes: Part II: potential mechanisms. *Circulation* 2002;**105**(15):1861–70.

64. Nichols GA, Gullion CM, Koro CE, Ephross SA, Brown JB. The incidence of congestive heart failure in type 2 diabetes: an update. *Diabetes Care* 2004;**27**(8):1879–84.

65. Stratton IM, Adler AI, Neil HA, Matthews DR, Manley SE, Cull CA *et al.* Association of glycaemia with macrovascular and microvascular complications of type 2 diabetes (UKPDS 35): prospective observational study. *BMJ* 2000;**321**(7258): 405–12.

66. Iribarren C, Karter AJ, Go AS, Ferrara A, Liu JY, Sidney S *et al.* Glycemic control and heart failure among adult patients with diabetes. *Circulation* 2001;**103**(22):2668–73.

67. Hockensmith ML, Estacio RO, Mehler P, Havranek EP, Ecder ST, Lundgren RA *et al.* Albuminuria as a predictor of heart failure hospitalizations in patients with type 2 diabetes. *J Card Fail* 2004;**10**(2):126–31.

68. Suskin N, McKelvie RS, Burns RJ, Latini R, Pericak D, Probstfield J *et al.* Glucose and insulin abnormalities relate to functional capacity in patients with congestive heart failure. *Eur Heart J* 2000;**21**(16):1368–75.

69. Pocock SJ, Wang D, Pfeffer MA, Yusuf S, McMurray JJ, Swedberg KB *et al.* Predictors of mortality and morbidity in patients with chronic heart failure. *Eur Heart J* 2006;**27**(1):65–75.

70. Held C, Gerstein HC, Yusuf S, Zhao F, Hilbrich L, Anderson C *et al.* Glucose levels predict hospitalization for congestive heart failure in patients at high cardiovascular risk. *Circulation* 2007;**115**(11):1371–5.

71. Eriksson H, Svardsudd K, Larsson B, Ohlson LO, Tibblin G, Welin L *et al.* Risk factors for heart failure in the general population: the study of men born in 1913. *Eur Heart J* 1989;**10**(7): 647–56.

72. Kenchaiah S, Gaziano JM, Vasan RS. Impact of obesity on the risk of heart failure and survival after the onset of heart failure. *Med Clin North Am* 2004;**88**(5):1273–94.

73. Suskin N, Sheth T, Negassa A, Yusuf S. Relationship of current and past smoking to mortality and morbidity in patients with left ventricular dysfunction. *J Am Coll Cardiol* 2001;**37**(6): 1677–82.

74. Piano MR. Alcoholic cardiomyopathy: incidence, clinical characteristics, and pathophysiology. *Chest* 2002;**121**(5):1638–50.

75. Slordal L, Spigset O. Heart failure induced by non-cardiac drugs. *Drug Saf* 2006;**29**(7):567–86.

76. Guglin M, Cutro R, Mishkin JD. Trastuzumab-induced cardiomyopathy. *J Card Fail* 2008;**14**(5):437–44.

77. Erdmann E, Wilcox RG. Weighing up the cardiovascular benefits of thiazolidinedione therapy: the impact of increased risk of heart failure. *Eur Heart J* 2008;**29**(1):12–20.

78. World Health Organization. Control of Chagas Disease. Geneva: World Health Organization: 2002.

79. Rassi A Jr, Rassi A, Rassi SG. Predictors of mortality in chronic Chagas disease: a systematic review of observational studies. *Circulation* 2007;**115**(9):1101–8.

80. Yusuf S, Sleight P, Pogue J, Bosch J, Davies R, Dagenais G. Effects of an angiotensin-converting-enzyme inhibitor, ramipril, on cardiovascular events in high-risk patients. The Heart Outcomes Prevention Evaluation Study Investigators. *N Engl J Med* 2000;**342**(3):145–53.

81. Psaty BM, Lumley T, Furberg CD, Schellenbaum G, Pahor M, Alderman MH et al. Health outcomes associated with various antihypertensive therapies used as first-line agents: a network meta-analysis. *JAMA* 2003;**289**(19):2534–44.

82. Dahlof B, Lindholm LH, Hansson L, Schersten B, Ekbom T, Wester PO. Morbidity and mortality in the Swedish Trial in Old Patients with Hypertension (STOP-Hypertension). *Lancet* 1991;**338**(8778):1281–5.

83. Kostis JB, Davis BR, Cutler J, Grimm RH Jr, Berge KG, Cohen JD et al. Prevention of heart failure by antihypertensive drug treatment in older persons with isolated systolic hypertension. SHEP Cooperative Research Group. *JAMA* 1997;**278**(3): 212–16.

84. Staessen JA, Fagard R, Thijs L, Celis H, Arabidze GG, Birkenhager WH et al. Randomised double-blind comparison of placebo and active treatment for older patients with isolated systolic hypertension. The Systolic Hypertension in Europe (Syst-Eur) Trial Investigators. *Lancet* 1997;**350**(9080):757–64.

85. Mochizuki S, Dahlof B, Shimizu M, Ikewaki K, Yoshikawa M, Taniguchi I et al. Valsartan in a Japanese population with hypertension and other cardiovascular disease (Jikei Heart Study): a randomised, open-label, blinded endpoint morbidity-mortality study. *Lancet* 2007;**369**(9571):1431–9.

86. Gueyffier F, Bulpitt C, Boissel JP, Schron E, Ekbom T, Fagard R et al. Antihypertensive drugs in very old people: a subgroup meta-analysis of randomised controlled trials. INDANA Group. *Lancet* 1999;**353**(9155):793–6.

87. Brown MJ, Palmer CR, Castaigne A, de Leeuw PW, Mancia G, Rosenthal T et al. Morbidity and mortality in patients randomised to double-blind treatment with a long-acting calcium-channel blocker or diuretic in the International Nifedipine GITS study: Intervention as a Goal in Hypertension Treatment (INSIGHT). *Lancet* 2000;**356**(9227):366–72.

88. Hansson L, Hedner T, Lund-Johansen P, Kjeldsen SE, Lindholm LH, Syvertsen JO et al. Randomised trial of effects of calcium antagonists compared with diuretics and beta-blockers on cardiovascular morbidity and mortality in hypertension: the Nordic Diltiazem (NORDIL) study. *Lancet* 2000;**356**(9227): 359–65.

89. ALLHAT Collaborative Research Group. Major cardiovascular events in hypertensive patients randomized to doxazosin vs chlorthalidone: the antihypertensive and lipid-lowering treatment to prevent heart attack trial (ALLHAT). *JAMA* 2000;**283**(15):1967–75.

90. Leenen FH, Smith DL, Farkas RM, Reeves RA, Marquez-Julio A. Vasodilators and regression of left ventricular hypertrophy. Hydralazine versus prazosin in hypertensive humans. *Am J Med* 1987;**82**(5):969–78.

91. Davis BR, Piller LB, Cutler JA, Furberg C, Dunn K, Franklin S et al. Role of diuretics in the prevention of heart failure: the Antihypertensive and Lipid-Lowering Treatment to Prevent Heart Attack Trial. *Circulation* 2006;**113**(18):2201–10.

92. Turnbull F, Neal B, Algert C, Chalmers J, Chapman N, Cutler J et al. Effects of different blood pressure-lowering regimens on major cardiovascular events in individuals with and without diabetes mellitus: results of prospectively designed overviews of randomized trials. *Arch Intern Med* 2005;**165**(12): 1410–19.

93. Dahlof B, Devereux RB, Kjeldsen SE, Julius S, Beevers G, de Faire U et al. Cardiovascular morbidity and mortality in the Losartan Intervention For Endpoint reduction in hypertension study (LIFE): a randomised trial against atenolol. *Lancet* 2002;**359**(9311):995–1003.

94. Julius S, Kjeldsen SE, Weber M, Brunner HR, Ekman S, Hansson L et al. Outcomes in hypertensive patients at high cardiovascular risk treated with regimens based on valsartan or amlodipine: the VALUE randomised trial. *Lancet* 2004;**363**(9426): 2022–31.

95. Berl T, Hunsicker LG, Lewis JB, Pfeffer MA, Porush JG, Rouleau JL et al. Cardiovascular outcomes in the Irbesartan Diabetic Nephropathy Trial of patients with type 2 diabetes and overt nephropathy. *Ann Intern Med* 2003;**138**(7):542–9.

96. Al Mallah MH, Tleyjeh IM, Abdel-Latif AA, Weaver WD. Angiotensin-converting enzyme inhibitors in coronary artery disease and preserved left ventricular systolic function: a systematic review and meta-analysis of randomized controlled trials. *J Am Coll Cardiol* 2006;**47**(8):1576–83.

97. Brenner BM, Cooper ME, de Zeeuw D, Keane WF, Mitch WE, Parving HH et al. Effects of losartan on renal and cardiovascular outcomes in patients with type 2 diabetes and nephropathy. *N Engl J Med* 2001;**345**(12):861–9.

98. Hyman DJ, Pavlik VN. Characteristics of patients with uncontrolled hypertension in the United States. *N Engl J Med* 2001;**345**(7):479–86.

99. Qureshi AI, Suri MF, Guterman LR, Hopkins LN. Ineffective secondary prevention in survivors of cardiovascular events in the US population: report from the Third National Health and Nutrition Examination Survey. *Arch Intern Med* 2001;**161**(13): 1621–8.

100. Boersma E, Mercado N, Poldermans D, Gardien M, Vos J, Simoons ML. Acute myocardial infarction. *Lancet* 2003;**361**(9360): 847–58.

101. Fox KM. Efficacy of perindopril in reduction of cardiovascular events among patients with stable coronary artery disease: randomised, double-blind, placebo-controlled, multicentre trial (the EUROPA study). *Lancet* 2003;**362**(9386):782–8.

102. Braunwald E, Domanski MJ, Fowler SE, Geller NL, Gersh BJ, Hsia J et al. Angiotensin-converting-enzyme inhibition in stable coronary artery disease. *N Engl J Med* 2004;**351**(20): 2058–68.

103. Dagenais GR, Pogue J, Fox K, Simoons ML, Yusuf S. Angiotensin-converting-enzyme inhibitors in stable vascular disease without left ventricular systolic dysfunction or heart failure: a combined analysis of three trials. *Lancet* 2006;**368**(9535): 581–8.

104. Kjekshus J, Pedersen TR, Olsson AG, Faergeman O, Pyorala K. The effects of simvastatin on the incidence of heart failure in patients with coronary heart disease. *J Card Fail* 1997;**3**(4): 249–54.

105. Lewis SJ, Moye LA, Sacks FM, Johnstone DE, Timmis G, Mitchell J et al. Effect of pravastatin on cardiovascular events in older patients with myocardial infarction and cholesterol levels in the average range. Results of the Cholesterol and Recurrent Events (CARE) trial. *Ann Intern Med* 1998;**129**(9):681–9.

106. Rubins HB, Robins SJ, Collins D, Fye CL, Anderson JW, Elam MB et al. Gemfibrozil for the secondary prevention of coronary heart disease in men with low levels of high-density lipoprotein cholesterol. Veterans Affairs High-Density Lipoprotein Cholesterol Intervention Trial Study Group. *N Engl J Med* 1999;**341**(6):410–18.

107. Afilalo J, Majdan AA, Eisenberg MJ. Intensive statin therapy in acute coronary syndromes and stable coronary heart disease: a comparative meta-analysis of randomised controlled trials. *Heart* 2007;**93**(8):914–21.

108. Scirica BM, Morrow DA, Cannon CP, Ray KK, Sabatine MS, Jarolim P et al. Intensive statin therapy and the risk of hospitalization for heart failure after an acute coronary syndrome in the PROVE IT-TIMI 22 study. *J Am Coll Cardiol* 2006;**47**(11): 2326–31.

109. Antithrombotic Trialists' Collaboration. Collaborative meta-analysis of randomised trials of antiplatelet therapy for prevention of death, myocardial infarction, and stroke in high risk patients. *BMJ* 2002;**324**(7329):71–86.

110. No authors listed. A randomized, controlled trial of aspirin in persons recovered from myocardial infarction. *JAMA* 1980;**243**(7):661–9.

111. Klimt CR, Knatterud GL, Stamler J, Meier P. Persantine-Aspirin Reinfarction Study. Part II. Secondary coronary prevention with persantine and aspirin. *J Am Coll Cardiol* 1986;**7**(2): 251–69.

112. Yusuf S, Zhao F, Mehta SR, Chrolavicius S, Tognoni G, Fox KK. Effects of clopidogrel in addition to aspirin in patients with acute coronary syndromes without ST-segment elevation. *N Engl J Med* 2001;**345**(7):494–502.

113. Vaur L, Gueret P, Lievre M, Chabaud S, Passa P. Development of congestive heart failure in type 2 diabetic patients with microalbuminuria or proteinuria: observations from the DIABHYCAR (type 2 DIABetes, Hypertension, CArdiovascular Events and Ramipril) study. *Diabetes Care* 2003;**26**(3): 855–60.

114. Alpert MA, Terry BE, Kelly DL. Effect of weight loss on cardiac chamber size, wall thickness and left ventricular function in morbid obesity. *Am J Cardiol* 1985;**55**(6):783–6.

115. Gahtan V, Goode SE, Kurto HZ, Schocken DD, Powers P, Rosemurgy AS. Body composition and source of weight loss after bariatric surgery. *Obes Surg* 1997;**7**(3):184–8.

116. Mohiuddin SM, Mooss AN, Hunter CB, Grollmes TL, Cloutier DA, Hilleman DE. Intensive smoking cessation intervention reduces mortality in high-risk smokers with cardiovascular disease. *Chest* 2007;**131**(2):446–52.

117. Critchley JA, Capewell S. Smoking cessation for the secondary prevention of coronary heart disease. *Cochrane Database of Systematic Reviews* 2003, Issue 4. Art. No.: CD003041. DOI: 10.1002/14651858.CD003041.pub2.

118. Barry E, Alvarez JA, Scully RE, Miller TL, Lipshultz SE. Anthracycline-induced cardiotoxicity: course, pathophysiology, prevention and management. *Expert Opin Pharmacother* 2007;**8**(8): 1039–58.

119. Schofield CJ, Dias JC. The Southern Cone Initiative against Chagas disease. *Adv Parasitol* 1999;**42**:1–27.

120. Villar JC, Villar LA, Marin-Neto JA, Ebrahim S, Yusuf S. Trypanocidal drugs for chronic asymptomatic Trypanosoma cruzi infection. *Cochrane Database of Systematic Reviews* 2002, Issue 1. Art. No.: CD003463. DOI: 10.1002/14651858.CD003463.

121. Marin-Neto JA, Rassi A Jr, Morillo CA, Avezum A, Connolly SJ, Sosa-Estani S et al. Rationale and design of a randomized placebo-controlled trial assessing the effects of etiologic treatment in Chagas' cardiomyopathy: the BENznidazole Evaluation For Interrupting Trypanosomiasis (BENEFIT). *Am Heart J* 2008; **156**(1):37–43.

122. World Health Organization. *Rheumatic Fever and Rheumatic Heart Disease*. Geneva: World Health Organization, 2004.

123. Jong P, Yusuf S, Rousseau MF, Ahn SA, Bangdiwala SI. Effect of enalapril on 12-year survival and life expectancy in patients with left ventricular systolic dysfunction: a follow-up study. *Lancet* 2003;**361**(9372):1843–8.

124. Kober L, Torp-Pedersen C, Carlsen JE, Bagger H, Eliasen P, Lyngborg K et al. A clinical trial of the angiotensin-converting-enzyme inhibitor trandolapril in patients with left ventricular dysfunction after myocardial infarction. Trandolapril Cardiac Evaluation (TRACE) Study Group. *N Engl J Med* 1995;**333**(25): 1670–6.

125. Exner DV, Dries DL, Waclawiw MA, Shelton B, Domanski MJ. Beta-adrenergic blocking agent use and mortality in patients with asymptomatic and symptomatic left ventricular systolic dysfunction: a post hoc analysis of the Studies of Left Ventricular Dysfunction. *J Am Coll Cardiol* 1999;**33**(4): 916–23.

126. Vantrimpont P, Rouleau JL, Wun CC, Ciampi A, Klein M, Sussex B et al. Additive beneficial effects of beta-blockers to angiotensin-converting enzyme inhibitors in the Survival and Ventricular Enlargement (SAVE) Study. SAVE Investigators. *J Am Coll Cardiol* 1997;**29**(2):229–36.

127. Australia/New Zealand Heart Failure Research Collaborative Group. Randomised, placebo-controlled trial of carvedilol in patients with congestive heart failure due to ischaemic heart disease. *Lancet* 1997;**349**(9049):375–80.

128. Dargie HJ. Effect of carvedilol on outcome after myocardial infarction in patients with left-ventricular dysfunction: the CAPRICORN randomised trial. *Lancet* 2001;**357**(9266):1385–90.

129. Doughty RN, Whalley GA, Walsh HA, Gamble GD, Lopez-Sendon J, Sharpe N. Effects of carvedilol on left ventricular remodeling after acute myocardial infarction: the CAPRICORN Echo Substudy. *Circulation* 2004;**109**(2):201–6.

130. Remme WJ, Riegger G, Hildebrandt P, Komajda M, Jaarsma W, Bobbio M et al. The benefits of early combination treatment of carvedilol and an ACE-inhibitor in mild heart failure and left ventricular systolic dysfunction. The carvedilol and ACE-inhibitor remodelling mild heart failure evaluation trial (CARMEN). *Cardiovasc Drugs Ther* 2004;**18**(1):57–66.

131. Colucci WS, Kolias TJ, Adams KF, Armstrong WF, Ghali JK, Gottlieb SS et al. Metoprolol reverses left ventricular remodel-

ing in patients with asymptomatic systolic dysfunction: the REversal of VEntricular Remodeling with Toprol-XL (REVERT) trial. *Circulation* 2007;**116**(1):49–56.

132. Pfeffer MA, McMurray JJ, Velazquez EJ, Rouleau JL, Kober L, Maggioni AP *et al.* Valsartan, captopril, or both in myocardial infarction complicated by heart failure, left ventricular dysfunction, or both. *N Engl J Med* 2003;**349**(20): 1893–906.

133. Dickstein K, Kjekshus J. Effects of losartan and captopril on mortality and morbidity in high-risk patients after acute myocardial infarction: the OPTIMAAL randomised trial. Optimal Trial in Myocardial Infarction with Angiotensin II Antagonist Losartan. *Lancet* 2002;**360**(9335):752–60.

134. Pitt B, Remme W, Zannad F, Neaton J, Martinez F, Roniker B *et al.* Eplerenone, a selective aldosterone blocker, in patients with left ventricular dysfunction after myocardial infarction. *N Engl J Med* 2003;**348**(14):1309–21.

135. Moss AJ, Brown MW, Cannom DS, Daubert JP, Estes M, Foster E *et al.* Multicenter automatic defibrillator implantation trial-cardiac resynchronization therapy (MADIT-CRT): design and clinical protocol. *Ann Noninvasive Electrocardiol* 2005;**10**(4 suppl):34–43.

136. Kadish A, Dyer A, Daubert JP, Quigg R, Estes NA, Anderson KP *et al.* Prophylactic defibrillator implantation in patients with nonischemic dilated cardiomyopathy. *N Engl J Med* 2004;**350**(21): 2151–8.

47 Management of overt heart failure

Paul J Hauptman[1] and Karl Swedberg[2]
[1]Saint Louis University School of Medicine, St Louis, MO, USA
[2]Sahlgrenska University Hospital/Östra, Göteborg, Sweden

Introduction

The heart may be exposed to various forms of injury brought about by ischemic, hemodynamic, metabolic or toxic insults. Progression to the clinical syndrome of congestive heart failure (CHF) occurs through a complex series of neurohormonal and hemodynamic interactions that results in a common cardiovascular phenotype, characterized by fluid overload, low cardiac output syndrome or a combination of both. Treatment paradigms developed over the past 20 years have increasingly focused on the attainment of long-term survival benefit rather than on improvements in presumptive surrogates for survival such as the hemodynamic profile. While symptom improvement is a goal of therapy, the relationship between symptom relief (for example, with diuretic therapy) and longevity is often non-linear; that is, interventions that may improve symptoms can have a negative or neutral effect on survival, while those that improve survival (for example, the beta-adrenergic receptor antagonists) may have neutral effects on important clinical markers like exercise tolerance.

Since the publication of the last edition of this chapter, the advent of device therapy (in particular implantable cardioverter defibrillators and biventricular pacemakers) has shifted the focus of management. However, the approach to the patient with heart failure must continue to be seen as multidimensional, multidisciplinary and predominantly pharmacologic. Given the morbidity and mortality associated with the condition, and its increasing prevalence, the need to define evidence-based medical therapies has become even more urgent. In this chapter we review contemporary standard-of-care approaches for both chronic and acute overt CHF with a focus on pharmacology, and offer an overview of new challenges ahead.

Evidence-Based Cardiology, 3rd edition. Edited by S. Yusuf, J.A. Cairns, A.J. Camm, E.L. Fallen, and B.J. Gersh. © 2010 Blackwell Publishing, ISBN: 978-1-4051-5925-8.

Pharmacologic therapy

Cardiac glycosides

Digitalis is the oldest of the drugs used in the treatment of CHF today. The main action of the drug is thought to be exerted by inhibition of the plasma membrane Na^+/K^+-ATPase, increasing intracellular concentrations of Na^+ and Ca^+. A variety of autonomic effects have been shown in acute experimental studies and sympatholytic effects have been described.

Acute effects in CHF

Older uncontrolled studies have suggested that digitalis produces beneficial hemodynamic effects in patients with decompensated heart failure, expressed as a decrease in pulmonary capillary wedge pressure, an increase in cardiac output, and a fall in heart rate.[1,2] It appears that the effect of digitalis on hemodynamics is dependent on the hemodynamic state of the patient. Whereas positive effects have been observed in decompensated heart failure, the effects in normal subjects are largely negligible.[3,4] Although the slowing of heart rate would be of benefit in diastolic heart failure without systolic dysfunction, there are limited data about this effect.[5] Acute administration of digitalis restores baroreceptor function and causes a decrease in sympathetic activity[6,7] though not all findings have been reproduced.[8]

Chronic digitalis therapy

The first double-blind placebo-controlled trial with chronic digoxin treatment was published in 1977.[9] Subsequently a series of small short-term trials provided conflicting data about digoxin efficacy,[10–13] with some studies suggesting favorable effects of digoxin on clinical heart failure symptoms, echocardiographic parameters, and exercise capacity, in particular in patients with more advanced left ventricular dysfunction.

In the first large study, the Captopril-Digoxin Multicenter Research Group trial, 300 patients with relatively mild heart failure were compared using captopril, digoxin or placebo. Digoxin and captopril were equally effective in preventing hospitalization or an increase in diuretic dosages. Although digoxin-treated patients showed a significant increase in ejection fraction, in contrast to the captopril group, digoxin did not improve exercise capacity as much as captopril. The German and Austrian Xamoterol Study Group investigated the effect of digoxin together with xamoterol and placebo. Digoxin improved clinical indices of heart failure but not exercise capacity.[14]

Several trials have used a withdrawal design to evaluate digoxin efficacy. In the PROVED trial a randomized double-blind withdrawal of digoxin was investigated in 88 patients with stable NYHA class II–III maintained on digoxin and diuretics.[15] More placebo patients had worsening heart failure with an increase in the need for diuretics and hospitalization, and an impairment in exercise capacity and LV function. In a similar study, the RADIANCE trial, 178 patients with CHF were investigated during digoxin withdrawal compared with maintained digoxin therapy;[16] both groups were also on angiotensin-converting enzyme (ACE) inhibitors. The results were similar to those of the PROVED trial, with placebo patients showing a statistically significant deterioration in cardiac function, hospitalization, quality of life and exercise capacity.

It should be noted that the withdrawal study design is inferior to prospective treatment studies and provides only inferential data about efficacy. In contrast, the Digitalis Investigators Group (DIG) study, the only survival study of digoxin, was a multicenter, prospective, randomized, placebo-controlled, double-blind trial in 7788 patients with mild to moderate heart failure and sinus rhythm.[5] Among the investigated patients, 6800 had signs of systolic dysfunction expressed as ejection fraction of <45%. The remaining patients might be considered to have had only diastolic dysfunction. There was no effect on the primary endpoint of all-cause mortality but digoxin significantly reduced the number of hospitalizations from worsening heart failure.

In clinical practice, the use of digoxin appears to be declining[17] as part of a secular trend as opposed to a reaction to the publication of the DIG trial results. However, other factors may be contributing. One substudy has garnered attention because of a putative increase in mortality in women assigned to receive digoxin.[18] Subsequently, data from the DIG trial supporting the relationship between serum digoxin concentration (measured at 4 hours post dose) and outcomes were published. A survival benefit was observed for serum digoxin concentrations of 0.5–0.8 ng/dL compared to a neutral effect for concentrations between 0.9 and 1.1 ng/dL and an increase in mortality for higher concentrations (greater than 1.1 ng/dL).[19] In an analysis that synthesized these two important observations, Adams *et al* determined that the increased mortality observed in women was likely an effect of higher serum digoxin concentrations, given that women tend to have smaller volumes of distribution of the drug than men.[20]

BOX 47.1 Documented value of digoxin

Proven indication: always acceptable **Level A**
Symptomatic left ventricular systolic heart failure and sinus rhythm on maximal medical therapy: symptomatic improvement, improved exercise capacity and decreased hospitalization for heart failure*

Acceptable indication but of uncertain efficacy and may be controversial **Level B**
CHF with atrial fibrillation: heart rate control

Acceptable indication but of uncertain efficacy and may be controversial **Level A**
Symptomatic heart failure due to diastolic dysfunction

Not proven: potentially harmful (contraindicated) **Level A**
Bradycardia and atrioventricular block
Significant ventricular arrhythmias
Renal dysfunction
Electrolyte disturbances, hypokalemia in particular

*Target serum digoxin level less than 1.0 ng/dL (see text for details)

Taken together, present data on digoxin suggest that this drug induces small but beneficial effects on cardiac function, morbidity, and symptoms. There is a neutral effect on all-cause mortality. However, the therapeutic window is narrow, and the potential risk for serious arrhythmias cannot be ignored. The need to monitor serum drug levels appears to be heightened by recent analyses and in that context practitioners must be vigilant about the possibility that drug–drug interactions may elevate digoxin concentration. Further, the applicability of the data derived from digoxin withdrawal trials to contemporary practice that includes beta-blockers is unclear; the efficacy of digoxin in stable patients with mild heart failure on combined ACE inhibition and beta-blocker has not been established.

Diuretics

Fluid retention is a consistent finding in patients with CHF. The need for reduction of blood volume in patients with edema was recognized several hundred years ago. Historically, drugs with mild diuretic effects, such as mercury salts, carbonic anhydrase inhibitors, and thiazides, have been used.

A more substantial and conventional way to achieve diuresis is the use of loop diuretics.[21] Compensatory fluid retention, as a response to lower cardiac output and reduced kidney perfusion,[22] might be of short-term benefit in restoring optimal preload in the earlier states of CHF. However, a further increase in intracavitary pressure increases wall stress in the myocardium with a parallel increase in oxygen consumption and energy expenditure.

In the classic physiologic description, the elevation of venous pressure shifts the hydrostatic balance across the capillary wall toward a net filtration of fluid to the extracellular space, and finally to the formation of edema. The decrease in renal blood flow that commonly accompanies heart failure stimulates the renin system, which leads to secretion of angiotensin and aldosterone. Other neurohormones that promote retention of sodium and water include vasopressin, norepinephrine, and prostaglandins.[23] In contrast, endogenous sodium excretion is promoted by natriuretic peptides and prostacyclin.

Neurohormonal and hemodynamic effects of loop diuretics

In patients with pulmonary edema, intravenous furosemide is normally followed by a prompt response and relief of symptoms. However, findings are not consistent regarding the mode of action of loop diuretics in the acute phase of decompensated heart failure. A reduction in filling pressures occurs even before diuresis is initiated[24–26] and has been attributed to vasodilation. However, acute arterial vasoconstriction has also been found, alone or in combination with venodilation,[27–29] potentially related, at least in part, to acute upregulation of neurohormones such as aldosterone. Similarly, cardiac output may increase, remain unchanged or decrease. Although furosemide is the most thoroughly tested loop diuretic, there are others available and commonly used, including bumetanide[30] and torsemide.[31]

Most long-term studies have involved a small number of patients and used a variety of drugs and doses; chronic neuroendocrine effects are less well studied. Oral furosemide treatment has been associated with a reduction in norepinephrine concentration and a profound increase in plasma renin activity, angiotensin, and plasma aldosterone concentration.[32,33]

Effects on clinical outcomes and survival

No prospective randomized study has been performed in the ACE inhibitor era examining the effect of diuretics on long-term survival. One meta-analysis of (small) randomized trials with active controls suggests that diuretics improve exercise capacity and the risk of worsening disease.[34] Further, despite concerns regarding the potential neurohormonal activation by diuretics, it should be kept in mind that studies showing positive survival effects of ACE inhibitors, beta-blockers or vasodilators in heart failure have all permitted diuretics as background treatment.

Clinical management

Diuretics reduce symptoms in CHF. The effect on symptoms has been formally tested in trials with furosemide and torsemide.[35] Further, it has been observed that the effects of ACE inhibitors may require the co-administration of diuretics.[36,37] Diuretics are also more effective in relieving edema and congestive symptoms than ACE inhibitors when given as single therapy.[38]

Through an increase in urinary excretion of electrolytes, diuretics are prone to induce metabolic abnormalities such as hypokalemia, hyponatremia, hypocalcemia, hypomagnesemia, and metabolic alkalosis.[39] The need for potassium supplements can be diminished by using potassium-sparing diuretics, such as amiloride or triamterine. However, ACE inhibitors act synergistically with potassium-sparing diuretics, which may produce hyperkalemia; diabetic patients with proteinuria and renal tubular acidosis are at particularly high risk. The addition of a potassium-sparing diuretic to a loop diuretic may further increase diuresis but in the case of spironolactone, the therapeutic effects seen in heart failure are likely mediated by aldosterone blockade rather than direct diuresis. Additionally, the diuretic effect of a loop diuretic can be augmented by other diuretics acting at different sites in the nephron, especially if clinically apparent diuretic resistance has developed. In particular, the combination of a loop diuretic with a thiazide enhances the diuretic effect, when the former is administered slightly after (e.g. 30 minutes) the latter.

Alternative to diuretic therapy: ultrafiltration

It is difficult to foresee a future situation when diuretics are no longer needed in the treatment of CHF. However, recent data using ultrafiltration show promise, albeit with an invasive approach that is likely to be limited to patients with significant or refractory edema or diuretic resistance. Specifically, the UNLOAD trial demonstrated that ultrafiltration led to greater weight loss ($5.0 \pm 3.1\,kg$) than diuretics alone (3.1 ± 3.5, $P = 0.001$) in a cohort of 200 patients hospitalized with symptomatic heart failure. Reductions in patient-reported dyspnea were the same. There were fewer subsequent heart failure hospitalizations at 90 days though it is important to highlight the fact that the trial had an open-label design. Mitigating this confounder to some degree was the companion finding of fewer unscheduled visits for heart failure during extended follow-up.[40]

Diuretics summary

The need for relief of edema and fluid retention and the generic status of most diuretics will prevent the initiation and completion of a classic placebo-controlled randomized long-term survival study. However, given concerns about the metabolic and neurohormonal effects of the diuretics and recognizing that peripheral edema is more a cosmetic nuisance than a life-threatening condition, it is advisable to keep the diuretic dosages as low as possible.

Aldosterone receptor blockers

Aldosterone plays an important role in the pathophysiology of heart failure, facilitating sodium retention and

---

BOX 47.2 Documented value of diuretics

Proven indication: always acceptable Level A
Symptomatic improvement in case of congestion. Improvement of exercise capacity

Acceptable indication but of uncertain efficacy and may be controversial Level B
Long-term treatment in conjunction with other drugs for heart failure, such as ACE inhibitors, vasodilators and beta-blockers

Not proven: potentially harmful (contraindicated) Level C
Heart failure without congestion or edema
Uncorrected pronounced hypokalemia or hyperuricemia

BOX 47.3 Documented value of aldosterone antagonists*

Proven indication: always acceptable Level A
Improvement of survival in severe CHF
Reduction of morbidity in severe heart failure
Improvement in survival with left ventricular dysfunction or heart failure early after myocardial infarction$

Acceptable indication but of uncertain efficacy and may be controversial Level B
Reduction of morbidity in mild to moderate heart failure
Reduction of mortality in mild to moderate heart failure

*Careful monitoring in patients at risk for hyperkalemia including diabetes, high-dose ACE inhibition and renal failure is required.
$This recommendation applies to eplerenone; all others apply to spironolactone.

---

potassium loss. Further, it activates the sympathetic nervous system, stimulates myocardial and vascular fibrosis, and is a component of the circulating renin–angiotensin–aldosterone system.[41–44]

Although aldosterone antagonists have diuretic effects, they differ from other diuretic agents in that they are neuroendocrine antagonists and thereby have a potential to be effective in the long-term treatment of patients with CHF. In particular, spironolactone was evaluated in the RALES study in which 1663 patients in NYHA class III or IV were randomized to active drug or placebo.[45] Spironolactone was initiated at 25 mg/day with adjustments to 12.5 or 50 mg depending on serum potassium. Ninety-five percent of the patients were on ACE inhibitors but only 11% had a background therapy of beta-blockers. The trial was discontinued early after a mean follow-up period of 24 months because of beneficial effect of spironolactone. There were 386 (46%) deaths in the placebo group and 284 (35%) in the spironolactone group; the relative risk attributed to spironolactone was 0.70 (95% confidence interval (CI) 0.60–0.82, $P < 0.001$) attributed mostly to a lower risk from sudden cardiac death. The RALES trial demonstrates that improved antagonism of the renin–angiotensin system by spironolactone reduces the risk of both morbidity and mortality in CHF. However, shortly after the publication of the RALES trial results, there was an apparent increase in admissions for hyperkalemia attributed to initiation of the drug,[46] highlighting the challenges of translating RCT data into sound clinical practice (e.g. appropriate patient selection and protocol-based monitoring of potassium levels).

Subsequently, in a different population (early post myocardial infarction (MI) with left ventricular dysfunction or heart failure), the selective aldosterone receptor blocker eplerenone was shown to reduce all-cause mortality and cardiovascular deaths, with effects most noticeable within the first 30 days following MI. This early effect suggests that the benefit may be mediated more by protection against hypokalemia than through inhibition of aldosterone. In fact, while cases of serious hyperkalemia were more common with study drug compared with placebo (5.5% versus 3.9%), the incidence of hypokalemia was decreased by more than half (from 8.4% to 3.1%).[47,48]

Vasodilators: acute therapy

Vasodilation reduces left ventricular afterload and preload and these beneficial effects were observed as early as 1956,[49,50] but it was not until the 1970s that the concept was widely accepted.[51,52] The first drugs used were pure vasodilators, such as nitroprusside, nitroglycerin, and phentolamine. Later, agents with combined effects were developed. Examples of combination therapies are the inotropic drugs with simultaneous vasodilation, such as milrinone, and the ACE inhibitors, both of which are reviewed in other sections of this chapter.

Reduction of afterload and preload in CHF improves left ventricular performance according to the Frank–Starling relation with less myocardial oxygen demand and increased cardiac output.[53,54] Further, vasodilation might theoretically reduce valvular regurgitation by means of afterload reduction and may improve organ dysfunction by acting directly on selected vascular beds, such as the coronary and renal vasculature.

Nitroglycerin, nitroprusside and, in the United States, nesiritide have been used for acute short-term vasodilation therapy in heart failure. However, the clinical trials data for these drugs are either limited or controversial.

Nitroglycerin
Nitroglycerin causes smooth muscle cell relaxation and vasodilation of arterial and venous vessels through action on guanylate cyclase and the generation of cyclic guanosine monophosphate.[55] Nitrates are conventionally used

topically or as an intravenous infusion; administration causes reduction in left ventricular filling pressures within 3–5 minutes, mainly by venodilation and lowering of preload.[56-61] Further, nitroglycerin reduces systemic vascular resistance and afterload, with ensuing improvement in cardiac output. It is also conceivable that nitrate therapy favorably affects myocardial perfusion and oxygen supply/demand ratio.[62,63] However, tolerance occurs early and may limit effectiveness.

Nitroprusside

Nitroprusside generates nitric oxide and nitrosothiols, which stimulate guanylate cyclase to increase intracellular cGMP. Smooth muscle cell relaxation is rapidly induced after administration. Sodium nitroprusside is converted to cyanide and is metabolized to thiocyanate, which may accumulate and lead to thiocyanate toxicity during prolonged nitroprusside therapy. Toxicity is rare during short-term administration ($<3\,\mu g/kg/min$ for less than 72 hours) in the absence of renal failure. As compared to nitroglycerin, nitroprusside is more potent and causes a more pronounced arterial vasodilation; there are minor effects on the renal and hepatosplanchnic vasculature.[59] In contrast to nitroglycerin, nitroprusside may induce a coronary steal phenomenon.[64] Owing to its potent vasodilation property, nitroprusside may cause adverse hypotension, especially in cases of inadequate filling pressure.

Nesiritide

Brain natriuretic factor, or nesiritide, was shown in early studies to lower filling pressures and improve patient report of symptoms. Colucci and investigators demonstrated a dose-dependent reduction in pulmonary capillary wedge pressure at 6 hours in a double-blinded placebo-controlled study.[65] Subsequently, the VMAC trial demonstrated improvements in PCWP at 3 hours compared to placebo (and comparable to nitroglycerin), with greater reductions compared to nitroglycerin (TNG) seen at 24 hours, perhaps reflecting tachyphylaxis to the nitrate therapy. Patient self-report of dyspnea also favored nesiritide.[66]

Following approval by the Food and Drug Administration in the United States, a series of controversial papers that included retrospectively reanalyzed published and unpublished data suggested that the drug might exacerbate renal dysfunction and worsen 30-day mortality rates.[67,68] The mechanism by which these effects occur was not clearly delineated but the impact on clinical practice was swift, leading to a marked decrease in use.[69] As a result, a panel of experts and the FDA reiterated that the major benefit is relief of dyspnea and the dose used to achieve this benefit is $0.01\,\mu g/kg/min$. In response to the concerns raised by the studies, a large randomized double-blinded outcomes clinical trial has been initiated. At the same time, other natriuretic peptides are either in clinical use (caperitide in Japan) or in clinical trials (ularitide, CD-NP).

It is important to note that data are lacking to support the use of nesiritide as an intermittent outpatient therapy[70] and in that context the data parallel what is known about the use of intermittent inotropic therapy.

Newer vasodilators

A number of other novel agents are in clinical trials for use in the acute phase including adenosine antagonists[71,72] and relaxin,[73] a naturally occurring peptide that modulates cardiovascular responses to pregnancy.[73] In addition, a direct myosin activator, CK1827452, will be studied both acutely using intravenous delivery and then, on conversion to oral formulation, chronically upon discharge, following the paradigm established in the EVEREST trial.

Effects of long-term vasodilator therapy

Nitrates and hydralazine Oral nitroglycerin and hydralazine have been studied, either alone or in combination. The effects on left ventricular function and hemodynamics are similar to the acute effects of vasodilators described above.[74,75]

Hydralazine was available as an antihypertensive agent when vasodilator therapy was adopted as a therapeutic strategy in CHF. Hydralazine acts as a dominant arterial vasodilator but has probably also mild inotropic properties, which might be due to a reflex activation of sympathetic activity.[76,77] This inotropic action might be responsible for a less favorable effect on myocardial oxygen consumption counteracting the unloading effects of vasodilation.[78,79]

The addition of a nitrate to hydralazine causes a greater effect on the reduction in filling pressures than can be achieved by hydralazine alone.[80] In view of the beneficial action of nitrates on coronary dynamics, a nitrate should be added to hydralazine therapy in patients with significant coronary artery disease.[81] However, despite the focus on direct venous and arterial vasodilation, current thinking about mechanism has focused on the nitrate component as a nitric oxide donor and hydralazine as an agent that mitigates nitrate tolerance through a complex mechanism mediated by NADH oxidase.[82] This mechanism has been used to explain the possible race-based differential clinical effect seen among African Americans compared with Caucasians, inferred from the first two V-HeFT trials.

V-HeFT-I was the first placebo-controlled clinical trial to study the effect of any vasodilator on survival in patients with chronic heart failure. The study randomized 642 patients with mild to moderate heart failure to placebo, prazosin or the combination of hydralazine and isosorbide dinitrate. Two years after randomization, the survival in the hydralazine-isosorbide treated group was significantly better than the placebo group ($P < 0.028$); for the entire follow-up, the difference trended toward significance ($P = 0.093$). Of note, the mortality rate in the prazosin group was not different from the placebo group.[83]

The second V-HeFT study compared the efficacy of hydralazine and isosorbide with that of enalapril. Two years after randomization, the all-cause mortality was 18% in the enalapril group as compared with 25% in the hydralazine-isosorbide group ($P = 0.016$). For the total follow-up, the difference was not significant ($P = 0.08$).[84]

A retrospective analysis of both V-HeFT-1 and V-HeFT-2 suggested that African Americans derived benefit from the hydralazine-nitrate combination, whereas Caucasians, presumably most of European descent, did not.[85] Conceptually, this analysis was based on a series of observations that suggested a relative deficiency of nitric oxide in African Americans, though the exact nature of the defect(s) has not been established.

To test this hypothesis, 1050 self-identified African Americans with NYHA class III or IV heart failure were randomized in a survival trial with a three times daily formulation of hydralazine and nitrate.[86,87] A composite endpoint was used, combining mortality, quality of life as measured on the Minnesota Living with Heart Failure Questionnaire and time to first hospitalization; each component was statistically significant in favor of the combination therapy. Most pronounced was the impact on mortality, which declined from 10.2% in placebo-treated patients to 6.2% in patients on active therapy. The cohorts were well managed, with high percentages on conventional treatment with ACE inhibitor, angiotensin receptor blocker and beta-blocker. The magnitude of this change parallels or exceeds almost all other double-blinded placebo-controlled trials and as such represents a significant achievement. However, while providing an opportunity to advance medical therapy for CHF, the controversial approval based on race by the US Food and Drug Adminstration and other factors such as three times daily therapy have negatively impacted its adoption by practitioners.

Calcium channel blockers The role for calcium channel blockers remains very limited in patients with CHF. With the first-generation calcium channel blocker nifedipine, vasodilatory effects are counterbalanced by negative inotropy and additional deleterious effects on hemodynamics, neurohormonal activation and, not surprisingly, disease progression.[88,89] The effects of diltiazem were unfavorable in patients with CHF in conjunction with myocardial infarction in a large placebo-controlled trial in 1237 patients.[90] Second-generation calcium channel blockers have not been extensively studied in patients with heart failure, but there are indications of a risk for clinical deterioration with drugs such as nisoldipine and nicardipine.[91,92] The second-generation calcium channel blocker felodipine caused vasodilation and an increase in cardiac output during 8 weeks of treatment in a placebo-controlled trial[93] but the effect on survival was neutral.[94]

Amlodipine, a third-generation calcium channel blocker, was investigated in the PRAISE trial.[95] Among more than 1100 patients with NYHA III–IV heart failure, the overall effect on mortality as well as on the combined endpoint mortality and hospitalization was neutral but there were significantly fewer endpoints in the non-ischemic group treated with amlodipine as compared to patients on placebo (22% vs 35%, $P < 0.001$). As a consequence, patients with non-ischemic etiology in NYHA class IIIb or IV heart failure (n = 1652) were randomized to placebo or amlodipine 10 mg/day.[96] There was no significant difference in all-cause or cardiac mortality and cardiac event rates between the two groups. The data from PRAISE and the felodipine trials suggest therapeutic neutrality; however, it is likely that both amlodipine and felodipine may be used safely to treat concomitant angina or hypertension in patients with CHF, if other proven drugs such as ACE inhibitors and beta-blockers are ineffective or not tolerated. All other drugs in this class are not indicated in any treatment algorithm for heart failure.

Other vasodilators Other potent vasodilators, such as prazosin and minoxidil, are not indicated in the short- or long-term management of CHF. Several other drugs with multiple effects including vasodilation have failed in clinical trials. For example, flosequinan, a vasodilator with a combined venous and arterial effect and possible positive inotropic and chronotropic effects, was associated with increased mortality in a large multicenter trial (PROFILE).[97] Additionally, the prostacyclin epoprostenol, which might improve hemodynamics, has been shown to have an adverse effect on mortality in severe heart failure.[98]

Drugs affecting the renin–angiotensin system

ACE inhibitors

ACE inhibitors were introduced for the treatment of heart failure within the last 25 years. Their potential value was

---

BOX 47.4 Documented value of vasodilators

Proven indication: always acceptable Level A
Short-term reduction of afterload in cases with acute heart failure
The combination hydralazine-isosorbide dinitrate can be used for long-term treatment in patients who do not tolerate ACE inhibitors or ARBs as add-on therapy in African American patients

Acceptable indication but of uncertain efficacy and may be controversial Level B
Third-generation calcium channel blockers may be used for symptomatic treatment of concomitant conditions such as angina pectoris or hypertension

Not proven: potentially harmful (contraindicated) Level C
Vasodilators other than hydralazine-isosorbide dinitrate and third-generation calcium channel blockers may increase mortality during long-term treatment
Treatment of patients with concomitant significant aortic or mitral stenosis

suggested by studies showing attenuated LV remodeling after myocardial infarction[99,100] and improved symptoms,[101] hemodynamics[102,103] and survival.[104] Multiple landmark studies have reported effects of ACE inhibitors on survival in patients at risk for heart failure and those with clinically manifest disease. In a similar way, these trials have demonstrated benefit across NYHA classes I–IV.[105] As a consequence, the use of ACE inhibitors is supported by all contemporary published clinical practice guidelines.

Effects on exercise capacity and hemodynamics An extensive review of these data[106] suggested that ACE inhibitors improve exercise capacity, consistent with changes in symptoms. In addition, ACE inhibitors were documented in early studies to induce beneficial hemodynamic responses. These effects included a vasodilatory effect and an increased cardiac output, increased stroke volume, and reduced pulmonary wedge pressure.[102,103]

Survival trials The first major trial, CONSENSUS, included 253 patients in NYHA class IV randomized to receive placebo or enalapril. After a follow-up of 6 months (primary objective), the overall mortality was reduced by 27% ($P = 0.003$). The number of days of hospital care was reduced and NYHA classification significantly improved with enalapril.[104] In the Studies of Left Ventricular Treatment (SOLVD) trial, 2569 patients with symptomatic heart failure NYHA class II–III received placebo or enalapril besides conventional heart failure therapy.[107] After an average follow-up of 41.4 months, mortality was significantly reduced from 40% to 35% ($P = 0.0036$), most notably reducing deaths attributed to progressive heart failure. Hospitalizations for heart failure were also reduced and symptoms and quality of life assessed by questionnaire were improved.[108]

The early post infarct cohort was examined in the Survival and Ventricular Enlargement (SAVE) trial, in which 2231 patients with ejection fraction of 40% or less, but without overt heart failure or symptoms of myocardial ischemia, were randomly assigned treatment with captopril or placebo.[109] Mortality from all causes was 20% in the captopril group and 25% in the placebo group (relative risk (RR) 19%, $P = 0.019$). In a similar evaluation (the TRACE study) with trandolapril, 1749 patients with left ventricular dysfunction were randomly assigned to treatment with placebo or active study drug.[110] Treatment was initiated 3–7 days from the onset of myocardial infarction. All-cause mortality in the placebo group was 42.3% and 34.7% in the trandolapril group, a 22% relative reduction of mortality ($P = 0.00065$). Finally, in the AIRE study, 2006 patients with clinical evidence of heart failure any time after the index infarction were randomly allocated to treatment with ramipril or placebo on day 3–10 from the onset of infarction.[111] Mortality from all causes at the end of the study was

17% in the ramipril group and 23% in the placebo group (RR 27%, $P = 0.002$) with a mean follow-up of 15 months. Taken together, these studies provide incontrovertible support for the use of ACE inhibitors in post-MI patients with left ventricular dysfunction.

Dose and class effects: clinical questions remain Uncertainties about the importance of dose of ACE inhibitor and class effects have stimulated debate and clinical evaluation. Two dose ranges of lisinopril were compared in the ATLAS trial. Patients with CHF (n = 3164) and ejection fraction <30% were randomized to a low dose of lisinopril (2.5–5.0 mg/day) or a high dose (32.5–35 mg/day) for a median of 45.7 months.[112] There were 717 deaths in the low-dose group versus 666 in the high-dose group (hazard ratio (HR) 0.92; $P = 0.128$) for the high dose. The combined endpoint of all-cause mortality or hospitalization for any reason showed a hazard ratio of 0.88 (95% CI 0.82–0.96, $P = 0.002$). The side effects and tolerability were similar in the two groups.

These findings indicate that patients with heart failure should generally be titrated up from low doses of an ACE inhibitor, but suggest that a difference in efficacy between intermediate and high doses of an ACE inhibitor is likely to be small. Thus, patients should be titrated to dose levels achieved in the clinical trials. The value of additional dose levels such as greater than 20 mg per day of lisinopril remains uncertain but can be viewed as supported in part by the results of the ATLAS trial.

With regard to the relative benefits of different ACE inhibitors, there are no large comparative studies that provide definitive evidence of the superiority of one ACE inhibitor over another. Nevertheless, it is widely acknowledged that these drugs differ in a number of fundamental respects: the ability to bind to tissue ACE, chemical structure, pharmacodynamics, pharmacokinetics and the supporting clinical trials data.[113] In an attempt to address the clinical relevance of different ACE inhibitors, Pilote and investigators compared 1-year survival among elderly post-MI patients using data from hospital discharge records and pharmacy databases in the province of Quebec, Canada.[114] Attempts were made to correct for the propensity to receive a particular ACE inhibitor and to the extent accomplished, the data suggest a significant difference among the seven options for ACE inhibitors available on the provincial formulary, favoring ramipril. These data support the concept but do not provide absolute confirmation that the different ACE inhibitors have different long-term clinical benefits.

Trials on prevention A reduced incidence of heart failure by ACE inhibitors has been demonstrated in several trials. In the prevention arm of the SOLVD study,[107] the incidence of heart failure and the number of hospitalizations were reduced and similar findings were reported in SAVE.[109] In an overview of ACE inhibitor trials,[108] the preventive potential of ACE inhibitors is clearly demonstrated.

Three landmark studies have been performed among patients at risk for heart failure: HOPE,[115] EUROPA[115] and PEACE.[116] These trials, when considered together, suggest a role for ACE inhibitors in heart failure prevention,[117] a topic covered in more detail elsewhere in this book.

Overall, it is clear that the number needed to treat to save one life in a year is significantly higher when heart failure prevention is the goal rather than treatment of established disease. Nevertheless, while the exact role for ACE inhibitors as a component of contemporary primary prevention is not absolutely clear, use of this class of drug in defined subgroups is highly justified. Those most at risk, including diabetics and hypertensives not at goal, should be strongly considered for ACE inhibitors as part of a comprehensive approach to risk factor modification.

Cost effectiveness In asymptomatic patients with left ventricular dysfunction after an acute myocardial infarction (SAVE), captopril was cost-effective in patients aged 50–80 years compared to other interventions.[119] Ramipril therapy for patients with clinical heart failure after acute myocardial infarction appears highly cost effective when assessed using data from the AIRE study.[120] ACE inhibitor treatment was also considered cost-effective in an economic evaluation of five independent studies.[121] For example, enalapril therapy for patients with heart failure was cost-effective in SOLVD. Given the fact that many of the ACE inhibitors are available in lower cost generic formulations, the cost effectiveness now even more strongly favors this class of drug.

Clinical perspective All patients with documented left ventricular systolic dysfunction (ejection fraction <35–40%) should be treated with an ACE inhibitor unless contraindications exist (including systolic blood pressure less than 80 mmHg, pronounced renal dysfunction, history of angioneurotic edema and important valve stenosis). Treatment should be continued long term. The dosage to be used should be titrated from a low dose and increased to the levels employed in clinical trials. If no hypotension or renal dysfunction develops, titration up to enalapril 10 mg 2×/day, captopril 50 mg 3×/day, ramipril 10 mg/day, trandolapril 4 mg/day and quinapril 10 mg 2×/day will be most effective.

Angiotensin II receptor (AT₁) antagonists

As ACE inhibition does not provide complete blockade from the synthesis of angiotensin II, a more effective blockade has been postulated by specific antagonism at the

---

BOX 47.5 Documented value of ACE inhibitors

Proven indication: always acceptable Level A
Symptomatic chronic heart failure and documented systolic myocardial dysfunction. Improved survival and reduced morbidity have been demonstrated. Symptoms will be attenuated and exercise capacity improved
Following acute myocardial infarction with clinical signs of heart failure or systolic dysfunction (ejection fraction <40%). Improved survival and reduced morbidity have been demonstrated
Prevention of cardiovascular events, including heart failure, in patients with atherosclerotic disease or in patients with diabetes mellitus and additional risk factors

Acceptable indication but of uncertain efficacy and may be controversial Level A
Heart failure from diastolic dysfunction

Not proven: potentially harmful (contraindicated) Level C
Treatment of patients with significant aortic or mitral stenosis
Treatment of patients with hypotension (systolic blood pressure <80 mmHg)
Treatment of patients with pronounced renal dysfunction

---

receptor (AT₁) level. One of the early ARB trials was ELITE-II, conducted in 3152 class II–IV patients with ejection fractions (EF) of <40%, randomized to losartan 50 mg/day or captopril 50 mg 3×/day.[122] There was no significant difference in all-cause mortality or sudden death (hazard ratio 1.13; 95% CI 0.95–1.35, $P = 0.16$). Significantly fewer patients in the losartan group discontinued study treatment because of adverse effects (9.7 vs 14.7%; $P < 0.001$). In the small RESOLVD trial, there were no differences between groups receiving candesartan and enalapril in exercise tolerance, ventricular function or symptomatic status over 43 weeks.[123] However, combined therapy with candasartan plus enalapril markedly reduced ventricular volumes and improved EF compared to either agent alone.

The major series of ARB trials began with Val-HeFT, a study of 5010 patients in class II–IV and EF of <40% randomized to placebo or valsartan.[124] Dose levels were increased to 160 mg twice a day. Background therapy with an ACE inhibitor was present in 93%. There was no effect on all-cause mortality (484 in the placebo group vs 495 in the valsartan group; RR 1.02, 95% CI 0.90–1.15, $P = 0.8$). In the other primary endpoint, mortality or hospitalization, there was a significant reduction from 801 (32.1%) to 723 (28.8%) (RR 0.87, 95% CI 0.79–0.96, $P = 0.009$).

The CHARM Program was designed to study the effects of candesartan in a broad spectrum of patients with CHF. Three component trials included patients with reduced systolic LV function (EF <40%) in two (CHARM-Alternative and CHARM-Added) and patients with preserved LV (EF >40%) in one (CHARM-Preserved). The primary outcome in each component trial was cardiovascular death or hospital admission for heart failure. In CHARM-Overall, the trials were combined and the effect on all-cause mortality was assessed.

Symptomatic patients with CHF intolerant to ACE inhibitors because of cough, symptomatic hypotension or renal dysfunction were included in CHARM-Alternative (n = 2028). Candesartan significantly reduced cardiovascular death or hospital admission for heart failure by 23% (P = 0.0004), whereas the rate of discontinuation of the study drug was similar to placebo.[125] In CHARM-Added (n = 2548), candesartan on top of ACE inhibitors significantly reduced the primary outcome of cardiovascular death or hospital admission for heart failure by 15% (P = 0.011). Hospitalizations for heart failure were also reduced significantly (P = 0.014).[126] In CHARM-Preserved (n = 3023), there was a non-significant effect on mortality. Hospitalizations for heart failure as reported by the investigators were reduced by 15% (P = 0.017).[127]

In all patients with symptomatic heart failure (n = 7599), irrespective of background ACE inhibitor or beta-blocker therapy, candesartan reduced all-cause mortality by 9% (P = 0.055), particularly among those with left ventricular systolic dysfunction (HR 0.88; P = 0.018).[128] Among these patients, the effects on mortality were seen early; the HRs were 0.67 and 0.82 (both P < 0.001) at 1 and 2 years respectively. Further, hospital admissions for heart failure were reduced significantly by 21% (P < 0.001).

ARB and background therapy

In the Val-HeFT trials, a *post-hoc* analysis suggested that the treatment effect with valsartan was attenuated by background beta-blocker therapy. This could not be confirmed in CHARM-Added where a similar effect of candesartan was observed regardless of background beta-blocker. In a meta-analysis, the effect of ARBs may be attenuated by background beta-blocker treatment.[129] In contrast, based on Val-HeFT and in particular CHARM-Added, the effect of valsartan and candesartan was additive on top of background ACE-inhibitor therapy with reduction of the composite primary outcome in both trials.

ARB summary

The trials with ARBs provide definitive proof that this class of drug can be used for treatment of patients with symptomatic heart failure who do not tolerate ACE inhibitors. The treatment effect is at least of similar magnitude as that achieved by ACE inhibitors. There is also an added, albeit modest effect on morbidity and mortality on top of ACE inhibitor therapy.

BOX 47.6 Documented value of angiotensin receptor blockers

Proven indication: always acceptable Level A
Symptomatic treatment of patients with heart failure who do not tolerate ACE inhibitors to improve morbidity and mortality

Acceptable indication: Level A
Add-on therapy in patients with heart failure on background therapy of ACE inhibitor

---

Non-digitalis inotropic drugs: short-term therapy but no long-term role

Vast efforts have been expended to develop drugs that might increase contractility or the state of inotropy. However, it has become increasingly evident that these drugs are associated with important negative effects in both the short and long term.

Inotropic agents differ according to their mode of action.[130] Several of these drugs increase the intracellular level of cyclic adenosine monophosphate (cAMP), either by receptor stimulation (beta-adrenergic agonists) or by decreasing cAMP breakdown (phosphodiesterase inhibitors). One class of agents affects intracellular calcium mechanisms by release of sarcoplasmic reticulum calcium or by increasing the sensitivity of contractile proteins to calcium. Further, there are inotropic drugs with multiple mechanisms of action.

Dobutamine

Drugs with beta-receptor agonist properties induce an increase in intracellular cAMP activity by stimulation of cellular receptors. Nearly 50 years ago, patients with cardiogenic shock were treated with beta-receptor agonists isoproterenol and norepinephrine.[131] It was realized that both drugs had potential negative effects, such as an increased risk for arrhythmias or, in the case of norepinephrine, untoward vasoconstriction. Dobutamine, a drug that is a modification of the isoproterenol molecule, has beta-1, beta-2 and alpha-1 adrenergic activity.[132] Dobutamine induces vasodilation in combination with an increase in contractility, leading to an increase in stroke volume and cardiac output.[133–135] An enhancement of contractility is usually associated with an increase in myocardial oxygen consumption.[136] Side effects, such as arrhythmias or an unfavorable blood pressure response, are usually modest. Dobutamine can only be administered intravenously, in doses from 2 μg/kg/min up to 20–25 μg /kg/min.[137] It has been noticed that dobutamine may decrease beta-receptor sensitivity,[138,139] and prolonged infusion over 96 hours has been associated with a decrease in the hemodynamic effect by as much as 50%[140] ("tachyphylaxis"). The role of dobutamine is limited to hemodynamic support for patients in or near a state of cardiogenic shock. The use of the drug on an intermittent basis is not recommended though it has been used continuously for palliation in end-stage patients.[141]

Dopamine

Dopamine is an adrenergic agonist with predominantly beta-1 receptor activity.[142,143] This drug increases contractility with minor effects on heart rate or blood pressure. At low doses (0.5–2.0 µg /kg/min), dopamine acts on dopaminergic receptors, while at doses above 5.0 µg /kg/min it has effects mediated through beta-1 receptors, and at higher doses also through alpha-receptors. Infusion at low doses causes dilation of smooth muscles in renal, mesenteric, and coronary arteries, leading to an increase in diuresis[144,145] though this therapy remains highly controversial.[146]

Milrinone

Through inhibition of cAMP breakdown, the phosphodiesterase inhibitors bypass the beta-receptor pathway. Milrinone, related to amrinone (which fell into disfavor because of thrombocytopenia), enhances myocardial contractility and has potent vasodilatory effects,[147–149] without thrombocytopenia.[150] Whereas short-term administration may improve myocardial performance and clinical condition in CHF,[149,151] the long-term effects of an oral formulation were discouraging. Specifically, in the PROMISE trial, 1088 class III–IV patients were given milrinone or placebo. There was a 28% increase in mortality in patients treated with milrinone (95% CI 1–61%, $P = 0.038$).[152]

Nevertheless, in those instances when an inotrope is required and selected, the choice of agent may be dictated, at least in part, by concomitant therapy with beta-blockers. In particular, use of milrinone should be strongly considered because the drug bypasses the beta-receptor. Indeed, Lowes and colleagues demonstrated that while dobutamine can bring about a comparable acute increase in cardiac index, it did so only at doses that are not usually used to treat heart failure: 15–20 µg /kg/minute.[153]

Other inotropic agents: a history marked by failure

The list of inotropes (or drugs with both inotropic and other effects) that have failed in clinical trials is large. Interested readers are referred to an earlier iteration of this chapter (second edition) and various clinical reviews for more detailed descriptions.[154,155] The list of drugs includes ibopamine (an orally active dopaminergic agonist), xamoterol (beta-adrenergic blocking and high partial agonist activity), pimobendan (multiple actions including phosphodiesterase [PDE] inhibition), milrinone (oral formulation), vesnarinone (multiple effects) and flosequinon (multiple effects). More recently, levosimendan and enoximone (see below) were extensively studied but also failed in pivotal studies. Although drug development efforts continue, as for example

with the novel drug CK-1827452, the goal of finding an inotropic drug that does not have proarrhythmic effects or increase energy expenditure may prove to be futile.

Levosimendan A calcium-sensitizing agent with properties similar to pimobendan, levosimendan looked very promising from the standpoint of hemodynamics and clinical outcomes in a number of early moderately sized clinical trials.[156–158] The drug and one active metabolite with a prolonged half-life demonstrate a novel mechanism of action: calcium-dependent binding to troponin C, facilitating and prolonging actin-myosin protein cross-bridge formation without an increase in calcium flux or energy requirement. In addition, vasodilation is achieved through smooth muscle cell relaxation. However, in two large multicenter international trials, the outcomes were mixed. While the drug attained its primary novel composite endpoint in the short-term REVIVE study,[159] safety issues including hypotension, ventricular tachycardia and atrial fibrillation were more apparent in the active study arm compared with placebo. In the companion SURVIVE trial in which the drug was compared to dobutamine,[160] there was no difference in survival through 180 days with only a 2% absolute difference between the two treatment groups. In retrospect, it was likely not realistic to expect that an infusion of an intravenous drug during a heart failure hospitalization would result in improved outcomes at 6 months. Currently, the lack of demonstrable efficacy, combined with concerns over safety, have stalled the clinical development program of this novel drug.

Enoximone In several Phase II/III trials, enoximone failed to achieve the primary endpoints. For example, in the EMOTE trial, enoximone did not significantly increase the likelihood of weaning from dobutamine versus placebo though there were favorable trends in time to death or reinitiation of intravenous inotrope. In the pivotal ESSENTIAL trial, the hazard ratio for time to first cardiovascular hospitalization or all-cause mortality was near unity and there were no differences in patient global assessments.[161]

Beta-adrenergic blockade

Clinicians have generally been cautious in using beta-blockers in patients with CHF, even though investigators in the early 1970s were already proposing a possible beneficial effect of beta-blockers in such cases.[162,163] Rigorous clinical trials data gathered during the last 15 years have incontrovertibly confirmed the beneficial role of beta-blockers in mild, moderate and severe heart failure.

Hemodynamic and neurohormonal effects
The short-term effects of beta-adrenergic blockade differ markedly from the long-term effects. After IV administra-

---

BOX 47.7 Documented value of inotropic drugs

Proven indication: always acceptable
Short-term improvement of symptoms in patients with severe heart failure **Level A**
Bridging towards more definitive surgical treatment, such as cardiac transplantation **Level C**

Acceptable indication but of uncertain efficacy and may be controversial Level B
Long-term treatment in chronic heart failure for patients with refractory symptoms in spite of maximal medical management.

Not proven: potentially harmful (contraindicated) Level B
Intermittent short-term treatment in chronic heart failure

---

tion, there is a rapid reduction in heart rate, contractility, and blood pressure, with ensuing fall in cardiac output.[164–166] Intraventricular volumes, stroke volume, and ejection fraction are unaffected.[164] Beta-blockers with vasodilating properties cause an acute reduction in afterload with reduction in filling pressures.[164–167]

During 1–3 months of treatment, positive diastolic effects have been observed and these effects probably precede full effects on cardiac systolic function.[165,168] During longer-term treatment (3–12 months), beta blockers induce myocardial improvement, as expressed by an increase in ejection fraction, cardiac output, and exercise capacity.[170–174] Eichhorn and colleagues documented decreases in echocardiographically measured indices of left ventricular function during the initiation phase of therapy but improvements thereafter.[171] Similar to ACE inhibitors, beta-blockers attenuate left ventricular remodeling.[169,175–177]

Acute administration of metoprolol causes a reflex increase in peripheral catecholamines without alteration of the transmyocardial gradient.[165] Some studies suggest a beneficial reduction in peripheral norepinephrine level.[178–182] A decrease in renin–angiotensin activity has been noted, while the levels of atrial natriuretic peptides might increase on a short-term basis.[175]

Effects on quality of life and hospitalizations

Studies have demonstrated a reduction of the need for hospitalizations with bisoprolol,[183] metoprolol,[184] and carvedilol,[185] improvement in quality of life[186] and both patient and physician global assessments of heart failure symptoms. However, quality of life scores were not improved in the US carvedilol studies or in the MERIT-HF study.[187–189]

Effects on survival

One of the first studies of beta-blockers in chronic heart failure showed a reduced mortality in patients treated by beta-blockade as compared with historical controls.[162] Not until 1993, when the MDC trial was published, did additional information on clinical outcome become available. This study demonstrated a 34% reduction in the combined endpoint deaths and need for heart transplantation ($P = 0.058$) in 383 patients with idiopathic dilated cardiomyopathy, treated with placebo or metoprolol.[186] A late follow-up of this study showed that this trend was maintained or possibly reinforced, regarding all-cause mortality and actual cardiac transplantations 3 years after randomization.[190] In the CIBIS study, bisoprolol was used in a placebo-controlled trial in 641 patients; overall there was a non-significant reduction in mortality (RR 0.80, 95% CI 0.56–1.15, $P = 0.22$).[191] Data from four pooled carvedilol studies in the USA were combined in an analysis that demonstrated a markedly lower mortality in the carvedilol group (22 of 696 [3.2%] vs 31 of 398 [7.8%] deaths; RR 65%, 95% CI 39–80, $P < 0.01$).[192] However, there was no statistically beneficial effect of carvedilol regarding survival in the smaller Australia–New Zealand trial of 415 patients with chronic heart failure of varying etiology.[193] None of the aforementioned trials was designed to specifically study mortality, and the number of events in each trial was relatively modest.

Subsequently, a series of landmark studies were prospectively designed to test the potential survival benefits of long-term beta-blockade. The first major study was CIBIS-II in which the beta-1 selective antagonist bisoprolol was tested versus placebo in 2647 patients in NYHA III–IV and an ejection fraction of <35.[183] Study drug was initiated at a dose of 1.25 mg/day and was progressively increased to 10 mg/day over 3 months. The study was stopped by the safety committee after a mean follow-up of 1.3 years. All-cause mortality was significantly lower with bisoprolol than with placebo (156 [11.8%] vs 228 [17.3%]; HR 0.66, 95% CI 0.54–0.81, $P < 0.0001$). There were significantly fewer sudden deaths among patients on bisoprolol than in those on placebo (3.6% vs 6.3%; HR 0.56, $P = 0.001$).

In the MERIT-HF trial, metoprolol controlled release/extended release (CR/XL) was compared in 3991 patients with chronic heart failure in NYHA class II–IV and an ejection fraction of <0.40. Background therapy including an ACE inhibitor or an ARB was present in 95% of the patients. Treatment was initiated with metoprolol CR/XL 12.5–25 mg/day and titrated for 6–8 weeks up to target dose of 200 mg/day. This study was also stopped early on the recommendation of the independent safety committee. At a mean follow-up time of 1 year, all-cause mortality was lower in the metoprolol group than in the placebo group: 145 (7.2% per patient-year of follow-up) versus 217 deaths (11.0%) (RR 0.66, 95% CI 0.53–0.81, $P = 0.0009$). There were fewer sudden deaths in the metoprolol CR/XL group than in the placebo group (79 vs 132; RR 0.59, $P = 0.0002$) and fewer deaths from worsening heart failure (30 vs 58; RR 0.51, $P = 0.0023$).[184]

The COPERNICUS trial was performed in 2289 patients with symptomatic chronic heart failure with symptoms at rest or at minimal exertion.[185] Carvedilol was initiated with 3.125 mg ×2/day and titrated to 25 mg ×2/day. There was a significant reduction in all-cause mortality from 190 (18.5% per patient-year) to 130 (11.4%) with a hazard ratio of 0.65 (95% CI 0.52–0.81, $P = 0.0001$). The effect was consistent among a number of prespecified subgroups. In particular, the outcomes in a high-risk subgroup, defined by multiple antecedent hospitalizations or recent need for intravenous inotrope or very low ejection fraction, were as favorable as in the main study cohort when examined during both early and late follow-up.[194] It is important to note that most if not all of these patients would have been excluded from the early beta-blocker trials (including the US Carvedilol trials).

In a *post-hoc* subgroup analysis of patients in the MERIT-HF study with similar characteristics as the patients in the COPERNICUS trial, including an EF of <0.25 and NYHA class III–IV, there was a comparable reduction in all-cause mortality (45 [11%] vs 72 [18%] deaths; HR 0.61, 95% CI 0.11–0.58, $P = 0.0086$).[195]

All three large beta-blocker studies (CIBIS-II, MERIT-HF, COPERNICUS) had been stopped early because of clear evidence of benefit. In contrast, in the BEST trial, the effects of the non-selective beta-blocker bucindolol compared with placebo in 2708 patients with CHF in NYHA class III–IV were modest and not statistically significant.[196] Bucindolol was initiated with 3 mg 2×/day and titrated up over 6–8 weeks to 50–100 mg 2×/day. The study was prematurely terminated by the safety committee. Mortality was reduced from 447 deaths to 409 deaths (RR 0.91, 95% CI 0.88–1.02, $P = 0.12$). In a subgroup analysis, there was a heterogeneous response among groups analyzed. For example, patients with NYHA class IV or ejection fraction below 20% did not appear to benefit. Furthermore, among African Americans there was a 17% excess mortality, suggesting a lack of benefit among these patients. However, these were *post-hoc* analyses and not prespecified endpoints. The analysis has raised interesting questions about the reasons for the lack of a significant overall survival benefit, including the particular drug studied, the dose used and the population under study. Of note, patients at highest risk for mortality had the most marked reductions in plasma norepinephrine levels, paralleling findings with the centrally acting sympatholytic agent moxonidine (see below).

Subsequently, a study of genetic polymorphisms for the beta-1 receptor has suggested that patients homozygos for beta(1)-arg 389 had large and statistically significant reductions in both mortality and the combination of mortality and hospitalizations compared with placebo (38% and 34% respectively). In contrast, carriers of beta(1)-gly 389 had no benefit.[197] This effect is presumably mediated through differences in signal transduction. Whether these observations will translate into meaningful clinical decision making and establish a pharmacogenomic approach to therapeutics remains to be seen.

Further in the SENIORS trial,[198] the beta-1 selective blocker nebivolol, which has the ancillary property of vasodilation mediated through nitric oxide modulation, was evaluated in a heterogeneous older cohort of patients (mean age 76) with 35% having an ejection fraction exceeding 35%. As with other trials, the drug was uptitrated (from 1.25 mg to 10 mg with mean dose of active study drug achieved at 7.7 mg). At a mean follow-up of 21 months, somewhat longer than most placebo-controlled beta-blocker trials, the combined primary endpoint of all-cause mortality or cardiovascular hospitalization was decreased from 35.3% to 31.1% (HR 0.86, 95% CI 0.74–0.99, $P = 0.039$). However, mortality alone was not statistically impacted (HR 0.88, 95% CI 0.71–1.08, $P = 0.21$). The mixed picture has many possible explanations, though the population studied most likely explains some, if not all, of the reasons underlying the modest effects.[199]

Comparison of beta-blockers

Given the variability in clinical data and the known differences among the beta-blockers in terms of receptor blockade, half-lives and lipophilicity, it is reasonable to assume that not all drugs in this class are appropriate for patients with heart failure. At present, only three beta-blockers can be recommended (bisoprolol, metoprolol succinate and carvedilol) though an argument can be made for nebivolol. Are there differences among these agents? The data are confined to comparisons of metoprolol tartrate and carvedilol. For example, an early crossover study suggested that there are differences with respect to receptor effects, while long-term clinical effects were comparable.[200]

This issue was further explored in the COMET trial in which carvedilol and metoprolol were compared in 3042 patients with NYHA class II–IV heart failure and a prior admission for cardiovascular reasons. The mean age was 62 years and mean ejection fraction was 0.26 (±0.07). At a mean follow-up of 58 months (longer than in the placebo-controlled trials because both arms received active therapy), the primary endpoint of all-cause mortality was favorably impacted by carvedilol (target dose 25 mg bid) over metoprolol tartrate (target dose 50 mg bid), with a HR of 0.83 (95% CI 0.74–0.93, $P = 0.0017$). Median survival was 1.4 years longer with carvedilol. There was also a trend toward improvement in the combination of all-cause mortality and all-cause hospitalization.[201]

The results of the trial were widely debated: was this a true difference or an issue related to dose or the formulation of metoprolol? At the very least, the results suggest that the concept of class effect is dubious, especially when COMET is also interpreted in the context of the BEST result which did not parallel the outcomes described for the other major beta-blocker trials.[202–204]

Beta blockers and ACE inhibitors in de novo heart failure: which to start first?

For *de novo* patients with heart failure or for established patients with heart failure who are ACE inhibitor and beta-blocker naïve, it is appropriate to ask which drug should be started first. The CIBIS 3 Trial randomized 1010 patients in open-label fashion to receive bisoprolol or enalapril for 6 months followed by combination therapy from months 6 to 24.[205] The two strategies appeared to be similar when the endpoints of all-cause mortality and all-cause hospitalization were analyzed in blinded fashion. In reality, the trial may not markedly affect practice, largely because of its design. First, beta-blocker trials were all performed in patients with background ACE inhibitor therapy, leading to the common practice of initial initiation of this drug followed by the beta-blocker. Second, *de novo* patients may present with fluid overload, in which case ACE inhibitor therapy is safer as a first line agent. Finally, current guidelines do not advocate a waiting period of 6 months before initiation of combination therapy for heart failure; rather, both the ACE inhibitors and beta-blockers should be used early during initiation of medical therapy.

Beta blockers in the post-MI setting: preventing heart failure

Data from several older large post myocardial infarction trials suggested that beta-blockers would be beneficial when symptoms of heart failure are present.[206–208] These findings were first extended prospectively in the CAPRICORN study, in which carvedilol or placebo was given to 1959 patients with a recent myocardial infarction and signs of left ventricular dysfunction (EF <40%)[209] in a study design conceptually similar to SAVE, AIRE, TRACE and EPHESUS. There was no effect on the primary endpoint of mortality or cardiovascular hospitalization (HR ratio 0.92, 95% CI 0.80–1.07), but there was a statistically significant reduction in all-cause mortality with 166 (15%) versus 151 (12%) deaths (HR 0.77, 95% CI 0.60–0.98, $P = 0.03$). The risk reduction was of similar magnitude compared with previous post myocardial infarction trials with beta-blockers.

Clinical perspective: drug titration and intolerance

Due to initial negative inotropic effects, treatment with beta-blocker requires a titration procedure. Experience from the clinical trials suggests that it is possible to initiate drug therapy with high tolerability. Patients with both marked hypotension and tachycardia, and/or expressing severe decompensation, may not tolerate beta-blockers.

BOX 47.8 Documented value of beta-blockers

Proven indication: always acceptable Level A
To improve long-term survival in patients with mild to severe heart failure
To improve cardiac function and symptoms in patients with symptomatic chronic heart failure, already on conventional treatment with ACE inhibitors (or ARBs), diuretics or digitalis
To improve outcomes in patients with acute myocardial infarction and left ventricular dysfunction with or without symptomatic heart failure
Symptomatic treatment of patients with heart failure who do not tolerate ACE inhibitors

Acceptable indication but of uncertain efficacy and may be controversial Level B
Symptomatic heart failure from diastolic dysfunction

Not proven: potentially harmful (contraindicated) Level C
Acute decompensated heart failure
CHF with pronounced hypotension and/or bradycardia

Clinical euvolemia remains critical at the time of initiation or dose uptitration. In cases with significant bronchospastic disease, beta-blockers should be used with caution, and a selective beta-blocker would be preferred.

Overall, reports of intolerance have been uncommon in randomized trials, comparable to those of ACE inhibitors, though it is important to note that the trial with the most pronounced mortality effect (the *post hoc* evaluation of data from the US Carvedilol family of trials) had an open-label run-in phase. The low starting doses with different beta-blockers have been: bisoprolol 1.25 mg/day; carvedilol 3.125–6.25 mg 2×/day; metoprolol 12.5–25 mg/day; and nebivolol 1.25 mg/day. Doses are increased every 1–2 weeks, until maintenance doses of full conventional beta-blockade are achieved.

Although resting basal heart rate probably is probably important, it has not been possible to adequately identify responders from non-responders to beta-blocker therapy.

Central nervous system modulators

Moxonidine

Reduction of sympathetic nervous system activity can also be achieved by stimulating receptors within the central nervous system. Studies in this area have been performed with clonidine[210] and moxonidine. Moxonidine has been documented in several Phase II and III trials. In a study over 12 weeks in 97 patients, Swedberg and co-workers demonstrated a significant attenuation of plasma norepinephrine levels.[211] With a sustained-release preparation of moxonidine, a more prolonged and effective reduction of plasma norepinephrine of the order of 40–50% was achieved within 3 weeks of initiation.[212] However, in a large Phase III trial with moxonidine sustained release (MOXCON), an early increase in death rate and adverse events in the moxonidine SR group led to premature termination of the trial because of safety concerns after 1934 patients had been entered.[213] Final analysis revealed 54 deaths (5.5%) in the moxonidine SR group and 32 deaths (3.1%) in the placebo group. Survival curves revealed a significantly ($P = 0.005$) worse outcome in the moxonidine SR group. Hospitalization for heart failure, acute myocardial infarction, and adverse events were also more frequent in the moxonidine SR group. This trial terminated the efforts to explore whether CNS inhibition of adrenergic activation could be an alternative to beta-adrenergic blockade in heart failure.

Antiarrhythmic drugs in heart failure

Although progressive pump dysfunction is a common cause of death in heart failure, sudden death is probably the most common reason, and has been considered responsible for 25–50% of all deaths.[214–217] The majority of sudden deaths are due to ventricular arrhythmias[218] rather than primary asystole (though in patients dying of pump dysfunction, terminal bradycardia is common). The issue of antiarrhythmic therapy in heart failure patients has therefore been of major interest.

However, while frequent and complex ventricular arrhythmias may be predictive of sudden death, left ventricular dysfunction is a more powerful predictor.[219] Unfortunately, most antiarrhythmics cause a depression of left ventricular function. Furthermore, these drugs may have proarrhythmic effects, especially in cases of left ventricular dysfunction, prolonged QT and metabolic abnormalities such as hypokalemia and low serum magnesium that may accompany acute or chronic diuretic therapy.

In the landmark CAST study the efficacy of antiarrhythmic drugs in patients with left ventricular dysfunction after myocardial infarction and with complex ventricular arrhythmias was evaluated. Patients who responded with attenuation of arrhythmias after drug testing were randomized to encainide, flecainide or moricizine. The results showed an increase in mortality in patients treated with the first two of these agents.[220]

Subsequently, interest in amiodarone, a class III antiarrhythmic drug with no or little negative inotropic effect, increased. However, despite a promising, albeit mixed set of results in smaller trials,[221–225] the SCD-HeFT trial suggested that the drug had no impact on survival when used for primary prevention of sudden death in patients with left ventricular dysfunction and heart failure.[226]

Similarly, sotalol, a beta-blocker with class III antiarrhythmic properties, has not been found to reduce deaths

---

BOX 47.9 Documented value of antiarrhythmic therapy in heart failure

Proven indication: always acceptable Level A
Beta-adrenergic blockade in euvolemic patients with chronic heart failure

Not proven: potentially harmful (contraindicated) Level A
Class I antiarrhythmic drugs in patients with asymptomatic ventricular arrhythmias and heart failure
Class III antiarrhythmic drugs in patients with asymptomatic ventricular arrhythmias or when used for primary prevention of sudden cardiac death

---

from ventricular arrhythmias. On the contrary, a study with the non-beta blocker isoform d-sotalol in postmyocardial patients had to be terminated in advance because of an increased mortality in the sotalol group.[227]

Without question, the most impressive effects on sudden deaths have been found in the large survival studies with beta-blockers. Consistent effects were found with all three agents: bisoprolol, metoprolol, and carvedilol.[183–185] In addition, both aldosterone antagonists (spironolactone and eplerenone) as well as the angiotensin receptor blocker candasartan have been shown to play a role in reduction of sudden death, the former likely mediated in part by protection against hypokalemia.[45,47,228] Implantable cardioverter defibrillators are also widely used for prevention of sudden death from ventricular arrhythmias. The appropriate indications and selection of patients for these therapeutic devices are dealt with elsewhere in this book.

Other pharmacologic approaches

Given the success of ACE inhibitors, beta-blockers and aldosterone antagonists, the search for effective therapies that antagonize the effects of other neurohormones or by extension cytokines and inflammatory mediators that are upregulated in heart failure has been an ongoing focus of drug development. Although the knowledge gained from negative trials can be significant, a plethora of recent studies has not led to meaningful changes for patients. We review data from three classes of drug that have failed to improve clinical outcomes and are not part of the contemporary treatment algorithm for patients with heart failure.

Anti-TNF therapy

Two anti-TNF therapies have failed in clinical studies, despite a wealth of basic, preclinical and early phase human studies that suggested a potential role for the anti-cytokine anti-inflammatory treatment paradigm. In the RENEWAL program, etanercept, a soluble TNF antagonist, was studied in two companion placebo-controlled trials (RECOVER and RENAISSANCE).[229] The former randomized patients to study drug in two different dosing regimens (25 mg once or twice weekly) versus placebo; the latter evaluated dosing at 25 mg twice or three times weekly. Clinical status, a composite of death, heart faile hospitalization, patient global assessment and NYHA class, was measured. However, the trial was stopped early when the relative risk for the combination of mortality and heart failure hospitalization crossed unity, suggesting a lack of benefit. Another agent, infliximab (a chimeric monoclonal antibody to TNF), was evaluated in advanced (NYHA III–IV) heart failure in two doses versus placebo.[230] A trend toward an increase in a combined endpoint of death or heart failure hospitalization at 28 weeks was observed.

Vasopressin antagonism

Vasopressin antagonists, both V2 and combined V1/V2 antagonists, have been studied. Most clinical data come from tolvaptan, an oral non-peptide V2-receptor antagonist. Preliminary data derived from ACTIV, a Phase II dose-ranging study, demonstrated that tolvaptan elicited a statistically significant change in body weight at all doses examined compared to placebo.[231] However, there were no differences in clinical outcomes such as death or hospitalization though the study was underpowered to detect such a difference.

The lowest dose from ACTIV was selected for EVEREST which randomized patients within 48 hours of admission to receive active drug versus placebo.[232,233] A short-term outcomes trial with endpoints of body weight on day 7 or discharge and scoring on a global visual analog scale (VAS) was embedded in a long-term survival study, as patients were continued on medical therapy on discharge. The endpoints were all-cause mortality (superiority and non-inferiority) and a composite of cardiovascular death or heart failure hospitalization (superiority). In the short-term trial, loss of weight favored tolvaptan, albeit with modest changes. There was no change on the global VAS though relief of dyspnea was greater with tolvaptan on day 1. There were no statistically significant differences in the primary endpoints of the long-term trial. These findings seriously jeopardize the concept that long-term vasopressin antagonism has a role in the management of chronic heart failure.

At least one other vaptan, lixivaptan, another oral non-peptide V2 selective agent[234] is in clinical trials.

Endothelin antagonism

Despite the fact that endothelin and precursors are elevated in heart failure and correlate with prognosis,[235] several endothelin antagonists have been tested and have failed in clinical trials. In particular, both oral bosentan for chronic heart failure[236] and intravenous tezosentan for acutely decompensated heart failure[237] have not improved outcomes. These trials have raised significant questions about therapeutic strategies that target particular neurohor-

mones, especially in light of the failures of other similar drug development programs.[238–240]

Adjunctive therapies

HMG CoA enzyme inhibitors

The HMG CoA enzyme inhibitor class ("statin") has been evaluated as a potential adjunct to heart failure management on the basis of retrospective data.[241] The proposed mechanisms of action include prevention of downstream ischemic events and an anti-inflammatory effect; however, clinically there is now a large prospective trial that has not confirmed the earlier favorable reports. In CORONA, 5011 patients with ischemic cardiomyopathy and NYHA class II–IV heart failure were randomized to receive rosuvastatin 10 mg versus placebo. Over a mean period of 32.8 months, a combined endpoint of cardiovascular death, non-fatal MI and non-fatal stroke was not significantly reduced (HR 0.92, 95% CI 0.83–1.02).[242] A secondary endpoint of cardiovascular hospitalizations was positive with a statistically significant reduction and there were no major safety concerns. The lack of a positive overall finding likely reflects the challenge of interpreting competing risks. In the case of statins, the impact of this class of drug on outcomes related to coronary artery disease is attenuated by the heightened importance of myocardial dysfunction and neurohormonal activation in patients with advanced heart failure. In addition, the lowering of LDL cholesterol may not necessarily be advantageous; the paradoxic observation that low cholesterol levels in chronic heart failure is associated with increased risk[243] is supported by CORONA.

Nevertheless, major questions remained including the possibility that the statins work by preventing ischemic complications in long-term survivors of dilated non-ischemic cardiomyopathy,[244] which was not addressed in CORONA. However, the GISSI-HF trial failed to demonstrate any difference between rosuvastatin and placebo in time to death or the combined endpoint of time to death or hospitalization for cardiovascular causes after 3.9 years of follow-up in over 4500 patients with chronic HF. Of note, there was a slight absolute reduction in mortality risk in patients randomized to receive omega-3 fatty acid supplementation, raising interesting questions about mechanism of action.[245]

Exercise rehabilitation

A large multicenter trial, HF-ACTION, demonstrated that a structured exercise program for patients with heart failure is safe.[246] However, there was only a nonsignificant trend in reduction of mortality or hospitalization due, perhaps in part, to the reduction in adherence to exercise over time. A variety of important secondary endpoints, such as health status as measured by the Kansas City Cardiomyopathy Questionnaire, may provide insight into other long term effects on outcomes.

Heart failure management

Physician or nurse-directed disease management has been increasingly recognized as an important component of heart failure care. Multiple studies have suggested that various interventions, including telemanagement, intensive discharge planning and other multidisciplinary interventions, can reduce overall costs and improve measurable outcomes in the quality of care.[247–251]

Device and surgical therapy

Implantable cardioverter defibrillators and biventricular pacing (cardiac resynchronization therapy)

In addition to a background of pharmacologic therapy, the addition of implantable cardioverter defibrillators (ICD) for primary prevention of sudden cardiac death and cardiac resynchronization therapy for mortality reduction in patients with symptomatic heart failure has dramatically impacted management approaches.[226,252–256] Defining appropriate candidates and providing meticulous longitudinal care are hallmarks of successful therapy, given the high degree of technical complexity, associated costs and impact on patients and patients' families.[257–259] The role of device therapy is covered in detail elsewhere in this book.

Ventricular assist devices

Support with ventricular assist and other circulatory support devices has been an area of considerable focus for the subgroup of patients with medically refractory and often near terminal heart failure. Different kinds of left ventricular mechanical assist devices (LVADs) have been studied for several years and they have been in clinical use since at least the early 1990s.[260] Newer and smaller generations of pumps are under clinical evaluation. They differ in size, flow patterns (centrifugal versus axial flow), method of implantation, durability, and intended clinical use (cardiogenic shock, post cardiotomy shock, bridge to transplant and destination). Long-term effects have been unclear.

In REMATCH (Randomized Evaluation of Mechanical Assistance for the Treatment of Congestive Heart failure), 129 patients with a mean age of 67 years and ejection fraction of 0.17 with advanced symptomatic heart failure (NYHA class IV) ineligible for transplantation were randomized to optimal medical management (mostly intravenous inotropic drugs) or LVAD (HeartMate).[261] Kaplan–Meier survival analysis showed a reduction of 48% in the risk of death from any cause in the group that received LVADs as compared with the medical therapy group (RR 0.52, 95% CI 0.34–0.78, $P = 0.001$). The rates of survival at 1 year were 52% in the device group and 25% in the medical therapy group ($P = 0.002$); the rates at 2 years were 23% and

8% ($P = 0.09$), respectively. The frequency of serious adverse events in the device group was nearly 2.4 times (95% CI 1.86–2.95) that in the medical therapy group, with a predominance of infection, bleeding, and malfunction of the device. Quality of life was significantly improved at 1 year in the device group assessed as SF-36 and Beck Depression Inventory but this was an unmatched survivors analysis.

In a more recent study, a newer generation axial flow pump (HeartMate 2) was assessed as a device for bridge to transplant. Three possible favorable outcomes were defined as transplant, recovery or ongoing support. Median survival on pump was 126 days (range 1–600 days) with 68% 1-year survival.[262] Other devices are under investigation; the focus is to define appropriate subgroups and to provide sustained support with a low incidence of thromboembolic and mechanical complications.

Key clinical challenges remain, highlighted by a report by Yacoub and colleagues in which the viability of LVAD weaning was demonstrated in a series of patients with non-ischemic cardiomyopathy at a mean of 320 ± 186 days of support facilitated by the use of the beta-2 agonist clenbuterol.[263] Of 15 patients examined, 11 were weaned; there was one death within 24 hours. To what degree this study has applicability to patients with long-standing advanced heart failure is not clear, nor is the durability of the recovery.

These studies demonstrate the viability of mechanical support and the fact that LVADs have the potential to prolong life and improve quality of life in severe heart failure. Based on REMATCH, treatment effect is limited in time although since publication of the trial results, refinements in the technology, patient selection and surgical technique have occurred. Important questions will require further study, including the degree to which long-term durability can be achieved, the identification of patients with a likelihood of recovery, the durability of that recovery, and cost-effectiveness.

Other surgical options

There are several surgical approaches to heart failure including revascularization, left ventricular reconstruction, cardiomyoplasty, constraining devices, mitral valvular repair and heart transplantation. Most of these techniques have not been subjected to rigorous evaluation in clinical trials, reflecting at least in part the difficulties inherent in defining control groups in surgical intervention trials.[264–266]

Heart failure with preserved left ventricular function

The evidence base for heart failure with preserved LV function is limited, reflecting uncertainties about the underlying heterogeneous pathophysiology, difficulties with trial design including standardization of definitions and endpoints, and lack of focused interest by industry. Nevertheless, recent trials have provided some important insight into several treatment options.

In the DIG trial, a subgroup of 988 patients had ejection fractions greater than 45%. Treatment with digoxin did not impact mortality but as in the main study group, hospitalizations were reduced by study drug. As mentioned in the section on angiotensin receptor blockers, candesartan did not impact mortality in CHARM-Preserved but hospitalizations were reduced.[127] Specifically, the composite primary endpoint of cardiovascular death or admission to hospital for CHF occurred in 22% of patients treated with candesartan and 24% of patients on placebo (HR 0.89, 95% CI 0.77–1.03, $P = 0.118$). The minor difference was driven entirely by a reduction in hospitalizations which, taken alone, reached statistical significance. A second large ARB trial, i-PRESERVED with irbesartan, failed to demonstrate a salutary effect of irbesartan versus placebo in over 4100 patients over the age of 59 with HF symptoms and left ventricular ejection fraction of at least 45%. The primary endpoint (a composite of death from any cause or hospitalization for HF, myocardial infarction, unstable angina, arrhythmia or stroke) was associated with a hazard ratio that was near unity.[267]

In the PEP-CHF study, patients with a diagnosis of heart failure treated with diuretics but demonstrating essentially preserved LV systolic function (EF 64% and 65% in placebo and active study arms respectively) were randomized to receive perindopril 4 mg or placebo for a period of at least 1 year. The cohort was elderly (mean age 76), predominantly female (55%) and hypertensive (prior hypertension in 79% and mean SBP at randomization approximately 139 mmHg). A high withdrawal rate at 1 year with crossover to open-label ACE inhibitor reduced the power of the study, though when analyzed at 1 year, the composite endpoint of all-cause mortality and unplanned heart failure hospitalization approached statistical significance, driven largely by a reduction in hospitalizations.

In the SENIORS trial with a novel beta blocker nebivolol,[198] approximately 35% of study patients had an ejection fraction over 35%; a proportion of these likely had preserved LVF. The effect on the primary endpoint of all-cause mortality or cardiovascular hospitalization was similar to the cohort with lower EFs; that is, ejection fraction did not appear to modify the effect of nebivolol. Nevertheless, the endpoint was largely driven by the reduction in hospitalizations.

What can one conclude about these trials and treatment approaches to patients with heart failure despite preserved or nearly preserved LVF? As in all patients, risk factor reduction including control of blood pressure is key. This concept has been supported by multiple clinical trials in hypertension among patients at risk for heart failure including the landmark SHEP trial in which antihyperten-

sive treatment in elderly patients with isolated systolic hypertension reduced heart failure events with a dramatic relative risk reduction of 0.51.[268] The potential utility of drugs in the ACE inhibitor, ARB and beta-blocker classes (especially those that have been shown to be effective in systolic heart failure) seems clear. Nevertheless, as outlined, clinical trial results are limited in scope and magnitude and as such do not permit the same high-level recommendations that are currently used in treatment guidelines for patients with systolic heart failure.

Challenges and controversies

Challenges for future clinical trials of therapeutics in heart failure

A key challenge for clinical trialists is the definition of endpoints in trials of both acutely decompensated and chronic heart failure. For the former, surrogates for mortality have not been well defined nor accepted. Although event rates are high, in-hospital mortality is under 5%, meaning that additional and often composite endpoints that include assessment of patient well-being need to be developed. For the latter, ACE inhibitors, beta-blockers and aldosterone blockers have seriously impacted power calculations and hence the ability of conventionally sized trials to detect meaningful differences in mortality. Further, non-pharmacologic trials (i.e. evaluation of devices) are limited in size by the expense and scope of the interventions. The need for trial designs that can pass regulatory requirements in the absence of survival endpoints is pivotal.

Heart failure monitoring

Acute
The role of invasive hemodynamic monitoring during hospitalization for decompensated heart failure was critically evaluated in the ESCAPE Trial in which 433 patients across 26 sites were randomized to receive usual clinical care or care supplemented by the placement of a pulmonary artery catheter.[269] Inotropic therapy was discouraged but not proscribed. The primary endpoint was days alive outside the hospital which did not differ between the two groups (HR 1.0); there were more adverse events in the group treated with the invasive approach. These results suggest that most patients can be managed without invasive hemodynamic monitoring in the acute setting.

Chronic
Multiple technologies have been considered for remote monitoring of patients with chronic heart failure, many using telemonitoring.[270–272] The range of options is significant from simple weight scales[273] to biomarkers[274] to inva-

sive physiologic monitors.[275] As a whole, the data have not been consistent or convincing.

For example, the use of the natriuretic peptides (BNP/NT-proBNP) for guiding treatment during follow-up has been supported by observational experience from large clinical trials[276] and more focused primary data from small controlled trials.[277] In the latter, 220 patients were randomized to control or treatment modifications based on target BNP concentrations <100 pg/mL. During a 15-month follow-up the primary endpoint of death or admissions for worsening heart failure was significantly reduced in the BNP-guided group. However, this group had an increase in non-heart failure-related admissions, largely negating the presumptive benefit of biomarker-based treatment. Further, the limited study size and open design make the results difficult to interpret. Other randomized trials are ongoing.[278]

In the example of chronic hemodynamic monitoring, the largest study to date using an implantable monitor of pulmonary capillary wedge pressure (COMPASS-HF) did not reach its primary endpoint.[279] The fact that outcomes were not favorably impacted raises questions about the underlying hypothesis that an improved hemodynamic profile is a key therapeutic goal. Nevertheless, despite these mixed results, interest remains in defining appropriate types and intensities of monitoring. In that context, it will be necessary to define the nature of clinical decision making in response to fluctuating or worsening markers of heart failure.

Performance measures

The standardization of heart failure care has been a focus of professional societies, health insurers and other stakeholders,[280,281] largely based on the recognition that there is great variability in the quality of care delivered to patients with heart failure.[282] Multiple initiatives have been developed[283] in attempt to improve quality. At the same time, the performance measures used to gauge quality may not in fact reflect outcomes,[284] an issue of enormous importance if hospitals and providers are to be judged by process measures related to the delivery of heart failure care.

Conclusion

In the pharmacologic treatment of CHF there are two main classes of drugs – ACE inhibitors and beta-blockers – with solid and consistent documentation for reduction of morbidity and mortality. Furthermore, aldosterone antagonists and hydralazine/nitrate in combination have demonstrated efficacy in defined subgroups. Several ARBs have a role, most clearly as a substitute when patients are not tolerating an ACE inhibitor (Table 47.1) and in some patients as add-on therapy. Ancillary approaches continue to be defined. The reader is also referred to the major published guidelines in Europe and the USA for additional background and classification of standard approaches to HF management.[285,286]

Table 47.1 Key recommendations

Aim of treatment	Class of drug	Level of evidence
Symptomatic improvement of congestion, improvement of exercise capacity	Diuretics	**Level A**
Reduction of mortality in mild to moderate heart failure	ACE inhibitors	**Level A**
	Beta-adrenergic blockers	**Level A**
Reduction of mortality in severe heart failure	ACE inhibitors	**Level A**
	Beta-adrenergic blockers	**Level A**
	Spironolactone	**Level A**
Reduction of mortality in patients not tolerating an ACE inhibitor	ARBs	**Level A**
Reduction of morbidity and symptoms in mild–severe heart failure	ACE inhibitors	**Level A**
	Beta-adrenergic blockers	**Level A**
	ARBs	**Level A**
	Spironolactone	**Level A**
	Digoxin	**Level A**
Short-term improvement of symptoms in patients with severe CHF	Non-digitalis inotropic drugs	**Level B**
Surgical treatment of end-stage CHF	Cardiac transplantation	**Level B**
Bridging towards heart transplantation in terminal heart failure	Left ventricular assist device	**Level B**

The challenges for the next decade are manifold. They include the need to: better define subgroups that benefit the most from different drug combinations; fulfill the mandate to ensure dissemination of the findings of clinical trials into practice; and develop appropriate metrics to gauge physician competencies in the treatment of patients with heart failure. In addition, the need to define strategies that can be used to translate and effectively implement clinical practice guidelines is significant, as many patients are not offered comprehensive contemporary treatments. Heart failure care must be structured, given its complexity and the importance of drug titration and close clinical follow-up. Finally, given an increasing prevalence, deleterious effects on patient morbidity and mortality and pronounced impact on the finances of healthcare systems, we need to continue to pursue a greater understanding of the mechanisms underlying cardiac failure and the methods that can be applied in order to prevent the development of and progression to symptomatic end-stage disease.

References

1. Ribner HS, Plucinski DA, Hsieh AM, Bresnahan D, Molteni A, Askenazi J, Lesch M. Acute effects of digoxin on total systemic vascular resistance in congestive heart failure due to dilated cardiomyopathy: a hemodynamic-hormonal study. *Am J Cardiol* 1985;**56**:896–904.

2. Gheorghiade M, St Clair J, St Clair C, Beller GA. Hemodynamic effects of intravenous digoxin in patients with severe heart failure initially treated with diuretics and vasodilators. *J Am Coll Cardiol* 1987;**9**:849–57.

3. Cohn K, Selzer A, Kersh ES, Karpman LS, Goldschlager N. Variability of hemodynamic responses to acute digitalization in chronic cardiac failure due to cardiomyopathy and coronary artery disease. *Am J Cardiol* 1975;**35**:461–8.

4. Braunwald E. Effects of digitalis on the normal and the failing heart. *J Am Coll Cardiol* 1985;**5**:51A–59A.

5. Digitalis Investigation Group The effect of digoxin on mortality and morbidity in patients with heart failure. *N Engl J Med* 1997;**336**:525–33.

6. Ferguson DW, Berg WJ, Sanders JS, Roach PJ, Kempf JS, Kienzle MG. Sympathoinhibitory responses to digitalis glycosides in heart failure patients. Direct evidence from sympathetic neural recordings. *Circulation* 1989;**80**:65–77.

7. Ferguson DW. Baroreflex-mediated circulatory control in human heart failure. *Heart Failure* 1990;**6**:3–11.

8. Goldsmith SR, Simon AB, Miller E. Effect of digitalis on norepinephrine kinetics in congestive heart failure. *J Am Coll Cardiol* 1992;**20**:858–63.

9. Dobbs SM, Kenyon WI, Dobbs RJ. Maintenance digoxin after an episode of heart failure: placebo-controlled trial in outpatients. *BMJ* 1977;**1**:749–52.

10. Lee DC, Johnson RA, Bingham JB, Leahy M, Dinsmore RE, Goroll AH *et al.* Heart failure in outpatients: a randomized trial of digoxin versus placebo. *N Engl J Med* 1982;**306**:699–705.

11. Guyatt GH, Sullivan MJ, Fallen EL, Tihal H, Rideout E, Halcrow S *et al.* A controlled trial of digoxin in congestive heart failure. *Am J Cardiol* 1988;**61**:371–5.

12. Haerer W, Bauer, U, Hetzel, M, Fehske J. Long-term effects of digoxin and diuretics in congestive heart failure. Results of a placebo-controlled randomized double-blind study. *Circulation* 1988;**78**:53.

13. Captopril-Digoxin Multicenter Research Group. Comparative effects of therapy with captopril and digoxin in patients with mild to moderate heart failure. *JAMA* 1988;**259**:539–44.

14. German and Austrian Xamoterol Study Group. Double-blind placebo-controlled comparison of digoxin and xamoterol in chronic heart failure. *Lancet* 1988;**1**:489–93.

15. Uretsky BF, Young JB, Shahidi FE, Yellen LG, Harrison MC, Jolly MK. Randomized study assessing the effect of digoxin withdrawal in patients with mild to moderate chronic congestive heart failure: results of the PROVED trial. PROVED Investigative Group. *J Am Coll Cardiol* 1993;**22**:955–962.

16. Packer M, Gheorghiade M, Young JB, Costantini PJ, Adams KF, Cody RJ *et al.* Withdrawal of digoxin from patients with chronic heart failure treated with angiotensin-converting-enzyme inhibitors. RADIANCE Study. *N Engl J Med* 1993;**329**:1–7.

17. Hussain Z, Swindle J, Hauptman PJ. Digoxin use and digoxin toxicity in the post-DIG trial era. *J Cardiac Fail* 2006;**12**:343–6.

18. Rathore SS, Wang Y, Krumholz HM. Sex-based differences in the effect of digoxin for the treatment of heart failure. *N Engl J Med* 2002;**347**:1403–11.

19. Rathore SS, Curtis JP, Wang Y, Bristow MR, Krumholz HM. Association of serum digoxin concentration and outcomes in patients with heart failure. *JAMA* 2003;**289**:871–8.

20. Adams KF Jr, Patterson JH, Gattis WA, O'Connor CM, Lee CR, Schwartz TA, Gheorghiade M. Relationship of serum digoxin concentration to mortality and morbidity in women in the digitalis investigation group trial: a retrospective analysis. *J Am Coll Cardiol* 2005;**46**:497–504.

21. Stason WB, Cannon PJ, Heinemann HO, Laragh JH. Furosemide. A clinical evaluation of its diuretic action. *Circulation* 1966;**34**:910–20.

22. Cody RJ, Ljungman S, Covit AB, Kubo SH, Sealey JE, Pondolfino K *et al.* Regulation of glomerular filtration rate in chronic congestive heart failure patients. *Kidney Int* 1988;**34**:361–7.

23. Francis GS, Goldsmith SR, Levine TB, Olivari MT, Cohn JN. The neurohumoral axis in congestive heart failure. *Ann Intern Med* 1984;**101**:370–7.

24. Lal S, Murtagh JG, Pollock AM, Fletcher E, Binnion PF. Acute haemodynamic effects of frusemide in patients with normal and raised left atrial pressures. *Br Heart J* 1969;**31**:711–17.

25. Stampfer M, Epstein SE, Beiser GD, Braunwald E. Hemodynamic effects of diuresis at rest and during intense upright exercise in patients with impaired cardiac function. *Circulation* 1968;**37**:900–11.

26. Magrini F, Niarchos AP. Hemodynamic effects of massive peripheral edema. *Am Heart J* 1983;**105**:90–7.

27. Francis GS, Siegel RM, Goldsmith SR, Olivari MT, Levine TB, Cohn JN. Acute vasoconstrictor response to intravenous furosemide in patients with chronic congestive heart failure. Activation of the neurohumoral axis. *Ann Intern Med* 1985;**103**:1–6.

28. Dikshit K, Vyden JK, Forrester JS, Chatterjee K, Prakash R, Swan HJ. Renal and extrarenal hemodynamic effects of furosemide in congestive heart failure after acute myocardial infarction. *N Engl J Med* 1973;**288**:1087–90.

29. Nelson GI, Ahuja RC, Silke B, Okoli RC, Hussain M, Taylor SH. Haemodynamic effects of frusemide and its influence on repetitive rapid volume loading in acute myocardial infarction. *Eur Heart J* 1983;**4**:706–11.

30. Verma SP, Silke B, Reynolds G, Muller P, Frais MA, Taylor SH. Immediate effects of bumetanide on systemic haemodynamics and left ventricular volume in acute and chronic heart failure. *Br J Clin Pharmacol* 1987;**24**:21–32.

31. Fiehring H AI. Influence of 10 mg torasemide iv and 20 mg furosemide iv on the intracardiac pressures in patients with heart failure at rest and during exercise. *Prog Pharmacol Clin Pharmacol* 1990;**8**:87–104.

32. Francis GS, Benedict C, Johnstone DE, Kirlin PC, Nicklas J, Liang CS *et al.* Comparison of neuroendocrine activation in patients with left ventricular dysfunction with and without congestive heart failure. A substudy of the Studies of Left Ventricular Dysfunction (SOLVD). *Circulation* 1990;**82**:1724–9.

33. Bayliss J, Norell M, Canepa-Anson R, Sutton G, Poole-Wilson P. Untreated heart failure: clinical and neuroendocrine effects of introducing diuretics. *Br Heart J* 1987;**57**:17–22.

34. Faris R, Flather M, Purcell H, Henein M, Poole-Wilson P, Coats A. Current evidence supporting the role of diuretics in heart failure: a meta analysis of randomised controlled trials. *Int J Cardiol* 2002;**82**:149–58.

35. Achhammer I. Long-term efficacy and tolerance of torasemide in congestive heart failure. *Prog Pharmacol Clin Pharmacol* 1990;**8**:127–36.

36. Odemuyiwa O, Gilmartin J, Kenny D, Hall RJ. Captopril and the diuretic requirements in moderate and severe chronic heart failure. *Eur Heart J* 1989;**10**:586–90.

37. Anand IS, Kalra GS, Ferrari R, Wahi PL, Harris PC, Poole-Wilson PA. Enalapril as initial and sole treatment in severe chronic heart failure with sodium retention. *Int J Cardiol* 1990;**28**:341–6.

38. Richardson A, Bayliss J, Scriven AJ, Parameshwar J, Poole-Wilson PA, Sutton GC. Double-blind comparison of captopril alone against frusemide plus amiloride in mild heart failure. *Lancet* 1987;**2**:709–11.

39. Cody RJ, Kubo SH, Pickworth KK. Diuretic treatment for the sodium retention of congestive heart failure. *Arch Intern Med* 1994;**154**:1905–14.

40. Costanzo MR, Guglin ME, Saltzberg MT, Jessup ML, Bart BA, Teerlink JR *et al.* Ultrafiltration versus intravenous diuretics for patients hospitalized for acute decompensated heart failure. *J Am Coll Cardiol* 2007;**49**:675–83.

41. Laragh JH. Hormones and the pathogenesis of congestive heart failure: vasopressin, aldosterone, and angiotensin II. Further evidence for renal-adrenal interaction from studies in hypertension and in cirrhosis. *Circulation* 1962;**25**:1015–23.

42. Swedberg K, Eneroth P, Kjekshus J, Wilhelmsen L. Hormones regulating cardiovascular function in patients with severe congestive heart failure and their relation to mortality. CONSENSUS Trial Study Group. *Circulation* 1990;**82**:1730–6.

43. Weber KT, Brilla CG. Pathological hypertrophy and cardiac interstitium. Fibrosis and renin-angiotensin-aldosterone system. *Circulation* 1991;**83**:1849–65.

44. Young M, Fullerton M, Dilley R, Funder J. Mineralocorticoids, hypertension, and cardiac fibrosis. *J Clin Invest* 1994;**93**:2578–83.

45. Pitt B, Zannad F, Remme WJ, Cody R, Castaigne A, Perez A, Palensky J, Wittes J. The effect of spironolactone on morbidity and mortality in patients with severe heart failure. Randomized Aldactone Evaluation Study Investigators. *N Engl J Med* 1999;**341**:709–17.

46. Juurlink DN, Mamdani MM, Lee DS, Kopp A, Austin PC, Laupacis A, Redelmeier DA. Rates of hyperkalemia after publication of the Randomized Aldactone Evaluation Study. *N Engl J Med* 2004;**351**:543–51.

47. Pitt B, Remme W, Zannad F *et al.* Eplerenone, a selective aldosterone blocker, in patients with left ventricular dysfunction after myocardial infarction. *N Engl J Med* 2003;**348**:1309–21.

48. Pitt B, White H, Nicolau J, Martinez F, Gheorghiade M, Aschermann M *et al.* Eplerenone reduces mortality 30 days after randomization following acute myocardial infarction in patients with left ventricular systolic dysfunction and heart failure. *J Am Coll Cardiol* 2005;**46**:425–31.

49. Eichna LW, Kessler RH, Sobol BJ. Hemodynamic and renal effects produced in congestive heart failure by the intravenous administration of a ganglionic blocking agent. *Trans Assoc Am Physicians* 1956;**69**:207–13.

50. Burch GE. Evidence for increased venous tone in chronic congestive heart failure. *AMA* 1956;**98**:750–66.

51. Zelis R, Mason DT, Braunwald E. A comparison of the effects of vasodilator stimuli on peripheral resistance vessels in normal subjects and in patients with congestive heart failure. *J Clin Invest* 1968;**47**:960–70.

52. Majid PA, Sharma B, Taylor SH. Phentolamine for vasodilator treatment of severe heart-failure. *Lancet* 1971;**2**:719–24.

53. Franciosa JA, Limas CJ, Guiha NH, Rodriguera E, Cohn JN. Improved left ventricular function during nitroprusside infusion in acute myocardial infarction. *Lancet* 1972;**1**:650–4.

54. Cohn JN, Franciosa JA. Vasodilator therapy of cardiac failure: (first of two parts). *N Engl J Med* 1977;**297**:27–31.

55. Tsai SC, Adamik R, Manganiello VC. Moss J Effects of nitroprusside and nitroglycerin on cGMP content and PGI2 formation in aorta and vena cava. *Biochem Pharmacol* 1989;**38**:61–5.

56. Lavine SJ, Campbell CA, Held AC, Johnson V. Effect of nitroglycerin-induced reduction of left ventricular filling pressure on diastolic filling in acute dilated heart failure. *J Am Coll Cardiol* 1989;**14**:233–41.

57. Mason DT, Braunwald E. The effects of nitroglycerin and amyl nitrite on arteriolar and venous tone in the human forearm. *Circulation* 1965;**32**:755–66.

58. Armstrong PW, Armstrong JA, Marks GS. Pharmacokinetic-hemodynamic studies of intravenous nitroglycerin in congestive cardiac failure. *Circulation* 1980;**62**:160–6.

59. Leier CV, Bambach D, Thompson MJ, Cattaneo SM, Goldberg RJ, Unverferth DV. Central and regional hemodynamic effects of intravenous isosorbide dinitrate, nitroglycerin and nitroprusside in patients with congestive heart failure. *Am J Cardiol* 1981;**48**:1115–23.

60. Flaherty JT, Reid PR, Kelly DT, Taylor DR, Weisfeldt ML, Pitt B. Intravenous nitroglycerin in acute myocardial infarction. *Circulation* 1975;**51**:132–9.

61. Ludbrook PA, Byrne JD, Kurnik PB, McKnight RC. Influence of reduction of preload and afterload by nitroglycerin on left ventricular diastolic pressure-volume relations and relaxation in man. *Circulation* 1977;**56**:937–43.

62. De Marco T, Chatterjee K, Rouleau JL, Parmley WW. Abnormal coronary hemodynamics and myocardial energetics in patients with chronic heart failure caused by ischemic heart disease and dilated cardiomyopathy. *Am Heart J* 1988;**115**:809–15.

63. Unverferth DV, Magorien RD, Lewis RP, Leier CV. The role of subendocardial ischemia in perpetuating myocardial failure in patients with nonischemic congestive cardiomyopathy. *Am Heart J* 1983;**105**:176–9.

64. Chiariello M, Gold HK, Leinbach RC, Davis MA, Maroko PR. Comparison between the effects of nitroprusside and nitroglycerin on ischemic injury during acute myocardial infarction. *Circulation* 1976;**54**:766–73.

65. Colucci WS, Elkayam U, Horton DP, Abraham WT, Bourge RC, Johnson AD *et al.* Intravenous nesiritide, a natriuretic peptide, in the treatment of decompensated congestive heart failure. Nesiritide Study Group. *N Engl J Med* 2000;**343**:246–53.

66. Intravenous nesiritide vs nitroglycerin for treatment of decompensated congestive heart failure: a randomized controlled trial. *JAMA* 2002;**287**:1531–40.

67. Sackner-Bernstein JD, Skopicki HA, Aaronson KD. Risk of worsening renal function with nesiritide in patients with acutely decompensated heart failure. *Circulation* 2005;**111**:1487–91.

68. Sackner-Bernstein JD, Kowalski M, Fox M, Aaronson K. Short-term risk of death after treatment with nesiritide for decompensated heart failure: a pooled analysis of randomized controlled trials. *JAMA* 2005;**293**:1900–5.

69. Hauptman PJ, Schnitzler MA, Swindle J, Burroughs TE. Use of nesiritide before and after publications suggesting drug-related risks in patients with acute decompensated heart failure. *JAMA* 2006;**296**:1877–84.

70. Cleland JG, Coletta AP, Clark AL. Clinical trials update from the American College of Cardiology 2007: ALPHA, EVEREST, FUSION II, VALIDD, PARR-2, REMODEL, SPICE, COURAGE, COACH, REMADHE, pro-BNP for the evaluation of dyspnoea and THIS-diet. *Eur J Heart Fail* 2007;**9**:740–5.

71. Coletta AP, Tin L, Loh PH, Clark AL, Cleland JG. Clinical trials update from the European Society of Cardiology heart failure meeting: TNT subgroup analysis, darbepoetin alfa, FERRIC-HF and KW-3902. *Eur J Heart Fail* 2006;**8**:547–9.

72. Greenberg B, Thomas I, Banish D, Goldman S, Havranek E, Massie BM *et al.* Effects of multiple oral doses of an A1 adenosine antagonist, BG9928, in patients with heart failure: results of a placebo-controlled, dose-escalation study. *J Am Coll Cardiol* 2007;**50**:600–6.

73. Teerlink JR, Metra M, Felker GM *et al.* Relaxin for the treatment of patients with acute heart failure (Pre-RELAX-AHF): a multicentre randomized, placebo-controlled, parallel-group, dose-finding phase IIb study. *Lancet* 2009;**373**:1429–39.

74. Chatterjee K, Ports TA, Brundage BH, Massie B, Holly AN, Parmley WW. Oral hydralazine in chronic heart failure: sustained beneficial hemodynamic effects. *Ann Intern Med* 1980;**92**:600–4.

75. Franciosa JA, Nordstrom LA, Cohn JN. Nitrate therapy for congestive heart failure. *JAMA* 1978;**240**:443–6.

76. Leier CV, Desch CE, Magorien RD, Triffon DW, Unverferth DV, Boudoulas H, Lewis RP. Positive inotropic effects of hydralazine in human subjects: comparison with prazosin in the setting of congestive heart failure. *Am J Cardiol* 1980;**46**:1039–44.

77. Rouleau JL, Chatterjee K, Benge W, Parmley WW, Hiramatsu B. Alterations in left ventricular function and coronary hemodynamics with captopril, hydralazine and prazosin in chronic ischemic heart failure: a comparative study. *Circulation* 1982;**65**:671–8.

78. Daly P, Rouleau JL, Cousineau D, Burgess JH, Chatterjee K. Effects of captopril and a combination of hydralazine and isosorbide dinitrate on myocardial sympathetic tone in patients with severe congestive heart failure. *Br Heart J* 1986;**56**: 152–7.

79. Magorien RD, Unverferth DV, Brown GP, Leier CV. Dobutamine and hydralazine: comparative influences of positive inotropy and vasodilation on coronary blood flow and myocardial energetics in nonischemic congestive heart failure. *J Am Coll Cardiol* 1983;**1**:499–505.

80. Massie B, Chatterjee K, Werner J, Greenberg B, Hart R, Parmley WW. Hemodynamic advantage of combined administration of hydralazine orally and nitrates nonparenterally in the vasodilator therapy of chronic heart failure. *Am J Cardiol* 1977;**40**: 794–801.

81. Packer M, Meller J, Medina N, Yushak M, Gorlin R. Provocation of myocardial ischemic events during initiation of vasodilator therapy for severe chronic heart failure. Clinical and hemodynamic evaluation of 52 consecutive patients with ischemic cardiomyopathy. *Am J Cardiol* 1981;**48**:939–46.

82. Munzel T, Kurz S, Rajagopalan S, Thoenes M, Berrington WR, Thompson JA *et al.* Hydralazine prevents nitroglycerin tolerance by inhibiting activation of a membrane-bound NADH oxidase. A new action for an old drug. *J Clin Invest* 1996;**98**: 1465–70.

83. Cohn JN, Archibald DG, Ziesche S, Franciosa JA, Harston WE, Tristani FE *et al.* Effect of vasodilator therapy on mortality in chronic congestive heart failure. Results of a Veterans Administration Cooperative Study. *N Engl J Med* 1986;**314**:1547–52.

84. Cohn JN, Johnson G, Ziesche S *et al.* A comparison of enalapril with hydralazine-isosorbide dinitrate in the treatment of chronic congestive heart failure. *N Engl J Med* 1991;**325**:303–10.

85. Carson P, Ziesche S, Johnson G, Cohn JN. Racial differences in response to therapy for heart failure: analysis of the vasodilator-heart failure trials. Vasodilator-Heart Failure Trial Study Group. *J Cardiac Fail* 1999;**5**:178–87.

86. Taylor AL, Ziesche S, Yancy C, Carson P, D'Agostino R Jr, Ferdinand K *et al.* Combination of isosorbide dinitrate and hydralazine in blacks with heart failure. *N Engl J Med* 2004;**351**: 2049–57.

87. Taylor AL, Ziesche S, Yancy CW, Carson P, Ferdinand K, Taylor M *et al.* Early and sustained benefit on event-free survival and heart failure hospitalization from fixed-dose combination of isosorbide dinitrate/hydralazine: consistency across subgroups in the African-American Heart Failure Trial. *Circulation* 2007; **115**:1747–53.

88. Elkayam U, Amin J, Mehra A, Vasquez J, Weber L, Rahimtoola SH. A prospective, randomized, double-blind, crossover study to compare the efficacy and safety of chronic nifedipine therapy with that of isosorbide dinitrate and their combination in the treatment of chronic congestive heart failure. *Circulation* 1990;**82**:1954–61.

89. Iida K, Matsuda M, Ajisaka R, Sugishita Y, Ito I, Takeda T *et al.* Effects of nifedipine on left ventricular systolic and diastolic function in patients with ischemic heart disease. Radionuclide angiocardiographic studies at rest and during exercise. *Japan Heart J* 1987;**28**:495–506.

90. Goldstein RE, Boccuzzi SJ, Cruess D, Nattel S. Diltiazem increases late-onset congestive heart failure in postinfarction patients with early reduction in ejection fraction. The Adverse Experience Committee; and the Multicenter Diltiazem Postinfarction Research Group. *Circulation* 1991;**83**:52–60.

91. Barjon JN, Rouleau JL, Bichet D, Juneau C, De Champlain J. Chronic renal and neurohumoral effects of the calcium entry blocker nisoldipine in patients with congestive heart failure. *J Am Coll Cardiol* 1987;**9**:622–30.

92. Gheorghiade M, Hall V, Goldberg D, Levine TB, Goldstein S. Long-term clinical and neurohormonal effects of nicardipine in patients with severe heart failure on maintenance therapy with angiotensin converting enzyme inhibitors. *J Am Coll Cardiol* 1991;**17**:274A.

93. Dunselman PH, Kuntze CE, van Bruggen A, Hamer JP, Scaf AH, Wessling H, Lie KI. Efficacy of felodipine in congestive heart failure. *Eur Heart J* 1989;**10**:354–64.

94. Cohn JN, Ziesche S, Smith R, Anand I, Dunkman WB, Loeb H et al. Effect of the calcium antagonist felodipine as supplementary vasodilator therapy in patients with chronic heart failure treated with enalapril: V-HeFT III. Vasodilator-Heart Failure Trial (V-HeFT) Study Group. *Circulation* 1997;**96**:856–63.

95. Packer M, O'Connor CM, Ghali JK, Pressler ML, Carson PE, Belkin RN et al. Effect of amlodipine on morbidity and mortality in severe chronic heart failure. Prospective Randomized Amlodipine Survival Evaluation Study Group. *N Engl J Med* 1996;**335**:1107–14.

96. Thackray S, Witte K, Clark AL, Cleland JG. Clinical trials update: OPTIME-CHF, PRAISE-2, ALL-HAT. *Eur J Heart Fail* 2000;**2**:209–12.

97. Packer M RJ, Swedberg K et al. Effect of flosequinan on survival in chronic heart failure. *Circulation* 1993;**88**:301.

98. Califf RM, Adams KF, McKenna WJ et al. A randomized controlled trial of epoprostenol therapy for severe congestive heart failure: The Flolan International Randomized Survival Trial (FIRST). *Am Heart J* 1997;**134**:44–54.

99. Sharpe N, Murphy J, Smith H, Hannan S. Treatment of patients with symptomless left ventricular dysfunction after myocardial infarction. *Lancet* 1988;**1**:255–9.

100. Pfeffer JM, Pfeffer MA. Angiotensin converting enzyme inhibition and ventricular remodeling in heart failure. *Am J Med* 1988;**84**:37–44.

101. Sharpe DN, Murphy J, Coxon R, Hannan SF. Enalapril in patients with chronic heart failure: a placebo-controlled, randomized, double-blind study. *Circulation* 1984;**70**:271–8.

102. DiCarlo L, Chatterjee K, Parmley WW, Swedberg K, Atherton B, Curran D, Cucci M. Enalapril: a new angiotensin-converting enzyme inhibitor in chronic heart failure: acute and chronic hemodynamic evaluations. *J Am Coll Cardiol* 1983;**2**:865–71.

103. Packer M, Medina N, Yushak M, Lee WH. Usefulness of plasma renin activity in predicting haemodynamic and clinical responses and survival during long term converting enzyme inhibition in severe chronic heart failure. Experience in 100 consecutive patients. *Br Heart J* 1985;**54**:298–304.

104. CONSENSUS Trial Study Group. Effects of enalapril on mortality in severe congestive heart failure. Results of the Cooperative North Scandinavian Enalapril Survival Study (CONSENSUS). *N Engl J Med* 1987;**316**:1429–35.

105. Flather MD, Yusuf S, Kober L, Pfeffer M, Hall A, Murray G et al. Long-term ACE-inhibitor therapy in patients with heart failure or left-ventricular dysfunction: a systematic overview of data from individual patients. ACE-Inhibitor Myocardial Infarction Collaborative Group. *Lancet* 2000;**355**:1575–81.

106. Narang R, Swedberg K, Cleland JG. What is the ideal study design for evaluation of treatment for heart failure? Insights from trials assessing the effect of ACE inhibitors on exercise capacity. *Eur Heart J* 1996;**17**:120–34.

107. SOLVD Investigators. Effect of enalapril on mortality and the development of heart failure in asymptomatic patients with reduced left ventricular ejection fractions. *N Engl J Med* 1992;**327**:685–91.

108. Rogers WJ, Johnstone DE, Yusuf S, Weiner DH, Gallagher P, Bittner VA et al. Quality of life among 5,025 patients with left ventricular dysfunction randomized between placebo and enalapril: the Studies of Left Ventricular Dysfunction. The SOLVD Investigators. *J Am Coll Cardiol* 1994;**23**:393–400.

109. Pfeffer MA, Braunwald E, Moye LA, Basta L, Brown EJ Jr, Cuddy TE et al. Effect of captopril on mortality and morbidity in patients with left ventricular dysfunction after myocardial infarction. Results of the survival and ventricular enlargement trial. The SAVE Investigators. *N Engl J Med* 1992;**327**:669–77.

110. Kober L, Torp-Pedersen C, Carlsen JE, Bagger H, Eliasen P, Lyngborg K et al. A clinical trial of the angiotensin-converting-enzyme inhibitor trandolapril in patients with left ventricular dysfunction after myocardial infarction. Trandolapril Cardiac Evaluation (TRACE) Study Group. *N Engl J Med* 1995;**333**:1670–6.

111. Acute Infarction Ramipril Efficacy (AIRE) Study Investigators. Effect of ramipril on mortality and morbidity of survivors of acute myocardial infarction with clinical evidence of heart failure. *Lancet* 1993;**342**:821–8.

112. Packer M, Poole-Wilson PA, Armstrong PW, Cleland JG, Horowitz JD, Massie BM et al. Comparative effects of low and high doses of the angiotensin-converting enzyme inhibitor, lisinopril, on morbidity and mortality in chronic heart failure. ATLAS Study Group. *Circulation* 1999;**100**:2312–18.

113. Furberg CD, Pitt B. Are all angiotensin-converting enzyme inhibitors interchangeable? *J Am Coll Cardiol* 2001;**37**:1456–60.

114. Pilote L, Abrahamowicz M, Rodrigues E, Eisenberg MJ, Rahme E. Mortality rates in elderly patients who take different angiotensin-converting enzyme inhibitors after acute myocardial infarction: a class effect? *Ann Intern Med* 2004;**141**:102–12.

115. Fox KM. Efficacy of perindopril in reduction of cardiovascular events among patients with stable coronary artery disease: randomised, double-blind, placebo-controlled, multicentre trial (the EUROPA study). *Lancet* 2003;**362**:782–8.

116. Braunwald E, Domanski MJ, Fowler SE, Geller NL, Gersh BJ, Hsia J et al. Angiotensin-converting-enzyme inhibition in stable coronary artery disease. *N Engl J Med* 2004;**351**:2058–68.

117. Dagenais GR, Pogue J, Fox K, Simoons ML, Yusuf S. Angiotensin-converting-enzyme inhibitors in stable vascular disease without left ventricular systolic dysfunction or heart failure: a combined analysis of three trials. *Lancet* 2006;**368**:581–8.

118. Paul SD, Kuntz KM, Eagle KA, Weinstein MC. Costs and effectiveness of angiotensin converting enzyme inhibition in patients with congestive heart failure. *Arch Intern Med* 1994;**154**:1143–9.

119. Tsevat J, Duke D, Goldman L, Pfeffer MA, Lamas GA, Soukup JR et al. Cost-effectiveness of captopril therapy after myocardial infarction. *J Am Coll Cardiol* 1995;**26**:914–19.

120. Martinez C BS. Cost effectiveness of ramipril therapy for patients with clinical evidence of heart failure after acute myocardial infarction. *Br J Clin Pract* 1995;**78**(suppl):26–32.

121. McMurray J, Davie A. The pharmacoeconomics of ACE inhibitors in chronic heart failure. *PharmacoEconomics* 1996;**9**:188–97.

122. Pitt B, Poole-Wilson PA, Segal R, Martinez FA, Dickstein K, Camm AJ et al. Effect of losartan compared with captopril on mortality in patients with symptomatic heart failure: randomised trial – the Losartan Heart Failure Survival Study ELITE II. *Lancet* 2000;**355**:1582–7.

123. McKelvie RS, Yusuf S, Pericak D, Avezum A, Burns RJ, Probstfield J et al. Comparison of candesartan, enalapril, and their

combination in congestive heart failure: randomized evaluation of strategies for left ventricular dysfunction (RESOLVD) pilot study. The RESOLVD Pilot Study Investigators. *Circulation* 1999;**100**:1056–64.

124. Cohn JN, Tognoni G. A randomized trial of the angiotensin-receptor blocker valsartan in chronic heart failure. *N Engl J Med* 2001;**345**:1667–75.

125. Granger CB, McMurray JJ, Yusuf S, Held P, Michelson EL, Olofsson B *et al*. Effects of candesartan in patients with chronic heart failure and reduced left-ventricular systolic function intolerant to angiotensin-converting-enzyme inhibitors: the CHARM-Alternative trial. *Lancet* 2003;**362**:772–6.

126. McMurray JJ, Ostergren J, Swedberg K, Granger CB, Held P, Michelson EL *et al*. Effects of candesartan in patients with chronic heart failure and reduced left-ventricular systolic function taking angiotensin-converting-enzyme inhibitors: the CHARM-Added trial. *Lancet* 2003;**362**:767–71.

127. Yusuf S, Pfeffer MA, Swedberg K, Granger CB, Held P, McMurray JJ *et al*. Effects of candesartan in patients with chronic heart failure and preserved left-ventricular ejection fraction: the CHARM-Preserved Trial. *Lancet* 2003;**362**:777–81.

128. Pfeffer MA, Swedberg K, Granger CB, Held P, McMurray JJ, Michelson EL *et al*. Effects of candesartan on mortality and morbidity in patients with chronic heart failure: the CHARM-Overall programme. *Lancet* 2003;**362**:759–66.

129. Dimopoulos K, Salukhe TV, Coats AJ, Mayet J, Piepoli M, Francis DP. Meta-analyses of mortality and morbidity effects of an angiotensin receptor blocker in patients with chronic heart failure already receiving an ACE inhibitor (alone or with a beta-blocker). *Int J Cardiol* 2004;**93**:105–11.

130. Feldman AM. Classification of positive inotropic agents. *J Am Coll Cardiol* 1993;**22**:1223–7.

131. Smith HJ, Oriol A, Morch J, McGregor M. Hemodynamic studies in cardiogenic shock. Treatment with isoproterenol and metaraminol. *Circulation* 1967;**35**:1084–91.

132. Tuttle RR, Mills J. Dobutamine: development of a new catecholamine to selectively increase cardiac contractility. *Circ Res* 1975;**36**:185–96.

133. Meyer SL, Curry GC, Donsky MS, Twieg DB, Parkey RW, Willerson JT. Influence of dobutamine on hemodynamics and coronary blood flow in patients with and without coronary artery disease. *Am J Cardiol* 1976;**38**:103–8.

134. Akhtar N, Mikulic E, Cohn JN, Chaudhry MH. Hemodynamic effect of dobutamine in patients with severe heart failure. *Am J Cardiol* 1975;**36**:202–5.

135. Leier CV, Webel J, Bush CA. The cardiovascular effects of the continuous infusion of dobutamine in patients with severe cardiac failure. *Circulation* 1977;**56**:468–72.

136. Pozen RG, DiBianco R, Katz RJ, Bortz R, Myerburg RJ, Fletcher RD. Myocardial metabolic and hemodynamic effects of dobutamine in heart failure complicating coronary artery disease. *Circulation* 1981;**63**:1279–85.

137. Leier CV, Unverferth DV, Kates RE. The relationship between plasma dobutamine concentrations and cardiovascular responses in cardiac failure. *Am J Med* 1979;**66**:238–42.

138. Colucci WS, Denniss AR, Leatherman GF, Quigg RJ, Ludmer PL, Marsh JD, Gauthier DF. Intracoronary infusion of dobutamine to patients with and without severe congestive heart failure. Dose-response relationships, correlation with circulat-

ing catecholamines, and effect of phosphodiesterase inhibition. *J Clin Invest* 1988;**81**:1103–10.

139. Bristow MR, Port JD, Hershberger RE, Gilbert EM, Feldman AM. The beta-adrenergic receptor-adenylate cyclase complex as a target for therapeutic intervention in heart failure. *Eur Heart J* 1989;**10**(suppl B):45–54.

140. Unverferth DA, Blanford M, Kates RE, Leier CV. Tolerance to dobutamine after a 72 hour continuous infusion. *Am J Med* 1980;**69**:262–6.

141. Hauptman PJ, Mikolajczak P, George A, Mohr CJ, Hoover R, Swindle J, Schnitzler MA. Chronic inotropic therapy in end-stage heart failure. *Am Heart J* 2006;**152**:1091–8.

142. Goldberg LI. Cardiovascular and renal actions of dopamine: potential clinical applications. *Pharmacol Rev* 1972;**24**:1–29.

143. Goldberg LI, Volkman PH, Kohli JD. A comparison of the vascular dopamine receptor with other dopamine receptors. *Annu Rev Pharmacol Toxicol* 1978;**18**:57–79.

144. Rajfer SI, Goldberg LI. Dopamine in the treatment of heart failure. *Eur Heart J* 1982;**3**(suppl D):103–6.

145. Lokhandwala MF, Barrett RJ. Cardiovascular dopamine receptors: physiological, pharmacological and therapeutic implications. *J Autonomic Pharmacol* 1982;**2**:189–215.

146. Denton MD, Chertow GM, Brady HR. "Renal-dose" dopamine for the treatment of acute renal failure: scientific rationale, experimental studies and clinical trials. *Kidney Int* 1996;**50**: 4–14.

147. Baim DS, McDowell AV, Cherniles J, Monrad ES, Parker JA, Edelson J *et al*. Evaluation of a new bipyridine inotropic agent – milrinone – in patients with severe congestive heart failure. *N Engl J Med* 1983;**309**:748–56.

148. Rettig GF, Schieffer HJ. Acute effects of intravenous milrinone in heart failure. *Eur Heart J* 1989;**10**(suppl C):39–43.

149. Klocke RK, Mager G, Kux A, Hopp HW, Hilger HH. Effects of a twenty-four-hour milrinone infusion in patients with severe heart failure and cardiogenic shock as a function of the hemodynamic initial condition. *Am Heart J* 1991;**121**:1965–73.

150. Kinney EL, Ballard JO, Carlin B, Zelis R. Amrinone-mediated thrombocytopenia. *Scand J Haematol* 1983;**31**:376–80.

151. Anderson JL. Hemodynamic and clinical benefits with intravenous milrinone in severe chronic heart failure: results of a multicenter study in the United States. *Am Heart J* 1991;**121**: 1956–64.

152. Packer M, Carver JR, Rodeheffer RJ, Ivanhoe RJ, DiBianco R, Zeldis SM *et al*. Effect of oral milrinone on mortality in severe chronic heart failure. The PROMISE Study Research Group. *N Engl J Med* 1991;**325**:1468–75.

153. Lowes BD, Tsvetkova T, Eichhorn EJ, Gilbert EM, Bristow MR. Milrinone versus dobutamine in heart failure subjects treated chronically with carvedilol. *Int J Cardiol* 2001;**81**:141–9.

154. Packer M. The development of positive inotropic agents for chronic heart failure: how have we gone astray? *J Am Coll Cardiol* 1993;**22**:119A–126A.

155. Ewy GA. Inotropic infusions for chronic congestive heart failure: medical miracles or misguided medicinals? *J Am Coll Cardiol* 1999;**33**:572–5.

156. Nieminen MS, Akkila J, Hasenfuss G, Kleber FX, Lehtonen LA, Mitrovic V *et al*. Hemodynamic and neurohumoral effects of continuous infusion of levosimendan in patients with congestive heart failure. *J Am Coll Cardiol* 2000;**36**:1903–12.

157. Slawsky MT, Colucci WS, Gottlieb SS, Greenberg BH, Haeusslein E, Hare J et al. Acute hemodynamic and clinical effects of levosimendan in patients with severe heart failure. Study Investigators. *Circulation* 2000;**102**:2222–7.

158. Follath F, Cleland JG, Just H, Papp JG, Scholz H, Peuhkurinen K et al. Efficacy and safety of intravenous levosimendan compared with dobutamine in severe low-output heart failure (the LIDO study): a randomised double-blind trial. *Lancet* 2002;**360**:196–202.

159. Cleland JG, Freemantle N, Coletta AP, Clark AL. Clinical trials update from the American Heart Association: REPAIR-AMI, ASTAMI, JELIS, MEGA, REVIVE-II, SURVIVE, and PROACTIVE. *Eur J Heart Fail* 2006;**8**:105–10.

160. Mebazaa A, Nieminen MS, Packer M, Cohen-Solal A, Kleber FX, Pocock SJ et al. Levosimendan vs dobutamine for patients with acute decompensated heart failure: the SURVIVE Randomized Trial. *JAMA* 2007;**297**:1883–91.

161. Cleland JG, Coletta AP, Lammiman M, Witte KK, Loh H, Nasir M, Clark AL. Clinical trials update from the European Society of Cardiology meeting 2005: CARE-HF extension study, ESSENTIAL, CIBIS-III, S-ICD, ISSUE-2, STRIDE-2, SOFA, IMAGINE, PREAMI, SIRIUS-II and ACTIVE. *Eur J Heart Fail* 2005;**7**:1070–5.

162. Swedberg K, Hjalmarson A, Waagstein F, Wallentin I. Prolongation of survival in congestive cardiomyopathy by beta-receptor blockade. *Lancet* 1979;**1**:1374–6.

163. Waagstein F, Hjalmarson A, Varnauskas E, Wallentin I. Effect of chronic beta-adrenergic receptor blockade in congestive cardiomyopathy. *Br Heart J* 1975;**37**:1022–36.

164. DasGupta P, Lahiri A. Can intravenous beta blockade predict long-term haemodynamic benefit in chronic congestive heart failure secondary to ischaemic heart disease? A comparison between intravenous and oral carvedilol. *Clin Invest* 1992;**70**(suppl 1):S98–104.

165. Andersson B, Lomsky M, Waagstein F. The link between acute haemodynamic adrenergic beta-blockade and long-term effects in patients with heart failure. A study on diastolic function, heart rate and myocardial metabolism following intravenous metoprolol. *Eur Heart J* 1993;**14**:1375–85.

166. Haber HL, Simek CL, Gimple LW, Bergin JD, Subbiah K, Jayaweera AR et al. Why do patients with congestive heart failure tolerate the initiation of beta-blocker therapy? *Circulation* 1993;**88**:1610–19.

167. Gilbert EM, Anderson JL, Deitchman D, Yanowitz FG, O'Connell JB, Renlund DG et al. Long-term beta-blocker vasodilator therapy improves cardiac function in idiopathic dilated cardiomyopathy: a double-blind, randomized study of bucindolol versus placebo. *Am J Med* 1990;**88**:223–29.

168. Andersson B, Caidahl K, di Lenarda A, Warren SE, Goss F, Waldenstrom A et al. Changes in early and late diastolic filling patterns induced by long-term adrenergic beta-blockade in patients with idiopathic dilated cardiomyopathy. *Circulation* 1996;**94**:673–82.

169. Hall SA, Cigarroa CG, Marcoux L, Risser RC, Grayburn PA, Eichhorn EJ. Time course of improvement in left ventricular function, mass and geometry in patients with congestive heart failure treated with beta-adrenergic blockade. *J Am Coll Cardiol* 1995;**25**:1154–61.

170. Woodley SL, Gilbert EM, Anderson JL, O'Connell JB, Deitchman D, Yanowitz FG et al. Beta-blockade with bucindolol in heart failure caused by ischemic versus idiopathic dilated cardiomyopathy. *Circulation* 1991;**84**:2426–41.

171. Eichhorn EJ, Bedotto JB, Malloy CR, Hatfield BA, Deitchman D, Brown M et al. Effect of beta-adrenergic blockade on myocardial function and energetics in congestive heart failure. Improvements in hemodynamic, contractile, and diastolic performance with bucindolol. *Circulation* 1990;**82**:473–83.

172. Bristow MR, O'Connell JB, Gilbert EM, French WJ, Leatherman G, Kantrowitz NE et al. Dose-response of chronic beta-blocker treatment in heart failure from either idiopathic dilated or ischemic cardiomyopathy. Bucindolol Investigators. *Circulation* 1994;**89**:1632–42.

173. Eichhorn EJ, Heesch CM, Risser RC, Marcoux L, Hatfield B. Predictors of systolic and diastolic improvement in patients with dilated cardiomyopathy treated with metoprolol. *J Am Coll Cardiol* 1995;**25**:154–62.

174. Metra M, Nardi M, Giubbini R, Dei Cas L. Effects of short- and long-term carvedilol administration on rest and exercise hemodynamic variables, exercise capacity and clinical conditions in patients with idiopathic dilated cardiomyopathy. *J Am Coll Cardiol* 1994;**24**:1678–87.

175. Australia-New Zealand Heart Failure Research Collaborative Group. Effects of carvedilol, a vasodilator-beta-blocker, in patients with congestive heart failure due to ischemic heart disease. *Circulation* 1995;**92**:212–18.

176. Groenning BA, Nilsson JC, Sondergaard L, Fritz-Hansen T, Larsson HB, Hildebrandt PR. Antiremodeling effects on the left ventricle during beta-blockade with metoprolol in the treatment of chronic heart failure. *J Am Coll Cardiol* 2000;**36**:2072 80.

177. Anonymous. Effects of metoprolol CR in patients with ischemic and dilated cardiomyopathy : the randomized evaluation of strategies for left ventricular dysfunction pilot study. *Circulation* 2000;**101**:378–84.

178. Andersson B, Blomstrom-Lundqvist C, Hedner T, Waagstein F. Exercise hemodynamics and myocardial metabolism during long-term beta-adrenergic blockade in severe heart failure. *J Am Coll Cardiol* 1991;**18**:1059–66.

179. Nemanich JW, Veith RC, Abrass IB, Stratton JR. Effects of metoprolol on rest and exercise cardiac function and plasma catecholamines in chronic congestive heart failure secondary to ischemic or idiopathic cardiomyopathy. *Am J Cardiol* 1990;**66**:843–8.

180. Eichhorn EJ, McGhie AL, Bedotto JB, Corbett JR, Malloy CR, Hatfield BA et al. Effects of bucindolol on neurohormonal activation in congestive heart failure. *Am J Cardiol* 1991;**67**:67–73.

181. Andersson B, Hamm C, Persson S, Wikstrom G, Sinagra G, Hjalmarson A, Waagstein F. Improved exercise hemodynamic status in dilated cardiomyopathy after beta-adrenergic blockade treatment. *J Am Coll Cardiol* 1994;**23**:1397–404.

182. Yoshikawa T, Handa S, Anzai T, Nishimura H, Baba A, Akaishi M et al. Early reduction of neurohumoral factors plays a key role in mediating the efficacy of beta-blocker therapy for congestive heart failure. *Am Heart J* 1996;**131**:329–36.

183. The CIBIS-II Investigators. Cardiac Insufficiency Bisoprolol Study II (CIBIS-II): a randomised trial. *Lancet* 1999;**353**:9–13.

184. The MERIT Investigators. Effect of metoprolol CR/XL in chronic heart failure: Metoprolol CR/XL Randomised Intervention

Trial in Congestive Heart Failure (MERIT-HF). *Lancet* 1999;**353**: 2001–7.

185. Packer M, Coats AJ, Fowler MB, Katus HA, Krum H, Mohacsi P *et al.* Effect of carvedilol on survival in severe chronic heart failure. *N Engl J Med* 2001;**344**:1651–8.

186. Waagstein F, Bristow MR, Swedberg K, Camerini F, Fowler MB, Silver MA *et al.* Beneficial effects of metoprolol in idiopathic dilated cardiomyopathy. Metoprolol in Dilated Cardiomyopathy (MDC) Trial Study Group. *Lancet* 1993;**342**:1441–6.

187. Colucci WS, Packer M, Bristow MR, Gilbert EM, Cohn JN, Fowler MB *et al.* Carvedilol inhibits clinical progression in patients with mild symptoms of heart failure. US Carvedilol Heart Failure Study Group. *Circulation* 1996;**94**:2800–6.

188. Packer M, Colucci WS, Sackner-Bernstein JD, Liang CS, Goldscher DA, Freeman I *et al.* Double-blind, placebo-controlled study of the effects of carvedilol in patients with moderate to severe heart failure. The PRECISE Trial. Prospective Randomized Evaluation of Carvedilol on Symptoms and Exercise. *Circulation* 1996;**94**:2793–9.

189. Hjalmarson A, Goldstein S, Fagerberg B, Wedel H, Waagstein F, Kjekshus J *et al.* Effects of controlled-release metoprolol on total mortality, hospitalizations, and well-being in patients with heart failure: the Metoprolol CR/XL Randomized Intervention Trial in congestive heart failure (MERIT-HF). MERIT-HF Study Group. *JAMA* 2000;**283**:1295–302.

190. Metoprolol in Dilated Cardiomyopathy (MDC) Trial Study Group. Three-year follow-up of patients randomised in the metoprolol in dilated cardiomyopathy trial. *Lancet* 1998;**351**: 1180–1.

191. CIBIS Investigators and Committees. A randomized trial of beta-blockade in heart failure. The Cardiac Insufficiency Bisoprolol Study (CIBIS). *Circulation* 1994;**90**:1765–3.

192. Packer M, Bristow MR, Cohn JN, Colucci WS, Fowler MB, Gilbert EM, Shusterman NH. The effect of carvedilol on morbidity and mortality in patients with chronic heart failure. U.S. Carvedilol Heart Failure Study Group. *N Engl J Med* 1996;**334**: 1349–55.

193. Australia/New Zealand Heart Failure Research Collaborative Group. Randomised, placebo-controlled trial of carvedilol in patients with congestive heart failure due to ischaemic heart disease. *Lancet* 1997;**349**:375–80.

194. Krum H, Roecker EB, Mohacsi P, Rouleau JL, Tendera M, Coats AJ *et al.* Effects of initiating carvedilol in patients with severe chronic heart failure: results from the COPERNICUS Study. *JAMA* 2003;**289**:712–18.

195. Goldstein S, Fagerberg B, Hjalmarson A, Kjekshus J, Waagstein F, Wedel H, Wikstrand J. Metoprolol controlled release/ extended release in patients with severe heart failure: analysis of the experience in the MERIT-HF study. *J Am Coll Cardiol* 2001;**38**:932–8.

196. Beta-Blocker Evaluation of Survival Trial Investigators. A trial of the beta-blocker bucindolol in patients with advanced chronic heart failure. *N Engl J Med* 2001;**344**:1659–67.

197. Liggett SB, Mialet-Perez J, Thaneemit-Chen S, Weber SA, Greene SM, Hodne D *et al.* A polymorphism within a conserved beta(1)-adrenergic receptor motif alters cardiac function and beta-blocker response in human heart failure. *Proc Natl Acad Sci USA* 2006;**103**:11288–93.

198. Flather MD, Shibata MC, Coats AJ, Van Veldhuisen DJ, Parkhomenko A, Borbola J *et al.* Randomized trial to determine the effect of nebivolol on mortality and cardiovascular hospital admission in elderly patients with heart failure (SENIORS). *Eur Heart J* 2005;**26**:215–25.

199. McMurray J. Making sense of SENIORS. *Eur Heart J* 2005;**26**:203–6.

200. Maack C, Elter T, Nickenig G, LaRosee K, Crivaro M, Stablein A *et al.* Prospective crossover comparison of carvedilol and metoprolol in patients with chronic heart failure. *J Am Coll Cardiol* 2001;**38**:939–46.

201. Poole-Wilson PA, Swedberg K, Cleland JG, Di Lenarda A, Hanrath P, Komajda M *et al.* Comparison of carvedilol and metoprolol on clinical outcomes in patients with chronic heart failure in the Carvedilol Or Metoprolol European Trial (COMET): randomised controlled trial. *Lancet* 2003;**362**:7–13.

202. Packer M. Do beta-blockers prolong survival in heart failure only by inhibiting the beta1-receptor? A perspective on the results of the COMET trial. *J Cardiac Fail* 2003;**9**:429–43.

203. Bristow MR, Feldman AM, Adams KF Jr, Goldstein S. Selective versus nonselective beta-blockade for heart failure therapy: are there lessons to be learned from the COMET trial? *J Cardiac Fail* 2003;**9**:444–53.

204. Massie BM. A comment on COMET: how to interpret a positive trial? *J Cardiac Fail* 2003;**9**:425–8.

205. Willenheimer R, van Veldhuisen DJ, Silke B, Erdmann E, Follath F, Krum H *et al.* Effect on survival and hospitalization of initiating treatment for chronic heart failure with bisoprolol followed by enalapril, as compared with the opposite sequence: results of the randomized Cardiac Insufficiency Bisoprolol Study (CIBIS) III. *Circulation* 2005;**112**:2426–35.

206. Herlitz J, Hjalmarson A, Holmberg S, Swedberg K, Vedin A, Waagstein F *et al. Development* of congestive heart failure after treatment with metoprolol in acute myocardial infarction. *Br Heart J* 1984;**51**:539–44.

207. Chadda K, Goldstein S, Byington R, Curb JD. Effect of propranolol after acute myocardial infarction in patients with congestive heart failure. *Circulation* 1986;**73**:503–10.

208. Olsson G, Rehnqvist N. Effect of metoprolol in postinfarction patients with increased heart size. *Eur Heart J* 1986;**7**:468–74.

209. Dargie HJ. Effect of carvedilol on outcome after myocardial infarction in patients with left-ventricular dysfunction: the CAPRICORN randomised trial. *Lancet* 2001;**357**:1385–90.

210. Manolis AJ, Olympios C, Sifaki M, Handanis S, Bresnahan M, Gavras I, Gavras H. Suppressing sympathetic activation in congestive heart failure. A new therapeutic strategy. *Hypertension.* 1995;**26**:719–24.

211. Swedberg K, Bergh CH, Dickstein K, McNay J, Steinberg M. The effects of moxonidine, a novel imidazoline, on plasma norepinephrine in patients with congestive heart failure. Moxonidine Investigators. *J Am Coll Cardiol* 2000;**35**:398–404.

212. Swedberg K, Bristow MR, Cohn JN, Dargie H, Straub M, Wiltse C, Wright TJ. Effects of sustained-release moxonidine, an imidazoline agonist, on plasma norepinephrine in patients with chronic heart failure. *Circulation* 2002;**105**:1797–803.

213. Cohn JN, Pfeffer MA, Rouleau J, Sharpe N, Swedberg K, Straub M *et al.* Adverse mortality effect of central sympathetic inhibition with sustained-release moxonidine in patients with heart failure (MOXCON). *Eur J Heart Fail* 2003;**5**:659–67.

214. Kannel WB, Plehn JF, Cupples LA. Cardiac failure and sudden death in the Framingham Study. *Am Heart J* 1988;**115**:869–75.

215. Kjekshus J. Arrhythmias and mortality in congestive heart failure. *Am J Cardiol* 1990;**65**:42I–48I.

216. Andersson B, Waagstein F. Spectrum and outcome of congestive heart failure in a hospitalized population. *Am Heart J* 1993;**126**:632–40.

217. Packer M. Sudden unexpected death in patients with congestive heart failure: a second frontier. *Circulation* 1985;**72**:681–5.

218. Stevenson WG, Stevenson LW, Middlekauff HR, Saxon LA. Sudden death prevention in patients with advanced ventricular dysfunction. *Circulation* 1993;**88**:2953–61.

219. Bigger JT Jr, Fleiss JL, Kleiger R, Miller JP, Rolnitzky LM. The relationships among ventricular arrhythmias, left ventricular dysfunction, and mortality in the 2 years after myocardial infarction. *Circulation* 1984;**69**:250–8.

220. Cardiac Arrhythmia Suppression Trial (CAST) Investigators. Preliminary report: effect of encainide and flecainide on mortality in a randomized trial of arrhythmia suppression after myocardial infarction. *N Engl J Med* 1989;**321**:406–12.

221. Doval HC, Nul DR, Grancelli HO, Perrone SV, Bortman GR, Curiel R. Randomised trial of low-dose amiodarone in severe congestive heart failure. Grupo de Estudio de la Sobrevida en la Insuficiencia Cardiaca en Argentina (GESICA). *Lancet* 1994;**344**:493–8.

222. Singh SN, Fletcher RD, Fisher SG, Singh BN, Lewis HD, Deedwania PC et al. Amiodarone in patients with congestive heart failure and asymptomatic ventricular arrhythmia. Survival Trial of Antiarrhythmic Therapy in Congestive Heart Failure. *N Engl J Med* 1995;**333**:77–82.

223. Julian DG, Camm AJ, Frangin G, Janse MJ, Munoz A, Schwartz PJ, Simon P. Randomised trial of effect of amiodarone on mortality in patients with left-ventricular dysfunction after recent myocardial infarction: EMIAT. European Myocardial Infarct Amiodarone Trial Investigators. *Lancet* 1997;**349**: 667–74.

224. Cairns JA, Connolly SJ, Roberts R, Gent M. Randomised trial of outcome after myocardial infarction in patients with frequent or repetitive ventricular premature depolarisations: CAMIAT. Canadian Amiodarone Myocardial Infarction *Arrhythmia Trial Investigators*. *Lancet* 1997;**349**:675–82.

225. Amiodarone Trials Meta-Analysis Investigators. Effect of prophylactic amiodarone on mortality after acute myocardial infarction and in congestive heart failure: meta-analysis of individual data from 6500 patients in randomised trials. *Lancet* 1997;**350**:1417–24.

226. Bardy GH, Lee KL, Mark DB, Poole JE, Packer DL, Boineau R et al. Amiodarone or an implantable cardioverter-defibrillator for congestive heart failure. *N Engl J Med* 2005;**352**:225–37.

227. Waldo AL, Camm AJ, deRuyter H, Friedman PL, MacNeil DJ, Pauls JF et al. Effect of d-sotalol on mortality in patients with left ventricular dysfunction after recent and remote myocardial infarction. The SWORD Investigators. Survival With Oral d-Sotalol. *Lancet* 1996;**348**:7–12.

228. Solomon SD, Wang D, Finn P, Skali H, Zornoff L, McMurray JJ et al. Effect of candesartan on cause-specific mortality in heart failure patients: the Candesartan in Heart failure Assessment of Reduction in Mortality and morbidity (CHARM) program. *Circulation* 2004;**110**:2180–3.

229. Mann DL, McMurray JJ, Packer M, Swedberg K, Borer JS, Colucci WS et al. Targeted anticytokine therapy in patients with chronic heart failure: results of the Randomized Etanercept Worldwide Evaluation (RENEWAL). *Circulation* 2004;**109**:1594–602.

230. Chung ES, Packer M, Lo KH, Fasanmade AA, Willerson JT. Randomized, double-blind, placebo-controlled, pilot trial of infliximab, a chimeric monoclonal antibody to tumor necrosis factor-alpha, in patients with moderate-to-severe heart failure: results of the anti-TNF Therapy Against Congestive Heart Failure (ATTACH) trial. *Circulation* 2003;**107**:3133–40.

231. Gheorghiade M, Gattis WA, O'Connor CM, Adams KF Jr, Elkayam U, Barbagelata A et al. Effects of tolvaptan, a vasopressin antagonist, in patients hospitalized with worsening heart failure: a randomized controlled trial. *JAMA* 2004;**291**: 1963–71.

232. Konstam MA, Gheorghiade M, Burnett JC Jr, Grinfeld L, Maggioni AP, Swedberg K et al. Effects of oral tolvaptan in patients hospitalized for worsening heart failure: the EVEREST Outcome Trial. *JAMA* 2007;**297**:1319–31.

233. Gheorghiade M, Konstam MA, Burnett JC Jr, Grinfeld L, Maggioni AP, Swedberg K et al. Short-term clinical effects of tolvaptan, an oral vasopressin antagonist, in patients hospitalized for heart failure: the EVEREST Clinical Status Trials. *JAMA* 2007; **297**:1332–43.

234. Abraham WT, Shamshirsaz AA, McFann K, Oren RM, Schrier RW. Aquaretic effect of lixivaptan, an oral, non-peptide, selective V2 receptor vasopressin antagonist, in New York Heart Association functional class II and III chronic heart failure patients. *J Am Coll Cardiol* 2006;**47**:1615–21.

235. Teerlink JR. Endothelins: pathophysiology and treatment implications in chronic heart failure. *Curr Heart Fail Rep* 2005;**2**:191–7.

236. Packer M, McMurray J, Massie BM, Caspi A, Charlon V, Cohen-Solal A et al. Clinical effects of endothelin receptor antagonism with bosentan in patients with severe chronic heart failure: results of a pilot study. *J Cardiac Fail* 2005;**11**:12–20.

237. McMurray JJ, Teerlink JR, Cotter G, Bourge RC, Cleland JG, Jondeau G et al. Effects of tezosentan on symptoms and clinical outcomes in patients with acute heart failure: the VERITAS randomized controlled trials. *JAMA* 2007;**298**: 2009–19.

238. Kalra PR, Moon JC, Coats AJ. Do results of the ENABLE (Endothelin Antagonist Bosentan for Lowering Cardiac Events in Heart Failure) study spell the end for non-selective endothelin antagonism in heart failure? *Int J Cardiol* 2002;**85**: 195–7.

239. Spieker LE, Luscher TF. Endothelin receptor antagonists in heart failure – a refutation of a bold conjecture? *Eur J Heart Fail* 2003;**5**:415–17.

240. Teerlink JR. Recent heart failure trials of neurohormonal modulation (OVERTURE and ENABLE): approaching the asymptote of efficacy? *J Cardiac Fail* 2002;**8**:124–7.

241. Horwich TB, MacLellan WR, Fonarow GC. Statin therapy is associated with improved survival in ischemic and non-ischemic heart failure. *J Am Coll Cardiol* 2004;**43**:642–8.

242. Kjekshus J, Apetrei E, Barrios V, Bohm M, Cleland JG, Cornel JH et al. Rosuvastatin in older patients with systolic heart failure. *N Engl J Med* 2007;**357**:2248–61.

243. Rauchhaus M, Clark AL, Doehner W, Davos C, Bolger A, Sharma R et al. The relationship between cholesterol and survival in patients with chronic heart failure. *J Am Coll Cardiol* 2003;**42**:1933–40.

244. Hedrich O, Jacob M, Hauptman PJ. Progression of coronary artery disease in non-ischemic dilated cardiomyopathy. *Coron Art Dis* 2004;**15**:291–7.

245. GISSI-HF Investigators. Effect of rosuvastatin in patients with chronic heart failure (the GISSI-HF trial): a randomised, double-blind, placebo-controlled trial. *Lancet* 2008;**373**:1231–39.

246. HF-ACTION Investigators. Efficacy and safety of exercise training n patients with chronic heart failure: HF-Action Randomized Controlled Trial. *JAMA* 2009;**372**:1439–50.

247. Rich MW, Beckham V, Wittenberg C, Leven CL, Freedland KE, Carney RM. A multidisciplinary intervention to prevent the readmission of elderly patients with congestive heart failure. *N Engl J Med* 1995;**333**:1190–5.

248. Stromberg A, Martensson J, Fridlund B, Levin LA, Karlsson JE, Dahlstrom U. Nurse-led heart failure clinics improve survival and self-care behaviour in patients with heart failure: results from a prospective, randomised trial. *Eur Heart J* 2003;**24**:1014–23.

249. Gohler A, Januzzi JL, Worrell SS, Osterziel KJ, Gazelle GS, Dietz R, Siebert U. A systematic meta-analysis of the efficacy and heterogeneity of disease management programs in congestive heart failure. *J Cardiac Fail* 2006;**12**:554–67.

250. Gonseth J, Guallar-Castillon P, Banegas JR, Rodriguez-Artalejo F. The effectiveness of disease management programmes in reducing hospital re-admission in older patients with heart failure: a systematic review and meta-analysis of published reports. *Eur Heart J* 2004;**25**:1570–95.

251. McAlister FA, Stewart S, Ferrua S, McMurray JJ. Multidisciplinary strategies for the management of heart failure patients at high risk for admission: a systematic review of randomized trials. *J Am Coll Cardiol* 2004;**44**:810–19.

252. Moss AJ, Zareba W, Hall WJ, Klein H, Wilber DJ, Cannom DS et al. Prophylactic implantation of a defibrillator in patients with myocardial infarction and reduced ejection fraction. *N Engl J Med* 2002;**346**:877–83.

253. Bristow MR, Saxon LA, Boehmer J, Krueger S, Kass DA, De Marco T et al. Cardiac-resynchronization therapy with or without an implantable defibrillator in advanced chronic heart failure. *N Engl J Med* 2004;**350**:2140–50.

254. Abraham WT, Fisher WG, Smith AL, Delurgio DB, Leon AR, Loh E et al. Cardiac resynchronization in chronic heart failure. *N Engl J Med* 2002;**346**:1845–53.

255. Cleland JG, Daubert JC, Erdmann E, Freemantle N, Gras D, Kappenberger L, Tavazzi L. The effect of cardiac resynchronization on morbidity and mortality in heart failure. *N Engl J Med* 2005;**352**:1539–49.

256. Curtis LH, Al-Khatib SM, Shea AM, Hammill BG, Hernandez AF, Schulman KA. Sex differences in the use of implantable cardioverter-defibrillators for primary and secondary prevention of sudden cardiac death. *JAMA* 2007;**298**:1517–24.

257. Carlson M, Wilkoff, BL, Maisel WH, Ellenbogen, KA, Saxon, LA, Prystowsky EN et al. Recommendations from the Heart Rhythm Society Task Force on Device Performance Policies and Guidelines. *Heart Rhythm* 2006;**3**:1251–72.

258. Sanders GD, Hlatky MA, Owens DK. Cost-effectiveness of implantable cardioverter-defibrillators. *N Engl J Med* 2005;**353**:1471–80.

259. Goldstein NE, Lampert R, Bradley E, Lynn J, Krumholz HM. Management of implantable cardioverter defibrillators in end-of-life care. *Ann Intern Med* 2004;**141**:835–8.

260. McCarthy PM, Smedira NO, Vargo RL, Goormastic M, Hobbs RE, Starling RC, Young JB. One hundred patients with the HeartMate left ventricular assist device: evolving concepts and technology. *J Thorac Cardiovasc Surg* 1998;**115**:904–12.

261. Rose EA, Gelijns AC, Moskowitz AJ, Heitjan DF, Stevenson LW, Dembitsky W et al. Long-term mechanical left ventricular assistance for end-stage heart failure. *N Engl J Med* 2001;**345**:1435–43.

262. Miller LW, Pagani FD, Russell SD, John R, Boyle AJ, Aaronson KD et al. Use of a continuous-flow device in patients awaiting heart transplantation. *N Engl J Med* 2007;**357**:885–96.

263. Birks EJ, Tansley PD, Hardy J, George RS, Bowles CT, Burke M et al. Left ventricular assist device and drug therapy for the reversal of heart failure. *N Engl J Med* 2006;**355**:1873–84.

264. McConnell PI, Michler RE. Surgical ventricular restoration and other surgical approaches to heart failure. *Curr Heart Fail Rep* 2004;**1**:21–9.

265. Joyce D, Loebe M, Noon GP, McRee S, Southard R, Thompson L et al. Revascularization and ventricular restoration in patients with ischemic heart failure: the STICH trial. *Curr Opin Cardiol* 2003;**18**:454–7.

266. Wu AH, Aaronson KD, Bolling SF, Pagani FD, Welch K, Koelling TM. Impact of mitral valve annuloplasty on mortality risk in patients with mitral regurgitation and left ventricular systolic dysfunction. *J Am Coll Cardiol* 2005;**45**:381–7.

267. Massie BM, Carson PE, McMurray JJ et al. Irbesartan in patients with heart failure and preserved ejection fraction. *N Engl J Med* 2008;**359**:2456–67.

268. Kostis JB, Davis BR, Cutler J, Grimm RH Jr, Berge KG, Cohen JD et al. Prevention of heart failure by antihypertensive drug treatment in older persons with isolated systolic hypertension. SHEP Cooperative Research Group. *JAMA* 1997;**278**:212–16.

269. Binanay C, Califf RM, Hasselblad V, O'Connor CM, Shah MR, Sopko G et al. Evaluation study of congestive heart failure and pulmonary artery catheterization effectiveness: the ESCAPE trial. *JAMA* 2005;**294**:1625–33.

270. Kashem A, Cross RC, Santamore WP, Bove AA. Management of heart failure patients using telemedicine communication systems. *Curr Cardiol Rep* 2006;**8**:171–9.

271. Yancy CW. Current approaches to monitoring and management of heart failure. *Rev Cardiovasc Med* 2006;**7**(suppl 1):S25–32.

272. Chaudhry SI, Phillips CO, Stewart SS, Riegel B, Mattera JA, Jerant AF, Krumholz HM. Telemonitoring for patients with chronic heart failure: a systematic review. *J Cardiac Fail* 2007;**13**:56–62.

273. Caldwell MA, Peters KJ, Dracup KA. A simplified education program improves knowledge, self-care behavior, and disease severity in heart failure patients in rural settings. *Am Heart J* 2005;**150**:983.

274. Troughton RW, Richards AM. BNP for clinical monitoring of heart failure. *Heart Fail Clin* 2006;**2**:333–43.

275. Pamboukian SV, Smallfield MC, Bourge RC. Implantable hemo-dynamic monitoring devices in heart failure. *Curr Cardiol Rep* 2006;**8**:187–90.

276. Olsson LG, Swedberg K, Cleland JG, Spark PA, Komajda M, Metra M *et al.* Prognostic importance of plasma NT-pro BNP in chronic heart failure in patients treated with a beta-blocker: results from the Carvedilol Or Metoprolol European Trial (COMET) trial. *Eur J Heart Fail* 2007;**9**:795–801.

277. Jourdain P, Jondeau G, Funck F, Gueffet P, Le Helloco A, Donal E *et al.* Plasma brain natriuretic peptide-guided therapy to improve outcome in heart failure: the STARS-BNP Multicenter Study. *J Am Coll Cardiol* 2007;**49**:1733–9.

278. Lainchbury JG, Troughton RW, Frampton CM, Yandle TG, Hamid A, Nicholls MG, Richards AM. NTproBNP-guided drug treatment for chronic heart failure: design and methods in the "BATTLESCARRED" trial. *Eur J Heart Fail* 2006;**8**:532–8.

279. Cleland JG, Coletta AP, Freemantle N, Velavan P, Tin L, Clark AL. Clinical trials update from the American College of Cardiology meeting: CARE-HF and the remission of heart failure, Women's Health Study, TNT, COMPASS-HF, VERITAS, CANPAP, PEECH and PREMIER. *Eur J Heart Fail.* 2005;**7**: 931–6.

280. Krumholz HM, Normand SL, Spertus JA, Shahian DM, Bradley EH. Measuring performance for treating heart attacks and heart failure: the case for outcomes measurement. *Health Affairs (Project Hope)* 2007;**26**:75–85.

281. Bonow RO, Bennett S, Casey DE Jr, Ganiats TG, Hlatky MA, Konstam MA *et al.* ACC/AHA Clinical Performance Measures for Adults with Chronic Heart Failure: a report of the American College of Cardiology/American Heart Association Task Force on Performance Measures (Writing Committee to Develop Heart Failure Clinical Performance Measures): endorsed by the Heart Failure Society of America. *Circulation* 2005;**112**: 1853–87.

282. Fonarow GC, Yancy CW, Heywood JT. Adherence to heart failure quality-of-care indicators in US hospitals: analysis of the ADHERE Registry. *Arch Intern Med* 2005;**165**:1469–77.

283. Fonarow GC, Abraham WT, Albert NM, Gattis Stough W, Gheorghiade M, Greenberg BH *et al.* Influence of a performance-improvement initiative on quality of care for patients hospitalized with heart failure: results of the Organized Program to Initiate Lifesaving Treatment in Hospitalized Patients With Heart Failure (OPTIMIZE-HF). *Arch Intern Med* 2007;**167**:1493–502.

284. Fonarow GC, Abraham WT, Albert NM, Stough WG, Gheorghiade M, Greenberg BH *et al.* Association between performance measures and clinical outcomes for patients hospitalized with heart failure. *JAMA* 2007;**297**:61–70.

285. Dickstein K, Coben-Solal A, Filippatos G *et al.* ESC Guidelines for the diagnosis and treatment of acute and chronic heart failure 2008 The Task Force for the Diagnosis and Treatment of Acute and Chronic Heart Failure 2008 of the European Sociaty of Cardiology. Developed in collaboration with the Heart Failure Association of the ESC (HFA) and endorsed by the European Sociaty of Intensive Care Medicine (ESICM). *Eur J Heart Fail* 2008;**10**:933–89.

286. Hunt SA, Abraham WT, Chin MH *et al.* 2009 Focused update incorporated into the ACC/AHA 2005 Guidelines for the Diagnosis and Management of Heart Failure in Adults. A Report of the American College of Cardiology Foundation/American Heart Association Task Force on Practice Guidelines Developed in Collaboration With the International Society for Heart and Lung Transplantation. *J Am Coll Cardiol* 2009;**53**(15): e1–e90.

48

Acute myocarditis and dilated cardiomyopathy

Leslie T Cooper Jr and Oyere K Onuma
Mayo Clinic College of Medicine, Rochester, MN, USA

Introduction and historic perspectives

"Is the inflammation of the heart always very sharp and acute, or does it not sometimes affect an insidious, hidden progress and which it appears, if not impossible, at least very difficult to distinguish?" Jean Corvisart, personal physician to Napoleon Bonaparte[1]

Myocarditis is usually defined by histologic criteria as inflammation of the myocardium, often with damage or injury to cardiac myocytes. The histologic Dallas criteria allow for two categories of myocarditis: active, in which myocyte damage is evident, and borderline, in which a cellular inflammatory infiltrate is not associated with myocyte injury or necrosis (Plate 48.1).[2] However, the diagnosis of myocarditis is frequently presumed if a compatible clinical scenario is associated with new abnormalities on non-invasive cardiac imaging and/or elevated serum biomarkers of cardiac injury. Clinically, myocarditis most often presents as an acute or occasionally fulminant illness with new-onset dilated cardiomyopathy (DCM). However, manifestations range from subclinical disease to sudden death, new-onset atrial or ventricular arrhythmias, complete heart block or an acute myocardial infarction-type syndrome. The known causes of myocarditis are as varied as the disease presentations and include infectious causes (including coxsackie B virus, parvovirus B19, adenovirus, *T. cruzi*), toxic agents, and cardiac manifestation of a systemic autoimmune disease (Box 48.1).

DCM is a common phenotype that results from many forms of myocardial injury and is both an acute and long-term consequence of viral myocarditis.[3] Usually a careful family history and a history of an antecedent viral prodrome in the weeks prior to cardiac symptoms permit the clinical distinction between familial and postviral cardiomyopathy. However, a small pedigree may confound the assessment of an inherited predisposition to DCM and inherited abnormalities of cytoskeletal proteins may actually predispose to more severe viral myocarditis, as is the case with Duchenne's muscular dystrophy and coxsackie B virus infection, both of which affect dystrophin. Therefore a clear distinction between primarily familial and primarily acquired DCM is not always possible.

This chapter focuses on primary DCM in which histologic evidence of myocarditis or persistent viral infection is present. In the USA, the estimated prevalence of all forms of DCM is 36.5 cases per 100 000.[4] DCM is important because it constitutes the leading cause (45%) of heart transplantation in the United States.[5] In a review of 1230 cases of initially unexplained DCM, only 9% were thought to be due to myocarditis when the Dallas criteria were applied.[6] Although standard histologic criteria for myocarditis are usually absent in chronic DCM, other markers of inflammation including ICAM, VCAM, and major histocompatability complex (MHC) antigen expression are present in up to 40% of cases.[7] Thus the prevalence of myocarditis in DCM varies widely depending on the histologic criteria used to establish the diagnosis.

Incidence, natural history and prognosis of acute myocarditis

The incidence of myocarditis in the community is unknown because many cases probably have minimal if any acute symptoms, and escape diagnosis only to present months or years later with a non-ischemic DCM. The incidence may also be underestimated due to the highly variable presentation of the disease which ranges from subclinical to fulminant heart failure, and includes sudden death, syncope, and acute myocardial infarction-like syndromes. Furthermore, the histologic diagnosis of patients with acute clinical symptoms and suspected myocarditis is confounded by a lack of sensitivity in the traditional Dallas Criteria.[8] For example, in the Myocarditis Treatment Trial, which used the Dallas criteria for study entry, only 10% of 2333 patients

Evidence-Based Cardiology, 3rd edition. Edited by S. Yusuf, J.A. Cairns, A.J. Camm, E.L. Fallen, and B.J. Gersh. © 2010 Blackwell Publishing, ISBN: 978-1-4051-5925-8.

BOX 48.1 Select etiologies of myocarditis

Infectious
- Viral – common
  - Parvovirus B19, increasing since 1994
  - Adenovirus, most common 1995 to 2005
  - Enterovirus (coxsackie B), decreasing since 2004
  - HCV (in Japan)
  - Human immunodeficiency virus
- Bacterial – consider in immunosuppressed hosts
  - Mycobacteria
  - Streptococcal sp.
  - *Treponema palladum*
  - *Borrelia burgdoferi*
- Fungal – consider in immunosuppressed hosts
  - *Aspergillus*
  - *Candida*
  - *Cryptococcus*
  - *Histoplasma*
  - *Coccidioides*
- Protozoal
  - *Trypanosoma cruzi*

Toxins
- Cocaine
- Anthracyclines
- Imatimib mesylate
- Interleukin-2

Hypersensitivity
- Clozapine
- Methyldopa
- Cephalosporins
- Penicillins
- Tricyclic antidepressants

Systemic/autoimmune
- Systemic lupus erythematosus
- Inflammatory bowel disease
- Giant cell myocarditis
- Sarcoidosis (idiopathic granulomatous myocarditis)
- Takayasu's arteritis
- Hypereosinophilic syndrome
- Endomyocardial eosinophilic diseases

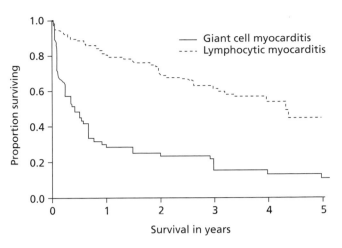

Figure 48.1 Transplant free survival of lymphocytic myocarditis versus giant cell myocarditis. Kaplan–Meier curves showing the duration of transplant-free survival from the onset of symptoms in 63 patients with giant cell myocarditis and 111 patients with lymphocytic myocarditis from the Myocarditis Treatment Trial. *P* < 0.001 by log-rank test. (Reproduced with permission from Cooper *et al.*[15])

transplant-free survival than borderline myocarditis.[12] In a Mayo Clinic series from the early 1990s by Grogan *et al*, the five-year survival in acute myocarditis was 56%, comparable to survival in patients with idiopathic DCM without myocarditis.[13] Immunoperoxidase based diagnostic criteria have higher sensitivity than the Dallas criteria and may have prognostic value.[14]

Histologic patterns that influence survival are limited to several uncommon disorders including giant cell myocarditis (GCM), acute necrotizing eosinophilic myocarditis, and cardiac sarcoidosis (CS).[15] The five-year transplant-free survival rate in GCM is less than 20% (Fig. 48.1).[16] In a large clinical series, subjects with either GCM or CS had a worse transplant-free survival than those with lymphocytic myocarditis.[17] Paradoxically, patients with the clinical pathologic entity of fulminant lymphocytic myocarditis, although severely ill at presentation with marked hemodynamic compromise, are more likely to recover than those with acute (2 weeks to 3 months duration) myocarditis who do not have a distinct viral prodrome.[18]

A few serologic and imaging biomarkers have been associated with poor clinical outcome. Higher concentrations of serologic markers such as Fas ligand (FasL) and interleukin 10 (IL-10) may predict increased mortality.[19,20] Right ventricular function on echocardiogram was an independent predictor of death or cardiac transplantation in a study of 23 patients with biopsy-confirmed myocarditis.[21] In this study, multivariate analysis revealed that right ventricular dysfunction as quantitated by right ventricular descent was the most powerful predictor of death or cardiac transplantation. In a separate study, Naqvi *et al* demonstrated that contractile reserve assessed by dobutamine

with suspected myocarditis and recent-onset DCM met these criteria.[9] The rate was somewhat higher at 17% in the European Study of Epidemiology and Treatment of Cardiac Inflammatory Diseases Study (ESETCID), which used less restrictive immunohistologic criteria.[10]

The prognosis in myocarditis is variable and depends partly on clinical, hemodynamic, and histologic variables. Presentation with syncope, heart block on EKG, lower left ventricular ejection fraction, and higher pulmonary artery pressures are associated with shorter transplant-free survival.[11] In the series from Massachusetts General Hospital, Dallas Criteria myocarditis was associated with shorter

echocardiography predicted left ventricular functional recovery in 22 patients with new-onset DCM, some of which may have been due to myocarditis.[22]

Pathogenesis of myocarditis

Studies in mouse and rat models of myocarditis have investigated the pathogenesis of autoimmune and viral myocarditis and enhanced our understanding of the relationship between direct viral injury and the host immune response to viral infection. Coxsackie B virus-induced myocarditis (CVB) is thought to progress in three temporal stages:

1 acute myocarditis characterized by viremia and a high fatality rate in animal models

2 subacute myocarditis with lymphocytic infiltrates in the myocardium, rising antibody titers and release of inflammatory cytokines including IL-1-beta, tumor necrosis factor (TNF)-alpha, interferon (IFN)-gamma and IL-2

3 chronic myocarditis characterized by fibrosis, progressive ventricular dilation and heart failure.[3]

It is this third stage of "chronic myocarditis" that is thought to result in "idiopathic" dilated cardiomyopathy.

Myocardial injury in CVB and encephalomyocarditis virus (ECMV) myocarditis occurs through several mechanisms.[23,24] Viral infection can lead within hours to days to myocyte death and release of sequestered intracellular antigens, which trigger an innate and adaptive immune response in the myocardium. Antibodies that cross-react with CVB, human cardiac myosin, and the beta-adrenergic receptor have been observed in cases of myocarditis. Cytokines, such as TNF-alpha, and autoantibodies associated with this inflammatory reaction impair cardiac myocyte contractility, and released cellular products such as major basic protein (MBP) can lead directly to myocyte cell death. T cell-deficient mice show a muted response or progression to myocarditis as compared to normal mice.[25] Long-term myocardial damage may also occur through an apoptotic mechanism, especially in the absence of active inflammation. In the Lewis rat model of autoimmune myocarditis, T cells also are a key mediator of myocardial damage. Myocardial damage may occur independently of any immune reaction. For example, protein products of the enteroviral genome, including viral protease 2a, can cleave host proteins, including dystrophin, and lead to cardiomyopathy.[26,27] Environmental variables such as selenium deficiency can affect viral virulence and individual susceptibility to cardiotopic viral infection.[28,29]

Genetic susceptibility to myocarditis is strongly suggested by animal models in which spontaneous myocarditis occurs.[30] A genetic component of DCM has also been well characterized in studies of familial association and linkage studies. Twenty to 40% of patients with DCM have a first-degree relative with some degree of left ventricular dysfunction.[31] A positive association of DCM with the MHC HLA DR4 has been identified in several independent studies. However, specific genes that predispose patients to myocarditis have not yet been identified.

Clinical presentation and diagnosis

The clinical presentation in myocarditis varies from asymptomatic ECG findings to cardiogenic shock or even sudden death. Although a non-specific viral prodrome with fevers, myalgias, and respiratory or gastrointestinal symptoms is classically associated with myocarditis, the published rates of reported symptoms are highly variable.[32] Cardiac symptoms include fatigue, decreased exercise tolerance, palpitations, precordial chest pain, and syncope. Of the 3055 patients in the ESETCID study, 72% had dyspnea, 33% had chest pain, and 18% had arrhythmic events.[10] Most studies of acute dilated cardiomyopathy and suspected myocarditis have a slight a male predominance. For example, 62% of the 111 patients enrolled in the Myocarditis Treatment Trial were male.[9]

Cardiac enzyme elevations are seen in a minority of patients with acute myocarditis and can help confirm the diagnosis. Standard markers of myocardial damage including troponin-I have a high specificity (89%) but limited sensitivity (34%) in the diagnosis of myocarditis, especially with a shorter duration (less than four weeks) of symptoms.[33] Clinical and experimental data suggest that cardiac troponin-I is increased much more frequently than creatnine kinase MB (CK-MB) in patients with myocarditis.[34] Other circulating biomarkers including cytokines, complement components and anti-heart antibodies have not been prospectively validated and are not in widespread clinical use.

Troponin I or T should be measured in suspected acute myocarditis (**Class I, Level C**).

The ECG in acute myocarditis may show sinus tachycardia with non-specific ST segment and T-wave abnormalities. Occasionally, the ECG changes are suggestive of an acute myocardial infarction and may include ST segment elevation in two or more contiguous leads (54%), widespread ST segment depressions (18%) and pathologic Q-waves (18–27%).[35] In a small proportion of patients, various degrees of heart block may occur. In the Myocarditis Treatment Trial, pacemaker implantation occurred in approximately 1% of subjects. Ventricular arrhythmias may also be present, but occur more commonly in cardiac sarcoidosis and giant cell myocarditis.[36]

An ECG should be performed in suspected acute myocarditis (**Class I, Level C**).

The most common echocardiographic features of acute myocarditis are unfortunately not specific; however, echocardiography is useful to exclude other causes of acute heart failure. Echocardiographic patterns of dilated, hypertrophic, restrictive, and ischemic cardiomyopathies have been described in histologically proven myocarditis. Segmental or global wall motion abnormalities can simulate myocardial infarction in myocarditis.[37] In the Myocarditis Treatment Trial, increased sphericity and left ventricular volume occurred in acute, active myocarditis. Left ventricular cavity size may be normal in very early myocarditis and increase over time due to remodeling. Fulminant myocarditis may be distinguished from acute myocarditis by echocardiographic criteria as suggested by Felker *et al.*[38] These authors performed echocardiography on 11 fulminant and 43 acute myocarditis patients at presentation and after six months. Patients with fulminant myocarditis had near normal LV diastolic dimensions with increased septal thickness at presentation, while those with acute myocarditis had increased diastolic dimensions but normal septal thickness.

An echocardiogram should be performed in suspected acute myocarditis (**Class I, Level C**).

Due to its availability and low risk, cardiac magnetic resonance imaging (CMR) is being used with increasing frequency as a diagnostic test in suspected acute myocarditis and may be used to localize sites for endomyocardial biopsies.[39,40] CMR may also be useful to differentiate ischemic from non-ischemic cardiomyopathy. McCrohon *et al* performed gadolinium-enhanced CMR in 90 patients with heart failure and LV systolic dysfunction, of whom 63 had idiopathic DCM. Subendocardial or transmural enhancement was seen in ischemic cardiomyopathy. In contrast, the DCM group had three patterns of enhancement: no enhancement, myocardial enhancement indistinguishable from the patients with CAD and patchy or longitudinal mid wall enhancement.[41] Results from similar studies suggest that diffuse and/or heterogeneous involvement with combined enhancement is highly suggestive of myocarditis. Histopathologic evaluation of biopsies directed by contrast CMR with delayed enhancement by Mahrholdt *et al* demonstrated active myocarditis in 19 of 21 patients. In contrast, only one in seven patients showed active myocarditis in biopsies guided by non-myocardial delayed enhancement (MDE) CMR.[42] Serial CMR using T1-weighted images with gadolinium have also been used to visualize the myocardial injury in myocarditis and track its progression.[43] The prognostic value of CMR to predict future cardiac events in acute myocarditis is under investigation.

CMR can be useful in suspected acute myocarditis (**Class IIa, Level C**).

The gold standard for the diagnosis of myocarditis is histopathology on endomyocardial biopsy (EMB). The histopathologic classification called the Dallas criteria[44] was used in the Myocarditis Treatment Trial and is widely cited, but the average incidence of positive right ventricular biopsy findings in acute dilated cardiomyopathy is only around 10%.[9,45] This is likely due to sampling error secondary to the patchy nature of myocardial inflammation[46] and interobserver variability.[8,47] Newer diagnostic criteria that rely on immunoperoxidase techniques are coming into broader clinical use. Expression of MHC antigens is a more sensitive marker than the Dallas criteria for myocardial inflammation, and this is detected using immunoperoxidase-based stains for HLA-ABC and HLA-DR antigens. Indeed, the sensitivity and specificity of MHC expression for detecting biopsy-proven myocarditis has been reported as high as 80%. Viral genomes can be detected using molecular methods like the polymerase chain reaction (PCR) to identify viral RNA and DNA from endomyocardial biopsy samples. The clinical value of viral genome analysis, immunoperoxidase stains, and transcriptome based biomarkers is being evaluated in ongoing clinical trials.

Currently, the risks of cardiac perforation and death associated with EMB preclude its routine use in the diagnosis of myocarditis. The 2007 AHA/ACCF/ESC scientific statement on the role of endomyocardial biopsy in cardiovascular disease lists 14 clinical scenarios in which EMB may be considered, and gives a class I recommendation to two of these 14 (Table 48.1).[49]

Management

Myocarditis presenting as acute DCM

Myocarditis should be treated according to the guidelines for the presenting clinical syndrome. For example, acute DCM should be managed according to the current AHA/ACCF, ESC, and HFSA guidelines.[48–51] The mainstay of therapy for acute myocarditis is supportive therapy for left ventricular dysfunction. Most patients will improve with standard heart failure regimen that includes ACE inhibitors or angiotensin receptor blockers, beta-blockers such as metoprolol or carvedilol, and diuretics, if needed. In patients who deteriorate despite optimal medical management, case series suggest a role for mechanical circulatory support such as ventricular assist devices or extracorporeal membrane oxygenation (ECMO) as a bridge to transplantation or recovery.[52,53]

Heart failure therapy

Angiotensin-converting enzyme inhibitors/angiotensin receptor blockers (ACEI/ARBs)

Although the utility of ACEI/ARBs in the treatment of symptomatic and asymptomatic heart failure with left ventricular dysfunction is well established, evidence for their specific use in myocarditis is limited to studies in animal models. Early treatment with captopril, starting on day 1

Table 48.1 The role of endomyocardial biopsy in 14 clinical scenarios

Scenario number	Clinical scenario	Level of evidence (A,B,C)	Class of recommendation (I, IIa, IIb, III)
1	New-onset heart failure of less than 2 weeks duration associated with a normal size or dilated left ventricle and hemodynamic compromise	B	I
2	New-onset heart failure of 2 weeks to 3 months duration associated with a dilated left ventricle, and new ventricular arrhythmias, Mobitz type II second- or third-degree heart block, or failure to respond to usual care within 1–2 weeks	B	I
3	Heart failure of greater than 3 months duration associated with a dilated left ventricle and new ventricular arrhythmias, second- or third-degree heart block, or failure to respond to usual care within 1–2 weeks	C	IIa
4	Heart failure associated with a dilated cardiomyopathy of any duration associated with suspected allergic reaction in addition to eosinophilia	C	IIa
5	Heart failure associated with suspected anthracycline cardiomyopathy	C	IIa
6	Heart failure associated with unexplained restrictive cardiomyopathy	C	IIa
7	Suspected cardiac tumors except for typical myxomas	C	IIa
8	Unexplained cardiomyopathy in children	C	IIa
9	New-onset heart failure of 2 weeks to 3 months duration associated with a dilated left ventricle, without new ventricular arrhythmias, Mobitz type II second- or third-degree heart block, and that responds to usual care within 1–2 weeks	B	IIb
10	Heart failure of greater than 3 months duration associated with a dilated left ventricle, without new ventricular arrhythmias, or Mobitz type 2 second- or third-degree heart block, and that responds to usual care within 1–2 weeks	C	IIb
11	Heart failure associated with unexplained hypertrophic cardiomyopathy	C	IIb
12	Suspected AVRD/C	C	IIb
13	Unexplained ventricular arrhythmias	C	IIb
14	Unexplained atrial fibrillation	C	III

AVRD/C, arrhythmogenic right ventricular dysplasia/cardiomyopathy
Reproduced with permission from Cooper et al.[49]

of infection, has beneficial effects in murine models of myocarditis in the reduction of inflammatory infiltrates, myocardial necrosis and calcification.[54] In a second study by Rezkalla et al, delayed captopril therapy, initiated 10 days after viral inoculation, was still found to result in a reduction of left ventricular mass and liver congestion.[55]

Studies of the ARB candersartan in a murine model of viral myocarditis showed a significant improvement in seven-day survival (60% versus 18%) in the candersartan group as compared to controls.[56] Studies in angiotensin receptor 1 (AT1) knockout mice demonstrate that AT1 signaling is important in the pathogenesis of viral cardiomyopathy through an NF-kB dependent pathway.[57] However, there are no specific studies of ACEI/ARBs in clinical myocarditis; therefore the applicability of these findings in human disease remains unknown. ACEI/ARBs should be used in patients with myocarditis and LVEF less than 40% (**Class I, Level C**).

Beta-adrenergic receptor blockers

The use of beta-blockers in murine models of myocarditis has been studied in acute, subacute and chronic models of myocarditis. In a murine model of coxsackie myocarditis using the BALB/C and DBA/2 strains of mice, carteolol, a non-selective beta-blocker, was shown to improve histopathologic measures including cell necrosis, cellular infiltration, reduction in wall thickness, fibrosis and clacification.[58] A previous study comparing metoprolol with saline in a murine model of acute coxsackie myocarditis resulted in increased mortality (60% vs 0%) in metoprolol-treated mice with an accompanying increase in the viral replication and myocyte necrosis.[59] Metoprolol treatment was started on the day of viral inoculation and continued for 10 days. These studies thus suggest that beta-blocker therapy, while useful in the management of chronic heart failure, may be harmful if initiated very early in acute myocarditis. Non-selective beta-blockers may be preferable. As with ACE inhibitors, there have been no trials of beta-blockers in human myocarditis. Recommendations for the use of beta-blockers in myocarditis rely on extrapolation from randomized trials of beta-adrenergic blocking drugs that demonstrated benefit for the treatment of heart failure with decreased left ventricular systolic function.

We recommend that beta-blockers that have been shown to improve mortality and heart failure symptoms should also be used in that subset of heart failure patients with myocarditis in accordance with current heart failure guidelines (**Class I, Level C**).

Aldosterone inhhibitors

In the Randomized Aldactone Evaluation Study (RALES), 1663 patients with severe heart failure, of whom 46% were non-ischemic in etiology, NYHA class III–IV and EF <35% were randomized to aldactone or placebo. The majority of the patients were concurrently on loop diuretics, ACE inhibitors and digitalis. There was a 30% reduction in the primary endpoint of all-cause mortality in the aldactone groups versus placebo, a 35% reduction in the rate of hospitalizations for worsening heart failure as well as a significant improvement in the symptoms of heart failure.

The risk reduction seen in reduction in hospitalizations may be related to the role of the aldosterone receptor antagonist in preventing myocardial fibrosis and decreasing sodium retention.[60] Aldosterone antgonists have not been studied in experimental or human myocarditis.

We recommend that aldosterone inhibitors that have been shown to improve mortality and heart failure symptoms should also be used in that subset of heart failure patients with myocarditis in accordance with current heart failure guidelines (**Class I, Level C**).

Digoxin

In a mouse model of viral myocarditis, digoxin worsened myocardial injury and increased mortality, possibly by increasing the production of proinflammatory cytokines in the myocardium.[61] There are no published studies evaluating digoxin for the specific treatment of myocarditis in human disease.

Therefore digoxin should be reserved for that subset of heart failiure patients with myocarditis who also have NYHA class II symptoms and other criteria set forth in the current heart failure guidelines (**Class I, Level C**).

Calcium channel blockers

In a study by Wang *et al*, amlodipine improved survival, heart weight to body weight ratio and the histopathologic grades of myocardial lesions in a murine model of viral myocarditis.[62] Diltiazem or verapamil may be used for rate control on patients with atrial fibrillation in whom beta-blockers have proven inadequate or are not tolerated.

There are no published data regarding the benefit or risk of calcium channel blockers in human myocarditis. Therefore, their use should be limited to other clinical indications for which their benefit has been demonstrated that might co-exist or develop concurrently with acute myocarditis, such as supraventricular tachycardia or hypertension. The lack of published data does not allow a recommendation for or against their use in acute myocarditis.

Specific therapy

Antiviral treatment

Data regarding the use of antiviral agents for the treatment of acute myocarditis is limited to animal models and small case series. In murine viral myocarditis, antiviral therapy with ribavarin and interferon-alpha was found to reduce the severity of myocardial lesions and mortality.[63,64] However, antiviral therapy was only effective if applied at the time of inoculation with the virus or soon thereafter, a timeline that is not practical in human cases of acute myocarditis. Antiviral therapy has been used in one case series of fulminant myocarditis[65] and therefore could be considered in laboratory-acquired cases or possibly institutional outbreaks. However, most cases of fulminant and acute myocarditis have a high rate of spontaneous improvement and in the absence of any human data, antiviral therapy cannot be recommended for the treatment of acute myocarditis at this time (**Class III, Level C**).

Antiviral therapy may be best utilized in patients with viral persistence in the setting of chronic dilated cardiomyopathy. In a study by Kuhl *et al*, 22 patients with persistent LV dysfunction, symptomatic heart failure and evidence of myocardial persistence of enteroviral or adenoviral genome by PCR were treated with beta-interferon for 24 weeks.[66] Viral clearance/eradication was achieved in all patients after antiviral treatment, with a significant increase in LV function and a significant decrease in LV dimensions in the treatment group. There have also been reports of treatment of enterovirus-induced cardiomyopathy with interferon-alpha[67]; however, no randomized trials of interferon treatment have been published. Pleconaril is being studied in an onging clinical trial for the treatment of enteroviral myocarditis in children (NCT00031512). An unpublished multicenter trial of beta-interferon for viral cardiomyopathy suggested a benefit for treatment of enteroviral and adenoviral but not parvovirus B19-related cardiomyopathy (**Class IIb, Level C**).

Immunosuppressive treatment

In an early study by Parillo *et al*, subjects with unexplained dilated cardiomyopathy were randomized to treatment with prednisone (initially 60 mg daily) or to placebo.[68] Subjects were categorized as reactive (patients with fibroblastic or immune deposition on EMB, with a positive gallium scan) or non-reactive if they lacked these features. Although patients in the prednisone group had a statistically larger chance at improvement in LVEF at three months, the increases in EF were small (4.3% in the treatment group) and were not sustained after the steroid dose was lowered at six or nine months. In the Myocarditis Treatment Trial, 111 patients with heart failure of less than two years' duration, histopathologic diagnosis of myocarditis according to the Dallas criteria and LVEF less than 45% were randomized to three treatment groups: prednisone and azathioprine, prednisone and ciclosporin, or placebo. Patients were treated for 24 weeks with concurrent conventional heart failure treatment. In the placebo and combined treatment groups, there was an improvement in the LVEF from an average of 25% to 34% and the combined endpoint of death or transplantation at five years was 56%. There was no significant change in LVEF in treated versus untreated patients and similarly, no significant difference in survival or need for cardiac transplantation between groups. A higher LVEF at baseline, less intensive conventional drug therapy at baseline, and a shorter duration of disease, but not the treatment assignment, were positive independent predictors of the LVEF at week 28.[9] These studies suggest that immunosuppression is not beneficial in the routine treatment of acute DCM due to lymphocytic myocarditis or unexplained DCM (**Class III, Level B**).

A recent meta-analysis of immunosuppression and immunomodulation trials found that trials performed in DCM of less than six months' duration were negative, while those in DCM of greater than six months duration were generally positive due to the large improvement in the placebo groups in subjects with acute myocarditis.[69] For example, in a trial of 84 patients with DCM of less than two years in duration and cardiomyocyte HLA expression on EMB, who were randomized to azathioprine and prednisone or placebo, Wojnicz *et al* showed an improvement in the secondary endpoints of LVEF, NYHA functional class, left ventricular volume and left ventricular end-diastolic diameter.[70] However, there was no difference in cardiac death, hospitalization or readmission rates. Today the use of immunosuppressive drugs for patients on optimal medical management with evidence of ongoing myocardial inflammation and persistent left ventricular dysfunction is controversial, and these should be considered for enrollment in clinical research trials when feasible (**Class IIb, Level B**).

Intravenous immunoglobulin (IVIG)

The antiviral and immunomodulatory effects of IVIG suggest that it might play a role in the management of viral and postviral autoimmune myocarditis. In the Immune Modulation for Acute Cardiomyopathy (IMAC) trial, patients with recent-onset myocarditis or dilated cardiomyopathy (less than six months) in duration were randomized to IVIG or placebo. Overall, there was an improvement in the LVEF at six months, from 25% to 40% in both cohorts, but there was no significant difference between the treatment group and placebo.[71] A recent systematic review that included IMAC and other smaller studies concluded that there is insufficient evidence to recommend its use in acute myocarditis in adults.[72] Therefore, the routine use of IVIG for acute myocarditis in adults is not recommended (**Class III, Level B**). However, case series suggest that IVIG confers benefit in acute pediatric myocarditis,[73,74] and its use is common in this clinical setting. Furthermore, the role of IVIG in chronic inflammatory cardiomyopathy remains to be determined.

Non-steroidal anti-inflammatory drugs

In several murine models, non-steroidal anti-inflammatory drugs (NSAIDS) have not shown any efficacy in the treatment of myocarditis, despite histologic evidence of inflammatory infiltrates in myocarditis. In fact, they may lead to increased mortality by exacerbating the inflammatory process in the myocardium and increasing the virulence of the infectious agent.[75–77]

The use of NSAIDS should be avoided in acute myocarditis (**Class III, Level C**).

Antiarrhythmics

Given the occurrence of both tachyarrhythmias and bradyarrhythmias in patients with myocarditis, patients with acute myocarditis should be hospitalized for ECG monitoring. Therapy for arrhythmias is supportive since they usually resolve after the acute phase of the disease. The 2006 ACC/AHA/ESC guidelines for the management of arrhythmias recommended that acute arrhythmic emergencies be managed conventionally in the setting of myocarditis.[78] Further recommendations for the management of arrhythmias in myocarditis are as follows.

- Temporary pacemakers should be considered in acute myocarditis for patients with symptomatic bradycardia or complete heart block (**Class I, Level C**).
- For patients with sustained supraventricular tachycardias (SVT) or symptomatic NSVT and acute myocarditis, the restoration of sinus rhythm is the recommended approach and antiarrhythmic therapy may be appropriate (**Class IIa, Level C**).
- For patients with life-threatening ventricular arrhythmias, ICD therapy may be appropriate if they are *not* in the acute phase of myocarditis and are on optimal medical therapy with reasonable prognosis for recovery of functional status (**Class IIa, Level C**).

- ICD implantation is *not* recommended for patients with acute myocarditis (**Class III, Level C**).

When antiarrhythmic therapy is indicated, amiodarone or dofetilide should be considered. Due to their proarrhythmic and negative inotropic effects, other class I and class III antiarrhythmics should be avoided in patients with acute myocarditis.

Mechanical support

In non-randomized case series and case reports, mechanical circulatory support has been shown to be an effective bridge to recovery or to transplantation in fulminant and acute myocarditis.[79,80] (**Class I, Level C**).

Cardiac transplantation

The overall five-year survival rate following cardiac transplantation is about 74%.[5] Although early case series suggested that cardiac transplantation for myocarditis was associated with a poorer survival and an increased risk of rejection, more recent and larger case series suggest that the overall survival for cardiac transplantation for myocarditis is similar to survival for other causes of cardiac transplantation.[5] Cardiac transplantation may be an effective treatment for myocarditis that is refractory to medical management and mechanical circulatory support (**Class I, Level C**).

Non-pharmacologic interventions

Exercise

Current recommendations with regard to the resumption of athletic activity are that athletes with a definite or presumed diagnosis of myocarditis refrain from competitive sports for a period of six months after the clinical onset of disease. Furthermore, the resumption of training should only occur if echocardiographic measures of LV function, wall motion and dimensions return to baseline in the absence of clinically relevant arrhythmias, a normal 12-lead ECG and normalization of serum biomarkers.[81] These recommendations are based on animal models in which exercise following acute myocarditis increases mortality. Therefore, we recommend that patients with acute myocarditis refrain from aerobic exercise for a period of months following the acute illness (**Class I, Level C**).

Prevention

There are no specific strategies for the prevention of myocarditis. However, the widespread use of vaccination in developed countries has made myocarditis secondary to measles, mumps, rubella, poliomyelitis and influenza quite rare. As such, vaccinations against other cardiotropic viruses may prevent viral myocarditis as shown in murine models.[82] At this time, there are no specific recommendations for the use of vaccinations to prevent viral myocarditis.

Specific etiologies of myocarditis and their management

Certain idiopathic or infectious causes of myocarditis have specific treatments. These are uncommon, but certain clinical clues can lead to a directed investigation and appropriate management.

Giant cell myocarditis

Giant cell myocarditis (GCM) is a rare but usually fatal autoimmune form of myocarditis, characterized by the presence of giant cells in the myocardium (Plate 48.2). Its pathogenesis is unknown; however, in animal models, a GCM-like inflammation is induced by immunization with cardiac myosin.[83] The clinical course is usually one of rapid deterioration in spite of usual clinical care, with frequent ventricular arrhythmias and complete heart block. The prognosis in GCM is significantly worse as compared to lymphocytic myocarditis, with a median survival of 5.5 months from the onset of symptoms and an 89% rate of death or cardiac transplant at five years.[16]

Management

Unlike acute lymphocytic myocarditis, transplant-free survival is prolonged in patients with acute GCM treated with a combination of ciclosporin and steroids. We recommend that immunosuppression that includes steroids and ciclosporin be used for patients with histologically proven, acute GCM of less than three months symptom duration (**Class I, Level C**). Despite a 20–25% rate of GCM recurrence in the allograft, transplantation is also an effective therapy for GCM. We recommend that heart transplantation be considered for patients with GCM who fail to respond to standard management of heat failure and immunosuppression (**Class I, Level C**).[16,84]

Hypersensitivity and eosinophilic myocarditis

Drug-induced hypersensitivity reactions can sometimes affect the myocardium. Numerous medications, including some antidepressants, antibiotics and antipsychotics, have been implicated in hypersensitivity myocarditis. Patients are generally older and are often on multiple medications and often present acutely with rash, fever, and occasionally liver function test abnormalities. ECG changes are similar to those with lymphocytic myocarditis, including sinus tachycardia, non-specific T-wave abnormalities and ST elevations.

Eosinophilic myocarditis is characterized by a predominantly eosinophilic infiltrate in the myocardium and may occur in association with systemic diseases such as hypereosinophilic syndrome (HES), Churg–Strauss syndrome and Löffler's endomyocardial fibrosis or in association with parasitic or helminthic or protozoal infections.[85–87] Clinical manifestations of eosinophilic myocarditis include endocardial fibrosis, fibrosis of the cardiac valves leading to regurgitation, right and left congestive heart failure and formation of thrombi on the endocardial surface. Acute necrotizing eosinophilic myocarditis is an aggressive form of eosinophilic myocarditis with acute onset and high mortality rates.

Management

In general, the treatment for eosinophilic myocarditis depends on the underlying cause and includes withdrawal of the offending agent, if known. High-dose corticosteroids may be beneficial in the setting of systemic disease-associated eosinophilic myocarditis, while surgical treatment may also play a role in the management of endomyocardial fibrosis (**Class IIa, Level C**).[15,88]

Lyme myocarditis

Myocarditis can occur in association with the infection by the spirochete *Borrelia burgdorferi* (Lyme disease). Lyme myocarditis should be suspected in patients who have a history of travel to the endemic regions or who give a history of a tick bite. Clinical presentation may include several degrees of atrioventricular conduction abnormalities, including transient or permanent heart block or cardiac arrhythmia.[89] The diagnosis of Lyme disease is confirmed by serologic testing but this does not establish the diagnosis of myocarditis. EMB, if indicated, may show a lymphocytic myocarditis with a prominent plasmacytic component and the organism may be visualized in the section with special stains. In a patient with suspected Lyme disease after a tick bite, the possibility of co-infection with *Ehrlichia* (ehrlichiosis) and *Babesia* (babesiosis) should be considered as both can also cause myocarditis. Serologic tests are available for both disorders.

Management

The treatment of Lyme myocarditis consists of supportive clinical care for left ventricular dysfunction and treatment of the underlying infection using appropriate antibiotics such as doxycycline and ceftriaxone. Permanent pacing may be required for symptomatic heart block (**Class IIa, Level C**).

Chagas' myocarditis

Trypanosoma cruzi infection in the heart can present as an acute myocarditis or as a chronic cardiomyopathy and is a leading cause of dilated cardiomyopathy and congestive heart failure in the endemic areas of rural Central or South America. Chagas' cardiomyopathy may present with symptoms of cardiac arrhythmia or heart block in 10–20% of infected persons. These symptoms may be related to congestive heart failure due to left ventricular dysfunction or ventricular arrhythmia resulting from progressive damage to the heart. An additional 20–30% of affected persons have asymptomatic cardiac involvement. The disease is clinically suspected if the patient has a strong history of environmental exposure, and the diagnosis is confirmed by serologic testing or polymerase chain reaction. The ECG may show evidence of conduction system disease including right bundle branch block or left anterior fascicular block. Echocardiography or contrast ventriculography may reveal a left ventricular apical aneurysm, regional wall motion abnormalities, or diffuse cardiomyopathy.

Management

There is no specific treatment for Chagas' cardiomyopathy. Antiparisitic treatments directed against *T. cruzi* may eradicate the disease in acute or subacute infection and congestive heart failure can be managed symptomatically with ACE inhibitors at high doses, diuretics and digoxin. Ventricular arrhythmias may respond to electrophysiology-guided treatments. Although heart transplantation for Chagas' cardiomyopathy has been successfully performed, reactivation of *T. cruzi* is common.[90] The best treatment is the institution of prevention measures. Improvements in housing and the use of pesticides may eradicate the reduviid bugs that transmit the disease, thus reducing infection and disease rates.

HIV myocarditis

Myocarditis is the most common cardiac pathologic finding at autopsy of HIV-infected patients, with prevalence as high as 70%. HIV-associated myocarditis is often characterized by a focal non-specific myocardial infiltrate in the presence of left ventricular dysfunction. HIV1-RNA has also been detected in the myocardial tissue of patients with acquired immunodeficiency syndrome (AIDS). Nevertheless, the pathogenesis of myocarditis and left ventricular dysfunction in immunocompromised patients is unclear, as the myocardial inflammation could be secondary to HIV itself, other opportunistic viruses and co-infections, or even due to the medications used in treatment. The prognosis for HIV-associated myocarditis is significantly poorer than that of lymphocytic myocarditis and in a large cardiomyopathy cohort, HIV-related myocarditis was the strongest predictor of death.[91]

Conclusion

Acute myocarditis presenting as dilated cardiomyopathy should be treated according to the current AHA/ACCF, ESC, and HFSA heart failure guidelines.[48–50] Arrhythmias should be managed according to the current ACC/AHA/ESC guideline.[77] Additionally patients should abstain from vigorous exercise for a period of up to six months, based on experimental data that indicates a greater mortality if animals exercise during the period of acute myocardial inflammation (**Class I**). If EMB reveals acute giant cell myocarditis, granulomatous or eosinophilic myocarditis, immunosuppressive treatment should be added (**Class I**). Mechanical circulatory support may provide a bridge to transplantation or recovery in patients with fulminant or acute myocarditis who deteriorate despite optimal medical management (**Class I**).

References

1. Abelmann WH. Viral myocarditis and its sequelae. *Annu Rev Med* 1973;**24**:145–52.
2. Aretz H, Billingham M, Edwards W *et al.* Myocarditis. A histopathologic definition and classification. *Am J Cardiovasc Pathol* 1986;**1**:3–14.
3. Cooper LT Jr. Myocarditis. *N Engl J Med* 2009;**360**(15):1526–38.
4. Codd M, Sugrue D, Gersh B, Melton L. Epidemiology of idiopathic dilated and hypertrophic cardiomyopathy. *Circulation* 1989;**80**:564–72.
5. Aurora P, Edwards LB, Christie J *et al.* Registry of the International Society for Heart and Lung Transplantation: eleventh official pediatric lung and heart–lung transplantation report 2008. *J Heart Lung Transplant* 2008;**27**(9):978–83.
6. Felker G, Thompson R, Hare J *et al.* Underlying causes and long-term survival in patients with initially unexplained cardiomyopathy. *N Engl J Med* 2000;**342**(15):1077–84.
7. Wojnicz R, Nowalany-Kozielska E, Wodniecki J *et al.* Immunohistological diagnosis of myocarditis. Potential role of sarcolemmal induction of the MHC and ICAM-1 in the detection of autoimmune mediated myocyte injury. *Eur Heart J* 1998;**19**(10):1564–72.
8. Baughman KL. Diagnosis of myocarditis: death of Dallas criteria. *Circulation* 2006;**113**(4):593–5.
9. Mason JW, O'Connell JB, Herskowitz A *et al.* A clinical trial of immunosuppressive therapy for myocarditis. *N Engl J Med* 1995;**333**(5):269–75.
10. Hufnagel G, Pankuweit S, Richter A, Schonian U, Maisch B. The European Study of Epidemiology and Treatment of Cardiac Inflammatory Diseases (ESETCID). First epidemiological results. *Herz* 2000;**25**(3):279–85.
11. McCarthy RE 3rd, Boehmer JP, Hruban RH *et al.* Long-term outcome of fulminant myocarditis as compared with acute (non-fulminant) myocarditis. *N Engl J Med* 2000;**342**(10):690–5.
12. Magnani JW, Danik HJ, Dec GW Jr, DiSalvo TG. Survival in biopsyproven myocarditis: a long-term retrospective analysis of the histopathologic, clinical, and hemodynamic predictors. *Am Heart J* 2006;**151**(2):463–70.
13. Grogan M, Redfield MM, Bailey KR *et al.* Long-term outcome of patients with biopsy-proved myocarditis: comparison with idiopathic dilated cardiomyopathy. *J Am Coll Cardiol* 1995;**26**(1):80–4.
14. Kindermann I, Kindermann M, Kandolf R, Klingel K, Bultmann B, Muller T *et al.* Predictors of outcome in patients with suspected myocarditis. [erratum appears in *Circulation* 2008 Sep 16; 118(12);e493]. *Circulation* 2008;**118**(6):639–48.
15. Cooper L, Zehr K. Biventricular assist device placement and immunosuppression as therapy for necrotizing eosinophilic myocarditis. *Nature Clin Pract Cardiovasc Med* 2005;**2**(10):544–9.
16. Cooper LT, Berry, G, Shabetai R. Giant cell myocarditis: natural history and treatment. *N Engl J Med* 1997;**336**:1860–66.
17. Davidoff R, Palacios I, Southern J, Fallon JT, Newell J, Dec GW. Giant cell versus lymphocytic myocarditis. A comparison of their clinical features and long-term outcomes. *Circulation* 1991;**83**(3):953–61.
18. Hare JM, Baughman KL. Fulminant and acute lymphocytic myocarditis: the prognostic value of clinicopathological classification. *Eur Heart J* 2001;**22**(4):269–70.
19. Sheppard R, Bedi M, Kubota T *et al.* Myocardial expression of fas and recovery of left ventricular function in patients with recent-onset cardiomyopathy. *J Am Coll Cardiol* 2005;**46**(6):1036–42.
20. Nishii M, Inomata T, Takehana H *et al.* Serum levels of interleukin-10 on admission as a prognostic predictor of human fulminant myocarditis. *J Am Coll Cardiol* 2004;**44**(6):1292–7.
21. Mendes LA, Dec GW, Picard MH, Palacios IF, Newell J, Davidoff R. Right ventricular dysfunction: an independent predictor of adverse outcome in patients with myocarditis. *Am Heart J* 1994;**128**(2):301–7.
22. Naqvi TZ, Goel RK, Forrester JS, Siegel RJ. Myocardial contractile reserve on dobutamine echocardiography predicts late spontaneous improvement in cardiac function in patients with recent onset idiopathic dilated cardiomyopathy. *J Am Coll Cardiol* 1999;**34**(5):1537–44.
23. Liu PP, Mason JW. Advances in the understanding of myocarditis. *Circulation* 2001;**104**(9):1076–82.
24. Matsumori A. Treatment options for myocarditis: what we know from experimental data nd how it translates to clinical trials. *Herz* 2007;**32**:452–6.
25. Huber SA, Job LP. Cellular immune mechanisms in Coxsackievirus group B, type 3 induced myocarditis in Balb/C mice. *Adv Exp Med Biol* 1983;**161**:491–508.
26. Badorff C, Lee G, Lamphear B *et al.* Enteroviral protease 2A cleaves dystrophin: evidence of cytoskeletal disruption in an aquired cardiomyopathy. *Nat Med* 1999;**5**:320–6.
27. Badorff C, Knowlton KU. Dystrophin disruption in enterovirus-induced myocarditis and dilated cardiomyopathy: from bench to bedside. *Med Microbiol Immunol* 2004;**193**(2–3):121–6.
28. Beck MA, Kolbeck PC, Rohr LH, Shi Q, Morris VC, Levander OA. Benign human enterovirus becomes virulent in selenium-deficient mice. *J Med Virol* 1994;**43**(2):166–70.
29. Cooper L, Virmani R, Chapman N *et al.* Report of a National Institutes of Health Sponsored Workshop on Inflammation and Immunity in Dilated Cardiomyopathy. *Mayo Clin Proc* 2006; **81**(2):199–204.

30. Taneja V, Cooper L, Behrens M *et al.* Spontaneous myocarditis mimicking human disease occurs in the presence of an appropriate MHC and non-MHC background in transgenic mice. *J Mol Cell Cardiol* 2007;**42**(6):1054–64.

31. Michels V, Moll P, Miller F *et al.* The frequency of familial dilated cardiomyopathy in a series of patients with idiopathic dilated cardiomyopathy. *N Engl J Med* 1992;**326**(2):77–82.

32. Magnani JW, Dec GW. Myocarditis: current trends in diagnosis and treatment. *Circulation* 2006;**113**(6):876–90.

33. Smith SC, Ladenson JH, Mason JW, Jaffe AS. Elevations of cardiac troponin I associated with myocarditis. Experimental and clinical correlates. *Circulation* 1997;**95**(1):163–8.

34. Lauer B, Niederau C, Kuhl U *et al.* Cardiac troponin T in patients with clinically suspected myocarditis. *J Am Coll Cardiol* 1997;**30**(5):1354–9.

35. Angelini A, Calzolari V, Calabrese F, Boffa GM, Maddalena F, Chioin R. Myocarditis mimicking acute myocardial infarction. *Heart* 2000;**84**(3):245–50.

36. Cooper LT. Giant cell and granulomatous myocarditis. *Heart Failure Clin* 2005;**1**(3):431–7.

37. Angelini A, Calzolari V, Calabrese F *et al.* Myocarditis mimicking acute myocardial infarction: role of endomyocardial biopsy in the differential diagnosis. *Heart* 2000;**84**(3):245–50.

38. Felker GM, Boehmer JP, Hruban RH *et al.* Echocardiographic findings in fulminant and acute myocarditis. *J Am Coll Cardiol* 2000;**36**(1):227–32.

39. Friedrich MG, Sechtem U, Schulz-Menger J *et al.* International Consensus Group on Cardiovascular Magnetic Resonance in Myocarditis. Cardiovascular magnetic resonance in myocarditis: A JACC White Paper. *J Am Coll Cardiol* 2009;**53**(17):1475–87.

40. Friedrich MG, Strohm O, Schulz-Menger J, Marciniak H, Luft FC, Dietz R. Contrast media-enhanced magnetic resonance imaging visualizes myocardial changes in the course of viral myocarditis. *Circulation* 1998;**97**(18):1802–9.

41. McCrohon JA, Moon JC, Prasad SK *et al.* Differentiation of heart failure related to dilated cardiomyopathy and coronary artery disease using gadolinium-enhanced cardiovascular magnetic resonance. *Circulation* 2003;**108**(1):54–9.

42. Mahrholdt H, Goedecke C, Wagner A *et al.* Cardiovascular magnetic resonance assessment of human myocarditis: a comparison to histology and molecular pathology. *Circulation* 2004;**109**(10):1250–8.

43. Abdel-Aty H, Boye P, Zagrosek A *et al.* Diagnostic performance of cardiovascular magnetic resonance in patients with suspected acute myocarditis: comparison of different approaches. *J Am Coll Cardiol* 2005;**45**(11):1815–22.

44. Aretz HT, Billingham ME, Edwards WD *et al.* Myocarditis. A histopathologic definition and classification. *Am J Cardiovasc Pathol* 1987;**1**(1):3–14.

45. Felker GM, Thompson RE, Hare JM *et al.* Underlying causes and long-term survival in patients with initially unexplained cardiomyopathy. *N Engl J Med* 2000;**342**(15):1077–84.

46. Hauck AJ, Kearney DL, Edwards WD. Evaluation of postmortem endomyocardial biopsy specimens from 38 patients with lymphocytic myocarditis: implications for role of sampling error. *Mayo Clin Proc* 1989;**64**(10):1235–45.

47. Shanes JG, Ghali J, Billingham ME *et al.* Interobserver variability in the pathologic interpretation of endomyocardial biopsy results. *Circulation* 1987;**75**(2):401–5.

48. Jessup M, Abraham WT, Casey DE *et al.* 2009 Focused Update: ACCF/AHA Guidelines for the Diagnosis and Management of Heart Failure in Adults. A Report of the American College of Cardiology Foundation/American Heart Association Task Force on Practice Guidelines: Developed in Collaboration With the International Society of Heart and Lung Transplantation 2009 Writing Group to Review New Evidence and Update the 2005 Guideline for the Management of Patients with Chronic Heart Failure Writing on Behalf of the 2005 Heart Failure Writing Committee. *Yancy Circulation* 2009;**119**:1977–2016.

49. Cooper LT, Baughman KL, Feldman AM *et al.* The role of endomyocardial biopsy in the management of cardiovascular disease: a scientific statement from the American Heart Association, the American College of Cardiology, and the European Society of Cardiology. *Circulation* 2007;**116**(19):2216–33.

50. Adams K, Lindenfeld J, Arnold J *et al.* Executive Summary: HFSA 2006 Comprehensive Heart Failure Practice Guideline. *J Cardiac Failure* 2006;**12**:10–38.

51. Swedberg K, Cleland J, Dargie HJ *et al.* Guidelines for the diagnosis and treatment of chronic heart failure (update 2005). *Eur Heart J* 2005;**26**:1115–40.

52. Farrar DJ, Holman WR, McBride LR *et al.* Long-term follow-up of thoratec ventricular assist device bridge-to-recovery patients successfully removed from support after recovery of ventricular function. *J Heart Lung Transplant* 2002;**21**(5):516–21.

53. Chen YS, Yu HY. Choice of mechanical support for fulminant myocarditis: ECMO vs. VAD? *Eur J Cardio-thorac Surg* 2005;**27**(5):931–2; author reply 2.

54. Rezkalla SH, Raikar S, Kloner RA. Treatment of viral myocarditis with focus on captopril. *Am J Cardiol* 1996;**77**(8):634–7.

55. Rezkalla S, Kloner RA, Khatib G, Khatib R. Effect of delayed captopril therapy on left ventricular mass and myonecrosis during acute coxsackievirus murine myocarditis. *Am Heart J* 1990;**120**(6 Pt 1):1377–81.

56. Saegusa S, Fei Y, Takahashi T *et al.* Oral administration of candesartan improves the survival of mice with viral myocarditis through modification of cardiac adiponectin expression. *Cardiovasc Drugs Therapy* 2007;**21**(3):155–60.

57. Yamamoto K, Shioi T, Uchiyama K, Miyamoto T, Sasayama S, Matsumori A. Attenuation of virus-induced myocardial injury by inhibition of the angiotensin II type 1 receptor signal and decreased nuclear factor-kappa B activation in knockout mice. *J Am Coll Cardiol* 2003;**42**(11):2000–6.

58. Tominaga M, Matsumori A, Okada I, Yamada T, Kawai C. Beta-blocker treatment of dilated cardiomyopathy. Beneficial effect of carteolol in mice. *Circulation* 1991;**83**:2021–8.

59. Rezkalla S, Kloner RA, Khatib G, Smith FE, Khatib R. Effect of metoprolol in acute coxsackievirus B3 murine myocarditis. *J Am Coll Cardiol* 1988;**12**(2):412–14.

60. Pitt B, Zannad F, Remme W *et al.* The effect of spironolactone on morbidity and mortality in patients with severe heart failure. Randomized Aldactone Evaluation Study Investigators. *N Engl J Med* 1999;**341**(10):709–17.

61. Matsumori A, Igata H, Ono K *et al.* High doses of digitalis increase the myocardial production of proinflammatory cytokines and worsen myocardial injury in viral myocarditis: a possible mechanism of digitalis toxicity. *Jpnese Circulation J* 1999;**63**(12):934–40.

62. Wang WZ, Matsumori A, Yamada T *et al.* Beneficial effects of amlodipine in a murine model of congestive heart failure induced

by viral myocarditis. A possible mechanism through inhibition of nitric oxide production. *Circulation* 1997;**95**(1):245–51.

63. Matsumori A, Crumpacker CS, Abelmann WH. Prevention of viral myocarditis with recombinant human leukocyte interferon alpha A/D in a murine model. *J Am Coll Cardiol* 1987;**9**(6):1320–5.

64. Okada I, Matsumori A, Matoba Y *et al.* Combination treatment with ribavarin and interferon for coxsackie B3 replication. *J Lab Clin Med* 1992;**120**:569–73.

65. Ray CG, Icenogle TB, Minnich LL, Copeland JG, Grogan TM. The use of intravenous ribavirin to treat influenza virus-associated acute myocarditis. *J Infect Dis* 1989;**159**(5):829–36.

66. Kuhl U, Pauschinger M, Schwimmbeck P *et al.* Interferon-beta treatment eliminates cardiotropic viruses and improves left ventricular function in patients with myocardial persistence of viral genomes and left ventricular dysfunction. *Circulation* 2003;**107**:2793–8.

67. Daliento L, Calabrese F, Tona F *et al.* Successful treatment of enterovirus-induced myocarditis with interferon-alpha. *J Heart Lung Transplant* 2003;**22**(2):214–17.

68. Parrillo J, Cunnion R, Epstein S *et al.* A prospective, randomized, controlled trial of prednisone for dilated cardiomyopathy. *N Engl J Med* 1989;**321**:1061–8.

69. Stanton C, Mookadam F, Cha S *et al.* Greater sympton duration predicts response to immunomodulatory therapy in dilated cardiomyopathy. *Int J Cardiol* 2008;**128**(1)38–41.

70. Wojnicz R, Nowalany-Kozielska E, Wojciechowska C *et al.* Randomized, placebo-controlled study for immunosuppressive treatment of inflammatory dilated cardiomyopathy: two-year follow-up results. *Circulation* 2001;**104**(1):39–45.

71. McNamara DM, Holubkov R, Starling RC *et al.* Controlled trial of intravenous immune globulin in recent-onset dilated cardiomyopathy. *Circulation* 2001;**103**(18):2254–9.

72. Hia CP, Yip WC, Tai BC, Quek SC. Immunosuppressive therapy in acute myocarditis: an 18 year systematic review. *Arch Dis Child* 2004;**89**(6):580–4.

73. Drucker NA, Colan SD, Lewis AB *et al.* Gamma-globulin treatment of acute myocarditis in the pediatric population. *Circulation* 1994;**89**(1):252–7.

74. Amabile N, Fraisse A, Bouvenot J, Chetaille P, Ovaert C. Outcome of acute fulminant myocarditis in children. *Heart* 2006;**92**(9):1269–73.

75. Khatib R, Reyes MP, Smith F, Khatib G, Rezkalla S. Enhancement of coxsackievirus B4 virulence by indomethacin. *J Lab Clin Med* 1990;**116**(1):116–20.

76. Costanzo-Nordin MR, Reap EA, O'Connell JB, Robinson JA, Scanlon PJ. A nonsteroid anti-inflammatory drug exacerbates Coxsackie B3 murine myocarditis. *J Am Coll Cardiol* 1985;**6**(5):1078–82.

77. Rezkalla S, Khatib R, Khatib G *et al.* Effect of indomethacin in the late phase of coxsackievirus myocarditis in a murine model. *J Lab Clin Med* 1988;**112**(1):118–21.

78. Zipes D, Camm A, Borggrefe M *et al.* ACC/AHA/ESC 2006 Guideline for Management of Patients with Ventricular Arrhythmias and the Prevention of Sudden Cardiac Death. *Circulation* 2006;**114**(10):e385–484.

79. Brilakis E, Olson L, Berry G *et al.* Survival outcomes of patients with giant cell myocarditis bridged to transplantation with ventricular assist devices. *ASAIO J* 2000;**46**:569–72.

80. Topkara VK, Dang NC, Barili F *et al.* Ventricular assist device use for the treatment of acute viral myocarditis. *J Thorac Cardiovasc Surg* 2006;**131**(5):1190–1.

81. Maron BJ, Ackerman MJ, Nishimura RA, Pyeritz RE, Towbin JA, Udelson JE. Task Force 4: HCM and other cardiomyopathies, mitral valve prolapse, myocarditis, and Marfan syndrome. *J Am Coll Cardiol* 2005;**45**(8):1340–5.

82. Matsumori A, Crumpacker CS, Abelmann WH, Kawai C. Virus vaccine and passive immunization for the prevention of viral myocarditis in mice. *Jpn Circ J* 1987;**51**(12):1362–4.

83. Kodama M, Matsumoto Y, Fujiwara M, Masani F, Izumi T, Shibata A. A novel experimental model of giant cell myocarditis induced in rats by immunization with cardiac myosin fraction. *Clin Immunol Immunopathol* 1990;**57**(2):250–62.

84. Cooper LT Jr, Hare JM, Tazelaar HD *et al.* Giant Cell Myocarditis Treatment Trial Investigators. Usefulness of immunosuppression for giant cell myocarditis. *Am J Cardiol* 2008;**102**(11):1535–9.

85. Corssmit EP, Trip MD, Durrer JD. Loffler's endomyocarditis in the idiopathic hypereosinophilic syndrome. *Cardiology* 1999;**91**(4):272–6.

86. Spodick DH. Eosinophilic myocarditis. *Mayo Clin Proc* 1997;**72**(10):996.

87. Corradi D, Vaglio A, Maestri R *et al.* Eosinophilic myocarditis in a patient with idiopathic hypereosinophilic syndrome: insights into mechanisms of myocardial cell death. *Human Pathol* 2004;**35**(9):1160–3.

88. Adsett M, West MJ, Galbraith A, Duhig E, Lange A, Palka P. Eosinophilic heart: marked left ventricular wall thickening and myocardial dysfunction improving with corticosteroid therapy. *Echocardiography* 2003;**20**(4):369–74.

89. McAlister HF, Klementowicz PT, Andrews C, Fisher JD, Feld M, Furman S. Lyme carditis: an important cause of reversible heart block. *Ann Intern Med* 1989;**110**(5):339–45.

90. de Carvalho VB, Sousa EF, Vila JH *et al.* Heart transplantation in Chagas' disease. 10 years after the initial experience. *Circulation* 1996;**94**(8):1815–17.

91. Pulerwitz TC, Cappola TP, Felker GM, Hare JM, Baughman KL, Kasper EK. Mortality in primary and secondary myocarditis. *Am Heart J* 2004;**147**(4):746–50.

49 Management of hypertrophic cardiomyopathy

Barry J Maron

Hypertrophic Cardiomyopathy Center, Minneapolis Heart Institute Foundation, Minneapolis, MN, USA

Over the last 50 years,[1] hypertrophic cardiomyopathy (HCM) has proven to be a genetic heart disease with heterogeneous phenotypic expression, unique pathophysiology, and a diverse clinical course caused by several distinct disease-provoking mutations in genes encoding proteins of the cardiac sarcomere.[2–12] HCM may cause disability and death at virtually any age, including early childhood and infancy, and is the most common cause of sudden death in the young (including competitive athletes).[13]

The first modern description of HCM was in 1958 by Teare.[14] Since then, our understanding of the diagnosis, natural history and management of this heterogeneous disease has evolved dramatically with the development of novel diagnostic tests and treatment modalities. Although literally thousands of papers have been published on HCM,[4] because this disease is relatively uncommon in cardiovascular practice and so diverse in its genetic substrate and clinical presentation, it has not been possible to develop large prospective and randomized clinical trials to test particular treatment modalities.[3] Therefore, most of the data available in HCM come from retrospective and observational studies often composed of relatively small numbers of patients that do not meet the evidence-based threshold achieved by the controlled trials carried out in patients with atherosclerotic coronary artery disease largely over the last 15–20 years. This is an important and unavoidable distinction that must be drawn between genetic heart diseases such as HCM and the much more common acquired coronary heart disease that essentially represents the core of cardiologic practice. For that fundamental reason, the guideline-assigned grades for the various treatments discussed here are usually Class IIa and IIb indications and C1 and C2 levels of evidence.

Indeed, the only truly randomized trials in the HCM literature include a cross-over drug comparison of a beta-blocker versus calcium channel blocker[15] and three pacemaker studies in the early 1990s in which individual patients acted as their own controls by virtue of alternating the pacing mode to either the on or off position.[16–18] Nevertheless, over the last 10–15 years the strategy of assembling multicenter populations from HCM centers of excellence has allowed for much larger HCM patient cohorts to be studied, thereby producing evidence concerning the disease that would not be possible with single institution populations.

Prevalence and epidemiology

A number of epidemiologic studies are now available showing that HCM occurs in at least 0.2% of the general population (e.g. 1:500).[8,19–22] This prevalence is greater than previously regarded, although HCM remains relatively uncommon in general cardiology practice.[23] This paradox strongly suggests that most individuals affected by HCM do not achieve clinical recognition. Furthermore, there is growing evidence that HCM is truly a global disease,[20] although to date the most intense interest and reporting of cases has been in North America, Western Europe and Asia (Japan and China). HCM occurs equally in the genders and has been reported in many racial groups, including African-Americans.[24]

Definition and nomenclature

HCM is characterized by a thickened but non-dilated left ventricle (LV) in the absence of another cardiac or systemic disease capable of producing the magnitude of hypertrophy evident (e.g. aortic valve stenosis, systemic hypertension, and some phenotypic expressions of athlete's heart).[2–8] For the past 35 years, the clinical diagnosis of HCM has usually been made by echocardiographic imaging.[3] Cardiovascular magnetic resonance (CMR) has an expand-

Evidence-Based Cardiology, 3rd edition. Edited by S. Yusuf, J.A. Cairns, A.J. Camm, E.L. Fallen, and B.J. Gersh. © 2010 Blackwell Publishing, ISBN: 978-1-4051-5925-8.

ing role in the non-invasive diagnosis of HCM. For example, CMR may visualize areas of segmental hypertrophy, specifically in the anterolateral free wall and LV apex, not reliably identified with echocardiography.[25]

Left ventricle morphology

Hypertrophy

The distribution of LV hypertrophy is characteristically asymmetric, in which some portion of the LV wall is thicker than other areas.[7] Frequently, the pattern of hypertrophy is strikingly heterogeneous, with contiguous segments of LV wall differing greatly in thickness. Hypertrophy may be diffuse, involving substantial portions of ventricular septum and LV free wall, including patients with the most substantial hypertrophy observed in any cardiac disease.[7] However, in about one-third of patients, LV hypertrophy may be relatively mild and confined to small areas of the chamber such as basal anterior septum or apex. Furthermore, genotype-phenotype studies in HCM families have documented the association of HCM mutant genes with near-normal or even normal LV wall thicknesses.[12,26] Therefore, virtually any LV wall thickness is compatible with the clinical and/or genetic diagnosis of HCM.

Histopathology

Cardiac muscle cells (myocytes) in ventricular septum and LV free wall have increased transverse diameter as well as bizarre shapes, often maintaining intercellular connections with several adjacent cells.[27,28] Frequently, these myocytes are arranged in a chaotic, disorganized pattern at oblique and perpendicular angles to each other; myofibrils within cardiac muscle cells may also be in disarray. Disorganized cardiac muscle cells occur in about 95% of patients dying of HCM and usually occupy substantial portions of the LV, about 33% of septum and 25% of free wall.[27,28]

Microvascular abnormalities of intramural coronary arteries are present in about 80% of patients studied at necropsy, most commonly in the ventricular septum.[29] These vessels commonly have thickened arterial walls due to increased intimal and/or medial components, associated with apparent luminal narrowing. This form of "small vessel disease" may be responsible for regional myocardial ischemia,[11] necrosis, and ultimately replacement fibrosis with grossly visible extensive (or even transmural) scars. It is likely that disorganized myocardial cells and architecture, as well as areas of replacement fibrosis dispersed throughout the LV wall, impair normal transmission of electrophysiologic impulses, predispose to disordered patterns and increased dispersion of electrical depolarization

and repolarization, and probably serve as an electrically unstable arrhythmogenic substrate with the potential to trigger lethal ventricular tachyarrhythmias and sudden death.[30] Myocardial disorganization and fibrosis could also contribute to diastolic dysfunction and progression of heart failure.

LV outflow obstruction

Dynamic subaortic obstruction in HCM is usually produced by systolic anterior motion (SAM) of the mitral valve, resulting in contact between mitral valve and ventricular septum.[6] Subaortic obstruction in HCM may fluctuate in response to a number of provocations (including exercise)[31,32] but represents true mechanical impedance to LV outflow. The markedly increased intraventricular pressures that result may be detrimental to LV function by increasing myocardial wall stress and oxygen demand. LV outflow tract obstruction (gradient ≥30 mmHg) is a proven determinant of progressive heart failure symptoms and cardiovascular death over many years[9] (9) (Fig. 49.1). Furthermore, fully 70% of an HCM cohort has the propensity to develop LV outflow obstruction either at rest or with physiologic exercise.[10]

Genetics

HCM is a Mendelian trait with an autosomal dominant pattern of inheritance. Molecular studies with clinical genotype-phenotype correlations have convincingly demonstrated that HCM is caused by mutations in any one of 11 genes, each encoding a protein component of the cardiac

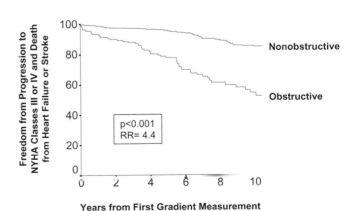

Figure 49.1 Long-term significance of LV outflow tract obstruction. Probability of progression to severe heart failure (NYHA III or IV) or death from heart failure or stroke among 224 patients with LV outflow tract obstruction (gradient at rest ≥30 mmHg), and 770 patients without obstruction. (From Maron et al[9] with permission of the Massachusetts Medical Society.)

sarcomere (of either the thick or thin filaments) with contractile, structural or regulatory functions.[12,26,33–38]

Two of the HCM-causing mutant genes, beta-myosin heavy chain and myosin-binding protein C, predominate in frequency. The other nine genes account for far fewer cases of HCM and include troponin T and I, regulatory and essential myosin light chains, titin, alpha-tropomyosin, alpha-actin, alpha-myosin heavy chain and muscle LIM protein (MLP). This genetic diversity is compounded by the considerable intragenic heterogeneity with over 400 mutations now identified (http://cardiogenomics.med. harvard.edu). The characteristic morphologic diversity of the HCM phenotype is largely attributable to the disease-causing mutations, but probably also to the influence of modifier genes and environmental factors on phenotypic expression.

Symptoms

Onset of heart failure symptoms often occurs in early adulthood between 20 and 40 years of age, although symptoms can become evident at any age, from young children to the elderly.[3,39,40] While some degree of heart failure is frequent in HCM, progression to severe functional limitation (i.e. NYHA class III–IV) is uncommon, occurring in about 10–15% of hospital-based patient populations.[3,4] The usual circumstance is characterized by exertional dyspnea and fatigue (and sometimes orthopnea and paroxysmal nocturnal dyspnea), indicative of elevated pulmonary venous pressures in the presence of intact or hyperdynamic systolic function. Such symptoms are related to diastolic dysfunction, outflow tract obstruction, microvascular myocardial ischemia, or a combination of these pathophysiologic variables. HCM patients may also experience syncope (or near-syncope), lightheadedness, palpitations, and chest pain, either typical of midsternal angina pectoris or with more atypical features.

Natural history

Overall patient population

Predicting clinical course and outcome for individual HCM patients continues to be challenging because of the marked variability and heterogeneity in disease expression, particularly for young patients with their long period of potential risk. Annual premature HCM-related mortality rates were initially reported to be 3–6% with the higher range in children.[5,41] However, these are now regarded as outdated estimates derived largely from highly selected HCM cohorts, skewed toward high-risk patients at tertiary referral centers. Greater insight into the clinical course of HCM has been achieved by analysis of unselected community-based patient populations, uncontaminated by tertiary center referral bias. These cohorts have allowed more realistic overall mortality rates of about 1%/year to be established, although somewhat higher for children (i.e. 2%/year)[3,40,41] (Fig. 49.2). Therefore, in adults, HCM does not add to total mortality over that expected for the general population and is compatible with normal life expectancy, often without significant disability or the necessity for major interventions.[3,39,40]

Risk stratification and sudden cardiac death

Demographics

Sudden death in HCM may occur at a wide range of ages, but most commonly during adolescence and young

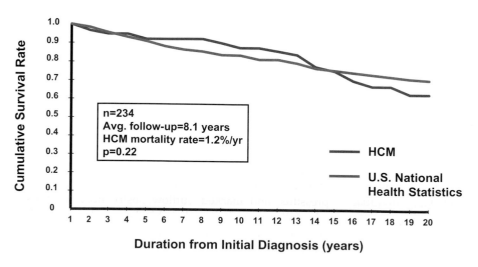

Figure 49.2 Cumulative survival in a community-based adult HCM population. Total mortality in 234 HCM patients (1%/year) does not differ significantly from that expected in general US population after adjustment for age, sex, and race. (From Maron et al,[40] reproduced with permission of the American Medical Association.)

adulthood, less than age 30–35 years of age.[3–6,41–45] Indeed, HCM is the most common cause of sudden cardiac death in young people and these events are arrhythmia-based due to primary ventricular tachycardia/fibrillation, with a predilection for the early morning hours.[30,45,46] Sudden death is often the initial disease manifestation in asymptomatic individuals, many of whom are undiagnosed during life. Although most patients die suddenly while sedentary or during normal/modest physical activity, an important proportion do so associated with vigorous exertion, including young competitive athletes in organized sports. This observation is the basis for the standard and prudent recommendation to disqualify young athletes with HCM from intense competitive sports to reduce their risk for sudden death, according to the guidelines of Bethesda Conference #36.[47]

Risk factors[3–5,30,43,44,48–54]

For secondary prevention, risk for sudden death is associated with prior cardiac arrest or sustained ventricular tachycardia. For primary prevention, one or more of the following clinical risk markers are relevant:

- family history of ≥1 premature HCM-related deaths, particularly if sudden and multiple
- unexplained recent syncope, particularly in the young and related to exertion
- hypotensive or attenuated blood pressure response to exercise
- multiple repetitive (or prolonged) non-sustained ventricular tachycardia on serial Holter (ambulatory) ECG monitoring
- massive LV hypertrophy (wall thickness ≥30 mm), most relevant to younger patients.

Each of these risk factors, taken individually, has potential limitations and all are encumbered with relatively low positive predictive value (of about 20%), although with high negative predictive accuracy. For example, the finding of non-sustained ventricular tachycardia (NSVT) on ambulatory Holter may be fraught with particular ambiguity.[48,53,54] A single brief isolated burst of NSVT on a random Holter ECG is no longer regarded as a risk factor which itself would trigger a primary prevention implanted cardioverter-defibrillator (ICD). However, long runs of NSVT (>10 beats) intuitively carry greater weight in these clinical circumstances. One potentially useful (but non evidence based) strategy utilized following identification of a short run of NSVT on the initial Holter ECG involves expanding the monitoring period to a total of six days by obtaining additional ECG recordings at about 1–2 week intervals.[53,54] This approach allows assembly of an extended profile of ectopy. Thus, a more measured assessment of an individual patient's day-to-day ventricular ectopy (including NSVT) is achieved, potentially clarifying the decision concerning a prophylactic ICD.

It has been proposed that certain mutations responsible for HCM could represent prognostic markers conveying either favorable or adverse outcome, including the risk for sudden death.[12,55] For example, early genotype-phenotype studies identified certain beta-myosin heavy chain and troponin T mutations to be associated with higher frequency of premature death compared to other mutations, such as those involving myosin-binding protein C or alpha-tropomyosin. More recently, however, the prognostic significance of disease-causing mutations for risk stratification and decision-making concerning treatment strategies has been questioned and de-emphasized.[37,38] Due to the substantial genetic heterogeneity in HCM and lack of compelling data, it is now evident that anticipating the future clinical course based on knowledge of the disease-causing mutation is untenable and has been largely abandoned in the management of individual patients.

While the presence of a subaortic gradient (≥30 mmHg at rest) is a strong determinant of progressive heart failure and cardiovascular death, the relationship is much less predictive of sudden cardiac death[9] and LV outflow obstruction should not be regarded as a primary risk marker.

Management

Treatment strategies in individual HCM patients are usually tailored along one of three major prognostic pathways: disabling symptoms due to heart failure, high risk for sudden death, and atrial fibrillation (Fig. 49.3).

Medical management of heart failure

Data dictating pharmacologic treatment of symptomatic HCM patients with heart failure are largely derived from clinical experience in selected patient subsets followed for relatively brief periods of time,[56] with the exception of one double-blind cross-over study in a small patient cohort.[15] When associated with normal or hyperdynamic LV function the response of heart failure symptoms to medical treatment is highly variable; hence, therapy is often tailored empirically to the individual requirements of symptomatic patients. Since the mid-1960s a variety of beta-adrenergic receptor-blocking drugs have been utilized extensively to relieve and control heart failure symptoms in patients with obstructive or non-obstructive HCM.[1] Verapamil may improve cardiac symptoms and exercise capacity (largely in non-obstructive patients) due to a beneficial effect on LV relaxation and filling, but should be avoided in the presence of elevated pulmonary venous pressures and marked outflow obstruction.[3] In patients who fail to benefit from beta-blockers and verapamil, an empiric trial may be initiated with disopyramide (in combination with a beta-blocker).[57]

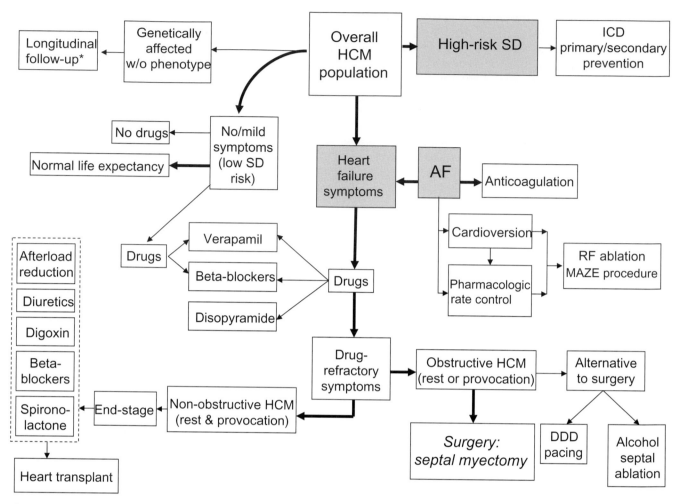

Figure 49.3 Current treatment strategies for patient subgroups within HCM disease spectrum. Management decisions usually proceed along three major prognostic pathways: disabling symptoms due to heart failure, high risk for sudden death, and atrial fibrillation. *No specific treatment or intervention indicated, except under exceptional circumstances. AF, atrial fibrillation; ICD, implantable cardioverter-defibrillator; RF, radiofrequency; SD, sudden death.

Alternatively, about 3% of HCM patients will manifest the "end-stage" of HCM in which progressive heart failure is associated with LV systolic dysfunction and often remodeling in the form of wall thinning and cavity dilation.[58] Drug therapy in these patients is similar to that employed for congestive heart failure in other cardiac diseases and may include the administration of beta-blockers, ACE inhibitors, angiotensin receptor blockers and diuretics, as well as possibly digoxin, spironolactone, warfarin, and ultimately heart transplant.

Prevention of sudden death

Historically, the management of high-risk HCM patients was first confined to prophylactic pharmacologic treatment with beta-blockers, verapamil, and antiarrhythmic agents (such as procainamide, quinidine, and subsequently amio-

darone). However, in HCM there are virtually no data supporting the efficacy of prophylactic drug treatment in preventing sudden death.[59]

When the level of risk for sudden death is judged by risk factor analysis to be unacceptably high and deserving of intervention, the ICD has proved to be the most effective available prophylactic treatment option, with the potential for absolute protection and alteration in the natural history of this disease by aborting potentially life-threatening ventricular tachyarrhythmias.[30,46,60] Unavoidably, all available ICD data in HCM are observational and by design nonrandomized, with patients accessed retrospectively and prospectively.[61–63]

The largest such study cohort is composed of 506 HCM patients in an international multicenter registry, all of whom had ICDs implanted for high-risk status, and were followed for an average period of about 3½ years (up to

16).[30] Appropriate device discharges (either defibrillation shocks or antitachycardia pacing) triggered by ventricular tachycardia/fibrillation occurred in 20% of patients with an overall annual discharge rate of 5.5%. Appropriate intervention rate was 11%/year for secondary and 4%/year for primary prevention. Of note, almost 30% of the young patients implanted at ≤20 years of age subsequently had appropriate ICD discharges at 18 ± 4 years of age. Therefore, the ICD has proven effective in HCM despite the often substantially increased cardiac mass characteristic of this disease, as well as the not infrequent occurrence of LV outflow tract obstruction. Furthermore, about 40% of those patients who received appropriate defibrillator therapy to terminate potentially lethal ventricular tachyarrhythmias in fact experienced multiple such interventions.

Medical treatment is not absolutely protective against the risk of sudden death in HCM. Indeed, in one large study, a substantial proportion of patients were taking amiodarone or other potentially antiarrhythmic drugs at the time of appropriate defibrillator interventions.[59]

There is general consensus and virtually no controversy that secondary sudden death prevention (i.e. with the ICD) is strongly warranted in those patients with fortuitous resuscitation from prior cardiac arrest (with documented ventricular fibrillation (VF)) or sustained and spontaneously occurring ventricular tachycardia (VT). While the presence of multiple clinical risk factors conveys greater comfort in judging increased risk for primary prevention,[43,44] it is also

obvious now that a single risk factor may often be sufficient evidence to justify a recommendation for a prophylactic ICD.[30] A large multicenter international registry found no difference in the likelihood of appropriate shocks when ICDs were implanted for either 1, 2 or ≥ 3 risk markers, and 35% of patients implanted for only one risk factor nevertheless experienced an appropriate shock (Fig. 49.4). Therefore, many investigators, particularly in the US, favor strong consideration of a prophylactic ICD even in the presence of only one major risk factor. Other (largely European) investigators are generally more conservative and restrictive in requiring two or more risk factors before raising consideration for a primary prevention ICD. Also, based on experience, both the end-stage phase and LV apical aneurysm (with regional myocardial scarring)[63] are subgroups at risk for sudden cardiac death and potentially warrant a prophylactic ICD as a bridge to heart transplantation.

While a single risk factor may be sufficient to trigger consideration for a prophylactic ICD, there are numerous clinical circumstances for which ambiguities and gray areas arise with respect to the presence, strength or number of risk factors.[30] For example, there are many elderly patients with a single risk factor (e.g. syncope) who may not be candidates for primary prevention, given that HCM-related sudden death is uncommon in this age group and survival to advanced age without complications itself generally declares lower risk status in HCM. Ultimately, many of the complex clinical scenarios involving only one risk factor

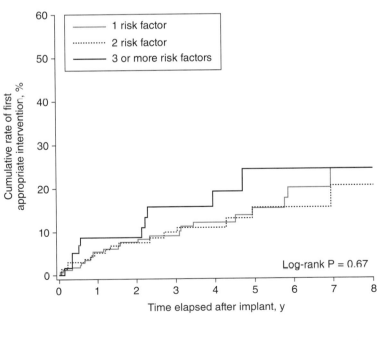

Figure 49.4 ICD therapy in HCM. Cumulative rates for first appropriate implantable defibrillator intervention in HCM patients with 1, 2 or ≥3 risk factors who had received devices for primary prevention. (From Maron et al,[30] reproduced with permission of the American Medical Association.)

NO. at risk								
1 risk factor	173	150	119	98	70	48	31	18	16
2 risk factor	143	123	95	71	53	34	28	16	6
3 or more risk factors	59	52	38	32	23	11	9	8	6

may require a measure of physician judgment in the context of the individual patient's clinical profile. Patient autonomy with full physician disclosure allows the fully informed HCM patient to contribute importantly to the resolution of such uncertainties which not infrequently arise in clinical situations with insufficient evidence-based data.[64,65] We also recognize that physician and patient attitudes toward ICDs (and access to such devices within respective healthcare systems) can vary considerably among countries and cultures, and thereby impact importantly on clinical decision making and the threshold for device implant in HCM.[66]

Crucial to understanding the role of the ICD within the broad HCM disease spectrum is an appreciation of certain demographic distinctions from ICD therapy in ischemic heart disease. The latter patients are of relatively advanced age at the time of implant (average about 65 years), often with severe and progressive heart failure as a consequence of prior myocardial infarction and LV dysfunction. In sharp contrast, ICDs in HCM often involve young asymptomatic patients with an extended period of risk for sudden death (mean age at implant and at first appropriate device intervention only 40 years). Therefore, although annual appropriate primary prevention intervention rates for HCM are lower than those reported in coronary artery disease,[67–69] they are nevertheless significant, since that experience must be placed in the context of a much younger patient population usually free of significant heart failure and noncardiac disease. Protected by the ICD, these patients could potentially survive many decades of productive life with few or no symptoms, even achieving normal or near-normal life expectancy if not encumbered by other major HCM-related or other disease complications.

The time interval between implant and first appropriate ICD intervention may be quite variable, with particularly long delays of up to 10 years not uncommon for the initial life-saving intervention.[30] This observation underscores the unpredictable timing of lethal arrhythmias and sudden death in HCM in which the ICD may remain dormant for substantial periods of time before it is ultimately required to intervene appropriately. Conversely, some appropriate shocks occur early after implant, not uncommonly even within the first 12 months.[70] The mechanisms underlying such earlier interventions are unresolved.

Indeed, the decision to prophylactically implant an ICD in an HCM patient is often fortuitously based on the precise time at which risk stratification is undertaken and high-risk status identified. Once potential risk is recognized, it becomes difficult and probably imprudent to temporize or delay potentially preventive treatment. Indeed, a patient identified as high risk at age 20 (and implanted with a device prophylactically) will still be young and at increased risk for an event at age 35, even if the ICD has not been triggered appropriately during that 15-year period. Consequently, once the decision to implant an ICD in a high-risk HCM patient is made it is likely to represent a life-long preventive measure.

Atrial fibrillation

Atrial fibrillation (AF) is the most common sustained arrhythmia in HCM, frequently accounts for unexpected hospital admissions and lost productivity, and often requires aggressive therapeutic intervention.[3] Data directly focused on the natural history and management of AF in HCM are limited, and essentially confined to one large retrospective study.[71] Consequently, treatment guidelines for AF in HCM are not infrequently translated from the experience in acquired cardiac diseases, particularly randomized trials such as AFFIRM.[72]

Paroxysmal episodes or chronic AF occur in about 25% of HCM patients, increasing in incidence with age, and linked to enlargement of the left atrium.[71] AF is reasonably well tolerated by about one-third of patients and has not proved to be an independent determinant of sudden cardiac death. It is associated with embolic stroke, progressive heart failure, disability and possibly heart failure-related death, particularly when associated with outflow obstruction at rest in patients <50 years of age. Paroxysmal AF only occasionally is responsible for acute clinical decompensation, requiring emergent electrical or pharmacologic cardioversion. Amiodarone is regarded as effective in reducing AF recurrences based on inferences from data in non-HCM patients. With chronic AF, beta-blockers and verapamil will usually control heart rate; atrioventricular (AV) node ablation with permanent ventricular pacing is rarely required to institute adequate drug therapy. In the absence of HCM-specific controlled data, AF management decisions regarding rate control versus conversion to sinus rhythm are generally made case by case, based upon the overall clinical profile, and the experience in patients with other cardiac diseases.

Because of the potential for clot formation and embolization, warfarin is indicated in HCM patients with AF. Since only one or two paroxysms of AF have been associated with risk for systemic thromboembolism in this disease, the threshold for initiation of anticoagulant therapy is low. However, such clinical decisions should be tailored to individual patients after considering obligatory lifestyle modifications, risk of hemorrhagic complications, and expectations for compliance. Some success in treating refractory AF complicating HCM has been reported in a small number of patients with the surgical MAZE procedure or by radiofrequency catheter ablation.[3]

Surgery

Based on a series of observational studies from many parts of the world over several decades, operation (surgical septal myectomy) is the primary treatment option for HCM patients with severe drug-refractory symptoms resulting in functional disability and associated with obstruction to LV outflow under basal conditions or with physiologic exercise (gradient ≥50 mmHg).[73–89] The primary objective of myectomy is reduction in heart failure-related symptoms and improved quality of life. Surgical myectomy is not recommended for asymptomatic or mildly symptomatic patients with outflow obstruction, as there is no evidence at present that prophylactic surgical relief of obstruction has greater long-term benefit with respect to survival or disease progression.

The most successful operative procedure has been the transaortic septal myectomy (Morrow procedure) in which a portion of muscle is resected from the basal septum (usually about 2–10 g).[90] More recently, at some centers, the myectomy has been extended much more distally within the septum.[86,91] Results achieved at several institutions with myectomy over the past 45 years have been excellent, with most patients afforded substantial symptomatic and hemodynamic benefit, but without important compromise in global LV function. Operative mortality has steadily decreased and is now considerably less than 1% at the most experienced centers.[89]

Long-term follow-up studies from surgical centers have demonstrated that basal outflow obstruction does not recur and heart failure is largely reversed by septal myectomy.[73–89] Symptoms are relieved long term in about 85% of patients, followed for up to 26 years, and overall survival has been reported to be 83% over a 10-year follow-up. In a observational study design, operated patients achieved the same longevity as the general population and had significantly better survival than non-operated patients with outflow obstruction (Fig. 49.5). Randomization of patients to surgery versus medical therapy is not practical or ethically feasible.

Alternatives to surgery

In the late 1990s, permanent dual-chamber pacing was promoted as an alternative to myectomy for patients with obstructive HCM and severe refractory symptoms.[16–18] However, several randomized double-blind, cross-over studies demonstrated that subjectively perceived symptomatic benefit from pacing was not accompanied by objective evidence of improved exercise capacity and appeared to largely represent a placebo effect.[16,18] These studies represent the few controlled investigations available addressing the treatment options for HCM patients since these study designs permitted assessment of patients blindly with the pacing mode on or off. While reduction in subaortic gradient may be induced by pacing in some patients, this benefit is more modest and inconsistent compared to that achieved with myectomy. Although selected patients

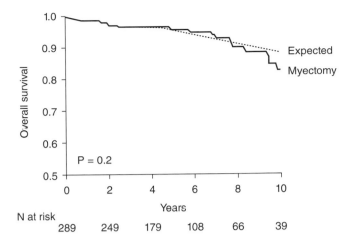

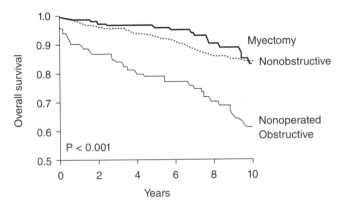

Figure 49.5 Long-term survival following surgical septal myectomy. (*Top panel*) Survival free from all-cause mortality after myectomy for obstructive HCM (n = 289) compared with age- and gender-matched US population. (*Bottom panel*) Survival free from all-cause mortality in three HCM patient subgroups: surgical myectomy (n = 289), non-operated with obstruction (n = 228), and non-obstructive (n = 820). Overall log-rank and myectomy vs non-operated obstructive HCM, *P* < 0.001. (From Ommen et al,[87] with permission of the American College of Cardiology.)

older than 65 years may more likely benefit from pacing, the overall role for this treatment modality in HCM has become particularly limited.

Percutaneous alcohol septal ablation may reduce LV outflow tract gradient and heart failure symptoms, by virtue of producing a large transmural septal infarct.[92] However, follow-up is necessarily short compared to myectomy (average 2–4 years vs up to 45 years for surgery) and the ultimate role of alcohol ablation in the treatment of patients with obstructive HCM is not yet definitively resolved. Observational studies show gradient and symptom relief from alcohol ablation to be similar although less complete and consistent compared to myectomy, with about 25% of ablation patients incurring major (even life-threatening) complications requiring repeated procedures due to unsatisfactory hemodynamic and symptomatic results.[89–91,93–97]

Table 49.1 Level of evidence for major management options in hypertrophic cardiomyopathy

	Class	Evidence
Surgical septal myectomy	I	C1
Percutaneous alcohol septal ablation	IIa	C2
Dual-chamber pacing	IIb	A
Genetic testing (for diagnosis)	I	C1
Genetic testing (for prognosis)	IIb	C2
Implantable cardioverter-defibrillator (primary and secondary sudden death prevention)	I	C1
Drug therapy for heart failure symptoms	IIa	C1
Control of atrial fibrillation (drugs/cardioversion)	IIa	C1
Heart transplantation (for end stage)	I	C2

Because percutaneous septal ablation has been perceived to be less invasive and more accessible than surgical myectomy, its penetration into cardiologic practice has been extensive, raising the possibility that the threshold for ablation is lower than for operation. Indeed, the American College of Cardiology/European Society of Cardiology expert consensus panel[3] placed surgical septal myectomy as the primary gold standard management option for patients with severe refractory symptoms and marked outflow obstruction. In those guidelines, alcohol ablation is regarded as an alternative treatment strategy for selected patients, i.e. those with co-morbidity or other medical factors which increase operative risk or who are adverse to surgical intervention.

However, long-term issues remain unresolved, most prominently the clinical significance of the alcohol-induced transmural scar (occupying about 10% of the LV wall) which represents a potentially unstable arrhythmogenic substrate and undoubtedly raises the risk for sudden cardiac death in some patients.[98] Reported procedural mortality for alcohol septal ablation at experienced centers ($\leq$2%) is higher than for HCM surgical centers (<1%). A prospective myectomy versus alcohol ablation trial, adequately powered to compare the key issue of long-term outcome, poses myriad practical problems which seem virtually insurmountable, and likely will never occur to resolve these issues.[99]

Conclusion

Hypertrophic cardiomyopathy is an important genetic heart disease, characterized by left ventricular hypertrophy, with a characteristically heterogeneous clinical presentation and course which greatly influences management strategies. Unavoidably, much of the available data concerning treatment options and decision making come from retrospective, observational studies, often composed of relatively small patient cohorts. Because randomized prospective studies are exceedingly uncommon, the level of evidence in HCM (and other genetic heart diseases) rarely reaches that achieved for patients with much more common coronary artery disease.

Treatment options in HCM target control of heart failure or atrial fibrillation, and prevention of sudden death. Heart failure is manifest largely as disability due to exertional dyspnea and is initially treated pharmacologically with a series of drugs (including beta-blockers, verapamil, disopyramide and possibly diuretics). Should limiting symptoms progress despite maximal medical therapy, and substantial obstruction LV outflow be present either at rest or with physiologic provocation, then invasive septal reduction is considered. In such disabled drug-refractory patients with obstructive HCM, surgical septal myectomy is the primary treatment option, with alcohol septal ablation an alternative for selected patients, particularly those of advanced age and/or with significant co-morbidity. Patients who progress to the "end-stage" phase with systolic dysfunction constitute the only HCM subset eligible for heart transplantation. Atrial fibrillation is managed by rate control or cardioversion and anticoagulation and possibly radiofrequency ablation in selected patients.

Recently, the ICD has been employed effectively in HCM, demonstrating that sudden death due to ventricular tachyarrhythmias can be prevented and the natural course of the disease importantly altered. The risk stratification algorithm employed in HCM has proved to be an efficacious and useful guide in selecting patients for defibrillator therapy, although likely incomplete. Management of individual HCM patients is predicated on targeting pathways of prognosis, i.e. heart failure (and progression to the end stage), atrial fibrillation or increased risk for sudden death risk.

References

1. Braunwald E, Lambrew CT, Rockoff SD *et al.* Idiopathic hypertrophic subaortic stenosis. I: A description of the disease based upon an analysis of 64 patients. *Circulation* 1964;**30**(suppl IV):3–217.
2. Maron BJ, Towbin JA, Thiene G *et al.* Contemporary definitions and classification of the cardiomyopathies. An American Heart Association Scientific Statement from the Council on Clinical Cardiology, Heart Failure and Transplantation Committee; Quality of Care and Outcomes Research and Functional Genomics and Translational Biology Interdisciplinary Working Groups; and Council on Epidemiology and Prevention. *Circulation* 2006;**113**:1807–16.
3. Maron BJ, McKenna WJ, Danielson GK *et al.* American College of Cardiology/European Society of Cardiology Clinical Expert Consensus Document on Hypertrophic Cardiomyopathy. A report of the American College of Cardiology Task Force on

Clinical Expert Consensus Documents and the European Society of Cardiology Committee for Practice Guidelines Committee to Develop an Expert Consensus Document on Hypertrophic Cardiomyopathy. *J Am Coll Cardiol* 2003;**42**:1687–713.

4. Maron BJ. Hypertrophic cardiomyopathy: a systematic review. *JAMA* 2002;**287**:1308–20.

5. Spirito P, Seidman, CE, McKenna WJ *et al.* The management of hypertrophic cardiomyopathy. *N Engl J Med* 1997;**336**:775–85.

6. Wigle ED, Rakowski H, Kimball BP *et al.* Hypertrophic cardiomyopathy. Clinical spectrum and treatment. *Circulation* 1995;**92**:1680–92.

7. Klues HG, Schiffers A, Maron BJ. Phenotypic spectrum and patterns of left ventricular hypertrophy in hypertrophic cardiomyopathy: morphologic observations and significance as assessed by two-dimensional echocardiography in 600 patients. *J Am Coll Cardiol* 1995;**26**:1699–708.

8. Maron BJ, Gardin, JM, Flack JM *et al.* Assessment of the prevalence of hypertrophic cardiomyopathy in a general population of young adults: echocardiographic analysis of 4111 subjects in the CARDIA Study. *Circulation* 1995;**92**:785–9.

9. Maron MS, Olivotto I, Betocchi S *et al.* Effect of left ventricular outflow tract obstruction on clinical outcome in hypertrophic cardiomyopathy. *N Engl J Med* 2003;**348**:295–303.

10. Maron MS, Olivotto I, Zenovich AG *et al.* Hypertrophic cardiomyopathy is predominantly a disease of left ventricular outflow tract obstruction. *Circulation* 2006;**114**:2232–9.

11. Cecchi F, Olivotto I, Gistri R *et al.* Coronary microvascular dysfunction and prognosis in hypertrophic cardiomyopathy. *N Engl J Med* 2003;**349**:1027–35.

12. Seidman JG, Seidman CE. The genetic basis for cardiomyopathy: from mutation identification to mechanistic paradigms. *Cell* 2001;**104**:557–67.

13. Maron BJ. Sudden death in young athletes. *N Engl J Med* 2003;**349**:1064–75.

14. Teare D. Asymmetrical hypertrophy of the heart in young athletes. *Br Heart J* 1958;**20**:1–8.

15. Gilligan DM, Chan WL, Joshi J *et al.* A double-blind, placebo-controlled crossover trial of nadolol and verapamil in mild and moderately symptomatic hypertrophic cardiomyopathy. *J Am Coll Cardiol* 1993;**21**:1672–9.

16. Maron BJ, Nishimura RA, McKenna WJ *et al.* Assessment of permanent dual-chamber pacing as a treatment for drug-refractory symptomatic patients with obstructive hypertrophic cardiomyopathy: a randomized, double-blind cross-over study (M-PATHY). *Circulation* 1999;**99**:2927–33.

17. Kappenberger L, Linde C, Daubert C *et al.* Pacing in hypertrophic obstructive cardiomyopathy: a randomized crossover study. *Eur Heart J* 1997;**18**:1249–56.

18. Nishimura RA, Trusty JM, Hayes DL *et al.* Dual-chamber pacing for hypertrophic cardiomyopathy: a randomized, double-blind cross-over study. *J Am Coll Cardiol* 1997;**29**:435–41.

19. Maron BJ, Mathenge R, Casey SA *et al.* Clinical profile of hypertrophic cardiomyopathy identified de novo in rural communities. *J Am Coll Cardiol* 1999;**33**:1590–5.

20. Maron BJ Hypertrophic cardiomyopathy: an important global disease (Editorial). *Am J Med* 2004;**116**:63–5.

21. Zou Y, Song L, Wang Z *et al.* Prevalence of idiopathic hypertrophic cardiomyopathy in China: a population-based echocardiographic analysis of 8080 adults. *Am J Med* 2004;**115**:14–18.

22. Agnarsson UT, Hardarson T, Hallgrimsson J, Sigfusson N. The prevalence of hypertrophic cardiomyopathy in men: an echocardiographic population screening study with a review of death records. *J Intern Med* 1992;**232**:499–506.

23. Maron BJ, Peterson EE, Maron MS, Peterson JE. Prevalence of hypertrophic cardiomyopathy in an outpatient population referred for echocardiographic study. *Am J Cardiol* 1994;**73**:577–80.

24. Maron BJ, Carney KP, Lever HM *et al.* Relationship of race to sudden cardiac death in competitive athletes with hypertrophic cardiomyopathy. *J Am Coll Cardiol* 2003;**41**:974–80.

25. Rickers C, Wilke NM, Jerosch-Herold M *et al.* Utility of cardiac magnetic resonance imaging in the diagnosis of hypertrophic cardiomyopathy. *Circulation* 2005;**112**:855–61.

26. Maron BJ, Niimura H, Casey SA *et al.* Development of left ventricular hypertrophy in adults with hypertrophic cardiomyopathy caused by cardiac myosin-binding protein C mutations. *J Am Coll Cardiol* 2001;**38**:315–21.

27. Maron BJ, Roberts WC. Quantitative analysis of cardiac muscle cell disorganization in the ventricular septum of patients with hypertrophic cardiomyopathy. *Circulation* 1979;**59**:689–706.

28. Maron BJ, Anan TJ, Roberts WC. Quantitative analysis of the distribution of cardiac muscle cell disorganization in the left ventricular wall of patients with hypertrophic cardiomyopathy. *Circulation* 1981;**63**:882–94.

29. Maron BJ, Wolfson JK, Epstein SE, Roberts WC. Intramural ("small vessel") coronary artery disease in hypertrophic cardiomyopathy. *J Am Coll Cardiol* 1986;**8**:545–57.

30. Maron BJ, Spirito P, Shen W-K *et al.* Implantable cardioverter-defibrillators and prevention of sudden cardiac death in hypertrophic cardiomyopathy. *JAMA* 2007;**298**:405–12.

31. Paz R, Jortner R, Tunick PA *et al.* The effect of the ingestion of ethanol on obstruction of the left ventricular outflow tract in hypertrophic cardiomyopathy. *N Engl J Med* 1997;**335**:938–41.

32. Gilligan DM, Chan WL, Ang EL, Oakley CM. Effects of a meal on hemodynamic function at rest and during exercise in patients with hypertrophic cardiomyopathy. *J Am Coll Cardiol* 1991;**18**:429–36.

33. Arad M, Benson DW, Perez-Atayde AR *et al.* Constitutively active AMP kinase mutations cause glycogen storage disease mimicking hypertrophic cardiomyopathy. *J Clin Invest* 2002;**109**:357–62.

34. Arad M, Maron BJ, Gorham JM *et al.* Glycogen storage diseases presenting as hypertrophic cardiomyopathy. *N Engl J Med* 2005;**352**:362–72.

35. Arad M, Penas-Lado M, Monserrat L *et al.* Gene mutations in apical hypertrophic cardiomyopathy. *Circulation* 2005;**112**:2805–11.

36. Maron BJ, Seidman JG, Seidman CE. Proposal for contemporary screening strategies in families with hypertrophic cardiomyopathy. *J Am Coll Cardiol* 2004;**44**:2125–32.

37. Ackerman MJ, Van Driest SL, Ommen SR *et al.* Prevalence and age dependence of malignant mutations in the beta-myosin heavy chain and troponin T genes in hypertrophic cardiomyopathy: a comprehensive outpatient perspective. *J Am Coll Cardiol* 2002;**39**:2042–8.

38. Van Driest SL, Ackerman MJ, Ommen SR *et al.* Prevalence and severity of "benign" mutations in the beta-myosin heavy chain,

cardiac troponin T, and alpha-tropomyosin genes in hypertrophic cardiomyopathy. *Circulation* 2002;**106**:3085–90.

39. Maron BJ, Casey SA, Hauser RG *et al.* Clinical course of hypertrophic cardiomyopathy with survival to advanced ages. *J Am Coll Cardiol* 2003;**42**:882–8.

40. Maron BJ, Casey SA, Poliac LC *et al.* Clinical course of hypertrophic cardiomyopathy in a regional United States cohort. *JAMA* 1999;**281**;650–5.

41. Maron BJ. Hypertrophic cardiomyopathy in childhood. *Ped Clin North Am* 2004;**51**;1305–1346.

42. Maron BJ, Olivotto I, Spirito P *et al.* Epidemiology of hypertrophic cardiomyopathy-related death. Revisited in a large non-referral-based patient population. *Circulation* 2000;**102**: 858–64.

43. Elliott PM, Poloniecki J, Dickie S *et al.* Sudden death in hypertrophic cardiomyopathy: identification of high risk patients. *J Am Coll Cardiol* 2000;**36**:2212–18.

44. Elliott PM, Gimeno Blanes JR, Mahon NG *et al.* Relation between severity of left ventricular hypertrophy and prognosis in patients with hypertrophic cardiomyopathy. *Lancet* 2001;**357**:420–4.

45. Maron BJ, Kogan J, Proschan MA *et al.* Circadian variability in the occurrence of sudden cardiac death in patients with hypertrophic cardiomyopathy. *J Am Coll Cardiol* 1994;**23**:1405–9.

46. Maron BJ, Shen W-K, Link MS *et al.* Efficacy of implantable cardioverter-defibrillators for the prevention of sudden death in patients with hypertrophic cardiomyopathy. *N Engl J Med* 2000;**342**:365–73.

47. Maron BJ, Zipes DP. 36th Bethesda Conference: Eligibility Recommendations for Competitive Athletes with Cardiovascular Abnormalities. *J Am Coll Cardiol* 2005;**45**:1312–75.

48. Monserrat L, Elliott PM, Gimeno JR *et al.* Nonsustained ventricular tachycardia in hypertrophic cardiomyopathy: an independent marker of sudden death risk in young patients. *J Am Coll Cardiol* 2003;**42**:873–9.

49. Spirito P, Bellone P, Harris KM *et al.* Magnitude of left ventricular hypertrophy predicts the risk of sudden death in hypertrophic cardiomyopathy. *N Engl J Med* 2000;**342**:1778–85.

50. Maki S, Ikeda H, Muro A *et al.* Predictors of sudden cardiac death in hypertrophic cardiomyopathy. *Am J Cardiol* 1998;**82**: 774–8.

51. Maron BJ, Piccininno M, Casey SA *et al.* Relation of extreme left ventricular hypertrophy to age in hypertrophic cardiomyopathy. *Am J Cardiol* 2003;**91**:626–8.

52. Olivotto I, Maron BJ, Montereggi A *et al.* Prognostic value of systemic blood pressure response during exercise in a community-based patient population with hypertrophic cardiomyopathy. *J Am Coll Cardiol* 1999;**33**:2044–51.

53. Adabag AS, Casey SA, Kuskowski MA *et al.* Spectrum and prognostic significance of arrhythmias on ambulatory Holter electrocardiogram in hypertrophic cardiomyopathy. *J Am Coll Cardiol* 2005;**45**:697–704.

54. Adabag AS, Maron BJ. Implications of arrhythmias and prevention of sudden death in hypertrophic cardiomyopathy. *Ann Noninvas Electrocardiol* 2007;**12**:171–80.

55. Maron BJ, Moller JH, Seidman CE *et al.* Impact of laboratory molecular diagnosis on contemporary diagnostic criteria for genetically transmitted cardiovascular diseases: hypertrophic cardiomyopathy, long-QT syndrome, and Marfan syndrome. *Circulation* 1998;**98**:1460–71.

56. Rydén L, Gadler F. Pharmacological therapy for hypertrophic cardiomyopathy: what is the evidence for success? *Eur Heart J* 2001;**3**(suppl L):L21–L25.

57. Sherrid MV, Barac I, McKenna WJ *et al.* Multicenter study of the efficacy and safety of disopyramide in obstructive hypertrophic cardiomyopathy. *J Am Coll Cardiol* 2005;**45**:1251–8.

58. Harris KM, Spirito P, Maron MS *et al.* Prevalence, clinical profile and significance of left ventricular remodeling in the end-stage phase of hypertrophic cardiomyopathy. *Circulation* 2006;**114**:216–25.

59. Melacini P, Maron BJ, Bobbo F *et al.* Evidence that pharmacological strategies lack efficacy for the prevention of sudden death in hypertrophic cardiomyopathy. *Heart* 2007;**93**:708–10.

60. Maron BJ, Estes NAM III, Maron MS, Almquist AK, Link MS, Udelson J. Primary prevention of sudden death as a novel treatment strategy in hypertrophic cardiomyopathy. *Circulation* 2003;**107**:2872–5.

61. Jayatilleke I, Doolan A, Ingles J *et al.* Long-term follow-up of implantable cardioverter defibrillator therapy for hypertrophic cardiomyopathy. *Am J Cardiol* 2004;**93**:1192–4.

62. Woo A, Monakier D, Harris L *et al.* Determinants of implantable defibrillator discharges in high-risk patients with hypertrophic cardiomyopathy. *Heart* 2007;**93**:1044–5.

63. Maron MS, Bos JM, Ackerman MJ *et al.* Left ventricular apical aneurysms: a novel under-recognized subgroup within the hypertrophic cardiomyopathy disease spectrum. *Circulation* 2006;**114**(suppl III):II-439.

64. Hauser RG, Maron BJ. Lessons from the failure and recall of an implantable cardioverter defibrillator. *Circulation* 2005;**112**:2040–2.

65. Maron BJ, Hauser RG. Past and future perspectives on the failure of pharmaceutical and medical device industries to protect the public health interests. *Am J Cardiol* 2007;**100**: 147–51.

66. Camm AJ, Nisam S. The utilization of the implantable defibrillator: a European enigma. *Eur Heart J* 2000;**21**:1998–2004.

67. Moss AJ, Zareba W, Hall WJ *et al*, for the MADIT II Investigators. Prophylactic implantation of a defibrillator in patients with myocardial infarction and reduced ejection fraction. *N Engl J Med* 2002;**346**:877–83.

68. Moss A, Hall J, Cannom D *et al*, for the Multicenter Automatic Defibrillator Implantation Trial Investigators. Improved survival with an implanted defibrillator in patients with coronary disease at high risk for ventricular arrhythmia. *N Engl J Med* 1996;**335**:1933–40.

69. Bardy GH, Lee KL, Mark DB *et al.* Amiodarone or an implantable cardioverter-defibrillator for congestive heart failure. *N Engl J Med* 2005;**352**:225–37.

70. Almquist AK, Hanna CA, Haas TS, Maron BJ. Significance of appropriate defibrillator shock 3 hours and 20 minutes following implantation in a patient with hypertrophic cardiomyopathy. *J Cardiovasc Electrophysiol* 2008;**19**(3):319–22.

71. Olivotto I, Cecchi F, Casey SA, Dolara A, Traverse JH, Maron BJ. Impact of atrial fibrillation on the clinical course of hypertrophic cardiomyopathy. *Circulation* 2001;**104**:2517–24.

72. Atrial Fibrillation Follow-up Investigation of Rhythm Management (AFFIRM) Investigators. A comparison of rate control and rhythm control in patients with atrial fibrillation. *N Engl J Med* 2002;**347**:1825–33.

73. Woo A, Williams WG, Choi R *et al.* Clinical and echocardiographic determinants of long-term survival following surgical myectomy in obstructive hypertrophic cardiomyopathy. *Circulation* 2005;**111**:2033–41.

74. Cohn LH, Trehan H, Collins JJ. Long term follow up of patients undergoing myotomy myectomy for obstructive hypertrophic cardiomyopathy. *Am J Cardiol* 1992;**70**:657–60.

75. Schulte HD, Bircks WH, Loesse B *et al.* Prognosis of patients with hypertrophic obstructive cardiomyopathy after transaortic myectomy. Late results up to twenty-five years. *J Thorac Cardiovasc Surg* 1993;**106**:709–17.

76. Seiler C, Hess OM, Schoenbeck M *et al.* Long term follow up of medical versus surgical therapy for hypertrophic cardiomyopathy: a retrospective study. *J Am Coll Cardiol* 1991;**17**:634–42.

77. McIntosh CL, Maron BJ. Current operative treatment of obstructive hypertrophic cardiomyopathy. *Circulation* 1988;**78**:487–95.

78. McCully RB, Nishimura RA, Tajik AJ *et al.* Extent of clinical improvement after surgical treatment of hypertrophic obstructive cardiomyopathy. *Circulation* 1996;**94**:467–71.

79. Robbins RC, Stinson EB. Long-term results of left ventricular myotomy and myectomy for obstructive hypertrophic cardiomyopathy. *J Thorac Cardiovasc Surg* 1996;**111**:586–94.

80. Schoendube FA, Klues HG, Reith S *et al.* Long-term clinical and echocardiographic follow-up after surgical correction of hypertrophic obstructive cardiomyopathy with extended myectomy and reconstruction of the subvalvular mitral apparatus. *Circulation* 1995;**92**(suppl II):II-122–II-127.

81. Theodoro DA, Danielson GK, Feldt RH *et al.* Hypertrophic obstructive cardiomyopathy in pediatric patients: Results of surgical treatment. *J Thorac Cardiovasc Surg* 1996;**112**:1589–99.

82. Yacoub MH. Surgical versus alcohol septal ablation for hypertrophic obstructive cardiomyopathy: the pendulum swings. *Circulation* 2005;**112**:450–2.

83. Ommen SR, Nishimura RA, Squires RW *et al.* Comparison of dual-chamber pacing versus septal myectomy for the treatment of patients with hypertrophic cardiomyopathy. A comparison of objective hemodynamic and exercise end points. *J Am Coll Cardiol* 1999;**34**:191–6.

84. Heric B, Lytle BW, Miller DP *et al.* Surgical management of hypertrophic obstructive cardiomyopathy: early and late results. *J Thorac Cardiovasc Surg* 1995;**110**:195–208.

85. Maron BJ. Surgery for hypertrophic obstructive cardiomyopathy: alive and quite well. *Circulation* 2005;**111**:2016–18.

86. Maron BJ, Dearani JA, Ommen SR *et al.* The case for surgery in obstructive hypertrophic cardiomyopathy. *J Am Coll Cardiol* 2004;**44**:2044–53.

87. Ommen SR, Maron BJ, Olivotto I *et al.* Long-term effects of surgical septal myectomy on survival in patients with obstructive hypertrophic cardiomyopathy. *J Am Coll Cardiol* 2005;**46**:470–6.

88. Maron BJ, Nishimura RA, Danielson GK. Pitfalls in clinical recognition and a novel operative approach for hypertrophic cardiomyopathy with severe outflow obstruction due to anomalous papillary muscle. *Circulation* 1998;**98**:2505–8.

89. Maron BJ. Controversies in cardiovascular medicine. Surgical myectomy remains the primary treatment option for severely symptomatic patients with obstructive hypertrophic cardiomyopathy. *Circulation* 2007;**116**:196–206.

90. Morrow AG, Lambrew CT, Braunwald E. Idiopathic hypertrophic subaortic stenosis: II. Operative treatment and the results of pre- and postoperative hemodynamic evaluations. *Circulation* 1964;**29**(suppl IV), **30**:IV-120–51.

91. Minekata K, Dearnai JA, Nishimura RA, Maron BJ, Danielson GK. Extended septal myectomy for hypertrophic obstructive cardiomyopathy with anomalous mitral papillary muscles or chordae. *J Thorac Cardiovasc Surg* 2004;**127**:481–9.

92. Fifer MA. Controversies in cardiovascular medicine. Most fully informed patients choose septal ablation over septal myectomy. *Circulation* 2007;**116**:207–16.

93. Alam M, Dokainish H, Lakkis N. Alcohol septal ablation for hypertrophic obstructive cardiomyopathy: a systematic review of published studies. *J Interv Cardiol* 2006;**19**:319–27.

94. Kimmelstiel CD, Maron BJ. Role of percutaneous septal ablation in hypertrophic obstructive cardiomyopathy. *Circulation* 2004;**109**:452–6.

95. Qin JX, Shirota T, Lever HM *et al.* Outcome of patients with hypertrophic obstructive cardiomyopathy after percutaneous transluminal septal myocardial ablation and septal myectomy surgery. *J Am Coll Cardiol* 2001;**38**:1994–2000.

96. van der Lee C, ten Cate FJ, Geleijnse ML *et al.* Percutaneous versus surgical treatment for patients with hypertrophic obstructive cardiomyopathy and enlarged anterior mitral valve leaflets. *Circulation* 2005;**112**:482–8.

97. Ralph-Edwards A, Woo A, McCrindle BW *et al.* Hypertrophic obstructive cardiomyopathy: comparison of outcomes after myectomy or alcohol ablation adjusted by propensity score. *J Thorac Cardiovasc Surg* 2005;**129**:351–8.

98. Valeti US, Nishimura RA, Holmes DR *et al.* Comparison of surgical septal myectomy and alcohol septal ablation with cardiac magnetic resonance imaging in patients with hypertrophic obstructive cardiomyopathy. *J Am Coll Cardiol* 2007;**49**:350–7.

99. Olivotto I, Ommen SR, Maron MS, Cecchi F, Maron BJ. Surgical myectomy versus percutaneous alcohol septal ablation for obstructive hypertrophic cardiomyopathy: will there ever be a randomized trial? *J Am Coll Cardiol* 2007;**50**:831–4.

50 Infective and infiltrative cardiomyopathies

Stavros Kounas and Perry M Elliott
The Heart Hospital, University College London, London, UK

Infective cardiomyopathies

Myocardial dysfunction is a well-recognized complication of viral, bacterial, fungal and parasitic infections. Worldwide, the most common infective myocarditis is Chagas' disease caused by *Trypanosoma cruzi*, a protozoan organism endemic in rural areas of South and Central America. In the Western world, viral myocarditis caused by enterovirus and adenovirus infection is the most common cause of inflammatory heart muscle disease.

Viral myocarditis

Until quite recently, enterovirus (Coxsackie B) and adenovirus were the most commonly implicated viruses in acute myocarditis in adults and children.[1-4] A causal association between enteroviruses and myocarditis was first suggested in studies showing a relationship between rising serum Coxsackie B antibody titers and acute symptomatic presentation.[3] Subsequently, enteroviral genome has been detected in myocardial biopsy samples of patients with myocarditis and dilated cardiomyopathy using polymerase chain reaction techniques.[4]

More recently, studies suggest that the frequency of enteroviral and adenoviral infection in patients with clinically suspected myocarditis and dilated cardiomyopathy has reduced. Instead, parvovirus B19 infection, which usually causes erythema infectiosum ("slapped cheek" *or* "fifth" disease), seems more common in adults.[5] Childhood parvovirus myocarditis has also been reported,[6] including four cases of sudden cardiac death.[7-10] Many other viruses have been implicated in myocarditis, including cytomegalovirus, hepatitis C virus, and herpes simplex virus[11-14] (see Table 50.1).

Evidence-Based Cardiology, 3rd edition. Edited by S. Yusuf, J.A. Cairns, A.J. Camm, E.L. Fallen, and B.J. Gersh. © 2010 Blackwell Publishing, ISBN: 978-1-4051-5925-8.

HIV-related cardiomyopathy

The human immunodeficiency virus (HIV) infection affects an estimated 39.5 million living people worldwide, with 4.3 million new cases in 2006.[15] Advances in treatment have substantially improved morbidity and mortality, but late cardiac complications are increasing as patients' survival improves.[16] These include myocardial dysfunction, pericardial effusion, endocarditis, malignancy and premature coronary disease. Observational data estimate the annual incidence of HIV-associated cardiomyopathy at 15.9 cases per 1000 HIV-positive patients.[13] Among children with vertically transmitted HIV infection the 2-year incidence of congestive heart failure was 4.7%.[17]

Pathogenesis of the heart muscle dysfunction in HIV infection is still poorly understood. Opportunistic infections, malnutrition and antiviral treatment have been implicated.[18] Some studies have also suggested a direct cardiotoxic effect of HIV and secondary effects caused by autoimmune responses against HIV and other cardiotropic viruses.[12,19] This latter hypothesis is supported by the demonstration of a high frequency of circulating cardiac specific autoantibodies in HIV positive patients in comparison to normal controls.[20]

Clinical presentation and diagnosis

Presentation of infective myocarditis varies enormously. Malaise, low-grade fever, chest pain, transient electrocardiographic changes (T-wave changes, ventricular extrasystoles), left ventricular dysfunction and biochemical signs of myocardial dysfunction are typical. In some cases, the clinical picture mimics acute myocardial infarction with ST segment elevation.[21] Other cases present with fulminant heart failure,[22] arrhythmias,[23] conduction disturbance[24] and sudden cardiac death.[25]

Although the echocardiogram is rarely entirely normal in myocarditis, the findings are non-specific. Evidence of impaired left ventricular systolic performance (with reduced fractional shortening and ejection fraction) is common. Regional wall motion abnormalities occur

Table 50.1 Studies showing viral genome persistence in patients with DCM or myocarditis

Study	Disease spectrum	Investigated viruses	Patients	Controls	Year
Weiss[55]	MC/DCM/controls	EV	1/5 (20%) MC, 0/11 (0%)DCM	0/21	1991
Keeling[56]	DCM/controls	EV	6/50 (12%)	13/75 (11%)	1992
Schwaiger[57]	DCM/controls	EV	6/19 (32%)	0/21	1993
Giacca[58]	DCM/MC/controls	EV	5/55 (9%)	0/21	1994
Pauschinger[59]	LVDF/controls	EV, ADV	(12+12)/94	0/14	1999
Fujioka[14]	DCM	EV, EBV,HHV, PVB, ADV, HCMV, HCV	9/26	–	2000
Bowles[60]	MC/DCM	EV, EBV, HHV, PVB, ADV, HCMV, influenza	239/624 (38%) MC 30/149 (20%)DCM	–	2003
Lotze[61]	DCM/controls	EV, ADV, PVB	38/52 (73%)	4/10 (40%)	2004
Fujioka[62]	DCM	EV, EBV, HHV, PVB, ADV	22/77 (29%)	–	2004
Kühl[5]	DCM	EV, ADV, PVB, HHV,EBV, HCMV, influenza	165/245 (67%)	–	2005
Mahrholdt[63]	MC	PVB, HHV, EV, EBV	82/87 (94%)	–	2006

EV,enteroviruses (coxsackieviruses, polioviruses, echoviruses); ADV, adenoviruses; HHV, human herpes viruses; EBV, Epstein–Barr virus; HCMV, human cytomegalovirus; PVB, parvoviruses; DCM, dilated cardiomyopathy; LVDF, left ventricular dysfunction; MC, myocarditis.

frequently. Left (or right) ventricular thrombus may be present. Evidence of left ventricular diastolic impairment may also be detected in myocarditis. Less often, right ventricular systolic and diastolic function may also be compromised. Echocardiography may show wall thickening caused by myocardial edema.[26]

Magnetic resonance imaging with gadolinium enahancement often demonstrates regions of signal enhancement.[27,28] Mild to severe persistent perfusion defects using thallium-201 myocardial scintigraphy may be present in the acute phase, with partial recovery on follow-up.[29]

Routine blood tests such as full blood count and erythrocyte sedimentation rate are usually unhelpful in confirming or refuting the diagnosis of myocarditis. In a study of 80 patients with suspected myocarditis, 35% had elevated troponin T levels. Troponin T levels greater than 0.1 ng/mL had a specificity of 94% and a positive predictive value of 93%, although the sensitivity for detecting myocarditis was low at 53%.[30] Similarly, troponin I has a high specificity (89%) for diagnosing myocarditis but a sensitivity of only 34%.[31] Creatine kinase and its cardiac isoform CK-MB are less sensitive and specific than troponin, and are not clinically useful as a screening test in suspected myocarditis. Autoantibodies directed against myocardial proteins such as myosin and the adenine nucleotide translocator protein are reported in myocarditis, and correlate with progressive ventricular dysfunction.[32,33]

Endomyocardial biopsy (EMB) theorectically provides the means for establishment of a pathologic diagnosis.[34] Only two clinical scenarios are class I indications: new-onset heart failure of less than 2 weeks' duration associated with a normal sized or dilated left ventricle and hemodynamic compromise; and new-onset heart failure of 2 weeks'

to 3 months' duration associated with a dilated left ventricle and new ventricular arrhythmias, second- or third-degree heart block, or failure to respond to usual care within 1 to 2 weeks. The rationale for these recommendations is that many patients presenting in this way have myocarditis and by determining the histologic type (lymphocytic, giant cell or necrotizing eosinophilic) prognostic information can be obtained and specific therapy initiated. The use of EMB to detect viral persistence is considered to be a research indication.

Management

General principles General principles of stabilization include afterload reduction, anticoagulation, diuresis and inotropic support. Patients with fulminant acute myocarditis may require intensive intravenous hemodynamic support. In severe cases, mechanical assist devices or extracorporeal membrane oxygenation may be necessary.[35–38] Following initial stabilization, treatment should follow standard heart failure guidelines. Patients with left ventricular enlargement may require anticoagulation with warfarin. Patients with intractable and deteriorating heart failure may require cardiac transplantation.

Immunotherapy (Table 50.2) Intravenous immunoglobulin has been extensively used in children with suspected myocarditis.[39] Evidence for its use includes case reports,[40,41] and case series[42,43] of children and adults with acute myocarditis. However, only one double-blind randomized controlled trial of immunoglobulin has been conducted. In 62 patients with recent-onset heart failure and unexplained dilated cardiomyopathy, intravenous immunoglobulin failed to

Table 50.2 Studies or case reports of immunotherapy with IV gammaglobulin (IVGG) for myocarditis

Author	Type of study	Patients	Results	Year
McNamara[44]	Randomized controlled trial	62	No difference in LVEF between patient and controls	2001
Ducker[42]	Retrospective case series	21	Better ventricular function at 12 months	1994
McNamara[43]	Uncontrolled trial	10	1 death – LVEF improved by 17% at 12 months for the 9 discharged	1997
Kishimoto[64]	Case series	9	LVEF improved 16% at follow up 12+/–5 days after treatment	2003
References[40,41,65–75]	Overall 13 cases	Case reports	10 cases showed LVEF improvement, one case with minimal improvement, 2 cases with no benefit from IVGG	1998–2004

LVEF, left ventricular ejection fraction.

improve all-cause mortality or left ventricular ejection fraction.[44] Furthermore, spontaneous improvement in left ventricular function occurred in both treatment and control groups.[44] A recent Cochrane Database review concluded that current evidence does not support the use of intravenous immunoglobulin for the management of presumed viral myocarditis and that "intravenous immunoglobulin for presumed viral myocarditis should not be part of routine practice"[45] (**Class IIb, Level B**).

Immunosuppression (Table 50.3) The hypothesis that immune responses to viral infection may cause the long-term sequelae of viral myocarditis has led to the use of immunosuppression to reduce the acute inflammatory response.[1,46] A potential danger of this approach is that immunosuppression might impair the ability of the host immune system to eradicate virus.[47] In mice, prednisolone increases mortality in animals with acute viral myocarditis.[48] Observational unrandomized case series in children have reported a beneficial effect of immunosuppression in children with myocarditis.[49–52] In the Myocarditis Treatment Trial, there was no difference in mortality or left ventricular function between the control group and the treatment groups (prednisolone plus either ciclosporin or azathioprine).[53] In another study of patients with major histocompatibility complex expression on endomyocardial biopsy samples randomized to prednisolone and azathioprine or placebo, there was improvement in left ventricular ejection fraction in the immunosuppressed group only, but no difference was observed in mortality, transplantation or rehospitalization rates over a 2-year follow-up period.[54] On the basis of the available data immunosuppression therapy is considered as a **Class IIa, Level C** recommendation for children with myocarditis. For adults the data are **Class IIb, Level B**.

Bacterial infections

Bacterial myocarditis is rare in the modern era but still occurs in high-risk groups such as immunosuppressed patients. Pathogenetic mechanisms include direct bacterial invasion with myocardial tissue destruction, abscess formation and toxin-related cardiac dysfunction. *Staphylococcus aureus* is the most common cause of bacterial myocarditis producing cardiac dysfunction, rhythm disturbances, and myocardial rupture with secondary purulent pericarditis.[81] *Corynebacterium diphtheriae* respiratory infections can proceed to myocardial involvement mediated by elaborated toxins and affecting predominantly the cardiac conducting system. Cardiac tuberculosis can produce miliary or nodular lesions[82] and has been associated with severe heart failure,[83] ventricular arrhythmias[84] and sudden cardiac death.[85] *Treponema whippleii* causing intestinal lipodystrophy or Whipple disease may affect cardiac valves, pericardium and myocardium.[86] Myocarditis can also be caused by *Clostridium* species.[87] *Brucella*,[88] *Mycoplasma, Chlamydia*,[89] *Salmonella*[90] and numerous other bacteria.

Therapy in the acute phase is supportive. Complete atrioventricular block should be treated with temporary or permanent transvenous pacing.[91] Antitoxins are available and should be used when appropriate. Specialized antibiotic regimens directed against the pathogen usually resolve the infection.

Rheumatic carditis

Rheumatic carditis is a common manifestation of acute rheumatic fever following group A streptococcal (GAS) infection of the tonsillopharynx.[92] The main pathogenetic process is a genetically predisposed autoimmune connective tissue damage, which affects primarily the cardiac valves.[93]

Table 50.3 Studies of immunosuppressive therapy for myocarditis

Reference	Type of study	Agent used	Patients	Results
Mason[53]	Multicenter randomized placebo-controlled	Prednisolone plus either ciclosporin or azathioprine	111	No difference in LVEF
Wojnicz[54]	Single-center randomized placebo-controlled	Prednisolone and azathioprine	84 DCM patients with increased HLA expression in EMB	No difference in composite endpoint of death, heart transplantation or hospital admissions. Statistically significant difference in LVEF
Parrilo[76]	Randomized trial	Prednisone	102	Small increase in LVEF. Marginal clinical benefit
Arbustini[77]	Observational series	6-month tapered steroid and azathioprine protocol	11 treated 9 not treated	10 year follow-up 6 deaths, 2 cardiac transplants, 3 survivals vs 3 deaths, 1 cardiac transplant, 5 survivals
Hosenpud[79]	Observational series	Prednisolone and azathioprine	6	No improvement in LV systolic function indices
Latham[80]	Observational series	Prednisone	52	No survival improvement
Chan[78]	Observational series	Prednisone	13 children	1 death, all survivors improved
Kleinert[49]	Observational series	Ciclosporin and prednisolone	29 children	Improved LV systolic function
Lee[50]	Retrospective review	Corticosteroids	34 children	Authors conclude excellent survival and recovery of LV function
Gagliardi[51]	Observational series	Ciclosporin and prednisone	114 children	Event free survival was 97% and 70% respectively for acute and borderline myocarditis respectively
Camargo[52]	Observational series	Four treatment groups In two prednisone was given with azathioprine or ciclosporin	68 children	According to authors immunosuppressive therapy with azathioprine or ciclosporin together with prednisone improves prognosis

LVEF, left ventricular ejection fraction; DCM, dilated cardiomyopathy; HLA, human leukocyte antigen; EMB, endomyocardial biopsy.

Diagnosis traditionally has been based on the constellation of symptoms and signs first introduced by Jones in 1944 and further updated in 1992.[94] The presence of two major or one major and two minor manifestations together with evidence of antecedent streptococcal infection implies a high probability of acute rheumatic fever.

Rheumatic carditis is seen usually within 3 weeks of GAS infection. Prevalence was estimated around 50% of acute RF cases based on clinical findings; however, using modern echocardiographic tools this proportion is somewhat higher.[95] Valvular dysfunction during the acute phase is typically seen as mitral and aortic valve regurgitation caused by ventricular dilation combined with leaflet restriction and thickening from active inflammation.[95] The tricuspid valve can also be affected but the pulmonary valve is spared. Overt heart failure is usually the consequence of acute valvular regurgitation with no significant myocardial contractile dysfunction detected in several series.[96,97] Parietal and visceral pericardial involvement with effusion is also rare. Moderate or severe carditis, recurrent rheumatic fever attacks or low educational level have been related to late valvular fibrosis and scarring causing debilitating hemodynamics and long-term morbidity.[98]

Cardiac troponin levels lie within the normal range, showing no myocardial necrosis despite the intense endocardial and connective tissue inflammation.[99] Acute phase reactants, like C-reactive protein or erythrocyte sedimentation rate, are high, reflecting the rheumatic activity and helping to establish the diagnosis.

Treatment during the acute phase is supportive and anti-inflammatory regimens with salicylates or steroids are dictated by the overall clinical picture. However, there is no convincing evidence supporting corticosteroid or immunoglobin administration during acute rheumatic carditis to prevent late valvular damage[100] (**Class III, Level B**). Antibiotics (penicillin or erythromycin in penicillin allergy) are mandatory to eradicate the causative agent. Secondary prevention to avoid recurrences should be implemented in patients without carditis for 5 years or until the age of 18, in those with mild mitral regurgitation for 10 years or until the age of 25, and life-long prevention is suggested for severe valve disease and after valve surgery.[101] However, the use of penicillin prophylaxis against recurrent rheumatic fever attacks has not always been efficient according to a recent Cochrane Database review (**Class IIb, Level C**). In the same review intramuscular penicillin injections every 2–3 weeks seem to be more effective than 4-week regimens or oral formulations.[102] (**Class IIa, Level C**).

Rickettsial-spirochetal infections

Myocarditis caused by *Coxiella burnetii* infection may be encountered during the course of Q fever. This may present with precordial pain or heart failure symptoms. The prognosis is generally poor.[103] Myocardial involvement with chest pain, elevated myocardial enzymes and depressed LV function has also been described with *Rickettsia rickettsii* infections, responsible for Rocky Mountain fever.[104] Spirochetal infections including syphilis and Lyme disease (*Borrelia burgdorferi*) can also cause myocarditis. Apart from aortitis, myocardial involvement with left ventricular aneurysms has been reported in secondary syphilis.[105] *Borrelia* infection usually has neurologic, joint and cutaneous manifestations (erythema migrans) with cardiac involvement appearing within 3 weeks in approximately 8% of cases.[106]

Fungal infections

Fungi, as opportunistic pathogens, can cause myocarditis in immunodeficient patients receiving chemotherapy, steroids or immunosuppressive therapy as well as patients with malignancies. The micro-organism may spread from neighboring lung or mediastinal foci or by hematogenous dissemination. Among the various fungal species, cardiac aspergillosis has several case reports in patients with aquired immunodeficiency syndrome and is associated with poor prognosis.[107]

Parasitic infections

Parasitic infections can present with a wide spectrum of cardiac manifestations and remain a major public health issue in developing countries. Helminths or protozoa have the ability to survive and multiply in a variety of mammalian cells including cardiomyocytes, in spite of the host's defensive immune mechanisms. This usually leads to chronic inflammatory responses that ultimately damage the heart muscle, conducting system and pericardial tissue. Chagas' disease, amebiasis, toxoplasmosis, cysticercosis, echinococcosis and trichinellosis are all parasitic infections that commonly affect the heart.[108] For a review of Chagas' disease see Chapter 51.

Infiltrative cardiomyopathies

A number of genetic and acquired disorders result in myocardial infiltration or excessive storage of various substances. Most are associated with extracardiac manifestations and often present exclusively in childhood. A relatively small number present with predominantly cardiac involvement in adults, most notably amyloidosis, hemochromatosis, and Anderson–Fabry disease.

Amyloidosis

Amyloidosis is caused by extracellular deposition in various tissues of proteinaceous material with a characteristic cross-beta sheet quaternary structure, in which strands from different monomers are aligned perpendicular to the axis of the fibril.[109] Amyloid deposits are characterized by a change in the fluorescence intensity (apple green birefringence) under polarized light microscopy of planar aromatic dyes such as Congo red and stain a characteristic color with sulfated alcian blue. The classification of amyloidosis is based on the different protein precursors that make up the amyloid fibrils. Amyloid protein deposition occurs in atria, ventricles, coronary vessels, conduction system and valves. The degree of cardiac involvement varies between each subtype. Hematologic disorders associated with excessive light chain (AL) immunoglobulin production are the most common cause of cardiac amyloid. Familial forms caused by the accumulation of mutant proteins (transthyretin or A-apolipoprotein) have variable cardiac involvement. Secondary amyloidosis, due to deposition of serum amyloid A protein associated with chronic inflammatory diseases, rarely affects the heart to a clinically significant degree.

AL amyloid

Deposition of clonal immunoglobin light chains (with or without multiple myeloma) is the most common cause of amyloidosis. Cardiac involvement occurs in up to 50% of patients with AL amyloid, but clinically isolated cardiac disease is seen in less than 5% of patients.[110] Myocardial wall thickening caused by extracellular deposits without myocyte hypertrophy results in stiff non-dilated ventricles and biatrial dilation.[111] Progressive dyspnea and profound fluid retention dominates the clinical picture. Low cardiac output causes weakness, fatigue and exercise intolerance. Typically, heart failure caused by cardiac infiltration is rapidly progressive with a median survival of less than 1 year.[112]

Chest discomfort or angina pectoris is common, but coronary angiography usually reveals normal epicardial arteries. Perivascular infiltrates and evidence of impaired myocardial flow reserve suggest small vessel disease as the underlying cause.[113] Obstructive intramural coronary amyloidosis has also been reported in autopsy series.[114] Small but persistent cardiac troponin elevations reflecting subtle ongoing myocardial necrosis are also reported.[115]

Syncope is caused by impaired cardiac output, arrhythmia and amyloid autonomic neuropathy.[116] Symptomatic supraventricular arrhythmias associated with atrial enlargement are frequent.[117] Infiltration of the atria may add to the risk for atrial fibrillation.[118] Infiltration of the sinus node and atrioventricular conduction system causes bradyarrhythmia and complete heart block.[119] Documented complex ventricular arrhythmias are rare, but may underlie some cases of sudden death; sudden death in advanced heart failure cases may also be caused by electromechanical dissociation.[120]

Cardiomegaly and pulmonary congestion with bilateral pleural effusions are seen at late stages on chest radiography. Cardiac troponins and B-type natriuretic peptide reflect the severity of cardiac involvement[121] and are associated with poor prognosis.[115,122] The resting 12-lead electrocardiogram (ECG) usually demonstrates low voltages (<5 mV in limb leads) or pseudo-infarction patterns with poor right precordial R-wave progression or inferior Q-waves.[123] Criteria for left ventricular hypertrophy are uncommon, probably because myocardial wall thickening is due to extracellular infiltration rather than true hypertrophy.[124] Atrial fibrillation occurs in 7–25% of patients and poses a significant risk of thromboembolism.[109] Ambulatory ECG monitoring reveals ventricular ectopics, couplets, and non-sustained ventricular tachycardia. Complex ventricular arrhythmias are considered harbingers of lethal arrhythmic events.[125] Sinus node dysfunction, supraventricular arrhythmias and atrioventricular conduction abnormalities may be evident.[119] Late potentials on signal-averaged ECG are common in patients with cardiac amyloidosis and predict sudden death independently of echocardiographic disease markers.[126] Electrophysiology studies may reveal subtle abnormalities of the His–Purkinje system not evident on surface ECG. HV prolongation is common, and is of prognostic significance in some series.[127]

Echocardiography typically shows that global indices of systolic function are preserved until the final stages of the disease. However, decreased longitudinal deformation is common and precedes the onset of heart failure symptoms[128] Two-dimensional echo findings in advanced cardiac amyloidosis are characteristic.[129] Increased biventricular wall thickness with concentric distribution is typical, although asymmetric septal hypertrophy with normal ejection fraction can be encountered. Dynamic left ventricular outflow tract obstruction is extremely unusual. Cardiac valves appear infiltrated and thick, the atria are dilated and the interatrial septum is often thickened. A small pericardial effusion is also common. The peculiar, granular texture of the affected myocardium has traditionally been described as an amyloid feature, but is difficult to quantify without digital image analysis. Transmitral Doppler recordings in advanced cases demonstrate a restrictive left ventricular filling pattern. Diastolic dysfunction indices are better prognostic markers than left ventricular wall thickness.[130]

Other imaging modalities such as cardiac magnetic resonance imaging are used to further assist morphologic description and tissue characterization. Subendocardial late gadolinium enhancement is considered to reflect the transmural distribution of amyloid deposits and cardiac amyloid load.[131] Abnormal gadolinium kinetics are also described, although the sensitivity of this observation is uncertain. Nuclear scans with ^{123}I-labeled serum amyloid P component are highly specific. The isotope localizes selectively in amyloid infiltrates and aids the diagnosis.[132] Other scintigraphic techniques have been used to demonstrate cardiac adrenergic denervation even before the development of clinically apparent heart disease.[133]

The diagnosis of amyloidosis requires a tissue biopsy. This need not be from the heart if the echocardiographic appearances are typical for cardiac amyloidosis. Fine-needle aspiration of the abdominal fat is positive for amyloid deposits in over 70% of patients with AL amyloidosis. If negative, endomyocardial biopsy has a very high sensitivity. Once confirmed, all patients with AL amyloid should be assessed for a plasma cell dyscrasia.

Management of cardiac amyloidosis is directed against symptoms of heart failure. Specific therapies designed to impede precursor production and fibril formation should be implemented whenever possible.[134] Diuretics, often in high dose, are the cornerstone of the palliative heart failure regimen. ACE or angiotensin II inhibitors should be introduced with extreme caution as they are often poorly tolerated and there are no data on their efficacy in cardiac amyloid. Aldosterone inhibitors might be helpful in advanced cases. Sensitivity to digoxin, attributed to enhanced drug binding on amyloid fibrils, demands cautious administration.[135] Although there are no data, the presence of atrial fibrillation in AL amyloidosis should always prompt anticoagulation with warfarin because of a very high rate of thromboembolism.

Management of the underlying amyloid disease process is based mainly on single-center experience with few randomized studies. In AL amyloidosis, progression of systemic disease contributes substantially to poor outcomes even when heart transplant is provided.[136] Heart transplantation followed by high-dose chemotherapy in combination with stem cell transplantation, is promising with short- to intermediate-term survival being now similar to patients receiving cardiac transplant for other indications.[137]

Familial amyloid

Hereditary amyloidosis is most commonly transmitted as an autosomal dominant trait with high penetrance, caused by mutations in the gene encoding transthyretin (TTR). More than 70 mutations in the transthyretin gene have been reported as amyloidogenic but one of the most common is a substitution of isoleucine for valine at position 122 which occurs in 4% of the black US population.[138] TTR amyloidoses usually present after the third decade of life with polyneuropathy and cardiomyopathy. Sometimes cardiac involvement is clinically confined to atrial arrhythmia and conduction disease. Despite significant myocardial infiltration, heart failure symptoms are less profound and survival is much better than AL amyloidosis.[139] Toxic light chain effects, absent in TTR amyloidosis, may explain the different clinical outcome.[140]

As transthyretin is produced by the liver, the definitive treatment of TTR amyloidosis is liver transplantation. Unfortunately, myocardial wall thickening progresses in some patients with TTR amyloid cardiomyopathy following liver transplantation, probably due to the continued deposition of wild-type transthyretin in the myocardium. Combined liver and heart transplantation or heart transplantation alone has been performed for TTR amyloidosis in small numbers. *In vitro* studies suggests that non-steroidal agents such as diflunisal can stabilize transthyretin.[141] Chemical stabilization to prevent TTR misfolding and decrease amyloidogenesis has also been successful in transgenic mice and human serum during recent *in vivo* studies.[142,143]

Senile cardiac amyloid (SCA)

In senile systemic amyloidosis, cardiomyopathy is caused by deposition of normal wild-type transthyretin. For unknown reasons, the disease nearly always affects elderly men above the age of 70. Presentation is with congestive heart failure, but the clinical course is considerably slower in comparison to other amyloid types (median survival from the onset of heart failure is 7.5 years).[144] Atrial fibrillation and bifascicular block on the ECG are common. Progression to complete AV block necessitating permanent pacemaker implantation is not infrequent. The echocardiographic appearances are indistinguishable from that seen in AL amyloidosis. As extracardiac involvement is rare in SCA, diagnosis usually requires endomyocardial biopsy. Cardiac symptoms predominate, with heart failure and conduction system abnormalities as main features. Atrial fibrillation and associated thromboembolic events are also frequent.[109]

There is no specific treatment for SCA, but as in familial amyloidosis, drugs that stabilize transthyretin are being evaluated.

Sarcoidosis

Sarcoidosis is a granulomatous disease of obscure etiology with multiorgan involvement. The lungs are most commonly involved but lymph nodes, skin, eyes, heart, nervous, musculoskeletal, renal and endocrine systems can be affected. The annual incidence peaks in the third and fourth decade of life and is higher in Japanese, Northern Europeans and African Americans, reaching 40 cases per 100 000 population.[145] Infective (*Mycobacterium tuberculosis*, *Mycoplasma*, *Corynebacteria*, and *Spirochaetes*), environmen-

tal (aluminum, clay) and genetic factors have been implicated in the pathogenesis. The histologic hallmark is the presence of non-caseating granulomas. The frequency of myocardial involvement in patients with sarcoid is difficult to determine, because it is frequently subclinical and patchy in nature. Post-mortem studies suggest that the heart is involved in at least 25% of patients with sarcoidosis[146] and that it accounts for as many as 13–25% of deaths.

Clinical manifestations

Clinical manifestations of sarcoid include congestive heart failure, conduction abnormalities, atrial and ventricular arrhythmias, pericardial effusion, valvular dysfunction and rarely sudden cardiac death. Right heart failure secondary to pulmonary hypertension is caused by extensive fibrotic lung sarcoidosis. Myocardial infiltration by sarcoid granulomata results in restrictive or dilated cardiomyopathy. The most common site is in the lateral wall of the left ventricle. Papillary muscle involvement is responsible for the most common valvulopathy, mitral regurgitation.[147] Granuloma formation in the basal interventricular septum may cause conduction abnormalities.[148] Ventricular arrhythmias are also frequent, generated by re-entry through surviving myocyte bundles around the scarred lesion.[149]

Abnormal Q-waves or repolarization abnormalities are common ECG findings. In one study, right bundle branch block was detected in 57% of patients, and third-degree atrioventricular block in 23–30%.[148,150] Several studies have examined the value of radionuclide scans using thallium-201, gallium-67 and technetium-99 isotopes in the diagnosis of cardiac sarcoid. Positron emission tomography (PET) may have better diagnostic accuracy.[151] Two-dimensional echocardiography may reveal regional wall motion abnormalities, increased LV dimensions, global systolic dysfunction, pericardial effusion, valvular abnormalities, LV aneurysms and raised pulmonary artery pressures.[152] The diagnostic role of magnetic resonance imaging (MRI) is rapidly expanding as regional myocardial enhancement representing focal inflammation or scarring[153] can be detected using contrast enhanced scans.

Demonstration of the typical granuloma on endomyocardial biopsy specimens is pathognomonic for cardiac sarcoidosis but the method lacks sensitivity.[154] In a study of 26 cases with strong clinical suspicion of cardiac sarcoidosis, right ventricular biopsy, with an average of four samples per patient, exhibited non-caseating granulomas diagnosis in only five individuals (19.2%).[154] In an older study, right-sided biopsies had a 63% sensitivity and left-sided 47%, with post-mortem autopsy as the gold standard.[155] The patchy myocardial infiltration with basal or left free lateral wall distribution may account for the low positive rates of endomyocardial biopsy as specimens are usually obtained from the apical septum.

Treatment

Patients with left ventricular systolic dysfunction caused by cardiac sarcoidosis have a poorer prognosis in comparison to idiopathic dilated cardiomyopathy controls.[156] Permanent pacing prevents bradyarrhythmia and ICDs can prevent sudden death by treating malignant arrhythmias.[157] Evidence on the efficacy of corticosteroids is scant and contradictory. Steroids may improve systolic function[158] but are probably most effective if initiated before the occurrence of dilated cardiomyopathy[159] (**Class IIa, Level C**). Some data suggest that steroids may not prevent ventricular arrhythmia[160] (**Class III, Level C**). Pulmonary involvement in advanced cases with progressive and severe heart failure in spite of optimal pharmacologic treatment often precludes cardiac transplantation as an option.[161] Recurrence in the cardiac allograft has been reported in some patients who have been transplanted.[162]

Hereditary hemochromatosis

Hereditary hemochromatosis (HH) is a common autosomal recessive disorder characterized by excessive iron deposition in parenchymal organs, including the liver, spleen, pancreas, endocrine glands and heart. In Caucasians, it has a prevalence of between 1 in 200 and 1 in 500, with an even higher prevalence in the Irish population. The most common form is caused by mutations in the HFE gene. Two common missense mutations account for the majority of disease: a change of cysteine at position 282 to tyrosine (C282Y); and a change of histidine at position 63 to aspartate (H63D). Between 80% and 100% patients of North European origin are C282Y homozygous. Lower rates of C282Y homozygosity occur in Mediterranean and Southern European populations. A minority (11%) of compound heterozygotes (C282Y/H63D) develop clinical symptoms of hemochromatosis. Disease caused by homozygous H63D mutations is very rare because of its much lower clinical penetrance. There are several rare forms of non-HFE-related HH. Juvenile hemochromatosis (HFE2) is the most common, presenting before the age of 30 with cardiac disease and hypogonadism. An autosomal dominant form linked to a mutation in the SLC11A3 gene has been described.[163]

Clinical manifestations

Clinical expression of HFE-related HH is variable. Most patients with classic disease present between the age of 40 and 60 with hyperpigmentation, diabetes mellitus and hepatomegaly. Cardiac disease has been reported on 52% of death certificates of patients with hemochromatosis,[164] and it is estimated that up to 35% of patients with hemochromatosis experience congestive cardiac failure and 36% develop arrhythmias.[165] However, the incidence of lethal cardiomyopathy is variable.[166] As clinical manifestations in HH can be subtle or delayed, a high index of suspicion and early intervention are crucial to avoid severe irreversible complications. Overt cardiac involvement, in the form of restrictive or dilated cardiomyopathy, is seen in late stages[167] as a consequence of chronic cardiac iron accumulation.

Diagnosis

The first-line investigations for HH are serum ferritin and fasting transferin saturation. Elevated ferritin is non-specific as it can be raised in many conditions including inflammatory and neoplastic disorders. However, in combination with transferin saturation, ferritin has a 97% negative predictive value for the diagnosis of HH. When both are elevated, genotyping rather than liver biopsy is recommended to confirm the diagnosis.[168]

Treatment

Treatment for hemochromatosis should be initiated before the emergence of any cardiac abnormalities. However, myocardial iron stores are difficult to assess with non-invasive methods as they correlate poorly with serum ferritin and serum iron levels.[169] Endomyocardial biopsy for direct pathologic examination can be used to measure cardiac iron, but advances in cardiac imaging with novel magnetic resonance techniques appear promising. T2-star sequences provide surrogates of myocardial iron load, allowing early diagnosis and proper treatment monitoring of cardiac hemochromatosis.[170] Regular venesection, until ferritin normalizes or patients become anemic, is the mainstay of therapy.[171] Most clinical features of the disease improve following treatment; in particular, cardiac involvement has been shown to improve[172] (**Class I, Level C**). There are some data showing that chelation therapy clears iron stores quickly and avoids complications of cardiac failure.[173]

Metabolic storage diseases

Metabolic storage diseases comprise a heterogeneous group of genetically determined enzyme deficiencies that result in accumulation of metabolic substrates in various cell types. The most common in clinical practice are the lysosomal storage disorders (LSD), a group of more than 40 diseases caused by a deficiency of lysosomal enzymes, membrane transporters and other proteins involved in lysosomal metabolism. Most are inherited as autosomal recessive traits except for Anderson–Fabry disease, glycogen storage disease (GSD) type IIb (Danon disease) and mucopolysaccharidosis (MPS) type II (Hunter disease). Cardiac disease is particularly important in glycogen storage diseases (Pompe and Danon disease), mucopolysaccharidoses and in glycosphingolipidoses (Anderson–Fabry disease).[174–175]

Pompe disease (acid maltase deficiency, glycogen storage disease IIa) presents as infantile, juvenile and adult variants, that differ with respect to age of onset, rate of disease progression and severity of tissue involvement. Massive cardiac hypertrophy and heart failure caused by myocardial glycogen deposition are characteristic of the infantile and childhood forms. LV outflow obstruction is described in about 6% of patients. The ECG typically shows wide high-voltage QRS complexes and a short PR interval with a pre-excitation pattern. The infantile form is usually fatal before 2 years of age due to cardiorespiratory failure. In the juvenile and adult-onset variants, disease is usually limited to skeletal muscle, with a slowly progressive proximal myopathy and respiratory muscle weakness.[176] Recombinant enzyme replacement in the infantile and childhood forms is associated with regression of LVH and improved survival.[177]

Danon disease is an X-linked disorder caused by deficiency of the lysosome-associated membrane protein type 2 (LAMP-2). The typical presentation includes skeletal myopathy, mental retardation and hypertrophic cardiomyopathy leading to death in affected males between the second and third decade. Heterozygous females have milder disease with later onset cardiomyopathy. The pathologic hallmark of the disease is the presence of intracytoplasmic vacuoles containing autophagic material and glycogen in cardiac and skeletal muscle cells.[178]

Glycogen storage disease type III results from deficient glycogen debrancher enzyme activity. There are two major GSD III subtypes explained by differences in tissue expression of the deficient enzyme: GSD IIIa, which affects both the liver and muscle, accounts for 80% of the cases, and GSD IIIb, affecting only the liver, for approximately 15% of all GSD III cases. Muscle weakness usually coincides with hepatomegaly, hypoglycemia, short stature, dyslipidemia, and occasionally slight mental retardation or facial abnormalities. However, muscle symptoms manifest in some cases long after liver disorders disappeared in childhood.[179] In the majority of GSD IIIa patients cardiac involvement is recognized as ventricular hypertrophy on ECG accompanied by abnormal echocardiographic features.[180] Creatine kinase level is usually increased in patients with skeletal muscle involvement; however, normal levels do not rule out the presence of muscle enzyme deficiency. Treatment for GSD III is primarily dietary and is aimed at maintaining normoglycemia. Liver transplantation to correct the related biochemical abnormalities is an option but with unclear efficacy with regard to muscle or cardiac disease.

Mucopolysaccharidoses

Mucopolysaccharidoses (MPS) are caused by a defect of intralysosomal degradation of acid mucopolysaccharides (glycosaminglycans). Seven main forms and several subtypes are described. Cardiac involvement is detectable in more than two-thirds of affected children, the most common abnormalities being mitral and aortic valve thickening. The prevalence of valve abnormalities ranges from 27% to 90% depending on disease subtype (highest frequency in MPS I, II and VI, lowest in type IV and III). Coronary involvement caused by intimal infiltration by storage cells is reported in more than 40% of patients, but rarely results in clinically evident myocardial ischemia. The aorta may also be affected. Left ventricular hypertrophy, dilated cardiomyopathy and endomyocardial fibroelastosis are described. Conduction system disease is also reported and sudden cardiac deaths are relatively frequent.[181]

Anderson–Fabry disease

Anderson–Fabry disease is an X-linked disorder caused by mutations in the gene encoding the lysosomal enzyme, alpha-galactosidase A. The resultant enzyme deficiency causes intracellular glycosphingolipid accumulation in nervous, renal, gastrointestinal, cutaneous and cardiac tissues. Cardiac involvement usually manifests in the third to fourth decades in hemizygote males and the fourth to fifth decades in heterozygote females.[182] An isolated cardiac variant has been reported, but careful investigations usually reveal subclinical involvement of other systems.[183]

Concentric left ventricular hypertrophy is most typical, although asymmetric septal hypertrophy occurs in approximately 10%. Left ventricular outflow tract obstruction is unusual.[184] Valve thickening results in mild to moderate valvular insufficiency.[185] Reduced coronary flow reserve measured with positron emission tomography may explain angina symptoms in the absence of obstructive coronary disease.[186] Supraventricular or ventricular arrhythmias and conduction abnormalities occur frequently in older patients.[187] The diagnosis in men is obtained by assessment of plasma and leukocyte alpha-galactosidase A activity. Diagnosis in females usually requires genetic analysis as heterozygote females often have enzyme activity levels within the lower normal range.[188] Multicenter randomized placebo-controlled studies have proved the safety and efficacy of enzyme replacement therapies in AFD (**Class I, Level B**). Accumulating data demonstrate encouraging symptomatic and functional amelioration of affected organs including the heart.[189]

References

1. Feldman AM, McNamara D. Myocarditis. *N Engl J Med* 2000;**343**(19):1388–98.
2. Coxsackie B5 virus infections during 1965. A report to the Director of the Public Health Laboratory Service from various laboratories in the United Kingdom. *BMJ* 1967;**4**(5579):575–7.
3. El-Hagrassy MM, Banatvala JE, Coltart DJ. Coxsackie-B-virus-specific IgM responses in patients with cardiac and other diseases. *Lancet* 1980;**2**(8205):1160–2.

4. Jin O, Sole MJ, Butany JW *et al.* Detection of enterovirus RNA in myocardial biopsies from patients with myocarditis and cardiomyopathy using gene amplification by polymerase chain reaction. *Circulation* 1990;**82**(1):8–16.

5. Kühl U, Pauschinger M, Noutsias M *et al.* High prevalence of viral genomes and multiple viral infections in the myocardium of adults with "idiopathic" left ventricular dysfunction. *Circulation* 2005;**111**(7):887–93.

6. Munro K, Croxson MC, Thomas S *et al.* Three cases of myocarditis in childhood associated with human parvovirus (B19 virus). *Pediatr Cardiol* 2003;**24**:473–5.

7. Dettmeyer R, Kandolf R, Baasner A *et al.* Fatal parvovirus B19 myocarditis in an 8-year-old boy. *J Forensic Sci* 2003;**48**:183–6.

8. Murry CE, Jerome KR, Reichenbach DD. Fatal parvovirus myocarditis in a 5-year-old girl. *Hum Pathol* 2001;**32**:342–5.

9. Rohayem J, Dinger J, Fischer R *et al.* Fatal myocarditis associated with acute parvovirus B19 and human herpesvirus 6 coinfection. *J Clin Microbiol* 2001;**39**:4585–7.

10. Zack F, Klingel K, Kandolf R *et al.* Sudden cardiac death in a 5-year-old girl associated with parvovirus B19 infection. *Forensic Sci Int* 2005;**155**:13–17.

11. Hofman P, Drici MD, Gibelin P *et al.* Prevalence of toxoplasma myocarditis in patients with the acquired immunodeficiency syndrome. *Br Heart J* 1993;**70**:376–81.

12. Herskowitz A, Wu TC, Willoughby SB *et al.* Myocarditis and cardiotropic viral infection associated with severe left ventricular dysfunction in late-stage infection with human immunodeficiency virus. *J Am Coll Cardiol* 1994;**24**:1025–32.

13. Barbaro G, Di LG, Grisorio B *et al.* Incidence of dilated cardiomyopathy and detection of HIV in myocardial cells of HIV-positive patients. Gruppo Italiano per lo Studio Cardiologico dei Pazienti Affetti da AIDS. *N Engl J Med* 1998;**339**:1093–9.

14. Fujioka S, Kitaura Y, Ukimura A *et al.* Evaluation of viral infection in the myocardium of patients with idiopathic dilated cardiomyopathy. *J Am Coll Cardiol* 2000;**36**(6):1920–6.

15. *UNAIDS/WHO epidemic update*, December 2006, www.unaids.org.

16. Bozzette SA, Ake CF, Tam HK *et al.* Cardiovascular and cerebrovascular events in patients treated for human immunodeficiency virus infection. *N Engl J Med* 2003;**348**(8):702–10.

17. Lipshultz SE, Easley KA, Orav EJ *et al.* Left ventricular structure and function in children infected with human immunodeficiency virus: the prospective P2C2 HIV Multicenter Study. Pediatric Pulmonary and Cardiac Complications of Vertically Transmitted HIV Infection (P2C2 HIV) Study Group. *Circulation* 1998;**97**(13):1246–56.

18. Currie PF, Boon NA. Immunopathogenesis of HIV-related heart muscle disease: current perspectives. *AIDS* 2000;**17**(suppl 1).S21–8.

19. Barbaro G, Di Lorenzo G, Grisorio B *et al.* Cardiac involvement in the acquired immunodeficiency syndrome: a multicenter clinical-pathological study. Gruppo Italiano per lo Studio Cardiologico dei pazienti affetti da AIDS Investigators. *AIDS Res Hum Retroviruses* 1998;**14**(12):1071–7.

20. Currie PF, Goldman JH, Caforio AL *et al.* Cardiac autoimmunity in HIV related heart muscle disease. *Heart* 1998;**79**(6):599–604.

21. Dec GW Jr, Waldman H, Southern J *et al.* Viral myocarditis mimicking acute myocardial infarction. *J Am Coll Cardiol* 1992;**20**(1):85–9.

22. Topkara VK, Dang NC, Barili F *et al.* Ventricular assist device use for the treatment of acute viral myocarditis. *J Thorac Cardiovasc Surg* 2006;**131**(5):1190–1.

23. Stankewicz MA, Clements SD Jr. Fulminant myocarditis presenting with wide complex tachycardia. *South Med J* 2004;**97**(10):1007–9.

24. Sato Y, Osaku A, Koyama S *et al.* Complete atrioventricular block associated with regional myocardial scarring in a patient with Coxsackie B2 myocarditis. *Jpn Heart J* 1989;**30**(6):935–41.

25. Theleman KP, Kuiper JJ, Roberts WC. Acute myocarditis (predominately lymphocytic) causing sudden death without heart failure. *Am J Cardiol* 2001;**88**(9):1078–83.

26. Hiramitsu S, Morimoto S, Kato S *et al.* Transient ventricular wall thickening in acute myocarditis: a serial echocardiographic and histopathologic study. *Jpn Circ J* 2001;**65**(10):863–6.

27. Friedrich MG, Strohm O, Schulz-Menger J *et al.* Contrast media-enhanced magnetic resonance imaging visualizes myocardial changes in the course of viral myocarditis. *Circulation* 1998;**97**(18):1802–9.

28. Mahrholdt H, Goedecke C, Wagner A *et al.* Cardiovascular magnetic resonance assessment of human myocarditis: a comparison to histology and molecular pathology. *Circulation* 2004;**109**(10):1250–8.

29. Kawamura Y, Morishita T, Yamazaki J *et al.* Evaluation of viral myocarditis in children by radionuclide method. *Ann Nucl Med* 1990;**4**(2):59–65.

30. Lauer B, Niederau C, Kuhl U *et al.* Cardiac troponin T in patients with clinically suspected myocarditis. *J Am Coll Cardiol* 1997;**30**:1354–9.

31. Smith SC, Ladenson JH, Mason JW *et al.* Elevations of cardiac troponin I associated with myocarditis. Experimental and clinical correlates. *Circulation* 1997;**95**:163–8.

32. Lauer B, Schannwell M, Kuhl U *et al.* Antimyosin autoantibodies are associated with deterioration of systolic and diastolic left ventricular function in patients with chronic myocarditis. *J Am Coll Cardiol* 2000;**35**:11–18.

33. Schultheiss HP, Schulze K, Dorner A. Significance of the adenine nucleotide translocator in the pathogenesis of viral heart disease. *Mol Cell Biochem* 1996;**163–164**:319–27.

34. Cooper LT, Baughman KL, Feldman AM *et al.* The role of endomyocardial biopsy in the management of cardiovascular disease: a scientific statement from the American Heart Association, the American College of Cardiology, and the European Society of Cardiology. *Circulation* 2007;**116**(19):2216–33.

35. Duncan BW, Hraska V, Jonas RA *et al.* Mechanical circulatory support in children with cardiac disease. *J Thorac Cardiovasc Surg* 1999;**117**:529–42.

36. Hetzer R, Loebe M, Potapov EV *et al.* Circulatory support with pneumatic paracorporeal ventricular assist device in infants and children. *Ann Thorac Surg* 1998;**66**:1498–506.

37. Levi D, Marelli D, Plunkett M *et al.* Use of assist devices and ECMO to bridge pediatric patients with cardiomyopathy to transplantation. *J Heart Lung Transplant* 2002;**21**:760–70.

38. McMahon AM, van Doorn C, Burch M *et al.* Improved early outcome for end-stage dilated cardiomyopathy in children. *J Thorac Cardiovasc Surg* 2003;**126**:1781–7.

39. Levi D, Alejos J. Diagnosis and treatment of pediatric viral myocarditis. *Curr Opin Cardiol* 2001;**16**:77–83.

40. Nigro G, Bastianon V, Colloridi V *et al.* Human parvovirus B19 infection in infancy associated with acute and chronic lymphocytic myocarditis and high cytokine levels: report of 3 cases and review. *Clin Infect Dis* 2000;**31**:65–9.

41. Tedeschi A, Airaghi L, Giannini S *et al.* High-dose intravenous immunoglobulin in the treatment of acute myocarditis. A case report and review of the literature. *J Intern Med* 2002;**251**:169–73.

42. Drucker NA, Colan SD, Lewis AB *et al.* Gamma-globulin treatment of acute myocarditis in the pediatric population. *Circulation* 1994;**89**:252–7.

43. McNamara DM, Rosenblum WD, Janosko KM *et al.* Intravenous immune globulin in the therapy of myocarditis and acute cardiomyopathy. *Circulation* 1997;**95**:2476–8.

44. McNamara DM, Holubkov R, Starling RC *et al.* Controlled trial of intravenous immune globulin in recent-onset dilated cardiomyopathy. *Circulation* 2001;**103**:2254–9.

45. Robinson J, Hartling L, Vandermeer B, Klassen TP. Intravenous immunoglobulin for presumed viral myocarditis in children and adults. *Cochrane Database of Systematic Reviews* 2005, Issue 1. Art. No.: CD004370. DOI: 10.1002/14651858.CD004370.pub2.

46. Magnani JW, Dec GW. Myocarditis: current trends in diagnosis and treatment. *Circulation* 2006;**113**:876–90.

47. Burch M. Immune suppressive treatment in paediatric myocarditis: still awaiting the evidence. *Heart* 2004;**90**:1103–4.

48. Tomioka N, Kishimoto C, Matsumori A *et al.* Effects of prednisolone on acute viral myocarditis in mice. *J Am Coll Cardiol* 1986;**7**:868–72.

49. Kleinert S, Weintraub RG, Wilkinson JL *et al.* Myocarditis in children with dilated cardiomyopathy: incidence and outcome after dual therapy immunosuppression. *J Heart Lung Transplant* 1997;**16**:1248–54.

50. Lee KJ, McCrindle BW, Bohn DJ *et al.* Clinical outcomes of acute myocarditis in childhood. *Heart* 1999;**82**:226–33.

51. Gagliardi MG, Bevilacqua M, Bassano C *et al.* Long term follow up of children with myocarditis treated by immunosuppression and of children with dilated cardiomyopathy. *Heart* 2004;**90**:1167–71.

52. Camargo PR, Snitcowsky R, da Luz PL *et al.* Favorable effects of immunosuppressive therapy in children with dilated cardiomyopathy and active myocarditis. *Pediatr Cardiol* 1995;**16**:61–8.

53. Mason JW, O'Connell JB, Herskowitz A *et al.* A clinical trial of immunosuppressive therapy for myocarditis. The Myocarditis Treatment Trial Investigators. *N Engl J Med* 1995;**333**:269–75.

54. Wojnicz R, Nowalany-Kozielska E, Wojciechowska C *et al.* Randomized, placebo-controlled study for immunosuppressive treatment of inflammatory dilated cardiomyopathy: two-year follow-up results. *Circulation* 2001;**104**:39–45.

55. Weiss LM, Movahed LA, Billingham ME *et al.* Detection of Coxsackievirus B3 RNA in myocardial tissues by the polymerase chain reaction. *Am J Pathol* 1991;**138**(2):497–503.

56. Keeling PJ, Jeffery S, Caforio AL *et al.* Similar prevalence of enteroviral genome within the myocardium from patients with idiopathic dilated cardiomyopathy and controls by the polymerase chain reaction. *Br Heart J* 1992;**68**(6):554–9.

57. Schwaiger A, Umlauft F, Weyrer K *et al.* Detection of enteroviral ribonucleic acid in myocardial biopsies from patients with idio-

pathic dilated cardiomyopathy by polymerase chain reaction. *Am Heart J* 1993;**126**(2):406–10.

58. Giacca M, Severini GM, Mestroni L *et al.* Low frequency of detection by nested polymerase chain reaction of enterovirus ribonucleic acid in endomyocardial tissue of patients with idiopathic dilated cardiomyopathy. *J Am Coll Cardiol* 1994;**24**(4):1033–40.

59. Pauschinger M, Bowles NE, Fuentes-Garcia FJ *et al.* Detection of adenoviral genome in the myocardium of adult patients with idiopathic left ventricular dysfunction. *Circulation* 1999;**99**(10):1348–54.

60. Bowles NE, Ni J, Kearney DL *et al.* Detection of viruses in myocardial tissues by polymerase chain reaction. evidence of adenovirus as a common cause of myocarditis in children and adults. *J Am Coll Cardiol* 2003;**42**:466–72.

61. Lotze U, Egerer R, Tresselt C *et al.* Frequent detection of parvovirus B19 genome in the myocardium of adult patients with idiopathic dilated cardiomyopathy. *Med Microbiol Immunol* 2004;**193**(2–3):75–82.

62. Fujioka S, Kitaura Y, Deguchi H *et al.* Evidence of viral infection in the myocardium of American and Japanese patients with idiopathic dilated cardiomyopathy. *Am J Cardiol* 2004;**94**(5):602–5.

63. Mahrholdt H, Wagner A, Deluigi CC *et al.* Presentation, patterns of myocardial damage, and clinical course of viral myocarditis. *Circulation* 2006;**114**(15):1581–90.

64. Kishimoto C, Shioji K, Kinoshita M *et al.* Treatment of acute inflammatory cardiomyopathy with intravenous immunoglobulin ameliorates left ventricular function associated with suppression of inflammatory cytokines and decreased oxidative stress. *Int J Cardiol* 2003;**91**:173–8.

65. Wang CY, Li Lu F, Wu MH *et al.* Fatal coxsackievirus A16 infection. *Pediatr Infect Dis J* 2004;**23**:275–6.

66. Takeda Y, Yasuda S, Miyazaki S *et al.* High-dose immunoglobulin G therapy for fulminant myocarditis. *Jpn Circ J* 1998;**62**:871–2.

67. Tsai YG, Ou TY, Wang CC *et al.* Intravenous gammaglobulin therapy in myocarditis complicated with complete heart block: report of one case. *Acta Paediatr Taiwan* 2001;**42**:311–13.

68. Shioji K, Matsuura Y, Iwase T *et al.* Successful immunoglobulin treatment for fulminant myocarditis and serial analysis of serum thiredoxin – a case report. *Circ J* 2002;**66**:977–80.

69. Stouffer GA, Sheahan RG, Lenihan DJ *et al.* The current status of immune modulating therapy for myocarditis: a case of acute parvovirus myocarditis treated with intravenous immunoglobulin. *Am J Med Sci* 2003;**326**(6):369–74.

70. Karaaslan S, Oran B, Caliskan U *et al.* Hemolysis after administration of high-dose immunoglobulin in a patient with myocarditis. *Turk J Haematol* 2003;**20**:237–40.

71. Khan MA, Das B, Lohe A *et al.* Neonatal myocarditis presenting as an apparent life threatening event. *Clin Pediatr (Phila)* 2003;**42**:649–52.

72. Kim HS, Sohn S, Park JY *et al.* Fulminant myocarditis successfully treated with high-dose immunoglobulin. *Int J Cardiol* 2004;**96**:485–6.

73. Braun JP, Schneider M, Dohmen P *et al.* Successful treatment of dilative cardiomyopathy in a 12-year-old girl using the calcium sensitizer levosimendan after weaning from mechanical

biventricular assist support. *J Cardiothorac Vasc Anest* 2004;**18**:772–4.

74. Abe S, Okura Y, Hoyano M *et al.* Plasma concentrations of cytokines and neurohumoral factors in a case of fulminant myocarditis successfully treated with intravenous immunoglobulin and percutaneous cardiopulmonary support. *Circ J* 2004;**68**:1223–6.

75. English RF, Janosly JE, Ettedgui JA, Webber SA. Outcomes for children with acute myocarditis. *Cardiol Young* 2004;**14**:488–93.

76. Parrillo JE, Cunnion RE, Epstein SE *et al.* A prospective, randomized, controlled trial of prednisone for dilated cardiomyopathy. *N Engl J Med* 1989;**321**(16):1061–8.

77. Arbustini E, Gavazzi A, Dal Bello B *et al.* Ten-year experience with endomyocardial biopsy in myocarditis presenting with congestive heart failure: frequency, pathologic characteristics, treatment and follow-up. *G Ital Cardiol* 1997;**27**(3):209–23.

78. Chan KY, Iwahara M, Benson LN *et al.* Immunosuppressive therapy in the management of acute myocarditis in children: a clinical trial. *J Am Coll Cardiol* 1991;**17**(2):458–60.

79. Hosenpud JD, McAnulty JH, Niles NR. Lack of objective improvement in ventricular systolic function in patients with myocarditis treated with azathioprine and prednisone. *J Am Coll Cardiol* 1985;**6**(4):797–801.

80. Latham RD, Mulrow JP, Virmani R *et al.* Recently diagnosed idiopathic dilated cardiomyopathy: incidence of myocarditis and efficacy of prednisone therapy. *Am Heart J* 1989;**117**(4):876–82.

81. Wasi F, Shuter J. Primary bacterial infection of the myocardium. *Front Biosci* 2003;**8**:s228–31.

82. Rose AG. Cardiac tuberculosis. A study of 19 patients. *Arch Pathol Lab Med* 1987;**111**(5):422–6.

83. López Gude MJ, Pérez de la Sota E, Cortina Romero JM *et al.* An unusual indication for cardiac transplantation: isolated myocardial tuberculosis. *J Heart Lung Transplant* 2006;**25**(1):128–30.

84. O'Neill PG, Rokey R, Greenberg S *et al.* Resolution of ventricular tachycardia and endocardial tuberculoma following antituberculosis therapy. *Chest* 1991;**100**(5):1467–9.

85. Biedrzycki OJ, Baithun SI. TB-related sudden death (TBRSD) due to myocarditis complicating miliary TB: a case report and review of the literature. *Am J Forensic Med Pathol* 2006;**27**(4):335–6.

86. Silvestry FE, Kim B, Pollack BJ *et al.* Cardiac Whipple disease: identification of Whipple bacillus by electron microscopy of a patient before death. *Ann Intern Med* 1997;**126**(3):214–16.

87. Kochman ML, Freedman N, Pine R *et al.* Fatal myocarditis due to Clostridium novyi type B in a previously healthy woman: case report and literature review. *Scand J Infect Dis* 2007;**39**(1):77–80.

88. Jubber AS, Gunawardana DR, Lulu AR. Acute pulmonary edema in Brucella myocarditis and interstitial pneumonitis. *Chest* 1990;**97**(4):1008–9.

89. Fairley CK, Ryan M, Wall PG *et al.* The organisms reported to cause infective myocarditis and pericarditis in England and Wales. *J Infect* 1996;**32**(3):223–5.

90. Wanby P, Olsen B. Myocarditis in a patient with salmonella and campylobacter enteritis. *Scand J Infect Dis* 2001;**33**(11):860–2.

91. Dung NM, Kneen R, Kiem N *et al.* Treatment of severe diphtheritic myocarditis by temporary insertion of a cardiac pacemaker. *Clin Infect Dis* 2002;**35**(11):1425–9.

92. Rullan E, Sigal LH. Rheumatic fever. *Curr Rheumatol Rep* 2001;**3**(5):445–52.

93. Guilherme L, Ramasawmy R, Kalil J. Rheumatic fever and rheumatic heart disease: genetics and pathogenesis. *Scand J Immunol* 2007;**66**(2–3):199–207.

94. Special Writing Group of the Committee on Rheumatic Fever, Endocarditis, and Kawasaki Disease of the Council on Cardiovascular Disease in the Young of the American Heart Association. Guidelines for the diagnosis of rheumatic fever: Jones criteria, 1992 update. *JAMA* 1992;**268**:2069–73.

95. Vasan RS, Shrivastava S, Vijayakumar M *et al.* Echocardiographic evaluation of patients with acute rheumatic fever and rheumatic carditis. *Circulation* 1996;**94**(1):73–82.

96. Essop MR, Wisenbaugh T, Sareli P. Evidence against a myocardial factor as the cause of left ventricular dilation in active rheumatic carditis. *J Am Coll Cardiol* 1993;**22**(3):826–9.

97. Kamblock J, Payot L, Iung B *et al.* Does rheumatic myocarditis really exists? Systematic study with echocardiography and cardiac troponin I blood levels. *Eur Heart J* 2003;**24**(9):855–62.

98. Meira ZM, Goulart EM, Colosimo EA *et al.* Long term follow up of rheumatic fever and predictors of severe rheumatic valvar disease in Brazilian children and adolescents. *Heart* 2005;**91**(8):1019–22.

99. Alehan D, Ayabakan C, Hallioglu O. Role of serum cardiac troponin T in the diagnosis of acute rheumatic fever and rheumatic carditis. *Heart* 2004;**90**(6):689–90.

100. Cilliers A, Manyemba J, Saloojee HH. Anti-inflammatory treatment for carditis in acute rheumatic fever. *Cochrane Database of Systematic Reviews* 2003, Issue 2. Art. No.: CD003176. DOI: 10.1002/14651858.CD003176.

101. Cilliers AM. Rheumatic fever and its management. *BMJ* 2006;**333**(7579):1153–6

102. Manyemba J, Mayosi BM. Penicillin for secondary prevention of rheumatic fever. *Cochrane Database of Systematic Reviews* 2002, Issue 3. Art. No.: CD002227. DOI: 10.1002/14651858.CD002227.

103. Fournier PE, Etienne J, Harle JR *et al.* Myocarditis, a rare but severe manifestation of Q fever: report of 8 cases and review of the literature. *Clin Infect Dis* 2001;**32**(10):1440–7.

104. Doyle A, Bhalla KS, Jones JM 3rd *et al.* Myocardial involvement in rocky mountain spotted fever: a case report and review. *Am J Med Sci* 2006;**332**(4):208–10.

105. Chino M, Minami T, Nishikawa K. Ruptured ventricular aneurysm in secondary syphilis. *Lancet* 1993;**342**(8876):935–6.

106. Nagi KS, Joshi R, Thakur RK. Cardiac manifestations of Lyme disease: a review. *Can J Cardiol* 1996;**12**(5):503–6.

107. Xie L, Gebre W, Szabo K *et al.* Cardiac aspergillosis in patients with acquired immunodeficiency syndrome: a case report and review of the literature. *Arch Pathol Lab Med* 2005;**129**(4):511–15.

108. Franco-Paredes C, Rouphael N, Méndez J *et al.* Cardiac manifestations of parasitic infections. Part 2: Parasitic myocardial disease. *Clin Cardiol* 2007;**30**(5):218–22.

109. Falk RH. Diagnosis and management of the cardiac amyloidoses. *Circulation* 2005;**112**(13):2047–60.

110. Dubrey SW, Cha K, Anderson J *et al.* The clinical features of immunoglobulin light-chain (AL) amyloidosis with heart involvement. *QJM* 1998;**91**(2):141–57.

111. Kushwaha SS, Fallon JT, Fuster V. Restrictive cardiomyopathy. *N Engl J Med* 1997;**336**(4):267–76.

112. Sanchorawala V, Wright DG, Seldin DC *et al.* An overview of the use of high-dose melphalan with autologous stem cell transplantation for the treatment of AL amyloidosis. *Bone Marrow Transplant* 2001;**28**(7):637–42.

113. Al Suwaidi J, Velianou JL, Gertz MA *et al.* Systemic amyloidosis presenting with angina pectoris. *Ann Intern Med* 1999;**131**(11):838–41.

114. Mueller PS, Edwards WD, Gertz MA. Symptomatic ischemic heart disease resulting from obstructive intramural coronary amyloidosis. *Am J Med* 2000;**109**(3):181–8.

115. Dispenzieri A, Kyle RA, Gertz MA *et al.* Survival in patients with primary systemic amyloidosis and raised serum cardiac troponins. *Lancet* 2003;**361**(9371):1787–9.

116. Chamarthi B, Dubrey SW, Cha K *et al.* Features and prognosis of exertional syncope in light-chain associated AL cardiac amyloidosis. *Am J Cardiol* 1997;**80**(9):1242–5.

117. Lévy S. Factors predisposing to the development of atrial fibrillation. *Pacing Clin Electrophysiol* 1997;**20**(10 Pt 2): 2670–4.

118. Röcken C, Peters B, Juenemann G *et al.* Atrial amyloidosis: an arrhythmogenic substrate for persistent atrial fibrillation. *Circulation* 2002;**106**(16):2091–7.

119. Eriksson P, Karp K, Bjerle P *et al.* Disturbances of cardiac rhythm and conduction in familial amyloidosis with polyneuropathy. *Br Heart J* 1984;**51**(6):658–62.

120. Falk RH, Rubinow A, Cohen AS. Cardiac arrhythmias in systemic amyloidosis: correlation with echocardiographic abnormalities. *J Am Coll Cardiol* 1984;**3**(1):107–13.

121. Iwanaga Y, Nishi I, Furuichi S *et al.* B-type natriuretic peptide strongly reflects diastolic wall stress in patients with chronic heart failure: comparison between systolic and diastolic heart failure. *J Am Coll Cardiol* 2006;**47**(4):742–8.

122. Dispenzieri A, Gertz MA, Kyle RA *et al.* Prognostication of survival using cardiac troponins and N-terminal pro-brain natriuretic peptide in patients with primary systemic amyloidosis undergoing peripheral blood stem cell transplantation. *Blood* 2004;**104**:1881–7.

123. Murtagh B, Hammill SC, Gertz MA *et al.* Electrocardiographic findings in primary systemic amyloidosis and biopsy-proven cardiac involvement. *Am J Cardiol* 2005;**95**(4):535–7.

124. Rahman JE, Helou EF, Gelzer-Bell R *et al.* Noninvasive diagnosis of biopsy-proven cardiac amyloidosis. *J Am Coll Cardiol* 2004;**43**(3):410–15.

125. Palladini G, Malamani G, Cò F, Pistorio A *et al.* Holter monitoring in AL amyloidosis: prognostic implications. *Pacing Clin Electrophysiol* 2001;**24**(8 Pt 1):1228–33.

126. Dubrey SW, Bilazarian S, LaValley M *et al.* Signal-averaged electrocardiography in patients with AL (primary) amyloidosis. *Am Heart J* 1997;**134**(6):994–1001.

127. Reisinger J, Dubrey SW, Lavalley M *et al.* Electrophysiologic abnormalities in AL (primary) amyloidosis with cardiac involvement. *J Am Coll Cardiol* 1997;**30**(4):1046–51.

128. Koyama J, Ray-Sequin PA, Falk RH. Longitudinal myocardial function assessed by tissue velocity, strain, and strain rate tissue Doppler echocardiography in patients with AL (primary) cardiac amyloidosis. *Circulation* 2003;**107**(19): 2446–52.

129. Picano E, Pinamonti B, Ferdeghini EM *et al.* Two-dimensional echocardiography in myocardial amyloidosis. *Echocardiography* 1991;**8**(2):253–9.

130. Klein AL, Hatle LK, Taliercio CP *et al.* Prognostic significance of Doppler measures of diastolic function in cardiac amyloidosis. A Doppler echocardiography study. *Circulation* 1991;**83**(3): 808–16.

131. Maceira AM, Joshi J, Prasad SK *et al.* Cardiovascular magnetic resonance in cardiac amyloidosis. *Circulation* 2005;**111**(2): 186–93.

132. Hawkins PN, Lavender JP, Pepys MB. Evaluation of systemic amyloidosis by scintigraphy with 123I-labeled serum amyloid P component. *N Engl J Med* 1990;**323**(8):508–13.

133. Tanaka M, Hongo M, Kinoshita O *et al.* Iodine-123 metaiodo-benzylguanidine scintigraphic assessment of myocardial sympathetic innervation in patients with familial amyloid polyneuropathy. *J Am Coll Cardiol* 1997;**29**(1):168–74.

134. Selvanayagam JB, Hawkins PN, Paul B *et al.* Evaluation and management of the cardiac amyloidosis. *J Am Coll Cardiol* 2007;**50**(22):2101–10.

135. Rubinow A, Skinner M, Cohen AS. Digoxin sensitivity in amyloid cardiomyopathy. *Circulation* 1981;**63**:1285–1288.

136. Dubrey SW, Burke MM, Hawkins PN *et al.* Cardiac transplantation for amyloid heart disease: the United Kingdom experience. *J Heart Lung Transplant* 2004;**23**(10):1142–53.

137. Maurer MS, Raina A, Hesdorffer C *et al.* Cardiac transplantation using extended-donor criteria organs for systemic amyloidosis complicated by heart failure. *Transplantation* 2007;**83**(5):539–45.

138. Jacobson DR, Pastore R, Pool S *et al.* Revised transthyretin Ile 122 allele frequency in African-Americans. *Hum Genet* 1996;**98**(2):236–8.

139. Dubrey SW, Cha K, Skinner M *et al.* Familial and primary (AL) cardiac amyloidosis: echocardiographically similar diseases with distinctly different clinical outcomes. *Heart* 1997;**78**(1):74–82.

140. Brenner DA, Jain M, Pimentel DR *et al.* Human amyloidogenic light chains directly impair cardiomyocyte function through an increase in cellular oxidant stress. *Circ Res* 2004;**94**: 1008–10.

141. Tojo K, Sekijima Y, Kelly JW *et al.* Diflunisal stabilizes familial amyloid polyneuropathy-associated transthyretin variant tetramers in serum against dissociation required for amyloidogenesis. *Neurosci Res* 2006;**56**(4):441–9.

142. Sekijima Y, Dendle MA, Kelly JW. Orally administered diflunisal stabilizes transthyretin against dissociation required for amyloidogenesis. *Amyloid* 2006;**13**(4):236–49.

143. Tagoe CE, Reixach N, Friske L *et al.* In vivo stabilization of mutant human transthyretin in transgenic mice. *Amyloid* 2007;**14**(3):227–36.

144. Ng B, Connors LH, Davidoff R *et al.* Senile systemic amyloidosis presenting with heart failure: a comparison with light chain-associated amyloidosis. *Arch Intern Med* 2005;**165**(12):1425–9.

145. Iannuzzi MC, Rybicki BA, Teirstein AS. Sarcoidosis. *N Engl J Med* 2007;**357**(21):2153–65.

146. Silverman KJ, Hutchins GM, Bulkley BH. Cardiac sarcoid: a clinicopathologic study of 84 unselected patients with systemic sarcoidosis. *Circulation* 1978;**58**(6):1204–11.

147. Bargout R, Kelly RF. Sarcoid heart disease: clinical course and treatment. *Int J Cardiol* 2004;**97**(2):173–82.

148. Roberts WC, McAllister HA Jr, Ferrans VJ. Sarcoidosis of the heart. A clinicopathologic study of 35 necropsy patients (group 1) and review of 78 previously described necropsy patients (group 11). *Am J Med* 1977;**63**(1):86–108.

149. Koplan BA, Soejima K, Baughman K *et al.* Refractory ventricular tachycardia secondary to cardiac sarcoid: electrophysiologic characteristics, mapping, and ablation. *Heart Rhythm* 2006;**3**(8):924–9.

150. Suzuki T, Kanda T, Kubota S *et al.* Holter monitoring as a noninvasive indicator of cardiac involvement in sarcoidosis. *Chest* 1994;**106**(4):1021–4.

151. Okumura W, Iwasaki T, Toyama T *et al.* Usefulness of fasting 18F-FDG PET in identification of cardiac sarcoidosis. *J Nucl Med* 2004;**45**(12):1989–98.

152. Lewin RF, Mor R, Spitzer S, Arditti A *et al.* Echocardiographic evaluation of patients with systemic sarcoidosis. *Am Heart J* 1985;**110**(1 Pt 1):116–22.

153. Smedema JP, Snoep G, van Kroonenburgh MP *et al.* Evaluation of the accuracy of gadolinium-enhanced cardiovascular magnetic resonance in the diagnosis of cardiac sarcoidosis. *J Am Coll Cardiol* 2005;**45**(10):1683–90.

154. Uemura A, Morimoto S, Hiramitsu S. Histologic diagnostic rate of cardiac sarcoidosis: evaluation of endomyocardial biopsies. *Am Heart J* 1999;**138**(2 Pt 1):299–302.

155. Sekiguchi M, Numao Y, Imai M *et al.* Clinical and histopathological profile of sarcoidosis of the heart and acute idiopathic myocarditis. Concepts through a study employing endomyocardial biopsy. I. Sarcoidosis. *Jpn Circ J* 1980;**44**:249–63.

156. Yazaki Y, Isobe M, Hiramitsu S *et al.* Comparison of clinical features and prognosis of cardiac sarcoidosis and idiopathic dilated cardiomyopathy. *Am J Cardiol* 1998;**82**(4):537–40.

157. Aizer A, Stern EH, Gomes JA *et al.* Usefulness of programmed ventricular stimulation in predicting future arrhythmic events in patients with cardiac sarcoidosis. *Am J Cardiol* 2005;**96**(2):276–82.

158. Shiotani H, Miyazaki T, Matsunaga K *et al.* Improvement of severe heart failure with corticosteroid therapy in a patient with myocardial sarcoidosis. *Jpn Circ J* 1991;**55**(4):393–6.

159. Yazaki Y, Isobe M, Hiroe M *et al.* Prognostic determinants of long-term survival in Japanese patients with cardiac sarcoidosis treated with prednisone. *Am J Cardiol* 2001;**88**(9):1006–10.

160. Winters SL, Cohen M, Greenberg S *et al.* Sustained ventricular tachycardia associated with sarcoidosis: assessment of the underlying cardiac anatomy and the prospective utility of programmed ventricular stimulation, drug therapy and an implantable antitachycardia device. *J Am Coll Cardiol* 1991;**18**(4):937–43.

161. Donsky AS, Escobar J, Capehart J *et al.* Heart transplantation for undiagnosed cardiac sarcoidosis. *Am J Cardiol* 2002;**89**(12):1447–50.

162. Yager JE, Hernandez AF, Steenbergen C *et al.* Recurrence of cardiac sarcoidosis in a heart transplant recipient. *J Heart Lung Transplant* 2005;**24**(11):1988–90.

163. Limdi JK, Crampton JR. Hereditary haemochromatosis. *QJM* 2004;**97**(6):315–24.

164. Yang Q, McDonnell SM, Khoury MJ *et al.* Hemochromatosis-associated mortality in the United States from 1979 to 1992: an analysis of multiple-cause mortality data. *Ann Intern Med* 1998;**129**(11):946–53.

165. Hanson EH, Imperatore G, Burke W. HFE gene and hereditary hemochromatosis: a HuGE review. Human Genome Epidemiology. *Am J Epidemiol* 2001;**154**(3):193–206.

166. Niederau C, Fischer R, Sonnenberg A *et al.* Survival and causes of death in cirrhotic and in noncirrhotic patients with primary hemochromatosis. *N Engl J Med* 1985;**313**(20):1256–62.

167. Hahalis G, Alexopoulos D, Kremastinos DT *et al.* Heart failure in beta-thalassemia syndromes: a decade of progress. *Am J Med* 2005;**118**(9):957–67.

168. Whitlock EP, Garlitz BA, Harris EL *et al.* Screening for hereditary hemochromatosis: a systematic review for the U.S. Preventive Services Task Force. *Ann Intern Med* 2006;**145**(3):209–23.

169. Kolnagou A, Economides C, Eracleous E *et al.* Low serum ferritin levels are misleading for detecting cardiac iron overload and increase the risk of cardiomyopathy in thalassemia patients. The importance of cardiac iron overload monitoring using magnetic resonance imaging T2 and T2*. *Hemoglobin* 2006;**30**(2):219–27.

170. Anderson LJ, Holden S, Davis B *et al.* Cardiovascular T2-star (T2*) magnetic resonance for the early diagnosis of myocardial iron overload. *Eur Heart J* 2001;**22**(23):2171–9.

171. Crosby WH. A history of phlebotomy therapy for hemochromatosis. *Am J Med Sci* 1991;**301**(1):28–31.

172. Candell-Riera J, Lu L, Serés L *et al.* Cardiac hemochromatosis: beneficial effects of iron removal therapy. An echocardiographic study. *Am J Cardiol* 1983;**52**(7):824–9.

173. Fabio G, Minonzio F, Delbini P *et al.* Reversal of cardiac complications by deferiprone and deferoxamine combination therapy in a patient affected by a severe type of juvenile hemochromatosis (JH). *Blood* 2007;**109**(1):362–4.

174. Guertl B, Noehammer C, Hoefler G. Metabolic cardiomyopathies. *Int J Exp Pathol* 2000;**81**(6):349–72.

175. Bos JM, Ommen SR, Ackerman MJ. Genetics of hypertrophic cardiomyopathy: one, two, or more diseases? *Curr Opin Cardiol* 2007;**22**(3):193–9.

176. van den Hout HPM, Hop W, van Diggelen OP *et al.* The natural course of infantile Pompe's disease: 20 original cases compared with 133 cases from the literature. *Pediatrics* 2003;**112**:332–40.

177. Klinge L, Straub V, Neudorf U *et al.* Safety and efficacy of recombinant acid alpha-glucosidase (rhGAA) in patients with classical infantile Pompe disease: results of a phase II clinical trial. *Neuromuscul Disord* 2005;**15**:24–31.

178. Sugie K, Yamamoto A, Murayama K *et al.* Clinicopathological features of genetically confirmed Danon disease. *Neurology* 2002;**58**(12):1773–8.

179. Ozen H. Glycogen storage diseases: new perspectives. *World J Gastroenterol* 2007;**13**(18):2541–53.

180. Moses SW, Wanderman KL, Myroz A *et al.* Cardiac involvement in glycogen storage disease type III. *Eur J Pediatr* 1989;**148**(8):764–6.

181. Mohan UR, Hay AA, Cleary MA *et al.* Cardiovascular changes in children with mucopolysaccharide disorders. *Acta Paediatr* 2002;**91**(7):799–804.

182. Mehta A, Ricci R, Widmer U *et al.* Fabry disease defined: baseline clinical manifestations of 366 patients in the Fabry Outcome Survey. *Eur J Clin Invest* 2004;**34**(3):236–42.

183. Linhart A, Elliott PM. The heart in Anderson-Fabry disease and other lysosomal storage disorders. *Heart* 2007;**93**(4):528–35.

184. Ommen SR, Nishimura RA, Edwards WD. Fabry disease: a mimic for obstructive hypertrophic cardiomyopathy? *Heart* 2003;**89**:929–30.

185. Linhart A, Palecek T, Bultas J *et al.* New insights in cardiac structural changes in patients with Fabry's disease. *Am Heart J* 2000;**139**:1101–8.

186. Elliott PM, Kindler H, Shah JS *et al.* Coronary microvascular dysfunction in male patients with Anderson-Fabry disease and the effect of treatment with alpha galactosidase A. *Heart* 2006;**92**(3):357–60.

187. Shah JS, Hughes DA, Sachdev B *et al.* Prevalence and clinical significance of cardiac arrhythmia in Anderson-Fabry disease. *Am J Cardiol* 2005;**96**(6):842–6.

188. Linthorst GE, Vedder AC, Aerts JM *et al.* Screening for Fabry disease using whole blood spots fails to identify one-third of female carriers. *Clin Chim Acta* 2005;**353**(1–2):201–3.

189. Eng CM, Guffon N, Wilcox WR *et al.* International Collaborative Fabry Disease Study Group. Safety and efficacy of recombinant human alpha-galactosidase A-replacement therapy in Fabry's disease. *N Engl J Med* 2001;**345**:9–16.

51

Chagas' heart disease

J Antonio Marin-Neto,[1] Anis Rassi Jr,[2] Benedito Carlos Maciel,[1] Marcus Vinicius Simões[1] and André Schmidt[1]

[1]Division of Cardiology, Medical School of Ribeirao Preto, University of Sao Paulo, Brazil
[2]Anis Rassi Hospital, Brazil

Historical perspective

Exactly one century ago Carlos Chagas discovered an entirely new infectious entity – Chagas disease, its etiologic agent – *Trypanosoma cruzi,* and the main mechanism of transmission of the disease, through the sting of *Triatominae* bugs.[1] By the early 1920s the most relevant syndrome of Chagas disease – cardiomyopathy – had been characterized, including its florid electrocardiographic disturbances.[2] However, during subsequent decades the disease was practically neglected and its epidemiologic significance was even refuted. Only in the 1950s, with the completion of systematic serologic and necropsy studies, did it became apparent that *T. cruzi* infection was responsible for the triad of cardiomyopathy, megaesophagus and megacolon which afflicted millions of people in Latin America.[3]

Definitions

Chagas' disease is characterized by acute and chronic phases. In the acute phase more than 90% of the patients have the unapparent form, while the remaining infected individuals show a febrile disease and rarely die because of myocarditis or encephalitis. During the chronic phase most patients remain for life with the indeterminate form. Others eventually show the cardiac, the digestive or the mixed form of organic involvement.[4] Cardiac and esophageal chagasic disease is further classified in stages (grades) (Fig. 51.1).

Although megaesophagus and megacolon produce typical clinical conditions in roughly 5–10% of patients, chronic Chagas' cardiomyopathy (CCC) is by far the most serious form of the disease.[5]

Evidence-Based Cardiology, 3rd edition. Edited by S. Yusuf, J.A. Cairns, A.J. Camm, E.L. Fallen, and B.J. Gersh. © 2010 Blackwell Publishing, ISBN: 978-1-4051-5925-8.

The long period of the indeterminate form – several decades before the appearance of clinically manifest disease – constitutes one of its most intriguing features.[6] Its traditional definition by a specialist panel in 1984 requires that asymptomatic patients with positive specific serology show no physical signs of disease, and no abnormalities in the ECG and in the radiologic assessment of the heart, esophagus and colon (barium swallowing and enema).[7] Although not adhering to such strict criteria (for instance, most studies do not allude to performing colon or esophageal X-rays) investigators using more sensitive diagnostic methods have described cardiac abnormalities in the majority of patients with the indeterminate form.[8] More significantly, patients with normal ECG and chest X-rays may have striking alterations in right ventricular biopsy specimens[9] and right ventricular contractile depression.[10] Also, these patients may have mild segmental or global left ventricular (LV) dysfunction as evaluated by the slope of the end-systolic pressure-dimension relationship.[11] In addition, independent of the clinical classification, the presence of minor LV wall motion abnormalities documented at baseline two-dimensional (2D) echocardiography in patients who have normal EKG and normal global systolic function is a predictor of deterioration of ventricular function during follow-up.[12]

Based on these findings, it has been proposed that seropositive chagasic patients who have minor LV wall motion abnormalities on 2D-echocardiography, despite normal ECG and chest X-rays, should be classified in the cardiac form of the disease. Conversely, patients with the indeterminate form of the disease should have normal global and segmental biventricular systolic function as documented by imaging techniques.[13] Whether every chagasic patient with normal ECG and chest X-rays should routinely undergo other cardiac tests is a distinct and controversial issue. Because the probability of survival of these patients is similar to that of the normal population, the current predominant view is that further initial evaluation is usually unnecessary. Subsequent follow-up of chagasic

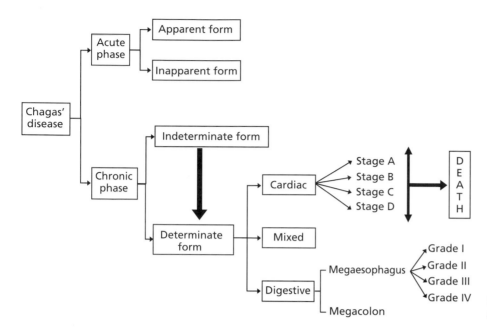

Figure 51.1 Chagas' disease: phases, forms, and stages.

patients with normal ECG should rely on annual history, physical examination and repeated ECG.[14]

Epidemiology

Transmission of *T. cruzi* is mainly vectoral, through the feces of infected bloodsucking insects of the family *Reduviidae* (subfamily *Triatominae*). Many case series reports have documented that the infection can also occur by blood transfusion, transplacental transmission, laboratory accident, organ transplantation and ingestion of *Triatominae*-contaminated food or drink.

Although cross-sectional epidemiologic studies assessing clinical manifestations and mortality rates have been reported in scattered areas of several South American countries, the actual prevalence of CCC is unknown, because no recent large-scale screening has been carried out. However, it is unquestionable that the global disease prevalence has steadily reduced. Recent rough estimates are in the range of 8–10 million people who have Chagas' disease in the Americas,[15,16] contrasting with the 1990 estimates of 16–18 million people infected.

In 1991 an initiative for the elimination of the transmission of Chagas' disease was launched in Argentina, Brazil, Bolivia, Chile, Paraguay and Uruguay, covering an area responsible for more than 65% of the global prevalence. As result, Uruguay (1997), Chile (1999) and Brazil (2006) declared themselves free of Chagas' disease transmission due to *Triatoma infestans*.[17] It is estimated that the incidence of new cases declined from 700 000/year in 1983 to 200 000/ year in 2000.[18] Other initiatives are now ongoing in other Latin American countries with results still pending. Nevertheless, CCC is by far the most common form of cardiomyopathy in Latin America countries. Further, because of modern migratory trends, it is likely to become ubiquitous.[19] This tendency can be exemplified by estimates, based on the prevalence of *T. cruzi* infection detected serologically (mostly Latin American immigrants), that 100 000–400 000 infected persons might be living in the United States.[20,21] The FDA recently issued strict surveillance of blood supply regarding *T. cruzi* infection, and in Europe, preventive measures have also been suggested.[22]

In the United States vector-borne transmission is rare[23] but Chagas seropositivity incidence among blood donors is increasing.[24] A recent survey by the American Red Cross, in facilities located in California and Arizona, identified 63 specimens from 61 donors among 148 969 blood donation specimens (nearly one in 2365 donations). Additionally, a systematic review of the literature providing evidence-based recommendations for the evaluation, counseling, and treatment of patients with chronic *T. cruzi* infection in the United States has recently been published.[14]

CCC has a high social impact.[25,26] Over 15 000 annual deaths can be attributed directly to this etiology and 667 000 disability-adjusted life years (DALYs) are lost annually.[18] Chagas' disease constitutes the third largest parasitic disease burden globally, after malaria and schistosomiasis.

Natural history and prognostic factors

There is sound experimental, pathologic, and clinical evidence that *T. cruzi* tissue parasitism produces organ damage acutely (immediately following infection) as well as decades later.[3] Acute infection is often asymptomatic or may be a self-limited febrile illness lasting 4–8 weeks. The case fatality rate in the acute phase is less than 5%, death occurring because of myocarditis and/or meningoencephalitis. Following the acute phase 30–40% of chronically infected individuals develop the clinical manifestations of cardiac and/or digestive disease, the majority 10–30 years after the initial infection.

Cardiac involvement typically produces conduction defects, ventricular arrhythmias, wall motion abnormalities, cardiac failure, pulmonary and systemic thromboembolic phenomena, and sudden death.[5] Megaesophagus and megacolon are also frequently diagnosed in chronic chagasic patients in Brazil, Argentina, and Chile, but not in Mexico, Colombia or Venezuela.[4] The hypothesis that different *T. cruzi* strains, coupled to genetic susceptibilities of infected individuals and to environmental factors, may cause this difference in morbidity has not been evaluated by appropriately designed studies.[27]

The natural history of CCC is relatively well known from observational studies conducted mainly in endemic areas of Brazil, Argentina, and Venezuela since the early 1940s. There is also a wealth of case series reports dealing with acute Chagas' disease acquired through non-vector transmission. Most of these investigations consist of longitudinal or cross-sectional observations of infected people in rural areas. Very few studies have been conducted using case–control populations of chagasic and non-chagasic people. There have also been some observational investigations focusing on the description and follow-up of hospital based cohorts.

Both the rural and the hospital-based studies have limitations. There is usually no adequate identification of cardiac involvement in the rural studies. Furthermore, because of the protracted course of heart involvement, from the acute phase to end-stage heart failure, no studies encompassing the whole span of the disease are available. Conversely, in hospital-based studies the disease is often well characterized but results could not be extended to the whole chagasic population. More recently, several longitudinal studies have been conducted on clinic-based populations at different referral centers in an attempt to establish predictors of death for patients with CCC.[28] These studies have analyzed clinical, radiologic, electrocardiographic, echocardiographic and Holter monitoring variables.

Prognosis in the acute phase

Case series using serologic tests in endemic areas have shown that in less than 10% of the acute cases were clinical manifestations sufficient to make a correct diagnosis.[29] This is a major deterrent for understanding the transition from the acute to the chronic phases. However, the scarce clinical data are in general agreement with findings from experimental models of Chagas' disease.

For the minority of patients in whom the clinical diagnosis was possible, cardiac involvement occurred in 90% of 313 successive cases reported in Bambuí (central Brazil). Of note, in 70–80%, cardiac enlargement was seen on chest X-rays, contrasting with only 50% of cases showing ECG abnormalities.[29] This is in disagreement with other reports showing a predominance of ECG alterations.[30] In the Bambuí study, the severity of myocarditis was inversely proportional to age, heart failure being more intense in children aged up to two years. Mortality in the acute phase, as seen in the 313 cases, was 8.3%. This was higher than the 3–5% reported in similar studies in other endemic areas in Brazil, Argentina, and Uruguay. The ECG was normal in 63.3% of the non-fatal cases and in only 14.3% of those who died in the acute phase. Seventy-five percent of all deaths were seen in children aged <3 years. Heart failure was the constant finding in all fatal cases, with or without concomitant encephalitis.[29]

The typical course of acutely manifested Chagas' disease includes disappearance of symptoms and signs of heart failure within 1–3 months and normalization of the ECG after one year of the infection. However, there is no evidence of spontaneous cure of the infection, as demonstrated by serial xenodiagnosis and serologic tests in studies of several hundreds of chagasic patients. Of 117 patients from Bambuí who were followed for up to 40 years after the acute infection, the development of CCC (based on clinical signs, ECG, and chest X-ray) occurred in 33.8%, 39.3%, and 58.1% for follow-up periods of 10–20 years, 21–30 years, and 31–40 years respectively.[29] In another review from the same cohort, for 268 patients whose acute phase of the disease had been diagnosed an average of 27 years before, the general mortality for the period was 13.8%.[29]

In contrast to the low mortality following the vectoral transmission, recent outbreaks of the disease, caused by ingestion of contaminated food or fluids, were associated with higher mortality rates, probably due to massive parasitic burden.[31]

Prognosis in the indeterminate form

The mechanisms responsible for preventing the progression of disease in more than 50% of cases (i.e. those with the indeterminate form) remain obscure. A 1–3% annual rate of appearance of CCC has been observed in several studies. Of 400 young adults followed for 10 years in São Felipe (north eastern Brazil), 91 (23%) developed ECG or chest X-ray abnormalities. Of note, eight deaths were recorded in that period, seven of them due to non-chagasic causes and only one occurring because of reactivation of myocarditis.[6]

Another longitudinal study in Bambuí contrasted the evolution of 885 young patients with indeterminate form to that of 911 chagasic patients with initially abnormal ECGs. Survival after 10 years was 97.4% and 61.3% respectively for the indeterminate group and the group with CCC.[32] A third longitudinal study in a rural Venezuelan community, with 47% prevalence of positive serology for Chagas' disease, followed 364 patients for a mean period of four years. Heart involvement appeared at a rate of 1.1% per year in seropositive individuals. Mortality was 3% in the four years of follow-up, CCC being the cause of death in 69% of all fatal cases.[33]

In 1973 a longitudinal study was initiated in Castro Alves (Bahia), a rural community in north east Brazil. In the initial cross-sectional study, of 644 individuals aged >10 years, 53.7% were seropositive. The population initially described in 1973–1974 was re-examined in 1977, 1980, and 1983. The overall rate of development of abnormal ECG was 2.57% in seropositive as compared to 1.25% per year in seronegative individuals, a relative risk of 2.0 for the same geographical area.[34] These results were obtained in chagasic populations with >50% of the patients aged <20 years. It is relevant that fewer indeterminate cases are found in the older age groups because of the evolving nature of the disease (that is, more aging patients presenting clinical signs of cardiac or digestive involvement).

Another study of 160 patients with the indeterminate form was conducted in São Paulo, Brazil, from 1979 to 1994. Patients were followed long term with repeated electrocardiographic and echocardiographic studies at regular intervals. After a mean follow-up of 8.2 years, 34 patients (21.3%) developed ECG changes. However, only in 15 of the 34 patients could the ECG changes be clearly attributed to CCC. In addition, LV ejection fraction remained normal in the entire population throughout the study, certainly contributing to the favorable outlook for these patients.[35] More recently, a longitudinal study in Argentina following 731 patients (mean age 44 years) with the indeterminate form of Chagas' disease for eight years found that 4.6% progressed to clinically manifest cardiomyopathy. Four patients (0.5%) died of cardiovascular causes during this period, but their cardiac status right before the death was not reported.[36] Finally, in the larger series of 4593 chagasic patients followed for an average of 5.3 years in Argentina, those with normal ECG showed a very low sudden cardiac mortality rate (0.004% per year).[37]

Prognosis of chronic Chagas cardiomyopathy

The evidence provided by the studies mentioned above shows that chagasic individuals with a normal ECG, in general, have a very good prognosis. In contrast, the appearance of ECG changes entails an unfavorable prognosis. In a community-based study in rural Brazil, right bundle brunch block and ventricular extrasystoles were each associated with 7–8-fold increase, and the two together with a 13-fold increase in risk of death over a seven-year period, as compared to the infected population with normal ECG.[38]

In another study of 107 chagasic patients followed for 10 years, a significant reduction in life expectancy, as compared to that of 22 control individuals, was detected only in patients with ECG or clinical changes. A mortality rate of 82% over the 10-year follow-up period was seen in the group of 34 patients with signs of heart failure at the beginning of the study. In contrast, a 65% 10-year survival was associated with ECG abnormalities but in the absence of signs of heart failure.[39] In a study of 160 cases, survival two years after the first episode of heart failure was only 33.4%.[40] Another study of 104 male chagasic patients admitted to hospital with heart failure revealed a mortality rate of 52% after five years. The strongest predictors of survival were reduced LV ejection fraction and maximal oxygen uptake during exercise.[41] The data support the concept that mortality associated with Chagas' disease strongly correlates with severity of myocardial dysfunction.

In a series of 42 patients with CCC in the United States, death occurred in 11 patients during a mean follow-up of nearly five years, always in association with global or regional LV dysfunction. Established or developing heart failure was a strong predictor of mortality but aborted sudden death or the presence of sustained ventricular tachycardia were not predictors for mortality in this series.[42] These results contrast with the evidence from 44 chagasic patients followed for a mean period of two years where ventricular tachycardia detected during exercise testing was a marker of increased risk of sudden death.[43] This discrepancy probably reflects the limitations of small number of patients and relatively short follow-up in both studies.

In a recent study of 424 patients with Chagas' heart disease in central Brazil, a mortality risk score based on extensive follow-up data was developed and validated in an external sample, after univariate and multivariate analysis. Six independent predictors of death were identified[44] (Fig. 51.2). Finally, a systematic review of all reports on prognostic factors using multivariate analysis in CCC confirmed that the risk of death is strongly related to the severity of disease, with markers of LV dysfunction, congestive heart failure and complex ventricular arrhythmias carrying the gravest prognosis.[28]

Risk Factor	Points
NYHA class III or IV	5
Cardiomegaly (chest x-ray)	5
Segmental or global WMA (2D echo)	3
Nonsustained VT (24h Holter)	3
Low QRS voltage (ECG)	2
Male sex	2

Total Points	Total Mortality		Risk
	5 years	10 years	
0 – 6	2%	10%	Low
7 – 11	18%	44%	Intermediate
12 – 20	63%	84%	High

Figure 51.2 Risk score for predicting death in chronic Chagas cardiomyopathy. NYHA, New York Heart Association; WMA, wall motion abnormality; VT, ventricular tachycardia.

Key points

- As long as patients remain in the indeterminate form, their prognosis is good. **Level C1**
- After 10 years almost 80% of patients remain with the indeterminate form of the disease and probably 50% of the entire population will have no signs of heart disease throughout their life span. **Level C1**
- There are no clues as to why some chagasic patients remain with the indeterminate form, while others sooner or later undergo severe organic damage.
- The prognosis of patients with Chagas' heart disease is predictable, despite the heterogeneity of clinical manifestations of the disease. **Level C1**
- By univariate analysis many variables indicate a poor prognosis. However, taking into account the relationship among variables (multivariate analysis), impaired LV dysfunction, NYHA class III/ IV, cardiomegaly, and non-sustained ventricular tachycardia are consistently and independently associated with higher mortality. **Level C1**
- The combination of non-sustained ventricular tachycardia (NSVT) and LV dysfunction is associated with a substantial increased risk of mortality when compared with patients without any of these risk markers. **Level C1**
- Once overt cardiac failure ensues the prognosis is poor and approaches 50% in four years. **Level C1**
- It is possible, but not proven by good evidence, that ventricular dysrhythmia and sudden death play a more prominent role in mortality due to Chagas' disease than in heart failure due to other etiologies. **Level C2**

Pathophysiology and pathogenetic mechanisms

Organ damage arising during the acute phase is closely related to parasite presence in targets such as the gastrointestinal tract, central nervous system and heart. High-grade parasitemia co-exists with lymphadenopathy, liver and spleen enlargement, markers of widespread immunologic reaction. As the parasitemia abates and the systemic inflammatory reaction subsides, silent relentless focal myocarditis ensues during the indeterminate phase.[45] In predisposed hosts, encompassing approximately 30–50% of the infected population, this chronic myocarditis may evolve to cumulative destruction of cardiac fibers and marked reparative fibrosis. The incessant myocarditis is eventually responsible for myocardial mass loss attaining critical degrees, thereby leading to regional and global ventricular remodeling and chamber dilation, and setting the anatomic substrate for malignant dysrhythmias. This hypothesis is based on several experimental animal models for CCC, but additional evidence has been provided by studies correlating clinical and pathologic findings in autopsied humans dying with all forms and stages of the disease.

The most intriguing challenge for understanding the pathogenesis of CCC lies in the complex host–parasite inter-relationship. In many patients, the myocardial aggression is controlled at low levels, remaining with the indeterminate form, whereas in others the development of fully blown CCC is triggered.[46]

Evidence from pathophysiologic studies in animal models and in humans points to four pathogenetic mechanisms producing myocardial damage in CCC.[45]

1. Cardiac autonomic disturbances

Intense neuronal depopulation has been demonstrated in several independent pathologic studies.[47,48] Also, abnormal autonomic cardiac regulation has been shown in many functional investigations, preceding the development of ventricular dysfunction.[10,49] Because of the dysautonomia, chagasic patients are deprived of the tonic inhibitory action normally exerted by the parasympathetic system on the sinus node, and also lack the vagally mediated mechanism to respond with rapid bradycardia or tachycardia to transient changes in blood pressure or venous return.[50,51] Although sympathetic denervation has also been shown in myocardial regions, even preceding perfusion defects and wall motion abnormalities,[52] on the basis of the striking parasympathetic impairment, the neurogenic theory postulated that a long-lasting autonomic imbalance would lead to a catecholamine-induced cardiomyopathy.[47,53]

However, various kinds of evidence militate against neurogenic derangements being a main pathogenetic mechanism.[45] First, even in endemic areas where cardiac denervation is readily detectable in some patients, its prevalence and intensity are highly variable. Second, no significant correlation seems to exist between parasympathetic denervation and the extent of myocardial dysfunction or the presence of dysrhythmia. Moreover, the typical chagasic cardiomyopathy is found in geographical regions where the disease is apparently caused by parasite strains devoid of neurotropism.[4] In such regions the typical chagasic digestive syndromes considered to be causally related to parasympathetic denervation of the esophagus and colon are rarely described. Third, no follow-up studies correlating autonomic regulation, myocardial function, and cardiac rhythm assessment have been reported in chagasic patients. Finally, the attractive hypothesis of autonomic impairment triggering sudden death has never been appropriately tested.

2. Microvascular disturbances

There is evidence from studies in experimental models of *T. cruzi* infection, as well as from pathologic and clinical investigations, that microvascular abnormalities causing ischemia contribute to the pathogenesis of CCC. In the experimental murine model of Chagas' disease, occlusive platelet thrombi in small epicardial and microcirculatory coronary vessels have been shown in concomitance with focal vascular constriction and spasm.[54,55] These abnormalities were partly reverted by long-term administration of verapamil, leading to attenuation of the myocardial damage and increased survival for the *T. cruzi* infected mice.[56]

Biopsy and autopsy histopathologic investigations in humans also showed microvascular abnormalities deemed responsible for the focal diffuse myocytolysis and extensive reparative fibrosis known to be related to transient ischemic disturbances of low intensity and short duration.[3,47,57–59]

From the clinical standpoint most chagasic patients have ischemic-like symptoms and ST changes and abnormal Q-waves indicative of regional myocardial fibrosis. They also have prominent LV localized dysynergy and striking myocardial perfusion defects in the absence of epicardial coronary artery obstruction.[60] Of note, these reversible ischemic defects are mostly seen in the apical and inferior-posterior LV segments, i.e. the regions where regional contractile dysfunction prevails in later stages of CCC.[52] In a recent study, 36 chagasic patients with normal coronary arteries were sequentially evaluated regarding progression of left ventricular dysfunction and myocardial perfusion disturbances over a mean period of 5.6 years. The results showed that the decrease of left ventricular ejection fraction over time was correlated to the increase of regional myocardial perfusion at rest, which is indicative of myocardial fibrosis. The appearance of new perfusion defects at rest at the final evaluation was topographically related to the presence of reversible ischemic perfusion defects at the initial scan.[61] Thus, microcirculatory ischemia could

represent an ancillary factor to potentiate and amplify the chronic inflammatory aggression to myocardial tissue, with coalescent microinfarctions leading to the development of aneurysms.[45]

3. Myocardial damage directly related to parasite persistence

Early in the natural history of CCC there is a low-grade but constant focal and diffuse inflammatory process, as shown by studies in experimental models[62] and in human necropsy (chagasics dead from other causes) and biopsy specimens.[9,63,64] Several independent investigators using immunohistochemistry, PCR and *in situ* hybridization methods described tissue *T. cruzi* antigens or its genomic material in the inflammatory foci, first in animal models[64,65] and later in humans.[65–70] There is also evidence of a direct correlation between organic parasite infection and the clinical expression of disease. Thus, *T. cruzi* genetic material could not be detected in the heart from patients who died without signs of cardiac involvement, but it was consistently found in heart specimens from patients with CCC.[69] Moreover, the persistence of *T. cruzi* is directly implicated in the pathology of the chronic phase, as shown by experimental models of Chagas' disease in which parasite load reduction by trypanocidal treatment resulted in attenuation of cardiomyopathy.[71,72] Conversely, in experimental models, enhancement of parasite burden results in exacerbation of the cardiomyopathy course.[73] Finally, in human CCC, during favorable conditions such as immunosuppression treatment to prevent transplant rejection or in patients with acquired immunodeficiency syndromes, intact amastigote parasites undertake active multiplication and cause reactivation of infection and striking recrudescence of myocarditis and esophagitis.[74–79]

4. Immune-mediated cardiac damage

Immunologic factors have been postulated to play a role in the pathogenesis of CCC. The demonstration of predominant mononuclear cells in the inflammatory infiltrates suggests a delayed hypersensitivity reaction, leading to immunoglobulin and complement deposition in myocardial tissue.[80,81] Experimental and clinical data from studies in CCC also show that several of the criteria required for an autoimmune pathogenesis have been fulfilled:[82]

• the identification of heart–*T. cruzi* cell cross-reactive T cell antigens with reproduction of pathobiologic changes by passive transfer of immune cells in murine models
• attenuation of the inflammatory process as a consequence of tolerance induction to myocardial antigens
• the induction of myocardial aggression after immunization with cardiac myosin

• the isolation of cardiac myosin autoreactive T cells in molecular mimicry with *T. cruzi* B13 protein from affected tissue

• *in vitro* immunization with B13 protein eliciting T cell clones cross-reactive with cardiac myosin

• immunization with *T. cruzi* ribosomal antigens inducing cross-reactive antibodies and heart conduction abnormalities

• similar cross-reactive autoantibodies present in sera from patients with CCC disease inducing arrhythmia in explanted hearts.

In summary, there is persuasive evidence of both parasite antigen-driven immunopathology and autoimmunity in cardiac inflammatory lesions. However, the nature of the essential antigen or antigens that elicit destructive immune responses remains elusive.[45]

Key points

• Cardiac dysautonomia is a well-characterized feature preceding myocardial damage, but its role is probably ancillary in the pathogenesis of CCC. **Level B**

• Microcirculatory derangements causing ischemia probably constitute important amplification mechanisms for the inflammatory myocardial aggression. **Level B**

• The low-grade but incessant myocarditis present in CCC is inextricably related to the parasite persistence, with superimposed antiparasite immunity and autoimmune reaction, but the mechanisms triggering exacerbated responses in some cases and deterring significant damage in others still remain to be elucidated. **Level B**

• A corollary of the parasite persistence hypothesis, with potential clinical implication, is that effective measures to control the parasite burden would probably reduce tissue damage and impact on the natural history of CCC.

Clinical features

Cardiac abnormalities may be detected in all phases or forms of Chagas' disease, but their clinical expression is highly variable (Table 51.1). The diagnosis of Chagas' disease in the acute phase is difficult because symptoms are easily mistaken for other infectious diseases and laboratory findings are non-specific, including leukocytosis with an absolute increase in lymphocyte count; ECG may show low-voltage, diffuse ST-T changes and first-degree atrioventricular block; chest X-ray shows variable degrees of cardiomegaly; serologic tests for *T. cruzi* infection are usually negative during the first weeks. In this setting, the diagnosis is based upon detection of circulating parasites by a variety of methods. The diagnosis of acute phase due to blood transfusion requires a high level of awareness, particularly in non-endemic areas This is also necessary for the increasing problem of recognizing reactivation of Chagas' disease in immunocompromised patients who have the chronic form.[79,83]

In the chronic phase, the relative prevalence of symptoms of cardiovascular and/or digestive involvement is variable in different geographical regions, and probably reflects the existence of diverse strains of *T. cruzi*, other environmental or host factors, and the type of laboratory and serologic testing.

Usually, cardiovascular symptoms and physical signs at this stage of the disease arise from three basic syndromes that may co-exist in the same patient: heart failure; cardiac dysrhythmia and thromboembolism (systemic and pulmonary). Of note, it is not uncommon for patients with marked ECG abnormalities to be asymptomatic hard workers, capable of performing strenuous physical exercise under laboratory conditions.[84] When symptoms

Table 51.1 A clinical and functional classification of Chagas' heart disease

	Clinical phase			
	Acute	**Indeterminate**	**Overt disease**	**Heart failure**
Symptoms	Fairly common	Absent	Minimal	Present
ECG changes	Common	Absent	RBBB, LAHB, AVB, PVCs	+ Q-waves, AF, VT
Heart size (X-rays)	Usually abnormal	Normal	Normal	Enlarged
RV function		May be depressed	Usually abnormal	Abnormal
LV diastolic function	?	Normal or mild abnormalities	Abnormal	Abnormal
LV systolic function	Abnormal	May have mild regional dysynergy	Segmental dysynergy	Global depression
Perfusion defects	?	?	Common	Common
Autonomic function	?	May be abnormal	May be abnormal	Usually abnormal
RV biopsy	Abnormal	May be abnormal	Abnormal	Abnormal

LV, left ventricle; RV, right ventricle; ECG, electrocardiogram; AVB, atrioventricular block; LAHB, left anterior hemiblock; RBBB, right bundle branch block; PVCs, premature ventricular complex; AF, atrial fibrillation; VT, ventricular tachycardia; ? = unknown.

occur they include edema, fatigue and exertional dyspnea, palpitations, dizziness, syncope and chest pain. Such manifestations are the expression of decreased cardiac reserve (including minor early signs of diastolic dysfunction), the presence of ventricular dysrhythmias, sinus node dysfunction, and high-degree atrioventricular block. Chest pain is usually atypical for myocardial ischemia but, in sporadic patients, mimics an acute coronary syndrome. It may also be related to esophageal mechanisms.[85,86]

ECG abnormalities are present in most patients with CCC, mainly in the form of conduction disturbances and ventricular arrhythmias.[5] In more advanced stages pathologic Q-waves and low voltage are found, compatible with extensive areas of myocardial fibrosis. The combination of right bundle branch block and left anterior hemiblock is very typical in CCC.

Many case series reports have documented the peculiar feature of striking segmental wall motion abnormalities in several hundreds of chronic chagasic patients.[87] The most characteristic lesion is the apical LV aneurysm. A few small retrospective studies have evaluated the correlation between ventricular arrhythmia and symptoms in CCC. It is apparent that complex ventricular dysrhythmia may occur in asymptomatic patients, but it is usually associated with poor LV function.[88] The aneurysms are also sources of emboli.[89,90]

Systemic and pulmonary embolism, arising from mural thrombi in the cardiac chambers, is a conspicuous complication of CCC, but post-mortem findings have shown that they are often overlooked: in 1345 necropsies on patients with CCC, 595 cases (44%) had cardiac thrombi and/or visceral thromboembolism. The presence of cardiac thrombi was related to severity of ventricular enlargement. Embolism most frequently involved lungs (36%), kidneys (36%), spleen (14%), and brain (10%).[88] Also, the incidence of cardiac thrombus was higher in cases of heart failure (36%) than in cases of sudden death (15%).

Congestive heart failure, in advanced stage, is more commonly expressed by prominent signs of systemic congestion, with less intense evidence of pulmonary congestion.[91,92] This peculiar feature of CCC is linked to early severe damage of the right ventricle (RV), a chamber frequently neglected in the clinical and echocardiographic evaluation of cardiac performance.[93] Isolated LV failure may also appear in early stages of cardiac decompensation.

Sudden death is the principal cause of death in CCC, accounting for about 55–65% of deaths, followed by pump failure (25–30%), and thromboembolism (10–15%). Sudden cardiac death can occur even in patients previously asymptomatic.[94] It is usually precipitated by physical exercise and associated with ventricular tachycardia and fibrillation or, more rarely, with complete atrioventricular (AV) block. Limited evidence from autopsy studies, in these patients,

indicates variable degrees of inflammatory and neuronal cardiac alterations.[95]

In spite of chest pain being a cardinal complaint in many chagasic patients, coronary angiography is usually normal.[96] However, functional abnormalities in the myocardial blood flow regulation have been described and all types of myocardial perfusion defects have been detected in several small groups of selected patients, possibly implying microvascular coronary disturbances, as discussed above.[52,60]

Cardiac autonomic dysfunction, mainly parasympathetic, has been shown by several independent studies in various groups of chagasic patients (including those with isolated digestive disease), whose response to various autonomic tests was compared to those of control subjects.[49,51,96–99] However, these abnormalities are neither correlated with any symptoms nor cause postural hypotension.[45,51]

Management

Etiologic treatment

Recent developments in basic biochemistry of the parasite allowed identification of potential targets for chemotherapy, such as protein prenylation, sterol, proteases and phospholipids metabolism.[99] However, only two currently available trypanocidal agents have been demonstrated to have acceptable efficacy and safety profiles: nifurtimox and benznidazole. Side effects, warranting discontinuation of therapy in roughly 10% of cases, include dermatitis, polyneuritis, leukopenia, gastrointestinal intolerance and central nervous system adverse symptoms. These untoward reactions are reversible with discontinuation of therapy. Benznidazole is considered the preferred drug at a dose of 5 mg/kg per day for 60 days; the dose in children up to age 12 is 10 mg/kg per day. Nifurtimox is given for 60–90 days at a dose of 8–10 mg/kg per day in adults and 15 mg/kg per day in children. Both drugs should be administered in divided doses at eight-hour intervals. Benznidazole can also be administered at 12-hour intervals.

Assessment of trypanocidal treatment efficacy is still hampered by methodologic issues. Parasitemia is readily demonstrated in the acute phase of Chagas' disease by direct examination of blood or buffy coat, hemoculture or xenodiagnosis but even without treatment, falls to undetectable levels by these methods within three months.[100,101] PCR techniques for detection of *T. cruzi* in blood are useful for monitoring the success of treatment in the acute phase, but also have low sensitivity in the chronic stages.[102] Hence, in the chronic phase of the disease documentation of cure should rely on negativation of IgG serologic tests. There is expert opinion that the length of time after successful treatment required for negative seroconversion is proportional to the duration of *T. cruzi* infection: 3–5 years for those treated in the acute phase, 5–10 years in those with <10 years, and 15–20 years in those with >10 years duration of infection.[103]

Trypanocidal therapy in the acute phase

There is consensus that in the acute phase, irrespective of the mechanism of transmission (vectorial, congenital, blood transfusion, transplantation, laboratory accident or oral), trypanocidal treatment is mandatory. Parasitologic and serologic cure is thought to occur in 60–85% of those treated in this phase.[102] Unfortunately, no long-term follow-up trials have evaluated the efficacy of trypanocidal therapy for the prevention of chronic organ damage in patients treated during the acute phase.

Trypanocidal therapy in the chronic phase

Etiologic treatment is unanimously recommended for chronic patients with reactivation of acute infection during immunosuppression, including those co-infected with *T. cruzi*/HIV.[104] This indication is supported by observational results of effective trypanocidal therapy for reduction of symptoms and parasitemia in small case series of chagasic patients who received various types of transplants.[105,106]

The prophylactic administration of trypanocidal drugs for women of reproductive age (as an attempt to reduce the possibility of congenital transmission), for anticipated immunosuppression in the future (pre-transplant), and for HIV infection with low CD4+ lymphocyte counts is more controversial.[107] Among experts there is a predominant trend toward recommendation of close monitoring for reactivation after solid organ or bone marrow transplants, and treatment only if infection is demonstrated, based on the concept that risk of reactivation depends strongly on the degree of immunosuppression.[108]

In the chronic phase, a small prospective non-randomized controlled trial suggested that etiologic treatment may impact favorably on prognosis. It involved 131 patients treated with benznidazole (5 mg/kg/day for 30 days) and 70 untreated patients with a mean follow-up period of eight years; progression of the disease was assessed by ECG changes: treated patients presented fewer ECG changes than control group (4.2% vs 30%) and less deterioration of clinical condition (2.1% vs 17%).[109] More recently the same group reported on a non-randomized, unblinded trial involving 566 patients followed for 10 years; the 283 patients treated with benznidazole (5 mg/kg per day for 30 days) were less likely to develop symptoms, ECG abnormalities, and deterioration of LV function. The study results are limited by missing data during follow-up (20% of patients), the lower than usually recommended treatment dose, and the non-randomized nature of the trial.[110]

Metanalysis of pooled data from observational studies showed that there is insufficient evidence, on the basis of results concerning hard clinical endpoints, to support the use of trypanocidal drugs for the treatment of chronic *T. cruzi* infection, especially if overt heart disease is present.[111] To resolve the current dilemma of treating or not treating adult patients with established CCC with trypanocidal drugs, a multicenter, randomized, placebo-controlled, double-blind study, the BENEFIT trial, is currently under way (http://clinicaltrials.gov/show/NCT00123916).

In asymptomatic patients with chronic Chagas' disease, pooled data derived from a systematic review found only five studies comparing groups of patients submitted to trypanocidal therapy against placebo (Table 51.2).

Table 51.2 General characteristic of randomized clinical trials evaluating trypanocidal therapy in chronic asymptomatic patients with Chagas' disease

Author, country (year)	Participants (% IP)	Interventions (*n* randomized) dose	Outcomes[a] (primary and secondary)
Andrade, Brazil (1996)	School children (90%)	Benznidazole (64) 7.5 mg/kg/day – 8 weeks vs placebo (65)	Seroconversion Antibody changes
Apt, Chile (1998)	Adults (70%)	Allopurinol (187) 8.5 mg/kg/day – 8 weeks vs itraconazole (217) 6 mg/kg/day – 16 weeks vs placebo[b] (165)	Seroconversion *n* positive xenodiagnosis ECG changes Side effects
Coura, Brazil (1997)	Adults (NA)	Benznidazole (26) 5 mg/kg/day – 4 weeks vs nifurtimox (27) 5 mg/kg/day – 4 weeks vs placebo (24)	*n* positive xenodiagnosis
Gianella, Bolívia (1997)	Adults (NA)	Allopurinol (20) 300 mg tid – 8 weeks vs placebo (20)	*n* positive xenodiagnosis
Sosa-Estani, Argentina (1998)	School children (95%)	Benznidazole (55) 5 mg/kg/day – 8 weeks vs placebo (51)	Seroconversion Antibody changes

[a] As stated by the authors in the report.
[b] Participants initially in placebo arm were re-allocated to one of the active arms after two months of treatment.
NA, information not available; IP, indeterminate phase. Reproduced with permission from Villar *et al.*[112]

A metanalysis of these non-randomized data, involving 756 patients, documented that host–parasite indices of disease were favorably modified by trypanocidal treatment but no results concerning hard clinical outcomes were available.[112] The most important finding in this review was that trypanocidal therapy with benznidazole improved parasite-related outcomes especially in children with asymptomatic *T. cruzi* infection, with approximately 60% apparent cure of infection as measured by conversion of Ig/IgG serologic tests to negative 3–4 years after the end of treatment (Fig. 51.3).[112] Another study, not included in the metanalysis, reported respectively 73% and 86% negativation of PCR and xenodiagnosis three years after treatment with nifurtimox in children.[113]

These studies, together with empiric clinical experience across Latin America, provided the basis for the current recommendation that early diagnosis should be sought and trypanocidal therapy implemented for all infected children.[103,114,115]

Key points

- Trypanocidal therapy is universally recommended in acute and congenital Chagas' disease, reactivation of acute infection and in early chronic Chagas' disease (children ≤12 years and people whose duration of infection is known or presumed to be <12 years). **Class I, Level B**
- In patients with chronic Chagas' disease with duration >12 years and no established disease (indeterminate form), treatment decisions must be based on an individual basis, only after thorough clinical assessment and with continuous monitoring of potential side effects. **Class IIa, Level C1**
- Until conclusive data are available, etiologic treatment should be considered optional for adults with remote *T. cruzi* infection and definite but not advanced cardiac manifestations. **Class IIb, Level C1**
- Trypanocidal agents may be administered for prevention of reactivation of infection in high-risk patients (e.g. anticipated immunossupression following organ transplantation recipients). **Class IIb, Level B**
- Treatment is contraindicated for patients with class IV heart failure, advanced megaesophagus before surgical intervention, severe renal and liver disease, and during pregnancy. **Class III, Level C2**

Management of rhythm disturbances

Management of rhythm disturbances in the chagasic patient is empirically similar to that recommended for other cardiomyopathies. However, chagasics patients have peculiar characteristics that may interfere with their treatment and deserve specific mention.

Complex ventricular dysrhythmia is the most important disturbance because of its impact on the risk of sudden death.[94] Data from Holter monitoring have shown that episodes of NSVT are present in approximately 40% of patients with mild wall motion abnormalities and in 90% of those with heart failure, an incidence that is higher than that observed in other cardiomyopathies.[83] Not infrequently, ventricular arrhythmias and atrioventricular conduction abnormalities or sinus node dysfunction co-exist in the same patient.

Sustained monomorphic ventricular tachycardia is another important feature of Chagas' heart disease.[116] It is reproducible during programmed ventricular stimulation in approximately 85% of patients, implying a re-entrant mechanism. The anatomic substrate for re-entrant ventricular tachycardia in CCC is the presence of fibrosis with impaired wall motion that is most frequently located at the LV inferolateral region.[117] Histologic analysis of the inferolateral segments showed non-uniform interstitial fibrosis level intermingled with surviving cardiac fibers arranged in random fashion.[118]

Although there is no evidence from randomized controlled trials that antiarrhythmic drugs prolong life or prevent sudden cardiac death in CCC, the use of empiric amiodarone is recommended as first-choice treatment by the guidelines of the Brazilian Society of Cardiology for patients with sustained and non-sustained ventricular tachycardia, particularly in the presence of myocardial dysfunction.[119] Amiodarone is a potent antiarrhythmic drug that markedly reduces the severity and complexity of ventricular arrhythmias, does not have significant negative inotropic properties, is well tolerated (when administered at low doses), has fewer proarrhythmic effects than class I agents, and may reduce total mortality and sudden cardiac death in patients with Chagas' disease according to some observational data. In a series that compared the survival of 34 patients with Chagas' disease and sustained ventricular tachycardia, treated with amiodarone, with an earlier matched cohort of 42 patients not treated or receiving class I agents, survival rate was significantly greater in the amiodarone group at one year (87 vs 57%), four years (65 vs 22%), and eight years (59 vs 7%).[93] In patients failing empiric amiodarone therapy, electrophysiologic guided antiarrhythmic therapy has been advocated by some authors.[120] Electrophysiologic study can also identify patients who may have a poor prognosis when treated with class III antiarrhythmic drugs and be an important tool for risk stratification and patient selection for implantable cardioverter-defibrillator (ICD) selection.[121] Implantation of a cardioverter-defibrillator has been advocated for patients with refractory and hemodynamically unstable sustained ventricular tachycardia or for survivors of sudden cardiac death.[122] In order to reduce frequent shocks, antiarrhythmic drug therapy is required in most patients because of the high prevalence of ambient atrial and ventricular arrhythmias.[88] However, there are no properly

I – Incidence of ECG abnormalities/ BZD - children

Study	BZD (n/N)	Plac (n/N)	Weight %	OR (95% CI)
Andrade	1/59	4/58	71	0.28 (0.05-1.69)
Sosa-Estani	1/40	1/41	29	1.03 (0.06-16.99)
Total	2/99	5/99	100	0.41 (0.09-1.85)

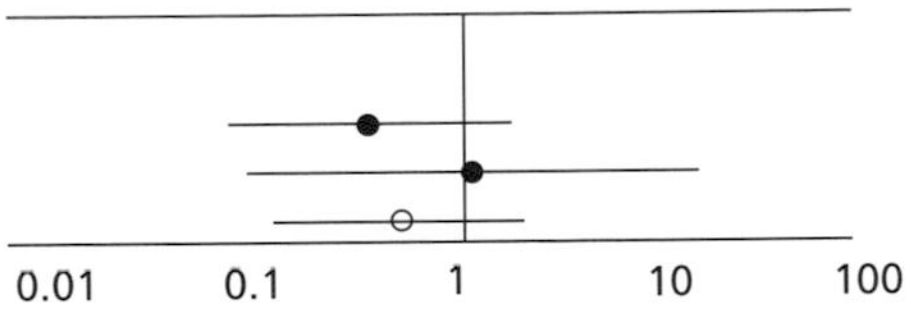

Heterogeneity test $\chi^2 = 0.58$ P = 0.45/Overall effect test Z=1.16 P = 0.2

II – Negative seroconversion/BZD – AT ELISA – children

Study	BZD (n/N)	Plac (n/N)	Weight %	OR (95% CI)
Andrade	37/58	3/54	57.8	12.35 (5.72-26.00)
Sosa-Estani	24/44	3/44	42.2	9.19 (3.73-22.64)
Total	61/102	6/98	100	10.91 (6.07-19.58)

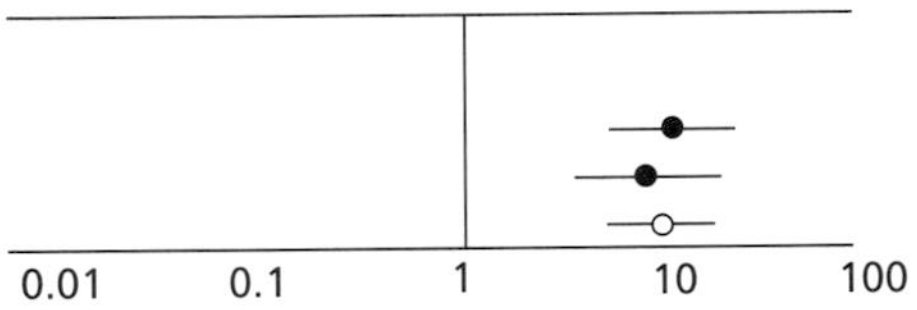

Heterogeneity test $\chi^2 = 0.24$ P = 0.63/Overall effect test Z=8.0 P = 0<0.001

III – Positive xenodiagnosis/all tests/All Avaliable studies

Study	BZD (n/N)	Plac (n/N)	Weight %	OR (95% CI)
Apt	22/336	9/165	32.6	1.21 (0.56-2.61)
Coura	10/193	23/67	28.0	0.07 (0.03-0.17)
Gianella	12/33	17/23	17.4	0.23 (0.08-0.66)
Sosa-Estani	2/42	22/43	22.0	0.10 (0.04-0.27)
Total	46/604	71/298	100	0.24 (0.15-0.37)

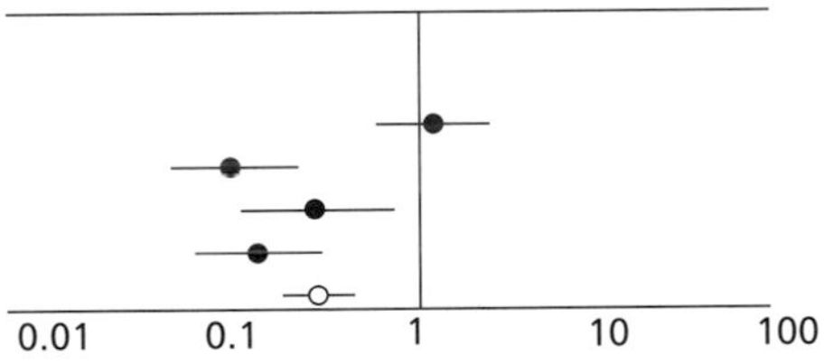

Heterogeneity test $\chi^2 = 27.72$ P <0.001/Overall effect test Z=-6.35 P = 0<0.001

IV – Antibody titers mean differences /All Avaliable studies (IIF)

Study (Weight %)	n TT/n Plac (Weight %)	All TT mean (sd)	Plac mean (sd)	SMD (95% CI)
Andrade	58/54 (48.4)	-1409 (1052)	-566 (1400)	0.68 (-1.06- - 0.30)
Gianella	13/17 (13.5)	-19.7 (317.5)	-30.1 (234.7)	0.04 (0.69-0.76)
Sosa-Estani	44/44 (38.1)	-1.40 (2.31)	0.17 (2.40)	-0.66 (-1.09- - 0.23)
Total	115/115 (100)			-0.58 (-0.84-0.31)

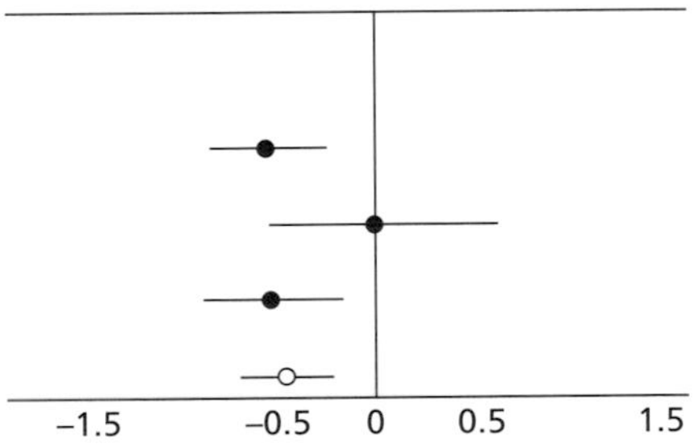

Heterogeneity test $\chi^2 = 3.20$ P =0.20/Overall effect test Z=-4.25 P <0.001

Figure 51.3 Overview of the effect, estimates for data on four outcomes pooled. Estimates are expressed as odds rations or standardized mean differences (SMD) and 95% confidence intervals using the fixed models statistical approach (95% CI fixed). Antibodies mean changes are given in the units originally reported by authors. A negative sign means reduction of levels after being treated. Adapted from Villar et al[112] with permission.

randomized controlled trials to ascertain whether pharmacologic or device therapy improves survival in CCC patients. Such a trial should urgently be conducted, and the indications for ICD therapy in patients with CCC should not be extrapolated from the results of randomized studies obtained in patients with other conditions, such as coronary artery disease or idiopathic dilated cardiomyopathy.[123]

Aneurysmectomy,[124] surgical ablation, transcoronary chemical ablation[125] and epicardial/endocardial catheter ablation[118,126] have been attempted in few patients, but neither efficacy nor impact on survival and arrhythmia recurrence is established.

Severe bradyarrhythmias are treated with pacemakers, as in other cardiac conditions, but the electrode should be placed in the subtricuspid area, not in the right ventricular apex, because apical fibrosis is common and may cause capture failure. The evidence for benefit of pacemaker implantation comes from limited case series reports with historic control series of patients in whom this treatment was not possible.[94]

The common association of sinus node or atrioventricular disturbances and ventricular complex dysrhythmia in the same patient may require pacemaker implantation associated with pharmacologic antiarrhythmic therapy. This management is regarded as prophylactic, although not based on unquestionable evidence.

In the later stages of CCC, with marked cardiac enlargement and heart failure, atrial fibrillation is common but the ventricular rate usually is not elevated because of conduction disturbances.

> ### Key points
>
> - Pharmacologic, surgical, and device-based strategies for the treatment of ventricular dysrhythmia in chagasic patients are empirical and not supported by any large randomized, controlled trial. **Level C2**

Treatment of congestive heart failure

Hemodynamic derangement in chronic chagasic patients with heart failure is similar to that reported in dilated cardiomyopathies of other etiologies. However, there are some peculiarities in the pathophysiology of CCC that may have therapeutic implications. For instance, there is usually marked predominance of systemic congestive manifestations over the pulmonary congestion symptoms and signs. Also, chagasic patients have striking conduction disturbances and tend to have symptomatic bradycardia, that may be aggravated with the use of digoxin, amiodarone, and beta-blockers. Congestive heart failure usually responds to routine management, including sodium restriction,

diuretics, digitalis, and angiotensin-converting enzyme (ACE) inhibitors. For patients with severe cardiac failure, higher doses of diuretics are usually necessary. Small observational studies have documented short-term hemodynamic beneficial effects of these agents and, to a lesser extent, improvement in exercise tolerance in chronic chagasic patients. However, no studies reported improvement in long-term hemodynamic or any hard clinical outcomes.

A prospective multicenter non-controlled trial assessed the impact of adding an ACE inhibitor to conventional therapy in 115 patients with heart failure (of whom 20 were chagasics). At the end of 12 weeks, irrespective of etiology, the NYHA functional class was significantly improved in most patients (85.2%).[127]

A single-blind, cross-over trial of ACE inhibitor and placebo for six weeks each, with a washout period of two weeks, was reported on 18 NYHA class IV chagasic patients.[128] Treatment with ACE inhibitor was associated with significant reduction in neurohumoral activation and amelioration of ventricular arrhythmias. These results indicate a potentially beneficial role for this class of drugs in controlling mechanisms triggering sudden death.

In a recent small trial designed to test the effect of beta-blocker therapy in addition to inhibition of the renin-angiotensin-aldosterone system, 42 chagasic patients NYHA classes I–III received enalapril (up-titrated to 20 mg bid) and spironolactone (25 mg qd).[129] The renin-angiotensin-aldosterone system inhibition was associated with improvement of quality of life score and reduction of neurohumoral activation assessed by brain natriuretic peptide (BNP) levels. Subsequently, 19 patients were randomly assigned to receive carvedilol (up-titrated to 25 mg bid) and 20 patients were allocated to placebo. Beta-blockade with carvedilol was associated to a trend toward LV ejection fraction (EF) increase, and was hemodynamically well tolerated, with no symptomatic bradycardia.

Thus, there is only very limited evidence suggesting benefit of drugs which reduce neurohormonal activation in Chagas' heart disease patients. No long-term controlled study has assessed the impact on survival of chagasic patients treated with ACE inhibitors, spironolactone or beta-blockers. Spironolactone is a theoretically attractive therapy because of the major role that cardiac fibrosis plays in the disease as well as the right heart failure. A randomized double-blind placebo-controlled study has been planned (CHARITY study) to investigate the impact of bisoprolol in a cohort of 500 patients with heart failure secondary to CCC (250 patients per arm), with a follow-up of two years.[130]

Surgical treatment

Procedures such as dynamic cardiomyoplasty and partial left ventriculectomy (Batista's surgery) are now abandoned and LV geometric reconstruction with apical aneurysmectomy is rarely indicated for chagasic patients. Severe mitral regurgitation, secondary to chamber dilation and to dysynergy of the posterior-inferior wall, contributes frequently to heart failure worsening. A recent retrospective report from a single center in Brazil showed promising results of the implantation of mitral prosthesis in 116 heart failure patients (three being chagasics).[131]

Cardiac transplantation has been performed in small series of patients with refractory heart failure due to CCC. However, transplantation is limited by socioeconomic factors in areas where the disease is endemic and by problems related to the obligatory immunosuppression. Chagas' disease reactivation with acute myocarditis and marked transitory LV systolic depression has previously been reported in small case series as a frequent complication in patients receiving the usual high dose of ciclosporin therapy.[76] Although the reactivation of infection was usually responsive to antiparasite therapy, the possibility of definitive damage to the allograft could not be ruled out and early concern was raised that this could represent a severe limitation or even a contraindication for heart transplantation in Chagas' disease. Nevertheless, the use of immunosuppression regimen with reduced ciclosporin dosing was reported to be effective in circumventing this limitation and the prophylactic treatment of the organ receptor with trypanocidal drugs previous to transplantation was considered not necessary.[105] However, a recent report indicated the occurrence of reactivation during the use of the new immunosuppressant, mycophenolate mofetil.[132]

The long-term impact of heart transplantation in chagasic patients has been described in a subgroup of a large cohort of 792 patients submitted to orthotopic heart transplantation in 16 centers in Brazil.[133] The mean overall follow-up period was 2.87 ± 3.0 years, and 117 patients with chronic CCC constituted the subgroup. The entire cohort population also included 407 patients with idiopathic dilated cardiomyopathy and 196 with ischemic heart disease. Among chagasic patients the reported criteria and contraindication for transplantation were similar to those used for non-chagasic patients, except for the detection of megacolon or megaesophagus, also considered a contraindication for transplantation. The survival rate of Chagas' disease patients at one and 12 years was respectively 76% and 46%. These survival rates were statistically better in comparison with the rest of the cohort group in which the respective survival rates were 72% and 27%. Reactivation of T. cruzi infection with myocarditis and meningoencephalitis was rarely reported, and was the cause of death in only 0.3% for the entire chagasic cohort.

A recent retrospective survey from a single center in Brazil reported on the later follow-up after cardiac transplantation, with average of 44.4 ± 55.2 months, in 285 patients of whom 59 had Chagas' disease. The late survival rates were similar in chagasic and non-chagasic patients. The reported T. cruzi infection reactivation rate in the initial 10 patients (with conventional ciclosporin dose regimen) was 2.3 episodes per patient. This rate was reduced to 0.25 episodes per patients in the subsequent series of patients for whom the ciclosporin dose was reduced.[105]

Even allowing for the poor control of other relevant characteristics of chagasic and non-chagasic patients in these retrospective observations, the limited available data suggest that heart transplantation is a valid therapeutic option in end-stage CCC, with an expected survival rate at least comparable to that of other patients.

Multisite pacing – cardiac resynchronization

This form of therapy is being widely used for treating chagasic patients, without any supporting evidence of benefit. In fact, there are several concerns about the use of cardiac resynchronization therapy in Chagas' disease patients that need to be resolved before any recommendation can be established. For instance, dysynergy caused by extensive fibrosis is likely to hamper resynchronizing. Also, QRS prolongation in chagasic patients are frequently related to right bundle branch block, and the effect of resynchronization in this setting has not been established.

Stem cell therapy

Preliminary preclinical studies in murine models suggest potential benefit of stem cell therapy in CCC.[134] Two months after treatment a significant reduction in inflammation and fibrosis was seen in recipients of the cell therapy compared to control untreated animals. Another recent observation demonstrated improvement of LV function four weeks after implantation of co-cultured mesenchymal stem cells and skeletal myoblasts in rats.[135]

To date, only one small non-randomized non-controlled clinical study reported the early results of bone marrow cell transplantation delivered by intracoronary injection in 28 chagasic patients with NYHA class III–IV heart failure. A significant increase in LV ejection fraction, assessed by echocardiography, was observed at 60 days after treatment when compared to baseline value (23.0 ± 9.0% vs 20.1 ± 6.8%, $P = 0.02$).[136] There was also improvement of symptoms and functional capacity. However, more studies are needed before this type of treatment can be recommended. A randomized placebo-controlled clinical trial, sponsored by the Brazilian Ministry of Health, is currently ongoing and will test the efficacy of autologous bone marrow derived mononuclear cell therapies in 300 patients with Chagas' heart disease.[137]

Prevention of thromboembolic events

There is very limited clinical information on the risk of embolism in patients with mural thrombosis or apical aneurysm. A recent study enrolled 305 patients to describe predictors of stroke in various cardiopathies, in a region where Chagas' disease is endemic.[138] Stroke was present in 32 (10.5%) patients, more commonly in chagasics (15.0%) than in other cardiopathies (6.3%; $P = 0.015$). At multivariate analysis only Chagas' disease, cardioversion and diabetes mellitus were predictors of stroke. A prospective cohort study in 1043 chronic chagasic patients found a global incidence of stroke of 5.6 per 1000 person-years. The mortality associated with the acute event was high (19.4%) and the five-year survival was 45%. Only the presence of cardiomyopathy by echocardiographic or radiologic criteria correlated with the occurrence of events.[139]

Because of the high incidence of thromboembolic phenomena in CCC, anticoagulants are recommended for patients with atrial fibrillation, previous embolism, and apical aneurysm with thrombus, even in the absence of controlled clinical trials demonstrating their efficacy. However, poor social and economic factors may limit the implementation of this therapy, because of the increased risk of bleeding. The use of small doses of acetylsalicylic acid could be a reasonable alternative for these patients.[140]

Figure 51.4 summarizes the cardiovascular interventions useful for the management of various stages of Chagas' heart disease (see Table 51.1 for an explanation of the stages of heart involvement in Chagas' disease).

Prevention

Preventive measures aiming at minimization of the medical and social burden imposed by Chagas' disease include interventions:

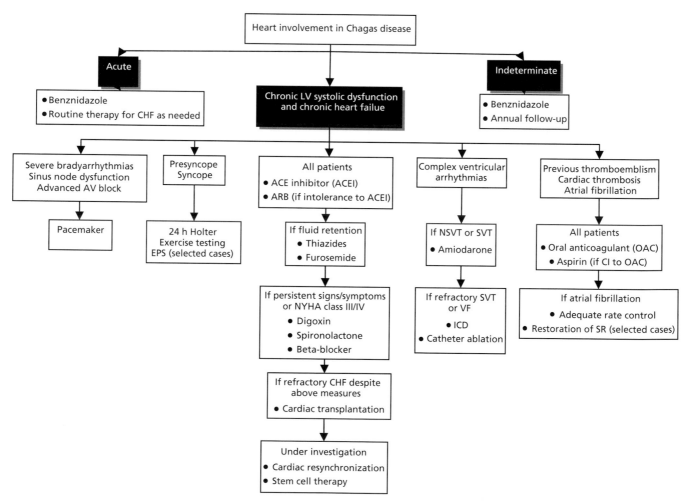

Figure 51.4 Treatment algorithm for patients with Chagas' disease. This treatment algorithm represents a summary of the main options available, which are usually empiric and not supported by large randomized controlled trials. ACEI, angiotensin-converting enzyme inhibitor; AV, atrioventricular; CHF, congestive heart failure; CI, contraindication; EPS, electrophysiologic study; ICD, implantable cardioverter-defibrillator; LV, left ventricular; NSVT, non-sustained ventricular tachycardia; NYHA, New York Heart Association; OAC, oral anticoagulant; SR, sinus rhythm; SVT, sustained ventricular tachycardia; VF, ventricular fibrillation.

- designed to prevent the transmission of the disease – primary prevention. The focus of this set of interventions is on the control of vectoral and blood transmission of the infection
- to reduce the chance of developing clinical illness (i.e. to prevent or inhibit disease in cases where infection has occurred) – secondary prevention, which includes trypanocidal therapy, aiming at eradication of *T. cruzi* not only to possibly prevent chronic organ damage, but also to interfere with the epidemiologic chain
- designed to limit human incapacity and to prevent morbidity and mortality, once disease has occurred – tertiary prevention.

References

1. Chagas C. Über eine neue Trypanosomiasis des Menschen. *Band XIII* 1909;5–7.
2. Chagas C, Vilella E. Cardiac form of American trypanosomiasis. *Mem Inst Oswaldo Cruz* 1922;**14**:5–61.
3. Laranja FS, Dias E, Nobrega G, Miranda A. Chagas' disease: a clinical, epidemiologic and pathologic study. *Circulation* 1956;**14**:1035–59.
4. Prata A. Clinical and epidemiological aspects of Chagas' disease. *Lancet Infect Dis* 2001;**1**:92–100.
5. Rassi A Jr, Rassi A, Little WC. Chagas' heart disease. *Clin Cardiol* 2000;**23**:883–9.
6. Dias JCP. The indeterminate form of human chronic Chagas' disease: a clinical epidemiological review. *Rev Soc Bras Med Trop* 1989;**22**:147–56.
7. First Annual Meeting of Applied Research in Chagas' Disease. Araxá MG. 1984. *Rev Soc Bras Med Trop* 1985;**18**:46.
8. Barreto ACP, Ianni BM. The undetermined form of Chagas' heart disease: concept and forensic implications. *São Paulo Med J* 1995;**13**:797–801.
9. Barreto ACP, Arteaga-Fernandez E. RV endomyocardial biopsy in chronic Chagas' disease. *Am Heart J* 1986;**111**:307–12.
10. Marin-Neto JA, Bromberg-Marin G, Pazin-Filho A, Simões MV, Maciel BC. Cardiac autonomic impairment and early myocardial damage involving the right ventricle are independent phenomena in Chagas' disease *Int J Cardiol* 1998;**65**:261–9.
11. Almeida-Filho OC, Maciel BC, Schmidt A, Pazin-Filho A, Marin-Neto JA. Minor segmental dyssynergy reflects extensive myocardial damage and global left ventricle dysfunction in chronic Chagas disease. *J Am Soc Echocardiogr* 2002;**156**:610–16.
12. Pazin-Filho A, Romano MM, Almeida-Filho OC *et al.* Minor segmental wall motion abnormalities detected in patients with Chagas' disease have adverse prognostic implications. *Braz J Med Biol Res* 2006;**394**:483–7.
13. Marin-Neto JA, Almeida Filho OC, Pazin-Filho A, Maciel BC. [Indeterminate form of Chagas' disease. Proposal of new diagnostic criteria and perspectives for early treatment of cardiomyopathy]. *Arq Bras Cardiol* 2002;**796**:623–7.
14. Bern C, Montgomery SP, Herwaldt BL *et al.* Evaluation and treatment of Chagas disease in the United States: a systematic review. *JAMA* 2007;**29818**:2171–81.
15. Kirchhoff LV. Changing epidemiology and approaches to therapy for Chagas disease. *Curr Infect Dis Rep* 2003;**51**:59–65.
16. Organizacion Panamericana de la Salud. Estimacion cuantitativa de la enfermedad de Chagas en las Americas. Montevideo, Uruguay: Organizacion Panamericana de la Salud, 2006:425–506.
17. Moncayo A, Ortiz Yanine MI. An update on Chagas disease human American trypanosomiasis. *Ann Trop Med Parasitol* 2006;**1008**:663–77.
18. Control of Chagas disease. *World Health Organ Tech Rep Ser* 2002;**905**:i-109.
19. Coura JR, Junqueira AC, Fernandes O, Valente SA, Miles MA. Emerging Chagas disease in Amazonian Brazil. *Trends Parasitol* 2002;**184**:171–6.
20. Hagar JM, Rahimtoola SH. Chagas' heart disease. *Curr Probl Cardiol* 1995;**2012**:825–924.
21. Leiby DA, Read EJ, Lenes BA *et al.* Seroepidemiology of Trypanosoma cruzi, etiologic agent of Chagas' disease, in US blood donors. *J Infect Dis* 1997;**1764**:1047–52.
22. Garraud O, Andreu G, Elghouzzi MH, Laperche S, Lefrere JJ. Measures to prevent transfusion-associated protozoal infections in non-endemic countries. *Travel Med Infect Dis* 2007;**52**:110–12.
23. Herwaldt BL, Grijalva MJ, Newsome AL *et al.* Use of polymerase chain reaction to diagnose the fifth reported US case of autochthonous transmission of Trypanosoma cruzi, in Tennessee, 1998. *J Infect Dis* 2000;**1811**:395–9.
24. Blood donor screening for chagas disease – United States, 2006–2007. *MMWR* 2007;**567**:141–3.
25. Dias JC, Silveira AC, Schofield CJ. The impact of Chagas disease control in Latin America: a review. *Mem Inst Oswaldo Cruz* 2002;**975**:603–12.
26. Morel CM, Lazdins J. Chagas disease. *Nat Rev Microbiol* 2003;**11**:14–15.
27. Miles MA, Cedillos RA, Povoa MM, de Souza AA, Prata A, Macedo V. Do radically dissimilar Trypanosoma cruzi strains zymodemes. cause Venezuelan and Brazilian forms of Chagas' disease. *Lancet* 1981;**8234**:1338–40.
28. Rassi A Jr, Rassi A, Rassi SG. Predictors of mortality in chronic Chagas disease: a systematic review of observational studies. *Circulation* 2007;**1159**:1101–8.
29. Dias JCP. Cardiopatia chagásica: história natural. In: Cançado JR, Chuster M (eds) Cardiopatia Chagásica. Belo Horizonte: Fundação Carlos Chagas de Pesquisa Médica, 1985.
30. Rassi A, Rassi A Jr, Rassi GG. Fase aguda. In: Brener Z, Andrade ZA, Barral-Netto M (eds) Trypanosoma cruzi e Doença de Chagas. Rio de Janeiro: Guanabara Koogan SA, 2000.
31. Benchimol Barbosa PR. The oral transmission of Chagas' disease: an acute form of infection responsible for regional outbreaks. *Int J Cardiol* 2006;**1121**:132–3.
32. Forichon E. Contribution aux Estimations de Morbidité et de Mortalité dans la Maladie de Chagas. Toulouse: Universiter Paul-Sabatier, 1974.
33. Puigbó JJ, Rhode JRN, Barrios HG, Yépez CG. A 4-year follow up study of a rural community with endemic Chagas' disease. *Bull WHO* 1968;**39**:341–8.
34. Mota EA, Guimaraes AC, Santana OO, Sherlock I, Hoff R, Weller TH. A nine year prospective study of Chagas' disease in

a defined rural population in northeast Brazil. *Am J Trop Med Hyg* 1990;**425**:429–40.

35. Ianni BM, Arteaga E, Frimm CC, Pereira Barretto AC, Mady C. Chagas' heart disease: evolutive evaluation of electrocardiographic and echocardiographic parameters in patients with the indeterminate form. *Arq Bras Cardiol* 2001;**771**:59–62.

36. Viotti R, Vigliano C, Lococo B *et al.* [Clinical predictors of chronic chagasic myocarditis progression]. *Rev Esp Cardiol* 2005;**589**:1037–44.

37. Manzullo EC, Chuit R. Risk of death due to chronic chagasic cardiopathy. *Mem Inst Oswaldo Cruz* 1999;**94**(suppl 1):317–20.

38. Maguire JH, Hoff R, Sherlock I *et al.* Cardiac morbidity and mortality due to Chagas' disease: prospective electrocardiographic study of a Brazilian community. *Circulation* 1987;**756**:1140–5.

39. Espinosa R, Carrasco HA, Belandria F *et al.* Life expectancy analysis in patients with Chagas' disease: prognosis after one decade 1973–1983. *Int J Cardiol* 1985;**81**:45–56.

40. Pugliese C, Lessa I, Santos FA. [Survival of decompensated chronic Chagas' myocardiopathy]. *Rev Inst Med Trop Sao Paulo* 1976;**183**:191–201.

41. Mady C, Cardoso RH, Barretto AC, da Luz PL, Bellotti G, Pileggi F. Survival and predictors of survival in patients with congestive heart failure due to Chagas' cardiomyopathy. *Circulation* 1994;**906**:3098–102.

42. Hagar JM, Rahimtoola SH. Chagas' heart disease in the United States. *N Engl J Med* 1991;**3251**:763–8.

43. de Paola AA, Gomes JA, Terzian AB, Miyamoto MH, Martinez Fo EE. Ventricular tachycardia during exercise testing as a predictor of sudden death in patients with chronic chagasic cardiomyopathy and ventricular arrhythmias. *Br Heart J* 1995;**743**:293–5.

44. Rassi A Jr, Rassi A, Little WC *et al.* Development and validation of a risk score for predicting death in Chagas' heart disease. *N Engl J Med* 2006;**3558**:799–808.

45. Marin-Neto JA, Cunha-Neto E, Maciel BC, Simoes MV. Pathogenesis of chronic Chagas heart disease. *Circulation* 2007;**1159**:1109–23.

46. Higuchi ML. Chronic chagasic cardiopathy: the product of a turbulent host-parasite relationship. *Rev Inst Med Trop São Paulo* 1997;**39**:53–60.

47. Köberle F. Chagas' heart disease and Chagas' syndromes: the pathology of American trypanosomiasis. *Adv Parasitol* 1968;**6**:63–116.

48. Lopes ER, Tafuri WL. Involvement of the autonomic nervous system in Chagas' heart disease. *Rev Soc Bras Med Trop* 1983;**16**:206–11.

49. Amorim DS, Manço JC, Gallo L Jr, Marin-Neto JA. Chagas' heart disease as an experimental model for studies of cardiac autonomic function in man. *Mayo Clin Proc* 1982;**57**:48–60.

50. Marin-Neto JA, Maciel BC, Gallo L Jr, Junqueira LF Jr, Amorim DS. Effect of parasympathetic impairment on the hemodynamic response to handgrip in Chagas' heart disease. *Br Heart J* 1986;**55**:204–8.

51. Amorim DS, Marin-Neto JA. Functional alterations of the autonomic nervous system in Chagas' heart disease. *São Paulo Med J* 1995;**113**:772–84.

52. Simões MV, Pintya AO, Bromberg-Marin G *et al.* Relation of regional sympathetic denervation and myocardial perfusion disturbances to wall motion impairment in Chagas' cardiomyopathy. *Am J Cardiol* 2000;**869**:975–81.

53. Oliveira JSM. A natural human model of intrinsic heart nervous system denervation: Chagas' cardiopathy. *Mem Inst Oswaldo Cruz* 1996;**91**:2117–24.

54. Rossi MA, Carobrez SG. Experimental Trypanosoma cruzi cardiomyopathy in BALB/c mice: histochemical evidence of hypoxic changes in the myocardium. *Br J Exp Pathol* 1985;**662**:155–60.

55. Factor SM, Cho S, Wittner M, Tanowitz H. Abnormalities of the coronary microcirculation in acute murine Chagas' disease. *Am J Trop Med Hyg* 1985;**342**:246–53.

56. Morris SA, Weiss LM, Factor SM, Bilezikian JP, Tanowitz HB, Wittner M. Verapamil ameliorates clinical, pathological and biochemical manifestations of the experimental chagasic cardiomyopathy in mice. *J Am Coll Cardiol* 1989;**14**:782–9.

57. Ferrans VJ, Milei J, Tomita Y, Storino RA. Basement membrane thickening in cardiac myocytes and capillaries in chronic Chagas' disease. *Am J Cardiol* 1988;**6113**:1137–40.

58. Morris SA, Tanowitz HB, Wittner M, Bilezikian JP. Pathophysiological insights into the cardiomyopathy of Chagas' disease. *Circulation* 1990;**826**:1900–9.

59. Rossi MA. Microvascular changes as a cause of chronic cardiomyopathy in Chagas' disease. *Am Heart J* 1990;**120**:233–6.

60. Marin-Neto JA, Marzullo P, Marcassa C *et al.* Myocardial perfusion abnormalities in chronic Chagas' disease. Assessment with thallium-201 scintigraphy. *Am J Cardiol* 1992;**69**:780–4.

61. Hiss FC, Lascala TF, Maciel BC, Marin-Neto JA, Simões MV. Changes in myocardial perfusion correlate with deterioration of left ventricular systolic function in chronic Chagas' cardiomyopathy. *Am Coll Cardiol Img* 2009;**2**:164–72.

62. Andrade ZA, Andrade SG, Sadigursky M *et al.* The indeterminate phase of Chagas' disease: ultrastructural characterization of cardiac changes in the canine model. *Am J Trop Med Hyg* 1997;**57**:328–36.

63. Lopes ER, Chapadeiro E, Andrade ZA, Almeida HO, Rocha A. [Pathological anatomy of hearts from asymptomatic Chagas disease patients dying in a violent manner]. *Mem Inst Oswaldo Cruz* 1981;**762**:189–97.

64. Carrasco-Guerra HA, Palacios-Pru E, Dagert de Scorza C *et al.* Clinical histochemical and ultrastructural correlation in septal endomyocardial biopsies from chronic chagasic patients. *Am Heart J* 1987;**113**:716–24.

65. Ben Younes-Chennoufi A, Hontebeyrie-Joskowicz M, Tricottet V *et al.* Persistence of Trypanosoma cruzi antigens in the inflammatory lesions of chronically infected mice. *Trans Roy Soc Trop Med Hyg* 1988;**82**:77–83.

66. Franco MF. Experimental carditis induced by Trypanosoma cruzi strain in guinea pigs: correlation between histopathology and the presence of T. cruzi antigens identified by indirect immunofluorescence. *Rev Soc Bras Med* 1990;**3**:187–9.

67. Higuchi ML, Brito T, Reis MM *et al.* Correlation between T. cruzi parasitism and myocardial inflammation in human chronic chagasic myocarditis: light microscopy and immunohistochemical findigns. *Cardiovasc Pathol* 1993;**2**:101–6.

68. Bellotti G, Bocchi EA, de Moraes AV *et al.* In vivo detection of Trypanosoma cruzi antigens in hearts of patients with chronic Chagas' heart disease. *Am Heart J* 1996;**1312**:301–7.

69. Jones EM, Colley DG, Tostes S, Lopes ER, Vnencak-Jones CL, McCurley TL. Amplification of a Trypanosoma cruzi DNA sequence from inflammatory lesions in human chagasic cardiomyopathy. *Am J Trop Med Hyg* 1993;**483**:348–57.

70. Añez N, Carrasco H, Parada H *et al.* Myocardial parasite persistence in chronic chagasic patients. *Am J Trop Med Hyg* 1999;**60**:726–32.

71. Andrade SG, Stocker-Guerret S, Pimentel AS, Grimaud JA. Reversibility of cardiac fibrosis in mice chronically infected with Trypanosoma cruzi, under specific chemotherapy. *Mem Inst Oswaldo Cruz* 1991;**862**:187–200.

72. Garcia S, Ramos CO, Senra JFV *et al.* Treatment with benznidazole during the chronic phase of experimental Chagas' disease decreases cardiac alterations. *Antimicrob Agents Chemother* 2005;**49**:1521–8.

73. Andrade ZA, Andrade SG, Sadigursky M. Enhancement of chronic Trypanosoma cruzi myocarditis in dogs treated with low doses of cyclophosphamide. *Am J Pathol* 1987;**1273**:467–73.

74. Silva JS, Rossi MA. Intensification of acute Trypanosoma cruzi myocarditis in BALB/c mice pretreated with low doses of cyclophosphamide or gamma irradiation. *J Exp Pathol Oxford* 1990;**711**:33–9.

75. Okumura M, Mester M, Iriya K, Amato N, V, Gama-Rodrigues J. Effects of immunosuppression and benzonidazole on Trypanosoma cruzi parasitism during experimental acute Chagas' disease. *Transplant Proc* 1994;**263**:1587–9.

76. Bocchi EA, Bellotti G, Mocelin AO *et al.* Heart transplantation for chronic Chagas' heart disease. *Ann Thorac Surg* 1996;**616**:1727–33.

77. Harms G, Feldmeier II. The impact of HIV infection on tropical diseases. *Infect Dis Clin North Am* 2005;**191**:121–35, ix.

78. Rassi A, Amato N, de Siqueira AF *et al.* [The influence of corticoids, in Chronic Chagas disease, administered in virtue of associated disorders]. *Rev Soc Bras Med Trop* 1997;**302**:93–9.

79. Simoes MV, Soares FA, Marin-Neto JA. Severe myocarditis and esophagitis during reversible long standing Chagas' disease recrudescence in immunocompromised host. *Int J Cardiol* 1995;**493**:271–3.

80. Andrade ZA. Immunopathology of Chagas disease. *Mem Inst Oswaldo Cruz* 1999;**94**(suppl 1):71–80.

81. Higuchi MD, Gutierrez PS, Aiello VD *et al.* Immunohistochemical characterization of infiltrating cells in human chronic chagasic myocarditis: comparison with myocardial rejection process. *Virchows Arch A Pathol Anat Histopathol* 1993;**423**:157–60.

82. Cunha-Neto E, Bilate AM, Hyland KV, Fonseca SG, Kalil J, Engman DM. Induction of cardiac autoimmunity in Chagas heart disease: a case for molecular mimicry. *Autoimmunity* 2006;**391**:41–54.

83. Simoes MV, Nonino A, Simoes BP, Almeida-Filho OC, Maciel BC, Marin-Neto JA. [Reagudization of Chagas myocarditis inducing exclusive right ventricular failure]. *Arq Bras Cardiol* 1994;**626**:435–7.

84. Gallo L Jr, Marin-Neto JA, Manço JC, Rassi A, Amorim DS. Abnormal heart rate responses during exercise in patients with Chagas' disease. *Cardiology* 1975;**60**:147–62.

85. Simoes MV, Dantas RO, Ejima FH, Meneghelli UG, Maciel BC, Marin-Neto JA. [Esophageal origin of precordial pain in chagasic patients with normal subepicardial coronary arteries]. *Arq Bras Cardiol* 1995;**642**:103–8.

86. Marin-Neto JA, Simões MV, Ayres-Neto EM *et al.* Studies of the coronary circulation in Chagas' heart disease. *São Paulo Med J* 1995;**113**:826–34.

87. Maciel BC, Almeida Filho OC, Schmidt A, Marin-Neto JA. Ventricular function in Chagas' heart disease. *Sao Paulo Med J* 1995;**1132**:814–20.

88. Rassi JA, Gabriel RA, Gabriel RS, Rassi JL, Rassi A. [Ventricular arrhythmia in Chagas disease. Diagnostic, prognostic, and therapeutic features]. *Arq Bras Cardiol* 1995;**654**:377–87.

89. Oliveira JSM, Araújo RRC, Mucillo G. Cardiac thrombosis and thromboembolism in chronic Chagas' heart disease. *Am J Cardiol* 1983;**52**:147–51.

90. Oliveira JS, Mello De Oliveira JA, Frederigue U Jr, Lima Filho EC. Apical aneurysm of Chagas's heart disease. *Br Heart J* 1981;**464**:432–7.

91. Marin-Neto JA, Andrade ZA. [Why is there predominance of right heart failure in Chagas' disease?] *Arq Bras Cardiol* 1991;**573**:181–3.

92. Prata A, Andrade Z, Guimarães AC. Chagas' heart disease. In: Shaper AG, Hutt MSR, Fejfar Z (eds) Cardiovascular Disease in the Tropics. London: British Medical Association, 1974.

93. Marin-Neto JA, Sousa AC, Maciel BC, Gallo JL, Iazigi N. [Radionuclide angiocardiographic evaluation of the effect of isosorbide dinitrate in patients with Chagas' disease]. *Arq Bras Cardiol* 1988;**515**:367–71.

94. Rassi A Jr, Rassi SG, Rassi A. Sudden death in Chagas' disease. *Arq Bras Cardiol* 2001;**76**:75–96.

95. Lopes ER. Sudden death in patients with Chagas disease. *Mem Inst Oswaldo Cruz* 1999;**94**(suppl 1):321–4.

96. Ribeiro AL, Moraes RS, Ribeiro JP *et al.* Parasympathetic dysautonomia precedes left ventricular systolic dysfunction in Chagas disease. *Am Heart J* 2001;**1412**:260–5.

97. Consolim-Colombo FM, Filho JA, Lopes HF *et al.* Decreased cardiopulmonary baroreflex sensitivity in Chagas' heart disease. *Hypertension* 2000;**366**:1035–9.

98. Soares Barreto-Filho JA, Consolim-Colombo FM, Ferreira LH, Martins Sobrinho CR, Guerra-Riccio GM, Krieger EM. Dysregulation of peripheral and central chemoreflex responses in Chagas' heart disease patients without heart failure. *Circulation* 2001;**1041**:1792–8.

99. Docampo R. Recent developments in the chemotherapy of Chagas disease. *Curr Pharm Des* 2001;**712**:1157–64.

100. Rassi A, Ferreira HO. Tentativas de tratamento especifico da fase aguda da doenca de Chagas com nifurtimox em esquema de duracao prolongada. *Rev Soc Bras Med Trop* 1971;**5**:235–62.

101. Borges-Pereira J, Junqueira AC, Santos LC, de Castro JA, de Araujo IB, Coura JR. [Xenodiagnosis in chronic Chagas' disease. I. The sensitivity of Panstrongylus megistus and Triatoma infestans]. *Rev Soc Bras Med Trop* 1996;**294**:341–7.

102. Britto C, Cardoso MA, Ravel C *et al.* Trypanosoma cruzi: parasite detection and strain discrimination in chronic chagasic patients from northeastern Brazil using PCR amplification of kinetoplast DNA and nonradioactive hybridization. *Exp Parasitol* 1995;**814**:462–71.

103. Rassi A, Luquetti AO. Specific treatment for *Trypanosoma cruzi* infection Chagas disease. In: Tyler KM, Miles MA (eds) American Trypanosomiasis. Boston: Kluwer Academic Publishers, 2003: 117–25.

104. Sartori AM, Ibrahim KY, Nunes Westphalen EV *et al.* Manifestations of Chagas disease American trypanosomiasis in patients with HIV/AIDS. *Ann Trop Med Parasitol* 2007;**1011**:31–50.

105. Fiorelli AI, Stolf NA, Honorato R *et al.* Later evolution after cardiac transplantation in Chagas' disease. *Transplant Proc* 2005;**376**:2793–8.

106. Maldonado C, Albano S, Vettorazzi L *et al.* Using polymerase chain reaction in early diagnosis of re-activated Trypanosoma cruzi infection after heart transplantation. *J Heart Lung Transplant* 2004;**2312**:1345–8.

107. Rassi A, Amato N, V, de Siqueira AF, Ferriolli FF, Amato VS, Rassi JA. [Protective effect of benznidazole against parasite reactivation in patients chronically infected with Trypanosoma cruzi and treated with corticoids for associated diseases]. *Rev Soc Bras Med Trop* 1999;**325**:475–82.

108. Riarte A, Luna C, Sabatiello R *et al.* Chagas' disease in patients with kidney transplants: 7 years of experience 1989–1996. *Clin Infect Dis* 1999;**293**:561–7.

109. Viotti R, Vigliano C, Armenti H, Segura E. Treatment of chronic Chagas' disease with benznidazole: clinical and serologic evolution of patients with long-term follow-up. *Am Heart J* 1994;**1271**:151–62.

110. Viotti R, Vigliano C, Lococo B *et al.* Long-term cardiac outcomes of treating chronic Chagas disease with benznidazole versus no treatment: a nonrandomized trial. *Ann Intern Med* 2006;**14410**:724–34.

111. Villar JC. Desenlaces clínicos de sujetos con infección crónica por Trypanosoma cruzi tratados o no con agentes tripanocidas. Un metaanálisis de estudios observacionales. *MEDUNAB* 2002;**5**:166–173.

112. Villar JC, Villar LA, Marin-Neto JA, Ebrahim S, Yusuf S. Trypanocidal drugs for chronic asymptomatic Trypanosoma cruzi infection. *Cochrane Database of Systematic Reviews* 2002, Issue 1. Art. No.: CD003463. DOI: 10.1002/14651858. CD003463.

113. Solari A, Ortiz S, Soto A *et al.* Treatment of Trypanosoma cruzi-infected children with nifurtimox: a 3 year follow-up by PCR. *J Antimicrob Chemother* 2001;**484**:515–19.

114. WHO Expert Committee. Control of Chagas Disease. WHO technical report series number 905. Geneva: World Health Organization, 2002.

115. Sosa-Estani S, Segura EL. Treatment of Trypanosoma cruzi infection in the undetermined phase. Experience and current guidelines of treatment in Argentina. *Mem Inst Oswaldo Cruz* 1999;**94**:363–5.

116. Mendoza I, Camardo J, Moleiro F *et al.* Sustained ventricular tachycardia in chronic chagasic myocarditis: electrophysiologic and pharmacologic characteristics. *Am J Cardiol* 1986;**576**:423–7.

117. Sosa E, Scanavacca M, d'Avila A *et al.* Endocardial and epicardial ablation guided by nonsurgical transthoracic epicardial mapping to treat recurrent ventricular tachycardia. *J Cardiovasc Electrophysiol* 1998;**93**:229–39.

118. d'Avila A, Splinter R, Svenson RH *et al.* New perspectives on catheter-based ablation of ventricular tachycardia complicating Chagas' disease: experimental evidence of the efficacy of near infrared lasers for catheter ablation of Chagas' VT. *J Interv Card Electrophysiol* 2002;**71**:23–38.

119. Scanavacca MI, Brito FS, Maia I. Diretrizes para avaliação e tratamento de pacientes com arritmias cardíacas. *Arq Bras Cardiol* 2002;**79**(suppl):V1–50.

120. Giniger AG, Retyk EO, Laino RA, Sananes EG, Lapuente AR. Ventricular tachycardia in Chagas' disease. *Am J Cardiol* 1992;**704**:459–62.

121. Leite LR, Fenelon G, Simoes A Jr, Silva GG, Friedman PA, de Paola AA. Clinical usefulness of electrophysiologic testing in patients with ventricular tachycardia and chronic chagasic cardiomyopathy treated with amiodarone or sotalol. *J Cardiovasc Electrophysiol* 2003;**146**:567–73.

122. Dubner S, Valero E, Pesce R *et al.* A Latin American registry of implantable cardioverter defibrillators: the ICD-LABOR study. *Ann Noninvasive Electrocardiol* 2005;**104**:420–8.

123. Rassi A Jr. Implantable cardioverter-defibrillators in patients with Chagas heart disease: misperceptions, many questions and the urgent need for a randomized clinical trial. *J Cardiovasc Electrophysiol* 2007;**18**(12):1241–3.

124. Milei J, Pesce R, Valero E, Muratore C, Beigelman R, Ferrans VJ. Electrophysiologic-structural correlations in chagasic aneurysms causing malignant arrhythmias. *Int J Cardiol* 1991;**321**:65–73.

125. de Paola AA, Gomes JA, Miyamoto MH, Fo EE. Transcoronary chemical ablation of ventricular tachycardia in chronic chagasic myocarditis. *J Am Coll Cardiol* 1992;**202**:480–2.

126. Sosa E, Scanavacca M, d'Avila A, Bellotti G, Pilleggi F. Radiofrequency catheter ablation of ventricular tachycardia guided by nonsurgical epicardial mapping in chronic Chagasic heart disease. *Pacing Clin Electrophysiol* 1999;**221**(Pt 1):128–30.

127. Batlouni M, Barretto AC, Armaganijan D *et al.* [Treatment of mild and moderate cardiac failure with captopril. A multicenter study]. *Arq Bras Cardiol* 1992;**585**:417–21.

128. Roberti RR, Martinez EE, Andrade JL *et al.* Chagas cardiomyopathy and captopril. *Eur Heart J* 1992;**137**:966–70.

129. Botoni FA, Poole-Wilson PA, Ribeiro AL *et al.* A randomized trial of carvedilol after renin-angiotensin system inhibition in chronic Chagas cardiomyopathy. *Am Heart J* 2007;**1534**: 544–8.

130. Quiros FR, Morillo CA, Casas JP, Cubillos LA, Silva FA. CHARITY: Chagas cardiomyopathy bisoprolol intervention study: a randomized double-blind placebo force-titration controlled study with Bisoprolol in patients with chronic heart failure secondary to Chagas cardiomyopathy [NCT00323973]. *Trials* 2006;**7**:21.

131. Buffolo E, Branco JN, Catani R. End-stage cardiomyopathy and secondary mitral insufficiency surgical alternative with prosthesis implant and left ventricular restoration. *Eur J Cardiothorac Surg* 2006;**29**(suppl 1):S266–S271.

132. Bacal F, Silva CP, Bocchi EA *et al.* Mycophenolate mofetil increased chagas disease reactivation in heart transplanted patients: comparison between two different protocols. *Am J Transplant* 2005;**58**:2017–21.

133. Bocchi EA, Fiorelli A. The paradox of survival results after heart transplantation for cardiomyopathy caused by Trypanosoma cruzi. First Guidelines Group for Heart Transplantation of the Brazilian Society of Cardiology. *Ann Thorac Surg* 2001;**716**:1833–8.

134. Soares MB, Lima RS, Rocha LL *et al.* Transplanted bone marrow cells repair heart tissue and reduce myocarditis in chronic chagasic mice. *Am J Pathol* 2004;**1642**:441–7.

135. Guarita-Souza LC, Carvalho KA, Woitowicz V *et al.* Simultaneous autologous transplantation of cocultured mesenchymal stem cells and skeletal myoblasts improves ventricular function in a murine model of Chagas disease. *Circulation* 2006; **1141**(suppl):I120–I124.

136. Vilas-Boas F, Feitosa GS, Soares MB *et al.* [Early results of bone marrow cell transplantation to the myocardium of patients with heart failure due to Chagas disease]. *Arq Bras Cardiol* 2006;**872**:159–66.

137. Tura BR, Martino HF, Gowdak LH *et al.* Multicenter randomized trial of cell therapy in cardiopathies – MiHeart Study. *Trials* 2007;**8**:2.

138. Oliveira-Filho J, Viana LC, Vieira-de-Melo RM *et al.* Chagas disease is an independent risk factor for stroke: baseline characteristics of a Chagas Disease cohort. *Stroke* 2005;**369**: 2015–17.

139. Sousa AS. Incidencia e escores de risco de acidente vascular encefalico cardioembolico em uma Coorte de 1043 pacientes com doencas de chagas: avaliacao do prognostico e proposta de estrategias de prevencao. Hospital Universitario Clementino Fraga Filho, doctoral thesis, 2003.

140. de Sousa AS, Xavier SS, de Freitas GR, Hasslocher-Moreno A. Prevention strategies of cardioembolic ischemic stroke in Chagas' disease. *Arq Bras Cardiol* 2008;**91**(5):306–10.

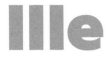

Specific cardiovascular disorders: pericardial disease

Bernard J Gersh, Editor

52 Pericardial disease: an evidence-based approach to clinical management

Faisal F Syed[1] and Bongani M Mayosi[2]
[1] Department of Cardiology, University of Newcastle-upon-Tyne, Newcastle, UK
[2] Department of Medicine, Groote Schuur Hospital and University of Cape Town, Cape Town, South Africa

This overview deals with the extent to which the clinical management of the common pericardial diseases (i.e. idiopathic pericarditis, purulent pericarditis, tuberculous pericarditis, and neoplastic pericarditis) is supported by evidence from well-designed prospective studies. The diagnosis of acute pericarditis is based on the presence of typical chest findings, history and the electrocardiogram. The echocardiogram is used to confirm and quantify an associated pericardial effusion. It is generally accepted that oral non-steroidal anti-inflammatory drugs (NSAIDs) or aspirin are effective in most patients with acute pericarditis. Colchicine added to an NSAID or aspirin or as monotherapy appears to shorten the duration of the initial attack, and reduce the risk of recurrent pericarditis. A preliminary study has highlighted the potential benefit of rosuvastatin as adjunctive therapy to NSAIDs in acute pericarditis. Corticosteroids are restricted to cases of autoimmune disease with early introduction of NSAIDs or colchicine during the tapering phase, because of their association with recurrent attacks of acute pericarditis on withdrawal. Recurrent pericarditis is treated with colchicine. Chronic idiopathic pericardial effusion, which is diagnosed on the basis of persistence of effusion for several months in populations with a low prevalence of tuberculosis, is treated by pericardiocentesis and pericardiectomy in the case of recurrence.

A specific cause of pericarditis, such as purulent, tuberculous or neoplastic pericarditis, must be sought in all patients with pericarditis who present with the following clinical features: a fever >38 °C, subacute course over several days or weeks, large effusion with an echo-free space >1 cm anterior to the heart on echocardiography, cardiac tamponade, and failure of aspirin or NSAID therapy within a week. In this context, diagnostic pericardiocentesis and other tests are required to make a specific diagnosis. Purulent pericarditis, which is diagnosed on the basis of a neutrophilic pericardial exudate in association with a positive microbiologic culture, requires treatment with antibiotics and pericardial drainage. Preliminary studies using intrapericardial thrombolysis show promise in reducing the incidence of pericardial adhesions and constriction.

A definite or proven diagnosis of tuberculous pericarditis is based on demonstration of tubercle bacilli in pericardial fluid or on histologic section of the pericardium. A probable or presumed diagnosis is based on proof of tuberculosis elsewhere in a patient with otherwise unexplained pericarditis, a lymphocytic pericardial exudate with elevated biomarkers of tuberculous infection, and/or appropriate response to a trial of antituberculosis chemotherapy. Treatment consists of four-drug therapy for at least two months (isoniazid, rifampicin, pyrazinamide, and ethambutol) followed by two drugs (isoniazid and rifampicin) for four months regardless of human immunodeficiency virus (HIV) status. It is uncertain whether adjunctive corticosteroids are effective in reducing mortality or pericardial constriction, and their safety in HIV-infected patients has not been established conclusively. Surgical resection of the pericardium is indicated for calcific constrictive pericarditis or persistent signs of constriction following a 6–8 trial of antituberculosis treatment in patients with non-calcific constrictive pericarditis.

The diagnosis of neoplastic pericarditis rests on sampling of pericardial fluid or tissue for pathologic examination. Treatment of neoplastic pericardial effusion is directed at the relief of immediate symptoms of pericarditis or tamponade, preventing reaccumulation, and the management of the underlying malignancy.

Introduction

A wide variety of conditions may result in pericardial disease, which presents clinically as acute pericarditis,

Evidence-Based Cardiology, 3rd edition. Edited by S. Yusuf, J.A. Cairns, A.J. Camm, E.L. Fallen, and B.J. Gersh. © 2010 Blackwell Publishing, ISBN: 978-1-4051-5925-8.

Table 52.1 Contemporary causes of large pericardial effusion

	South Africa Reuter *et al* 2006[1] (n 233, 1995–2001)	Italy Imazio *et al* 2007[2] (n 453, 1996–2004)
Tuberculous pericarditis	162 (69.5%)	17 (3.7%)
Neoplastic pericarditis	22 (9.4%)	23 (5.1%)
Autoimmune aetiology	12 (5.2%)	33 (7.3%)
Purulent/septic pericarditis	5 (2.2%)	3 (0.7%)
Idiopathic or other causes	32 (13.7%)	377 (83.2%)

pericardial effusion or constrictive pericarditis. The etiologic spectrum depends on the epidemiologic setting of the patient. For example, in industrialized countries, most cases of pericarditis are idiopathic, whereas tuberculosis accounts for the majority of patients in the developing world (Table 52.1).[1,2] In many cases, pericardial disease is associated with a known condition (e.g. malignancy) or underlying cardiac disease, which prove to be the cause of pericardial disease. In patients with no apparent cause of the pericardial syndrome, the presence of inflammatory signs is predictive of acute pericarditis; on the other hand, a large effusion without inflammatory signs or tamponade is predictive of chronic idiopathic pericardial effusion.[3] Tamponade without inflammatory signs is suspicious for neoplastic pericardial effusion. In patients living in tuberculosis-endemic regions, a pericardial effusion without apparent cause is likely to be tuberculous until proven otherwise. The prognosis of pericardial disease is related to the underlying disease, being especially poor in patients with malignancy.[3]

This overview deals with the clinical management of the common pericardial diseases, including idiopathic pericarditis, purulent pericarditis, tuberculous pericarditis, and neoplastic pericarditis. We examine the extent to which existing treatments are supported by evidence from well-designed prospective studies. The findings reported here are based on a comprehensive search of electronic databases and bibliographies of articles on pericarditis.

Idiopathic pericarditis

Epidemiology

Acute idiopathic pericarditis accounts for 80–90% of primary acute pericardial disease (i.e. pericardial syndrome without apparent cause at initial clinical evaluation) in Western countries.[2,4,5] Incidence has been estimated at 28 per 100 000 per year, but the influence of the tested population, mode of presentation and seasonal and geographic variation of viral infections is significant.[6] Acute pericarditis is responsible for ~1% of presentations to emergency departments with electrocardiographic ST elevation, but at least an additional 10% of patients are diagnosed in the absence of electrocardiographic criteria.[7,8]

Etiology

The etiology of idiopathic pericarditis is presumed to be viral or autoimmune. However, in a French study of 136 patients diagnosed with idiopathic pericarditis after standard investigations and pericardiocentesis, serologic antibody evaluation and viral culture of throat swabs yielded alternative diagnoses in 39 (29%); the commonest causes were *Coxiella burnetii* (n = 10), enterovirus (n = 8), Mycoplasma infection (n = 4) and autoimmunity (high antinuclear antibody titer, n = 3).[9] Previously unsuspected hypothyroidism was diagnosed in an additional 14 patients through routine measurement of thyroid-stimulating hormone. The use of more sophisticated methods for examining pericardial fluid and tissue, such as tumor markers, fluorescence-activated cell sorting, polymerase chain reaction and immunohistochemistry, as in the Marburg Pericarditis Registry, means that less than 5% of cases are labeled as idiopathic and a much higher proportion of cases are found to be viral or autoimmune.[10]

Diagnosis

Acute pericarditis is the occurrence of two or more of the following: characteristic chest pain, pericardial friction rub (pathognomonic of acute pericarditis), and an electrocardiogram showing characteristic ST segment elevation or typical serial changes. Transthoracic echocardiography is recommended for all patients.[10,11] Cardiac tamponade is an indication for therapeutic pericardiocentesis. Diagnostic pericardiocentesis is recommended if an infective or malignant cause of effusion is suspected.[10,11] Although there are no absolute clinical differentiators, a history of malignancy or autoimmune illness, high fever with rigors, skin rash or weight loss point to a specific disease. Blood tests may reveal renal failure while a markedly raised white cell count suggests purulent pericarditis.[11]

A recent prospective evaluation of 453 patients identified fever >38 °C (odds ratio (OR) 3.56), subacute course (3.97), large effusion or tamponade (2.15), and failure of aspirin or NSAID therapy (2.50) as predictive of a specific cause being present (noted in 76 patients (17 %)) with identified diagnoses of autoimmune, neoplastic, tuberculous or bacterial pericarditis.[2] In another prospective study of 130 patients, the presence of inflammatory signs (characteristic chest pain, pericardial friction rub, fever or typical electro-cardiographic changes) in the absence of an identified cause of moderate to large effusion predicted the diagnosis of idiopathic pericarditis (OR 5.4), whereas when these were not present, tamponade predicted neoplasia (OR 2.9).[12] This is in stark contrast to tuberculosis and HIV-endemic areas where the majority of effusions are caused by tuberculosis.[13] The presence of features suggestive of a specific cause should prompt the clinician to investigate the patient further for an infective, neoplastic or autoimmune cause of the pericarditis.

Management

When none of the above features are present to suggest high risk and the presence of autoimmune, neoplastic, tuberculous or bacterial pericarditis, management in a day case unit has been shown to be safe as long as these low-risk patients are observed for a few hours while preliminary investigations are being undertaken and closely followed up thereafter to ensure response to treatment.[8] Acute pericarditis can therefore be triaged based on clinical and echocardiographic criteria and those with high-risk features admitted and thoroughly investigated[2] (**Class I, Level C1**).

It is generally accepted that bed rest and oral NSAIDs are effective in most patients with acute pericarditis, although there are no controlled trials.[4,10,14] Ibuprofen has been recommended over indometacin due to its better side effect profile, larger dose range and anecdotal efficacy.[10,14] Ketorolac is an extremely potent analgesic agent which has been reported to cause rapid resolution of symptomatic acute pericarditis in an uncontrolled study of 20 patients.[15] However, before using expensive NSAIDs, it is appropriate to consider aspirin.[16] In a prospective uncontrolled study of 254 patients with uncomplicated acute pericarditis, aspirin given at a dose of 800 mg every 6–8 hours for 7–10 days (in conjunction with misoprostol or omeprazole for gastric protection) with gradual tapering over 2–3 weeks resulted in a favorable response in 87%.[8] Although similar in presentation to responders, those 33 of 254 patients with poor response to aspirin (defined as persistence of fever, a new pericardial effusion, or worsening of general illness after seven days) were shown to have a higher incidence of autoimmune (39% versus 2%) and tuberculous pericarditis (18% versus 0%). The differences in etiology of pericarditis between responders and non-responders probably explain the reduced incidence of recurrent pericarditis (10% versus 61%) and constriction by one year in responders (0.5% versus 9%).[8] In view of this evidence, response to a trial of aspirin or NSAID can be taken as predictive of good prognosis and no further investigation is routinely required. Conversely, failure of aspirin or NSAID therapy should prompt further investigation for a specific cause of pericarditis[2,8] (**Class I, Level C1**).

A randomized open-label trial of COlchicine for acute PEricarditis (COPE study) in 120 patients with pericarditis due to idiopathic, viral, postpericardiectomy and connective tissue disease demonstrated on intention-to-treat analysis that a three-month course of colchicine in addition to a 3–4 week course of aspirin reduced symptom persistence at 72 hours (from 37% to 12%, $P = 0.003$) and recurrence rate at 18 months (32% to 11%, $P = 0.004$, number needed to treat (NNT) = 5).[17] No serious adverse effects of colchicine were seen but the drug had to be discontinued in 8% of patients due to diarrhea. The results of this trial will be supplemented with a larger trial of colchicine versus placebo currently underway.[18] Colchicine (0.5 mg bd)[10] added to an NSAID/aspirin (**Class I, Level B**) or as monotherapy (**Class IIa, Level C2**) appears to be effective for the initial attack and prevention of recurrences of acute pericarditis.

A preliminary study has highlighted the potential benefits of rosuvastatin as adjunctive therapy to NSAIDs in acute pericarditis.[19] The rationale for the use of statins in this setting is based on their known anti-inflammatory effects, as shown by the lowering of C-reactive protein (CRP) independently of their lipid-lowering effect.[19] Fifty five consecutive patients with a first episode of acute pericarditis were randomized to either indometacin plus placebo or indometacin plus rosuvastatin 10 mg, with treatment continued for a week after inflammatory markers normalized. The addition of rosuvastatin resulted in significantly earlier normalization of CRP levels (5.0 versus 6.0 days, $P = 0.022$), ST segment deviation (3.5 vs 4.5 days, $P = 0.001$), pericardial effusion (4.5 vs 5.5 days, $P = 0.001$) and erythrocyte sedimentation rate (ESR) (5.0 vs 6.0 days, $P = 0.022$). These promising results need to be confirmed in larger studies before application to clinical practice (**Class IIb, Level B**).

Corticosteroids are effective in acute pericarditis but observational data suggest that their use in this setting is associated with an increased risk of recurrence.[16,20] The pain and any associated fever, leukocytosis, and other inflammatory factors resolve rapidly with high-dose corticosteroid administration (e.g. 1–1.5 mg/kg/day), only to return during tapering to a low dose of the steroid.[16] Prospective data from the COPE trial add to these observations.[17] Patients in both arms of the study with aspirin intolerance or contraindication (n = 19, 16%) were treated with corticosteroids for a similar duration to aspirin. Steroid use was an independent risk factor for recurrence on multivariate analysis (OR 4.30, 95% confidence interval (CI) 1.21–15.25). Therefore corticosteroids are restricted to cases of autoimmune or connective tissue disease with early introduction of NSAIDs or colchicine during the tapering phase (**Class IIa, Level C2**).[10] Intrapericardial triamcinolone is one way of reducing systemic side effects which have been shown to be effective in up to 93% of patients with autoimmune pericardial effusion[21] (**Class I, Level C2**).

Recurrent pericarditis

Recurrent pericarditis is the most troublesome complication of acute pericarditis. The criteria for the diagnosis of recurrent pericarditis are a documented first attack of acute pericarditis, and evidence of either recurrence or continued activity of pericarditis despite therapy.[22] Recurrent pericarditis, which affects about 20% of cases,[20,22] is diagnosed in the presence of chest pain and one or more of the following: pericardial friction rub, electrocardiographic changes, echocardiographic evidence of pericardial effusion, and raised inflammatory markers.[22,23] Approximately 40% have multiple attacks and 10% have more than five attacks over several years, although attacks tend to become progressively less severe.[20] The disease process can continue for up to 43 years (mean 5.4 years), with symptom-free periods ranging from one month to 39 years (median three months), but in most it gradually "burns out" after 10 years.[24] Despite this, prognosis is good: cardiac tamponade and pericardial constriction are very rare, myocardial disease is not seen, and atrial fibrillation is an uncommon transient feature of exacerbations.[23–25]

There is no single consistent etiologic factor but evidence of ongoing viral infection, prior corticosteroid use, autoimmunity and familial clustering have all been variably reported.[16,20] Antinuclear antibodies have been reported in approximately 55% and a new diagnosis of connective tissue disease in 10% of 61 patients with recurrent idiopathic pericarditis.[24] Where patients from Mediterranean countries are over-represented, familial Mediterranean fever has been reported in 4%.[26]

In the assessment of patients with recurrence, evaluation for connective tissue disease is appropriate but complex diagnostic procedures, such as invasive endomyocardial or pericardial sampling, are usually not justified.[16,20]

The open-label COlchicine for REcurrent pericarditis (CORE) study randomized 84 consecutive patients with first recurrence of idiopathic, autoimmune or viral pericarditis to aspirin or aspirin and a six-month course of colchicine.[22] On intention-to-treat analysis, treatment with colchicine significantly decreased 18-month recurrence from 51% to 24% ($P = 0.02$, NNT 4) and symptom persistence at 72 hours from 31% to 10% ($P = 0.03$).[10] Colchicine (2 mg/day for one or two days, followed by 1 mg/day)[10] can be recommended as effective therapy for recurrent pericarditis (**Class I, Level B**). Prednisolone was substituted in 30 patients with aspirin contraindication and on multivariate analysis this was an independent risk factor for further recurrences (OR 2.9, 95% CI 1.1–8.3). These findings confirm uncontrolled studies reporting on the use of colchicine as first-line therapy for recurrence[25,27,28] and the deleterious effects of corticosteroids in attenuating its effectiveness[26] and increasing the risk of further recurrence.[20,25] A sustained response on discontinuation of colchicine is

Table 52.2 Therapeutic strategies previously evaluated in recurrent pericarditis (after failure of NSAID)

Study	Patients (n)	Therapeutic strategy evaluated	Remission rate
Fowler[23]	9	Pericardiectomy	2/9 (22%)
Hatcher[32]	24	Pericardiectomy	20/24 (83%)
Asplen[33]	2	Azathioprine	2/2 (100%)
Imazio[25]	2	Azathioprine	2/2 (100%)
Melchior[34]	2	High-dose methylprednisolone as pulse therapy	2/2 (100%)
Marcolongo[35]	12	High-dose prednisolone with aspirin	11/12 (92%)
Peterlana[36]	4	High-dose intravenous immunoglobulin	3/4 (75%)
Tona[37]	2	High-dose intravenous immunoglobulin	2/2 (100%)

seen in 60%, although recurrences are minor and resolve with reinstitution of colchicine (**Class IIa, Level C2**).[28] Relapse on colchicine can be managed effectively in the majority with reinstitution of NSAIDs.[28] Patients with recurrent pain despite NSAIDs and colchicine are challenging yet there is a paucity of evidence to guide management. Corticosteroids are recommended in European guidelines only in patients with poor general condition or frequent crises 10 (**Class IIa, Level C2**). An extended course of low-dose steroids may be superior to regimes utilizing a high dose initially. A nonrandomized retrospective comparison reported a significantly increased risk of recurrence with a higher dose: 33 of 51 patients taking prednisone 1.0 mg/kg/day suffered a recurrence by mean followup of 58 months as compared to 16 of 49 taking 0.2–0.5 mg/kg/day by 54 months (hazards ratio 3.6, $P < 0.001$). Some of this may be related to premature withdrawal of therapy as the higher dose was associated with significantly increased toxicity (osteoporosis and Cushing's syndrome reported in 24% vs 2%).[28a] (**Class IIa, Level C1**) Claims of effectiveness have been made in small uncontrolled studies for pericardiectomy, azathioprine, chloroquine, and intravenous immunoglobulin (Table 52.2) (**Class IIb, Level C2**).

Chronic idiopathic pericardial effusion

Patients with large pericardial effusion of no apparent cause which persists for more than three months constitute 3% of pericarditis and 70% of large chronic effusions in the West.[29] The main concern is the occurrence of tamponade, reported in 30–40% of cases, at times with unexpected decompensation after being asymptomatic for several years.[29,30] For this reason, drainage is recommended even in the absence of tamponade (**Class IIa, Level C1**). Lasting remission is seen in 33–75% after therapeutic pericardiocentesis alone and 95% after extended catheter drainage.[30] Pericardiectomy offers long-term success whether carried out initially or after failure of percutaneous drainage.[29–31] Survival rates are similar to the background population[30] but a late appearance of malignancy has been reported in 5–10% of cases at 6–80 months following diagnosis.[29,30]

Purulent pericarditis

Epidemiology

Purulent pericarditis is now rare in the developed world, comprising 0.7–5% of pericardial effusions[2,12,38,39] and less than 1% of cases undergoing pericardiectomy.[40–42] In Western series, the most common reported organisms have been staphylococci, streptococci and pneumococci when the predominant associated lesions are empyema (50%) or pneumonia (33%).[43] In a series where over 50% of patients had compromised immunity or thoracic surgery, *Staphylococcus aureus* (30%) and fungi (20%) have predominated.[44] In another unselected retrospective series anaerobes originating from the oropharynx were most commonly found.[45] Seeding may be hematogenous but contiguous spread from less common sites such as the retropharyngeal space, cardiac valves, and below the diaphragm must be excluded.[46] *Neisseria meningitidis* may involve the pericardium in two ways: either through initiating an immune-mediated sterile effusion[47,48] or by direct infection and purulent reaction.[49] The modern era of iatrogenic and HIV-associated immunosuppression has witnessed more unusual organisms and presentations.[50–54]

Diagnosis

A prodrome of 3–10 days precedes presentation with fever, cough, chest pain and tachycardia.[43,44] Pericardial rub is present in 35–45% of patients and tamponade in 40–80%. However, when pericardial involvement is secondary, the underlying sepsis predominates the illness and its outcome.[55] This may partly explain why as many as 30–40% of patients are diagnosed post mortem[43,44] and also stresses the importance of identifying associated foci, with the use of adjunctive investigations as indicated.

Blood tests are in keeping with sepsis whilst radiographic cardiomegaly (75%), lung field shadowing (50%) and pleural effusions (30%) are common. Electrocardiography is usually typical of myopericarditis but may be normal in 10–30% of patients. Echocardiography confirms the presence of effusion; however, in patients with sepsis this is not proof in itself of pericardial infection.[56] Suspicion of purulent pericarditis is an indication for urgent pericardiocentesis,[10] which is diagnostic.[57] The fluid may be frankly purulent. A low pericardial to serum glucose ratio (mean 0.3) and raised pericardial fluid white cell count with high proportion of neutrophils (mean cell count 2.8 per μl, 92% neutrophils) differentiate from tuberculous (ratio 0.7, count 1.7 per μl, 50% neutrophils) and neoplastic (ratio 0.8, count 3.3 per μl, 55% neutrophils) pericarditis.[58] Fluid should be sent for bacterial, fungal and tuberculous studies, blood cultures drawn and other samples taken as guided by the clinical presentation.

Management

Purulent pericarditis should be managed aggressively as mortality is universal if untreated, whereas with comprehensive therapy 85% have been reported to survive the episode and have good long-term outcome.[43] Intravenous antimicrobial therapy should be started empirically until microbiologic results are available. Effective pericardial drainage is crucial.[10] There are no prospective studies comparing one modality over another in purulent pericarditis. Retrospective comparisons with unselected cases feature purulent pericarditis rarely and in small numbers. Central to the choice of modality is the fact that purulent effusions are often heavily loculated and likely to reaccumulate rapidly. Subxiphoid pericardiostomy and rinsing of the pericardial cavity is recommended.[10] This allows more complete drainage of the effusion as loculations can be manually lyzed at the time of surgery. In a Zimbabwean report of 21 cases of purulent pericarditis managed as such, under local anesthesia in most cases, there was one recurrence of effusion (5%), one case of constriction (5%), and four deaths (20%)[59] (**Class IIa, Level C2**).

Intrapericardial thrombolysis through a percutaneous catheter has attempted to address the problems encountered with loculations restricting adequate drainage. Ten studies have reported a total of 35 patients with purulent pericardial effusion treated with percutaneous intrapericardial thrombolysis.[57,60–68] Intrapericardial thrombolysis did not alter systemic clotting parameters and was associated with regression or disappearance of intrapericardial fibrin strands, improvement in hemodynamic status and prevention of constriction. Treatment failure was reported in two patients. Reported complications were intrapericardial haemorrhage (n = 2) and mortality from ongoing sepsis (n = 1). A controlled study of intrapericardial urokinase in 60 patients with tuberculous pericarditis and 34 with purulent pericarditis reported a 13% incidence of intrapericardial haemorrhage.[69] An adequately designed study is required to evaluate the safety and effectiveness of this promising therapy in selected patients with purulent effusion and subacute constriction (**Class IIb, Level C2**). Pericardiectomy is recommended for dense adhesions, loculated or thick purulent effusion, recurrence of tamponade, persistent infection, and progression to constriction, with up to 8% surgical mortality (**Class IIa, Level C2**).[10] Duration of antimicrobial therapy has to be individualized (**Class IIa, Level C2**).

Tuberculous pericarditis

Epidemiology

Tuberculous pericarditis accounts for less than 5% of pericardial disease in the developed world.[2,4,5] By contrast, tuberculosis is the cause of large pericardial effusions in over 90% of HIV-infected[70-72] and 50–70% of non-HIV infected individuals who live in tuberculosis-endemic regions and communities.[72,70] The disease can occur at any age[73,74] and men are more frequently affected than women, though occasionally a greater proportion of female patients has been reported.[75-78] Clinical presentations are as pericardial effusion (80% of cases), effusive-constrictive pericarditis (15%) or constrictive pericarditis (5%).[79] Tuberculous pericarditis is a serious condition with a mortality of 17–40%; constriction occurs in a similar proportion of cases following tuberculous pericardial effusion.[80]

Tuberculous pericardial effusion

Tuberculous pericardial effusion should be suspected in all instances of pericarditis without a rapidly self-limiting course. Onset is insidious and presentation is with non-specific systemic symptoms, such as fever, night sweats, fatigue, and weight loss.[13] Chest pain, cough, and breathlessness are common, although severe pericardial pain of acute onset characteristic of idiopathic pericarditis is unusual. Right upper abdominal aching owing to liver congestion is also common. In African patients with tuberculous pericardial effusions, evidence of chronic cardiac compression mimicking heart failure is the most common presentation and 10% present with clinical tamponade.[75] While there is marked overlap between the physical signs of pericardial effusion and constrictive pericarditis, the presence of a pericardial friction rub and increased cardiac dullness extending to the right of the sternum favor a clinical diagnosis of pericardial effusion.[81]

Diagnosis

The chest radiograph, which shows an enlarged cardiac shadow in almost all cases,[82] demonstrates features of active pulmonary tuberculosis in 30% of cases and pleural effusion in 40–60% of cases.[75,82-85] The electrocardiogram is abnormal in virtually all cases, usually in the form of non-specific ST T-wave changes.[86] The PR segment deviation

and ST segment elevation characteristic of acute pericarditis are found in only 9–11% of cases. Atrial fibrillation is usually transient. Echocardiographic findings of effusion with fibrinous strands on the visceral pericardium are typical but not specific for a tuberculous aetiology.[87,88] Imaging by CT scanning or MRI can also be used to provide incremental information to echocardiography.[89-91] In addition to features of pericardial disease (i.e. pericardial effusion and thickening of the pericardium), CT of the chest shows typical changes in mediastinal lymph nodes (i.e. enlargement >10 mm with matting and hypodense centers and sparing of hilar lymph nodes) in almost all cases which resolve on treatment.[89] MRI has the added advantage of assessing the extent of pericardial inflammation[91,92] and myocardial involvement.[93,94]

A "definite or proven" diagnosis of tuberculous pericarditis is based on the demonstration of tubercle bacilli in pericardial fluid or on histologic section of the pericardium, and a "probable or presumptive" diagnosis is made when there is proof of tuberculosis elsewhere in a patient with unexplained pericarditis, a lymphocytic pericardial exudate with elevated adenine deaminase (ADA), interferon-gamma (IFN-γ) or lysozyme levels, and/or an appropriate response to antituberculosis chemotherapy.[13] A protocol for the evaluation of a patient with suspected tuberculous pericardial effusion in tuberculosis-endemic and non-endemic communities and regions of the world is presented in Table 52.3.[13,80]

A new diagnostic index score has been developed to predict the diagnosis of tuberculous pericarditis in patients living in an endemic area.[1] Independently predictive of tuberculous pericarditis (with diagnostic index score) were fever (1), night sweats (1), weight loss (2), globulin level >40 g/L (3) and peripheral leukocyte count <10 × 10^9/L(3). A total score of ≥6 indicates tuberculous pericarditis with 86% sensitivity and 85% specificity, which proved to have better diagnostic efficiency than culture or pericardial histology in this study.[1]

Management

In patients living in non-endemic areas, there is no justification for starting antituberculosis treatment empirically when systematic investigation fails to yield a diagnosis of tuberculous pericarditis; such patients should be treated as chronic idiopathic pericardial effusion (as indicated above)[85] (**Class I, Level C1**). By contrast, in tuberculosis endemic regions and communities, after exclusion of other causes of pericardial effusion such as malignancy (**Class I, Level B**), a regimen consisting of rifampicin, isoniazid, pyrazinamide and ethambutol for at least two months, followed by isoniazid and rifampicin (total of six months of therapy), has been shown to be highly effective in treating patients with extrapulmonary tuberculosis; treatment for nine months or

Table 52.3 A step-wise protocol for the evaluation of suspected tuberculous pericardial effusion[13,80]

Stage 1: Initial non-invasive evaluation	Chest radiograph may reveal changes suggestive of pulmonary tuberculosis in 30% of cases.
	Echocardiogram: the presence of a large pericardial effusion with frond-like projections, and thick "porridge-like" fluid is suggestive of an exudate but not specific for a tuberculous etiology.
	CT scan and/or MRI of the chest are alternative imaging modalities where available: for evidence of pericardial effusion and thickening (>3 mm), and typical mediastinal and tracheobronchial lymphadenopathy (>10 mm, hypodense centers, matting), with sparing of hilar lymph nodes.
	Culture of sputum, gastric aspirate and/or urine should be considered in all patients.
	Right scalene lymph node biopsy if pericardial fluid is not accessible and lymphadenopathy present.
	Tuberculin skin test is not helpful in adults regardless of the background prevalence of tuberculosis.
Stage 2: Pericardiocentesis	*Therapeutic pericardiocentesis* is absolutely indicated in the presence of cardiac tamponade.
	Diagnostic pericardiocentesis should be considered in all patients with suspected tuberculous pericarditis, and the following tests performed on the pericardial fluid:
	Direct inoculation of the pericardial fluid into double strength liquid Kirchner culture medium (or equivalent medium) at the bedside, and culture for *M. tuberculosis*.
	Biochemical tests to distinguish between an exudate and a transudate (fluid and serum protein; fluid and serum LDH).
	White cell analysis and count, and cytology: a lymphocytic exudate favours TB pericarditis.
	Indirect tests for tuberculous infection: adenosine deaminase (ADA), interferon-gamma (IFN-γ) or lysozyme assay.
Stage 3: Pericardial biopsy	*"Therapeutic" biopsy*: as part of surgical drainage in patients with severe tamponade relapsing after pericardiocentesis or requiring open drainage of pericardial fluid for whatever reason.
	Diagnostic biopsy: in areas where TB is endemic, a diagnostic biopsy is not required prior to commencing empiric antituberculosis treatment. In areas where TB is not endemic, a diagnostic biopsy is recommended in patients with >3 weeks of illness and without etiologic diagnosis having been reached by other tests.
Stage 4: Empiric antituberculosis chemotherapy	*Tuberculosis endemic in the population*: trial of empiric antituberculosis chemotherapy is recommended for exudative pericardial effusion, after excluding other causes such as malignancy, uremia, and trauma.
	Tuberculosis not endemic in the population: when systematic investigation fails to yield a diagnosis of tuberculous pericarditis, there is no justification for starting antituberculosis treatment empirically.

longer gives no better results, but has the disadvantages of increased cost and poor compliance.[95] Short-course chemotherapy is also highly effective in curing tuberculosis in HIV-infected patients[96] (**Class I, Level A**).

The role of routine pericardiotomy at the outset has been studied in a trial of 122 consenting participants randomized to complete open drainage by substernal pericardiotomy and biopsy under general anesthesia on admission or percutaneous pericardiocentesis as required to control symptoms and signs.[75] Complete open drainage abolished the need for repeat pericardiocentesis (relative risk (RR) 0.04; 95% CI 0.00–0.64, *P* = 0.02) but did not significantly influence the need for pericardiectomy for subsequent constriction (RR 0.39; 95% CI, 0.08–1.91; *P* = 0.20) or the risk of death as a result of pericarditis (RR 1.29; 95% CI 0.30–5.49; *P* = 0.70).[97] Therefore, routine open drainage by substernal pericardiotomy is not recommended (**Class III, Level B**).

Preliminary reports have identified two interventions that may reduce the incidence of constriction in tuberculous pericarditis. First, extended pericardial drainage with an indwelling pigtail catheter has been reported to be safe and associated with a low rate of constrictive pericarditis at two years (1.7 %) in a series of 118 patients with tuber-

culous pericardial effusion in Africa, a significant proportion of whom were HIV positive.[98] Second, a small controlled study of intrapericardial urokinase in 60 patients with tuberculous pericarditis and 34 with purulent pericarditis reported a 67% reduction in the risk of constriction in the total group of patients with infectious pericarditis (*P* < 0.001).[69] Intrapericardial hemorrhage was seen in 13% of the treatment group but no deaths were associated with the intervention. The effectiveness of extended intrapericardial drainage and intrapericardial urokinase in reducing the risk of constriction in tuberculous pericarditis requires further evaluation in randomized controlled studies (**Class IIb, Level C2**).

Tuberculous pericardial constriction

Prior to the introduction of effective tuberculosis chemotherapy, up to 50% of patients with effusive tuberculous pericarditis progressed to the constrictive stage of the disease.[99] The introduction of rifampicin-based antituberculosis treatment in the 1970s resulted in reduction of the incidence of constriction to 17–40% in patients with effusive tuberculous pericarditis.[81,85]

Constriction generally develops within six months of presentation with effusive pericarditis.[100,101] The presentation is highly variable, ranging from asymptomatic to severe constriction. The diagnosis is often missed on cursory clinical examination (see Table 53.2). The diastolic lift (pericardial knock) which coincides with a high-pitched early diastolic sound and sudden inspiratory splitting of the second heart sound are subtle but specific physical signs, which are found in 21–45% of patients.

Diagnosis

Most patients with constrictive pericarditis in South Africa have the subacute variety, in which a thick fibrinous exudate fills the pericardial sac, compressing the heart and causing a circulatory disturbance. As a result, calcification of the pericardium is absent in the majority and 75% have increased cardiothoracic ratio.[76] It is uncommon to find concomitant pulmonary tuberculosis. Non-specific but generalized T-wave changes are seen in most cases, while low-voltage complexes occur in about 30% of cases. Atrial fibrillation occurs in less than 5% of cases, is persistent, and usually occurs with a calcified pericardium. As with tuberculous pericardial effusion, the electrocardiogram is useful only in drawing attention to the presence of a cardiac abnormality. Echocardiography is particularly valuable in confirming the diagnosis of subacute constrictive pericarditis. Typically, a thick fibrinous exudate is seen in the pericardial sac and is associated with diminished movements of the surface of the heart, normal-sized chambers, absence of valvular heart disease, and absence of myocardial hypertrophy.[76] In time, the pericardial exudate condenses into a thick skin surrounding the heart, which usually, but not always, can be distinguished from myocardium. CT and MRI of the heart offer the advantage of better imaging of the pericardium with more accurate measurement of pericardial thickening.[102] This is important as tuberculous pericardial constriction is almost always associated with pericardial thickening; reports of constriction in the face of normal pericardial thickness have not included tuberculosis as a cause.[103] Contrast MRI has the added advantage of identifying ongoing pericardial and myocardial inflammation. Cardiac catheterization usually confirms the diagnosis.

Management

In a prospective study of 143 patients in Africa with clinical signs of pericardial constriction treated with antituberculosis therapy, only 25% required pericardiectomy for persistent or worsening constriction during the follow-up of two years.[76] These benefits were maintained up to 10 years.[104] The treatment of tuberculous pericardial constriction therefore involves the use of standard antituberculosis drugs for

six months (**Class I, Level C1**). Pericardiectomy is recommended if the patient's condition is static hemodynamically or deteriorates after 4–8 weeks of antituberculosis therapy (**Class I, Level C2**). If, however, the disease is associated with pericardial calcification, a marker of chronic disease, surgery should be undertaken earlier under antituberculosis drug cover. Perioperative mortality ranges from 7% to 11%[105–107] (**Class I, Level C2**).

Effusive constrictive tuberculous pericarditis

Effusive constrictive pericarditis is a common presentation in Southern Africa; preliminary studies suggest that it can be demonstrated in 50% of patients with suspected tuberculous pericardial effusion when right atrial pressure is monitored during pericardiocentesis.[108] Conventional assessment is less sensitive but in addition to physical signs of pericardial effusion, a diastolic knock may be detected on palpation and an early third heart sound on auscultation, while echocardiography may show a pericardial effusion between thickened pericardial membranes, with fibrinous pericardial bands apparently causing loculation of the effusion.[13]

The treatment of effusive constrictive pericarditis is problematic because pericardiocentesis does not relieve the impaired filling of the heart and surgical removal of the fibrinous exudate coating the visceral pericardium is not possible. Antituberculosis drugs should be given and the patient monitored clinically and by echocardiography for development of constrictive pericarditis (**Class I, Level C2**).

Steroids

The role of adjunctive corticosteroids in the management of tuberculous pericarditis has been reviewed systematically by Mayosi and others.[97,109] Four randomized controlled trials with a total of 469 participants have assessed the impact of oral steroids on mortality in tuberculous pericarditis.[75,76,99,110] Three of the trials (including 411 participants) tested adjunctive oral steroid use in participants with suspected tuberculous pericarditis in the pre-HIV era.[75,76,99] Fewer participants died in the intervention group, but the potentially large reduction in mortality was not statistically significant (RR 0.65, 95% CI 0.36–1.16, $P = 0.14$). A similarly promising but non-significant trend was found for other important clinical outcomes including the need for pericardiectomy for constriction (RR 0.85, 95% CI 0.51–1.42) and the need for repeat pericardiocentesis for cardiac tamponade (RR 0.45, 95% CI 0.20–1.05, $P = 0.07$). When a combined end-point of death or persisting symptoms and signs of pericardial disease at two years follow-up was considered, participants on steroids for pericardial effusion were significantly more likely to be cured at 24 months (i.e. alive and symptom free) than participants on placebo (RR

0.48, 95% CI 0.29–0.80, *P* = 0.04). This promising effect was not statistically significant in a sensitivity analysis of the worst case scenario in which all participants lost to follow-up in each group were assumed to have died (12/105 lost in treatment group, 7/116 in placebo group; sensitivity analysis assuming all died: RR 0.78, 95% CI 0.52–1.118, *P* = 0.1).

One trial with 58 HIV-infected individuals,[110] which was analyzed separately from the non-HIV studies, also showed a potentially large reduction in mortality of 50%, but this was not statistically significant (RR 0.50, 95% CI 0.19–1.28, *P* = 0.15).[97,111] There was no increase in opportunistic infections or malignancy associated with adjunctive steroid use in this small study with 18 months of follow-up.

It is clear from the meta-analysis that adjunctive oral steroids could potentially have large beneficial effects on the major clinically significant outcomes in tuberculous pericarditis (i.e. death, constriction, cardiac tamponade), but the published trials are too small to be conclusive (**Class IIa, Level B**). The effectiveness of intrapericardial instillation of corticosteroids was also examined in a randomized trial of 57 patients with tuberculous pericarditis.[109] There was no significant effect found on major clinical outcomes in this small study which was probably underpowered for major clinical events such as mortality (**Class IIb, Level B**).

Neoplastic pericarditis

Epidemiology

In developed countries, neoplastic pericarditis accounts for 5–7% of presentations with acute pericardial disease[2,4,5] and 30–60% of patients undergoing drainage of pericardial effusions.[112,113] Metastases are 40 times more common than primary cardiac tumors; mesothelioma, the most common of the primary tumors, is almost always incurable.[10] The common malignancies giving rise to symptomatic neoplastic effusions are bronchogenic (51%), hematologic (24%), gastrointestinal (9%), breast (8%) cancer, and melanoma (11%);[39,113] lymphoma and Kaposi's sarcoma are the predominant forms of neoplastic effusions in patients with AIDS.[111] Pericardial involvement may be the first manifestation of malignancy in 22–55% of cases of neoplastic pericardial effusion with or without cardiac tamponade.[114,115] Survival is principally determined by the underlying malignancy with median survival times ranging from 22 days for adenocarcinoma of unknown origin, 3.0–3.6 months for bronchogenic carcinoma, 3.2 months for Kaposi's sarcoma, 3.7–16.4 months for other solid malignancies, 4.9–17 months for hematologic malignancies, 6.2 months for primary effusion lymphoma, and 8.8–14.5 months for breast carcinoma.[116–120]

Diagnosis

Demonstration of neoplastic pericarditis requires sampling of pericardial fluid for cytologic examination and/or pericardial tissue for histology. Cytology has a high specificity (100%) but variable sensitivity (67–92%) which is higher with adenocarcinoma and lower with mesothelioma and lymphoma.[121 123] Cytologic analysis can be supplemented with immunocytochemistry which offers the added advantage of identifying cellular lineage, though is dependent on the markers used;[124,125] in one study the origins of 85% of metastatic carcinomas were correctly identified using a sequential panel of six antibodies.[125] Similarly, techniques such as flow cytometry and telomerase repeat amplification protocol (TRAP) in situ have yet to be proven in neoplastic pericardial disease per se.[126,127]

Histologic analysis of pericardial tissue in adjunction to cytologic analysis increases sensitivity. Studies delineating the stages leading up to targeted biopsy under pericardioscopy have reported incremental sensitivities from 54–65% with cytology alone, 71–75% with subxiphoid biopsy and cytology, to 92–97% with addition of pericardioscopic epicardial biopsy.[128,129] Increasing the number of targeted epicardial biopsies increases yield.[130] In contrast, blind pericardial biopsy has a lower sensitivity to cytology alone (45–55%).[113,122]

In the majority, clinical presentation, chest radiography, electrocardiography and echocardiography indicate only the presence of significant pericardial disease.[122] CT and MR imaging may be useful in providing evidence of malignancy elsewhere and further detail on pericardial and myocardial involvement.[131] The diagnosis of neoplastic pericarditis therefore rests on adequate sampling of pericardial fluid or tissue for pathologic examination. However, only 40–55% of malignancy-related effusions are shown to be secondary to neoplastic pericardial spread when investigated invasively.[122,129] Other causes include radiation pericarditis in 3–18% and idiopathic pericardial effusions in 30%.

Management

Treatment of neoplastic pericardial effusion is directed at the relief of immediate symptoms of pericarditis or tamponade, preventing reaccumulation, and diagnosis and management of the underlying cancer.[132] Pericardiocentesis is recommended for diagnosis in suspected neoplastic pericardial effusion, and as a therapeutic intervention in the presence of cardiac tamponade (**Class I, Level C2**). The great challenge is to prevent recurrence of malignant pericardial effusion. There are three strategies that have been used: (1) intrapericardial instillation of cytostatic/sclerosing agents (Table 52.4), (2) intrapericardial or external radiation therapy, and (3) mechanical drainage by pericardiocentesis with indwelling catheter, subxiphoid pericardiotomy or

Table 52.4 Recent prospective experience of intrapericardial therapy in preventing recurrent neoplastic effusion (limited to those distinguishing outcome of pericardial disease)

Study	Intrapericardial therapy	No. of patients	Malignancy	Success at preventing recurrence (%)	Stated complications
Lashevski[133]	Minocycline	14	Varied	93	Pericarditis (n = 7)
Liu[134]	Doxycycline	10	Varied	90	Pericarditis (n = 7)
Martinoni et al[117]	Thiotepa	33	Varied	91	Nil
Bishiniotis[135]	Thiotepa	19	Breast	100	Nil
Colleoni[136]	Thiotepa	23	Varied	83	Leukopenia (n = 1), leukopenia + thrombocytopenia (n = 1)
Maisch[137]	Cisplatin	42	Varied	83 (lung 96, breast 63)	Myocardial ischemia (n = 1)
Tomkowski et al[138]	Cisplatin	46	Varied	93	AF (n = 7), non-constricting pericardial sclerosis (n = 5)
Bischiniotis[139]	Cisplatin	25	Lung adenocarcinoma	96	AF (n = 3), NSVT (n = 2), non-constricting pericardial sclerosis (n = 4)
Moriya[140]	Carboplatin	10	NSCLC	80	Nil
Kunitoh[132a]	Bleomycin	38	Lung unspecified	77%#	Pain (n = 11*), Infection (n = 3*), Bleeding (n = 2), cardiac dysfunction (n = 1), pericardial constriction (n = 1), transient fever (n = 2)
Marayuma et al[141]	Bleomycin	22	NSCLC	95	Pericardial constriction (n = 1)
Liu[134]	Bleomycin	10	Varied	90	Nil
Yano[142]	Bleomycin	7	NSCLC	71	Nil
Kaira[143]	Mitomycin C	8	NSCLC	75	Nil
Lee[144]	Mitomycin C	20	Varied	70	Pericardial constriction (n = 1)
Kawashima[145]	Aclarubicin	5	Breast and lung	100	Nil
Musch[146]	Mitoxantrone	16	Varied	94	Nil
Norum[147]	Mitoxantrone	5	Breast and ovarian	60	Nil
Dempke[148]	32P-colloid	36	Varied	95	Nil
Toh[149]	Autologous IL-2 activated tumor-infiltrating lymphocytes	4	Varied	100	Low-grade fever (n = 4)

NSCLC, non-small cell lung carcinoma; AF, atrial fibrillation; NSVT, non-sustained ventricular tachycardia; IL-2, interleukin 2. # using 6 month data; * no different from controls.

pleuropericardiotomy with drainage of malignant pericardial effusion into the pleural space. Vaitkus and colleagues report a statistically superior effect of indwelling pericardial catheters, intrapericardial sclerosis, subxiphoid or percutaneous balloon pericardiotomy and pericardiectomy over pericardiocentesis alone (**Class IIb, Level C2**).[132] In the treatment of lung cancer-associated moderate to large pericardial effusions, intrapericardial instillation of bleomycin following pericardial drainage was not demonstrated to be superior to drainage alone in a randomised trial of 80 patients. Survival at two months free of effusion was 29% in the bleomycin group compared to 46% in controls (one-sided $P = 0.086$). There was no difference in symptom palliation, survival was equally low at 6 months (27% vs 31%), and rates of repeat pericardiocentesis were not reported.[132a]

In choosing the appropriate strategy for the management of the patient with neoplastic pericardial effusion, it is important to note, first, that the treatment of neoplastic pericardial effusion is palliative as the prognosis is ultimately determined by the underlying disease. Second, there are no good randomized studies to guide the management strategy in this field. Finally, the management of the patient must be individualized and will depend on the experience and available therapeutic options in a particular center, and the preferences of the patient and relatives.

References

1. Reuter H, Burgess L, van Vuuren W, Doubell A. Diagnosing tuberculous pericarditis. *QJM* 2006;**99**:827–39.
2. Imazio M, Cecchi E, Demichelis B *et al*. Indicators of poor prognosis of acute pericarditis. *Circulation* 2007;**115**:2739–44.
3. Soler Soler J, Sagrista Sauleda J, Permanyer Miralda G. Management of pericardial effusion. *Heart* 2001;**86**:235–240.
4. Permanyer-Miralda G, Sagrista-Sauleda J, Soler-Soler J Primary acute pericardial disease: a prospective series of 231 consecutive patients. *Am J Cardiol* 1985;**56**:623–30.

5. Zayas R, Anguita M, Torres F et al. Incidence of specific etiology and role of methods for specific etiologic diagnosis of primary acute pericarditis. Am J Cardiol 1995;**75**:378–82.

6. Imazio M, Cecchi E, Demichelis B et al. Myopericarditis versus viral or idiopathic acute pericarditis. Heart 2008;**94**(4):498–501.

7. Brady WJ, Perron AD, Martin ML, Beagle C, Aufderheide TP. Cause of ST segment abnormality in ED chest pain patients. Am J Emerg Med 2001;**19**:25–28.

8. Imazio M, Demichelis B, Parrini I et al. Day-hospital treatment of acute pericarditis: a management program for outpatient therapy. J Am Coll Cardiol 2004;**43**:1042–6.

9. Levy PY, Corey R, Berger P et al. Etiologic diagnosis of 204 pericardial effusions. Medicine (Baltimore) 2003;**82**:385–91.

10. Maisch B, Seferovic PM, Ristic AD et al. Guidelines on the diagnosis and management of pericardial diseases executive summary; The Task force on the diagnosis and management of pericardial diseases of the European society of cardiology. Eur Heart J 2004;**25**:587–610.

11. Lange RA, Hillis LD. Clinical practice. Acute pericarditis. N Engl J Med 2004;**351**:2195–202.

12. Sagrista-Sauleda J, Merce J, Permanyer-Miralda G, Soler-Soler J Clinical clues to the causes of large pericardial effusions. Am J Med 2000;**109**:95–101.

13. Mayosi BM, Burgess LJ, Doubell AF. Tuberculous pericarditis. Circulation 2005;**112**:3608–16.

14. Schifferdecker B, Spodick DH. Nonsteroidal anti-inflammatory drugs in the treatment of pericarditis. Cardiol Rev 2003;**11**:211–17.

15. Arunsalam S, Siegel RJ. Rapid resolution of symptomatic acute pericarditis with ketorolac tromethamine: a parenteral nonsteroidal antiinflammatory agent. Am Heart J 1883;**125**:1455–8.

16. Shabetai R. Recurrent pericarditis: recent advances and remaining questions. Circulation 2005;**112**:1921–3.

17. Imazio M, Bobbio M, Cecchi E et al. Colchicine in addition to conventional therapy for acute pericarditis: results of the COlchicine for acute PEricarditis (COPE) trial. Circulation 2005;**112**:2012–16.

18. Imazio M, Cecchi E, Ierna S, Trinchero R. Investigation on Colchicine for Acute Pericarditis: a multicentre randomised placebo-controlled trial evaluating the clinical benefits of colchicine as adjunct to conventional threapy in the treatment and prevention of pericarditis; study design and rationale. J Cardiovasc Med (Hagerstown) 2007;**8**:613–17.

19. Di Pasquale P, Cannizzaro S, Fasullo S et al. The combination of indomethacin and statin versus indomethacin and placebo in patients with first episode of acute pericarditis: preliminary findings. Clin Sci (Lond) 2007;**113**:443–8.

20. Soler-Soler J, Sagrista-Sauleda J, Permanyer-Miralda G. Relapsing pericarditis. Heart 2004;**90**:1364–8.

21. Maisch B, Ristic AD, Pankuweit S. Intrapericardial treatment of autoreactive pericardial effusion with triamcinolone; the way to avoid side effects of systemic corticosteroid therapy. Eur Heart J 2002;**23**:1503–8.

22. Imazio M, Bobbio M, Cecchi E et al. Colchicine as first-choice therapy for recurrent pericarditis: results of the CORE (COlchicine for REcurrent pericarditis) trial. Arch Intern Med 2005;**165**:1987–91.

23. Fowler NO, Harbin AD. Recurrent acute pericarditis: follow-up study of 31 patients. J Am Coll Cardiol 1986;**7**:300–5.

24. Brucato A, Brambilla G, Moreo A et al. Long-term outcomes in difficult-to-treat patients with recurrent pericarditis. Am J Cardiol 2006;**98**:267–71.

25. Imazio M, Demichelis B, Parrini I et al. Management, risk factors, and outcomes in recurrent pericarditis. Am J Cardiol 2005;**96**:736–9.

26. Artom G, Koren-Morag N, Spodick DH et al. Pretreatment with corticosteroids attenuates the efficacy of colchicine in preventing recurrent pericarditis: a multi-centre all-case analysis. Eur Heart J 2005;**26**:723–7.

27. Millaire A, de Groote P, Decoulx E, Goullard L, Ducloux G. Treatment of recurrent pericarditis with colchicine. Eur Heart J 1994;**15**:120–4.

28. Adler Y, Finkelstein Y, Guindo J et al. Colchicine treatment for recurrent pericarditis. A decade of experience. Circulation 1998;**97**:2183–5.

28a. Imazio M, Brucato A, Cumetti D et al. Corticosteroids for recurrent pericarditis: high versus low doses: a nonrandomized observation. Circulation 2008;**118**:667–71.

29. Sagristà-Sauleda J, Angel J, Permanyer-Miralda G, Soler-Soler J. Long-term follow-up of idiopathic chronic pericardial effusion. N Engl J Med 1999;**341**:2054–9.

30. Tsang TS, Barnes ME, Gersh BJ, Bailey KR, Seward JB. Outcomes of clinically significant idiopathic pericardial effusion requiring intervention. Am J Cardiol 2003;**91**:704–7.

31. Loire R, Goineau P, Fareh S, Saint-Pierre A. Apparently idiopathic chronic pericardial effusion. Long-term outcome in 71 cases. Arch Mal Coeur Vaiss 1996;**89**:835–41.

32. Hatcher CR Jr, Logue RB, Logan WD Jr, Symbas PN, Mansour KA, Abbott OA. Pericardiectomy for recurrent pericarditis. J Thorac Cardiovasc Surg 1971;**62**:371–8.

33. Asplen CH, Levine HD. Azathioprine therapy of steroid responsive pericarditis. Am Heart J 1970;**80**:109–11.

34. Melchior TM, Ringsdal V, Hildebrandt P, Torp-Pedersen C. Recurrent acute idiopathic pericarditis treated with intravenous methylprednisolone given as pulse therapy. Am Heart J 1992;**123**(4 Pt 1):1086–8.

35. Marcolongo R, Russo R, Lavender F, Noventa F, Agostini C. Immunosuppressive therapy prevents recurrent pericarditis. J Am Coll Cardiol 1995;**26**:1276–9.

36. Peterlana D, Puccetti A, Simeoni S, Tinazzi E, Corrocher R, Lunardi C. Efficacy of intravenous immunoglobulin in chronic idiopathic pericarditis: report of four cases. Clin Rheumatol 2005;**24**:18–21.

37. Tona F, Bellotto F, Laveder F, Meneghin A, Sinagra G, Marcolongo R. Efficacy of high-dose intravenous immunoglobulins in two patients with idiopathic recurrent pericarditis refractory to previous immunosuppressive treatment. Ital Heart J 2003;**4**:64–8.

38. Becit N, Unlu Y, Ceviz M, Kocogullari CI, Kocak H, Gurlertop Y. Subxiphoid pericardiostomy in the management of pericardial effusions: case series analysis of 368 patients. Heart 2005;**91**:785–90.

39. Allen KB, Faber LP, Warren WH, Shaar CJ. Pericardial effusion: subxiphoid pericardiostomy versus percutaneous catheter drainage. Ann Thorac Surg 1999;**67**:437–40.

40. Nataf P, Cacoub P, Dorent R et al. Results of subtotal pericardiectomy for constrictive pericarditis. Eur J Cardiothorac Surg 1993;**7**:252–5; discussion 255–6.

41. Ling LH, Oh JK, Schaff HV *et al.* Constrictive pericarditis in the modern era: evolving clinical spectrum and impact on outcome after pericardiectomy. *Circulation* 1999;**100**:1380–6.

42. Bertog SC, Thambidorai SK, Parakh K *et al.* Constrictive pericarditis: etiology and cause-specific survival after pericardiectomy. *J Am Coll Cardiol* 2004;**43**:1445–52.

43. Sagrista Sauleda J, Barrabés JA, Permanyer Miralda G, Soler Soler J Purulent pericarditis: review of a 20-year experience in a general hospital. *J Am Coll Cardiol* 1993;**22**:1661–5.

44. Rubin RH, Moellering RC Jr. Clinical, microbiologic and therapeutic aspects of purulent pericarditis. *Am J Med Sci* 1975;**59**:68.

45. Brook I, Frazier EH. Microbiology of acute purulent pericarditis. A 12-year experience in a military hospital. *Arch Intern Med* 1996;**156**:1857–60.

46. Goodman LJ. Purulent pericarditis. *Curr Treat Options Cardiovasc Med* 2000;**2**:343–50.

47. Morse JR, Oretsky MI, Hudson JAM. Pericarditis as a complication of meningococcal meningitis. *Ann Intern Med* 1971; **74**(2):212–17.

48. Pierce HI, Cooper EB. Meningococcal pericarditis: clinical features and therapy in five patients. *Arch Intern Med* 1972;**129**:918.

49. Falcao SN, Tsutsui JM, Ramires FJ *et al.* The role of echocardiography in diagnosis and management of isolated meningococcal pericarditis. *Echocardiography* 2007;**24**:263–6.

50. Franco-Paredes C, Rouphael N, Mendez J *et al.* Cardiac manifestations of parasitic infections part 1: overview and immunopathogenesis. *Clin Cardiol* 2007;**30**:195–9.

51. Louw A, Tikly M. Purulent pericarditis due to co-infection with Streptococcus pneumoniae and Mycobacterium tuberculosis in a patient with features of advanced HIV infection. *BMC Infect Dis* 2007;**7**:12.

52. Leang B, Lynen L, Lim K, Jacques G, Van Esbroeck M, Zolfo M. Disseminated nocardiosis presenting with cardiac tamponade in an HIV patient. *Int J STD AIDS* 2004;**15**:839–40.

53. Xie L, Gebre W, Szabo K, Lin JH. Cardiac aspergillosis in patients with acquired immunodeficiency syndrome: a case report and review of the literature. *Arch Pathol Lab Med* 2005;**129**:511–15.

54. Uzoigwe C. Campylobacter infections of the pericardium and myocardium. *Clin Microbiol Infect* 2005;**11**:253–5.

55. Kan B, Ries J, Normark BH *et al.* Endocarditis and pericarditis complicating pneumococcal bacteraemia, with special reference to the adhesive abilities of pneumococci: results from a prospective study. *Clin Microbiol Infect* 2006;**12**:338–44.

56. Caksen H, Uzum K, Yuksel S, Basriustunbas H, Ozturk MK, Narin N. Cardiac findings in childhood staphylococcal sepsis. *Jpn Heart J* 2002;**43**:9–11.

57. Cakir O, Gurkan F, Balci AE, Eren N, Dikici B. Purulent pericarditis in childhood: ten years of experience. *J Pediatr Surg* 2002;**37**:1404–8.

58. Ben-Horin S, Bank I, Shinfeld A, Kachel E, Guetta V, Livneh A. Diagnostic value of the biochemical composition of pericardial effusions in patients undergoing pericardiocentesis. *Am J Cardiol* 2007;**99**:1294–7.

59. Sinzobahamvya N. Results of subxiphoid pericardiostomy in pericardial effusion. *Acta Chir Belg* 1988;**88**:175–8.

60. Winkler WB, Karnik R, Slany J. Treatment of exudative fibrinous pericarditis with intrapericardial urokinase. *Lancet* 1994;**344**:1541–2.

61. Defouilloy C, Meyer G, Slama Mea. Intrapericardial fibrinolysis: a useful treatment in the management of purulent pericarditis. *Intensive Care Med* 1997;**23**:117.

62. Juneja R, Kothari SS, Saxena A *et al.* Intrapericardial streptokinase in purulent pericarditis. *Arch Dis Child* 1999;**80**:275.

63. Bridgman PG. Failure of intrapericardial streptokinase in purulent pericarditis. *Intensive Care Med* 2001;**27**:942.

64. Keersmaekers T, Elshot SR, Sergeant PT. Primary bacterial pericarditis. *Acta Cardiol* 2002;**57**:387–9.

65. Ustunsoy H, Celkan MA, Sivrikoz MC, Kazaz H, Kilinc M. Intrapericardial fibrinolytic therapy in purulent pericarditis. *Eur J Cardiothorac Surg* 2002;**22**:373–6.

66. Reznikoff CP, Fish JT, Coursin DB. Pericardial infusion of tissue plasminogen activator in fibropurulent pericarditis. *J Intensive Care Med* 2003;**18**:47–51.

67. Ekim H, Demirbag R. Intrapericardial streptokinase for purulent pericarditis. *Surg Today* 2004;**34**:569–72.

68. Tomkowski WZ, Gralec R, Kuca P, Burakowski J, Orlowski T, Kurzyna M. Effectiveness of intrapericardial administration of streptokinase in purulent pericarditis. *Herz* 2004;**29**:802–5.

69. Cui HB, Chen XY, Cui CC *et al.* Prevention of pericardial constriction by transcatheter intrapericardial fibrinolysis with urokinase. *Chin Med Sci J* 2005;**20**:5–10.

70. Cegielski JP, Ramiya K, Lallinger GJ, Mtulia IA, Mbaga IM. Pericardial disease and human immunodeficiency virus in Dar es Salaam, Tanzania. *Lancet* 1990;**335**:209–12.

71. Maher D, Harries AD. Tuberculous pericardial effusion: a prospective clinical study in a low-resource setting – Blantyre, Malawi. *Int J Tuberculosis Lung Dis* 1997;**1**:358–64.

72. Reuter H, Burgess LJ, Doubell AF. Epidemiology of pericardial effusions at a large academic hospital in South Africa. *Epidemiol Infect* 2005;**133**:393–9.

73. Spodick DH. Tuberculous pericarditis. *AMA Arch Intern Med* 1956;**98**:737–49.

74. Schepers GW. Tuberculous pericarditis. *Am J Cardiol* 1962;**9**: 248–76.

75. Strang JI, Kakaza HH, Gibson DG *et al.* Controlled clinical trial of complete open surgical drainage and of prednisolone in treatment of tuberculous pericardial effusion in Transkei. *Lancet* 1988;**2**:759–64.

76. Strang JI, Kakaza HH, Gibson DG, Girling DJ, Nunn AJ, Fox W. Controlled trial of prednisolone as adjuvant in treatment of tuberculous constrictive pericarditis in Transkei. *Lancet* 1987;**2**:1418–22.

77. Hugo-Hamman CT, Scher H, De Moor MM. Tuberculous pericarditis in children: a review of 44 cases. *Pediatr Infect Dis J* 1994;**13**:13–18.

78. Komsuoglu B, Goldeli O, Kulan K, Gedik Y. Tuberculous pericarditis in north-east Turkey. An echocardiographic study. *Acta Cardiol* 1994;**49**:157–63.

79. Mayosi BM, Wiysonge CS, Ntsekhe M *et al.* Clinical characteristics and initial management of patients with tuberculous pericarditis in the HIV era: the Investigation of the Management of Pericarditis in Africa (IMPI Africa) registry. *BMC Infect Dis* 2006;**6**:2.

80. Syed FF, Mayosi BM. A modern approach to tuberculous pericarditis. *Prog Cardiovasc Dis* 2007;**50**:218–36.

81. Strang JI. Tuberculous pericarditis in Transkei. *Clin Cardiol* 1984;**7**:667–70.

82. Reuter H, Burgess LJ, Doubell AF. The role of chest radiography in diagnosing patients with tuberculous pericarditis. *Cardiovasc J S Afr* 2005;**16**:108–11.

83. Ortbals DW, Avioli LV. Tuberculous pericarditis. *Arch Intern Med* 1979;**139**:231–4.

84. Fowler NO. Tuberculous pericarditis. *JAMA* 1991;**266**:99–103.

85. Sagrista-Sauleda J, Permanyer-Miralda G, Soler-Soler J. Tuberculous pericarditis: ten year experience with a prospective protocol for diagnosis and treatment. *J Am Coll Cardiol* 1988;**11**:724–8.

86. Smedema JP, Katjitae I, Reuter H et al. Twelve-lead electrocardiography in tuberculous pericarditis. *Cardiovasc J S Afr* 2001;**12**:31–4.

87. George S, Salama AL, Uthaman B, Cherian G. Echocardiography in differentiating tuberculous from chronic idiopathic pericardial effusion. *Heart* 2004;**90**:1338–9.

88. Liu PY, Li YH, Tsai WC et al. Usefulness of echocardiographic intrapericardial abnormalities in the diagnosis of tuberculous pericardial effusion. *Am J Cardiol* 2001;**87**:1133–5, A10.

89. Cherian G, Habashy AG, Uthaman B, Cherian JM, Salama A, Anim JT. Detection and follow-up of mediastinal lymph node enlargement in tuberculous pericardial effusions using computed tomography. *Am J Med* 2003;**114**:319–22.

90. Gulati GS, Sharma S. Pericardial abscess occurring after tuberculous pericarditis: image morphology on computed tomography and magnetic resonance imaging. *Clin Radiol* 2004;**59**:514–19.

91. Hayashi H, Kawamata H, Machida M, Kumazaki T. Tuberculous pericarditis: MRI features with contrast enhancement. *Br J Radiol* 1998;**71**:680–2.

92. Ha JW, Lee JD, Ko YG et al. Images in cardiovascular medicine. Assessment of pericardial inflammation in a patient with tuberculous effusive constrictive pericarditis with 18F-2-deoxyglucose positron emission tomography. *Circulation* 2006;113:e4–5.

93. Rodriguez E, Soler R, Juffe A, Salgado L. CT and MR findings in a calcified myocardial tuberculoma of the left ventricle. *J Comput Assist Tomogr* 2001;**25**:577–9.

94. Khera G, Chowdhury V, Singh S, Dixit R. Magnetic resonance imaging of effusive constrictive pericarditis. *Indian Heart J* 2005;**57**:780–2.

95. Combs DL, O'Brien RJ, Geiter LJ. USPHS Tuberculosis Short-Course Chemotherapy Trial 21: effectiveness, toxicity and acceptability: the report of final results. *Ann Intern Med* 1990;**112**:397–406.

96. Perriens JH, St Louis ME, Mukadi YB et al. Pulmonary tuberculosis in HIV-infected patients in Zaire: a controlled trial of treatment for either 6 or 12 months. *N Engl J Med* 1995;**332**:779–85.

97. Mayosi BM. Interventions for treating tuberculous pericarditis. *Cochrane Database of Systematic Reviews* 2002, Issue 4. Art. No.: CD000526. DOI: 10.1002/14651858.CD000526.

98. Reuter H, Burgess LJ, Louw VJ, Doubell AF. The management of tuberculous pericardial effusion: experience in 233 consecutive patients. *Cardiovasc J S Afr* 2007;**18**:20–5.

99. Schrire V. Experience with pericarditis at Groote Schuur Hospital, Cape Town: an analysis of one hundred and sixty cases studied over a six-year period. *S Afr Med J* 1959;**33**:810–17.

100. Komsuoglu B, Gedik Y, Duman E. Tuberculous pericarditis in north-east Turkey. An echocardiographic study. *Mater Med Pol* 1989;**21**:141–2.

101. Bahn GL. Tuberculous pericarditis. *J Infect* 1980;**2**:360–4.

102. Wang ZJ, Reddy GP, Gotway MB, Yeh BM, Hetts SW, Higgins CB. CT and MR imaging of pericardial disease. *Radiographics* 2003;**23**:S167–80.

103. Talreja DR, Edwards WD, Danielson GK et al. Constrictive pericarditis in 26 patients with histologically normal pericardial thickness. *Circulation* 2003;**108**:1852–7.

104. Strang JI, Nunn AJ, Johnson DA, Casbard A, Gibson DG, Girling DJ. Management of tuberculous constrictive pericarditis and tuberculous pericardial effusion in Transkei: results at 10 years follow-up. *QJM* 2004;**97**:525–35.

105. Bashi VV, John S, Ravikumar E, Jairaj PS, Shyamsunder K, Krishnaswami S. Early and late results of pericardiectomy in 118 cases of constrictive pericarditis. *Thorax* 1988;**43**:637–41.

106. Cinar B, Enc Y, Goksel O et al. Chronic constrictive tuberculous pericarditis: risk factors and outcome of pericardiectomy. *Int J Tuberc Lung Dis* 2006;**10**:701–6.

107. Chowdhury UK, Subramaniam GK, Kumar AS et al. Pericardiectomy for constrictive pericarditis: a clinical, echocardiographic, and hemodynamic evaluation of two surgical techniques. *Ann Thorac Surg* 2006;**81**:522–9.

108. Syed FF, Russell JW, Ntsekhe M, Mayosi BM. An early invasive approach to the investigation of suspected tuberculous pericardial effusion: initial lessons from the Investigation of the Management of PericarditIs (IMPI) Cohort Study. *Cardiovasc J S Afr* 2007;**18**:121.

109. Reuter H, Burgess LJ, Louw VJ, Doubell AF. Experience with adjunctive corticosteroids in managing tuberculous pericarditis. *Cardiovasc J S Afr* 2006;**17**:233–8.

110. Hakim JG, Ternouth I, Mushangi E, Siziya S, Robertson V, Malin A. Double blind randomised placebo controlled trial of adjunctive prednisolone in the treatment of effusive tuberculous pericarditis in HIV seropositive patients. *Heart* 2000;**84**:183–8.

111. Ntsekhe M, Hakim J Impact of human immunodeficiency virus infection on cardiovascular disease in Africa. *Circulation* 2005;**112**:3602–7.

112. Tsang TS, Enriquez-Sarano M, Freeman WK et al. Consecutive 1127 therapeutic echocardiographically guided pericardiocenteses: clinical profile, practice patterns, and outcomes spanning 21 years. *Mayo Clin Proc* 2002;**77**:429–36.

113. McDonald JM, Meyers BF, Guthrie TJ, Battafarano RJ, Cooper JD, Patterson GA. Comparison of open subxiphoid pericardial drainage with percutaneous catheter drainage for symptomatic pericardial effusion. *Ann Thorac Surg* 2003;**76**:811–15; discussion 816.

114. Imazio M, Demichelis B, Parrini I et al. Relation of acute pericardial disease to malignancy. *Am J Cardiol* 2005;**95**:1393–4.

115. Ben-Horin S, Bank I, Guetta V, Livneh A. Large symptomatic pericardial effusion as the presentation of unrecognized cancer: a study in 173 consecutive patients undergoing pericardiocentesis. *Medicine (Baltimore)* 2006;**85**:49–53.

116. Girardi LN, Ginsberg RJ, Burt ME. Pericardiocentesis and intrapericardial sclerosis: effective therapy for malignant pericardial effusions. *Ann Thorac Surg* 1997;**64**:1422–8.

117. Martinoni A, Cipolla CM, Cardinale D, Civelli M, Lamantia G, Colleoni M, Fiorentini C. Long-term results of intrapericardial chemotherapeutic treatment of malignant pericardial effusions with thiotepa. *Chest* 2004;**126**:1412–16.

118. Cullinane CA, Paz IB, Smith D, Carter N, Grannis FW Jr. Prognostic factors in the surgical management of pericardial

effusion in the patient with concurrent malignancy. *Chest* 2004;**125**:1328–34.

119. Boulanger E, Gerard L, Gabarre J *et al.* Prognostic factors and outcome of human herpesvirus 8-associated primary effusion lymphoma in patients with AIDS. *J Clin Oncol* 2005;**23**:4372–80.

120. Gross JL, Younes RN, Deheinzelin D, Diniz AL, Silva RA, Haddad FJ. Surgical management of symptomatic pericardial effusion in patients with solid malignancies. *Ann Surg Oncol* 2006;**13**:1732–8.

121. Wiener HG, Kristensen IB, Haubek A, Kristensen B, Baandrup U. The diagnostic value of pericardial cytology. An analysis of 95 cases. *Acta Cytol* 1991;**35**(2):149–53.

122. Wilkes JD, Fidias P, Vaickus L, Perez RP. Malignancy-related pericardial effusion. 127 cases from the Roswell Park Cancer Institute. *Cancer* 1995;**76**:1377–87.

123. Meyers DG, Meyers RE, Prendergast TW. The usefulness of diagnostic tests on pericardial fluid. *Chest* 1997;**111**:1213–21.

124. Politi E, Kandaraki C, Apostolopoulou C, Kyritsi T, Koutselini H. Immunocytochemical panel for distinguishing between carcinoma and reactive mesothelial cells in body cavity fluids. *Diagn Cytopathol* 2005;**32**:151–5.

125. Pomjanski N, Grote HJ, Doganay P, Schmiemann V, Buckstegge B, Bocking A. Immunocytochemical identification of carcinomas of unknown primary in serous effusions. *Diagn Cytopathol* 2005;**33**:309–15.

126. Bardales RH, Stanley MW, Schaefer RF, Liblit RL, Owens RB, Surhland MJ. Secondary pericardial malignancies: a critical appraisal of the role of cytology, pericardial biopsy, and DNA ploidy analysis. *Am J Clin Pathol* 1996;**106**:29–34.

127. Zendehrokh N, Dejmek A. Telomere repeat amplification protocol (TRAP) in situ reveals telomerase activity in three cell types in effusions: malignant cells, proliferative mesothelial cells, and lymphocytes. *Mod Pathol* 2005;**18**:189–96.

128. Nugue O, Millaire A, Porte H, de Groote P, Guimier P, Wurtz A, Ducloux G. Pericardioscopy in the etiologic diagnosis of pericardial effusion in 141 consecutive patients. *Circulation* 1996;**94**:1635–41.

129. Porte HL, Janecki-Delebecq TJ, Finzi L, Metois DG, Millaire A, Wurtz AJ. Pericardoscopy for primary management of pericardial effusion in cancer patients. *Eur J Cardiothorac Surg* 1999;**16**:287–91.

130. Seferovic PM, Ristic AD, Maksimovic R, Tatic V, Ostojic M, Kanjuh V. Diagnostic value of pericardial biopsy: improvement with extensive sampling enabled by pericardioscopy. *Circulation* 2003;**107**:978–83.

131. Chiles C, Woodard PK, Gutierrez FR, Link KM. Metastatic Involvement of the Heart and Pericardium: CT and MR Imaging. *Radiographics* 2001;**21**:439–49.

132. Vaitkus PT, Herrmann HC, LeWinter MM. Treatment of malignant pericardial effusion. *JAMA* 1994;**272**:59–64.

132a. Kunitoh H, Tamura T, Shibata T *et al.* A randomised trial of intrapericardial bleomycin for malignant pericardial effusion with lung cancer (JCOG9811). *Br J Cancer* 2009;**100**:464–69.

133. Lashevsky I, Ben Yosef R, Rinkevich D, Reisner S, Markiewicz W. Intrapericardial minocycline sclerosis for malignant pericardial effusion. *Chest* 1996;**109**:1452–4.

134. Liu G, Crump M, Goss PE, Dancey J, Shepherd FA. Prospective comparison of the sclerosing agents doxycycline and bleomy-

cin for the primary management of malignant pericardial effusion and cardiac tamponade. *J Clin Oncol* 1996;**14**:3141–7.

135. Bishiniotis TS, Antoniadou S, Katseas GP, Mouratidou D, Litos AG, Balamoutsos N. Malignant cardiac tamponade in women with breast cancer treated by pericardiocentesis and intrapericardial administration of triethylenethiophosphoramide (thiotepa). *Am J Cardiol* 2000;**86**:362–4.

136. Colleoni M, Martinelli G, Beretta F *et al.* Intracavitary chemotherapy with thiotepa in malignant pericardial effusions: an active and well-tolerated regimen. *J Clin Oncol* 1998;**16**: 2371–6.

137. Maisch B, Ristic AD, Pankuweit S, Neubauer A, Moll R. Neoplastic pericardial effusion. Efficacy and safety of intrapericardial treatment with cisplatin. *Eur Heart J* 2002;**23**:1625–31.

138. Tomkowski WZ, Wisniewska J, Szturmowicz M *et al.* Evaluation of intrapericardial cisplatin administration in cases with recurrent malignant pericardial effusion and cardiac tamponade. *Support Care Cancer* 2004;**12**:53–7.

139. Bischiniotis TS, Lafaras CT, Platogiannis DN, Moldovan L, Barbetakis NG, Katseas GP. Intrapericardial cisplatin administration after pericardiocentesis in patients with lung adenocarcinoma and malignant cardiac tamponade. *Hellenic J Cardiol* 2005;**46**:324–9.

140. Moriya T, Takiguchi Y, Tabeta H *et al.* Controlling malignant pericardial effusion by intrapericardial carboplatin administration in patients with primary non-small-cell lung cancer. *Br J Cancer* 2000;**83**:858–62.

141. Maruyama R, Yokoyama H, Seto T *et al.* Catheter drainage followed by the instillation of bleomycin to manage malignant pericardial effusion in non-small cell lung cancer: a multi-institutional phase II trial. *J Thorac Oncol* 2007;**2**:65–8.

142. Yano T, Yokoyama H, Inoue T, Takanashi N, Asoh H, Ichinose Y. A simple technique to manage malignant pericardial effusion with a local instillation of bleomycin in non-small cell carcinoma of the lung. *Oncology* 1994;**51**:507–9.

143. Kaira K, Takise A, Kobayashi G *et al.* Management of malignant pericardial effusion with instillation of mitomycin C in non-small cell lung cancer. *Jpn J Clin Oncol* 2005;**35**:57–60.

144. Lee LN, Yang PC, Chang DB *et al.* Ultrasound guided pericardial drainage and intrapericardial instillation of mitomycin C for malignant pericardial effusion. *Thorax* 1994;**49**:594–5.

145. Kawashima O, Kurihara T, Kamiyoshihara M, Sakata S, Ishikawa S, Morishita Y. Management of malignant pericardial effusion resulting from recurrent cancer with local instillation of aclarubicin hydrochloride. *Am J Clin Oncol* 1999;**22**:396–8.

146. Musch E, Gremmler B, Nitsch J, Rieger J, Malek M, Chrissafidou A. Intrapericardial instillation of mitoxantrone in palliative therapy of malignant pericardial effusion. *Onkologie* 2003;**26**:135–9.

147. Norum J, Lunde P, Aasebo U, Himmelmann A. Mitoxantrone in malignant pericardial effusion. *J Chemother* 1998;**10**: 399–404.

148. Dempke W, Firusian N. Treatment of malignant pericardial effusion with 32P-colloid. *Br J Cancer* 1999;**80**:1955–7.

149. Toh U, Fujii T, Seki N, Niiya F, Shirouzu K, Yamana H. Characterization of IL-2-activated TILs and their use in intrapericardial immunotherapy in malignant pericardial effusion. *Cancer Immunol Immunother* 2006;**55**:1219–27.

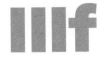

Specific cardiovascular disorders: valvular heart disease

Bernard J Gersh, Editor

53 Rheumatic heart disease: prevention and acute treatment

Bongani M Mayosi and Patrick J Commerford
Division of Cardiology, Department of Medicine, Groote Schuur Hospital and University of Cape Town, Cape Town, South Africa

Introduction

Rheumatic fever is the most important cause of acquired heart disease in children and young adults worldwide. Initiated by an oropharyngeal infection with group A beta-hemolytic streptococci (GAS) and following a latent period of approximately 3 weeks, the illness is characterized by an inflammatory process primarily involving the heart, joints, and central nervous system. Pathologically, the inflammatory process causes damage to collagen fibrils and connective tissue ground substance (fibrinoid degeneration) and thus rheumatic fever is classified as a connective tissue or collagen vascular disease. It is the destructive effect on the heart valves that leads to the important effects of the disease, with serious hemodynamic disturbances causing cardiac failure or embolic phenomena resulting in significant morbidity and mortality at a young age.

A number of recent systematic reviews have summarized the effectiveness of primary and secondary prevention of rheumatic fever and the treatment of the acute attack.[1-3] The evidence from randomized controlled clinical trials, while dated, is in favor of the effectiveness of antibiotics in the primary (or the treatment of pharyngitis caused by group A streptococci) and secondary prevention of rheumatic fever.[1,2] In the treatment of the acute attack, most publications have been observational studies with only a small minority of poorly designed randomized trials.[3]

Epidemiology

In the developed countries of the world, the incidence of rheumatic fever has fallen markedly during the last century. For example, in the USA the incidence per 100 000 was 100 at the start of the last century, 45–65 between 1935 and 1960, and is currently estimated to be approximately 10 cases per 100 000.[4] This decrease in rheumatic fever incidence preceded the introduction of antibiotics and is a reflection of improved socio-economic standards, less overcrowded housing and improved access to medical care. The current prevalence of rheumatic heart disease in the USA and Japan, 0.6–0.7 per 1000 population, contrasts sharply with that in the developing countries of Africa and Asia where rates as high as 30 per 1000 have been reported.[5] As GAS pharyngitis and rheumatic fever are causally related, both diseases share similar epidemiologic features.[4] The age of first infection is commonly between 6 and 15 years. Also, the risk for developing rheumatic fever is highest in situations where GAS is more common, for example where people live in crowded conditions.[6]

Pathogenesis

Clinical, epidemiologic, and immunologic observations tend to strongly support the causative role of untreated GAS pharyngitis in rheumatic fever.[6,7] Beyond this, however, the pathogenesis of acute rheumatic fever (ARF) and clinical heart disease remains unclear and several important and unexplained observations render the management of this important disease extremely difficult. These are:
- individual variability of susceptibility to GAS pharyngitis
- individual variability of development of symptomatic GAS pharyngitis
- individual variability of development of acute rheumatic fever after an episode of GAS pharyngitis
- individual variation in the development of carditis and chronic rheumatic heart disease after an attack of acute rheumatic fever
- the development of chronic rheumatic heart disease (RHD) in patients who have no definite history of acute rheumatic fever.

Evidence-Based Cardiology, 3rd edition. Edited by S. Yusuf, J.A. Cairns, A.J. Camm, E.L. Fallen, and B.J. Gersh. © 2010 Blackwell Publishing, ISBN: 978-1-4051-5925-8.

Streptococcal skin infection (impetigo) is considered not to cause rheumatic fever. However, a report of acute rheumatic fever following streptococcal wound infection[8] and the high prevalence of pyoderma with relative paucity of streptococcal pharyngitis in some communities with a high incidence of rheumatic fever has raised questions about the link between streptococcal skin infection and rheumatic fever.[9] While effective antibiotic treatment virtually abolishes the risk of rheumatic fever, in situations of untreated epidemic GAS pharyngitis up to 3% of patients develop it.[1,7] Worryingly, as many as a third of patients who develop rheumatic fever do so after virtually asymptomatic GAS and in more recent outbreaks, 58% denied preceding symptoms.[10] This does not augur well for the primary prevention of rheumatic fever where prompt diagnosis of GAS pharyngitis and treatment are essential.

The virulence of the streptococcal infection is dependent on the organisms' M protein serotype which determines the antigenic epitopes which are shared with human heart tissue, especially sarcolemmal membrane proteins and cardiac myosin.[11] It is these variations in virulence, as a result of M protein variation, which are thought to explain the occasional outbreaks of rheumatic fever in areas of previously low incidence.[12] Other factors influencing the risk for rheumatic fever are the magnitude of the immune response and the persistence of the organism during the convalescent phase of the illness.[7]

Evidence suggests that host factors play a role in the risk for rheumatic fever. In patients who have suffered an attack of rheumatic fever, the incidence of a repeat attack is approximately 50%. A specific B-cell alloantigen has been found to be present in 99% of patients with rheumatic fever versus 14% of controls.[13] Certain HLA antigens appear to be associated with increased risk for rheumatic fever. Approximately 60–70% of patients worldwide are positive for HLA-DR3, DR4, DR7, DRW53 or DQW2.[14] Such genetic markers for rheumatic fever risk may be useful to identify those in need of GAS prophylaxis. However, in view of the frequency with which these markers occur, they are unlikely to be of practical benefit in the short term.

Clinical features

While there is no specific clinical, laboratory or other test to confirm conclusively a diagnosis of rheumatic fever, the diagnosis is usually made using the clinical criteria first formulated in 1944 by Duckett Jones[15] and recently modified by the World Health Organization (WHO).[16] The diagnosis is suggested if, in the presence of preceding GAS infection, two major criteria (carditis, chorea, polyarthritis, erythema marginatum, and subcutaneous nodules) or one major and two minor criteria (fever, arthralgia, elevated erythrocyte sedimentation rate, elevated C-reactive protein

or a prolonged PR interval on ECG) are present. Evidence of preceding GAS infection, essential for the diagnosis, may be obtained from throat swab culture (only positive in approximately 11% of patients at the time of diagnosis of acute rheumatic fever[3]) or by demonstrating a rising titer of antistreptococcal antibodies, either antistreptolysin O (ASO) or antideoxyribonuclease B (anti-DNase B).

There has been concern that strict application of the Jones criteria may result in underdiagnosis of rheumatic fever in endemic areas. particularly in the case of recurrent episodes.[17] During recurrence of rheumatic activity in a patient with pre-existing RHD, the carditis may precipitate heart failure but may not be possible to diagnose because of lack of information on previous cardiac findings or because valve replacement surgery has been performed. The new WHO criteria thus recommend that a diagnosis of a recurrence of ARF in a patient with pre-existing RHD is possible on the basis of minor manifestations and evidence of recent streptococcal infection.[16] Doctors should recognize that the published criteria are guidelines, and are particularly useful in epidemiologic investigations where diagnostic rigor is essential. It is appropriate for clinical judgment to be applied and to supersede guidelines particularly in parts of the world where ARF remains common.[17]

Prevention

The most recent recommendations on the prevention of rheumatic fever have been published by the WHO.[16]

Prevention of rheumatic fever may be considered to be either prevention of the initial attack (primary prevention) or prevention of recurrent attacks (secondary prevention). *True primary prevention* of rheumatic fever depends more on socio-economic than medical factors. Upgrading housing and other aspects of poverty eradication will do more to eradicate the disease than antibiotic prophylaxis.

Primary prevention

Prevention of the initial attack of rheumatic fever depends on the prompt recognition of GAS pharyngitis and its effective treatment. While it has been demonstrated that therapy initiated as long as 9 days after the onset of GAS pharyngitis can prevent an attack of rheumatic fever,[18] early treatment reduces both the morbidity and the period of infectivity.

The first report of the use of penicillin for the treatment of GAS pharyngitis and prevention of most attacks of rheumatic fever was published in 1950.[18] Over the following 40 years, attention focused on accurate diagnosis and treatment of GAS pharyngitis. A single dose of intramuscular benzathine penicillin G became the most common mode of treatment and avoided problems of non-compliance. Subsequently, as a result of the pain and possibility of allergic reaction associated with benzathine penicillin G, oral penicillin became the treatment of choice[19] and remains so today[20] (**Class I, Level A**). In situations where compliance with a 10-day course of oral penicillin would be unreliable, a single dose of intramuscular benzathine penicillin G would be preferred (dosage 1.2 million u if >27 kg, otherwise 600 000 u).[21]

Early studies established a 10-day course of oral penicillin as optimal[22,23] and this has been supported in more recent studies.[24,25] Shorter treatment periods are associated with significant decreases in bacteriologic cure while longer courses of treatment do not increase cure rate. Current recommendations[26] for oral penicillin therapy in children cite a dose of 250 mg two or three times daily. These recommendations are based on trials (Table 53.1) of 250 mg given two, three or four times daily resulting in equivalent cure rates[27–30] (**Class I, Level A**). A dose of 750 mg penicillin once a day yielded significantly worse results than 250 mg three times daily when compared in a randomized study.[31] There is no evidence available for optimal doses of penicillin in adults but 500 mg two to three times daily is currently recommended.[26]

Over the past decade, many trials have been published comparing penicillin VK to a variety of other antimicrobial agents, most commonly cephalosporins and macrolides. This has been prompted by the reported increase in treatment failures with penicillin. It has been suggested that treatment failure rates of up to 38% are possible. This contention, however, has been thoroughly investigated in a study by Markowitz et al[32] in which treatment failure rates of penicillin were compared between two time periods, 1953–1979 and 1980–1993. Of the almost 2800 patients with GAS serotyping, treatment failures ranged between 10.5% and 17%, with no significant difference between each time period. It was thus concluded that the overreporting of treatment failures was due to problems with the design of the individual studies.

An increased bacteriologic cure rate for streptococcal pharyngitis by cephalosporins was demonstrated in a meta-analysis of 19 randomized comparisons of a variety of cephalosporins with 10 days of oral penicillin therapy.[33] Throat swab cultures were used to determine the presence of GAS and clearance after treatment. The results showed a statistically significant advantage of cephalosporins for which a bacteriologic cure rate of 92% was reported versus 84% for penicillin. The corresponding clinical cure rates were 95% and 89% respectively. It is suggested that the resistance of cephalosporins to penicillinase-producing anaerobes and staphylococci present in the pharyngeal flora may explain these findings. This difference in efficacy would mean that 12–13 patients would require cephalosporin treatment to potentially prevent one penicillin bacteriologic treatment failure (**Class II, Level A**). More recently, a multicenter comparison of 10-day therapy with cefibuten oral suspension (9 mg/kg/d in one dose) and penicillin V (25 mg/kg/d in three divided doses)[34] revealed a bacteriologic cure rate of 91% versus 80% respectively (corresponding clinical cure rates were 97% v 89%). Shorter courses of selected cephalosporins[35] (4 or 5 days) have been shown to be effective but current recommendations[26] suggest that further study of these regimens is required before their adoption.

The cephalosporins offer statistically significant advantages over penicillin in controlled clinical trials. It remains to be demonstrated, however, whether this statistical benefit can be translated into clinical or epidemiologic benefit in regions where the disease is endemic. Given the financial constraints on healthcare resources of developing nations and the considerable cost difference, it would seem that this is unlikely in the foreseeable future. Greater benefit is likely to be achieved by concerted efforts to identify, treat, and ensure compliance in large numbers of patients with the established, albeit inferior, penicillin schedules[1,21] (**Class II, Level A**).

In patients allergic to penicillin, erythromycin has been shown to have an equivalent cure rate.[36] The recommended dosage for erythromycin estolate is 20–40 mg/kg/d in 2–4 divided doses and for erythromycin ethylsuccinate, it is 40 mg/kg/d in 2–4 divided doses, both for 10 days[37] (**Class I, Level A**). The efficacy of erythromycin estolate is superior to that of erythromycin ethylsuccinate and is associated with fewer gastrointestinal tract side effects.[38] GAS strains resistant to erythromycin have been reported in some parts of the world.[39]

Thus, penicillin V remains the treatment of choice in non-penicillin allergic patients as it has a long record of efficacy and is probably the most cost-effective option.[1]

Appropriate antibiotic therapy in children with streptococcal pharyngitis should result in a clinical response

Table 53.1 Cure rates for various penicillin dosage schedules used in treatment of streptococcal pharyngitis

Reference	Agent/dose	Bacteriologic cure rate (%)
Gerber et al[30]	Pen V 250 mg 2× daily ×10 days	82
	Pen V 250 mg 3× daily ×10 days	71.5
Gerber et al[31]	Pen V 750 mg once daily ×10 days	78
	Pen V 250 mg 3× daily ×10 days	92
Vann & Harris[28]	Potassium Pen G 80 000 u 2× daily ×10 days	88
Spitzer & Harris[29]	Pen V 500 mg 2× daily ×10 days	83
	Pen V 250 mg 3× daily ×10 days	84

within 24 hours – most children will become culture negative within the first or second day of treatment.[40] After completion of therapy, only patients who have persistent or recurring symptoms or those at an increased risk for recurrence require repeat throat swab culture. If symptomatic patients are still harboring GAS in the oropharynx, a second course of antibiotics, preferably with another agent (amoxicillin clavulanate, cephalosporins, clindamycin or penicillin and rifampicin), is recommended.[26] Failure to eradicate GAS occurs more frequently following the administration of oral penicillin than intramuscular benzathine penicillin G.[41] Further treatment of asymptomatic patients, who are frequently chronic GAS carriers, is only indicated for those with previous rheumatic fever or their family members.

Secondary prevention

Following an initial attack of rheumatic fever, there is a high risk of recurrent attacks which increase the likelihood of cardiac damage and continuous antibiotic therapy is required[42] (**Class I, Level A**). This is especially important as GAS infections need not be symptomatic to trigger a recurrence of rheumatic fever nor does optimal GAS treatment preclude a recurrence. It is recommended that patients who have suffered either proven attacks of rheumatic fever or Sydenham's chorea be given long-term prophylaxis following the initial treatment to eradicate the pharyngeal GAS organisms. Recommendations regarding the duration of such prophylaxis are largely empiric and based on observational studies.

The duration of prophylaxis should be individualized and take into account the socio-economic conditions and risk of exposure to GAS for that patient. Individuals who have suffered carditis, with or without valvular involvement, are at higher risk for recurrent attacks[43,44] and should receive prophylaxis well into adulthood and perhaps for life. If valvular heart disease persists then prophylaxis should be lifelong.[16] Those patients who have not suffered rheumatic carditis can receive prophylaxis until 21 years of age or 5 years after the last attack.[45]

The choice of prophylactic agent has to be made with due regard for the likelihood of compliance with a regimen over a period of many years. Therefore, despite associated pain, which can be ameliorated by using lidocaine as a diluent,[46] intramuscular injection of benzathine penicillin G is the method of choice in most situations.[2,42] The recommended dose is 1.2 million u every 3–4 weeks. A comparison of 3-weekly ($n = 90$) versus 4-weekly ($n = 63$) benzathine penicillin prophylaxis[47] demonstrated the superiority of the 3-weekly dosage. The only prophylaxis failure in the 3-weekly dosage group was due to partial compliance, versus five true failures in the 4-weekly dosage group. A long-term follow-up study[48] for a mean period of 6.4 years

(range 1–12 years) in 249 consecutively randomized patients to 3- or 4-weekly regimens further supported the former schedule (0.25% versus 1.29% prophylaxis failures respectively) (**Class II, Level A**). Assays for penicillin levels in blood have also shown that 4-weekly dosage did not provide adequate drug levels throughout the intervening period between doses.[49] Therefore, only those considered at low risk should receive a 4-weekly dose.

Oral prophylaxis has been shown to be less effective than intramuscular penicillin G prophylaxis, even when compliance is optimal.[1,42,43] Penicillin V 250 mg twice daily for adults and children is the recommended dose. No published data exist on other penicillins, macrolides or cephalosporins for secondary prophylaxis of rheumatic fever. However, erythromycin, at a dose of 250 mg twice daily, is usually recommended for those allergic to penicillin.

Patients who have either had mechanical prosthetic valves inserted and/or who are in atrial fibrillation require warfarin anticoagulation. This is a situation which may necessitate the use of an oral prophylaxis regimen. In such patients intramuscular injections of penicillin may carry the risk of hematoma formation, especially in patients rendered asthenic as a consequence of their underlying illness. This important circumstance is, as far as we are aware, not addressed in the literature.

Acute management

The aim of the acute treatment of a proven attack of rheumatic fever is to suppress the inflammatory response and so minimize the effects on the heart and joints, to eradicate the GAS from the pharynx, and provide symptomatic relief.

The long-standing recommendation of bedrest would appear to be appropriate, mainly in order to lessen joint pain. The duration of bedrest should be individually determined but ambulation can usually be started once the fever has subsided and acute phase reactants are returning towards normal. Strenuous exertion should be avoided, especially for those with carditis (**Level C**).

Even though throat swabs taken during the acute attack of rheumatic fever are rarely positive for GAS, it is advisable for patients to receive a 10-day course of penicillin V (or erythromycin if penicillin allergic). Although conventional, this strategy is untested. Thereafter, secondary prophylaxis should commence as described in the previous section[21] (**Level C**).

The choice of anti-inflammatory agent is between salicylates and corticosteroids. A meta-analysis of trials comparing these two agents was published in 1995.[50] In this review, a total of 130 publications from 1949 onwards were assessed. While 11 studies had been randomized, only five[51–55] (Table 53.2) fulfilled the meta-analysis criteria of:

Table 53.2 Randomized trials of acute rheumatic fever treatment

Reference	Number of patients analyzed	Agent/dose	Apical murmur present at 1 year (%)
Combined Rheumatic Fever Study Group[51]	57	Prednisone 60 mg/d ×21 d then taper vs ASA 50 mg/lb/d ×9 wk, then taper	Steroids 57.1% vs ASA 37%
Combined Rheumatic Fever Study Group[52]	73	Prednisone 3 mg/lb/d ×7 d then taper vs ASA 50 mg/lb/d ×6 wk	Steroids 25.3% vs ASA 32.1%
Dorfman et al[53]	129	Hydrocortisone 250 mg then taper and/or ASA to 20–30 mg%	Steroids 12.5% vs ASA 34.4%
Rheumatic Fever Working Party[54]	497	ACTH 80–120 u and taper vs cortisone 300 mg and taper vs ASA 60 mg/lb/d and taper	Steroids 48.6% vs ASA 44%
Stolzer et al[55]	128	ASA 30–60 mg/lb/d ×6 wk vs cortisone 50–300 mg/d vs ACTH 20–120 mg/d	Steroids 26.3% vs ASA 34.6%

- adequate case definition by the Jones criteria
- proper randomization to either salicylates or some form of corticosteroid
- non-overlap of subjects between studies
- follow-up for at least a year for assessment of the presence of an apical systolic murmur suggesting structural cardiac damage as a result of carditis.

The trials varied in the use of steroid agent used –cortisone, ACTH or prednisone. The largest study of the five selected for the meta-analysis was that of the Rheumatic Fever Working Party where ACTH, cortisone, and aspirin were compared in a trial involving 505 children in the USA and United Kingdom.[54] This study found no long-term advantage to be associated with either therapy. While apical systolic murmurs disappeared more rapidly in the steroid-treated groups, the prevalence of a cardiac murmur at 1-year follow-up was the same as for the salicylate-treated group. The erythrocyte sedimentation rate was found to normalize and nodules resolved faster in the steroid group.

When the five studies were examined in the meta-analysis, it was found that the advantage of corticosteroids over salicylates, in preventing the development of a pathologic apical systolic murmur after 1 year of treatment, was not statistically significant (estimated odds ratio 0.88; 95% confidence interval (CI) 0.53–1.46). A more recent systematic review of the effectiveness of anti-inflammatory agents (steroids, aspirin or immunoglobulins) for preventing or reducing further heart valve damage in patients with acute rheumatic fever came to a similar conclusion[56] (**Class II, Level B**).

All these trials may be criticized on two important points. First, the method used to assess cardiac involvement was clinical with the development or persistence of an apical systolic murmur the usual criterion. It could be argued that observer error and interobserver variability of clinical methodology could invalidate the results and that the question should be re-examined using modern non-invasive techniques. It has, however, been shown that, at least during the acute phase of the illness, transthoracic two-dimensional echocardiography with color flow imaging does not add significantly to the clinical evaluation of the degree of cardiac involvement.[57] The second point relates to the duration of follow-up. Lack of clinical evidence of cardiac involvement at 1 or 2 years following the initial attack of acute rheumatic fever is no guarantee that the important sequelae of valvular incompetence or stenosis will not develop in the ensuing decades.

Appropriate dosages of anti-inflammatory agents are aspirin 100 mg/kg/d in four or five divided doses or prednisone 1–2 mg/kg/d. Patients with severe cardiac involvement appear to respond more promptly to corticosteroids.[58]

The duration of therapy must be gauged from the severity of the attack, the presence of carditis, and the rate of response to treatment. Milder attacks with little or no carditis may be treated with salicylates for approximately a month or until inflammation has subsided, as assessed by clinical and laboratory evidence. More severe cases may require 2–3 months of steroid therapy before this can be gradually weaned. Up to 5% of patients may still have rheumatic activity despite treatment at 6 months. Occasionally a "rebound" of inflammatory activity can occur when anti-inflammatory therapy is reduced and may require salicylate treatment.

Alternative non-steroidal anti-inflammatory agents have not been adequately assessed in trials and would only be of benefit in individuals allergic to or intolerant of aspirin.

A prospective randomized controlled trial demonstrated no benefit for intravenous immunoglobulin over placebo when administered during the first episode of rheumatic fever.[56,59] In patients whose initial attack of rheumatic fever is inadequately treated, there is a high risk that the rheumatic activity will continue and result in valvular incompetence, most commonly of the mitral valve. The end result of an ongoing rheumatic process with deteriorating valvu-

Table 53.3 Randomized trials of acute rheumatic fever treatment

Agent	Dose	Route	Duration
Primary prevention			
Benzathine penicillin G	600 000 u if ≤27 kg, 1 200 000 u if >27 kg	Intramuscular injection	Once
Penicillin V	Children 250 mg, 2–3× daily	Oral	10 days
	Adults 500 mg 2–3× daily		
Erythromycin estolate	20–40 mg/kg/d 2–4× daily (max 1 g/d)	Oral	10 days
Secondary prevention (prevention of recurrent attacks)[a]			
Benzathine penicillin G	1 200 000 u every 3 weeks (low risk, every 4 weeks)	Intramuscular injection	
Penicillin V	250 mg 2× daily	Oral	
Erythromycin	250 mg 2× daily	Oral	

Treatment of the acute attack of rheumatic fever
- Bedrest
- Salicylates 100 mg/kg/d in 4–5 doses (in severe attacks with cardiac involvement, prednisone 1–2 mg/kg/d)
- Valve repair/replacement surgery for severe valve dysfunction

lar function is heart failure. Experience has shown that in such cases prompt surgical management[60] is the sole option and can result in the survival of up to 90% of patients.[61,62] It has been suggested that the reduction in cardiac workload following valve surgery results in a settling of the rheumatic process – akin to the beneficial effect observed for bedrest (**Class II, Level C**).

Conclusion

While questions regarding the pathogenesis of rheumatic fever remain, sufficient evidence is available to offer guidance on the appropriate prevention and acute treatment of this common illness (Table 53.3).[1,2] It must be remembered that as most sufferers of this disease are in poor socioeconomic environments and in countries where resources are scarce, the regimens used must be cost-effective and chosen with a view to maximizing patient compliance. A study of the effect of a 10-year education program on the reduction of rheumatic fever incidence[64] demonstrated what can be achieved by a structured approach to community education, patient identification, and effective diagnosis and treatment. This intervention resulted in a 78% reduction in the incidence of rheumatic fever within 10 years. Much could be achieved through the establishment of similar programs where rheumatic fever is rife.[64]

References

1. Robertson KA, Volmink JA, Mayosi BM. Antibiotics for the primary prevention of acute rheumatic fever: a meta-analysis. *BMC Cardiovasc Disord* 2005;**5**:11.

2. Manyemba J, Mayosi BM. Intramuscular penicillin is more effective than oral penicillin in secondary prevention of rheumatic fever-a systematic review. *S Afr Med J* 2003;**93**:212–18.

3. Cilliers A, Manyemba J, Saloojee HH. Anti-inflammatory treatment for carditis in acute rheumatic fever. *Cochrane Database of Systematic Reviews* 2003, Issue 2. Art. No.: CD003176. DOI: 10.1002/14651858.CD003176.

4. Carapetis JR, Steer AC, Mulholland EK, Weber M. The global burden of group A streptococcal diseases. *Lancet Infect Dis* 2005;**5**:685–94.

5. Marijon E, Ou P, Celermajer DS, Ferreira B, Mocumbi AO, Jani D *et al.* Prevalence of Rheumatic Heart Disease Detected by Echocardiographic Screening. *N Engl J Med* 2007;**357**:470–6.

6. Carapetis J, McDonald M, Wilson NJ. Acute rheumatic fever. *Lancet* 2005;**366**:155–68.

7. Siegel AC, Johnson EE, Stollerman GH. Controlled studies of streptococcal pharyngitis in a pediatric population. 1. Factors related to the attack rate of rheumatic fever. *N Engl J Med* 1961;**265**:559–65.

8. Popat K, Riding W. Acute rheumatic fever following streptococcal wound infection. *Postgrad Med J* 1976;**52**:165–70.

9. McDonald M, Currie BJ, Carapetis JR. Acute rheumatic fever: a chink in the chain that links the heart to the throat? *Lancet Infect Dis* 2004;**4**:240–5.

10. Dajani AS. Current status of nonsuppurative complications of Group A streptococci. *Pediatr Infect Dis J* 1991;**10**:S25–7.

11. Dale JB, Beachey EH. Sequence of myosin cross-reactive epitopes of streptococcal M protein. *J Exp Med* 1986;**164**:1785–90.

12. Schwartz B, Facklam RR, Breiman RF. Changing epidemiology of group A streptococcal infection in the U.S.A. *Lancet* 1990;**336**:1167–71.

13. Khanna AK, Buskirk DR, Williams RC *et al.* Presence of non-HLA B cell antigen in rheumatic fever patients and their families as defined by a monoclonal antibody. *J Clin Invest* 1989;**83**:1710–16.

14. Haffejee I. Rheumatic fever and rheumatic heart disease: the current state of its immunology, diagnostic criteria and prophylaxis. *Quart J Med* 1992;**84**:641–58.

15. Jones TD. Diagnosis of rheumatic fever. *JAMA* 1944;**126**:481–4.

16. WHO Technical Report Series No. 923. *Rheumatic Fever and Rheumatic Heart Disease: Report of a WHO Expert Panel, Geneva 29 October –1 November 2001*. Geneva: WHO, 2004.

17. Commerford PJ, Mayosi BM. Acute rheumatic fever. *Medicine* 2006;**34**:239–43.

18. Denny FW, Wannamaker LW, Brink WR, Rammelkamp CH Jr, Custer EA. Prevention of rheumatic fever: treatment of the preceding streptococci infection. *JAMA* 1950;**143**:151–3.

19. Gerber MA, Markowitz M. Management of streptococcal pharyngitis reconsidered. *Pediatr Infect Dis* 1984;**4**:518–26.

20. Nelson JD, McCracken GH Jr, Streptococcal infections (editorial). *Pediatr Infect Dis J Newsletter* 1993;**12**:12.

21. Mayosi BM. Protocols for antibiotic use in primary and secondary prevention of rheumatic fever. *S Afr Med J* 2006;**96**(3 Pt 2):240.

22. Wannamaker LW, Rammelkamp CR Jr, Denny FW *et al.* Prophylaxis of acute rheumatic fever by the treatment of the preceding streptococcal infection with varying amounts of depot penicillin. *Am J Med* 1951;**10**:673–95.

23. Breese BB. Treatment of beta haemolytic streptococcal infections in the home: relative value of available methods. *JAMA* 1953;**152**:10–14.

24. Schwartz RH, Wientzen RL, Pedreira F *et al.* Penicillin V for group A streptococcal pharyngotonsillitis: a randomised trial of seven vs. ten day therapy. *JAMA* 1981;**246**:1790–5.

25. Gerber MA, Randolf MF, Chanatry J *et al.* Five vs. ten days of penicillin V therapy for streptococcal pharyngitis. *Am J Dis Child* 1987;**141**:224–7.

26. Dajani A, Taubert K, Ferrieri P *et al.* Treatment of acute streptococcal pharyngitis and prevention of rheumatic fever: a statement for health professionals. *Paediatrics* 1995;**96**:758–64.

27. Breese BB, Disney FA, Talpey WB. Penicillin in streptococcal infections: total dose and frequency of administration. *Am J Dis Child* 1965;**110**:125–30.

28. Vann RL, Harris BA. Twice a day penicillin therapy for streptococcal upper respiratory infections. *South Med J* 1972;**65**:203–5.

29. Spitzer TG, Harris BA. Penicillin V therapy for streptococcal pharyngitis: comparison of dosage schedules. *South Med J* 1977;**70**:41–2.

30. Gerber MA, Spadaccini LJ, Wright LL, Deutsch L, Kaplan EL. Twice daily penicillin in the treatment of streptococcal pharyngitis. *Am J Dis Child* 1985;**139**:1145–8.

31. Gerber MA, Randolf MF, DeMeo K, Feder HM, Kaplan EL. Failure of once-daily penicillin therapy for streptococcal pharyngitis. *Am J Dis Child* 1989;**143**:153–5.

32. Markowitz M, Gerber MA, Kaplan EL. Treatment of streptococcal pharyngotonsillitis: reports of penicillin's demise are premature. *J Pediatr* 1993;**123**:679–85.

33. Pichichero ME, Margolis PA. A comparison of cephalosporins and penicillins in the treatment of group A beta-haemolytic streptococcal pharyngitis: a meta analysis supporting the concept of microbial copathogenicity. *Pediatr Infect Dis J* 1991;**10**:275–81.

34. Pichichero ME, McLinn SE, Gooch WM IIIrd *et al.* Cefibuten vs. penicillin V in group A beta-haemolytic streptococcal pharyngitis. Members of the Cefibuten Pharyngitis International Study Group. *Pediatr Infect Dis J* 1995;**14**:S102–7.

35. Aujard Y, Boucot I, Brahimi N, Chiche D, Bingen E. Comparative efficacy and safety of four-day cefuroxime axetil and ten day penicillin treatment of group A beta-haemolytic streptococcal pharyngitis in children. *Pediatr Infect Dis J* 1995;**14**:295–300.

36. Shapera RM, Hable KA, Matsen JM. Erythromycin therapy twice daily for streptococcal pharyngitis: a controlled comparison with erythromycin or penicillin phenoxymethyl four times daily or penicillin G benzathine. *JAMA* 1973;**226**:531–5.

37. Derrick CW, Dillon HC. Erythromycin therapy for streptococcal pharyngitis. *Am J Dis Child* 1976;**130**:175–8.

38. Ginsberg CM, McCracken GH Jr, Crow SD *et al.* Erythromycin therapy for group A streptococcal pharyngitis. Results of a comparative study of the estolate and ethylsuccinate formulations. *Am J Dis Child* 1984;**138**:536–9.

39. Seppala H, Missinen A, Jarvinen H *et al.* Resistance to erythromycin in group A streptococci. *N Engl J Med* 1992;**326**:292–7.

40. Krober MS, Bass JW, Michels GN. Streptococcal pharyngitis placebo controlled double-blind evaluation of clinical response to penicillin therapy. *JAMA* 1985;**253**:1271–4.

41. Feinstein AR, Wood HF, Epstein JA *et al.* A controlled study of three methods of prophylaxis against streptococcal infection in a population of rheumatic children. *N Engl J Med* 1959;**260**:697–702.

42. Manyemba J, Mayosi BM. Penicillin for secondary prevention of rheumatic fever. *Cochrane Database of Systematic Reviews* 2002, Issue 3. Art. No.: CD002227. DOI: 10.1002/14651858.CD002227.

43. Majeed HA, Yousof AM, Khuffash FA *et al.* The natural history of acute rheumatic fever in Kuwait: a prospective six year follow up report. *J Chronic Dis* 1986;**39**:361–9.

44. Kuttner AG, Mayer FE. Carditis during second attacks of rheumatic fever – its incidence in patients without clinical evidence of cardiac involvement in their initial rheumatic episode. *N Engl J Med* 1963;**268**:1259–61.

45. Berrios X, delCampo E, Guzman B, Bisno AL. Discontinuing rheumatic fever prophylaxis in selected adolescents and young adults. *Ann Intern Med* 1993;**118**:401–6.

46. Amir J, Ginat S, Cohen YH *et al.* Lidocaine as a diluent for administration of benzathine penicillin G. *Pediatr Infect Dis J* 1998;**17**:890–3.

47. Lue HC, Wu MH, Hseih KH *et al.* Rheumatic fever recurrences: controlled study of 3-week versus 4-week benzathine penicillin prevention programs. *J Pediatr* 1986;**108**:299–304.

48. Lue HC, Wu MH, Wang JK *et al.* Long-term outcome of patients with rheumatic fever receiving benzathine penicillin G prophylaxis every three weeks versus every four weeks. *J Pediatr* 1994;**125**:812–16.

49. Kaplan EL, Berrios X, Speth J *et al.* Pharmacokinetics of benzathine penicillin G: serum levels during the 28 days after intramuscular injection of 1 200 000 units. *J Pediatr* 1989;**115**:146–50.

50. Albert DA, Harel L, Karrison T. The treatment of rheumatic carditis: a review and meta-analysis. *Medicine (Baltimore)* 1995;**74**:1 12.

51. Combined Rheumatic Fever Study Group (RFSG). A comparison of the effect of prednisone and acetylsalicylic acid on the incidence of residual rheumatic carditis. *N Engl J Med* 1960;**262**:895–902.

52. Combined Rheumatic Fever Study Group (RFSG). A comparison of short-term intensive prednisone and acetyl salicylic acid therapy in the treatment of acute rheumatic fever. *N Engl J Med* 1965;**272**:63–70.

53. Dorfman A, Gross JI, Lorincz AE. The treatment of acute rheumatic fever. *Pediatrics* 1961;**27**:692–706.

54. Rheumatic Fever Working Party (RFWP) of the MRC, Great Britain, and the Subcommittee of Principal Investigators of the American Council on Rheumatic Fever and Congenital Heart Disease, American Heart Association. The treatment of acute rheumatic fever in children: a cooperative clinical trial of ACTH, cortisone and aspirin. *Circulation* 1955;**11**:343–71.

55. Stolzer BL, Houser HB, Clark EJ. Therapeutic agents in rheumatic carditis. *Arch Intern Med* 1955;**95**:677–88.

56. Cilliers A, Manyemba J, Saloojee HH. Anti-inflammatory treatment for carditis in acute rheumatic fever. *Cochrane Database of Systematic Reviews* 2003, Issue 2. Art. No.: CD003176. DOI: 10.1002/14651858.CD003176.

57. Vasan RS, Shrivastava S, Vijayakumar M *et al.* Echocardiographic evaluation of patients with acute rheumatic fever and rheumatic carditis. *Circulation* 1996;**94**:73–82.

58. Czoniczer G, Amezcua F, Pelargonio S, Massel BF. Therapy of severe rheumatic carditis: comparison of adrenocortical steroids and aspirin. *Circulation* 1964;**29**:813–19.

59. Voss LM, Wilson NJ, Neutze JM *et al.* Intravenous immunoglobulin in acute rheumatic fever: a randomized controlled trial. *Circulation* 2001;**103**:401–6.

60. Lewis BS, Geft IL, Milo S, Gotsman MS. Echocardiography and valve replacement in the critically ill patient with acute rheumatic carditis. *Ann Thorac Surg* 1979;**27**:529–35.

61. Barlow JB, Kinsley RH, Pocock WA. Rheumatic fever and rheumatic heart disease. In: Barlow JB, ed. *Perspectives on the Mitral Valve*. Philadelphia: FA Davis, 1987.

62. Essop MR, Nkomo VT. Rheumatic and nonrheumatic valvular heart disease: epidemiology, management, and prevention in Africa. *Circulation* 2005;**112**:3584–91.

63. Bach JF, Chalons S, Forier E *et al.* 10-year educational programme aimed at rheumatic fever in two French Caribbean islands. *Lancet* 1996;**347**:644–8.

64. Robertson KA, Volmink JA, Mayosi BM. Towards a uniform plan for the control of rheumatic fever and rheumatic heart disease in Africa – the Awareness Surveillance Advocacy Prevention (A.S.A.P.) Programme. *S Afr Med J* 2006;**96**(3 Pt 2): 241–5.

Blase A Carabello
Baylor College of Medicine, Houston, TX, USA

Introduction

In mitral valve disease, symptomatic status, ventricular functional status, and the kind of operation which will ultimately be performed all affect the indication for valve surgery. This chapter will integrate these aspects into a strategy for surgical correction. It should be noted that in surgery for valve disease there are few large controlled trials of therapy. Indeed, in the most recent (2006) AHA/ACC Guidelines for the Management of Patients with Valvular Heart Disease no recommendation is based on a level of evidence "A."[1] Most knowledge of the response of valve disease to surgery accrues from reports of surgical outcome in both selected and unselected patients.

Mitral regurgitation

Surgical objectives

Like all valvular lesions, mitral regurgitation imposes a hemodynamic overload on the heart. Ultimately, this overload can only be corrected by surgically restoring valve competence. For valve surgery in general, the timing of surgery has two opposing tenets. First, since surgery has an operative risk and, if a prosthesis is inserted, imposes the risks inherent to valve prosthesis, surgery should be delayed for as long as possible. Second, surgery which is delayed until the hemodynamic overload has caused irreversible left ventricular dysfunction will result in a suboptimal outcome. In some patients, far advanced left ventricular dysfunction may militate against operating at all.

Evidence-Based Cardiology, 3rd edition. Edited by S. Yusuf, J.A. Cairns, A.J. Camm, E.L. Fallen, and B.J. Gersh. © 2010 Blackwell Publishing, ISBN: 978-1-4051-5925-8.

The timing of valve surgery is made even more complex in mitral regurgitation since frequently valve repair rather than valve replacement can be effected. Because valve repair does not involve the use of a valvular prosthesis and because it also helps to preserve left ventricular function, it is applicable at the two ends of the spectrum of mitral regurgitation. Repair might be considered in asymptomatic patients with normal left ventricular function because the disease could be cured then without the need for intense follow-up and without the use of a valve prosthesis.[2] At the other end of the spectrum, patients with severe impairment of left ventricular function who might not be candidates for mitral valve replacement with chordal disruption might have a good result from mitral valve repair.[3] However, for most patients, mitral valve surgery is performed for the relief of symptoms or for prevention of worsening of asymptomatic left ventricular dysfunction.

Etiology

The mitral valve apparatus consists of the mitral valve annulus, the valve leaflets, the chorda tendineae, and the papillary muscles. Abnormalities of any of these structures may cause mitral regurgitation. The common causes of mitral regurgitation include infective endocarditis, the mitral valve prolapse syndrome with myxomatous degeneration of the valve, spontaneous chordal rupture, rheumatic heart disease, collagen disease such as Marfan's syndrome and coronary artery disease leading to papillary muscle ischemia or necrosis. These etiologies of mitral regurgitation are important especially with regard to surgical correction. For instance, the spontaneous rupture of a posterior chorda tendinea leads to mitral valve repair in almost 100% of cases. On the other hand, severe rheumatic deformity of the valve which has led to mitral regurgitation may be irreparable, necessitating mitral valve replacement.

Pathophysiology

Hemodynamic phases of mitral regurgitation

Figure 54.1 depicts the pathophysiologic phases of mitral regurgitation.[4] In the acute phase, such as might occur with spontaneous chordal rupture, there is sudden volume overload on both the left ventricle and left atrium. The regurgitant volume, together with the venous return from the pulmonary veins, distends both chambers. Distension of the left ventricle increases use of the Frank–Starling mechanism by which increased sarcomere stretch increases end-diastolic volume modestly and also increases left ventricular stroke work. The new orifice for left ventricular ejection (the regurgitant pathway) facilitates left ventricular emptying and end-systolic volume decreases. Acting in concert, these two effects increase ejection fraction and total stroke volume. However, as shown in Figure 54.1, panel A, if only 50% of the total stroke volume is ejected into the aorta there is a net loss of 30% of the initial forward stroke volume. At the same time, volume overload on the left atrium increases left atrial pressure. At this point, the patient suffers from low output and pulmonary congestion and appears to be in left ventricular failure although left ventricular muscle function is either normal or even augmented by sympathetic reflexes. Acute severe mitral regurgitation may lead to shock and pulmonary edema, requiring intra-aortic balloon counterpulsation and urgent mitral valve repair or replacement. However, if the patient can be maintained in a relatively stable condition, he or she may then enter the chronic compensated phase (Fig. 54.1, panel B) within 3–6 months.

In the chronic compensated phase of mitral regurgitation, eccentric cardiac hypertrophy, in which sarcomeres are laid down in series, allows enlargement of the left ventricle, enhancing its total volume pumping capacity. Total stroke volume is increased, allowing normalization of forward stroke volume. Enlargement of the left atrium accommodates the volume overload at a lower pressure, eliminating pulmonary congestion. In this phase the patient may be remarkably asymptomatic, able to perform normal daily activities, and can even engage in sporting events of modest physical demands.[5]

The patient may remain in the compensated phase for months or years. However, eventually the persistent volume overload leads to a decline in left ventricular function (Fig. 54.1, panel C). A loss of myofibrils or an insensitivity to cyclic AMP may be responsible, at least in part, for loss of left ventricular contractility.[6,7] In this phase, left ventricular end-systolic volume increases because reduced force of contraction results in poor left ventricular emptying, forward stroke volume falls, and left ventricular dilation may worsen the mitral regurgitation. At this time there is re-elevation of the left atrial pressure, resulting again in pulmonary congestion. Of note, the still favorable

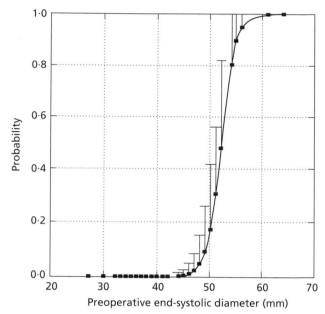

Figure 54.1 (a) Normal hemodynamic state compared to acute mitral regurgitation (AMR). In AMR, total stroke volume and ejection performance increase as preload is increased and afterload is reduced. However, forward stroke volume is reduced and left atrial pressure is increased. (b) AMR compared to chronic compensated mitral regurgitation (CCMR). In CCMR, increased end-diastolic volume permitted by eccentric hypertrophy increases both total and forward stroke volume. Enlargement of atrium and ventricle allows increased volume to be accommodated at lower filling pressure. Increase in afterload toward normal in this state of compensation reduces ejection performance slightly. (c) Chronic decompensated mitral regurgitation (CDMR) compared with CCMR contractile function is reduced and afterload is increased in CDMR. Both reduce ejection performance and forward cardiac output. There is further cardiac dilation in CDMR, leading to worsening mitral regurgitation, further compromising pump function by reducing forward stroke volume and increasing filling pressure. CF, contractile function; EDV, end-diastolic volume; EF, ejection fraction; ESS, end-systolic stress; ESV, end-systolic volume; FSV, forward stroke volume; LA, left atrial pressure; N, normal hemodynamic state; RF, regurgitant fraction; SL, sarcomere length. (Reproduced with permission from Carabello.[4])

loading conditions of mitral regurgitation (increased preload and normal afterload) permit a "normal" ejection fraction even though left ventricular dysfunction has developed.

Importance of the mitral valve apparatus

Although the contribution of the mitral valve apparatus to left ventricular function was noted by Rushmer and Lillehei decades ago,[8,9] its physiologic significance and impact on patient care have only recently received widespread appreciation. It is quite clear that the mitral valve apparatus has a wider role than to simply prevent mitral regurgitation. Rather, the apparatus is an integral part of the left ventricular internal skeleton. In early systole, tugging on the apparatus by the chorda tendineae may shorten the major axis while lengthening the minor axis, in turn augmenting preload there during ejection systole. In addition, the apparatus helps to maintain the normal and efficient ellipsoid shape of the left ventricle.

Transsection of the chordae causes an immediate fall in left ventricular function.[10] Until the importance of chordal preservation during mitral valve surgery was recognized, ejection fraction almost always fell following surgery. This fall was attributed to increased afterload from surgical closure of the low-impedance pathway which preoperatively had facilitated ejection into the left atrium. However, it is now clear that closure of the same low-impedance pathway in which chordal integrity is maintained results in no fall in ejection fraction or only a modest decline, suggesting that the increased postoperative load theory is not the sole mechanism for why ejection fraction falls.[3] In fact, chordal preservation can actually effect a lowering of systolic wall stress (afterload) instead of an increase as left ventricular radius decreases following surgery (stress = pressure × radius/2× thickness).[11] Thus, chordal integrity should be maintained whenever possible[12–14]; in fact, a randomized study demonstrated that maintenance of just the posterior apparatus lowers mortality and leads to superior postoperative function compared to posterior and anterior chordal transection.[15]

Apart from the benefits on left ventricular function, if mitral valve repair instead of a replacement can be performed, operative mortality is lower (Fig. 54.2), postoperative survival is better and the need for anticoagulation is removed while thromboembolism remains low.[13,16–18] Long-term outcome is excellent and repairs are durable. In one study only seven of 162 patients required reoperation a mean of 17 years after repair.[19] Even if the mitral valve is so badly damaged that a mitral valve prosthesis must be inserted, chordal preservation, especially of the posterior chords, can usually be performed resulting in better ventricular function than if all the chords were removed.[12]

Unfortunately, despite recognition of the importance of the mitral valve apparatus, mitral repair is only performed in about 50% of all operations for mitral regurgitation, varying from 0% in some institutions to 90% in others.

Indications for surgery

Severity of mitral regurgitation

Under most circumstances only severe mitral regurgitation is corrected surgically. Mild to moderate regurgitation (regurgitant fraction <40%) neither causes symptoms nor leads to left ventricular dysfunction even over a protracted period of time in the absence of other cardiac disease. Severity is difficult to ascertain by physical examination alone, especially in acute mitral regurgitation. As noted above, in acute mitral regurgitation there has been no time for cardiac dilation to occur. Thus, palpation of the precordium does not reveal a hyperdynamic left ventricular impulse. Although the murmur of mitral regurgitation is present, severity cannot be gauged from its intensity. In most cases of severe mitral regurgitation an S3 should be present. This finding does not necessarily indicate heart failure but may simply be the result of a large regurgitant volume filling the left ventricle under a higher than usual left atrial pressure. In chronic mitral regurgitation there should be evidence on physical examination of an enlarged hyperdynamic left ventricle unless the patient's size or habitus makes physical examination difficult. Failure to find evidence of an enlarged heart suggests that the mitral regurgitation is neither severe enough or chronic enough to cause left ventricular enlargement.

In chronic severe mitral regurgitation, the chest radiograph should also show cardiac enlargement and the electrocardiogram is likely to demonstrate left atrial abnormality and left ventricular hypertrophy.

In most cases, quantitation of regurgitant severity is estimated during echocardiography with Doppler interrogation of the mitral valve. In acute mitral regurgitation, transthoracic echocardiography may underestimate regurgitant severity.[20] In such cases, transesophageal echocardiography is helpful. It should be noted that Doppler flow studies visually demonstrate blood flow velocity across the mitral valve and not true flow. Because of this, both under- and overestimation of regurgitant severity is possible. Flow mapping, which expresses the regurgitant jet in terms relative to left atrial size, has been used extensively. However, limitations of this method are well known and the technique is semiquantitative at best.[20,21] Other methods, such as the proximal isovelocity surface area, have been employed experimentally and in clinical investigation.[23–25] In using proximal isovelocity surface area to estimate regurgitation flow, the area of convergence of the regurgitant jet on the ventricular side of the mitral valve is measured at the point of aliasing. By multiplying proximal

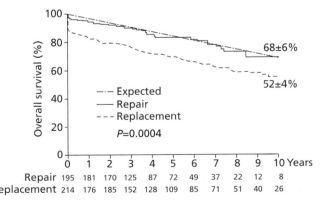

Figure 54.2 Postoperative survival following mitral valve repair is compared to that of mitral valve replacement.

isovelocity surface area by the known aliasing velocity, actual flow is obtained, which should be a better indication of regurgitant severity and even outcome. Indeed, in one prospective study a regurgitant orifice area of >0.4 cm^2 predicted a poorer prognosis than when orifice area was smaller.[26] However, the convergence pattern is often difficult to pinpoint clinically and is not applicable in many cases. As with mitral valve repair, practice varies from center to center with some centers routinely accurately quantifying the severity of disease[27] while others rely upon a visual estimation.

When regurgitation severity is in doubt because of discordance between left ventricular size and the regurgitant signal, i.e. a small left ventricle and left atrium suggesting mild disease and a Doppler signal suggesting severe disease, the issue often can be resolved at cardiac catheterization. During cardiac catheterization, hemodynamics and a left ventriculogram give additional although also imperfect information about the degree of mitral regurgitation. The left ventriculogram, unlike the Doppler study, visualizes actual flow of contrast media from the left ventricle into the left atrium. Care must be taken to inject enough contrast agent (at least 60 mL) to opacify both the enlarged left ventricle and left atrium of mitral regurgitation. Coronary arteriography is also performed at cardiac catheterization if there is any suspicion of an ischemic etiology for mitral regurgitation or when risk factors for coronary disease co-exist.

Acute mitral regurgitation

In almost all cases of severe acute mitral regurgitation, the patient is symptomatic. The acute hemodynamic changes noted above cause decreased forward output and sudden left atrial hypertension, resulting in pulmonary congestion, reduced forward flow, and the symptoms of dyspnea, orthopnea, exercise intolerance, and fatigue. Vasodilator therapy may be successful in alleviating symptoms by preferentially increasing forward flow while simultaneously decreasing left ventricular size, partially restoring mitral valve competence.[28] If vasodilators fail or if the patient is so severely decompensated that hypotension contraindicates the use of vasodilators, intra-aortic balloon counterpulsation is necessary. In such cases surgery should follow soon after. This is especially true for the patient with ischemic mitral regurgitation. Such patients may have a volatile course with initially mild heart failure which progresses unpredictably in severity. These patients require close follow-up.[29,30] In milder cases where symptoms can be relieved by medical therapy, patients should be given a trial of medical therapy during which they may enter the compensated chronic phase. In such cases, patients may then become asymptomatic for months or years. However, one study suggests that such patients are at risk for sudden death.[31] If confirmed, this would indicate that relief of symptoms with medical therapy might be masking hemodynamic or electrical instability and thus be dangerous.

Chronic mitral regurgitation

Symptomatic disease The onset of symptoms of congestive heart failure or a more subtle decrease in exercise tolerance is usually indicative of a change in physiologic status which usually has important clinical significance. The onset of new atrial fibrillation is also probably indicative of a significant change in disease status. Further, atrial fibrillation by itself leads to increased morbidity and decreased cardiac output. In most cases, the onset of symptoms or persistent atrial fibrillation is an indication for mitral valve surgery even when objective indicators of left ventricular function do not show advancement to dysfunction. Early surgery in the mildly symptomatic patient is especially indicated when there is a high probability that mitral valve repair can be effected. In this circumstance there is no need to delay longer, waiting for more severe symptoms or the onset of more apparent left ventricular dysfunction. A valve repair will allow improvement in lifestyle while at the same time avoiding the risks of a prosthesis. Early surgery may be especially important when mitral regurgitation is due to a flail leaflet because this condition may be associated with a modest increase in the risk of sudden death.[32] If preoperative evaluation indicates repair is unlikely, close follow-up of the patient is indicated. If symptoms continue to worsen or if left ventricular dysfunction develops, mitral competence should be restored.

In the patient with mild symptoms and normal left ventricular function, transesophageal echocardiography to determine valve anatomy is crucial. This procedure is the best preoperative test to define whether or not repair can be performed or if replacement will be necessary.

Assessment of left ventricular function A major goal in the management of the patient with mitral regurgitation is to correct the lesion prior to the development of irreversible left ventricular contractile dysfunction. Unfortunately, contractility is difficult to measure clinically. Standard ejection phase indices such as ejection fraction, which are used to gauge left ventricular function in most cardiac diseases, are confounded by the abnormal loading conditions present in mitral regurgitation, necessitating alterations in the way these indexes are used.[33] Because ejection fraction is augmented by increased preload in mitral regurgitation,[34] the value for ejection fraction should be supernormal in the face of normal contractility. A "normal" ejection fraction for the patient with mitral regurgitation is probably 0.65–0.75. Indeed, Enriquez-Sarano and colleagues have demonstrated that once the ejection fraction falls to less than 0.60 in patients with mitral regurgitation, long-term mortality is increased, suggesting that left ventricular dysfunction has already developed at that threshold for ejection fraction.[35]

End-systolic dimension, which is less dependent upon preload, has also been developed as an important indicator of left ventricular dysfunction in this disease. Wisenbaugh *et al* noted that when end-systolic dimension exceeded 45 mm, outcome following surgery was compromised.[36] This figure or its angiographic equivalent has been found to be predictive in other studies.[37,38] However, more recent studies have suggested that for ejection fraction to be predictably normal following surgery, end-systolic dimension should not exceed 40 mm, now the new ACC/AHA guideline for operation.[39] Careful evaluation of the patient with mitral regurgitation with history and physical examination augmented with serial echocardiograms should avoid the situation in which unrecognized left ventricular dysfunction develops. Yearly follow-up is probably adequate as long as the ejection fraction exceeds 0.65 and the end-systolic dimension is less than 35 mm. If the ejection fraction is lower or the end-systolic dimension is higher, more frequent follow-up is indicated. When the ejection fraction approaches 0.60 or when the end-systolic dimension approaches 40 mm, surgery should be contemplated.

Indications for surgery in the asymptomatic patient with mitral regurgitation

Patients with normal left ventricular function At first glance, the asymptomatic patient with mitral regurgitation who has normal left ventricular function would not seem to require surgery. In this patient, surgery will neither improve lifestyle nor prevent reversible left ventricular dysfunction from developing imminently. However, patients with flail leaflet may become symptomatic within the next year[32] and may be at some increased risk for sudden death. In other cases where it is apparent that the severity of mitral regurgitation will eventually necessitate surgery, it could be argued that if mitral valve repair could be performed, little is to be gained by waiting. This circumstance is much like atrial septal defect where at low operative mortality (less than 1%) the defect can be repaired without the use of a prosthesis before unwanted sequelae develop (in the case of atrial septal defect, persistent atrial arrhythmias and pulmonary hypertension; in the case of mitral regurgitation, left ventricular dysfunction). If this approach is taken it must be clear that repair rather than replacement can be effected. If the asymptomatic patient with normal ventricular function is ultimately treated with a prosthesis when a repair had been anticipated, it should be considered a complication of surgery since the unwanted risks of a prosthesis could have been at least temporarily avoided.

Asymptomatic patients with left ventricular dysfunction It is the asymptomatic patient with left ventricular dysfunction at whom serial follow-up is aimed. If left ventricular dysfunction has developed (ejection fraction <0.6, end-systolic dimension >40 mm), surgery should be performed to prevent further irreversible left ventricular dysfunction even if surgery entails a prosthetic valve. Since left ventricular dysfunction has already been indicated by noninvasive testing in such patients, every effort should be made to spare at least part of the mitral valve apparatus to prevent a further decline in left ventricular function postoperatively. Indeed, a recent prospective but non-randomized study demonstrated that when patients undergo corrective surgery either at the onset of symptoms or when left ventricular dysfunction occurs using these points of demarcation, the outcome is excellent.[40]

Asymptomatic elderly patients Patients with mitral regurgitation over the age of 75 are at increased risk for operative death and a poor outcome. This is especially true if mitral valve replacement instead of repair is performed or if concomitant coronary disease, a consequence of aging, is present.[13,41] However, recent reports indicate improved results in octogenarians undergoing mitral valve surgery, especially when preoperative left ventricular function has been avoided and when mitral valve repair has been employed.[42,43] A summary of indications for surgery is shown in Table 54.1.

Establishment of symptom status

Because of the insidious nature of mitral valve disease, patients may subtly alter their lifestyle to maintain their asymptomatic status. Thus, history alone may fail to identify this gradual decline in exercise tolerance. Therefore, in patients with mitral valve disease, formal exercise testing is useful to objectively quantify changes in exercise tolerance over the time of follow-up and to separate truly asymptomatic patients from those who avoid situations which produce symptoms.

Far advanced disease

Occasionally patients reach the first attention of the physician in severe congestive heart failure with far advanced

Table 54.1 Indications for mitral surgery in asymptomatic patients with severe non-ischemic mitral regurgitation

Repair likely	Repair unlikely
Patient with flail leaflet	–
Patient with persistent atrial fibrillation	–
Patient with EF < 0.60 or ESD > 40 mm	Patient with EF < 0.60 or ESD > 40 mm

ESD, end-systolic minor axis dimension; EF, ejection fraction.

left ventricular dysfunction. Many patients in this category may benefit from surgery because correction of mitral regurgitation will lower left atrial pressure and perhaps increase forward output. However, in such cases postoperative left ventricular function will remain depressed and lifespan is likely to be shortened. It is often difficult to decide whether left ventricular dysfunction is so far advanced that surgery should not be performed. The answer to this question is predicated upon what kind of operation is contemplated. If repair with sparing of most chordal structures can be performed, patients with an ejection fraction as low as 30% can survive surgery with postoperative ejection performance maintained at this relatively low level.[3] However, for patients with an ejection fraction <40% in whom only mitral valve replacement can be performed, operative mortality might be prohibitive. Wisenbaugh has further suggested that if the end-systolic dimension exceeds 50 mm in patients with rheumatic mitral regurgitation, postoperative risk is extremely high whether repair can be effected or not.[36]

Ischemic and cardiomyopathic (functional) mitral regurgitation

In primary mitral regurgitation as discussed above, valve pathology causes regurgitation, inducing a volume overload that damages the left ventricle, i.e. "the valve makes the heart sick." However, in functional mitral regurgitation, either from ischemic ventricular damage from coronary disease or from dilated cardiomyopathy, wall motion abnormalities and annular dilation lead to papillary muscle displacement, causing a normal valve to leak, i.e. "the heart makes the valve sick." Because there are already other serious cardiac abnormalities present, the outcome of surgical correction for functional mitral regurgitation is worse than with primary mitral regurgitation[44,45] and guidelines for surgery are not well developed. As noted above, there is no obligatory fall in ejection fraction after mitral valve repair so even patients with very low ejection fraction may benefit from surgery.[46] However, while some have found good results with surgery in this group of patients,[47] there is no proof that such surgery prolongs life and even studies of quality of life have been disappointing.[48,49] Common sense indicates that surgery should be performed when ischemic mitral regurgitation has caused shock or intractable pulmonary congestion.

Medical therapy

Apart from the use of prophylactic antibiotics against infective endocarditis in very specific patients, there is no proven medical therapy for chronic mitral regurgitation. While vasodilators are effective in treating the acute disease, no large long-term trials have been performed to examine their effect in chronic disease. The trials which have been performed differ regarding benefit from this therapy.[50,51] Further, since afterload is not typically elevated in chronic mitral regurgitation, the physiologic underpinnings for vasodilators used for afterload reduction are less clear.

Summary

Patients with acute mitral regurgitation with severe hemodynamic instability require surgical correction. In less severe situations, medical therapy may allow the patient to enter the chronic compensated phase in which surgery can be delayed.

When symptoms develop in chronic mitral regurgitation, they are usually an indication for valve surgery. This is especially true if left ventricular dysfunction is developing or if it is certain that a mitral valve repair can be performed. In asymptomatic patients with normal ventricular function, surgery should only be contemplated when there is certainty of repair. On the other hand, if left ventricular dysfunction is developing, surgery should be performed to prevent further deterioration whether or not a repair can be effected.

Mitral stenosis

Etiology and pathophysiology

Most mitral stenosis in adults is acquired through rheumatic heart disease. In developed countries it typically appears in women in their fourth or fifth decades. In developing nations, where the rheumatic process appears to be more aggressive, stenosis may develop in adolescence or early adulthood.

As mitral stenosis worsens, a gradient develops between the left atrium and left ventricle during diastole. At the same time the stenotic valve impairs left ventricular filling, limiting cardiac output. The combination of pulmonary congestion caused by left atrial hypertension and diminished forward cardiac output caused by inflow obstruction mimics the hemodynamics of left ventricular failure even though the left ventricle itself is usually spared from the rheumatic process, especially in developed countries.[52] However, in approximately one-third of patients, left ventricular ejection performance is reduced despite no impairment in contractility.[53] Reduced ejection fraction is caused by reduced preload from the impairment of left ventricular filling and from increased left ventricular afterload secondary to reflex systemic vasoconstriction in the face of decreased cardiac output. Ejection performance may return to normal shortly after mitral stenosis is relieved.[54]

Although the left ventricle is usually spared from direct involvement in this disease, the right ventricle experiences pressure overload because it supplies the hemodynamic force propelling blood across the stenotic mitral valve. Thus, as left atrial pressure rises, pulmonary pressure and right ventricular pressure also must increase, placing a pressure overload on the right ventricle. For unclear reasons, as the disease progresses, reversible pulmonary vasoconstriction develops, leading to a worsening of pulmonary hypertension and eventually to right ventricular failure.

Indications for surgery

In most cases, mitral stenosis can be relieved by balloon valvotomy which offers results comparable to open commissurotomy, as shown in a randomized trial.[55] Surgery is reserved for those cases in which valve anatomy is unfavorable for balloon valvotomy or in which balloon valvotomy has been attempted and failed. Although in some instances open surgical commissurotomy can be successful even though balloon valvotomy was predicted to be unsuccessful, the unfavorable anatomy for balloon valvotomy will also be unfavorable for commissurotomy, necessitating valve replacement. Thus when surgery is anticipated, the risks and complications of a prosthesis should also be anticipated.

The timing of surgery for mitral stenosis can largely be predicated on symptomatic status as shown in Figure 54.3.[56] Once more than New York Heart Association (NYHA) class II symptoms develop, mortality increases abruptly and surgery should be performed before class III symptoms appear. Additionally, some studies indicate that the presence of pulmonary hypertension substantially increases operative risk[38,57] and thus surgery should be contemplated in patients who develop asymptomatic pulmonary hypertension (pulmonary artery systolic pressure >50 mmHg). When surgery precedes severe pulmonary hypertension, operative mortality, even with the insertion of a prosthesis, is 1–3%.

The most difficult situation for timing surgery arises in the young woman who wishes to bear children. In such patients in whom balloon valvotomy has already been ruled out because of unfavorable valve anatomy, the choice of prosthetic valve becomes quite difficult. If a mechanical valve is placed, it will require anticoagulation which is problematic during pregnancy. Administration of warfarin causes a particularly high incidence of fetal malformation, especially when used during the first trimester. It can be substituted by daily injections of heparin but serious thrombotic complications have occurred in such circumstances, suggesting that this therapy is inadequate at least in some cases.[58] On the other hand, if a bioprosthesis is placed in a young woman it is likely to degenerate within a decade or sooner, forcing the patient to have a reoperation attended by increased surgical risk. There is no correct solution to this dilemma and the prosthesis which is eventually inserted is chosen after lengthy consultation between both the patient and surgeon.

Summary

In most cases, mitral stenosis can be treated successfully with balloon valvotomy. However, if this procedure is unfeasible, open commissurotomy or valve replacement is indicated for greater than NYHA class II symptoms or for the development of pulmonary hypertension.

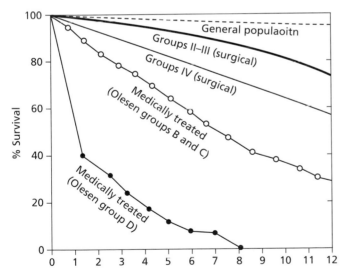

Figure 54.3 Comparison of surgically treated patients with medically treated patients with mitral stenosis. Groups II, III, and IV equivalent to NYHA classifications II, III, and IV are approximately similar to the groups represented by letters B, C, and D, respectively. Class IV patients had better improved survival when treated surgically than did class D patients who were treated medically. Class II and III patients also had better survival when treated surgically than did the patients in groups B and C, although the difference is not as dramatic. (Reproduced with permission from Roy & Gopinath.[56])

References

1. Bonow R, Carabello BA, Kanu C, de Leon AC Jr, Faxon DP, Freed MD *et al*. ACC/AHA 2006 guidelines for the management of patients with valvular heart disease: a report of the American College of Cardiology/American Heart Association Task Force on Practice Guidelines (Writing Committee to Revise the 1998 Guidelines for the Management of Patients With Valvular Heart Disease): developed in collaboration with the Society of Cardiovascular Anesthesiologists: endorsed by the Society of Cardiovascular Angiography and Interventions and the Society of Thoracic Surgeons. *Circulation* 2006;**114**(5):e84–231.
2. Carabello BA. Timing of surgery for mitral regurgitation in asymptomatic patients. *Choices Cardiol* 1991;**5**:137–8.
3. Goldman ME, Mora F, Guarino T, Fuster V, Mindich BP. Mitral valvuloplasty is superior to valve replacement for preservation

of left ventricular function. An intraoperative two-dimensional echocardiographic study. *J Am Coll Cardiol* 1987;**10**:568–75.

4. Carabello BA. Mitral regurgitation, Part 1. basic pathophysiologic principles. *Mod Concepts Cardiovasc Dis* 1988;**57**:53–8.

5. Cheitlin MD, Douglas PS, Parmley WW. 26th Bethesda Conference: recommendations for determining eligibility for competition in athletes with cardiovascular abnormalities. Task Force 2: acquired valvular heart disease. *J Am Coll Cardiol* 1994;**24**:874–80.

6. Urabe Y, Mann DL, Kent RL *et al.* Cellular and ventricular contractile dysfunction in experimental canine mitral regurgitation. *Circ Res* 1992;**70**:131–47.

7. Mulieri LA, Leavitt BJ, Martin BJ, Haeberle JR, Alpert NR. Myocardial force-frequency defect in mitral regurgitation heart failure is reversed by forskolin. *Circulation* 1993;**88**:2700–4.

8. Rushmer RF. Initial phase of ventricular systole: asynchronous contraction. *Am J Physiol* 1956;**184**:188–94.

9. Lillehei CW, Levy MJ, Bonnabeau RC. Mitral valve replacement with preservation of papillary muscles and chordae tendineae. *J Thorac Cardiovasc Surg* 1964;**47**:532–43.

10. Hansen DE, Cahill PD, DeCampli WM *et al.* Valvular-ventricular interaction: importance of the mitral apparatus in canine left ventricular systolic performance. *Circulation* 1986;**73**:1310–20.

11. Rozich JD, Carabello BA, Usher BW *et al.* Mitral valve replacement with and without chordal preservation in patients with chronic mitral regurgitation. Mechanisms for differences in postoperative ejection performance. *Circulation* 1992;**86**:1718–226.

12. David TE, Burns RJ, Bacchus CM, Druck MN. Mitral valve replacement for mitral regurgitation with and without preservation of chordae tendineae. *J Thorac Cardiovasc Surg* 1984;**88**:718–25.

13. Enriguez-Sarano M, Schaff HV, Orszulak TA *et al.* Valve repair improves the outcome of surgery for mitral regurgitation. A multivariate analysis. *Circulation* 1995;**91**:1022–8.

14. Duran CG, Pomar JL, Revuelta JM *et al.* Conservative operation for mitral insufficiency: critical analysis supported by postoperative hemodynamic studies in 72 patients. *J Thorac Cardiovasc Surg* 1980;**79**:326–37.

15. Horskotte D, Schulte HD, Bircks W, Strauer BE. The effect of chordal preservation on late outcome after mitral valve replacement: a randomized study. *J Heart Valve Dis* 1993;**2**:150–8.

16. Cohn LH, Couper GS, Aranki SF *et al.* Long-term results of mitral valve reconstruction for regurgitation of the myxomatous mitral valve. *Cardiovasc Surg* 1994;**107**:143–51.

17. Cosgrove DM, Chavez AM, Lytle BW *et al.* Results of mitral valve reconstruction. *Circulation* 1986;**74**(suppl I):I-82–I-87.

18. Wells FC. Conservation and surgical repair of the mitral valve. In: Wells FC, Shapiro LM, eds. Mitral Valve Disease, 2nd edn. London: Butterworths, 1996: 114–34.

19. Braunberger E, Deloche A, Berrebi A, Abdallah F, Celestin JA, Meimoun P *et al.* Very long-term results (more than 20 years) of valve repair with carpentier's techniques in nonrheumatic mitral valve insufficiency. *Circulation* 2001;**104**(12 Suppl 1): I8–11.

20. Castello R, Fagan L Jr, Lenzen P, Pearson AC, Labovitz AJ. Comparison of transthoracic and transesophageal echocardiography for assessment of left-sided valve regurgitation. *Am J Cardiol* 1991;**68**:1677–80.

21. Smith MD, Kwan OL, Spain MG, DeMaria AN. Temporal variability of color Doppler jet areas in patients with aortic and mitral regurgitation. *Am Heart J* 1992;**123**:953–60.

22. Slater J, Gindea AJ, Freedberg RS *et al.* Comparison of cardiac catheterization and Doppler echocardiography in the decision to operate in aortic and mitral valve disease. *J Am Coll Cardiol* 1991;**17**:1026–36.

23. Recusani F, Bargiggia GS, Yoganathan AP *et al.* A new method for quantification of regurgitant flow rate using color Doppler flow imaging of the flow convergence region proximal to a discrete orifice: an in vitro study. *Circulation* 1991;**83**:594–604.

24. Utsunomiya T, Ogawa T, Doshi R *et al.* Doppler color flow 'proximal isovelocity surface area' method for estimating volume flow rate: effects of orifice shape and machine factors. *J Am Coll Cardiol* 1991;**17**:1103–11.

25. Vandervoort PM, Rivera JM, Mele D *et al.* Application of color Doppler flow mapping to calculate effective regurgitant orifice area: an in vitro study and initial clinical observations. *Circulation* 1993;**88**:1150–6.

26. Enriquez-Sarano M, Avierinos JF, Messika-Zeitoun D *et al.* Quantitative determinants of the outcome of asymptomatic mitral regurgitation. *N Engl J Med* 2005;**352**:875–83.

27. Enriquez-Sarano M, Miller FA Jr., Hayes SN *et al.* Effective mitral regurgitant orifice area: clinical use and pitfalls of the proximal isovelocity surface area method. *J Am Coll Cardiol* 1995;**25**(3):703–9.

28. Yoran C, Yellin EL, Becker RM *et al.* Mechanisms of reduction of mitral regurgitation with vasodilator therapy. *Am J Cardiol* 1979;**43**:773–7.

29. Nishimura RA, Schaff HV, Shub C *et al.* Papillary muscle rupture complicating acute myocardial infarction: analysis of 17 patients. *Am J Cardiol* 1983;**51**:373–7.

30. Nishimura RA, Schaff HV, Gersh BJ, Holmes DR Jr, Tajik AJ. Early repair of mechanical complications after acute myocardial infarction. *JAMA* 1986;**256**:47–50.

31. Grigioni F, Enriquez-Sarano M, Ling LH *et al.* Sudden death in mitral regurgitation due to flail leaflet. *J Am Coll Cardiol* 1999;**34**:2078–85.

32. Ling LH, Enriquez-Sarano M, Seward JB *et al.* Clinical outcome of mitral regurgitation due to flail leaflet. *N Engl J Med* 1996;**335**:1417–23.

33. Eckberg DL, Gault JH, Bouchard RL, Karliner JS, Ross J Jr. Mechanics of left ventricular contraction in chronic severe mitral regurgitation. *Circulation* 1973;**47**:1252–9.

34. Wisenbaugh T, Spann JF, Carabello BA. Differences in myocardial performance and load between patients with similar amounts of chronic aortic versus chronic mitral regurgitation. *J Am Coll Cardiol* 1984;**3**:916–23.

35. Enriquez-Sarano M, Tajik AJ, Schaff HV *et al.* Echocardiographic prediction of survival after surgical correction of organic mitral regurgitation. *Circulation* 1994;**90**:830–7.

36. Wisenbaugh T, Skudicky D, Sareli P. Prediction of outcome after valve replacement for rheumatic mitral regurgitation in the era of chordal preservation. *Circulation* 1994;**89**:191–7.

37. Zile Mr, Gaasch Wh, Carroll JD, Levine HF. Chronic mitral regurgitation: predictive value of preoperative echocardiographic indexes of left ventricular function and wall stress. *J Am Coll Cardiol* 1984;**3**:235–42.

38. Crawford MH, Souchek J, Oprian CA *et al.* Determinants of survival and left ventricular performance after mitral valve replacement. Department of Veterans Affairs Cooperative Study on Valvular Heart Disease. *Circulation* 1990;**81**:1173–81.

39. Matsumura T, Ohtaki E, Tanaka K, Misu K, Tobaru T, Asano R *et al.* Echocardiographic prediction of left ventricular dysfunction after mitral valve repair for mitral regurgitation as an indicator to decide the optimal timing of repair. *J Am Coll Cardiol* 2003;**42**:458–63.

40. Rosenhek R, Rader F, Klaar U *et al.* Outcome of watchful waiting in asymptomatic severe mitral regurgitation. *Circulation* 2006;**113**:2238–44.

41. Nair CK, Biddle WP, Kaneshige A *et al.* Ten-year experience with mitral valve replacement in the elderly. *Am Heart J* 1992;**124**:154–9.

42. Nagendran J, Norris C, Maitland A, Koshal A, Ross DB. Is mitral valve surgery safe in octogenarians? *Eur J Cardiothorac Surg* 2005;**28**:83–7.

43. DiGregorio V, Zehr KJ, Orszulak TA *et al.* Results of mitral surgery in octogenarians with isolated nonrheumatic mitral regurgitation. *Ann Thorac Surg* 2004;**78**:807–13.

44. Connolly MW, Gelbfish JS, Jacobowitz IJ *et al.* Surgical results for mitral regurgitation from coronary artery disease. *J Thorac Cardiovasc Surg* 1986;**91**:379–88.

45. Akins CW, Hilgenberg AD, Buckley MJ *et al.* Mitral valve reconstruction versus replacement for degenerative or ischemic mitral regurgitation. *Ann Thorac Surg* 1994;**58**:668–75.

46. Bolling SF. Mitral reconstruction in cardiomyopathy. *J Heart Valve Dis* 2002;**11**(suppl 1):S26–31.

47. Gazoni LM, Kern JA, Swenson BR, Dent JM, Smith PW, Mulloy DP *et al.* A change in perspective: results for ischemic mitral valve repair are similar to mitral valve repair for degenerative disease. *Ann Thorac Surg* 2007;**84**(3):750–7; discussion 758.

48. Wu AH, Aaronson KD, Bolling SF, Pagani FD, Welch K, Koelling TM. Impact of mitral valve annuloplasty on mortality risk in patients with mitral regurgitation and left ventricular systolic dysfunction. *J Am Coll Cardiol* 2005;**45**:381–7.

49. Mihaljevic T, Lam BK, Rajeswaran J, Takagaki M, Lauer MS, Gillinov AM *et al.* Impact of mitral valve annuloplasty combined with revascularization in patients with functional ischemic mitral regurgitation. *J Am Coll Cardiol* 2007;**49**(22):2191–201.

50. Schon HR, Schroter G, Barthel P, Schomig A. Quinapril therapy in patients with chronic mitral regurgitation. *J Heart Valve Dis* 1994;**3**:303–12.

51. Wisenbaugh T, Sinovich V, Dullabh A, Sareli P. Six month pilot study of captopril for mildly symptomatic, severe isolated mitral and isolated aortic regurgitation. *J Heart Valve Dis* 1994;**3**:197–204.

52. Hildner FJ, Javier RP, Cohen LS *et al.* Myocardioal dysfunction associated with valvular heart disease. *Am J Cardiol* 1972;**30**:319–26.

53. Gash AK, Carabello Ba, Cepin D, Spann JF. Left ventricular ejection performance and systolic muscle function in patients with mitral stenosis. *Circulation* 1983;**67**:148–54.

54. Fawzy ME, Choi WB, Mimish L, Sivandam V, Lingamanaicker J, Khan A, Patel A, Khan B. Immediate and long-term effect of mitral balloon valvotomy on left ventricular volume and systolic function in severe mitral stenosis. *Am Heart J* 1996;**132**(2 Pt 1):356–60.

55. Reyes VP, RAju BS, Wynne J *et al.* Percutaneous balloon valvuloplasty compared with open surgical commissurotomy for mitral stenosis. *N Engl J Med* 1994;**331**:961–7.

56. Roy SB, Gopinath N. Mitral stenosis. *Circulation* 1968;**38**(1, suppl V):V68–76.

57. Vincens JJ, Temizer D, Post JR, Edmunds LH Jr, Herrmann HC. Long term outcome of cardiac surgery in patients with mitral stenosis and severe pulmonary hypertension. *Circulation* 1995;**92**(suppl):II-137–II-142.

58. Sbarouni E, Oakley CM. Outcome of pregnancy in women with valve prosthesis. *Br Heart J* 1994;**71**:196–201.

Surgical indications in aortic valve disease

Sunil Mankad,[1] Heidi M Connolly[1] and Shahbudin H Rahimtoola[2]

[1] Mayo Clinic, Rochester, MN, USA

[2] Keck School of Medicine at University of Southern California, Los Angeles, CA, USA

Introduction

Evidence-based management of patients with aortic valve disease is limited by the absence of prospective randomized trials of surgery versus medical therapy. Furthermore, the small number of prospective, randomized trials of medical treatment in aortic valve disease have provided conflicting results. However, retrospective studies provide extremely useful data which are important in the management of patients. Sir Thomas Lewis pointed out over 80 years ago the inadequacy of knowledge of prognosis in patients with heart disease and proposed a system for prospective follow-up of patients, which we now call "databases" or "registries". The latter are, of course, the major evidence used in this chapter to delineate the indications for surgery and also influenced the recently updated American College of Cardiology (ACC) and American Heart Association (AHA) *Guidelines for the Management of Patients with Valvular Heart Disease*,[1] and the European Society of Cardiology (ESC) *Guidelines on the Management of Patients with Valvular Heart Disease*[2] which provide a framework upon which clinical decisions can be based. However, the guidelines must be put in perspective. The ACC/AHA guidelines had 124 pages and 1066 references. Of their 324 recommendations, only one (0.3%) was based on level of evidence A and 242 (74.7%) were based on level of evidence C. The ESC guidelines had 32 pages and 232 references. Of the 64 recommendations, none (0%) had level of evidence A and 58 (90.6%) were based on level of evidence C.

Aortic valve stenosis

Etiology

A wide variety of disorders may produce aortic valve obstruction.[3] However, those that result in severe stenosis in adults are:
- congenital
- acquired
- calcific (degenerative)
- autoimmune
- rheumatic.

The most common cause of aortic stenosis (AS) in younger adults is a congenital bicuspid valve, which is found in approximately 1% of the general population. In most patients aged 40–64 years, the severely stenotic aortic valve is bicuspid. In patients aged ≥65 years, 90% of severely stenotic valves are tricuspid. Non-rheumatic calcified valves are thought to be "degenerative" but recent data suggest that calcification and obstruction may be the result of an autoimmune reaction to antigens present in the valve,[4] and that the initial process may be an atherosclerotic lesion.[5,6] Early lesions are similar to atherosclerosis, with prominent accumulation of "atherogenic" lipoprotein, including low-density lipoprotein (LDL) and lipoprotein(a), evidence of LDL oxidation, an inflammatory cell infiltrate, and microscopic calcification. In late lesions, there are more prominent accumulation of lipid cells and extracellular matrix.[7] Rheumatic heart disease is still common in developing countries.

Grading the degree of stenosis

The natural history of AS is variable depending on the degree of stenosis and the rate at which it progresses. Cardiac catheterization and echocardiographic–Doppler ultrasound studies indicate the systolic pressure gradient increases on an average by 10–15 mmHg per year. The

Evidence-Based Cardiology, 3rd edition. Edited by S. Yusuf, J.A. Cairns, A.J. Camm, E.L. Fallen, and B.J. Gersh. © 2010 Blackwell Publishing, ISBN: 978-1-4051-5925-8.

10–15 mmHg increase is not linear but a stepwise function with periods of steady state interspersed by an increase in gradient. The range of progression is also wide. Data suggest that the progression of AS may be related to cardiovascular risk factors[8] and the rate of progression may be more rapid if marked leaflet calcification is noted by echocardiography.[9] However, even some patients with only modest calcification may progress very rapidly, making careful follow-up essential.

The systolic gradient across the stenotic aortic valve is dependent on the following:
- the stroke volume (not the cardiac output because the gradient and valve area are a per beat, and not a per minute, function)
- the systolic ejection period
- the systolic pressure in the ascending aorta.

The stenotic valve area is inversely related to the square root of the mean systolic gradient. Thus, measurement of valve area is an important part of the assessment of the severity of AS. The valve area may decrease by as much as $0.12 \pm 0.19\,cm^2$ per year.[10]

Valve area is related to body surface area and is larger in bigger individuals, probably because of the need for a larger stroke volume and cardiac output. The normal aortic valve area ranges from 3 to 4 cm^2. It is reduced to half its size before a systolic gradient occurs.[11] The orifice area has to be reduced to one-third of its size before significant hemodynamic changes are seen;[12] gradients increase precipitously after that. The obvious clinical problem is that in an individual patient with AS, one usually does not know the valve area prior to the onset of disease.

Cardiac magnetic resonance imaging (MRI) and computed tomography (CT) are emerging tools in assessment of patients with AS.[13,14] However, echocardiography remains the primary diagnostic tool and initial procedure used to confirm the presence and determine the severity of AS.[15] In an experienced center the severity of AS determined by Doppler echocardiography correlates well with the severity determined by cardiac catheterization.[16] A comprehensive echocardiographic-Doppler examination in AS should include assessment of the aortic valve peak and mean gradient as well as aortic valve area.[17] When the clinical picture does not correlate with the hemodynamic data obtained by Doppler echocardiography, re-evaluation by cardiac catheterization is indicated.

Several series suggest B-type natriuretic peptide (BNP) is useful in assessing severity of aortic stenosis and identifying patients at high risk for cardiovascular events. It has been found that BNP is regulated by systolic and diastolic load, suggesting that myocardial stretch modulates BNP.[18]

The outcome of patients with severe AS was described by Ross and Braunwald[19] after review of seven autopsy studies published before 1955, and also by Horstkotte and Loogen[20] reporting on 55 patients (10 of whom were

Table 55.1 Survival, according to symptoms, of patients with "severe" aortic stenosis

Symptoms	Average survival	
	Autopsy data[a] (years)	Post cardiac catheterization[b] (months)
Overall	3	23
Angina[c]	5	45
Syncope	3	27
Heart failure	<2	11

[a] Data from Ross and Braunwald.[19]
[b] Data from Horstkotte and Loogen.[20]
[c] Angina in patients with AS occurs even in those without associated obstructive CAD.

asymptomatic) with aortic valve area of <0.8 cm^2 by cardiac catheterization who refused surgery. The findings are shown in Table 55.1. The mortality of symptomatic patients with "severe" AS from eight studies[21] is given in Table 55.2.

Mild aortic stenosis

AS is best considered a disease continuum with resulting overlap of specific cut-off values. Nevertheless, a defined classification template is useful clinically. The ACC/AHA valve guidelines revised severity criteria[1] are shown in Table 55.3. This document defines mild AS as an aortic valve area >1.5 cm^2, peak aortic valve jet velocity by Doppler echocardiography <3.0 m/sec, and mean gradient <25 mmHg. In two studies, patients with aortic valve area >1.5 cm^2 by catheterization had no mortality on follow-up. At the end of 10 years, in one study 8% had severe stenosis, and in the other 15% had a cardiac event. At the end of 20 years, AS had become severe in only 20% and continued to be mild in 63%.[20,21]

Moderate aortic stenosis

Moderate AS is defined as a valve area of >1.0–1.5 cm^2, peak aortic valve jet velocity by Doppler echocardiography 3.0–4.0 m/sec, and mean gradient 25–40 mmHg. In one study in which patients were followed after cardiac catheterization, the one-year and 10-year mortality was 3% and 15%, respectively, and at 10 years 65% of patients had had a cardiac event.[21]

Severe aortic stenosis

Several criteria have been used to define severe AS. The guidelines provided by the ACC and AHA Committee on Valvular Heart Disease[1] describe severe AS as an aortic

Table 55.2 Mortality of symptomatic patients with "severe" aortic stenosis[21]

Authors	Year of publication	Patients (n)	Mortality follow-up time (years)					
			1	2	3	5	10	11
Frank et al[29]	1973	15			36%	52%	90%	
Rapaport[96]	1975					62%	80%	
Chizner et al[97]	1980	23	26%	48%		64%		94%
Schwarz et al[40]	1982	19			79%			
O'Keefe et al[98]	1987	50	43%	63%	75%			
Turina et al[99]	1987	50	40%					
Kelly et al[100]	1988	39	38%					
Horstkotte et al[20]	1988	35			82%			

Table 55.3 ACC/AHA recommendations for classification of aortic stenosis[1]

Parameter	Mild	Moderate	Severe
Jet velocity (m/sec)	<3.0	3.0–4.0	>4.0
Mean gradient (mmHg)	<25	25–40	>40
Valve area (cm^2)	>1.5	1.0–1.5	<1.0
Valve area index (cm^2 per m^2)			<0.6

valve area ≤1.0 cm^2 and a mean aortic pressure gradient, in the setting of normal cardiac output, of >40 mmHg. Although controversial, this definition was supported by data from a large multicenter database (492 patients) which suggested that the one-year mortality of those with aortic valve areas after catheter balloon valvuloplasty for calcific AS of ≤0.7 cm^2 versus that of those with valve areas >0.7 cm^2 was 37% versus 42%, respectively.[22] Kennedy and co-workers[23] reported on 66 patients with aortic valve areas of 0.7–1.2 cm^2 (0.92 ± 0.15 cm^2), normal left ventricular volumes and ejection fraction, whose average age was 67 years. In an average follow-up of 35 months, 21% died and 32% had valve replacement; at four years, the actuarial incidence of death or valve replacement was 41%.[23] Thus, these studies show that patients with aortic valve areas of 0.7–1.0 cm^2 have an outcome without valve replacement that is not benign, and is not consonant with moderate stenosis; these patients should be considered as having severe AS.

Natural history

The duration of the asymptomatic period after the development of severe AS is variable. Pellikka et al recently added to their previous work and reported the long term (5.4 ± 4.0 years) follow-up of 622 patients (aged 72 ± 11 years) with asymptomatic, hemodynamically significant AS (peak jet velocity 4 m/sec by Doppler echocardiography).[24] They found that most patients developed symptoms related to AS with the probability of remaining symptom-free at one, two and five years being 82%, 67%, and 33%, respectively. Furthermore, the one-, two- and five-year probabilities of remaining free of aortic valve surgery or cardiac death were 80%, 63%, and 25%, respectively with the risk of sudden death of approximately 1%/year. Patients having a peak velocity of ≥4.5 m/sec had a higher likelihood of developing symptoms (relative risk, 1.34) or having aortic valve surgery or cardiac death (relative risk, 1.48). In another study of 123 asymptomatic adults with varying grades of severity of AS (aged 63 ± 16 years),[10] the actuarial probability of death or aortic valve surgery was 7 ± 5% at one year, 38 ± 8% at three years and 74 ± 10% at five years. The event rate at two years for aortic jet velocity by Doppler ultrasound of >4.0 m/s (peak gradient by Doppler ultrasound >64 mmHg) was 79 ± 18%, for a velocity of 3.0–4.0 m/s (peak gradient 36–64 mmHg) was 66 ± 13%, and for a velocity of <3.0 m/s (peak gradient of <36 mmHg) was 16 ± 16%.[10] Thus, the duration of the asymptomatic period, particularly in those aged ≥60 years, is probably very short and the course of these patients is not benign.[25,26] However, it should be remembered that it can be difficult to ascribe with certainty a cardiac cause of death if the patients died in their own communities far from the referral center.

Paul Dudley White in 1951[27] credited the first recorded occurrence of sudden death from AS to T. Bonet in 1679.[28] In the past 70 years the reported incidence of sudden death in AS from eight series has ranged from 1% to 21%. Ross and Braunwald,[19] after reviewing seven autopsy series published before 1955, concluded the incidence was 3–5%. The data reported by Pellikka et al[24] suggest the risk of sudden death in asymptomatic patients with AS is approximately 1%/year. The incidence of sudden death in symptomatic adult patients has been 33% (one in three) in one series[29] and 30% (three of ten) in another series.[20] The development of symptoms of angina, syncope or heart failure changes the prognosis of the patient with AS. Average survival after the onset of symptoms is <2–3 years and careful clinical monitoring for the development of symptoms and progressive disease is paramount.

Management

Medical management

For many years, the standard of care has been to provide antibiotic prophylaxis against infective endocarditis in patients with significant AS.[1] However, recently published AHA guidelines for the prevention of infective endocarditis have created significant controversy and no longer recommend antibiotic prophylaxis for AS based on lack of proven efficacy, risk of adverse reactions and poor cost-effectiveness unless the patient has had prior endocarditis, has a prosthetic valve, or has additional complex cardiac lesions that are high risk for the development of endocarditis.[30] Patients who have had rheumatic fever should still receive antibiotic prophylaxis against recurrences of rheumatic fever[1,31] (**Class I, Level B**; recommendation classes and levels of evidence are as noted in Box 55.1).

Unfortunately, there are no medical treatments proven to delay the progression of AS. AS shares similar atherosclerotic risk factors with coronary artery disease (CAD). Retrospective, observational studies have suggested that both statin therapy and possibly angiotensin-converting enzyme inhibition (ACEI) are effective in slowing progression of AS.[32–35] However, no prospective trials assessing the efficacy of ACEI in AS exist and the two largest

prospective, randomized trials looking at statin therapy in this setting have yielded conflicting results.[36,37] Thus, further prospective trials with longer follow-up and assessment of these treatment strategies in mild or moderate AS are needed. Evaluation and modification of cardiovascular risk factors to prevent concurrent CAD as recommended by current guidelines is the best approach for now.

Surgical management

Surgery is recommended for severe symptomatic AS and is the only specific and direct therapy for most adults with severe AS. Rarely, in young patients, the aortic valve is suitable for balloon or surgical valvotomy. Recently, the results of transcatheter implantation of a balloon-expandable stent valve using a femoral arterial approach in 50 patients with severe AS at high risk for conventional open heart surgery have been published.[38] The procedure was successful in 86% of patients and 30-day mortality was 12% in this high-risk cohort. With further refinement, percutaneous valve replacement may become an alternative to conventional open heart surgery in selected high-risk patients with severe symptomatic AS but in most adults, surgery for AS means aortic valve replacement (AVR).[31,39] AVR is indicated for symptomatic patients with severe AS (**Class I, Level B**), although there are no prospective randomized trials of surgery versus no surgery in severe symptomatic AS, and there are unlikely to be any in the future.

In severe symptomatic AS, AVR results in an improvement of survival even with normal preoperative left ventricular function.[20,40] Schwartz *et al*[39] compared the results of AVR with medical treatment during the same time period in patients with severe symptomatic AS and normal LV systolic function at a single center. They demonstrated significant survival benefit with AVR (Fig. 55.1). Horskotte and Loogen further demonstrated the poor prognosis of medical treatment in severe symptomatic AS with a mean survival of only 23 ± 5 months and a five-year probability of survival of only 18 ± 7% in patients who refused AVR.[20] In patients who refused surgery, mean survival after the occurrence of angina pectoris was 45 ± 13 months, after syncope 27 ± 15 months, and after first occurrence of left heart failure 11 ± 10 months.[20] These differences in survival between those treated medically and surgically are so large that there is a great deal of confidence that AVR significantly improves the survival of those with severe, symptomatic AS (**Class I, Level B**).

The operative mortality of valve replacement is ≤5%.[39,41,42] Data from the Euro Heart Survey demonstrate that operative mortality rates have dropped to 2.7% and 4.3%, for AVR and AVR+ coronary bypass surgery, respectively.[43] Furthermore, in patients without other co-morbid conditions, the risk of AVR is ≤2% in experienced and skilled

> **BOX 55.1** Recommendation classes and levels of evidence
>
> **Class I**: Conditions for which there is evidence and/or general agreement that a given procedure or treatment is useful and effective.
>
> **Class II**: Conditions for which there is conflicting evidence and/or a divergence of opinion about the usefulness/efficacy of a procedure or treatment.
>
> **Class IIa**: Weight of evidence or opinion is in favor of usefulness/efficacy.
>
> **Class IIb**: Usefulness/efficacy is less well established by evidence/opinion.
>
> **Class III**: Conditions for which there is evidence and/or general agreement that the procedure/treatment is not useful, and in some cases, may be harmful.
>
> **Level of Evidence A**: Data derived from multiple randomized clinical trials or meta-analyses
>
> **Level of Evidence B**: Data derived from a single randomized clinical trial or large non-randomized studies
>
> **Level of Evidence C**: Consensus of opinion of the experts and/or small studies, retrospective studies, registries

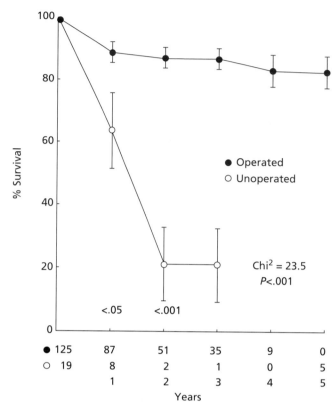

Figure 55.1 Aortic valve replacement is associated with a survival benefit in patients with severe symptomatic aortic stenosis. (From Schwarz et al[40] with permission.) Open circles, unoperated; closed circles, operated.

centers.[44] The operative mortality in those ≥70 years is increased, averaging 8% for AVR and 13% for those undergoing AVR and associated coronary bypass surgery;[39] however, operative mortality is also dependent on co-morbidities.[45] Patients with associated CAD should have coronary artery bypass grafting at the same time as AVR, because it results in a lower operative mortality (4.0% vs 9.4%) and better 10-year survival (49% vs 36%).[44] This was in spite of the fact that those who underwent coronary bypass surgery had more CAD (34% had three-vessel disease, 11% had left main artery disease, and 38% had single-vessel disease) than those who did not undergo coronary bypass surgery (13% had three-vessel disease, 1% had left main disease, and 65% had single-vessel disease).[44] Although this approach to CAD is generally approved, there are no randomized trials to support these recommendations. The presence of CAD, its site and severity can be estimated best by selective coronary angiography, which should be performed in all patients 35 years of age or older who are being considered for aortic valve surgery, and in those aged <35 years if they have left ventricular dysfunction, symptoms or signs suggesting CAD, or they have two or more risk factors for premature CAD (excluding gender).[39] The incidence of associated CAD will vary con-

siderably depending on the prevalence of CAD in the population;[21,39] in general, in persons 50 years of age or older it is about 50%.[39] Normal preoperative left ventricular function remains normal postoperatively if perioperative myocardial damage has not occurred.[46] Left ventricular hypertrophy regresses toward normal;[46,47] after two years, the regression continues at a slower rate up to 10 years after AVR.[47] In patients with excessive preoperative left ventricular hypertrophy,[48] the hypertrophy may regress slowly or not at all. Preoperatively, these patients have a small left ventricular cavity, severe increase in wall thickness, and "supernormal" ejection fraction; this occurs in 42% of women and 14% of men aged ≥60 years.[48] After AVR their clinical picture often resembles that of hypertrophic cardiomyopathy without outflow obstruction, which is a difficult clinical condition to treat, both in the early postoperative period and after hospital discharge;[48] therefore, surgery should be performed prior to development of excessive hypertrophy. Surviving patients are functionally improved.[39]

After AVR, the 10-year survival is ≥60% and 15-year survival is about 45%.[39,49] One half or more of the late deaths are not related to the prosthesis but to associated cardiac abnormalities and other co-morbid conditions.[49] Thus, the late survival will vary in different subgroups of patients. The older patients (≥60 years) have a 12-year actuarial survival of ≥60%.[50] Data from the Karolinska Institute in Sweden have provided an interesting perspective on the long-term survival after AVR in patients with AS aged ≥65 years. They compared the relative survival of the patient who has undergone AVR with another age- and sex-matched person in the same population. Relative survival refers to survival of patients compared to age- and gender-matched people in the population. Patients under the age of 65 had a relative survival of 81% which is significantly lower than 100%, and is also lower than that of those aged ≥65 years. On the other hand, patients who underwent AVR at age ≥65 had a relative survival of 94% at the end of 10 years and this was not significantly different from 100% (Fig. 55.2). These data indicate that survival following AVR for AS in patients aged ≥65 is not significantly different from age- and sex-matched individuals in the population without AS; and the late relative survival of patients aged ≥65 years is much better than that of patients aged <65. Thus, surgery should not be denied to those ≥60–65 years old and should be performed early.[50–52]

Patients who present with heart failure related to AS should undergo surgery as soon as possible. Medical treatment in hospital prior to surgery is reasonable to improve the perioperative risk, but ACE inhibitors should be used with great caution and in such a dosage that hypotension is avoided. Selected critically ill patients with left ventricular systolic dysfunction and severe AS may benefit from cautious administration of sodium nitroprusside therapy.[53]

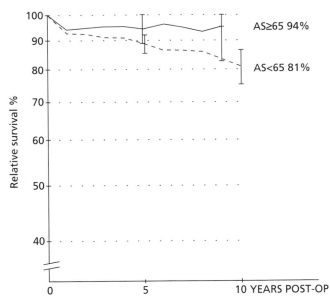

Figure 55.2 Relative survival rates for patients operated on for pure AS. Patients are stratified according to age: <65 years old (dashed line) or ≥65 years old (solid line) with vertical bars indicating 95% confidence limits. Patients aged ≥65 who underwent AVR for AS obtained a normalized survival pattern after operation. POST-OP, postoperatively; AS, aortic stenosis; AVR, aortic valve replacement. (From Lindblom *et al*[51] with permission.)

BOX 55.2 Results of valve replacement in patients with severe aortic valve stenosis

- Improved symptoms and survival in symptomatic patients, especially in those with left ventricular systolic dysfunction, clinical heart failure, and in those aged ≤65 years
- Improvement in left ventricular systolic dysfunction, which normalizes in two thirds of patients
- Regression of left ventricular hypertrophy
- Improvement in functional class, more marked in those with severe symptoms preoperatively

BOX 55.3 Factors predictive of a less favorable outcome

- Extent and severity of associated co-morbid conditions
- Presence and severity of clinical heart failure preoperatively
- Severe associated coronary artery disease
- Severity of depression of preoperative left ventricular ejection fraction
- Duration of preoperative left ventricular systolic dysfunction
- Extent of preoperative irreversible myocardial damage
- Skill and experience of operating and other associated professional teams
- Extent of perioperative myocardial damage
- Complications of a prosthetic heart valve

However, this study is problematic. The goal was to study cardiac output by the Fick principle after 24 hours, but O_2 consumption was not measured but obtained from a nomogram that has no data on O_2 consumption in heart failure before and after treatment. The patients were made hypotensive and the one-month mortality was 25%. We strongly discourage the use of nitroprusside unless the patient is very hypertensive and needs intravenous therapy for control of hypertension and with the caveat that hypotension must be avoided. If heart failure does not respond satisfactorily and rapidly to medical therapy, surgery becomes a matter of considerable urgency.[39] Catheter balloon valvuloplasty has a very limited role in adults with calcific AS and carries a mortality risk of >10%. In addition, restenosis and clinical deterioration occur within 6–12 months. In adults with AS, balloon valvuloplasty is not a substitute for AVR but can be a bridge procedure in selected patients.[54] It may improve hemodynamics and make them better candidates for AVR. The results of valve replacement in patients with severe AS and preoperative left ventricular systolic dysfunction and the factors predictive of reduced postoperative survival, persistent left ventricular systolic dysfunction, and persistence of symptoms are summarized in Boxes 55.2 and 55.3.[21,39,40,45–47,49–51,55–57]

Surgical mortality for AS patients with heart failure has declined: 25 years ago the operative mortality was <20%[57] but in the current era it is ≤10%.[55] Although this is higher than in patients without heart failure, late outcome in those who survive the operation is excellent and is far superior to that which can be expected with medical therapy. Patients who survive operation have an 84% seven-year survival.[56] Survival in those without associated CAD is greater than in those with CAD (69% vs 39% five-year survival, $P = 0.02$).[55] Left ventricular function improves in most patients after AVR, and becomes normal in two-thirds of the patients, unless there was irreversible preoperative myocardial damage (Fig. 55.3).[55,57] In addition, operative survivors are functionally much improved, and left ventricular hypertrophy and left ventricular dilation, if present preoperatively, regress toward normal.[57] Despite the excellent results of AVR in patients with severe AS who are in heart failure, these results are not as good as for those who are not in heart failure; therefore, it is important to recognize that surgery should not be delayed until heart failure develops (**Class I, Level B**).

Six percent of older patients with AS present in cardiogenic shock.[54] The hospital mortality in such patients is near 50%. The subsequent mortality is also very high if the patients have not had their AS relieved.[54] Thus, these patients need to be managed aggressively by medical therapy[53] and emergency surgery with or without catheter balloon valvuloplasty as a "bridge" procedure.[54]

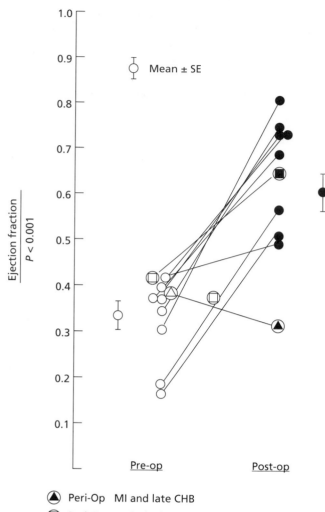

Figure 55.3 Change in LV EF for each individual patient with severe AS and LV systolic dysfunction. After AVR the LV EF improved from 0.34 to 0.63. All but one patient showed an improvement in LV EF; the only patient who showed deterioration in EF suffered a perioperative MI and had a complete heart block; and the only patient who showed only a relatively small increase in EF had had a MI prior to AVR. Note that LV EF normalized in two-thirds of the patients and in the two patients with the lowest ejection fraction (0.18 and 0.19), LV EF normalized in both. These data indicate that there is probably no lower limit of EF at which time patients with AS become inoperable. This also indicates that the lower the EF, the more urgent the need for AVR. AS, aortic stenosis; LV, left ventriclular; EF, ejection fraction; AVR, aortic valve replacement; MI, myocardial infarction. (From Smith *et al*[57] with permission.)

Low gradient aortic stenosis

Patients with severe left ventricular systolic dysfunction, low aortic valve gradient, and small calculated aortic valve area represent a difficult clinical problem. There is controversy regarding the best management of these patients, in part related to the difficulty differentiating patients with true severe AS from patients with moderate AS and severe left ventricular dysfunction. A small gradient across the valve may be associated with a small calculated aortic

valve area that would be in a range indicating severe AS. There are at least two possible causes for this clinical circumstance. First, there is a small or reduced stroke volume and a normal or near normal systolic ejection time; thus, the gradient is small and the calculated aortic valve area correctly indicates severe AS. The second consideration is that the stroke volume is reduced, and thus the valve needs to open only to a small extent to allow the left ventricle to eject the small stroke volume. The calculated aortic valve area accurately reflects the extent to which the valve has opened but overestimates the severity of AS. Use of a provocative test using an inotropic agent, such as dobutamine,[58–60] may allow one to make the correct differentiation between the two. Dobutamine increases systolic flow per second owing to increases in stroke volume or shortening of ejection time or both. In the first circumstance described above, dobutamine will result in an increase in gradient but the calculated valve area remains more or less unchanged. On the other hand, in the second circumstance described above, the gradient may or may not increase with dobutamine but the calculated valve area increases significantly, indicating that the stenosis is not severe. When the dobutamine test is used in the catheterization laboratory, it is important to measure cardiac output and simultaneous left ventricular and aortic pressures both before and during dobutamine infusion. Alternatively, the gradient and valve area may be assessed by echocardiography/Doppler during dobutamine infusion; however, one needs to be certain that cardiac output has increased significantly with dobutamine (**Class IIa, Level B**).

Differentiating these two patient groups with AS may impact management decision and affects the operative outcome.[59] A multicenter study reported that the surgical mortality is related to contractile reserve, which was determined during echocardiographic-Doppler investigation and described as an increase in stroke volume ≥20%.[61] The presence of contractile reserve in this high-risk AS subset impacts surgical outcome.[62] The absence of LV contractile reserve in patients with low-gradient AS identifies a group of patients who have a higher AVR mortality compared to those with contractile reserve[59] (Fig. 55.4). However, if these patients survive surgery, their left ventricular ejection fraction increases in the majority of cases and the concept that surgery should be contraindicated in the absence of contractile reserve with dobutamine stimulation is incorrect.[63] BNP has been demonstrated to be significantly higher in patients with truly severe low-gradient AS compared to patients with pseudosevere low-gradient AS. BNP was also demonstrated to predict survival of the whole cohort and in patients undergoing AVR.[64]

Aortic valve replacement in asymptomatic AS

In view of the dismal natural history of symptomatic patients with severe AS, the excellent outcome after

Patient Survival (%)

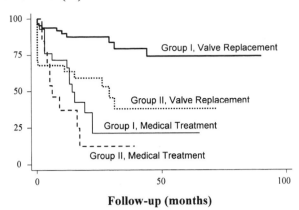

Figure 55.4 Importance of contractile reserve in low-gradient, low-EF severe aortic stenosis. Kaplan–Meier survival estimates by group are shown; improvement in three-year survival with AVR was significant in group I but not significant in group II; survival duration under medical therapy was not different between groups. According to Cox proportional hazard analysis, two parameters were independently associated with long-term survival: AVR (hazard ratio 0.30; 95% CI 0.17–0.53; $P = 0.001$) and LV contractile reserve (hazard ratio 0.40; 95% CI 0.23–0.69; $P = 0.001$). Group I patients *did* and Group II patients *did not* demonstrate contractile reserve with dobutamine on echo/Doppler evaluation. EF, ejection fraction; AVR, aortic valve replacement. (From Monin et al[61] with permission.)

surgery, and the uncertain natural history of the asymptomatic patient, it is reasonable to recommend AVR in select asymptomatic patients in centers with the appropriate skill and experience. Recently, a large retrospective review of 622 asymptomatic patients with hemodynamically significant AS followed for over five years was published by Pellikka *et al*[24] which demonstrated that most patients with asymptomatic, hemodynamically significant AS will develop symptoms within five years and that sudden death occurred in ≈1%/year. They found that age, chronic renal failure, inactivity, and aortic valve velocity by Doppler echocardiography independently were predictive of all-cause mortality. The combined risk of surgery and late complications of AVR must be weighed against the risk of sudden death. There is no consensus about AVR in the truly asymptomatic patient. Clearly, if the patient has left ventricular dysfunction, obstructive CAD or other valve disease that needs surgery, and has severe AS, then AVR should be performed. Some would recommend AVR in all asymptomatic patients with severe AS, while others would recommend it in all those with aortic valve area of ≤0.70 cm^2 and in selected patients only with aortic valve area of 0.71–1.0 cm^2.

Exercise testing should be avoided in symptomatic patients with AS but it may have a role in risk-stratifying asymptomatic AS patients.[25] In a small series, Amato and colleagues reported no serious exercise-related complications.[25] All patients in this series had documented no coronary artery disease by angiography prior to performing the exercise test. During follow-up, 6% of the asymptomatic patients (4/66) experienced sudden death; all had a positive exercise test and an aortic valve area of ≤0.6 cm^2. The exercise test was considered positive if there was a horizontal or down-sloping ST segment depression of ≥1 mm in men or ≥2 mm in women, or an up-sloping ST segment depression of ≥3 mm in men, measured 0.08 seconds after the J point. The exercise test was also considered positive if precordial chest pain or near syncope occurred, if the ECG showed a complex ventricular arrhythmia or if systolic blood pressure failed to rise by ≥20 mmHg during exercise compared with baseline.

Lancellotti *et al* evaluated the prognostic importance of quantitative Doppler exercise supine bicycle echocardiography in a group of patients (n = 69) with severe asymptomatic AS.[65] In multivariate Cox regression analysis, an increase in the mean transaortic pressure gradient by ≥18 mmHg during exercise, an abnormal exercise test (defined as having ≥1 of the following: angina, dyspnea, 2 mm ST depression 0.08 sec after the J point, fall or small (<20 mmHg) rise in systolic blood pressure, or significant arrhythmias), and an aortic valve area <0.75 cm^2 were independent predictors of cardiac events in follow-up (15 ± 7 months).

It must be emphasized that this is a controversial issue. Some cardiologists advise against exercise testing in any patient with severe AS, especially when the extent of coronary artery disease is not known. The recommendations of the ACC/AHA[1] and European Society of Cardiology Guidelines[2] for AVR in severe AS are shown in Tables 55.4 and 55.5.

Chronic aortic valve regurgitation

Etiology

The causes of chronic aortic regurgitation (AR) are:[66,67]
- aortic root/annular dilation
- congenital bicuspid valve
- previous infective endocarditis
- rheumatic
- in association with other diseases – aortitis, drug-related valve disease and others.

In developed countries, aortic root/annular dilation and congenital bicuspid valve are the commonest causes of severe chronic AR.

Natural history

Chronic aortic valve regurgitation is a condition of combined volume and pressure overload. With progression of the disease, compensatory hypertrophy and recruitment of

Table 55.4 ACC/AHA recommendations for AVR in aortic stenosis[1]

	Class	Level of evidence
AVR is indicated for symptomatic patients with severe AS	**I**	**B**
AVR is inidicated for patients with severe AS undergoing CABG, surgery on the aorta or other heart valves	**I**	**C**
AVR is recommended for patients with severe AS and LV systolic dysfunction (EF < 0.50)	**I**	**C**
AVR is reasonable for patients with moderate AS undergoing CABG or surgery on the aorta or other heart valves	**IIa**	**B**
AVR may be considered for asymptomatic patients with severe AS and abnormal response to exercise (e.g. development of symptoms or asymptomatic hypotension)	**IIb**	**C**
AVR may be considered for adults with severe asymptomatic AS if there is a high likelihood of rapid progression (age, calcification, and CAD) or if surgery might be delayed at the time of symptom onset	**IIb**	**C**
AVR may be considered in patients undergoing CABG who have mild AS when there is evidence, such as moderate to severe valve calcification, that progression may be rapid	**IIb**	**C**
AVR may be considered for asymptomatic patients with extremely severe AS (aortic valve area less than 0.6 cm², mean gradient greater than 60 mmHg, and jet velocity greater than 5.0 m per second) when the patient's expected operative mortality is 1.0% or less	**IIb**	**C**
AVR is not useful for the prevention of sudden death in asymptomatic patients with AS who have none of the findings listed under the Class IIa/IIb recommendations	**III**	**B**

Table 55.5 European Society of Cardiology Recommendations for AVR in severe aortic stenosis[65]

	Class of recommendation	Level of evidence
Patients with severe AS and any symptoms	**I**	**B**
Patients with severe AS undergoing coronary artery bypass surgery, surgery of the ascending aorta, or on another valve	**I**	**C**
Asymptomatic patients with severe AS and abnormal exercise test showing symptoms on exercise	**I**	**C**
Asymptomatic patients with severe AS and abnormal exercise test showing fall in blood pressure below baseline	**IIa**	**C**
Asymptomatic patients with severe AS and moderate-to-severe valve calcification, and a rate of peak velocity progression ≥ 0.3m/sec/year	**IIa**	**C**
AS with low gradient (<40 mmHg) and LV dysfunction with contractile reserve	**IIa**	**C**
Asymptomatic patients with severe AS and abnormal exercise test showing complex ventricular arrhythmias	**IIb**	**C**
Asymptomatic patients with severe AS and excessive LV hypertrophy (≥15 mm) unless this is due to hypertension	**IIb**	**C**
AS with low gradient (<40 mmHg) and LV dysfunction without contractile reserve	**IIb**	**C**

preload reserve permit the left ventricle to maintain normal global LV systolic pump function despite the elevated afterload. The majority of patients remain asymptomatic throughout the compensated phase, which may last decades. The natural history of chronic aortic valve regurgitation can be divided into three different eras: the era of syphilis, the era of rheumatic fever/carditis, and the current era of non-invasive quantification of left ventricular function.

Era of syphilis
Prior to availability of antibiotics, the duration from syphilis infection to death was 20 years.[68] The duration of the asymptomatic AR was five years in 60% of patients and the five-year survival was 95%. Once symptoms had developed, the 10-year survival ranged from 40% to 60%. Heart failure was associated with a one-year survival of 30–50%, and 10-year survival of 6%. In a study of 161 patients reported in 1935, the 10-year survival after the onset of heart failure had developed was 34% but was 66% in those treated with arsenic.[68] Syphilis still occurs, but current therapy is cheap and efficacious if diagnosed early. Syphilitic AR is uncommon.

Era of rheumatic fever/carditis
Although the incidence of rheumatic valve disease is low in developed countries, rheumatic heart disease remains

Table 55.6 Outcomes of patients with severe aortic regurgitation

Outcome	Incidence
Asymptomatic patients with normal left ventricular systolic function[69–75,101]	
Progression to symptoms and/or left ventricular systolic dysfunction	2.4–5.7% per year (average 3.8% per year)
Progression to asymptomatic left ventricular dysfunction	
– follow-up at 12-month intervals[c(69)]	0.9% per year
– follow-up at 6-month intervals[c(73)]	3.4% per year
sudden death	0.1% per year
Asymptomatic patients with left ventricular systolic dysfunction[102,103]	
Progression to cardiac symptoms	>25% per year
Symptomatic patients[66,96,104,105]	
Mortality rate	Average >10% per year
Angina	>10% per year
Heart failure	>20% per year

[a] see text for details.

Table 55.7 Likelihood of symptoms of left ventricular dysfunction or death

Left ventricular end-diastolic dimension	
≥70 mm	10% per year
<70 mm	2% per year
Left ventricular end-systolic dimension	
≥50 mm	19% per year
End-systolic dimension >25 mm/m^2	8% per year
40–49 mm	6% per year
<40 mm	0% per year

the most common form of valve disease in many parts of the world. Moreover, some people now domiciled in the developed world have had their initial attack(s) of acute rheumatic fever whilst living in developing countries.

Following the episode of acute rheumatic fever, a murmur is characteristically detected after approximately 10 years.[68] The average interval from detection of a murmur to development of symptoms is 10 years and the percentage of patients remaining symptom free 10 years after detection of the murmur is 50%.[68] Rheumatic AR most commonly occurs in conjunction with mitral valve disease.

Current era

In the current era, patients with AR are followed clinically, with non-invasive tests including echocardiography/Doppler, and radionuclide angiogram to assess left ventricular ejection fraction (EF) or after invasive studies such as cardiac catheterization with angiography. Reported outcomes are shown in Table 55.6. As outlined in Table 56.6,[66,69–75] the natural history of patients with chronic AR depends on the presence or absence of symptoms and on the status of the left ventricle. In asymptomatic patients with normal left ventricular function, data would suggest the progression to symptoms and/or left ventricular systolic dysfunction in approximately 4% per year. Sudden death occurs very rarely, 0.1% per year, and asymptomatic left ventricular dysfunction occurs at a rate of 1–3% per year, depending on the frequency of follow-up.

There are limited data on asymptomatic patients with AR and reduced left ventricular systolic function. Available data would suggest that most of these patients will develop symptoms warranting surgery within 2–3 years, at an average rate of >25% per year. Similarly, limited data are available on the natural history of symptomatic patients with severe AR. These patients have a poor prognosis despite medical therapy, with reported mortality rates of 10% and 20% per year in patients with angina and heart failure, respectively.

Important limitations of some of the studies in the literature must be kept in mind. For example, the "natural history" group in one study was composed of several subsets of patients[74] and 36% of this group was on medication for symptoms. Another concern is the true rate of the development of asymptomatic left ventricular dysfunction.[69] At least 25% of patients who develop left ventricular systolic dysfunction do so before they have symptoms, thus emphasizing the need for regular quantitative assessment of left ventricular systolic function at follow-up in asymptomatic patients with severe AR and previously normal left ventricular systolic function. More recent studies indicate a poor outcome of symptomatic patients with medical therapy, even among those with preserved systolic function (Table 55.7).[70,76]

Sir William Broadbent stated 100 years ago that "The *age* of the patient at the time when the lesion is acquired is the most important consideration in prognosis …".[77] In asymptomatic patients with normal left ventricular systolic function, the independent predictors of symptoms, left ventricular systolic dysfunction, and death by multivariate analysis were: older age, decreasing resting left ventricular EF at rest, and left ventricular dimension on M-mode echocardiography.[69] Importantly, most of these dimensions were obtained in the United States, and American women have smaller body surface area and thus smaller left ventricular dimensions than men, in the absence of valve disease, or in the presence of AR, even when they become symptomatic.[78] Thus, recommendations for intervention based on left ventricular dimension alone will not be applicable to most women and almost certainly will not be applicable to populations of smaller body size. The left ventricular dimension should be corrected to body surface area.[79] Patients also develop symptoms and/or left ventricular systolic dysfunction at a faster rate if their initial left ventricular end-diastolic volume is ≥150 mL/m² when compared to those with volumes <150 mL/m².[74] Older age also appears to increase the annual mortality.[79]

Management

This chapter discusses indications for intervention in patients with chronic severe AR. It should be mentioned that acute severe AR usually causes sudden severe symptoms of heart failure or cardiogenic shock. The sudden large regurgitant volume load is imposed on a normal size left ventricle causing marked elevation in left ventricular end-diastolic pressure and left atrial pressure. Echocardiography is invaluable in determining the severity and etiology of aortic valve regurgitation.[15] The etiology of acute aortic valve regurgitation may have an important impact on the treatment, which is usually emergency surgery.

Medical management

Angina is a recognized symptom in patients with severe AR and is a result of a relative reduction of myocardial blood flow because of an increased demand and/or associated obstructive CAD.[39] The treatment options are to reduce the degree of AR, reduce the myocardial demand or revascularize the myocardium. Clinical heart failure is treated with traditional therapy, including digitalis, diuretics, and ACEI. Parenteral inotropic and vasodilator therapy may be needed for those in severe heart failure.[80] Ultimately the only direct method to reduce the amount of AR is with AVR or valve repair.

Arterial dilators

The role of arterial dilators in chronic, severe, asymptomatic AR is controversial, partly because some of the patients in several of the studies that demonstrated benefit were symptomatic and/or had associated systemic hypertension. Therapy with vasodilating agents should improve forward stroke volume and reduce regurgitant volume and these effects might then translate into reductions in left ventricular end-diastolic volume, wall stress, and afterload, resulting in preservation of left ventricular systolic function and reduction in left ventricular mass. These effects have been observed in small numbers of patients receiving hydralazine.[81] In a trial of 80 patients treated with digitalis, diuretics, and hydralazine over two years, medical therapy produced very minor improvements in left ventricular size and function.[82] Side effects associated with long-term use of hydralazine seriously impaired compliance and only 46% of the patients completed the trial. Hydralazine is rarely used currently.

Inconsistent results have been reported with ACEI, depending on the degree of reduction in arterial pressure

and end-diastolic volume. In an acute study in the catheterization laboratory, 20 patients with severe AR were randomized to either oral nifedipine or oral captopril.[83] Nifedipine produced a reduction of regurgitant fraction but captopril did not. Nifedipine produced a greater increase of forward stroke volume and cardiac output and a greater fall of systemic vascular resistance. This study showed that, acutely, nifedipine was superior to an ACEI. A subsequent six-month randomized trial of a small number of patients showed that the results with captopril were similar to placebo, demonstrating no significant changes in left ventricular dimensions.[84]

The role of long-acting nifedipine on *patient outcome* was evaluated by Scognamiglio et al in a prospective, randomized trial of 143 asymptomatic patients with chronic severe AR, and normal left ventricular systolic function; 69 patients were randomized to long-acting nifedipine and 74 patients to digoxin. The patients underwent clinical and echocardiographic evaluation at six-month intervals. At six years, the need for AVR was 34 ± 6% in the digoxin-treated group and 15 ± 3% in the nifedipine-group, $P < 0.001$ (see Fig. 55.4).[73] Thus, for every 100 patients treated with nifedipine, 19 fewer AVRs were needed at the end of six years (see Fig. 56.4). Compared to the digoxin group, the nifedipine-treated group demonstrated a reduction in left ventricular volume and mass. Ejection fraction, left ventricular volumes and mass all increased during follow-up in the digoxin arm of the trial. Normal left ventricular EF was noted after AVR in 12 of 16 patients (75%) in the digoxin group and all six patients in the nifedipine group who had an abnormal left ventricular EF before surgery. This randomized trial demonstrates that arteriolar dilator therapy with long-acting nifedipine delays the need for AVR in asymptomatic patients with severe AR and normal left ventricular systolic function. The same group has more recently reported a favorable recovery of left ventricular systolic function following AVR in patients with reduced left ventricular EF from chronic severe AR treated with nifedipine.[85]

Evangelista and colleagues studied 95 patients with asymptomatic severe AR and normal left ventricular systolic function who were randomly assigned to open label nifedipine (20 mg every 12 hours), enalapril (20 mg per day) or no treatment.[86] In contrast to the findings of Scognamiglio et al,[71,73] they found that neither nifedipine nor enalapril reduced or delayed the need for AVR in patients with asymptomatic severe AR and normal left ventricular systolic function. In this study vasodilator therapy was not found to reduce the aortic regurgitant volume, decrease the size of the left ventricle, or improve left ventricular systolic function. This study has major flaws with respect to methodology (many patients did not have severe AR), very small numbers of patients (32 in the nifedipine arm of whom seven were lost to follow-up within a few months),

Table 55.8 ACC/AHA recommendations for vasodilator treatment in severe AR[1]

	Class of recommendation	Level of evidence
Vasodilator therapy is indicated for chronic therapy in patients with severe aortic regurgitation who have symptoms or LV dysfunction whn surgery is not recommended because of additional cardiac or non cardiac factors	I	B
Vasodilator therapy is reasonable for short-term therapy to improve the hemodynamic profile of patients with severe heart failure symptoms and severe LV systolic dysfunction before proceeding with AVR	IIa	C
Vasodilator therapy may be considered for long-term therapy in asymptomatic patients with severe aortic regurgitation who have LV dilation but have normal LV systolic function	IIb	C
Vasodilator therapy is not indicated for long-term therapy in asymptomatic patients with mild-moderate aortic regurgitation and normal LV systolic function	III	B
Vasodilator therapy is not indicated for long-term therapy in asymptomatic patients with LV systolic dysfunction who are otherwise candidates for AVR	III	C
Vasodilator therapy is not indicated for long-term therapy in symptomatic either normal LV function or mild-moderate LV systolic dysfunciton who are otherwise candidates for AVR	III	C

and the type as well as dosing of nifedipine used. Nevertheless, there is now less confidence about the role of arterial vasodilators in chronic severe AR and the current ACC/AHA (Table 55.8) and ESC guidelines have downplayed the use of arterial vasodilators.

Surgical management

Surgery for primary AR should only be considered when the degree of regurgitation is severe. However, the presence of severe AR does not mandate surgery. The critical issue is to choose the best time for surgical intervention. Aortic valve repair or AVR should be performed in symptomatic patients irrespective of left ventricular function. Postoperative survival is better after AVR in symptomatic patients with normal or mildly impaired left ventricular systolic function than in those with greater impairment of left ventricular systolic function.[87]

Recently, an important study has documented the long-term outcome of surgically treated AR.[88] One hundred and seventy patients with severe isolated chronic AR had AVR between 1982 and 2002 according to predefined protocol. Patients were divided into two groups depending on their preoperative clinical status: Group A ("early" surgery) included asymptomatic patients and those in NYHA functional class II with "moderate degrees" of LV dysfunction (EF 45–50% and/or end-systolic diameters 50–55 mm) and Group B ("too late" surgery) included patients with either severe symptoms (NYHA functional classes III and IV) or in NYHA functional class I/II with an left ventricular EF <45% or a left ventricular end-systolic diameter >55 mm. Follow-up was 10 ± 6 years (1–22 years). Survival up to 22 years was significantly better in Group A patients. Both groups showed significant increases in left ventricular EF,

reductions in left ventricular end-diastolic diameter and left ventricular end-systolic diameter and improvement in NYHA functional class (Table 55.9). The authors concluded: "Early operation as defined in the guidelines improves long-term survival in patients with chronic AR".

Extreme left ventricular dilation (end-diastolic dimension >80 mm) associated with AR occurs primarily in men and is often associated with left ventricular dysfunction. Extreme left ventricular dilation, however, is not a marker of irreversible left ventricular dysfunction. Operative risk and late postoperative survival are acceptable in these patients.[89]

Chaliki et al reconfirmed the excess mortality rates of AVR in patients with severe AR and markedly reduced left ventricular EF.[90] Importantly, they demonstrated that EF increases significantly and that most patients have improved survival without recurrence of heart failure after AVR. Bhudia et al have demonstrated a dramatic reduction in operative mortality in this group of patients over the last 30 years.[91] Thus, even in patients with severe left ventricular systolic dysfunction, the risk of surgery and postoperative medical therapy for heart failure are usually less than the risk of long-term medical management.

After AVR, patients with normal preoperative left ventricular systolic function have reduction in left ventricular volumes and hypertrophy.[88] In the majority of patients with normal preoperative left ventricular systolic function, there is an eventual increase in EF after AVR, presumably because of a reduction of myocardial stress.[88] Left ventricular hypertrophy continues to decline for up to 5–8 years in those with normal preoperative left ventricular systolic function, but at a slower rate after 18–24 months.[46,92] Most patients are symptomatically improved and are in NYHA class I (Boxes 55.4, 55.5).[39]

Table 55.9 Long-term outcome after aortic valve replacement for aortic regurgitation

	Group A ("Early" Surgery)	Group B ("Too Late" Surgery)	*P* value
Patient, n	60	110	–
Hospital mortality	3 (5%)	9 (8%)	0.5
Later mortality	7/57 (12%)	37/101 (37%)	0.001
Survival*(%) at:			
5 years	90 ± 4	75 ± 8	
10 years	86 ± 5	64 ± 5	
15 years	78 ± 7	53 ± 6	0.009
LVEDD (mm)			
Preoperative	71 ± 7	75 ± 8	0.001
Postoperative (1 yr)	53 ± 6	59 ± 12	0.0001
P value	0.0001	0.0001	
LVESD (mm)			
Preoperative	48 ± 6	55 ± 10	0.0001
Postoperative (1 yr)	38 ± 6	44 ± 14	0.0001
P value	0.0001	0.0001	
LVEF (%)			
Preoperative	54 ± 7	42 ± 10	0.0001
Postoperative (1 yr)	57 ± 9	47 ± 16	0.0001
P value	0.023	0.0001	
Preoperative NYHA functional class			
I	43%	25%	
II	57%	15%	
III	–	32%	
IV	–	29%	
End of follow-up NYHA functional class			

LVEDD, left ventricular end-diastolic dimension; LVEF, left ventricular ejection fraction; LVESD, left ventricular end-systolic dimension; NYHA, New York Heart Association.

*Best-case scenario: 2 patients lost to follow-up considered to be alive. Data from Tornos *et al.*[88]

BOX 55.4 Results of valve replacement in patients with severe chronic aortic valve regurgitation

- Improved survival in those with mild to moderate impairment of left ventricular systolic function and in those with severe left ventricular enlargement irrespective of their symptomatic status
- Improvement in left ventricular systolic dysfunction; function normalizes if the dysfunction is of ≤12 months' duration preoperatively
- Regression of left ventricular hypertrophy
- Improvement in functional class, particularly in those with preoperative mild to moderate impairment and in those with preoperative left ventricular dysfunction

BOX 55.5 Factors predictive of a less favorable outcome after AVR for AR

- Extent and severity of associated co-morbid conditions
- Severe obstructive coronary artery disease
- Presence and severity of clinical heart failure preoperatively
- Severity of depression of preoperative LVEF
- Duration of preoperative left ventricular systolic dysfunction
- Extent of preoperative irreversible myocardial damage
- Severity of increase in left ventricular end-diastolic and end-systolic size (left ventricular end-diastolic and end-systolic volumes of ≥210 and ≥110 ml/m², respectively, or end-diastolic and end-systolic dimensions of ≥80 mm and ≥60 mm, respectively)
- Skill and experience of operating and associated professional teams, for example, anesthetists
- Extent of perioperative myocardial damage
- Complications of a prosthetic heart valve

After AVR in those with abnormal preoperative left ventricular systolic function (EF 0.25–0.49), there is a reduction of heart size and left ventricular end-diastolic pressure, end-diastolic and end-systolic volumes and hypertrophy.[88] Generally, left ventricular EF improves or normalizes only if the EF was abnormal for ≤12 months prior to surgery.[92] Early after AVR, there may be a reduction in EF. The left ventricular end-diastolic volume has not yet decreased but the regurgitant volume has been eliminated; this causes a decline in EF. An early decrease in left ventricular end-diastolic dimension is a good indicator of functional success of AVR as the magnitude of reduction in end-diastolic dimension after operation correlates with the magnitude of late increase in EF.[1] Moreover, unless there is a perioperative complication, most patients are symptomatically improved and are in NYHA class I or II after AVR for chronic AR.[39] In those with severe symptoms and severe reduction of EF or severe left ventricular dilation preoperatively, the operative mortality can still be relatively low although survival as well as the beneficial effects on left ventricular function and functional class are less marked.[93,94]

The current status of aortic valve repair prevents recommending this as an early prophylactic procedure. It is difficult to determine which aortic valves will be amenable to repair and repair is feasible only in a minority of cases even at experienced and skilled centers. The rate of recurrent AR requiring reoperation is at a level that decreases the enthusiasm for this procedure in asymptomatic patients with minimal left ventricular enlargement.[95]

Aortic valve replacement in asymptomatic AR

Aortic valve surgery for asymptomatic patients with AR is controversial. AVR is indicated in the setting of left ventricular dysfunction with an EF ≤0.50[92] and in the setting of severe left ventricular dilation (end-diastolic dimension >70 mm, end-systolic dimension >50 mm, or left ventricular systolic dimension/body surface area ≥0.25 mm/m²), even if the EF is normal. Ideally, the threshold values of end-diastolic and end-systolic dimension recommended for AVR in asymptomatic patients should be adjusted to body surface area. It has been demonstrated that a left ventricular end-systolic dimension corrected for body surface area (left ventricular systolic dimension/body surface area) of ≥25 mm/m² is associated with increased mortality when followed conservatively.[1,79,89] Aortic valve surgery for asymptomatic patients with severe AR is also recommended for when these patients are being referred for cardiac surgery for associated conditions such as CAD, thoracic aortic aneurysmal disease, or another valve lesion. Asymptomatic patients who do not have severe left ventricular dilation and those who do not have left ventricular dysfunction at rest or exercise should not have surgery for chronic AR, and can be safely followed. The current ACC/AHA and European guidelines for AVR in patients with AR are shown in Tables 55.10 and 55.11.

Table 55.10 ACC/AHA guidelines for AVR in AR[1]

	Class of recommendation	Level of evidence
AVR is indicated for symptomatic patients with severe aortic regurgitation irrespective of LV systolic function	I	B
AVR is indicated for asymptomatic patients with chronic severe aortic regurgitation and LV systolic dysfunction (EF ≤50% at rest)	I	B
AVR is indicated for patiens with chronic severe AR while undergoing CABG or surgery on the aorta or other valves	I	C
AVR is reasonable for asymptomatic patients with severe aortic regurgition with normal LV systolic function (EF >50%) but with severe dilation of the LV (end-diastolic dimension >75 mm or end-systolic dimension >55 mm)	IIa	B
AVR may be considered in patients with moderate AR while undergoing surgery on the ascending aorta or CABG	IIb	C
AVR may be considered in asymptomatic patients with severe aortic regurgitation and normal LV systolic function (EF >50%) when the degree of LV dilation exceeds an end-diastolic dimension of 70 mm or end-systolic dimension of 50 mm, when there is evidence of progressive LV dilation, declining exercise tolerance, or abnormal hemodynamic responses to exercise	IIb	C
AVR is not indicated for asymptomatic patients with mild, moderate, or severe AR and normal LV systolic function at rest (EF >50%) when the degree of dilation is not moderate or severe (end-diastolic dimension <70 mm or end-systolic dimension <50 mm)	III	B

Table 55.11 European Society of Cardiology recommendations for surgery in severe aortic regurgitation[65]

	Class of recommendation	Level of evidence
Symptomatic patients (dyspnea, NYHA class II, III, IV or angina)	I	B
Asymptomatic patients with resting LVEF ≤50%	I	B
Patients undergoing CABG or surgery of ascending aorta, or on another valve	I	C
Asymptomatic patients with resting LVEF >50% with severe LV dilation: end-diastolic dimension >70 mm or end-systolic dimension >50 mm (or >25 mm/m² BSA)	IIa	C

Conclusion

The timing of AVR in aortic valve disease remains one of the more important decisions in cardiology. Although operative mortality has diminished with improvement in surgical techniques, the risk of AVR and the presence of an aortic valve prosthesis still outweigh the benefits in most patients without symptoms or evidence of LV remodeling/dysfunction. The regular use of imaging techniques, especially echocardiography, plays an important role not only in quantifying the severity of the valve lesion but also in assessing LV geometry and function. A careful evaluation of evidence based on good studies and data from excellent databases is paramount in making decisions about surgical intervention in patients with aortic valve disease.

References

1. Bonow R, Carabello B, Kanu C et al. ACC/AHA Guidelines for the management of patients with valvular heart disease. A report of the American College of Cardiology/American Heart Association Task Force on Practice Guidelines (Writing Committee to Revise the 1998 Guidelines for the Management of Patients with Valvular Heart Disease). *Circulation* 2006;**114**: 84–231.
2. Vahanian A, Baumgartner H, Bax J et al. Guidelines on the management of valvular heart disease: The Task Force on the Management of Valvular Heart Disease of the European Society of Cardiology. *Eur Heart J* 2007;**28**:230–68.
3. Rahimtoola S. *Aortic Valve Stenosis*. St. Louis: CV Mosby, 1997.
4. Olsson N, Dalsgaaro C, Haegerstrand A, Rosenqvist M, Ryden L, Nilson J. Accumulation of T lymphocytes and expression of interluken-2 receptors in nonrheumatic stenotic aortic valves. *J Am Coll Cardiol* 1994;**23**:1162–70.
5. Otto C. Aortic stenosis – listen to the patient, look at the valve. *N Engl J Med* 2000;**343**:652–4.
6. Otto C, Kuusisto J, Reichenbach D, Gown A, O'Brien K. Characterization of the early lesion of 'degenerative' valvular aortic stenosis. Histological and immunohistochemical studies. *Circulation* 1994;**90**:844–53.
7. Freeman R, Otto C. Spectrum of calcific aortic valve disease pathogenesis, disease progression, and treatment strategies. *Circulation* 2005;**111**:3316–26.
8. Pohle K, Maffert R, Ropers D et al. Progression of aortic valve calcification: association with coronary atherosclerosis and cardiovascular risk factors. *Circulation* 2001;**104**:1927–32.
9. Bahler R, Desser D, Finkelhor R, Brener S, Youssefi M. Factors leading to progression in valvular aortic stenosis. *Am J Cardiol* 1999;**84**:1044–8.
10. Otto C, Burwask I, Legget M et al. Prospective study of asymptomatic valvular aortic stenosis: clinical, echocardiographic, and exercise predictors of outcome. *Circulation* 1997;**95**: 2262–70.
11. Rahimtoola S. The problem of valve prosthesis-patient mismatch. *Circulation* 1978;**58**:20–4.
12. Tobin J Jr, Rahimtoola S, Blundell P, Swan H. Percentage of left ventricular stroke workloss: a simple hemodynamic concept for estimation of severity in valvular aortic stenosis. *Circulation* 1967;**35**:868–79.
13. Kupfahl C, Honold M, Meindhardt G et al. Evaluation of aortic stenosis by cardiovascular magnetic resonance imaging: comparison with established routine clinical techniques. *Heart* 2004;**90**:893–901.
14. Messika-Zeitoun D, MC MA, Detaint D et al. Evaluation and clinical implications of aortic valve calcification measured by electron-beam computed tomography. *Circulation* 2004;**110**: 356–62.
15. Cheitlin M, Alpert J, Armstrong W et al. ACC/AHA Guidelines for the Clinical Application of Echocardiography. A report of the American College of Cardiology/American Heart Association Task Force on Practice Guidelines (Committee on Clinical Application of Echocardiography). Developed in colloboration with the American Society of Echocardiography. *Circulation* 1997;**95**:1686–744.
16. Currie P, Seward J, Reeder G et al. Continuous-wave Doppler echocardiographic assessment of severity of calcific aortic stenosis: a simultaneous Doppler-catheter correlative study in 100 adult patients. *Circulation* 1985;**71**:1162–9.
17. Rahimtoola S. "Prophylactic" valve replacement for mild aortic valve disease at time of surgery for other cardiovascular disease? No. *J Am Coll Cardiol* 1999;**33**:2009–15.
18. Vanderheyden M, Goethals M, Verstreken S et al. Wall stress modulates brain natriuretic peptide production in pressure overload cardiomyopathy. *J Am Coll Cardiol* 2004;**44**:2349–54.
19. Ross J Jr, Braunwald E. Aortic stenosis. *Circulation* 1968;**36**: 61–7.

20. Horstkotte D, Loogen F. The natural history of aortic valve stenosis. *Eur Heart J* 1988;**9**:57–64.

21. Rahimtoola S. Perspective on Valvular Heart Disease: Update II. New York: Elsevier, 1991.

22. O'Neill W. Predictors of long-term survival after percutaneous aortic valvuloplasty: report of the Mansfield Scientific Balloon Aortic Valvuloplasty registry. *J Am Coll Cardiol* 1991;**17**:193–8.

23. Kennedy K, Nishimura R, Holmes DJ, Bailey K. Natural history of moderate aortic stenosis. *J Am Coll Cardiol* 1991;**17**:313–19.

24. Pellikka P, Sarano M, Nishimura R *et al*. Outcome of 622 adults with asymptomatic, hemodynamically significant aortic stenosis during prolonged follow-up. *Circulation* 2005;**111**: 3290–5.

25. Amato M, Moffa P, Werner K, Ramires J. Treatment decision in asymptomatic aortic valve stenosis: role of exercise testing. *Heart* 2001;**86**:361–2.

26. Rosenhek R, Binder T, Porenta G *et al*. Predictors of outcome in severe, asymptomatic aortic stenosis. *N Engl J Med* 2000;**343**: 611–17.

27. White P. Heart Disease, 4th edn. New York: Macmillan, 1951.

28. Bonet T. *Sepulchretum, sire Anatomia Practica*. Geneva: Leonard Chouet. 4th edn. New York: Macmillan, 1951.

29. Frank S, Johnson A, Ross JJ. Natural history of valvular aortic stenosis. *Br Heart J* 1973;**35**:41–6.

30. Wilson W, Taubert K, Gewitz M *et al*. Prevention of Infective Endocarditis. Guidelines From the American Heart Association. A Guideline From the American Heart Association Rheumatic Fever, Endocarditis, and Kawasaki Disease Committee, Council on Cardiovascular Disease in the Young, and the Council on Clinical Cardiology, Council on Cardiovascular Surgery and Anesthesia, and the Quality of Care and Outcomes Research Interdisciplinary Working Group. *Circulation* 2007;**115**:1–19.

31. Rahimoola S. *Aortic Valve Stenosis*, 10th edn. York: McGraw-Hill, 2001.

32. Bellamy M, Pellikka P, Klarich K, AJ AT, Enriquez-Sarano M. Association of cholesterol levels, hydroxymethylglutaryl coenzyme-A reductase inhibitor treatment, and progression of aortic stenosis in the community. *J Am Coll Cardiol* 2002;**40**: 1723–30.

33. Novaro G, Tiong I, Pearce G, Lauer M, Sprecher D, Griffin B. Effect of hydroxymethylglutaryl coenzyme a reductase inhibitors on the progression of calcific aortic stenosis. *Circulation* 2001;**104**:2205–9.

34. O'Brien K, Probstfield J, Caulfield M *et al*. Angiotensin-converting enzyme inhibitors and change in aortic valve calcium. *Arch Intern Med* 2005;**165**:858–62.

35. Rosenhek R, Rader F, Loho N *et al*. Statins but not angiotensin-converting enzyme inhibitors delay progression of aortic stenosis. *Circulation* 2004;**110**:1291–5.

36. Cowell S, Newby D, Prescott R *et al*. A randomized trial of intensive lipid-lowering therapy in calcific aortic stenosis. *N Engl J Med* 2005;**352**:2389–97.

37. Moura L, Ramos S, Zamorano J *et al*. Rosuvastatin affecting aortic valve endothelium to slow the progression of aortic stenosis. *J Am Coll Cardiol* 2007;**49**:554–61.

38. Webb J, Pasupati S, Humphries K *et al*. Percutaneous transarterial aortic valve replacement in selected high-risk patients with aortic stenosis. *Circulation* 2007;**116**:755–63.

39. Rahimtoola S. *Aortic Valve Regurgitation*, 9th edn. New York: McGraw-Hill, 1998.

40. Schwarz F, Banmann P, Manthey J *et al*. The effect of aortic valve replacement on survival. *Circulation* 1982;**66**:1105–10.

41. Edwards F, Peterson E, Coombs L *et al*. Prediction of operative mortality after valve replacement surgery. *J Am Coll Cardiol* 2001;**37**:885–92.

42. Sethi GK, Miller DC, Souchek J *et al*. Clinical, hemodynamic and angiographic predictors of operative mortality in patients undergoing single valve replacement. *J Thorac Cardiovasc Surg* 1987;**93**:884–7.

43. Lung B, Baron G, Butchart E *et al*. A prospective survey of patients with valvular heart disease in Europe: the Euro Heart Survey on Valvular Heart Disease. *Eur Heart J* 2003;**24**:1231–43.

44. Mullany C, Elveback E, Frye R *et al*. Coronary artery disease and its management: influence on survival in patients undergoing aortic valve replacement. *J Am Coll Cardiol* 1987;**10**:66–72.

45. Rahimtoola S. Lessons learned about the determinants of the results of valve surgery. *Circulation* 1988;**78**:1503–7.

46. Pantely G, Morton M, Rahimtoola S. Effects of successful uncomplicated valve replacement on ventricular hypertrophy, volume, and performance in aortic stenosis and aortic incompetence. *J Thorac Cardiovasc Surg* 1978;**75**:383–91.

47. Monrad E, Hess O, Murakami T, Nonogi H, Corin W, Krayenbuehl H. Time course of regression of left ventricular hypertrophy after aortic valve replacement. *Circulation* 1988;**77**: 1345–55.

48. Carroll J, Carroll EP, Feldman T *et al*. Sex-associated differences in left ventricular function in aortic stenosis of the elderly. *Circulation* 1992;**86**:1099–107.

49. Hammermeister K, Sethi G, Henderson W, Oprian C, Kim T, Rahimtoola S. A comparison of outcomes in men 11 years after heart-valve replacement with a mechanical valve or bioprosthesis. *N Engl J Med* 1993;**328**:1289–96.

50. Murphy E, Lawson R, Starr A, Rahimtoola S. Severe aortic stenosis in patients 60 years of age and older: left ventricular function and ten-year survival after valve replacement. *Circulation* 1981;**64**:184–8.

51. Lindblom D, Lindblom U, Qvist J, Lundström H. Long-term relative survival rates after heart valve replacement. *J Am Coll Cardiol* 1990;**15**:566–73.

52. Sprigings D, Forfar J. How should we manage symptomatic aortic stenosis in the patient who is 80 or older? *Br Heart J* 1995;**74**:481–4.

53. Khot U, Novaro G, Popovic Z *et al*. Nitroprusside in critically ill patients with left ventricular dysfunction and aortic stenosis. *N Engl J Med* 2003;**348**:1756–63.

54. Rahimtoola S. Catheter balloon valvuloplasty for severe calcific aortic stenosis: a limited role. *J Am Coll Cardiol* 1994;**23**: 1076–8.

55. Connolly H, Oh J, Orszulak T *et al*. Aortic valve replacement for aortic stenosis with severe left ventricular dysfunction. Prognostic indicators. *Circulation* 1997;**95**:2395–400.

56. Rahimtoola S, Starr A. Valvular Surgery. New York: Grune and Stratton, 1982.

57. Smith N, McAnulty J, Rahimtoola S. Severe aortic stenosis with impaired left ventricular function and clinical heart failure: results of valve replacement. *Circulation* 1978;**58**:255–64.

58. deFilippi C, Willett D, Brickner M *et al.* Usefulness of dobutamine echocardiography in distinguishing severe from nonsevere valvular aortic stenosis in patients with depressed left ventricular function and low transvalvular gradients. *Am J Cardiol* 1995;**75**:191–4.

59. Monin J, Monchi M, Gest V, Duval-Moulin A, Dubois-Rande J, Gueret P. Aortic stenosis with severe left ventricular dysfunction and low transvalvular pressure gradients: risk stratification by low-dose dobutamine echocardiography. *J Am Coll Cardiol* 2001;**37**:2101–7.

60. Nishimura R, Grantham J, Connolly H, Schaff H, Higano S, Holmes D Jr. Low-output, low-gradient aoratic stenosis in patients with depressed left ventricular systolic function: the clinical utility of the dobutamine challenge in the catheterization laboratory. *Circulation* 2002;**106**:809–13.

61. Monin J, Quéré J, Monchi M *et al.* Low-gradient aortic stenosis: operative risk stratification and predictors for long-term outcome: a multicenter study using dobutamine stress hemodynamics. *Circulation* 2003;**108**:319–24.

62. Connolly H, Oh J, Schaff H *et al.* Severe aortic stenosis with low transvalvular gradient and severe left ventricular dysfunction: result of aortic valve replacement in 52 patients. *Circulation* 2000;**101**:1940–6.

63. Quere J-P, Monin J-L, Levy F *et al.* Influence of preoperative left ventricular contractile reserve on postoperative ejection fraction in low-gradient aortic stenosis. *Circulation* 2006;**113**: 1738–44.

64. Bergler-Klein J, Mundigler G, Pibarot P *et al.* B-type natriuretic peptide in low-flow, low-gradient aortic stenosis: relationship to hemodynamics and clinical outcome: results from the Multicenter Truly or Pseudo-Severe Aortic Stenosis (TOPAS) study. *Circulation* 2007;**115**:2848–55.

65. Lancellotti P, Lebois F, Simon M, Tombeux C, Chauvel C, Pierard L. Prognostic importance of quantitative exercise Doppler echocardiography in asymptomatic valvular aortic stenosis. *Circulation* 2005;**112**(9 suppl):I377–82.

66. Rahimoola S. *Aortic Valve Regurgitation*, 10th edn. New York: McGraw-Hill, 2001.

67. Rahimtoola S. *Aortic Valve Regurgitation*. St. Louis: CV Mosby, 1997.

68. McKay C, Rahimtoola S. *Natural History of Aortic Regurgitation*. New York: Kluwer, 1980.

69. Bonow R, Lakatos E, Maron B, Epstein S. Serial long-term assessment of the natural history of asymptomatic patients with chronic aortic regurgitation and normal left ventricular systolic function. *Circulation* 1991;**84**:1625–35.

70. Ishii K, Hirota Y, Suwa M, Kita Y, Onaka H, Kawamura K. Natural history and left ventricular response in chronic regurgitation. *Am J Cardiol* 1996;**78**:357–61.

71. Scognamiglio R, Fasoli G, Dalla Volta S. Progression of myocardial dysfunction in asymptomatic patients with severe aortic insufficiency. *Clin Cardiol* 1986;**9**:151–6.

72. Scognamiglio R, Fasoli G, Ponchia A, Dalla Volta S. Long-term nifedipine unloading therapy in asymptomatic patients with chronic severe aortic regurgitation. *J Am Coll Cardiol* 1990;**16**:424–9.

73. Scognamiglio R, Rahimtoola S, Fasoli G, Nistri S, Dalla Volta S. Nifedipine in asymptomatic patients with severe aortic

74. Siemienczuk D, Greenberg B, Morris C *et al.* Chronic aortic insufficiency: factors associated with progression to aortic valve replacement. *Ann Intern Med* 1989;**110**:587–92.

75. Tornos M, Olona M, Permanyer-Miralda G *et al.* Clinical outcome of severe asymptomatic chronic aortic regurgitation. A long-term prospective follow-up study. *Am Heart J* 1995;**130**:333–9.

76. Aronow W, Ahn C, Kronzon I, Nanna M. Prognosis of patients with heart failure and unoperated severe aortic valvular regurgitation and relation to ejection fraction. *Am J Cardiol* 1994;**74**:286–8.

77. Broadbent W, Broadbent F. Aortic Incompetence. London: Baillière, Tindall & Cox, 1987.

78. Klodas E, Enriquez-Sarano M, Tajik A, Mullany C, Bailey K, Seward J. Surgery for aortic regurgitation in women: contrasting indications and outcomes compared with men. *Circulation* 1996;**94**:2472–8.

79. Dujardin K, Enriquez-Sarano M, Schaff H, Bailey K, Seward J, Tajik A. Mortality and morbidity of aortic regurgitation in clinical practice. A long-term follow-up study. *Circulation* 1999;**99**:1851–7.

80. Rahimtoola S. Management of heart failure in valve regurgitation. *Clin Cardiol* 1992;**15**:22–7.

81. Rahimtoola S. Vasodilator therapy in chronic, severe aortic regurgitation. *J Am Coll Cardiol* 1990;**16**:430–2.

82. Greenberg B, Massie B, Bristow J *et al.* Long-term vasodilator therapy of chronic aortic insufficiency: a randomized double-blind, placebo-controlled clinical trial. *Circulation* 1988;**78**:92–103.

83. Röthlisberger C, Sareli P, Wisenbaugh T. Comparison of single-dose nifedipine and captopril for chronic severe aortic regurgitation. *Am J Cardiol* 1993;**72**:799–804.

84. Wisenbaugh T, Sinovich V, Dullabh A, Sareli P. Six month pilot study of captopril for mildly symptomatic, severe isolated mitral and isolated aortic regurgitation. *J Heart Valve Dis* 1994;**3**:197.

85. Scognamiglio R, Negut C, Palisi M, Fasoli G, Dalla-Volta S. Long-term survival and functional results after aortic valve replacement in asymptomatic patients with chronic severe aortic regurgitation and left ventricular dysfunction. *J Am Coll Cardiol* 2005;**45**:1025–30.

86. Evangalista A, Tornos P, Sambola A, Permanyer-Miralda G, Soler-Soler J. Long-term vasodilator therapy in patients with severe aortic regurgitation. *N Engl J Med* 2005;**353**: 1342–9.

87. Greves J, Rahimtoola S, Clinic M *et al.* Preoperative criteria predictive of late survival following valve replacement for severe aortic regurgitation. *Am Heart J* 1981;**101**:300–8.

88. Tornos P, Sambola A, Permanyer-Miralda G, Evangalista A, Gomez Z, Soler-Soler J. Long-term outcome of surgically treated aortic regurgitation: influence of guideline adherence toward early surgery. *J Am Coll Cardiol* 2006;**47**:1012–17.

89. Klodas E, Enriquez-Sarano M, Tajik A, Mullany C, Bailey K, Seward J. Optimizing timing of surgical correction in patients with severe aortic regurgitation: role of symptoms. *J Am Coll Cardiol* 1997;**30**:746–52.

73. (cont.) regurgitation and normal left ventricular function. *N Engl J Med* 1994;**331**:689–95.

90. Chaliki H, Mohty D, Avierinos JF et al. Outcomes after aortic valve replacement in patients with severe aortic regurgitation and markedly reduced left ventricular function. *Circulation* 2002;**106**:2687–93.

91. Bhudia S, McCarthy P, Kumpati G et al. Improved outcomes after aortic valve surgery for chronic aortic regurgitation with severe left ventricular dysfunction. *J Am Coll Cardiol* 2007;**49**: 1465–71.

92. Bonow R, Dodd J, Maron B et al. Long-term serial changes in left ventricular function and reversal of ventricular dilatation after valve replacement for chronic aortic regurgitation. *Circulation* 1988;**78**:1108–20.

93. Clark D, McAnulty J, Rahimtoola S. Valve replacement in aortic insufficiency with left ventricular dysfunction. *Circulation* 1980;**61**:411–21.

94. Klodas E, Enriquez-Sarano M, Tajik A, Mullany C, Bailey K, Seward J. Aortic regurgitation complicated by extreme left ventricular dilation: long-term outcome after surgical correction. *J Am Coll Cardiol* 1996;**28**(3):670–7.

95. Izumoto H, Kawazoe K, Ishibashi K et al. Aortic valve repair in dominant aortic regurgitation. *Jpn J Thorac Cardiovasc Surg* 2001;**49**:355–9.

96. Rapaport E. Natural history of aortic and mitral valve disease. *Am J Cardiol* 1975;**35**:221–7.

97. Chizner M, Pearle D, deLeon A. The natural history of aortic stenosis in adults. *Am Heart J* 1980;**99**:419–24.

98. O'Keefe J Jr, Vlietstra R, Bailey K, Holmes D Jr. Natural history of candidates for balloon aortic valvuloplasty. *Mayo Clin Proc* 1987;**62**:986–91.

99. Turina J, Hess O, Sepulcri F, Krayenbuehl H. Spontaneous course of aortic valve disease. *Eur Heart J* 1987;**8**:471–83.

100. Kelly T, Rothbart R, Cooper C, Kaiser D, Smucker M, Gibson R. Comparison of outcome of asymptomatic to symptomatic patients older than 20 years of age with valvular aortic stenosis. *Am J Cardiol* 1988;**61**(1):123–30.

101. Henry W, Bonow R, Rosing D, Epstein S. Observations on the optimum time for operative intervention for aortic regurgitation. II. Serial echocardiographic evaluation of asymptomatic patients. *Circulation* 1980;**61**:484–92.

102. Bonow R. Radionuclide angiography in the management of asymptomatic aortic regurgitation. *Circulation* 1991;**84**: I.296–I.302.

103. McDonald I, Jelinek V. Serial M-mode echocardiography in severe chronic aortic regurgitation. *Circulation* 1980;**62**:1291–6.

104. Hegglin R, Scheu H, Rothlin M. Aortic insufficiency. *Circulation* 1968;**38**:V77–V92.

105. Spagnuolo M, Kloth H, Taranta A, Doyle F, Pasternack B. Natural history of rheumatic aortic regurgitation. Criteria predictive of death, congestive heart failure, and angina in young patients. *Circulation* 1971;**34**:368–80.

56 Non-surgical aortic valve therapy: balloon valvuloplasty and transcatheter aortic valve replacement

Robert H Boone and John G Webb

St Paul's Hospital, University of British Columbia, Vancouver, British Columbia, Canada

Surgical valve replacement is the current standard of care for many patients with degenerative valve disease. In appropriate candidates outcomes are excellent and benefit is durable. Nevertheless, surgical valve replacement may not be ideal for all patients and the search for less invasive options has been aggressively pursued.

There was initial enthusiasm for balloon aortic valvuloplasty as a palliative alternative for patients with severe aortic stenosis who were at high operative risk. However, multiple series have shown that although valvuloplasty can be completed with acceptable risk, it provides only short-term symptomatic benefit without improved survival. Nevertheless, valvuloplasty may have a role in temporary palliation or as a bridge to, or component of, a more definitive therapy.

Transcatheter aortic valve replacement is a new therapy which is progressing rapidly, and preliminary experience suggests it may be a viable alternative to conventional surgical valve replacement while avoiding the need for median sternotomy and cardiopulmonary bypass. In selected high-risk patients mortality and morbidity may be superior to outcomes anticipated with conventional surgery. However, current information is primarily from relatively small, single-center registries. Larger, multicenter and randomized evaluations are needed.

Introduction

There are three primary causes of aortic stenosis (AS): congenitally bicuspid valves with superimposed calcification, rheumatic valve disease, and calcific disease of a trileaflet valve. Calcific AS is the most frequent expression of valvu-

lar heart disease in the Western world, is the leading indication for valve replacement, and its prevalence increases with increasing age. Community data document the prevalence of moderate or severe AS at 0.6%, 1.4% and up to 4.6% in patients aged 55–64, 65–74, and ≥75 years, respectively.[1] Surgical aortic valve replacement (AVR) is the preferred treatment strategy for symptomatic patients, but has limitations in the presence of co-morbidities, including advanced age, which increase the operative risk.

Pathophysiology and natural history

The early valve lesions of AS show features similar to atherosclerosis with lipid accumulation and accompanying inflammatory cells and calcification. Myofibroblasts play a central role in the process, and it is believed these cells differentiate into an osteoblast-like cell phenotype which in turn promotes formation of the calcified nodules and bone.[2] The calcification process occurs over decades and causes reduced leaflet mobility, which leads to increased transvalvular pressure gradients, left ventricular outflow obstruction, and systolic pressure overload. The left ventricular wall thickens to maintain chamber size, wall stress and ejection fraction,[3] which is both beneficial and detrimental. Hypertrophied myocardium has less coronary flow per gram and less vasodilator reserve which makes it vulnerable to ischemia, even in the absence of epicardial coronary disease.[4–6] Ischemic stress can be greater in the hypertrophied heart, which must be considered during transcatheter aortic valve replacement (TAVR) where transient left ventricular outflow obstruction and rapid pacing are procedurally required.

The natural history of adult AS consists of a prolonged latent period during which morbidity and mortality are very low. As the calcification process continues, the transvalvular gradient increases and eventually the cardinal symptoms of AS are experienced: angina, syncope and

Evidence-Based Cardiology, 3rd edition. Edited by S. Yusuf, J.A. Cairns, A.J. Camm, E.L. Fallen, and B.J. Gersh. © 2010 Blackwell Publishing, ISBN: 978-1-4051-5925-8.

heart failure. The outlook changes dramatically once symptoms are present, and average survival is 2–3 years.[7–9] Progression from mild AS to severe AS is variable, but once moderate stenosis is present the average rate of progression is a decrease in aortic valve area (AVA) of 0.1cm^2/year.[10] Once symptoms are present the risk of sudden death is high and AVR must be considered.[11]

Aortic valve replacement indications and risk

Surgical AVR may offer survival and symptom benefit, and can be performed at low risk with excellent and durable results in most patient groups. The current American College of Cardiology (ACC)/American Heart Association (AHA) valvular heart disease guideline recommendations for AVR are provided in Table 56.1 and, simply stated, give a Class I recommendation to surgical aortic valve replacement for patients with severe AS in combination with symptoms, left ventricular ejection fraction (LVEF) <50%, or concomitant coronary bypass, aortic or heart valve surgery. In the developing arena of transcatheter aortic valve replacement (TAVR), such guidelines do not exist, and the understanding of surgical risk is fundamental to the process of patient selection.

Among those centers reporting within the Society of Thoracic Surgeons (STS) database (1998–2005) the average perioperative mortality was 3–4% for isolated AVR, and 5–7% for AVR plus coronary artery bypass grafts (CABG).[12] In patients ≥70 years of age, other large series report a 5–15% operative mortality for isolated AVR, and rates are higher in the presence of co-morbidities or the need for additional cardiac procedures.[13–20]

Beyond mortality, morbidity is a significant risk with surgical AVR. For very elderly patients, postoperative stay is more than tw weeks, most are discharged to nursing care or rehabilitation facilities, and rehospitalization within one

Table 56.1 ACC/AHA recommended indications for AVR in patients with AS[37]

Indication	Class[1]	Level of evidence[2]
Severe AS[3] and symptoms	I	B
Severe AS, undergoing CABG	I	C
Severe AS, undergoing aortic or other valve surgery	I	C
Severe AS and EF <50%	I	C
Moderate AS,[4] undergoing CABG, aortic or other valve surgery	IIa	B
Asymptomatic, severe AS, and abnormal exercise response[5]	IIb	C
Asymptomatic, severe AS, and features suggesting rapid progression[6] or potential delay of surgery at the time of symptom onset	IIb	C
Mild AS, undergoing CABG, and features suggesting rapid progression[6]	IIb	C
Asymptomatic, extremely severe AS[7], and expected operative mortality <1%	IIb	C
Asymptomatic, no findings listed above	III	B

ACC, American College of Cardiology; AHA, American Heart Association; AVR, aortic valve replacement; AS, aortic stenosis; CABG, coronary artery bypass grafting; EF, ejection fraction; AVA, aortic valve area.

[1] Definitions for recommendation:

Class I: Conditions for which there is evidence and/or general agreement that the procedure or treatment is beneficial, useful, and effective.

Class II: Conditions for which there is conflicting evidence and/or a divergence of opinion about the usefulness/efficacy of a procedure or treatment: IIA Weight of evidence/opinion is in favor of usefulness/efficacy; IIB Usefulness/efficacy is less well established by evidence/opinion.

Class III: Conditions for which there is evidence and/or general agreement that the procedure/treatment is not useful/effective and in some cases may be harmful.

[2] Definitions for level of evidence:

A: Data derived from multiple randomized clinical trials.

B: Data derived from a single randomized trial or non-randomized studies.

C: Only consensus opinion of experts, case studies or standard of care.

[3] Severe AS: AVA <1cm^2, AVA index <0.6cm^2/m^2, mean gradient >40mmHg, and/or jet velocity >4m/s.[37]

[4] Moderate AS: AVA 1.5–1cm^2, mean gradient 25–40mmHg, and/or jet velocity 3–4m/s.[37]

[5] Development of symptoms or asymptomatic hypotension.

[6] Age, calcification, and CAD.

[7] AVA <0.6cm^2, mean gradient >60mmHg, and jet velocity >5m/s.

month is required for >20%.[21,22] Nevertheless, some series show excellent outcomes.[23]

The increased risk of morbidity and mortality may lead patients, or their physicians, to hesitate when considering surgical options. Iung *et al*[24] performed a cross-sectional survey of patients with valvular heart disease presenting to 92 European hospitals or clinics over a three-month period in 2001, and found that 9.8% of those with aortic stenosis who had guideline indications for surgery were not offered intervention. Subsequently they looked at elderly patients with AS (age >75 yrs), and found that 33% of those with indications for surgery were not offered intervention.[25] Others found that 40–60% of elderly patients with severe symptomatic AS were not offered intervention.[26,27] Patient refusal of surgery has been a consistent reason for conservative management despite the one-, five- and 10-year survivals of 60%, 32%, and 18% respectively of medical therapy.[28]

The growing series of successful TAVR procedures have been performed in an elderly cohort of "high-risk" or non-surgical candidates. This classification has been based on the clinical opinion of senior surgeons in high-volume centers and the use of objective risk calculators as defined by the European System for Cardiac Operative Risk Evaluation (EuroSCORE)[29,30] and/or the Society of Thoracic Surgeons (STS) database.[31] Both EuroSCORE and STS provide an estimate of mortality at 30 days or hospital discharge for patients undergoing CABG and/or valve surgery.

The EuroSCORE model considers 17 clinical risk factors, and was developed in a 13 302 patient cohort with validation in a 1479 patient cohort. It was subsequently tested in a North American cohort of 401 684 patients where the predicted mortality was almost identical to the observed mortality (predicted 3.994%, observed 3.992%). The STS model was developed from the STS National Adult Cardiac Surgery Database which collects information on cardiac surgery morbidity and mortality from 497 participating member sites throughout the United States.[31] The 11 STS models predict both 30-day mortality and major morbidity, are updated and reported annually, and allow comparisons between the observed and predicted outcomes in an effort to improve quality of care. An alternative risk model for patients undergoing valve surgery has been published by Ambler *et al*.[32] It was developed and validated using the database of the Society of Cardiothoracic Surgeons of Great Britain and Ireland, but remains less well utilized. All groups have facilitated risk calculations by providing on-line calculators: 66.89.112.110/STSWebRiskCalc/, euroscore.org/calc.html and www.ucl.ac.uk/stats/research/riskmodel/.

An objective assessment of individual risk has been commonly used to define TAVR eligibility.[33] Published case series have seen average logistic EuroSCOREs >20.[34,35] Furthermore, the inclusion criteria for upcoming randomized trials will likely have an objective risk measurement, with possible thresholds being in the range of logistic EuroSCORE >20 or STS score >10.

Balloon valvuloplasty

Percutaneous balloon aortic valvuloplasty (PBAV) was first performed by Cribier in 1985, with the first three patient series published in 1986.[36] Subsequently there have been many reports of the effectiveness and durability of PBAV, and in reviewing the literature for this chapter we collected 50 publications documenting results from over 2400 patients. Most procedures were performed in elderly patients with calcific AS who were considered either non-operative candidates or of high operative risk. All reports are case series (**Level C1**), and PBAV has never been subjected to a large-scale randomized trial. The discussion below is not a formal systematic review, but is based on a comprehensive and representative sample of English-language publications. We will not discuss the evidence for PBAV in young patients with congenital AS where it remains a Class I therapeutic option.[37]

The 27-center Mansfield Investigational Device Exemption Protocol employed standardized protocols with definite inclusion and exclusion criteria to study aortic valvuloplasty.[38] Patient recruitment occurred from December 1986 through November 1987. The data collected from 492 patients undergoing PBAV were pooled to create the Mansfield Scientific Balloon Aortic Valvuloplasty Registry.[38–45] Subsequently, the NHLBI Balloon Valvuloplasty Registry was organized, and enrolled 674 patients from 24 centers between 1987 and 1989, generating reports on early and late procedure results.[46,47] The Cribier group in France[48–52] and the Duke University Medical Center group[53–55] have also contributed significant numbers of patients to this literature.

To support PBAV as a therapeutic option, we must consider the ability of the procedure to do what it claims: reduce the transaortic pressure gradient. Table 56.2 outlines the changes in AVA and mean transaortic gradient (MG) reported in a variety of series. Most reports show the AVA increases to between 0.8 and 1 cm², and the largest series found AVA increased <0.4 cm² in 77% of patients.[47] However, in 13% of this cohort there was either no change or <0.1 cm² improvement in AVA. Similarly, 13% of the Mansfield group had an unsuccessful procedure (procedural/in-hospital death, AVR within seven days, or <40% change in AVA).[42] It is clear that PBAV is successful in reducing the transaortic gradient in most, but not all patients with critical AS secondary to calcific disease.

Another measure of procedural success is symptom status, and all series report significant initial improvement. We present a representative sample of the available data in

Table 56.2 Summary of hemodynamic effectiveness and procedural complications of percutaneous aortic balloon valvuloplasty

Reference	Number of patients	Average age (yrs)	Hemodynamic outcomes					Complication rate (excluding in-hospital mortality)				In-hospital mortality
			Baseline AVA (cm²)	Final AVA (cm²)	Baseline MG (mmHg)	Final MG (mmHg)		Overall	Vascular	Aortic insufficiency	Stroke	
NHLBI Registry[47]	674	78 ± 9	0.5 ± 0.2	0.8 ± 0.3	55 ± 2¹	29 ± 13		25%	7%	1%	3%	10.2%
Mansfield Scientific Registry[42]	492	79 ± 8.4	0.5 ± 0.18	0.82 ± 0.3	59.8 ± 23	29.5 ± 13.4		20.5%	11%	2.1%	2.2%	7.5%
Letac et al.[50]	218		0.52 ± 0.18	0.93 ± 0.33				15%	13%		1.8%	4.6%
Agarwal et al.[57]	212	82 ± 8	0.61 ± 0.19	1.2 ± 0.3	44 ± 18	18 ± 9		~18%	13.5%	0.4%	1.1%	8%
Knutz et al.[104]	205	78 ± 10	0.6 ± 0.2	0.9 ± 0.3	55 ± 19	30 ± 12		12.7%	9.9%	1%	0%	4.4%
Lewin et al.[105]	125	12 ± 4	0.6 ± 0.2	1.0 ± 0.3	70 ± 26	30 ± 13		9%	4%	0%	3%	10%
Letac et al.[51]	92	84 ± 3.7	0.48 ± 0.16	0.91 ± 0.35	71 ± 27	27 ± 15		16.1%	15%	1.1%	1.1%	6.5%
Klein et al.[63]	78	78 ± 11	0.47 ± 0.15	0.83 ± 0.27	50 ± ¹6	29 ± 14		22%	20%	0%	0%	5.5%
Berland et al.[52]	55	77 ± 9			66 ± 24	28 ± 14		14.5	12.7	0%	1.8	

AVA, aortic valve area; MG, mean transaortic gradient.

Table 56.3. The NHLBI registry found symptom improvement in 75% of survivors at 30-days, and 60–85% of survivors report symptom improvement at follow-up out to 24 months. Davidson *et al* [56] report LVEF was the only independent predictor of overall symptom improvement at 3 months, and found less than 50% of those with an ejection fraction (EF) <45% had symptom improvement. Taken in aggregate, the data suggests the majority of survivors have some initial symptom improvement.

However, the result is not durable, and most patients will see symptom recurrence with time. Agarwal *et al*[57] report that the mean duration of symptom relief after

Table 56.3 Summary of studies reporting symptom response to percutaneous aortic balloon valvuloplasty, sorted by duration of follow-up

Reference	Number of patients	Age (yrs)	Follow-up duration (months)	Symptom response
NHLBI Registry[47]	674	78 ± 9	30 days	75% of survivors (86%) improved 1 NYHA class (or remained class I) 53% experienced at least a quartile improvement in functional status score
Davidson[56]	81		3	65.4% of patients had sustained symptom improvement LVEF was the only independent predictor of overall status at 3 months: • EF >45% : 84% improvement in symptoms • EF <45% : <50% had symptom improvement
Block[59]	90	79 ± 1	5.5 ± 0.3	Baseline → follow-up: NYHA I: 1% → 16% NYHA II: 1% → 20% NYHA III: 25% → 11% NYHA IV: 73% → 25%
O'Neill[44]	492	79 ± 8.4	Median 7 range 0 – 18.8	66% had subjective improvement of symptoms for >6 months Baseline → follow-up: NYHA I: 4% → 26% NYHA II: 14% → 42% NYHA III: 45% → 26% NYHA IV: 36% → 6%
Safian[60]	170	77 ± 5	9.1	60.6% subjective improvement 25.9% had recurrent symptoms and had either medical therapy (n = 11, 25%), AVR (n = 17, 38.6%), or repeat PBAV (n = 16, 36.4%)
Lewin[105]	125		12 ± 4	76.3% of survivors (57.6%) had sustained symptom improvement
Letac[51]	92	84 ± 3.7	13 ± 5	84% of survivors (45.8%) had significantly improved dyspnea Baseline → follow-up: NYHA II or IV: 86 → 20% Angina: 55 → 32% CCS III or IV: 27 → 9%
Otto[46]	674	78 ± 9	48	Survivors at 2 years (35%): 61% report improved symptoms 11% NYHA class I or II Functional status score: Baseline: 47 ± 27 6 months: 63 ± 29 5 weeks: 58 ± 30 3 years: 57 ± 31 Patients reporting any limitation to activity: Baseline: 79% After procedure: 76% 3 years: 73%
Agarwal[57]	212	82 ± 8	32 ± 18	Duration of symptom alleviation after the first, second, and third BAV procedures were 18 ± 3, 15 ± 4, and 10 ± 3 months, respectively

NYHA, New York Heart Association; AVR, aortic valve replacement; LVEF, left ventricular ejection fraction; LV, left ventricle; PBAV, percutaneous balloon aortic valvuloplasty; PG, peak gradient.

PBAV was 18 ± 3 months. Upon repeat investigation, most patients with recurrent symptoms are found to have restenosis (defined as ≥50% loss in the AVA gained by PBAV), and this is assumed to be the cause of recurrent symptoms. The rate of restenosis has been reported to vary between 25% and 47% at six months[58–60] and up to 80% at 15 months.[61] Postprocedure AVA can be influenced by a variety of procedural modifications[42,47] and although initially thought to alter prognosis,[57–60] these techniques have not been found to change rates of restenosis or survival in larger series.[39]

Reported periprocedural complication rates range from 9% to 25% (see Table 57.2). The nature of periprocedural complications as reported in the NHLBI Registry can be found in Table 57.4. Procedural morbidity and in-hospital mortality decreases with increased procedural experience and equipment refinements.[50,62] Interestingly, the two most recent PBAV series report periprocedural complication rates of 22% and 18%.[57,63] Although Klein et al[63] do report a trend toward a decrease in procedural complications over time, these complication rates are not significantly less than that reported in the Mansfield Registry. Periprocedural stroke and aortic insufficiency are uncommon complications (see Table 56.2).

The final analysis of PBAV must consider its effectiveness in altering the natural history of the disease. Mortality rates address this question directly, and are presented in Table 56.5. One- and two-year survival ranged from 75% to 38% (average 65%) and 28% to 60% (average 35%), respectively. These rates are not significantly different from the one- and two-year survival of elderly patients with untreated AS (60% and 40%, respectively)[9,28] and suggest PBAV alone does not alter the natural history of AS for most patients.

Many authors employed multivariate techniques to identify clinical, historical and/or hemodynamic factors that might be significantly associated with PBAV outcome. These results are presented in Table 56.5 and consistently show older age, low EF, and worse baseline NYHA class are all associated with a poor prognosis. In the largest series, Otto et al defined a "lower risk" subgroup (normal LVEF and mild functional limitation) who had a three-year survival of 36% as opposed to 17% in the rest of the group.[46]

Table 56.4 Comparison of periprocedural complications between PBAV and TAVR procedures

Complications[1]	NHLBI BAV Registry[4/*] % (n)	Core valve[34]† % (n)	Edwards Lifesciences[35]* % (n)
Death	3 (17)	6 (5)	2 (1)
Patients with any severe complication	25 (167)	26 (22)	16 (8)
Specific complications:			
Hemodynamic			
Cardiac tamponade	1 (10)	7 (6)	0
Mechanical circulatory support[2]	2 (11)[2]	69 (60)[2]	0[2]
Acute aortic valvular insufficiency	1 (6)	2 (2)	0
Cardiogenic shock	2 (15)	–	–
Valve malposition	–	2 (2)	4 (2)
Valve embolization	–	0	4 (2)
Emergent cardiac surgery	0	6 (6)	0
Neurologic			
Vasovagal reaction	5 (36)	–	–
Stroke	2 (13)	10 (9)	4 (2)
AV block requiring pacing	4 (30)	NR	2 (1)
Vascular			
Emergency vascular intervention[3]	5 (33)	NR	6 (3)
Transfusion required	20 (136)	NR	18 (9)[4]
Arterial rupture	0	NR	8 (4)

AV, atrioventricular; NR, not reported; n/r, not recorded; –, not applicable.
[1] Complications at time of procedure or within 24 hours (*), and within 48 hours (†).
[2] Mechanical support was procedurally required for all 69% (n=60) in the Core Valve group, unplanned IABP was inserted for support in the PBAV series. IABP, intra-aortic balloon pump.
[3] Intervention defined as surgery or endovascular procedure beyond that normally required for the procedure.
[4] % (number) of patients requiring >3 units packed red blood cells.

Table 56.5 Summary of studies reporting long-term outcome of percutaneous aortic balloon valvuloplasty sorted by duration of follow-up

Reference	Number of patients	Patient age (years)	Mean follow-up (months)	Mortality	Actuarial survival	Incidence of AVR post PBAV	Incidence of repeat PBAV	Event-free survival	Predictors of outcome
NHLBI Registry[47]	674	78 ± 9	30 day	14%	–	–	–	–	30-day mortality associated with: hypotension and NYHA class IV (risk ratio, 4.4), blood urea nitrogen >10.7 mmol/L (risk ratio, 3.7), use of an antiarrhythmic (risk ratio, 2.9), and cardiac output less than 3.0 L/min (risk ratio, 2.4)
O'Neill et al.[44]	492	–	7	24%	1y: 64%	16.6% AVR & PBAV together	16.6% AVR & PBAV together	1y: 43%	Independent predictors of long-term survival (discriminate function analysis): age, initial cardiac output, initial left ventricular systolic pressures, initial left ventricular end-diastolic pressures, presence of coronary artery disease, NYHA class, number of balloon inflations and final valve area: predict 1-yr survival 20–80% Postprocedure variables predicting worse prognosis: low LVEF, CAD, multiple balloon inflations
Letac et al.[50]	144	74 ± 11	8	16.7%	–	14.6%	14.5%	–	–
Davidson et al.[53]	170	78	8.3	20.6%	–	12.4%	7.6%	1y: 62%	Independent variables significantly associated with event-free survival in multivariate model: LV end-diastolic diameter, CHF at baseline, and age. BUT, when compared to predictive ability of baseline EF alone: no difference. Suggest baseline EF only important prognostic variable EF >45% predicted good outcome (cardiac survival 80% at 1 yr)
Safian et al.[60]	170	77 ± 5	9.1 ± 5.5	18.2%	1y: 74%	2.9%	8.8%	1y: 50%	–
Lewin et al.[105]	125	76	12 ± 4	38%	1y: 62%	6.9%	13.9%	–	Mortality associated with: baseline EF, CO, severe HF
Klein et al.[63]	78	78 ± 11	122 patient years	87%	1y: 38% 2y: 32% 3y: 20% 5y: 13%	22%	6.4%	–	Multivariate analysis showed that advancing age was the strongest predictor of mortality, while controling for gender, diabetes, and baseline LVEF, mean aortic pressure, and aortic valve index. For each 10-year increase in age, the relative hazard was 2.0 (95% CI 1.2–3.3; $P = 0.005$). No other demographic, clinical or baseline hemodynamic variables were independent predictors of mortality after PBAV

Study	N	Age							
Otto et al.[46]	674	78 ± 9	18 ± 15	1y: 45%, 2y: 65%, 3y: 77%	1y: 55%, 2y: 35%, 3y: 23%	20%	15%	—	Independent predictors of survival: baseline functional status, baseline cardiac output, renal function, cachexia, female gender, left ventricular systolic function, and mitral regurgitation A "lower-risk" subgroup (28% of the study population), defined by normal left ventricular systolic function and mild clinical functional limitation, had a 3-year survival of 36% compared with 17% in the remainder of the study group PBAV + AVR: survival was 88% and 71% at 30 days and 2 yrs respectively
Kuntz et al.[104]	205	78 ± 10	24 ± 12	30%	1y: 75%, 2y: 60%	27.8%	20.5%	Event free survival: 18% Predicted: 1y: 50% 2y: 25%	Independent variables significantly associated with event-free survival in multivariate model: • Baseline aortic systolic pressure (<110 mmHg. RR 2.03 (1.33,3.08) vs >=140 mmHg) • Pulmonary capillary wedge pressure (>25 mmHg. RR 1.73 (1.18,2.55) vs <=18 mmHg) • Reduction in peak aortic gradient (< 40%. RR 1.75 (1.17,2.63) >=55%)
Agarwal et al.[57]	212	82 ± 8	32 ± 18	1y: 36%, 2y: 72%, 5y: 86%	1y: 64%, 2y: 28%, 5y: 14%	5%	24%	—	Independent variables significantly associated with postdischarge mortality in multivariate model: women and multiple PBAV procedures (protective), and Charleston Co-Morbidity Index and chronic renal insufficiency (harmful)
Lieberman et al.[54,55]	165	—	46.8	66.7%	1y: 64%, 2y: 48%, 3y: 37%	24%	19%	1y: 40%, 2y: 19%, 3y: 6%	Independent variables significantly associated with adverse prognosis in multivariate Cox proportional hazards model: younger age and a lower LVEF Actuarial survival by treatment group: PBAV only: 1y: 44%, 2y: 21%, 3y: 13% PBAV*2: 1y: 77%, 2y: 61%, 3y: 37% PBAV + AVR: 1y: 98%, 2y: 92%, 3y: 83%

AVR, aortic valve replacement; PBAV, percutaneous balloon aortic valvuloplasty; NR, not reported; m, month; y, year; LV, left ventricle; EF, ejection fraction; NYHA, New York Heart Association; CO, cardiac output; CHF, congestive heart failure.

Given the early benefit but limited durability of PBAV, some investigators proposed that patients with restenosis be considered for repeat valvuloplasty. Table 56.5 provides details on the incidence of such treatment (roughly 5–20%), but the outcomes were most carefully considered in the three separate series.[40,49,57] Each series has shown a second procedure is efficacious in reducing AVA and symptoms, but none was able to find factors that would point to an increased durability of a second procedure. Although patients who underwent repeat procedures had higher three-year survival rates than those with a single procedure,[54,57] there was a decrease in the duration of symptom relief with each subsequent dilation.[57] Several reports have highlighted the success of PBAV followed by AVR where two-year survival can be as high as 92%.[54] This is an attractive strategy but has limited applicability as it is unclear how delaying definitive treatment would improve operative risk for the majority of patients. In fact, the AHA/ACC guidelines give a Class III recommendation to the concept of PBAV as an alternative to AVR.[37]

Despite the problems with PBAV, the current AHA/ACC guidelines recognize the possibility that it may have a limited therapeutic role, and the following situations are given Class IIB recommendations.

1 Aortic balloon valvotomy might be reasonable as a bridge to surgery in hemodynamically unstable adult patients with AS who are at high risk for AVR.

2 Aortic balloon valvotomy might be reasonable for palliation in adult patients with AS in whom AVR cannot be performed because of serious co-morbid conditions.[37]

Additionally, several groups have reported that PBAV can be used to successfully treat patients with cardiogenic shock secondary to severe AS.[64,65] Similarly, PBAV can be used to reduce the risk of non-cardiac surgery when a stepwise approach using AVR is not possible.[66,67]

In an attempt to address the significant problem of limited durability with PBAV, newer studies have focused on the mechanisms of restenosis. PBAV improves leaflet mobility by fracturing calcified nodules and creating cleavage planes within collagenous stroma.[68,69] Feldman et al[70] suggest that the process of restenosis following PBAV is histologically distinct from that of calcified valves not having undergone PBAV. They found granulation tissue, fibrosis, and ossification present within the leaflets of valves treated with PBAV, suggesting an active process of osteoblast-mediated calcification. This lead Pedersen et al to perform a 20-patient pilot study of external beam radiation applied 3–5 days following PBAV in elderly patients with calcific AS (the RADAR pilot trial).[71] They found one-year restenosis rates of 21–30% in a dose-responsive manner. This is substantially less than the 15-month 80% restenosis rates found by Letac et al[61] and offers an interesting option for the future of PBAV techniques.

In summary, PBAV is successful in reducing left ventricular outflow obstruction in most patients with severe calcific AS. However, the results are not durable, and the long-term survival resembles that of the natural history of critical AS. We conclude that PBAV currently has a limited role in palliation of some patients with critical AS, and surgical AVR remains the treatment of choice. However, new therapies targeting post-PBAV restenosis offer promise and may lead to expanded indications in the elderly population. Furthermore, the future role of PBAV may be influenced by the development of TAVR as discussed below.

Transcatheter heart valve

Andersen et al pioneered the development of a balloon-expandable aortic valve, reporting experience with a porcine model in 1992.[72] Subsequently, others demonstrated the feasibility of percutaneous prosthetic valve delivery.[73–77] In 2000, Bonhoeffer et al described the first-in-man experience of a successfully implanted catheter-based stent valve in a pulmonary conduit.[78] In 2002, Cribier et al demonstrated the feasibility of aortic valve implantation in man using an antegrade approach via the femoral vein and transseptal puncture,[79] following which we described the development of a retrograde approach via the femoral artery.[80] Subsequently, the experience and technology for transcatheter aortic valve replacement (TAVR) have evolved rapidly, and will be discussed below. Like the PBAV literature, the evidence for these procedures is limited to case series (**Level C1**), but randomized trials are under way.

Balloon-expandable aortic valve

The currently available SAPIEN™ valve (Edwards Lifesciences LLC, Irvine, CA) consists of three bovine pericardial leaflets hand-sewn to a stainless steel, tubular, slotted, balloon expandable stent (Fig. 56.1). There is a fabric sealing cuff that covers the bottom portion of the stent and is intended to form a seal against the aortic annulus. Currently the valve is available in 20, 23 and 26mm diameter sizes. The SAPIEN™ valve replaces the Cribier–Edwards equine valve that was used for the majority of the published experience with balloon-expandable valves described below. As of late October 2007, 494 patients have been treated with this prosthesis.

The procedure for TAVR with balloon-expandable stents utilizes three approaches: transvenous, transarterial and transapical.

Transvenous procedure

Following the first successful human TAVR by Cribier in 2002, a formal European registry was initiated (I-REVIVE

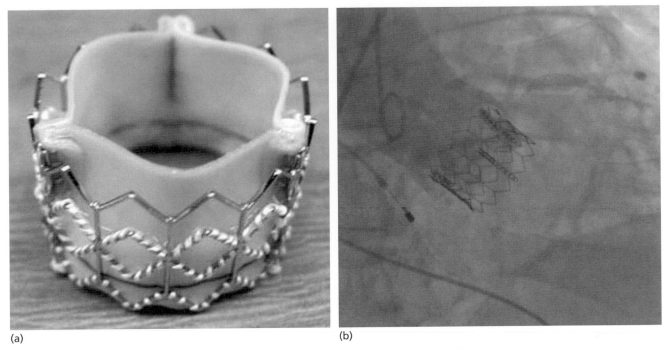

(a)   (b)

Figure 56.1 (a) The SAPIEN™ balloon-expandable aortic valve. (b) Aortogram showing the implanted valve.

or Initial Registry of EndoVascular Implantation of Valves in Europe) for patients with critical AS and no surgical options. A single-center registry was also established by the group in Rouen for high-risk patients who had been refused surgery (RECAST or Registry of Endovascular Critical Aortic Stenosis Treatment). The results of the initial 36 patients enrolled in these registries by Cribier were reported in 2006.[81] The majority of patients (79%) had a transvenous antegrade approach. Stent placement was successful in 75%, with failures secondary to embolization of the stent valve, hemodynamic instability, and inability to cross the native aortic valve. Postprocedure hemodynamics showed a significant decrease in MG (from 37 to 9 mmHg), increase in AVA (from 0.6 to 1.7 cm²), and paravalvular aortic insufficiency was graded moderate to severe in 63% of patients. There was a high rate of procedure-related in-hospital complications (26%), and an additional 10 patients died in the subsequent six months. Nevertheless, extended follow-up demonstrated sustained normal bioprosthetic valve function for over three years. This experience provided proof that TAVR could be performed with a durable result, but it became clear that the transvenous antegrade approach was technically complex and unpredictable.[82]

Transarterial procedure
The early attempts with the transarterial retrograde approach encountered a number of difficulties which included: arterial access issues related to the need for large sheaths and catheters, passage of large-diameter prosthesis

around the aortic arch, difficulty crossing the stenotic aortic valve from the retrograde direction, and the use of standard valvuloplasty balloons for stent deployment which was only sporadically successful.[83] An important advance was the 2006 publication by Webb et al of an 18-patient series of high-risk elderly patients (logistic EuroSCORE 26%) in whom a reproducible transarterial approach had been developed.[80] Procedural advancements included the development of arterial access equipment and techniques and a steerable guiding catheter used to actively direct the prosthesis through the tortuous aorta and retrograde through the aortic valve. Transarterial TAVR was successful in 14 of 18 patients, and there were no intraprocedural deaths. Thirty-day mortality was 11.1% with two early deaths related to procedural complications: one due to iliac artery perforation, and the other likely due to inadvertent obstruction of the left main coronary ostium by a displaced native aortic valve leaflet excrescence.

Recently Webb et al have published a 50-patient series which confirmed the success of the transarterial approach.[35] Valve implantation was successful in 86% of patients with an intraprocedural mortality of 2%. Mortality at 30 days was 12%, which compared favorably to a logistic EuroSCORE estimate of 28%. With experience, procedural success increased from 76% in the first 25 patients to 96% in the second half of this experience, and 30-day mortality fell from 16% to 8%. There were significant improvements in AVA, left ventricular ejection fraction, mitral regurgitation and functional class, and all were maintained at one year (Fig. 56.2). An 85-patient series by our group confirm and

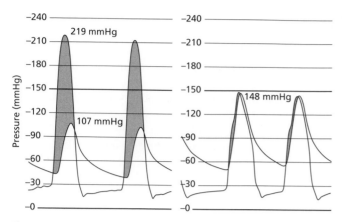

Figure 56.2 Hemodynamic results before and after transcatheter aortic valve replacement with the SAPIEN™ valve. (a) Preprocedure simultaneous left ventricular and femoral artery peak to peak gradient was 108 mmHg and mean gradient was 108; calculated aortic valve area was 0.43 cm² using the Gorlin formula. (b) Postprocedure peak to peak gradient was 3 mmHg.

improve the above findings.[84] Importantly, procedural success increased to 91%, and 30-day mortality was 11% in the group with a mean logistic EuroSCORE of 31%. None of the patients had moderate or severe aortic insufficiency, and although mild paravalvular aortic regurgitation was common, it remained stable with no clinical consequences at one year. Furthermore, at a median follow-up of 359 days there was no structural valve deterioration, endocarditis or late valve embolization. Survival at one, six and 12 months was 89%, 84% and 77% respectively. Our largest series of combined transfemoral (n = 113) and transapical (n = 55) procedures was recently published.[85] Thirty-day mortality mortality was further reduced: transfemoral 8% vs transapical 18.2% (P = 0.07, overall 30-day mortality of 11.3%), and evidence of a learning curve continued with mortality falling from 14.3% to 8.3% between the first and second half of the series. (From 12.3% to 3.6% (P = 0.16) in transfemoral patients and from 25% to 11.1% (P = 0.30) in transapical patients.) Functional class improved over the year following the procedure (P < 0.001). Survival at 1 year was 74%, with the bulk of late re-admissions and mortality occurring as a function of co-morbidities rather than procedure or valve-related events. The 1-year survival of 74% compares favourably with the reported 1-year survivals of 51% and 66% in elderly patients with aortic stenosis who were not considered to be surgical candidates or who declined surgery (respectively).[86]

Edwards Lifesciences (unpublished data) has maintained a worldwide registry of patients treated with TAVR. In September 2007, the SAPIEN™ valve received CE mark in the European community and as of May, 2009 there have been over 2500 SAPIEN™ implants world wide. The SOURCE registry contains data on over 1000 implants. These data confirm the structural and hemodynamic integrity of the valve with follow-up to one year, and the transfemoral (n = 459 patients) 30-day mortality was 6.3% with 93.3% of the cohort having a logistic EuroScore of >20% (mean 33.3%). One-year survival was approximately 75%.

The demonstrated safety and feasibility of the transarterial approach has lead to the development of a randomized clinical trial: the PARTNER (Placement of AoRTic TraNscathetER Valves) Trial. This prospective, randomized, controlled, multicenter pivotal trial will evaluate the safety and effectiveness of the SAPIEN™ Transcatheter Heart Valve in a stratified population of 600 patients with symptomatic severe aortic stenosis. One cohort will consist of high-risk surgery patients (operative mortality estimated at >15% and STS ≥10) randomized to either transarterial aortic valve implantation or surgical aortic valve replacement. The second cohort will consist of inoperable patients (cardiologist and two cardiovascular surgeons agree that the probability of death or serious, irreversible morbidity should exceed 50%) randomized to medical therapy or TAVR. The primary outcome is one-year mortality, and enrolment began in 2007.

Transapical approach

Some patients are poorly suited to the transarterial procedure due to femoral, iliac or aortic size, tortuousity or atheroma. Direct balloon catheter implantation of experimental prostheses through the left ventricular apex was used by our group in early studies of percutaneous valve implantation,[77] and was subsequently trialed extensively in animals.[87] The first human applications utilized a median sternotomy with cardiopulmonary bypass[88] but this has been supplanted by the current approach of intercostal thoracotomy without cardiopulmonary bypass.[89–90] The procedure is performed by a combined team of interventional cardiologists and cardiac surgeons in an operating room or catheterization laboratory using fluoroscopy and echocardiographic guidance with the patient under general anesthesia.[88,91–93]

The transapical approach avoids problems related to arterial access, and the short distance from the LV apex to the aortic valve may facilitate antegrade crossing and prosthesis positioning. However, disadvantages include the need for a thoracotomy, chest tube, apical repair, and the possibility of injury to the mitral apparatus. Experience with this procedure is limited. As of October 2007, 193 procedures had been performed in seven centers in Canada, Europe and the United States with a 30-day mortality of 18% in a high-risk cohort (source: Edwards Lifesciences LLC, unpublished data). The largest experience from four centers in Europe and North America was recently published and highlights the success of this approach. Fifty-nine patients with average logistic EuroSCORE of 26.8 ± 13.5% underwent transapical TAVR. Thirty-day mortality was 13.6%, and actuarial survival 75.7 ± 5.9% at a follow-up interval of 110 ± 77 days (range 1–255 days).[91]

A slightly larger series of 61 patients showed six- and 12-month survival of 74.4 ± 6.6% and 70.5 ± 7.3%, respectively.[94] This procedural success was recently replicated by Walther et al.[95] where procedural success was 92.8% in a cohort of 168 patients. Thirty-day and 6-month mortality was 16% and 30% respectively.

Self-expanding aortic valve

The CoreValve ReValving™ System (CoreValve Inc, Irvine, CA) is delivered using a transcatheter procedure, but the prosthesis is self-expanding rather than balloon expandable. When the restraining sheath is retracted the nitinol stent alloy expands to its predetermined shape, forming a tubular rigid frame with a trileaflet pericardial tissue valve attached with PTFE sutures. It measures 50mm in axial length and incorporates three distinct areas of radial force. The lower portion has a high radial force and implants within the subannular region. The middle portion contains the valve leaflets and is tapered so as to be unopposed to the aorta and coronary sinuses, thereby allowing normal flow and access to the coronary ostia through the stent struts. The upper portion is flared and anchors the prosthesis against the ascending aorta with low radial force while providing longitudinal stability.[96] The valve is currently available in two sizes depending on the diameter of the ascending aorta (<35mm or <45mm) with one aortic annular diameter (23mm). Initially the delivery system was 24Fr, but subsequently evolved to 21Fr with a more recent 18Fr iteration.[34,96] Following PBAV, the CoreValve ReValving™ System is correctly positioned in a transaortic position and the over-riding sheath slowly withdrawn. Initially, valve implantation required femoral–femoral cardiopulmonary support due to obstruction of transvalvular flow during valve release, but recent cases have been performed without this support.

As of early 2007, over 168 CoreValve procedures had been performed.[34] Initial procedures were performed in India with procedural success but poor clinical outcomes. The first case report from Germany was published in 2005[97] and the first series of 25 elderly patients (mean age 80.3 ± 5.4) was published in 2006.[96] Valve implantation was successful in 88% patients. Mean transvalvular gradients were significantly reduced (44 to 12mmHg), and postprocedure aortic regurgitation grade was unchanged. However, major in-hospital adverse events occurred in 32%, and in-hospital mortality was 20% in this high-risk group with a median logistic EuroSCORE of 11%.

A more recent report describes 86 cases performed using the newer 21Fr and 18Fr systems.[34] The group had a mean age of 81.3 ± 5.2 (21Fr) and 83.4 ± 6.7 years (18Fr), and a mean logistic EuroSCORE of 23.4 ± 13.5% (21Fr) and 19.1 ± 11.1% (18Fr). The valve was successfully implanted in 88% of patients, with a marked reduction in mean trans-

valvular gradient (44 to 9mmHg) and no change in aortic regurgitation. Periprocedural major adverse cardiovascular and cerebral events were reported in 26% of patients within the first 48 hours after device implantation, primarily driven by stroke (10%) and tamponade (7%). Procedural mortality was 6%, and overall 30-day mortality was 12% which was a significant improvement over the earlier case series. The most recent series of 1243 patients shows 30-day mortality has decreased to 6.7% (Logistic EUROscore 22.9 ± 4.1%), and post-procedure pacemaker implant was required in 12%.[98] Importantly, the 18Fr system has allowed transition to a percutaneous approach under local anaesthesia without hemodynamic support.[34]

Evidence around procedural issues

Paravalvular insufficiency

Mild paravalvular aortic regurgitation (PVAR) is commonly found with the current transcatheter valves, but for the most part does not appear to have major clinical consequences.[35,80] Severe leaks are uncommon but can occur. Accurate aortic annulus sizing has played a key role in minimizing paravalvular leak. Complicating sizing is variability in annular measurements obtained with the available imaging modalities and the apparent demonstration by multislice cardiac computed tomography that at least a portion of patients have an aortic annulus that is oval rather than round.[99]

PVAR can sometimes be reduced with redilation. Our center found 31 of 124 (26%) balloon-expandable valves were redilated for significant PVAR at the time of the initial procedure.[100] It appeared that cautious redilation appeared safe (no embolizations or persistent worsening of valvular insufficiency) and effective at reducing PVAR, and that oversizing the valve and using less compliant balloons may prove to be useful in reducing PVAR.

Learning curve

Transcatheter aortic valve implantation is a relatively complex procedure in which technical errors are not well tolerated and mortality may ensue. Like the previously outlined experience for PBAV, TAVR outcomes clearly improve with improvements in equipment, techniques and experience.[34,35] Consequently, cautious dissemination appears prudent. Formal educational programs, virtual simulators and proctoring have been utilized and appear helpful. Regional centers of expertise may be desirable to optimize outcomes.

Long-term follow-up

Early experience demonstrated an acute improvement in left ventricular systolic function.[101] Unlike the experience with PBAV, longer term follow-up has confirmed that this is sustained and associated with a sustained improvement

Table 56.6 Comparison of outcomes between PBAV and TAVR procedures

	NHLBI BAV Registry[46,47]	CoreValve[34]	Edwards Lifesciences[35]
Demographics			
Number of patients	674	86	50
Age (years)	78 ± 9	82 ± 6	82 ± 7
Follow-up (days)	3 years	30	359
Mortality:			
Logistic EuroSCORE	NR	21.7 ± 12.6%	28%
Mortality (30 days)	14%	12%	12%
Survival (1 year)	55%	n/a	81%
Survival (2 year)	35%	n/a	70%[1]
Hemodynamic:			
Aortic valve area (cm²)	0.57 → 0.78→ 0.65	0.6 → NR → n/a	0.6 → 1.7 → 1.6
(Baseline → post procedure → 6 month follow-up)			
Mean gradient (mmHg)	55 → 29 → 43[2]	43.7 → ~8[3] → ~7[3,4]	46 → 11 → 11
(Baseline → post procedure → 6 month follow-up)			
Symptoms:			
Symptom improvement	~75% NYHA III or IV	NHYA class 2.85 ± 0.73	70% NYHA III
(Baseline → 1 year)	→	→	→
	~30% NYHA III or IV[5]	NYHA class 1.85 ± 0.6	82.3% NYHA I or II
			17.7% NYHA III

IQR, interquartile range; n/a, not applicable; NR, not reported; NYHA, New York Heart Association dyspnea classification
[1] 2-year survival data taken from Pasupati et al.[102]
[2] Only 157 of 674 completed 6-month echocardiographic follow-up.
[3] VALUES are estimated from figure in paper, exact valves not provided in text.
[4] 30-day follow-up, 6-month data not available.
[5] Only 214 of 674 completed 1-year follow-up.

Table 56.7 Screening for transcatheter valve replacement

Questions to be answered	Evaluation	Comments
Should the patient have conventional AVR?	Surgical consult	Estimated operative mortality <20% Acceptable morbidity
What is the annulus diameter?	Echocardiogram	Valves are specific to a range of diameters Transesophageal echocardiogram if transthoracic parasternal long axis dimensions are borderline
Is percutaneous access adequate?	Iliofemoral angiogram with calibrated measurement catheter, CT or MR	Assess lumen diameter, tortuousity and calcification
Is the aortic root adequate?	Aortic root angiogram with calibrated measurement catheter, CT or MR	Assess abnormal root, potential for coronary obstruction
Is the ascending aorta diameter suitable?	CT or MR	Relevant to the CoreValve device
Is there LV dysfunction?	Echocardiogram or left ventricular angiogram	Increases risk of myocardial ischemia during implantation
Is there the potential for ischemia?	Coronary angiogram	Is there increased risk of ischemia during implantation. Is revascularization required?
Is there anemia or a clotting disorder?	Hemoglobin concentration, platelet count, partial thromboplastin time, prothrombin time	There is a risk of blood loss from access sites
Is there renal dysfunction?	Serum creatinine, glomerular filtration rate	Contrast nephropathy and transient hypotension can occur
Are there anesthetic concerns?	Anesthetic consult	Intubation and ventilation may be utilized
Are expectations realistic?	History, family support, co-morbidities	Do co-morbidities permit a reasonable quality and duration of life?

CT, computed tomography; MR, magnetic resonance.

in mitral insufficiency and functional class.[35,102] *In vitro* valve testing of currently available devices anticipates durability in excess of 10 years and structural valve deterioration has not been reported. However, only one report has documented late survival beyond one year in a significant number of patients, and follow-up beyond three years has only been reported in a few patients to date.[35,81] Zajarias and Cribier (REF) recently published a review of over 4000 transcatheter valve replacement procedures highlighting the lack of re-stenosis or prosthetic valve dysfunction over mid-term follow-up. Futhermore, a small series by Ussia *et al.* have shown a striking improvements in physical and physical and mental quality of life scores 5 months following transcatheter aortic valve replacement.[103]

Non-surgical aortic valve therapy compared

TAVR procedures are technically complex and evolving rapidly. Table 56.6 provides a comparison of the outcomes from PBAV and the two currently available TAVR devices.

Recommendations

- Surgical aortic valve replacement is currently the treatment of choice for patients with symptomatic critical aortic stenosis (**Class I, Level B**).
- In symptomatic patients with critical aortic stenosis who are felt to be of high surgical risk (EuroSCORE >15, STS >10), TAVR may be a reasonable alternative (**Class IIa, Level C1**).
- Current prosthesis size limits the procedure to patients whose annulus is appropriate (≥18 mm or ≤26 mm diameter).
- Patients with excessively bulky native valve leaflets in close proximity to a coronary ostium may be at risk of coronary occlusion.
- Selection between transarterial or transapical access should take into account local expertise, current more favorable outcomes with the transfemoral approach and the advantages of transapical access in the presence of arterial and aortic access limitations.
- A variety of patient factors may increase procedural risk and should be considered individually: obstructive coronary artery disease, reduced ejection fraction, chronic renal insufficiency, immobility.
- Percutaneous balloon aortic valvuloplasty may be a reasonable therapeutic alternative for patients with symptomatic critical AS in the following settings if they are NOT CANDIDATES for either transcatheter or surgical aortic valve replacement:
  - bridge to surgical AVR or TAVR in hemodynamically unstable patients (**Class IIa, Level C1**)
  - anticipated survival of <3 years (**Class IIb, Level C1**)
  - severe and/or disabling conditions that would limit the ability to undergo postoperative rehabilitation (**Class IIb, Level C1**).

Procedural complications have been compared previously and can be reviewed in Table 56.4. These comparisons form the basis for the recommendations below, but patient selection needs to be individualized. Table 56.7 is provided for reference and outlines some of the issues to be addressed for individualization.

Conclusion

Critical AS is a common problem and patients are often elderly and not well suited to surgery. For those with multiple co-morbidities and at high risk for morbidity and mortality from open heart surgery with cardiopulmonary bypass, therapeutic options are limited. Medical therapy provides no survival advantage and has limited efficacy for symptom control. PBAV can be performed with some periprocedural morbidity and modest symptom control, but is limited in durability and does not alter the natural history of the disease process. It is early in the development of TAVR technology, but in a relatively short period of time it has become clear that the procedure can reduce symptoms and potentially improve longevity with a periprocedural morbidity and mortality rate that continues to improve. This technology offers a viable therapeutic alternative to patients at high risk for traditional surgical AVR. A potential role in routine management of lower risk aortic stenosis remains speculative and restraint remains desirable.

References

1. Nkomo VT, Gardin JM, Skelton TN *et al.* Burden of valvular heart diseases: a population-based study. *Lancet* 2006;**368**(9540): 1005–11.
2. Freeman RV, Otto CM. Spectrum of calcific aortic valve disease: pathogenesis, disease progression, and treatment strategies. *Circulation* 2005;**111**(24):3316–26.
3. Gunther S, Grossman W. Determinants of ventricular function in pressure-overload hypertrophy in man. *Circulation* 1979;**59**(4):679–88.
4. Bache RJ, Vrobel TR, Ring WS *et al.* Regional myocardial blood flow during exercise in dogs with chronic left ventricular hypertrophy. *Circ Res* 1981;**48**(1):76–87.
5. Gaasch WH, Zile MR, Hoshino PK *et al.* Tolerance of the hypertrophic heart to ischemia. Studies in compensated and failing dog hearts with pressure overload hypertrophy. *Circulation* 1990;**81**(5):1644–53.
6. Marcus ML, Doty DB, Hiratzka LF *et al.* Decreased coronary reserve: a mechanism for angina pectoris in patients with aortic stenosis and normal coronary arteries. *N Engl J Med* 1982;**307**(22):1362–6.
7. Pellikka PA, Sarano ME, Nishimura RA *et al.* Outcome of 622 adults with asymptomatic, hemodynamically significant aortic stenosis during prolonged follow-up. see comment. *Circulation* 2005;**111**(24):3290–5.

8. Ross J Jr. Braunwald E. Aortic stenosis. *Circulation* 1968;**38**(1 suppl):61–7.

9. Turina J, Hess O, Sepulcri F *et al.* Spontaneous course of aortic valve disease. *Eur Heart J* 1987;**8**(5):471–83.

10. Rosenhek R, Binder T, Porenta G *et al.* Predictors of outcome in severe, asymptomatic aortic stenosis. *N Engl J Med* 2000;**343**(9):611–17.

11. Otto CM. Valvular aortic stenosis: disease severity and timing of intervention. *J Am Coll Cardiol* 2006;**47**(11):2141–51.

12. Society of Thoracic Surgeons National Cardiac Surgery Database. STS Spring 2006 Report – Executive Summary. Available at: www.sts.org/documents/pdf/STS-ExecutiveSummarySpring2006.pdf. Accessed Aug 2007.

13. Alexander KP, Anstrom KJ, Muhlbaier LH *et al.* Outcomes of cardiac surgery in patients > or = 80 years: results from the National Cardiovascular Network. *J Am Coll Cardiol* 2000;**35**(3):731–8.

14. Asimakopoulos G, Edwards MB, Taylor KM. Aortic valve replacement in patients 80 years of age and older: survival and cause of death based on 1100 cases: collective results from the UK Heart Valve Registry. *Circulation* 1997;**96**(10): 3403–8.

15. Dalrymple-Hay MJ, Alzetani A, Aboel-Nazar S *et al.* Cardiac surgery in the elderly. *Eur J Cardiothorac Surg* 1999;**15**(1): 61–6.

16. Kolh P, Kerzmann A, Honore C *et al.* Aortic valve surgery in octogenarians: predictive factors for operative and long-term results. *Eur J Cardiothorac Surg* 2007;**31**(4):600–6.

17. Kolh P, Kerzmann A, Lahaye L *et al.* Cardiac surgery in octogenarians; peri-operative outcome and long-term results. *Eur Heart J* 2001;**22**(14):1235–43.

18. Langanay T, De Latour B, Ligier K *et al.* Surgery for aortic stenosis in octogenarians: influence of coronary disease and other comorbidities on hospital mortality. *J Heart Valve Dis* 2004;**13**(4):545–52; discussion 52–3.

19. Suttie SA, Jamieson WRE, Burr LH *et al.* Elderly valve replacement with bioprostheses and mechanical prostheses. Comparison by composites of complications. *J Cardiovasc Surg* 2006;**47**(2):191–9.

20. Vahanian A, Baumgartner H, Bax J *et al.* Guidelines on the management of valvular heart disease: The Task Force on the Management of Valvular Heart Disease of the European Society of Cardiology. *Eur Heart J* 2007;**28**(2):230–68.

21. Goodney PP, Stukel TA, Lucas FL *et al.* Hospital volume, length of stay, and readmission rates in high-risk surgery. see comment.. *Ann Surg* 2003;**238**(2):161–7.

22. Hara H, Pedersen WR, Ladich E *et al.* Percutaneous balloon aortic valvuloplasty revisited: time for a renaissance? *Circulation* 2007;**115**(12):e334–8.

23. Sundt TM, Bailey MS, Moon MR *et al.* Quality of life after aortic valve replacement at the age of >80 years. *Circulation* 2000;**102**(19 suppl 3):III70–4.

24. Iung B, Baron G, Butchart EG *et al.* A prospective survey of patients with valvular heart disease in Europe: The Euro Heart Survey on Valvular Heart Disease. *Eur Heart J* 2003;**24**(13): 1231–43.

25. Iung B, Cachier A, Baron G *et al.* Decision-making in elderly patients with severe aortic stenosis: why are so many denied surgery? *Eur Heart J* 2005;**26**(24):2714–20.

26. Bouma BJ, van Den Brink RB, van Der Meulen JH *et al.* To operate or not on elderly patients with aortic stenosis: the decision and its consequences. *Heart* 1999;**82**(2):143–8.

27. Varadarajan P, Kapoor N, Bansal RC *et al.* Clinical profile and natural history of 453 non-surgically managed patients with severe aortic stenosis. *Ann Thorac Surg* 2006;**82**(6):2111–15.

28. Pai RG, Kapoor N, Bansal RC *et al.* Malignant natural history of asymptomatic severe aortic stenosis: benefit of aortic valve replacement. *Ann Thorac Surg* 2006;**82**(6):2116–22.

29. Nashef SA, Roques F, Michel P *et al.* European system for cardiac operative risk evaluation (EuroSCORE). *Eur J Cardiothorac Surg* 1999;**16**(1):9–13.

30. Nashef SAM, Roques F, Hammill BG *et al.* Validation of European System for Cardiac Operative Risk Evaluation (EuroSCORE) in North American cardiac surgery. *Eur J Cardiothorac Surg* 2002;**22**(1):101–5.

31. Shroyer ALW, Coombs LP, Peterson ED *et al.* The Society of Thoracic Surgeons: 30-day operative mortality and morbidity risk models. *Ann Thorac Surg* 2003;**75**(6):1856–64; discussion 1864–5.

32. Ambler G, Omar RZ, Royston P *et al.* Generic, simple risk stratification model for heart valve surgery. *Circulation* 2005;**112**(2):224–31.

33. Vassiliades TA Jr, Block PC, Cohn LH *et al.* The clinical development of percutaneous heart valve technology: a position statement of the Society of Thoracic Surgeons (STS), the American Association for Thoracic Surgery (AATS), and the Society for Cardiovascular Angiography and Interventions (SCAI) Endorsed by the American College of Cardiology Foundation (ACCF) and the American Heart Association (AHA). *J Am Coll Cardiol* 2005;**45**(9):1554–60.

34. Grube E, Schuler G, Buellesfeld L *et al.* Percutaneous aortic valve replacement for severe aortic stenosis in high-risk patients using the second- and current third-generation self-expanding CoreValve prosthesis: device success and 30-day clinical outcome. *J Am Coll Cardiol* 2007;**50**(1):69–76.

35. Webb J, Pasupati S, Humphries K *et al.* Percutaneous transarterial aortic valve replacement in selected high-risk patients with aortic stenosis. *Circulation* 2007;**116**(7):755–63.

36. Cribier A, Savin T, Saoudi N *et al.* Percutaneous transluminal valvuloplasty of acquired aortic stenosis in elderly patients: an alternative to valve replacement? *Lancet* 1986;**1**(8472): 63–7.

37. Bonow RO, Carabello BA, Kanu C *et al.* ACC/AHA 2006 guidelines for the management of patients with valvular heart disease: a report of the American College of Cardiology/American Heart Association Task Force on Practice Guidelines (Writing Committee to Revise the 1998 Guidelines for the Management of Patients With Valvular Heart Disease): developed in collaboration with the Society of Cardiovascular Anesthesiologists: endorsed by the Society for Cardiovascular Angiography and Interventions and the Society of Thoracic Surgeons. *Circulation* 2006;**114**(5):e84–231.

38. O'Neill WW. Seminar on Balloon Aortic Valvuloplasty – I: Introduction. *J Am Coll Cardiol* 1991;**17**(1):187–8.

39. Bashore TM, Davidson CJ. Follow-up recatheterization after balloon aortic valvuloplasty. Mansfield Scientific Aortic Valvuloplasty Registry Investigators. *J Am Coll Cardiol* 1991; **17**(5):1188–95.

40. Ferguson JJ, Garza RA. Efficacy of multiple balloon aortic valvuloplasty procedures. The Mansfield Scientific Aortic Valvuloplasty Registry Investigators. *J Am Coll Cardiol* 1991; **17**(6):1430–5.

41. Isner JM. Acute catastrophic complications of balloon aortic valvuloplasty. The Mansfield Scientific Aortic Valvuloplasty Registry Investigators. *J Am Coll Cardiol* 1991;**17**(6): 1436–44.

42. McKay RG. The Mansfield Scientific Aortic Valvuloplasty Registry: overview of acute hemodynamic results and procedural complications. *J Am Coll Cardiol* 1991;**17**(2):485–91.

43. Nishimura RA, Holmes DR Jr, Michela MA. Follow-up of patients with low output, low gradient hemodynamics after percutaneous balloon aortic valvuloplasty: the Mansfield Scientific Aortic Valvuloplasty Registry. *J Am Coll Cardiol* 1991;**17**(3):828–33.

44. O'Neill WW. Predictors of long-term survival after percutaneous aortic valvuloplasty: report of the Mansfield Scientific Balloon Aortic Valvuloplasty Registry. *J Am Coll Cardiol* 1991;**17**(1):193–8.

45. Reeder GS, Nishimura RA, Holmes DR Jr. Patient age and results of balloon aortic valvuloplasty: the Mansfield Scientific Registry experience. The Mansfield Scientific Aortic Valvuloplasty Registry Investigators. *J Am Coll Cardiol* 1991;**17**(4): 909–13.

46. Otto CM, Mickel MC, Kennedy JW et al. Three-year outcome after balloon aortic valvuloplasty. Insights into prognosis of valvular aortic stenosis. *Circulation* 1994;**89**(2):642–50.

47. NBVR Participants. Percutaneous balloon aortic valvuloplasty. Acute and 30-day follow-up results in 674 patients from the NHLBI Balloon Valvuloplasty Registry. *Circulation* 1991;**84**(6): 2383–97.

48. Eltchaninoff H, Cribier A, Tron C et al. Balloon aortic valvuloplasty in elderly patients at high risk for surgery, or inoperable. Immediate and mid-term results. *Eur Heart J* 1995;**16**(8): 1079–84.

49. Koning R, Cribier A, Asselin C et al. Repeat balloon aortic valvuloplasty. *Catheterization Cardiovasc Diagn* 1992;**26**(4): 249–54.

50. Letac B, Cribier A, Koning R et al. Results of percutaneous transluminal valvuloplasty in 218 adults with valvular aortic stenosis. *Am J Cardiol* 1988;**62**(9):598–605.

51. Letac B, Cribier A, Koning R et al. Aortic stenosis in elderly patients aged 80 or older. Treatment by percutaneous balloon valvuloplasty in a series of 92 cases. *Circulation* 1989;**80**(6): 1514–20.

52. Berland J, Cribier A, Savin T et al. Percutaneous balloon valvuloplasty in patients with severe aortic stenosis and low ejection fraction. Immediate results and 1-year follow-up. *Circulation* 1989;**79**(6):1189–96.

53. Davidson CJ, Harrison JK, Pieper KS et al. Determinants of one-year outcome from balloon aortic valvuloplasty. *Am J Cardiol* 1991;**68**(1):75–80.

54. Lieberman EB, Bashore TM, Hermiller JB et al. Balloon aortic valvuloplasty in adults: failure of procedure to improve long-term survival. *J Am Coll Cardiol* 1995;**26**(6):1522–8.

55. Lieberman EB, Wilson JS, Harrison JK et al. Aortic valve replacement in adults after balloon aortic valvuloplasty. *Circulation* 1994;**90**(5 Pt 2):II205–8.

56. Davidson CJ, Harrison JK, Leithe ME et al. Failure of balloon aortic valvuloplasty to result in sustained clinical improvement in patients with depressed left ventricular function. *Am J Cardiol* 1990;**65**(1):72–7.

57. Agarwal A, Kini AS, Attanti S et al. Results of repeat balloon valvuloplasty for treatment of aortic stenosis in patients aged 59 to 104 years. *Am J Cardiol* 2005;**95**(1):43–7.

58. Bernard Y, Etievent J, Mourand JL et al. Long-term results of percutaneous aortic valvuloplasty compared with aortic valve replacement in patients more than 75 years old. *J Am Coll Cardiol* 1992;**20**(4):796–801.

59. Block PC, Palacios IF. Clinical and hemodynamic follow-up after percutaneous aortic valvuloplasty in the elderly. *Am J Cardiol* 1988;**62**(10 Pt 1):760–3.

60. Safian RD, Berman AD, Diver DJ et al. Balloon aortic valvuloplasty in 170 consecutive patients. *N Engl J Med* 1988;**319**(3): 125–30.

61. Letac B, Cribier A, Eltchaninoff H et al. Evaluation of restenosis after balloon dilatation in adult aortic stenosis by repeat catheterization. *Am Heart J* 1991;**122**(1 Pt 1):55–60.

62. Block PC. The "experience curve" for percutaneous aortic valvuloplasty. Report from the Mansfield Scientific Aortic Valvuloplasty Registry. *Circulation* 1988;**78**(suppl II):II-531.

63. Klein A, Lee K, Gera A et al. Long-term mortality, cause of death, and temporal trends in complications after percutaneous aortic balloon valvuloplasty for calcific aortic stenosis. *J Intervent Cardiol* 2006;**19**(3):269–75.

64. Desnoyers MR, Salem DN, Rosenfield K et al. Treatment of cardiogenic shock by emergency aortic balloon valvuloplasty. *Ann Intern Med* 1988;**108**(6):833–5.

65. Moreno PR, Jang IK, Newell JB et al. The role of percutaneous aortic balloon valvuloplasty in patients with cardiogenic shock and critical aortic stenosis. *J Am Coll Cardiol* 1994;**23**(5): 1071–5.

66. Hayes SN, Holmes DR Jr, Nishimura RA et al. Palliative percutaneous aortic balloon valvuloplasty before noncardiac operations and invasive diagnostic procedures. *Mayo Clinic Proc* 1989;**64**(7):753–7.

67. Roth RB, Palacios IF, Block PC. Percutaneous aortic balloon valvuloplasty: its role in the management of patients with aortic stenosis requiring major noncardiac surgery. *J Am Coll Cardiol* 1989;**13**(5):1039–41.

68. Safian RD, Mandell VS, Thurer RE et al. Postmortem and intraoperative balloon valvuloplasty of calcific aortic stenosis in elderly patients: mechanisms of successful dilation. *J Am Coll Cardiol* 1987;**9**(3):655–60.

69. McKay RG, Safian RD, Lock JE et al. Balloon dilatation of calcific aortic stenosis in elderly patients: postmortem, intraoperative, and percutaneous valvuloplasty studies. *Circulation* 1986;**74**(1):119–25.

70. Feldman T, Glagov S, Carroll JD. Restenosis following successful balloon valvuloplasty: bone formation in aortic valve leaflets. *Catheterization Cardiovasc Diagn* 1993;**29**(1):1–7.

71. Pedersen WR, Van Tassel RA, Pierce TA et al. Radiation following percutaneous balloon aortic valvuloplasty to prevent restenosis (RADAR pilot trial). *Catheterization Cardiovasc Intervent* 2006;**68**(2):183–92.

72. Andersen HR, Knudsen LL, Hasenkam JM. Transluminal implantation of artificial heart valves. Description of a new

expandable aortic valve and initial results with implantation by catheter technique in closed chest pigs. *Eur Heart J* 1992;**13**(5):704–8.

73. Boudjemline Y, Agnoletti G, Bonnet D *et al.* Percutaneous pulmonary valve replacement in a large right ventricular outflow tract: an experimental study. *J Am Coll Cardiol* 2004;**43**(6):1082–7.

74. Cribier A, Eltchaninoff H, Bash A *et al.* Trans-catheter implantation of balloon-expandable prosthetic heart valves. Early results in an animal model. *Circulation* 2001;**104**(suppl 2):I552.

75. Lutter G, Kuklinski D, Berg G *et al.* Percutaneous aortic valve replacement: an experimental study. I. Studies on implantation. *J Thorac Cardiovasc Surg* 2002;**123**(4):768–76.

76. Sochman J, Peregrin JH, Pavcnik D *et al.* Percutaneous transcatheter aortic disc valve prosthesis implantation: a feasibility study. *Cardiovasc Intervent Radiol* 2000;**23**(5):384–8.

77. Webb JG, Munt B, Makkar RR *et al.* Percutaneous stent-mounted valve for treatment of aortic or pulmonary valve disease. *Catheterization Cardiovasc Intervent* 2004;**63**(1):89–93.

78. Bonhoeffer P, Boudjemline Y, Saliba Z *et al.* Percutaneous replacement of pulmonary valve in a right-ventricle to pulmonary-artery prosthetic conduit with valve dysfunction. *Lancet* 2000;**356**(9239):1403–5.

79. Cribier A, Eltchaninoff H, Bash A *et al.* Percutaneous transcatheter implantation of an aortic valve prosthesis for calcific aortic stenosis: first human case description. *Circulation* 2002;**106**(24):3006–8.

80. Webb JG, Chandavimol M, Thompson CR *et al.* Percutaneous aortic valve implantation retrograde from the femoral artery. *Circulation* 2006;**113**(6):842–50.

81. Cribier A, Eltchaninoff H, Tron C *et al.* Treatment of calcific aortic stenosis with the percutaneous heart valve: mid-term follow-up from the initial feasibility studies: the French experience. *J Am Coll Cardiol* 2006;**47**(6):1214–23.

82. Sakata Y, Syed Z, Salinger MH *et al.* Percutaneous balloon aortic valvuloplasty: antegrade transseptal vs. conventional retrograde transarterial approach. *Catheterization Cardiovasc Intervent* 2005;**64**(3):314–21.

83. Hanzel GS, Harrity PJ, Schreiber TL *et al.* Retrograde percutaneous aortic valve implantation for critical aortic stenosis. *Catheterization Cardiovasc Intervent* 2005;**64**(3):322–6.

84. Pasupati S, Humphries K, Altwegg L *et al.* Transarterial percutaneous aortic valve PAV. Insertion: Canadian single centre experience. *Am J Cardiol* 2007;**100**(8(suppl I)):56L.

85. Webb JG, Altwegg L, Boone RH *et al.* Transcatheter Aortic Valve Implantation. Impact on Clinical and Valve-Related Outcomes. *Circulation* 2009;**119**:3009–16.

86. Kojodjojo P, Gohil N, Barker D *et al.* Outcomes of elderly patients aged 80 and over with symptomatic, severe aortic stenosis: impact of patient's choice of refusing aortic valve replacement on survival. *Q J Med* 2008;**101**(7):567–73.

87. Walther T, Dewey T, Wimmer-Greinecker G *et al.* Transapical approach for sutureless stent-fixed aortic valve implantation: experimental results. *Eur J Cardiothorac Surg* 2006;**29**(5):703–8.

88. Walther T, Mohr FW. Aortic valve surgery: time to be open-minded and to rethink. *Eur J Cardiothorac Surg* 2007;**31**(1):4–6.

89. Ye J, Cheung A, Lichtenstein SV *et al.* Transapical aortic valve implantation in humans. see comment. *J Thorac Cardiovasc Surg* 2006;**131**(5):1194–6.

90. Ye J, Cheung A, Lichtenstein SV *et al.* Six-month outcome of transapical transcatheter aortic valve implantation in the initial seven patients. see comment.. *Eur J Cardiothorac Surg* 2007;**31**(1):16–21.

91. Walther T, Simon P, Dewey T *et al.* Transapical minimally invasive aortic valve implantation: multicenter experience. *Circulation* 2007;**116**(11 suppl):I240–5.

92. Antunes MJ. Off-pump aortic valve replacement with catheter-mounted valved stents. Is the future already here? *Eur J Cardiothorac Surg* 2007;**31**(1):1–3.

93. Huber CH, von Segesser LK. Direct access valve replacement (DAVR) – are we entering a new era in cardiac surgery? *Eur J Cardiothorac Surg* 2006;**29**(3):380–5.

94. Walther T, Falk V, Borger MA *et al.* Transapical aortic valve implantation at one year. *Circulation* 2007;**116**(suppl II):543.

95. Walther T. Transapical aortic valve implantation: Traverse Feasibility Study. *Transcatheter Cardiovascular Therapeutics*. Washington, DC, 13 October 2008.

96. Grube E, Laborde JC, Gerckens U *et al.* Percutaneous implantation of the CoreValve self-expanding valve prosthesis in high-risk patients with aortic valve disease: the Siegburg first-in-man study. *Circulation* 2006;**114**(15):1616–24.

97. Grube E, Laborde JC, Zickmann B *et al.* First report on a human percutaneous transluminal implantation of a self-expanding valve prosthesis for interventional treatment of aortic valve stenosis. *Catheterization Cardiovasc Intervent* 2005;**66**(4):465–9.

98. Laborde JC. Transcatheter aortic valve implantation with the CoreValve ReValving device. *Transcatheter Cardiovascular Therapeutics*. Washington, DC, 12 October 2008.

99. Wood D, Mayo J, Pasupati S *et al.* The Role of Multislice Computed Tomography in the Assessment of Transcatheter Aortic Valve Replacement. Transcatheter Cardiovascular Therapeutics, Washington DC, 2007.

100. Pasupati S, Sinhal A, Humphries K *et al.* Re-dilation of Balloon Expandable Aortic Valves BEAV. What do we know? *Am J Cardiol* 2007;**100**(8 suppl I):57L.

101. Bauer F, Eltchaninoff H, Tron C *et al.* Acute improvement in global and regional left ventricular systolic function after percutaneous heart valve implantation in patients with symptomatic aortic stenosis. *Circulation* 2004;**110**(11):1473–6.

102. Pasupati S, Humphries K, AlAli A *et al.* Balloon Expandable Aortic Valve BEAV. Implantation. The first 100 Canadian patients. *Circulation* 2007;**116**(suppl II):357b.

103. Ussia GP, Mule M, Barbanti M *et al.* Quality of life assessment after percutaneous aortic valve implantation. 2009:ehp171.

104. Kuntz RE, Tosteson AN, Berman AD *et al.* Predictors of event-free survival after balloon aortic valvuloplasty. *N Engl J Med* 1991;**325**(1):17–23.

105. Lewin RF, Dorros G, King JF *et al.* Percutaneous transluminal aortic valvuloplasty: acute outcome and follow-up of 125 patients. *J Am Coll Cardiol* 1989;**14**(5):1210–17.

57 Balloon valvuloplasty: mitral valve

Zoltan G Turi

Division of Cardiology, Cooper University Hospital, Camden, NJ, USA

Introduction and historical perspective

Percutaneous balloon mitral valvuloplasty (PBMV) represents part of an evolution from early, primitive cardiac surgical techniques to the modern era of percutaneous valve interventions. This evolution began with Elliot Cutler advancing a knife retrograde through the apex of the left ventricle of a beating heart in 1923.[1] Neither he nor Henry Suttar, who performed what today would be considered an antegrade fingertip commissurotomy in England 2 years later,[2] received the expected accolades. In part this reflected disagreement over the role of mitral valve obstruction in defining the spectrum of mitral stenosis (MS). Sir Thomas Lewis' statement that valvotomy was based on an "erroneous idea, namely that the valve is the chief source of the trouble"[3] has few proponents in the modern era. Nevertheless, because of the broad spectrum of cardiac and non-mitral valvular involvement resulting from rheumatic carditis and valvulitis,[4] relieving mitral valve obstruction largely palliates rather than cures patients with MS.

Some 20 years after the initial attempts to relieve mitral obstruction, the surgical experience in World War II battlefield hospitals with closed heart procedures led to the application of newly learned techniques to civilian use. Although early results were confounded by significant morbidity and mortality, closed mitral valvotomy became a routine procedure for severe MS by the 1950s and 1960s, and is still performed in many parts of the world where the disease is endemic and medical facilities are limited. Large series[5,6] have claimed good long-term results, but lack of systematic follow-up or comprehensive objective data obscures the actual restenosis rate and survival. In a Mayo Clinic retrospective analysis[7] there was a 79% 10-year and a 55% 20-year survival rate with reoperation in 34% by 10 years; however, nearly a quarter of patients were lost to follow-up and severity of disease at baseline could only be estimated. A more recent evaluation of a 36-year experience included a 44% rate of repeat surgery by 12 years.[8] Open commissurotomy, with the potential advantages of direct vision, has supplanted closed procedures in industrial nations.[9] Controversy remains as to its superiority,[10–12] with the advantages of direct vision favoring cases where thrombus is present. The relative role of open commissurotomy versus mitral valve replacement with or without chordal preservation has been explored with somewhat equivocal results.[13] Mitral valve replacement has higher periprocedural and postoperative event rates including mortality, but superior freedom from repeat mitral valve intervention; when the chordae to at least one leaflet are preserved, the outcomes of mitral valve replacement are superior (**Level C**).

The percutaneous approach

Following the initial percutaneous structural heart disease interventions of Rashkind with balloon atrial septostomy,[14] a device designed by Inoue to inflate sequentially across the septum (Fig. 57.1) was instead adapted for PBMV.[15] After initially demonstrating its ability to split fused commissures in the operating room,[16] the first percutaneous PBMV was performed in 1982.[17] After several small series demonstrated feasibility,[18,19] a number of alternative techniques were developed, including large single balloons,[18] two cylindrical balloons used in parallel over two guidewires[20] through a single or two transseptal punctures,[21] a monorail technique for using two balloons,[22] a retrograde technique that avoided the transseptal approach[23] and a percutaneous metal commissurotome.[24] The initial technique and device developed by Inoue, with scant

Evidence-Based Cardiology, 3rd edition. Edited by S. Yusuf, J.A. Cairns, A.J. Camm, E.L. Fallen, and B.J. Gersh. © 2010 Blackwell Publishing, ISBN: 978-1-4051-5925-8.

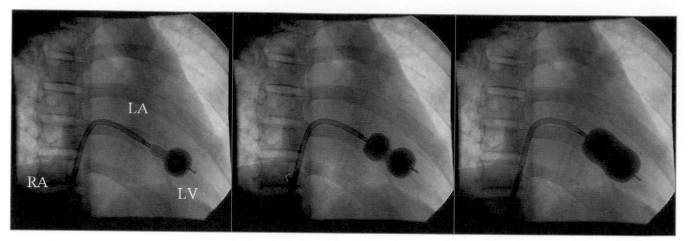

Figure 57.1 Deployment of the Inoue balloon via the transseptal approach. The catheter has been advanced across the interatrial septum from the right atrium (RA) into the left atrium (LA) and then into the left ventricle (LV) across the stenotic mitral valve. The balloon is designed to inflate distally first (left frame), then to be pulled back against the mitral valve after which the proximal portion inflates (center frame), centering the balloon across the valve. As additional volume is injected into the balloon, full inflation occurs, ideally causing splitting of the commissures (right frame).

modification, remains the predominant (and only US FDA approved) approach.

PBMV typically results in a doubling of the mitral valve area (on average from 1.0 cm^2 to 2.0 cm^2) with a 50% reduction in gradient and an 80–95% success rate, the latter defined as the mitral valve area increasing to >1.5 cm^2 and left atrial pressure decreasing to <18 mmHg without major complications.[25] Overall, the results are highly operator dependent with a steep learning curve.[26,27] As a result, the ACC/AHA guidelines[25] emphasize that the decision to proceed to PBMV must take into consideration the experience of the operators involved (**Class I, Level B**).

Mechanism of balloon commissurotomy and Pathophysiology

In general, balloon valvuloplasty, regardless of the valve being dilated, has three possible mechanisms for relief of obstruction: stretching of the valve orifice, splitting of fused commissures, and cracking of valvular calcifications. In the case of PBMV, the mechanisms[28] responsible for the benefits seen arise from the substantial radial force[29] exerted by the enlarging balloon. This stretches the mitral annulus, has the capacity to split fused commissures, and occasionally results in cracking of calcifications. The stretching mechanism has been described in the intraoperative setting.[30] The splitting of commissures[31] and cracking of calcification[32] have been demonstrated by direct observation in excised valves. The largely successful nature of PBMV is derived virtually exclusively from commissural splitting of rheumatically fused leaflets.[33] Balloon dilation procedures dependent on the other two mechanisms, such as balloon valvuloplasty for calcific aortic stenosis[34] or bio-

prosthetic valves,[35] have poor short- and long-term results. Thus non-rheumatic MS secondary to calcification of the mitral annulus, leaflets or subvalvular apparatus, such as seen with elevated hyperparathyroid levels (e.g. patients on dialysis), lends itself poorly to balloon dilation (**Level C**).

Successful splitting of the commissures results in decreased gradient and improved mitral valve area, and typically leads to significant clinical and hemodynamic improvement. This occurs progressively, with reduction in gradient, left atrial pressure and pulmonary artery pressures continuing over a 3-year period.[36] It is important to consider that relief of mitral valve obstruction will typically increase left ventricular volume loading secondary to facilitated left atrial emptying. In the relatively underfilled ventricle seen with "pure" MS this is typically well tolerated, although some degree of left ventricular dysfunction in patients with rheumatic heart disease may be present even without concomitant valvular regurgitation. In patients with concomitant mitral or aortic insufficiency, the left ventricle may become volume loaded after PBMV. Thus, although the gradient may be substantially reduced, left heart filling pressures may rise and be accompanied by failure of clinical improvement or actual deterioration.

Indications

Balloon valvuloplasty is primarily indicated for moderate to severe MS (Table 57.1) and is the procedure of choice for symptomatic patients if the valve anatomy is suitable and there is neither left atrial thrombus nor greater than mild mitral insufficiency (**Class I, Level A**). The guidelines incorporate evidence that PBMV is beneficial for patients with MS and pulmonary hypertension (**Class I**) or atrial fibrillation (AF) (**Class II, Level B**). The guidelines have been expanded to include mild MS under limited circumstances (**Class II, Level C**).

Preprocedure evaluation and prediction of outcomes

A variety of anatomic and physiologic factors determine suitability for PBMV. Anatomic features that correlate with procedural success as well as long-term outcomes have been described since the early development of PBMV.[37] These include characteristics of the valve leaflets, annulus and subvalvular apparatus. Although there are major limitations, the most commonly used has been a scoring system described by Wilkins and colleagues[38] that incorporates thickening, mobility and calcification of the valve leaflets as well as disease of the subvalvular apparatus (Table 57.2). This, the so-called MGH (Massachusetts General Hospital) scoring system, assigns up to four points for the most severe disease for each characteristic, with a maximum of 16 points. Ideal valves have a score of eight or less, and echo scores >12 have been predictive of poor short- and long-term outcomes[39] (Fig. 57.2) (**Level B**).

Intermediate and long-term event-free survival has correlated well with the echo score, as well as the immediate postprocedure hemodynamics[39–42] (see Fig. 57.2). Five-year event free survival is negligible in patients with echo scores of 12 or greater, but approximately two-thirds in those with favorable valve morphology (**Level B**).

While the correlation between the echo score and initial as well as long-term outcomes has been good, the MGH scoring system has been criticized because it is semiquantitative, does not include important anatomic elements

such as the nature of commissural fusion, and because one element of the score, leaflet mobility, correlates more strongly with outcome (r value = 0.67) than the complete score. Valve calcification alone predicts a fourfold increase in cardiac complications and a 26% increase in 6-year mortality.[43] Anatomic features such as a funnel-shaped subvalvular apparatus and eccentric commissural fusion[44] are not included in the score, nor is severe fusion and calcification

Table 57.1 Indications for percutaneous balloon mitral valvuloplasty, incorporating modifications from the 2006 ACC/AHA guidelines.[25] Note that the presence of pulmonary hypertension in asymptomatic patients is now a Class I indication. The effect of exercise has been incorporated. Pulmonary hypertension is assumed to be secondary to mitral stenosis. Where the guidelines specify valve morphology favorable for PBMV, the table lists an echo score ≤8 using the MGH scoring system. It should be noted that a boundary effect likely exists, and the scoring system has significant limitations so the guidelines do not specify either a specific scoring system or an absolute threshold. AF, atrial fibrillation: LA, left atrium; MR, mitral insufficiency; MVA, mitral valve area; PA, pulmonary artery systolic pressure.

Symptoms	MVA	Score	Other	Class
+	≤1.5 cm²	≤8		I
–	≤1.5 cm²	≤8	PA > 50 mmHg or 60 ex	I
II	≤1.5 cm²	>8	PA > 60 mmHg	IIa
III–IV	≤1.5 cm²	>8	High risk for surgery	IIa
–	≤1.5 cm²	≤8	New onset AF	IIb
+	>1.5 cm²	≤8	PA > 60, PAW > 25, MVG > 15 EX	IIb
III–IV	≤1.5 cm²	>8	Low risk for surgery	IIb
			LA thrombus, severe MR	III

Table 57.2 The Wilkins–Weyman echocardiographic scoring system of mitral valve characteristics

Grade	Mobility	Subvalvar thickening	Thickening	Calcification
1	Highly mobile valve with only leaflet tips restricted	Minimal thickening just below the mitral leaflets	Leaflets near normal in thickness (4–5 mm)	A single area of increased echo brightness
2	Leaflet mid and base portions have normal mobility	Thickening of chordal structures extending up to one third of the chordal length	Midleaflets normal, considerable thickening of margins (5–8 mm)	Scattered areas of brightness confined to leaflet margins
3	Valve continues to move forward in diastole, mainly from the base	Thickening extending to the distal third of the chords	Thickening extending through the entire leaflet (5–8 mm)	Brightness extending into the midportion of the leaflets
4	No or minimal forward movement of the leaflets in diastole	Extensive thickening and shortening of all chordal structures extending down to the papillary muscles	Considerable thickening of all leaflet tissue (>8–10 mm)	Extensive brightness throughout much of the leaflet tissue

The total echocardiographic score was derived from an analysis of mitral leaflet mobility, valar and subvalvar thickening, and calcification which were graded form 0 to 4 according to the above criteria. The total possible score ranges from 0 to 16.
(Reprinted by kind permission of the BMJ Publishing Group from reference.)[38]

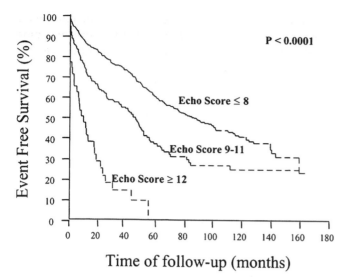

Figure 57.2 Survival free of repeat balloon dilation or mitral valve replacement in 879 patients undergoing percutaneous balloon mitral valvuloplasty with echo scores of ≤8, 9–11, and ≥12. (Reproduced from Palacios[39] with permission of the American Heart Association, Inc.)

of the commissures[45]; all are strong negative predictors of outcome.[46] In the case of calcification, valve area varied inversely in 223 patients: $0.9 \, cm^2$ in those with no calcification versus 0.8, 0.7 and $0.6 \, cm^2$ respectively in those with grade 1, 2 and 3 calcium ($P < 0.05$).[47] A number of other scoring systems have been proposed, some of which appear to have a strong correlation with outcomes,[48] including an echocardiographic system assessing characteristics of leaflets and the subvalvular apparatus that correlates with PBMV-induced mitral regurgitation.[49] Perhaps the most compelling reason for routinely deriving the MGH echo score is to allow for comparison with known data: most PBMV trials have incorporated this system to define baseline severity of disease. As such, an echo score ≤8 is commonly interpreted as representing the ideal valve anatomy for PBMV described in the ACC/AHA guidelines[25] (see Table 57.1).

Besides anatomic features, a number of other factors appear to predict acute and longer term results. The presence of AF is an independent risk factor for adverse outcomes in several datasets.[50] A recent analysis of a 531-patient cohort with long-term follow-up demonstrated inferior acute results (1.87 v $2.0 \, cm^2$ mitral valve area (MVA) and higher restenosis rates (33% v 23% at 10 years, 66% v 54% at 15 years)[51] in patients with AF. Age[39,52] and severity of stenosis as defined by hemodynamics and functional class[53] correlate with outcomes based on multivariate analyses (**Level C**).

Physiologic determinants of outcome may include the presence of left ventricular volume loading or dysfunction with or without concomitant valvular or myocardial disease. PBMV in the setting of more than mild mitral insufficiency

is an independent predictor of adverse events at long-term follow-up.[39] Increase of mitral regurgitation by one grade is common after PBMV, occurring in some 33% of patients; an additional 13% increased by two grades or more.[54] Superimposed on pre-existing mitral insufficiency, developing postprocedure mitral regurgitation of 3+ or greater is therefore a significant risk, the latter being an independent predictor of adverse outcomes as well.[39] In contrast, PBMV in the setting of mild to moderate aortic insufficiency (AI) is usually well tolerated. Comparing outcomes in 315 patients with mild or moderate AI versus 361 patients without AI, the only significant difference in outcomes was a higher rate of aortic valve replacement in patients with moderate AI, albeit at a mean of 4.1 years after PBMV[55] (**Level C**).

Transesophageal echocardiography

Routine preprocedure transesophageal echocardiography (TEE) has become the standard of care and has been raised to a **Class I, Level C** indication. Essential is the increased sensitivity for detection of left atrial thrombus,[56] as well as aspects of mitral valve morphology and regurgitation; however, the subvalvular apparatus is better interrogated with transthoracic echo. It should be noted that left atrial thrombus occurs outside the appendage in 43% of patients with rheumatic heart disease.[57] Although left atrial thrombus is primarily seen in patients in AF, it has been reported in approximately 2% of severe MS patients in sinus rhythm.[58] Based on a study of 100 patients referred for PBMV, there is a significant increased risk of left atrial thrombus in the presence of spontaneous echo contrast.[59] However, with successful resolution of the gradient, and perhaps with the detergent effect of any periprocedural mitral insufficiency, resolution of spontaneous echo contrast corresponds with relief of mitral obstruction.[60] An increasing body of evidence has also demonstrated increased coagulability in patients with mitral valve stenosis.[61] Finally, other structural abnormalities such as the presence of vegetations or ruptured chordae can be detected by TEE with much higher sensitivity than surface echo.

Cardiac catheterization

Cardiac catheterization to assess hemodynamics is indicated only if the non-invasive evaluation is equivocal in assessing valve anatomy and physiology, ventricular function and pulmonary hypertension (**Level C**). Patients with angina, objective evidence of ischemia or known coronary artery disease should have coronary angiography before PBMV; coronary angiography for risk factors alone is not required (**Level C**). A new element in the guidelines is a **Class IIb** indication for so-called "drive-by" coronary angiography regardless of whether patients meet these criteria if they do require a hemodynamic study because of equivocal non-invasive data; there is no evidence base for this recommendation, however (**Level C**).

The severity of MS can be determined by multiple methods including gradient, valve area as derived from multiple techniques, and finally the pulmonary artery pressure. It is important to consider that each technique is fraught with significant potential for inaccuracy. Importantly, the gradient is highly flow dependent, and is thus a poor proxy for severity of disease. It is particularly likely to lead to overestimation of severity of MS in the setting of poor heart rate control. Patients with new onset of AF are highly prone to having the extent of MS judged severe when it is mild or moderate, since these patients usually have poor initial rate control combined with loss of the contribution of atrial contraction to atrial emptying. Because tachycardia disproportionately shortens the diastolic filling period, they also have disproportionately high gradients and far worse symptoms than their MS would otherwise warrant. Inappropriate intervention in these patients, when heart rate control or cardioversion would suffice, is a classic error in management of MS. In contrast, excessive bradycardia or dehydration (such as occurs when a patient is maintained without fluids pending catheterization for an extensive period of time) can lead to gross underestimation of severity of MS. The use of pulmonary artery wedge pressures as proxy for left atrial pressure leads to overestimation of the gradient and underestimation of the mitral valve area because of the delayed decompression of wedge pressure across the high resistance of the pulmonary vascular bed.[62]

Contraindications

The ACC/AHA guidelines specifically cite left atrial thrombus and greater than mild mitral regurgitation as absolute contraindications and suggest that severe calcification and severe subvalvular disease are relative contraindications.

Left atrial thrombus

Several studies have explored chronic oral anticoagulation followed by repeat TEE to assess for thrombus resolution prior to PBMV. The rate of resorption is highly variable; the ACC/AHA guidelines recommend anticoagulation for 3 months. However, a prospective survey found resorption at 6 months in only one-quarter of 219 candidates for PBMV[63]; resorption was predicted by absence of spontaneous echo contrast, small thrombus size, and anticoagulation to an INR of 2.5 or greater. If clot remains present, we generally would avoid PBMV in favor of surgery since avoiding the left atrial appendage with guidewires and balloons, while usually feasible, takes significant additional skill, and even in the best of hands cannot be guaranteed. Nevertheless, Chen and colleagues[64] have described a large series of patients with apparent organized left atrial appendage clot who underwent uncomplicated PBMV despite documented left atrial appendage thrombus. We believe that clot elsewhere in the left atrium remains an absolute contraindication, although novel algorithms such as placing distal protection devices in both internal carotid arteries have been described[65] (**Level C**).

Mitral regurgitation

A comparison of 25 patients with moderate mitral regurgitation and 25 age- and gender-matched patients with mild or no regurgitation demonstrated an increased incidence of severe insufficiency post procedure in the former.[66] However, these patients had much higher echo scores and twice as frequently had severe calcification. While 20% of those with initially moderate mitral regurgitation developed severe regurgitation, hemodynamic improvement overall was similar, as was the incidence of postprocedure mitral valve replacement. Even patients with mild mitral regurgitation tend to have less favorable anatomy at baseline and lower event-free survival but a similar success rate[67] (**Level C**).

Severe calcification

Balloon dilation of a symmetric fused and severely calcified and essentially immobile mitral apparatus as well as attempted dilation of a severely calcified mitral annulus are largely futile. Thus patients with symmetric severely fused commissures may not respond at all.[45,68] In contrast, those with asymmetric calcification are prone to leaflet tearing or rupture due to asymmetric application of force to the less diseased commissure or leaflet.[69] While high echo score alone does not predict the occurrence of severe post-PBMV mitral regurgitation,[70] one component, severe calcification, does.[71] In general, greater degree of calcification predicts less successful improvement in valve area, higher periprocedural complications, and lower event-free survival.[43] Nevertheless, when the risk of surgery is prohibitive, growing experience with predominantly elderly patients with high echo scores and poor overall morphology has shown moderate improvement in hemodynamics and palliation of symptoms at the cost of high morbidity and mortality[72] (**Level C**).

Procedure

Except for a small cohort of patients, virtually all PBMV has been performed via the antegrade transseptal route.

The retrograde approach avoids the need for transseptal puncture, an advantage that is offset by the need to introduce relatively large hardware into the arterial circulation and to advance a balloon retrograde across the submitral apparatus over a guidewire, potentially causing entrapment in the subvalvular apparatus. Nevertheless, the success rates and intermediate term follow-up of retrograde PBMV have been comparable to the antegrade approach (88% success in a 441-patient cohort) with the usual finding of outcomes correlating with the MGH echo score.[73] A small, 72-patient, single-site non-randomized comparison found no significant difference in outcomes between the antegrade Inoue technique and retrograde approaches except for increase in mitral insufficiency with the latter, but the study was underpowered to assess trends in postprocedure adverse events.[74]

The Inoue technique is virtually unchanged since the mid-1980s. In a review of 19 series reporting results in a total of 7091 patients, the overall success rate was 93%.[75] Success was variably defined, and in some studies the definition included patients with severe iatrogenic mitral insufficiency, atrial septal defect or embolic events, but typically included a doubling of valve area. The principal features of the Inoue device are a balloon with a stretchable distal shaft to facilitate transseptal passage, a nylon mesh over a latex balloon that allows for variable inflation of the distal and proximal portions to promote straddling of the mitral valve (see Fig. 57.1), and a compliance curve that allows the balloon to dilate predictably over at least a 4 mm range of sizes. The device lends itself to a stepwise dilation technique, with repetitive inflations at progressively increasing balloon sizes.[76] After each inflation, residual gradient, hemodynamics including blood pressure and left atrial pressure, and echocardiographic data are assessed; if residual MS is still substantial and mitral insufficiency has not increased, repeat inflation with the balloon inflated to a larger size is performed. No formal evidence base exists comparing this stepwise technique to a single inflation at the calculated optimal balloon size based on patient height and body surface area. The compliance curve of the Inoue balloon results in an exponential rise in radial force within a mm of its maximal size and is a risk factor for post-PBMV mitral insufficiency[77] (**Level C**).

PBMV is typically performed with continuous TEE or, more recently, intracardiac echocardiographic guidance.[78] The benefits include continuous monitoring for periprocedural mitral insufficiency, tamponade, and spontaneous echo contrast.[79] TEE is useful as an aid to optimize transseptal puncture[80] with decreased procedure time, mitral insufficiency, and residual atrial septal defects described in a randomized study of fluoroscopy plus TEE versus fluoroscopy without echo during PBMV.[81] The evidence base provided by these studies is not compelling, with the latter study including a 60% rate of major complications in the non-TEE group, suggesting limited experience on the part of the operators. Surface two-dimensional echo is sensitive enough to detect increasing mitral regurgitation during PBMV in most patients, and is an excellent tool for early appreciation of tamponade. A randomized prospective study comparing TEE with intracardiac echo guidance found equal utility to facilitate transseptal puncture, but otherwise superior imaging with TEE[82] (**Level B**).

Alternative techniques

Cylindrical balloons

The first alternative technique to the Inoue device was a single large cylindrical balloon[18] but this gave way early to two parallel cylindrical balloons[20] with the rationale that two balloons better distributed lateral pressure along the planes of the commissures. Anecdotal results comparing single cylindrical (non-Inoue) versus double balloon inflations demonstrated superior acute gradient reduction with two balloons deployed in parallel.[19] More formal but non-randomized comparison also suggested superior results with the double balloon technique.[27,83,84] Additional confirmation came from an *in vitro* study of operatively excised fused mitral valves that demonstrated superior splitting and increase in valve area.[33]

Relatively few operators still perform cylindrical balloon valvuloplasty of the mitral valve. Disadvantages have included the need to dilate the septum to accommodate the bulk of hardware when two balloons are used, as well as risk of adverse events including "harpooning" of a balloon through the apex of the ventricle, in part due to a "water melon seed" effect with balloon inflation. Nevertheless, cylindrical balloon series have had relatively good results, including an extraordinary 4832 patient experience in 120 centers across China claiming a 99.3% success rate with virtually no complications, and a low 5.2% restenosis rate at a mean 32 months follow-up, likely suggesting significant problems with data collection.[85] Nevertheless, PBMV studies using cylindrical balloons have been generally good when the anatomy was favorable.[86] This is particularly true with a monorail system that simplifies the double balloon technique and has potential cost advantages as well.[22] Regardless of technology used, the results are dependent on anatomic suitability. Thus, a 145-patient cylindrical balloon trial by Cohen *et al*[53] revealed only 51% 5-year freedom from mitral valve replacement, redilation or death in a setting where patients had unfavorable anatomic features. Many of the cylindrical balloon studies occurred early in the development of PBMV and suffered from incomplete follow-up, non-overlapping endpoints, and lack of serial hemodynamic measurements for assessing hemodynamic results and restenosis.

Inoue versus cylindrical balloons

A large number of studies have compared the Inoue technique to double balloons.[87] Generally, the former has greater simplicity, resulting in shorter procedure times. The Inoue balloon, unlike cylindrical balloons, is self-centering across the mitral valve (see Fig. 57.1) and does not predispose to the occasional catastrophic left ventricular apex perforations seen with cylindrical devices.[88] Because of its low-profile passage over a specially designed stainless steel guidewire across the septum, avoiding the need for balloon dilation of the septum itself, the rate of iatrogenic atrial septal defect with the Inoue balloon is substantially lower[89] (≤2.5% v approximately 10% for the double balloon technique[27]) (**Level B**). Several randomized trials have compared Inoue and double balloon techniques[90,91] and demonstrated similar outcomes. It is likely that an easier procedure with lower complication rates (the Inoue technique) is a trade-off for slightly greater mitral regurgitation,[92,93] possibly because the distal portion of the balloon is oversized and may traumatize the subvalvular apparatus. There are also suggestive data that the double balloon technique, by virtue of the lateralization of forces, is advantageous in less favorable anatomy. One example is the result of dilation of asymmetrically fused commissures: where the Inoue technique has been used, this led to significant risk of mitral regurgitation[69] whereas with double balloon use this has been less common.[94] Other findings, primarily from non-randomized or historical comparisons, reflect inferiority of the double balloon technique compared to Inoue, including longer procedure times, higher risk of left ventricular perforation[95-98] and higher complication rates[91,97] although the latter may reflect operator learning curves with this more complex procedure (**Level C**).

A percutaneous metallic mitral valvulotome, designed to mimic the Tubbs dilator used by surgeons for closed commissurotomy but delivered percutaneously via a transseptal route, was highly effective.[24] Its theoretic advantages included the ability to resterilize most of the valvulotome assembly, a potentially important cost benefit in developing countries. The technique was challenging and had a significant complication rate. Randomized comparisons[99] suggested a somewhat lower success rate and higher complication rate, though this device had the steepest learning curve of the PBMV technologies and is no longer available (**Level B**).

Balloon Versus Open and Closed Surgical Commissurotomy

Randomized trials comparing balloon and surgical commissurotomy began early in the development phase of the percutaneous technique. Because blind dilation of the valve with blunt instruments, typically via the retrograde approach through the left ventricular apex with instruments like the Tubbs dilator, was the standard procedure in countries where MS was prevalent, the early randomized trials compared balloon and closed commissurotomy. In these trials, surgeons were typically highly experienced while the operators performing PBMV were in their learning curve. In 1988 we randomized 40 patients with relatively ideal anatomy and severe MS[100]; these patients were followed with serial invasive and non-invasive testing. There were similar hemodynamic improvements in both groups through 7 years (Fig. 57.3), with one cardiovascular death and a 25% clinical restenosis rate.[101] The actual 3-year restenosis rate (26% in the balloon group and 35% in the surgical group), as defined by a 50% loss of the gain and a valve area <1.5 cm^2, is significantly higher than the repeat intervention rate because restenosis and functional class do not correlate strongly. Thus it is likely that restenosis rates in trials that have not done formal follow-up hemodynamics or non-invasive testing underestimate the true severity of disease during follow-up.

Two other studies compared balloon and closed commissurotomy with shorter non-invasive follow-up only; these demonstrated PBMV to be superior[102] or similar to closed commissurotomy.[103] These studies had relatively unaggressive dilation, with relatively small postprocedure mitral valve areas. A 90-patient three-arm study by Ben Farhat and colleagues compared PBMV with closed and open commissurotomy and demonstrated superior acute results for PBMV (2.2 ± 0.4 cm^2) than for closed commissurotomy (1.6 ± 0.4 cm^2) and a 7-year actuarial restenosis rate of 7% v 37%.[104] Thus, PBMV is at least equal and probably superior to closed mitral commissurotomy (**Level A**).

The hypothesis that open commissurotomy would be superior to PBMV and closed commissurotomy was based on the potential benefits of direct vision, including surgical splitting and remodeling of the subvalvular apparatus, neither of which is a feature of closed commissurotomy or PBMV. A prospective series of 100 open mitral commissurotomy patients had data analyzed specifically to compare to the then reported results of PBMV and concluded that the latter was inferior to the 2.9 cm^2 they reported for open commissurotomy.[105] While these exceptional results were laudable, they likely were impacted by measurement technique as well, and exceed the results reported by others.[10] In our randomized prospective comparison of 60 patients with balloon or open commissurotomy, patients undergoing PBMV had superior mitral valve areas at 3 years,[36] findings that were sustained through 7-year follow-up (see Fig. 57.3).[106] A possible explanation for the superior results of PBMV is the benefit of hemodynamic and echocardiographic feedback to the operator in the catheterization laboratory during stepwise dilation that allows for optimizing inflations, feedback that is less avail-

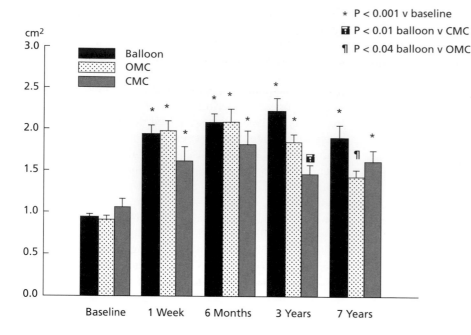

Figure 57.3 Mitral valve area at baseline, 1 week, 6 months, 3 and 7 years after balloon dilation, closed (CMC) or open (OMC) mitral commissurotomy, in prospective randomized trials conducted in Hyderabad, India.[36,100]

able to the surgeon. Ben Farhat and colleagues, in the three-arm trial referred to earlier, found similar results through 7 years for both PBMV and open commissurotomy, in contrast to the inferior results for closed commissurotomy. Thus, PBMV is equal or superior to closed or open commissurotomy, acutely and at long-term follow-up (**Class I, Level A**).

Restenosis

Early mitral restenosis is likely secondary to a suboptimal result[107] although the possibility of a repeat bout of rheumatic fever and carditis should be considered, particularly in endemic areas.[108] Progressive thickening and calcification of the leaflets and subvalvular apparatus are considered the likely mechanisms of longer term restenosis, with pathologic evidence not supporting commissural refusion.[109] Similar to the results of repeat valve surgery,[110] balloon dilation for mitral valve restenosis after surgical commissurotomy has had inferior results.[111] Thus, patients have had less symptomatic improvement,[112] lower success rate (with only 51% having valve area >1.5 cm^2),[113] a higher incidence of subsequent mitral valve replacement (20% by 4 years)[113] and a twofold[114] to 10-fold[115] increase in restenosis rates at 5 years for patients with prior surgical commissurotomy. Similarly, patients with restenosis after PBMV have had lower success rates and less improvement in mitral valve area.[116] However, the poorer outcomes appear to be related to a deterioration in valve morphology at the time of redilation, with results similar to those predictable by the echo scores of patients undergoing *de novo* dilation.[113,117,118] Thus PBMV is appropriate first-line therapy in

restenosis patients with suitable anatomy (**Class II, Level C**).

Pulmonary hypertension

The improvement in hemodynamics after PBMV includes not only gradient reduction and improvement in mitral valve area, but also a progressive decrease in pulmonary artery pressure and pulmonary vascular resistance.[119] Even in patients with severe pulmonary hypertension, a marker for overall MS severity, there is parallel postprocedure improvement in hemodynamics,[120] a phenomenon that continues through 3 years of follow-up[36] (**Class II, Level B**).

Pregnancy

A number of studies have reported successful PBMV in pregnant women with initial results identical to the superior valve areas seen in non-pregnant patients in the same age groups.[121,122] In order to avoid the radiation exposure to the fetus, the procedure has been done with echo guidance only, although appropriate shielding of the fetus is adequate in most instances[123] (**Class II, Level C**).

Tricuspid insufficiency

Song and colleagues compared PBMV to mitral valve surgery and tricuspid valve repair for 92 patients with severe MS and severe functional tricuspid insufficiency.[124] The 7-year event-free survival was 77% in the PBMV-only group versus 95% for the operated group (**Class II, Level C**).

Bioprosthesis

A number of case reports have described balloon dilation of bioprosthetic mitral valves,[125–127] although the acute hemodynamic benefits, potential for complications, and long-term outcomes are questionable. Histologically, bioprosthetic valves resemble calcific native aortic stenosis and balloon dilation is of limited effectiveness.[128] Intraoperative balloon dilation, examining the morphology of severely stenosed bioprosthetic valves before and after balloon dilation, appeared "completely ineffectual" with leaflet tearing and cuspal perforation.[129]

Complications

The rate of complications is inversely proportional to operator experience with a steep learning curve associated with the procedure.[26,27] The NHLBI reported substantially lower rates of all major complications except acute mitral insufficiency at centers performing more than 25 cases and in the second year that sites enrolled patients; a willingness to attempt PBMV in higher risk subsets in the second year may explain the mitral insufficiency. The ACC/AHA guidelines emphasize that the decision to proceed to PBMV must take into consideration the experience of the operators involved (**Level B**).

Overall mortality has been approximately 1%, most commonly related to tamponade from transseptal catheterization[130] but also from fenestration of the left ventricular apex. Tamponade has been reported in a range of <1–4% of PBMVs, the latter level reported in both a 146-patient series from the Beth Israel Hospital in Boston[53] and the 738-patient NHLBI Mitral Valvuloplasty Registry.[27] Besides transseptal puncture and balloon "harpooning," catheter manipulation in the left atrium has also been implicated. In an analysis of 10 cases of tamponade in a 903-patient PBMV series,[88] Joseph et al demonstrated the following etiologies: perforation during transseptal puncture (2), harpooning of the left ventricular apex (3), perforation by an apical guidewire (2), stitch perforation caused by low transseptal puncture of the posterior wall of the right atrium (2), and temporary pacing-induced perforation of the right ventricle (1). There was an inverse relationship between frequency of tamponade and operator experience.

Other complications include severe mitral insufficiency (1–6%) and cerebrovascular accident and thromboembolism (up to 4%). Disturbingly, magnetic resonance imaging detected new hyperintensivity foci suggestive of periprocedural cerebral infarcts in 18 of 63 post-PBMV patients[131] although only one had relegatable symptoms. Clot in the left atrium had not been detected on TEE in these patients. Thus, embolization may be common even if not clinically apparent. The probable sources, besides intracavitary clot, are catheter-induced thrombus formation and showers of calcium; the latter has been associated with rare but catastrophic coronary artery occlusion.[132]

Atrial septal defects were a significant source of complications early in the development of technologies for PBMV, in part arising from tearing of the septum during balloon dilation to allow catheter passage, inadvertent proximal deployment of cylindrical balloons or withdrawal of winged balloons retrograde through the septum. Residual left to right flow is seen in >90% of patients[133] though the majority resolve within 3 months. Persistent left to right shunting is likely related to size of the hole and the residual gradient across the mitral valve. Because the Inoue balloon does not require balloon dilation of the septum and proximal inflation is unlikely given its self-centering method, a comparison of Inoue and double or bifoil balloon techniques demonstrated substantial reduction in residual shunt with the former.[134] The presence of a residual atrial septal defect does decompress the left atrium after PBMV and leads to overestimation of the mitral valve area because of lowering of the mitral valve gradient by left to right transseptal flow.[135]

Postprocedure management

Oral anticoagulation is indicated in MS patients in AF, known clot in the left atrium or a history of prior embolic disease (**Class I, Level A**). When the left atrium is enlarged at 55 mm or greater, or in the presence of spontaneous echo contrast,[59] the guidelines suggest that anticoagulation be considered in the setting of severe MS (**Class II, Level B**). However, there is little evidence base regarding continuation of anticoagulation in the latter patients after PBMV.

Patients with successful PBMV and therefore decompression of the left atrium have been shown to have some involution of left atrial size[136] with about a one-third reduction in left atrial volume, although this phenomenon is less pronounced in patients with AF. Cardioversion after PBMV has been recommended predicated on successful maintenance of sinus rhythm in patients operated for MS routinely shocked during recovery from cardioplegic arrest.[137] Successful post-PBMV cardioversion has correlated strongly with duration of pre-PBMV AF.[138] In a recent study using an inclusion threshold of left atrial size <60 mm, two-thirds of patients undergoing cardioversion remained in sinus rhythm 12 months after PBMV[139] (**Class II, Level C**).

Conclusion

Percutaneous balloon mitral valvuloplasty is both safe and effective. Short-term results in ideal patients include a doubling of the mitral valve area and a relatively low complication rate, with freedom from reintervention at 7–10 years of >50% (**Level A**). Less favorable outcomes are seen in patients with significant thickening and calcification of the leaflets and subvalvular apparatus, as well as older patients and those in AF (**Level C**). The procedure has a steep learning curve and success and complication rates are directly related to operator experience (**Level B**). Based on a sizable evidence base of randomized controlled trials, PBMV is the treatment of choice for patients with rheumatic MS and suitable valve anatomy who require intervention (**Class I, Level A**).

References

1. Cutler EC, Levine SA. Cardiotomy and valvulotomy for mitral stenosis. Experimental observations and clinical notes concerning an operated case with recovery. *Boston Med Surg J* 1923;**188**:1023–7.

2. Suttar HS. The surgical treatment of mitral stenosis. *BMJ* 1925;**2**:603–6.

3. Lewis T. *Diseases of the Heart*, 3rd edn. London: Macmillan, 1943:130.

4. Raju BS, Turi ZG. Rheumatic fever. In: Libby P, Bonow RO, Mann DL, Zipes DP, eds. Braunwald's Heart Disease: *A Textbook of Cardiovascular Medicine*. Philadelphia: Elsevier, 2008:2079–86.

5. John S, Bashi VV, Jairaj PS *et al.* Closed mitral valvotomy: early results and long-term follow- up of 3724 consecutive patients. *Circulation* 68:891–896, 1983.

6. Toumbouras M, Panagopoulos F, Papakonstantinou C *et al.* Long-term surgical outcome of closed mitral commissurotomy. *J Heart Valve Dis* 1995;**4**:247–50.

7. Rihal CS, Schaff HV, Frye RL *et al.* Long-term follow-up of patients undergoing closed transventricular mitral commissurotomy: a useful surrogate for percutaneous balloon mitral valvuloplasty? *J Am Coll Cardiol* 1992;**20**:781–6.

8. Tutun U, Ulus AT, Aksoyek AI *et al.* The place of closed mitral valvotomy in the modern cardiac surgery era. *J Heart Valve Dis* 2003;**12**:585–91.

9. Choudhary SK, Dhareshwar J, Govil A *et al.* Open mitral commissurotomy in the current era: indications, technique, and results. *Ann Thorac Surg* 2003;**75**:41–6.

10. Scalia D, Rizzoli G, Campanile F *et al.* Long-term results of mitral commissurotomy. *J Thorac Cardiovasc Surg* 1993;**105**:633–42.

11. Villanova C, Melacini P, Scognamiglio R *et al.* Long-term echocardiographic evaluation of closed and open mitral valvulotomy. *Int J Cardiol* 1993;**38**:315–21.

12. Hickey MS, Blackstone EH, Kirklin JW *et al.* Outcome probabilities and life history after surgical mitral commissurotomy: implications for balloon commissurotomy. *J Am Coll Cardiol* 1991;**17**:29–42.

13. Glower DD, Landolfo KP, Davis RD *et al.* Comparison of open mitral commissurotomy with mitral valve replacement with or without chordal preservation in patients with mitral stenosis. *Circulation* 1998;**98**:II120–II123.

14. Rashkind WJ, Miller WW. Creation of an atrial septal defect without thoracotomy. *JAMA* 1966;**196**:991.

15. Inoue K, Kitamura F, Chikusa H *et al.* Atrial septostomy by a new balloon catheter. *Jpn Circ J* 1981;**45**:730–8.

16. Inoue K, Nakamura T, Kitamura F. Nonoperative mitral commissurotomy by a new balloon catheter. *Jpn Circ J* 1982;**46**:877.

17. Inoue K, Owaki T, Nakamura T *et al.* Clinical application of transvenous mitral commissurotomy by a new balloon catheter. *J Thorac Cardiovasc Surg* 1984;**87**:394–402.

18. Lock JE, Khalilullah M, Shrivastava S *et al.* Percutaneous catheter commissurotomy in rheumatic mitral stenosis. *N Engl J Med* 1985;**313**:1515–18.

19. Palacios I, Block PC, Brandi S *et al.* Percutaneous balloon valvotomy for patients with severe mitral stenosis. *Circulation* 1987;**75**:778–84.

20. al Zaibag M, Ribeiro PA, Al Kasab S *et al.* Percutaneous double-balloon mitral valvotomy for rheumatic mitral-valve stenosis. *Lancet* 1986;**1**:757–61.

21. Grifka RG, O'Laughlin MP, Nihill MR *et al.* Double-transseptal, double-balloon valvuloplasty for congenital mitral stenosis. *Circulation* 1992;**85**:123–9.

22. Bonhoeffer P, Esteves C, Casal U *et al.* Percutaneous mitral valve dilatation with the Multi-Track System. *Catheter Cardiovasc Interv* 1999;**48**:178–83.

23. Stefanadis C, Stratos C, Pitsavos C *et al.* Retrograde nontransseptal balloon mitral valvuloplasty. Immediate results and long-term follow-up. *Circulation* 1992;**85**:1760–7.

24. Cribier A, Eltchaninoff H, Koning R *et al.* Percutaneous mechanical mitral commissurotomy with a newly designed metallic valvulotome: immediate results of the initial experience in 153 patients. *Circulation* 1999;**99**:793–9.

25. Bonow RO, Carabello BA, Chatterjee K *et al.* ACC/AHA 2006 guidelines for the management of patients with valvular heart disease: a report of the American College of Cardiology/American Heart Association Task Force on Practice Guidelines (Writing Committee to Revise the 1998 Guidelines for the Management of Patients with Valvular Heart Disease) developed in collaboration with the Society of Cardiovascular Anesthesiologists endorsed by the Society for Cardiovascular Angiography and Interventions and the Society of Thoracic Surgeons. *J Am Coll Cardiol* 2006;**48**:e1–148.

26. Sanchez PL, Harrell LC, Salas RE *et al.* Learning curve of the Inoue technique of percutaneous mitral balloon valvuloplasty. *Am J Cardiol* 2001;**88**:662–7.

27. National Heart, Lung, and Blood Institute Balloon Valvuloplasty Registry Participants. Multicenter experience with balloon mitral commissurotomy. NHLBI Balloon Valvuloplasty Registry Report on immediate and 30-day follow-up results. *Circulation* 1992;**85**:448–61.

28. Block PC, Palacios IF, Jacobs ML *et al.* Mechanism of percutaneous mitral valvotomy. *Am J Cardiol* 1987;**59**:178–9.

29. Matsuura Y, Fukunaga S, Ishihara H *et al.* Mechanics of percutaneous balloon valvotomy for mitral valvular stenosis. *Heart Vessels* 1988;**4**:179–83.

30. Nabel E, Bergin PJ, Kirsh MM. Morphological analysis of balloon mitral valvuloplasty; intra-operative results. *J Am Coll Cardiol* 1990;**15**:97A.

31. Kaplan JD, Isner JM, Karas RH et al. In vitro analysis of mechanisms of balloon valvuloplasty of stenotic mitral valves. Am J Cardiol 1987;**59**:318–23.

32. McKay RG, Lock JE, Safian RD et al. Balloon dilation of mitral stenosis in adult patients: postmortem and percutaneous mitral valvuloplasty studies. J Am Coll Cardiol 1987;**9**:723–31.

33. Ribeiro PA, al Zaibag M, Rajendran V et al. Mechanism of mitral valve area increase by in vitro single and double balloon mitral valvotomy. Am J Cardiol 1988;**62**:264–9.

34. Lieberman EB, Bashore TM, Hermiller JB et al. Balloon aortic valvuloplasty in adults: failure of procedure to improve long-term survival. J Am Coll Cardiol 1995;**26**:1522–8.

35. Kirwan C, Richardson G, Rothman MT. Is there a role for balloon valvuloplasty in patients with stenotic aortic bioprosthetic valves? Catheter Cardiovasc Interv 2004;**63**:251–3.

36. Reyes VP, Raju BS, Wynne J et al. Percutaneous balloon valvuloplasty compared with open surgical commissurotomy for mitral stenosis. N Engl J Med 1994;**331**:961–7.

37. Reid CL, McKay CR, Chandraratna PA et al. Mechanisms of increase in mitral valve area and influence of anatomic features in double-balloon, catheter balloon valvuloplasty in adults with rheumatic mitral stenosis: a Doppler and two-dimensional echocardiographic study. Circulation 1987;**76**:628–36.

38. Wilkins GT, Weyman AE, Abascal VM et al. Percutaneous balloon dilatation of the mitral valve: an analysis of echocardiographic variables related to outcome and the mechanism of dilatation. Br Heart J 1988;**60**:299–308.

39. Palacios IF, Sanchez PL, Harrell LC et al. Which patients benefit from percutaneous mitral balloon valvuloplasty? Prevalvuloplasty and postvalvuloplasty variables that predict long-term outcome. Circulation 2002;**105**:1465–71.

40. Palacios IF, Sanchez PL, Harrell LC et al. Which patients benefit from percutaneous mitral balloon valvuloplasty? Prevalvuloplasty and postvalvuloplasty variables that predict long-term outcome. Circulation 2002;**105**:1465–71.

41. Hernandez R, Banuelos C, Alfonso F et al. Long-term clinical and echocardiographic follow-up after percutaneous mitral valvuloplasty with the Inoue balloon. Circulation 1999;**99**:1580–6.

42. Dean LS, Mickel M, Bonan R et al. Four-year follow-up of patients undergoing percutaneous balloon mitral commissurotomy. A report from the National Heart, Lung, and Blood Institute Balloon Valvuloplasty Registry. J Am Coll Cardiol 1996;**28**:1452–7.

43. Zhang HP, Allen JW, Lau FY et al. Immediate and late outcome of percutaneous balloon mitral valvotomy in patients with significantly calcified valves. Am Heart J 1995;**129**:501–6.

44. Tanaka S, Watanabe S, Matsuo H et al. Over 10 years clinical outcomes in patients with mitral stenosis with unilateral commissural calcification treated with catheter balloon commissurotomy: single-center experience. J Cardiol 2008;**51**:33–41.

45. Fatkin D, Roy P, Morgan JJ et al. Percutaneous balloon mitral valvotomy with the Inoue single- balloon catheter: commissural morphology as a determinant of outcome. J Am Coll Cardiol 1993;**21**:390–7.

46. Miche E, Fassbender D, Minami K et al. Pathomorphological characteristics of resected mitral valves after unsuccessful valvuloplasty. J Cardiovasc Surg 1996;**37**:475–81.

47. Wei T, Zeng C, Chen F et al. Influence of commissural calcification on the immediate outcomes of percutaneous balloon mitral valvuloplasty. Acta Cardiol 2003;**58**:411–15.

48. Zhang HP, Ruiz CE, Allen JW et al. A novel prognostic scoring system to predict late outcome after percutaneous balloon valvotomy in patients with severe mitral stenosis. Am Heart J 1997;**134**:772–8.

49. Padial LR, Abascal VM, Moreno PR et al. Echocardiography can predict the development of severe mitral regurgitation after percutaneous mitral valvuloplasty by the Inoue technique. Am J Cardiol 1999;**83**:1210–13.

50. Ben Farhat M, Betbout F, Gamra H et al. Predictors of long-term event-free survival and of freedom from restenosis after percutaneous balloon mitral commissurotomy. Am Heart J 2001;**142**:1072–9.

51. Fawzy ME, Shoukri M, Osman A et al. Impact of atrial fibrillation on immediate and long-term results of mitral balloon valvuloplasty in 531 consecutive patients. J Heart Valve Dis 2008;**17**:141–8.

52. Neumayer U, Schmidt HK, Fassbender D et al. Early (three-month) results of percutaneous mitral valvotomy with the Inoue balloon in 1,123 consecutive patients comparing various age groups. Am J Cardiol 2002;**90**:190–3.

53. Cohen DJ, Kuntz RE, Gordon SP et al. Predictors of long-term outcome after percutaneous balloon mitral valvuloplasty. N Engl J Med 1992;**327**:1329–35.

54. Abascal VM, Wilkins GT, Choong CY et al. Mitral regurgitation after percutaneous balloon mitral valvuloplasty in adults: evaluation by pulsed Doppler echocardiography. J Am Coll Cardiol 1988;**11**:257–63.

55. Sanchez-Ledesma M, Cruz-Gonzalez I, Sanchez PL et al. Impact of concomitant aortic regurgitation on percutaneous mitral valvuloplasty: Immediate results, short-term, and long-term outcome. Am Heart J 2008;**156**:361–6.

56. Kronzon I, Tunick PA, Glassman E et al. Transesophageal echocardiography to detect atrial clots in candidates for percutaneous transseptal mitral balloon valvuloplasty. J Am Coll Cardiol 1990;**16**:1320–2.

57. Blackshear JL, Odell JA. Appendage obliteration to reduce stroke in cardiac surgical patients with atrial fibrillation. Ann Thorac Surg 1996;**61**:755–9.

58. Davison G, Greenland P. Predictors of left atrial thrombus in mitral valve disease. J Gen Intern Med 1991;**6**:108–12.

59. Rittoo D, Sutherland GR, Currie P et al. A prospective study of left atrial spontaneous echo contrast and thrombus in 100 consecutive patients referred for balloon dilation of the mitral valve. J Am Soc Echocardiogr 1994;**7**:516–27.

60. Fatkin D, Roy P, Sindone A et al. Rapid onset and dissipation of left atrial spontaneous echo contrast during percutaneous balloon mitral valvotomy. Am Heart J 1998;**135**:609–13.

61. Wang J, Xie X, He H et al. Hypercoagulability existing in the local left atrium of patient with mitral stenosis. Chin Med J (Engl) 2003;**116**:1198–202.

62. Schoenfeld MH, Palacios IF, Hutter AM, Jr et al. Underestimation of prosthetic mitral valve areas: role of transseptal catheterization in avoiding unnecessary repeat mitral valve surgery. J Am Coll Cardiol 1985;**5**:1387–92.

63. Silaruks S, Thinkhamrop B, Kiatchoosakun S et al. Resolution of left atrial thrombus after 6 months of anticoagulation in

candidates for percutaneous transvenous mitral commissurotomy. *Ann Intern Med* 2004;**140**:101–5.

64. Chen WJ, Chen MF, Liau CS *et al.* Safety of percutaneous transvenous balloon mitral commissurotomy in patients with mitral stenosis and thrombus in the left atrial appendage. *Am J Cardiol* 1992;**70**:117–19.

65. Blake JW, Hanzel GS, O'Neill WW. Neuro-embolic protection during percutaneous balloon mitral valvuloplasty. *Catheter Cardiovasc Interv* 2007;**69**:52–5.

66. Zhang HP, Gamra H, Allen JW *et al.* Balloon valvotomy for mitral stenosis associated with moderate mitral regurgitation. *Am J Cardiol* 1995;**75**:960–3.

67. Alfonso F, Macaya C, Hernandez R *et al.* Early and late results of percutaneous mitral valvuloplasty for mitral stenosis associated with mild mitral regurgitation. *Am J Cardiol* 1993;**71**:1304–10.

68. Tuzcu EM, Block PC, Griffin B *et al.* Percutaneous mitral balloon valvotomy in patients with calcific mitral stenosis: immediate and long-term outcome. *J Am Coll Cardiol* 1994;**23**:1604–9.

69. Miche E, Bogunovic N, Fassbender D *et al.* Predictors of unsuccessful outcome after percutaneous mitral valvulotomy including a new echocardiographic scoring system. *J Heart Valve Dis* 1996;**5**:430–5.

70. Feldman T, Carroll JD, Isner JM *et al.* Effect of valve deformity on results and mitral regurgitation after Inoue balloon commissurotomy. *Circulation* 1992;**85**:180–7.

71. Herrmann HC, Lima JA, Feldman T *et al.* Mechanisms and outcome of severe mitral regurgitation after Inoue balloon valvuloplasty. North American Inoue Balloon Investigators. *J Am Coll Cardiol* 1993;**22**:783–9.

72. Tuzcu EM, Block PC, Griffin BP *et al.* Immediate and long-term outcome of percutaneous mitral valvotomy in patients 65 years and older. *Circulation* 1992;**85**:963–71.

73. Stefanadis CI, Stratos CG, Lambrou SG *et al.* Retrograde non-transseptal balloon mitral valvuloplasty: immediate results and intermediate long-term outcome in 441 cases – a multicenter experience. *J Am Coll Cardiol* 1998;**32**:1009–16.

74. Iakovou I, Pavlides G, Voudris V *et al.* Outcome of percutaneous mitral balloon valvuloplasty: comparison of the inoue and retrograde non-transseptal techniques. A single-center experience. *J Invasive Cardiol* 2002;**14**:522–6.

75. Glazier JJ, Turi ZG. Percutaneous balloon mitral valvuloplasty. *Prog Cardiovasc Dis* 1997;**40**:5–26.

76. Feldman T, Carroll JD, Herrmann HC *et al.* Effect of balloon size and stepwise inflation technique on the acute results of Inoue mitral commissurotomy. Inoue Balloon Catheter Investigators. *Cathet Cardiovasc Diagn* 1993;**28**:199–205.

77. Yamabe T, Nagata S, Ishikura F *et al.* Influence of intraballoon pressure on development of severe mitral regurgitation after percutaneous transvenous mitral commissurotomy. *Cathet Cardiovasc Diagn* 1994;**31**:270–6.

78. Liu Z, McCormick D, Dairywala I *et al.* Catheter-based intracardiac echocardiography in the interventional cardiac laboratory. *Catheter Cardiovasc Interv* 2004;**63**:63–71.

79. Goldstein SA, Campbell A, Mintz GS *et al.* Feasibility of on-line transesophageal echocardiography during balloon mitral valvulotomy: experience with 93 patients. *J Heart Valve Dis* 1994;**3**:136–48.

80. Ballal RS, Mahan EF, Nanda NC *et al.* Utility of transesophageal echocardiography in interatrial septal puncture during percutaneous mitral balloon commissurotomy. *Am J Cardiol* 1990;**66**:230–2.

81. Ramondo A, Chirillo F, Dan M *et al.* Value and limitations of transesophageal echocardiographic monitoring during percutaneous balloon mitral valvotomy. *Int J Cardiol* 1991;**31**:223–33.

82. Chiang CW, Huang HL, Ko YS. Echocardiography-guided balloon mitral valvotomy: transesophageal echocardiography versus intracardiac echocardiography. *J Heart Valve Dis* 2007;**16**:596–601.

83. Shrivastava S, Mathur A, Dev V *et al.* Comparison of immediate hemodynamic response to closed mitral commissurotomy, single-balloon, and double-balloon mitral valvuloplasty in rheumatic mitral stenosis. *J Thorac Cardiovasc Surg* 1992;**104**:1264–7.

84. Al Kasab S, Ribeiro PA, Sawyer W. Comparison of results of percutaneous balloon mitral valvotomy using consecutive single (25 mm) and double (25 mm and 12 mm) balloon techniques. *Am J Cardiol* 1989;**64**:1385–7.

85. Chen CR, Cheng TO. Percutaneous balloon mitral valvuloplasty by the Inoue technique: a multicenter study of 4832 patients in China. *Am Heart J* 1995;**129**:1197–203.

86. Iung B, Cormier B, Ducimetiere P *et al.* Functional results 5 years after successful percutaneous mitral commissurotomy in a series of 528 patients and analysis of predictive factors. *J Am Coll Cardiol* 1996;**27**:407–14.

87. Turi ZG. Balloon valvuloplasty: mitral valve. In: Yusuf S, Cairns JA, Camm AJ, Fallen EL, Gersh BJ, eds. *Evidence Based Cardiology*. London: BMJ Books, 1998: 853–70.

88. Joseph G, Chandy ST, Krishnaswami S *et al.* Mechanisms of cardiac perforation leading to tamponade in balloon mitral valvuloplasty. *Cathet Cardiovasc Diagn* 1997;**42**:138–46.

89. Thomas MR, Monaghan MJ, Metcalfe JM *et al.* Residual atrial septal defects following balloon mitral valvuloplasty using different techniques. A transthoracic and transoesophageal echocardiography study demonstrating an advantage of the Inoue balloon. *Eur Heart J* 1992;**13**:496–502.

90. Kang DH, Park SW, Song JK *et al.* Long-term clinical and echocardiographic outcome of percutaneous mitral valvuloplasty: randomized comparison of Inoue and double-balloon techniques. *J Am Coll Cardiol* 2000;**35**:169–75.

91. Park SJ, Kim JJ, Park SW *et al.* Immediate and one-year results of percutaneous mitral balloon valvuloplasty using Inoue and double-balloon techniques. *Am J Cardiol* 1993;**71**:938–43.

92. Sharma S, Loya YS, Desai DM *et al.* Percutaneous mitral valvotomy using Inoue and double balloon technique: comparison of clinical and hemodynamic short term results in 350 cases. *Cathet Cardiovasc Diagn* 1993;**29**:18–23.

93. Arora R, Kalra GS, Murty GS *et al.* Percutaneous transatrial mitral commissurotomy: immediate and intermediate results. *J Am Coll Cardiol* 1994;**23**:1327–32.

94. Rodriguez L, Monterroso VH, Abascal VM *et al.* Does asymmetric mitral valve disease predict an adverse outcome after percutaneous balloon mitral valvotomy? An echocardiographic study. *Am Heart J* 1992;**123**:1678–82.

95. Trevino AJ, Ibarra M, Garcia A *et al.* Immediate and long-term results of balloon mitral commissurotomy for rheumatic mitral stenosis: comparison between Inoue and double-balloon techniques. *Am Heart J* 1996;**131**:530–6.

96. Zhang HP, Gamra H, Allen JW *et al.* Comparison of late outcome between Inoue balloon and double-balloon techniques for percutaneous mitral valvotomy in a matched study. *Am Heart J* 1995;**130**:340–4.

97. Fu XY, Zhang DD, Schiele F *et al.* [Complications of percutaneous mitral valvuloplasty; comparison of the double balloon and the Inoue techniques]. *Arch Mal Coeur Vaiss* 1994;**87**: 1403–11.

98. Rihal CS, Nishimura RA, Reeder GS *et al.* Percutaneous balloon mitral valvuloplasty: comparison of double and single (Inoue) balloon techniques. *Cathet Cardiovasc Diagn* 1993;**29**:183–90.

99. Guerios EE, Bueno RR, Nercolini DC *et al.* Randomized comparison between Inoue balloon and metallic commissurotome in the treatment of rheumatic mitral stenosis: immediate results and 6-month and 3-year follow-up. *Catheter Cardiovasc Interv* 2005;**64**:301–11.

100. Turi ZG, Reyes VP, Raju BS *et al.* Percutaneous balloon versus surgical closed commissurotomy for mitral stenosis. A prospective, randomized trial. *Circulation* 1991;**83**:1179–85.

101. Raju PR, Turi ZG, Raju BS *et al.* Percutaneous balloon versus closed mitral commissurotomy: 7 year follow-up of a randomized trial. *J Am Coll Cardiol* 1996;**27**:259A.

102. Patel JJ, Shama D, Mitha AS *et al.* Balloon valvuloplasty versus closed commissurotomy for pliable mitral stenosis: a prospective hemodynamic study *J Am Coll Cardiol* 1991;**18**:1318–22.

103. Arora R, Nair M, Kalra GS *et al.* Immediate and long-term results of balloon and surgical closed mitral valvotomy: a randomized comparative study. *Am Heart J* 1993;**125**:1091–4.

104. Ben Farhat M, Ayari M, Maatouk F *et al.* Percutaneous balloon versus surgical closed and open mitral commissurotomy: seven-year follow-up results of a randomized trial [see comments]. *Circulation* 1998;**97**:245–50.

105. Antunes MJ, Vieira H, Ferrao de Oliveira J. Open mitral commissurotomy: the 'golden standard'. *J Heart Valve Dis* 2000; **9**:472–7.

106. Turi ZG, Raju BS, Farkas S *et al.* Percutaneous balloon mitral commissurotomy is superior to open surgical commissurotomy at long term follow-up. *J Am Coll Cardiol* 1998;**31**:74A.

107. Langerveld J, Thijs Plokker HW, Ernst SM *et al.* Predictors of clinical events or restenosis during follow-up after percutaneous mitral balloon valvotomy. *Eur Heart J* 1999;**20**:519–26.

108. Nigri A, Alessandri N, Martuscelli E *et al.* Rheumatic fever recurrence: a possible cause of restenosis after percutaneous mitral valvuloplasty. *Ital Heart J* 2001;**2**:845–7.

109. Tsuji T, Ikari Y, Tamura T *et al.* Pathologic analysis of restenosis following percutaneous transluminal mitral commissurotomy. *Catheter Cardiovasc Interv* 2002;**57**:205–10.

110. Suri RK, Pathania R, Jha NK *et al.* Closed mitral valvotomy for mitral restenosis: experience in 113 consecutive cases. *J Thorac Cardiovasc Surg* 1996;**112**:727–30.

111. Fawzy ME, Hassan W, Shoukri M *et al.* Immediate and long-term results of mitral balloon valvotomy for restenosis following previous surgical or balloon mitral commissurotomy. *Am J Cardiol* 2005;**96**:971–5.

112. Davidson CJ, Bashore TM, Mickel M *et al.* Balloon mitral commissurotomy after previous surgical commissurotomy. The National Heart, Lung, and Blood Institute Balloon Valvuloplasty Registry participants. *Circulation* 1992;**86**:91–9.

113. Jang IK, Block PC, Newell JB *et al.* Percutaneous mitral balloon valvotomy for recurrent mitral stenosis after surgical commissurotomy. *Am J Cardiol* 1995;**75**:601–5.

114. Cohen JM, Glower DD, Harrison JK *et al.* Comparison of balloon valvuloplasty with operative treatment for mitral stenosis. *Ann Thorac Surg* 1993;**56**:1254–62.

115. Medina A, de Lezo JS, Hernandez E *et al.* Mitral restenosis: the Cordoba-Las Palmas experience. In: Cheng TO, ed. *Percutaneous Balloon Valvuloplasty.* New York: Igaku-Shoin, 1992: 294–304.

116. Pathan AZ, Mahdi NA, Leon MN *et al.* Is redo percutaneous mitral balloon valvuloplasty (PMV) indicated in patients with post-PMV mitral restenosis? *J Am Coll Cardiol* 1999;**34**:49–54.

117. Peixoto EC, Peixoto RT, Borges IP *et al.* Influence of the echocardiographic score and not of the previous surgical mitral commissurotomy on the outcome of percutaneous mitral balloon valvuloplasty. *Arq Bras Cardiol* 2001;**76**:473–82.

118. Chmielak Z, Ruzyllo W, Demkow M *et al.* Late results of percutaneous balloon mitral commissurotomy in patients with restenosis after surgical commissurotomy compared to patients with 'de-novo' stenosis. *J Heart Valve Dis* 2002;**11**:509–16.

119. Fawzy ME, Hassan W, Stefadouros M *et al.* Prevalence and fate of severe pulmonary hypertension in 559 consecutive patients with severe rheumatic mitral stenosis undergoing mitral balloon valvotomy. *J Heart Valve Dis* 2004;**13**:942–7.

120. Alfonso F, Macaya C, Hernandez R *et al.* Percutaneous mitral valvuloplasty with severe pulmonary artery hypertension. *Am J Cardiol* 1993;**72**:325–30.

121. Esteves CA, Munoz JS, Braga S *et al.* Immediate and long-term follow-up of percutaneous balloon mitral valvuloplasty in pregnant patients with rheumatic mitral stenosis. *Am J Cardiol* 2006;**98**:812–16.

122. Nercolini DC, Rocha Loures BR, Eduardo GE *et al.* Percutaneous mitral balloon valvuloplasty in pregnant women with mitral stenosis. *Catheter Cardiovasc Interv* 2002;**57**:318–22.

123. Mangione JA, Cristovao SA, Maior GI *et al.* Percutaneous mitral valvuloplastry in a pregnant woman guided only by the transesophageal echocardiography. *Arq Bras Cardiol* 2007;**88**: e62–e65.

124. Song H, Kang DH, Kim JH *et al.* Percutaneous mitral valvuloplasty versus surgical treatment in mitral stenosis with severe tricuspid regurgitation. *Circulation* 2007;**116**:I246–250.

125. Hurst FP, Caravalho J Jr, Wisenbaugh TW. Prosthetic mitral valvuloplasty. *Catheter Cardiovasc Interv* 2004;**63**:503–6.

126. Fernandez JJ, DeSando CJ, Leff RA *et al.* Percutaneous balloon valvuloplasty of a stenosed mitral bioprosthesis. *Cathet Cardiovasc Diagn* 1990;**19**:39–41.

127. Cox DA, Friedman PL, Selwyn AP *et al.* Improved quality of life after successful balloon valvuloplasty of a stenosed mitral bioprosthesis. *Am Heart J* 1989;**118**:839–41.

128. Waller BF, McKay C, VanTassel J *et al.* Catheter balloon valvuloplasty of stenotic porcine bioprosthetic valves: Part II: Mechanisms, complications, and recommendations for clinical use. *Clin Cardiol* 1991;**14**:764–72.

129. Lin PJ, Chang JP, Chu JJ *et al.* Balloon valvuloplasty is contra-indicated in stenotic mitral bioprostheses. *Am Heart J* 1994;**127**:724–6.

130. Schoonmaker FW, Vijay NK, Jantz RD. Left atrial and ventricular transseptal catheterization review: losing skills. *Cathet Cardiovasc Diagn* 1987;**13**:233–8.

131. Rocha P, Qanadli SD, Strumza P *et al.* Brain "embolism" detected by magnetic resonance imaging during percutaneous mitral balloon commissurotomy. *Cardiovasc Intervent Radiol* 1999;**22**:268–73.

132. Powell BD, Holmes DR Jr, Nishimura RA *et al.* Calcium embolism of the coronary arteries after percutaneous mitral balloon valvuloplasty. *Mayo Clin Proc* 2001;**76**:753–7.

133. Arora R, Jolly N, Kalra GS *et al.* Atrial septal defect after balloon mitral valvuloplasty: a transesophageal echocardiographic study. *Angiology* 1993;**44**:217–21.

134. Thomas MR, Monaghan MJ, Metcalfe JM *et al.* Residual atrial septal defects following balloon mitral valvuloplasty using different techniques. A transthoracic and transoesophageal echo-cardiography study demonstrating an advantage of the Inoue balloon. *Eur Heart J* 1992;**13**:496–502.

135. Petrossian GA, Tuzcu EM, Ziskind AA *et al.* Atrial septal occlusion improves the accuracy of mitral valve area determination following percutaneous mitral balloon valvotomy. *Cathet Cardiovasc Diagn* 1991;**22**:21–4.

136. Stefadouros MA, Fawzy ME, Malik S *et al.* The long-term effect of successful mitral balloon valvotomy on left atrial size. *J Heart Valve Dis* 1999;**8**:543–50.

137. Kahn DR, Kirsh MM, Ferguson PW *et al.* Cardioversion after mitral valve operations. *Circulation* 1967;**35**:I82–I85.

138. Kavthale SS, Fulwani MC, Vajifdar BU *et al.* Atrial fibrillation: how effectively can sinus rhythm be restored and maintained after balloon mitral valvotomy? *Indian Heart J* 2000;**52**:568–73.

139. Krittayaphong R, Chotinaiwatarakul C, Phankingthongkum R *et al.* One-year outcome of cardioversion of atrial fibrillation in patients with mitral stenosis after percutaneous balloon mitral valvuloplasty. *Am J Cardiol* 2006;**97**:1045–50.

58 Valve repair and choice of valve

Shafie S Fazel and Tirone E David
Peter Munk Cardiac Center, Toronto General Hospital, University of Toronto, Toronto, Canada

Introduction

The ideal replacement cardiac valve is yet to be developed. The ideal valve would be easy to implant, would be non-thrombogenic, would last the patient's lifetime, and in children it would grow with the child. Currently available mechanical and biologic heart valves are imperfect and heart valve repair should always be considered prior to replacement.

This chapter reviews the information on the surgical management of heart valve disease excluding transcatheter therapies. The heterogeneity of heart valve disease and the variability of outcome of complex procedures make the design and execution of randomized clinical trials difficult. The majority of the present evidence is derived from single-center reports. Our recommendations reflect the position of the American College of Cardiology and American Heart Association (ACC/AHA) 2006 Practice Guidelines.[1]

Nomenclature and definitions

Since the publication of the *Guidelines for Reporting Morbidity and Mortality After Cardiac Valvular Operations* approved by the Society of Thoracic Surgeons and the American Association for Thoracic Surgery in 1988, and revised in 1996,[2] surgical journals require that authors conform to those guidelines, which are presented in Box 58.1.

Natural history and indications for surgery

The ACC/AHA 2006 guidelines contain a comprehensive review of the natural history of heart valve disease and the

indications for surgery.[1] This information is also covered in Chapters 53–55, and 81.

Valve repair

Aortic valve repair

The morphologic characteristics and function of the aortic valve are interrelated to the aortic root and are best described as a single functional unit. The aortic root is the anatomic segment that connects the left ventricle with the ascending aorta and has four components: aortoventricular junction or aortic annulus, aortic cusps, aortic sinuses or sinuses of Valsalva, and sinotubular junction. Although the aortic cusps are the most important component of the aortic valve, aortic insufficiency (AI) can occur in patients with normal aortic cusps that have dilation of the sinotubular junction and/or aortic annulus.

Congenital aortic stenosis used to be managed by means of open surgical valvotomy but this procedure has been largely replaced by transcatheter valvotomy (see Chapter 56). Acquired aortic stenosis is not suitable for aortic valve repair.

Patients with AI are potential candidates for aortic valve repair and the aortic cusps are the most important determinant of reparability.[3,4] If the cusps are thin and mobile and have smooth free margins, the feasibility of aortic valve repair is high. Calcified, fibrotic or excessively over-stretched cusps preclude aortic valve repair. Aortic insufficiency caused by prolapse of a single cusp in patients with tricuspid aortic valves is uncommon but repairable. Prolapse of one cusp in patients with bicuspid aortic valve is common and is also suitable for repair.[5] Aortic valve repair frequently is needed in combination with aortic valve-sparing operations.[6] However, isolated repair of the aortic valve is not routinely carried out given the durability of contemporary mechanical and bioprosthetic valves (**Class I, Level C**).

Evidence-Based Cardiology, 3rd edition. Edited by S. Yusuf, J.A. Cairns, A.J. Camm, E.L. Fallen, and B.J. Gersh. © 2010 Blackwell Publishing, ISBN: 978-1-4051-5925-8.

BOX 58.1 Guidelines for reporting morbidity and mortality after cardiac valvular operations

Operative mortality

This is defined as death within the index hospitalization or within 30 days of the operation.

Structural valve deterioration

This is defined as any change in function (including a decrease in New York Heart Association functional class) of an operated valve resulting from an intrinsic abnormality of the valve that causes either stenosis or regurgitation. This definition, however, does not include deterioration because of infection or thrombosis of the valve as determined by reoperation, autopsy or clinical investigations. The term includes changes that are intrinsic to the valve such as wear, fracture, poppet escape, calcification, leaflet tear, stent creep, and suture line disruption of components of an operated valve.

Non-structural dysfunction

This is defined as any abnormality resulting in stenosis or regurgitation at the operated valve that is not intrinsic to the valve itself. Again, this term is exclusive of thrombosis and/or infection but includes entrapment by pannus, tissue or suture; paravalvular leak; inappropriate sizing or positioning; residual leak or obstruction; and clinically important hemolytic anemia.

Valve thrombosis

This includes any thrombosis, in the absence of infection, attached to or near an operated valve that occludes part of the blood flow path or that interferes with the function of the valve.

Embolism

This is any embolic event that occurs in the absence of infection after the immediate perioperative period (when anesthesia-induced unconsciousness is completely reversed). Importantly, a neurologic event includes any new, temporary or permanent focal or global neurologic deficit, but does not include psychomotor deficits elicited by specialized testing. Patients who do not awaken or who awaken after operation with a new stroke are excluded from tabulations of valve-related morbidity. A peripheral embolic event is also tabulated under this definition.

Bleeding event (formerly anticoagulant hemorrhage)

This is any episode of major internal or external bleeding that causes death, hospitalization or permanent injury or that requires blood transfusion. Notably, this definition applies also to patients who are not taking anticoagulants or antiplatelet agents.

Operated valvular endocarditis

This is defined as an infection involving an operated valve. It is based on the traditional criteria including an appropriate combination of positive blood cultures, clinical signs, and/or autopsy or operative findings. Importantly, morbidity associated with endocarditis, such as valve thrombosis, thrombotic embolus, bleeding event or paravalvular leak, is included under this category and is not included in other categories of morbidity.

Note added in proof: these guidelines have recently been updated. See Atkins CW *et al. J Thorac Cardiovasc Surg* 2008;**135**(4):732–8.

Patients with aortic root aneurysm often have normal or minimally stretched aortic cusps and reconstruction of the aortic root with preservation of the native aortic cusps is feasible. Most patients with aortic root aneurysms have normally functioning aortic valve or mild AI. If the AI is severe, the cusps may be thinned and overstretched, or have stress fenestrations along the commissural areas. These valves are not suitable for repair. Patients with ascending aortic aneurysm and AI often have dilated sinotubular junction and normal or minimally altered aortic cusps. The AI is central and caused by outward displacement of the commissures of the aortic valve.

Aortic valve-sparing operations are usually feasible in patients with aortic root aneurysms without AI or with AI and fairly normal aortic cusps as well as in patients with ascending aortic aneurysm and AI due to dilated sinotubular junction. These operations can be classified into three types[7,8]:

• replacement of the ascending aorta with downsizing of the sinotubular junction

• replacement of diseased aortic sinuses (one, two or all three sinuses – in the latter group the procedure is also referred to as a root remodeling or Yacoub procedure)[9]

• full root replacement with reimplantation of the aortic valve in a tube graft (David procedure).[10]

Aortic valve-sparing operations are technically demanding. They can be applied to aortic dissection that extends into the root,[11] Marfan's syndrome patients with aortic root aneurysms,[9,10] in patients with bicuspid aortic valves[5,12] and in patients with aortic root aneurysms of unknown etiology. The competing options for dealing with aortic root and ascending aortic aneurysms are the composite valve graft (mechanical or bioprosthetic valve in a Dacron graft or a biologic valve conduit such as aortic valve homograft or xenograft)[13,14] and aortic valve replacement and supracoronary replacement of the ascending aorta.[15,16]

The long-term outcomes of aortic valve-sparing operations in patients with ascending aortic aneurysms are excellent.[17] Reoperation rate at 10 years after replacement of the ascending aorta with reduction of the diameter of the sinotubular junction is only 3%, which is better than the results of valve replacement (Fig. 58.1). However, if the surgeon is not familiar with aortic cusp repair, presence of an eccen-

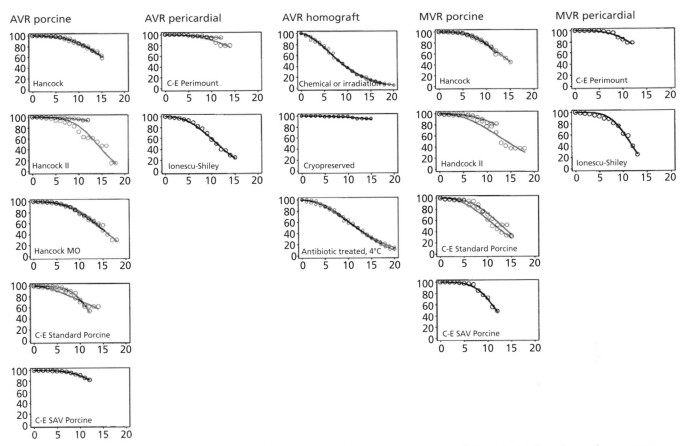

Figure 58.1 Freedom from structural valve deterioration. If data from more than two reports were available, only data from the two largest reports were included. (Modified from Grunkemeier *et al.*[110])

tric AI jet at preoperative echocardiography should alert him or her to other concomitant aortic valve pathology and the need for more complex surgery.

Aneurysm of the sinuses of Valsalva requires either a remodeling or a reimplantation procedure. Long-term results indicate a reoperation rate of about 10% at 10 years for progressive AI[18] with the remodeling technique. In our own experience, return of moderate to severe AI occurred in 15% of patients at 10 years.[6] This rate is suboptimal in young patients but may be acceptable in an older patient population.[5] In patients with dilated aortic annuli, further strategies to stabilize the annulus should be employed.[19] Otherwise, these patients, and patients with connective tissue disorders such as Marfan's syndrome, will have progressive annular dilation, which would cause AI again.[6,20] The reimplantation technique allows stabilization of the annulus within the cylindrical graft and avoids moderate to severe AI in 94% of patients at 10 years.[21,22] Some question the appropriateness of preserving the aortic valve in patients with Marfan's syndrome, but valve repair is safe and durable in this patient population.[6,23] Composite valve graft replacement of the valve and aortic root remains the gold standard across most centers given the reproducibility of the procedure (**Class I, Level C**).

Mitral valve repair

The mitral valve, which includes the annulus, leaflets, chorda tendineae, papillary muscles, and left ventricular wall, may become dysfunctional for a variety of reasons.[24] Rheumatic heart disease causes fibrosis of all components of the mitral valve with resulting mitral stenosis (MS) and/or regurgitation (MR) (see Chapter 53). Myxomatous mitral valve disease typically causes MR because of elongated/ruptured chordae and redundant and prolapsing leaflets. Ischemic functional MR is caused by infarction of the left ventricular wall that tethers the mitral leaflets. This causes an increase in the septolateral dimension of the annulus toward the posteromedial commissure or may result in leaflet prolapse due to papillary muscle rupture and/or fibrosis and elongation. Non-ischemic functional MR is caused by global left ventricular and mitral annular dilation.

Rheumatic mitral valve disease

Mitral balloon valvotomy, in the MS patient without MR and with low echocardiographic calcium scores, is the first line of intervention (see Chapter 57). Patients with moderate distortion of mitral valvular anatomy, but in whom the anterior leaflet and chordae tendineae still appear to be pliable, may be candidates for open mitral commissurotomy and repair. However, in patients in whom there is severe distortion of the valve apparatus preoperatively, mitral valve replacement is more appropriate. Repair of rheumatic MR has been relatively successful but may be attempted by experienced surgeons only if the mitral apparatus is not significantly damaged (**Class IIa, Level C**).

The failure of mitral valve repair in patients with rheumatic disease is related to progressive primary valve disease, leaflet fibrosis and retraction.[25] Valve repair in this population is not as durable as valve repair in patients with non-rheumatic disease. Freedom from reoperation is approximately 70–85% at 5–10 years of follow-up.[26-29] A recent meta-analysis, however, demonstrated superior survival of patients with repair as compared to replacement.[30] If a patient has an indication for anticoagulation, serious consideration should be given to mechanical mitral valve replacement (**Class IIa, Level C**). In this context, we emphasize the critical importance of preserving the chordae tendineae[31-35] (**Class I, Level C**).

Myxomatous or degenerative mitral valve disease

The two major subcategories as initially defined by Carpentier are: myxomatous degeneration where typically the valve leaflets are redundant with elongated chordae, and fibroelastic deficiency which occurs in the older patient with minimal thickening of the leaflet.[36] In the extreme form of myxomatous degeneration, the so-called "Barlow's disease" of the mitral valve, there is also atrialization of the posterior mitral annulus that may have bearing on the technique of repair.[37] Valve repair for these patients involves resection of the prolapsing segment,[38] replacement and/or transposition of the chorda if necessary, and mitral valve annuloplasty.[39,40] Mitral valve repair for degenerative mitral disease may be possible in greater than 90% of cases in experienced hands with excellent results and is recommended (**Class I, Level C**).

Several groups have reported long-term survival outcomes of mitral valve repair in comparison with mitral valve replacement.[41-44] In broad terms, repair provides better survival and clinical outcomes than replacement, but more often than not, patients who undergo mitral valve replacement are sicker. The longest follow-up on mitral valve repair to date shows a freedom from reoperation of 92% at 20 years.[45] At our center, freedom from reoperation ranged from 88% to 96% at 10 years depending on the prolapsing leaflet. Anterior leaflet prolapse or bileaflet prolapse portends worse outcome.[46,47] Results of the edge-to-edge repair in a somewhat younger but similar patient population (with an incomplete follow-up) documented a freedom from reoperation of 96% at 10 years.[48] The superior results obtained in the repair of the mitral valve in myxomatous disease,[46] given the natural history of asymptomatic but severe MR,[49] argues for early surgical intervention (**Class IIa, Level C**). Caution and judgement, however, must be exercised when the mitral valve is affected by rheumatic disease, if MR is caused by complex valvular abnormalities that include anterior leaflet prolapse, or if the surgical team has inadequate experience with valve repair.

Endocarditis

Mitral valve replacement had been the standard surgical therapy for patients with mitral valve endocarditis but repair is feasible depending on the degree of tissue destruction.[50-52] A recent pooled analysis of the reported series demonstrated low rates of early and late repeat mitral valve surgery after mitral valve repair for endocarditis.[53] The principles of mitral valve repair in endocarditis are to remove all infected tissue and to avoid implantation of foreign material. Autologous pericardium, which may be fixed with glutaraldehyde, or bovine pericardium can be used in place of prosthetic annuloplasty rings.

Ischemic mitral regurtitation (IMR)

The role of mitral valve replacement versus repair in chronic IMR is controversial.[54] Mitral replacement is typically reserved for patients with higher preoperative risk factors and co-morbidity at experienced centers.[55-57] Although the results of mitral valve repair appear to be superior to mitral valve replacements in early follow-up, these differences disappear and possibly reverse in longer follow-up.[55-57] This suggests that mitral valve replacement may be the procedure of choice at centers that have limited experience with mitral valve repair (**Class IIa, Level C**).

The most common technique of mitral valve repair for IMR is undersized annuloplasty. Considering the asymmetric alteration in the mitral valve annulus, some advocate the use of a rigid and geometric ring that reduces the septal-lateral annular dimension in particular in the posteromedial segment.[58] Clinical outcomes do not support the use of a complete over a partial ring[59] but given that the intertrigonal region dilates over time, it is reasonable to suggest that complete rings are likely to provide better long-term durability.[60,61] Most support the use of a rigid ring,[62] although concerns that rigid ring annuloplasty may adversely affect LV function remain.[63,64] The long-term result of mitral repair for IMR is poor with return of significant MR in nearly 30% of patients.[59] Perhaps an undersized annuloplasty does not fully address the multifaceted alterations in the mitral apparatus of a patient with IMR.[24] We have clinically introduced Levine's concept of severing secondary chordae tendineae.[65,66] Our initial results are encouraging.[65]

Non-ischemic mitral regurgitation

The principal repair techniques are undersized annuloplasty and the edge-to-edge repair. Correction of severe

MR in end-stage heart failure is safe.[67,68] In spite of symptomatic benefit, no survival benefit is currently apparent.[69,70] Importantly, the Acorn clinical trial confirmed the impact of MR repair alone on patient symptoms and also documented progressive decline in left ventricular volume in a randomized trial setting[71] (**Class IIa, Level B**). The results of the edge-to-edge technique in patients with LV dysfunction have been somewhat mixed.[72,73]

Tricuspid valve repair

Commonly, tricuspid regurgitation (TR) occurs as a result of left heart pathology. In these instances, the tricuspid apparatus is normal, but dilation of the tricuspid annulus results in significant regurgitation. Organic tricuspid valve disease is less common. Functional TR may be repaired by suture annuloplasty (De Vega procedure) or by ring annuloplasty. Ring annuloplasty provides superior long-term outcomes[74-76] (**Class IIa, Level C**). Plication of the posterior leaflet (bicuspidalization) is now rarely performed.[77]

Valve replacement

Types of heart valves

The two main categories of valves are mechanical and tissue valves. Within the former category, three principal valve types are available: caged-ball valves, single tilting disc valves, and bileaflet valves. Tissue valves may also be divided in to three major subtypes: xenografts, homografts, and pulmonary autograft. Xenograft valves are either porcine aortic valves or constructed pericardial valves. Xenograft valves can also be subdivided into stented and stentless.

Randomized clinical trials: mechanical versus biologic

Two randomized clinical trials have compared the outcome of aortic and mitral valve replacement. The Edinburgh Heart Valve Trial[78-80] enrolled patients between 1975 and 1979 and the Department of Veterans Affairs Trial[81-83] enrolled patients between 1977 and 1982. Both of these trials compared the Bjork–Shiley tilting disk valve to the first-generation Hancock or Carpentier–Edwards porcine valve. Although these valves are no longer used in North America, certain principles of valve behavior may be distilled from these two trials.

Edinburgh Heart Valve Trial

In this study, a total of 541 men and women undergoing either aortic or mitral valve replacement were included. The major finding of this trial was the lack of survival benefit for a particular valve type at 20 years. Porcine valves had a substantially higher structural valve deterioration and reoperation rate. Bioprosthesis had structural valve deterioration 12–14 years after implantation in the aortic position and 8–10 years after implantation in the mitral position. The bleeding rates were substantially higher with the mechanical valves, implanted in the aortic but not in the mitral position.

Department of Veterans Affairs Trial

This multicenter trial enrolled a total of 575 men only. It showed that patients randomized to receive a mechanical valve had improved survival after aortic valve replacement (AVR) but not after mitral valve replacement (MVR). Importantly, differences in mortality started to diverge after 10 years. As with the Edinburgh trial, porcine valves had substantially higher primary valve failure. The outcome in the two groups at 15 years is summarized in Table 58.1.

Differences between the trials

In the Edinburgh trial, the linearized rates of major hemorrhage requiring hospital admission and/or blood transfusions were 1.5% per year in the porcine group and 2% per year in the mechanical valve group. In the VA trial the linearized bleeding rates were 2.5% per year in the porcine group and 4.3% in the mechanical group. Higher intensity of anticoagulation in the USA likely accounts for this difference.[84] In the contemporary data from the Stroke Prevention in Atrial Fibrillation III[85] trial with international normalized ratio (INR) of 2.0–3.0, the incidence of bleeding was 1.5% per year. The linearized rates of thromboembolism were not different between the two types of valve.

New developments in valve prostheses

Since the above two trials were concluded, other single-center or multi-center but non-randomized studies have been published documenting the performance of newer biologic and mechanical prostheses in terms of structural valve deterioration[86-98] (Fig. 58.1) and patient survival.[90,99-109] These are reviewed in Table 58.2 and Table 58.3. Most biologic valves are now treated with anticalcification agents, undergo zero-pressure fixation, have a lower profile, and are hemodynamically superior to the older valves. These advances have generally meant longer durability of the bioprosthetic valves. At the same time, new mechanical valve designs such as the bileaflet design have improved the hemodynamic performance. By and large, the majority of the valves that have received FDA approval based on 800 patient-years of experience are similar in terms of valve function and valve durability (see Fig. 58.1) and risk of complications (Fig. 58.2). Leaders in the field have generalized the comparison of the various valves by

Table 58.1 Probability of an outcome event at 15 years after valve replacement

| | Aortic valve replacement | | *P*-value | Mitral valve replacement | | *P*-value |
	Mechanical **n = 198**	**Bioprosthetic** **n = 196**		**Mechanical** **n = 88**	**Bioprosthesis** **n = 93**	
Death from any cause	66 ± 3%	79 ± 3%	0.02	81 ± 4%	79 ± 4%	0.3
Any valve-related complication	65 ± 4%	66 ± 5%	0.26	73 ± 6%	81 ± 5%	0.56
Systemic embolism	18 ± 4%	18 ± 4%	0.66	18 ± 5%	22 ± 5%	0.96
Bleeding	51 ± 4%	30 ± 4%	0.0001	53 ± 7%	31 ± 6%	0.01
Endocarditis	7 ± 2%	15 ± 5%	0.45	11 ± 4%	17 ± 5%	0.37
Valve thrombosis	2 ± 1%	1 ± 1%	0.33	1 ± 1%	1 ± 1%	0.95
Perivalvular regurgitation	8 ± 2%	2 ± 1%	0.09	17 ± 5%	7 ± 4%	0.05
Reoperation	10 ± 3%	29 ± 5%	0.004	25 ± 6%	50 ± 8%	0.15
Primary valve failure	0 ± 0%	23 ± 5%	0.0001	5 ± 4%	44 ± 8%	0.0002

n, number of patients randomized; *P*, significance of difference between mechanical and bioprosthetic valve groups.
From Hammermeister *et al.*[81]

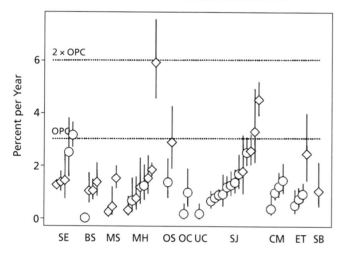

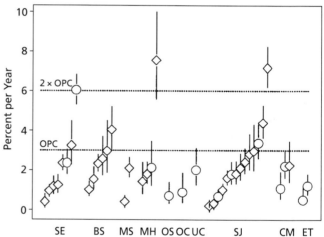

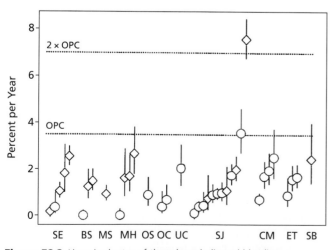

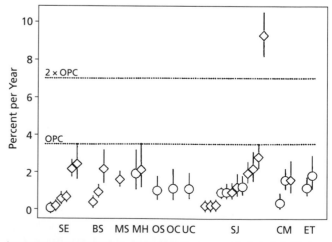

Figure 58.2 Linearized rates of thromboembolic and bleeding complications from major mechanical valve replacement data for AVR and MVR are shown. (Modified from Grunkemeier *et al.*[110]) OPC (objective performance criteria) are used by the FDA to approve new values; the upper confidence interval should not cross twice the OPC rate for approval. Circles indicate that only late events were included. SE, Starr Edwards; BS, Björk-Shiley; MS, Monostrut; MH, Medtronic Hall; OS, Omniscience; OC, Omnicarbon; UC, Ultracar; SJ, St Jude; CM, Carbomedics; ET, Edwards Tekna or Duromedics; SB, Sorin Bicarbon.

Table 58.2 Structural valve deterioration. Modified from Bonow et al.[1]

Author, reference	Type of PHV	Number of valves		Time of SVD estimate, y	Age, y	Freedom from SVD, %	
		AVR	MVR			AVR	MVR
Jamieson et al[92]	Carpentier–Edwards standard porcine bioprosthesis	572	509	10	30–59	81 ± 4	78 ± 5
					>60	91 ± 3	71 ± 9
Cohn et al[89]	Hancock porcine bioprosthesis (includes 146 combined AVR + MVR procedures)	971	708	15	≤40	68 ± 9	68 ± 10
					41–69	86 ± 2	84 ± 13
					≥70	94 ± 3	84 ± 10
Jones et al[95]	Hancock or Carpentier–Edwards porcine bioprosthesis (includes 88 combined AVR + MVR procedures)	610	528	10	<40	46 ± 7	47 ± 8
					40–49	60	48 ± 8
					50–59	79	61
					60–69	92 ± 2	80 ± 6
Burdon et al[87]	Hancock I and Hancock modified orifice porcine bioprosthesis	857	793	15	16–39	33 ± 7	37 ± 6
					40–49	54 ± 10	38 ± 12
					50–59	57 ± 6	38 ± 5
					60–69	73 ± 6	61 ± 15
					>70	93 ± 3	62 ± 6
Burr et al[88]	Carpentier–Edwards standard porcine bioprosthesis (similar results were obtained with Carpentier–Edwards supra-annular porcine bioprosthesis)	574	500	7	<65	94 ± 1	88 ± 2
					65–69	98 ± 1	90 ± 4
					70–79	100	95 ± 3
					≥80	100	100
				13–15	<65	62 ± 8	37 ± 7
					65–69	98 ± 3	63 ± 8
					70–79	95 ± 5	74 ± 19
					≥80	100	–
Pelletier et al[96]	Carpentier–Edwards standard (302 AVR, 324 MVR) improved annulus (97 AVR, 135 MVR), supra-annular (52 AVR, 88 MVR) porcine bioprostheses (includes 121 combined AVR + MVR and 5 combined MVR + TVR procedures)	451	547	10	<45	70	55
					45–54	84	64
					55–64	84	69
					≥65	93	95
Cosgrove et al[91]	Carpentier–Edwards pericardial aortic bioprosthesis	310	–	10	<65	88.6	–
					≥65	95.5	–
Pelletier et al[97]	Carpentier–Edwards pericardial aortic bioprosthesis	416	–	10	<60	86.3	–
					60–69	95.3	–
					≥70	100	–
Cohn et al[90]	Hancock modified orifice porcine aortic valve	843	–	10	≤50	57	–
					51–69	77	–
					≥70	96	–
				15	≤50	16	–
					51–69	54	–
					≥70	87	–
Banbury et al[86]	Carpentier–Edwards pericardial aortic bioprosthesis	267	–	15	45	58	–
					55	70	–
					65	82	–
					75	91	–
Jamieson et al[94]	Medtronic Intact porcine bioprosthesis	836	332	12	51–60	92 ± 3	90 ± 3
					61–70	96 ± 2	
					>70	98 ± 1	97 ± 3

Table 58.3 Long-term mortality after AVR. Modified from Rahimtoola.[111]

Author, reference	Type of PHV	No. of patients	Mortality	
			at yr	%
Orszulak et al[107]	Starr–Edwards	1,100	10	40.4
			15	55.1
			20	68.8
Lindblom et al[104]	Bjork–Shiley	1,753	10	30*
			15	46*
Lund et al[106]	St Jude	694	10	42 ± 5
Butchart et al[99]	Medtronic Hall	736	10	36
			15	55
Peterseim et al[108]	St Jude	412	10	50 ± 6
	C-E porcine	429	10	46 ± 3
Yun et al[109]	Hancock porcine	652	12	49 ± 2
	Hancock MO porcine	561	12	58 ± 3
	C-E porcine	389	12	56 ± 7
Jamieson et al[102]	C-E supra-annular porcine	1,335	10	40.6 ± 2.1
			12	45.8 ± 2.8
Cohn et al[90]	Hancock MO porcine	843	10	48 ± 2*
			15	72 ± 3*
Khan et al[103]	Hancock porcine/Hancock MO porcine	243	10	45*
			15	64*
Frater et al[101]	C-E pericardial	267	14	60.7 ± 3.1*
David et al[100]	Hancock II porcine	670	10	39 ± 2
			15	53 ± 3

* Excluding operative mortality.

AVR, aortic valve replacement; C-E, Carpentier–Edwards; MO, modified orifice; PHV, prosthetic heart valve.

concluding that patient-related factors are more important than valve-related factors.[110,111]

Stentless xenograft valves

Conventional porcine and bovine pericardial valves, which are mounted on a stent, cause some degree of obstruction with persistent gradients that may be clinically important.[112] Stentless xenograft valves were developed to provide superior hemodynamics[113] which may not necessarily be evident at rest.[114] Stentless valve implantation appears to be associated with greater left ventricular mass regression and improved survival.[115,116] Long-term follow-up on the Toronto SPV bioprostheis, however, has demonstrated suboptimal durability with a freedom from reoperation of 69% at 12 years.[117]

Aortic homograft

Aortic valve homograft has been used with satisfactory results since 1962.[118–121] Cryopreservation is the preferred technique of valve preservation during storage[122–124] (see Fig. 58.1). Freedom from reoperation for structural valve deterioration at 15 years of follow-up is age dependent (0–20 years of age, 47%; 21–60 years of age, 80%; >60 years

of age, 94%).[121] Aortic valve homograft is an excellent choice for patients with active valve endocarditis, particularly with aortic root abscess.[121,125–127] Aortic valve homograft may be used as a full root replacement, as a root inclusion or in the subcoronary position. When the homograft is used as a full root replacement, better long-term durability and valve function are obtained, but neo-root dilation may occur in patients with annuloaortic ectasia.[128,129] The recreation of normal aortic root anatomy may be difficult with the subcoronary technique, and emphasizes the importance of surgical expertise.[124] Reoperation on homografts is technically difficult because of extensive calcification.[130]

Pulmonary autograft

Aortic valve homograft has high failure rates in the younger patient. The Ross procedure was developed to overcome this limitation in 1967.[131,132] In the pioneer series, the mean age at time of operation was 32 years and the majority of the patients received the autograft in the subcoronary position and not as a root inclusion or root replacement. Twenty years after operation, survival was 61%, freedom from autograft replacement was 75%, and freedom from replacement of homograft in the pulmonary position was 80%.[133] Others have also reported excellent outcome with this operation.[134–137] A subset of patients developed AI, likely because of technical difficulties of placing the valve in the subcoronary position, as with the experience with aortic valve homograft.[133] Surgeons adopted the root inclusion or the root replacement, because the technique was more reproducible.[138] Stabilization of the aortic annulus and downsizing of the sinotubular junction provide improved results.[138]

Given the superior performance of today's bioprostheses, the lifespan of the patient has to be judged to be greater than 20 years for the patient to derive benefit from the Ross procedure. Relative contraindications to this procedure have been proposed:

- multiple valve disease
- Marfan's syndrome
- variety of autoimmune diseases such as systemic lupus erythematosus, rheumatoid arthritis, acute rheumatic fever, ankylosing spondylysis, Reiter's syndrome, Libman–Sachs endocarditis
- dilated aortic root and/or annulus.[139–141]

ACC/AHA guidelines

The use of biologic prostheses is increasing. The ACC/AHA guidelines documented five principal reasons for this observation:

1 current bioprostheses have longer durability

2 the risk of reoperation has continued to decrease with time

3 patients receiving AVR are now more likely to be older than in the previous era

4 young patients are more reluctant to accept the risks of anticoagulation and the restraints that the therapy places on lifestyle

5 recent non-randomized trials have now suggested an apparent survival benefit for patients receiving bioprosthesis.

The most recent guidelines regarding prosthesis choice for aortic valve replacement (Table 58.4), mitral valve repair (Table 58.5) and mitral valve replacement (Table 58.6) are summarized.

Conclusion

Valve repair, when feasible, remains the best option only in experienced hands. Valve replacement remains quite reproducible from center to center with excellent long-term results and should be, in most instances, the procedure of choice. The currently available biologic valves have very good durability. As a result, there will most likely be a decrease in the age cut-off at which patients are recom-

Table 58.4 Major criteria for valve selection in aortic valve replacement (AVR)

Class of recommendation	Level of evidence
Class I	
A mechanical prosthesis is recommended for AVR in patients with a mechanical valve in the mitral or tricuspid position	C
A bioprosthesis is recommended for AVR in patients of any age who will not take warfarin or who have major medical contraindications to warfarin therapy	C
Class IIa	
Patient preferences is a reasonable consideration in the selection of aortic valve operation and valve prosthesis. A mechanical prosthesis is reasonable for AVR in patients under 65 years of age. A bioprosthesis is reasonable for AVR in patients under 65 years of age who elect to receive this valve for lifestyle considerations after detailed discussion of the risks of anticoagulation versus the likelihood that a second AVR may be necessary in the future	C
A bioprosthesis is reasonable for AVR in patients aged 65 years or older without risk factors for thromboembolism	C
Aortic valve replacement with a homograft is reasonable for patients with active prosthetic valve endocarditis	C
Class IIb	
A bioprosthetic might be considered for AVR in a woman of child-bearing age	C

Table 58.5 Major criteria for mitral valve (MV) repair

Class of recommendation	Level of evidence
Class I	
Degenerative mitral valve disease: MV repair is recommended when anatomically possible for patients who fulfill clinical indications, only by surgeons who are experts in mitral valve repair	C
Rheumatic mitral valve disease: percutaneous or surgical commissurotomy is indicated when anatomically possible for treatment of severe mitral valve stenosis, when clinically indicated	C
Class IIa	
Functional mitral valve regurgitation: MV repair is recommended in patients who fulfill clinical indications, only by surgeons who are experts in mitral valve repair, and only in patients who are clinically stable	C

Table 58.6 Major criteria for mitral valve (MV) replacement

Class of recommendation	Level of evidence
Class I	
A bioprosthesis is indicated for MV replacement in a patient who will not take warfarin, or has a clear contraindication to warfarin therapy	C
Class IIa	
A mechanical prosthesis is reasonable for MV replacement in patients under 65 years of age with long-standing atrial fibrillation	C
A bioprosthesis is reasonable for MV replacement in patients 65 years of age or older	C
A bioprosthesis is reasonable for MV replacement in patients under 65 years of age in sinus rhythm who elect to receive this valve for lifestyle considerations after detailed discussions of the risks of anticoagulation versus the likelihood that a second MV replacement may be necessary in the future	C

mended to have a biologic valve substitute. The pulmonary autograft and the homograft will continue to occupy a specialized niche, but will not become routine given the inherent complexity of the procedures. Stentless valves and biologic aortic roots are increasingly used, but the long-term data on their durability remain to be seen. Valve surgery is rapidly evolving and new technologies now allow implantation of a bioprosthetic valve in a stent using catheter-based techniques or transapical approach. Simplified mitral valve repair with percutaneous edge-to-edge techniques or annular cinching is under clinical trials. There is no evidence to allow proper evaluation of these new techniques. Although these procedures may be widely used in the future, they have not been discussed here. Advances in tissue-engineering techniques may finally allow the manufacture of the perfect living valve prosthesis.

References

1. Bonow RO, Carabello BA, Kanu C *et al.* ACC/AHA 2006 guidelines for the management of patients with valvular heart disease: a report of the American College of Cardiology/American Heart Association Task Force on Practice Guidelines (Writing Committee to Revise the 1998 Guidelines for the Management of Patients With Valvular Heart Disease): developed in collaboration with the Society of Cardiovascular Anesthesiologists: endorsed by the Society for Cardiovascular Angiography and Interventions and the Society of Thoracic Surgeons. *J Am Coll Cardiol* 2006;**48**(3):e1–148.

2. Edmunds LH Jr, Clark RE, Cohn LH, Grunkemeier GL, Miller DC, Weisel RD. Guidelines for reporting morbidity and mortality after cardiac valvular operations. Ad Hoc Liaison Committee for Standardizing Definitions of Prosthetic Heart Valve Morbidity of the American Association for Thoracic Surgery and The Society of Thoracic Surgeons. *J Thorac Cardiovasc Surg* 1996;**112**(3):708–11.

3. Yacoub MH, Cohn LH. Novel approaches to cardiac valve repair: from structure to function: Part II. *Circulation* 2004;**109**(9):1064–72.

4. Yacoub MH, Cohn LH. Novel approaches to cardiac valve repair: from structure to function: Part I. *Circulation* 2004;**109**(8):942–50.

5. Aicher D, Langer F, Kissinger A, Lausberg H, Fries R, Schafers HJ. Valve-sparing aortic root replacement in bicuspid aortic valves: a reasonable option? *J Thorac Cardiovasc Surg* 2004;**128**(5):662–8.

6. David TE, Feindel CM, Webb GD, Colman JM, Armstrong S, Maganti M. Long-term results of aortic valve-sparing operations for aortic root aneurysm. *J Thorac Cardiovasc Surg* 2006;**132**(2):347–54.

7. Hopkins RA. Aortic valve leaflet sparing and salvage surgery: evolution of techniques for aortic root reconstruction. *Eur J Cardiothorac Surg* 2003;**24**(6):886–97.

8. Miller DC. Valve-sparing aortic root replacement: current state of the art and where are we headed? *Ann Thorac Surg* 2007;**83**(2):S736–S739.

9. Sarsam MA, Yacoub M. Remodeling of the aortic valve anulus. *J Thorac Cardiovasc Surg* 1993;**105**(3):435–8.

10. David TE, Feindel CM. An aortic valve-sparing operation for patients with aortic incompetence and aneurysm of the ascending aorta. *J Thorac Cardiovasc Surg* 1992;**103**(4):617–21.

11. Kallenbach K, Pethig K, Leyh RG, Baric D, Haverich A, Harringer W. Acute dissection of the ascending aorta: first results of emergency valve sparing aortic root reconstruction. *Eur J Cardiothorac Surg* 2002;**22**(2):218–22.

12. Alsoufi B, Borger MA, Armstrong S, Maganti M, David TE. Results of valve preservation and repair for bicuspid aortic valve insufficiency. *J Heart Valve Dis* 2005;**14**(6):752–8.

13. Gott VL, Greene PS, Alejo DE, Cameron DE, Naftel DC, Miller DC *et al.* Replacement of the aortic root in patients with Marfan's syndrome. *N Engl J Med* 1999;**340**(17):1307–13.

14. Kallenbach K, Pethig K, Schwarz M, Milz A, Haverich A, Harringer W. Valve sparing aortic root reconstruction versus composite replacement – perioperative course and early complications. *Eur J Cardiothorac Surg* 2001;**20**(1):77–81.

15. Sundt TM, III, Mora BN, Moon MR, Bailey MS, Pasque MK, Gay WA Jr. Options for repair of a bicuspid aortic valve and ascending aortic aneurysm. *Ann Thorac Surg* 2000;**69**(5):1333–7.

16. Yun KL, Miller DC, Fann JI, Mitchell RS, Robbins RC, Moore KA *et al.* Composite valve graft versus separate aortic valve and ascending aortic replacement: is there still a role for the separate procedure? *Circulation* 1997;**96**(9 suppl):II–75.

17. David TE, Feindel CM, Armstrong S, Maganti M. Replacement of the ascending aorta with reduction of the diameter of the sinotubular junction to treat aortic insufficiency in patients with ascending aortic aneurysm. *J Thorac Cardiovasc Surg* 2007;**133**(2):414–18.

18. Yacoub MH, Gehle P, Chandrasekaran V, Birks EJ, Child A, Radley-Smith R. Late results of a valve-preserving operation in patients with aneurysms of the ascending aorta and root. *J Thorac Cardiovasc Surg* 1998;**115**(5):1080–90.

19. Erasmi AW, Sievers HH, Bechtel JF, Hanke T, Stierle U, Misfeld M. Remodeling or reimplantation for valve-sparing aortic root surgery? *Ann Thorac Surg* 2007;**83**(2): S752–S756.

20. Miller DC. Valve-sparing aortic root replacement in patients with the Marfan syndrome. *J Thorac Cardiovasc Surg* 2003;**125**(4): 773–8.

21. Kallenbach K, Leyh RG, Salcher R, Karck M, Hagl C, Haverich A. Acute aortic dissection versus aortic root aneurysm: comparison of indications for valve sparing aortic root reconstruction. *Eur J Cardiothorac Surg* 2004;**25**(5):663–70.

22. Leyh RG, Fischer S, Kallenbach K, Kofidis T, Pethig K, Harringer W *et al*. High failure rate after valve-sparing aortic root replacement using the "remodeling technique" in acute type A aortic dissection. *Circulation* 2002;**106**(12 suppl 1):I229–I233.

23. Karck M, Kallenbach K, Hagl C, Rhein C, Leyh R, Haverich A. Aortic root surgery in Marfan syndrome: comparison of aortic valve-sparing reimplantation versus composite grafting. *J Thorac Cardiovasc Surg* 2004;**127**(2):391–8.

24. Fazel SS, Ihlberg L, David TE. Mitral valve reconstruction in the failing heart. *Scand J Surg* 2007;**96**(2):111–20.

25. Gometza B, Al Halees Z, Shahid M, Hatle LK, Duran CM. Surgery for rheumatic mitral regurgitation in patients below twenty years of age. An analysis of failures. *J Heart Valve Dis* 1996;**5**(3):294–301.

26. Chauvaud S, Fuzellier JF, Berrebi A, Deloche A, Fabiani JN, Carpentier A. Long-term (29 years) results of reconstructive surgery in rheumatic mitral valve insufficiency. *Circulation* 2001;**104**(12 suppl 1):I12–I15.

27. Galloway AC, Colvin SB, Baumann FG, Grossi EA, Ribakove GH, Harty S *et al*. A comparison of mitral valve reconstruction with mitral valve replacement: intermediate-term results. *Ann Thorac Surg* 1989;**47**(5):655–62.

28. Grossi EA, Galloway AC, Miller JS, Ribakove GH, Culliford AT, Esposito R *et al*. Valve repair versus replacement for mitral insufficiency: when is a mechanical valve still indicated? *J Thorac Cardiovasc Surg* 1998;**115**(2):389–94.

29. Yau TM, El Ghoneimi YA, Armstrong S, Ivanov J, David TE. Mitral valve repair and replacement for rheumatic disease. *J Thorac Cardiovasc Surg* 2000;**119**(1):53–60.

30. Shuhaiber J, Anderson RJ. Meta-analysis of clinical outcomes following surgical mitral valve repair or replacement. *Eur J Cardiothorac Surg* 2007;**31**(2):267–75.

31. David TE, Uden DE, Strauss HD. The importance of the mitral apparatus in left ventricular function after correction of mitral regurgitation. *Circulation* 1983;**68**(3 Pt 2):II76–II82.

32. David TE, Burns RJ, Bacchus CM, Druck MN. Mitral valve replacement for mitral regurgitation with and without preservation of chordae tendineae. *J Thorac Cardiovasc Surg* 1984;**88**(5 Pt 1):718–25.

33. DeAnda A Jr, Komeda M, Nikolic SD, Daughters GT, Ingels NB, Miller DC. Left ventricular function, twist, and recoil after mitral valve replacement. *Circulation* 1995;**92**(9 suppl): II458–II466.

34. Lee EM, Shapiro LM, Wells FC. Importance of subvalvular preservation and early operation in mitral valve surgery. *Circulation* 1996;**94**(9):2117–23.

35. Moon MR, DeAnda A Jr, Daughters GT, Ingels NB, Miller DC. Effects of chordal disruption on regional left ventricular torsional deformation. *Circulation* 1996;**94**(9 suppl): II143–II151.

36. Fornes P, Heudes D, Fuzellier JF, Tixier D, Bruneval P, Carpentier A. Correlation between clinical and histologic patterns of degenerative mitral valve insufficiency: a histomorphometric study of 130 excised segments. *Cardiovasc Pathol* 1999;**8**(2): 81–92.

37. Eriksson MJ, Bitkover CY, Omran AS, David TE, Ivanov J, Ali MJ *et al*. Mitral annular disjunction in advanced myxomatous mitral valve disease: echocardiographic detection and surgical correction. *J Am Soc Echocardiogr* 2005;**18**(10):1014–22.

38. Carpentier A. Cardiac valve surgery – the "French correction". *J Thorac Cardiovasc Surg* 1983;**86**(3):323–37.

39. David TE, Bos J, Rakowski H. Mitral valve repair by replacement of chordae tendineae with polytetrafluoroethylene sutures. *J Thorac Cardiovasc Surg* 1991;**101**(3):495–501.

40. David TE. Update on mitral valve repair. *Ann Thorac Surg* 1995;**59**(5):1257–8.

41. Gillinov AM, Faber C, Houghtaling PL, Blackstone EH, Lam BK, Diaz R *et al*. Repair versus replacement for degenerative mitral valve disease with coexisting ischemic heart disease. *J Thorac Cardiovasc Surg* 2003;**125**(6):1350–62.

42. Lee EM, Shapiro LM, Wells FC. Superiority of mitral valve repair in surgery for degenerative mitral regurgitation. *Eur Heart J* 1997;**18**(4):655–63.

43. Mohty D, Orszulak TA, Schaff HV, Avierinos JF, Tajik JA, Enriquez-Sarano M. Very long-term survival and durability of mitral valve repair for mitral valve prolapse. *Circulation* 2001;**104**(12 suppl 1):I1–I7.

44. Yacoub M, Halim M, Radley-Smith R, McKay R, Nijveld A, Towers M. Surgical treatment of mitral regurgitation caused by floppy valves: repair versus replacement. *Circulation* 1981;**64**(2 Pt 2):II210–II216.

45. Braunberger E, Deloche A, Berrebi A, Abdallah F, Celestin JA, Meimoun P *et al*. Very long-term results (more than 20 years) of valve repair with carpentier's techniques in nonrheumatic mitral valve insufficiency. *Circulation* 2001;**104**(12 suppl 1):I8–11.

46. David TE, Ivanov J, Armstrong S, Rakowski H. Late outcomes of mitral valve repair for floppy valves: Implications for asymptomatic patients. *J Thorac Cardiovasc Surg* 2003;**125**(5): 1143–52.

47. David TE, Ivanov J, Armstrong S, Christie D, Rakowski H. A comparison of outcomes of mitral valve repair for degenerative disease with posterior, anterior, and bileaflet prolapse. *J Thorac Cardiovasc Surg* 2005;**130**(5).1242–9.

48. De Bonis M, Lorusso R, Lapenna E, Kassem S, De Cicco G, Torracca L *et al*. Similar long-term results of mitral valve repair for anterior compared with posterior leaflet prolapse. *J Thorac Cardiovasc Surg* 2006;**131**(2):364–70.

49. Enriquez-Sarano M, Avierinos JF, Messika-Zeitoun D, Detaint D, Capps M, Nkomo V *et al*. Quantitative determinants of the outcome of asymptomatic mitral regurgitation. *N Engl J Med* 2005;**352**(9):875–83.

50. Lee EM, Shapiro LM, Wells FC. Conservative operation for infective endocarditis of the mitral valve. *Ann Thorac Surg* 1998;**65**(4):1087–92.

51. Muehrcke DD, Cosgrove DM III, Lytle BW, Taylor PC, Burgar AM, Durnwald CP *et al*. Is there an advantage to repairing infected mitral valves? *Ann Thorac Surg* 1997;**63**(6): 1718–24.

52. Sternik L, Zehr KJ, Orszulak TA, Mullany CJ, Daly RC, Schaff HV. The advantage of repair of mitral valve in acute endocarditis. *J Heart Valve Dis* 2002;**11**(1):91–7.

53. Feringa HH, Shaw LJ, Poldermans D, Hoeks S, van der Wall EE, Dion RA *et al*. Mitral valve repair and replacement in endocarditis: a systematic review of literature. *Ann Thorac Surg* 2007;**83**(2):564–70.

54. Miller DC. Ischemic mitral regurgitation redux – to repair or to replace? *J Thorac Cardiovasc Surg* 2001;**122**(6):1059–62.

55. Al Radi OO, Austin PC, Tu JV, David TE, Yau TM. Mitral repair versus replacement for ischemic mitral regurgitation. *Ann Thorac Surg* 2005;**79**(4):1260–7.

56. Gillinov AM, Wierup PN, Blackstone EH, Bishay ES, Cosgrove DM, White J *et al*. Is repair preferable to replacement for ischemic mitral regurgitation? *J Thorac Cardiovasc Surg* 2001;**122**(6): 1125–41.

57. Grossi EA, Goldberg JD, LaPietra A, Ye X, Zakow P, Sussman M *et al*. Ischemic mitral valve reconstruction and replacement: Comparison of long-term survival and complications. *J Thorac Cardiovasc Surg* 2001;**122**(6):1107–24.

58. Daimon M, Fukuda S, Adams DH, McCarthy PM, Gillinov AM, Carpentier A *et al*. Mitral valve repair with Carpentier-McCarthy-Adams IMR ETlogix annuloplasty ring for ischemic mitral regurgitation: early echocardiographic results from a multi-center study. *Circulation* 2006;**114**(1 suppl):I588–I593.

59. McGee EC Jr, Gillinov AM, Blackstone EH, Rajeswaran J, Cohen G, Najam F *et al*. Recurrent mitral regurgitation after annuloplasty for functional ischemic mitral regurgitation. *J Thorac Cardiovasc Surg* 2004;**128**(6):916–24.

60. Gorman JH III, Gorman RC, Jackson BM, Enomoto Y, John-Sutton MG, Edmunds LH Jr. Annuloplasty ring selection for chronic ischemic mitral regurgitation: lessons from the ovine model. *Ann Thorac Surg* 2003;**76**(5):1556–63.

61. Hueb AC, Jatene FB, Moreira LF, Pomerantzeff PM, Kallas E, de Oliveira SA. Ventricular remodeling and mitral valve modifications in dilated cardiomyopathy: new insights from anatomic study. *J Thorac Cardiovasc Surg* 2002;**124**(6): 1216–24.

62. Spoor MT, Geltz A, Bolling SF. Flexible versus nonflexible mitral valve rings for congestive heart failure: differential durability of repair. *Circulation* 2006;**114**(1 suppl):I67–I71.

63. David TE, Komeda M, Pollick C, Burns RJ. Mitral valve annuloplasty: the effect of the type on left ventricular function. *Ann Thorac Surg* 1989;**47**(4):524–7.

64. Okada Y, Shomura T, Yamaura Y, Yoshikawa J. Comparison of the Carpentier and Duran prosthetic rings used in mitral reconstruction. *Ann Thorac Surg* 1995;**59**(3):658–62.

65. Borger MA, Murphy PM, Alam A, Fazel S, Maganti M, Armstrong S *et al*. Initial results of the chordal-cutting operation for ischemic mitral regurgitation. *J Thorac Cardiovasc Surgery* 2007;**133**(6):1483–92.

66. Levine RA, Schwammenthal E. Ischemic mitral regurgitation on the threshold of a solution: from paradoxes to unifying concepts. *Circulation* 2005;**112**(5):745–58.

67. Bolling SF, Deeb GM, Brunsting LA, Bach DS. Early outcome of mitral valve reconstruction in patients with end-stage cardiomyopathy. *J Thorac Cardiovasc Surg* 1995;**109**(4):676–82.

68. Bolling SF, Pagani FD, Deeb GM, Bach DS. Intermediate-term outcome of mitral reconstruction in cardiomyopathy. *J Thorac Cardiovasc Surg* 1998;**115**(2):381–6.

69. Wu AH, Aaronson KD, Bolling SF, Pagani FD, Welch K, Koelling TM. Impact of mitral valve annuloplasty on mortality risk in patients with mitral regurgitation and left ventricular systolic dysfunction. *J Am Coll Cardiol* 2005;**45**(3):381–7.

70. Bishay ES, McCarthy PM, Cosgrove DM, Hoercher KJ, Smedira NG, Mukherjee D *et al*. Mitral valve surgery in patients with severe left ventricular dysfunction. *Eur J Cardiothorac Surg* 2000;**17**(3):213–21.

71. Acker MA, Bolling S, Shemin R, Kirklin J, Oh JK, Mann DL *et al*. Mitral valve surgery in heart failure: insights from the Acorn Clinical Trial. *J Thorac Cardiovasc Surg* 2006;**132**(3):568–77.

72. Bhudia SK, McCarthy PM, Smedira NG, Lam BK, Rajeswaran J, Blackstone EH. Edge-to-edge (Alfieri) mitral repair: results in diverse clinical settings. *Ann Thorac Surg* 2004;**77**(5):1598–606.

73. De Bonis M, Lapenna E, La Canna G, Ficarra E, Pagliaro M, Torracca L *et al*. Mitral valve repair for functional mitral regurgitation in end-stage dilated cardiomyopathy: role of the "edge-to-edge" technique. *Circulation* 2005;**112**(9 suppl): I402–I408.

74. Tang GH, David TE, Singh SK, Maganti MD, Armstrong S, Borger MA. Tricuspid valve repair with an annuloplasty ring results in improved long-term outcomes. *Circulation* 2006;**114**(1 suppl):I577–I581.

75. McCarthy PM, Bhudia SK, Rajeswaran J, Hoercher KJ, Lytle BW, Cosgrove DM *et al*. Tricuspid valve repair: durability and risk factors for failure. *J Thorac Cardiovasc Surg* 2004;**127**(3): 674–85.

76. Rivera R, Duran E, Ajuria M. Carpentier's flexible ring versus De Vega's annuloplasty. A prospective randomized study. *J Thorac Cardiovasc Surg* 1985;**89**(2):196–203.

77. Nakano S, Kawashima Y, Hirose H, Matsuda H, Shimazaki Y, Taniguchi K *et al*. Evaluation of long-term results of bicuspidalization annuloplasty for functional tricuspid regurgitation. A seventeen-year experience with 133 consecutive patients. *J Thorac Cardiovasc Surg* 1988;**95**(2):340–5.

78. Bloomfield P, Kitchin AH, Wheatley DJ, Walbaum PR, Lutz W, Miller HC. A prospective evaluation of the Bjork-Shiley, Hancock, and Carpentier-Edwards heart valve prostheses. *Circulation* 1986;**73**(6):1213–22.

79. Bloomfield P, Wheatley DJ, Prescott RJ, Miller HC. Twelve-year comparison of a Bjork-Shiley mechanical heart valve with porcine bioprostheses. *N Engl J Med* 1991;**324**(9):573–9.

80. Oxenham H, Bloomfield P, Wheatley DJ, Lee RJ, Cunningham J, Prescott RJ *et al*. Twenty year comparison of a Bjork-Shiley mechanical heart valve with porcine bioprostheses. *Heart* 2003;**89**(7):715–21.

81. Hammermeister K, Sethi GK, Henderson WG, Grover FL, Oprian C, Rahimtoola SH. Outcomes 15 years after valve replacement with a mechanical versus a bioprosthetic valve:

final report of the Veterans Affairs randomized trial. *J Am Coll Cardiol* 2000;**36**(4):1152–8.

82. Hammermeister KE, Henderson WG, Burchfiel CM, Sethi GK, Souchek J, Oprian C *et al.* Comparison of outcome after valve replacement with a bioprosthesis versus a mechanical prosthesis: initial 5 year results of a randomized trial. *J Am Coll Cardiol* 1987;**10**(4):719–32.

83. Hammermeister KE, Sethi GK, Henderson WG, Oprian C, Kim T, Rahimtoola S. A comparison of outcomes in men 11 years after heart-valve replacement with a mechanical valve or bioprosthesis. Veterans Affairs Cooperative Study on Valvular Heart Disease. *N Engl J Med* 1993;**328**(18):1289–96.

84. Hirsh J, Levine MN. The optimal intensity of oral anticoagulant therapy. *JAMA* 1987;**258**(19):2723–6.

85. Adjusted-dose warfarin versus low-intensity, fixed-dose warfarin plus aspirin for high-risk patients with atrial fibrillation: Stroke Prevention in Atrial Fibrillation III randomised clinical trial. *Lancet* 1996;**348**(9028):633–8.

86. Banbury MK, Cosgrove DM III, White JA, Blackstone EH, Frater RW, Okies JE. Age and valve size effect on the long-term durability of the Carpentier-Edwards aortic pericardial bioprosthesis. *Ann Thorac Surg* 2001;**72**(3):753–7.

87. Burdon TA, Miller DC, Oyer PE, Mitchell RS, Stinson EB, Starnes VA *et al.* Durability of porcine valves at fifteen years in a representative North American patient population. *J Thorac Cardiovasc Surg* 1992;**103**(2):238–51.

88. Burr LH, Jamieson WR, Munro AI, Miyagishima RT, Janusz MT, Ling H *et al.* Structural valve deterioration in elderly patient populations with the Carpentier-Edwards standard and supra-annular porcine bioprostheses: a comparative study. *J Heart Valve Dis* 1992;**1**(1):87–91.

89. Cohn LH, Collins JJ Jr, DiSesa VJ, Couper GS, Peigh PS, Kowalker W *et al.* Fifteen-year experience with 1678 Hancock porcine bioprosthetic heart valve replacements. *Ann Surg* 1989;**210**(4):435–42.

90. Cohn LH, Collins JJ Jr, Rizzo RJ, Adams DH, Couper GS, Aranki SF. Twenty-year follow-up of the Hancock modified orifice porcine aortic valve. *Ann Thorac Surg* 1998;**66**(6 suppl):S30–S34.

91. Cosgrove DM, Lytle BW, Taylor PC, Camacho MT, Stewart RW, McCarthy PM *et al.* The Carpentier-Edwards pericardial aortic valve. Ten-year results. *J Thorac Cardiovasc Surg* 1995;**110**(3):651–62.

92. Jamieson WR, Rosado LJ, Munro AI, Gerein AN, Burr LH, Miyagishima RT *et al.* Carpentier-Edwards standard porcine bioprosthesis: primary tissue failure (structural valve deterioration) by age groups. *Ann Thorac Surg* 1988;**46**(2):155–62.

93. Jamieson WR, Tyers GF, Janusz MT, Miyagishima RT, Munro AI, Ling H *et al.* Age as a determinant for selection of porcine bioprostheses for cardiac valve replacement: experience with Carpentier-Edwards standard bioprosthesis. *Can J Cardiol* 1991;**7**(4):181–8.

94. Jamieson WR, Lemieux MD, Sullivan JA, Munro IA, Metras J, Cartier PC. Medtronic Intact porcine bioprosthesis experience to twelve years. *Ann Thorac Surg* 2001;**71**(5 suppl):S278–S281.

95. Jones EL, Weintraub WS, Craver JM, Guyton RA, Cohen CL, Corrigan VE *et al.* Ten-year experience with the porcine bioprosthetic valve: interrelationship of valve survival and patient survival in 1,050 valve replacements. *Ann Thorac Surg* 1990;**49**(3):370–83.

96. Pelletier LC, Carrier M, Leclerc Y, Dyrda I, Gosselin G. Influence of age on late results of valve replacement with porcine bioprostheses. *J Cardiovasc Surg (Torino)* 1992;**33**(5):526–33.

97. Pelletier LC, Carrier M, Leclerc Y, Dyrda I. The Carpentier-Edwards pericardial bioprosthesis: clinical experience with 600 patients. *Ann Thorac Surg* 1995;**60**(2 suppl):S297–S302.

98. Pomar JL, Jamieson WR, Pelletier LC, Gerein AN, Castella M, Brownlee RT. Mitroflow pericardial bioprosthesis: clinical performance to ten years. *Ann Thorac Surg* 1995;**60**(2 suppl):S305–S309.

99. Butchart EG, Li HH, Payne N, Buchan K, Grunkemeier GL. Twenty years' experience with the Medtronic Hall valve. *J Thorac Cardiovasc Surg* 2001;**121**(6):1090–100.

100. David TE, Ivanov J, Armstrong S, Feindel CM, Cohen G. Late results of heart valve replacement with the Hancock II bioprosthesis. *J Thorac Cardiovasc Surg* 2001;**121**(2):268–77.

101. Frater RW, Furlong P, Cosgrove DM, Okies JE, Colburn LQ, Katz AS *et al.* Long-term durability and patient functional status of the Carpentier-Edwards Perimount pericardial bioprosthesis in the aortic position. *J Heart Valve Dis* 1998;**7**(1):48–53.

102. Jamieson WR, Burr LH, Tyers GF, Miyagishima RT, Janusz MT, Ling H *et al.* Carpentier-Edwards supraannular porcine bioprosthesis: clinical performance to twelve years. *Ann Thorac Surg* 1995;**60**(2 suppl):S235–S240.

103. Khan SS, Chaux A, Blanche C, Kass RM, Cheng W, Fontana GP *et al.* A 20-year experience with the Hancock porcine xenograft in the elderly. *Ann Thorac Surg* 1998;**66**(6 suppl):S35–S39.

104. Lindblom D. Long-term clinical results after aortic valve replacement with the Bjork-Shiley prosthesis. *J Thorac Cardiovasc Surg* 1988;**95**(4):658–67.

105. Lindblom D. Long-term clinical results after mitral valve replacement with the Bjork-Shiley prosthesis. *J Thorac Cardiovasc Surg* 1988;**95**(2):321–33.

106. Lund O, Nielsen SL, Arildsen H, Ilkjaer LB, Pilegaard HK. Standard aortic St. Jude valve at 18 years: performance profile and determinants of outcome. *Ann Thorac Surg* 2000;**69**(5):1459–65.

107. Orszulak TA, Schaff HV, Puga FJ, Danielson GK, Mullany CJ, Anderson BJ *et al.* Event status of the Starr-Edwards aortic valve to 20 years: a benchmark for comparison. *Ann Thorac Surg* 1997;**63**(3):620–6.

108. Peterseim DS, Cen YY, Cheruvu S, Landolfo K, Bashore TM, Lowe JE *et al.* Long-term outcome after biologic versus mechanical aortic valve replacement in 841 patients. *J Thorac Cardiovasc Surg* 1999;**117**(5):890–7.

109. Yun KL, Miller DC, Moore KA, Mitchell RS, Oyer PE, Stinson EB *et al.* Durability of the Hancock MO bioprosthesis compared with standard aortic valve bioprostheses. *Ann Thorac Surg* 1995;**60**(2 suppl):S221–S228.

110. Grunkemeier GL, Li HH, Naftel DC, Starr A, Rahimtoola SH. Long-term performance of heart valve prostheses. *Curr Probl Cardiol* 2000;**25**(2):73–154.

111. Rahimtoola SH. Choice of prosthetic heart valve for adult patients. *J Am Coll Cardiol* 2003;**41**(6):893–904.

112. Pibarot P, Dumesnil JG. Prosthesis-patient mismatch: definition, clinical impact, and prevention. *Heart* 2006;**92**(8):1022–9.

113. David TE, Ropchan GC, Butany JW. Aortic valve replacement with stentless porcine bioprostheses. *J Card Surg* 1988; **3**(4):501–5.

114. Cohen G, Christakis GT, Joyner CD, Morgan CD, Tamariz M, Hanayama N *et al*. Are stentless valves hemodynamically superior to stented valves? A prospective randomized trial. *Ann Thorac Surg* 2002;**73**(3):767–75.

115. Borger MA, Carson SM, Ivanov J, Rao V, Scully HE, Feindel CM *et al*. Stentless aortic valves are hemodynamically superior to stented valves during mid-term follow-up: a large retrospective study. *Ann Thorac Surg* 2005;**80**(6):2180–5.

116. Lehmann S, Walther T, Kempfert J, Leontjev S, Rastan A, Falk V *et al*. Stentless versus conventional xenograft aortic valve replacement: midterm results of a prospectively randomized trial. *Ann Thorac Surg* 2007;**84**(2):467–72.

117. David TE, Feindel CM, Armstrong S, Bos J, Ivanov J. Aortic valve replacement with Toronto SPV bioprosthesis: excellent patient survival but poor valve survival. *J Thorac Cardiovasc Surg* 2008;**135**(1):19–24.

118. Ross DN. Homograft replacement of the aortic valve. *Lancet* 1962;**2**:487.

119. Barratt-Boyes BG, Roche AH, Whitlock RM. Six year review of the results of freehand aortic valve replacement using an antibiotic sterilized homograft valve. *Circulation* 1977;**55**(2): 353–61.

120. Byrne JG, Karavas AN, Mihaljevic T, Rawn JD, Aranki SF, Cohn LH. Role of the cryopreserved homograft in isolated elective aortic valve replacement. *Am J Cardiol* 2003;**91**(5):616–19.

121. O'Brien MF, Harrocks S, Stafford EG, Gardner MA, Pohlner PG, Tesar PJ *et al*. The homograft aortic valve: a 29-year, 99.3% follow up of 1,022 valve replacements. *J Heart Valve Dis* 2001;**10**(3):334–44.

122. O'Brien MF, McGiffin DC, Stafford EG, Gardner MA, Pohlner PF, McLachlan GJ *et al*. Allograft aortic valve replacement: long-term comparative clinical analysis of the viable cryopreserved and antibiotic 4 degrees C stored valves. *J Card Surg* 1991;**6**(4 suppl):534–43.

123. Daly RC, Orszulak TA, Schaff HV, McGovern E, Wallace RB. Long-term results of aortic valve replacement with nonviable homografts. *Circulation* 1991;**84**(5 suppl):III81–III88.

124. Lund O, Chandrasekaran V, Grocott-Mason R, Elwidaa H, Mazhar R, Khaghani A *et al*. Primary aortic valve replacement with allografts over twenty-five years: valve-related and procedure-related determinants of outcome. *J Thorac Cardiovasc Surg* 1999;**117**(1):77–90.

125. Dearani JA, Orszulak TA, Schaff HV, Daly RC, Anderson BJ, Danielson GK. Results of allograft aortic valve replacement for complex endocarditis. *J Thorac Cardiovasc Surg* 1997;**113**(2): 285–91.

126. Donaldson RM, Ross DM. Homograft aortic root replacement for complicated prosthetic valve endocarditis. *Circulation* 1984;**70**(3 Pt 2):I178–I181.

127. Haydock D, Barratt-Boyes B, Macedo T, Kirklin JW, Blackstone E. Aortic valve replacement for active infectious endocarditis in 108 patients. A comparison of freehand allograft valves with mechanical prostheses and bioprostheses. *J Thorac Cardiovasc Surg* 1992;**103**(1):130–9.

128. Palka P, Harrocks S, Lange A, Burstow DJ, O'Brien MF. Primary aortic valve replacement with cryopreserved aortic allograft: an echocardiographic follow-up study of 570 patients. *Circulation* 2002;**105**(1):61–6.

129. Athanasiou T, Jones C, Jin R, Grunkemeier GL, Ross DN. Homograft implantation techniques in the aortic position: to preserve or replace the aortic root? *Ann Thorac Surg* 2006;**81**(5):1578–85.

130. Sundt TM III, Rasmi N, Wong K, Radley-Smith R, Khaghani A, Yacoub MH. Reoperative aortic valve operation after homograft root replacement: surgical options and results. *Ann Thorac Surg* 1995;**60**(2 suppl):S95–S99.

131. Ross DN. Replacement of aortic and mitral valves with a pulmonary autograft. *Lancet* 1967;**2**(7523):956–8.

132. Ross DN, Radley-Smith R, Somerville J. Pulmonary autograft replacement for severe aortic valve disease. *Br Heart J* 1969;**31**(6):797–8.

133. Chambers JC, Somerville J, Stone S, Ross DN. Pulmonary autograft procedure for aortic valve disease: long-term results of the pioneer series. *Circulation* 1997;**96**(7):2206–14.

134. Elkins RC. The Ross operation: a 12-year experience. *Ann Thorac Surg* 1999;**68**(3 suppl):S14–S18.

135. Kouchoukos NT, Davila-Roman VG, Spray TL, Murphy SF, Perrillo JB. Replacement of the aortic root with a pulmonary autograft in children and young adults with aortic-valve disease. *N Engl J Med* 1994;**330**(1):1–6.

136. Melo JQ, Abecasis M, Neves JP, Canada M, Ribeiras R, Parreira L *et al*. What are the limits for the Ross operation? *Cardiovasc Surg* 1996;**4**(4):526–9.

137. Jaggers J, Harrison JK, Bashore TM, Davis RD, Glower DD, Ungerleider RM. The Ross procedure: shorter hospital stay, decreased morbidity, and cost effective. *Ann Thorac Surg* 1998;**65**(6):1553–7.

138. Sievers HH, Hanke T, Stierle U, Bechtel MF, Graf B, Robinson DR *et al*. A critical reappraisal of the Ross operation: renaissance of the subcoronary implantation technique? *Circulation* 2006;**114**(1 suppl):I504–I511.

139. Kouchoukos NT. Aortic allografts and pulmonary autografts for replacement of the aortic valve and aortic root. *Ann Thorac Surg* 1999;**67**(6):1846–8.

140. David TE, Omran A, Ivanov J, Armstrong S, de Sa MP, Sonnenberg B *et al*. Dilation of the pulmonary autograft after the Ross procedure. *J Thorac Cardiovasc Surg* 2000;**119**(2):210–20.

141. de Sa M, Moshkovitz Y, Butany J, David TE. Histologic abnormalities of the ascending aorta and pulmonary trunk in patients with bicuspid aortic valve disease: clinical relevance to the Ross procedure. *J Thorac Cardiovasc Surg* 1999;**118**(4):588–94.

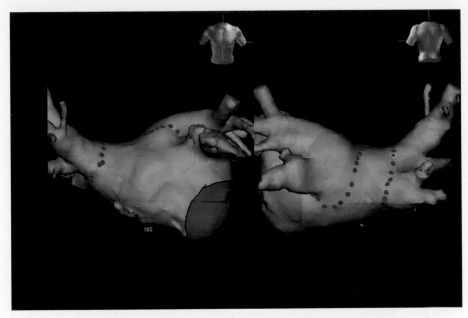

Plate 38.1 Typical lesion set used to perform pulmonary vein isolation. The figure shows an ESI/NavX reconstruct of the left atrium in two views. On the left is an anteroposterior view; on the right is a posteroanterior view. The RF lesion points are represented by the red dots. It can be appreciated that ablation is performed encircling the right- and left-sided veins as two separate units. The ablation points are distant from the ostia of the pulmonary veins, thereby minimizing the risk of pulmonary vein stenosis. The above representation is the usual minimal ablation set in most electrophysiology laboratories; additional ablation may be performed along the posterior LA wall, LA roof, mitral isthmus (from the left inferior pulmonary vein to the mitral valve), along the interatrial septum and also in areas where complex fractionated atrial electrograms are observed.

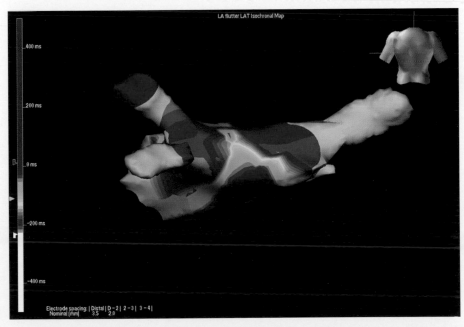

Plate 38.2 Atypical flutter in a patient following previous RF ablation for atrial fibrillation. An ESI/NavX electroanatomic activation map of the tachycardia in the same patient. This demonstrates activation breaking through the roof of the left atrium, where a region of slow conduction was observed. Ablation at this point terminated the tachycardia.

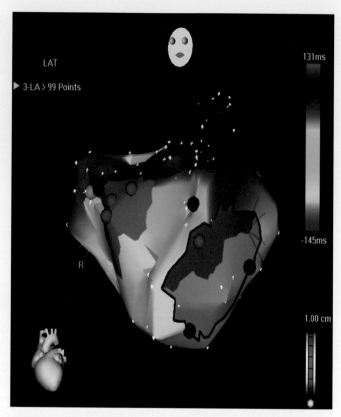

Plate 38.3 Atypical flutter in a patient following previous RF ablation for atrial fibrillation. Carto electroanatomic activation map of the tachycardia in the same patient. This demonstrates a gap between the right superior PV and a septal scar in gray. Such gaps between an area of scar and an anatomical boundary can facilitate atypical atrial flutter in patients following left atrial ablation.

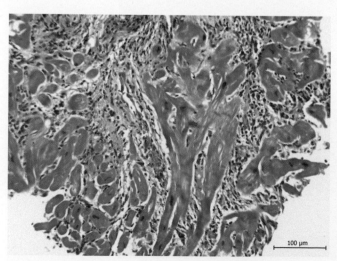

Plate 48.1 Lymphocytic myocarditis. A mixed inflammatory infiltrate with lymphocytes associated with damaged myocytes. Granulomas and giant cells are absent. (Courtesy of Dylan Miller MD.)

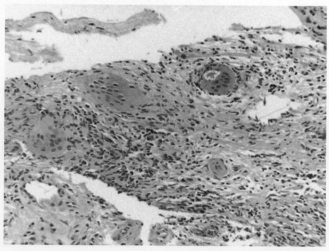

Plate 48.2 Giant cell myocarditis. Multinucleated giant cells are seen in association with a lymphocytic infiltrate and extensive myocyte damage.

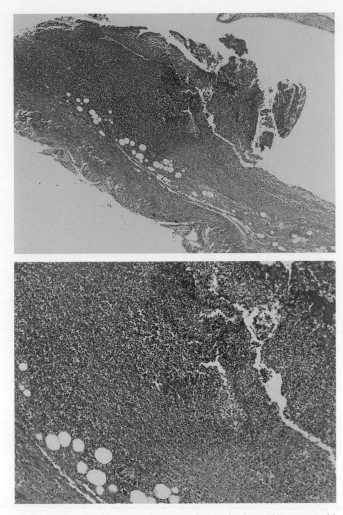

Plate 59.1 Histopathology of an excised mitral valve demonstrating distortion of normal valve architecture and intense inflammation.

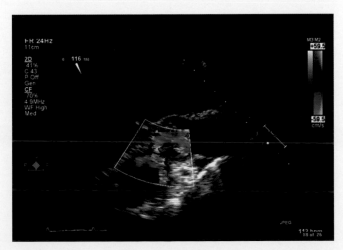

Plate 59.2 A TEE view demonstrating color flow between the aorta and right ventricle.

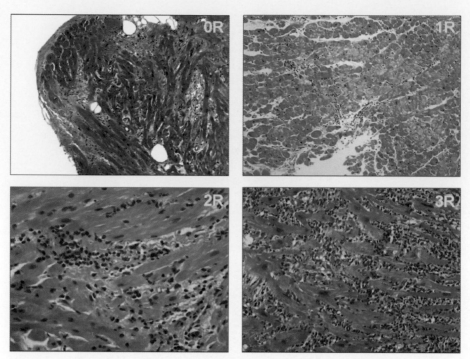

Plate 68.1 Cell-mediated rejection – 2004 ISHLT grading.

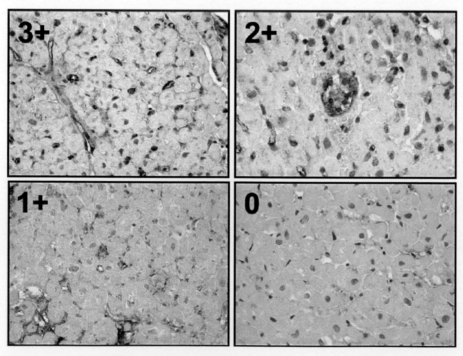

Plate 68.2 Antibody-mediated rejection with intensity of C4d staining, 0 to 3+.

f patients and their risk factors for endocarditis
o major changes in the microbiologic causation
rdits.[9] In the contemporary, multinational study,
ational Collaboration on Endocarditis or ICE reg-
1179 patients with definite native or prosthetic
is), 32% cases were attributable to *S. aureus*, 18%
reptococci, 11% enterococci, 11% coagulase-neg-
hylococci, 5% other streptococcal species, 2%
K gram-negative bacteria, 2% fungi, and 2%
oup.[10] Among those with *S. aureus* endocarditis,
associated infection accounted for 39% of

, the microbiology of prosthetic valve endocar-
) has changed. Whereas coagulase-negative
ccal infection (such as *S. epidermidis*) was previ-
most common causative species, a recent, large
6 cases of definite PVE found that *S. aureus*
s the predominant cause of infection, with coag-
ive staphylococci accounting for 16.9%.[11]

nesis

ing valvular or endocardial condition, such as
e prolapse with regurgitation, degenerative
disease (including bicuspid aortic valve) and
heart disease, is a major host factor related to
t of IE. Endothelial damage and denudation of
lium exposes the underlying basement mem-
osters platelet and fibrin deposition, a process
spontaneously in individuals with valvular
se. These deposits are called non-bacterial
endocarditis and form the nidus for vegetations
g of bacteremia. The ability of micro-organisms
denuded endothelium is another factor related
ent of IE. The classic lesion of endocarditis, the
s thus made up of fibrin, platelets, inflamma-
d micro-organisms, adherent to the endothe-
heart (Plate 59.1).

s of endocarditis is dependent on findings of
ith an organism associated with endocarditis
of endocardial involvement. Because these
lings may not be sought unless the possibility
itis is considered, careful attention to the
ry and physical examination is critical to the
nosis. The clinical presentation of IE is highly
can range from chronic fatigue with low-
o acute heart failure due to new, severe val-
tation. While the virulence of the organism
acuity of presentation, the onset of infection

in most cases is quickly followed by the onset of symptoms. Most patients with endocarditis develop symptoms within two weeks of bacteremia.[12] In general, four processes contribute to the clinical presentation of endocarditis: (1) infection on the valve, including the local intracardiac complications; (2) septic or aseptic embolization to distant organs; (3) continuous bacteremia, often with metastatic foci of infection; and (4) circulating immune complexes and other immunopathologic factors.[8]

Approximately 85% patients present with fever, although this finding may not be present in immunosuppressed states and in patients who have previously been on antibiotic therapy. Non-specific symptoms such as chills (42–75%), sweats (25%), anorexia (25–55%), weight loss (25–35%), malaise (25–40%), dyspnea (20–40%), and cough (25%) are common. In addition, predisposing conditions or risk factors for the development of endocarditis, including a history of structural heart disease, injection drug use or recent invasive procedure, should be sought in the patient's history.

Evidence of a *new or changing* regurgitant murmur in the presence of fever of undetermined origin should prompt further, objective evaluation for possible endocarditis. Embolic phenomena, a common extracardiac complication of endocarditis, may present with localizing symptoms.[8] The patient should be carefully examined for any peripheral stigmata of endocarditis such as petechiae, splinter hemorrhages, Janeway lesions (10%), Osler nodes (10–25%) and Roth spots. Many of these findings are immune mediated. Although Janeway lesions, Osler nodes, and Roth spots are more specific abnormalities for endocarditis, they may occur in other conditions and their low frequency in cases of proven endocarditis limits their diagnostic utility for this condition.

Laboratory testing

Blood cultures

Blood cultures remain the definitive microbiologic procedure for the diagnosis of IE. Continuous and low-grade bacteremia makes it unnecessary to await fever spikes or chills to obtain blood cultures and the first two blood cultures yield an etiologic agent in 90% of cases.[13] In antibiotic-naïve patients, it is recommended that at least three blood culture sets from separate venepunctures should be obtained over the first 24 hours, which will increase the yield to more than 95% in cases of untreated endocarditis with continuous bacteremia (**Class I, Level A**). Finally, each culture media bottle should be inoculated with at least 10 mL of blood to increase the number of colony-forming units per culture (**Class I, Level B**). The results of blood cultures should be interpreted based on the specific micro-organisms identified as well as the recognized, constant nature of bacteremia in endocarditis.

PART III

59 Infective endocarditis

Zainab Samad and Andrew Wang
Duke University Medical Center, Durham, NC, USA

Introduction and historical perspective

Infective endocarditis (IE) is a non-contagious, microbial infection of the valves and endocardium of the heart. The disease was first described by a French physician, Jean Francois Fernel, in his book *Medicina* in 1554.[1] Almost 300 years later, in 1885, Sir William Osler gave a comprehensive account of endocarditis in three Gulstonian lectures.[2] Osler astutely noted the host factors which predisposed to developing endocarditis, describing it *"as a primary disease of the lining membrane of the heart or its valves, either attacking persons in previous good health or more often attacking the debilitated and dissipated and those with old valve lesions."*

Nomenclature

Initially known as bacterial endocarditis, infective endocarditis (IE) is the current nomenclature used since fungi are recognized as potential causative organisms.[3] Infection of arteriovenous shunts, arterio-arterial shunts (such as patent ductus arteriosus), and coarctation of the aorta, although known as infectious endarteritis, are clinically and pathologically similar to infective endocarditis. Endocarditis is classified as acute or subacute based on the rapidity of progression and presentation of the illness prior to diagnosis, factors related to both the virulence of the causative organism and host immune response. Acute endocarditis develops over days to weeks with marked toxicity and a course involving valvular destruction, extracardiac complications and, if untreated, death. In contrast, subacute endocarditis follows an indolent course, progressing slowly

over weeks to months, cau... tion and rarely metastatic cations.[4] Native valve end... native cardiac valves, whe... tis involves a biologic or ... prosthetic repair materia... thetic valve endocarditis... (within 12 months of val... than 12 months after imp... ditis is defined as develo... more than 48 hours befo... consistent with endoca... refers to an infection... as a permanent pacema... defibrillator, the infectio... with IE.

Incidence and epi...

The incidence of IE vari... ulation reported in Fra... Philadelphia.[6] This rang... to differences in predis... factors, such as injectio... valve endocarditis incr... 30/100000 after 30 ye... patient with endocardi... related to the decreas... disease (the major pre... rian times)[7] and increa... vular disease in the agi... diagnosed in men, wi... ratios of 1.7:1.[8]

In earlier eras, strep... nant cause of native... delivery of healthcare... sive procedures and...

graphics... have led... of endoca... the Intern... istry (n =... endocard... viridans s... ative sta... non-HAC... HACEK g... healthcare... cases.[10]

Similar... ditis (PV... staphyloc... ously the... study of ... (23.0%) wa... ulase-nega...

Pathoge...

A pre-exist... mitral val... aortic valv... congenital... developme... the endoth... brane and ... that occurs... heart disea... thrombotic... in the settin... to adhere to... to developn... vegetation,... tory cells a... lium of the...

Diagnosi...

The diagnos... bacteremia ... and evidenc... objective fin... of endocard... patient's his... eventual dia... variable, an... grade fever ... vular regurg... can influenc...

Evidence-Based Cardiology, 3rd edition. Edited by S. Yusuf, J.A. Cairns, A.J. Camm, E.L. Fallen, and B.J. Gersh. © 2010 Blackwell Publishing, ISBN: 978-1-4051-5925-8.

59 Infective endocarditis

Zainab Samad and Andrew Wang
Duke University Medical Center, Durham, NC, USA

Introduction and historical perspective

Infective endocarditis (IE) is a non-contagious, microbial infection of the valves and endocardium of the heart. The disease was first described by a French physician, Jean Francois Fernel, in his book *Medicina* in 1554.[1] Almost 300 years later, in 1885, Sir William Osler gave a comprehensive account of endocarditis in three Gulstonian lectures.[2] Osler astutely noted the host factors which predisposed to developing endocarditis, describing it *"as a primary disease of the lining membrane of the heart or its valves, either attacking persons in previous good health or more often attacking the debilitated and dissipated and those with old valve lesions."*

Nomenclature

Initially known as bacterial endocarditis, infective endocarditis (IE) is the current nomenclature used since fungi are recognized as potential causative organisms.[3] Infection of arteriovenous shunts, arterio-arterial shunts (such as patent ductus arteriosus), and coarctation of the aorta, although known as infectious endarteritis, are clinically and pathologically similar to infective endocarditis. Endocarditis is classified as acute or subacute based on the rapidity of progression and presentation of the illness prior to diagnosis, factors related to both the virulence of the causative organism and host immune response. Acute endocarditis develops over days to weeks with marked toxicity and a course involving valvular destruction, extracardiac complications and, if untreated, death. In contrast, subacute endocarditis follows an indolent course, progressing slowly over weeks to months, causing less severe valvular destruction and rarely metastatic infection or extracardiac complications.[4] Native valve endocarditis involves any of the four native cardiac valves, whereas prosthetic valve endocarditis involves a biologic or mechanical valve replacement or prosthetic repair material (e.g. annuloplasty ring). Prosthetic valve endocarditis is further classified into early (within 12 months of valve replacement) and late (greater than 12 months after implantation). Nosocomial endocarditis is defined as developing in a patient hospitalized for more than 48 hours before the onset of signs or symptoms consistent with endocarditis. Cardiac device infection refers to an infection of an intracardiac device such as a permanent pacemaker or implantable cardioverter-defibrillator, the infection of which may also be associated with IE.

Incidence and epidemiology

The incidence of IE varies regionally from 2.6/100 000 population reported in France[5] to 11.6/100 000 population in Philadelphia.[6] This range of incidence has been attributed to differences in predisposing cardiac conditions or risk factors, such as injection drug use. The incidence of native valve endocarditis increases with age and exceeds 14.5–30/100 000 after 30 years of age. The average age of the patient with endocarditis has increased over time, likely related to the decreased prevalence of rheumatic heart disease (the major predisposing cardiac condition in Oslerian times)[7] and increased prevalence of degenerative valvular disease in the aging population. IE is more commonly diagnosed in men, with studies showing male-to-female ratios of 1.7:1.[8]

In earlier eras, streptococcal species were the predominant cause of native valve IE. However, changes in the delivery of healthcare, with increasing exposure to invasive procedures and devices, and the changing demo-

Evidence-Based Cardiology, 3rd edition. Edited by S. Yusuf, J.A. Cairns, A.J. Camm, E.L. Fallen, and B.J. Gersh. © 2010 Blackwell Publishing, ISBN: 978-1-4051-5925-8.

graphics of patients and their risk factors for endocarditis have led to major changes in the microbiologic causation of endocarditis.[9] In the contemporary, multinational study, the International Collaboration on Endocarditis or ICE registry (n = 1179 patients with definite native or prosthetic endocarditis), 32% cases were attributable to *S. aureus*, 18% viridans streptococci, 11% enterococci, 11% coagulase-negative staphylococci, 5% other streptococcal species, 2% non-HACEK gram-negative bacteria, 2% fungi, and 2% HACEK group.[10] Among those with *S. aureus* endocarditis, healthcare-associated infection accounted for 39% of cases.[10]

Similarly, the microbiology of prosthetic valve endocarditis (PVE) has changed. Whereas coagulase-negative staphylococcal infection (such as *S. epidermidis*) was previously the most common causative species, a recent, large study of 556 cases of definite PVE found that *S. aureus* (23.0%) was the predominant cause of infection, with coagulase-negative staphylococci accounting for 16.9%.[11]

Pathogenesis

A pre-existing valvular or endocardial condition, such as mitral valve prolapse with regurgitation, degenerative aortic valve disease (including bicuspid aortic valve) and congenital heart disease, is a major host factor related to development of IE. Endothelial damage and denudation of the endothelium exposes the underlying basement membrane and fosters platelet and fibrin deposition, a process that occurs spontaneously in individuals with valvular heart disease. These deposits are called non-bacterial thrombotic endocarditis and form the nidus for vegetations in the setting of bacteremia. The ability of micro-organisms to adhere to denuded endothelium is another factor related to development of IE. The classic lesion of endocarditis, the vegetation, is thus made up of fibrin, platelets, inflammatory cells and micro-organisms, adherent to the endothelium of the heart (Plate 59.1).

Diagnosis

The diagnosis of endocarditis is dependent on findings of bacteremia with an organism associated with endocarditis and evidence of endocardial involvement. Because these objective findings may not be sought unless the possibility of endocarditis is considered, careful attention to the patient's history and physical examination is critical to the eventual diagnosis. The clinical presentation of IE is highly variable, and can range from chronic fatigue with low-grade fever to acute heart failure due to new, severe valvular regurgitation. While the virulence of the organism can influence acuity of presentation, the onset of infection

in most cases is quickly followed by the onset of symptoms. Most patients with endocarditis develop symptoms within two weeks of bacteremia.[12] In general, four processes contribute to the clinical presentation of endocarditis: (1) infection on the valve, including the local intracardiac complications; (2) septic or aseptic embolization to distant organs; (3) continuous bacteremia, often with metastatic foci of infection; and (4) circulating immune complexes and other immunopathologic factors.[8]

Approximately 85% patients present with fever, although this finding may not be present in immunosuppressed states and in patients who have previously been on antibiotic therapy. Non-specific symptoms such as chills (42–75%), sweats (25%), anorexia (25–55%), weight loss (25–35%), malaise (25–40%), dyspnea (20–40%), and cough (25%) are common. In addition, predisposing conditions or risk factors for the development of endocarditis, including a history of structural heart disease, injection drug use or recent invasive procedure, should be sought in the patient's history.

Evidence of a *new or changing* regurgitant murmur in the presence of fever of undetermined origin should prompt further, objective evaluation for possible endocarditis. Embolic phenomena, a common extracardiac complication of endocarditis, may present with localizing symptoms.[8] The patient should be carefully examined for any peripheral stigmata of endocarditis such as petechiae, splinter hemorrhages, Janeway lesions (10%), Osler nodes (10–25%) and Roth spots. Many of these findings are immune mediated. Although Janeway lesions, Osler nodes, and Roth spots are more specific abnormalities for endocarditis, they may occur in other conditions and their low frequency in cases of proven endocarditis limits their diagnostic utility for this condition.

Laboratory testing

Blood cultures

Blood cultures remain the definitive microbiologic procedure for the diagnosis of IE. Continuous and low-grade bacteremia makes it unnecessary to await fever spikes or chills to obtain blood cultures and the first two blood cultures yield an etiologic agent in 90% of cases.[13] In antibiotic-naïve patients, it is recommended that at least three blood culture sets from separate venepunctures should be obtained over the first 24 hours, which will increase the yield to more than 95% in cases of untreated endocarditis with continuous bacteremia (**Class I, Level A**). Finally, each culture media bottle should be inoculated with at least 10 mL of blood to increase the number of colony-forming units per culture (**Class I, Level B**). The results of blood cultures should be interpreted based on the specific micro-organisms identified as well as the recognized, constant nature of bacteremia in endocarditis.

Other laboratory data, although useful clues, are not diagnostic due to their lack of specificity. Hematologic parameters are often abnormal. A normocytic, normochromic anemia (70–90%), thrombocytopenia (5–15%) and leukocytosis (30%) dominate the peripheral blood picture. The differential cell count is usually normal, but there may be a neutrophil predominance. The erythrocyte sedimentation rate (ESR) and C-reactive protein concentrations are usually elevated.[13] Rheumatoid factor assay is positive in up to half of the cases, especially if the illness is protracted.[14] Urinalysis may demonstrate microscopic hematuria and mild proteinuria. Red blood cell casts and heavy proteinuria can be seen in patients with immune complex glomerulonephritis.[8,13]

Electrocardiography

Although the electrocardiogram lacks sufficient sensitivity and specificity for the diagnosis of endocarditis, electrocardiographic abnormalities commonly occur in patients with endocarditis (26% in one cohort) and are associated with invasive infection and increased in-hospital mortality. The presence of atrioventricular heart block in a patient with IE is diagnostic of the presence of a ring abscess, typically of the aortic valve with invasion posteriorly toward the atrioventricular conduction system. Meine *et al* found that 53% of patients with invasive infection had EKG changes and about a third of the patients with EKG conduction abnormalities died during hospitalization in their cohort of 137 patients with definite endocarditis.[15]

Diagnostic criteria for IE

Diagnostic criteria developed by Petersdorf and Pellitier in 1977[13] and subsequently by Von Reyn in 1981[16] have been replaced by the Duke Criteria, first proposed in 1994,[17] which incorporated echocardiographic findings and isolation of "typical" micro-organisms into the case definitions. Several comparative studies of the Von Reyn and Duke Criteria in various cohorts established the superior sensitivity of the Duke criteria.[18–25] Recent modifications of the Duke criteria have added more specificity to the schema[26] (Table 59.1). In addition to their diagnostic utility in clinical

Table 59.1 The modified Duke Criteria and case definitions of infective endocarditis

Modified Duke Criteria	Case definitions

Major Criteria
Blood culture positive for IE
Typical microbes consistent with IE from 2 separate blood cultures: viridans streptococci, *Strep bovis*, HACEK group, *Staph aureus*, community-acquired enterococci in absence of another focus; or
 	
Micro-organisms consistent with IE from persistently positive blood cultures defined as follows: at least 2 blood cultures drawn >12 h apart or all of three or majority of >4 separate blood cultures
 	
Single positive blood culture for *Coxiella burnetti* or antiphase IgG antibody titer >1:800
 	
Evidence of endocardial involvement
 	
Echo positive for IE defined as follows:
  Oscillating intracardiac mass on valve or supporting structure
  Abscess
  New partial dehiscence of prosthetic valve
 	
New valvular regurgitation
 	
Minor criteria
 	
Predisposition; predisposing heart condition or injection drug use
 	
Fever, temperature > 38 °C
 	
Vascular phenomena, major arterial emboli, septic pulmonary infarcts, mycotic aneurysm, intracranial hemorrhage, conjunctival hemorrhage, and Janeway lesions
 	
Immunologic phenomena; glomerulonephritis, Osler's nodes, Roth's spots, rheumatoid factor
 	
Microbiologic evidence: positive blood cultures but does not meet a major criterion as noted above, or serologic evidence of active infection with organism consistent with causing IE
	Definitive Infective Endocarditis
	Pathologic criteria
	1. Micro-organisms demonstrated by culture or histologic examination of a vegetation, a vegetation that has embolized or an intracardiac abscess specimen; or
	2. Pathologic lesions; vegetation or intracardiac abscess confirmed by histologic examination showing active endocarditis
	
	Clinical criteria
	1. 2 major criteria; or
	2. 1 major and 3 minor criteria; or
	3. 5 minor criteria
	
	Possible Infective Endocarditis
	1. 1 major criterion and 1 minor criterion; or
	2. 3 minor criteria
	
	Rejected
	1. Firm alternative diagnosis explaining evidence of infective endocarditis; or
	2. Resolution of infective endocarditis syndrome with antibiotic therapy for ≤4 days; or
	3. No pathologic evidence of infective endocarditis at surgery or autopsy, with antibiotic therapy for < 4 days; or
	4. Does not meet criteria for possible infective endocarditis, as above

Adapted from Li[8].

care, these criteria provide a common case definition for studies of this condition.

Echocardiography and other cardiac imaging modalities

Echocardiography provides not only non-invasive evidence of endocardial infection that, as described above, is among the major diagnostic criteria for endocarditis, but also important hemodynamic information regarding the presence and severity of valvular regurgitation. It is of fundamental importance in detecting vegetations, visualized as "echogenic distinct masses" from the adjacent valve with "independent motion", from the valve itself (Fig. 59.1).

The diagnostic utility of transthoracic echocardiography (TTE) for suspected IE is highest in patients with intermediate to high likelihood of this disease[27] (e.g. a patient with a new or changed heart murmur and bacteremia). Hence, TTE should be performed in all patients with suspected IE (**Class I, Level A**). However, the diagnostic sensitivity of TTE for the visualization of an intracardiac vegetation or abscess is limited, ranging from 40% to 80%, and thus the diagnosis of endocarditis cannot be "ruled out" on the basis of a negative study.

Transesophageal echocardiography (TEE) has greater spatial resolution than TTE and thus is more sensitive than TTE for the detection of intracardiac vegetations As a result, TEE should be performed in patients with a high likelihood of IE and a negative TTE[28,29] (**Class I, Level A**) (Plate 59.2). Although TTE and TEE have been found to have concordant results in approximately half of patients with suspected endocarditis, TEE results in additional diagnostic information in a high percentage, particularly those with prosthetic valves.[30] Specific subsets of patients

in which TEE should be performed, even as the primary imaging modality (without TTE) include those with prosthetic heart valves and suspected endocarditis (**Class I, Level B**) and those with persistent staphylococcal bacteremia without known source (**Class IIa, Level B**) or nosocomial staphylococcal bacteremia (**Class IIb, Level C**). For instance, TEE has been shown to be a cost-effective method for determining the duration of antibiotic therapy (two weeks vs four weeks) compared to empiric duration in patients with intravascular catheter associated *S. aureus* bacteremia.[31] TEE has a high sensitivity and specificity (87% and 95%, respectively) and therefore should be performed in patients with endocarditis when perivalvular abscess is suspected (**Class I, Level A**).[32]

Cardiac magnetic resonance imaging with contrast appears promising for the detection of perivalvular abscesses, thrombus associated with vegetations, valvular complications and aortocameral fistulas, although temporal resolution may limit its use for detection of vegetation (**Level C**). Cardiac computed tomography has also been used to detect aortic root abscess. However, clinical experience with these techniques in IE patients is limited and their operating characteristics (sensitivity and specificity) in comparison to echocardiography are not well defined.[33–35]

Routine coronary angiography is recommended in patients over age 55 prior to surgery for IE or in those at high risk for coronary artery disease.

Treatment

The management of IE has evolved over the last few decades with improvements in diagnostic capabilities and therapy.[17,32] Rapid diagnosis, early risk stratification, institution of appropriate bactericidal therapy, and prompt recognition and treatment of complications are key elements in a good outcome. Central to the care of these complex patients is the involvement and close collaboration of multiple interdisciplinary teams including the general medicine team, infectious diseases specialists, cardiologists, and cardiothoracic surgeons.

Antibiotic therapy

Antibiotic therapy has improved survival in IE by 70–80%, and has been shown to reduce the incidence of complications of endocarditis. Although the choice of antimicrobial therapy is mainly guided by the infecting organism and its antibiotic susceptibilities, there are three basic tenets of treatment that are aimed at eradicating the infecting organism from vegetations.

First, a prolonged course of antibiotic treatment (4–6ix weeks) is necessary to eradicate infection because bacterial concentration within vegetations is as high as 10^9 to

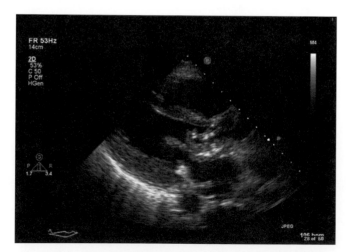

Figure 59.1 TTE parasternal long axis view demonstrating a large vegetation on the ventricular aspect of the anterior mitral valve leaflet extending into the left ventricular outflow tract.

10^{11}CFU/gram of tissue and organisms deep within vegetations are inaccessible to phagocytic cells[36,37] (**Class I, Level A**). Consensus dictates that the counting of days for recommended duration of treatment should begin on the first day of negative blood cultures in cases where blood cultures had been positive previously (**Class IIa, Level B**). For patients who undergo valve replacement for endocarditis, the postoperative course of antibiotics should be similar to that prescribed for PVE rather than native valve endocarditis. If the excised native valve tissue is culture negative, then the recommended duration of treatment for PVE should be given after subtracting the duration of antibiotics administered prior to valve replacement surgery (**Class IIa, Level C**).[38]

Second, parenteral administration of antibiotic therapy is necessary to achieve adequate drug levels required to eradicate infection (**Class I, Level A**). Parenteral therapy is typically initiated in the hospital setting, and the patient may be transitioned to outpatient parenteral antibiotic therapy for the remaining duration after an initial period of observation to assess for clinical response to therapy (e.g. clearance of bacteremia, absence of complications). Oral therapy for endocarditis has been described in certain situations but is not recommended, particularly for left-sided endocarditis[39,40] (**Class IIb, Level B**).

Third, because of rising antimicrobial resistance amongst organisms, combination therapy typically involving a beta-lactam and aminoglycoside antibiotic is recommended. Combination therapy has been shown to reduce the duration of bacteremia in *S. aureus* endocarditis[41] although this more rapid resolution of bacteremia was not associated with an improved clinical response or outcome. While administering combination therapy, both antibiotics should be given temporally close together so that maximum synergistic killing effect is obtained.[38] In addition, careful monitoring of the dosage and renal function should be performed, as combination therapy has been associated with a higher rate of renal dysfunction.[41]

Initial choice of therapy should be guided by clinical findings and microbiologic evidence. Antibiotic therapy should only be administered after obtaining at least three sets of blood cultures, since a high percentage of "culture-negative" endocarditis may be attributable to prior antibiotic therapy. In uncomplicated cases with a subacute course, treatment can be delayed up to 48 hours till the results of the initial blood cultures are available. In cases complicated by sepsis, valvular dysfunction, conduction disturbances or embolic phenomena, empiric antimicrobial therapy should be initiated after obtaining blood cultures.[42] Clinical efficacy studies support the use of antibiotics regimens described in the American Heart Association (AHA) and European Society of Cardiology (ESC) scientific statements. Specific recommendations of the AHA and ESC for antimicrobial treatment of native and prosthetic valve endocarditis, based on common causative micro-organisms, are shown in Tables 59.2–59.7.[38,42]

Surgical treatment: indications and outcome

Surgical intervention for endocarditis may be performed in either the acute or active phase of infection or after the eradication of infection. Surgery during the active phase is generally considered for those patients in whom the likelihood of cure with antibiotic therapy alone is low or in whom severe complications of endocarditis have occurred or will likely occur. Surgery after eradication of infection is predominantly performed for adverse hemodynamic effects of valvular regurgitation that results from valve damage. In native valve endocarditis, heart failure due to valvular regurgitation, which often develops and progresses rapidly due to ongoing valvular damage and the lack of ventricular adaptation in the acute setting, is a primary indication for urgent surgical intervention (**Class I, Level B**). In the absence of overt heart failure symptoms, hemodynamic evidence of severe regurgitation (such as premature closure of the mitral valve in severe aortic regurgitation or pulmonary hypertension in severe mitral regurgitation) should also prompt surgical intervention since valvular regurgitation, or rarely stenosis, is a mechanical or structural complication of endocarditis that will not improve with antimicrobial therapy alone. For mitral valve regurgitation, surgical repair of the native valve without replacement of the valve with a prosthesis has been reported in a number of case series.[43,44] However, the role of repair has not been evaluated in controlled studies and its feasibility will be limited by the extent of infection and valvular damage as well as the experience of the surgeon. Because embolic complications often involve the central nervous system and may worsen neurologic function after cardiopulmonary bypass, the timing of surgery after a cerebral embolic infarct is controversial. One recent study found that neurologic deterioration did not occur among patients with IE who experienced transient ischemic attacks or asymptomatic emboli, even if surgery was performed acutely (median 9 days after cerebrovascular complication) (**Class IIb, Level C**). Overall mortality as well as neurologic death were independently associated with lower Glasgow Coma Scale, and valve surgery had a survival benefit.[45] Regarding persistent bacteremia as an indication for surgery, it is important to recognize that certain micro-organisms, particularly *S. aureus*, may be associated with prolonged bacteremia (up to 10 days) after initiation of antibiotic therapy. Because of possible difficulty in eradicating infection from prosthetic materials, all cases of prosthetic valve endocarditis should receive surgical consultation. Other indications for surgery are described in Box 59.1.

With valve conservation and improved surgical techniques, the surgical mortality rates have declined over time with recent reported rates in the range of 7–14%.[46,47] The

Table 59.2 Native valve endocarditis: Strep species

Antibiotic susceptibility	AHA/ACC antibiotic	duration	ESC antibiotic	duration
Penicillin-susceptible viridans streptococci and *Strep bovis* (MIC <0.12 μg/mL)	Aqueous crystalline penicillin G sodium 12–18 million U/24 h IV either continuously or in 4–6 doses Or Ceftriaxone sodium 2 g/24 h IV/IM in 1 dose Or Vancomycin hydrochloride 30 mg.kg per 24 h IV in 2 equally divided doses not to exceed 2 g/24 h unless concentrations in serum are inappropriately low	4 weeks	Penicillin G 12–20 million U/24 h IV in 4–6 divided doses (4 weeks) Or Ceftriaxone 2 g/24 h IV in 1 dose (4 weeks) Or Vancomycin 30 mg/kg per 24 h IV in 2 doses Or Penicillin G 12–20 million U/24 h IV in 4–6 divided doses for 4 weeks + gentamicin 3 mg/kg per 24 h IV (max 240 mg/g) divided in 2 or 3 doses for 2 weeks	4 weeks
Relatively resistant strains of viridans streptococci and *Strep bovis* MIC >0.12 μg/ mL <0.5 μg/mL	Aqueous crystalline penicillin G sodium 24 million U/24 h IV either continuously or in 4–6 divided doses (4 weeks) Or Ceftriaxone sodium 2 g/24 h IV/IM in 1 dose (4 weeks) Plus Gentamicin sulfate 3 mg/kg per 24 h IV/IM in 1 dose or in 2–3 equally divided doses (2 weeks)	4 weeks	Penicillin G 20–24 million U/24 h IV in 4–6 divided doses (4 weeks) Or Ceftriaxone 2 g/24 h IV/IM in 1 dose (4 weeks) Plus Gentamicin 3 mg/kg per 24 h IV (max. 240 mg/d) divided in 2–3 doses for the first 2 weeks Followed by Cefriaxone 2 g/24 h IV/IM for additional 2 weeks for a total treatment course of 6 weeks Or Vancomycin 30 mg/kg per 24 h IV in 2 doses for 4 weeks	4 weeks

Adapted from Baddour et al,[38] Sexton,[77] Karchmer.[78]

Table 59.3 Prosthetic valve endocarditis: *Strep* species

Antibiotic susceptibility	AHA/ACC antibiotic duration		ESC antibiotic duration	
Penicillin susceptible viridans streptococci and *Strep bovis* (MIC < 0.12 µg/mL)	Aqueous crystalline penicillin G sodium 24 million U/24h IV either continuously or in 4–6 doses (6 weeks)	6 weeks	Penicillin G 20–24 million U/24h IV in 4–6 divided doses for 4 weeks	6 weeks
	Or		Or	
	Ceftriaxone sodium 2 g/24h IV/IM in 1 dose for 6 weeks		Ceftriaxone 2 g/24h IV in 1 dose for 4 weeks	
	With or without		Plus	
	Gentamicin sulfate 3 mg/kg per 24h IV/IM in 1 dose for 2 weeks		Gentamicin 3 mg/kg per 24h IV (max 240 mg/d) divided in 2 or 3 doses for 2 weeks	
	Or		Followed by	
	Vancomycin hydrochloride 30 mg/kg per 24h IV in 2 equally divided doses not to exceed 2 g/24h unless concentration in serum are inappropriately low for 6 weeks		Cefriaxone 2 g/24h IV/IM for additional 2 weeks for a total treatment course of 6 weeks	
			Or	
			Vancomycin 30 mg/kg per 24h IV in 2 doses for 4 weeks	
Relatively resistant strains of viridans streptococci and *Strep bovis* MIC >0.12 ug/mL	Aqueous crystalline penicillin G sodium 24 million U/24h IV either continuously or in 4–6 doses (6 weeks)	6 weeks	Penicillin G 20–24 million U/24h IV in 4–6 divided doses for 4 weeks	6 weeks
	Or		Or	
	Ceftriaxone sodium 2 g/24h IV/IM in 1 dose for 6 weeks		Ceftriaxone 2 g/24h IV in 1 dose for 4 weeks	
	Plus		Plus	
	Gentamicin sulfate 3 mg/kg per 24h IV/IM in 1 dose for 6 weeks		Gentamicin 3 mg/kg per 24h IV (max 240 mg/d) divided in 2 or 3 doses for 2 weeks	
	Or		Followed by	
	Single drug treatment		Cefriaxone 2 g/24h IV/IM for additional 2 weeks for a total treatment course of 6 weeks	
	Vancomycin hydrochloride 30 mg/kg per 24h IV in 2 equally divided doses not to exceed 2 g/24h unless concentration in serum are inappropriately low for 6 weeks		Or	
			Vancomycin 30 mg/kg per 24h IV in 2 doses for 4 weeks	

Adapted from Baddour et al,[38] Sexton,[77] Karchmer.[78]

Table 59.4 Native valve endocarditis: enterococci

Antibiotic susceptibility	AHA/ACC antibiotic duration		ESC antibiotic duration	
Enterococci strains susceptible to penicillin, gentamicin, and vancomycin	Gentamicin sulfate 3 mg/kg per 24 h IV/IM in 3 equally divided doses for 4–6 wks Plus one of the following: Aqueous crystalline penicillin G sodium 18–30 million U/24 h IV either continuously or in 6 equally divided doses for 4–6 wks Or Ampicillin sodium 12 g/24 h IV in 6 equally divided doses for 4–6 wks Or Vancomycin hydrochloride 30 mg/kg per 24 h IV in 2 equally divided doses for 6 wks; not to exceed 2 g/24 h unless concentrations in serum are inappropriately low	4–6 weeks	One of the following: Aqueous crystalline penicillin G sodium 16–20 million U/24 h IV in 4–6 equally divided doses for 4 wks Plus Gentamicin 3 mg/kg per 24 h IV divided in 2 doses for 4 wks Or Vancomycin 30 mg/kg per 24 h IV in 2 divided doses for 6 wks Plus Gentamicin 3 mg/kg per 24 h IV divided in 2 doses for 6 wks	4 – 6 wks
Enterococci strains resistant to penicillin and susceptible to aminoglycoside and vancomycin	*B-Lactamase producing* One of the following: Gentamicin sulfate 3 mg/kg per 24 h IV/IM in 3 equally divided doses for 6 wks Plus either Ampicillin–sulbactam 12 g/24 h IV in 4 equally divided doses for 6 wks Or Vancomycin* hydrochloride 30 mg/kg per 24 h IV in 2 equally divided doses for 6 wks; not to exceed 2 g/24 h unless concentrations in serum are inappropriately low *Intrinsic penicillin resistance* Vancomycin* 30 mg/kg per 24 h IV in 2 divided doses for 6 wks Plus Gentamicin sulfate 3 mg/kg per 24 h IV/IM in 3 equally divided doses for 6 wks	6 weeks	Vancomycin* 30 mg/kg per 24 h IV in 2 divided doses for 6 wks Plus Gentamicin 3 mg/kg per 24 h IV divided in 2 doses for 6 wks	6 wks

Adapted from Baddour et al,[38] Sexton,[77] Karchmer.[78]

Table 59.5 Prosthetic valve endocarditis: enterococci

Antibiotic susceptibility	AHA antibiotic duration		ESC antibiotic duration	
Enterococci strains susceptible to penicillin and vancomycin	Aqueous crystalline penicillin G 18–30 million U/24h IV either continuously or in 6 equally divided doses for 6 wks Or Ampicillin sodium 12 g/24h IV in 6 equally divided doses for 6 wks Or Vancomycin* hydrochloride 30 mg/kg per 24h IV in 2 equally divided doses for 6 wks; not to exceed 2 g/24h unless concentrations in serum are inappropriately low Plus Gentamicin sulfate 3 mg/kg per 24h IV/IM in 3 equally divided doses for 6 weeks	6 weeks	Aqueous crystalline penicillin G 16–20 million U/24h IV in 4–6 equally divided doses for 6 wks Or Vancomycin* 30 mg/kg per 24h IV in 2 divided doses for 6 wks Plus Gentamicin sulfate 3 mg/kg per 24h IV/IM in 3 equally divided doses for 6 weeks	6 weeks
Enterococci strains resistant to penicillin and susceptible to aminoglycoside and vancomycin	*Intrinsic penicillin resistance* Penicillin/ampicillin MIC 32 μg/mL: Vancomycin 30 mg/kg per 24h IV in 2 divided doses for 6 wks Plus Gentamicin sulfate 3 mg/kg per 24h IV/IM in 3 equally divided doses for 6 wks *B-Lactamase producing* One of the following: Ampicillin-sulbactam 12 g/24h IV in 4 equally divided doses for 6 wks Or Vancomycin hydrochloride 30 mg/kg per 24h IV in 2 equally divided doses for 6 wks; not to exceed 2 g/24h unless concentrations in serum are inappropriately low Plus Gentamicin sulfate 3 mg/kg per 24h IV/IM in 3 equally divided doses for 6 wks	6 weeks	Vancomycin 30 mg/kg per 24h IV in 2 divided doses for 6 wks Plus Gentamicin 3 mg/kg per 24h IV divided in 2 doses for 6 wks	6 weeks

Adapted from Baddour et al,[38] Sexton,[77] Karchmer.[78]

Table 59.6 Native valve endocarditis: *Staph* species

Antibiotic susceptibility	AHA/ACC antibiotic duration		ESC antibiotic duration	
Methicillin susceptible	Nafcillin or oxacillin 12 g/24 h IV in 4 or 6 equally divided doses for 6 wks	6 weeks	Oxacillin or nafcillin 8 to 12 g/24 h IV in 4 equally divided doses for 4 wks	4–6 weeks
	Plus		Plus	
	Optional addition of gentamicin sulfate 3 mg/kg per 24 h IV/IM in 2 or 3 equally divided doses for 3 to 5 days		Gentamicin 3 mg/kg per 24 h IV (maximum 240 mg/d), divided in 3 doses for 3–5 days	
	Or		Or	
	Cefazolin 6 g/24 h IV in 3 equally divided doses for 6 wks		Vancomycin 30 mg/kg per 24 h IV in 2 doses for 4–6 wks	
	Plus		Plus	
	Optional addition of gentamicin sulfate 3 mg/kg per 24 h IV/IM in 2 or 3 equally divided doses for 3 to 5 days		Gentamicin 3 mg/kg per 24 h IV (maximum 240 mg/d), divided in 3 doses for 3–5 days	
Methicillin resistant	Vancomycin hydrochloride 30 mg/kg per 24 h IV in 2 equally divided doses for 6 wks; not to exceed 2 g/24 h unless concentrations in serum are inappropriately low	6 weeks	Vancomycin 30 mg/kg per 24 h IV in 2 doses for 6 wks	6 weeks

Adapted from Baddour *et al*,[38] Sexton,[77] Karchmer.[78]

Table 59.7 Prosthetic valve endocarditis: *Staph* species

Antibiotic susceptibility	AHA/ACC antibiotic duration		ESC antibiotic duration	
Methicillin susceptible	One of the following:	6 weeks	One of the following:	6–8 weeks
	Nafcillin or oxacillin* 12 g/24 h IV in 6 divided doses for 6 wks		Oxacillin or nafcillin 8 to 12 g/24 h IV in 4 divided doses for 6–8 wks	
	Or		Or	
	Cefazolin 6 g/24 h IV in 3 divided doses for 6 wks		Vancomycin 30 mg/kg per 24 h IV in 2 doses for 4 to 6–8 wks	
	Or		Plus	
	Vancomycin 30 mg/kg per 24 h IV in 2 divided doses for 6 wks		Gentamicin 3 mg/kg per 24 h IV (maximum 240 mg/d), divided in 3 doses for 2 wks	
	Plus		Plus	
	Rifampin 900 mg/24 h IV/PO in 3 divided doses for 6 wks		Rifampin 900 mg/24 h IV in 3 divided doses for 6–8 wks	
	Plus			
	Gentamicin sulfate 3 mg/kg per 24 h IV/IM in 2 or 3 divided doses for 2 wks			
Methicillin resistant strains	Vancomycin 30 mg/kg per 24 h IV in 2 divided doses for 6 wks	6 weeks	Vancomycin 30 mg/kg per 24 h IV in 2 doses for 6–8 wks	6–8 weeks
	Plus		Plus	
	Rifampin 900 mg/24 h IV/PO in 3 divided doses for 6 wks		Rifampin 900 mg/24 h IV in 3 divided doses for 6–8 wks	
	Plus		Plus	
	Gentamicin 3 mg/kg per 24 h IV/IM in 2 or 3 divided doses for 2 wks		Gentamicin 3 mg/kg per 24 h IV (maximum 240 mg/d), divided in 3 doses for 6–8 wks	

Adapted from Baddour *et al*,[38] Sexton,[77] Karchmer.[78]

optimal timing of surgery in the setting of active endocarditis has not been well evaluated. In patients with serious, life-threatening complications of endocarditis, surgery should be performed urgently. A number of case series have shown that surgery in the active phase of endocarditis can be performed with acceptable risk and without an obvious risk of prosthetic valve infection.[48]

An understanding of outcomes with surgical treatment of endocarditis is influenced by the inherent selection bias

---

BOX 59.1 Surgical indications in native valve infective endocarditis

Class I recommendation
- Heart failure (**Level B**)
- Aortic regurgitation or mitral regurgitation with evidence of elevated left ventricular end-diastolic or left atrial pressure (**Level B**)
- Fungal endocarditis or highly resistant organism (left-sided IE with *S. marcescens* and *Pseudomonas* species, persistent infection with blood cultures positive despite 1 week of antibiotic therapy, or 1 or more embolic event during first 2 weeks of therapy (**Level B**)
- Echocardiographic evidence of valve dehiscence, perforation, rupture, fistula or large perivalvular abscess (**Level B**)

Class IIa recommendation
- Recurrent emboli and persistent vegetations despite appropriate antibiotic treatment (**Level B**)

Class IIb recommendation
- Mobile, large(>10mm) vegetation with or without emboli (**Level C**)

Adapted from Bonow *et al.*[29]

---

in observational cohorts and the lack of randomized, controlled trials for this therapy. One recent, retrospective study of 513 cases of complicated, left-sided endocarditis found that valve surgery was independently associated with reduced six-month mortality (hazard ratio (HR) 0.40; 95% confidence interval (CI) 0.18–0.91; $P = 0.03$) in propensity-matched subgroups. Patients with moderate to severe heart failure appeared to derive the greatest benefit from surgery, whereas surgical treatment had a neutral effect on mortality for patients without heart failure[49] (Fig. 59.2). Other factors which have been related to a survival benefit from surgery include patients with aortic valve disease and prosthetic endocarditis.[50]

This differential effect of surgery on outcome depending on the presence or absence of complications may simply reflect that surgery confers the greatest clinical benefit or absolute risk reduction for patients at highest risk, but demonstrating a benefit for patients at lower risk is more challenging. Along these lines, when propensity score adjustment is used to assess the effect of surgery on outcome of endocarditis as compared to medical therapy alone, studies have shown differing results, including survival benefit,[49] neutral effect,[51] and poorer survival[52] associated with surgery. These contrasting results likely reflect significant differences in the study cohorts, the clinical variables collected and included in the analyses, statistical methodologies, and the time points for the survival endpoint.

Complications and outcome

In the absence of appropriate therapy, endocarditis typically progresses to the development of various intra- and

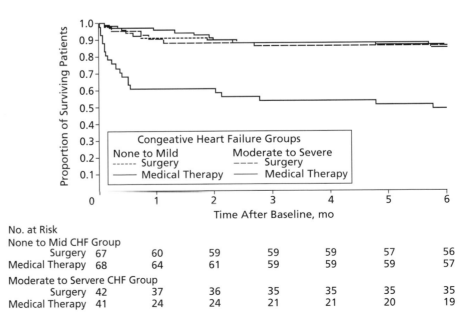

Figure 59.2 Kaplan-Meir survival curve relating the effect of congestive heart failure to time to death among propensity-matched patients receiving medical therapy or surgery. (From Vikram *et al*[49] with permission.)

No. at Risk

None to Mid CHF Group							
Surgery	67	60	59	59	59	57	56
Medical Therapy	68	64	61	59	59	59	57
Moderate to Severe CHF Group							
Surgery	42	37	36	35	35	35	35
Medical Therapy	41	24	24	21	21	20	19

extracardiac complications. Heart failure or pulmonary edema is probably the most common complication, occurring in about a third to one half of patients with IE, as well as the most frequent indication for urgent surgery. Heart failure occurs as a result of valvular destruction and ensuing insufficiency or, in rare cases of large vegetations, as a result of valvular stenosis. Heart failure complicates aortic valve endocarditis more frequently than mitral or tricuspid endocarditis and may result in the setting of moderate, rather than severe, regurgitation, particularly in case of involvement of the aortic valve,[53] since the left ventricle is unable to compensate for the acute increase in preload and afterload in this condition.

Medical therapy alone is generally insufficient in managing endocarditis complicated by heart failure, particularly in the setting of severe or progressive valvular regurgitation. Surgery should be prompt and unnecessary delays avoided (**Class III, Level C**).[42]

Paravalvular abscess complicates 30–40% cases of IE[32] and is a result of invasive infection that spreads generally along contiguous tissue planes, particularly with aortic valve infection. In the International Collaboration on Endocarditis (ICE) cohort, 22% cases of definite aortic valve endocarditis were complicated by a periannular abscess. These patients were more likely to have prosthetic valves and coagulase-negative staphylococcal infection. Transesophageal echocardiography is the diagnostic test of choice when an abscess is suspected clinically. An abscess is diagnosed by TEE as the visualization of a "thickened area" or "mass with a heterogeneous echogenic or echolucent appearance".[32] Rarely, antibiotic therapy may be used to treat an intracardiac abscess, though this treatment alone is generally reserved for patients who are poor surgical candidates. The vast majority of patients with an intracardiac abscess require cardiac surgery for debridement (**Class I, Level C**) as evidenced in a recent large study in which 86% of patients with periannular abscess underwent surgery.[54] In addition, surgery represents the gold standard for the diagnosis of abscess.

In rare cases, due to high intravascular pressures and progressive burrowing infection, these perivalvular cavities can form fistulous connections (aorto-atrial or aorto-ventricular), and even myocardial perforation (Plate 59.2). Fistula formation complicated endocarditis in 1.6% cases of native valve endocarditis and 3.5% cases of PVE in a cohort of 4681 cases of IE. These occurred with similar frequency in the three sinuses of Valsalva and among all the cardiac chambers. Despite surgical intervention (87%), the mortality rate in this group of patients was 41%.[54] The development of cavitary fistulas thus heralds a poor outcome and must prompt surgical intervention.

Embolic phenomena frequently complicate the clinical course in endocarditis. Although clinical signs of embolization manifest in approximately one-third of patients with IE,[55] atleast another third of patients have silent embolism.[56] In the majority of cases, embolic events occur before the initiation of antibiotic therapy, whereas only 7% of events occur after treatment has begun.[57] In a subset of 66 patients with embolic complications among 178 patients with endocarditis, the most frequent sites of embolic events were central nervous system (41%), lungs (18%), spleen (21%), peripheral artery (14%), and kidney (12%).[58]

Factors including vegetation size, mobility, and location as well as the causative organism have been associated with the likelihood of embolic event. Vegetations larger than 10 mm in greatest diameter pose an increased risk of embolization.[57,59] Causative organisms such as *S. aureus* and *Strep. bovis* confer an independent risk of embolization.[60] Also, there is a 2–3 times higher frequency of embolism in endocarditis caused by enterococci, *Abiotrophia* spp, fastidious gram-negative organisms (HACEK) and fungi as compared to streptococci.[61,62] In addition to causing infarction of distal vascular beds, embolic events may result in metastatic sites of infection.

Cerebral embolization occurs in 10–35% and is at times complicated by meningitis, brain abscess or intracerebral hemorrhage. In the ICE cohort, stroke complicated endocarditis in 15% of patients.[63] The risk of stroke dramatically decreases with initiation of antibiotic therapy. Findings from the ICE merged database suggested a 65% reduction in stroke incidence by week two of initiating antimicrobial therapy.[63] Given the low incidence of embolic events after initiation of antibiotic therapy, routine screening for emboli in patients with IE is not recommended (**Class IIb, Level C**). However, patients with persistent fever or bacteremia or localizing symptoms of possible infarction should undergo computed tomographic imaging with radiographic contrast for the diagnosis of embolic complications.

Embolic events have been found to be an independent predictor of in-hospital death in endocarditis.[64] In patients who experience recurrent embolic events, particularly if occurring after initiation of antibiotic therapy, surgical treatment is indicated (**Class IIa, Level C**). For the prevention of embolic events, surgery may be considered for patients with endocarditis who have large (greater than 10 mm), mobile vegetations, especially with involvement of left-sided heart valves (**Class IIb, Level C**).

The issue of anticoagulation in patients with endocarditis remains controversial. There is no demonstrable benefit of anticoagulation in native valve endocarditis. In patients with PVE, continuation of oral anticoagulation or switching to intravenous heparin has been advocated by some experts, while others have recommended discontinuation of all anticoagulation in patients with *S. aureus* endocarditis and recent stroke until completion of two weeks of antibiotic therapy,[65] presumably to avoid hemorrhagic transformation.[66] Regarding antiplatelet therapy with aspirin, no beneficial effect on outcome has been found, and aspirin therapy has been associated with a higher risk of bleeding complications in IE (**Class III, Level A**).[67,68]

Mortality in native valve endocarditis

The six-month mortality estimate from various reports is approximately 27%.[69,70] Such unacceptably high mortality rates despite therapeutic and diagnostic advances have lead many investigators to risk stratify patients with endocarditis. Amongst host factors, age, female sex, presence of diabetes mellitus, APACHE II score, elevated white blood cell count, serum creatinine level >2 mg/dL, and lower serum albumin have been associated with poor outcomes. Moderate to severe congestive heart failure, periannular abscess formation, vegetation length >10 mm, absence of surgical therapy, and infection with virulent organisms, particularly *S. aureus*, are disease factors related to embolic events and death.[57,64,69,71,72]

Mortality in prosthetic valve endocarditis

Medical progress has similarly allowed the in-hospital mortality rates of PVE to fall from 50–60% in earlier series[73] to approximately 23% as reported in a recent large, multinational study.[11] Studies have found that long-term survival after the active phase of infection is similar for early and late PVE (74% and 82% survival at four-year follow-up).[74]

Heart failure severity was the only predictor of death among 66 patients with PVE, in the Veterans Affairs Co-operative Study on Valvular Heart Disease.[75] More recently, results of the International Collaboration on Endocarditis-Prospective Cohort Study (ICE-PCS) confirmed that complications of heart failure, persistent bacteremia, abscess, and stroke are important, independent prognostic factors in PVE. In addition, older age, healthcare-associated infection and *S. aureus* infection were factors associated with a higher mortality.[11] Recent guidelines support the use of surgery for PVE associated with these complications.[29]

Prevention

Over the past few decades, the efficacy of antimicrobial prophylaxis in preventing IE has been questioned. Recently, after an extensive review of all available literature and consensus of experts, the American Heart Association published updated guidelines for IE prophylaxis.[76] These guidelines have concluded that endocarditis was more likely to result from bacteremia associated with daily activities than with a dental procedure. Antibiotic prophylaxis, even if 100% effective, is estimated to prevent only an extremely small number of cases of endocarditis. These

> **BOX 59.2** Conditions warranting antimicrobial prophylaxis
>
> - Prosthetic cardiac valve or prosthetic device used for valve repair
> - History of endocarditis
> - Unrepaired cyanotic CHD, including palliative shunts and conduits
> - Repaired CHD with prosthetic materiel (whether placed surgically or catheter based) in the first six months following the procedure
> - Repaired CHD with residual defect at the site or adjacent to site of prosthetic material
> - Cardiac transplant recipients who develop valvulopathy
>
> Adapted from Wilson *et al.*[76]

recommendations surmised that antibiotic prophylaxis should not be prescribed solely on the basis of an increased life-time risk of endocarditis but on the basis of cardiac conditions associated with highest risk of an adverse outcome from endocarditis.[76]

Conditions that warrant IE prophylaxis prior to dental procedures, and procedures on respiratory tract, skin and musculoskeletal structures are listed in Box 59.2 (**Class I, Level C**). The American Heart Association no longer recommends prophylaxis before gastrointestinal or genitourinary procedures solely for the prevention of IE.[76]

References

1. Fye WB. Jean Francois Fernel. Clin Cardiol 1997;**20**(12):1037–8.
2. Osler W, Fye B. *William Osler's Collected Papers on the Cardiovascular System.* Birmingham: Classics of Medicine Library, 1988.
3. Millar BC, Moore JE. Emerging issues in infective endocarditis. *Emerg Infect Dis* 2004;**10**(6):1110–16.
4. Zipes DP, Braunwald E. *Braunwald's Heart Disease : A Textbook of Cardiovascular Medicine*, 7th edn. Philadelphia: Elsevier Saunders, 2005: xxi.
5. Delahaye F, Goulet V, Lacassin F *et al*. Characteristics of infective endocarditis in France in 1991. A 1-year survey. *Eur Heart J* 1995;**16**(3):394–401.
6. Berlin JA, Abrutyn E, Strom BL *et al*. Incidence of infective endocarditis in the Delaware Valley, 1988–1990. *Am J Cardiol* 1995;**76**(12):933–6.
7. Rabinovich S, Evans J, Smith IM *et al*. A long-term view of bacterial endocarditis. 337 cases 1924 to 1963. *Ann Intern Med* 1965;**63**:185–98.
8. Li JS, Corey GR, Fowler VG. Infective endocarditis. In: Topol EJ, Califf RM (eds) *Textbook of Cardiovascular Medicine*. Philadelphia: Lippincott Williams & Wilkins, 2007: xxix.
9. Cabell CH, Abrutyn E. Progress toward a global understanding of infective endocarditis. Lessons from the International Collaboration on Endocarditis. *Cardiol Clin* 2003;**21**(2):147–58.

10. Fowler VG Jr, Miro JM, Hoen B *et al.* Staphylococcus aureus endocarditis: a consequence of medical progress. *JAMA* 2005;**293**(24):3012–21.

11. Wang A, Athan E, Pappas PA *et al.* Contemporary clinical profile and outcome of prosthetic valve endocarditis. *JAMA* 2007;**297**(12):1354–61.

12. Tzukert AA, Leviner E, Sela M. Prevention of infective endocarditis: not by antibiotics alone. A 7-year follow-up of 90 dental patients. *Oral Surg Oral Med Oral Pathol* 1986;**62**(4):385–8.

13. Pelletier LL Jr, Petersdorf RG. Infective endocarditis: a review of 125 cases from the University of Washington Hospitals, 1963–72. *Medicine (Baltimore)* 1977;**56**(4):287–313.

14. Williams RC Jr, Kunkel HG. Rheumatoid factor, complement, and conglutinin aberrations in patients with subacute bacterial endocarditis. *J Clin Invest* 1962;**41**:666–75.

15. Meine TJ, Nettles RE, Anderson DJ *et al.* Cardiac conduction abnormalities in endocarditis defined by the Duke criteria. *Am Heart J* 2001;**142**(2):280–5.

16. Von Reyn CF, Levy BS, Arbeit RD *et al.* Infective endocarditis: an analysis based on strict case definitions. *Ann Intern Med* 1981;**94**(4 pt 1):505–18.

17. Durack DT, Lukes AS, Bright DK. New criteria for diagnosis of infective endocarditis: utilization of specific echocardiographic findings. Duke Endocarditis Service. *Am J Med* 1994;**96**(3): 200–9.

18. Andres E, Baudoux C, Noel E *et al.* The value of the Von Reyn and the Duke diagnostic criteria for infective endocarditis in internal medicine practice. A study of 38 cases. *Eur J Intern Med* 2003;**14**(7):411–14.

19. Perez-Vazquez A, Farinas MC, Garcia-Palomo JD *et al.* Evaluation of the Duke criteria in 93 episodes of prosthetic valve endocarditis: could sensitivity be improved? *Arch Intern Med* 2000;**160**(8):1185–91.

20. Stockheim JA, Chadwick EG, Kessler S *et al.* Are the Duke criteria superior to the Beth Israel criteria for the diagnosis of infective endocarditis in children? *Clin Infect Dis* 1998;**27**(6):1451–6.

21. Heiro M, Nikoskelainen J, Hartiala JJ *et al.* Diagnosis of infective endocarditis. Sensitivity of the Duke vs von Reyn criteria. *Arch Intern Med* 1998;**158**(1):18–24.

22. Sekeres MA, Abrutyn E, Berlin JA *et al.* An assessment of the usefulness of the Duke criteria for diagnosing active infective endocarditis. *Clin Infect Dis* 1997;**24**(6):1185–90.

23. Martos-Perez F, Reguera JM, Colmenero JD. Comparable sensitivity of the Duke criteria and the modified Beth Israel criteria for diagnosing infective endocarditis. *Clin Infect Dis* 1996;**23**(2): 410–11.

24. Olaison L, Hogevik H. Comparison of the von Reyn and Duke criteria for the diagnosis of infective endocarditis: a critical analysis of 161 episodes. *Scand J Infect Dis* 1996;**28**(4):399–406.

25. Hoen B, Selton-Suty C, Danchin N *et al.* Evaluation of the Duke criteria versus the Beth Israel criteria for the diagnosis of infective endocarditis. *Clin Infect Dis* 1995;**21**(4):905–9.

26. Li JS, Sexton DJ, Mick N *et al.* Proposed modifications to the Duke criteria for the diagnosis of infective endocarditis. *Clin Infect Dis* 2000;**30**(4):633–8.

27. Lindner JR, Case RA, Dent JM *et al.* Diagnostic value of echocardiography in suspected endocarditis. An evaluation based on the pretest probability of disease. *Circulation* 1996;**93**(4):730–6.

28. Erbel R, Rohmann S, Drexler M *et al.* Improved diagnostic value of echocardiography in patients with infective endocarditis by transoesophageal approach. A prospective study. *Eur Heart J* 1988;**9**(1):43–53.

29. Bonow RO, Carabello BA, Chatterjee K *et al.* ACC/AHA 2006 guidelines for the management of patients with valvular heart disease: a report of the American College of Cardiology/American Heart Association Task Force on Practice Guidelines (Writing Committee to Revise the 1998 Guidelines for the Management of Patients with Valvular Heart Disease) developed in collaboration with the Society of Cardiovascular Anesthesiologists endorsed by the Society for Cardiovascular Angiography and Interventions and the Society of Thoracic Surgeons. *J Am Coll Cardiol* 2006;**48**(3):e1–148.

30. Roe MT, Abramson MA, Li J *et al.* Clinical information determines the impact of transesophageal echocardiography on the diagnosis of infective endocarditis by the duke criteria. *Am Heart J* 2000;**139**(6):945–51.

31. Rosen AB, Fowler VG Jr, Corey GR *et al.* Cost-effectiveness of transesophageal echocardiography to determine the duration of therapy for intravascular catheter-associated Staphylococcus aureus bacteremia. *Ann Intern Med* 1999; **130**(10):810–20.

32. Daniel WG, Mugge A, Martin RP *et al.* Improvement in the diagnosis of abscesses associated with endocarditis by transesophageal echocardiography. *N Engl J Med* 1991;**324**(12): 795–800.

33. Cowan JC, Patrick D, Reid DS. Aortic root abscess complicating bacterial endocarditis. Demonstration by computed tomography. *Br Heart J* 1984;**52**(5):591–3.

34. Allum C, Knight C, Mohiaddin R *et al.* Images in cardiovascular medicine. Use of magnetic resonance imaging to demonstrate a fistula from the aorta to the right atrium. *Circulation* 1998;**97**(10):1024.

35. Akins EW, Slone RM, Wiechmann BN *et al.* Perivalvular pseudoaneurysm complicating bacterial endocarditis: MR detection in five cases. *AJR* 1991;**156**(6):1155–8.

36. Hamburger M, Stein L. Streptococcus viridans subacute bacterial endocarditis; two week treatment schedule with penicillin. *JAMA* 1952;**149**(6):542–5.

37. Durack DT, Beeson PB. Experimental bacterial endocarditis. II. Survival of a bacteria in endocardial vegetations. *Br J Exp Pathol* 1972;**53**(1):50–3.

38. Baddour LM, Wilson WR, Bayer AS *et al.* Infective endocarditis: diagnosis, antimicrobial therapy, and management of complications: a statement for healthcare professionals from the Committee on Rheumatic Fever, Endocarditis, and Kawasaki Disease, Council on Cardiovascular Disease in the Young, and the Councils on Clinical Cardiology, Stroke, and Cardiovascular Surgery and Anesthesia, American Heart Association: endorsed by the Infectious Diseases Society of America. *Circulation* 2005;**111**(23): e394–434.

39. Fuller RE, Hayward SL. Oral antibiotic therapy in infective endocarditis. *Ann Pharmacother* 1996;**30**(6):676–8.

40. Heldman AW, Hartert TV, Ray SC *et al.* Oral antibiotic treatment of right-sided staphylococcal endocarditis in injection drug users: prospective randomized comparison with parenteral therapy. *Am J Med* 1996;**101**(1):68–76.

41. Korzeniowski O, Sande MA. Combination antimicrobial therapy for Staphylococcus aureus endocarditis in patients addicted to parenteral drugs and in nonaddicts: a prospective study. *Ann Intern Med* 1982;**97**(4):496–503.

42. Horstkotte D, Follath F, Gutschik E *et al.* Guidelines on prevention, diagnosis and treatment of infective endocarditis executive summary; the task force on infective endocarditis of the European Society of Cardiology. *Eur Heart J* 2004;**25**(3):267–76.

43. Doukas G, Oc M, Alexiou C *et al.* Mitral valve repair for active culture positive infective endocarditis. *Heart* 2006;**92**(3):361–3.

44. Feringa HH, Shaw LJ, Poldermans D *et al.* Mitral valve repair and replacement in endocarditis: a systematic review of literature. *Ann Thorac Surg* 2007;**83**(2):564–70.

45. Thuny F, Avierinos JF, Tribouilloy C *et al.* Impact of cerebrovascular complications on mortality and neurologic outcome during infective endocarditis: a prospective multicentre study. *Eur Heart J* 2007;**28**(9):1155–61.

46. d'Udekem Y, David TE, Feindel CM *et al.* Long-term results of surgery for active infective endocarditis. *Eur J Cardiothorac Surg* 1997;**11**(1):46–52.

47. Jassal DS, Neilan TG, Pradhan AD *et al.* Surgical management of infective endocarditis: early predictors of short-term morbidity and mortality. *Ann Thorac Surg* 2006;**82**(2):524–9.

48. Guerra JM, Tornos MP, Permanyer-Miralda G *et al.* Long term results of mechanical prostheses for treatment of active infective endocarditis. *Heart* 2001;**86**(1):63–8.

49. Vikram HR, Buenconsejo J, Hasbun R *et al.* Impact of valve surgery on 6-month mortality in adults with complicated, left-sided native valve endocarditis: a propensity analysis. *JAMA* 2003;**290**(24):3207–14.

50. Vlessis AA, Hovaguimian H, Jaggers J *et al.* Infective endocarditis: ten-year review of medical and surgical therapy. *Ann Thorac Surg* 1996;**61**(4):1217–22.

51. Cabell CH, Abrutyn E, Fowler VG Jr *et al.* Use of surgery in patients with native valve infective endocarditis: results from the International Collaboration on Endocarditis Merged Database. *Am Heart J* 2005;**150**(5):1092–8.

52. Tleyjeh IM, Ghomrawi HM, Steckelberg JM *et al.* The impact of valve surgery on 6-month mortality in left-sided infective endocarditis. *Circulation* 2007;**115**(13):1721–8.

53. Sexton DJ, Spelman D. Current best practices and guidelines. Assessment and management of complications in infective endocarditis. *Cardiol Clin* 2003;**21**(2):273–82, vii–viii.

54. Anguera I, Miro JM, Cabell CH *et al.* Clinical characteristics and outcome of aortic endocarditis with periannular abscess in the International Collaboration on Endocarditis Merged Database. *Am J Cardiol* 2005;**96**(7):976–81.

55. De Castro S, Magni G, Beni S *et al.* Role of transthoracic and transesophageal echocardiography in predicting embolic events in patients with active infective endocarditis involving native cardiac valves. *Am J Cardiol* 1997;**80**(8):1030–4.

56. Snygg-Martin U, Gustafsson L, Rosengren L *et al.* Cerebrovascular complications in patients with left-sided infective endocarditis are common: a prospective study using magnetic resonance imaging and neurochemical brain damage markers. *Clin Infect Dis* 2008;**47**(1):23–30.

57. Thuny F, Di Salvo G, Belliard O *et al.* Risk of embolism and death in infective endocarditis: prognostic value of echocardiog-

58. Di Salvo G, Habib G, Pergola V *et al.* Echocardiography predicts embolic events in infective endocarditis. *J Am Coll Cardiol* 2001;**37**(4):1069–76.

59. Tischler MD, Vaitkus PT. The ability of vegetation size on echocardiography to predict clinical complications: a meta-analysis. *J Am Soc Echocardiogr* 1997;**10**(5):562–8.

60. Vilacosta I, Graupner C, San Roman JA *et al.* Risk of embolization after institution of antibiotic therapy for infective endocarditis. *J Am Coll Cardiol* 2002;**39**(9):1489–95.

61. Steckelberg JM, Murphy JG, Ballard D *et al.* Emboli in infective endocarditis: the prognostic value of echocardiography. *Ann Intern Med* 1991;**114**(8):635–40.

62. Salgado AV, Furlan AJ, Keys TF *et al.* Neurologic complications of endocarditis: a 12-year experience. *Neurology* 1989;**39**(2 Pt 1):173–8.

63. Dickerman SA, Abrutyn E, Barsic B *et al.* The relationship between the initiation of antimicrobial therapy and the incidence of stroke in infective endocarditis: an analysis from the ICE Prospective Cohort Study (ICE-PCS). *Am Heart J* 2007;**154**(6):1086–94.

64. Chu VH, Cabell CH, Benjamin DK Jr *et al.* Early predictors of in-hospital death in infective endocarditis. *Circulation* 2004;**109**(14):1745–9.

65. Tornos P, Almirante B, Mirabet S *et al.* Infective endocarditis due to Staphylococcus aureus: deleterious effect of anticoagulant therapy. *Arch Intern Med* 1999;**159**(5):473–5.

66. Salem DN, Daudelin HD, Levine HJ *et al.* Antithrombotic therapy in valvular heart disease. *Chest* 2001;**119**(1 suppl):207S–219S.

67. Anavekar NS, Tleyjeh IM, Anavekar NS *et al.* Impact of prior antiplatelet therapy on risk of embolism in infective endocarditis. *Clin Infect Dis* 2007;**44**(9):1180–6.

68. Chan KL, Dumesnil JG, Cujec B *et al.* A randomized trial of aspirin on the risk of embolic events in patients with infective endocarditis. *J Am Coll Cardiol* 2003;**42**(5):775–80.

69. Wallace SM, Walton BI, Kharbanda RK *et al.* Mortality from infective endocarditis: clinical predictors of outcome. *Heart* 2002;**88**(1):53–60.

70. Hasbun R, Vikram HR, Barakat LA *et al.* Complicated left-sided native valve endocarditis in adults: risk classification for mortality. *JAMA* 2003;**289**(15):1933–40.

71. Cabell CH, Pond KK, Peterson GE *et al.* The risk of stroke and death in patients with aortic and mitral valve endocarditis. *Am Heart J* 2001;**142**(1):75–80.

72. Miro JM, Anguera I, Cabell CH *et al.* Staphylococcus aureus native valve infective endocarditis: report of 566 episodes from the International Collaboration on Endocarditis Merged Database. *Clin Infect Dis* 2005;**41**(4):507–14.

73. Wilson WR, Jaumin PM, Danielson GK *et al.* Prosthetic valve endocarditis. *Ann Intern Med* 1975;**82**(6):751–6.

74. Castillo JC, Anguita MP, Torres F *et al.* Long-term prognosis of early and late prosthetic valve endocarditis. *Am J Cardiol* 2004;**93**(9):1185–7.

75. Grover FL, Cohen DJ, Oprian C *et al.* Determinants of the occurrence of and survival from prosthetic valve endocarditis. Experi-

ence of the Veterans Affairs Cooperative Study on Valvular Heart Disease. *J Thorac Cardiovasc Surg* 1994;**108**(2):207–14.

76. Wilson W, Taubert KA, Gewitz M *et al*. Prevention of infective endocarditis: guidelines from the American Heart Association: a guideline from the American Heart Association Rheumatic Fever, Endocarditis, and Kawasaki Disease Committee, Council on Cardiovascular Disease in the Young, and the Council on Clinical Cardiology, Council on Cardiovascular Surgery and Anesthesia, and the Quality of Care and Outcomes Research Interdisciplinary Working Group. *Circulation* 2007;**116**(15): 1736–54.

77. Sexton DJ. Anti-microbial therapy of native valve endocarditis. *UptoDate* Version 16.1; 2008.

78. Karchmer AW. Anti-microbial therapy of prosthetic valve endocarditis. *UptoDate* Version 16.1; 2008.

60 Antithrombotic therapy after heart valve replacement

Jack C J Sun and John W Eikelboom
McMaster University, Hamilton, Ontario, Canada

Introduction and historical perspective

Valvular heart disease affects more than 100 million patients worldwide and is a growing problem because of the increasing survival of patients with rheumatic heart disease in the developing world and the growing burden of degenerative valve disease in the aging population.[1-2] Prosthetic valve replacement is the only definitive treatment for valvular heart disease and is performed in about 100 000 patients each year in North America.[3] Thromboembolism is one of the most important complications of prosthetic heart valves and although the thrombogenicity of newer valves is less than with older valves, all patients undergoing valve replacement surgery require antithrombotic therapy.

This chapter reviews the evidence for antithrombotic therapy in patients with prosthetic heart valves and makes treatment recommendations based on the strength and quality of the evidence. The class of evidence reflects opinion about the usefulness of the treatment, and balances the positive effects of treatment against the negative effects on patient-important outcomes. Class I recommendations are strong and indicate that the benefits of the treatment outweigh the risks. Class II recommendations are weak and suggest that there are differences between patients in the balance of the benefits and risks of treatment. Class III recommendations indicate that the treatment does not have any benefits or that the risks outweigh the benefits. The level of evidence reflects the quality of the evidence. Level A is high-quality evidence from well-conducted randomized controlled trials or meta-analyses of well-conducted randomized trials with clear results. Level B is evidence from randomized trials or overviews of randomized trials that have significant limitations. Level C1 is evidence from high-quality and persuasive cohort studies, case–control studies or case series while Level C2 is lower quality evidence from non-randomized studies or opinions of experts.

Nomenclature and definitions

Mechanical valves

Mechanical heart valves comprise three major components: an occluder (closure mechanism), housing and sewing ring.[4] There are three main types of mechanical valves: caged ball, single leaflet/tilting disk and bileaflet valves (Figure 60.1). All mechanical valves have some degree of regurgitant flow that acts as a "washing jet" to prevent thrombus formation on the surfaces of the valve.

Caged-ball valves

The first prosthetic heart valve was the Starr–Edwards caged-ball valve introduced in 1960.[5] The original version of the Starr–Edwards valve had a silicone rubber (Silastic) ball or poppet that freely moved within the confines of a three-strut alloy cage (Fig. 60.1a). Subsequent models had a metal ball and a four-strut cage. The free ball design theoretically prevents thrombus growth from the sewing ring onto the occluder[6] but the ball generates a large wake of stagnant flow that may account for the high risk of thromboembolism associated with caged-ball valves.[7] The Starr–Edwards valve was the "gold standard" against which new mechanical valves were compared for more than 20 years.[8]

Single leaflet/tilting disk valves

Single leaflet/tilting disk valves consist of a major orifice and a minor orifice. The single tilting disk enables central

Evidence-Based Cardiology, 3rd edition. Edited by S. Yusuf, J.A. Cairns, A.J. Camm, E.L. Fallen, and B.J. Gersh. © 2010 Blackwell Publishing, ISBN: 978-1-4051-5925-8.

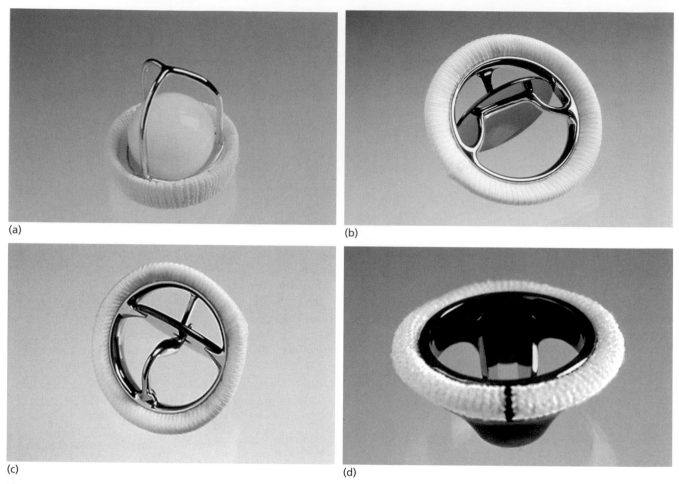

Figure 60.1 Different models of mechanical valves. (a) Starr–Edwards caged ball (courtesy of Edwards Lifesciences LLC, Irvine, California). (b) Bjork–Shiley tilting disk (courtesy of Sorin Group of Canada Inc.). (c) Medtronic Hall tilting disk (©Medtronic Inc. Printed with permission.). (d) St Jude Medical bileaflet (courtesy of Sorin Group of Canada Inc.).

flow of blood, which may reduce the risk of thromboembolism compared to the circumferential blood flow of caged-ball valves. Single tilting disk valves appear to be associated with a slightly higher risk of thromboembolism than bileaflet mechanical valves, possibly because they have a region of stagnant blood flow located adjacent to the wall immediately downstream from the minor orifice and because the regurgitant washing jet volume is lower than for bileaflet valves.[7]

The first successful tilting disk valve was the Bjork–Shiley valve introduced in 1969.[9] This valve consists of a single leaflet of pyrolytic carbon held in place by large inflow and small outflow alloy struts encircled by a Teflon sewing ring[6] (Fig. 60.1b). The Bjork–Shiley convexoconcave valve was withdrawn in 1986 because of several cases of strut fracture and embolization of the disk.[6] Figure 60.1c displays the Medtronic Hall single leaflet/tilting disk valve. Table 60.1 lists other models of single leaflet/tilting disk valves.

Bileaflet valves

The St Jude Medical valve introduced in 1977[10] was the first bileaflet valve and is the single most commonly implanted mechanical valve. Made of pyrolytic carbon coated with graphite, it consists of two leaflets hinged on a ring (Fig 60.1d). Encircling this structure is a sewing ring. The bileaflet valves listed in Table 60.1 have a similar design. Bileaflet valves provide symmetric, relatively non-turbulent, central blood flow.[6]

Bioprosthetic valves

Most bioprosthetic valves are porcine or made from bovine pericardium that is fashioned into valve leaflets. The valves are preserved in glutaraldehyde and mounted on a frame or stent made of metal or plastic covered with fabric that acts as the sewing ring.[11] Bioprosthetic valves mimic native heart valves more closely than mechanical valves because they have unobstructed central flow which provides excel-

Table 60.1 Models of prosthetic valves

Type of valve	Model name
Mechanical	
Caged ball	Starr–Edwards
	Magovern–Cromie
	Smeloff–Cutter
Single leaflet/ tilting disk	Bjork–Shiley
	Medtronic–Hall
	Omniscience, Omnicarbon
	Sorin Allcarbon
	Beall
	Cooley–Cutter
	Cross–Jones
	Gott Daggett
	Harken
	Kay–Shiley
	Starr–Edwards Disc
	AorTech Ultracor
	Wada–Cutter
Bileaflet	St. Jude Medical
	ATS Open Pivot
	Carbomedics Standard, TopHat, Orbis, Optiform
	Edwards Duromedics, Tekna, Mira
	Medtronic Parallel
	MCRI On-X, Conform-X
	Sorin Bicarbon
Bioprosthetic	
Porcine	Medtronic Hancock Standard, Hancock II, Hancock MO, MO II, MI, Mosaic, Ultra
	Carpentier–Edwards, SAV
	St. Jude Medical Biocor
	Tissuemed
	Angell–Shiley
Pericardial	Carpentier–Edwards Perimount
	Sorin Mitroflow, Pericarbon
	Ionescu–Shiley Standard, Low Profile
	Hancock
	Labcor–Santiago
Stentless	CryoLife stentless porcine
	Edwards Prima Plus stentless porcine
	Medtronic Freestyle Aortic Root porcine
	St. Jude Medical Toronto stentless porcine
	St. Jude Medical Quattro Valve

lent hemodynamics. The surfaces of bioprosthetic valves also are less thrombogenic than mechanical valves and do not require lifelong anticoagulant therapy. Porcine and pericardial (bovine) valves do not differ importantly in thrombogenicity.

Porcine bioprosthetic valves

Porcine valves are the most widely used bioprosthetic valves.[8] The first commercial porcine valve was the Hancock

valve introduced in 1970. Figure 60.2a displays the Medtronic valve and Figure 60.2b displays a freestyle model consisting of a porcine valve housed within its native aorta. Table 60.1 lists other types of porcine valves.

Bovine pericardial bioprosthetic valves

Bovine pericardial valves have several theoretic advantages over porcine valves. The valve leaflets are larger, which accommodates shrinkage over the life of the valve; leaflet opening is more complete and symmetric, which improves valve hemodynamics; and the collagen content of the valves is higher, which improves valve durability. The Carpentier–Edwards Perimount valve (Fig. 60.2c) is the only pericardial valve presently available in North America. It is unclear whether the theoretic advantages of pericardial over porcine valves translate into improved outcomes for patients. Bovine valves appear to be at least as durable as contemporary porcine valves.[12,13]

Oral anticoagulants

Vitamin K antagonists (VKAs) are the only oral anticoagulants available for clinical use and warfarin is the most widely used VKA in North America. Other VKAs commonly used in Europe include acenocoumarol and phenprocoumon. VKAs are challenging to use in clinical practice because they have a slow onset and offset, narrow therapeutic window, and variable dose response and are subject to numerous food and drug interactions.[14] Thus close laboratory monitoring of the anticoagulant effect of VKAs is required. The international normalized ratio (INR) is a standardized method of reporting the intensity of anticoagulant therapy with VKAs adopted in 1982.[15,16] Studies completed prior to 1982 often reported anticoagulant intensity based on the ratio of the patient's plasma value to that of plasma from a healthy control and it is difficult to compare these results with subsequent studies that reported anticoagulant intensity based on the INR.

Starting dose of VKA for patients requiring oral anticoagulant therapy

One randomized trial has studied the optimal starting dose of VKA for patients who have undergone valve replacement. Ageno *et al* randomized, in an open-label fashion, 197 patients after heart valve replacement to an initial 2.5 mg (n = 84) versus 5 mg dose of warfarin (n = 113).[17] The INR was measured daily and the dose of warfarin was adjusted according to the result of the INR in the 5 mg starting dose group. The dose of warfarin was not modified in the 2.5 mg group until day 3 and then only if the INR was less than 1.5 or greater than 3.0. The primary outcome of the study was the proportion of patients with an INR of >2.6 within 6 days of surgery. A greater percentage of patients in the 5 mg than the 2.5 mg group had an INR level

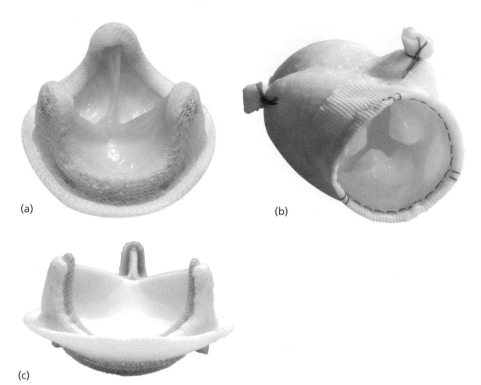

(a)

(b)

(c)

Figure 60.2 Different models of bioprosthetic valves. (a) Medtronic HK II Ultra porcine. (b) Medtronic Freestyle porcine (©Medtronic Inc. Printed with permission.). (c) Carpentier–Edwards Perimount bovine pericardial (courtesy of Edwards Lifesciences LLC, Irvine, California).

>2.6 within 6 days of surgery (42% v 26%, $P < 0.05$). There was no difference in the rate of bleeding between the two groups although the study was not powered for clinical outcomes (Level A).

Incidence, natural history and prognosis

Thromboembolism after mechanical valve replacement without antithrombotic therapy

Information concerning the risk of thromboembolism after mechanical valve replacement in patients not treated with anticoagulants primarily comes from small case series of patients who had a contraindication to VKAs. Cannegieter and colleagues performed a systematic review in which they examined the risk of thromboembolism and bleeding in patients with mechanical heart valves.[18] Included in the review were seven studies involving 460 patients who did not receive oral anticoagulant therapy. During 1225 patient-years of follow-up the rates of thromboembolism per 100 patient-years were (95% confidence intervals (CI) in parentheses): valve thrombosis 1.8 (0.9–3.0), major embolism 4.0 (2.9–5.2), total embolism 8.6 (7.0–10.4). The risk thromboembolism was reduced by more than 75% in a parallel group of patients who received VKA therapy (**Level C1**).

Thromboembolism after bioprosthetic valve replacement

The largest study of thromboembolism risk after bioprosthetic valve replacement is by Heras and colleagues who followed 816 patients with aortic, mitral or combined aortic and mitral bioprosthetic valves for a median of 8.6 years.[19] The rate of thromboembolism during the first 10 days among patients who did not receive any antithrombotic therapy was approximately 50% for aortic valves and 60% for mitral valves. Patients who were commenced immediately postoperatively on VKA therapy had higher rates of thromboembolism during the first 10 days (aortic 41%, mitral 55%) compared with between day 11 and 30 (aortic 3.6%, mitral 10%) and after day 30 (aortic 1.9% per year, mitral 2.4% per year) (**Level C2**). The unexpectedly high rate of early thromboembolism in the study by Heras and colleagues is unexplained and is inconsistent with other reports. Multiple small cases series of patients with bioprosthetic valves have reported thromboembolism rates of between 0.7% and 2.8% per patient-year during long-term follow-up ranging from 18 months to 6 years.[20–21,22,23,24,25,26] Most patients in the latter studies received oral anticoagulants, antiplatelet therapy or a combination of anticoagulants and antiplatelet therapy for 2–3 months after surgery (**Level C2**).

Pathophysiology

Factors that contribute to the thrombogenicity of prosthetic heart valves include altered blood flow and hemostatic activation caused by endothelial injury during surgery or exposure of artificial surfaces (sutures, sewing ring, occluder and valve housing) to the circulating blood.[27] Because almost all prosthetic valves are stented, they have a smaller effective orifice area than the native valve that results in a transvalvular flow gradient. Stagnant flow may also result from growth of endocardial tissue (pannus) into the leaflets or valve mechanism. Endothelialization of foreign surfaces occurs over a period of about 3 months after which the risk of thrombosis decreases.[21]

Antithrombotic therapy

In this section, we review the evidence for the benefits and risks of antithrombotic therapy in patients with prosthetic heart valves and make recommendations based on the usefulness of the treatment and the quality of the evidence. We focus on the results of high-quality studies (randomized controlled trials and meta-analyses of randomized controlled trials) whenever available and consider lower quality studies only when there are no high-quality studies.

Mechanical valves

Acute

Possible approaches to antithrombotic therapy immediately after mechanical heart valve replacement include aspirin, oral VKA therapy with or without initial "bridging" unfractionated heparin (UFH) or low molecular weight heparin (LMWH) therapy, or aspirin in combination with oral VKA therapy.

Oral VKA therapy There are no randomized trials comparing oral anticoagulation to placebo (or no anticoagulation) in the immediate postoperative period. A systematic review by Kulik *et al* of primarily observational studies comparing different initial anticoagulation strategies involving 3056 patients who received VKA therapy immediately after surgery[28] revealed an absolute rate of thromboembolism of 0.9% and a bleeding rate of 3.3% during the first 30 days (**Level C1**).

Oral VKA + LMWH There are no randomized trials comparing VKA plus LMWH to VKA alone in patients with a mechanical heart valve. A prospective observational "before-and-after" study by Talwar and colleagues compared initial LMWH plus oral VKA therapy to VKA therapy alone in 538 patients.[29] Group A (n = 245) consisted of con-

secutive patients undergoing mechanical valve replacement over a 2-year period who were started on VKAs on postoperative day 1. Group B (n = 293) consisted of consecutive patients undergoing mechanical valve replacement over a subsequent 2-year period who received enoxaparin 1 mg/kg started 6 hours after surgery, repeated every 12 hours, in combination with VKA therapy (started day one) and continued until the INR was therapeutic. The target INR was 2.5 (range 2.5–3.5) for patients with a mitral valve replacement (MVR) or multiple mechanical valves and 2.0 (range 2.0–3.0) for patients with an aortic valve replacement (AVR). All patients received aspirin 150 mg daily and were followed for 6 months. The incidence of prosthetic valve thrombosis (PVT) was significantly lower in patients who received enoxaparin compared with those who did not receive enoxaparin (6.1% v 2.0%, P = 0.01) and there was no significant difference in bleeding (**Level C1**).

Three observational studies reviewed by Kulik and colleagues involving a total of 168 patients who received oral anticoagulation in combination with LMWH showed a rate of thromboembolism of 0.6% and bleeding 4.8% during the first 30 days after surgery[30] (**Level C2**).

Oral VKA therapy + UFH There have been no randomized trials comparing the combination of VKA therapy and UFH with VKA therapy alone in patients with a mechanical heart valve. Kulik *et al* reviewed seven observational studies involving 2535 patients who received oral anticoagulation and intravenous UFH postoperatively and reported thromboembolism rates of 1.1% and bleeding 7.2% during the first 30 days.[30] Bleeding data were available from only two studies (n = 261) (**Level C2**).

Oral VKA therapy + UFH versus oral VKA therapy + LMWH There have been no randomized comparisons between UFH and LMWH for immediate postoperative anticoagulation in patients with mechanical heart valves receiving VKA therapy but UFH and LMWH have been compared in observational studies.

Montalescot and colleagues studied 208 consecutive patients undergoing mechanical heart valve replacement.[30] The first 106 patients were treated with intravenous UFH as soon as postoperative chest tube drainage had decreased to acceptable levels (approximately 2 days after surgery) and were switched from intravenous to subcutaneous UFH three times daily in conjunction with oral VKAs starting on postoperative day 6. The target activated partial thromboplastin time (APTT) was 1.5–2.5 times control for both intravenous and subcutaneous heparin therapies. The next 102 patients were treated with LMWH (enoxaparin or nadroparin) immediately after surgery and were started on oral VKAs on postoperative day 6. LMWH doses were titrated according to anti-Xa levels (target 0.5–1.0 IU/mL). In both groups, intravenous or subcutaneous anticoagulation was discontinued once the INR was therapeutic. One patient treated with UFH suffered a TIA while there were no thromboembolic events in the LMWH group. There were two major bleeds in each treatment group (**Level C2**).

Fanikos and colleagues compared 29 patients receiving postoperative LMWH to 34 retrospectively matched patients who had received UFH.[31] In both groups treatment was continued until the INR was therapeutic. One patient in the LMWH group and four in the UFH group died within 90 days of discharge. There were two (6%) thromboembolic events in the UFH group and none in the LMWH group. Three patients in each group experienced major bleeding (**Level C2**).

Long-term

Possible approaches to long-term antithrombotic therapy after mechanical heart valve replacement include antiplatelet therapy alone, oral VKA therapy alone or antiplatelet therapy in combination with oral VKA therapy.

Oral VKA alone There have been no randomized studies comparing the VKA therapy with placebo or no VKA therapy in patients with mechanical prosthetic heart valves. However, there is a widespread belief that lifelong anticoagulation is necessary, based on the inherent thrombogenicity of mechanical valves and the results of studies of the natural history of thromboembolism in patients with mechanical valves who did not receive anticoagulation (see Incidence, natural history and prognosis above) (**Level C2**).

Oral VKA versus antiplatelet therapy Only one randomized trial has compared oral VKA therapy to antiplatelet therapy for the long-term management of patients with mechanical heart valves. Mok *et al*[32] treated patients with either Starr–Edwards or Bjork–Shiley valves with warfarin (target INR range 1.8–2.5) for the first 6 months after surgery. After 6 months, patients were randomized to continue warfarin (n = 97) or to switch to dipyridamole-aspirin (dipyridamole 75 mg twice daily and aspirin 650 mg once daily) (n = 81) or pentoxifylline-aspirin (pentoxifylline 400 mg twice daily and aspirin 650 mg daily) (n = 76). Follow-up was continued for a mean of 24 months in the warfarin group and approximately 18 months in each of the antiplatelet groups.

The incidence of thromboembolism was significantly lower in the warfarin group compared to the dipyridamole-aspirin and pentoxifylline-aspirin groups (4.1% v 13.6% v 10.5% respectively, $P < 0.05$). Rates of bleeding were higher in the warfarin group compared to the dipyridamole-aspirin and pentoxifylline-aspirin groups (5.2% v 0% v 1.3% respectively) (**Level B**).

Optimal intensity of anticoagulation In 1995 Cannegieter and colleagues published the results of a cohort study in which they examined the relationship between thromboembo-

lism, bleeding, anticoagulant intensity and type of mechanical valve.[33] The study included retrospective and prospective data on 1608 patients with mechanical prosthetic valves treated with oral VKA therapy who were monitored by regional anticoagulation clinics. The target INR was 3.6–4.8 and patients were followed for up to 6 years. The number of thromboembolic events and major bleeding episodes were recorded as well as the most recent INR prior to the event (to a maximum of 8 days before). The study included patients with mechanical aortic (59.8%), mitral (30.2%), and combined aortic and mitral (9.8%) valves. Valve types included tilting disk (76.7%), bileaflet (19.6%), and caged-ball or caged-disk valves (3.0%). Follow-up was 6475 patient-years and 123 254 INR measurements. INRs were within the target range 61% of the time, below therapeutic range 31% of the time, and above therapeutic range 8% of the time.

The lowest rates of bleeding and thromboembolism occurred when the INR was between 2.5 and 4.9 (2 per 100 patient-years). The incidence of thromboembolic events increased significantly when the INR was below 2.5 and bleeding increased sharply when the INR was greater than 4.9. The rates of thromboembolism were higher for valves in the mitral compared to the aortic position (0.9 and 0.5 per 100 patient-years respectively), and were still higher in patients with two mechanical valves (1.2 per 100 patient-years). Caged-ball and caged-disk valves were the most thrombogenic (2.5 per 100 patient-years), followed by tilting disk valves (0.7 per 100 patient-years) and bileaflet valves (0.5 per 100 patient-years). *P*-values were not reported for the comparisons of thromboembolism rates between valve in the aortic compared with the mitral position or between different valve types (**Level C1**).

Two open-label randomized controlled trials have tested the hypothesis that a lower target INR level is safe and effective for patients with a bileaflet mechanical valve in the aortic position. The AREVA trial[34] randomized 380 patients with a St Jude bileaflet mechanical valve (81%) or Omniscience single leaflet/tilting disk valve (19%) to receive VKA therapy with a target INR range of 2.0–3.0 (n = 188) or 3.0–4.5 (n = 192). Patients were followed for an average of 2.2 years and the majority (96%) had a mechanical aortic valve replacement. Rates of thromboembolism were similar in both groups (5.3% v 4.7%, $P = 0.78$) but those with a lower intensity target INR group had fewer non-major hemorrhages (12.2% v 22.9%, $P < 0.01$) and a non-significant reduction in major hemorrhages (6.9% v 9.9%, $P = 0.29$) (**Level B**).

The GELIA trial[35] randomized 2735 patients 3 months after surgery for a St Jude bileaflet mechanical valve replacement to one of three target INR ranges: 2.0–3.5, 2.5–4.0 or 3.0–4.5. Most patients had a mechanical aortic valve (74%) and there were 6801 patient-years of follow-up. Rates of thromboembolic events and clinically important bleeding were not significantly different in the three groups. The overall incidence of thromboembolic events for patients with an AVR was 0.53 per patient-year of follow-up and for patients with a MVR was 1.64 per patient-year of follow-up (**Level A**).

A meta-analysis of 35 (mostly observational) studies reported the incidence of thromboembolic and hemorrhagic events in 23 145 patients with mechanical valves and found that patients had significantly fewer thromboembolic events when the target INR was at least 3.0 compared to less than 3.0.[36] Among patients with a mechanical aortic valve, those targeted with higher-intensity VKA therapy had an incidence of valve thrombosis of 0.87 compared with 1.16 per 1000 patient-years in the low-intensity group (relative risk (RR) 0.75, 95% CI 0.50–1.13, $P = 0.13$). The incidence of thromboembolism was 9.83 per 1000 patient-years versus 13.09 per 1000 patient-years favoring the higher intensity therapy (RR 0.75, 95% CI 0.70–0.81, $P < 0.01$) but at the cost of more bleeding (14.89 versus 12.06 per 1000 patient-years, RR 1.23, 95% CI 1.16–1.31, $P < 0.01$). Among patients with a mechanical mitral valve the incidence of adverse events (thromboembolism or bleeding) was 29.76 per 1000 patient-years in the high-intensity group compared with 35.33 per 1000 patient-years in the lower intensity group (RR 0.84, 95% CI 0.79–0.89, $P < 0.001$) (**Level C1**).

Self-monitoring of oral anticoagulation The Early Self-Controlled Anticoagulation Trial (ESCAT I) randomized 600 patients with mechanical heart valves to self-management (n = 305) or conventional management (n = 295) of anticoagulation.[37] The target INR range for all patients was 2.5–4.5. After a mean follow-up period of 38 months, the conventional monitoring group had mean INRs consistently around 2.0 and anticoagulation was frequently subtherapeutic. The self-monitoring group tended to be subtherapeutic for the first 6–8 weeks, but was consistently within the therapeutic range thereafter. Complications leading to hospital admission during the study were significantly lower in the self-monitoring group compared with conventionally monitored patients (9.5% v 15.3%, $P = 0.03$) (**Level B**).

The ESCAT II study randomized 2673 patients with mechanical heart valves to self-monitoring of the INR, targeting a range of 2.5–4.5 (n = 1346) versus 1.8–2.8 for aortic valves or 2.5–3.5 for mitral and combined aortic and mitral valves (n = 1327).[38,39] The majority of the valves were St Jude Medical (49%) or Medtronic Hall (47%) valves and 81% were in the aortic position. Patients were followed for 24 months. The proportion of patients requiring hospital admission was similar between the low- and high-intensity groups (0.19% v 0.37% per patient-year, $P = $ NS) as was the rate of bleeding (1.42% v 1.52% per patient-year, $P = $ NS) (**Level A**).

Oral VKA therapy combined with antiplatelet therapy The results of the three largest randomized studies and a meta-analysis of randomized controlled trials comparing oral VKA therapy versus oral VKA in combination with antiplatelet therapy are summarized below.

Turpie and colleagues randomized 370 patients with a mechanical (76%) or tissue (24%) valve treated with warfarin (target INR range 3.0–4.5) to receive low-dose aspirin (100 mg daily) or placebo for a median of 2.5 years.[40] Patients receiving both aspirin and warfarin experienced less major systemic embolism or death from vascular causes (1.9% v 8.5% per year, relative risk reduction (RRR) 77%, $P < 0.001$) and less all-cause death (2.8% v 7.4%, RRR 63%, $P = 0.01$). There were more bleeding events in the dual therapy group (35% v 22%, relative risk increase (RRI) 55%, $P = 0.02$) but major bleeding was not significantly increased (12.9% v 10.3%, RRI 27%, $P = 0.43$) (**Level A**).

Meschengieser and colleagues randomized 503 patients with a mechanical heart valve to receive low-dose aspirin (100 mg per day) plus low-intensity warfarin (target INR 2.5–3.5) (n = 258) or high-intensity warfarin alone (target INR 3.5–4.5) (n = 245) using an open-label design.[41] Types of valves included single leaflet tilting disk (65%), Starr–Edwards caged ball (26%) and St Jude bileaflet (5%) with the remaining types unknown. During a median follow-up of 23 months, median INRs for both groups were within the respective target INR ranges. Rates of thromboembolism were similar: 2.7% in the combined aspirin and warfarin group and 2.8% in the high-intensity warfarin group ($P = 0.7$). There was an excess of major bleeding in patients receiving combined anticoagulant and antiplatelet therapy (4.5% v 2.3%, $P = 0.11$) but the difference was not statistically significant (**Level B**).

Laffort and colleagues[42] randomized 229 patients with a mechanical St Jude bileaflet valve in the mitral position to receive oral anticoagulation (target INR 2.5–3.5) plus aspirin (200 mg per day) (n = 109) or oral anticoagulation alone (target INR 2.5–3.5) (n = 120) using an open-label design. Transesophageal echocardiogram was performed at 9 days, 5 months, and 1 year. The group receiving combined therapy had significantly fewer thromboembolic events (9% v 25%, $P = 0.004$) and fewer valvular thrombi seen on echocardiogram (5% v 13%, $P = 0.03$), but more major hemorrhage (19.2% v 8.3%, $P = 0.02$) due to an excess number of gastrointestinal bleeds (7% v 0%, $P = 0.003$) (**Level B**).

The Cochrane Collaboration published a systematic review and meta-analysis of 11 studies involving 2428 patients comparing oral anticoagulation plus antiplatelet therapy with anticoagulation alone in patients with prosthetic heart valves in 2003.[43] Studies were eligible for inclusion if they were randomized, followed patients for at least 1 year, and reported thromboembolism, death and major bleeding. The addition of antiplatelet therapy to oral anti-

embolism is highest during the first 3 months after prosthetic valve replacement surgery.

References

1. Nkomo VT, Gardin JM, Skelton TN *et al.* Burden of valvular heart diseases: a population-based study. *Lancet* 2006;**368**: 1005–11.
2. Carapetis JR, Steer AC, Mulholland EK *et al.* The global burden of group A streptococcal diseases. *Lancet Infect Dis* 2005;**5**: 685–94.
3. American Heart Association. Heart Disease and Stroke Statistics – 2006 Update. Dallas, Texas: American Heart Association, 2006. http://www.americanheart.org/downloadable/heart/1136308 648540Statupdate2006.pdf (accessed July 2007).
4. Butany J, Ahluwalia MS, Munroe C *et al.* Mechanical heart valve prostheses: identification and evaluation. *Cardiovasc Pathol* 2003;**12**:322–44.
5. Starr A, Edwards M. Mitral replacement: clinical experience with a ball valve prosthesis. *Ann Surg* 1961;**154**:726–40.
6. Grunkemeier GL, Li HH, Naftel DC *et al.* Long-term performance of heart valve prostheses. *Curr Prob Cardiol* 2000;**25**:75–154.
7. Yoganathan AP, He Z, Jones SC. Fluid mechanics of heart valves. *Annu Rev Biomed Eng* 2004;**6**:331–62.
8. Jamieson WRE. *Advanced Technologies for Cardiac Valvular Replacement, Transcatheter Innovations and Reconstructive Surgery.* Surgical Technology International XV. San Francisco: Universal Medical Press, 2006.
9. Bjork VO. A new tilting disc valve prosthesis. *Scand J Thorac Cardiovasc Surg* 1969;**3**:1–10.
10. Emery RW, Mettler E, Nicoloff DM. A new cardiac prosthesis: the St. Jude Medical cardiac valve: in vivo results. *Circulation* 1979;**60**:48–54.
11. Butany J, Fayet C, Ahluwalia MS *et al.* Biological replacement heart valves: identification and evaluation. *Cardiovasc Pathol* 2003;**12**:119–39.
12. Marchand M, Aupart M, Norton R *et al.* Twelve-year experience with Carpentier–Edwards PERIMOUNT pericardial valve in the mitral position: a multicenter study. *J Heart Valve Dis* 1998; **7**:292–8.
13. Gao G, Wu Y, Grunkemeier Gl *et al.* Durability of pericardial versus porcine aortic valves. *J Am Coll Cardiol* 2004;**44**:384–8.
14. Berkowitz SD. Antithrombotic therapy after prosthetic cardiac valve implantation: potential novel antithrombotic therapies. *Am Heart J* 2001;**142**:7–13.
15. Bussey HI. An overview of anticoagulants, antiplatelet agents, and the combination in patients with mechanical heart valves. *J Heart Valve Dis* 2004;**13**:319–24.
16. Ansell J, Hirsh J, Poller L *et al*, for the Seventh ACCP Conference on Antithrombotic and Thrombolytic Therapy. The pharmacology and management of the Vitamin K antagonists. *Chest* 2004;**126**:204S-233S.
17. Ageno W, Turpie AGG, Steidl L *et al.* Comparison of a daily fixed 2.5-mg warfarin dose with a 5-mg international normalized ratio adjusted, warfarin dose initially following heart valve replacement. *Am J Cardiol* 2001;**88**:40–4.
18. Cannegieter SC, Rosendaal FR, Briet E. Thromboembolic and bleeding complications in patients with mechanical heart valve prostheses. *Circulation* 1994;**89**:635–41.
19. Heras M, Chesebro JH, Fuster V *et al.* High risk of thromboemboli early after bioprosthetic cardiac valve replacement. *J Am Coll Cardiol* 1995;**25**:1111–19.
20. David TE, Ho WIC, Christakis GT. Thromboembolism in patients with aortic porcine bioprostheses. *Ann Thorac Surg* 1985;**40**:229–33.
21. Spencer FC, Grossi EA, Culliford AT *et al.* Experiences with 1643 porcine prosthetic valves in 1492 patients. *Ann Surg* 1986;**203**:691–9.
22. Louagie Y, Noirhomme P, Aranguis E *et al.* Use of the Carpentier-Edwards porcine bioprosthesis: assessment of a patient selection policy. *J Thorac Cardiovasc Surg* 1992;**104**:1013–24.
23. Gallo I, Ruiz B, Duran CMG. Five- to eight-year follow-up of patients with the Hancock cardiac bioprosthesis. *J Thorac Cardiovasc Surg* 1983;**86**:897–902.
24. Babin-Ebell J, Schmidt W, Eigel P *et al.* Aortic bioprosthesis without early anticoagulation – risk of thromboembolism. *Thorac Cardiovasc Surg* 1995;**43**:212–14.
25. Revuelta JM, Duran CM. Performance of the Ionescu-Shiley pericardial valve in the aortic position: 100 months clinical experience. *Thorac Cardiovasc Surg* 1986;**34**:247–51.
26. Hartz RS, Fisher EB, Finkelmeier B *et al.* An eight-year experience with porcine bioprosthetic cardiac valves. *J Thorac Cardiovasc Surg* 1986;**91**:910–17.
27. Berkowitz SD. Antithrombotic therapy after prosthetic cardiac valve implantation: potential novel antithrombotic therapies. *Am Heart J* 2002;**142**:7–13.
28. Kulik A, Rubens FD, Wells PS *et al.* Early postoperative anticoagulation after mechanical valve replacement: a systematic review. *Ann Thorac Surg* 2006;**81**:770–81.
29. Talwar S, Kapoor CK, Velayoudam D, Kumar AS. Anticoagulation protocol and early prosthetic valve thrombosis. *Indian Heart J* 2004;**56**:225–8.
30. Montalescot G, Polle V, Collet JP *et al.* Low molecular weight heparin after mechanical heart valve replacement. *Circulation* 2000;**101**:1083–6.
31. Fanikos J, Tsilimingras K, Kucher N *et al.* Comparison of efficacy, safety, and cost of low-molecular-weight heparin with continuous-infusion unfractionated heparin for initiation of anticoagulation after mechanical prosthetic valve implantation. *Am J Cardiol* 2004;**93**:247–50.
32. Mok CK, Boey J, Wang R *et al.* Warfarin versus dipyridamole-aspirin and pentoxifylline-aspirin for the prevention of prosthetic heart valve thromboembolism: a prospective randomized clinical trial. *Circulation* 1985;**5**:1059–63.
33. Cannegieter SC, Rosendaal FR, Wintzen AR *et al.* Optimal oral anticoagulant therapy in patients with mechanical heart valves. *N Engl J Med* 1995;**333**:11–17.
34. Acar J, Iung B, Boissel JP *et al.* AREVA: multicenter randomized comparison of low-dose versus standard-dose anticoagulation in patients with mechanical prosthetic heart valves. *Circulation* 1996;**94**:2107–12.
35. Hering D, Piper C, Bergemann R *et al.* Thromboembolic and bleeding complications following St. Jude Medical valve replacement. *Chest* 2005;**127**:53–9.

36. Vink R, Kraaijenhagen RA, Hutten BA *et al.* The optimal intensity of Vitamin K antagonists in patients with mechanical heart valves. *J Am Coll Cardiol* 2003;**42**:2042–8.

37. Koertke H, Minami K, Bairaktaris A *et al.* INR self-management following mechanical heart valve replacement. *J Thromb Thrombolysis* 2000;**9**:S41–5.

38. Koertke H, Zittermann A, Minami K *et al.* Low-dose international normalized ratio self-management: a promising tool to achieve low complication rates after mechanical heart valve replacement. *Ann Thorac Surg* 2005;**79**:1909–14.

39. Koertke H, Zittermann A, Tenderich G *et al.* Low-dose oral anticoagulation in patients with mechanical heart valve prostheses: final report from the early self-management anticoagulation trial II. *Eur Heart J* 2007;**28**:2479–84.

40. Turpie A, Gent M, Laupacis A *et al.* A comparison of aspirin and placebo in patients treated with warfarin after heart-valve replacement. *N Engl J Med* 1993;**329**:524–9.

41. Meschengieser SS, Fondevila CG, Frontroth J *et al.* Low-intensity oral anticoagulation plus low-dose aspirin versus high-intensity oral anticoagulation alone: a randomized trial in patients with mechanical prosthetic heart valves. *J Thorac Cardiovasc Surg* 1997;**113**:910–16.

42. Laffort P, Roudaut, Roques X *et al.* Early and long-term (one-year) effects of the association of aspirin and oral anticoagulant on thrombi and morbidity after replacement of the mitral valve with the St. Jude Medical prosthesis. *J Am Coll Cardiol* 2000;**35**:739–46.

43. Little SH, Massel DR. Antiplatelet and anticoagulation for patients with prosthetic heart valves. *Cochrane Database of Systematic Reviews* 2003, Issue 4. Art. No.: CD003464. DOI: 10.1002/14651858.CD003464..

44. Blair KL, Hatton AC, White WD *et al.* Comparison of anticoagulation regimens after Carpentier-Edwards aortic or mitral valve replacement. *Circulation* 1994;**90**:214–19.

45. Moinuddeen K, Quin J, Shaw R *et al.* Anticoagulation is unnecessary after biological aortic valve replacement. *Circulation* 1998;**98**(19S):95II–98II.

46. Turpie AGG, Gunstensen J, Hirsh J *et al.* Randomised comparison of two intensities of oral anticoagulant therapy after tissue heart valve replacement. *Lancet* 1988;**1**:1242–5.

47. Di Marco, F, Giordan M, Gerosa G. Early antithrombotic therapy after aortic valve replacement with tissue valves: when the practice diverges from the guidelines. *J Thorac Cardiovasc Surg* 2006;**131**:1223.

48. CTSNet Editors, Valve Technology Center. Anticoagulation therapy after aortic tissue valve replacement: Final results, 2004. www.ctsnet.org/file/AnticoagulationSurveyFinalResults SlidesPDF.pdf (accessed July 2007).

49. Vaughan P, Waterworth PD. An audit of anticoagulation practice among UK cardiothoracic consultant surgeons following valve replacement/repair. *J Heart Valve Dis* 2005;**14**:576–82.

50. Aramendi JI, Mestres CA, Martinez-Leon J *et al.* Triflusal versus oral anticoagulation for primary prevention of thromboembolism after bioprosthetic valve replacement (trac): prospective, randomized, co-operative trial. *Eur J Cardio-thorac Surg* 2005;**27**:854–60.

51. Aramendi JL, Agredo J, Llorente A *et al.* Prevention of thromboembolism with Ticlopidine shortly after valve repair or replacement with a bioprosthesis. *J Heart Valve Dis* 1998;**7**:610–14.

52. Gherli T, Colli A, Fragnito C *et al.* Comparing warfarin with aspirin after biological aortic valve replacement: a prospective study. *Circulation* 2004;**110**:496–500.

53. Di Marco F, Grendene S, Feltrin G *et al.* Antiplatelet therapy in patients receiving aortic bioprostheses: a report of clinical and instrumental safety. *J Thorac Cardiovasc Surg* 2007;**133**:1597–603.

54. Khaja M, Quin J, Shaw R *et al.* Anticoagulation is unnecessary after biological aortic valve replacement. *Circulation* 1998;**98**(19S):95II–98II.

55. Sundt TM, Zehr KJ, Dearani JA *et al.* Is early anticoagulation with warfarin necessary after bioprosthetic aortic valve replacement? *J Thorac Cardiovasc Surg* 2005;**129**:1024–31.

56. Jamieson WRE, Moffatt-Bruce SD, Skarsgard P *et al.* Early antithrombotic therapy for aortic valve bioprostheses: is there an indication for routine use? *Ann Thorac Surg* 2007;**83**:549–57.

57. Goldsmith I, Lip GYH, Mukundan S *et al.* Experience with low-dose aspirin as thromboprophylaxis for the Tissuemed porcine aortic bioprosthesis: a survey of five years' experience. *J Heart Valve Dis* 1998;**7**:574–9.

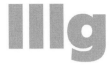

Specific cardiovascular disorders: other conditions

Bernard J Gersh and Salim Yusuf , Editors

61 Stroke

Brian H Buck,[1,2] Ashfaq Shuaib[2] and Craig Anderson[3]

[1]Grey Nuns Community Hospital, Edmonton, Alberta, Canada
[2]University of Alberta, Edmonton, Alberta, Canada
[3]The George Institute for International Health, University of Sydney and the Royal Prince Alfred Hospital, Sydney, Australia

Management of acute ischemic stroke

Brian H Buck, Ashfaq Shuaib

Introduction

Epidemiology

Worldwide, stroke is the second most common cause of death after coronary heart disease (CHD)[1] and accounts for 4.38 million deaths annually, with almost three million of those in developing countries. Most strokes are not fatal[2] and consequently mortality data underestimate the true global burden of stroke which is chronic disability.[3] Stroke is the sixth most common cause of disability-adjusted life years (DALYs).[4] More than 80% of strokes occur in the 14% of the population aged 65 and older[5] and 20–25% of individuals will have a stroke if they live until 85 years.[6] Consequently the incidence of stroke and socioeconomic burden is expected to increase globally and particularly in Western countries, where there is expected to be a shift in the age distribution of the population towards older ages. By 2030 stroke is projected to be the fourth most common cause of reduced DALYs.[7]

Estimates of the incidence of stroke come from a number of population-based epidemiologic studies. One of the largest studies to examine the incidence of vascular disease including stroke is the Oxford Vascular Study (OXVASC) in which >91 000 individuals were followed over a three-year period in Oxfordshire, United Kingdom (UK). The rate per 1000 population per year of first-ever incident cerebrovascular events was 2.27 (95% confidence interval

(CI) 2.09–2.45) which was higher than event rates in the coronary and peripheral vascular beds[5] (Table 61.1). Event rates rose steeply with age with 80% of strokes occurring in the 14% of the study population aged 65 and older. Long-term trends in stroke incidence have been reported over a 20-year period in Oxfordshire. The age-specific incidence of stroke has fallen by 40% largely due to increased use of preventive medications and risk factor modifications.[8]

Nomenclature, definitions

Stroke is divided broadly into either ischemic or hemorrhagic types with ischemic strokes accounting for the majority of stroke (>80%).[9] The treatment of these stroke subtypes is dramatically different and as a result, one of the first steps in managing stroke patients is to evaluate them for the presence of hemorrhage. Clinical features of hemorrhagic and ischemic stroke overlap and as a result, the distinction is often made with hyperacute computed tomography (CT) imaging. Specialized magnetic resonance imaging (MRI) sequences are more sensitive than CT to acute and chronic hemorrhage and better at detecting early ischemia and are becoming more commonly used for the early diagnosis of stroke.[10]

Ischemic strokes can be further classified based on clinical findings and the results of investigations into subtypes. The value of identifying stroke subtype is that identifying the most likely mechanism of vessel occlusion helps guide early treatment and subsequent investigations. The Trial of Org 10172 in Acute Stroke Treatment (TOAST) criteria is one of the most widely employed classification systems for ischemic stroke.[11] Ischemic stroke, based on the presumed pathophysiologic mechanism of occlusion, is subdivided into small vessel occlusion ("lacunes"), large artery atherosclerosis (embolus or thrombosis) and cardioembolic. The TOAST criteria also recognize that a proportion of ischemic stroke will remain cryptogenic in etiology or will result

Evidence-Based Cardiology, 3rd edition. Edited by S. Yusuf, J.A. Cairns, A.J. Camm, E.L. Fallen, and B.J. Gersh. © 2010 Blackwell Publishing, ISBN: 978-1-4051-5925-8.

Table 61.1 Incidence of first and recurrent stroke compared to ischemic heart disease and peripheral vascular disease in Oxford Vascular Study population[5]

		Total number*	Rate† (95% CI)
Cerebrovascular events	Ischemic stroke	550	2.01 (1.85–2.19)
	Intracerebral hemorrhage	41	0.15 (0.11–0.20)
	Subarachnoid hemorrhage	27	0.10 (0.07–0.14)
	Transient ischemic attack	300	1.10 (0.98–1.23)
	All events	918	3.36 (3.14–3.58)
Coronary vascular events	Sudden cardiac death	163	0.60 (0.51–0.7)
	STEMI	159	0.58 (0.49–0.68)
	NSTEMI	316	1.16 (1.03–1.29)
	Unstable angina	218	0.80 (0.70–0.91)
	All coronary events	856	3.13 (2.93–3.35)
Peripheral vascular events	All events	188	0.69 (0.59–0.79)

STEMI, ST segment elevation acute myocardial infarction; NSTEMI, non-ST segment elevation acute myocardial infarction.

*Number of events during 3 years.

†Number of events per 1000 population per year.

Reproduced from Donnan and colleagues[95] with permission.

Table 61.2 Acute stroke management strategies of proven benefit (**Level A**)

Intervention	Outcome	RRR	ARR	NNT	Reference
Stroke unit	Death or dependency	9% (4–14%)	5.6%	18	96
Thrombolysis with 3 hours of symptom onset (IV tPA)	Minimal or no disability at 3 months	30%	11–13%	7–9	46
ASA	Recurrent stroke	24%	0.5%	200	74
Decompressive hemicraniectomy for malignant MCA infarct (within 48 hours)	Survival with favorable outcome	68%	51%	2	91

RRR, relative risk reduction; ARR, absolute risk reduction; NNT, numbers needed to treated; IV tPA, intravenous tissue plasminogen activator; ASA, acetylsalicylic acid; MCA, middle cerebral artery.

from some combination of mechanisms or other causes such as dissection or a vasculitis.

There are two subtypes of hemorrhagic stroke: intracerebral hemorrhage (ICH) and subarachnoid hemorrhage (SAH). Primary ICH is more common (about 8% of total strokes) and is most often caused by hypertensive small vessel disease which causes the rupture of small lipohyalinotic aneurysms.[12] SAH accounts for about 5% of strokes and is usually caused by the rupture of saccular aneurysms within the subarachnoid space. The acute management of ICH frequently involves admission to an intensive care unit and management of increased intracranial pressure, a discussion of which is beyond the scope of the current chapter (see American Heart Association guidelines for detailed review[13]). With the exception of a recently reported negative Phase III trial of hemostasis with recombinant activated factor VII,[14] treatments for ICH have not been subjected to large randomized trials. There are no therapies for ICH with Level A evidence and in general, the evidence guiding therapy for ICH is less established. Acute ischemic

stroke treatments with Level A evidence are summarized in Table 61.2.

Acute stroke management

Prehospital management

The treatment of acute ischemic stroke (AIS) is exquisitely time sensitive and the speed and accuracy of evaluating and managing patients are important in optimizing patient outcomes. Based on data extrapolated from experimental studies of ischemic stroke, with each minute that passes there is a loss of 1.9 million neurons.[15] Accordingly, timely reperfusion of ischemic brain is the primary goal of most acute stroke therapies.

The narrow time window for the delivery of reperfusion therapies such as intravenous (IV) recombinant tissue plasminogen activator (tPA) necessitates the development of stroke-specific prehospital algorithms to ensure the timely transport of patients to hospitals capable of providing acute stroke care. The most time-efficient means for stroke patients to seek medical care is by activating Emergency Medical Services (EMS) by calling 911 or the equivalent "immediate" EMS response phone service. Compared to patients who contact their primary physician or hospital directly, stroke patients who call EMS are more likely to arrive within the three-hour time window.[16] Currently only about half of patients with signs and symptoms of acute stroke will use EMS to first access medical care.[17] The decision to call 911 either by patients or other bystanders is influenced by the knowledge that stroke is a serious and treatable disease.[18] There is evidence that patients transported to hospitals through the activation of emergency stroke pathways receive neurologic attention sooner, more frequently are treated with tPA, and have better outcomes[19] (**Level C1**).

Early recognition of stroke by EMS paramedics helps ensure that patients are provided with appropriate initial stabilization and therapy, and advance notice is provided to the receiving emergency department. Diagnosis of stroke in the prehospital setting can be facilitated by the use of validated prehospital screening tools (**Class I, Level B**) such as the Los Angeles Prehospital Stroke Screen[20] and the Cincinnati Prehospital Stroke Scale.[21] Once a diagnosis of stroke is made, patients with acute symptoms that may eligible for fibrinolytic therapy can then be transported to the closest facility that provides emergency stroke care. In rural areas where long distances prevent timely transport of patients to specialized stroke centers, telestroke systems can facilitate the safe delivery of intravenous tPA administration[22–24] (**Class IIa, Level B**).

Emergency management

The initial management of acute stroke patients most often occurs in the emergency department (ED) of hospitals. A number of conditions can mimic stroke including seizures, tumors, infection, hypoglycemia and other metabolic abnormalities. Stroke mimics are common and 13–31% of patients initially diagnosed with acute stroke in the emergency room have other conditions.[25,26] Early brain imaging of stroke patients is required to help make decisions about the emergency management. A non-contrast enhanced CT (NCCT) scan is recommended to exclude non-vascular causes of neurologic symptoms and identify brain hemorrhage (**Class I, Level A**). NCCT will often show early signs of brain ischemia and identify arterial occlusion; however, the interobserver agreement for these early infarction signs on NCCT is general poor (κ statistic range 0.14–0.78).[27] NCCT (performed within 14 hours of symptom onset) will reveal brain parenchymal abnormalities in up to 94% of ischemic stroke patients[28]; however, the sensitivity decreases at earlier time points. In the first six hours the sensitivity of NCCT is 66% (range, 20–87%) with a specificity of 87% (range, 56–100%).[27] At under three hours, which is the time window for treatment with intravenous fibrinolytics, the diagnostic sensitivity of NCCT has been reported as low as 7% (range 3–14%).[10]

The sensitivity of MRI with diffusion-weighted susceptibility images (DWI) is greater than NCCT for the detection of acute stroke (83% vs 26%).[10] DWI MRI sequences measure the degree of free diffusion of water molecules. With cerebral ischemia and subsequent cytotoxic edema, water diffusion becomes restricted and will result in abnormal DWI signal[29] that can be seen within minutes of stroke onset.[30] Case–control studies have suggested that the use of MRI with DWI may improve the safety and efficacy outcomes of fibrinolytic therapy[31]; however, at present there is insufficient evidence to recommend the routine use of MRI for the initial management of acute stroke (**Class II, Level C**).

Early infarction signs such as extent of brain parenchymal hypoattenuation, hyperattenuation within the intracranial artery, and swelling in the affected hemisphere increase the risk of poor functional outcome (overall odds ratio (OR) 3.11; 95% CI 2.77–3.49) but do predict response to fibrinolytic therapy.[27] Other than the identification of intracerebral hemorrhage, no finding on NCCT should preclude treatment of AIS patients with tPA within three hours of symptom onset (Class IIb, Level A).

General supportive care

There are few data from clinical trials to guide initial medical care of acute stroke patients. It is generally agreed that ventilatory assistance should be provided to patients with decreased level of consciousness or bulbar dysfunction compromising the airway. Supplemental oxygen should be provided to prevent hypoxia but in general most stroke patients do not need or benefit from routine oxygen supplementation.[32] Furthermore, increasing brain tissue oxygenation with hyperbaric oxygen therapy has been the focus of a Cochrane review and the authors concluded that there was no evidence of clinical benefit.[33]

Fever in the setting of acute stroke has been consistently associated with stroke severity, infarct size and poor neurologic outcomes[34,35] and should be treated with antipyretics such as acetaminophen (**Class I, Level C**). In experimental studies, small elevations in ischemic brain temperature have a large impact on the extent of ischemic neuronal injury.[36] A few small trials have examined whether prophylactic antipyretic use improves clinical outcomes. These studies have shown a small mean decrease in body temperature in treated patients but without any clear benefit on clinical outcomes. There is both experimental and clinical evidence to suggest that more aggressive lowering of body temperature (induced hypothermia) can protect the brain after cardiac arrest.[37] The value of induced hypothermia in stroke is not yet established but is the focus of ongoing investigations.

Hyperglycemia is commonly detected in acute stroke patients[38] and has been associated with poor outcomes and increased odds of symptomatic intracerebral hemorrhage (OR 1.75 per 100 mg/dL increase in admission glucose, 95% CI 0.61–0.95), independent of fibrinolytic treatment.[39] Hyperglycemia is thought to increase hemorrhage by provoking anaerobic metabolism, lactic acidosis, and free radical production, resulting in membrane lipid peroxidation and cell lysis in ischemic brain tissue.[40] A randomized clinical trial (GIST-UK) of aggressive treatment of hyperglycemia in acute stroke with glucose-potassium-insulin infusions found lower blood pressures and blood glucose in treated patients but no differences in stroke outcomes[41] (**Level A**). In all stroke patients, monitoring of blood glucose is recommended and persistent extreme hyperglycemia should be treated with insulin (**Class II, Level C**). Hypoglycemia can result in brain injury and mimic stroke symptoms and should be corrected as part of the emergency management of stroke patients (**Class I, Level C**).

Acute management of blood pressure

The goal of blood pressure (BP) management in acute stroke is to maximize perfusion to the ischemic penumbra while minimizing the risk of hemorrhagic transformation. Both high and low blood pressures are associated with poor outcomes.[42] Data from the IST trial showed that early death increased by 17.9% for every 10 mm Hg of systolic blood pressure (SBP) below 150 mm Hg and by 3.8% for every 10 mm Hg SBP above 150 mm Hg, suggesting a "U shaped" curve.[43] The optimal blood pressure in the setting of acute stroke remains poorly defined with little clinical trial evidence to guide decisions about blood pressure thresholds. Current guidelines for blood pressure management are largely empirically derived.[44]

BP elevation is often seen in the first minutes to hours after the onset of focal cerebral ischemia[45] and represents a compensatory reaction to vascular occlusion. Targets for the treatment of hypertension depend on whether the patient is a potential candidate for fibrinolytic therapy. A systolic blood pressure >185 mm Hg or a diastolic blood pressure >110 mm Hg is a contraindication to intravenous administration of tPA, which is based on the criteria for the NINDS trial[46] rather than experimental data. Patients with blood pressures above this level should be treated prior to starting lytic therapy (**Class I, Level B**).

There is a theoretic basis for not being overly aggressive with BP lowering in the hyperacute phase of ischemic stroke. Cerebral autoregulation is disrupted by acute ischemia and subsequent tissue acidosis and in turn leads to maximal vasodilation.[47] As a result, with vascular occlu-

sion, overly aggressive treatment of blood pressure could reduce cerebral blood flow (CBF) through stenotic and collateral vessels[48] and cause tissue in the ischemic penumbra to progress to infarction. As a result, AIS patients not receiving tPA therapy should be treated with antihypertensive medications only when blood pressure exceeds 220/120 mm Hg.[44] This blood pressure upper limit corresponds to a mean arterial pressure of around 150 mm Hg, which is the normal upper limit of cerebral autoregulation (**Class II, Level C**).

In acute stroke, tolerating elevated blood pressures in order to maintain CBF ("permissive hypertension") needs to be balanced with the potentially harmful effects of severe hypertension. Acute blood pressure elevation in stroke may increase the risk of ICH and worsen cerebral edema. However, the benefits of early BP reduction have yet to be confirmed in large clinical trials. Only five trials and a total of 218 patients were identified in a recent systematic review of blood pressure alterations in acute stroke and the conclusion was that data were too limited to assess the effect of BP modulation on clinical outcomes.[49]

Intravenous thrombolysis

Within the first hours after the onset of stroke symptoms, most patients with persistent arterial occlusion will have brain tissue that is hypoperfused and functionally inactive.[50] Hypoperfused brain tissue that has not been irreversibly damaged is termed ischemic penumbra. Penumbral tissue is present in almost all stroke patients at under three hours but after three hours the number of patients with salvable penumbra rapidly diminishes.[51]

Early vessel recanalization and cerebral reperfusion is goal of most acute stroke therapies and it is the most effective means to salvage penumbral tissue and improve clinical outcomes. A meta-analysis of pooled data from 53 studies of acute stroke therapies that reported recanalization rates found that good functional outcomes at three months were more frequent in recanalized than in non-recanalized patients (OR 0.24, 95% CI 0.16–0.35) with no difference in symptomatic hemorrhage[52] (**Level B**).

Currently the only approved and recommended reperfusion therapy for AIS is thrombolysis with intravenous tPA administered within three hours of symptom onset (**Class I, Level A**). Intravenous tPA was approved for use in AIS by the US Food and Drug Administration in 1996 based partly on the National Institute of Neurologic Disease and Stroke (NINDS) tPA Stroke Study.[46] In the study, 624 patients with ischemic stroke were treated with placebo or tPA (0.9 mg/kg IV, maximum 90 mg; 10% given as a bolus with the remainder given over one hour) within three hours of symptom onset and almost half of patients were treated within 90 minutes. The NINDS study was conducted in two parts. The primary endpoint in part I was neurologic improvement in 24 hours as indexed by an improvement of ≥4 points on the National Institutes of Health Stroke Scale (NIHSS) (Table 61.3) or complete neurologic recovery. Part II of the study used a global test statistic to assess clinical outcome at three months, with favorable outcome defined as a complete or nearly complete neurologic recovery. The trial showed no group difference in percentages of patients with neurologic improvement at 24 hours. At three months, however, tPA treatment resulted in a 32% relative (12% absolute) increase in the proportion of patients with minimal or no disability.[46] The major risk of treatment with tPA is symptomatic hemorrhage, which in the NINDS trial occurred in 6.4% of treated patients compared to 0.6% in the placebo group. Despite the increased hemorrhage risk, there was no difference in the three-month mortality between the tPA-treated and placebo groups (17% vs 20%, respectively). Recently a large prospective, open-label, observational study of 6438 patients from 14 countries confirmed that tPA is safe, with hemorrhage rates comparable to clinical trials, when used within three hours of stroke onset following protocols, even in centers with little prior experience in treating acute stroke patients.[53]

In addition to the NINDS trial, there have been a number of other trials of intravenous fibrinolytic agents in stroke. These trials all had important differences from the NINDS trial, including the use of higher doses of tPA,[54] the randomization of patients beyond three hours,[54–57] and treatment with other fibrinolytics such as streptokinase along with antithrombotic drugs.[58–60] Streptokinase trials were halted prematurely due to high hemorrhage rates and its use is not recommended (**Class III, Level A**). Intention to treat analysis of data pooled from randomized trials of tPA in stroke patients treated up to six hours (NINDS, ECASS-I, ECASS-II and ATLANTIS) has highlighted the important relationship between time to initiate treatment and clinical outcomes.[54–57] Combined data from 2775 stroke patients treated in more than 300 hospitals in 18 countries was used to analyze the relationship between tPA benefit and time to treatment.[61] This study showed that the odds ratio for favorable outcome at three months and adjusted for baseline clinical features decreases as time to treatment increases (Fig. 61.1). The odds of a favorable outcome was greatest in the 0–90 minute interval (1.2, 95% CI 1.8–4.5). The beneficial effect of tPA extended beyond three hours to 270 minutes at which point the lower confidence interval for the odds ratio crosses unity (see Fig. 61.1).

The recently completed ECASS-3 trial provides new data on the tPA treatment in an extended time window.[61a] The trial randomized ischemic stroke patients (n = 821) between 3 and 4.5 hours after symptom onset to treatment with IV tPA or standard medical care. The tPA dosing regimen and enrollment criteria were similar to the current guidelines for treating stroke patients within 3 hours. More patients

Table 61.3 National Institutes of Health Stroke Scale (NIHSS) used to measure the severity of stroke deficit. Total NIHSS score is calculated by adding scores on the 11 items

Tested item	Title	Responses and scores
1A	Level of consciousness	0 – alert 1 – drowsy 2 – obtunded 3 – coma/unresponsive
1B	Orientation questions (2)	0 – answers both correctly 1 – answers one correctly 2 – answers neither correctly
1C	Response to commands (2)	0 – performs both tasks correctly 1 – performs one task correctly 2 – performs neither
2	Gaze	0 – normal horizontal movements 1 – partial gaze palsy 2 – complete gaze palsy
3	Visual fields	0 – no visual field defect 1 – partial hemianopia 2 – complete hemianopia 3 – bilateral hemianopia
4	Facial movement	0 – normal 1 – minor facial weakness 2 – partial facial weakness 3 – complete unilateral palsy
5	Motor function (arm) a. Left b. Right	0 – no drift 1 – drift before 5 seconds 2 – falls before 10 seconds 3 – no effort against gravity 4 – no movement
6	Motor function (leg) a. Left b. Right	0 – no drift 1 – drift before 5 seconds 2 – falls before 5 seconds 3 – no effort against gravity 4 – no movement
7	Limb ataxia	0 – no ataxia 1 – ataxia in 1 limb 2 – ataxia in 2 limbs
8	Sensory	0 – no sensory loss 1 – mild sensory loss 2 – severe sensory loss
9	Language	0 – normal 1 – mild aphasia 2 – severe aphasia 3 – mute or global aphasia
10	Articulation	0 – normal 1 – mild dysarthria 2 – severe dysarthria
11	Extinction or inattention	0 – absent 1 – mild (loss 1 sensory modality) 2 – severe (loss 2 modalities)

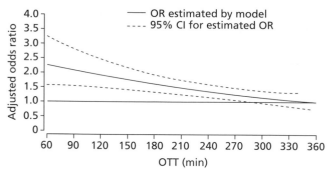

Figure 61.1 Model estimating odds ratio for favorable outcome at 3 months in rt-PA treated patients compared with controls by OTT. Adjusted for age, baseline glucose concentration, baseline NIHSS measurement, baseline diastolic blood pressure, previous hypertension, and interaction between age and baseline NIHSS measurement. (From Hack et al. [61] with permission).

treated with tPA had good outcomes (no or minimal disability) than with placebo (52.4% vs 45.2%; odds ratio, 1.34; 95% CI, 1.02 to 1.76; $P = 0.04$) although the degree of benefit was less than that of patient enrolled from 0 to 3 hours in the NINDS study. The tPA treated group had higher rates of symptomatic intracranial hemorrhage (2.4% vs 0.2%) but this did not result in any increase in mortality. ECASS-3 provides further evidence that although the benefits of tPA are attenuated at later time points, IV tPA therapy can be administered safely from 3 to 4.5 hours in select patients and improves clinical outcomes (**Class I, Level B**).[61b]

Recent studies have examined whether specialized stroke MRI sequences that include DWI and images of brain perfusion can identify ischemic stroke patients with penumbral tissue who may benefit from perfusion with IV tPA beyond three hours.[62,63] These studies show that patients with large regions of hypoperfusion and relatively small areas of tissue infarction (i.e. large amounts of penumbral tissue) may safely be given tPA beyond three hours. The subset of patients with large amounts of penumbral tissue and early reperfusion shows the greatest improvement in clinical outcomes.[63] The value of MRI selection of stroke patients for IV tPA therapy beyond three hours has yet to be replicated in larger Phase III trials.

Other reperfusion therapies that are currently being evaluated in clinical trials include alternative fibrinolytic agents such as reteplase, desmoteplase, and tenecteplase, and augmenting IV tPA with transcranial Doppler.[64] At present, there are insufficient data to support the use of any of these reperfusion approaches (**Class III, Level C**).

Intra-arterial thrombolysis

Endovascular methods of achieving vessel recanalization in AIS include mechanical and pharmacologic approaches.[65] Intra-arterial (IA) delivery of fibrinolytic agents offers the potential advantage of more rapid removal of thrombus compared to intravenous approaches as agents are infused at high concentration in close proximity to sites of occlusion with a microcatheter system. IA therapies, at least in theory, may expand the time window for reperfusion therapy by reducing or eliminating systemic exposure to fibrinolytic agents.

The only randomized trial to assess the efficacy and safety of IA fibrinolytic therapy was the Prolyse in Acute Cerebral Thromboembolism Trial (PROACT-II).[66] In PROACT-II, 180 patients with acute stroke of less than six hours and angiographically confirmed occlusion of the middle cerebral artery (MCA) were randomized to receive IA recombinant prourokinase (r-proUK) plus heparin or heparin alone. The primary outcome was the proportion of patients with mild or no neurologic disability at 90 days. Based on an intention to treat analysis, 40% of r-proUK treated patients had good outcomes, which was significantly better than the 25% of control patients. Rates of partial or full recanalization were also markedly higher in the r-proUK group than controls (66% versus 18%). Mortality rates were around 25% for both groups. Symptomatic hemorrhage rates were, however, higher in the r-proUK patients compared to controls (10% vs 2% respectively).

The only other randomized data of IA fibrinolytics come from the recently published MELT trial.[67] In this study, conducted in Japan prior to the availability of IV tPA, ischemic stroke patients presenting within six hours were randomized to IA UK or placebo. The trial was halted prematurely largely over ethical concerns about the randomization once IV tPA was approved for use in Japan. The incomplete MELT dataset, however, when pooled with other trials of r-proUK, further supports a benefit of IA fibrinolytics in AIS.[68]

In addition to pharmacologic approaches to recanalization, there have been a number of endovascular approaches to treat intracranial or extracranial occlusions that do not involve the delivery of fibrinolytics (see Molina and Saver[65] for review). At present, the only devices approved by the FDA for the revascularization of patients with AIS are the Merci Retriever device (Concentric Medical) and the Penumbra System (Penumbra Inc.) aspiration catheter. While these devices can achieve high rates of vessel recanalization when used in AIS,[69,70] they lack any evidence of improved clinical outcomes from randomized controlled trials.

The treatment of acute stroke with endovascular therapies suffers a number of important limitations that prevent their widespread adoption. Endovascular procedures require substantially more infrastructure support, there are insufficient numbers of neurointerventionalists, treatment is limited to more proximal vessel occlusions, and time to initiate therapy is longer than IV fibrinolysis. Current guidelines recognize the value of IA fibrinolysis as a treatment option for patients with major anterior circulation stroke within six hours of symptom onset and up to 24 hours for vertebrobasilar occlusion (**Class I, Level B**). IA therapies should not take precedence over the administration of IV tPA to eligible patients.

Anticoagulants

There is no evidence that urgent anticoagulation with either unfractionated or low molecular weight heparin (LMWH) reduces the rate of recurrent stroke, improves neurologic outcomes or can be used either along with or in place of IV tPA (**Class III, Level A**). The largest study of anticoagulation in AIS was the International Stroke Trial (IST).[71] This was a randomized, open-label trial, which compared the safety and efficacy of acetylsalicylic acid (ASA) and subcutaneous heparin (5000 or 12500 IU) in 19435 patients. Neither heparin regimen offered any clinical advantage over ASA. The higher dose of heparin was associated with an excess of morbidity and mortality. *Post hoc* analysis of the IST data examined stroke patients with atrial fibrillation and presumed cardiac embolism. Even in this subgroup of patients, the absolute risk of recurrent stroke in the first 14 days was relatively low (3.9%) and there was no net benefit to use of heparin.[72] Other trials have similarly found no benefit of emergency anticoagulation for AIS behond prevention of deep vein thrombosis and pulmonary embolism.[73]

Antiplatelet agents

ASA has been evaluated for the treatment of AIS in two large randomized controlled trials (CAST and IST) and one smaller trial (MAST).[58,71,74] In the CAST trial (n = 21106), patients with acute ischemic stroke were randomized within 48 hours to ASA or placebo. There was a small but significant reduction in mortality amongst ASA-allocated patients (relative risk reduction (RRR) 14%, absolute risk reduction (ARR) 0.6%) and patients treated with ASA had significantly fewer recurrent strokes than patients in the placebo arm (1.6% vs 2.1%, respectively). ASA was associated with slightly more (0.2%) recurrent hemorrhagic strokes but this did not affect overall mortality, as ASA patients were less likely to be dead or dependent at discharge (11.4 fewer per 1000).

Meta-analysis of nine trials (n = 41399) confirmed that acute ASA treatment was associated with a significant decrease in death or dependency at the end of follow-up (OR 0.94; 95% CI 0.91–0.98) and increased odds of making a complete recovery from the stroke (OR 1.06; 95% CI 1.01–1.11).[75] For every 1000 ischemic stroke patients treated with ASA within 48 hours, there were 13 more patients alive and independent at follow-up and 10 additional patients made a complete recovery. In addition, per 1000 ASA treated patients there was reduction of seven recurrent ischemic strokes and one pulmonary embolus but at a cost of two excess symptomatic intracranial hemorrhages. Based on these data, ASA

is recommended for all ischemic stroke patients within 48 hours of stroke onset provided there are no strong contraindications, and hemorrhagic stroke has been excluded (**Class I, Level A**). In patients treated with fibrinolytic therapy, ASA should not be given in the first 24 hours.

Neuroprotection

The development of neuroprotective therapies that attenuate the cascade of pathophysiologic events that occur with ischemia in acute stroke has been disappointing. A large number of neuroprotective agents have been developed based on animal models of focal ischemia but all have failed in translation to clinical practice.[76] Most recently, the results of a large trial using NXY-059 was reported. The initial NXY-059 trial suggested the drug was safe and effective in improving stroke outcomes[77] but a subsequent Phase III trial found no evidence of efficacy.[78] The failure to develop neuroprotective agents using current paradigms has led researchers to explore different strategies such as prehospital delivery of neuroprotective drugs.[79] Currently, no neuroprotective therapy is recommended for treating stroke (**Class III, Level A**).

Preventing early complications

Stroke care units

The intervention that has the greatest potential to improve outcomes of stroke patients is the establishment of specialized stroke care units (SCU). A recent Cochrane analysis pooled data from 31 trials and a total of 6936 patients examining the benefits of routine management of stroke patients in SCUs.[80] Stroke patients who received organized care in a SCU had significantly lower odds of being dead or dependent at follow-up (OR 0.82; 95% CI 0.73–0.92; $P = 0.001$) than patients receiving care on general medical wards. Subgroup analyses showed that stroke patients benefit regardless of sex, age or stroke severity. Based on data extrapolated from a community-based epidemiologic study, it is estimated that the establishment of SCUs has the potential to prevent death and disability for 50 patients per 1000 strokes compared to six per 1000 for tPA treatment and four per 1000 with ASA therapy.[81]

The precise components of an SCU that account for the benefit in functional outcomes are not well delineated. It is established that SCUs that occupy a separate physical space are associated with better outcomes than care provided by mobile stroke teams in general wards.[82] Likely interventions that are important for improved outcomes include early mobilization, better blood pressure control, and prevention of complications such as deep venous thrombosis through closer adherence to current evidence-based guidelines. All stroke patients should be admitted to

SCUs (**Class I, Level A**). Stroke units ideally should be geographically distinct, with well-defined protocols that address common problems such as early mobilization, screening for dysphagia, treatment of infections with antibiotics, and subcutaneous administration of anticoagulants for deep vein thrombosis (DVT) prophylaxis.

Venous thromboembolism

Venous thromboembolism is an important cause of morbidity in stroke patients. The risk of venous thromboembolism in patients with AIS approaches that of surgical patients and without thromboprophylaxis, about 20% of patients will develop pulmonary embolus (PE) and 1–2% of stroke patients will have a fatal PE. Unfractionated heparin is associated with an 81% reduction in deep vein thrombosis and 58% reduction in PE with a small increased risk of hemorrhagic transformation of the infarct.[83] The recently completed PREVAIL trial showed that thromboprophylaxis with LMWH may further reduce the risk of venous thromboembolism by 43% compared to unfractionated heparin; however, most (95%) of the DVT detected in the trial were asymptomatic.[84] Current guidelines recommend thromboprophylaxis for all ischemic stroke patients with anticoagulants (**Class I, Level A**) although there is still controversy about whether LMWH or unfractionated heparin is superior.

Acute neurologic complications

Many patients with ischemic stroke will worsen during the first 24–48 hours after stroke onset. The main neurologic causes of early worsening are the development of intracerebral hemorrhage and space-occupying cerebral edema and, less commonly, seizures. The risk of hemorrhagic transformation of ischemic stroke is increased with fibrinolytic drugs, anticoagulation or antiplatelet agents. Hemorrhage after ischemic stroke can be petechial, which is often asymptomatic, or result in hematoma formation that increases intracranial pressure and results in neurologic decline. There are currently no proven therapies for the treatment of hemorrhagic transformation. Seizures occur in about 3% of stroke patients within the first 24 hours.[85] Prophylactic anticonvulsant therapy is not recommended (**Class III, Level C**).

About 10% of patients with supratentorial infarction will develop life-threatening, space-occupying brain edema ("malignant infarction") usually on the second to fifth day after stroke.[86] The prognosis of patients with malignant MCA territory infarctions is poor, with mortality rates of around 80%[87] and no effective medical therapy. There is evidence from three European randomized trials (DECIMAL, DESTINY and HAMLET) that suggests that decompressive surgery improves functional outcomes in patients with malignant MCA infarction[88–90] (**Level A**).

Pooled data from these three trials (n = 93) showed that patients in the decompressive surgery group (treated within 48 hours, mean age 45) were more likely than controls to survive their stroke, free of severe disability (75% vs 24%; pooled ARR 51%; 95% CI 34–69).[91] Surgery in these trials was performed within 48 hours of stroke onset and the NNT = 4 for survival with a moderate deficit or better. These results highlight that decompressive hemicraniectomy increases survival at a cost of more survivors with at least moderate deficits. The timing of surgery and the clinical characteristics of patients' most likely to benefit are still not well established. Decompressive hemicraniectomy is usually reserved for younger patients and after discussion about the potential outcomes, including survival with moderate to severe disability (**Class II, Level B**).

The only other clear indication for surgery in acute stroke is for space-occupying cerebellar infarction (**Class I, Level B**). In about 11–25% of cerebellar stroke the edema becomes space occupying within the posterior fossa, and brainstem compression and acute obstructive hydrocephalus result.[92] The indications for surgical intervention in cerebellar strokes are a decreased level of consciousness and/or clinical signs of brainstem compression. The management involves the insertion of an external ventricular drain (EVD) and/or suboccipital decompressive craniectomy; however, the optimal procedure is controversial.[93] While the efficacy is not supported by clinical trials, case series have established decompressive surgical evacuation of space-occupying cerebellar infarction as a potentially lifesaving procedure.[94]

Conclusion

Over the past decade, there have been significant advances in our knowledge of the epidemiology, pathophysiology, and treatment of acute stroke. Management of acute stroke has emerged from a long period of therapeutic nihilism, largely the result of the recognition that, with emergent evaluation and treatment, ischemic brain can be salvaged and patient outcomes improved.

Perhaps the most significant advance in acute stroke management is the development of specialized stroke units. From a population health perspective, stroke care units have the potential to be widely implemented and benefits can extend to almost all stroke patients. Stroke units provide an opportunity to implement evidence-based treatment pathways focused on salvaging penumbral tissue, preventing post-stroke complications, initiating secondary prevention regimens, and promoting recovery through early rehabilitation. Compared to stroke units, no other acute stroke treatment strategy has the potential to have such a large impact on saving lives and reducing long-term dependency.

Almost all patients with AIS can benefit from the early administration of ASA. ASA is the only medical therapy proven to improve stroke outcomes, prevent recurrent stroke, and reduce stroke mortality. In comparison, the narrow time window for administration of IV tPA limits the potential benefit to only a small percentage of stroke patients. IV tPA remains, however, the only approved reperfusion therapy and when administered within three hours of symptom onset, results in a more than 30% increase in the number of patients returning to their pre-morbid level of functioning.

Novel neuroimaging methods and new strategies to open occluded vessels offer the potential to extend the therapeutic window for reperfusion of penumbral tissue although at present there is a paucity of evidence to support the expanded use of these treatment approaches. The challenge of the next decades will be to expand the availability of those acute stroke therapies with well-established evidence of efficacy to help offset the predicted rise in stroke-related morbidity and mortality expected over the next decades.

Secondary prevention of stroke

Craig Anderson

Introduction

With an estimated 20 million events occurring in the world each year, stroke is ranked as the sixth leading cause of global disease burden.[97] Although declines in stroke incidence are emerging,[98–100] aging and adverse lifestyle changes in populations will further intensify the impact of stroke and re-emphasize the importance of prevention and management strategies.[101] Patients who experience a stroke or transient ischemic attack (TIA) are at substantial risk of a further serious vascular event (recurrent stroke, myocardial infarction or death from vascular cause). The risks of recurrent stroke are about 10% in the first week, 14% at one month, and 20% by three months after onset.[102,103] Thereafter, the annual risks of recurrent stroke and myocardial infarction are around 5% and 2–3%, respectively.[104] Given that 30–40% of patients with ischemic stroke have had a preceding TIA or minor stroke,[105] and accumulating evidence indicates benefits from early assessment and management,[106,107] TIAs serve as an important opportunity to intervene to prevent stroke.

This section reviews current evidence-based medical and surgical strategies used in reducing the risk of recurrent stroke and other vascular events after an ischemic stroke or TIA, or an intracerebral hemorrhage. Approaches to the prevention of subarachnoid hemorrhage or rarer forms of stroke, such as arterial dissection, are not considered.

Diagnosis of stroke and transient ischemic attack

Stroke is a clinical diagnosis, as outlined in a standard definition, of "rapidly developing clinical signs of focal (or global) disturbance of cerebral function with symptoms lasting 24 hours or longer (or leading to death), with no apparent cause other than vascular origin".[108] The term TIA refers to acute stroke symptoms (and signs) of the brain or eye that resolve within 24 hours.[109] However, the advent of modern neuroimaging and use of thrombolysis for acute ischemic stroke has called into question the usefulness of the definition of TIA with a 24-hour time window for clinical decision making in the first few hours after the onset of symptoms.[110] Even so, TIA remains a useful concept, both clinically and epidemiologically, as it does not rely on brain imaging and is a well-accepted diagnosis all over the world.

Pathologically, stroke generally occurs as a result of either ischemia or hemorrhage. Ischemic stroke, which accounts for about 80% of strokes in "white" populations, may occur via various mechanisms that include cardio-embolism (20–25% in Western population, e.g. secondary to atrial fibrillation (AF), valvular heart disease or patent foramen ovale), large-vessel atherosclerosis (approximately 50%, e.g. *in situ* occlusion of intracerebral arteries, or artery-to-artery embolism from carotid atheroma or aortic plaques), small vessel disease (10–20%; lacunar stroke) and, more rarely, secondary to arterial dissection, hematologic or other disorders. In black African-Americans, Hispanics and Asians, the proportion of lacunar ischemic strokes is increased and the proportion of cardioembolic strokes is decreased. In addition, the distribution of atheroma also differs between ethnic groups: Caucasians tend to have the disease around the extracranial carotid vessels, whereas intracranial large vessel disease is more common in Asian populations.[111–114] However, it is often difficult to assign an exact single etiologic mechanism in a case of ischemic stroke because of non-specific or overlapping risk factors, clinical features and underlying pathology. Hemorrhagic stroke includes primary intracerebral hemorrhage occurring in 10–15% of non-Asian and 20–40% of Asian cases (due mainly to spontaneous rupture of an intracerebral vessel)[114] and subarachnoid hemorrhage in 5–8% (due mainly to rupture of an intracranial aneurysm),[115] which are both associated with a worse prognosis than ischemic stroke.

Blood pressure-lowering therapy

Elevated blood pressure (BP) is the single most important reversible risk factor for both first-ever and recurrent (secondary) stroke,[116–119] with near continuous associations between risk and usual levels of BP, without threshold. The association attenuates with increasing age, but remains strongly positive at all ages, across different ethnic populations,[118,120,121] and is greater for intracerebral hemorrhage than ischemic stroke.[118,121]

Substantial evidence indicates beneficial effects of lowering BP after stroke or TIA (**Class I, Level A**). Randomized trials support the observational data in demonstrating that a modest (e.g. 8/4 mm Hg) average reduction in BP is associated with a 20–25% reduction in the risk of serious vascular events.[118,119] From the trials in which there was about a 5% annual risk of vascular events among control group patients, BP-lowering treatment produces an absolute reduction of 1%, or 10 vascular events avoided per 1000 patients treated per year.[119,122] Meta-analyses of all the trials of BP lowering among different types of patients, including those with stroke or TIA, indicate that the degree of BP lowering is far more important than the particular BP-lowering agent used in determining the size of the benefit in reducing the risks of stroke, myocardial infarction and all other vascular outcomes including heart failure[122] (**Class I, Level A**). Among the agents that inhibit the renin-angiotensin system, though, evidence is emerging that angiotension receptor blockers (ARBs) are better tolerated and may be modestly superior to angiotensin-converting enzyme (ACE) inhibitors in preventing stroke[123–125] (**Class IIa, Level A**).

Who should be treated?

The relative benefits of BP-lowering treatment after stroke or TIA are similar irrespective of different characteristics of patients including the initial level of BP, age, and pathologic type of stroke[122] (**Class I, Level A**). BP-lowering therapy should, therefore, be commenced in almost all patients with a stroke or TIA, irrespective of whether or not they would be considered "hypertensive" according to standard definitions (**Class I, Level A**). However, in very old patients with consistently low levels of BP (i.e. below 130 systolic), it would seem reasonable to consider withholding such therapy, given the risks associated with hypotension, including dizziness and falls, and less certainty regarding the net benefit of treatment at such low levels (**Class IIb, Level C**).

How soon to commence treatment after a stroke or TIA?

With a paucity of randomized data, and observational studies showing U- or J-shaped associations between levels of BP and the risk of a poor outcome after ischemic stroke, there is much uncertainty about the effects of early intensive BP lowering with intravenous agents in the acute phase of stroke,[126,127] including intracerebral hemorrhage.[128]

Therefore, various guidelines recommend that such treatment be avoided in the first 24–48 hours, unless the BP is very high (systolic >180–220 mm Hg or diastolic >110–120 mm Hg), and depending on whether the stroke is hemorrhagic or rtPA is being used for cerebral ischemia[129] (**Class IIb, Level B**). Otherwise, BP-lowering treatment should be started promptly within the first week in almost all patients with mild- or non-disabling stroke, to not only maximize efficacy but also adherence. Although direct evidence of benefit is lacking,[123,130] trials have not shown any excess in adverse effects related to potential cerebral hypoperfusion due to impaired cerebral auto-regulation worsening cerebral ischemia, from such an approach (**Class IIb, Level B**).

How low should the BP be lowered?

Secondary analyses of the Perindopril Protection against Recurrent Stroke Study (PROGRESS) trial[131] indicate that the lowest risk of recurrent stroke occurs in patients with the lowest levels of BP during follow-up. However, the intensity of treatment (use of an ACE inhibitor alone or in combination with a diuretic) in PROGRESS was determined by the randomizing clinician, who took into account the various characteristics of patients, including the level of BP, at baseline. Thus, the lower risks seen in patients with lower BP levels during follow-up may not necessarily have been due entirely to the treatment. Moreover, PROGRESS and most other trials of BP lowering have tested a specific agent(s) added onto a background of standard care and/or have included patients whose BP had been stabilized (usually less than 160 mm Hg systolic and 90 mm Hg diastolic) prior to randomization. Therefore, as shown in the recently completed Ongoing Telmisartan Alone and in Combination with Ramipril Global Endpoint Trial (ONTARGET) study,[120] the benefit of additional BP lowering at levels below 140 mm Hg systolic in patients with cardiovascular disease, including a history of stroke, has yet to be determined.

It seems reasonable, therefore, to be more aggressive with treatment in those patients with initially high levels, with the aim of achieving target levels of 130/80 mm Hg, as recommended in most current guidelines (**Class I, Level A**). Moreover, since most of the evidence of benefit specifically in patients with stroke or TIA has come from either a thiazide alone or the combination of a thiazide with an ACE inhibitor, similar such therapy is recommended (**Class I, Level A**). Ultimately, though, the choice of agent(s) will likely to depend on the patient's age, associated co-morbid factors and treatment, tolerance, adherence issues, and cost (**Class I, Level A**). Such treatment is recommended for as long as the benefits are considered worthwhile for the patient, and even in those who are very elderly (over 80 years of age)[132] (**Class I, Level A**).

Antiplatelet therapy

Strong evidence exists for the benefits of long-term antiplatelet therapy, with relative reduction of about one-fifth in serous vascular events (including stroke), in patients with prior stroke or TIA[133,134] (**Class I, Level A**). With about an average 7% annual rate of vascular events among patients in the control groups of the relevant trials, this effect translates into an absolute reduction of about 14 vascular events per 1000 patients treated per year. The absolute excess risk of major bleeding in the trials was less than one intracranial hemorrhage, and 102 serious extracranial hemorrhages per 1000 patients treated per year. Thus, the overall benefits of antiplatelet therapy greatly outweigh the bleeding risks, so the therapy is appropriate for all patients with ischemic stroke or TIA unless there are specific contraindications, such as aspirin sensitivity, or if anticoagulation to reduce the risk of cardioembolic events is considered more appropriate (**Class I, Level A**). Patients with recent gastrointestinal or other major bleeding, or with symptoms suggestive of active peptic ulceration, should generally not receive antiplatelet drugs, although the addition of a proton pump inhibitor can reduce upper gastrointestinal adverse effects[135] (**Class IIa, Level A**). It seems reasonable and safe to use them in patients with a history of intracerebral hemorrhage if they are at high risk of future ischemic vascular events, for example in those with ischemic heart disease or prior ischemic stroke[136] (**Class IIb, Level C**).

How soon to commence antiplatelet therapy after an ischemic stroke or TIA?

Two large randomized trials which between them included nearly 40 000 patients showed a net benefit from aspirin 160–300 mg daily commenced within 48 hours of acute ischemic stroke[137] (**Class I, Level A**). A CT is recommended to exclude intracerebral hemorrhage before commencing aspirin. However, significant proportions of the patients included in these two trials were given aspirin prior to CT, and were later shown to have had an intracerebral hemorrhage, but they did not experience any adverse effects of the treatment. Thus, it is probably safe to give low-dose aspirin to patients with a mild disabling stroke or TIA should there be a delay in obtaining a CT (**Class IIa, Level A**). In situations where the CT shows a hemorrhagic transformation of an ischemic stroke, which is often the situation with large MCA cardioembolic cerebral infarcts, it is probably wise to wait for 1–2 weeks before commencing antiplatelet therapy (**Class IIb, Level C**).

Which single antiplatelet agent to use?

Until recently, aspirin has been the undisputed gold standard antiplatelet agent for the long-term prevention of atherothrombotic events.[134] The optimal dose for both efficacy and tolerability has been established as low, anything from 30 mg to 300 mg daily[134,138] (**Class I, Level A**). Gastrointestinal side effects such as gastritis and hemorrhage are more common in older people, and with higher doses and longer duration of treatment with aspirin (**Class I, Level A**). In one study, treatment with dipyridamole alone was found to reduce the risk of major vascular events by a similar amount as aspirin,[139] while clopidogrel was shown to be slightly superior to aspirin in the trial of Clopidogrel versus Aspirin in Patients at Risk of Ischemic Events (CAPRIE), which overall reducing the risk of stroke and other major vascular events by about 10%, from about 6.0% (aspirin) to 5.4% (clopidogrel) per year, in a broad group of patients with a history of cardiovascular disease[140,141] (**Class I, Level A**). There was no statistically significant difference in the subset of patients with previous ischemic stroke in CAPRIE, with an average annual event rate of 7.2% for clopidogrel versus 7.7% for aspirin, for a relative risk reduction of about 7.3%. However, a meta-analysis confirms a modest superiority of clopidogrel over aspirin, but also differences in their side effect profile[141,142] (**Class I, Level A**). While aspirin produces more upper gastrointestinal adverse effects, clopidogrel produces more diarrhea and skin rash, and a very small risk of thrombocytopenia and thrombotic thrombocytopenic purpura. Moreover, prior to the availability of generic versions, clopidogrel has been substantially more expensive than aspirin, so it is generally recommended as an alternative to aspirin in patients who are genuinely intolerant or allergic to aspirin.[142] In the meta-analyses, dipyridamole and trifusal have not been shown to clearly reduce vascular events, and may be inferior, compared with aspirin alone[134] (**Class I, Level A**).

Does a combination of antiplatelet agents offer benefits over aspirin alone?

Clinical trials have shown that, in long-term secondary prevention, the combination of aspirin and clopidogrel is associated with a higher risk of bleeding complications, most importantly intracranial hemorrhage, than either agent alone, which offsets any modest additional benefit in terms of reducing vascular events[143,144] (**Class I, Level A**). However, in subgroup analysis of these studies, data showing a reduction in embolic signals seen on transcranial Doppler ultrasound in patients with severe carotid stenosis,[145] and the benefit seen in acute coronary syndromes,[146,147] suggest that such combination therapy may be beneficial very early after ischemic stroke or TIA when the risk of recurrence is very high.[106,148]

Two randomized trials which included nearly 6000 patients with ischemic stroke or TIA have both shown that the combination of low-dose (25 mg) aspirin and dipyridaomle (specifically modified-release dipyridamole 200 mg) twice daily reduces the risk of vascular events by about one-fifth compared with aspirin alone, without an increase in the risk of major bleeding[139,149] (**Class I, Level A**). The benefits of adding dypiridamole were independent of gender, history of ischemic heart disease, and dose of aspirin (**Class I, Level A**). Most recently, the Prevention Regime for Effectively avoiding Second Strokes (PRoFESS) trial which involved nearly 20 000 patients showed that the aspirin-dipyridamole combination regime offered comparable overall efficacy in preventing future serious vascular events to clopidogrel alone in patients with recent ischemic stroke, although statistically it failed to demonstrate a non-inferior difference of 7.5%.[150] Thus, it is appropriate to consider the addition of dipyridamole to aspirin (or use of the marketed aspirin and extended-release dipyridamole combination pill) for modest superior beneficial effect over aspirin for secondary prevention, so long as clinicians and patients consider the additional absolute benefit and increased costs to be worthwhile (**Class I, Level A**). Patients should be warned about the potential for dipyridamole-related headache, which may occur in up to a third of people taking the medication, but which usually settles after a few weeks.

Anticoagulation

Valvular and non-valvular AF (including paroxysmal AF and atrial flutter) are major risk factors for stroke, although the former is now uncommon in developed countries due to low rates of rheumatic heart disease. Non-valvular AF predisposes to the formation of intracardiac thrombi, mainly within the atria, which can embolize to the brain and other organs. AF affects about 1% of the population, with the prevalence increasing sharply with age from 0.5% in those aged 50–59 years to about 9% in those over the age of 70 years.[151] AF is associated with a fivefold increase in stroke risk, and the strokes tend to be larger, more disabling and have a worse prognosis.[152] Overall, the annual risk of stroke in the setting of AF is about 5%, but rates vary from less than 2% to more than 10% according to the presence of one or more clinical characteristics such as congestive cardiac failure, hypertension, older age (≥75 years), diabetes, and a history of stroke or TIA[153] (**Class I, Level A**).

Substantial evidence indicates that warfarin is highly efficacious in preventing stroke (and other vascular and embolic events) in patients with AF, even in people up to 85 years and over[154] (**Class I, Level A**). Several systematic reviews and meta-analyses of randomized trials of antithrombotic agents in patients with non valvular AF[155–157] show that adjusted-dose warfarin (with an average achieved international normalized ratio (INR) of about 2.5) reduces the risk of stroke by about two-thirds, whereas aspirin reduces the risk of stroke by about one-fifth. In direct comparison, adjusted-dose warfarin was substantially more efficacious than antiplatelet therapy (including aspirin and clopidogrel).[158] Excess risks of intracranial hemorrhage and major extracranial hemorrhage with warfarin are small, about 1–2% and less than 0.3% per year, respectively. Therefore, since patients with co-existing AF and a prior ischemic stroke or TIA are at very high risk of recurrent stroke (about 12% per year), the absolute benefit in these patients is substantial, about 70 strokes prevented per 1000 patients treated for a year with warfarin compared to about 50 strokes prevented per 1000 patients treated a year for aspirin. Thus, for most patients with ischemic stroke or TIA that is related to AF, the benefits of adjusted-dose warfarin with a target INR of around 2.5 far outweigh the risks, provided there are no major contraindications and good monitoring of the INR can be organized (**Class I, Level A**).

Which patients should not be treated with warfarin?

Contraindications to warfarin include an active source of gastrointestinal bleeding, alcoholic liver disease, dementia, prior major hemorrhage, and an inability to ensure regular monitoring of INR (**Class IIb, Level C**). *Post hoc* analysis of trials[159] suggests an increased risk of intracerebral hemorrhage in patients with extensive cerebral white matter disease ("leukoaraiosis") and in older people with a high tendency to fall[160] (**Class IIb, Level C**). In some of these situations, warfarin can still be justified as the estimated net benefit from reducing the risk of future ischemic stroke far outweighs the potential hazards of bleeding. For patients unable or unwilling to take warfarin, aspirin is a reasonable but less effective alternative (**Class I, Level A**).

When to start treatment?

There is no randomized evidence to support the early (within the first 1–2 weeks) use of anticoagulation following an ischemic stroke that is related to AF in order to prevent recurrent cardioembolic events. Given that AF-related ischemic strokes tend to be larger and more likely to have *in situ* micro-hemorrhage due to cerebral reperfusion, consideration should be given to early use of anticoagulation increasing the risk of hemorrhagic transformation of the infarct while the risks of recurrent ischemic stroke are around 5% in the first two weeks after the initial event[161] (**Class IIb, Level C**). It is recommended, therefore, to wait 1–2 weeks before commencing warfarin, although it seems reasonable to commence such treatment earlier in patients who have experienced a small ischemic stroke or TIAs, or in situations where the embolic risk is considered to be extremely high. In the latter case, LMWH may be used as a bridge before the therapeutic effect of warfarin is achieved (**Class IIb, Level C**).

What is the target INR?

Data from both randomized trials and observational studies suggest that the optimal target INR is about 2.5. Below 2.0, the risks of both ischemic stroke and extracranial bleeding increase, while above 3.0 there is an increased risk of major bleeding, death and hospitalization[162-164] (**Class I, Level A**).

What are the benefits of combining antiplatelet therapy with warfarin?

Randomized trials and observational data indicate that the combination of aspirin (or other antiplatelet agent) and warfarin should generally be avoided because of an increased risk of major bleeding[165] (**Class I, Level A**). However, in situations where the risk of cardio-emboli is particularly high, such as with mechanical heart values, the potential benefits outweigh the increased risks of bleeding[166] (**Class I, Level A**).

Are there any benefits of anticoagulation in patients without AF?

In patients with a presumed non-cardio-embolic source of an ischemic stroke or TIA, that is in those with presumed or established large artery atheromatous disease of the intra or extracranial vessels, there is no evidence of a benefit of oral anticoagulation (mainly warfarin, with target INRs in the range of 1.4–4.5) over antiplatelet therapy (mainly aspirin) and an increase in the risk of hemorrhage[167-170] (**Class I, Level A**).

Cholesterol-lowering therapy

The relation between serum cholesterol and stroke is complex due largely to the diversity of stroke pathogenesis, with qualitatively different associations of serum cholesterol with the risks of ischemic and hemorrhagic stroke.[171-175] Elevated serum cholesterol is an important risk factor for ischemic stroke, more so in Western populations than in Asian populations,[175] whereas a weak inversion association is apparent between serum cholesterol and the risk of intracerebral hemorrhage. Part of the latter association may relate to the confounding influence of heavy alcohol consumption which tends to lower cholesterol levels.[176]

Evidence from systematic reviews of randomized trials shows that reducing total (and more importantly low-density lipoprotein (LDL)) cholesterol with a 3-hydrozy-3-methylglutaryl co-enzyme A reductase inhibitor (statin) significantly reduces the risks of major cardiovascular events, including stroke, across a wide range of lipid levels in patients with high cardiovascular risk (**Class I, Level A**). Relative risk reductions are proportional to the absolute reduction in LDL cholesterol, such that a 1 mmol reduction is associated with almost a one-quarter reduction in the risk of coronary events, and about a 15% reduction in the risk of stroke, over about five years of treatment[177] (**Class I, Level A**). Two major randomized controlled trials have specifically evaluated the benefits of statin therapy against placebo by including patients with a history of ischemic stroke or TIA. In the Heart Protection Study (HPS)[178] undertaken in a broad population of patients with high cardiovascular risk, simvastatin 40 mg per day, which reduced LDL cholesterol by 1 mmol/L, resulted in about a 20% reduction in major vascular events and non-significantly by a similar amount for ischemic stroke. In the Stroke Prevention by Aggressive Reduction in Cholesterol Levels (SPARCL),[179] specifically undertaken in patients with principally ischemic stroke, atorvastatin 80 mg daily, which reduced LDL cholesterol by 1.4 mmol/L, was associated with about a 25% reduction in major vascular events, including a significant 20% reduction in the risk of recurrent ischemic stroke, as well as a 30% reduction in the risk of coronary events. In contrast to a meta-analysis of randomized trials which did not find a specific effect of treatment on hemorrhagic stroke,[180] both of these trials showed a slight increase in the risk of intracerebral hemorrhage. Secondary analysis of SPARCL has shown that hemorrhagic stroke was more frequent in those patients with a hemorrhagic stroke at entry, in men, with older age, and in those high BP levels during follow-up. However, there was no relationship between hemorrhage risk and baseline LDL cholesterol level or the most recent LDL cholesterol level in treated patients.[181] In the trials, the average annual risk of serious vascular events among patients in the placebo groups was about 6%, so that the observed one-fifth relative reduction equates to an absolute reduction of about 12 vascular events avoided per 1000 patients treated by year.

Who should be and should not be treated?

The randomized evidence indicates that statin therapy should be used routinely in most patients with a history of ischemic stroke or TIA, since the trials demonstrated substantial benefits in patients whose baseline total cholesterol level was greater than 3.5 mmol/L or LDL cholesterol levels of greater than 2.6 mmol/L, which would account for most patients with vascular disease in developing countries (**Class I, Level A**). Moreover, there are benefits in terms of the prevention of not only recurrent ischemic stroke but also myocardial infarction, indicating that underlying coronary artery disease is common in patients with cerebrovascular disease (**Class I, Level A**). As statins are expensive, the cost–benefit ratio is likely to be favorable in those patients without frailty or major non-vascular co-morbidity who are likely to derive the most benefit from the avoidance of future vascular events.

What statin and at what dose?

Systematic overviews of trials and observational studies indicate that greater benefits can be derived from larger degrees of cholesterol lowering[175,177,181] (**Class I, Level A**). While direct comparisons of different intensities of statin-based cholesterol-lowering regimes have been undertaken in patients with coronary heart disease,[182–184] the benefit of intensive cholesterol lowering has not been reliably established in patients with ischemic stroke and is potentially complicated by an increase in the frequency of myalgia and gastrointestinal symptoms. In the absence of direct evidence, it seems reasonable to use standard doses of statins in patients with ischemic stroke or TIA, reserving an increase in dose and/or combining with other lipid-lowering agents in those people with a persistently abnormal lipid profile and high risk of large vessel atheromatous ischemic events.

When to start therapy after ischemic stroke or TIA?

There is no definite evidence that statins, through any non-lipid lowering (antithrombotic) effects, offer benefits in the acute phase of ischemic stroke or early after TIA.[148] However, as statins are safe and well tolerated, and treatments commenced in hospital are likely to lead to better compliance, it seems reasonable to commence a statin within a few days after the onset of ischemic stroke or TIA (**Class IIb, Level C**). As statins are expensive, they should be ceased in those patients with significant stroke-related disability and/or who require long-term residential care, where it is unlikely that quality of life will be improved by avoiding recurrent stroke and other vascular events.

Carotid revascularization

Atherosclerotic disease of the extracranial vessels is an important cause of stroke, particularly in Caucasian populations, where the atheromatous narrowing at, or around, the origin of the internal carotid artery accounts for up to 50% of "large artery" ischemic stroke and TIA. Patients with higher degrees of carotid stenosis are at higher risks of ipsilateral ischemic stroke, but they are also more likely to have advanced atheroma elsewhere in the body, especially the heart.

Carotid stenosis carries a risk of embolization from the atheromatous plaque debris or thrombus which may block a more distal vessel in the cerebral circulation. Carotid stenosis rarely causes stroke due to low flow (i.e. hemodynamic compromise), only doing so if the underlying stenosis is very severe (>95% stenosis), and even then there appears to be a reduced risk of ipsilateral

stroke on medical treatment,[185,186] possibly due to the presence of good collateral circulation. Most of the strokes that occur in the first few years after a minor stroke or TIA in patients with carotid stenosis are ischemic, and they occur in the territory of the "symptomatic" vessel. The risk of stroke is related to the severity of stenosis and is time dependent.[187] The risk of stroke is highest in the first few days after a TIA, remains fairly high for the next year and then falls. Overall, the risks of stroke are approximately 10% for the first month, 15% for the subsequent year, 5% for the second year and 2% thereafter.[188,189] The high early risk of stroke is probably caused by plaque "activation". Atheromatous plaques are typically slow growing or quiescent for long periods but may develop ruptures or fissures, which trigger platelet activation and thrombus formation. Ulcerated carotid plaques are more likely than smooth plaques to be associated with coronary vascular events, suggesting the plaque activation is a systemic phenomenon.[190]

Who benefits from carotid endarterectomy?

Several randomized trials including the North American Symptomatic Carotid Endarterectomy Trial (NASCET) and the European Carotid Surgery Trial (ECST) have shown that the addition of carotid endarterectomy to best medical therapy is beneficial in reducing the absolute risk of stroke or death over the next few years by about 16% for patients with severe (≥70%) and 8% for patients with moderate (50–69%) degrees of symptomatic carotid stenosis,[191] and of some benefit (5%) in patients with neurologically asymptomatic severe (60–99%) carotid stenosis.[192] Furthermore, the durability of carotid endarterectomy in preventing ipsilateral ischemic stroke has been shown up to 13 years of follow-up[188] (**Class I, Level A**). However, the benefits of carotid endarterectomy are dependent on two important caveats, first that the surgical complication rate undertaken by experienced surgeons must be low (<5%) and second that the measurement of the degree of stenosis is robust. Conventional angiography carries a 1% risk of stroke, and one out of every five of these is disabling.[193] Modern non-invasive carotid imaging such as MRI, CT, and duplex and Doppler ultrasound avoids the risk associated with conventional intra-arterial catheter carotid angiography, but it is important that reliable images are obtained in order to avoid operating on patients with false-positive scans, or denying benefits of the intervention to those with false-negative scans.[194] Moreover, carotid ultrasound alone will not identify important lesions of the intracranial arteries where aneurysms and stenosis of intracranial vessels exist in about 2% and 5% of patients symptomatic with extracranial stenosis, respectively.

A systematic review of the randomized data provides information about the effects of treatment according to different patient characteristics (**Class I, Level A**). The benefit of surgery appears greatest in the elderly, in men, after stroke compared with TIA, decreased with time from the last ischemic event, and tended to be greater in patients with ulcerated plaques than in those with smooth plaques[192] (**Class I, Level A**). In particular, the subgroup in whom the benefit of surgery was highest was patients who were randomized within two weeks of an ischemic event, again emphasizing the need for rapid assessment and treatment of patients with stroke and TIA to identify those with carotid stenosis (**Class I, Level A**).

Is carotid stenting more effective than carotid endarterectomy?

The last decade has witnessed a rapid growth in the use of percutaneous, transluminal stenting techniques for carotid stenosis, in part to avoid some of the drawbacks (i.e. admission to hospital, general anesthetic, incision in the neck) and complications associated with endarterectomy, and in part due to the awareness and accessibility of the carotid to such treatment. Initial endovascular techniques primarily used angioplasty, which was randomly evaluated in the Carotid and Vertebral Artery Transluminal Angioplasty Study (CAVATAS) involving over 500 patients, most of whom had symptomatic carotid stenosis. The results showed 30-day outcomes were comparable between the randomized groups[195]; the rate of death or any major stroke was 9.9% after surgery and 10.0% after angioplasty. However, analysis of the other risks confirmed that angioplasty was safer than surgery in terms of minor morbidity and reduced hospital length of stay, but was associated with a higher rate of (asymptomatic) restenosis during follow-up.

Subsequently, there have been several more randomized trials that have compared the safety and efficacy of endovascular techniques by means of angioplasty or stenting with carotid endarterectomy, involving a total of 3.227 patients.[196] Overall, the results to date suggest similar risks of early stroke (about 5–8%) or death (about 1%), although among the individual larger trials, the results vary from favoring stenting (SAPPHIRE[197]), equivalence (CAVATAS[195] and SPACE[198]), to favoring endarterectomy (EVA-35[199]). However, the characteristics of patients and the revascularization techniques used varied across the studies. Long-term follow-up data suggest that there are no significant differences between the treatments in preventing stroke or death, but there are wide confidence intervals around the effect estimates and significant heterogeneity across studies (**Class I, Level A**). Endovascular procedures clearly reduce the risk of local complications (e.g. cranial nerve injury and hematoma) but may be associated with a greater risk of silent cerebral ischemic lesions detected on MRI irrespec-

tive of whether or not a distal embolic protection device was used.[200,201] Despite the presence of such lesions, though, one study has shown similar risk of cognitive changes between endarterectomy and stenting.[202] Finally, as well as advancing age,[203] unfavorable anatomic aspects of the carotid artery, such as calcification, great vessel origin stenosis, tortuosity and the severity of the stenosis may make stenting of the carotid artery more difficult and hazardous[204] (**Class IIa, Level A**).

What is the appropriate timing of carotid revascularization after ischemic stroke or TIA?

Histologic examination of carotid endarterectomy specimens has highlighted certain features such as the presence of a large lipid-rich necrotic core, a thin overlying fibrous cap, an inflammatory infiltrate, neovasculature growth, and intraplaque hemorrhage, which support the "vulnerable plaque" theory to produce an embolic source of thrombosis.[205,206] In the meta-analysis of the trials, the benefits of carotid endarterectomy were highest in patients randomized within two weeks of an ischemic event[192] (**Class I, Level A**). Thus, it is probably best to perform carotid endarterectomy early (within the first few weeks) of a non- or mildly disabling ischemic stroke or TIA. Conversely, early use of carotid stenting appears more hazardous[199,207] and should be reserved for when the patient is stable several weeks or more after the onset of the event (**Class IIa, Level B**).

Conclusion

Major progress has been made in the evidence base supporting approaches to the prevention of second stroke. Several key points emerge.
- Given continuous associations of risk factors and stroke rates, effective prevention of stroke involves the management of the patient as a *whole* person defined by their absolute risk of future major vascular events rather than by a single variable defined by a particular threshold level of BP or cholesterol.
- BP-lowering therapy is pivotal to the prevention of recurrent stroke in all patients with cerebrovascular disease, irrespective of BP levels, age and other characteristics.
- Aspirin (optimal dose 30–300 mg) is cheap, safe, familiar and acceptable as the antiplatelet agent of first choice for patients with vascular disease, but clopidogrel and the combination of low-dose aspirin and dypridamole provide comparable modest additional benefit over aspirin.
- Warfarin is indicated in patients with a cardiac (embolic) source of stroke including AF unless there are contraindications or the risk of stroke is low, in which case aspirin is recommended.

• Cholesterol-lowering therapy with statins is safe, well tolerated and effective in preventing major vascular events including stroke in all high-risk individuals irrespective of baseline cholesterol levels.

• Carotid endarterectomy or stenting is indicated for patients with severe carotid artery stenosis who have had symptoms of retinal or brain ischemia appropriate to the stenosis, and are willing to undergo a small but definite risk of death or disability related to the procedure undertaken by an experienced proceduralist.

References

1. Murray CJL, Lopez AD. Mortality by cause for eight regions of the world: Global Burden of Disease Study. *Lancet* 1997;**349**(9061):1269–76.

2. Bamford J, Sandercock P, Dennis M, Burn J, Warlow C. A prospective study of acute cerebrovascular disease in the community: the Oxfordshire Community Stroke Project – 1981–86. 2. Incidence, case fatality rates and overall outcome at one year of cerebral infarction, primary intracerebral and subarachnoid haemorrhage. *J Neurol Neurosurg Psychiatry* 1990;**53**(1):16–22.

3. Wolfe CD. The impact of stroke. *Br Med Bull* 2000;**56**(2): 275–86.

4. Murray CJL, Lopez AD. Global mortality, disability, and the contribution of risk factors: Global Burden of Disease Study. *Lancet* 1997;**349**(9063):1436–42.

5. Rothwell PM, Coull AJ, Silver LE *et al.* Population-based study of event-rate, incidence, case fatality, and mortality for all acute vascular events in all arterial territories (Oxford Vascular Study). *Lancet* 2005;**366**(9499):1773–83.

6. Bonita R. Epidemiology of stroke. *Lancet* 1992;**339**(8789): 342–4.

7. Lopez AD, Mathers CD, Ezzati M, Jamison DT, Murray CJ. Global and regional burden of disease and risk factors, 2001: systematic analysis of population health data. *Lancet* 2006;**367**(9524):1747–57.

8. Rothwell PM, Coull AJ, Giles MF *et al.* Change in stroke incidence, mortality, case-fatality, severity, and risk factors in Oxfordshire, UK from 1981 to 2004 (Oxford Vascular Study). *Lancet* 2004;**363**(9425):1925–33.

9. Wolf PA. Epidemiology of stroke. In: Mohr JP, Choi DW, Grotta JC, Weir B, Wolf PA (eds) *Stroke: Pathophysiology, Diagnosis and* Management, 4th edn. Philadelphia: Churchill Livingstone, 2004.

10. Chalela JA, Kidwell CS, Nentwich LM *et al.* Magnetic resonance imaging and computed tomography in emergency assessment of patients with suspected acute stroke: a prospective comparison. *Lancet* 2007;**369**(9558):293–8.

11. Adams HP Jr, Bendixen BH, Kappelle LJ *et al.* Classification of subtype of acute ischemic stroke. Definitions for use in a multicenter clinical trial. TOAST. Trial of Org 10172 in Acute Stroke Treatment. *Stroke* 1993;**24**(1):35–41.

12. Auer RN, Sutherland GR. Primary intracerebral hemorrhage: pathophysiology. *Can J Neurol Sci* 2005;**32**(suppl 2):S3–12.

13. Broderick J, Connolly S, Feldmann E *et al.* Guidelines for the Management of Spontaneous Intracerebral Hemorrhage in Adults: 2007 Update: A Guideline From the American Heart Association/American Stroke Association Stroke Council, High Blood Pressure Research Council, and the Quality of Care and Outcomes in Research Interdisciplinary Working Group: The American Academy of Neurology affirms the value of this guideline as an educational tool for neurologists. *Stroke* 2007;**38**(6):2001–23.

14. Mayer SA, Brun NC, Begtrup K *et al.* Efficacy and safety of recombinant activated Factor VII for acute intracerebral hemorrhage. *N Engl J Med* 2008;**358**(20):2127–37.

15. Saver JL. Time is brain – quantified. *Stroke* 2006;**37**(1):263–6.

16. Barsan WG, Brott TG, Broderick JP, Haley EC, Levy DE, Marler JR. Time of hospital presentation in patients with acute stroke. *Arch Intern Med* 1993;**153**(22):2558–61.

17. Wein TH, Staub L, Felberg R *et al.* Activation of emergency medical services for acute stroke in a nonurban population: the T.L.L. Temple Foundation Stroke Project. *Stroke* 2000;**31**(8): 1925–8.

18. Mikulik R, Bunt L, Hrdlicka D, Dusek L, Vaclavik D, Kryza J. Calling 911 in response to stroke. A nationwide study assessing definitive individual behavior. *Stroke* 2008;**39**(6):1844–9.

19. de la Ossa NP, Sanchez-Ojanguren J, Palomeras E *et al.* Influence of the stroke code activation source on the outcome of acute ischemic stroke patients. *Neurology* 2008;**70**(15):1238–43.

20. Kidwell CS, Starkman S, Eckstein M, Weems K, Saver JL. Identifying stroke in the field : prospective validation of the Los Angeles Prehospital Stroke Screen (LAPSS). *Stroke* 2000; **31**(1):71–6.

21. Kothari RU, Pancioli A, Liu T, Brott T, Broderick J. Cincinnati Prehospital Stroke Scale: reproducibility and validity. *Ann Emerg Med* 1999;**33**(4):373–8.

22. Audebert HJ, Kukla C, Vatankhah B *et al.* Comparison of tissue plasminogen activator administration management between telestroke network hospitals and academic stroke centers: the Telemedical Pilot Project for Integrative Stroke Care in Bavaria/ Germany. *Stroke* 2006;**37**(7):1822–7.

23. Hess DC, Wang S, Hamilton W *et al.* REACH: clinical feasibility of a rural telestroke network. *Stroke* 2005;**36**(9):2018–20.

24. Schwab S, Vatankhah B, Kukla C *et al.* Long-term outcome after thrombolysis in telemedical stroke care. *Neurology* 2007;**69**(9):898–903.

25. Hand PJ, Kwan J, Lindley RI, Dennis MS, Wardlaw JM. Distinguishing between stroke and mimic at the bedside: the Brain Attack Study. *Stroke* 2006;**37**(3):769–75.

26. Norris JW, Hachinski VC. Misdiagnosis of stroke. *Lancet* 1982;**1**(8267):328–31.

27. Wardlaw JM, Mielke O. Early signs of brain infarction at CT: observer reliability and outcome after thrombolytic treatment – systematic review. *Radiology* 2005;**235**(2):444–53.

28. Moulin T, Cattin F, Crepin-Leblond T *et al.* Early CT signs in acute middle cerebral artery infarction: predictive value for subsequent infarct locations and outcome. *Neurology* 1996;**47**(2):366–75.

29. Warach S, Gaa J, Siewert B *et al.* Acute human stroke studied by whole brain echo planar diffusion-weighted magnetic resonance imaging. *Ann Neurol* 1995;**37**(2):231–41.

30. Hjort N, Christensen S, Solling C *et al.* Ischemic injury detected by diffusion imaging 11 minutes after stroke. *Ann Neurol* 2005;**58**(3):462–5.

31. Schellinger PD, Thomalla G, Fiehler J *et al.* MRI-based and CT-based thrombolytic therapy in acute stroke within and beyond established time windows: an analysis of 1210 patients. *Stroke* 2007;**38**(10):2640–5.

32. Ronning OM, Guldvog B. Should stroke victims routinely receive supplemental oxygen? A quasi-randomized controlled trial. *Stroke* 1999;**30**(10):2033–7.

33. Bennett MH, Wasiak J, Schnabel A, Kranke P, French C. Hyperbaric oxygen therapy for acute ischaemic stroke. *Cochrane Database of Systematic Reviews* 2005, Issue 3. Art. No.: CD004954. DOI: 10.1002/14651858.CD004954.pub2.

34. Hajat C, Hajat S, Sharma P. Effects of poststroke pyrexia on stroke outcome: a meta-analysis of studies in patients. *Stroke* 2000;**31**(2):410–14.

35. Reith J, Jorgensen HS, Pedersen PM *et al.* Body temperature in acute stroke: relation to stroke severity, infarct size, mortality, and outcome. *Lancet* 1996;**347**(8999):422–5.

36. Busto R, Dietrich WD, Globus MY, Valdes I, Scheinberg P, Ginsberg MD. Small differences in intraischemic brain temperature critically determine the extent of ischemic neuronal injury. *J Cereb Blood Flow Metab* 1987;**7**(6):729–38.

37. Hypothermia after Cardiac Arrest Study. Mild therapeutic hypothermia to improve the neurologic outcome after cardiac arrest. *N Engl J Med* 2002;**346**(8):549–56.

38. Scott JF, Robinson GM, French JM, O'Connell JE, Alberti KG, Gray CS. Prevalence of admission hyperglycaemia across clinical subtypes of acute stroke. *Lancet* 1999;**353**(9150):376–7.

39. Bruno A, Levine SR, Frankel MR *et al.* Admission glucose level and clinical outcomes in the NINDS rt-PA Stroke Trial. *Neurology* 2002;**59**(5):669–74.

40. Lindsberg PJ, Roine RO. Hyperglycemia in acute stroke. *Stroke* 2004;**35**(2):363–4.

41. Gray CS, Hildreth AJ, Sandercock PA *et al.* Glucose-potassium-insulin infusions in the management of post-stroke hyperglycaemia: the UK Glucose Insulin in Stroke Trial (GIST-UK). *Lancet Neurol* 2007;**6**(5):397–406.

42. Castillo J, Leira R, Garcia MM, Serena J, Blanco M, Davalos A. Blood pressure decrease during the acute phase of ischemic stroke is associated with brain injury and poor stroke outcome. *Stroke* 2004;**35**(2):520–6.

43. Leonardi-Bee J, Bath PM, Phillips SJ, Sandercock PA. Blood pressure and clinical outcomes in the International Stroke Trial. *Stroke* 2002;**33**(5):1315–20.

44. Adams HP Jr, del Zoppo G, Alberts MJ *et al.* Guidelines for the Early Management of Adults With Ischemic Stroke: A Guideline From the American Heart Association/American Stroke Association Stroke Council, Clinical Cardiology Council, Cardiovascular Radiology and Intervention Council, and the Atherosclerotic Peripheral Vascular Disease and Quality of Care Outcomes in Research Interdisciplinary Working Groups: The American Academy of Neurology affirms the value of this guideline as an educational tool for neurologists. *Stroke* 2007;**38**(5):1655–711.

45. Broderick J, Brott T, Barsan W *et al.* Blood pressure during the first minutes of focal cerebral ischemia. *Ann Emerg Med* 1993;**22**(9):1438–43.

46. The National Tissue Institute of Neurological Disorders and Stroke rt-PA Stroke Study Group. National Institute of Neurological D, Stroke rt PASSG. Tissue plasminogen activator for acute ischemic stroke. *N Engl J Med* 1995;**333**(24):1581–8.

47. Pannier JL, Weyne J, Leusen I. Effects of changes in acid-base composition in the cerebral ventricles on local and general cerebral blood flow. *Eur Neurol* 1971;**6**(1):123–6.

48. Mori S, Sadoshima S, Fujii K, Ibayashi S, Iino K, Fujishima M. Decrease in cerebral blood flow with blood pressure reductions in patients with chronic stroke. *Stroke* 1993;**24**(9):1376–81.

49. Geeganage C, Bath PMW. Interventions for deliberately altering blood pressure in acute stroke. *Cochrane Database of Systematic Reviews* 2008, Issue 4. Art. No.: CD000039. DOI: 10.1002/14651858.CD000039.pub2.

50. Baron JC. Mapping the ischaemic penumbra with PET: implications for acute stroke treatment. *Cerebrovasc Dis* 1999;**9**(4):193–201.

51. Darby DG, Barber PA, Gerraty RP *et al.* Pathophysiological topography of acute ischemia by combined diffusion-weighted and perfusion MRI. *Stroke* 1999;**30**(10):2043–52.

52. Rha J-H, Saver JL. The impact of recanalization on ischemic stroke outcome: a meta-analysis. *Stroke* 2007;**38**(3):967–73.

53. Wahlgren N, Ahmed N, Dávalos A *et al.* Thrombolysis with alteplase for acute ischaemic stroke in the Safe Implementation of Thrombolysis in Stroke-Monitoring Study (SITS-MOST): an observational study. *Lancet* 2007;**369**(9558):275–82.

54. Hacke W, Kaste M, Fieschi C *et al.* Intravenous thrombolysis with recombinant tissue plasminogen activator for acute hemispheric stroke. The European Cooperative Acute Stroke Study (ECASS). *JAMA* 1995;**274**(13):1017–25.

55. Hacke W, Kaste M, Fieschi C *et al.* Randomised double-blind placebo-controlled trial of thrombolytic therapy with intravenous alteplase in acute ischaemic stroke (ECASS II). *Lancet* 1998;**352**(9136):1245–51.

56. Clark WM, Wissman S, Albers GW *et al.* Recombinant tissue-type plasminogen activator (alteplase) for ischemic stroke 3 to 5 hours after symptom onset: the ATLANTIS Study: a randomized controlled trial. *JAMA* 1999;**282**(21):2019–26.

57. Clark WM, Albers GW, Madden KP, Hamilton S. The rtPA (Alteplase) 0- to 6-Hour Acute Stroke Trial, Part A (A0276g): results of a double-blind, placebo-controlled, multicenter study. *Stroke* 2000;**31**(4):811–16.

58. Multicentre Acute Stroke Trial – Italy (MAST-I) Group. Randomised controlled trial of streptokinase, aspirin, and combination of both in treatment of acute ischaemic stroke. *Lancet* 1995;**346**(8989):1509–14.

59. Donnan GA, Davis SM, Chambers BR *et al.* Streptokinase for acute ischemic stroke with relationship to time of administration: Australian Streptokinase (ASK) Trial Study Group. *JAMA* 1996;**276**(12):961–6.

60. Multicenter Acute Stroke Trial – Europe Study. Thrombolytic therapy with streptokinase in acute ischemic stroke. *N Engl J Med* 1996;**335**(3):145–50.

61. Hacke W, Donnan G, Fieschi C *et al.* Association of outcome with early stroke treatment: pooled analysis of ATLANTIS, ECASS, and NINDS rt-PA stroke trials. *Lancet* 2004;**363**(9411):768–74.

61a. Hacke W, Kaste M, Bluhmki E, Brozman M, Davalos A, Guidetti D *et al.* Thrombolysis with alteplase 3 to 4.5 hours after acute ischemic stroke. *N Engl J Med* 2008;**359**(13):1317–29.

61b. Del Zoppo GJ, Saver JL, Jauch EC, Adams HP, Jr. Expansion of the Time Window for Treatment of Acute Ischemic Stroke With

Intravenous Tissue Plasminogen Activator. A Science Advisory From the American Heart Association/American Stroke Association. *Stroke* 2009;May 28.

62. Albers GW, Thijs VN, Wechsler L E *et al.* Magnetic resonance imaging profiles predict clinical response to early reperfusion: the diffusion and perfusion imaging evaluation for understanding stroke evolution (DEFUSE) study. *Ann Neurol* 2006;**60**(5):508–17.

63. Davis SM, Donnan GA, Parsons MW *et al.* Effects of alteplase beyond 3h after stroke in the Echoplanar Imaging Thrombolytic Evaluation Trial (EPITHET): a placebo-controlled randomised trial. *Lancet Neurol* 2008;**7**(4):299–309.

64. Alexandrov AV, Molina CA, Grotta JC *et al.* Ultrasound-enhanced systemic thrombolysis for acute ischemic stroke. *N Engl J Med* 2004;**351**(21):2170–8.

65. Molina CA, Saver JL. Extending reperfusion therapy for acute ischemic stroke: emerging pharmacological, mechanical, and imaging strategies. *Stroke* 2005;**36**(10):2311–20.

66. Furlan A, Higashida R, Wechsler L *et al.* Intra-arterial prourokinase for acute ischemic stroke. The PROACT II study: a randomized controlled trial. Prolyse in Acute Cerebral Thromboembolism. *JAMA* 1999;**282**(21):2003–11.

67. Ogawa A, Mori E, Minematsu K *et al.* Randomized trial of intraarterial infusion of urokinase within 6 hours of middle cerebral artery stroke: the Middle Cerebral Artery Embolism Local Fibrinolytic Intervention Trial (MELT) Japan. *Stroke* 2007;**38**(10):2633–9.

68. Saver JL. Intra-arterial fibrinolysis for acute ischemic stroke: the message of MELT. *Stroke* 2007;**38**(10):2627–8.

69. Smith WS, Sung G, Saver J *et al.* Mechanical thrombectomy for acute ischemic stroke: final results of the Multi MERCI Trial. *Stroke* 2008;**39**(4):1205–12.

70. Bose A, Henkes H, Alfke K *et al.* The Penumbra System: a mechanical device for the treatment of acute stroke due to thromboembolism. *Am J Neuroradiol* 2008:**29**(7):1409–13.

71. International Stroke Trial Collaborative Group. The International Stroke Trial (IST): a randomised trial of aspirin, subcutaneous heparin, both, or neither among 19435 patients with acute ischaemic stroke. *Lancet* 1997;**349**(9065):1569–81.

72. Saxena R, Lewis S, Berge E, Sandercock PAG, Koudstaal PJ. Risk of early death and recurrent stroke and effect of heparin in 3169 patients with acute ischemic stroke and atrial fibrillation in the International Stroke Trial. *Stroke* 2001;**32**(10):2333–7.

73. Adams HP Jr. Emergent use of anticoagulation for treatment of patients with ischemic stroke. *Stroke* 2002;**33**(3):856–61.

74. Chen Z-M. CAST: randomised placebo-controlled trial of early aspirin use in 20000 patients with acute ischaemic stroke. *Lancet* 1997;**349**(9066):1641–9.

75. Sandercock PAG, Counsell C, Gubitz GJ, Tseng MC. Antiplatelet therapy for acute ischaemic stroke. *Cochrane Database of Systematic Reviews* 2008, Issue 3. Art. No.: CD000029. DOI: 10.1002/14651858.CD000029.pub2.

76. Gladstone DJ, Black SE, Hakim AM. Toward wisdom from failure: lessons from neuroprotective stroke trials and new therapeutic directions. *Stroke* 2002;**33**(8):2123–36.

77. Lees KR, Zivin JA, Ashwood T *et al.* NXY-059 for acute ischemic stroke. *N Engl J Med* 2006;**354**(6):588–600.

78. Shuaib A, Lees KR, Lyden P *et al.* NXY-059 for the treatment of acute ischemic stroke. *N Engl J Med* 2007;**357**(6):562–71.

79. Saver JL, Kidwell C, Eckstein M, Starkman S, for the F-MAGPTI. Prehospital neuroprotective therapy for acute stroke: results of the Field Administration of Stroke Therapy-Magnesium (FAST-MAG) Pilot Trial. *Stroke* 2004;**35**(5):e106–8.

80. Stroke Unit Trialists' Collaboration. Organised inpatient (stroke unit) care for stroke. *Cochrane Database of Systematic Reviews* 2007, Issue 4. Art. No.: CD000197. DOI: 10.1002/14651858.CD000197.pub2.

81. Gilligan AK, Thrift AG, Sturm JW, Dewey HM, Macdonell RAL, Donnan GA. Stroke units, tissue plasminogen activator, aspirin and neuroprotection: which stroke intervention could provide the greatest community benefit? *Cerebrovasc Dis* 2005;**20**(4):239–44.

82. Langhorne P, Dey P, Woodman M *et al.* Is stroke unit care portable? A systematic review of the clinical trials. *Age Ageing* 2005;**34**(4):324–30.

83. Sandercock PA, van den Belt AG, Lindley RI, Slattery J. Antithrombotic therapy in acute ischaemic stroke: an overview of the completed randomised trials. *J Neurol Neurosurg Psychiatry* 1993;**56**(1):17–25.

84. Sherman DG, Albers GW, Bladin C *et al.* The efficacy and safety of enoxaparin versus unfractionated heparin for the prevention of venous thromboembolism after acute ischaemic stroke (PREVAIL Study): an open-label randomised comparison. *Lancet* 2007;**369**(9570):1347–55.

85. Szaflarski JP, Rackley AY, Kleindorfer DO *et al.* Incidence of seizures in the acute phase of stroke: a population-based study. *Epilepsia* 2008;**49**(6):974–81.

86. Frank JI. Large hemispheric infarction, deterioration, and intracranial pressure. *Neurology* 1995;**45**(7):1286–90.

87. Hacke W, Schwab S, Horn M, Spranger M, De Georgia M, von Kummer R. "Malignant" middle cerebral artery territory infarction: clinical course and prognostic signs. *Arch Neurol* 1996;**53**(4):309–15.

88. Hofmeijer J, Amelink GJ, Algra A *et al.* Hemicraniectomy after middle cerebral artery infarction with life-threatening Edema trial (HAMLET). Protocol for a randomised controlled trial of decompressive surgery in space-occupying hemispheric infarction. *Trials* 2006;**7**:29.

89. Juttler E, Schwab S, Schmiedek P *et al.* Decompressive Surgery for the Treatment of Malignant Infarction of the Middle Cerebral Artery (DESTINY): a randomized, controlled trial. *Stroke* 2007;**38**(9):2518–25.

90. Vahedi K, Vicaut E, Mateo J *et al.* Sequential-design, multicenter, randomized, controlled trial of early decompressive craniectomy in malignant middle cerebral artery infarction (DECIMAL Trial). *Stroke* 2007;**38**(9):2506–17.

91. Vahedi K, Hofmeijer J, Juettler E *et al.* Early decompressive surgery in malignant infarction of the middle cerebral artery: a pooled analysis of three randomised controlled trials. *Lancet Neurol* 2007;**6**(3):215–22.

92. Horwitz NH, Ludolph C. Acute obstructive hydrocephalus caused by cerebellar infarction. Treatment alternatives. *Surg Neurol* 1983;**20**(1):13–19.

93. Kudo H, Kawaguchi T, Minami H, Kuwamura K, Miyata M, Kohmura E. Controversy of surgical treatment for severe cerebellar infarction. *J Stroke Cerebrovasc Dis* 2007;**16**(6):259–62.

94. Hornig CR, Rust DS, Busse O, Jauss M, Laun A. Space-occupying cerebellar infarction. Clinical course and prognosis. *Stroke* 1994;**25**(2):372–4.

95. Donnan GA, Fisher M, Macleod M, Davis SM. Stroke. *Lancet* 2008;**371**(9624):1612–23.

96. Hankey GJ, Warlow CP. Treatment and secondary prevention of stroke: evidence, costs, and effects on individuals and populations. *Lancet* 1999;**354**(9188):1457–63.

97. Murray C, Lopez A. *The Global Burden of Disease: a comprehensive assessment of mortality and disability from diseases, injuries and risk factors in 1990 and projected to 2020.* Boston: Harvard School of Public Health, 1996.

98. Rothwell PM, Coull AJ, Giles MF, for the Oxford Vascular Study. Change in stroke incidence, mortality, case-fatality, severity and risk factors in Oxfordshire, UK from 1981 to 2004 (Oxford Vascular Study). *Lancet* 2004;**363**:1925–33.

99. Anderson CS, Carter KN, Hackett ML *et al*, on behalf of the Auckland Regional Community Stroke (ARCOS) Study Group. Trends in stroke incidence in Auckland, New Zealand, during 1981 to 2003. *Stroke* 2005;**36**:2087–93.

100. Islam S, Anderson CS, Hankey G *et al*. Trends in the incidence and outcome of stroke in Perth, Western Australia, 1989 to 2001: the Perth Community Stroke Study. *Stroke* 2008;**39**: 776–82.

101. Tobias M, Cheung J, Carter K, Feigin V, Anderson CS. Stroke surveillance: population-based estimates and projections for New Zealand. *Aust NZ J Pub Health* 2007;**31**:520–5.

102. Johnston SC, Gress DR, Browner WS, Sidney S. Short-term prognosis after emergency departmenet diagnosis of TIA. *JAMA* 2000;**284**:2901–6.

103. Coull AJ, Lovett JK, Rothwell PM. Population based study of early risk of stroke after transient ischemic attack and minor stroke: implications for public education and organisation of services. *BMJ* 2004;**328**:326–8.

104. Van Wijk I, Kappelle LJ, van Gijn J *et al*. Long-term survival and vascular event risk after transient ischemic attack or minor ischemic stroke: a cohort study. *Lancet* 2005;**365**: 2098–104.

105. Rothwell PM, Warlow CO. Timing of TIAs preceding stroke: time window for prevention is very short. *Neurology* 2005;**64**: 817–20.

106. Rothwell PM, Giles MF, Chandratheva A *et al*. Effect of urgent treatment of transient ischemic attack and minor stroke on early recurrent stroke (EXPRESS study): a prospective population-based sequential comparison. *Lancet* 2007;**370**: 1432–42.

107. Lavallée PC, Mesenuei E, Abboud H *et al*. A transient ischemic attack clinic with round-the-clock access (SOS-TIA): feasibility and effects. *Lancet* 2007;**6**:953–60.

108. WHO MONICA Project Principal Investigators. The World Health Organisation MONICA project (Monitoring Trends and Determinants in Cardiovascular Disease): a major international collaboration. *J Clin Epidemiol* 1988;**41**:105–14.

109. Warlow C, Dennis M, van Gijn J *et al*. Stroke: a practical guide to management. Oxford, Blackwell Science, 1996.

110. Albers GW, Caplan LR, Easton JD *et al*. Transient ischemic attack – proposal for a new definition. *N Engl J Med* 2002;**347**: 1713.

111. Wang KS, Li H, Lam WWM, Chan YL, Kay R. Progression of middle cerebral artery occlusive disease and its relationship with further vascular events after stroke. *Stroke* 2002;**33**: 532–6.

112. Arenillas JF, Molina CA, Montaner J *et al*. Progression and clinical recurrent of symptomatic middle cerebral artery stenosis: a long-term follow-up transcranial doppler ultrasound study. *Stroke* 2001;**32**:2898–904.

113. Wityk RJ, Lehman D, Klag M, Coresh J, Ahn H, Litt B. Race and sex differences in the distribution of cerebral atherosclerosis. *Stroke* 1996;**27**:1974–80.

114. Zhang L, Yang J, Hong Z *et al*. Proportion of different subtypes of stroke in China. *Stroke* 2003;**34**:2091–6.

115. Australasian Co-operative Research on Subarachnoid Hemorrhage Study Group. Epidemiology of aneurysmal subarachnoid hemorrhage in Australia and New Zealand: incidence and case fatality from the Australasian Co-operative Research on Subarachnoid Hemorrhage Study (ACROSS). *Stroke* 2000;**31**: 1843–50.

116. Ezzati M, van der Horn S, Rodgers A, Lopez AD, Mathers CD, Murray CJ, and the Comparative Risk Assessment Collaborative Group. Estimates of global and regional potential health gains from reducing multiple major risk factors. *Lancet* 2003;**362**: 271–80.

117. MacMahon S, Peto R, Cutler J, Collins R, Sorlie P. Blood pressure, stroke, and coronary heart disease. Part 1, prolonged differences in blood pressure: prospective observational studies corrected for regression dilution bias. *Lancet* 1990;**335**: 765–74.

118. Lawes CML, Bennett DA, Feigin VL, Rodgers A. Blood pressure and stroke: an overview of published reviews. *Stroke* 2004;**35**:1024–33.

119. Rashid P, Leonardi-Bee J, Bath P. Blood pressure reduction and secondary prevention of stroke and other vascular events: a systematic review. *Stroke* 2003;**34**:2741–8.

120. Prospective Studies Collaboration. Age-specific relevance of usual blood pressure to vascular mortality: a meta-analysis of individual data for one million adults in 61 prospective studies. *Lancet* 2002;**360**:1903–13.

121. Asia Pacific Cohort Studies Collaboration. Blood pressure and cardiovascular disease in the Asia Pacific region. *J Hypertens* 2003;**21**:707–16.

122. Blood Pressure Lowering Treatment Trialists' Collaboration. Effects of different blood-pressure-lowering regimens on major cardiovascular events: results of prospectively-designed overviews of randomized trials. *Lancet* 2003;**362**:1527–35.

123. Yusuf S, on behalf of the PRoFESS Study Group. Randomized trial of telmisartan therapy to prevent recurrent therapy strokes and major vascular events among 20,332 individuals with recent stroke. The PRoFESS trial. Presented at the XVIIth European Stroke Conference in Nice, 14 May 2008 (www.phri.ca/profess.htm).

124. ONTARGET Investigators. Telmisartan, ramipril, or both in patients at high risk for vascular events. *N Engl J Med* 2008;**358**: 1547–59.

125. Reboldi G, Angeli F, Cavallini C, Gentile G, Mancia G, Verdecchia P. Comparison between angiotensin-converting enzyme inhibitors and angiotensin receptor blockers on the risk of myocardial infarction, stroke and death: a meta-analysis. *J Hypertens* 2008;**26**:1282–9.

126. Willmot M, Leonardi-Bee J, Bath PM. High blood pressure in acute stroke and subsequent outcome: a systematic review. *Hypertension* 2004;**43**:18–24.

127. Leonardi-Bee J, Bath PMW, Phillips SJ, Sandercock PAG, for the IST Collaborative Group. Blood pressure and clinical outcomes in the International Stroke Trial. *Stroke* 2002;**33**: 1315–20.

128. Anderson CS, Huang Y, Wang JG et al, for the INTERACT Investigators. Intensive blood pressure reduction in acute cerebral hemorrhage trial (INTERACT): a randomised pilot trial. *Lancet Neurol* 2008;**7**:391–9.

129. Broderick J, Connolly S, Feldmann E et al. Guidelines for the management of spontaneous intracerebral hemorrhage in adults: 2007 update: a guideline from the American Heart Association / American Stroke Association Stroke Council, High Blood Pressure Research Council, and the Quality of Care and Outcomes in Research Interdisciplinary Working Group. *Stroke* 2007;**38**:2001–3.

130. Schrader J, Luders S, Kulschewski A et al. The ACCESS Study: evaluation of acute candesartan cilexetil therapy in stroke survivors. *Stroke* 2003;**34**:1699–703.

131. Arima H, Chalmers J, Woodward M et al. Lower target blood pressures are safe and effective for the prevention of recurrent stroke: the PROGRESS trial. PROGRESS Collaborative Group. *J Hypertens* 2006;**4**:1201–8.

132. Beckett NS, Peters R, Fletcher AE et al. Treatment of hypertension in patients 80 years of age or older. *N Engl J Med* 2008;**358**: 1887–98.

133. Antiplatelet Trialists' Collaboration. Collaborative overview of randomised trials of antiplatelet therapy in various categories of patients. *BMJ* **1994**; 308: 81–106. [Published erratum appears *BMJ* 1994;**308**:1540.].

134. Antithrombotic Trialists' Collaboration. Collaborative meta-analysis of randomized trials of antiplatelet therapy for prevention of death, myocardial infarction, and stroke in high risk patients. *BMJ* 2002;**324**:71–86.

135. Chan FK, Ching JY, Hung LC et al. Clopidogril versus aspirin and esomeprazole to prevent recurrent ulcer bleeding. *N Engl J Med* 2005;**352**:238–44.

136. Foerch C, Sitzer M, Steinmetz H, Neumann-Haefelin T for the Aubeitsgruppe Schlaganfall Hessen. Pretreatment with antiplatelet agents is not independently associated with unfavorable outcome in intracerebral hemorrhage. *Stroke* 2006;**37**: 165–67.

137. Chen ZM, Sandercock P, Pan HC et al, on behalf of the CAST and IST Collaborative Groups. Indications for early aspirin use in acute ischemic stroke: a combined analysis of 40,000 randomized patients from the Chinese Acute Stroke Trial and the International Stroke Trial. *Stroke* 2000;**31**:1240–9.

138. Algra A, van Gijn J. Aspirin at any dose above 30 mg offers only modest protection after cerebral ischemia. *J Neurol Neurosurg Psychiatry* 1996;**60**:197–9.

139. Diener HC, Cunha L, Forbes C, Sivenius J, Smets P, Lowenthal A. European Stroke Prevention Study 2. Dipyridamole and acetylsalicylic acid in the secondary prevention of stroke. *J Neurol Sci* 1996;**143**:1–13.

140. CAPRIE Steering Committee. A randomized, blinded, trial of clopidogrel versus aspirin in patients at risk of ischemic events (CAPRIE). *Lancet* 1996;**348**:1329–39.

141. Hankey GJ, Sudlow CLM, Dunbabin DW. Thienopyridines or aspirin to prevent stroke and other serious vascular events in patients at high risk of vascular disease. *Stroke* 2000;**31**: 1779–84.

142. Hankey G, Sudlow CLM, Dunbabin DW. Thienopyridine derivatives (ticlopidine, clopidogrel) versus aspirin for preventing stroke and other serious vascular events in high vascular risk patients. *Cochrane Database of Systematic Reviews* 2000, Issue 1. Art. No.: CD001246. DOI: 10.1002/14651858.CD001246.

143. Diener HC, Bogousslavsky J, Brass LM et al. Aspirin and clopidogrel compared with clopidogrel alone after recent ischemic stroke or transient ischemic attack in high-risk patients (MATCH): randomized, double-blind, placebo-controlled trial. *Lancet* 2004;**364**:331–7.

144. Bhatt DL, Fox KA, Hacke W et al. Clopidogrel and aspirin versus aspirin alone for the prevention of atherothrombotic events. *N Engl J Med* 2006;**354**:1706–17.

145. Markus HS, Droste DW, Kaps M et al. Dual antiplatelet therapy with clopidogrel and aspirin in symptomatic carotid stenosis evaluated using doppler embolic signal detection: the Clopridogrel and Aspiriin for Reduction of Emboli in Symptomatic Carotid Stenosis (CARESS) trial. *Circulation* 2005;**111**:2233–40.

146. Chen ZM, Jiang LX, Chen YP et al. Addition of clopidogril to aspirin in 45,852 patients with acute myocardial infarction: randomized placebo-controlled trial. *Lancet* 2005;**366**:1607–21.

147. Yusuf S, Zhao F, Mehta SR, Chrolavicius S, Tognoni G, Fox KK. Effects of clopidogrel in addition to aspirin in patients with acute coronary syndromes without ST-segment elevation. *N Engl J Med* 2001;**345**:494–502.

148. Kennedy J, Hill MD, Ryckborst KJ, Eliasziw M, Demchuk AM, Buchan AM, for the FASTER Investigators. Fast assessment of stroke and transient ischemic attack to prevent early recurrence (FASTER): a randomized controlled pilot trial. *Lancet Neurol* 2007;**6**:961–9.

149. ESPRIT Study Group. Aspirin plus dipyridamole versus aspirin alone after cerebral ischemic of arterial origin (ESPRIT): randomized controlled trial. *Lancet* 2006;**367**:1665–73.

150. Sacco R, for the PRoFESS Study Group. Prevention Regimen For Effectively avoiding Second Strokes: the PRoFESS trial. Presentation at the European Stroke Conference, Nice, 14 May 2008 (www.phri.ca/profess.htm).

151. Kannel WB, Abbott RD, Savage DD, McNamara PM. Coronary heart disease and atrial fibrillation: the Framingham Study. *Am Heart J* 1983;**106**:389–96.

152. Wolf PA, Abbott RD, Kannel WB. Atrial fibrillation as an independent risk factor for stroke: the Framingham study. *Stroke* 1991;**22**:983–8.

153. Cage BF, Waterman AD, Shannon W, Boechler M, Rich MW, Radford MJ. Validation of clinical classification schemes for predicting stroke: results from the National Registry of Atrial Fibrillation. *JAMA* 2001;**285**:2864–70.

154. Mant J, Hobbs FDR, Fletcher K et al on behalf of the BAFTA Investigators and the Midland Research Practices Network (MidReC). Warfarin versus aspirin for stroke prevention in an elderly community population with atrial fibrillation (the Birmingham Atrial Fibrillation Treatment of the Aged Study, BAFTA): a randomized controlled trial. *Lancet* 2007;**370**: 493–503.

155. Hart RG, Pearce LA, Agullar MI. Meta-analysis: antithrombotic therapy to prevent stroke in patients who have nonvalvular atrial fibrillation. *Ann Intern Med* 2007;**146**:857–67.

156. Aguilar MI, Hart R. Oral anticoagulants for preventing stroke in patients with non-valvular atrial fibrillation and no previous history of stroke or transient ischemic attacks. *Cochrane Database of Systematic Reviews* 2005, Issue 3. Art. No.: CD001927. DOI: 10.1002/14651858.CD001927.pub2.

157. Saxena R, Koudstaal PJ. Anticoagulants for preventing stroke in patients with nonrheumatic atrial fibrillation and a history of stroke or transient ischaemic attack. *Cochrane Database of Systematic Reviews* 2004, Issue 2. Art. No.: CD000185. DOI: 10.1002/14651858.CD000185.pub2.

158. Connolly S, Progue J, Hart R *et al.* Clopidogrel plus aspirin versus oral anticoagulation for atrial fibrillation in the Atrial fibriallation Clopidogrel Trial with Irbesartan for prevention of Vascular Events (ACTIVE W): a randomised controlled trial. *Lancet* 2006;**367**:1903–12.

159. Stroke Prevention in Reversible Ischemia Trial (SPIRIT) Study Group. A randomised trial of anticoagulants versus aspirin after cerebral ischemia of presumed arterial origin. *Ann Neurol* 1997;**42**:857–65.

160. Levine MN, Raskob G, Beyth RJ, Kearon C, Schulman S. Hemorrhagic complications of anticoagulant treatment: the Seventh ACCP Conference on Antithrombotic and Thrombolytic Therapy. *Chest* 2004;**126**(3 suppl):287S–310S.

161. Saxena R, Lewis S, Berge E, Sandercock PAG, Koudstaal PJ. Risk of early death and recurrent stroke and effect of heparin in 3169 patients with acute ischemic stroke and atrial fibrillation in the International Stroke Trial. *Stroke* 2001;**32**:2333–7.

162. Hylek EM, Go AS, Chang Y *et al.* Effect of intensity of oral anticoagulation on stroke severity and mortality in atrial fibrillation. *N Engl J Med* 2003;**349**:1019–26.

163. Singer DE, Albers GW, Dalen JE, Go AS, Halperin JL, Manning WJ. Antithrombotic therapy in atrial fibriallation; the Seventh ACCP Conference on Antithrombotic and Thrombolytic Therapy. *Chest* 2004; **126**(3 suppl): 429S–456S.

164. Odén A, Fahlén M, Hart RG. Optimal INR for prevention of stroke and death in atrial fibrillation. *Thrombosis Res* 2006,**117**: 493–9.

165. Hart RG, Benavente O, Pearce L. Increased risk of intracranial hemorrhage when aspirin is combined with warfarin: a meta-analysis and hypothesis. *Cerebrovasc Dis* 1999;**9**:215–17.

166. Salem DN, Stein PD, Al Ahmad A *et al.* Antithrombotic therapy in valvular heart disease – native and prosthetic: the Seventh ACCP Conference on Antithrombotic and Thrombolytic Therapy. *Chest* 2004;**126**(3 suppl):457S–482S.

167. Sandercock PAG, Mielke O, Liu M, Counsell C. Anticoagulants for preventing recurrence following presumed non-cardioembolic ischaemic stroke or transient ischaemic attack. *Cochrane Database of Systematic Reviews* 2003, Issue 1. Art. No.: CD000248. DOI: 10.1002/14651858.CD000248.

168. Chimowitz MI, Lynn MJ, Howlett-Smith H *et al.* Comparison of warfarin and aspirin for symptomatic intracranial arterial stenosis. *N Engl J Med* 2005;**352**:1305–16.

169. Mohr JP, Thompson JLP, Lazar RM *et al*, for the Warfarin-Aspirin Recurrent Stroke Study Group. A comparison of warfarin and aspirin for the prevention of recurrent ischemic stroke. *N Engl J Med* 2001;**345**:1444–57.

170. ESPRIT Study Group. Medium intensity oral anticoagulants versus aspirin after cerebral ischemia of arterial origin (ESPRIT): a randomized controlled trial. *Lancet Neurol* 2007;**6**: 115–24.

171. Neaton JD, Blackburn H, Jacobs D. Serum cholesterol level and mortality findings for men screened in the Multiple Risk Factor Intervention Trial. *Arch Intern Med* 1992;**152**:1490–500.

172. Yano K, Reed DM, MacLean CJ. Serum cholesterol and hemorrhagic stroke in the Honolulu Heart Program. *Stroke* 1989;**20**: 1460–5.

173. Iribarren C, Jacobs DR, Sadler M, Claxton AJ, Sidney S. Low total serum cholesterol and intracerebral hemorrhagic stroke: is the association confined to elderly men? The Kaiser Permanente Medical Care Program. *Stroke* 1996;**27**:1993–8.

174. Iso H, Jacobs DRJ, Wentworth D, Neaton JD, Cohen JD. Serum cholesterol levels and six-year mortality from stroke in 350 977 men screened for the Multiple Risk Factor Intervention Trial. *N Engl J Med* 1989;**320**:904–10.

175. Eastern Stroke and Coronary Heart Disease Collaborative Research Group. Blood pressure, cholesterol, and stroke in eastern Asia. *Lancet* 1998;**352**:1801–7.

176. Suh I, Jee SH, Kim HC, Nam CM, Kim IS, Appel LJ. Low serum cholesterol and hemorrhagic stroke in men: Korea Medical insurance Corporation Study. *Lancet* 2001;**357**:922–5.

177. Cholesterol Treatment Trialists' (CTT) Collaborators. Efficacy and safety of cholesterol-lowering treatment: prospective meta-analysis of data from 90,056 participants in 14 randomised trials of statins. *Lancet* 2005;**366**:1267–78.

178. Heart Protection Study Collaborative Group. MRC/BHF Heart Protection Study of cholesterol lowering with simvastatin in 20,536 high-risk individuals: a randomized placebo controlled trial. *Lancet* 2002;**360**:7–22.

179. Stroke Prevention by Aggressive Reduction in Cholesterol Levels (SPARCL) Investigators. High-dose atorvastatin after stroke or transient ischemic attack. *N Engl J Med* 2006;**355**: 549–59.

180. Amarenco P, Labreuche J, Lavallée P, Touboul PJ. Statins in stroke prevention and carotid atherosclerosis: systematic review and up-to-date meta-analysis. *Stroke* 2004;**35**:2902–9.

181. Goldstein LB, Amarenco P, Szarek M *et al*, on behalf of the SPARCL Investigators. Hemorrhagic stroke in the Stroke Prevention by Aggressive Reduction in Cholesterol Levels study. *Neurology* 2008;**70**:2364–70.

182. Cannon CP, Braunwald E, McCabe CH *et al.* Intensive versus moderate lipid lowering with statins after acute coronary syndromes. *N Engl J Med* 2004;**350**:1495–504.

183. Pedersen TR, Faergeman O, Kaselein JJ *et al.* High-dose atorvastatin vs usual-dose simvastatin for secondary prevention after myocardial infarction: the IDEAL study: a randomized controlled trial. *JAMA* 2005;**294**:2437–45.

184. Schwartz GG, Olsson AG, Ezekowitz MD *et al.* Effects of atorvastatin on early recurrent ischemic events in acute coronary syndromes: the MIRACL study: a randomized controlled trial. *JAMA* 2001;**285**:1711–18.

185. Morgenstern LB, Fox AJ, Sharpe BL, Eliasziw M, Barnett HJM, Grotta JC for the North American Symptomatic Carotid Endarterectomy Trial (NASCET) Group. The risks and benefits of carotid endarterectomy in patients with near occlusion of the carotid artery. *Neurology* 1997;**48**:911–15.

186. Rothwell PM, Warlow CP for the European Carotid Surgery Trialists' Collaborative Group. Low risk of ischemic stroke in patients with collapse of the internal carotid artery distal to severe carotid stenosis: cerebral protection due to low poststenotic flow. *Stroke* 2000;**31**:622–30.

187. Rothwell PM, Gibson R, Warlow CP on behalf of the European Carotid Surgery Trialists' Collaborative Group. Interrelation between plaque surface morphology and degree of stenosis on carotid angiograms and the risk of ischemic stroke in patients with symptomatic carotid stenosis. *Stroke* 2000;**31**: 615–21.

188. European Carotid Surgery Trialists' Collaborative Group. Randomised trial of endarterectomy for recently symptomatic carotid stenosis: final results of the MRC European Carotid Surgery Trial (ECST). *Lancet* 1998;**351**:1379–87.

189. North American Symptomatic Carotid Endarterectomy Trial Collaborators. Benefit of carotid endarterectomy in patients with symptomatic, moderate or severe stenosis. *N Engl J Med* 1998;**339**:1415–25.

190. Rothwell PM, Villagra R, Gibson R, Donders RC, Warlow CP. Evidence of a chronic systemic cause of instability of atherosclerotic plaques. *Lancet* 2000;**355**:19–24.

191. Rothwell PM, Elisziw M, Gutnikov SA et al, for the Carotid Endarterectomy Trialists' Collaboration. Pooled analysis of individual patient data from randomized controlled trials of endarterctomy for symptomatic carotid stenosis. *Lancet* 2003;**361**:107–16.

192. Rothwell PM, Eliasziw M, Gutnikov SA, Warlow CP, Barnett HJ, for the Carotid Endarterectomy Trialists' Collaboration. Endarterectomy for symptomatic carotid stenosis in relation to clinical subgroups and timing of surgery. *Lancet* 2004;**363**: 915–24.

193. Hankey GJ, Warlow CP, Molyneuz AJ. Complications of cerebral angiography for patients with mild carotid territory ischemia being considered for carotid endarterectomy. *J Neurol Neurosurg Psychiatry* 1990;**53**:542–8.

194. Eliasziw M, Rankin RN, Fox AJ, Haynes RB, Barnett HJM, for the North American Symptomatic Carotid Endarterectomy Trial (NASCET) Group. Accuracy and prognostic consequences of ultrasonography in identifying severe carotid artery stenosis. *Stroke* 1995;**26**:1747–52.

195. CAVATAS Investigators. Endovascular versus surgical treatment in patients with carotid stenosis in the Carotid and Vertebral Artery Transluminal Angioplasty Study: a randomised trial. *Lancet* 2001;**357**:1729–37.

196. Ederle J, Featherstone R, Brown MM. Percutaneous transluminal angioplasty and stenting for carotid artery stenosis. *Cochrane Database of Systematic Reviews* 2007, Issue 4. Art. No.: CD000515. DOI: 10.1002/14651858.CD000515.pub3.

197. Yadav JS, Wholey MH, Kuntz RE et al. Protected carotid-artery stenting versus endarterectomy in high-risk patients. *N Engl J Med* 2004;**351**:1493–501.

198. Ringleb PA, Allenberg J, Berger J et al, for the SPACE Collaborative Group. 30 day results from the SPACE trial of stent-protected angioplasty versus carotid endarterectomy in symptomatic patients: a randomized non-inferiority trial. *Lancet* 2006;**368**:1239–47.

199. Mas JL, Chatellier G, Beyssen B et al, for the EVA-35 Investigators. Endarterectomy versus stenting in patients with severe carotid stenosis. *N Engl J Med* 2006;**355**:1660–71.

200. Maleux G, Demaerel P, Verbeken E et al. Cerebral ischemia after filter-protected carotid artery stenting is common and cannot be predicted by the presence of substantial amount of debris captured by the filter device. *Am J Neuroradiol* 2006;**27**: 830–33.

201. Tedsco MM, Lee JT, Dalman RL et al. Postprocedural microembolic events following carotid surgery and carotid angioplasty and stenting. *J Vasc Surg* 2007;**46**:244–50.

202. Witt K, Borsch K, Daniels C et al. Neuropsychological consequences of endarterectomy and endovascular angioplasty with stent placement for treatment of symptomatic carotid stenosis; a prospective randomised study. *J Neurol* 2007;**254**:1524–32.

203. Stringele R, Berger J, Alfke K et al, for the SPACE Investigators. Clinical and angiographic risk factors for stroke and death within 30 days after carotid endarterectomy and stent-protected angioplasty: a subanalysis of the SAPCE study. *Lancet Neurol* 2008;**7**:216–22.

204. Lam RC, Lin SC, DeRubertis B, Hynecek R, Kent KC, Faries PL. The impact of increasing age on anatomic factors affecting carotid angioplasty and stenting. *J Vasc Surg* 2007;**45**:875–80.

205. Spagnoli LG, Mauriello A, Sangiorgi G et al. Extracranial thrombotically active carotid plaque as a risk factor for ischemic stroke. *JAMA* 2004;**292**:1845–52.

206. Redgrave JN, Lovett JK, Gallagher PJ, Rothwell PM. Histological assessment of 526 symptomatic carotid plaques in relation to the nature and timing of ischemic symptoms: the Oxford Plaque Study. *Circulation* 2006;**113**:2320–8.

207. Topakian R, Strasak AM, Sonnberger J et al. Timing of stenting of symptomatic carotid stenosis is predictive of 30-day outcome. *Eur J Neurol* 2007;**14**:672–8.

62 Heart disease and pregnancy

Rachel M Wald[1] and Samuel C Siu[2]

[1]Toronto General Hospital and Mount Sinai Hospital, University Health Network, University of Toronto, Toronto, Ontario, Canada

[2]London Health Science Centre, University of Western Ontario, London, Ontario, Canada

Introduction

Women with heart disease comprise approximately 1% of the population in obstetric referral centers.[1] The majority of pregnant women with heart disease seen at referral centers have congenital or rheumatic lesions.[1,2] Other important but less frequently encountered conditions include cardiac arrhythmias, peripartum cardiomyopathy, hypertrophic cardiomyopathy and coronary artery disease. Most current management recommendations have been based on expert opinion and/or retrospective series. To date, there has been only one large multicenter study to prospectively ascertain maternal and fetal outcomes in women with cardiac disease. This Canadian study also derived and validated a risk index for the prediction of maternal cardiac complications during pregnancy.[1]

With the exception of patients with pulmonary vascular obstructive disease, Marfan syndrome with aortopathy, peripartum cardiomyopathy, severe aortic stenosis or mechanical heart valves, maternal death during pregnancy in women with heart disease is rare.[1-6] However, pregnant women with heart disease do remain at risk for cardiac, obstetric, and fetoneonatal complications.[1,2,7-9] Commonly encountered complications include congestive heart failure (CHF) and arrhythmia.[1,2,9,10]

Cardiovascular physiology and pregnancy

Increases in blood volume, red cell mass, and heart rate result in a 50% antepartum increase in cardiac output.[11]

Increases in left ventricular (LV) volume are present by 14 weeks gestation and reach maximum levels early in the third trimester but contractility remains in the normal range. Gestational hormones, circulating prostaglandins, and the low-resistance vascular bed in the placenta result in decreased peripheral vascular resistance and blood pressure. During labor and delivery, there are additional increases in cardiac output and oxygen consumption. Immediately following delivery, relief of caval compression and autotransfusion from the emptied uterus result in a transient increase in cardiac output. Most of the hemodynamic changes of pregnancy have resolved by the second postpartum week but complete return to baseline may not occur until six months after delivery.

Outcomes associated with specific cardiac lesions

Congenital heart lesions

Volume overload lesions

Left-to-right shunts The effect of increased cardiac output on the volume-loaded right ventricle (RV) in atrial septal defect (ASD) or LV in ventricular septal defect (VSD) and patent ductus arteriosus (PDA) is counterbalanced by a decrease in peripheral vascular resistance during pregnancy. Therefore, pregnancy and delivery are well tolerated in the absence of pulmonary hypertension.[1,12-15] In a recent overview, significant arrhythmia requiring therapy was reported in 1/123 pregnancies with ASD (0.8%) and in no pregnancies with VSD; there were no reports of CHF.[9] Paradoxic embolization may be encountered, albeit infrequently, if systemic vasodilation and/or elevation of pulmonary resistance promotes transient right-to-left shunting (particularly in the setting of an ASD).

Atrioventricular septal defect (AVSD), a more complex form of septal defect, may be less well tolerated in preg-

Evidence-Based Cardiology, 3rd edition. Edited by S. Yusuf, J.A. Cairns, A.J. Camm, E.L. Fallen, and B.J. Gersh. © 2010 Blackwell Publishing, ISBN: 978-1-4051-5925-8.

nancy as compared with simpler defects described above. A recent retrospective review of 48 pregnancies reported postpartum persistence of NYHA class deterioration, arrhythmias and worsening of pre-existing left atrioventricular valvular regurgitation in 23%, 19% and 17%, respectively.[16]

Regurgitant valves Significant pulmonary regurgitation (PR) is commonly seen after tetralogy of Fallot (TOF) repair, particularly if a transannular patch was applied. Sequelae of severe PR include RV dilation and dysfunction. From a retrospective review of 82 successful pregnancies (including 20 pregnancies in women with unrepaired TOF), cardiovascular events occurred in six women (14%) and included supraventricular arrhythmia, CHF, pulmonary hypertension and pulmonary embolus. In 5/6 women, cardiovascular complications were associated with the following: severe PR with RV dilation, RV hypertension and peripartum LV dysfunction.[17] Another study of 50 pregnancies in women with corrected TOF found cardiac complications in 12% of pregnancies, consisting of CHF, arrhythmia or both.[18]

Important congenital tricuspid valve insufficiency is commonly related to structural disease, such as Ebstein anomaly. Apical displacement of the tricuspid valve results in atrialization of the RV and commensurate compromise in functional RV size. A diminutive functional RV may not be able to accommodate the increased stroke volume of pregnancy, resulting in worsening tricuspid insufficiency, raised right atrial pressure and right-to-left shunting across the atrial septum. A study of 111 pregnancies in women with Ebstein anomaly did not find any serious maternal complications but did note increased risk of prematurity and fetal loss; birth weight was significantly lower in those born to cyanotic women.[19]

Both mitral and aortic regurgitation during pregnancy are generally well tolerated, even if severe, due to reduced antenatal systemic vascular resistance resulting in reduced afterload. Symptoms usually respond to medical therapy.[20,21]

Pressure overload lesions: left heart

Left ventricular outflow tract obstruction When aortic stenosis (AS) complicates pregnancy it is usually due to a bicuspid aortic valve (BAV), which may also be associated with aortic coarctation and/or ascending aortopathy. Subvalvular and supravalvular AS have similar hemodynamic consequences to valvular AS. Women with symptomatic AS should delay pregnancy until after surgical correction[20] (**Class I, Level C2**). Women with moderate or severe AS continue to be at increased risk for pulmonary edema or arrhythmia during pregnancy, even if they are asymptomatic prior to conception.[1,12,22,23] Contemporary studies report either no or low maternal mortality despite including a significant number of women with severe AS.[23–25] Antena-

tal percutaneous balloon valvuloplasty for symptomatic AS is preferable to cardiac surgery which carries substantial fetal mortality (**Class I, Level C1**).[22,26–29] In the absence of prosthetic valve dysfunction or residual AS, those with a tissue prosthesis usually tolerate pregnancy well. Pregnancy has not been clearly shown to accelerate degeneration of bioprosthetic or homograft valves.[30,31] In two reports, 24 completed pregnancies in women post Ross operation (pulmonary autograft aortic valve replacement) were described and no cardiac complications were reported during pregnancy; one woman developed a dilated cardiomyopathy six months after delivery unrelated to aortic valve dysfunction.[32,33]

Pregnancy in a woman with a mechanical valve prosthesis carries increased risk of valve thrombosis as a result of the prothombotic state of pregnancy. Thrombosis risk during pregnancy is also influenced by valve type (more likely in older-generation valves), position (greater in the mitral as compared with the aortic position), prenatal level of valve function, and type of anticoagulation used.[34]

Coarctation of the aorta In 308 pregnancies reported in four contemporary studies, the only maternal death occurred as a result of dissection in a woman with Turner syndrome who had previously undergone coarctation repair.[1,12,35,36] In uncorrected coarctation, satisfactory control of upper body hypertension may lead to excessive hypotension below the coarctation site, compromising the fetus. Intrauterine growth restriction and premature labor are more common. Following coarctation repair, the risk of dissection and rupture is reduced but not eliminated.[35,37] Medical therapy with beta-blockade may reduce aortic wall stress but its clinical efficacy has not been formally studied in pregnancy. Pregnant women with repaired coarctation are at increased risk for pregnancy-induced hypertension, likely as a result of abnormal aortic compliance.[1,12,35]

Aortopathies Life-threatening aortic complications of Marfan syndrome are primarily due to aortic dissection resulting from medial aortopathy which often manifests as aortic dilation. Risk is increased in pregnancy due to hemodynamic stress and perhaps hormonal effects. A prospective study of 45 pregnancies in 21 patients reported no increase in obstetric complications or significant change in aortic root size in patients with normal aortic roots. Importantly, in the eight patients with a dilated aortic root (>40 mm) or prior aortic root surgery, 3/9 pregnancies were complicated by aortic dissection in two and rapid aortic dilation in one. Of note, beta-blockade therapy was withheld during pregnancy in the majority of women in this study.[38] A later prospective study of 33 pregnancies in 23 women with Marfan syndrome reported favorable outcomes with aortic root diameter <45 mm and no previous history of dissection. There was a small but statistically significant increase in aortic root diameter during pregnancy in women with an initial diameter >40 mm as compared with those <40 mm.[39] Surgical repair should be offered to women prior to conception if the aortic root diameter is >40–45 mm,[20] though this is unlikely to normalize the risk of dissection thereafter.[40] Thus, patients with aortic root involvement should receive preconception counseling emphasizing their risk, and in early pregnancy should be offered termination (**Class 1, Level C1**) In contrast, women with normal aortic root diameter may tolerate pregnancy well, though there remains a possibility of dissection even with normal aortic dimensions. Serial echocardiography should be used to identify progressive aortic root dilation during pregnancy and for six months post partum.[41] Despite the absence of trials specifically evaluating beta-blocker therapy in pregnancy, the potential benefit likely outweighs the relatively small risk of use of this medication during pregnancy (**Class 1, Level C2**).

Less is known about risk factors for dissection in pregnant women with a dilated aorta in the context of a BAV, although this complication has been reported in the pregnant population.[42] The histologic features of aortopathy related to a BAV are similar to what has been described in Marfan syndrome.[43] Some have suggested that management guidelines as described for Marfan syndrome should be applied to those with aortopathy related to a BAV (**Class IIa, Level C2**).[20,42]

With assisted reproductive technology, women with Turner syndrome can now become pregnant. These women are at particular risk of dissection, relatively early in life,[44] even in the absence of recognized aortic root pathology or hypertension.[45] Pregnancy appears to significantly increase the risk of cardiovascular mortality.[46]

Pressure overload lesions: right heart
Pulmonary stenosis Unlike aortic stenosis, pulmonary stenosis (PS) is not associated with significant cardiovascular complications during pregnancy.[1,12,25] Two recent studies examining 68 women have reported no major cardiac complications.[47,48] One study also reported hypertension, thromboembolism and premature delivery in 15%, 4%, and 17% of pregnancies respectively.[48] Balloon valvuloplasty during pregnancy is feasible if symptoms of PS progress (**Class I, Level C2**).

Pulmonary vascular obstructive disease Maternal mortality in Eisenmenger syndrome continues to be high and is approximately 30% in each pregnancy.[5] Most complications occur at term and during the first week post partum. Current consensus is to advise against conception and to offer termination in the event of a pregnancy[49] (**Class I, Level C1**). The vasodilation associated with pregnancy will increase the magnitude of right-to-left shunting, exacerbating maternal cyanosis with adverse effect on fetal outcome. Consequently, these women are particularly sensitive to volume depletion and hypotension, situations which augment right-to-left shunting resulting in worsening cyanosis, hypoxemia and vasoconstriction. Overall, spontaneous abortion is common, intrauterine growth restriction is seen in 30% of pregnancies, and preterm labor is frequent. The high perinatal mortality rate (28%) is largely due to prematurity.

In an overview of 125 pregnancies in patients with Eisenmenger syndrome, primary and secondary pulmonary hypertension, maternal mortality was uniformly high at 36%, 30%, and 56% respectively.[5] The overall neonatal mortality was 13%.

Cyanotic heart disease: unrepaired and repaired
In the absence of pulmonary hypertension, mortality associated with pregnancy is rare in women with uncorrected cyanotic congenital heart disease (CHD) although morbidity may be substantial.[50] The usual pregnancy-associated fall in systemic vascular resistance and rise in cardiac output exacerbate right-to-left shunting, leading to increased maternal hypoxemia and cyanosis. A study examining the outcomes of 96 pregnancies in 44 women with a variety of cyanotic congenital heart defects reported a high rate of maternal cardiac events (32%) and prematurity (37%) as well as a low livebirth rate (43%).[50] The lowest livebirth rate (12%) was observed in mothers with arterial oxygen saturation ≤85%.

Abnormalities of the systemic ventricle: systemic right ventricle and functional single ventricle
Transposition of the great arteries: systemic right ventricle The original repair for ventriculo-arterial discordance or complete transposition of the great arteries (TGA) was the atrial switch procedure (Mustard or Senning operation). Contemporary surgical management has replaced the atrial switch procedure with the arterial switch operation (Jatene procedure). Virtually all published data regarding pregnancy in women with TGA are derived from women after atrial redirection. As the morphologic RV supports the systemic circulation, tricuspid regurgitation, RV dilation and RV dysfunction are commonly seen. Additional sequelae may include sinus node dysfunction, atrial tachyarrhythmia and baffle leak/obstruction.

Two retrospective studies of pregnancy post atrial redirection in 68 women (139 pregnancies) were recently published. The most commonly reported complications were arrhythmias (13–22%), CHF (7–15%) and maternal death/transplant (8%).[51,52] When serial echocardiography was utilized to examine impact of pregnancy on the systemic RV after the Mustard operation, progressive RV dilation occurred in 5/18 women (21%) and worsening RV function was noted in 4/21 (25%) women during pregnancy. At a mean follow-up 33 months after delivery, the RV remained enlarged in all five women (100%) and the RV dysfunction persisted in three-quarters of women (75%).[53] Although these data suggest that pregnancy may affect subsequent systemic RV function, these observations require confirmation using more objective and reproducible methods of RV quantification.

Women managed with an arterial switch operation have only recently reached child-bearing age and there are no published case series examining this population. However, in the absence of ventricular dysfunction, coronary obstruction, or other important residua or sequelae, a good outcome may be anticipated.

In congenitally corrected transposition, characterized by atrioventricular and ventriculo-arterial discordance (double discordance), the morphologic RV supports the systemic circulation. Consequently, tricuspid regurgitation and RV dilation and dysfunction are frequently seen. In two large studies of 105 pregnancies in 41 women, the most common complication was CHF (9–16%) and no maternal deaths were reported.[54,55]

Fontan palliation: functional single ventricle By surgically redirecting systemic venous return to the pulmonary arteries in those with single ventricle physiology, the Fontan palliation decreases volume overload on the systemic ventricle and reduces or eliminates cyanosis. However, there remains an inherent limitation in the heart's ability to augment cardiac output. Long-term sequelae may include arrhythmia, ventricular dysfunction, protein-losing enteropathy and thromboembolic events. As the 10-year survival following the Fontan operation is only 60–80%, it is important that long-term maternal prognosis be discussed during preconception counseling.

In the largest series of pregnant women with Fontan palliation published to date, 33 pregnancies in 14 mothers were reviewed. The single cardiac complication reported in this study was supraventricular tachycardia in one woman.[56] In two subsequent studies examining 14 pregnancies in nine women, maternal cardiac complications included atrial tachyarrhythmia (three women), symptomatic ventricular dysfunction (two women), and right heart failure (two women); the rate of premature birth was high.[57,58] There have been no reported maternal deaths.[59]

Rheumatic heart disease

Mitral stenosis (MS) is the most common rheumatic valvular lesion encountered during pregnancy. The hypervolemia and tachycardia associated with pregnancy exacerbate the impact of mitral valve obstruction. The resultant elevation in left atrial pressure increases the likelihood of atrial

fibrillation.[21] Thus, even patients with mild to moderate MS, who are asymptomatic prior to pregnancy, may develop atrial fibrillation and heart failure during the antepartum and peripartum periods, contributing to substantial morbidity[1,12,25,60] Atrial fibrillation is a frequent precipitant of CHF in pregnant patients with MS. In a study of 80 pregnancies (moderate or severe MS in 47%), the first episode of pulmonary edema occurred at a mean gestational age of 30 weeks and occurred in the setting of atrial tacharhythmias in 20%.[60]

Percutaneous mitral valvuloplasty should be considered in patients with functional class III or IV symptoms despite optimal medical therapy and hospitalization[61–63] (**Class I, Level C1**).

Pregnant women whose dominant lesion is rheumatic AS have a similar outcome to those with congenital AS.

Peripartum cardiomyopathy

Peripartum cardiomyopathy is diagnosed by otherwise unexplained LV systolic dysfunction presenting during the last antepartum month or in the first five postpartum months.[64] Proposed echocardiographic criteria of LV systolic dysfunction include ejection fraction <45%, fractional shortening <30%, and end-diastolic dimension >2.7 cm/m^2.[65] This entity can manifest as CHF, arrhythmia or embolic events. Many affected women will show improvement in functional status and ventricular function post partum, but others may have persistent or progressive dysfunction. The relapse rate during subsequent pregnancies is substantial in women with evidence of persisting cardiac enlargement or LV dysfunction. In a multicenter survey examining the outcomes of 60 pregnancies in women with peripartum cardiomyopathy diagnosed during a prior pregnancy, 44% of women with persistent LV systolic dysfunction (ejection fraction <50%) developed symptoms of CHF during subsequent pregnancies, with an associated mortality rate of 19%. In contrast, symptoms of CHF developed in 21% of women with normalized LV systolic function (ejection fraction ≥50%) and none of this group died.[4] For women who are planning on another pregnancy, angiotensin-converting enzyme inhibitors should be avoided due to their teratogenic effects.[66] In another survey of 100 pregnancies in women with peripartum cardiomyopathy and no subsequent pregnancies, the majority of cases (75%) were diagnosed in the first month postpartum; normalization of LV systolic function occurred in 54% and was more likely if ejection fraction was >30% at diagnosis.[67] These authors suggest that the criteria for diagnosis of peripartum cardiomyopathy based on timing of presentation may be unnecessarily restrictive as those with "pregnancy-associated cardiomyopathy" diagnosed earlier in pregnancy are indistinguishable in terms of baseline characteristics and outcome.[67] Women with peripartum cardiomyopathy and significant residual LV dysfunction are advised against further pregnancies (**Class I, Level C1**).

Hypertrophic cardiomyopathy

In patients who have either resting or provocable LV outflow tract obstruction, the degree of LV outflow tract obstruction during pregnancy is variable and is a result of interplay between increases in preload (which reduces severity of obstruction) and decreases in afterload (which worsens obstruction). Diastolic dysfunction magnifies preload dependence of cardiac output and may result in worsening symptoms even in the absence of LV outflow tract obstruction.

Maternal outcomes are often good, though several deaths have been reported, and serious complications (CHF, tachyarrhythmias, syncope) may occur, especially in women with preconceptual symptoms, and in those with substantial LV diastolic and/or systolic dysfunction or significant LV outflow tract obstruction. In a multicenter retrospective review of 199 pregnancies, there were two sudden deaths in women known to be at high risk who were counseled against pregnancy (one with severe LV outflow tract obstruction and symptomatic heart failure and one with a malignant family history); clinical decompensation during pregnancy occurred in 15% and was significantly associated with prepregnancy functional class.[68] In a recent single-center retrospective review of 271 pregnancies, there were no maternal deaths and >90% of women with cardiac symptoms during pregnancy experienced cardiac symptoms prior to pregnancy; symptomatic deterioration occurred in <10%.[69] Fetal outcomes are good. Beta-blockers may be used, as in the non-pregnant state. Dual-chamber pacing may be of value in patients with symptoms refractory to medical therapy (**Class IIb, Level C2**). The role of septal alcohol ablation or surgical myectomy during pregnancy has not been defined.

Coronary artery disease

The risk of myocardial infarction (MI) appears to be increased by pregnancy. A study examining hospital discharge data of >23 million pregnancies between 2000 and 2002 determined that the incidence of pregnancy-related acute MI in pregnancy was 6.2/100 000 deliveries with a mortality rate of 0.35/100 000 deliveries.[70] Of 859 cases of acute MI related to pregnancy reviewed, 73% occurred during pregnancy and 27% occurred post partum necessitating readmission to hospital. The risk of acute MI was 3–4 times higher in pregnancy as compared with the published incidence of MI among reproductive-aged women. Risk factors for MI included advanced maternal age, hypertension, diabetes mellitus, smoking, thrombophilia, need for transfusion and postpartum infection. Earlier studies demonstrating lower incidences of MI may relate to better ascertainment in recent studies, improved diagnosis related to widespread troponin use, or increased number of pregnancies in older women.[71,72] Guidelines for the cardiopulmonary resuscitation of the pregnant patient have been recently published.[73]

Diagnosis of infarction may be confounded peripartum because of release of CK-MB isoenzyme from the uterus.[74] Thrombolysis is not contraindicated[75] but the diagnosis of coronary thrombosis as opposed to other causes of coronary occlusion cannot be routinely assumed; if immediately available, coronary angiography with the option of primary angioplasty should be considered, especially as other causes of myocardial ischemia/infarction are more frequent in or aggravated by pregnancy. These may include coronary artery dissection, coronary artery embolism, vascular complications of vasoactive obstetric therapies (e.g. ergot derivatives, prostaglandins), and collagen vascular diseases. The long-term residua of childhood Kawasaki disease include coronary artery stenoses and aneurysms, which may become symptomatic during pregnancy. Cocaine abuse must be considered in any young person with an acute coronary event.[75] Fetal exposure to radiation from routine coronary angiography is <5 mGy (<500 mrad).[76] Adverse fetal consequences of this amount of radiation are extremely small or negligible.

Management

Risk stratification and counseling

Risk stratification and counseling of women with heart disease is best accomplished prior to conception. The data required for risk stratification can be acquired readily from a thorough cardiovascular history and examination (including percutaneous oximetry, when appropriate), 12-lead electrocardiogram, and transthoracic echocardiogram. In counseling, the following four areas should be considered: identification of the risk factors for maternal and fetoneonatal complications, recurrence risk of CHD in offspring, anepartum management, and peripartum management.

Risk stratification

Definition of the underlying cardiac lesion is the first step of risk stratification and determining management. Review of prior catheterization and operative reports may be necessary to clarify the diagnosis and define the nature of residua and sequelae such as ventricular function, pulmonary pressure, severity of obstructive lesions, persistence of shunts, and presence of hypoxemia. Almost all patients can be stratified into low-, intermediate-, or high-risk groups using a risk index (Table 62.1), with additional risk data supplemented by results of lesion-specific studies (**Class I,**

Table 62.1 Risk factors for maternal cardiac adverse events during pregnancy (adapted from Siu *et al.*[1])

Adverse maternal cardiac event	Maternal risk factors
Pulmonary edema Arrhythmia Stroke Death	**General*** NYHA functional classification III or IV or cyanosis Systemic ventricular ejection fraction <40% Left heart obstruction (mitral valve area <2 cm², aortic valve area <1.5 cm², peak left ventricular outflow gradient >30 mmHg) Cardiac event (arrhythmia, stroke, pulmonary edema) prior to pregnancy **Lesion specific** As discussed in the text

* The general risk factors can be used to create a maternal risk index for adverse cardiac events related to pregnancy: 0 risk factors <5% risk, 1 risk factor ~ 27% risk, ≥2 risk factors ~ 75% risk

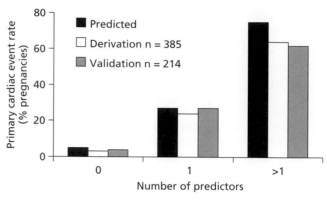

Figure 62.1 The frequency of maternal cardiac complications (pulmonary edema, cardiac arrhythmia, stroke, or cardiac death), as predicted by the number of risk factors, observed in the derivation and validation groups (n = number of pregnancies). (From Siu *et al.*[1]).

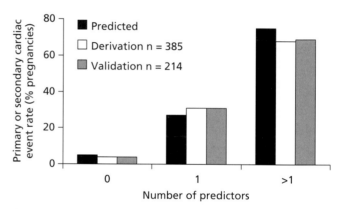

Figure 62.2 The frequency of any primary or secondary cardiac events (deterioration in maternal functional class, need for urgent cardiac interventions during the ante- or postpartum periods, pulmonary edema, cardiac arrhythmia, stroke, or cardiac death), as predicted by the number of risk factors, observed in the derivation and validation groups (n = number of pregnancies). (From Siu *et al.*[1]).

Level C1). Poor functional status (NYHA >II) or cyanosis, systemic ventricular systolic dysfunction, left heart obstruction, and history of cardiac events prior to pregnancy (arrhythmia, stroke or pulmonary edema) are independent predictors of maternal cardiac complications.[1]

The four above-mentioned risk factors are the components of a risk index and have been prospectively validated (see Table 62.1). The risk of a cardiac event (cardiac death, stroke, pulmonary edema or arrhythmia) during pregnancy increases with the number of predictors present during the antepartum evaluation (Fig. 62.1).[1] Pregnancies with 0, 1 or >1 predictor correspond to low, intermediate or high-level risk, respectively. The above-mentioned predictors were also predictive of the combined endpoint of cardiac event (as defined above), deterioration of maternal functional class during pregnancy or need for an urgent cardiac intervention during the ante- or postpartum periods (Fig. 62.2). This risk index, together with lesion-specific risk estimates, can be applied at the time of preconception counseling or during pregnancy. If lesion-specific and index estimates of maternal cardiac risk are discordant, then the higher of the two risk estimates should be applied. Furthermore, if no lesion-specific data are present or the lesion was not included in current risk indices, it may be prudent to assume an intermediate level of risk.

In a subsequent single-center retrospective study examining women with CHD, the global predictors of risk as listed above were again validated, and subpulmonary ventricular dysfunction and severe pulmonary regurgitation were proposed as additional predictors of adverse cardiac outcomes.[10]

Identification of potentially treatable risk factors is crucial. Both maternal and fetal outcomes are improved by surgery to correct cyanosis, which should be undertaken prior to conception when possible.[13] Similarly, patients with symptomatic obstructive lesions should undergo intervention prior to pregnancy[20] (**Class I, Level C1**). A systematic overview of the outcome of cardiovascular surgery performed during pregnancy reported a maternal and fetal mortality of 6% and 30% respectively.[77] Planning for valve replacement prior to pregnancy nessesitates weighing the need for ongoing anticoagulation with a mechanical valve against the likelihood of early reoperation if a tissue valve is used. For women with AS, an attractive alternative is the pulmonary autograft.

Table 62.2 Maternal risk factors for fetoneonatal adverse events during pregnancy (adapted from Siu *et al.*[1,7])

Adverse neonatal events	Maternal risk factors
	Cardiac
Premature birth	NYHA functional classification III or
Small-for-gestational-age	IV, or cyanosis
birthweight	Left heart obstruction (mitral valve
Respiratory distress syndrome	area <2 cm², aortic valve area
Intraventricular hemorrhage	<1.5 cm², peak left ventricular
Death (fetal or neonatal)	outflow gradient >30 mm Hg
	General
	Maternal age <20 or >35 years
	Anticoagulant therapy
	Smoking during pregnancy
	Multiple gestation pregnancy
	Obstetric
	Premature delivery/premature
	membrane rupture
	Incompetent cervix
	Cesarean section
	Intrauterine growth retardation
	Bleeding >12 weeks gestation
	Febrile illness
	Uterine/placental abnormalities

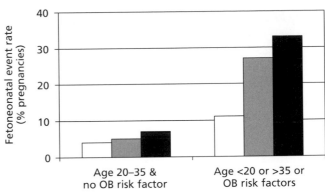

Figure 62.3 The frequency of fetoneonatal complications in two groups defined by the presence or absence of maternal noncardiac characteristics (obstetric high-risk characteristics, smoking, use of anticoagulation, multiple gestation, and maternal age). Control group is represented by white bars. Heart disease group with neither left heart obstruction nor poor functional class/cyanosis is in gray. Heart disease group with left heart obstruction or poor functional class/cyanosis is in black.

Additional associated risk factors that may complicate pregnancy include prosthetic valves and conduits, anticoagulant therapy, and the use of teratogenic drugs such as warfarin and angiotensin-converting enzyme inhibitors.

Maternal life expectancy and ability to care for a child need to be considered. A patient with limited physical capacity or with a condition that may result in premature maternal death should be advised of her potential inability to look after her child. Women whose condition imparts a high likelihood of fetal complications, such as those with cyanosis or on anticoagulants, must be apprised of these added risks.

Some of the same factors that are predictive of maternal cardiac risk (poor maternal functional class or cyanosis, left heart obstruction) are also predictors of fetoneonatal complications. Furthermore, there is an interaction between baseline obstetric and cardiac characteristics in determining fetoneonatal outcomes (Table 62.2, Fig. 62.3).[1,7] Women with heart disease and additional obstetrical risk factors (such as very young or advanced maternal age, or smoking) are at the highest risk of fetoneonatal complications. Obstetrical outcomes such as premature labor, pregnancy induced hypertension, and postpartum hemorrhage have been examined in only a few studies to date.[1,7,12,24,48]

Recurrence risk of congenital heart disease

The *risk of recurrence of CHD in offspring* should be addressed in the context of ~0.5% risk in the general population. The risk with a first-degree relative affected increases about 10-fold. A multicenter study examining offspring of patients with major congenital heart defects who survived cardiac surgery described an overall recurrence rate of 4% in their offspring.[78] The type of CHD seen in offspring can differ from the lesion seen in the mother.[79] Recurrence risk of CHD in offspring varies by lesion and in some reports is as low as 0.6% in association with maternal TGA[9] and as high as 18% in the presence of maternal LV outflow tract obstruction.[80] Certain conditions such as Marfan syndrome and 22q11 deletion syndrome are autosomal dominant, conferring a 50% recurrence risk in her offspring. BAV may also be transmitted in a familial or autosomal dominant pattern. Patients with CHD who reach reproductive age should be offered formal genetic counseling so that they are fully informed of the mode of inheritance and recurrence risk as well as the prenatal diagnosis options available to them (**Class I, Level C1**). Preventive strategies to decrease the incidence of congenital defects such as preconception use of multivitamins containing folic acid can be discussed at the time of such counseling[81] (**Class I, Level B**). Antepartum fetal echocardiography should be offered to pregnant women with CHD and will exclude major congenital lesions (**Class I, Level C1**).[82] Pediatric cardiac assessment is of additional diagnosic utility even if the fetal echocardiogram was normal.[83]

Antepartum management

General principles Women with heart disease who are at intermediate or high risk for complications should be

Table 62.3 Management of pregnancy in women with heart disease

All patients
- Define the lesion, the residua and the sequelae
- Assess functional status
- Determine predictors of risk: general and lesion specific
- Eliminate teratogens
- Arrange genetic counseling when relevant
- Consider consultation with a regional center
- Assess need for endocarditis prophylaxis during labor and delivery

Intermediate and high-risk patients
- Arrange management at a regional center for high-risk pregnancy
- Consider antepartum interventions to reduce pregnancy risk
- Engage a multidisciplinary team, as appropriate
- Consider a multidisciplinary case conference
- Develop and disseminate a management plan
- Anticipate vaginal delivery in almost all cases, unless there are obstetric contraindications
- Consider early epidural anesthesia
- Modify labor and delivery to reduce cardiac work
- Plan postpartum monitoring

managed in a high-risk pregnancy unit by a multidisciplinary team from obstetrics, cardiology, anesthesia, and pediatrics (**Class I, Level C2**) (Table 62.3). When dealing with a complex problem the medical team should meet early in the pregnancy, develop and distribute a written management plan. Consultation at a regional referral center should be encouraged with subsequent management at a community hospital setting for women who are confirmed to be in a "low-risk" group.

Activity limitation and hospital admission by mid second trimester may be advisable in some women with structural cardiac lesions and NYHA III or IV symptoms. Gestational hypertension, hyperthyroidism, infection and anemia should be identified early and treated vigorously.

For patients with functionally significant MS, beta-adrenergic blockers should be used to control heart rate (**Class I, Level C1**). Digitalis is often ineffective in blunting pregnancy-induced tachycardia. Diuretics should be used cautiously in the treatment of pulmonary congestion or right heart failure as aggressive diuresis may lead to decreased uteroplacental perfusion. Some have advocated for the use of anticoagulation prophylaxis in the presence of severe MS and an enlarged left atrium, even in the absence of an atrial tachyarrhythmia, due to the hypercoagulability inherent in pregnancy.[84] Rheumatic fever penicillin prophylaxis should continue as in the non-pregnant state.[20] We also offer empiric therapy with beta-adrenergic blockers to patients with coarctation or Marfan syndrome or those with dilated aorta in the presence of a BAV (**Class IIa, Level C2**).

Special circumstances

Arrhythmias The pregnant state may increase arrhythmia propensity related to several factors including altered hormonal milieu, enhanced sympathetic tone and cardiac chamber dilation.[85] Premature atrial or ventricular beats are common in normal pregnancy; sustained tachyarrhythmias have also been reported. Women with a previous history of arrhythmia are at increased risk of recurrence during pregnancy. Adverse fetal and neonatal outcomes have been related to recurrent arrhythmia during pregnancy.[86] In a recent overview, women at particular risk of arrhythmia were those with atrial redirection surgery (for transposition), those after Fontan repair, and those with AVSD.[9]

Pharmacologic treatment is usually reserved for patients with frequent or sustained episodes, particularly if poorly tolerated and/or in the presence of structural cardiac abnormalities. Sustained tachyarrhythmias such as atrial flutter or atrial fibrillation should be treated promptly, avoiding teratogenic antiarrhythmic drugs. Electrical cardioversion is safe in pregnancy. Digoxin and beta-adrenergic blockers are antiarrhythmic drugs of choice in view of their known safety profiles (**Class I, Level C1**).[20,87] Quinidine, adenosine, sotalol, and lidocaine are generally considered "safe" but published data on their use during pregnancy are more limited. Amiodarone is more problematic and standard texts classify it as contraindicated in pregnancy, although there are case reports describing successful use with careful follow-up; it is not teratogenic, but may impair neonatal thyroid function.[88,89] Pregnancies in women with implantable cardioverter-defibrillators were associated with favorable maternal and fetal outcomes.[90]

Anticoagulation for mechanical heart valve In a systematic overview of pregnancy outcomes in women with prosthetic heart valves, the overall pooled maternal mortality was 2.9% and was mostly related to valve thrombosis.[3] The choices of anticoagulants include oral warfarin, unfractionated heparin, and low molecular weight heparin (LMWH). Warfarin is easier to administer and is effective but has the associated risk of embryopathy during organogenesis, and fetal intracranial bleeding can occur throughout pregnancy. Although the incidence of embryopathy was lowest when a daily warfarin dose of ≤5mg was utilized,[91] there are ongoing concerns about neurodevelopmental abnormalities from intracranial bleeding. Fetal intracranial hemorrhage during vaginal delivery is a risk with warfarin unless it has been stopped for at least two weeks. Adjusted-dose subcutaneous unfractionated heparin has no teratogenic effects, as the drug does not cross the placenta, but there is risk of maternal thrombocytopenia and osteoporosis. Claims of inadequate effectiveness of heparin in patients with mechanical heart valves have been countered by arguments that inadequate doses were used. LMWH has better bioavailability and has been suggested as an alternative to adjusted-dose unfractionated heparin, particularly in the context of meticulously monitored plasma anti-Xa levels.

In the absence of systematic data on the optimal anticoagulation regimen in pregnant women with mechanical heart valves, current practice guidelines are all based on expert opinion and are not in agreement with one another.[20,92,93] The American College of Chest Physicians (ACCP) recommends that either LMWH or unfractionated heparin be used throughout pregnancy with dose adjustments based on careful monitoring; the European Society of Cardiology does not endorse the use of LMWH during pregnancy for women with prosthetic heart valves.[20,92,93] Some have proposed alternative strategies for patients deemed at "higher risk" as compared to those deemed to be at "lower risk" for thromboembolism.[34] The practice within our group is based on ACCP guidelines with LMWH at least during the first trimester. Monitoring of both peak and trough levels of anti-Xa may be necessary to ensure adequate anticoagulation in women with mechanical heart valves receiving LMWH.[34] Adjunctive use of low-dose aspirin should also be considered.[20,92,93] Aspirin in low dose is safe for the fetus, even at term[94] (**Class I, Level B**) although high maternal doses may promote premature fetal ductus arteriosus closure.

Eisenmenger syndrome If a woman with Eisenmenger syndrome does not accept counseling to terminate or presents late in pregnancy, meticulous antepartum management is necessary including early hospitalization, supplemental oxygen and possibly empiric anticoagulation (**Class IIa, Level C2**). The efficacy of nitric oxide therapy in these patients has yet to be demonstrated. Experience with targeted pulmonary vasodilator therapy is limited to case reports, which suggest that agents may improve pulmonary pressures.[95–98]

Hypertension in pregnancy Mild pre-existing hypertension may not require pharmacotherapy in pregnancy, as fetal outcomes are unaffected, maternal blood pressure falls lower than baseline during the first 20 weeks of gestation, and excessive lowering of maternal blood pressure may compromise placental perfusion.[99] Therapy should be initiated or reinstituted if moderate-to-severe hypertension develops (systolic BP ≥150–160, diastolic BP ≥100–110 or both) or there is target organ damage. A recent meta-analysis of 46 randomized trials evaluating antihypertensive therapy in women with mild-to-moderate hypertension (140–169 mm Hg systolic, 90–109 mm Hg diastolic) during pregnancy did not find any significant difference in fetal outcome or risk of developing superimposed gestational hypertension with proteinuria (pre-eclampsia), although

the risk of developing severe hypertension was halved in treated women.[100] If treatment is indicated, drug therapy established as safe includes methyldopa, hydralazine, labetalol and other beta-blockers, and nifedipine (**Class I, Level C1**).[101,102] As there are no clear benefits of one class of medication over another, choice of an antihypertensive should be based on the potential for side effects and the experience of the prescribing clinician with a particular drug.[103] Diuretics are indicated for the management of volume overload in renal failure or CHF and may be used as adjuncts in the management of pre-existing (chronic) hypertension, but should be avoided in gestational hypertension (pre-eclampsia), which is a volume-contracted state.[99,104] Due to increased risk of fetopathy, angiotensin-converting enzyme inhibitors, and angiotensin-receptor blocking agents by extension, are not considered safe at any point during pregnancy (**Class I, Level C1**).

Gestational hypertension with proteinuria (pre-eclampsia) is treated effectively only by delivery of the fetus and placenta. Delay in delivery to allow maturation of the fetus can often be accomplished if the syndrome is mild, the patient is under very close surveillance in a hospital or obstetric day unit, and pregnancy is terminated as soon as further benefit to the fetus is unlikely or maternal safety is compromised.[99]

Management during labor and delivery

Vaginal delivery is recommended, with cesarean delivery for cardiac indications reserved for aortic dissection, Marfan syndrome with dilated aortic root, and failure to switch from warfarin to heparin within two weeks prior to labor. Preterm induction is rarely indicated, but once fetal lung maturity is assured a planned induction is preferred in high-risk situations so that appropriate support will be available. There is no consensus on the use of invasive hemodynamic peripartum monitoring. We commonly utilize intra-arterial monitoring and often use central venous pressure monitoring as well in cases where there are concerns about the interpretation and deleterious effects of a sudden drop in systemic blood pressure (severe AS, pulmonary hypertension or moderate or severe systemic ventricular systolic dysfunction). The utility of an indwelling pulmonary artery catheter has not been studied during pregnancy, and it is rarely utilized; risk may be increased with complex anatomy such as atrial baffles or in the setting of pulmonary hypertension because of possible pulmonary infarction or rupture.

Heparin anticoagulation is discontinued 12–24 hours prior to induction or reversed with protamine if spontaneous labor develops, and can usually be resumed 6–12 hours post partum. According to current guidelines,[105] routine prophylactic antibiotic therapy is not indicated but has been recommended by some because of the possibility of bacteremia during labor and delivery, particularly in the setting of a complicated delivery.[21]

Epidural anesthesia with adequate volume preloading is the technique of choice (**Class I, Level C2**). Epidural fentanyl is particularly advantageous in cyanotic patients with shunt lesions as it does not lower peripheral vascular resistance. In the presence of a shunt, air and particulate filters should be placed in all intravenous lines.

Labor is conducted in the left lateral decubitus position to attenuate hemodynamic fluctuations associated with contractions in the supine position. A shortened second stage of labor will reduce need for maternal expulsive efforts. As hemodynamics do not approach baseline for many days after delivery, those patients at intermediate or high risk may require monitoring for a minimum of 72 hours post partum. Patients with Eisenmenger syndrome require longer close postpartum observation, since mortality risk persists for seven days or more.

Conclusion

With important exceptions, most women with cardiac disease can be expected to do well during pregnancy with appropriate management based on systematic risk stratification. A preconceptual cardiac evaluation is of great value as baseline testing can be arranged, medications can be reviewed and revised if need be, pregnancy-related risk stratification can be established and interventions can be planned prior to pregnancy, when necessary. Pregnancies deemed to be at intermediate or high risk should be managed and delivered in a tertiary care setting. An antepartum multidisciplinary conference to co-ordinate management should take place if complex care is anticipated. If intervention is required during pregnancy, a percutaneous approach, if at all possible, should be undertaken and cardiac surgery should be avoided. In some cardiac conditions, conception should be avoided and in the event of pregnancy, termination should be offered; these include pulmonary vascular obstructive disease, Marfan syndrome with aortopathy, and peripartum cardiomyopathy with residual ventricular dysfunction (**Class I, Level C1**).

References

1. Siu SC, Sermer M, Colman JM *et al*. Prospective multicenter study of pregnancy outcomes in women with heart disease. *Circulation* 2001;**104**:515–21.
2. Avila WS, Rossi EG, Ramires JA *et al*. Pregnancy in patients with heart disease: experience with 1,000 cases. *Clin Cardiol* 2003;**26**:135–42.
3. Chan WS, Anand S, Ginsberg JS. Anticoagulation of pregnant women with mechanical heart valves: a systematic review of the literature. *Arch Intern Med* 2000;**160**:191–6.
4. Elkayam U, Tummala PP, Rao K *et al*. Maternal and fetal outcomes of subsequent pregnancies in women with peripartum cardiomyopathy. *N Engl J Med* 2001;**344**:1567–71.
5. Weiss BM, Zemp L, Seifert B, Hess OM. Outcome of pulmonary vascular disease in pregnancy: a systematic overview from 1978 through 1996. *J Am Coll Cardiol* 1998;**31**:1650–7.
6. Pyeritz R. Maternal and fetal complications of pregnancy in the Marfan syndrome. *Am J Med* 1981;**71**:784–90.
7. Siu SC, Colman JM, Sorensen S *et al*. Adverse neonatal and cardiac outcomes are more common in pregnant women with cardiac disease. *Circulation* 2002;**105**:2179–84.
8. Kaemmerer H, Bauer U, Stein JI *et al*. Pregnancy in congenital cardiac disease: an increasing challenge for cardiologists and obstetricians – a prospective multicenter study. *Z Kardiol* 2003;**92**:16–23.
9. Drenthen W, Pieper PG, Roos-Hesselink JW *et al*. Outcome of pregnancy in women with congenital heart disease: a literature review. *J Am Coll Cardiol* 2007;**49**:2303–11.
10. Khairy P, Ouyang DW, Fernandes SM, Lee-Parritz A, Economy KE, Landzberg MJ. Pregnancy outcomes in women with congenital heart disease. *Circulation* 2006;**113**:517–24.
11. Elkayam U, Gleicher N. Hemodynamics and cardiac function during normal pregnancy and the puerperium. In: Elkayam U, Gleicher N (eds) Cardiac Problems in Pregnancy: Diagnosis and Management of Maternal and Fetal Disease. New York: Wiley-Liss, 1998: 3–19.
12. Siu SC, Sermer M, Harrison DA *et al*. Risk and predictors for pregnancy-related complications in women with heart disease. *Circulation* 1997;**96**:2789–94.
13. Shime J, Mocarski EJ, Hastings D, Webb GD, McLaughlin PR. Congenital heart disease in pregnancy: short- and long-term implications. *Am J Obstet Gynecol* 1987;**156**:313–22.
14. Zuber M, Gautschi N, Oechslin E, Widmer V, Kiowski W, Jenni R. Outcome of pregnancy in women with congenital shunt lesions. *Heart* 1999;**81**:271–5.
15. Actis Dato GM, Rinaudo P, Revelli A *et al*. Atrial septal defect and pregnancy: a retrospective analysis of obstetrical outcome before and after surgical correction. *Minerva Cardioangiol* 1998;**46**:63–8.
16. Drenthen W, Pieper PG, van der Tuuk K *et al*. Cardiac complications relating to pregnancy and recurrence of disease in the offspring of women with atrioventricular septal defects. *Eur Heart J* 2005;**26**:2581–7.
17. Veldtman GR, Connolly HM, Grogan M, Ammash NM, Warnes CA. Outcomes of pregnancy in women with tetralogy of Fallot. *J Am Coll Cardiol* 2004;**44**:174–80.
18. Meijer JM, Pieper PG, Drenthen W *et al*. Pregnancy, fertility, and recurrence risk in corrected tetralogy of Fallot. *Heart* 2005;**91**:801–5.
19. Connolly H, Warnes C. Ebstein's anomaly: outcome of pregnancy. *J Am Coll Cardiol* 1994;**23**:1194–8.
20. Bonow RO, Carabello BA, Kanu C *et al*. ACC/AHA 2006 guidelines for the management of patients with valvular heart disease: a report of the American College of Cardiology/American Heart Association Task Force on Practice Guidelines

(writing committee to revise the 1998 Guidelines for the Management of Patients With Valvular Heart Disease): developed in collaboration with the Society of Cardiovascular Anesthesiologists: endorsed by the Society for Cardiovascular Angiography and Interventions and the Society of Thoracic Surgeons. *Circulation* 2006;**114**:e84–231.

21. Elkayam U, Bitar F. Valvular heart disease and pregnancy part I: native valves. *J Am Coll Cardiol* 2005;**46**:223–30.

22. Lao T, Sermer M, MaGee L, Farine D, Colman J. Congenital aortic stenosis and pregnancy – a reappraisal. *Am J Obstet Gynecol* 1993;**169**:540–5.

23. Silversides CK, Colman JM, Sermer M, Farine D, Siu SC. Early and intermediate-term outcomes of pregnancy with congenital aortic stenosis. *Am J Cardiol* 2003;**91**:1386–9.

24. Yap SC, Drenthen W, Pieper PG *et al.* Risk of complications during pregnancy in women with congenital aortic stenosis. *Int J Cardiol* 2008;**126**(2):240–6.

25. Hameed A, Karaalp IS, Tummala PP *et al.* The effect of valvular heart disease on maternal and fetal outcome of pregnancy. *J Am Coll Cardiol* 2001;**37**:893–9.

26. Myerson SG, Mitchell AR, Ormerod OJ, Banning AP. What is the role of balloon dilatation for severe aortic stenosis during pregnancy? *J Heart Valve Dis* 2005;**14**:147–50.

27. Bhargava B, Agarwal R, Yadav R, Bahl VK, Manchanda SC. Percutaneous balloon aortic valvuloplasty during pregnancy: use of the Inoue balloon and the physiologic antegrade approach. *Cathet Cardiovasc Diagn* 1998;**45**:422–5.

28. Banning AP, Pearson JF, Hall RJ. Role of balloon dilatation of the aortic valve in pregnant patients with severe aortic stenosis. *Br Heart J* 1993;**70**:544–5.

29. Arnoni RT, Arnoni AS, Bonini RC *et al.* Risk factors associated with cardiac surgery during pregnancy. *Ann Thorac Surg* 2003;**76**:1605–8.

30. North RA, Sadler L, Stewart AW, McCowan LM, Kerr AR, White HD. Long-term survival and valve-related complications in young women with cardiac valve replacements. *Circulation* 1999;**99**:2669–76.

31. Salazar E, Espinola N, Roman L, Casanova JM. Effect of pregnancy on the duration of bovine pericardial bioprostheses. *Am Heart J* 1999;**137**:714–20.

32. Yap SC, Drenthen W, Pieper PG *et al.* Outcome of pregnancy in women after pulmonary autograft valve replacement for congenital aortic valve disease. *J Heart Valve Dis* 2007;**16**:398–403.

33. Dore A, Somerville J. Pregnancy in patients with pulmonary autograft valve replacement. *Eur Heart J* 1997;**18**:1659–62.

34. Elkayam U, Bitar F. Valvular heart disease and pregnancy: part II: prosthetic valves. *J Am Coll Cardiol* 2005;**46**:403–10.

35. Beauchesne LM, Connolly HM, Ammash NM, Warnes CA. Coarctation of the aorta: outcome of pregnancy. *J Am Coll Cardiol* 2001;**38**:1728–33.

36. Vriend JW, Drenthen W, Pieper PG *et al.* Outcome of pregnancy in patients after repair of aortic coarctation. *Eur Heart J* 2005;**26**:2173–8.

37. Plunkett MD, Bond LM, Geiss DM. Staged repair of acute type I aortic dissection and coarctation in pregnancy. *Ann Thorac Surg* 2000;**69**:1945–7.

38. Rossiter JP, Repke JT, Morales AJ, Murphy EA, Pyeritz RE. A prospective longitudinal evaluation of pregnancy in the Marfan syndrome. *Am J Obstet Gynecol* 1995;**173**:1599–606.

39. Meijboom LJ, Vos FE, Timmermans J, Boers GH, Zwinderman AH, Mulder BJ. Pregnancy and aortic root growth in the Marfan syndrome: a prospective study. *Eur Heart J* 2005;**26**: 914–20.

40. McDermott CD, Sermer M, Siu SC, David TE, Colman JM. Aortic dissection complicating pregnancy following prophylactic aortic root replacement in a woman with Marfan syndrome. *Int J Cardiol* 2007;**120**:427–30.

41. Shores J, Berger K, Murphy E, Pyeritz R. Progression of aortic dilatation and the benefit of long-term B-adrenergic blockade in Marfan's syndrome. *N Engl J Med* 1994;**330**:1335–41.

42. Immer FF, Bansi AG, Immer-Bansi AS *et al.* Aortic dissection in pregnancy: analysis of risk factors and outcome. *Ann Thorac Surg* 2003;**76**:309–14.

43. Nistri S, Sorbo MD, Basso C, Thiene G. Bicuspid aortic valve: abnormal aortic elastic properties. *J Heart Valve Dis* 2002;**11**:369–73;discussion 373–4.

44. Gravholt CH, Landin-Wilhelmsen K, Stochholm K *et al.* Clinical and epidemiological description of aortic dissection in Turner's syndrome. *Cardiol Young* 2006;**16**:430–6.

45. Lin AE, Lippe BM, Geffner ME *et al.* Aortic dilation, dissection, and rupture in patients with Turner syndrome. *J Pediatr* 1986;**109**:820–6.

46. Practice Committee of the American Society for Reproductive Medicine. Increased maternal cardiovascular mortality associated with pregnancy in women with Turner syndrome. *Fertil Steril* 2006;**86**:S127–8.

47. Hameed AB, Goodwin TM, Elkayam U. Effect of pulmonary stenosis on pregnancy outcomes – a case-control study. *Am Heart J* 2007;**154**:852–4.

48. Drenthen W, Pieper PG, Roos-Hesselink JW *et al.* Non-cardiac complications during pregnancy in women with isolated congenital pulmonary valvar stenosis. *Heart* 2006;**92**:1838–43.

49. Kiely D, Elliot C, Webster V, Stewart P. Pregnancy and pulmonary hypertension: new approaches to the management of a life-threatening condition. In: Steer P, Gatzoulis M, Baker P (eds) Heart Disease and Pregnancy. London: RCOG Press, 2006: 79–95.

50. Presbitero P, Somerville J, Stone S, Aruta E, Spiegelhalter D, Rabajoli F. Pregnancy in cyanotic congenital heart disease. Outcome of mother and fetus. *Circulation* 1994;**89**:2673–6.

51. Drenthen W, Pieper PG, Ploeg M *et al.* Risk of complications during pregnancy after Senning or Mustard (atrial) repair of complete transposition of the great arteries. *Eur Heart J* 2005;**26**:2588–95.

52. Canobbio MM, Morris CD, Graham TP, Landzberg MJ. Pregnancy outcomes after atrial repair for transposition of the great arteries. *Am J Cardiol* 2006;**98**:668–72.

53. Guedes A, Mercier LA, Leduc L, Berube L, Marcotte F, Dore A. Impact of pregnancy on the systemic right ventricle after a Mustard operation for transposition of the great arteries. *J Am Coll Cardiol* 2004;**44**:433–7.

54. Connolly HM, Grogan M, Warnes CA. Pregnancy among women with congenitally corrected transposition of great arteries. *J Am Coll Cardiol* 1999;**33**:1692–5.

55. Therrien J, Barnes I, Somerville J. Outcome of pregnancy in patients with congenitally corrected transposition of the great arteries. *Am J Cardiol* 1999;**84**:820–4.

56. Canobbio MM, Mair DD, van der Velde M, Koos BJ. Pregnancy outcomes after the Fontan repair. *J Am Coll Cardiol* 1996;**28**:763–7.

57. Hoare JV, Radford D. Pregnancy after fontan repair of complex congenital heart disease. *Aust N Z J Obstet Gynaecol* 2001;**41**:464–8.

58. Drenthen W, Pieper PG, Roos-Hesselink JW *et al.* Pregnancy and delivery in women after Fontan palliation. *Heart* 2006;**92**:1290–4.

59. Walker F. Pregnancy and the various forms of the Fontan circulation. *Heart* 2007;**93**:152–4.

60. Silversides CK, Colman JM, Sermer M, Siu SC. Cardiac risk in pregnant women with rheumatic mitral stenosis. *Am J Cardiol* 2003;**91**:1382–5.

61. Desai DK, Adanlawo M, Naidoo DP, Moodley J, Kleinschmidt I. Mitral stenosis in pregnancy: a four-year experience at King Edward VIII Hospital, Durban, South Africa. *Br J Obstet Gynaecol* 2000;**107**:953–8.

62. Mangione JA, Lourenco RM, dos Santos ES *et al.* Long-term follow-up of pregnant women after percutaneous mitral valvuloplasty. *Catheter Cardiovasc Interv* 2000;**50**:413–17.

63. de Souza JA, Martinez EE Jr, Ambrose JA *et al.* Percutaneous balloon mitral valvuloplasty in comparison with open mitral valve commissurotomy for mitral stenosis during pregnancy. *J Am Coll Cardiol* 2001;**37**:900–3.

64. Pearson GD, Veille JC, Rahimtoola S *et al.* Peripartum cardiomyopathy: National Heart, Lung, and Blood Institute and Office of Rare Diseases (National Institutes of Health) workshop recommendations and review. *JAMA* 2000;**283**:1183–8.

65. Sliwa K, Fett J, Elkayam U. Peripartum cardiomyopathy. *Lancet* 2006;**368**:687–93.

66. Cooper WO, Hernandez-Diaz S, Arbogast PG *et al.* Major congenital malformations after first-trimester exposure to ACE inhibitors. *N Engl J Med* 2006;**354**:2443–51.

67. Elkayam U, Akhter MW, Singh H *et al.* Pregnancy-associated cardiomyopathy: clinical characteristics and a comparison between early and late presentation. *Circulation* 2005;**111**:2050–5.

68. Autore C, Conte MR, Piccininno M *et al.* Risk associated with pregnancy in hypertrophic cardiomyopathy. *J Am Coll Cardiol* 2002;**40**:1864–9.

69. Thaman R, Varnava A, Hamid MS *et al.* Pregnancy related complications in women with hypertrophic cardiomyopathy. *Heart* 2003;**89**:752–6.

70. James AH, Jamison MG, Biswas MS, Brancazio LR, Swamy GK, Myers ER. Acute myocardial infarction in pregnancy: a United States population-based study. *Circulation* 2006;**113**:1564–71.

71. Ladner HE, Danielsen B, Gilbert WM. Acute myocardial infarction in pregnancy and the puerperium: a population-based study. *Obstet Gynecol* 2005;**105**:480–4.

72. Macarthur A, Cook L, Pollard JK, Brant R. Peripartum myocardial ischemia: a review of Canadian deliveries from 1970 to 1998. *Am J Obstet Gynecol* 2006;**194**:1027–33.

73. 2005 American Heart Association Guidelines for Cardiopulmonary Resuscitation and Emergency Cardiovascular Care. Part 10.8: Cardiac Arrest Associated With Pregnancy. *Circulation* 2005;**112**:IV-150–153.

74. Leiserowitz GS, Evans AT, Samuels SJ, Omand K, Kost GJ. Creatine kinase and its MB isoenzyme in the third trimester and the peripartum period. *J Reprod Med* 1992;**37**:910–16.

75. Roth A, Elkayam U. Acute myocardial infarction associated with pregnancy. *Ann Intern Med* 1996;**125**:751–62.

76. Colletti PM, Lee K. Cardiovascular imaging in the pregnant patient. In: Elkayam U, Gleicher N (eds) Cardiac Problems in Pregnancy. New York: Wiley-Liss, 1998:33–6.

77. Weiss BM, von Segesser LK, Alon E, Seifert B, Turina MI. Outcome of cardiovascular surgery and pregnancy: a systematic review of the period 1984–1996. *Am J Obstet Gynecol* 1998;**179**:1643–53.

78. Burn J, Brennan P, Little J *et al.* Recurrence risks in offspring of adults with major heart defects: results from first cohort of British Collaborative study. *Lancet* 1998;**351**:311–16.

79. Whittemore R, Wells JA, Castellsague X. A second-generation study of 427 probands with congenital heart defects and their 837 children. *J Am Coll Cardiol* 1994;**23**:1459–67.

80. Nora JJ, Nora AH. Maternal transmission of congenital heart diseases: new recurrence risk figures and the questions of cytoplasmic inheritance and vulnerability to teratogens. *Am J Cardiol* 1987;**59**:459–63.

81. Czeizel A. Reduction of urinary tract and cardiovascular defects by periconceptional multivitamin supplementation. *Am J Med Genet* 1996;**62**:179–83.

82. Rychik J, Ayres N, Cuneo B *et al.* American Society of Echocardiography guidelines and standards for performance of the fetal echocardiogram. *J Am Soc Echocardiogr* 2004;**17**:803–10.

83. Thangaroopan M, Wald RM, Silversides CK *et al.* Incremental diagnostic yield of pediatric cardiac assessment after fetal echocardiography in the offspring of women with congenital heart disease: a prospective study. *Pediatrics* 2008;**121**:e660–5.

84. Hameed A, Akhter MW, Bitar F *et al.* Left atrial thrombosis in pregnant women with mitral stenosis and sinus rhythm. *Am J Obstet Gynecol* 2005;**193**:501–4.

85. Mak S, Harris L. Arrhythmia in pregnancy In: Wilansky S, Willerson J (eds) Heart Disease in Women. Philadelphia: Churchill Livingstone, 2002: 497–514.

86. Silversides CK, Harris L, Haberer K, Sermer M, Colman JM, Siu SC. Recurrence rates of arrhythmias during pregnancy in women with previous tachyarrhythmia and impact on fetal and neonatal outcomes. *Am J Cardiol* 2006;**97**:1206–12.

87. Khalil A. Cardiac drugs in pregnancy. In: Steer P, Gatzoulis M, Baker P (eds) Heart Disease and Pregnancy. London: RCOG Press, 2006:7 9–95.

88. Magee LA, Downar E, Sermer M, Boulton BC, Allen LC, Koren G. Pregnancy outcome after gestational exposure to amiodarone in Canada. *Am J Obstet Gynecol* 1995;**172**:1307–11.

89. Bartalena L, Bogazzi F, Braverman LE, Martino E. Effects of amiodarone administration during pregnancy on neonatal thyroid function and subsequent neurodevelopment. *J Endocrinol Invest* 2001;**24**:116–30.

90. Natale A, Davidson T, Geiger M, Newby K. Implantable cardioverter-defibrillators and pregnancy: a safe combination? *Circulation* 1997;**96**:2808–12.

91. Vitale N, De Feo M, De Santo LS, Pollice A, Tedesco N, Cotrufo M. Dose-dependent fetal complications of warfarin in pregnant women with mechanical heart valves. *J Am Coll Cardiol* 1999;**33**:1637–41.

92. Bates SM, Greer IA, Hirsh J, Ginsberg JS. Use of antithrombotic agents during pregnancy: the Seventh ACCP Conference on Antithrombotic and Thrombolytic Therapy. *Chest* 2004;**126**: 627S–644S.

93. Task Force on the Management of Cardiovascular Diseases During Pregnancy. Expert consensus document on management of cardiovascular diseases during pregnancy. *Eur Heart J* 2003;**24**:761–81.

94. CLASP (Collaborative Low-dose Aspirin Study in Pregnancy) Collaborative Group. CLASP: a randomised trial of low-dose aspirin for the prevention and treatment of pre-eclampsia among 9364 pregnant women. *Lancet* 1994;**343**:619–29.

95. Lynch TD, Laffey JG. Sildenafil for pulmonary hypertension in pregnancy? *Anesthesiology* 2006;**104**:382; author reply 383.

96. Monnery L, Nanson J, Charlton G. Primary pulmonary hypertension in pregnancy; a role for novel vasodilators. *Br J Anaesth* 2001;**87**:295–8.

97. Huang S, DeSantis ER. Treatment of pulmonary arterial hypertension in pregnancy. *Am J Health Syst Pharm* 2007;**64**:1922–6.

98. Elliot CA, Stewart P, Webster VJ *et al.* The use of iloprost in early pregnancy in patients with pulmonary arterial hypertension. *Eur Respir J* 2005;**26**:168–73.

99. Report of the National High Blood Pressure Education Program Working Group on High Blood Pressure in Pregnancy. *Am J Obstet Gynecol* 2000;**183**:S1–S22.

100. Abalos E, Duley L, Steyn DW, Henderson-Smart DJ. Antihypertensive drug therapy for mild to moderate hypertension during pregnancy. *Cochrane Database of Systematic Reviews* 2007, Issue 1. Art. No.: CD002252. DOI: 10.1002/14651858.CD002252.pub2.

101. Magee LA, Ornstein MP, von Dadelszen P. Fortnightly review: management of hypertension in pregnancy. *BMJ* 1999;**318**: 1332–6.

102. Magee LA, Schick B, Donnenfeld AE *et al.* The safety of calcium channel blockers in human pregnancy: a prospective, multicenter cohort study. *Am J Obstet Gynecol* 1996;**174**:823–8.

103. Duley L, Henderson-Smart DJ, Meher S. Drugs for treatment of very high blood pressure during pregnancy. *Cochrane Database of Systematic Reviews* 2006, Issue 3. Art. No.: CD001449. DOI: 10.1002/14651858.CD001449.pub2.

104. Collins R, Yusuf S, Peto R. Overview of randomised trials of diuretics in pregnancy. *BMJ (Clin Res Ed)* 1985;**290**:17–23.

105. Wilson W, Taubert KA, Gewitz M *et al.* Prevention of infective endocarditis: guidelines from the American Heart Association: a guideline from the American Heart Association Rheumatic Fever, Endocarditis, and Kawasaki Disease Committee, Council on Cardiovascular Disease in the Young, and the Council on Clinical Cardiology, Council on Cardiovascular Surgery and Anesthesia, and the Quality of Care and Outcomes Research Interdisciplinary Working Group. *Circulation* 2007;**116**: 1736–54.

Adult congenital heart disease

Elisabeth Bédard and Michael A Gatzoulis
Royal Brompton Hospital, London, UK

Introduction: prevalence of congenital heart disease

Congenital heart disease (CHD) is defined as a cardiovascular abnormality that is present from birth, and approximately 4–10 liveborn infants per 1000 are affected.[1,2] However, the true prevalence may be much higher, as these estimates often exclude bicuspid aortic valve and prolapse of the mitral valve, the most common cardiac malformations.[1] A more accurate estimation has been reported to be around 50 per 1000 live births.[1] Table 63.1 summarizes the recently reported incidence of the common congenital heart defects.[2] The great successes of pediatric cardiac care in the past 25 years have resulted in a marked increase in adult patients with CHD. About 85% of children with CHD are now expected to survive into adulthood.[3] The most recent epidemiologic study, conducted in Quebec, Canada, revealed that the prevalence of adults with CHD was 4.09 per 1000 for the year 2000, representing an increase of 85% compared with 1985, while this increase was only 22% in children for the same period.[4] The authors extrapolated their results to the US population and estimated that about 900 000 adults had CHD in the year 2000 in the USA.

Most early interventions carried out on patients with CHD have not been curative and a significant proportion of them will need further surgery or experience various complications such as arrhythmia and heart failure. Their cardiovascular disease is complex and their management poses a real challenge, requiring expert cardiologic care. Indeed, initial assessment of suspected CHD, follow-up of patients with CHD of moderate severity and complex lesions as well as risk assessment for non-cardiac surgery

and pregnancy should ideally take place in a tertiary adult care center. However, there are currently not enough such specialists worldwide. Education on the principles of CHD for a broader professional audience is therefore imperative to improve the lifetime care of this population.[5] Primary care physicians, general adult cardiologists, obstetricians, surgeons and anesthesiologists should also be aware of the various issues in the general medical management of CHD because most patients will also need local follow-up for economic, social and geographic reasons.[6,7]

This chapter provides key clinical information and guidelines for the management of adults with CHD.[7a]

Etiology

Genetic basis of CHD

In recent years, there have been tremendous advances not only in diagnosis and treatment of CHD but also in our knowledge of the etiologies of CHD. Improvements in genetic techniques have resulted in identification of several loci and genes associated with CHD. In their extensive review of the current genetic basis for congenital heart defects, Pierpont *et al*[1] emphasized the reasons why it is very important to determine whether there is an underlying genetic abnormality:

- other organ systems may be involved
- it may provide prognostic information
- there may be significant risks of transmission to the offspring
- genetic testing in other family members may be appropriate.

A *chromosome* deletion can be identified by fluorescence *in situ* hybridization (FISH) in some syndromes associated with heart defects. For example, a 22q11 deletion is present in ~90% of patients with DiGeorge syndrome, which is characterized by cardiac defects (such as aortic arch anomalies, truncus arteriosus, tetralogy of Fallot (TOF) or ven-

Evidence-Based Cardiology, 3rd edition. Edited by S. Yusuf, J.A. Cairns, A.J. Camm, E.L. Fallen, and B.J. Gersh. © 2010 Blackwell Publishing, ISBN: 978-1-4051-5925-8.

Table 63.1 Incidence per 10 000 live births

Lesion	Median
Bicuspid aortic valve (BAV)	92.4
Ventricular septal defect (VSD)	28.3
Patent ductus arteriosus (PDA)	5.7
Atrial septal defect (ASD)	5.6
Pulmonary stenosis (PS)	5.3
Aortic coarctation	3.6
Tetralogy of Fallot (TOF)	3.6
Atrioventricular septal defect (AVSD)	3.4
Complete transposition of the great arteries (d-TGA)	3.0
Aortic valve stenosis (AS)	2.6

Modified with permission from Hoffman and Kaplan.[2]

Table 63.2 Definite or possible risk factors associated with CHD in offspring

	RR of any defect	Common lesions
Maternal illness		
Phenylketonuria	>6	TOF, VSD, PDA, single ventricle
Pregestational diabetes	3.1–18	Dextrocardia, heterotaxy, TGA, AVSD, VSD, PDA, conotruncal defects
Febrile illness	1.82.9	R- and L-sided obstructive defect, tricuspid atresia, coarctation of the aorta, VSD
Influenza	2.1	Aortic coarctation, VSD, TGA, R and L-sided obstructive defect
Maternal rubella	–	PDA, PV abnormalities, peripheral PS, VSD
Maternal drug exposure		
Vitamin A	0.5–9.2	Outflow tract defects, cranial neural crest defect, PS
Retinoids	–	Any defects
Anticonvulsants	4.2	Any defects
Indometacin tocolysis	–	PDA
Ibuprofen	1.86	TGA, AVSD (Down syndrome), VSD, BAV
Sulfasalazine	3.4	Any defects
Thalidomide	–	VSD, ASD, conotruncal defects
Marijuana	1.9–2.4	VSD, Ebstein's anomaly
Alcohol	§	§
Maternal environmental exposure		
Organic solvents	2.0–5.6	AVSD, PS, conotruncal defects, Ebstein's anomaly, TGA

Modified with permission from Jenkins et al.[8]
–Not available.
§Inconclusive data on CHD.
R, Right; L, Left; PV, pulmonary valve.

tricular septal defect (VSD)), specific facial features, palate anomalies, hypoplasia of the thymus, aplasia or hypoplasia of the parathyroid glands, and psychiatric disorders. The 22q11 deletion syndrome is an autosomal dominant syndrome which carries a 50% risk of transmission from an affected parent to the offspring.[1] Therefore, FISH testing should be considered for patients with such cardiac defects, especially if one of the other features of the 22q11 deletion syndrome listed above is present.[1] A chromosome microdeletion (7q11.23) is also found in ~90% of patients with Williams syndrome, which is associated with supravalvular aortic stenosis (AS) and often supravalvular or peripheral pulmonary stenosis (PS). Mutations in various single genes have been found in several syndromes, namely Holt–Oram, Alagille, Char, Noonan, LEOPARD, CHARGE association, Ellis–van Creveld and Marfan. Single-gene disorders can also result in non-syndromic congenital heart defects, such as familial congenital atrial septal defect (ASD) and atrioventricular block (AVB).[1] However, a more complex combination of multiple genetic alterations and environmental factors instead of a single gene mutation is likely to be the cause in many cases of non-syndromic CHD.[1] Our knowledge of the association between CHD and genetic alterations will continue to grow with ongoing research and current availability of genetic testing.

Non-inherited risk factors for CHD

During the past decade, there has been an increase in epidemiologic literature concerning modifiable risk factors that may have an adverse effect on the fetal heart,[8] especially with an exposure during the first pregnancy trimester and the 3 months before conception (Table 63.2).[8]

We now provide information on specific lesions.

Atrial septal defect

Anatomic findings and pathophysiology

Interatrial communications are common and can be classified in four types: ostium secundum defects, the most common, are located within the region of the fossa ovalis; ostium primum, part of an atrioventricular septal defect (AVSD), includes a common atrioventricular junction with a trileaflet left atrioventricular valve (AVV); superior sinus venosus defects are frequently associated with partial anomalous pulmonary vein return; and coronary sinus defects are characterized by a deficiency in the roof between the coronary sinus and the left atrium (Fig. 63.1). The size of the defect and the ventricular diastolic filling pressures (right and left) determine the degree of left-to-right shunting. A Qp:Qs ratio greater than 1.5/1.0 or the presence of right heart dilation is considered an indication for closure.[9]

Clinical presentation

Dyspnea and fatigue on exertion are the most common symptoms in adults. Patients can also present with palpitations from atrial fibrillation or flutter, which rarely occurs before 40 years of age.[10,11] On examination, a right ventricular lift and a wide and fixed splitting of the second heart sound are distinctive clinical signs of ASD. A pulmonary ejection systolic murmur and a mid-diastolic rumble reflect increased flow through the pulmonary and tricuspid valves.

Diagnostic evaluation

Electrocardiogram
The ECG in ASD can reveal sinus rhythm, atrial fibrillation or atrial flutter, rightward axis deviation in secundum ASD (leftward or extreme right in primum ASD), prolonged PR interval, and right bundle branch block pattern (RBBB).[12–14] In superior sinus venosus defect, sinus node dysfunction may lead to inverted P-waves in inferior leads.[10,15,16]

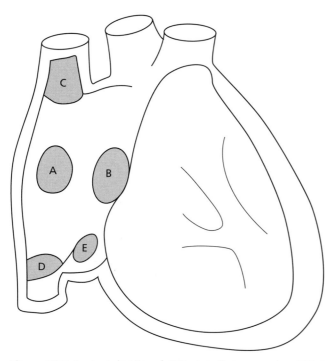

Figure 63.1 Anatomic location of ASDs. A, indicates secundum ASD; B, ostium primum ASD or partial AV septal defect; C, superior sinus venosus ASD; D, inferior sinus venosus ASD; E, coronary sinus ASD.

Chest radiography
Signs of increased pulmonary blood flow,[17,18] as well as enlarged central pulmonary arteries, cardiomegaly (right heart dilation), and small aortic knuckle from chronic low systemic cardiac output, are present in significant defects.[10]

Exercise testing
Useful to document exercise capacity when there is discrepancy between symptoms and clinical findings, or to show changes in oxygen saturation in patients with mild or moderate pulmonary arterial hypertension (PAH) (**Class IIa, Level C**).

Echocardiography
Transthoracic echocardiogram (TTE) usually demonstrates the location, shape and size of the defect and its septal margins.[19] TTE can also provide the direction of the shunt, an estimation of the shunt ratio (Qp:Qs)[20] and an estimation of the pulmonary artery pressures (PAP) from the Doppler velocity of the tricuspid regurgitation (TR). An enlarged right ventricle (RV),[21] with or without paradoxic septal motion.[22] might be the only initial findings of a significant ASD. Transesophageal echocardiogram may better visualize the pulmonary venous return, and is used to guide device closure of the defect.

Cardiac magnetic resonance imaging (CMR)
Cardiac magnetic resonance imaging is the modality of choice to assess right ventricular size and function. Pulmonary venous return can also be accurately demonstrated.[23]

Management

Indications for ASD closure are shown in Table 63.3.[7a,10] Most centers favor percutaneous closure when the anatomy is suitable.[24,25] Device closure is safe (complication rate less than 1%) and effective, and minimizes hospital stay.[26] It

Table 63.3 ASD closure

Indications
ASD associated with RA and RV enlargement, with or without symptoms (**Class I, Level B**)
Paradoxic embolism (**Class IIa, Level C**)
Documented orthodeoxia-platypnea (**Class IIa, Level B**)

Contraindications
Advanced pulmonary arterial hypertension (PAH) (**Class III, Level B**)
Pregnancy (defer closure for 6 months after delivery) (**Level C**)
Severe left ventricular dysfunction (**Level C**)

RA, Right atrium.

Table 63.4 Complications of ASD
Arrhythmias[11,28]
Atrial flutter or fibrillation
Bradyarrhythmia
Impaired functional capacity[31,32]
Right heart failure
PAH (if large, unrestrictive defect)
Cerebrovascular events from paradoxic embolism (uncommon)

also improves RV size and function[27] and exercise capacity,[24] as does surgical closure. However, surgical closure is required for patients with ostium primum and sinus venosus ASDs (**Class I, Level B**), as well as ostium secundum defects with one or more of the following features: stretched diameter >36–40 mm, inadequate atrial septal rims to allow device deployment, or proximity of the defect to the AVV, coronary sinus or vena cavae[10,25] (**Class IIa, Level C**).

Outcomes and complications

Normal long-term survival has been reported after surgical ASD closure when patients were operated on before 25 years of age.[28] Nevertheless, benefits (reduced morbidity and mortality) have also been demonstrated with surgical ASD closure compared with medical treatment in patients over 40 years of age.[29,30] The risk of developing late atrial flutter or fibrillation is clearly higher if surgical repair is performed after 40 years of age.[11] Other complications are summarized in Table 63.4.

Ventricular septal defect

Anatomic findings and pathophysiology

Ventricular septal defect (VSD) is a very common congenital heart malformation (up to 53.2 per 1000 liveborn infants).[33] VSDs are classified into (1) perimembranous, (2) muscular, and (3) double committed subarterial (Fig. 63.2). In perimembranous VSDs, part of the rim of the defect is formed by part of the central fibrous body, which is between the leaflets of an AVV and an arterial valve. Muscular VSDs possess completely muscular rims. Finally, double committed subarterial VSDs are present when the aortic and pulmonary valves are contiguous in the roof of the defect.[34]

The magnitude of and direction of flow through the VSD are determined by the size of the defect, the right and left ventricular pressures, and the pulmonary vascular resistance. In small (restrictive) VSDs, there is a significant

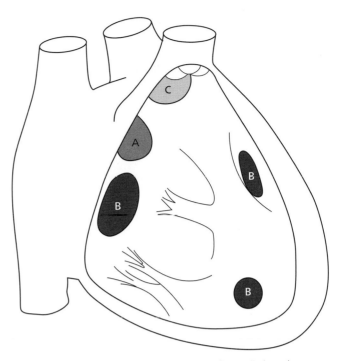

Figure 63.2 Anatomic location of VSDs. A, indicates perimembranous VSD; B, muscular VSDs; C, doubly committed and subarterial VSD.

pressure gradient between the left and right ventricles. In large non-restrictive VSDs, the pulmonary pressures are at or close to systemic levels. With the development of pulmonary vascular disease, the degree of left-to-right shunting decreases and then reverses, leading to Eisenmenger syndrome.

Clinical presentation

Patients with small VSDs are usually asymptomatic. Moderately restrictive and large VSDs can cause dyspnea on exertion, and/or palpitations if arrhythmias arise. As mentioned above, non-restrictive VSDs can lead to Eisenmenger syndrome. On examination, a holosystolic murmur is heard on the left sternal edge, which is loudest and may be accompanied by a thrill in small defects. In moderate and large defects, the apical impulse is laterally displaced. There is a widely split second heart sound that varies with respiration. With large shunts, a diastolic rumble of increased mitral flow may be heard. Large non-restrictive VSDs may have signs of PAH, including a RV heave and a loud P2.

Diagnostic evaluation

Electrocardiogram

In small VSDs, the ECG is usually normal. In moderate VSDs, ECG may reveal left atrial hypertrophy and signs of left ventricular overload. In large non-restrictive VSDs with PAH, the QRS axis shifts to the right and right atrial/ventricular hypertrophy is present. Following surgical repair, RBBB is found in 29–65% of patients more than 25 years after surgery[35,36] and 0.7–3.5% may develop late complete AVB.[36,37]

Chest radiography

Small VSDs have normal chest X-rays. Pulmonary plethora and cardiomegaly are present with larger defects. When significant PAH develops, the chest X-ray shows dilated central pulmonary arteries and right heart enlargement.

Echocardiography

The size and location of VSDs can be accurately assessed by TTE.[38,39] Shunt ratio (Qp:Qs) and PAP can be estimated[20] and, most importantly, hemodynamic consequences such as left ventricular enlargement or hypertrophy can be ascertained. Associated lesions should be sought (aortic regurgitation (AR), right or left ventricular outflow tract obstruction). Transesophageal or three-dimensional echocardiography may be occasionally required when the TTE quality is poor.[40]

Cardiac catheterization

Cardiac catheterization is useful when non-invasive data are inconclusive and further information is needed (**Class IIa**), such as assessment of pulmonary vascular resistance, magnitude of shunts, and pulmonary vasoreactivity (**Level B**).

Management

Table 63.5 summarizes the indications for VSD closure.[7a] Surgical closure in the current era carries low perioperative mortality risk (less than 1%),[41] with a low risk of AVB requiring permanent pacemaker (0.7–3%).[37,41,42] Transcatheter closure is currently in the investigational stage and should be considered only in selected cases of muscular and perimembranous VSDs (**Class IIb, Level C**). Butera *et al* recently reported their 38.5 months follow-up of 104 patients who underwent percutaneous closure of perimembranous VSDs, and the occlusion rate reached 99% at follow-up. However, pacemaker implantation for complete AVB occurred in 5.6% (all in patients <6 years old).

Outcomes and complications

Small restrictive VSDs with normal PVR have an excellent prognosis.[43] Twenty-five year survival rate decreases with increasing size of the VSD (small, 96%; moderate, 86%; large, 61%; Eisenmenger, 42%).[44] Following surgical closure in patients without previous PAH, life expectancy should be close to normal. Even small VSDs, in unoperated patients or as residual defects following surgery, can lead to

Table 63.5 VSD closure

Indications

Left-to-right shunt (Qp:Qs) >2 by echocardiography, CMR or cardiac catheterization and evidence of LV volume overload (**Class I, Level B**)

Left-to-right shunt (Qp:Qs) >1.5:1 with pulmonary artery pressure < two-thirds of systemic pressure and PVR < two-thirds of systemic vascular resistance (**Class IIa, Level B**)

Left-to-right shunt (Qp:Qs) >1.5:1 in the presence of LV systolic or diastolic dysfunction (**Class IIa, Level B**)

Regardless of the size:

History of endocarditis (**Class I, Level C**)

May be considered in patients with aortic regurgitation (**Level C**)

Contraindications

Advanced PAH (**Class III, Level B**)

Pregnancy (defer closure for 6 months after delivery) (**Level C**)

LV, left ventricle; EF, ejection fraction.

Table 63.6 Complications of VSDs

Arrhythmias[47]

Atrial fibrillation

Ventricular arrhythmias, sudden cardiac death

Aortic regurgitation

Endocarditis

LV dysfunction (in large defects)

PAH and Eisenmenger syndrome (if large, unrestrictive defect)

complications such as endocarditis, aortic regurgitation or arrhythmias.[45,46] Other possible complications of VSDs are listed in Table 63.6.

Atrioventricular septal defect

Anatomic findings and pathophysiology

The morphologic hallmark of an AVSD is a common atrioventricular junction, with abnormalities of the AVV. In complete AVSD, there is a common AVV with five leaflets, while in partial AVSD (ostium primum ASD), the AVV is divided into two orifices (Fig. 63.3). The left AVV has three leaflets (mural leaflet, inferior and superior bridging leaflets). In complete AVSD, there is usually a primum ASD and a large VSD. In partial AVSD, only a primum ASD is present. Other common features include an inlet-to-outlet disproportion of the left ventricle and unwedged position of the aortic valve, which result in an elongated left ventricular outflow tract (LVOT) ("goose neck deformity"), predisposing to subaortic obstruction. Septal chordal

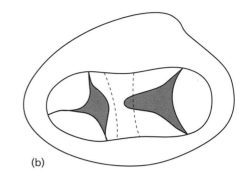

Figure 63.3 Complete and partial AVSDs. A illustrates common valvar orifice (a, superior bridging leaflet; b, left mural leaflet; c, inferior bridging leaflet; d, right inferior leaflet; e, right antero-superior leaflet). B illustrates separate right and left valvar orifices.

(a)　　　(b)

attachments of the left AVV contribute to this complication.[48] The conduction system is also abnormal in patients with AVSD, leading to an increased risk of AVB.[49]

Complete AVSD is associated with abnormal karyotype in 49% of cases diagnosed in fetal life (39% having trisomy 21),[51] while some surgical series report Down syndrome in up to 73% of patients undergoing complete AVSD repair.[52]

Complete AVSDs have a significant degree of left-to-right shunting through the primum ASD and the large VSD, leading to left ventricular enlargement and early PAH. Partial AVSDs (with only a primum ASD) will usually have similar pathophysiology to other isolated interatrial shunts, unless the left AVV is very dysplastic, leading to severe stenosis and/or regurgitation.

Clinical presentation

The clinical presentation relates to the morphology of the defect. Large left-to-right shunts and severe left AVV regurgitation will present with congestive heart failure (CHF) in infancy and will develop PAH and cyanosis. Adults with unrepaired complete AVSDs may present with exercise intolerance and fatigue, Eisenmenger syndrome (see below), palpitations from atrial arrhythmias or bradycardia from complete AVB. Examination may reveal cyanosis and clubbing, right ventricular impulse, increased pulmonary component of the second sound, variable ejection systolic murmurs, mid-diastolic murmur in large left-to-right shunt, and pansystolic murmur with left AVV regurgitation. Isolated ostium primum ASDs will share the clinical features of ASDs described above but may also have signs of left AVV dysfunction.

Diagnostic evaluation

Electrocardiogram
Left axis deviation, RBBB, and first-degree AVB are common ECG findings in patients with AVSD.[53,54] Atrial fibrillation can also be present.[53]

Chest radiography
Cardiomegaly from left heart dilation usually present in patients with large VSD and/or significant left AVV regurgitation. Large primum ASD will give rise to right heart enlargement and increased pulmonary vascular markings. Patients with Eisenmenger syndrome will have dilated central pulmonary arteries and peripheral pruning.

Echocardiography
Diagnosis of AVSD can accurately be made by TTE.[55] The following features should be assessed.[56–58]
- Abnormal configuration of the AVVs are at the same level.
- Left AVV has three leaflets.
- May have some degree of regurgitation.
- Presence of ASD and VSD, and the magnitude of left-to-right shunting.
- Estimated right ventricular systolic pressure.
- Inlet-to-outlet disproportion with elongated LVOT and possible LVOT obstruction.
- Abnormal position of the papillary muscles.
- Left ventricular size and function.

Cardiac magnetic resonance
This provides detailed morphologic information and accurately estimates the size of the VSD.[59]

Cardiac catheterization and angiography
Echocardiography and CMR have replaced cardiac catheterization for the diagnostic and preoperative evaluation of AVSDs. However, cardiac catheterization may be necessary to assess formally the pulmonary vascular resistance and vasoreactivity (**Class IIa, Level B**).

Management

Patients with complete AVSD should have early surgical correction (including repair of the AVV[60,61]) within the first few months of life to prevent pulmonary vascular disease. Most patients who present with partial AVSDs in later life

Table 63.7 Late complications of VSDs

Left AVV regurgitation
LVOT obstruction
Complete AVB
Pulmonary vascular disease
Atrial or ventricular arrhythmias
Left AVV stenosis
Right AVV stenosis/regurgitation
Residual VSD
Aortic regurgitation

Modified with permission from Craig.[50]

(>40 years old) will also benefit from surgical repair.[62] However, patients with irreversible pulmonary vascular disease and/or Eisenmenger syndrome should usually be treated medically (see below). Indications of reintervention in adults include:[7a]

- significant left AVV regurgitation or stenosis with symptoms, atrial or ventricular arrhythmias, a progressive increase in LV dimensions or deterioration of LV function (**Class I, Level B**)
- significant LVOT obstruction (**Class I, Level B**)
- residual ASD or VSD with significant left-to-right shunting (**Class I, Level B**)
- complete AVB (pacemaker implantation) (**Class IIa, Level B**).

Outcomes and complications

Without surgical repair, only 4% of patients with complete AVSD will survive beyond 5 years of age.[63] Conversely, the 10-year survival rate in patients following complete AVSD repair is 83%[60] and 93% after partial AVSD repair.[64] Table 63.7 summarizes late complications of AVSD, including the most common, left AVV regurgitation (10% of patients).[50,60,64]

Left ventricular outflow tract obstruction and bicuspid aortic valve

Anatomic findings and pathophysiology

Left ventricular outflow tract obstructions (LVOTOs) comprise a group of stenotic lesions which may be located at the subvalvar, valvar or supravalvar level. Significant LVOTO creates an increase in afterload, resulting in elevated end-diastolic left ventricular pressure and concentric hypertrophy.

Subvalvar aortic stenosis (SAS)
Fixed SAS ranges from discrete fibrous membrane (91% of cases) to tunnel-like fibromuscular band.[65,66] Nearly

one-quarter of patients also have bicuspid aortic valve (BAV).[65] Other associated cardiac defects include VSD, coarctation of the aorta and Shone syndrome (parachute mitral valve, mitral stenosis, SAS, aortic coarctation, BAV). SAS is usually progressive; AR is common but usually mild.[67]

Congenital valvar AS
Abnormal valve and cusp formation may result in unicuspid, bicuspid, trileaflet bicommissural or rarely quadricuspid valves. Fifty-four percent of patients with significant AS requiring surgery have congenitally malformed valves, of which more than 90% are bicuspid.[68] The estimated incidence of BAV in the general population is 1–2%, affecting more males than females.[69] The high incidence (37%) of BAV in first-degree relatives suggests an autosomal dominant inheritance with reduced penetrance.[70] BAV is associated with abnormal aortic root tissue structure, including medial disease,[71] explaining why patients may develop aortic root dilation and aortic dissection.

Supravalvar AS (SVAS)
SVAS is the less common LVOTO. The morphologic feature of this condition is aortic narrowing at the level of the sinotubular junction. The entire ascending aorta may be involved and, less commonly, the aortic arch and peripheral arteries.[66] SVAS is frequently associated with Williams syndrome, which is characterized by intellectual impairment, elfin facies, short stature and, often, peripheral pulmonary artery stenosis. A mutation of elastin gene on chromosome 7q11.23 has been detected in most patients,[72] irrespective of the form of SVAS (autosomal dominant form, sporadic form or associated with Williams syndrome).

Clinical presentation

Symptoms may develop in childhood or adulthood, depending on the degree of obstruction. Patients with significant LVOTO (subvalvar, valvar or supravalvar) may present with dyspnea, angina, syncope, congestive heart failure or signs of endocarditis. The following signs may be found on examination.
- Slow-rising, diminished carotid pulse
- Apex-to-carotid delay (severe)
- Sustained apical impulse
- Ejection click (with BAV, if valve pliable, or with dilated aortic root)
- Diminished aortic component of S2, paradoxic splitting if severe
- S4, S3 if ventricular dysfunction
- Crescendo-decrescendo systolic murmur, late peaking if severe
- Diastolic murmur if AR present

Diagnostic evaluation

Electrocardiogram

Left axis deviation, left ventricular hypertrophy, T-wave inversion with ST segment depression in lateral leads and left atrial enlargement.

Chest radiography

Cardiomegaly (mild, unless significant AR and/or left ventricular dysfunction are present), dilation of ascending aorta (common with BAV), calcifications of the aortic valve.

Echocardiography

Modality of choice to identify and quantify the severity and level of LVOTO (**Class I, Level B**). Peak instantaneous Doppler velocity and gradient help to determine prognosis and guide the timing of intervention.[73,74] Aortic root diameter, left ventricular size/hypertrophy, and systolic/diastolic function should also be assessed.

Exercise stress testing

May be useful if the patient anticipates athletic participation or pregnancy, if clinical findings differ from non-invasive measurements, or in asymptomatic young adults with a mean Doppler gradient greater than 40 mmHg or a peak Doppler gradient greater than 64 mmHg (**Class IIa, Level C**).

CMR and CT angiography

Both helpful for visualizing the entire intrathoracic aorta and detect associated lesions (**Class IIa, Level C**).

Cardiac catheterization and angiography

Cardiac catheterization is useful before aortic valve replacement (AVR):[75]

• when non-invasive imaging is suboptimal or discordant with the clinical evaluation (**Class I, Level C**)

• to determine if there is co-existent coronary artery disease (CAD) (**Class I, Level B**)

• to identify the origin of coronary arteries when a Ross procedure (see below) is contemplated, if non-invasive imaging is inadequate (**Class I, Level C**).

Management

SAS

Surgical resection is the treatment of choice, but the timing of intervention remains controversial. Some authors advocate an early aggressive approach to prevent AR,[65,76,77] while others consider the significant risk of recurrence and are more conservative. Table 63.8 proposes some indications for operative resection.[66,74]

Congenital valvar AS

There are currently no proven medical treatments to delay the disease process in patients with AS. It is reasonable to use beta-blockers for dilation of the ascending aorta.[66] Management and recommendations for AVR in adults with valvar AS are discussed in Chapter 55.[75] Table 63.8 summarizes the indications for balloon valvotomy in adolescents and young adults with congenital valvar AS.[75] When valve replacement is required, the Ross procedure may be

Table 63.8 Indications for intervention in patients with LVOTO

Subaortic stenosis	Congenital valvar aortic stenosis	Supravalvar AS
Surgical resection should be considered for:	Balloon valvotomy should be considered for adolescents and young adults with pliable valve, fusion of commissures and[1]:	Surgical resection should be considered for:
Significant AS and development of symptoms or	Significant AS and development of symptoms (**Class I, Level C**) or	Significant AS and development of symptoms (**Class I, Level B**)
Doppler-derived estimated peak gradient ≥50 mmHg (**Class I, Level C**) or	Peak echo Doppler gradient >70–80 mmHg or peak-to-peak catheter gradient >60 mmHg (**Class I, Level C**) or	Doppler-derived mean gradient >50 mmHg or peak gradient >70 mmHg) (**Class I, Level B**)
Doppler-derived peak gradient <50 mmHg and LV ejection fraction <55% or LV end-systolic diameter >50 mm (**Class I, Level C**)	Ischemic ECG changes at rest or on exercise with peak to peak catheter gradient >50 mmHg (**Class I, Level C**) or	Doppler-derived mean gradient <50 mmHg and LVH (**Class I, Level C**)
Moderate/severe AR (**Class I, Level C**)	Peak to peak catheter gradient >50 mmHg in patients who wish to do competitive sports (**Class IIa, Level C**)	LV systolic dysfunction (**Class I, Level C**)
VSD		Wish to participate in competitive sports (**Class I, Level C**)
Contemplating pregnancy (**Class IIb, Level C**)		Contemplating pregnancy (**Class I, Level C**)
Wish to participate in competitive sports (**Class IIb, Level C**)		

[1] Indications for surgical aortic valve replacement in adults with valvar AS are discussed in Chapter 55.
LVH, left ventricular hypertrophy.

Table 63.9 Complications of LVOTO (SAS, BAV, SVAS)

Endocarditis
Aortic regurgitation
Recurrent AS after surgical or balloon intervention in BAV, or
    following surgical resection in SAS
Aortic root dilation or dissection (BAV)
Sudden cardiac death
Left ventricular failure

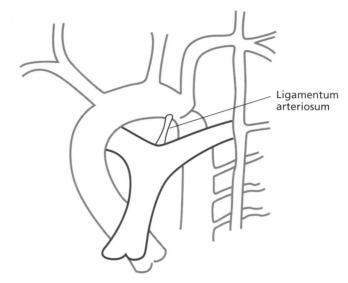

Ligamentum arteriosum

Figure 63.4 Aortic coarctation.

considered (particularly for young women of reproductive age).

Outcomes and complications

SAS

Recurrence rates following surgical resection vary and are probably close to 15%.[65,78,79] Risk factors for recurrence include proximity of the obstructive lesion to the aortic valve and severe obstruction.[78] Infective endocarditis and AR are other complications of SAS. AR may develop despite surgical resection of the SAS.[66]

Congenital valvar AS

It has been suggested that the 3 year-mortality for symptomatic patients with AS, not undergoing surgery, is approximately 75%.[80] In asymptomatic patients, however, the risk of sudden cardiac death is less than 1%/year, even in hemodynamically significant AS.[73] Complications for patients with LVOTO are listed in Table 63.9.

Coarctation of the aorta

Anatomic findings and pathophysiology

Coarctation of the aorta is a localized narrowing usually located just below the origin of the left subclavian artery (LSCA), in the region of the ligamentum arteriosum (Fig. 63.4). Less commonly, a diffuse form with tubular hypoplasia may involve the aortic arch or the aorta distal to the LSCA. Aortic medial abnormalities may be present.[71] Extensive arterial collaterals often develop through the intercostal, subclavian, internal thoracic and scapular arteries to supply the lower body. Aortic coarctation is more frequent in men than women (1.5:1).[66] The reported incidence of BAV in patients with coarctation varies from 27% to 85%.[81–83] Coarctation may also occur in conjunction with VSD, mitral valve abnormalities, intracranial aneurysms (in up to 10% of patients[84]) and Turner syndrome.

Clinical presentation

Adults are most often asymptomatic and diagnosis is suspected after fortuitous systemic arterial hypertension or murmurs are found. Other possible clinical presentations include headache, epistaxis, intracranial hemorrhage, leg fatigue on exertion, CHF, angina and aortic dissection.[85] Physical examination classically reveals:
• upper body systemic hypertension (blood pressure should be taken in the right arm)
• blood pressure drop between upper and lower extremities
• delayed and weak femoral pulses
• palpable arteries over the scapulae or lateral chest wall
• systolic thrill in suprasternal notch
• sustained apex (pressure overload)
• loud aortic component of S2
• ejection click if BAV ± ejection systolic murmur
• continuous murmurs over the back (collaterals).

Diagnostic evaluation

Electrocardiogram

The ECG may show left atrial and ventricular hypertrophy.

Chest radiography

The so-called "3" sign (double contour in the region of descending aorta) and rib notching (erosion of the postero-inferior border of third to ninth ribs, caused by intercostal collaterals) are two characteristic features on the chest X-ray. The ascending aorta may appear dilated, and overall heart size is normal in the majority of patients.[85]

Echocardiography

Continuous wave Doppler assessment of the distal aortic arch via the suprasternal notch provides peak pressure gradient through the coarctation. Velocities proximal and distal to the stenosis should be included in an expanded Bernouilli equation to avoid overestimation of the gradient.[86] Doppler systolic velocities may be affected by lesion length,[87] presence of collateral flow,[86,88] and aortic compliance.[89] Diastolic velocities should therefore also be measured; the presence of a diastolic tail (elevated diastolic velocities) correlates with significant aortic coarctation.[90–92] TTE can also show LVH, associated BAV or dilated ascending aorta.

CMR and CT angiography

CMR and CT angiography are the imaging modalities of choice to evaluate coarctation before and after surgical or transcatheter intervention (site, extent and severity[93] of stenosis, presence of aneurysms,[94] anatomy of intracranial vessels, and extent of collateral network).

Cardiac catheterization and angiography

A peak-to-peak catheter gradient ≥20 mmHg is generally accepted as *significant coarctation*.[66] Cardiac catheterization is mainly employed for catheter intervention and for screening the coronary arteries.

Management

Timing of intervention or reintervention (surgery or angioplasty ± stent) in adults with coarctation may be challenging. Nevertheless, intervention should be considered when:
- peak-to-peak catheter gradient is greater than or equal to 20 mmHg across the coarctation (**Class I, Level C**)
- peak-to-peak catheter gradient is less than 20 mmHg across the coarctation in the presence of significant coarctation demonstrated by imaging studies, with radiologic evidence of significant collateral flow.[7a,95]

The presence of symptoms, systemic hypertension (at rest or with 24-hour monitoring) or LVH should be considered in the intervention decision-making process.

Surgical repair may involve end-to-end anastomosis, interposition graft, patch aortoplasty (abandoned because of the high incidence of aneurysms), ascending to descending aorta conduit repair (for complex/hypoplastic aortic arch) and subclavian flap repair (for neonates). Balloon angioplasty represents an alternative with encouraging results, although more aneurysm formation is reported compared with surgery.[96] The incidence of aneurysm seems to decrease substantially with primary stent implantation, however.[97] Catheter interventions appear to be safe and effective, and thus should be considered for simple native and recurrent coarctation (with catheter gradient >20 mmHg) (**Class I, Level B**).

Table 63.10 Residua following repair of coarctation

Persistent systemic hypertension
Recoarctation
Aneurysm of the aorta
Coronary artery disease
AS/AR (if BAV present)
Endocarditis/endarteritis
Rupture of aortic or cerebral aneurysm
Postsurgical repair paraplegia (rare)

Outcomes and complications

Seventy-five percent of unoperated patients will have died by 46 years of age.[66,98] Estimated 30-year survival following repair is 72%.[99]

Patent ductus arteriosus

Anatomic findings and pathophysiology

The patent ductus arteriosus (PDA) is a blood vessel that connects the descending aorta (just distal to the LSCA) to the proximal left pulmonary artery (Fig. 63.5). In fetal life, this structure is vital as it carries the blood from the right ventricle to the descending aorta, bypassing the lungs. The ductus normally closes soon after birth. When it remains patent, it can lead to left-to-right shunting with increased pulmonary flow and left heart volume overload.

Clinical presentation

Patients with small PDAs are asymptomatic and present with a murmur. Moderate and large PDAs may cause exercise intolerance, palpitations secondary to onset of atrial fibrillation, or even CHF. Eisenmenger syndrome can occur with long-standing left-to-right shunting through a large PDA. With moderate to large PDAs, the physical examination may reveal:
- bouncy pulses, wide pulse pressure, low diastolic pressure
- prominent ventricular impulse
- occasional paradoxic S2
- continuous "machinery" murmur in the upper left sternal edge, radiating to the back
- diastolic rumble
- in patients with Eisenmenger syndrome (see below), differential cyanosis (cyanosis and clubbing of toes but not fingers), usually no murmurs.

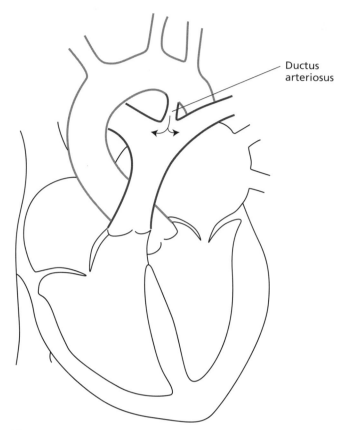

Figure 63.5 Patent ductus arteriosus.

Diagnostic evaluation

Electrocardiogram
Moderate and large PDAs may show left atrial enlargement and LVH. Atrial fibrillation may also occur.

Chest radiography
Significant shunting may lead to cardiomegaly from left heart enlargement, increased pulmonary vascular markings and dilated central pulmonary arteries.

Echocardiography
TTE may confirm the diagnosis, clarify the PDA size and degree of shunting, assess the left ventricular size and function, and estimate the right ventricular pressure from peak velocity of the tricuspid insufficiency. PAP curve can also be obtained from the PDA Doppler flow velocity signal.[100]

CMR and CT angiography
These modalities may be useful to clarify some anatomic variations such as ductus arteriosus aneurysm,[101] vascular ring and right aortic arch.[102]

Cardiac catheterization and angiography
Cardiac catheterization allows assessment of pulmonary vascular resistance and pulmonary vasoreactivity before transcatheter closure.

Table 63.11 Closure of PDA

Indications
Significant left-to-right shunting and left heart enlargement
(**Class I, Level C**)
Prior endarteritis (**Class I, Level C**)

Debatable indications
Tiny silent PDAs to eliminate the risk of endarteritis (**Class IIa, Level C**)
Patients with PAH and a net left-to-right shunt (**Class IIa, Level C**)

Contraindication
Eisenmenger's syndrome (**Class III, Level C**)

Management

Transcatheter closure has become the procedure of choice. Table 63.11 summarizes indications for PDA closure.[7a,103–106] Surgical closure is reserved for PDAs that are not suitable for transcatheter approach, often because they are too large (**Class I, Level C**) or distorted (**Class I, Level B**).

Outcomes and complications

Patients with silent PDAs or PDAs closed in infancy have normal life expectancy. Prognosis worsens in the presence of pulmonary vascular disease. Complications of PDAs include CHF, arrhythmias, pulmonary vascular disease, endarteritis, and aneurysm of the ductus arteriosus.

Pulmonary valve stenosis

Anatomic findings and pathophysiology

The most common form of RV outflow tract (OT) obstruction is the typical dome-shaped pulmonary valve stenosis, characterized by fusion of the pulmonary valve leaflets and narrowed central orifice. The valve is usually mobile and associated with medial abnormalities and dilation of the pulmonary trunk. PVS may be associated with Noonan, Williams, Alagille, Keutel or rubella syndromes.[1,107]

Clinical presentation

Most patients with mild to moderate PVS are asymptomatic. Severe PVS may cause exertional dyspnea and fatigue, chest pain, palpitations and syncope. Mild cyanosis reflects high right atrial (RA) pressure with right-to-left shunt through a patent foramen ovale (PFO). Physical examination depends on the severity of the PVS. Findings in patients with severe PVS include:

- increased "a" wave
- RV lift
- thrill along the left sternal edge
- widely split S2 with reduced or absent P2
- short S1-to-ejection click interval or no ejection click
- right-sided S4
- long systolic ejection murmur, late peak.

Diagnostic evaluation

Electrocardiogram
Right axis deviation, RA enlargement and RV hypertrophy may be detected on ECG.

Chest radiography
Dilation of the main (and left) pulmonary arteries is common.[108] Cardiomegaly secondary to right heart enlargement occurs if there is right ventricular failure.

Echocardiography
Echocardiography, the imaging modality of choice, assesses morphology and mobility of PVS, severity of stenosis, RV size and function, and associated lesions.

Management
Table 63.12 summarizes the recommendations for percutaneous balloon valvuloplasty in patients with PVS.[7a] The procedure has excellent 10-year outcomes,[109] which are comparable to surgical valvotomy,[110] and is considered successful if the post-valvuloplasty Doppler gradient is <30 mmHg. Patients with dysplastic PV may need surgical valvectomy and PV replacement (PVR). PVR (with bioprosthesis or homograft) is also required when there is significant pulmonary regurgitation (PR).

Outcomes and complications
The 25-year surgery-free survival in unoperated patients with PV gradient >50 mmHg is only 31%, compared with

Table 63.12 Indications for balloon valvuloplasty in adolescents and young adults with PS

Asymptomatic patients with peak Doppler gradient >60 mmHg or mean gradient >40 mmHg and less than moderate PR (**Class I, Level B**)

Symptomatic patients with peak Doppler gradient >50 mmHg or mean gradient >30 mmHg and less than moderate PR (**Class I, Level C**)

Surgical therapy is recommended for dysplastic PV, hypoplastic pulmonary annulus, severe PR, subvalvular PS or supravalvular PS (**Class I, Level C**)

Modified from Bonow *et al.*[75]

96% in patients with gradient <25 mmHg.[111] Prognosis following repair is excellent, with a near-normal life expectancy.[111] Late complications after pulmonary valvotomy are residual PS, PR with progressive RV dilation that may require PVR, and arrhythmias.

Ebstein anomaly of the tricuspid valve

Anatomic findings and pathophysiology
Ebstein anomaly of the tricuspid valve (TV) is composed of[112]:
- downward (apical) displacement of the septal and often the mural leaflet
- adherence of the septal and mural leaflets to the underlying myocardium
- dilation of the "atrialized" portion of the RV
- redundant, malformed anterior leaflet.

The abnormal TV leads to variable degrees of tricuspid regurgitation which compromises further forward pulmonary blood flow and exaggerates right heart enlargement. ASD or PFO have been reported in up to 94% of patients.[112] Other associated lesions include multiple accessory atrioventricular pathways, pulmonary stenosis or atresia, BAV, coarctation, VSD, congenitally corrected transposition of the great arteries, and left-sided heart abnormalities.[112,113]

Clinical presentation
Symptoms depend on anatomic severity, associated defects and degree of right-to-left shunting. Patients may present with cyanosis, right heart failure, exercise intolerance, palpitations secondary to arrhythmias and sudden cardiac death. Physical examination may reveal:
- cyanosis ± digital clubbing in patients with right-to-left shunting
- large V-wave is rare despite severe TR
- widely split S1 and S2 and added sounds are common
- holosystolic murmur of TR
- hepatomegaly.

Diagnostic evaluation

Pulse oximetry
Pulse oximetry (at rest and/or during exercise) is useful in the evaluation of Ebstein anomaly (**Class IIa, Level C**).

Electrocardiogram
Tall P-waves secondary to RA enlargement, first-degree AVB, RBBB, low QRS voltage, and delta wave secondary to accessory pathway are common ECG features associated with Ebstein anomaly. Supraventricular tachyarrhythmias and atrial fibrillation can also occur.

Chest radiography

Cardiomegaly from right heart enlargement with globular cardiac silhouette, and small aortic knuckle from chronic low systemic blood flow are typical findings.

Echocardiography

The anatomy of the abnormal TV, the RV size and function, and the associated lesions should all be assessed by echocardiography. An apical displacement of the septal leaflet from the insertion of the mitral valve by >8 mm/m² is characteristic of Ebstein anomaly.[112]

Outcomes and complications

The actuarial survival for all live-born patients with Ebstein anomaly is 67% at 1 year and 59% at 10 years[114] but some patients survive to their 70s. Complications may include:
- arrhythmias (supraventricular tachycardia from accessory pathways, atrial flutter or fibrillation, and ventricular tachycardia)
- cyanosis
- right heart failure
- paradoxic embolism
- endocarditis
- sudden cardiac death.

Management

Tachyarrhythmias secondary to accessory pathways should be treated with catheter ablation (**Class IIa, Level B**), although success rates are lower and the risk of recurrence higher compared to patients with normal cardiac morphology.[115,116] TV surgery (repair or replacement with RA plasty and a MAZE procedure; Table 63.13) has evolved and encouraging mid-term results are now reported.[112]

For high-risk patients with impaired RV function, a bidirectional cavopulmonary shunt has been proposed,[117] although many would advocate transplantation (**Level C**).

Table 63.13 Indications for tricuspid valve surgery in patients with Ebstein anomaly

Symptomatic patients despite medical treatment (**Class I, Level B**)

Progressive right heart enlargement/reduced RV systolic function/early RV failure (**Class I, Level B**)

Significant cyanosis (**Class I, Level B**)

Paradoxic emboli (**Class I, Level B**)

May be considered in patients with recurrent supraventricular tachycardia despite medical and catheter ablative therapy (**Level C**)

Tetralogy of Fallot

Anatomic findings and pathophysiology

Tetralogy of Fallot (TOF) is the most common cyanotic heart defect. As Etienne-Louis Arthur Fallot described in 1888, this malformation is composed of four morphologic characteristics: VSD (usually large), aorta over-riding the ventricular septum, obstruction of the RVOT, and RV hypertrophy. However, the essential anatomic features of TOF are the anterocephalad deviation of the outlet septum and hypertrophy of the septoparietal trabeculations, creating obstruction of the RVOT. The PV is often small and bicuspid. Pulmonary artery hypoplasia and pulmonary branch stenosis may also occur. The degree of aortic override varies widely and >50% may come from the RV (so-called double-outlet RV). The magnitude of the right-to-left shunting depends on the severity of the RVOT obstruction.

TOF can be associated with other malformations, such as right aortic arch (~25%), ASD, AVSD, and coronary arterial anomalies. Indeed, the left anterior descending coronary artery arises anteriorly from the right coronary artery and

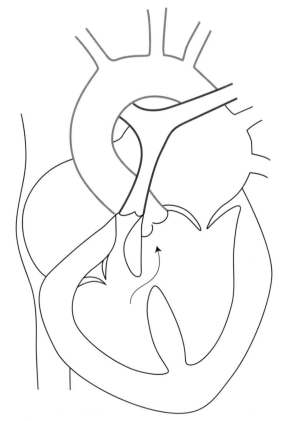

Figure 63.6 Tetralogy of Fallot.

crosses the RV outflow in about 3% of cases. It has been suggested that between 8% and 35% of patients with TOF have a 22q11 deletion (see above, *Genetic basis of CHD*)[1]; screening should therefore be offered (**Class I, Level C**).

Clinical presentation

Most adults will have had previous repair in childhood and present with late symptoms related to complications (see below), such as exertional dyspnea, palpitations, syncope or heart failure. Unoperated patients invariably develop cyanosis. On examination, blood pressure and brachial pulse may be difficult to take on the side of a previous Blalock–Taussig shunt. Unless TR or RV failure develops, the jugular venous pressure will be normal. A right ventricular lift is often present. On auscultation, a residual RVOT obstruction and/or an increased flow due to PR will create an ejection systolic murmur on the pulmonary area. Diastolic murmurs of AR (related to aortic root dilation) and/or PR can also be noted. The pulmonary component of the second sound is often not audible.

Diagnostic evaluation

Electrocardiogram

Patients who underwent surgery commonly have RBBB. Right axis deviation and RV hypertrophy are other common findings. Atrial tachyarrhythmia can occur in up to one-third of patients who had previous repair.[118] Ventricular tachycardia and sudden cardiac death are relatively uncommon.[119] and risk factors include QRS duration >180 ms, QRS prolongation over time and increased QT dispersion.[119–121] Incidence of atrial and ventricular arrhythmias seems to decrease after PVR for chronic PR in patients with previous repair.[122]

Chest radiography

A right-sided aortic arch is noted in ~25% of patients. Dilation of the ascending aorta[123,124] and/or central pulmonary arteries may be present. Cardiomegaly can be the result of:
• significant pulmonary and/or tricuspid regurgitation with RV enlargement
• significant residual VSD, aortic regurgitation or LV dysfunction with related LV dilation.

Echocardiography

Most important observations should include[125]:
• assessment of RV size and function
• RVOT imaging for assessment of residual PS and PR, including continuous-wave Doppler velocities
• detection and quantification of TR, and estimation of RV systolic pressure
• assessment of left ventricular size and function
• measurement of aortic root and detection of AR.

Exercise testing

Objective functional capacity and decline in exercise capacity over time are useful for predicting prognosis[126] and defining optimal timing of intervention.[125]

CMR

CMR can accurately assess right and left ventricular size and function, identify RVOT aneurysms or akinetic regions and quantify PR. RV volume measurements may help to determine the optimal timing for PVR, as RV end-diastolic volume >160–170 mL/m^2 does not normalize after surgery.[127,128] CMR with late gadolinium enhancement can detect the presence of ventricular fibrosis, which is a marker of adverse outcome.[129] CMR also demonstrates pulmonary artery and aortic anomalies.

Cardiac catheterization and angiography

Non-invasive imaging nowadays provides most important information. However, coronary anomalies, atherosclerosis, systemic–pulmonary collaterals, residual shunts and presence of PAH can all be documented by cardiac catheterization.[107]

Management

Surgical strategies have evolved and a transatrial-transpulmonary approach (with a limited RV incision) is now widely employed to relieve the RVOT obstruction and close the VSD. Although still controversial, early primary repair, rather than a staged approach with initial arterial-to-pulmonary shunt, is favored in many centers. Unoperated adults should still be considered for late repair to improve quality of life and prognosis.[130,131] Indications for

---

Table 63.14 Indications for reintervention in TOF

Severe PR associated with:
   Symptoms or deterioration in exercise capacity (**Class I, Level B**)
   RV enlargement/dysfunction (**Class IIa, Level B**)
   Moderate or severe TR (**Class IIa, Level C**)
   Development of clinical arrhythmias (atrial or ventricular) (**Class IIa, Level C**)

Residual RVOT obstruction (valvular or subvalvular) with:
   Peak echocardiography gradient >50 mmHg (**Class IIa, Level C**)
   RV/LV pressures > 0.67 (**Class IIa, Level C**)
   Residual VSD with Qp:Qs >1.5:1 (**Class IIa, Level B**)
   Significant AR with LV enlargement/dysfunction (**Class IIa, Level C**)
Should be considered in patients with aortic root enlargement (>55 mm) (**Level C**)

Table 63.15 Late complications after TOF repair

Residual PR
Residual RVOT obstruction
RV dysfunction/RVOT aneurysm
LV dysfunction
AR ± aortic root dilation
Endocarditis
Atrial tachyarrhythmia
Sustained VT/sudden death
Heart block (uncommon)

reintervention in patients who underwent a previous surgical correction are listed in Table 63.14.[7a,125] Recently, percutaneous PVR has been used with good initial success in selected patients with postoperative pulmonary homograft or conduit stenosis and/or regurgitation.[132]

Outcomes and complications

Nearly 70% of patients die before 10 years of age without surgery.[133] Survival rates after repair are 86% and 85% at 32 and 36 years.[131,134] Sudden death occurs in up to 6% of patients in late follow-up.[134] Older age at the time of repair is consistently a marker of poor prognosis. Table 63.15 summarizes late complications after TOF repair.

Transposition of the great arteries

Complete TGA (d-TGA)

Anatomic findings and pathophysiology

In complete TGA, the aorta arises from the morphologic right ventricle (on the right and anterior in 95% of cases) and the pulmonary artery arises from the morphologic left ventricle (ventriculoarterial discordance). The two great vessels are parallel to each other, without their usual crossover arrangement. The pulmonary and systemic circulations are running in parallel; this is incompatible with life unless there is a communication (ASD, VSD or PDA) between the two circulations. Complete TGA is associated with VSD (~40–45%), LVOTO (~25%), and aortic coarctation (~5%).[135]

Clinical presentation

Almost all adults with complete TGA have had prior repair, but some with a large VSD reach adulthood with Eisenmenger physiology. Clinical presentation in adult patients who had previous surgery are related to late complications (see below) and include palpitations, dyspnea on exertion, CHF, syncope, sudden death, and signs of endocarditis.

Management options and late complications

Atrial switch procedure (Senning and Mustard procedures) The blood from the systemic venous return is redirected through the mitral valve into the subpulmonary left ventricle, and the pulmonary venous blood is redirected through the TV into the subaortic morphologic right ventricle. In the Senning operation,[136] the atrial baffle is made of autologous tissue while in the Mustard procedure, synthetic material or pericardium is used to create the baffle. Senning operations seem to have better long-term outcomes, with a 25-year survival rate of 91% compared with 76% in patients with previous Mustard procedure.[137] Late complications following either procedure are summarized in Table 63.16.[138]

Arterial switch procedure This procedure conveys anatomic repair by switching the great arteries and including the coronaries to their normal position. This operation, performed within the first month of life, has the advantage of restoring a systemic left ventricle. Survival rates at 15 years are 88%.[151] Nearly 10% of patients will require reoperation.[151] Long-term complications include pulmonary artery stenosis, dilation of the neo-aortic root with aortic regurgitation, and coronary ostia stenosis.

Rastelli procedure This procedure is used for patients with combination of TGA, LVOTO and a large VSD. An intracardiac baffle tunnels the LV through the VSD to the aorta, and an extracardiac conduit is inserted between the RV and the pulmonary artery. The LV becomes the systemic ventricle, but late complications such as conduit stenosis, atrial and ventricular arrhythmias or ventricular failure (right and left) may occur.

Congenitally corrected TGA (cc-TGA)

Anatomic findings

In this condition, the RA communicates with the morphologic LV, which is connected to the PA, and the LA enters the morphologic RV, which is connected to the aorta (double discordance). The RV is therefore the systemic ventricle. cc-TGA may be associated with several other malformations such as VSD (70%), PS (40%), abnormalities of the systemic AVV (Ebstein like – 90%), abnormalities of the conduction system (complete AVB), and dextrocardia.[138]

Clinical presentation

Adult patients with cc-TGA may develop CHF with exertional dyspnea, palpitations, syncope secondary to complete AVB, or cyanosis (if LVOTO and VSD are present). Physical examination depends on presence of associated lesions and complications. The ECG may show left axis deviation, Q-waves in right precordial leads and absence

Table 63.16 Complications following atrial switch procedures and their management

Complications	Management
Tachyarrhythmias: atrial re-entry tachycardia (flutter) Develops in 14% of patients[139] Predictor of sudden cardiac death[140] and marker of RV dysfunction[141]	Restore sinus rhythm Antiarrhythmic drugs with caution (risk of bradyarrhythmia) Radiofrequency ablation (success rate ~70%)[142]
Bradyarrhythmias: sinus node dysfunction and AVB (less common) Nearly 48% develop sinus node dysfunction[143] ~11% need a pacemaker[139]	Pacemaker implantation (may be technically difficult) (**Class I, Level B**)
Sudden death Reported in ~4–7% of patients[137,139,144]	Implantable cardiac defibrillator (ICD) implantation (**Level C**)
Systemic ventricular dysfunction Common late complication	No large prospective studies available Beta-blockers may improve exercise capacity and prevent RV remodeling[145]; use with caution (risk of bradyarrhythmia) (**Level C**) No proven effect with ACE inhibitors[146]; may be used empirically (**Level C**) Consider arterial switch conversion preceded by LV reconditioning (PA banding) in selected young patients; less favourable outcomes in adults[147,148] (**Level C**) Consider transplantation in selected cases with end-stage heart failure
Tricuspid regurgitation	TV replacement in some cases with severe TR (**Class I, Level B**); less useful if due to annular dilation[138]
Baffle obstruction SVC obstruction more common than IVC	Percutaneous balloon dilation and stenting[149] (**Class IIa, Level B**); surgery if not amenable to percutaneous treatment (**Class I, Level B**)
Significant baffle leak	Percutaneous or surgical closure (**Class IIa, Level B**); surgery if not amenable to percutaneous treatment (**Class I, Level B**)
PAH Occurs in ~7% of patients[150]	Consider advanced pulmonary vasodilator therapy (**Level C**)

of Q-waves in left precordial leads, and prominent Q-waves in inferior leads. In TGA (complete or congenitally corrected), a small vascular pedicle is the rule on chest radiograph because of the parallel arrangement of the vessels.

Outcomes, complications and management

Twenty-five percent of unoperated patients have developed CHF by 45 years of age (isolated cc-TGA), compared with 67% if associated lesions are present.[152] Long-term complications include:

- RV dysfunction and CHF
- systemic AVV regurgitation
- complete AVB (3% risk per year)
- arrhythmias (atrial and ventricular)
- sudden cardiac death
- endocarditis.

Patients with severe left AVV (tricuspid) regurgitation should be considered for tricuspid valve replacement, ideally before significant systemic RV dysfunction occurs (**Class I, Level B**). Double-switch procedures, combining an atrial switch with either an arterial switch or Rastelli repair (in cases in which the left ventricle is functioning at systemic pressures), have been performed in young patients with encouraging early outcomes (**Class I, Level B**), but reinterventions are common and long-term survival rates are not available.[153]

Univentricular physiology and the Fontan procedure

Nomenclature, anatomic findings, and pathophysiology

Although some patients with univentricular hearts may survive into their sixth decade without operation,[154] most of them presenting in adulthood will have had previous surgical interventions. This section focuses on patients with the Fontan circulation.

Univentricular heart or "single ventricle" Despite controversial nomenclature and classification, the term "univentricular heart" usually refers to several congenital cardiac defects in which a biventricular repair is not possible,[155] such as tricuspid and mitral atresia, double-inlet ventricle, hypoplastic left heart syndrome, heterotaxy syndromes, etc. The pathophysiology of the univentricular heart depends on the underlying anatomy and physiology; the most favorable involves an unrestrictive ASD, a well-balanced systemic and pulmonary circulation and preserved ventricular function.[155]

Palliative procedures as a prelude for the Fontan operation (neonatal period)
- Arterial-to-pulmonary shunt: performed in patients with severe pulmonary obstruction.
- Blalock–Taussig shunt: end-to-side anastomosis of the subclavian and pulmonary artery.
- Modified Blalock–Taussig shunt: tube graft connecting the subclavian artery to the ipsilateral pulmonary artery.
- Waterston shunt: connection between the ascending aorta and the pulmonary artery.
- Potts shunt: connection between the descending aorta and the left pulmonary artery.
- Pulmonary artery banding: initial palliation for infants with unrestricted pulmonary blood flow.

Second- stage palliation (~4–12 months of age) Bidirectional Glenn shunt: end-to-side anastomosis of the superior vena cava to the right PA. Older patients may have had a classic Glenn (end-to-end anastomosis of the SVC to the disconnected right PA).

Fontan operation (usually 18 months to 4 years of age or later) Consists of a connection of the systemic venous return to the PAs without the interposition of a subpulmonary ventricle. In the classic Fontan repair (no longer used), the RA was anastomosed to the PA via a valved conduit.[156] Many adults today will have had a modified Fontan, in which the right atrium was directly anastomosed to the PA.[157]

Total cavopulmonary connection (TCPC) (Fig. 63.7) Currently, TCPC is the surgical technique of choice. It combines a bidirectional Glenn (see above), together with a connection of the inferior vena cava to the PA by a lateral tunnel[158] or an extracardiac conduit. A fenestration is also created between the tunnel conduit and the pulmonary atrium to allow a right-to-left shunting, which helps the immediate postoperative course and can be closed later with a catheter approach.[159]

Clinical presentation of adults with Fontan circulation
Adults with Fontan physiology often present with the clinical picture related to the long-term sequelae of this

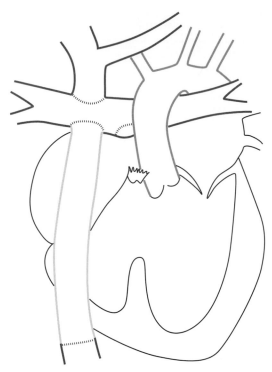

Figure 63.7 Univentricular physiology and total cavopulmonary connection.

procedure (see below). Physical examination reveals elevated non-pulsatile jugular venous pressure with prominent A-wave, and single (often accentuated) second sound. Heart murmurs are normally not present. If the patient has a dominant left ventricle, the ECG will show left axis deviation, tall and broad P-wave, and left ventricular strain, while a dominant right ventricle will create superior frontal QRS axis and right ventricular hypertrophy.[155] Intra-atrial re-entry tachycardia (or atypical atrial flutter) is common, and sinus node dysfunction can also occur following the Fontan procedure.[160] Chest radiograph and echocardiogram also depend on the initial anatomic defect.

Outcomes
Earlier studies reported a 10-year survival of ~70% following initial Fontan operations.[161,162] Modified Fontans with lateral tunnel or extracardiac conduit seem to have better outcomes, with a 10-year survival ranging between 85% and 94%.[163,164] In a recent study from a single center, the 15-year survival after atriopulmonary connection was 81% versus 94% for lateral tunnel.[165]

Complications and their management (Table 63.17)
Supraventricular tachycardias (SVT, most often intra-atrial re-entry tachycardia) are a major cause of late morbidity[166]; incidence increases with time. The 15-year freedom from SVT is 61% for atriopulmonary connections versus 87% for the lateral tunnel technique.[165] Transcatheter

Table 63.17 Complications

Tachyarrhythmias (often intra-atrial re-entry tachycardia)
Bradyarrhythmias: sinus node dysfunction
Thromboembolic events
Hepatic dysfunction
Protein-losing enteropathy
Cyanosis
Pulmonary arteriovenous malformations
Obstruction of pulmonary veins (giant RA or aorta)
Residual interatrial communication
Systemic venous collateralization
Hepatic venous connection to the coronary sinus or LA
Ventricular dysfunction and failure
Obstruction or leaks in the Fontan pathway

Table 63.18 Common causes of Eisenmenger syndrome

Simple lesions
VSD
ASD
PDA
Aortopulmonary window
Total or partial anomalous pulmonary venous return

Complex lesions
AVSD
Truncus arteriosus
Univentricular heart with unobstructed pulmonary blood flow
TGA with large ventricular or arterial shunt

radiofrequency ablation is the treatment of choice, although recurrence is common.[167] When tachyarrhythmias occur, underlying hemodynamic lesions such as obstruction of the Fontan pathway should be excluded[155] (**Class I, Level C**). Patients with failing Fontan should be considered for reoperation (**Class I, Level C**). Revision of the circuit to an extracardiac conduit or lateral tunnel, in combination with MAZE procedure, can be useful in selected cases.[168] Heart transplantation may be considered for severe ventricular dysfunction or protein-losing enteropathy (**Class IIb, Level C**).

Eisenmenger syndrome

Definition, classification, and pathophysiology

Eisenmenger syndrome represents the extreme end of the spectrum of pulmonary PAH in patients with CHD.[169] It consists of PAH with reversed (right-to-left) or bidirectional shunting and cyanosis.[170] Patients who develop Eisenmenger syndrome have a large communication at atrial, ventricular or arterial level with consequent increase in pulmonary blood flow, resulting with time in pulmonary vascular disease.

Clinical presentation

Most patients with Eisenmenger syndrome have shortness of breath and exercise intolerance.[31,171] Palpitations, chest pain, edema or syncope may occur. Patients can also present with symptoms related to one of the complications of Eisenmenger syndrome (see below). Examination depends on the underlying defect, but physical findings usually include:
- central cyanosis
- clubbing

- RV lift
- loud P2 ± pulmonary ejection click
- holosystolic murmur of TR or PR may be present.

Diagnostic evaluation

Electrocardiogram
The ECG may show right axis deviation, RA enlargement and RV hypertrophy. Arrhythmias may occur.

Chest radiography
Central pulmonary arteries are most often dilated or aneurysmal, and calcifications may be present. Chest radiogram may also reveal cardiomegaly due to right atrial and ventricular enlargement.

Digital oximetry
Pulse oximetry, both with and without supplemental oxygen therapy, should be assessed at least yearly (**Class I, Level C**).

Echocardiography
Echocardiography should:
- specify the underlying defect and anatomy
- estimate RV systolic pressure
- determine the level, size and direction of shunting.

Exercise testing
The 6-minute walk test and cardiopulmonary exercise testing with peak oxygen consumption can both be used to assess functional capacity. Exercise-induced desaturation provides prognostic information[31,169] and helps to assess response to advanced therapies (**Class IIa, Level C**).

CMR and CT angiography
CMR allows a more precise visualization of the anatomy, while CT angiography is useful to exclude the possibility of pulmonary embolism and assess the lung parenchyma.

Cardiac catheterization and angiography

Cardiac catheterization in patients with Eisenmenger syndrome may be useful to confirm the diagnosis and evaluate severity of PAH. Furthermore, it can assess the pulmonary vascular resistance and determine vasoreactivity; the latter seems to have prognostic value[172] (**Class I, Level C**).

Laboratory testing

Full blood count, electrolytes, urea, creatinine, liver function tests and uric acid should be part of the routine laboratory assessment (**Class I, Level C**). Secondary erythrocytosis facilitates tissue oxygenation.[169] Moreover, iron status should be carefully evaluated by measurement of transferrin saturation and ferritin. Indeed, iron deficiency is common in patients with Eisenmenger syndrome, whereas the classic microcytosis and hypochromia are often absent.[169,173,174] Iron deficiency in this population has been associated with decreased exercise tolerance and increased risk of stroke.[175,176]

Outcomes and complications

Actuarial survival of patients with Eisenmenger syndrome has been reported to be 75%, 70%, and 55% at the age of 30, 40, and 50 years respectively.[171] Eisenmenger syndrome is a multiorgan disease (Table 63.19).

Table 63.19 Complications of Eisenmenger syndrome

Hematologic complications
Secondary erythrocytosis
Hyperviscosity symptoms (may be due to iron deficiency)
Headache, altered mentation, blurred vision, paresthesia, myalgia
Thrombocytopenia
Iron deficiency

Bleeding complications
Hemoptysis, pulmonary hemorrhage, cerebral bleeding, epistaxis

Thrombotic and thromboembolic events
Intrapulmonary thrombosis
Cerebrovascular accidents
Arrhythmias (supraventricular or ventricular) and sudden cardiac death

Viral and bacterial infections
Endocarditis
Cerebral abcess
Pneumonia

Renal dysfunction
Glomerular abnormalities
Hyperuricemia and gout
Gallstones and cholecystitis
Hypertrophic osteoarthropathy

Management

The main goal is to avoid complications. The following general recommendations apply.
- Iron deficiency should be treated with iron supplementation (**Class I, Level B**).
- Routine phlebotomy is contraindicated (**Class III**). Phlebotomy should be restricted to patients with hemoglobin greater than 20 g/dL and hematocrit greater than 65%, associated with severe hyperviscosity symptoms, in the absence of dehydration and iron deficiency (**Class I, Level C**).
- Anemia and dehydration should be avoided and treated promptly (**Class I, Level C**).
- Contraception advice should be provided and pregnancy strongly discouraged (risk of death reported as 30–50%) (**Class I, Level B**).
- Strenuous exercise and chronic high altitude should be avoided (**Class I, Level C**).
- Anticoagulation should be discussed with the patient (**Level C**).
- Long-term nocturnal oxygen may have a role for selected patients[177] (**Level C**).
- Vaccination: flu shot annually + Pneumovax every 5 years (**Level C**).
- Non-selective endothelin receptor antagonist (such as bosentan) or phosphodiesterase inhibitors (such as sildenafil) should be considered for patients in WHO functional class ≥III[172,178–180] (**Class IIa, Level C**).

Arrhythmias in adult congenital heart disease

Arrhythmias represent one of the most common long-term complications in patients with CHD, posing new challenges in terms of management. Rhythm anomalies can be part of the natural history of the underlying defect itself, but most of them arise from consequences of surgical interventions or from long-standing abnormal hemodynamics. Specific arrhythmias associated with CHD and their management[181] are summarized below and in Table 63.20.

Intra-atrial re-entrant tachycardia (IART)

Intra-atrial re-entrant tachycardia is the most common arrhythmia in this population. The mechanism is a macrore-entry circuit within the atrium, usually occurring years after surgical intervention involving the right atrial tissue. This "atypical" atrial flutter is more frequent in patients with previous *Mustard* and *Senning* procedures, or classic *Fontan* operations (severe dilation and scarring of the RA), but it can also occur even after simple ASD closure. Atrial rates are usually between 150 and 250 per minute

Table 63.20 Most frequent arrhythmias in CHD lesions

CHD/arrhythmia	IART	WPW	Atrial fibrillation	VT	Sinus node dysfunction	AV block
ASD	x		x		x	
AVSD			x			x
TOF	x		x	x		
Mustard/Senning	x		x	x	x	
cc-TGA		x	x	x		x
Fontan	x		x		x	
AS/coarctation			x			
Ebstein	x	x	x	x		

and 1:1 AV conduction can lead to severe symptoms such as syncope and even cardiac arrest. Therapeutic options include[181]:

- acute episode can be terminated with electrical cardioversion, antiarrhythmic drugs or overdrive pacing
- long-term antiarrhythmic drug therapy: often ineffective
- catheter ablation[182]: often used as an early intervention. Good short- to mid-term success, reduces the frequency of episodes, but relatively high recurrence rates have been reported
- pacemaker implantation: used for patients with tachy-brady syndrome; decrease in IART frequency by addressing bradycardia and by incorporating antitachycardia pacing facility
- surgical ablation with a modified right atrial MAZE operation: low rates of recurrence but associated with surgical risks; often performed in patients who already have other surgical indications.

Re-entrant tachycardia secondary to accessory pathways

Wolff–Parkinson–White syndrome occurs in ~20% of patients with *Ebstein anomaly*. About half of them have multiple accessory pathways. Even if the success rate is lower than in the general population, catheter ablation remains the procedure of choice for Wolff–Parkinson–White syndrome in Ebstein patients.[181]

Atrial fibrillation

Congenital heart disease conditions associated with left atrial pressure and/or volume overload predispose to atrial fibrillation. Mitral valve abnormalities (or left AVV in the setting of an AVSD), AS, left ventricular dysfunction (or systemic right ventricular dysfunction in the setting of a cc-TGA) with elevated end-diastolic pressures, and unrepaired single ventricle are such defects. General management of atrial fibrillation is the same as for other groups. Early intervention to improve or restore target hemodynamic lesions should be encouraged.

Ventricular tachycardia

Ventricular tachycardia and sudden cardiac death have become a major issue in selected patients with CHD reaching adulthood. Macrore-entrant circuits in the regions of a previous surgical scar can occur following a ventriculotomy or patching for a VSD. Other mechanisms that might be involved in arrhythmogenesis are severe ventricular dysfunction and/or hypertrophy with fibrosis. *TOF, aortic valve disease, cc-TGA* with systemic RV dysfunction, *Eisenmenger syndrome*, and severe *Ebstein anomaly* are lesions with increased risk of VT.

Sinus node dysfunction

Sinus node dysfunction late after surgical repair is the most common cause of sinus bradycardia in patients with CHD. *Mustard, Senning, Glenn,* and *Fontan* operations can all be associated with sinus node dysfunction. Pacemaker implantation is indicated if the bradycardia is associated with symptoms. *Left atrial isomerism* is associated with absence of sinus node and atrial or junctional escape rhythm with bradycardia.

AV block

Congenitally corrected TGA and *AVSD* both carry an intrinsic risk of developing complete AVB with time. Complete AVB can also result from surgical trauma following VSD closure, resection of LVOTO or replacement/repair of an AVV. Postoperative AVB is often transient, but pacemaker implantation is indicated if it does not recover within 7–10 days from surgery.

References

1. Pierpont ME, Basson CT, Benson DW Jr, Gelb BD, Giglia TM, Goldmuntz E *et al*. Genetic basis for congenital heart defects: current knowledge: a scientific statement from the American Heart Association Congenital Cardiac Defects Committee, Council on Cardiovascular Disease in the Young: endorsed by the American Academy of Pediatrics. *Circulation* 2007;**115**(23):3015–38.

2. Hoffman JI, Kaplan S. The incidence of congenital heart disease. *J Am Coll Cardiol* 2002;**39**(12):1890–900.

3. Nieminen HP, Jokinen EV, Sairanen HI. Late results of pediatric cardiac surgery in Finland: a population-based study with 96% follow-up. *Circulation* 2001;**104**(5):570–5.

4. Marelli AJ, Mackie AS, Ionescu-Ittu R, Rahme E, Pilote L. Congenital heart disease in the general population: changing prevalence and age distribution. *Circulation* 2007;**115**(2):163–72.

5. Gatzoulis MA. Adult congenital heart disease: education, education, education. *Nat Clin Pract Cardiovasc Med* 2006;**3**(1):2–3.

6. Mackie AS, Pilote L, Ionescu-Ittu R, Rahme E, Marelli AJ. Health care resource utilization in adults with congenital heart disease. *Am J Cardiol* 2007;**99**(6):839–43.

7. Gurvitz MZ, Inkelas M, Lee M, Stout K, Escarce J, Chang RK. Changes in hospitalization patterns among patients with congenital heart disease during the transition from adolescence to adulthood. *J Am Coll Cardiol* 2007;**49**(8):875–82.

7a. Warnes CA, Williams RG, Bashore TM, Child JS, Connolly HM, Dearani JA *et al*. ACC/AHA 2008 Guidelines for the Management of Adults With Congenital Heart Disease: Executive Summary. A Report of the American College of Cardiology/American Heart Association Task Force on Practice Guidelines (Writing Committee to Develop Guidelines for the Management of Adults With Congenital Heart Disease) Developed in Collaboration With the American Society of Echocardiography, Heart Rhythm Society, International Society for Adult Congenital Heart Disease, Society for Cardiovascular Angiography and Interventions, and Society of Thoracic Surgeons. *J Am Coll Cardiol* 2008;**52**(23):1890–947.

8. Jenkins KJ, Correa A, Feinstein JA, Botto L, Britt AE, Daniels SR *et al*. Noninherited risk factors and congenital cardiovascular defects: current knowledge: a scientific statement from the American Heart Association Council on Cardiovascular Disease in the Young: endorsed by the American Academy of Pediatrics. *Circulation* 2007;**115**(23):2995–3014.

9. Therrien J, Warnes C, Daliento L, Hess J, Hoffmann A, Marelli A *et al*. Canadian Cardiovascular Society Consensus Conference 2001 update: recommendations for the management of adults with congenital heart disease part III. *Can J Cardiol* 2001;**17**(11):1135–58.

10. Webb G, Gatzoulis MA. Atrial septal defects in the adult: recent progress and overview. *Circulation* 2006;**114**(15):1645–53.

11. Gatzoulis MA, Freeman MA, Siu SC, Webb GD, Harris L. Atrial arrhythmia after surgical closure of atrial septal defects in adults. *N Engl J Med* 1999;**340**(11):839–46.

12. Carmichael DB, Forrester RH, Inmon TW, Mattingly TW, Pollock BE, Walker WJ. Electrocardiographic and hemodynamic correlation in atrial septal defect. *Am Heart J* 1956;**52**(4):547–61.

13. Toscano Barboza E, Brandenburg RO, Swan HJ. Atrial septal defect; the electrocardiogram and its hemodynamic correlation in 100 proved cases. *Am J Cardiol* 1958;**2**(6):698–713.

14. Heller J, Hagege AA, Besse B, Desnos M, Marie FN, Guerot C. "Crochetage" (notch) on R wave in inferior limb leads: a new independent electrocardiographic sign of atrial septal defect. *J Am Coll Cardiol* 1996;**27**(4):877–82.

15. Davia JE, Cheitlin MD, Bedynek JL. Sinus venosus atrial septal defect: analysis of fifty cases. *Am Heart J* 1973;**85**(2):177–85.

16. Attenhofer Jost CH, Connolly HM, Danielson GK, Bailey KR, Schaff HV, Shen WK *et al*. Sinus venosus atrial septal defect: long-term postoperative outcome for 115 patients. *Circulation* 2005;**112**(13):1953–8.

17. Simon M. The pulmonary vasculature in congenital heart disease. *Radiol Clin North Am* 1968;**6**(3):303–17.

18. Egeblad H, Berning J, Efsen F, Wennevold A. Non-invasive diagnosis in clinically suspected atrial septal defect of secundum or sinus venosus type. Value of combining chest x-ray, phonocardiography, and M-mode echocardiography. *Br Heart J* 1980;**44**(3):317–21.

19. Chau AK, Leung MP, Yung T, Chan K, Cheung Y, Chiu S. Surgical validation and implications for transcatheter closure of quantitative echocardiographic evaluation of atrial septal defect. *Am J Cardiol* 2000;**85**(9):1124–30.

20. Vargas Barron J, Sahn DJ, Valdes-Cruz LM, Lima CO, Goldberg SJ, Grenadier E *et al*. Clinical utility of two-dimensional doppler echocardiographic techniques for estimating pulmonary to systemic blood flow ratios in children with left to right shunting atrial septal defect, ventricular septal defect or patent ductus arteriosus. *J Am Coll Cardiol* 1984;**3**(1):169–78.

21. Radtke WE, Tajik AJ, Gau GT, Schattenberg TT, Giuliani ER, Tancredi RG. Atrial septal defect: echocardiographic observations. Studies in 120 patients. *Ann Intern Med* 1976;**84**(3):246–53.

22. Lieppe W, Scallion R, Behar VS, Kisslo JA. Two-dimensional echocardiographic findings in atrial septal defect. *Circulation* 1977;**56**(3):447–56.

23. Prasad SK, Soukias N, Hornung T, Khan M, Pennell DJ, Gatzoulis MA *et al*. Role of magnetic resonance angiography in the diagnosis of major aortopulmonary collateral arteries and partial anomalous pulmonary venous drainage. *Circulation* 2004;**109**(2):207–14.

24. Brochu MC, Baril JF, Dore A, Juneau M, De Guise P, Mercier LA. Improvement in exercise capacity in asymptomatic and mildly symptomatic adults after atrial septal defect percutaneous closure. *Circulation* 2002;**106**(14):1821–6.

25. Inglessis I, Landzberg MJ. Interventional catheterization in adult congenital heart disease. *Circulation* 2007;**115**(12):1622–33.

26. Du ZD, Hijazi ZM, Kleinman CS, Silverman NH, Larntz K. Comparison between transcatheter and surgical closure of secundum atrial septal defect in children and adults: results of a multicenter nonrandomized trial. *J Am Coll Cardiol* 2002;**39**(11):1836–44.

27. Veldtman GR, Razack V, Siu S, El-Hajj H, Walker F, Webb GD *et al*. Right ventricular form and function after percutaneous atrial septal defect device closure. *J Am Coll Cardiol* 2001;**37**(8):2108–13.

28. Murphy JG, Gersh BJ, McGoon MD, Mair DD, Porter CJ, Ilstrup DM et al. Long-term outcome after surgical repair of isolated atrial septal defect. Follow-up at 27 to 32 years. *N Engl J Med* 1990;**323**(24):1645–50.

29. Konstantinides S, Geibel A, Olschewski M, Gornandt L, Roskamm H, Spillner G et al. A comparison of surgical and medical therapy for atrial septal defect in adults. *N Engl J Med* 1995;**333**(8):469–73.

30. Attie F, Rosas M, Granados N, Zabal C, Buendia A, Calderon J. Surgical treatment for secundum atrial septal defects in patients >40 years old. A randomized clinical trial. *J Am Coll Cardiol* 2001;**38**(7):2035–42.

31. Diller GP, Dimopoulos K, Okonko D, Li W, Babu-Narayan SV, Broberg CS et al. Exercise intolerance in adult congenital heart disease: comparative severity, correlates, and prognostic implication. *Circulation* 2005;**112**(6):828–35.

32. Helber U, Baumann R, Seboldt H, Reinhard U, Hoffmeister HM. Atrial septal defect in adults: cardiopulmonary exercise capacity before and 4 months and 10 years after defect closure. *J Am Coll Cardiol* 1997;**29**(6):1345–50.

33. Roguin N, Du ZD, Barak M, Nasser N, Hershkowitz S, Milgram E. High prevalence of muscular ventricular septal defect in neonates. *J Am Coll Cardiol* 1995;**26**(6):1545–8.

34. Soto B, Becker AE, Moulaert AJ, Lie JT, Anderson RH. Classification of ventricular septal defects. *Br Heart J* 1980;**43**(3):332–43.

35. Roos-Hesselink JW, Meijboom FJ, Spitaels SE, Van Domburg R, Van Rijen EH, Utens EM et al. Outcome of patients after surgical closure of ventricular septal defect at young age: longitudinal follow-up of 22–34 years. *Eur Heart J* 2004;**25**(12):1057–62.

36. Moller JH, Patton C, Varco RL, Lillehei CW. Late results (30 to 35 years) after operative closure of isolated ventricular septal defect from 1954 to 1960. *Am J Cardiol* 1991;**68**(15):1491–7.

37. Andersen HO, de Leval MR, Tsang VT, Elliott MJ, Anderson RH, Cook AC. Is complete heart block after surgical closure of ventricular septum defects still an issue? *Ann Thorac Surg* 2006;**82**(3):948–56.

38. Capelli H, Andrade JL, Somerville J. Classification of the site of ventricular septal defect by 2-dimensional echocardiography. *Am J Cardiol* 1983;**51**(9):1474–80.

39. Sutherland GR, Godman MJ, Smallhorn JF, Guiterras P, Anderson RH, Hunter S. Ventricular septal defects. Two dimensional echocardiographic and morphological correlations. *Br Heart J* 1982;**47**(4):316–28.

40. Kardon RE, Cao QL, Masani N, Sugeng L, Supran S, Warner KG et al. New insights and observations in three-dimensional echocardiographic visualization of ventricular septal defects: experimental and clinical studies. *Circulation* 1998;**98**(13):1307–14.

41. Nygren A, Sunnegardh J, Berggren H. Preoperative evaluation and surgery in isolated ventricular septal defects: a 21 year perspective. *Heart* 2000;**83**(2):198–204.

42. Tucker EM, Pyles LA, Bass JL, Moller JH. Permanent pacemaker for atrioventricular conduction block after operative repair of perimembranous ventricular septal defect. *J Am Coll Cardiol* 2007;**50**(12):1196–200.

43. Gabriel HM, Heger M, Innerhofer P, Zehetgruber M, Mundigler G, Wimmer M et al. Long-term outcome of patients with ventricular septal defect considered not to require surgical closure during childhood. *J Am Coll Cardiol* 2002;**39**(6):1066–71.

44. Kidd L, Driscoll DJ, Gersony WM, Hayes CJ, Keane JF, O'Fallon WM et al. Second natural history study of congenital heart defects. Results of treatment of patients with ventricular septal defects. *Circulation* 1993;**87**(2 suppl):I38–51.

45. Neumayer U, Stone S, Somerville J. Small ventricular septal defects in adults. *Eur Heart J* 1998;**19**(10):1573–82.

46. Gersony WM, Hayes CJ, Driscoll DJ, Keane JF, Kidd L, O'Fallon WM et al. Bacterial endocarditis in patients with aortic stenosis, pulmonary stenosis, or ventricular septal defect. *Circulation* 1993;**87**(2 suppl):I121–6.

47. Wolfe RR, Driscoll DJ, Gersony WM, Hayes CJ, Keane JF, Kidd L et al. Arrhythmias in patients with valvar aortic stenosis, valvar pulmonary stenosis, and ventricular septal defect. Results of 24-hour ECG monitoring. *Circulation* 1993;**87**(2 suppl):I89–101.

48. Suzuki K, Ho SY, Anderson RH, Becker AE, Neches WH, Devine WA et al. Morphometric analysis of atrioventricular septal defect with common valve orifice. *J Am Coll Cardiol* 1998;**31**(1):217–23.

49. Feldt RH, DuShane JW, Titus JL. The atrioventricular conduction system in persistent common atrioventricular canal defect: correlations with electrocardiogram. *Circulation* 1970;**42**(3):437–44.

50. Craig B. Atrioventricular septal defect: from fetus to adult. *Heart* 2006;**92**(12):1879–85.

51. Huggon IC, Cook AC, Smeeton NC, Magee AG, Sharland GK. Atrioventricular septal defects diagnosed in fetal life: associated cardiac and extra-cardiac abnormalities and outcome. *J Am Coll Cardiol* 2000;**36**(2):593–601.

52. Al-Hay AA, MacNeill SJ, Yacoub M, Shore DF, Shinebourne EA. Complete atrioventricular septal defect, Down syndrome, and surgical outcome: risk factors. *Ann Thorac Surg* 2003;**75**(2):412–21.

53. Hynes JK, Tajik AJ, Seward JB, Fuster V, Ritter DG, Brandenburg RO et al. Partial atrioventricular canal defect in adults. *Circulation* 1982;**66**(2):284–7.

54. Fournier A, Young ML, Garcia OL, Tamer DF, Wolff GS. Electrophysiologic cardiac function before and after surgery in children with atrioventricular canal. *Am J Cardiol* 1986;**57**(13):1137–41.

55. Silverman NH, Zuberbuhler JR, Anderson RH. Atrioventricular septal defects: cross-sectional echocardiographic and morphologic comparisons. *Int J Cardiol* 1986;**13**(3):309–31.

56. Sulafa AK, Tamimi O, Najm HK, Godman MJ. Echocardiographic differentiation of atrioventricular septal defects from inlet ventricular septal defects and mitral valve clefts. *Am J Cardiol* 2005;**95**(5):607–10.

57. Smallhorn JF. Cross-sectional echocardiographic assessment of atrioventricular septal defect: basic morphology and preoperative risk factors. *Echocardiography* 2001;**18**(5):415–32.

58. Sittiwangkul R, Ma RY, McCrindle BW, Coles JG, Smallhorn JF. Echocardiographic assessment of obstructive lesions in atrioventricular septal defects. *J Am Coll Cardiol* 2001;**38**(1):253–61.

59. Parsons JM, Baker EJ, Anderson RH, Ladusans EJ, Hayes A, Qureshi SA et al. Morphological evaluation of atrioventricular septal defects by magnetic resonance imaging. *Br Heart J* 1990;**64**(2):138–45.

60. Najm HK, Coles JG, Endo M, Stephens D, Rebeyka IM, Williams WG *et al.* Complete atrioventricular septal defects: results of repair, risk factors, and freedom from reoperation. *Circulation* 1997;**96**(9 suppl):II-311–5.

61. Wetter J, Sinzobahamvya N, Blaschczok C, Brecher AM, Gravinghoff LM, Schmaltz AA *et al.* Closure of the zone of apposition at correction of complete atrioventricular septal defect improves outcome. *Eur J Cardiothorac Surg* 2000;**17**(2):146–53.

62. Bergin ML, Warnes CA, Tajik AJ, Danielson GK. Partial atrioventricular canal defect: long-term follow-up after initial repair in patients > or = 40 years old. *J Am Coll Cardiol* 1995;**25**(5): 1189–94.

63. Berger TJ, Blackstone EH, Kirklin JW, Bargeron LM Jr, Hazelrig JB, Turner ME Jr. Survival and probability of cure without and with operation in complete atrioventricular canal. *Ann Thorac Surg* 1979;**27**(2):104–11.

64. El-Najdawi EK, Driscoll DJ, Puga FJ, Dearani JA, Spotts BE, Mahoney DW *et al.* Operation for partial atrioventricular septal defect: a forty-year review. *J Thorac Cardiovasc Surg* 2000; **119**(5):880–9; discussion 9–90.

65. Brauner R, Laks H, Drinkwater DC Jr, Shvarts O, Eghbali K, Galindo A. Benefits of early surgical repair in fixed subaortic stenosis. *J Am Coll Cardiol* 1997;**30**(7):1835–42.

66. Aboulhosn J, Child JS. Left ventricular outflow obstruction: subaortic stenosis, bicuspid aortic valve, supravalvar aortic stenosis, and coarctation of the aorta. *Circulation* 2006;**114**(22): 2412–22.

67. Oliver JM, Gonzalez A, Gallego P, Sanchez-Recalde A, Benito F, Mesa JM. Discrete subaortic stenosis in adults: increased prevalence and slow rate of progression of the obstruction and aortic regurgitation. *J Am Coll Cardiol* 2001;**38**(3):835–42.

68. Roberts WC, Ko JM. Frequency by decades of unicuspid, bicuspid, and tricuspid aortic valves in adults having isolated aortic valve replacement for aortic stenosis, with or without associated aortic regurgitation. *Circulation* 2005;**111**(7):920–5.

69. Fedak PW, Verma S, David TE, Leask RL, Weisel RD, Butany J. Clinical and pathophysiological implications of a bicuspid aortic valve. *Circulation* 2002;**106**(8):900–4.

70. Huntington K, Hunter AG, Chan KL. A prospective study to assess the frequency of familial clustering of congenital bicuspid aortic valve. *J Am Coll Cardiol* 1997;**30**(7):1809–12.

71. Niwa K, Perloff JK, Bhuta SM, Laks H, Drinkwater DC, Child JS *et al.* Structural abnormalities of great arterial walls in congenital heart disease: light and electron microscopic analyses. *Circulation* 2001;**103**(3):393–400.

72. Keating MT. Genetic approaches to cardiovascular disease. Supravalvular aortic stenosis, Williams syndrome, and long-QT syndrome. *Circulation* 1995;**92**(1):142–7.

73. Pellikka PA, Sarano ME, Nishimura RA, Malouf JF, Bailey KR, Scott CG *et al.* Outcome of 622 adults with asymptomatic, hemodynamically significant aortic stenosis during prolonged follow-up. *Circulation* 2005;**111**(24):3290–5.

74. Gersony WM. Natural history of discrete subvalvar aortic stenosis: management implications. *J Am Coll Cardiol* 2001;**38**(3): 843–5.

75. Bonow RO, Carabello BA, Kanu C, de Leon AC Jr, Faxon DP, Freed MD *et al.* ACC/AHA 2006 guidelines for the management of patients with valvular heart disease: a report of the American College of Cardiology/American Heart Association Task Force on Practice Guidelines (Writing Committee to Revise the 1998 Guidelines for the Management of Patients With Valvular Heart Disease): developed in collaboration with the Society of Cardiovascular Anesthesiologists: endorsed by the Society for Cardiovascular Angiography and Interventions and the Society of Thoracic Surgeons. *Circulation* 2006;**114**(5): e84–231.

76. Coleman DM, Smallhorn JF, McCrindle BW, Williams WG, Freedom RM. Postoperative follow-up of fibromuscular subaortic stenosis. *J Am Coll Cardiol* 1994;**24**(6):1558–64.

77. Rizzoli G, Tiso E, Mazzucco A, Daliento L, Rubino M, Tursi V *et al.* Discrete subaortic stenosis. Operative age and gradient as predictors of late aortic valve incompetence. *J Thorac Cardiovasc Surg* 1993;**106**(1):95–104.

78. Geva A, McMahon CJ, Gauvreau K, Mohammed L, del Nido PJ, Geva T. Risk factors for reoperation after repair of discrete subaortic stenosis in children. *J Am Coll Cardiol* 2007;**50**(15): 1498–504.

79. de Vries AG, Hess J, Witsenburg M, Frohn-Mulder IM, Bogers JJ, Bos E. Management of fixed subaortic stenosis: a retrospective study of 57 cases. *J Am Coll Cardiol* 1992;**19**(5):1013–17.

80. Carabello BA. Evaluation and management of patients with aortic stenosis. *Circulation* 2002;**105**(15):1746–50.

81. Tawes RL Jr, Berry CL, Aberdeen E. Congenital bicuspid aortic valves associated with coarctation of the aorta in children. *Br Heart J* 1969;**31**(1):127–8.

82. Scovil JA, Nanda NC, Gross CM, Lombardi AC, Gramiak R, Lipchick EO *et al.* Echocardiographic studies of abnormalities associated with coarctation of the aorta. *Circulation* 1976;**53**(6): 953–6.

83. Edwards JE. The congenital bicuspid aortic valve. *Circulation* 1961;**23**:485–8.

84. Connolly HM, Huston J 3rd, Brown RD Jr, Warnes CA, Ammash NM, Tajik AJ. Intracranial aneurysms in patients with coarctation of the aorta: a prospective magnetic resonance angiographic study of 100 patients. *Mayo Clin Proc* 2003;**78**(12): 1491–9.

85. Glancy DL, Morrow AG, Simon AL, Roberts WC. Juxtaductal aortic coarctation. Analysis of 84 patients studied hemodynamically, angiographically, and morphologically after age 1 year. *Am J Cardiol* 1983;**51**(3):537–51.

86. Marx GR, Allen HD. Accuracy and pitfalls of Doppler evaluation of the pressure gradient in aortic coarctation. *J Am Coll Cardiol* 1986;**7**(6):1379–85.

87. Teirstein PS, Yock PG, Popp RL. The accuracy of Doppler ultrasound measurement of pressure gradients across irregular, dual, and tunnellike obstructions to blood flow. *Circulation* 1985;**72**(3):577–84.

88. Houston AB, Simpson IA, Pollock JC, Jamieson MP, Doig WB, Coleman EN. Doppler ultrasound in the assessment of severity of coarctation of the aorta and interruption of the aortic arch. *Br Heart J* 1987;**57**(1):38–43.

89. Tacy TA, Baba K, Cape EG. Effect of aortic compliance on Doppler diastolic flow pattern in coarctation of the aorta. *J Am Soc Echocardiogr* 1999;**12**(8):636–42.

90. Tan JL, Babu-Narayan SV, Henein MY, Mullen M, Li W. Doppler echocardiographic profile and indexes in the evaluation of aortic coarctation in patients before and after stenting. *J Am Coll Cardiol* 2005;**46**(6):1045–53.

91. Carvalho JS, Redington AN, Shinebourne EA, Rigby ML, Gibson D. Continuous wave Doppler echocardiography and coarctation of the aorta: gradients and flow patterns in the assessment of severity. *Br Heart J* 1990;**64**(2):133–7.

92. Lim DS, Ralston MA. Echocardiographic indices of Doppler flow patterns compared with MRI or angiographic measurements to detect significant coarctation of the aorta. *Echocardiography* 2002;**19**(1):55–60.

93. Nielsen JC, Powell AJ, Gauvreau K, Marcus EN, Prakash A, Geva T. Magnetic resonance imaging predictors of coarctation severity. *Circulation* 2005;**111**(5):622–8.

94. Parks WJ, Ngo TD, Plauth WH Jr, Bank ER, Sheppard SK, Pettigrew RI *et al.* Incidence of aneurysm formation after Dacron patch aortoplasty repair for coarctation of the aorta: long-term results and assessment utilizing magnetic resonance angiography with three-dimensional surface rendering. *J Am Coll Cardiol* 1995;**26**(1):266–71.

95. Kaemmerer H. Aortic coarctation and interrupted aortic arch. *Diagn Manage Adult Congen Heart Dis* 2003:253–64.

96. Cowley CG, Orsmond GS, Feola P, McQuillan L, Shaddy RE. Long-term, randomized comparison of balloon angioplasty and surgery for native coarctation of the aorta in childhood. *Circulation* 2005;**111**(25):3453–6.

97. Chessa M, Carrozza M, Butera G, Piazza L, Negura DG, Bussadori C *et al.* Results and mid-long-term follow-up of stent implantation for native and recurrent coarctation of the aorta. *Eur Heart J* 2005;**26**(24):2728–32.

98. Campbell M. Natural history of coarctation of the aorta. *Br Heart J* 1970;**32**(5):633–40.

99. Cohen M, Fuster V, Steele PM, Driscoll D, McGoon DC. Coarctation of the aorta. Long-term follow-up and prediction of outcome after surgical correction. *Circulation* 1989;**80**(4):840–5.

100. Becker TE, Ensing GJ, Darragh RK, Caldwell RL. Doppler derivation of complete pulmonary artery pressure curves in patent ductus arteriosus. *Am J Cardiol* 1996;**78**(9):1066–9.

101. Taneja K, Gulati M, Jain M, Saxena A, Das B, Rajani M. Ductus arteriosus aneurysm in the adult: role of computed tomography in diagnosis. *Clin Radiol* 1997;**52**(3):231–4.

102. Zachary CH, Myers JL, Eggli KD. Vascular ring due to right aortic arch with mirror-image branching and left ligamentum arteriosus: complete preoperative diagnosis by magnetic resonance imaging. *Pediatr Cardiol* 2001;**22**(1):71–3.

103. Schneider DJ, Moore JW. Patent ductus arteriosus. *Circulation* 2006;**114**(17):1873–82.

104. Yamaki S, Mohri H, Haneda K, Endo M, Akimoto H. Indications for surgery based on lung biopsy in cases of ventricular septal defect and/or patent ductus arteriosus with severe pulmonary hypertension. *Chest* 1989 Jul;**96**(1):31–9.

105. Pas D, Missault L, Hollanders G, Suys B, De Wolf D. Persistent ductus arteriosus in the adult: clinical features and experience with percutaneous closure. *Acta Cardiol* 2002;**57**(4):275–8.

106. Epting CL, Wolfe RR, Abman SH, Deutsch GH, Ivy D. Reversal of pulmonary hypertension associated with plexiform lesions in congenital heart disease: a case report. *Pediatr Cardiol* 2002;**23**(2):182–5.

107. Bashore TM. Adult congenital heart disease: right ventricular outflow tract lesions. *Circulation* 2007;**115**(14):1933–47.

108. Chen JT, Robinson AE, Goodrich JK, Lester RG. Uneven distribution of pulmonary blood flow between left and right lungs in isolated valvular pulmonary stenosis. *Am J Roentgenol Rad Ther Nucl Med* 1969;**107**(2):343–50.

109. Jarrar M, Betbout F, Farhat MB, Maatouk F, Gamra H, Addad F *et al.* Long-term invasive and noninvasive results of percutaneous balloon pulmonary valvuloplasty in children, adolescents, and adults. *Am Heart J* 1999;**138**(5 Pt 1):950–4.

110. O'Connor BK, Beekman RH, Lindauer A, Rocchini A. Intermediate-term outcome after pulmonary balloon valvuloplasty: comparison with a matched surgical control group. *J Am Coll Cardiol* 1992;**20**(1):169–73.

111. Hayes CJ, Gersony WM, Driscoll DJ, Keane JF, Kidd L, O'Fallon WM *et al.* Second natural history study of congenital heart defects. Results of treatment of patients with pulmonary valvar stenosis. *Circulation* 1993;**87**(2 suppl):I28–37.

112. Attenhofer Jost CH, Connolly HM, Dearani JA, Edwards WD, Danielson GK. Ebstein's anomaly. *Circulation* 2007;**115**(2):277–85.

113. Attenhofer Jost CH, Connolly HM, O'Leary PW, Warnes CA, Tajik AJ, Seward JB. Left heart lesions in patients with Ebstein anomaly. *Mayo Clin Proc* 2005;**80**(3):361–8.

114. Celermajer DS, Bull C, Till JA, Cullen S, Vassillikos VP, Sullivan ID *et al.* Ebstein's anomaly: presentation and outcome from fetus to adult. *J Am Coll Cardiol* 1994;**23**(1):170–6.

115. Chetaille P, Walsh EP, Triedman JK. Outcomes of radiofrequency catheter ablation of atrioventricular reciprocating tachycardia in patients with congenital heart disease. *Heart Rhythm* 2004;**1**(2):168–73.

116. Cappato R, Schluter M, Weiss C, Antz M, Koschyk DH, Hofmann T *et al.* Radiofrequency current catheter ablation of accessory atrioventricular pathways in Ebstein's anomaly. *Circulation* 1996;**94**(3):376–83.

117. Quinonez LG, Dearani JA, Puga FJ, O'Leary PW, Driscoll DJ, Connolly HM *et al.* Results of the 1.5-ventricle repair for Ebstein anomaly and the failing right ventricle. *J Thorac Cardiovasc Surg* 2007;**133**(5):1303–10.

118. Roos-Hesselink J, Perlroth MG, McGhie J, Spitaels S. Atrial arrhythmias in adults after repair of tetralogy of Fallot. Correlations with clinical, exercise, and echocardiographic findings. *Circulation* 1995;**91**(8):2214–19.

119. Gatzoulis MA, Balaji S, Webber SA, Siu SC, Hokanson JS, Poile C *et al.* Risk factors for arrhythmia and sudden cardiac death late after repair of tetralogy of Fallot: a multicentre study. *Lancet.* 2000;**356**(9234):975–81.

120. Gatzoulis MA, Till JA, Somerville J, Redington AN. Mechanoelectrical interaction in tetralogy of Fallot. QRS prolongation relates to right ventricular size and predicts malignant ventricular arrhythmias and sudden death. *Circulation* 1995;**92**(2):231–7.

121. Gatzoulis MA, Till JA, Redington AN. Depolarization-repolarization inhomogeneity after repair of tetralogy of Fallot. The substrate for malignant ventricular tachycardia? *Circulation* 1997;**95**(2):401–4.

122. Therrien J, Siu SC, Harris L, Dore A, Niwa K, Janousek J *et al.* Impact of pulmonary valve replacement on arrhythmia propensity late after repair of tetralogy of Fallot. *Circulation* 2001;**103**(20):2489–94.

123. Tan JL, Gatzoulis MA, Ho SY. Aortic root disease in tetralogy of Fallot. *Curr Opin Cardiol* 2006;**21**(6):569–72.

124. Niwa K, Siu SC, Webb GD, Gatzoulis MA. Progressive aortic root dilatation in adults late after repair of tetralogy of Fallot. *Circulation* 2002;**106**(11):1374–8.

125. Gatzoulis M. Tetralogy of Fallot. *Diagn Manage Adult Congen Heart Dis* 2003:315–26.

126. Giardini A, Specchia S, Tacy TA, Coutsoumbas G, Gargiulo G, Donti A *et al.* Usefulness of cardiopulmonary exercise to predict long-term prognosis in adults with repaired tetralogy of Fallot. *Am J Cardiol* 2007;**99**(10):1462–7.

127. Therrien J, Provost Y, Merchant N, Williams W, Colman J, Webb G. Optimal timing for pulmonary valve replacement in adults after tetralogy of Fallot repair. *Am J Cardiol* 2005;**95**(6):779–82.

128. Oosterhof T, van Straten A, Vliegen HW, Meijboom FJ, van Dijk AP, Spijkerboer AM *et al.* Preoperative thresholds for pulmonary valve replacement in patients with corrected tetralogy of Fallot using cardiovascular magnetic resonance. *Circulation* 2007;**116**(5):545–51.

129. Babu-Narayan SV, Kilner PJ, Li W, Moon JC, Goktekin O, Davlouros PA *et al.* Ventricular fibrosis suggested by cardiovascular magnetic resonance in adults with repaired tetralogy of fallot and its relationship to adverse markers of clinical outcome. *Circulation* 2006;**113**(3):405–13.

130. Hu DC, Seward JB, Puga FJ, Fuster V, Tajik AJ. Total correction of tetralogy of Fallot at age 40 years and older: long-term follow-up. *J Am Coll Cardiol* 1985;**5**(1):40–4.

131. Nollert G, Fischlein T, Bouterwek S, Bohmer C, Dewald O, Kreuzer E *et al.* Long-term results of total repair of tetralogy of Fallot in adulthood: 35 years follow-up in 104 patients corrected at the age of 18 or older. *Thorac Cardiovasc Surg* 1997;**45**(4):178–81.

132. Khambadkone S, Coats L, Taylor A, Boudjemline Y, Derrick G, Tsang V *et al.* Percutaneous pulmonary valve implantation in humans: results in 59 consecutive patients. *Circulation* 2005;**112**(8):1189–97.

133. Bertranou EG, Blackstone EH, Hazelrig JB, Turner ME, Kirklin JW. Life expectancy without surgery in tetralogy of Fallot. *Am J Cardiol* 1978;**42**(3):458–66.

134. Murphy JG, Gersh BJ, Mair DD, Fuster V, McGoon MD, Ilstrup DM *et al.* Long-term outcome in patients undergoing surgical repair of tetralogy of Fallot. *N Engl J Med* 1993;**329**(9):593–9.

135. Hornung TS, Derrick GP, Deanfield JE, Redington AN. Transposition complexes in the adult: a changing perspective. *Cardiol Clin* 2002;**20**(3):405–20.

136. Senning A. Surgical correction of transposition of the great vessels. *Surgery* 1959;**45**(6):966–80.

137. Lange R, Horer J, Kostolny M, Cleuziou J, Vogt M, Busch R *et al.* Presence of a ventricular septal defect and the Mustard operation are risk factors for late mortality after the atrial switch operation: thirty years of follow-up in 417 patients at a single center. *Circulation* 2006;**114**(18):1905–13.

138. Warnes CA. Transposition of the great arteries. *Circulation* 2006;**114**(24):2699–709.

139. Gelatt M, Hamilton RM, McCrindle BW, Connelly M, Davis A, Harris L *et al.* Arrhythmia and mortality after the Mustard procedure: a 30-year single-center experience. *J Am Coll Cardiol* 1997;**29**(1):194–201.

140. Kammeraad JA, van Deurzen CH, Sreeram N, Bink-Boelkens MT, Ottenkamp J, Helbing WA *et al.* Predictors of sudden cardiac death after Mustard or Senning repair for transposition of the great arteries. *J Am Coll Cardiol* 2004;**44**(5):1095–102.

141. Gatzoulis MA, Walters J, McLaughlin PR, Merchant N, Webb GD, Liu P. Late arrhythmia in adults with the mustard procedure for transposition of great arteries: a surrogate marker for right ventricular dysfunction? *Heart* 2000;**84**(4):409–15.

142. Kanter RJ, Papagiannis J, Carboni MP, Ungerleider RM, Sanders WE, Wharton JM. Radiofrequency catheter ablation of supraventricular tachycardia substrates after Mustard and Senning operations for d-transposition of the great arteries. *J Am Coll Cardiol* 2000;**35**(2):428–41.

143. Dos L, Teruel L, Ferreira IJ, Rodriguez-Larrea J, Miro L, Girona J *et al.* Late outcome of Senning and Mustard procedures for correction of transposition of the great arteries. *Heart* 2005;**91**(5):652–6.

144. Wilson NJ, Clarkson PM, Barratt-Boyes BG, Calder AL, Whitlock RM, Easthope RN *et al.* Long-term outcome after the mustard repair for simple transposition of the great arteries. 28-year follow-up. *J Am Coll Cardiol* 1998;**32**(3):758–65.

145. Doughan AR, McConnell ME, Book WM. Effect of beta blockers (carvedilol or metoprolol XL) in patients with transposition of great arteries and dysfunction of the systemic right ventricle. *Am J Cardiol* 2007;**99**(5):704–6.

146. Hechter SJ, Fredriksen PM, Liu P, Veldtman G, Merchant N, Freeman M *et al.* Angiotensin-converting enzyme inhibitors in adults after the Mustard procedure. *Am J Cardiol* 2001;**87**(5):660–3, A11.

147. Helvind MH, McCarthy JF, Imamura M, Prieto L, Sarris GE, Drummond-Webb JJ *et al.* Ventriculo-arterial discordance: switching the morphologically left ventricle into the systemic circulation after 3 months of age. *Eur J Cardiothorac Surg* 1998;**14**(2):173–8.

148. Poirier NC, Mee RB. Left ventricular reconditioning and anatomical correction for systemic right ventricular dysfunction. *Semin Thorac Cardiovasc Surg Pediatr Card Surg Annu* 2000;**3**:198–215.

149. Santoro G, Ballerini L, Bialkowski J, Bermudez-Canete R. Stent implantation for post-Mustard systemic venous obstruction. *Eur J Cardiothorac Surg* 1998;**14**(3):332–4.

150. Ebenroth ES, Hurwitz RA, Cordes TM. Late onset of pulmonary hypertension after successful Mustard surgery for d-transposition of the great arteries. *Am J Cardiol* 2000;**85**(1):127–30, A10.

151. Losay J, Touchot A, Serraf A, Litvinova A, Lambert V, Piot JD *et al.* Late outcome after arterial switch operation for transposition of the great arteries. *Circulation* 2001;**104**(12 suppl 1):I121–6.

152. Graham TP Jr, Bernard YD, Mellen BG, Celermajer D, Baumgartner H, Cetta F *et al.* Long-term outcome in congenitally corrected transposition of the great arteries: a multi-institutional study. *J Am Coll Cardiol* 2000;**36**(1):255–61.

153. Langley SM, Winlaw DS, Stumper O, Dhillon R, De Giovanni JV, Wright JG *et al.* Midterm results after restoration of the morphologically left ventricle to the systemic circulation in patients with congenitally corrected transposition of the great arteries. *J Thorac Cardiovasc Surg* 2003;**125**(6):1229–41.

154. Ammash NM, Warnes CA. Survival into adulthood of patients with unoperated single ventricle. *Am J Cardiol* 1996;**77**(7):542–4.

155. Khairy P, Poirier N, Mercier LA. Univentricular heart. *Circulation* 2007;**115**(6):800–12.

156. Fontan F, Baudet E. Surgical repair of tricuspid atresia. *Thorax* 1971;**26**(3):240–8.

157. Kreutzer G, Galindez E, Bono H, De Palma C, Laura JP. An operation for the correction of tricuspid atresia. *J Thorac Cardiovasc Surg* 1973;**66**(4):613–21.

158. de Leval MR, Kilner P, Gewillig M, Bull C. Total cavopulmonary connection: a logical alternative to atriopulmonary connection for complex Fontan operations. Experimental studies and early clinical experience. *J Thorac Cardiovasc Surg* 1988;**96**(5):682–95.

159. Lemler MS, Scott WA, Leonard SR, Stromberg D, Ramaciotti C. Fenestration improves clinical outcome of the fontan procedure: a prospective, randomized study. *Circulation* 2002;**105**(2):207–12.

160. Cohen MI, Wernovsky G, Vetter VL, Wieand TS, Gaynor JW, Jacobs ML et al. Sinus node function after a systematically staged Fontan procedure. *Circulation* 1998;**98**(19 suppl):II352–8; discussion II8–9.

161. Driscoll DJ, Offord KP, Feldt RH, Schaff HV, Puga FJ, Danielson GK. Five- to fifteen-year follow-up after Fontan operation. *Circulation* 1992;**85**(2):469–96.

162. Fontan F, Kirklin JW, Fernandez G, Costa F, Naftel DC, Tritto F et al. Outcome after a "perfect" Fontan operation. *Circulation* 1990;**81**(5):1520–36.

163. Nakano T, Kado H, Tachibana T, Hinokiyama K, Shiose A, Kajimoto M et al. Excellent midterm outcome of extracardiac conduit total cavopulmonary connection: results of 126 cases. *Ann Thorac Surg* 2007;**84**(5):1619–25; discussion 25–6.

164. Giannico S, Hammad F, Amodeo A, Michielon G, Drago F, Turchetta A et al. Clinical outcome of 193 extracardiac Fontan patients: the first 15 years. *J Am Coll Cardiol* 2006;**47**(10):2065–73.

165. d'Udekem Y, Iyengar AJ, Cochrane AD, Grigg LE, Ramsay JM, Wheaton GR et al. The Fontan procedure: contemporary techniques have improved long-term outcomes. *Circulation* 2007;**116**(11 suppl):I157–64.

166. Gatzoulis MA, Munk MD, Williams WG, Webb GD. Definitive palliation with cavopulmonary or aortopulmonary shunts for adults with single ventricle physiology. *Heart* 2000;**83**(1):51–7.

167. Triedman JK, Alexander ME, Love BA, Collins KK, Berul CI, Bevilacqua LM et al. Influence of patient factors and ablative technologies on outcomes of radiofrequency ablation of intraatrial re-entrant tachycardia in patients with congenital heart disease. *J Am Coll Cardiol* 2002;**39**(11):1827–35.

168. Mavroudis C, Deal BJ, Backer CL. The beneficial effects of total cavopulmonary conversion and arrhythmia surgery for the failed Fontan. *Semin Thorac Cardiovasc Surg Pediatr Card Surg Annu* 2002;**5**:12–24.

169. Diller GP, Gatzoulis MA. Pulmonary vascular disease in adults with congenital heart disease. *Circulation* 2007;**115**(8):1039–50.

170. Wood P. The Eisenmenger syndrome or pulmonary hypertension with reversed central shunt. I. *BMJ.* 1958;**2**(5098):701–9.

171. Cantor WJ, Harrison DA, Moussadji JS, Connelly MS, Webb GD, Liu P et al. Determinants of survival and length of survival in adults with Eisenmenger syndrome. *Am J Cardiol* 1999;**84**(6):677–81.

172. Galie N, Beghetti M, Gatzoulis MA, Granton J, Berger RM, Lauer A et al. Bosentan therapy in patients with Eisenmenger syndrome: a multicenter, double-blind, randomized, placebo-controlled study. *Circulation* 2006;**114**(1):48–54.

173. Spence MS, Balaratnam MS, Gatzoulis MA. Clinical update: cyanotic adult congenital heart disease. *Lancet* 2007;**370**(9598):1530–2.

174. Kaemmerer H, Fratz S, Braun SL, Koelling K, Eicken A, Brodherr-Heberlein S et al. Erythrocyte indexes, iron metabolism, and hyperhomocysteinemia in adults with cyanotic congenital cardiac disease. *Am J Cardiol* 2004;**94**(6):825–8.

175. Perloff JK, Marelli AJ, Miner PD. Risk of stroke in adults with cyanotic congenital heart disease. *Circulation* 1993;**87**(6):1954–9.

176. Broberg CS, Bax BE, Okonko DO, Rampling MW, Bayne S, Harries C et al. Blood viscosity and its relationship to iron deficiency, symptoms, and exercise capacity in adults with cyanotic congenital heart disease. *J Am Coll Cardiol* 2006;**48**(2):356–65.

177. Sandoval J, Aguirre JS, Pulido T, Martinez-Guerra ML, Santos E, Alvarado P et al. Nocturnal oxygen therapy in patients with the Eisenmenger syndrome. *Am J Respir Crit Care Med* 2001;**164**(9):1682–7.

178. Michelakis ED, Tymchak W, Noga M, Webster L, Wu XC, Lien D et al. Long-term treatment with oral sildenafil is safe and improves functional capacity and hemodynamics in patients with pulmonary arterial hypertension. *Circulation* 2003;**108**(17):2066–9.

179. D'Alto M, Vizza CD, Romeo E, Badagliacca R, Santoro G, Poscia R et al. Long term effects of bosentan treatment in adult patients with pulmonary arterial hypertension related to congenital heart disease (Eisenmenger physiology): safety, tolerability, clinical, and haemodynamic effect. *Heart* 2007;**93**(5):621–5.

180. Humpl T, Reyes JT, Holtby H, Stephens D, Adatia I. Beneficial effect of oral sildenafil therapy on childhood pulmonary arterial hypertension: twelve-month clinical trial of a single-drug, open-label, pilot study. *Circulation* 2005;**111**(24):3274–80.

181. Walsh EP, Cecchin F. Arrhythmias in adult patients with congenital heart disease. *Circulation* 2007;**115**(4):534–45.

182. Walsh EP. Interventional electrophysiology in patients with congenital heart disease. *Circulation* 2007;**115**(25):3224–34.

64 Venous thromboembolic disease

Lori-Ann Linkins and Clive Kearon

Henderson Hospital and McMaster University, Hamilton, Ontario, Canada

Introduction and historical perspective

Venous thromboembolic disease includes deep vein thrombosis (DVT) and pulmonary embolism (PE). The first recorded case of thrombosis of the lower limb is believed to be found in the Hindu medicine writings of Susruta, an Indian healer who lived around 800 BC, where he described a patient with a "swollen and painful leg, which was difficult to treat".[1] While only a few thrombosis specialists will be familiar with Susruta's contribution to the field, all are familiar with the contributions of Rudolph Virchow. Virchow, a Prussian physician born in 1821, is credited with coining the term "embolism" after discovering the relationship between a blood clot that forms within a blood vessel (thrombus), and a blood clot that breaks loose from the original and travels through the bloodstream to occlude the pulmonary vessels (embolus).[1] In addition, Virchow was the first to identify the pathogenic triad for thrombosis: stasis, vessel wall damage, and hypercoagulability. Virchow's triad has stood the test of time and today, it is still the foundation upon which prevention and treatment of venous thromboembolism (VTE) is based.

The first randomized trial for the treatment of VTE was performed by Barritt and Jordan in 1960.[2] They showed that treatment of PE with heparin and oral anticoagulants reduced the risk of recurrent PE and reduced mortality compared with no anticoagulant therapy (Table 64.1). Since then, there has been considerable progress in the development of new anticoagulants (e.g. low molecular weight heparin (LMWH), fondaparinux) for the prevention and treatment of VTE. Unfortunately, despite these advances, VTE remains a leading cause of morbidity and mortality.

In this chapter, we will briefly review the natural history and pathogenesis of VTE and provide an overview of evidence-based management of VTE divided into three categories: diagnosis, treatment, and prevention.

Nomenclature and definitions

Proximal deep vein thrombosis is defined as a DVT that involves the popliteal and more proximal veins. *Distal deep vein thrombosis* is defined as a DVT that is confined to the calf veins (including the calf trifurcation).

Incidence, natural history and prognosis

Venous thromboembolism is rare before the age of 16 years, probably because the immature coagulation system is resistant to thrombosis. However, the risk of VTE increases exponentially with advancing age (i.e. 1.9-fold per decade), rising from an annual incidence of approximately 30/100 000 at 40 years, to 90/100 000 at 60 years, and 260/100 000 at 80 years.[3–5]

DVT usually starts in the calf veins.[6] When DVT causes symptoms, over 80% involve the popliteal or more proximal veins.[6,7] However, if venography is used to diagnose DVT in asymptomatic high-risk patients (e.g. following orthopedic surgery) only about one-third of venous thrombi are proximal. The majority of isolated calf DVT will undergo spontaneous lysis; however, 20% of these thrombi subsequently extend to involve the proximal veins, usually within a week of presentation.[8] Non-extending calf DVT rarely causes PE, whereas proximal DVT often does.[9] The majority (70%) of patients with symptomatic proximal DVT have asymptomatic PE and vice versa.[10] Only about 25% of patients with symptomatic PE have symptoms or signs of DVT.[11]

It is estimated that 10% of symptomatic PE cause death within an hour of onset[12] and that, left untreated, about one-third of patients with initially non-fatal PE will have a fatal recurrence.[2] Untreated, symptomatic proximal DVT progresses to symptomatic PE in about one half of cases

Evidence-Based Cardiology, 3rd edition. Edited by S. Yusuf, J.A. Cairns, A.J. Camm, E.L. Fallen, and B.J. Gersh. © 2010 Blackwell Publishing, ISBN: 978-1-4051-5925-8.

Table 64.1a Landmark trials in the prevention and treatment of acute venous thromboembolism

Study	Populat.	Intervention Active	Intervention Control	Outcome	Efficacy Active	Efficacy Control	Relative risk	95% CI
Prevention								
Sevitt & Gallagher[163]	Hip Fracture	OA	Untreated	DVT/PE	4/150 (2.7%)	43/150 (29%)	0.09	0.02–0.25
Kakkar et al[139]	Surgical	LD heparin	Untreated	Fatal PE	2/2045 (0.10%)	16/2075 (0.77%)	0.13	0.01–0.5
PEP[154]	Surgical	Aspirin#	Placebo#	DVT/PE*	105/6679 (1.6%)	165/6677 (2.5%)	0.64	0.50–0.81
Turpie et al[145]	Surgical	Fondaparinux	LMWH	DVT/PE**	182/2682 (6.8%)	371/2703 (13.7%)	0.49	0.42–0.59
Gardlund et al[155]	Medical	LD Heparin	Untreated	fatal PE	15/5776 (0.3%)	16/5917 (0.3%)	0.96	0.48–1.9
Acute treatment								
Barritt & Jordan[2]	PE	Heparin, OA	Untreated	PE	0/16 (0%)	10/19 (53%)	0	–
UPET[164]	PE	Urokinase	No urokinase	Death	6/82 (7.3%)	7/78 (9.0%)	0.82	0.24–2.7
Gallus et al[85]	DVT/PE	~4d Heparin	~10d Heparin	DVT/PE	5/139 (3.6%)	6/127 (4.7%)	0.76	0.19–2.9
Hull et al[86]	DVT	5d Heparin	10d Heparin	DVT/PE	7/99 (7.1%)	7/10 (7.0%)	1.01	0.31–3.2
Brandjes et al[165]	DVT	Heparin IV	No heparin	DVT/PE	4/60 (6.7%)	12/60 (20%)	0.33	0.08–1.0
Prandoni et al[74]	DVT/PE	LMWH	Heparin	DVT/PE	14/360 (3.9%)	15/360 (4.2%)	0.93	0.46–1.9
Hull et al[166]	DVT	LMWH	Heparin	DVT/PE	6/213 (2.8%)	15/219 (6.8%)	0.41	0.13–1.1
Levine et al[167]	DVT	Outpatient LMWH	Heparin	DVT/PE	13/247 (5.3%)	17/253 (6.7%)	0.78	0.36–1.7
Koopman et al[168]	DVT	Outpatient LMWH	Heparin	DVT/PE	14/202 (6.9%)	17/198 (8.6%)	0.81	0.38–1.7
Columbus study[169]	DVT/PE	LMWH	Heparin, IV	DVT/PE	27/510 (5.3%)	25/511 (4.9%)	1.08	0.64–1.8
Kearon et al[75]	DVT/PE	Heparin, SC^	LMWH	DVT/PE	13/345 (3.8%)	12/352 (3.4%)	1.11	0.51–2.4
Matisse DVT[76]	DVT	Fondaparinux	LMWH	DVT/PE	43/1098 (3.9%)	45/1107 (4.1%)	0.96	0.64–1.5
Matisse PE[82]	PE	Fondaparinux	Heparin, IV	DVT/PE	43/1103 (3.9%)	56/1110 (5.0%)	0.77	0.52–1.1

Continued on p. 1034

Table 64.1b Landmark trials in the long-term treatment of venous thromboembolism

Study	Populat.	Intervention		Outcome	Efficacy		Relative risk	95% CI
		Active	Control		Active	Control		
Long-term treatment								
Hull et al[13]	DVT	OA	L.D. heparin	DVT/PE	0/33 (0%)	9/35 (26%)	0.0	0.0–0.5
Hull et al[97]	DVT	INR~2.1	INR~3.2	DVT/PE	1/47 (2.1%)	1/49 (2.0%)	1.04	0.01–80
British Thoracic Society[18]	DVT/PE	4 weeks	3 months	DVT/PE	28/358 (7.8%)	14/354 (4.0%)	1.78	1.03–4.0
Schulman et al[15]	DVT	6 weeks	6 months	DVT/PE	80/443 (18.1%)	43/454 (9.5%)	1.91	1.33–2.8
Schulman et al[105]	2nd DVT/PE	Indefinite	6 months	DVT/PE	3/116 (2.6%)	23/111 (21%)	0.12	0.02–0.40
Lee et al[111]	Cancer	LMWH 6 months	LMWH 5 days/OA 6 months	DVT/PE	27/336 (8.0%)	53/336 (15.8%)	0.51	0.33–0.79
Kearon et al[104]	DVT/PE unprovoked	OA 1 year	OA 3 months	DVT/PE	1/79 (1.3%)	17/83 (20%)	0.06	0.01–0.45
Kearon et al[123]	DVT/PE unprovoked	OA INR 1.5–1.9	OA INR 2.0–3.0	DVT/PE	16/369 (4.3%)	6/369 (1.6%)	2.67	1.06–6.7
Ridker et al[170]	DVT/PE unprovoked	OA INR 1.5–2.0	Placebo	DVT/PE	14/255 (5.5%)	37/253 (14.6%)	0.38	0.21–0.68
Agnelli et al[101]	DVT unprovoked	OA 9 months	Nothing	DVT/PE	21/134 (15.7%)	21/133 (15.8%)	0.99	0.57–1.7
PREPIC I[125]	DVT	IVC filter	No IVC filter	DVT/PE at 2 years	37/178 (20.8%)	29/187 (15.5%)	1.34	0.86–2.08
PREPIC II[126]	DVT	IVC filter	No IVC filter	at 8 years	58/159 (36.4%)	55/155 (35.4%)	1.03	0.77–1.4

Populat., population studied; 95% CI, 95% confidence interval of relative risk; OA, oral anticoagulants; LD, low-dose subcutaneous heparin; DVT, deep vein thrombosis; PE, pulmonary embolism; LMWH, low molecular weight heparin; IVC, inferior vena caval filter; * secondary outcome measure; ** DVT detected on mandatory bilateral venography; # additional prophylaxis used: heparin 18%, LMWH 26% and compression stockings 30%; ^ fixed, weight-adjusted dose without laboratory monitoring.

and, in general, the risk of recurrent VTE is highest within days or weeks of an acute event.[13] The risk of recurrent VTE remains elevated in patients with thrombosis that was unprovoked or associated with persistent risk factors (e.g. malignancy, congenital hypercoagulable states) compared to those in whom VTE was associated with a transient risk factor (e.g. surgery).[14–19]

Pathophysiology

Venous thrombi are composed primarily of fibrin and red blood cells. They form when the following elements are present: venous stasis, vessel wall damage, and hypercoaguability (Virchow's triad). Classification of risk factors for VTE according to this pathogenic triad remains valuable.

Venous stasis

The importance of venous stasis as a risk factor for VTE is demonstrated by the fact that most DVT associated with stroke affect the paralyzed leg,[20] and most DVT associated with pregnancy affect the left leg,[21] the iliac veins of which are prone to extrinsic compression by the pregnant uterus and the right common iliac artery.

Vessel wall damage

Venous endothelial damage, usually as a consequence of accidental injury, manipulation during surgery (e.g. hip replacement) or iatrogenic injury, is an important risk factor for VTE. Hence, three-quarters of proximal DVT which complicate hip surgery occur in the operated leg[22] and thrombosis is common with indwelling venous catheters.[23]

Hypercoagulability

A complex balance of naturally occurring coagulation and fibrinolytic factors, and their inhibitors, serves to maintain blood fluidity and hemostasis. Inherited or acquired changes in this balance predispose to thrombosis. The most important inherited biochemical disorders associated with VTE are due to:
- defects in the naturally occurring inhibitors of coagulation including deficiencies of antithrombin, protein C or protein S
- resistance to activated protein C caused by factor V Leiden
- a mutation in the 3′ untranslated region of the prothrombin gene (G20210A) which is associated with a 25% increase in prothrombin levels.

The first three of these disorders are rare in the normal population (combined prevalence of <1%), have a combined prevalence of 5% in patients with a first episode of VTE[24] and are associated with a 10 to 40-fold increase in the risk of

VTE.[25] The factor V Leiden mutation is common, occurring in 5% of Caucasians and 20% of patients with a first episode of VTE (i.e. fourfold increase in VTE risk).[25,26] The prothrombin gene mutation occurs in 2% of Caucasians and about 5% of those with a first episode of VTE (i.e. 2.5-fold increase in risk).[25–27] Hyperhomocysteinemia, due to hereditary and acquired factors, is also associated with VTE.[28]

Elevated levels of a number of coagulation factors (I, II, VIII, IX, XI) are associated with thrombosis in a "dose-dependent" manner.[29–31] It is probable that such elevations are often inherited, with strong evidence for this with factor VIII.[29] Prothrombotic abnormalities of the fibrinolytic system have questionable importance.

Acquired hypercoagulable states include estrogen therapy, antiphospholipid antibodies (anticardiolipin antibodies and/or lupus anticoagulants), systemic lupus erythematosus, malignancy, combination chemotherapy, and surgery.[3] Patients who develop immunologically related heparin-induced thrombocytopenia (HIT) also have a very high risk of developing arterial and venous thromboembolism.[32] Unlike the congenital abnormalities, acquired risk factors are often transient, which has important implications for the duration of anticoagulant prophylaxis and treatment.

Combinations of risk factors and risk stratification

The risk of developing VTE depends on the prevalence and severity of risk factors (Box 64.1).[3]

BOX 64.1 Risk factors for venous thromboembolism

Patient factors
Previous venous thromboembolism*
Age over 40
Pregnancy, puerperium
Marked obesity
Inherited hypercoagulable state

Underlying condition and acquired factors
Malignancy*
Estrogen therapy
Cancer chemotherapy
Paralysis*
Prolonged immobility
Major trauma*
Lower limb injuries*
Heparin-induced thrombocytopenia
Antiphospholipid antibodies

Type of surgery
Lower limb orthopedic surgery*
General anesthesia >30 min

*Common major risk factors for venous thromboembolism

Diagnosis

Objective testing for DVT and PE is important because clinical assessment alone is unreliable. Failure to diagnose VTE exposes patients to the risk of fatal PE. However, inappropriate use of anticoagulants exposes patients to the risk of serious bleeding complications including fatal hemorrhage.

Diagnosis of deep vein thrombosis

Venography is the criterion standard for the diagnosis of DVT.[7,33] However, because of its invasive nature, technical demands, costs, and risks associated with contrast media, non-invasive tests have been developed, of which venous ultrasound imaging (VUI) and D-dimer testing are the most important.

Clinical assessment

Although clinical assessment cannot unequivocally confirm or exclude DVT, clinical evaluation using empiric assessment or a structured clinical model (Table 64.2) can stratify patients as having a low (5% prevalence), moderate (25%

Table 64.2 Clinical model for determining clinical suspicion of DVT[171]

Variables	Points
Active cancer (treatment ongoing or within previous 6 months or palliative)	1
Paralysis, paresis or recent plaster immobilization of the lower extremities	1
Recently bedridden >3 days or major surgery within the previous 12 weeks requiring general or regional anesthesia	1
Localized tenderness along the distribution of the deep venous system	1
Entire leg swollen	1
Calf swelling 3 cm > asymptomatic side (measured 10 cm below tibial tuberosity)	1
Pitting edema confined to the symptomatic leg	1
Collateral superficial veins (non-varicose)	1
Previously documented deep vein thrombosis	1
Alternative diagnosis as likely or greater than that of DVT	-2

Total points (pretest probability for DVT):
Score >2:   High
Score 1–2:   Moderate
Score 0:   Low

NOTE: In patients with symptoms in both legs, the more symptomatic leg is used.

prevalence) or high (60% prevalence) probability of DVT.[34] Such categorization is useful in guiding the performance and interpretation of objective testing.[34–38]

Venous ultrasound imaging (VUI)

With this modality, pressure is applied to the proximal veins with an ultrasound probe to determine compressibility.[7,39] Incompressibility of a vein is considered diagnostic for DVT. VUI has a sensitivity for proximal DVT of 97% and a specificity of 94% in symptomatic patients which, on average, translates into a positive predictive value of 97% and a negative predictive value of 98% for proximal DVT.[7,40]

The utility of VUI for diagnosing calf vein thrombosis is more controversial. VUI is technically more difficult to perform in the calf and some studies have reported the accuracy of this approach to be poor (e.g. sensitivity of 70%).[7,40] Recently, investigators have proposed that a single complete compression ultrasound that includes examination of the calf veins should be used to exclude DVT. Studies using this method have reported an incidence of VTE of 0.5% during 3 months follow-up after a negative examination, establishing that negative VUI that includes the calf veins excludes VTE.[41–43] However, this method has the potential to diagnose calf DVT that would have spontaneously lysed without treatment and to yield false-positive results, thereby exposing patients to the risk of bleeding due to anticoagulant therapy without clear benefit.

At most centers, if DVT cannot be excluded by a normal proximal VUI in combination with other results (e.g. low clinical probability or normal D-dimer (Table 64.3)) treatment is withheld and a follow-up VUI is performed after 1 week to detect extending calf vein thrombosis (2% of patients).[7] If the second VUI examination is normal, the risk of symptomatic VTE during the next 6 months is less than 2%.[7]

The accuracy of VUI in asymptomatic postoperative patients who have a high risk for DVT is poor with a sensitivity for proximal DVT of only 62%,[7] and such screening is not recommended in patients who have received prophylaxis.[44]

Computed tomographic (CT) venography and magnetic resonance (MR) venography

The limitations of VUI in diagnosing DVT in certain clinical settings, e.g. isolated pelvic DVT and asymptomatic patients, has stimulated interest in alternative imaging modalities such as CT venography and MR venography. In one review of studies comparing CT venography with VUI, the sensitivity and specificity were reported as 89–100% and 94–100%, respectively, for all DVT.[45] However, the majority of the studies included in the review were case series and given the cost, exposure to radiation, and limited availability of CT venography, it is unlikely that this modality will play an important role in the diagnosis of DVT.

Table 64.3 Diagnostic tests which confirm or exclude DVT

Diagnostic test	Confirms DVT	Excludes DVT
First acute DVT		
Venography	Intraluminal filling defect	No intraluminal filling defect; all deep veins seen
Venous ultrasound	Non-compressible at CFV, PopV or C-tri	Fully compressible proximal veins **AND**
		a) low cPTP for DVT **OR**
		b) normal D-dimer with sensitivity ≥85% **OR**
		c) normal ultrasound on repeat testing at day 7
		Normal whole-leg ultrasound
D-dimer		Normal D-dimer with sensitivity >98% **OR**
		Normal D-dimer with sensitivity > 85% **AND**
		a) low cPTP **OR**
		b) negative proximal ultrasound
Recurrent DVT		
Venography	Intraluminal filling defect	No intraluminal filling defect; all deep veins seen
Venous ultrasound	New non-compressible CFV or PopV **OR**	Normal **OR**
	4.0 mm increase in diameter of CFV or PopV compared with recent previous test	≤1 mm increase in diameter of CFV or PopV compared with recent previous test **AND** remains unchanged on repeat ultrasound testing on day 2 and day 7
D-dimer		Normal D-dimer with sensitivity >98%
		Normal D-dimer with sensitivity >85% **AND**
		a) low cPTP **OR**
		b) ≤1 mm increase in diameter of CFV or PopV

CFV, common femoral vein; PopV, popliteal vein; C-tri, calf vein trifurcation; cPTP, clinical pretest probability.

Magnetic resonance venography can be performed with injection of gadolinium or without any contrast (MR direct thrombus imaging). A recent meta-analysis of studies comparing MR venography with conventional venography reported a pooled sensitivity of 92% and specificity of 95% of MR venography for proximal DVT.[46] However, there was significant heterogeneity between the studies and, therefore, these pooled estimates should be interpreted with caution. MR direct thrombus imaging looks promising, but has only been evaluated in a single accuracy study to date.[47] As with CT venography, cost and availability will inhibit the widespread use of MR for diagnosis of DVT.

D-dimer blood testing

D-dimer is formed when cross-linked fibrin is broken down by plasmin and levels are usually elevated with DVT and/or PE. Normal levels can help to exclude VTE, but elevated D-dimer levels are non-specific and have low positive predictive value.[48,49] D-dimer tests differ markedly as diagnostic procedures for VTE. A normal result with a very sensitive (i.e. 98%) D-dimer assay excludes VTE on its own.[48–50] However, very sensitive D-dimer tests have low specificity (40%) which limits their utility because of high false-positive rates.[50] In order to exclude DVT and/or PE, a normal result with a less sensitive D-dimer assay (i.e. 85%) needs to be combined with either a low clinical probability or another objective test that has negative predictive value but is also non-diagnostic on its own (see Table 64.3).[35,38,51–53] As less sensitive D-dimer assays are more specific (70%), they yield fewer false-positive results. Specificity of D-dimer decreases with aging[54] and with co-morbid illness such as cancer.[55] Consequently, D-dimer testing has limited value in the diagnosis of VTE in hospitalized patients and is unhelpful in the early postoperative period.

Diagnosis of recurrent DVT

Persistent abnormalities of the deep veins are common following DVT.[7,56] Therefore, diagnosis of recurrent DVT requires evidence of new clot formation. Tests that can diagnose or exclude recurrent DVT are noted in Table 64.3.[7,56,57]

Diagnosis of pulmonary embolism

Pulmonary angiography is the criterion standard for the diagnosis of PE, but it has similar limitations to venography.[58]

Computed tomographic pulmonary angiography (CTPA)

Computed tomographic pulmonary angiography (also known as spiral or helical CT) with peripheral injection of contrast dye is the current standard diagnostic test for PE.[59–62] Helical CT technology has rapidly advanced from use of single detector scanners to use of progressively larger numbers of detectors (termed multidetector CT), which enable more detailed examination of the pulmonary arteries.

Current evidence suggests that CTPA is non-diagnostic in 6% of patients, and that among adequate examinations, sensitivity is 83%, specificity is 96%, positive predictive value is 86% and negative predictive value is 95%.[59] Accuracy varies according to the size of the largest pulmonary artery involved: positive predictive value was 97% for pulmonary emboli in the main or lobar artery, 68% for segmental arteries, and 25% for subsegmental arteries. Predictive values were also influenced by clinical assessment of pulmonary embolism probability: positive predictive value is 96% with high, 92% with intermediate, and 58% with low clinical probability (8% of patients); negative predictive value is 96% with low, 89% with intermediate, and 60% with high clinical probability (5% of patients).[59]

The ability of CTPA to exclude pulmonary embolism has also been evaluated in management studies in which anticoagulant therapy was withheld in patients with negative CTPA.[61] More recent studies suggest that less than 2% of patients with a negative CTPA for pulmonary embolism will return with symptomatic VTE during follow-up.[60–62] Taken together, these observations suggest the following:
- intraluminal filling defects in lobar or larger pulmonary arteries are generally diagnostic for PE
- a good-quality normal CTPA excludes PE if clinical suspicion is low or moderate
- intraluminal defects confined to segmental pulmonary arteries are generally diagnostic for PE if clinical suspicion is moderate or high, but should be considered non-diagnostic if suspicion is low or there are discordant findings (e.g. negative D-dimer)
- intraluminal defects confined to subsegmental pulmonary arteries are non-diagnostic and patients with such findings require further testing.

CTPA delivers a substantial dose of radiation to the chest, which increases the risk of cancer. For this reason, CTPA should be used selectively, particularly in younger women.[63]

Magnetic resonance angiography (MRA)
Gadolinium-enhanced pulmonary MRA offers advantages over CTPA in that it can be performed on patients with an allergy to iodinated contrast media and it avoids exposure to radiation. However, only a limited number of small studies evaluating MRA for diagnosis of PE have been performed.[64] In addition, a warning has been issued by the Federal Drug Administration about an increased risk of nephrogenic systemic fibrosis in patients with severe renal insufficiency (glomerular filtration rate <30 mL/min) who

are exposed to gadolinium. Like CTPA, MRA is able to identify alternative pulmonary diagnoses, and can be extended to look for concomitant DVT.

Ventilation-perfusion lung scanning
In the past, the imaging modality typically used to investigate patients with suspected PE was a ventilation-perfusion lung scan. More recently, CTPA has supplanted this imaging modality, although lung scanning is still used, particularly when CTPA is contraindicated because of renal failure or associated radiation exposure to the chest (e.g. in young women). A normal perfusion scan excludes PE[65,66] but is found in a minority (10–40%) of patients.[11,54,67] Perfusion defects are non-specific; only about one-third of patients with defects have PE.[67,68] The probability that a perfusion defect is due to PE increases with size and number of defects, and the presence of a normal ventilation scan ("mismatched" defect).[67,68] A lung scan with mismatched segmental or larger perfusion defects is termed "high probability."[68] A single mismatched defect is associated with a prevalence of PE of 80%.[69] Three or more mismatched defects are associated with a prevalence of PE of 90%.[69] Lung scan findings are highly age dependent with a relatively high proportion of normal scans, and a low proportion of non-diagnostic scans, in younger patients.[54]

Clinical assessment
As with suspected DVT, clinical assessment is useful at categorizing probability of PE (Table 64.4).[37,70]

D-dimer testing
As previously discussed when considering diagnosis of DVT, a normal D-dimer result, alone[50] or in combination with another negative test,[49,62,70,71] can be used to exclude PE (Table 64.5).

Management of patients with non-diagnostic combinations of non-invasive tests for PE
Patients with non-diagnostic imaging for PE at presentation have, on average, a prevalence of PE of 20% and therefore further investigations to exclude this diagnosis are required.[39,67] The first step is to perform imaging investigations (venous ultrasound, venography) to look for DVT. If DVT is confirmed, it can be concluded that the patient's symptoms are due to PE. If imaging studies are negative for DVT, we recommend one of the following management approaches (Table 64.5):
- withhold anticoagulants and perform serial venous ultrasounds to check for evolving proximal DVT (after 1 and 2 weeks)
- perform CTPA or lung scanning if either of these tests has not been performed, or
- repeat CTPA after 24 hours (to reduce the risk of contrast-induced nephrotoxicity).

If serial VUI for DVT (two additional tests a week apart) is negative, the subsequent risk of recurrent VTE during the next 3 months is less than 1%[11,70] which is similar to that after a normal pulmonary angiogram.[58]

Treatment

Anticoagulants are the mainstay of treatment for VTE. The objectives of anticoagulant therapy are to prevent extension and potentially fatal embolization of the initial thrombus, and to prevent recurrent VTE (early and late).

Acute treatment of VTE

Low molecular weight heparin for a minimum of 5 days, administered by subcutaneous injection on an outpatient basis, has become standard practice for initial treatment of patients with an uncomplicated DVT and normal renal function[72] (**Class I, Level A**). Many trials have established that weight-adjusted LMWH (without laboratory monitoring) is as safe and effective as adjusted-dose unfractionated intravenous heparin (UFH) for the treatment of acute VTE[73] (see Table 64.1). Alternatives to LMWH include twice-daily subcutaneous UFH (with or without laboratory monitoring) and fondaparinux administered once daily by subcutaneous injection (without laboratory monitoring)[74–76] (see Table 64.1) (**Class I, Level A**). If unmonitored subcutaneous UFH is used it should be administered in weight-adjusted doses (i.e. 333 units/kg initially followed by 250 units/kg every 12 hours).[75] Patients with severe renal impairment or those who are considered at high risk for bleeding should be treated in hospital with intravenous UFH titrated according to activated partial thromboplastin

Table 64.4 Model for determining clinical suspicion of PE[71,172]

Variables	Points
Clinical signs and symptoms of deep vein thrombosis (minimum leg swelling and pain with palpation of the deep veins)	3.0
An alternative diagnosis is less likely than pulmonary embolism	3.0
Heart rate >100 beats/min	1.5
Immobilization or surgery in the previous 4 weeks	1.5
Previous deep vein thrombosis/pulmonary embolism	1.5
Hemoptysis	1.0
Malignancy (treatment ongoing or within previous 6 months or palliative)	1.0

Total points (pretest probability for PE):
Score <4: PE unlikely*
Score ≥4: PE likely**

* low;
** score of 4 or 5 = moderate, score of 6 or higher = high.

Table 64.5 Diagnostic tests which confirm or exclude PE

Diagnostic test	Confirms PE	Excludes PE
Pulmonary angiography	Intraluminal filling defect	No intraluminal filling defect
CTPA	Intraluminal filling defect in *lobar or main PA* **OR**	Negative good-quality study **AND** a) cPTP is low or moderate **OR** b) cPTP is high, but negative bilateral leg ultrasounds
	Intraluminal filling defect in *segmental PA* **AND** cPTP is moderate or high **OR** Non-diagnostic study **AND** confirmed DVT	Non-diagnostic study **AND** normal bilateral leg ultrasound **AND** a) low cPTP **OR** b) normal D-dimer with sensitivity >85% **OR** c) negative bilateral leg ultrasound at 7 & 14 days
Ventilation-perfusion scan	High-probability scan **AND** cPTP moderate or high **OR** Non-diagnostic study **AND** confirmed DVT	Normal **OR** Non-diagnostic study **AND** normal bilateral leg ultrasound **AND** a) low cPTP **OR** b) normal D-dimer with sensitivity >85%
D-dimer		Normal D-dimer with sensitivity >98% **OR** normal D-dimer with sensitivity >85% **AND** low cPTP

PA, pulmonary artery; CTPA, computed tomographic pulmonary angiography; cPTP, clinical pretest probability.

time corresponding to plasma heparin levels from 0.3 to 0.7 IU/mL anti-Xa activity by the amidolytic assay[77] (**Class II, Level C**). Patients with thrombosis associated with HIT or with a past history of HIT should be treated with danaparoid, argatroban or lepirudin[78–80] (**Class I, Level C**).

A similar approach can be used for the initial treatment of PE, including treatment as an outpatient, as long as the patient is hemodynamically stable[72,81,82] (**Class I, Level A**). No trials have specifically randomized acute PE patients to be treated either in hospital or at home. However, in one randomized controlled trial comparing fixed-dose UFH and LMWH, 39% (52/134) of patients who had PE were treated entirely at home[75] (see Table 64.1). Further support for the safety of this approach is derived from two observational studies in which 30% of patients with PE were treated with LMWH at home.[83,84] Patients with severe symptoms and signs, and particularly if there is evidence of hemodynamic compromise, should be assessed for thrombolytic therapy (discussed below).

For both DVT and PE, the currently recommended approach to is to start treatment with a vitamin K antagonist (e.g. warfarin) concurrently with LMWH (or UFH or fondaparinux) at the time of diagnosis.[72,85,86] Two trials performed in hospitalized patients showed that starting warfarin at a dose of 5 mg, compared to 10 mg, is associated with less excessive anticoagulation.[87,88] A similar study in outpatients failed to demonstrate an advantage to starting warfarin at a dose of 5 mg compared with 10 mg.[89] Observational studies have shown that lower VKA maintenance doses are required in older patients, women, and those with impaired nutrition and vitamin K deficiency.[90,91] Taken together, these data suggest that warfarin can usually be started at a dose of 10 mg in younger (e.g. less than 60 years) otherwise healthy outpatients, and at a dose of 5 mg in older patients and those who are hospitalized.

Idraparinux, a long-acting inhibitor of factor Xa which is administered subcutaneously once weekly, has recently been shown to be as effective as standard therapy for the first 3–6 months of treatment for DVT, but is less effective than standard therapy in patients with PE.[92]

Ximelagatran, an oral direct thrombin inhibitor, has been shown to be effective for the acute and long-term treatment of VTE, but is not used because of hepatic toxicity.[93]

Recommendation

- LMWH (or UFH or fondaparinux) and a vitamin K antagonist should be started on the day of diagnosis. LMWH (or UFH or fondaparinux) should be stopped once the international normalization ration (INR) is 2.0 or above for at least 24 hours and the patient has received a minimum of 5 days of treatment (**Class I, Level C**).

Subacute and long-term treatment of VTE

A randomized trial of patients with DVT which compared 3 months of warfarin (INR 3.0–4.0) with low-dose UFH after initial treatment with full-dose UFH established the necessity for prolonged oral anticoagulation after initial heparin therapy[13] (see Table 64.1). Prolonged high-dose subcutaneous UFH[94] and, subsequently, LMWH (50–75% of acute treatment dose) were shown to be as effective as warfarin therapy.[95,96] In the 1970s it was recognized that, because of differences in the responsiveness of thromboplastins to oral anticoagulants, a prothrombin time ratio of 2.0 reflected a much more intense level of anticoagulation in North America than in Europe. This prompted a comparison of two intensities of warfarin therapy (corresponding to mean INRs of 2.1 and 3.2) for the treatment of DVT[97] (see Table 64.1). This study found that the lower intensity of oral anticoagulation was as effective as the higher intensity but caused less bleeding.

Duration of anticoagulant treatment of VTE

During the last decade, a series of well-designed studies have helped to define the optimal duration of anticoagulation. The findings can be summarized as follows.

- Shortening the duration of anticoagulation from 3 or 6 months to 4 or 6 weeks results in a doubling of the frequency of recurrent VTE during 1–2 years of follow-up[15,16,18,19] (**Class I, Level A**).
- Patients with VTE provoked by a transient risk factor have a lower (about one-third) risk of recurrence than those with an unprovoked VTE or a persistent risk factor[14,15,17–19,98] (**Class I, Level A**).
- Risk of recurrent VTE after 3 months of anticoagulant therapy for VTE *provoked* by a transient risk factor is about 3% in the first year and 10% in the first 5 years after stopping anticoagulant therapy[17–19,98–100] (**Class I, Level A**).

Recommendation

Three months of anticoagulation is adequate treatment for VTE provoked by a transient risk factor. **Class I, Level A**

- Risk of recurrent VTE after 3 months of anticoagulant therapy for *unprovoked* VTE is about 10% in the first year and 30% in the first 5 years after stopping anticoagulant therapy[15,17,99,101,102] (**Class I, Level A**).
- After 3 months of anticoagulation, recurrent DVT is at least as likely to affect the contralateral leg (**Class I, Level A**); this suggests that "systemic" rather than "local" (including inadequate treatment) factors are responsible for recurrences after 3 months of treatment.[103]
- Extending duration of anticoagulation beyond 3 months to 6 or 12 months may delay, but ultimately not reduce the risk of recurrence if anticoagulant therapy is then stopped.[101,102]

- Oral anticoagulants targeted at an INR of ~2.5 are very effective (risk reduction ≥90%) at preventing recurrent unprovoked VTE after the first 3 months of treatment[104,105] (**Class I, Level A**).

Recommendation

Patients with unprovoked DVT should receive anticoagulant therapy for a minimum of three months. **Class I, Level A** After three months, these patients should be assessed for indefinite anticoagulant therapy. Calculation of the risk to benefit ratio of indefinite anticoagulant therapy for an individual patient should include evaluation of risk of bleeding, quality of anticoagulant monitoring, and patient preference. **Class I, Level A** Patients who remain on long-term anticoagulant therapy should be reassessed at periodic intervals to ensure the risk to benefit ratio remains in favour of anticoagulant therapy. **Class I, Level C**

- A second episode of VTE is associated with an increased risk of recurrence (RR 1.5)[106–108] (**Class I, Level A**).

Recommendation

Patients with a second episode of unprovoked VTE should be assessed for indefinite anticoagulant therapy. **Class I, Level A**

- An isolated distal DVT (provoked or unprovoked) is associated with a low risk of recurrence (2% in the first year) compared to proximal DVT or PE (6% in the first year).[15,99]

Recommendation

Three months of anticoagulant therapy is adequate for patients with unprovoked isolated distal DVT. **Class I, Level B**

- Risk of recurrence is about threefold higher in patients with active cancer.[14,109,110]
- Long-term treatment with LMWH is more effective than warfarin in patients with VTE associated with cancer.[111]

Recommendation

Patients with VTE and cancer should be treated with LMWH for the first 3 to 6 months of long-term anticoagulant therapy. **Class I, Level B**. Anticoagulant therapy should be continued with a vitamin K antagonist or LMWH indefinitely or until the cancer is resolved.

- Men appear to have about a 50% higher risk of recurrent VTE than women.[112]
- Risk of recurrence appears to be somewhat higher in patients with antiphospholipid antibodies[104,107,113] and in patients with inherited thrombophilias.[17,114–116]
- Other risk factors for recurrence may include: elevated levels of clotting factors VIII, IX, XI and homocysteine, and

deficiencies of protein C and protein S; elevated D-dimer levels after stopping anticoagulant therapy[117]; residual DVT on ultrasound[118]; and presence of the post-thrombotic syndrome. Currently, these factors do not have clear implications for duration of treatment.[119]

Bleeding during anticoagulant therapy

Risk of bleeding on anticoagulants differs markedly among patients depending on the prevalence of risk factors (e.g. age greater than 75; previous gastrointestinal bleeding or stroke; renal failure; anemia; antiplatelet therapy; malignancy; poor anticoagulant control).[120,121] Approximately 13% of episodes of major bleeding during the first 3 months of anticoagulant therapy are fatal and greater than 50% of intracranial bleeds are fatal.[122] The risk of major bleeding in younger patients (e.g. less than 60 years) who do not have risk factors for bleeding and have good anticoagulant control (target INR 2–3) is about 1% per year.[90,123,124] The risk of major bleeding is expected to be as much as 10-fold higher in patients with multiple risk factors for bleeding.[120,121]

Inferior vena caval filters

No randomized trial or prospective cohort study has evaluated inferior vena caval filters as sole therapy in patients with DVT (i.e. without concurrent anticoagulant therapy). Permanent inferior vena caval filter insertion as an adjunct to anticoagulant therapy has been evaluated in a single large randomized controlled trial of patients with acute DVT who were considered to be at high risk for PE.[125] The findings of this study, which were reported after 2 years[125] and 8 years,[126] indicated that filters decrease the rate of PE, increase the rate of DVT, and have no effect on overall rate of VTE or mortality. Indirectly, this study supports the use of vena caval filters to prevent PE in patients with acute DVT and/or PE who cannot be anticoagulated (i.e. bleeding), but does not support more liberal use of filters (**Class I, Level C**). Patients should receive a course of anticoagulation if this subsequently becomes safe, which should be continued for the same duration as for similar patients who do not have an inferior vena caval filter.

Thrombolytic therapy

Systemic thrombolytic therapy accelerates the rate of resolution of DVT and PE, which can be life-saving for patients with PE and hemodynamic compromise.[127,128] However, the cost of thrombolytic therapy is a twofold or greater increase in frequency of major bleeding, and probably a greater increase in intracranial bleeding.[127,129,130] Right ventricular dysfunction on echocardiography, right ventricular dilation on echocardiography or CTPA, elevated troponin levels, and elevated brain natriuretic hormone levels are associated with increased early mortality in patients with acute PE.[131–136] Thrombolytic therapy may reduce the risk of the prothrombotic syndrome following DVT, but this does not appear to justify its associated risks.[130] Catheter-based treatments (i.e. thrombolytic therapy or removal of thrombus) require further evaluation before they can be recommended.

Recommendation

Patients with PE and hemodynamic compromise should be treated with thrombolytic therapy unless they have a high risk of bleeding. **Class I, Level B**. Thrombolytic therapy may also be given to selected high-risk patients without hypotension who are judged to have a high risk of dying from PE and have a low risk of bleeding. **Class II, Level B**

Prevention

Postoperative fatal PE is rarely preceded by symptomatic DVT.[137] Consequently, primary prophylaxis is the best way to prevent fatal PE. Use of primary prophylaxis is strongly supported by cost-effectiveness analyses, which indicate that it reduces overall costs in addition to reducing morbidity.[138]

Postoperative patients: pharmacologic prophylaxis

Surgical patients can be categorized as at low, moderate or high risk of VTE depending upon the type of surgery and patient-related risk factors (Table 64.6).

Low-dose unfractionated heparin has been shown to reduce postoperative DVT and fatal PE by two-thirds.[139] LMWH is more effective (odds ratio 0.83) than low-dose UFH following orthopedic surgery and is associated with a similar frequency of bleeding.[140] An additional 3 or 4 weeks of LMWH after hospital discharge further reduces the frequency of symptomatic VTE after orthopedic surgery.[141-143] At a minimum, extended prophylaxis after major orthopedic surgery is recommended for the highest risk patients (i.e. previous VTE, active malignancy). Warfarin (target INR 2–3 for about 7–10 days) is less effective than LMWH at preventing DVT that are detected by venography soon after orthopedic surgery[144] but appears to be similarly effective at preventing symptomatic VTE over a 3-month period.[142-144] Fondaparinux has been shown to be more effective than LMWH following major orthopedic surgery, but causes marginally more bleeding.[145]

Table 64.6 Risk stratification for postoperative VTE, frequency of VTE without prophylaxis, and recommendations[144]

	Venographic DVT*		Pulmonary embolism		Recommended prophylaxis
	Calf	Proximal	Symptomatic	Fatal	
Low risk <40 years of age and uncomplicated surgery and no additional risk factors	2%	0.4%	0.2%	<0.01%	Early mobilization
Moderate risk Minor surgery in patients with additional risk factors Surgery in patients 40–60 years old with no additional risk factors	20%	5%	2%	0.5%	Low-dose UFH (q12h) LMWH (~3000 U per day) GCS or IPC
High risk Surgery in patients >60 years or age 40–60 with additional risk factors Major surgery in patients with malignancy or previous VTE Knee/hip surgery or heparin-induced thrombocytopenia	50%	15%	5%	2%	LMWH (>3000 U per day) Warfarin (INR 2–3) Fondaparinux IPC/GCS and low-dose UFH or LMWH

*Asymptomatic DVT detected by surveillance bilateral venography.

Low-dose UFH: 5000 U of subcutaneous unfractionated heparin preoperatively, and twice or three times daily postoperatively.

LMWH: subcutaneous low molecular weight heparin; higher doses (e.g. ~4000 U once daily with a preoperative start or ~3000 U twice daily with a postoperative start) are used in high-risk patients than in moderate-risk patients (~3000 U daily with a preoperative start).

GCS: graduated compression stockings, alone or in combination with pharmacologic methods.

IPC devices: intermittent pneumatic compression devices, alone or in combination with graduated compression stockings and/or pharmacologic methods.

Warfarin: usually started postoperatively and adjusted to achieve an INR of 2.0–3.0.

Fondaparinux: postoperative start at dose of 2.5 mg subcutaneous daily.

Recently, two new oral anticoagulants have received approval in Canada and Europe for prophylaxis following hip and knee arthroplasty. Dabigatran etexilate, an oral direct thrombin inhibitor, given at a dose of 220 mg once-daily has been evaluated in 3 randomized trials and found to be non-inferior to enoxaparin 40 mg once-daily.[146–148] Rivaroxaban, an oral Factor Xa inhibitor, given at dose of 10 mg once-daily, has been evaluated in 4 randomized trials and found to be superior to enoxaparin 40 mg once-daily and enoxaparin 30 mg twice-daily.[149–152]

There is evidence that aspirin reduces the risk of postoperative VTE by one-third.[153] A study of over 17 000 patients, mostly following hip fracture repair, confirmed these findings, including a reduction in fatal PE (0.27% v 0.65%) during the month following surgery.[154] However, as warfarin, LMWH and fondaparinux are expected to be more effective (at least a two-thirds reduction in VTE), aspirin alone is not recommended during the initial postoperative period.[144] Indirect evidence suggests that a month of aspirin therapy following a short period of prophylaxis with anticoagulant therapy (e.g. 10 days) is likely to be beneficial in patients who undergo major orthopedic surgery.[143,154]

Medical patients: pharmacologic prophylaxis

The evidence that short-term prophylaxis with low-dose UFH prevents clinically important VTE in immobilized medical patients is less convincing, partly because it has been less extensively studied in this population and because there is concern that medical patients remain at high risk of VTE after prophylaxis is stopped.[144,155,156] In recent years, three large randomized controlled trials have shown that LMWH (enoxaparin 40 mg or dalteparin 5000 IU subcutaneously once daily for 10 days) and fondaparinux (2.5 mg once daily) reduce the rate of VTE by about 50% (range 45–63%) compared with placebo in acutely ill medical patients.[157–159]

Mechanical VTE prophylaxis

Graduated compression stockings prevent postoperative VTE in moderate-risk patients (risk reduction of 68%)[160] and intermittent pneumatic compression devices prevent postoperative VTE in high-risk orthopedic patients.[144,161,162] Mechanical methods of prophylaxis should be used in patients who have a moderate or high risk of VTE if anticoagulants are contraindicated (e.g. neurosurgical patients).[144]

> ### Recommendation
>
> Primary prophylaxis with anticoagulants and/or mechanical methods should be used in hospitalized patients who have a moderate or high risk of VTE **Class I, Level A**

Conclusion

Venous thromboembolism is a leading cause of morbidity and mortality in both inpatients and outpatients. Objective testing for VTE is essential because clinical assessment alone is unreliable. Failure to diagnose VTE exposes patients to the risk of fatal PE. However, inappropriate use of anticoagulants exposes patients to the risk of serious bleeding complications, including fatal hemorrhage. Current treatment for acute VTE consists of LMWH or UFH or fondaparinux for a minimum of 5 days, usually administered by subcutaneous injection, as an outpatient in stable patients. A vitamin K antagonist is started the same day and continued for a length of time determined by the individual patient's risk factors for recurrent VTE, risk factors for bleeding, and patient preferences. In general, VTE associated with a reversible risk factor is treated for 3 months, VTE associated with active cancer is treated indefinitely, and unprovoked proximal DVT or PE is treated for a minimum of 3 months and often indefinitely, if anticoagulant therapy is well tolerated and associated with a low risk of bleeding. Patients with confirmed PE and hemodynamic compromise should be treated with thrombolytic therapy unless they have a high risk of bleeding. Most hospitalized patients should receive pharmacologic or mechanical prophylaxis for VTE.

References

1. Cervantes J, Rojas G. Virchow's legacy: deep vein thrombosis and pulmonary embolism. *World J Surg* 2005;**29**(suppl 1):S30–S34.
2. Barritt DW, Jordan SC. Anticoagulant drugs in the treatment of pulmonary embolism. A controlled trial. *Lancet* 1960;**1**:1309–12.
3. Anderson FA Jr, Spencer FA. Risk factors for venous thromboembolism. *Circulation* 2003;**107**(23 suppl 1):I9–16.
4. White RH. The epidemiology of venous thromboembolism. *Circulation* 2003;**107**(23 suppl 1):I4–I8.
5. Heit JA, Silverstein MD, Mohr DN, Petterson TM, O'Fallon WM, Melton LJ III. Risk factors for deep vein thrombosis and pulmonary embolism: a population-based case-control study. *Arch Intern Med* 2000;**160**(6):809–15.
6. Cogo A, Lensing AW, Prandoni P, Hirsh J. Distribution of thrombosis in patients with symptomatic deep vein thrombosis. Implications for simplifying the diagnostic process with compression ultrasound. *Arch Intern Med* 1993;**153**(24):2777–80.
7. Kearon C, Julian JA, Newman TE, Ginsberg JS. Noninvasive diagnosis of deep venous thrombosis. McMaster Diagnostic Imaging Practice Guidelines Initiative. *Ann Intern Med* 1998;**128**(8):663–77.
8. Lagerstedt CI, Olsson CG, Fagher BO, Oqvist BW, Albrechtsson U. Need for long-term anticoagulant treatment in symptomatic calf-vein thrombosis. *Lancet* 1985;**2**(8454):515–18.

9. Moser KM, LeMoine JR. Is embolic risk conditioned by location of deep venous thrombosis? *Ann Intern Med* 1981;**94**(4 pt 1):439–44.

10. Hull RD, Hirsh J, Carter CJ, Jay RM, Dodd PE, Ockelford PA *et al.* Pulmonary angiography, ventilation lung scanning, and venography for clinically suspected pulmonary embolism with abnormal perfusion lung scan. *Ann Intern Med* 1983; **98**(6):891–9.

11. Wells PS, Ginsberg JS, Anderson DR, Kearon C, Gent M, Turpie AG *et al.* Use of a clinical model for safe management of patients with suspected pulmonary embolism. *Ann Intern Med* 1998;**129**(12):997–1005.

12. Stein PD, Henry JW. Prevalence of acute pulmonary embolism among patients in a general hospital and at autopsy. *Chest* 1995;**108**(4):978–81.

13. Hull R, Delmore T, Genton E, Hirsh J, Gent M, Sackett D *et al.* Warfarin sodium versus low-dose heparin in the long-term treatment of venous thrombosis. *N Engl J Med* 1979;**301** (16):855–8.

14. Prandoni P, Lensing AW, Cogo A, Cuppini S, Villalta S, Carta M *et al.* The long-term clinical course of acute deep venous thrombosis. *Ann Intern Med* 1996;**125**(1):1–7.

15. Schulman S, Rhedin AS, Lindmarker P, Carlsson A, Larfars G, Nicol P *et al.* A comparison of six weeks with six months of oral anticoagulant therapy after a first episode of venous thromboembolism. Duration of Anticoagulation Trial Study Group. *N Engl J Med* 1995;**332**(25):1661–5.

16. Kearon C, Ginsberg JS, Anderson DR, Kovacs MJ, Wells P, Julian JA *et al.* Comparison of 1 month with 3 months of anticoagulation for a first episode of venous thromboembolism associated with a transient risk factor. *J Thromb Haemost* 2004;**2**(5):743–9.

17. Baglin T, Luddington R, Brown K, Baglin C. Incidence of recurrent venous thromboembolism in relation to clinical and thrombophilic risk factors: prospective cohort study. *Lancet* 2003;**362**(9383):523–6.

18. Research Committee of the British Thoracic Society. Optimum duration of anticoagulation for deep-vein thrombosis and pulmonary embolism. *Lancet* 1992;**340**(8824):873–6.

19. Levine MN, Hirsh J, Gent M, Turpie AG, Weitz J, Ginsberg J *et al.* Optimal duration of oral anticoagulant therapy: a randomized trial comparing four weeks with three months of warfarin in patients with proximal deep vein thrombosis. *Thromb Haemost* 1995;**74**(2):606–11.

20. Turpie AG, Levine MN, Hirsh J, Carter CJ, Jay RM, Powers PJ *et al.* Double-blind randomised trial of Org 10172 low-molecular-weight heparinoid in prevention of deep-vein thrombosis in thrombotic stroke. *Lancet* 1987;**1**(8532):523–6.

21. Ray JG, Chan WS. Deep vein thrombosis during pregnancy and the puerperium: a meta-analysis of the period of risk and the leg of presentation. *Obstet Gynecol Surv* 1999;**54**(4):265–71.

22. Cruickshank MK, Levine MN, Hirsh J, Turpie AG, Powers P, Jay R *et al.* An evaluation of impedance plethysmography and 125I-fibrinogen leg scanning in patients following hip surgery. *Thromb Haemost* 1989;**62**(3):830–4.

23. Merrer J, De JB, Golliot F, Lefrant JY, Raffy B, Barre E *et al.* Complications of femoral and subclavian venous catheterization in critically ill patients: a randomized controlled trial. *JAMA* 2001;**286**(6):700–7.

24. Heijboer H, Brandjes DP, Buller HR, Sturk A, ten Cate JW. Deficiencies of coagulation-inhibiting and fibrinolytic proteins in outpatients with deep-vein thrombosis. *N Engl J Med* 1990;**323**(22):1512–16.

25. Kearon C, Crowther M, Hirsh J. Management of patients with hereditary hypercoagulable disorders. *Annu Rev Med* 2000;**51**:169–85.

26. Emmerich J, Rosendaal FR, Cattaneo M, Margaglione M, De Stefano V, Cumming T *et al.* Combined effect of factor V Leiden and prothrombin 20210A on the risk of venous thromboembolism – pooled analysis of 8 case-control studies including 2310 cases and 3204 controls. Study Group for Pooled-Analysis in Venous Thromboembolism. *Thromb Haemost* 2001;**86**(3): 809–16.

27. Poort SR, Rosendaal FR, Reitsma PH, Bertina RM. A common genetic variation in the 3′-untranslated region of the prothrombin gene is associated with elevated plasma prothrombin levels and an increase in venous thrombosis. *Blood* 1996;**88**(10): 3698–703.

28. den Heijer M, Lewington S, Clarke R. Homocysteine, MTHFR and risk of venous thrombosis: a meta-analysis of published epidemiological studies. *J Thromb Haemost* 2005;**3**(2):292–9.

29. Tsai AW, Cushman M, Rosamond WD, Heckbert SR, Tracy RP, Aleksic N *et al.* Coagulation factors, inflammation markers, and venous thromboembolism: the longitudinal investigation of thromboembolism etiology (LITE). *Am J Med* 2002;**113**(8): 636–42.

30. Meijers JC, Tekelenburg WL, Bouma BN, Bertina RM, Rosendaal FR. High levels of coagulation factor XI as a risk factor for venous thrombosis. *N Engl J Med* 2000;**342**(10): 696–701.

31. Van Hylckama Vlieg A, van der Linden IK, Bertina RM, Rosendaal FR. High levels of factor IX increase the risk of venous thrombosis. *Blood* 2000;**95**(12):3678–82.

32. Warkentin TE, Levine MN, Hirsh J, Horsewood P, Roberts RS, Gent M *et al.* Heparin-induced thrombocytopenia in patients treated with low-molecular-weight heparin or unfractionated heparin. *N Engl J Med* 1995;**332**(20):1330–5.

33. Hull R, Hirsh J, Sackett DL, Taylor DW, Carter C, Turpie AG *et al.* Clinical validity of a negative venogram in patients with clinically suspected venous thrombosis. *Circulation* 1981;**64**(3): 622–5.

34. Wells PS, Anderson DR, Bormanis J, Guy F, Mitchell M, Gray L *et al.* Value of assessment of pretest probability of deep-vein thrombosis in clinical management. *Lancet* 1997;**350**(9094): 1795–8.

35. Wells PS, Anderson DR, Rodger M, Forgie M, Kearon C, Dreyer J *et al.* Evaluation of D-dimer in the diagnosis of suspected deep-vein thrombosis. *N Engl J Med* 2003;**349**(13):1227–35.

36. Anand SS, Wells PS, Hunt D, Brill-Edwards P, Cook D, Ginsberg JS. Does this patient have deep vein thrombosis? *JAMA* 1998;**279**(14):1094–9.

37. Chunilal SD, Eikelboom JW, Attia J, Miniati M, Panju AA, Simel DL *et al.* Does this patient have pulmonary embolism? *JAMA* 2003;**290**(21):2849–58.

38. Wells PS, Owen C, Doucette S, Fergusson D, Tran H. Does this patient have deep vein thrombosis? *JAMA* 2006;**295**(2):199–207.

39. Kearon C, Ginsberg JS, Hirsh J. The role of venous ultrasonography in the diagnosis of suspected deep venous thrombosis

and pulmonary embolism. *Ann Intern Med* 1998;**129**(12): 1044–9.

40. Goodacre S, Sampson F, Thomas S, van Beek EJ, Sutton A. Systematic review and meta-analysis of the diagnostic accuracy of ultrasonography for deep vein thrombosis. *BMC Med Imaging* 2005;**5**:6.

41. Stevens SM, Elliott CG, Chan KJ, Egger MJ, Ahmed KM. Withholding anticoagulation after a negative result on duplex ultrasonography for suspected symptomatic deep venous thrombosis. *Ann Intern Med* 2004;**140**(12):985–91.

42. Elias A, Mallard L, Elias M, Alquier C, Guidolin F, Gauthier B *et al.* A single complete ultrasound investigation of the venous network for the diagnostic management of patients with a clinically suspected first episode of deep venous thrombosis of the lower limbs. *Thromb Haemost* 2003;**89**(2):221–7.

43. Schellong SM, Schwarz T, Halbritter K, Beyer J, Siegert G, Oettler W *et al.* Complete compression ultrasonography of the leg veins as a single test for the diagnosis of deep vein thrombosis. *Thromb Haemost* 2003;**89**(2):228–34.

44. Robinson KS, Anderson DR, Gross M, Petrie D, Leighton R, Stanish W *et al.* Ultrasonographic screening before hospital discharge for deep venous thrombosis after arthroplasty: the post-arthroplasty screening study. A randomized, controlled trial. *Ann Intern Med* 1997;**127**(6):439–45.

45. Kanne JP, Lalani TA. Role of computed tomography and magnetic resonance imaging for deep venous thrombosis and pulmonary embolism. *Circulation* 2004;**109**(12 suppl 1):I15–I21.

46. Sampson FC, Goodacre SW, Thomas SM, van Beek EJ. The accuracy of MRI in diagnosis of suspected deep vein thrombosis: systematic review and meta-analysis. *Eur Radiol* 2007;**17**(1):175–81.

47. Fraser DG, Moody AR, Morgan PS, Martel AL, Davidson I. Diagnosis of lower-limb deep venous thrombosis: a prospective blinded study of magnetic resonance direct thrombus imaging. *Ann Intern Med* 2002 ;**136**(2):89–98.

48. Kelly J, Rudd A, Lewis RR, Hunt BJ. Plasma D-dimers in the diagnosis of venous thromboembolism. *Arch Intern Med* 2002;**162**(7):747–56.

49. Stein PD, Hull RD, Patel KC, Olson RE, Ghali WA, Brant R *et al.* D-dimer for the exclusion of acute venous thrombosis and pulmonary embolism: a systematic review. *Ann Intern Med* 2004;**140**(8):589–602.

50. Perrier A, Desmarais S, Miron MJ, de Moerloose P, Lepage R, Slosman D *et al.* Non-invasive diagnosis of venous thromboembolism in outpatients. *Lancet* 1999;**353**(9148):190–5.

51. Bernardi E, Prandoni P, Lensing AW, Agnelli G, Guazzaloca G, Scannapieco G *et al.* D-dimer testing as an adjunct to ultrasonography in patients with clinically suspected deep vein thrombosis: prospective cohort study. The Multicentre Italian D-dimer Ultrasound Study Investigators Group. *BMJ* 1998;**317**(7165):1037–40.

52. Kearon C, Ginsberg JS, Douketis J, Crowther M, Brill-Edwards P, Weitz JI *et al.* Management of suspected deep venous thrombosis in outpatients by using clinical assessment and D-dimer testing. *Ann Intern Med* 2001;**135**(2):108–11.

53. Fancher TL, White RH, Kravitz RL. Combined use of rapid D-dimer testing and estimation of clinical probability in the diagnosis of deep vein thrombosis: systematic review. *BMJ* 2004;**329**(7470):821.

54. Righini M, Goehring C, Bounameaux H, Perrier A. Effects of age on the performance of common diagnostic tests for pulmonary embolism. *Am J Med* 2000;**109**(5):357–61.

55. Lee AY, Julian JA, Levine MN, Weitz JI, Kearon C, Wells PS *et al.* Clinical utility of a rapid whole-blood D-dimer assay in patients with cancer who present with suspected acute deep venous thrombosis. *Ann Intern Med* 1999;**131**(6):417–23.

56. Prandoni P, Cogo A, Bernardi E, Villalta S, Polistena P, Simioni P *et al.* A simple ultrasound approach for detection of recurrent proximal-vein thrombosis. *Circulation* 1993;**88**(4 Pt 1):1730–5.

57. Rathbun SW, Whitsett TL, Raskob GE. Negative D-dimer result to exclude recurrent deep venous thrombosis: a management trial. *Ann Intern Med* 2004;**141**(11):839–45.

58. Stein PD, Athanasoulis C, Alavi A, Greenspan RH, Hales CA, Saltzman HA *et al.* Complications and validity of pulmonary angiography in acute pulmonary embolism. *Circulation* 1992;**85**(2):462–8.

59. Stein PD, Fowler SE, Goodman LR, Gottschalk A, Hales CA, Hull RD *et al.* Multidetector computed tomography for acute pulmonary embolism. *N Engl J Med* 2006;**354**(22):2317–27.

60. van Belle A, Buller HR, Huisman MV, Huisman PM, Kaasjager K, Kamphuisen PW *et al.* Effectiveness of managing suspected pulmonary embolism using an algorithm combining clinical probability, D-dimer testing, and computed tomography. *JAMA* 2006;**295**(2):172–9.

61. Quiroz R, Kucher N, Zou KH, Kipfmueller F, Costello P, Goldhaber SZ *et al.* Clinical validity of a negative computed tomography scan in patients with suspected pulmonary embolism: a systematic review. *JAMA* 2005;**293**(16):2012–17.

62. Roy PM, Colombet I, Durieux P, Chatellier G, Sors H, Meyer G. Systematic review and meta-analysis of strategies for the diagnosis of suspected pulmonary embolism. *BMJ* 2005;**331** (7511):259.

63. Einstein AJ, Henzlova MJ, Rajagopalan S. Estimating risk of cancer associated with radiation exposure from 64-slice computed tomography coronary angiography. *JAMA* 2007; **298**(3):317–23.

64. Pedersen MR, Fisher MT, van Beek EJ. MR imaging of the pulmonary vasculature – an update. *Eur Radiol* 2006;**16**(6):1374–86.

65. Hull RD, Raskob GE, Coates G, Panju AA. Clinical validity of a normal perfusion lung scan in patients with suspected pulmonary embolism. *Chest* 1990;**97**(1):23–6.

66. Kipper MS, Moser KM, Kortman KE, Ashburn WL. Longterm follow-up of patients with suspected pulmonary embolism and a normal lung scan. Perfusion scans in embolic suspects. *Chest* 1982;**82**(4):411–15.

67. PIOPED Investigators. Value of the ventilation/perfusion scan in acute pulmonary embolism. Results of the prospective investigation of pulmonary embolism diagnosis (PIOPED). *JAMA* 1990;**263**(20):2753–9.

68. Hull RD, Hirsh J, Carter CJ, Raskob GE, Gill GJ, Jay RM *et al.* Diagnostic value of ventilation-perfusion lung scanning in patients with suspected pulmonary embolism. *Chest* 1985; **88**(6):819–28.

69. Stein PD, Henry JW, Gottschalk A. Mismatched vascular defects. An easy alternative to mismatched segmental equivalent defects for the interpretation of ventilation/perfusion lung scans in pulmonary embolism. *Chest* 1993;**104**(5):1468–71.

70. Wells PS, Anderson DR, Rodger M, Stiell I, Dreyer JF, Barnes D et al. Excluding pulmonary embolism at the bedside without diagnostic imaging: management of patients with suspected pulmonary embolism presenting to the emergency department by using a simple clinical model and d-dimer. *Ann Intern Med* 2001;**135**(2):98–107.

71. Kearon C, Ginsberg JS, Douketis J, Turpie AG, Bates SM, Lee AY et al. An evaluation of D-dimer in the diagnosis of pulmonary embolism: a randomized trial. *Ann Intern Med* 2006;**144**(11):812–21.

72. Buller HR, Agnelli G, Hull RD, Hyers TM, Prins MH, Raskob GE. Antithrombotic therapy for venous thromboembolic disease: the Seventh ACCP Conference on Antithrombotic and Thrombolytic Therapy. *Chest* 2004;**126**(3 suppl):401S–28S.

73. van Dongen CJ, van den Belt AGM, Prins MH, Lensing AWA. Fixed dose subcutaneous low molecular weight heparins versus adjusted dose unfractionated heparin for venous thromboembolism. *Cochrane Database of Systematic Reviews* 2004, Issue 4. Art. No.: CD001100. DOI: 10.1002/14651858.CD001100.pub2.

74. Prandoni P, Carnovali M, Marchiori A. Subcutaneous adjusted-dose unfractionated heparin vs fixed-dose low-molecular-weight heparin in the initial treatment of venous thromboembolism. *Arch Intern Med* 2004;**164**(10):1077–83.

75. Kearon C, Ginsberg JS, Julian JA, Douketis J, Solymoss S, Ockelford P et al. Comparison of fixed-dose weight-adjusted unfractionated heparin and low-molecular-weight heparin for acute treatment of venous thromboembolism. *JAMA* 2006;**296**(8):935–42.

76. Buller HR, Davidson BL, Decousus H, Gallus A, Gent M, Piovella F et al. Fondaparinux or enoxaparin for the initial treatment of symptomatic deep venous thrombosis: a randomized trial. *Ann Intern Med* 2004;**140**(11):867–73.

77. Raschke RA, Reilly BM, Guidry JR, Fontana JR, Srinivas S. The weight-based heparin dosing nomogram compared with a "standard care" nomogram. A randomized controlled trial. *Ann Intern Med* 1993;**119**(9):874–81.

78. Chong BH, Gallus AS, Cade JF, Magnani H, Manoharan A, Oldmeadow M et al. Prospective randomised open-label comparison of danaparoid with dextran 70 in the treatment of heparin-induced thrombocytopaenia with thrombosis: a clinical outcome study. *Thromb Haemost* 2001;**86**(5):1170–5.

79. Greinacher A, Janssens U, Berg G, Bock M, Kwasny H, Kemkes-Matthes B et al. Lepirudin (recombinant hirudin) for parenteral anticoagulation in patients with heparin-induced thrombocytopenia. Heparin-Associated Thrombocytopenia Study (HAT) investigators. *Circulation* 1999;**100**(6):587–93.

80. Lewis BE, Wallis DE, Berkowitz SD, Matthai WH, Fareed J, Walenga JM et al. Argatroban anticoagulant therapy in patients with heparin-induced thrombocytopenia. *Circulation* 2001;**103**(14):1838–43.

81. Aujesky D, Perrier A, Roy PM, Stone RA, Cornuz J, Meyer G et al. Validation of a clinical prognostic model to identify low-risk patients with pulmonary embolism. *J Intern Med* 2007;**261**(6):597–604.

82. Buller HR, Davidson BL, Decousus H, Gallus A, Gent M, Piovella F et al. Subcutaneous fondaparinux versus intravenous unfractionated heparin in the initial treatment of pulmonary embolism. *N Engl J Med* 2003;**349**(18):1695–702.

83. Kovacs MJ, Anderson D, Morrow B, Gray L, Touchie D, Wells PS. Outpatient treatment of pulmonary embolism with dalteparin. *Thromb Haemost* 2000;**83**(2):209–11.

84. Beer JH, Burger M, Gretener S, Bernard-Bagattini S, Bounameaux H. Outpatient treatment of pulmonary embolism is feasible and safe in a substantial proportion of patients. *J Thromb Haemost* 2003;**1**(1):186–7.

85. Gallus A, Jackaman J, Tillett J, Mills W, Wycherley A. Safety and efficacy of warfarin started early after submassive venous thrombosis or pulmonary embolism. *Lancet* 1986;**2**(8519):1293–6.

86. Hull RD, Raskob GE, Rosenbloom D, Panju AA, Brill-Edwards P, Ginsberg JS et al. Heparin for 5 days as compared with 10 days in the initial treatment of proximal venous thrombosis. *N Engl J Med* 1990;**322**(18):1260–4.

87. Harrison L, Johnston M, Massicotte MP, Crowther M, Moffat K, Hirsh J. Comparison of 5-mg and 10-mg loading doses in initiation of warfarin therapy. *Ann Intern Med* 1997;**126**(2):133–6.

88. Crowther MA, Ginsberg JB, Kearon C, Harrison L, Johnson J, Massicotte MP et al. A randomized trial comparing 5-mg and 10-mg warfarin loading doses. *Arch Intern Med* 1999;**159**(1):46–8.

89. Kovacs MJ, Rodger M, Anderson DR, Morrow B, Kells G, Kovacs J et al. Comparison of 10-mg and 5-mg warfarin initiation nomograms together with low-molecular-weight heparin for outpatient treatment of acute venous thromboembolism. A randomized, double-blind, controlled trial. *Ann Intern Med* 2003;**138**(9):714–19.

90. Ansell J, Hirsh J, Poller L, Bussey H, Jacobson A, Hylek E. The pharmacology and management of the vitamin K antagonists: the Seventh ACCP Conference on Antithrombotic and Thrombolytic Therapy. *Chest* 2004;**126**(3 suppl):204S–33S.

91. Garcia D, Regan S, Crowther M, Hughes RA, Hylek EM. Warfarin maintenance dosing patterns in clinical practice: implications for safer anticoagulation in the elderly population. *Chest* 2005;**127**(6):2049–56.

92. Buller HR, Cohen AT, Davidson B, Decousus H, Gallus AS, Gent M et al. Idraparinux versus standard therapy for venous thromboembolic disease. *N Engl J Med* 2007;**357**(11):1094–104.

93. Schulman S, Lundstrom T, Walander K, Billing CS, Eriksson H. Ximelagatran for the secondary prevention of venous thromboembolism: a complementary follow-up analysis of the THRIVE III study. *Thromb Haemost* 2005;**94**(4):820–4.

94. Hull R, Delmore T, Carter C, Hirsh J, Genton E, Gent M et al. Adjusted subcutaneous heparin versus warfarin sodium in the long-term treatment of venous thrombosis. *N Engl J Med* 1982;**306**(4):189–94.

95. van der Heijden JF, Hutten BA, Büller HR, Prins MH. Vitamin K antagonists or low-molecular-weight heparin for the long term treatment of symptomatic venous thromboembolism. *Cochrane Database of Systematic Reviews* 2001, Issue 3. Art. No.: CD002001. DOI: 10.1002/14651858.CD002001.

96. Iorio A, Guercini F, Pini M. Low-molecular-weight heparin for the long-term treatment of symptomatic venous thromboembolism: meta-analysis of the randomized comparisons with oral anticoagulants. *J Thromb Haemost* 2003;**1**(9):1906–13.

97. Hull R, Hirsh J, Jay R, Carter C, England C, Gent M et al. Different intensities of oral anticoagulant therapy in the treatment

of proximal-vein thrombosis. *N Engl J Med* 1982;**307**(27): 1676–81.

98. Pini M, Aiello S, Manotti C, Pattacini C, Quintavalla R, Poli T et al. Low molecular weight heparin versus warfarin in the prevention of recurrences after deep vein thrombosis. *Thromb Haemost* 1994;**72**(2):191–7.

99. Pinede L, Ninet J, Duhaut P, Chabaud S, Demolombe-Rague S, Durieu I et al. Comparison of 3 and 6 months of oral anticoagulant therapy after a first episode of proximal deep vein thrombosis or pulmonary embolism and comparison of 6 and 12 weeks of therapy after isolated calf deep vein thrombosis. *Circulation* 2001;**103**(20):2453–60.

100. Pinede L, Duhaut P, Cucherat M, Ninet J, Pasquier J, Boissel JP. Comparison of long versus short duration of anticoagulant therapy after a first episode of venous thromboembolism: a meta-analysis of randomized, controlled trials. *J Intern Med* 2000;**247**(5):553–62.

101. Agnelli G, Prandoni P, Santamaria MG, Bagatella P, Iorio A, Bazzan M et al. Three months versus one year of oral anticoagulant therapy for idiopathic deep venous thrombosis. Warfarin Optimal Duration Italian Trial Investigators. *N Engl J Med* 2001;**345**(3):165–9.

102. Agnelli G, Prandoni P, Becattini C, Silingardi M, Taliani MR, Miccio M et al. Extended oral anticoagulant therapy after a first episode of pulmonary embolism. *Ann Intern Med* 2003; **139**(1):19–25.

103. Lindmarker P, Schulman S. The risk of ipsilateral versus contralateral recurrent deep vein thrombosis in the leg. The DURAC Trial Study Group. *J Intern Med* 2000;**247**(5):601–6.

104. Kearon C, Gent M, Hirsh J, Weitz J, Kovacs MJ, Anderson DR et al. A comparison of three months of anticoagulation with extended anticoagulation for a first episode of idiopathic venous thromboembolism. *N Engl J Med* 1999;**340**(12):901–7.

105. Schulman S, Granqvist S, Holmstrom M, Carlsson A, Lindmarker P, Nicol P et al. The duration of oral anticoagulant therapy after a second episode of venous thromboembolism. The Duration of Anticoagulation Trial Study Group. *N Engl J Med* 1997;**336**(6):393–8.

106. Murin S, Romano PS, White RH. Comparison of outcomes after hospitalization for deep venous thrombosis or pulmonary embolism. *Thromb Haemost* 2002;**88**(3):407–14.

107. Schulman S, Svenungsson E, Granqvist S. Anticardiolipin antibodies predict early recurrence of thromboembolism and death among patients with venous thromboembolism following anticoagulant therapy. Duration of Anticoagulation Study Group. *Am J Med* 1998;**104**(4):332–8.

108. Schulman S, Wahlander K, Lundstrom T, Clason SB, Eriksson H. Secondary prevention of venous thromboembolism with the oral direct thrombin inhibitor ximelagatran. *N Engl J Med* 2003;**349**(18):1713–21.

109. Heit JA, Mohr DN, Silverstein MD, Petterson TM, O'Fallon WM, Melton LJ III. Predictors of recurrence after deep vein thrombosis and pulmonary embolism: a population-based cohort study. *Arch Intern Med* 2000;**160**(6):761–8.

110. Palareti G, Legnani C, Cosmi B, Guazzaloca G, Pancani C, Coccheri S. Risk of venous thromboembolism recurrence: high negative predictive value of D-dimer performed after oral anticoagulation is stopped. *Thromb Haemost* 2002;**87**(1):7–12.

111. Lee AY, Levine MN, Baker RI, Bowden C, Kakkar AK, Prins M et al. Low-molecular-weight heparin versus a coumarin for the prevention of recurrent venous thromboembolism in patients with cancer. *N Engl J Med* 2003;**349**(2):146–53.

112. McRae S, Tran H, Schulman S, Ginsberg J, Kearon C. Effect of patient's sex on risk of recurrent venous thromboembolism: a meta-analysis. *Lancet* 2006;**368**(9533):371–8.

113. Schulman S, Lindmarker P, Holmstrom M, Larfars G, Carlsson A, Nicol P et al. Post-thrombotic syndrome, recurrence, and death 10 years after the first episode of venous thromboembolism treated with warfarin for 6 weeks or 6 months. *J Thromb Haemost* 2006;**4**(4):734–42.

114. Ho WK, Hankey GJ, Quinlan DJ, Eikelboom JW. Risk of recurrent venous thromboembolism in patients with common thrombophilia: a systematic review. *Arch Intern Med* 2006;**166**(7):729–36.

115. Palareti G, Legnani C, Cosmi B, Valdre L, Lunghi B, Bernardi F et al. Predictive value of D-dimer test for recurrent venous thromboembolism after anticoagulation withdrawal in subjects with a previous idiopathic event and in carriers of congenital thrombophilia. *Circulation* 2003;**108**(3):313–18.

116. Christiansen SC, Cannegieter SC, Koster T, Vandenbroucke JP, Rosendaal FR. Thrombophilia, clinical factors, and recurrent venous thrombotic events. *JAMA* 2005;**293**(19):2352–61.

117. Palareti G, Cosmi B, Legnani C, Tosetto A, Brusi C, Iorio A et al. D-dimer testing to determine the duration of anticoagulation therapy. *N Engl J Med* 2006;**355**(17):1780–9.

118. Prandoni P, Lensing AW, Prins MH, Bernardi E, Marchiori A, Bagatella P et al. Residual venous thrombosis as a predictive factor of recurrent venous thromboembolism. *Ann Intern Med* 2002;**137**(12):955–60.

119. Kearon C. Duration of therapy for acute venous thromboembolism. *Clin Chest Med* 2003;**24**(1):63–72.

120. Beyth RJ, Quinn LM, Landefeld CS. Prospective evaluation of an index for predicting the risk of major bleeding in outpatients treated with warfarin. *Am J Med* 1998;**105**(2):91–9.

121. Gage BF, Yan Y, Milligan PE, Waterman AD, Culverhouse R, Rich MW et al. Clinical classification schemes for predicting hemorrhage: results from the National Registry of Atrial Fibrillation (NRAF). *Am Heart J* 2006;**151**(3):713–19.

122. Linkins LA, Choi PT, Douketis JD. Clinical impact of bleeding in patients taking oral anticoagulant therapy for venous thromboembolism: a meta-analysis. *Ann Intern Med* 2003; **139**(11):893–900.

123. Kearon C, Ginsberg JS, Kovacs MJ, Anderson DR, Wells P, Julian JA et al. Comparison of low-intensity warfarin therapy with conventional-intensity warfarin therapy for long-term prevention of recurrent venous thromboembolism. *N Engl J Med* 2003;**349**(7):631–9.

124. Levine MN, Raskob G, Beyth RJ, Kearon C, Schulman S. Hemorrhagic complications of anticoagulant treatment: the Seventh ACCP Conference on Antithrombotic and Thrombolytic Therapy. *Chest* 2004;**126**(3 suppl):287S–310S.

125. Decousus H, Leizorovicz A, Parent F, Page Y, Tardy B, Girard P et al. A clinical trial of vena caval filters in the prevention of pulmonary embolism in patients with proximal deep-vein thrombosis. Prevention du Risque d'Embolie Pulmonaire par Interruption Cave Study Group. *N Engl J Med* 1998;**338**(7): 409–15.

126. Eight-year follow-up of patients with permanent vena cava filters in the prevention of pulmonary embolism: the PREPIC (Prevention du Risque d'Embolie Pulmonaire par Interruption Cave) randomized study. *Circulation* 2005;**112**(3):416–22.

127. Wan S, Quinlan DJ, Agnelli G, Eikelboom JW. Thrombolysis compared with heparin for the initial treatment of pulmonary embolism: a meta-analysis of the randomized controlled trials. *Circulation* 2004;**110**(6):744–9.

128. Jerjes-Sanchez C, Ramirez-Rivera A, de Lourdes GM, Arriaga-Nava R, Valencia S, Rosado-Buzzo A *et al.* Streptokinase and heparin versus heparin alone in massive pulmonary embolism: a randomized controlled trial. *J Thromb Thrombolysis* 1995;**2**(3):227–9.

129. Dong BR, Yue J, Liu GJ, Wang Q, Wu T. Thrombolytic therapy for pulmonary embolism. *Cochrane Database of Systematic Reviews* 2006, Issue 2. Art. No.: CD004437. DOI: 10.1002/14651858. CD004437.pub2.

130. Watson L, Armon MP. Thrombolysis for acute deep vein thrombosis. *Cochrane Database of Systematic Reviews* 2004, Issue 3. Art. No.: CD002783. DOI: 10.1002/14651858.CD002783.pub2.

131. Konstantinides S, Geibel A, Olschewski M, Kasper W, Hruska N, Jackle S *et al.* Importance of cardiac troponins I and T in risk stratification of patients with acute pulmonary embolism. *Circulation* 2002;**106**(10):1263–8.

132. Giannitsis E, Katus HA. Risk stratification in pulmonary embolism based on biomarkers and echocardiography. *Circulation* 2005;**112**(11):1520–1.

133. Scridon T, Scridon C, Skali H, Alvarez A, Goldhaber SZ, Solomon SD. Prognostic significance of troponin elevation and right ventricular enlargement in acute pulmonary embolism. *Am J Cardiol* 2005;**96**(2):303–5.

134. Douketis JD, Leeuwenkamp O, Grobara P, Johnston M, Sohne M, Ten WM *et al.* The incidence and prognostic significance of elevated cardiac troponins in patients with submassive pulmonary embolism. *J Thromb Haemost* 2005;**3**(3):508–13.

135. Goldhaber SZ. Echocardiography in the management of pulmonary embolism. *Ann Intern Med* 2002;**136**(9):691–700.

136. Schoepf UJ, Kucher N, Kipfmueller F, Quiroz R, Costello P, Goldhaber SZ. Right ventricular enlargement on chest computed tomography: a predictor of early death in acute pulmonary embolism. *Circulation* 2004;**110**(20):3276–80.

137. Collins R, Scrimgeour A, Yusuf S, Peto R. Reduction in fatal pulmonary embolism and venous thrombosis by perioperative administration of subcutaneous heparin. Overview of results of randomized trials in general, orthopedic, and urologic surgery. *N Engl J Med* 1988;**318**(18):1162–73.

138. Salzman EW, Davies GC. Prophylaxis of venous thromboembolism: analysis of cost effectiveness. *Ann Surg* 1980;**191**(2):207–18.

139. Kakkar VV, Corrigan TP, Fossard DP, Sutherland I, Thirwell J. Prevention of fatal postoperative pulmonary embolism by low doses of heparin. Reappraisal of results of international multicentre trial. *Lancet* 1977;**1**(8011):567–9.

140. Koch A, Bouges S, Ziegler S, Dinkel H, Daures JP, Victor N. Low molecular weight heparin and unfractionated heparin in thrombosis prophylaxis after major surgical intervention: update of previous meta-analyses. *Br J Surg* 1997;**84**(6):750–9.

141. Eikelboom JW, Quinlan DJ, Douketis JD. Extended-duration prophylaxis against venous thromboembolism after total hip or knee replacement: a meta-analysis of the randomised trials. *Lancet* 2001;**358**(9275):9–15.

142. Douketis JD, Eikelboom JW, Quinlan DJ, Willan AR, Crowther MA. Short-duration prophylaxis against venous thromboembolism after total hip or knee replacement: a meta-analysis of prospective studies investigating symptomatic outcomes. *Arch Intern Med* 2002;**162**(13):1465–71.

143. Kearon C. Duration of venous thromboembolism prophylaxis after surgery. *Chest* 2003;**124**(6 Suppl):386S–92S.

144. Geerts WH, Pineo GF, Heit JA, Bergqvist D, Lassen MR, Colwell CW *et al.* Prevention of venous thromboembolism: the Seventh ACCP Conference on Antithrombotic and Thrombolytic Therapy. *Chest* 2004;**126**(3 suppl):338S–400S.

145. Turpie AG, Bauer KA, Eriksson BI, Lassen MR. Fondaparinux vs enoxaparin for the prevention of venous thromboembolism in major orthopedic surgery: a meta-analysis of 4 randomized double-blind studies. *Arch Intern Med* 2002;**162**(16):1833–40.

146. Ginsberg JS, Davidson BL, Comp PC, Francis CW, Friedman RJ, Huo MH *et al.* Oral thrombin inhibitor dabigatran etexilate vs North American enoxaparin regimen for prevention of venous thromboembolism after knee arthroplasty surgery. *J Arthroplasty* 2009;**24**(1):1–9.

147. Eriksson BI, Dahl OE, Rosencher N, Kurth AA, van Dijk CN, Frostick SP *et al.* Dabigatran etexilate versus enoxaparin for prevention of venous thromboembolism after total hip replacement: a randomised, double-blind, non-inferiority trial. *Lancet* 2007;**370**(9591):949–56.

148. Eriksson BI, Dahl OE, Rosencher N, Kurth AA, van Dijk CN, Frostick SP *et al.* Oral dabigatran etexilate vs. subcutaneous enoxaparin for the prevention of venous thromboembolism after total knee replacement: the RE-MODEL randomized trial. *J Thromb Haemost* 2007;**5**(11):2178–85.

149. Eriksson BI, Borris LC, Friedman RJ, Haas S, Huisman MV, Kakkar AK *et al.* Rivaroxaban versus enoxaparin for thromboprophylaxis after hip arthroplasty. *N Engl J Med* 2008;**358**(26):2765–75.

150. Lassen MR, Ageno W, Borris LC, Lieberman JR, Rosencher N, Bandel TJ *et al.* Rivaroxaban versus enoxaparin for thromboprophylaxis after total knee arthroplasty. *N Engl J Med* 2008;**358**(26):2776–86.

151. Kakkar AK, Brenner B, Dahl OE, Eriksson BI, Mouret P, Muntz J *et al.* Extended duration rivaroxaban versus short-term enoxaparin for the prevention of venous thromboembolism after total hip arthroplasty: a double-blind, randomised controlled trial. *Lancet* 2008;**372**(9632):31–9.

152. Turpie AG, Lassen MR, Davidson BL, Bauer KA, Gent M, Kwong LM *et al.* Rivaroxaban versus enoxaparin for thromboprophylaxis after total knee arthroplasty (RECORD4): a randomised trial. *Lancet* 2009;**373**(9676):1673–80.

153. Antiplatelet Trialists' Collaboration. Collaborative overview of randomised trials of antiplatelet therapy – III: Reduction in venous thrombosis and pulmonary embolism by antiplatelet prophylaxis among surgical and medical patients. *BMJ* 1994;**308**(6923):235–46.

154. No authors listed. Prevention of pulmonary embolism and deep vein thrombosis with low dose aspirin: Pulmonary Embolism Prevention (PEP) trial. *Lancet* 2000;**355**(9212):1295–302.

155. Gardlund B. Randomised, controlled trial of low-dose heparin for prevention of fatal pulmonary embolism in patients with

infectious diseases. The Heparin Prophylaxis Study Group. *Lancet* 1996;**347**(9012):1357–61.

156. Dentali F, Douketis JD, Gianni M, Lim W, Crowther MA. Meta-analysis: anticoagulant prophylaxis to prevent symptomatic venous thromboembolism in hospitalized medical patients. *Ann Intern Med* 2007;**146**(4):278–88.

157. Samama MM, Cohen AT, Darmon JY, Desjardins L, Eldor A, Janbon C et al. A comparison of enoxaparin with placebo for the prevention of venous thromboembolism in acutely ill medical patients. Prophylaxis in Medical Patients with Enoxaparin Study Group. *N Engl J Med* 1999;**341**(11):793–800.

158. Leizorovicz A, Cohen AT, Turpie AG, Olsson CG, Vaitkus PT, Goldhaber SZ. Randomized, placebo-controlled trial of dalteparin for the prevention of venous thromboembolism in acutely ill medical patients. *Circulation* 2004;**110**(7):874–9.

159. Cohen AT, Davidson BL, Gallus AS, Lassen MR, Prins MH, Tomkowski W et al. Efficacy and safety of fondaparinux for the prevention of venous thromboembolism in older acute medical patients: randomised placebo controlled trial. *BMJ* 2006;**332**(7537):325–9.

160. Wells PS, Lensing AW, Hirsh J. Graduated compression stockings in the prevention of postoperative venous thromboembolism. A meta-analysis. *Arch Intern Med* 1994;**154**(1):67–72.

161. Hull RD, Raskob GE, Gent M, McLoughlin D, Julian D, Smith FC et al. Effectiveness of intermittent pneumatic leg compression for preventing deep vein thrombosis after total hip replacement. *JAMA* 1990;**263**(17):2313–17.

162. Hull R, Delmore TJ, Hirsh J, Gent M, Armstrong P, Lofthouse R et al. Effectiveness of intermittent pulsatile elastic stockings for the prevention of calf and thigh vein thrombosis in patients undergoing elective knee surgery. *Thromb Res* 1979;**16**(1–2):37–45.

163. Sevitt S, Gallagher NG. Prevention of venous thrombosis and pulmonary embolism in injured patients. A trial of anticoagulant prophylaxis with phenindione in middle-aged and elderly patients with fractured necks of femur. *Lancet* 1959;**2**:981–9.

164. Urokinase pulmonary embolism trial. Phase 1 results: a cooperative study. *JAMA* 1970;**214**(12):2163–72.

165. Brandjes DP, Heijboer H, Buller HR, de Rijk M, Jagt H, ten Cate JW. Acenocoumarol and heparin compared with acenocoumarol alone in the initial treatment of proximal-vein thrombosis. *N Engl J Med* 1992;**327**(21):1485–9.

166. Hull RD, Raskob GE, Pineo GF, Green D, Trowbridge AA, Elliott CG et al. Subcutaneous low-molecular-weight heparin compared with continuous intravenous heparin in the treatment of proximal-vein thrombosis. *N Engl J Med* 1992;**326**(15):975–82.

167. Levine M, Gent M, Hirsh J, Leclerc J, Anderson D, Weitz J et al. A comparison of low-molecular-weight heparin administered primarily at home with unfractionated heparin administered in the hospital for proximal deep-vein thrombosis. *N Engl J Med* 1996;**334**(11):677–81.

168. Koopman MM, Prandoni P, Piovella F, Ockelford PA, Brandjes DP, van der Meer J et al. Treatment of venous thrombosis with intravenous unfractionated heparin administered in the hospital as compared with subcutaneous low-molecular-weight heparin administered at home. The Tasman Study Group. *N Engl J Med* 1996;**334**(11):682–7.

169. Low-molecular-weight heparin in the treatment of patients with venous thromboembolism. The Columbus Investigators. *N Engl J Med* 1997;**337**(10):657–62.

170. Ridker PM, Goldhaber SZ, Danielson E, Rosenberg Y, Eby CS, Deitcher SR et al. Long-term, low-intensity warfarin therapy for the prevention of recurrent venous thromboembolism. *N Engl J Med* 2003;**348**(15):1425–34.

171. Wells PS, Hirsh J, Anderson DR, Lensing AW, Foster G, Kearon C et al. A simple clinical model for the diagnosis of deep-vein thrombosis combined with impedance plethysmography: potential for an improvement in the diagnostic process. *J Intern Med* 1998;**243**(1):15–23.

172. Wells PS, Anderson DR, Rodger M, Ginsberg JS, Kearon C, Gent M et al. Derivation of a simple clinical model to categorize patients probability of pulmonary embolism: increasing the models utility with the SimpliRED D-dimer. *Thromb Haemost* 2000;**83**(3):416–20.

65 Peripheral arterial disease

Catherine McGorrian and Sonia S Anand
McMaster University, Hamilton, Ontario, Canada

Introduction

Peripheral arterial disease (PAD) is usually defined as arterial disease which affects the arterial vasculature outside the heart. Aortic, renal and cerebral vascular diseases are addressed elsewhere in this text; therefore this chapter will focus on peripheral arterial disease of the lower extremities, distal to the aortic bifurcation.

The underlying pathologic abnormality of PAD of the lower extremities is obstruction of arterial flow, most commonly caused by atherosclerosis. However, other causes of arterial obstruction must also be entertained during diagnosis and include inflammatory diseases such as arteritis, entrapment syndromes, aneurysms and thrombosis *in situ* or thromboembolism. Atherosclerosis is a disease which primarily affects the intimal layer of elastic arteries, with the formation initially of a fatty streak, caused by adhesion molecule-dependent infiltration of the intima of mononuclear leukocytes, potentiated by chemoattractant chemokines. The leukocytes then become lipid laden, becoming macrophage foam cells, and the fatty streak is formed. Smooth muscle cells also infiltrate the plaque, with varying degrees of collagen formation. The resultant lipid-rich lesion, which is separated from the lumen of the artery only by a fibrous cap, can either rupture into the artery's lumen, triggering a thrombotic cascade and resulting in atherothrombosis and infarction, or become organized and ultimately even calcified, causing local obstruction to distal blood flow or stenosis.

PAD is an insidious condition, usually having a gradual onset and long latency before symptoms arise. It is associated with an increased risk of cardiovascular morbidity and mortality, and therefore evidence of PAD should direct health professionals to ensure that aggressive cardiovascular secondary prevention strategies are implemented.

Evidence-Based Cardiology, 3rd edition. Edited by S. Yusuf, J.A. Cairns, A.J. Camm, E.L. Fallen, and B.J. Gersh. © 2010 Blackwell Publishing, ISBN: 978-1-4051-5925-8.

Epidemiology and natural history

The prevalence of PAD depends on the age of the population surveyed and the method of diagnosis. The most commonly used method of PAD diagnosis is the Ankle Brachial Index (ABI). Data from several population-based studies indicate that PAD prevalence ranges between 3% and 10%, and increases to 15–20% among individuals over 70 years of age.[1-3] The annual incidence of intermittent claudication is greater among men than women, and is reported as 4.1–12.9/1000 men and 3.3–8.2/1000 women aged 55 and over attending a primary care setting.[4] The primary symptom of PAD of the lower extremities is limb claudication which is defined by a history of muscular leg pain on exercise that is relieved by a short rest. Claudication occurs when a stenosis in the artery restricts blood flow to the distal extremity to such an extent that when the person exercises and tissue oxygen demand increases, blood flow velocity cannot increase enough to cross the stenosis in adequate amounts to prevent tissue ischemia. Critical ischemia occurs when the arterial stenosis is so severe that blood flow is insufficient at rest, and the person has "rest pain", which is initially resolved by placing the limb in a dependent position.

While the clinical interventions among patients with PAD traditionally focused on the impact of the arterial disease on the limbs, more recently the emphasis has shifted towards the risk of cardiovascular (CV) complications such as fatal and non-fatal myocardial infarction, and stroke faced by individuals with PAD. With respect to morbidity in the affected leg(s), only 1–3.3% of patients with intermittent claudication require amputation over a five-year period.[5] However, some subgroups of PAD patients remain at higher risk of further limb pathology. Specifically, 25% of patients with critical limb ischemia require amputation as the primary treatment[5]; patients who present with premature onset of PAD (i.e. at an age of ≤45 years) have an increased need for repeat limb intervention[6] and those who continue to smoke after their PAD diagnosis

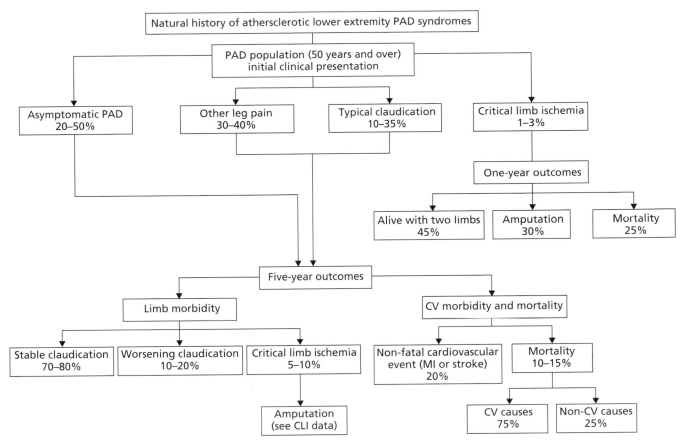

Figure 65.1 Natural history of atherosclerotic lower limb PAD over five years. PAD, peripheral arterial disease; CLI, critical limb ischemia; CV, cardiovascular; MI, myocardial infarction. (From Hirsch et al.[18], with permission.)

have a worse prognosis for limb-related morbidity.[7] A more ominous threat to patients with PAD is their poor CV prognosis, as approximately 40–60% of patients with PAD have concurrent coronary artery disease (CAD) and cerebrovascular disease. The annual major adverse cardiovascular event rate (myocardial infarction, ischemic stroke and vascular death) in PAD patients is 5–7%, with a five-year probability of a major non-fatal or fatal CV complication of 30–35%, and there is a 70% mortality rate after 15 years. A low ABI has also been shown to have a high specificity for future cardiovascular events, including stroke and myocardial infarction.[8] Figure 65.1 shows the natural history of atherosclerotic lower limb PAD.

Risk factors

Risk factors for PAD are similar to the major risk factors of atherosclerosis, although the relative impact of each risk factor varies somewhat. The major risk factors for PAD include male sex, tobacco exposure, advancing age, dyslipidemia, diabetes, and hypertension.

Male sex is reported as a PAD risk factor, as there are more men than women with PAD in younger age groups, which is likely due to the greater prevalence of smoking among men than women. However, because of the increased life span of women compared with men, and the increased incidence of PAD with increasing age, the overall incidence of PAD is actually similar in both sexes (Fig. 65.2). *Tobacco exposure* is the major risk factor for PAD, with the risk in current smokers being 2.3 times that of non-smokers.[9] In one population-based study, the prevalence of current or former smoking in persons with PAD with an ABI of less than 0.9 was 85% in men and 47% in women,[10] which results in a population attributable risk of tobacco exposure for PAD of 50–76%.[9] Furthermore, the degree of tobacco exposure has a dose–response relationship with PAD risk, increasing with increasing pack-years of smoking. Other risk factors for the development of PAD include *increasing age* (see Fig. 65.1), *dyslipidemia*, *diabetes* (increase in PAD risk of 2–4-fold[3]), *hypertension* (increase in PAD risk of 2–4-fold[11]), *impaired renal function* (increase in PAD risk of threefold in women with a creatinine clearance of <30mL/min/ 1.73m^2[12]),

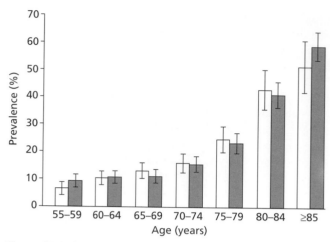

Figure 65.2 The age- and sex-specific prevalence of PAD (and 95% CI) according to age for men (white bars) and women (shaded bars). (From Meijer et al[10], with permission.)

Risk factor*	Point
Age	+1 point for every increase in age by 5 years, starting at age 55 (i.e. 1 point for age 60–64, +2 for 65–69, etc.)
Smoking	0 for never smoked, +2 for ever smoked
Hypertension	0 for no hypertension, +1 for adequately treated hypertension, +3 for inadequately treated hypertension

Score	Prevalence of ABI <0.9
0–3	7.0%
4	11.9%
5	14.5%
6	17.5%
7	19.3%
8	23.5%
9	25.9%
10	24.3%
11	25.1%
12	31.1%
≥13	40.6%

Figure 65.3 The PREVALENT Risk Score. *Risk factors were examined using a stepwise multiple logistic regression model in 7454 subjects, which consistently removed gender, diabetes, hypercholesterolaemia, positive family history and body-mass index. (Adapted from Bendermacher et al.[16], with permission.)

and *prior history of coronary artery disease* (increase in PAD risk of 1.5-fold[11]). Dyslipidemia is a well-recognized risk factor, with an association between decreased ABI and increased total cholesterol and decreasing HDL cholesterol shown in the Cardiovascular Health Study.[13] Similarly, a trend towards decreased ABI with higher triglyceride levels was noted, though this did not persist in multivariate analysis.[13] Persons with diabetes mellitus are at particular risk of developing PAD, with a relative risk of 2–4 times that of non-diabetics.[10] For every 1% increase in HbA1C in type 2 diabetes, the risk of PAD increases by 28%.[14] Diabetics are also much more likely to develop further PAD complications, with a risk of major amputation 7–15 times greater than non-diabetics with PAD. This is likely due to the peripheral sensory neuropathy associated with diabetic foot conditions, meaning that diabetics often present later, as their disease has been asymptomatic. Diabetes also causes rheologic changes, with increased blood coagulability, and a greater predisposition to acute and subacute thrombotic episodes, and increased vascular inflammation with calcification of the intima and more widespread vascular disease.

The Framingham investigators have reported that age, sex, cholesterol, hypertension, cigarette smoking, diabetes and pre-existing CAD are associated with increased risk of intermittent claudication, and have developed and published an intermittent claudication risk score based on these risk factors.[15] Bendermacher et al[16] have also developed a prediction rule to guide general and family practitioners with regard to which patients to screen for PAD, based on age, smoking status and hypertension (Fig. 65.3).

Diagnosis

Despite the prognostic importance of asymptomatic as well as symptomatic PAD, it is underdiagnosed in routine medical practice.[17] The initial clinical assessment for PAD is a history and physical examination. A history of intermittent claudication is useful in raising the suspicion of PAD, and symptoms are usually assessed by asking the person about the presence of exercise-induced calf pain, not present at rest, and which is relieved within 10 minutes by rest. The most recent ACC/AHA guidelines for the management of PAD[18] recommend a vascular "review of symptoms" in every clinical history, where people are asked routinely about leg symptoms on exertion, rest pain in the lower leg or foot, and the presence of poorly healing leg or foot wounds. However, reliance on symptoms alone significantly underestimates the true prevalence of PAD. Persons with PAD may have atypical symptoms, or even no symptoms,[10,17] and reliance on a classic history of claudication alone for screening purposes will miss 85–90% of PAD diagnoses.[17] Persons with PAD are more than twice as likely as those without PAD to have a history of myocardial infarction, angina, congestive heart failure, stroke or transient ischemic attack[13] and therefore PAD screening must be considered in these patients.

Physical examination is an important part of the PAD evaluation, and a number of bedside tests can be performed. The most useful positively predictive clinical features for screening asymptomatic persons for PAD are a positive history of claudication (likelihood ratio (LR) for PAD 3.3, 95% confidence interval (CI) 2.3–4.8), listening for a femoral, iliac or popliteal bruit (LR 4.8, 95% CI 2.4–9.5, for the presence of one bruit at rest) and palpation for a pulse abnormality (femoral, popliteal, dorsalis pedis or posterior tibial; LR 3.1, 95% CI 1.4–6.6). For people with symptomatic PAD, clinical features such as cool skin (L 5.9, 95% CI 4.1–8.6), the presence of a bruit (LR 5.6, 95% CI 4.7–6.7, for the presence of one bruit at rest), and a pulse abnormality (LR 4.7, 95% CI 2.2–9.9) are positive predictors of PAD.[19] However, reliance on a pulse abnormality alone can overestimate the incidence of PAD.[1] A scoring system for PAD risk using arterial Doppler signals has been published[20] and is useful for identifying those patients who require further testing with an ABI test. Commonly, patients with intermittent claudication are classified using either the Rutherford or the Fontaine staging approach. The Rutherford staging is currently recommended[5] (Table 65.1).

Ankle Brachial Index

The ABI is a simple bedside test which can be rapidly performed, and which is most often used in epidemiologic studies to assess the presence of PAD (Fig. 65.4). The ABI is useful for both diagnosis and assessment of the efficacy of therapeutic interventions, and has been shown to have a high sensitivity and specificity for PAD, with a sensitivity of +90% and specificity of 95% for detecting angiographically significant disease with an ABI of 0.9 or less.[21] An ABI

Table 65.1 Classification of peripheral arterial disease: Rutherford categories

Grade	Category	Clinical description
0	0	Asymptomatic
I	1	Mild claudication
I	2	Moderate claudication
I	3	Severe claudication
II	4	Ischemic rest pain
III	5	Minor tissue loss
III	6	Major tissue loss

Reproduced with permission from Schmieder FA, Comerota AJ. *Am J Cardiol* 2001;**87**(12, suppl 1);3–13.

of <0.9 has typically been used to diagnose PAD in large epidemiologic studies, and is recommended as the cut-off by both the American Heart Association[18] and the Transatlantic Inter-Society (TASC) guidelines.[5] Furthermore, the presence of a low ABI is highly specific for adverse CV prognosis, although its sensitivity is low. For example, a low ABI (<0.8–0.9) has a sensitivity and specificity for the prediction of incident CAD of 16.5% and 92.7%, of incident stroke of 16.0% and 92.2%, and of CV mortality of 41.0% and 87.9% respectively.[8] The ABI shows a U-shaped relationship with both all-cause and cardiovascular mortality (Fig. 65.5), with both ABIs of <0.9 and >1.4 associated with increased risk.[22] Higher ABIs >1.4 are associated with abnormal calcification of the arterial wall and resultant non-compressibility of the vessel, such as is common in diabetes.

Performing an ABI

With the patient in a supine position, the brachial systolic pressure is taken in both arms and the highest pressure recorded. Some recommend that the pressure be recorded ideally with a handheld 5 or 10 mHz Doppler ultrasound[17] though use of a stethoscope is acceptable, as long as the methods are consistent over time. Then the systolic pressure at the ankle, in both the anterior tibial and dorsalis pedis arteries, is determined using a 10–12 cm sphygmomanometer cuff around the ankle and the Doppler, and the highest pressure is recorded. The ABI is the ankle pressure divided by the brachial pressure. If the ankle arteries are non-compressible (such as in patients with diabetes mellitus or the very elderly) the ankle toe index can be a more informative test of distal disease, with an index of <0.70 indicating PAD. Some patients, in particular those with iliac disease, may not have a detectable abnormality on the ABI at rest, but complain of symptoms on exercise. The abnormality in these patients may only become apparent on exercise, as the inflow velocity increases, so a treadmill or plantarflexion test may be performed, with the ABI measurement repeated after exercise. Other useful non-invasive testing includes segmental Doppler pressure measurements, which uses a cuff method to identify pressure drops along the lower limbs, to try and isolate the lesion. However, weaknesses of this test are the possibility of missing iliac lesions, and the difficulty in interpreting results in the very old or diabetic subjects.

Treadmill testing

Treadmill testing is particularly useful for identifying PAD in patients in whom the disease is suspected but who have no reduction in ABI at rest. This is sometimes the case in patients with isolated iliac lesions. The procedure requires an initial measurement of either the ABI or full segmental Doppler leg pressures at rest. The patient is then asked to

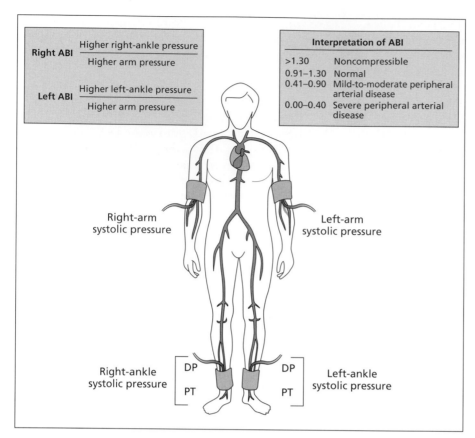

Figure 65.4 Measurement of the Ankle Brachial Index. Systolic blood pressure is measured in both brachial arteries, and in the posterior tibial and dorsalis pedis arteries using a Doppler ultrasound device. The higher of the pedal systolic pressures is chosen on each side, and the higher of the two brachial pressures is chosen. The ABI for each side is calculated by dividing the ankle pressure by the arm pressure. (Reproduced with permission from Hiatt WR. *N Engl J Med* 2001; **344**(21):1608–21.)

Within Figure 65.4:

Right ABI = Higher right-ankle pressure / Higher arm pressure

Left ABI = Higher left-ankle pressure / Higher arm pressure

Interpretation of ABI	
>1.30	Noncompressible
0.91–1.30	Normal
0.41–0.90	Mild-to-moderate peripheral arterial disease
0.00–0.40	Severe peripheral arterial disease

Right-arm systolic pressure
Left-arm systolic pressure
Right-ankle systolic pressure
Left-ankle systolic pressure
DP PT DP PT

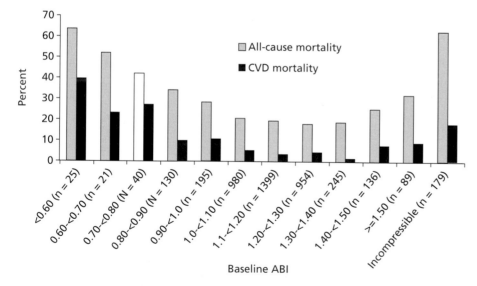

Figure 65.5 All-cause and CVD mortality in a population-based cohort of American Indians, showing the "U" shaped relationship with ABI. (Reproduced from Resnick *et al*[22], with permission.)

walk (typically on a motorized treadmill with a programmed schedule, such as at 3.2 km/h (2 mph), 10–12% grade) for a maximum of five minutes or until maximal claudication pain occurs, unless another reason to stop such as coronary ischemia arises. Following this, the ankle pressure is again measured. A decrease in ABI of 15–20% is diagnostic of PAD. For patients who are uncomfortable using a treadmill, especially older patients, a six-minute

walk test along a corridor can also be an effective exercise modality

Diagnostic imaging

This is usually reserved for patients in whom an intervention is being planned or to follow up graft patency. Historically, the gold standard for diagnosis of PAD has been conventional angiography, but because of its invasive and labor-intensive nature and the risks associated with it, non-invasive imaging tools are frequently used.

The primary use of *angiography* is detection of disease in the arterial tree in persons in whom an intervention is being planned, such as those with critical ischemia or severe intermittent claudication symptoms unresponsive to lifestyle or medical therapy. The advantages of angiography are that definition of the vascular tree is optimized, and hemodynamic parameters may be measured directly. However, as an invasive procedure, angiography carries risks of contrast nephropathy and/or anaphylaxis, access site bleeding or hematoma, atheroembolism, and rarely vascular disruption with dissection or rupture. It is therefore best reserved for carefully chosen patients.

Duplex ultrasound is used to identify exact lesion sites in persons with symptoms or an abnormal ABI, and also has utility in venous graft surveillance post peripheral bypass procedures. The sensitivity and specificity for detecting lesions are high, reported as 94% by one meta-analysis.[23] Duplex ultrasound is especially powerful when using color-guided methods. However, it is labor intensive and requires a high level of technical expertise.

Contrast computed tomographic (CT) angiography is a further option for imaging the peripheral arterial system. Previously hampered by poorer image quality and slow scanning times, the new generation of multidetector array CT scanners offer high-quality images at high imaging speeds, although image reconstruction can be time consuming. Multidetector row spiral CT angiography (CTA) has been shown to provide sufficient clinical information, although at lower therapeutic confidence, when compared with digital subtraction angiography (DSA). It has excellent sensitivity and specificity for depicting arterial occlusions (sensitivity and specificity of 88.6% and 97.7%) and stenoses of at least 75% (92.2% and 96.8% respectively).[24] A meta-analysis of CTA compared with DSA showed sensitivity and specificity of detecting a stenosis >50% for CTA of 92% and 93%, respectively.[25] Another study randomized patients to either contrast MR angiography or multi-detector row CTA and found similar clinical utilities, but decreased costs in the CTA group.[26] However, the limitations of CTA include difficulty in interpretation of images in which there is a high degree of scatter caused by highly calcified vascular segments, the potential for renal impairment due to contrast injections, and the exposure to ionizing radiation.

Contrast-enhanced magnetic resonance (MR) angiography is an alternative to CTA and has the clear advantage of providing a "road map" of the arterial system of the lower limbs. Again, it is operator dependent, of limited use in patients with a contrast allergy, pacemaker or cardiac stent, and is expensive. Nevertheless, it has been shown to have better diagnostic accuracy than duplex US and to have similar accuracy to DSA, with sensitivity and specificity of greater than 90% quoted for stenoses of >50% in studies using three-dimensional gadolinium-enhanced methods.[27]

Therapeutics

Therapy for PAD can be divided into general lifestyle measures, measures aimed at improving symptoms, and measures to optimize secondary prevention of CV events. Therapies mentioned will be graded as per the *Evidence Based Cardiology* grading system. We will also discuss emerging therapies and the evidence for these to date.

Lifestyle measures

Smoking cessation

Our understanding of the effects of smoking cessation in PAD patients comes primarily from observational studies, as there have been no prospective randomized controlled trials (RCTs) of smoking cessation and its effects on CVD outcomes in patients with PAD. Nevertheless, reports show that smoking cessation is associated with improvements in claudication symptoms, reduced rest pain, improved graft patency rates post lower limb bypass procedures, and decreased risk of death, MI or amputation. Patients who have undergone lower extremity bypass surgery also have a higher rate of major amputation if they are heavy smokers ($\geq$15 cigarettes per day) compared with more moderate smokers (21% amputation rate vs 2%, $P < 0.001$).[28] Smoking cessation rates have also been associated with reduced mortality in an RCT of small infrarenal aneurysm outcomes,[29] where the mortality benefit in the surgical vs surveillance group could be explained by the 12-fold increase in the odds of smoking cessation in the surgical group.[30]

Smoking cessation can be difficult to achieve, but effective interventions include physician guidance (2% of patients advised by their physician to quit had remained off cigarettes at one year[31]) and cessation aids including nicotine replacement therapy, varenicline (Champix™), bupropion, and other antidepressant therapies.

Simple physician advice to quit smoking in a brief clinical encounter has been shown to increase quit rates by 5%.[32] Nicotine replacement therapy (NRT) has been shown to be up to 13% effective in achieving adherence to non-smoking at one year,[31] with a meta-analysis of data from 16 RCTs of transdermal NRT patches reporting an odds ratio (OR) for 12-month abstinence of 1.75 (95% CI 1.49–2.05).[33] An increase in success for smoking cessation of 50–70% with all types of NRT was reported in a Cochrane review and meta-analysis of 132 trials by Stead *et al*.[34] Bupropion (Zyban™), an atypical antidepressant agent, has been found to be superior to placebo and NRT, with 12-month abstinence rates of 30%, although there was a high with-drawal rate from therapy (11%) and an unusually high quit rate in the placebo group.[35] A second RCT also found that bupropion doubled the success of smoking cessation, with an odds ratio of abstinence at 12 months for bupropion of 2.78 (95% CI 1.70–4.63), compared with placebo and usual care.[36] However, bupropion should not be used in patients with epilepsy, and only used with great caution in patients with low seizure thresholds.

A newer agent which has recently entered the market-place is varenicline tartrate (Champix™), a partial nicotine receptor agonist. A Phase II RCT comparing varenicline to placebo demonstrated significantly higher quit rates of 14.4% with varenicline, compared with 4.9% for placebo, $P = 0.002$.[37] This was followed by a Phase III study which showed continuous abstinence rates for 9–52 weeks were significantly higher among patients receiving varenicline (21.9%) or bupropion (16.1%) compared to placebo (8.4%).[38] Varenicline is reasonably well tolerated, with better adher-ence rates than for bupropion, although larger and longer term trials of varenicline are needed.

Smoking cessation aids have been shown to be cost effec-tive, with cost per life-year saved less for smoking cessation aids than for other secondary prevention steps commonly used post myocardial infarction (Fig. 65.6).

Recommendations

- Smoking cessation in all patients, to reduce PAD symptoms and future adverse CVD events (**Class 1, Level C1**).
- Use of smoking cessation aids such as physician advice, NRT, bupropion or varenicline to aid in quitting (**Class 1, Level B**).

Exercise

Patients with PAD benefit from a regular exercise program to optimize walking ability and maximal walking time.[39] A meta-analysis of 21 trials of walking therapy found that walking to near maximal pain, for 30 minutes and as part of a program lasting more than six months, increased the distance to onset of claudication pain by 179% (225.3 m) and the distance to maximal claudication pain by 122% (397.5 m).[40] Resistance training is not as beneficial as regular walking to near maximal pain threshold for 30 minutes at least four times a week, and supervised programs have been shown to be more beneficial than non-supervised, although there are nevertheless benefits to be gained from the home-based programs. There is also preliminary evi-dence from two small RCTs (n = 35[41] and n = 67[42]) which

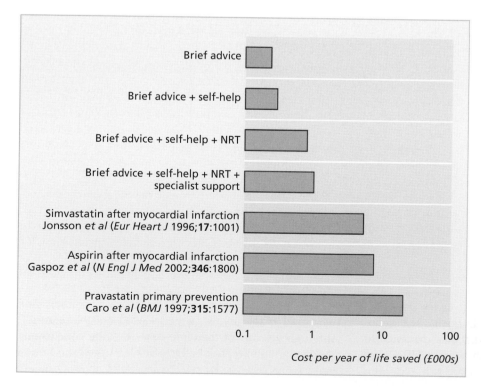

Figure 65.6 Cost effectiveness of smoking cessation strategies post MI when compared with other routine secondary prevention methods. (Reproduced with permission from Parrott S, Godfrey C. *BMJ* 2004;**328**:947–9.)

suggests that arm ergonometry may be as successful as treadmill training in increasing initial claudication distance and maximal walking distance. This may offer an exercise alternative to those with severely reduced mobility.

Although one theory is that walking induces angiogenesis and collateral growth around the occluded or stenosed area, it is actually more likely that the benefits are due to improvements in muscle tone with muscle hypertrophy, improved endothelial function and altered gait.[18] It was also shown in one trial that exercise therapy was more beneficial for walking times than percutaneous revascularization therapies[43] although this has not been replicated elsewhere. Exercise training for patients with PAD is optimally supervised by an exercise physiologist, physical therapist or nurse, in the setting of a cardiac rehabilitation program or similar,[18] with the option of further non-invasive monitoring, since these patients may have concomitant cardiac disease. Supervised exercise sessions are typically scheduled three times a week, for a period of three months, with 30–60-minute sessions each time.[5] Exercise also has further benefits in that it can improve dyslipidemia, hypertension and risk of type 2 diabetes mellitus, as well as reducing overall adiposity and Body Mass Index.

Recommendations

- A graded supervised exercise program should be advised to improve walking distance and other cardiovascular risk factors in patients with PAD (**Class 1, Level B**).
- There is less evidence to support home-based exercise programs (**Class IIa, Level B**).
- Arm ergonometry may be an acceptable alternative to walking-based programs (**Class IIa, Level B**).

Therapies for secondary event prevention

As discussed, patients with PAD are at very high risk of adverse vascular events elsewhere in the arterial tree, such as MI and stroke. Diabetes, hypertension and elevated cholesterol are not only etiologic factors in the pathogenesis of PAD, they also contribute to high rates of CV events among patients with established PAD. Therefore, it is generally accepted that control of etiologic risk factors will result in improved cardiovascular prognosis. Below we present evidence to support this practice.

Glycemic control in patients with diabetes

Control of blood glucose is advisable in patients with diabetes, to reduce the risk of adverse CVD events. The Steno-2 trial[44] randomized 160 type 2 diabetes patients to conventional or intensive control with a target HBA1C of <6.5%, in conjunction with tight blood pressure and lipid

control with a mean follow-up of 13.3 years. It reported reduced risks of cardiovascular mortality (hazard ratio (HR) 0.43, 95% CI 0.19–0.94, $P = 0.04$) and of cardiovascular events (HR 0.41, 95% CI 0.25–0.67, $P < 0.001$) with intensive glycemic control. However, a conflicting message has been given by the ACCORD study, in which an increase in total mortality was noted in the intensive control intervention arm, which aimed to reduce HBA1C in type 2 diabetes patients to <6.4%.[45] Further analysis of the ACCORD results is awaited.

The major trials of strict diabetic control in both type 1[46] and type 2[47] diabetes mellitus were not sufficiently powered nor designed to examine changes in PAD symptoms or outcomes, with the latter study showing no significant reduction in amputation from PAD in the intensive control group. Nevertheless, the results showing improvements in micro- and macrovascular conditions have been widely extrapolated and, in keeping with the American Diabetes Association recommendations among patients with established diabetes, it is reasonable to aim for a HbA1C of <7% in patients with PAD.[48]

Recommendation

- Persons with PAD should aim for optimal glycemic control, with HbA1C maintained at <7%, using medication, weight control and exercise (**Class I, Level C**).

Antihypertensive agents

Two trials have recently shown clear benefit of antihypertensive therapy in PAD patients. HOPE-PAD[49] examined the incidence of PAD within the HOPE RCT and the effects of ramipril within PAD groups. In total, of the 9541 patients in HOPE, 1715 had symptomatic PAD and a further 2118 had PAD by ABI criteria (ABI <0.9). Ramipril was associated with a significant relative risk reduction (RRR) in fatal CVD events, non-fatal MI and non-fatal stroke, with a RRR of 0.75 (95% CI 0.61–0.92) in persons with symptomatic PAD. The Appropriate Blood Pressure Control in Diabetes trial[50] randomized patients with diabetes to usual care (moderate blood pressure control) or intensive blood pressure control with enalapril and nisoldipine, and found that intensive control in the PAD subgroup (n = 53) had a protective effect on cardiovascular events, even for those patients with lower ABIs, who had more events in the control group.

There is, however, a paucity of data on the effects of antihypertensive agents on the symptoms and progression of PAD itself, and a Cochrane meta-analysis only identified two small trials, involving perindopril and verapamil.[51] Although we cannot therefore draw definite conclusions on the possible beneficial effects of blood pressure lowering, the findings in the HOPE-PAD trial, in conjunction with the growing body of evidence recommending antihypertensive agents (and ACE inhibitors in particular) in secondary prevention, would indicate that we should recommend intensive blood pressure lowering in this high-risk group. There has historically been a concern that lowering blood pressure will concomitantly lower limb perfusion pressure, and possibly worsen limb ischemic symptoms. However, a meta-analysis of the effects of beta-blockers on limb symptoms showed no consistent concern with their use in PAD,[52] and the JNC 7 recommendations for treatment of hypertension have suggested that all antihypertensive agents are suitable for use in PAD, depending also of course on patient-specific factors.[53] Nevertheless, in patients with critical ischemia unresponsive to medical therapy, some clinicians will replace a beta-blocker with an alternative antihypertensive agent.

Recommendation

- Antihypertensive agents should be administered to PAD patients to reduce risk of secondary CVD events, to aim for a blood pressure of less than 140/90 in non-diabetic persons and less than 130/80 for diabetic persons (**Class I, Level A**).

Lipid-lowering regimens

Use of HMG co-enzyme A reductase inhibitors (statins) and other lipid-lowering agents has been a cornerstone of coronary and cerebral atherosclerotic disease management for a number of years. The Heart Protection Study which had a large representation of patients with PAD demonstrated that use of simvastatin in PAD patients even with normal levels of LDL cholesterol was associated with a reduction in recurrent non-fatal MI, stroke and also a lowering in mortality.[54] The impact of lipid lowering on intermittent claudication in PAD patients was examined in a large meta-analysis (pooling data from 19 studies with 10049 patients).[55] Patients in the lipid-lowering arm were found to have statistically significant improvements in total walking distance and pain-free walking distance, though no improvement in ABI, when a number of smaller trials assessing these outcomes were pooled, with improvements in either total mortality or total cardiovascular events. However, these analyses are a little difficult to extrapolate to clinical practice, as so many different lipid-lowering modalities were used in the component trials.

Looking at the fibrate group specifically, a trial of gemfibrozil in coronary heart disease has previously shown reductions in non-fatal MI and CVD death in persons with low HDL levels.[56] However, a trial of bezafibrate in PAD patients has shown that although claudication severity improved in the fibrate group, there was no effect on mortality or cardiovascular events, despite a reduction in non-fatal coronary events.[57] Niacin is used in patients with CVD and low HDL. Studies have shown that niacin therapy is safe in PAD and raises HDL, but data on long-term CVD benefits are sparse, and a recent study which used carotid intima-media thickness (IMT) as a surrogate for CVD events in niacin and statin combination therapy showed only a non-significant trend to reduction in carotid IMT.[58]

Similarly, in HMG co-enzyme inhibitor or statin trials, statin use has been found in a number of small randomized studies to be associated with improvements in claudication times.[59–61] The Heart Protection Study randomized patients with vascular disease or diabetes to simvastatin 40 mg or placebo, and had a large number of patients with PAD (n = 6748).[54] This study showed that the simvastatin group had a 19% RRR and a 6.3% absolute risk reduction (ARR) of major vascular events, and this effect persisted even in the patients who did not have high levels of LDL cholesterol at baseline.

Recommendations

- Statins are first-choice lipid-lowering therapy in patients with PAD to reduce the risk of secondary vascular events, regardless of initial cholesterol level (**Class I, Level A**).
- Statins may also improve pain-free walking time and six-minute walk test performance in patients with symptomatic PAD, regardless of initial cholesterol level (**Class IIa, Level A**).
- Fibrate therapy may be used as second-line therapy to decrease CVD events (**Class IIa, Level B**).
- Niacin can be used to raise HDL in PAD patients, but there are no convincing data to support a benefit in CVD outcomes (**Class IIa, Level A**).

Antiplatelet therapies

Antiplatelet therapies include acetylsalicylic acid or aspirin, dipyridamole, thromboxane antagonists including picotamide, and the thienopyridine group (ticlodipine and clopidogrel). From the Antiplatelet Trialists' Collaboration, 287 studies were included in a meta-analysis[62] to examine the effects of antiplatelet therapies in those with vascular disease. In data pooled from 42 trials of 9214 patients with PAD, antiplatelet agents were found to be associated with an odds reduction of serious vascular events of 23% (standard error 8%, $P = 0.001$), for patients with intermittent claudication, post vascular bypass operations or undergoing percutaneous therapies. Similarly, Anand and Tran noted an odds reduction in vascular events with antiplatelet therapy (aspirin, ticlodipine, picotamide, dipyridamole or aspirin + dipyridamole) vs control of 23% (95% CI 7.9–35.5, $P < 0.004$).[63]

Aspirin is an inhibitor of platelet cyclo-oxygenase and thromboxane production. Collins *et al* performed a meta-analysis examining antiplatelet agents vs placebo after infra-inguinal bypass grafting[64] and combined data from seven trials, six of which studied aspirin or an aspirin/dipyridamole combination. Antiplatelet therapy was associated with an odds reduction for mortality of 30% (95% CI 5–49%), for graft occlusion of 57% (95% CI 33–73%), and a non-significant increase of bleeding side effects (OR 1.82, 95% CI 0.43–7.73). Data on aspirin dosing have not specifically addressed optimum dose in PAD patients, but the Antiplatelet Trialists' Collaboration data would suggest that a dose of between 75 and 150 mg daily would achieve maximum efficacy with a lower risk of bleeding.[65]

Antiplatelet agents and aspirin have also been shown to have a role in maintaining the patency of vessels after lower extremity bypass or percutaneous angioplasty procedures. The 1994 meta-analysis by the Antiplatelet Trialists' Collaboration[65] pooled data on 3226 patients with intermittent claudication or who had undergone lower extremity bypass or percutaneous angioplasty, and found graft occlusion rates of 16% with antiplatelet therapy (mainly aspirin, or aspirin and dipyridamole in combination) vs 25% with control, resulting in a proportional reduction of occlusion of 43% (SD 8%, 2P < 0.0001). Collins *et al*[64] also examined graft patency after lower extremity bypass surgery in studies which had greater than 12 months of follow-up, and found an odds reduction of 64% (95% CI 34–68%) for graft occlusion in the antithrombotic group (seven trials of antiplatelet therapy, three trials of oral anticoagulant therapy) vs the control group. Analyses from the Cochrane Group also suggest that antiplatelet agents are superior to placebo in maintaining vessel patency post surgical bypass.[66] A subgroup analysis of a large trial comparing oral anticoagulants (OAC) to antiplatelet therapy suggests that OAC may be superior in maintaining patency of venous grafts[67] whereas antiplatelet agents may be preferable in artificial grafts.[68] However, in light of the excess risk of bleeding with OAC vs antiplatelet agents observed in the WAVE trial,[69] the decision to use OAC over aspirin in patients with venous grafts to improve patency must be made on an indivdual patient basis. For percutaneous revascularization, there is no significant difference in occlusion rates with aspirin vs oral anticoagulants.[70] Aspirin has also been shown to reduce the rate of peripheral bypass surgery in a large RCT of aspirin vs control over 60.2 months in healthy participants (RR for surgery 0.54, 95% CI 0.30–0.95, P = 0.03: data from the Physicians Health Study[71]).

Thienopyridines (clopidogrel and ticlodipine) have been shown in meta-analyses to be effective in reducing postoperative occlusion and need for revascularization in patients undergoing lower limb interventions,[72] and to have a

mortality benefit in patients with intermittent claudication.[73] The thienopyridines block adenosine diphosphate-mediated platelet activation, and therefore they may have a different efficacy to aspirin in secondary prevention. This theory was examined by a Cochrane Collaboration study, which performed a meta-analysis of pooled data from four studies and 22 565 patients at high risk of secondary vascular events.[74] Two of these studies (CAPRIE[75] and Schoop[76]) randomized patients with PAD. From the pooled data, the thienopyridine group had a reduced odds of a serious vascular event (OR 0.91, 95% CI 0.84–0.98) and a decreased odds of major hemorrhage (OR 0.71, 95% CI 0.59–0.86), though an increased risk of skin rash and neutropenia (most associated with ticlodipine).[74] Within CAPRIE alone, which compared aspirin 325 mg daily with clopidogrel 75 mg daily, the overall RR comparing clopidogrel to aspirin was 8.7% (95% CI 0.3–16.5%), although given their higher baseline risk, the PAD patients had a greater RRR with clopidogrel than the other at-risk vascular subgroups (RRR 23.8%, 95% CI 8.9–36.2%).[75] However, in the CHARISMA trial,[77] the use of dual antiplatelet therapy (i.e. aspirin and clopidogrel) was not significantly more effective in the prevention of CVD than aspirin alone (RR of stroke, MI or CV death 0.93, 95% CI 0.83–1.05) and was associated with an increase in severe and moderate bleeding complications (RR for severe bleeding with dual therapy 1.25, 95% CI 0.97–1.61) in patients with atherosclerotic CVD and high CVD risk.

At present, there seems to be no clear role for regular or extended-release dipyridamole alone in PAD. Early trials examined dipyridamole in conjunction with aspirin in maintaining patency of lower extremity bypass grafts/percutaneous procedures, and suggested that this was an advantageous combination. However, in terms of secondary prevention, the Antiplatelet Trialists' Collaboration suggested that the combination of aspirin plus dipyridamole was not superior to aspirin alone.[62] A Cochrane meta-analysis[78] included data from 27 studies which randomized people with vascular disease to dipyridamole and found that dipyridamole was not superior to control in preventing CVD death, and was only superior to control in preventing CVD events in patients with cerebral ischemia.

There has been interest in the use of antiplatelet agents in the treatment of intermittent claudication. Ticlodipine has been investigated in a small blinded placebo-controlled trial for improvements in ABI and walking times; an improvement was shown but the trial numbers were small (n = 151) and the placebo group had worse ABIs and walking times at baseline.[79] Another trial (n = 296) randomized patients to aspirin and dipyridamole, ticlodipine or xanthinol nicotinate, and found again that the ABI improved with aspirin/dipyridamole and ticlodipine, but not with xanthinol.[80]

- Patients with PAD, including patients who have undergone peripheral vascular bypass or percutaneous revascularization procedures, should take lifelong antiplatelet therapy with aspirin 75–150 mg per day. Clopidogrel 75 mg per day is a useful alternative, as demonstrated in the CAPRIE trial (**Class I, Level A**).
- There is no additional benefit in using aspirin in conjunction with clopidogrel for the long-term management of PAD patients (**Class IIb, Level A**).
- There is no additional benefit in using aspirin in conjunction with dipyridamole in PAD patients, unless there is a concomitant history of cerebrovascular disease (**Class IIb, Level A**).

Vitamin K antagonists

Oral anticoagulants, like antiplatelet agents, have a theoretically appealing role in PAD, both in preventing vascular occlusion and preventing other systemic athero-thrombotic events. A meta-analysis by the WAVE investigators has shown that OAC are better than placebo at reducing mortality and graft occlusion, but have an increased risk of major bleeding.[81] Comparing oral anticoagulants with aspirin showed no benefit for mortality or graft occlusion in the oral anticoagulation group above that achieved with aspirin, again at an increased risk of bleeding. Most recently, the WAVE trial, which evaluated combined OAC and antiplatelet therapy in 2161 patients with PAD, showed that combined therapy was not superior to treatment with antiplatelet therapy alone for the combined outcome of fatal and non-fatal cardiovascular events (RR for combination therapy 0.91, 95% CI 0.74–1.12, $P = 0.37$). Combined OAC and antiplatelet therapy was associated with a substantially higher risk of life-threatening bleeding complications (RR 3.41, 95% CI 1.84–6.35, $P < 0.0001$).[69] Therefore, oral anticoagulation for secondary prevention in PAD should only be used if there is a supplemental indication for anticoagulation, such as atrial fibrillation.

- OAC should not be used routinely in patients with PAD, without a secondary indication (**Class II, Level A**).

Therapies aimed at the circulatory disease itself

Aside from the lifestyle measures, therapies aiming to improve the circulation to the affected limb(s) and to ameliorate symptoms may be pharmacologic, percutaneous or surgical.

Pharmacologic treatments for intermittent claudication

The TASC II guidelines[5] suggest two medications for the amelioration of intermittent claudication symptoms – cilostazol and naftidrofuryl – and discuss the lack of evidence supporting others such as pentoxifylline.

Pentoxifylline is thought to act by decreasing blood viscosity and increasing erythrocyte flexibility. It has long been used for intermittent claudication symptoms, but the evidence regarding its efficacy is sparse and it does not have a large safety record. Girolami et al[39] examined 13 RCTs of pentoxifylline vs placebo in intermittent claudication and found that mean walking distance was improved on pentoxifylline (increase in mean walking distance of 43.8 m, 95% CI 14.1–73.6 m). In another meta-analysis (of 11 trials, n = 612), Hood et al[82] similarly found that pentoxifylline increased pain-free walking distance (weighted mean difference 29.4 m, 95% CI 13.0–45.9 m) and absolute claudication time (weighted mean difference 48.4 m, 95% CI 18.3–78.6 m) compared with placebo. Whilst smaller trials have shown benefits for pentoxifylline, a larger RCT (n = 471 patients in the pentoxifylline vs placebo arm) showed no difference between pentoxyifylline and placebo.[83] At present, the TASC group suggests that there is insufficient evidence to use pentoxifylline in intermittent claudication.[5]

Naftidrofuryl is a serotonin antagonist, which is thought to work by promoting aerobic metabolism in oxygen-depleted tissues and by reducing platelet and erythrocyte aggregation. It has been shown to reduce disease-related limitations in quality of life when compared with placebo in a meta-analysis of three RCTs (n = 754)[84] and to increase pain-free walking distance in another meta-analysis.[85] However, like pentoxifylline, the absolute increases in walking distances achieved with naftidrofuryl are small (increase in mean total walking distance with naftidrofuryl 71.2 m, 95% CI 13.3–129.0 m).[39]

Cilostazol is a phosphodiesterase III inhibitor, which inhibits platelet activation and relaxes vascular smooth muscle. A 2002 meta-analysis synthesized the results of six randomized trials of cilostazol vs control (n = 1751), and reported that cilostazol increased maximal treadmill walking, with improvements in the Walking Impairment Questionnaire and also in health-related quality of life.[86] A Cochrane meta-analysis synthesized data from eight trials and reported that cilostazol was associated with an improvement in initial claudication distance (ICD) and absolute claudication distance (ACD), with a weighted mean difference in ICD of 31.1 m (95% CI 21.4–40.9 m) with cilostazol.[87] Cilostazol is contraindicated in patients with congestive cardiac failure, although the safety analysis in the Cochrane review did not show any increase in CV events with cilostazol. One study also compared cilostazol directly with pentoxifylline and found that cilostazol significantly reduced ACD, whereas the effects of pentoxifylline were similar to those of placebo.[83] Serious adverse events and withdrawals from therapy were similar in the two treatment groups, although the incidence of minor side effects was greater in the cilostazol group.

Other agents

Other agents which have been proposed for use in intermittent claudication include buflomedil, arteriolar vasodilators, and prostaglandins. Buflomedil is a vasodilator which also has antiplatelet actions. However, a Cochrane review could only find appropriate data on 127 patients with improvements in pain-free walking distance with buflomedil, leading to concerns about safety and publication bias.[88] Vasodilators such as calcium channel blockers have been used in an attempt to increase local blood flow, but there is scant evidence for their use. Intravenous prostaglandin infusions have been used in critical limb ischemia, and an oral prostaglandin called beraprost has been investigated but the trials in intermittent claudication are negative to date.[5] There has also been interest in angiogenic growth factors, but again the trials have not proved conclusive. In relation to the treatment of critical limb ischemia, the TASC group suggests that treatments like vasodilators, naftidrofuryl, pentoxifylline and unfractionated heparin have no proven benefit.

Recommendations

- Cilostazol is recommended for use in intermittent claudication to improve ICD and ACD, although side effects are common (**Class I–IIa, Level A**).
- Naftidrofuryl can be used as an alternative to cilostazole, although there is less evidence regarding its use (**Class IIa, Level A**).
- There is currently insufficient evidence to recommend the use of pentoxifylline, buflomedil, vasodilators and oral prostaglandins in intermittent claudication (**Class III, Level B**).

Surgical

Percutaneous angioplasty Percutaneous angioplasty (PCA) is an appealing therapy for peripheral arterial disease, but it is far from a cure-all. The AHA/ACC guidelines suggest that only certain patients be considered for percutaneous therapies, these being patients who have not responded to exercise or pharmacotherapies, patients who have a severe disability with their claudication symptoms, patients in whom other co-conditions are not also limiting exercise tolerance, and patients with a focal lesion amenable to percutaneous treatment.[18] One chief difficulty is that patients with severe PAD frequently have multiple or long lesions which are not suitable for angioplasty, with only 10% of participants screened in one trial of PCA vs medical therapy found to be suitable for PCA.[89] Furthermore, it has been shown in one trial only that exercise therapy was more beneficial for walking times than percutaneous therapies.[43]

There is a paucity of data regarding direct comparisons of PCA with medical and lifestyle therapies for PAD. Whyman randomized 62 patients to medical therapy or PCA + medical therapy, reporting that at six months follow-up, the PCA patients had higher mean ABI (0.88, standard error 0.03, vs 0.74, standard error 0.03; $P < 0.01$) and higher quality of life scores.[89] Another study examined 56 patients with stable claudication who were randomized to PCA vs exercise therapy, and found that while the PCA group made short-term improvements in ABI, at six years follow-up there was no difference between the groups with respect to ABI and maximal walking distance.[90] Spronk *et al* compared functional capacity and quality of life scores in five studies of exercise therapy and three of PCA, and found that while ABIs were higher in the PCA groups at six months, there was no difference in reported quality of life.[91]

Focal lesions of the iliac arteries can cause both peripheral claudication symptoms and Leriche's syndrome, where a terminal aorta lesion causes erectile dysfunction and buttock claudication. Endovascular stenting can be recommended for TASC type lesions A to B of the iliac arteries (short stenoses <3 cm long, not extending into the superficial femoral artery) in patients who are persistently symptomatic despite optimal medical and lifestyle therapies.[5] The iliac arteries are particularly prone to disruption and dissection, and primary stenting (without prior balloon angioplasty) is usually recommended. Infrainguinal disease is more technically challenging, with common femoral disease being associated with poorer endovascular outcomes due to acute vessel closure or late restenosis. Superficial femoral artery disease is commonly diffuse and not amenable to stent placement, and stents in the arterial portion within the adductor canal can be subject to extra strain and torsion, predisposing to stent fractures. Balloon angioplasty has traditionally been the percutaneous treatment of choice in the superficial femoral artery, with stents reserved for "bail out" in case of dissection or acute vessel closure. However, techniques have improved and stenting is becoming more commonplace. A recent RCT of superficial femoral artery PCA vs nitinol stent implantation in 104 patients reported better ABIs and better maximal treadmill walking distance at 12 months in the stent group (387 vs 267 m, $P = 0.04$).[92]

Although the use of antiproliferative drug-eluting stents has effectively reduced in-stent restenosis in coronary revascularization, the results with sirolimus-eluting stents in superficial femoral peripheral arterial interventions have been mixed. However, in the preliminary THUNDER (Local Taxane with Short Exposure for Reduction of

Restenosis in Distal Arteries) trial,[93] a randomized, double-blind study of 154 patients who underwent percutaneous femoropopliteal angioplasty interventions, 17 of whom also required nitinol stent implantation. 48 patients were randomized to a paclitaxel-coated balloon; 52 to a usual balloon, with paclitaxel in the contrast medium; and 54 received usual care. The paclitaxel balloon (but not the paclitaxel contrast) group saw significant reductions both in mean late lumen loss and target lesion revascularization (2/48 (4%) with the paclitavel balloon vs 20/54 (37%) in the control group, $P < 0.001$) at six months follow-up. Whilst further studies are needed, this suggests potential for future improvements in peripheral PCA.

Atherectomy devices, including laser atherectomy, extraction atherectomy and cutting balloon atherectomy, have been proposed for use in superficial femoral lesions, including chronic total occlusions. However, the published randomized controlled data for atherectomy are not indicative of benefit above balloon angioplasty, and cutting balloons have recently been recalled. Laser atherectomy has shown promising results in observational studies and registries but a RCT is awaited. Therefore, the use of these devices must be viewed with appropriate caution.

Recommendations

- PCA is recommended for patients with aorto-iliac disease which is disabling and refractory to medical and lifestyle therapies, and technically amenable to PCA (**Class I, Level B**).
- Endovascular stenting can be recommended in aorto-iliac disease as either primary or bail-out therapy (**Class I, Level B**).
- PCA can be used in patients with femoral, popliteal or tibial disease which is disabling and refractory to medical and lifestyle therapies, and technically amenable to PCA (**Class IIa, Level C**). There is less information on the use of primary stenting in this group.
- The usefulness of atherectomy devices and/or cutting balloons is not established from the literature.

Surgical revascularization Surgical revascularization is subject to the same caveats as percutaneous therapies, in that it should only be undertaken if the symptoms are severely limiting, and if medical and lifestyle therapies have not achieved sufficient improvement. Aorto-bifemoral bypass procedures are considered the standard of care for aorto-iliac occlusive disease where the patient is refractory to medical and exercise therapy, and where symptoms are sufficient to warrant further treatment. One metasynthesis of outcomes post aorto-iliac bypass procedures found an operative mortality rate of 3.3%, with a systemic morbidity rate of 8.3% for procedures in studies started since 1975. Limb-based patency rates at five and 10 years

were 91.0% and 86.8% respectively for patients with claudication and 87.5% and 81.8% for patients with critical limb ischemia.[94] Tobacco smoking is associated with worse patency rates. A synthesis of four RCTs (which randomized patients to different types of grafts) and 12 prospective studies of the influence of smoking on graft patency in lower limb arterial revascularization reported that ongoing smoking was associated with a 3.09-fold (95% CI 2.34–4.08, $P < 0.0001$) increase in graft failure, with a dose–response effect with increasing numbers of cigarettes smoked.[95] Infrainguinal procedures also have worse five-year graft patency rates, ranging from 29% to 62%, with worse rates associated with prosthetic grafts below the knee and with continued smoking. Procedures involving the tibioperoneal trunk and tibial vessels are associated with the greatest postoperative morbidity and tissue loss. Other studies have also shown that venous grafts have better long-term patency than prosthetic (polytetrafluoroethylene coated) grafts, with the long saphenous vein being the graft of choice. A requirement for infrainguinal surgical bypass procedures is a patent and uncompromised inflow artery.

Postoperatively, clinical surveillance programs are advised up to two years postoperatively, with regular clinical review with ABI and a vascular history noted. Patients should also be treated with long-term antiplatelet therapy. Cohort studies have identified factors which can be associated with decreased long-term patency such as female sex, redo procedures, diabetes mellitus and African-American ethnicity, as well as the technical expertise of the surgeon.

Comparisons between surgical and percutaneous therapies are limited by the differing profiles and anatomy of patients who are referred for these procedures. Feinglass *et al* examined outcomes in a prospective cohort of patients who underwent percutaneous transluminal angioplasty (PTA) or surgery or medical therapy, and reported that mean walking distances and ABIs were improved in the interventional groups.[96] The BASIL study[97] randomized 452 patients with severe limb ischemia to surgery or PTA and found similar outcomes in both groups, with amputation-free survival at six months in 60 surgical vs 48 PTA patients (HR 1.07, 95% CI 0.72–1.60), with PTA noted to be less costly than surgical bypass procedures. Other studies have noted the superior cost effectiveness of PTA vs surgery.

Recommendations

- Aorto-iliac disease which is disabling and refractory to medical and exercise therapy can be treated with aorto-iliac bypass procedures, if PTA is not appropriate (**Class I, Level B**).
- Infrainguinal bypass procedures can be used in cases of severe ischemia, and should be performed using autologous vein grafts as first choice, with artifical grafts used as a second option (**Class IIa, Level B**).

Special considerations: critical limb ischemia and acute limb ischemia

Critical limb ischemia (CLI) is said to occur when the patient has symptoms of ischemic rest pain for at least two weeks or an ischemic ulcer or gangrene, with the ankle pressure usually below 50 mmHg. In this situation, a multidisciplinary approach is needed, and perfusion needs to be restored using either surgical or percutaneous approaches. Intravenous vasodilator prostaglandins, such as ilioprost and PGE-1, are sometimes used in patients with CLI, although the trials of these drugs have typically had small sample sizes. The most recent large trial randomized 1560 patients with CLI to PGE-1, and noted that there was a short-term reduction in death, amputation and major CV events, but that this effect became less at six months follow-up.[98] A meta analysis of PGE-1 studies also showed improved survival with PGE-1.[99] Oral iloprost (a synthetic PGI-2 analog) has not been shown to improve time to major amputation or stroke or death up to 12 months. The usual secondary prevention steps as outlined above should also be taken. The treatment priorities are to alleviate pain, to heal the ulcer and prevent further tissue loss, with the aim of improving the patient's quality of life and long-term survival.

Acute limb ischemia (ALI) is a surgical emergency and can be characterized by some (or all) of the Five "Ps": Pain in the affected limb, Pallor, Pulselessness, Paresthesia and Paralysis. The aims in ALI are to restore circulatory flow, relieve ischemia and prevent further thrombus propagation. Patients are treated with heparin and may receive catheter-delivered thrombolysis or surgical embolectomy. Urokinase is the thrombolytic agent of choice, as streptokinase is associated with a lower efficacy and more bleeding complications. Furthermore, there is no role for systemic thrombolysis, as this is also associated with higher bleeding rates and lower efficacy. Both catheter-delivered thrombolysis and surgical embolectomy have a potential role, with no significant difference in limb salvage or death up to one year,[100,101] albeit with higher rates of stroke and major bleeding associated with thrombolysis therapy (in one meta-analysis, the OR for excess bleeding with thrombolysis vs vascular surgery was 2.95; 95% CI 1.62–5.32, $P = 0.001$[100]). The TOPAS (Thrombolysis Or Peripheral Arterial Surgery) trial[101] was a large multicenter randomized trial of catheter-delivered urokinase compared with surgery for ALI of <14 days duration: again, there was no significant difference in amputation rates or death up to one year, but an increase in major bleeding with thrombolysis (12.5% vs 5.5%, $P = 0.005$). The STILE trial again showed similar limb salvage rates between the catheter-delivered thrombolysis group and the surgical group, and even a one-year mortality benefit in the thrombolysis group

(84% vs 58%, $P = 0.01$), although the study numbers were small.[102] A further subgroup analysis of the STILE data noted that native artery occlusions had a poorer amputation-free survival with thrombolysis than with surgery.

Recommendations

- Intravenous prostaglandins can be a useful adjunct to therapy in CLI (**Class IIa, Level A**).
- There is no role for oral prostaglandin agents in CLI (**Class III, Level A**).
- All patients with ALI should be treated with heparin (**Class I, Level C**).
- Revascularization is a priority in ALI, and can be performed using surgical or endovascular techniques or with catheter-directed thrombolysis with urokinase if the occlusion is less than 14 days duration (**Class I, Level A**).

Conclusion

PAD of the lower extremities is primarily due to atherosclerosis and is increasing in prevalence worldwide. PAD is a frequently underdiagnosed and when present, indicates that patients are at high risk of future cardiovascular complications. The mainstay of treatment for intermittent claudication is smoking cessation and supervised exercise, as well as aggressive CV prevention therapies including antiplatelet therapy, blood pressure and lipid-lowering therapies, as well as tight glucose control among diabetics for secondary prevention. Percutaneous catheter-based therapies and surgical bypass procedures should be reserved for highly selected patients with severe limb ischemia in whom medical and lifestyle therapies have not succeeded.

References

1. Criqui M, Fronek A, Barrett-Connor E, Klauber M, Gabriel S, Goodman D. The prevalence of peripheral arterial disease in a defined population. *Circulation* 1985;**71**:510–15.
2. Hiatt W, Hoag S, Hammam RF. Effect of diagnostic criteria on the prevalence of peripheral arterial disease. The San Luis valley diabetes study. *Circulation* 1995;**91**:1472–9.
3. Selvin E, Erlinger T. Prevalence of and risk factors for peripheral arterial disease in the United States: Results from the national health and nutrition examination survey, 1999–2000. *Circulation* 2004;**110**:738–43.
4. Meijer WT, Cost B, Bernsen RMD, Hoes AW. Incidence and management of intermittent claudication in primary care in the Netherlands. *Scand J Primary Health Care* 2002;**20**:33–4.
5. Norgren L, Hiatt WR, Dormandy JA, Nehler MR, Harris KA, Fowkes FGR. Inter-society consensus for the management of

peripheral arterial disease (TASC II). *Eur J Vasc Endovasc Surg* 2007;**33**:S1–S75.

6. Valentine R, Jackson MR, Modrall J, McIntyre KE, Clagett G. The progressive nature of peripheral arterial disease in young adults: A prospective analysis of white men referred to a vascular surgery service. *J Vasc Surg* 1999;**30**:436–45.

7. Krupski WC. The peripheral vascular consequences of smoking. *Ann Vasc Surg* 1991;**5**:291.

8. Doobay A, Anand SS. Sensitivity and specificity of the ankle-brachial index to predict future cardiovascular outcomes: a systematic review. *Arterioscler Thromb Vasc Biol* 2005;**25**:1463–9.

9. Willigendael EM, Teijink JAW, Bartelink ML *et al.* Influence of smoking on incidence and prevalence of peripheral arterial disease. *J Vasc Surg* 2004;**40**:1158–65.

10. Meijer WT, Hoes AW, Rutgers D, Bots ML, Hofman A, Grobbee DE. Peripheral arterial disease in the elderly: the Rotterdam study. *Arterioscler Thromb Vasc Biol* 1998;**18**:185–92.

11. Lane J, Vittinghoff E, Lane K, Hiramoto J, Messina L. Risk factors for premature peripheral vascular disease: Results for the national health and nutritional survey, 1999–2002. *J Vasc Surg* 2006;**44**:319–25.

12. O'Hare AM, Vittinghoff E, Hsia J, Shlipak MG. Renal insufficiency and the risk of lower extremity peripheral arterial disease: Results from the heart and Estrogen/Progestin replacement study (HERS). *J Am Soc Nephrol* 2004;**15**:1046–51.

13. Newman AB, Siscovich, Manolio TA *et al.* Ankle-arm index as a marker of atherosclerosis in the cardiovascular health study. cardiovascular heart study (CHS) collaborative research group. *Circulation* 1993;**88**:837–45.

14. Selvin E, Marinopoulos S, Berkenblit G *et al.* Meta-analysis: glycosylated hemoglobin and cardiovascular disease in diabetes mellitus. *Ann Intern Med* 2004;**141**:421–31.

15. Murabito JM, D'Agostino RB, Silbershatz H, Wilson PWF. Intermittent claudication: a risk profile from the Framingham heart study. *Circulation* 1997;**96**:44–9.

16. Bendermacher BLW, Teijink JAW, Willigendael EM *et al.* A clinical prediction model for the presence of peripheral arterial disease – the benefit of screening individuals before initiation of measurement of the ankle–brachial index: an observational study. *Vasc Med* 2007;**12**:5–11.

17. Hirsch A, Criqui M, Treat-Jacobson D *et al.* Peripheral arterial disease detection, awareness, and treatment in primary care. *JAMA* 2001;**286**:1317–24.

18. Hirsch A, Haskal Z, Hertzer N *et al.* ACC/AHA 2005 guidelines for the management of patients with peripheral arterial disease (lower extremity, renal, mesenteric, and abdominal aortic): executive summary. A collaborative report from the American Association for Vascular Surgery/Society for Vascular Surgery, Society for Cardiovascular Angiography and Interventions, Society for Vascular Medicine and Biology, Society of Interventional Radiology, and the ACC/AHA Task Force on Practice Guidelines (Writing Committee to Develop Guidelines for the Management of Patients with Peripheral Arterial Disease): endorsed by the American Association of Cardiovascular and Pulmonary Rehabilitation; National Heart, Lung, and Blood Institute; Society for Vascular Nursing; TransAtlantic Inter-Society Consensus; and Vascular Disease Foundation. *J Am Coll Cardiol* 2006;**47**:1239–312.

19. Khan N, Rahim S, Anand S, Simel D, Panju A. Does the clinical examination predict lower extremity peripheral arterial disease? *JAMA* 2006;**295**:536–46.

20. Farkouh M, Oddone E, Simel D. Improving the clinical examination for a low ankle-brachial index. *Int J Angiol* 2002;**11**:41–5.

21. Fowkes F. The measurement of atherosclerotic peripheral arterial disease in epidemiological surveys. *Int J Epidemiol* 1988;**17**:248–54.

22. Resnick H, Lindsay R, McDermott M *et al.* Relationship of high and low ankle brachial index to all-cause and cardiovascular disease mortality: the Strong Heart Study. *Circulation* 2004;**109**:733–9.

23. Koelemay MJ, den Hartog D, Prins MH, Kromhout JG, Legemate DA, Jacobs MJ. Diagnosis of arterial disease of the lower extremities with duplex ultrasonography. *Br J Surg* 1996;**83**:404–9.

24. Martin M, Tay K, Flak B *et al.* Multidetector CT angiography of the aortoiliac system and lower extremities: a prospective comparison with digital subtraction angiography. *AJR* 2003;**180**:1085–91.

25. Heijenbrok-Kal M, Kock MJM, Hunink MGM. Lower extremity arterial disease: multidetector CT angiography meta-analysis. *Radiology* 2007;**245**(2):433–9.

26. Ouwendijk R, deVries M, Pattynama PT *et al.* Imaging peripheral arterial disease: a randomized controlled trial comparing contrast-enhanced MR angiography and multi-detector row CT angiography. *Radiology* 2005;**236**:1094–103.

27. Koelemay MJW, Lijmer JG, Stoker J, Legemate DA, Bossuyt PMM. Magnetic resonance angiography for the evaluation of lower extremity arterial disease: A meta-analysis. *JAMA* 2001;**285**:1338–45.

28. Lassila R, Lepantalo M. Cigarette smoking and the outcome after lower limb arterial surgery. *Acta Chir Scand* 1988;**154**:635–40.

29. UK Small Aneurysm Trial Participants. Mortality results for randomised controlled trial of early elective surgery or ultrasonographic surveillance of small abdominal aortic aneurysms. *Lancet* 1998;**352**:1649–55.

30. Merali FS, Anand SS. Vascular viewpoint. *Vasc Med* 2002;**7**:249–50.

31. Law M, Tang JL. An analysis of the effectiveness of interventions intended to help people stop smoking. *Arch Intern Med* 1995;**155**:1933–41.

32. Russell MA, Wilson C, Taylor C, Baker CD. Effect of general practitioners' advice against smoking. *BMJ* 1979;**2**:231–5.

33. Myung SK, Yoo K, Oh SW *et al.* Meta-analysis of studies investigating one-year effectiveness of transdermal nicotine patches for smoking cessation. *Am J Health Syst Pharm* 2007;**64**:2471–6.

34. Stead LF, Perera R, Bullen C, Mant D, Lancaster T. Nicotine replacement therapy for smoking cessation. *Cochrane Database of Systematic Reviews* 2008, Issue 1. Art. No.: CD000146. DOI: 10.1002/14651858.CD000146.pub3.

35. Jorenby DE, Leischow SJ, Nides MA *et al.* A controlled trial of sustained-release bupropion, a nicotine patch, or both for smoking cessation. *N Engl J Med* 1999;**340**:685–91.

36. Tonstad S, Farsang C, Klaene G *et al.* Bupropion SR for smoking cessation in smokers with cardiovascular disease: a multicentre, randomised study. *Eur Heart J* 2003;**24**:946–55.

37. Nides M, Oncken C, Gonzales D *et al.* Smoking cessation with varenicline, a selective {alpha}4beta2 nicotinic receptor partial agonist: Results from a 7-week, randomized, placebo- and bupropion-controlled trial with 1-year follow-up. *Arch Intern Med* 2006;**166**:1561–8.

38. Gonzales D, Rennard SI, Nides M *et al.* Varenicline, an {alpha}4beta2 nicotinic acetylcholine receptor partial agonist, vs sustained-release bupropion and placebo for smoking cessation: a randomized controlled trial. *JAMA* 2006;**296**:47–55.

39. Girolami B, Bernardi E, Prins MH *et al.* Treatment of intermittent claudication with physical training, smoking cessation, pentoxifylline, or nafronyl: a meta-analysis. *Arch Intern Med* 1999;**159**:337–45.

40. Gardner AW, Poehlman ET. Exercise rehabilitation programs for the treatment of claudication pain. A meta-analysis. *JAMA* 1995;**274**:975–80.

41. Treat-Jacobson D, Bronas UG, Leon AS. Abstract 2760: Both arm ergometry and treadmill exercise training improve walking distance in peripheral arterial disease (PAD) patients with claudication. *Circulation* 2006;**114**:II-577–a.

42. Walker RD, Nawaz S, Wilkinson CH, Saxton JM, Pockley AG, Wood RFM. Influence of upper- and lower-limb exercise training on cardiovascular function and walking distances in patients with intermittent claudication. *J Vasc Surg* 2000;**31**:662–9.

43. Perkins JMT, Collin J, Creasy TS, Fletcher EWL, Morris PJ. Exercise training versus angioplasty for stable claudication. long and medium term results of a prospective, randomised trial. *Eur J Vasc Endovasc Surg* 1996;**11**:409–13.

44. Gaede P, Lund-Andersen H, Parving HH, Pedersen O. Effect of a multifactorial intervention on mortality in type 2 diabetes. *N Engl J Med* 2008;**358**:580–91.

45. National Heart Lung and Blood institute. ACCORD Blood Sugar Treatment Strategy Announcement. Available at http://www.nhlbi.nih.gov/health/prof/heart/other/accord/index.htm.

46. Diabetes Control and Complications Trial/Epidemiology of Diabetes Interventions and Complications (DCCT/EDIC) Study Research Group. Intensive diabetes treatment and cardiovascular disease in patients with type 1 diabetes. *N Engl J Med* 2005;**353**:2643–53.

47. UK Prospective Diabetes Study Group. Intensive blood-glucose control with sulphonylureas or insulin compared with conventional treatment and risk of complications in patients with type 2 diabetes (UKPDS 33). *Lancet* 1998;**352**:837–53.

48. American Diabetes Association. Peripheral arterial disease in people with diabetes (consensus statement). *Diabetes Care* 2003;**26**:3333(9).

49. Ostergren J, Sleight P, Dagenais G *et al.* Impact of ramipril in patients with evidence of clinical or subclinical peripheral arterial disease. *Eur Heart J* 2004;**25**:17–24.

50. Mehler PS, Coll JR, Estacio R, Esler A, Schrier RW, Hiatt WR. Intensive blood pressure control reduces the risk of cardiovascular events in patients with peripheral arterial disease and type 2 diabetes. *Circulation* 2003;**107**:753–6.

51. Lip GYH, Makin AJ. Treatment of hypertension in peripheral arterial disease. *Cochrane Database of Systematic Reviews* 2003, Issue 2. Art. No.: CD003075. DOI: 10.1002/14651858.CD003075.

52. Radack K, Deck C. Beta-adrenergic blocker therapy does not worsen intermittent claudication in subjects with peripheral arterial disease. A meta-analysis of randomized controlled trials. *Arch Intern Med* 1991;**151**:1769–76.

53. Chobanian AV, Bakris GL, Black HR *et al.* The seventh report of the joint national committee on prevention, detection, evaluation, and treatment of high blood pressure: the JNC 7 report. *JAMA* 2003;**289**(19):2560–72. Erratum in *JAMA* 2003;**290**(2):197.

54. Heart Protection Study Collaborative Group. MRC/BHF heart protection study of cholesterol lowering with simvastatin in 20536 high-risk individuals: a randomised placebo controlled trial. *Lancet* 2002;**360**:7–22.

55. Aung PP, Maxwell H, Jepson RG, Price J, Leng GC. Lipid-lowering for peripheral arterial disease of the lower limb. *Cochrane Database of Systematic Reviews* 2007, Issue 4. Art. No.: CD000123. DOI: 10.1002/14651858.CD000123.pub2.

56. Rubins HB, Robins SJ, Collins D *et al.* Gemfibrozil for the secondary prevention of coronary heart disease in men with low levels of high-density lipoprotein cholesterol. *N Engl J Med* 1999;**341**:410–18.

57. Meade T, Zuhrie R, Cook C, Cooper J. Bezafibrate in men with lower extremity arterial disease: randomised controlled trial. *BMJ* 2002;**325**:1139.

58. Taylor AJ, Sullenberger LE, Lee HJ, Lee JK, Grace KA. Arterial biology for the investigation of the treatment effects of reducing cholesterol (ARBITER) 2: a double-blind, placebo-controlled study of extended-release niacin on atherosclerosis progression in secondary prevention patients treated with statins. *Circulation* 2004;**110**:3512–17.

59. Mohler ER III, Hiatt WR, Creager MA, for the Study Investigators. Cholesterol reduction with atorvastatin improves walking distance in patients with peripheral arterial disease. *Circulation* 2003;**108**:1481–6.

60. McDermott MM, Guralnik JM, Greenland P *et al.* Statin use and leg functioning in patients with and without lower-extremity peripheral arterial disease. *Circulation* 2003;**107**:757–61.

61. Aronow WS, Nayak D, Woodworth S, Ahn C. Effect of simvastatin versus placebo on treadmill exercise time until the onset of intermittent claudication in older patients with peripheral arterial disease at six months and at one year after treatment. *Am J Cardiol* 2003;**92**:711–12.

62. Antiplatelet Trialists Collaboration. Collaborative meta-analysis of randomised trials of antiplatelet therapy for prevention of death, myocardial infarction, and stroke in high risk patients. *BMJ* 2002;**324**:71–86.

63. Tran H, Anand SS. Oral antiplatelet therapy in cerebrovascular disease, coronary artery disease, and peripheral arterial disease. *JAMA* 2004;**292**:1867–74.

64. Collins TC, Souchek J, Beyth RJ. Benefits of antithrombotic therapy after infrainguinal bypass grafting: a meta-analysis. *Am J Med* 2004;**117**:93–9.

65. Antiplatelet Trialists' Collaboration. Collaborative overview of randomised trials of antiplatelet therapy – II: Maintenance of vascular graft or arterial patency by antiplatelet therapy. *BMJ* 1994;**308**:159–68.

66. Dörffler-Melly J, Büller HR, Koopman MM, Prins MH. Antithrombotic agents for preventing thrombosis after infrainguinal arterial bypass surgery. *Cochrane Database of Systematic Reviews* 2003, Issue 2. Art. No.: CD000536. DOI: 10.1002/14651858.CD000536.

67. Dutch Bypass Oral Anticoagulants or Aspirin (BOA) Study Group. Efficacy of oral anticoagulants compared with aspirin after infrainguinal bypass surgery (the Dutch Bypass Oral Anticoagulants or Aspirin Study): a randomised trial. *The Lancet* 2000;**355**:346–51.

68. Brown J, Lethaby A, Maxwell H, Wawrzyniak AJ, Prins MH. Antiplatelet agents for preventing thrombosis after peripheral arterial bypass surgery. *Cochrane Database of Systematic Reviews* 2008, Issue 4. Art. No.: CD000535. DOI: 10.1002/14651858. CD000535.pub2.

69. Warfarin Antiplatelet Vascular Evaluation Trial Investigators. Oral anticoagulant and antiplatelet therapy and peripheral arterial disease. *N Engl J Med* 2007;**357**:217–27.

70. Dörffler-Melly J, Koopman MM, Prins MH, Büller HR. Antiplatelet and anticoagulant drugs for prevention of restenosis/reocclusion following peripheral endovascular treatment. *Cochrane Database of Systematic Reviews* 2005, Issue 1. Art. No.: CD002071. DOI: 10.1002/14651858.CD002071.pub2.

71. Goldhaber SZ, Manson JE, Stampfer MJ *et al*. Low-dose aspirin and subsequent peripheral arterial surgery in the physicians' health study. *Lancet* 1992;**340**:143–5.

72. Girolami B. Antiplatelet therapy and other interventions after revascularisation procedures in patients with peripheral arterial disease: a meta-analysis. *Eur J Vasc Endovasc Surg* 2000; **19**:370.

73. Girolami B. Antithrombotic drugs in the primary medical management of intermittent claudication: a meta-analysis. *Thromb Haem* 1999;**81**:715.

74. Hankey G, Sudlow CLM, Dunbabin DW. Thienopyridine derivatives (ticlopidine, clopidogrel) versus aspirin for preventing stroke and other serious vascular events in high vascular risk patients. *Cochrane Database of Systematic Reviews* 2000, Issue 1. Art. No.: CD001246. DOI: 10.1002/14651858. CD001246.

75. CAPRIE Steering Committee. A randomised, blinded, trial of clopidogrel versus aspirin in patients at risk of ischaemic events (CAPRIE). *Lancet* 1996;**348**:1329–39.

76. Schoop W. Open randomised study comparing ticlopidine with acetylsalicylic acid in the prevention of contralateral thrombosis in patients initially presenting with unilateral thrombosis. Internal Report. Guildford: Sanofi, 1983.

77. Bhatt DL, Fox KAA, Hacke W *et al*. Clopidogrel and aspirin versus aspirin alone for the prevention of atherothrombotic events. *N Engl J Med* 2006;**354**:1706–17

78. De Schryver E, Algra A, van Gijn J. Dipyridamole for preventing stroke and other vascular events in patients with vascular disease. *Cochrane Database of Systematic Reviews* 2007, Issue 3. Art. No.: CD001820. DOI: 10.1002/14651858.CD001820. pub3.

79. Balsano F, Coccheri S, Libretti A *et al*. Ticlodipine in the treatment of intermittent claudication: a 21-month double-blind trial. *J Lab Clin Med* 1989;**114**:84–91.

80. Giansante C, Calabrese S, Fisicaro M, Fiotti N, Mitri E. Treatment of intermittent claudication with antiplatelet agents. *J Int Med Res* 1990;**18**:400–7.

81. WAVE Investigators. The effects of oral anticoagulants in patients with peripheral arterial disease: rationale, design, and baseline characteristics of the warfarin and antiplatelet vascu-

lar evaluation (WAVE) trial, including a meta-analysis of trials. *Am Heart J* 2006;**151**:1–9.

82. Hood SC, Moher D, Barber GG. Management of intermittent claudication with pentoxifylline: meta-analysis of randomized controlled trials. *CMAJ* 1996;**155**:1053–9.

83. Dawson DL, Cutler BS, Hiatt WR *et al*. A comparison of cilostazol and pentoxifylline for treating intermittent claudication. *Am J Med* 2000;**109**:523–30.

84. Spengel F. Findings of the Naftidrofuryl in Quality of Life (NIQOL) European study program. *Int Angiol* 2002;**21**:20.

85. Lehert P, Comte S, Gamand S, Brown TM. Naftidrofuryl in intermittent claudication: a retrospective analysis. *J Cardiovasc Pharmacol* 1994;**23**:S48.

86. Regensteiner JG, Ware JE, McCarthy WJ *et al*. Effect of cilostazol on treadmill walking, community-based walking ability, and health-related quality of life in patients with intermittent claudication due to peripheral arterial disease: Meta-analysis of six randomized controlled trials. *J Am Geriatr Soc* 2002; **50**:1939–46.

87. Robless P, Mikhailidis DP, Stansby GP. Cilostazol for peripheral arterial disease. *Cochrane Database of Systematic Reviews* 2008, Issue 1. Art. No.: CD003748. DOI: 10.1002/14651858. CD003748.pub3.

88. de Backer TLM, Bogaert M, Vander Stichele R. Buflomedil for intermittent claudication. *Cochrane Database of Systematic Reviews* 2008, Issue 1. Art. No.: CD000988. DOI: 10.1002/14651858. CD000988.pub3.

89. Whyman MR. Randomised controlled trial of percutaneous transluminal angioplasty for intermittent claudication. *Eur J Vasc Endovasc Surg* 1996;**12**:167.

90. Perkins JM, Collin J, Creasy TS, Fletcher EW, Morris PJ. Exercise training versus angioplasty for stable claudication: Long and medium term results of a prospective, randomised trial. *Eur J Vasc Endovasc Surg* 1996;**11**:409–13.

91. Spronk S, Bosch JL, Veen HF, den Hoed PT, Hunink MGM. Intermittent claudication: functional capacity and quality of life after exercise training or percutaneous transluminal angioplasty – systematic review. *Radiology* 2005;**235**:833–42.

92. Schillinger M, Sabeti S, Loewe C *et al*. Balloon angioplasty versus implantation of nitinol stents in the superficial femoral artery. *N Engl J Med* 2006;**354**:1879–88.

93. Tepe G, Zeller T, Albrecht T *et al*. Local delivery of paclitaxel to inhibit restenosis during angioplasty of the leg. *N Engl J Med* 2008;**358**:689–99.

94. de Vries SO, Hunink MGM. Results of aortic bifurcation grafts for aortoiliac occlusive disease: a meta-analysis. *J Vasc Surg* 1997;**26**:558–69.

95. Willigendael E, Teijink J, Bartelink M, Peters R, Büller H, Prins M. Smoking and the patency of lower extremity bypass grafts: a meta-analysis. *J Vasc Surg* 2005;**42**(1):67–74.

96. Feinglass J, McCarthy WJ, Slavensky R, Manheim LM, Martin GJ. Functional status and walking ability after lower extremity bypass grafting or angioplasty for intermittent claudication: results from a prospective outcomes study. *J Vasc Surg* 2000;**31**:93–103.

97. BASIL Trial Participants. Bypass surgery versus angioplasty in severe ischaemia of the leg (BASIL): multicentre, randomised controlled trial. *Lancet* 2005;**366**:1925.

98. ICAI Study Group. Prostanoids for chronic critical leg isch-emia: a randomized, controlled, open-label trial with prosta-glandin E1. *Ann Intern Med* 1999;**130**:412–21.

99. Creutzig A. Meta-analysis of randomised controlled prosta-glandin E1 studies in peripheral arterial occlusive disease stages III and IV. *VASA* 2004;**33**:137.

100. Palfreyman SJ. A systematic review of intra-arterial thrombo-lytic therapy for lower-limb ischaemia. *Eur J Vasc Endovasc Surg* 2000;**19**:143.

101. Ouriel K. A comparison of recombinant urokinase with vascu-lar surgery as initial treatment for acute arterial occlusion of the legs. Thrombolysis or Peripheral Arterial Surgery (TOPAS) Investigators. *N Engl J Med* 1998;**338**:1105.

102. Ouriel K. A comparison of thrombolytic therapy with operative revascularization in the initial treatment of acute peripheral arterial ischemia. *J Vasc Surg* 1994;**19**:1021.

66 Cardiac risk in those undergoing non-cardiac surgery

Ameeth Vedre and Kim A Eagle
University of Michigan, Ann Arbor, MI, USA

Introduction and historical perspective

The prevalence of cardiovascular disease increases with age, and it is estimated that the number of persons older than 65 years in the United States will increase 25–35% over the next 30 years.[1] The number of non-cardiac surgical procedures performed in older persons will increase from the current 6 million to nearly 12 million per year, and nearly a fourth of these – major intra-abdominal, thoracic, vascular, and orthopedic procedures – have been associated with significant perioperative cardiovascular morbidity and mortality.[2]

Guidelines on the assessment and management of perioperative cardiovascular risk for patients undergoing noncardiac surgery were published by American College of Cardiology/American Heart Association (ACC/AHA) Task Force in 1996 and updated in 2002 and 2006 and revised in 2007.[2-4] Guidelines published in 2006 by the ACC/AHA focused the management from non-invasive risk stratification to risk reduction through strategies such as the use of perioperative beta-blockade.

Assessment of preoperative risk for non-cardiac surgery

The range of risk seen in current practice was illustrated in a retrospective study of 663665 adults with no contraindications to beta-blockers who underwent major non-cardiac surgery in 2000 and 2001 at 329 hospitals in the United States. Orthopedic and abdominal surgery accounted for 70% of cases. In-hospital mortality in patients not treated with beta-blockers increased progressively from 1.4% to 7.4% according to a preoperative assessment of risk using the revised Goldman Cardiac Risk Index[5,6] (**Level C1**).

Evidence-Based Cardiology, 3rd edition. Edited by S. Yusuf, J.A. Cairns, A.J. Camm, E.L. Fallen, and B.J. Gersh. © 2010 Blackwell Publishing, ISBN: 978-1-4051-5925-8.

Eagle *et al* retrospectively studied 254 consecutive patients presenting to the nuclear cardiology laboratory for dipyridamole-thallium imaging before proposed vascular surgery.[7] Logistic regression analysis identified five clinical predictors of postoperative cardiac events in patients undergoing major vascular surgery: Q-waves on the ECG, history of angina, ventricular ectopy requiring treatment, diabetes mellitus requiring therapy other than diet, and age above 70 years (**Level C1**).

A subsequent validation study by Vanzetto added three more clinical predictors to the Eagle criteria which were ischemic ST segment abnormalities on resting ECG, hypertension with severe left ventricular hypertrophy and history of heart failure (HF). This author also identified two independent dipyridamole-thallium test predictors of ischemic events: thallium redistribution and ischemic ECG changes during or after dipyridamole infusion[8] (**Level C1**).

Fleisher and Eagle[9] emphasized six factors in a further report, the first five of which are also in the revised Goldman Cardiac Risk Index,[6] and are all associated with increased cardiac risk in patients undergoing non-cardiac surgery, including vascular surgery (**Level C1**).

- Ischemic heart disease (angina or prior MI)
- Heart failure
- High-risk surgery (including intraperitoneal, intrathoracic, and suprainguinal vascular procedures)
- Diabetes mellitus (especially requiring insulin)
- Renal insufficiency
- Poor functional status (defined as the inability to walk four blocks or climb two flights of stairs)

General approach to the patient

Preoperative cardiac evaluation must be carefully tailored to the circumstances that have prompted the consultation and the nature of the proposed surgery. Given an acute surgical emergency, preoperative evaluation might have to be limited to rapid bedside assessment including assessment of vital signs, volume status, basic metabolic panel and electrocardiogram (ECG)[2,10] (**Class I, Level B**). The physician should review available patient data, obtain a history, and perform a physical examination pertinent to the patient's problem and the proposed surgery.

History and physical examination

Cardiac conditions such as prior angina, recent or past MI, HF, symptomatic arrhythmias, and history of a pacemaker or implantable cardioverter defibrillator (ICD) should be identified. Modifiable risk factors for coronary heart disease (CHD) should be recorded along with evidence of associated diseases, such as peripheral vascular disease, cerebrovascular disease, diabetes mellitus, renal impairment, and chronic pulmonary disease (Table 66.1).

- *Major* predictors, when present, mandate intensive management, which may result in delay or cancellation of surgery unless it is urgent.
- *Intermediate* predictors are well-validated markers of enhanced risk of perioperative cardiac complications and justify careful assessment of the patient's current status.

Table 66.1 Clinical predictors of increased perioperative cardiovascular risk (myocardial infarction, congestive heart failure, death)

Major
Unstable coronary syndromes
   Recent myocardial infarction* with evidence of important ischemic risk by clinical symptoms or non-invasive study
   Unstable or severe† angina (Canadian class III or IV)
Decompensated congestive heart failure
Significant arrhythmias
   High-grade atrioventricular block
   Symptomatic ventricular arrhythmias in the presence of underlying heart disease
   Supraventricular arrhythmias with uncontrolled ventricular rate
Severe valvular disease

Intermediate
Mild angina pectoris (Canadian class I or II)
Prior myocardial infarction by history or pathologic Q-waves
Compensated or prior congestive heart failure
Diabetes mellitus
Chronic renal insufficiency

Minor
Advanced age
Abnormal electrocardiogram (left ventricular hypertrophy, left bundle branch block, ST-T abnormalities)
Rhythm other than sinus (e.g. atrial fibrillation)
Low functional capacity (e.g. inability to climb one flight of stairs with a bag of groceries)
History of stroke
Uncontrolled systemic hypertension

Reproduced with permission from Eagle *et al.*[2]

- *Minor* predictors are recognized markers for cardiovascular disease that have not been proven to independently increase perioperative risk.[2]

A careful cardiovascular examination should include an assessment of vital signs (including measurement of blood pressure in both arms), carotid pulse, contour and bruits, jugular venous pressure and pattern, auscultation of the lungs, precordial palpation, cardiac auscultation and examination of the extremities for edema and vascular integrity.[2] The history should also seek to determine the patient's functional capacity (Table 66.2).

An assessment of an individual's capacity to perform a spectrum of common daily tasks has been shown to correlate well with maximum oxygen uptake by treadmill testing[10] (**Level C**).

A patient classified as high risk owing to age or known CAD but who is asymptomatic and runs for 30 minutes daily may need no further evaluation. In contrast, a sedentary patient without a history of cardiovascular disease but with clinical factors that suggest increased perioperative risk may benefit from a more extensive preoperative evaluation (**Class II, Level C1**).

Management of co-morbid conditions

The stress of non-cardiac surgery may raise heart rate and blood pressure and has been associated with a high incidence of symptomatic and asymptomatic myocardial ischemia in patients with known vascular disease.

Associated conditions often heighten the risk of anesthesia and may complicate cardiac management. The most common of these conditions are discussed below.

If significant pulmonary disease is suspected by history or physical examination, determination of functional capacity, response to bronchodilators, and/or evaluation for the presence of carbon dioxide retention through arterial blood gas analysis may be justified[2] (**Class I, Level C1**).

Management of blood glucose levels in the perioperative period may be difficult. Fragile diabetic patients need careful treatment with adjusted doses or infusions of short-acting insulin based on frequent blood sugar determinations. Historically, it has been acceptable to maintain relatively high glucose levels perioperatively to avoid the attendant risks of hypoglycemic episodes. However, aggressive perioperative glucose control in coronary bypass surgery patients by a continuous, intravenous insulin infusion was superior to intermittent subcutaneous insulin administration in significantly reducing postoperative wound infection.[11] Similar benefit may occur surrounding non-cardiac surgery[12] (**Class I, Level C**).

Anemia imposes a stress on the cardiovascular system that may exacerbate myocardial ischemia and aggravate HF.[13] Preoperative transfusion, when used appropriately in patients with advanced CAD and/or HF, may reduce peri-

Table 66.2 Estimated energy requirement for various activities*

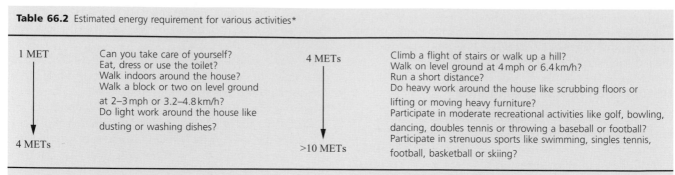

1 MET	Can you take care of yourself? Eat, dress or use the toilet? Walk indoors around the house? Walk a block or two on level ground at 2–3 mph or 3.2–4.8 km/h? Do light work around the house like dusting or washing dishes?	4 METs	Climb a flight of stairs or walk up a hill? Walk on level ground at 4 mph or 6.4 km/h? Run a short distance? Do heavy work around the house like scrubbing floors or lifting or moving heavy furniture? Participate in moderate recreational activities like golf, bowling, dancing, doubles tennis or throwing a baseball or football?
4 METs		>10 METs	Participate in strenuous sports like swimming, singles tennis, football, basketball or skiing?

MET, metabolic equivalent. Reproduced with permission from Eagle et al.[2] *Adapted from the Duke Activity Status Index and AHA Exercise Standards.

operative cardiac morbidity (**Class II, Level C1**). Hematocrits less than 28% are associated with an increased incidence of perioperative ischemia and postoperative complications in patients undergoing prostate and vascular surgery[14,15] (**Level B**).

Due to high risk for the development of further decompensation and death during the perioperative period, patients facing high-stress surgery who have acute coronary syndromes (e.g. unstable angina or decompensated HF of ischemic origin) and stable patients with likelihood of advanced multivessel coronary artery disease, with or without left ventricular dysfunction, will benefit from coronary angiography[2] (**Class II, Level B**). If the non-cardiac surgery is truly urgent, intra-aortic balloon bump counterpulsation as a means of providing short-term myocardial protection in addition to maximal medical therapy[4] (**Class I, Level C1**).

If the patient does not demonstrate unstable symptoms, the identification of known or symptomatic stable CAD or risk factors for CAD can guide the need for further diagnostic evaluation or changes in perioperative management (**Class I, Level C**). In determining the extent of the preoperative evaluation, it must be remembered that testing should not be performed unless the results would affect perioperative management. These management changes include cancellation of surgery because of prohibitive risk compared with benefit, delay of surgery for further medical management, coronary interventions before non-cardiac surgery, and utilization of an intensive care unit.

Multiple studies have demonstrated an increased incidence of reinfarction after non-cardiac surgery if the prior MI was within 6 months of the operation and especially within 6–12 weeks[16,17] (**Level C1**). Severe hypertension of a chronic nature, e.g. diastolic blood pressure higher than 110 mmHg, should be controlled before any elective non-cardiac surgery.[2] The Study of Perioperative Ischemia Research Group trial (POISE), in which patients had continuous perioperative electrocardiographic monitoring, showed that a history of hypertension was one of five independent predictors of postoperative ischemia and one of three independent predictors of increased postoperative mortality.[18] Patients with a history of hypertension had

almost twice the risk of postoperative myocardial ischemia and almost four times the risk of postoperative death compared with patients without hypertension in the first 48 hours postoperatively[19] (**Level B**).

For patients who present for non-cardiac surgery with signs or symptoms of HF, the goal of the preoperative evaluation should be identification of the underlying disease processes and assessment of the severity of systolic and diastolic dysfunction (**Class I, Level B**). Ischemic cardiomyopathy is of greatest concern because the patient has a substantial risk for developing further ischemia, leading to myocardial necrosis and potentially a downward spiral. In such patients, a pulmonary artery catheter or intraoperative transesophageal echocardiography may be helpful[4] (**Level C1**). Since both severe stenotic and/or regurgitant valve disease can cause or complicate heart failure, clarification of underlying valve function is important when suspected based on the history of physical exam (**Class II, Level C**).

The presence of critical aortic stenosis is associated with a very high risk of cardiac decompensation in patients undergoing elective non-cardiac surgery. The presence of any of the classic triad of angina, syncope, and heart failure in a patient with aortic stenosis should alert the clinician to the need for further evaluation and potential interventions, usually valve replacement. However, many patients with severe or critical aortic stenosis may be asymptomatic, and preoperative patients with aortic systolic murmurs warrant a careful history and physical examination and often further evaluation. There are several case series of patients with critical aortic stenosis demonstrating that, when necessary, non-cardiac surgery can be performed with acceptable risk[20] (**Class I, Level C1**).

Decision to undergo diagnostic testing

Several groups have published meta-analyses examining the various preoperative diagnostic tests (Table 66.3). Mantha and colleagues demonstrated good predictive values of ambulatory electrocardiographic monitoring, radionuclide angiography, dipyridamole-thallium imaging, and dobutamine stress echocardiography[21] (**Level C2**).

Table 66.3 Recommendations for use of ancillary tests in patients undergoing non-cardiac surgery

Indication	Class I (indicated)	Class IIa	Class IIb	Class III (not indicated)
Preoperative 12-lead rest ECG	1. Recent episode of chest pain or ischemic equivalent in clinically intermediate- or high-risk patients scheduled for an intermediate- or high-risk operative procedure.	1. Asymptomatic persons with diabetes mellitus.	1. Patients with prior coronary revascularization. 2. Asymptomatic male older than 45 yr or female older than 55 yr with two or more atherosclerotic risk factors. 3. Prior hospital admission for cardiac causes.	1. As a routine test in asymptomatic subjects undergoing low-risk operative procedures.
Preoperative non-invasive evaluation of left ventricular function	1. Patients with current or poorly controlled heart failure.	1. Patients with prior heart failure and patients with dyspnea of unknown origin.		1. As a routine test of left ventricular function in patients without prior heart failure.
Exercise or pharmacological stress testing	1. Diagnosis of adult patients with intermediate pretest probability of CAD. 2. Prognostic assessment of patients undergoing initial evaluation for suspected or proven CAD; evaluation of subjects with significant change in clinical status. 3. Demonstration of proof of myocardial ischemia before coronary revascularization. 4. Evaluation of adequacy of medical therapy; prognostic assessment after an acute coronary syndrome	1. Evaluation of exercise capacity when subjective assessment is unreliable.	1. Diagnosis of CAD patients with high or low pretest probability; those with resting ST depression less than 1 mm, those undergoing digitalis therapy, and those with ECG criteria for left ventricular hypertrophy. 2. Detection of restenosis in high-risk asymptomatic subjects within the initial months after PCI.	1. For *exercise* stress testing, diagnosis of patients with resting ECG abnormalities that preclude adequate assessment, e.g. pre-excitation syndrome, electronically paced ventricular rhythm, rest ST depression greater than 1 mm, or left bundle branch block. 2. Severe co-morbidity likely to limit life expectancy or candidacy for revascularization. 3. Routine screening of asymptomatic men or women without evidence of CAD. 4. Investigation of isolated ectopic beats in young patients.
Coronary angiography in perioperative evaluation before (or after) non-cardiac surgery	Patients with suspected or known CAD:	1. Multiple markers of intermediate clinical risk† and planned vascular surgery (non-invasive testing should be considered first).	1. Perioperative MI.	1. Low-risk* non-cardiac surgery with known CAD and no high-risk results on non-invasive testing.

Continued on p. 1072

Table 66.3 *Continued*

Indication	Class I (indicated)	Class IIa	Class IIb	Class III (not indicated)
	1. Evidence for high risk of adverse outcome based on noninvasive test results.		2. Medically stabilized class III or IV angina and planned low-risk or minor* surgery.	2. Asymptomatic after coronary revascularization with excellent exercise capacity (greater than or equal to 7 METs).
	2. Angina unresponsive to adequate medical therapy.	2. Moderate to large region of ischemia on non-invasive testing but without high-risk features and without lower LVEF.		3. Mild stable angina with good left ventricular function and no high-risk non-invasive test results.
	3. Unstable angina, particularly when facing intermediate-risk* or high-risk* non-cardiac surgery.	3. Non-diagnostic non-invasive test results in patients of intermediate clinical risk† undergoing high-risk* non-cardiac surgery.		4. Non-candidate for coronary revascularization owing to concomitant medical illness, severe left ventricular dysfunction (e.g., LVEF less than 0.20), or refusal to consider revascularization.
	4. Equivocal non-invasive test results in patients at high clinical risk† undergoing high-risk* surgery.	4. Urgent non-cardiac surgery while convalescing from acute MI.		5. Candidate for liver, lung, or renal transplantation older than 40yr as part of evaluation for transplantation, unless non-invasive testing reveals high risk for adverse outcome.

CAD, coronary artery disease; ECG, electrocardiogram; HF, heart failure; LVEF, left ventricular ejection fraction; MET, metabolic equivalent; MI, myocardial infarction; PCI, percutaneous coronary intervention.Reproduced with permission from Eagle *et al.*[2], and from Fleisher LA, Eagle KA. Anesthesia and non-cardiac surgery in patients with heart disease. In: Lily LS, ed. *Braunwald's heart disease review and assessment*, 7th edn. Philadelphia: Elsevier Saunders, 2005.

Shaw and co-workers also demonstrated excellent predictive values for both dipyridamole-thallium imaging and dobutamine stress echocardiography[22] (**Level C1**).

Type of surgery

Cardiac complications after non-cardiac surgery are a reflection of factors specific to the patient, the operation, and the circumstances under which the operation is undertaken. To the extent that preoperative cardiac evaluation reliably predicts postoperative cardiac outcomes, it may lead to interventions that lower perioperative risk, decrease long-term mortality or alter the surgical decision-making process (**Class I**).

When, for example, surgery in asymptomatic individuals is undertaken with the objective of prolonging life (e.g. elective repair of aortic aneurysm) or preventing a future stroke (e.g. carotid endarterectomy), the decision to intervene must be made with the expectation that the patient will live long enough to benefit from the prophylactic intervention.

For elective surgery, cardiac risk can be stratified according to a number of factors, including the magnitude of the surgical procedure. Some operations are simply more dangerous than others (Table 66.4). Backer *et al*[16] encountered no cardiac complications after 288 ophthalmologic procedures in 195 patients with a prior history of MI compared with a reinfarction rate of 6.1% for a number of non-ophthalmologic surgeries at the same center (**Level C1**). In general, major vascular, thoracic, abdominal and/or emergency surgeries are placed into a moderate- or high-risk category, while orthopedic, breast, prostate, ophthalmologic, and endoscopic procedures are considered lower risk.

The AHA/ACC Task Force on Perioperative Evaluation of Cardiac Patients Undergoing Non-cardiac Surgery has proposed an algorithm (Fig. 66.1) for decisions regarding the need for further evaluation. First, the clinician must evaluate the urgency of the surgery and the appropriateness of a formal preoperative assessment. Next, he or she must determine whether the patient has had a previous revascularization procedure or coronary evaluation. Patients with unstable

Table 66.4 Cardiac risk* stratification for non-cardiac surgical procedures

High (reported cardiac risk often >5%)
Emergency major operations, particularly in elderly people
Aortic and other major vascular
Peripheral vascular
Anticipated prolonged surgical procedures associated with large fluid shifts and/or blood loss

Intermediate (reported cardiac risk generally <5%)
Carotid endarterectomy
Head and neck
Intraperitoneal and intrathoracic
Orthopedic
Prostate

Low†(reported cardiac risk generally <1%)
Endoscopic procedures
Superficial procedure
Cataract
Breast

Reproduced with permission from Eagle *et al.*[2]
* The American College of Cardiology National Database Library defines "recent MI" as greater than 7 days but less than or equal to 1 month (30 days); acute MI is within 7 days.
† May include "stable" angina in patients who are usually sedentary. Campeau L. Grading of angina pectoris. *Circulation* 1976;**54**:522–23.

coronary syndromes should be identified, and appropriate treatment should be instituted. The decision to have further testing depends on the interaction of the clinical risk factors, surgery-specific risk, and functional capacity.

Implementation of the ACC/AHA guidelines into clinical practice has been demonstrated to be effective in reducing use of preoperative stress myocardial imaging (44.3% versus 20.6%; $P < 0.05$) and coronary revascularization (7.7% versus 0.8%; $P < 0.05$) in patients undergoing elective vascular surgery. During the intervention period, there was a significant decrease in the incidence of cardiac complications (from 11.3% to 4.5%) and an increase in event-free survival at 1 year after surgery (from 91.3 to 98.2%).[23] Froehlich and colleagues compared 102 historical control patients with 94 patients directly after guideline implementation and 104 patients later after guideline implementation.[24] Resource utilization and costs were reduced after guideline implementation, and the effect was sustained for 2 years (**Level C1**).

Perioperative beta-blocker therapy

Studies on the outcomes of perioperative beta-blockade have initially shown benefits, but recently a few randomized trials have not shown a beneficial effect.

BOX 66.1 Recommendations for beta-blocker therapy during perioperative medical therapy

Class I
1. Beta-blockers should be continued in patients undergoing surgery who are receiving beta-blockers to treat angina, symptomatic arrhythmias, hypertension **or** other ACC/AHA Class I guideline indications.
2. Beta-blockers should be given to patients undergoing vascular surgery at high cardiac risk owing to the finding of ischemia on preoperative testing (**Level B**).

Class IIa
1. Beta-blockers are probably recommended for patients undergoing vascular surgery in which preoperative assessment identifies coronary heart disease (**Level B**).
2. Beta-blockers are probably recommended for patients in whom preoperative assessment for vascular surgery identifies high cardiac risk as defined by the presence of multiple clinical risk factors* (**Level B**).
3. Beta-blockers are probably recommended for patients in whom preoperative assessment identifies coronary heart disease or high cardiac risk as defined by the presence of multiple clinical risk factors* and who are undergoing intermediate- or high-risk procedures as defined in these guidelines (**Level B**).

Class IIb
1. Beta-blockers may be considered for patients who are undergoing intermediate- or high-risk procedures as defined in these guidelines, including vascular surgery, in whom preoperative assessment identifies intermediate cardiac risk as defined by the presence of a single clinical risk factor* (**Level C**).
2. Beta-blockers may be considered in patients undergoing vascular surgery with low cardiac risk (as defined in these guidelines) who are not currently on beta-blockers (**Level C**).

Class III
1. Beta-blockers should not be given to patients undergoing surgery who have absolute contraindications to beta-blockade (**Level C**).

* Clinical risk factors. High cardiac risk includes patients with major and intermediate clinical predictors. Care should be taken in applying recommendations on beta-blocker therapy to patients with decompensated heart failure, non-ischemic cardiomyopathy, high-degree AV block, or severe valvular heart disease in the absence of coronary heart disease.

As per the ACC/AHA 2007 guideline update by Fleisher *et al*, Box 66.1 shows the recommendations for beta-blocker therapy during perioperative medical therapy.[3,4]

Since publication of the ACC/AHA focused update on perioperative beta-blocker therapy, several randomized trials have been published that have not demonstrated the efficacy of these agents. Despite several meta-analyses, some

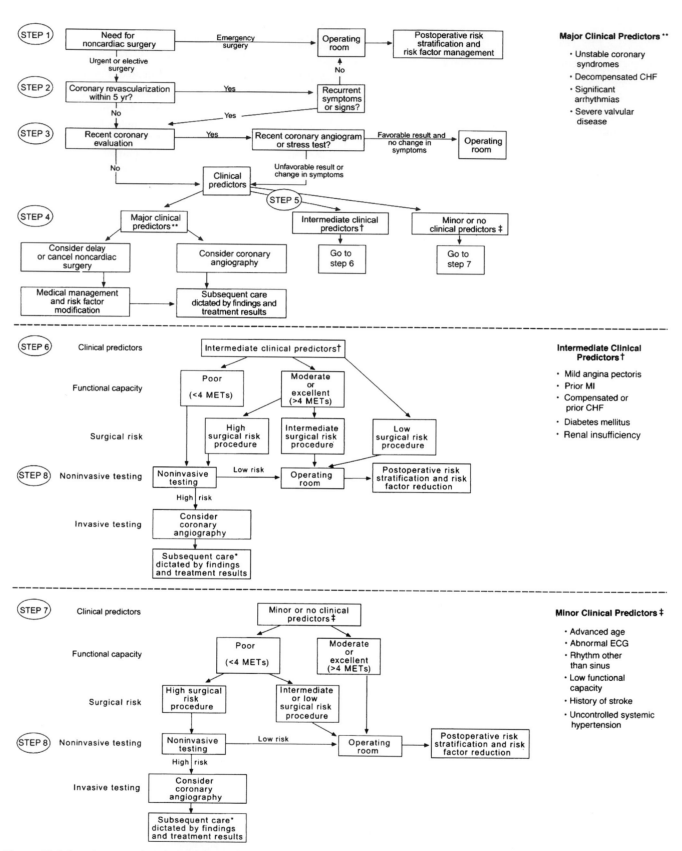

Figure 66.1 Stepwise approach to preoperative cardiac assessment. Steps are discussed in text.
*Subsequent care may include cancellation or delay of surgery, coronary revascularization followed by non-cardiac surgery or intensified care.
(Reproduced with permission from Eagle *et al.*[2])

of which reached conflicting conclusions, there are still very few randomized trials of this issue.[4] Randomized controlled trials are still needed to explore the observation that there may be some harm associated with beta-blocker therapy in low-risk patients[25] (**Level C**). In fact, studies involving the shorter-acting agent metoprolol have shown lower or no efficacy[26,27] (**Level C1, B**). In summary, the best approach on how to protect patients medically from cardiovascular complications during non-cardiac surgery is still unknown.

Several randomized trials examined the effect of perioperative beta-blockers on cardiac events surrounding surgery. Poldermans *et al* examined the effect of bisoprolol on patients undergoing vascular surgery and in patients at high risk for perioperative cardiac complications who were scheduled for vascular surgery[28] (**Level C1**). The Multicenter Study of Perioperative Ischemia Research Group[27,29] reported on 200 patients undergoing general surgery randomized to a combination of intravenous and oral atenolol versus placebo for 7 days. Although they found no difference in perioperative MI or death, they reported significantly fewer episodes of ischemia by Holter monitoring in the atenolol versus placebo groups (24% versus 39%, respectively; $P = 0.03$). They then conducted follow-up on these patients after discharge and documented fewer deaths in the atenolol group over the subsequent 6 months (1% versus 10%; $P < 0.001$) (**Level B**).

In POISE[30] (Perioperative Ischemia) trial 8351 patients with, or at risk of, atherosclerotic disease who were undergoing non-cardiac surgery were randomly assigned to receive extended-release metoprolol succinate. Fewer patients in the metoprolol group than in the placebo group had a myocardial infarction (176 [4.2%] vs 239 [5.7%] patients; 0.73, 0.60–0.89; $P = 0.0017$). However, there were more deaths in the metoprolol group than in the placebo group (129 [3.1%] vs 97 [2.3%] patients; 1.33, 1.03–1.74; $P = 0.0317$). More patients in the metoprolol group than in the placebo group had a stroke (41 [1.0%] vs 19 [0.5%] patients; 2.17, 1.26–3.74; $P = 0.0053$).

These data indicate that although perioperative extended-release metoprolol reduced the risk of myocardial infarction, cardiac revascularization, and clinically significant atrial fibrillation 30 days after randomization compared with placebo, the drug also resulted in a significant excess risk of death and non fatal stroke probably due to excess dose leading to hypotension and with it more infections, stroke and noncardiac death. POISE study group authors highlighted the risk in assuming a perioperative β-blocker regimen has benefit without substantial harm, and the importance and need for large randomized trials in the perioperative setting (**Class 1, Level A**).[30]

Recent meta analysis of 33 trials determined that β blockers were not associated with any significant reduction in the risk of all-cause mortality, cardiovascular mortality, or heart failure, but were associated with a decrease in non-fatal myocardial infarction and decrease in myocardial ischemia (**Class 1, Level A**).[31]

Limitations in the perioperative beta-blocker literature include the following: few randomized trials have examined the role of perioperative beta-blocker therapy, there is particularly a lack of trials that focus on high-risk patients and there is a lack of studies to determine the role and type of beta-blockers in intermediate- and low-risk populations.

Perioperative statin therapy

Lipid lowering has proven to be highly effective in the secondary prevention of cardiac events. The bulk of this evidence applies to hydroxymethylglutaryl coenzyme A (HMG-CoA) reductase inhibitors or statin therapy.[4]

Durazzo *et al*[32] randomly assigned 100 patients to receive 20 mg atorvastatin or placebo once a day for 45 days, irrespective of their serum cholesterol concentration. Vascular surgery was performed on average 30 days after randomization, and patients were prospectively followed up over 6 months. The cardiovascular events studied were death from cardiac cause, non-fatal myocardial infarction, unstable angina, and stroke. During the 6-month follow-up, primary endpoints occurred in 17 patients: four in the atorvastatin group (incidence of 8%) and 13 in the placebo group (incidence of 26%) ($P = 0.31$). The risk for an event was compared between the groups with the Kaplan–Meier method, as event-free survival after vascular surgery. Patients given atorvastatin exhibited a significant decrease in the rate of cardiac events, compared with the placebo group, within 6 months after vascular surgery. Outcome measures included death from cardiac causes, non-fatal acute myocardial infarction, ischemic stroke, and unstable angina. Rate of event-free survival at 6 months (180 days) was 91.4% in the atorvastatin group and 73.5% in the placebo group ($P = 0.018$).

BOX 66.2 Recommendations for perioperative statin therapy

Class I
1. For patients currently taking statins and scheduled for non-cardiac surgery, statins should be continued (**Level B**).

Class IIa
1. For patients undergoing vascular surgery with or without clinical risk factors, statin use is reasonable (**Level B**).

Class IIb
1. For patients with at least one clinical risk factor who are undergoing intermediate-risk procedures, statins may be considered (**Level C**).

Short-term treatment with atorvastatin significantly reduces the incidence of major adverse cardiovascular events after vascular surgery (**Class II, Level B**).

Kapoor et al[33] carried out an exhaustive meta-analysis to determine the strength of evidence for using statins during the perioperative period to reduce the risk of cardiovascular events. There were 18 studies included: two randomized trials (n = 177), 15 cohort studies (n = 799 632), and one case–control study (n = 480) which assessed whether statins provide perioperative cardiovascular protection. Twelve studies enrolled patients undergoing non-cardiac vascular surgery, four enrolled patients undergoing coronary bypass surgery, and two enrolled patients undergoing various surgical procedures. In the randomized trials the summary odds ratio (OR) for death or acute coronary syndrome during the perioperative period with statin use was 0.26 (95% confidence interval (CI) 0.07–0.99) and the summary odds ratio in the cohort studies was 0.70 (95% CI 0.57–0.87). Results in retrospective cohort studies were larger (OR 0.65, 95% CI 0.50–0.84) than those in the prospective cohorts (OR 0.91, 95% CI 0.65–1.27), and dose, duration, and safety of statin use were not reported. The authors concluded that the evidence base for routine administration of statins to reduce perioperative cardiovascular risk was inadequate.

The evidence so far accumulated suggests a protective effect of perioperative statin use on cardiac complications during non-cardiac surgery (**Level C1**). Most of these data are observational and identify patients in whom time of initiation of statin therapy and duration of statin therapy are unclear. Furthermore, statin dose, target or achieved low-density lipoprotein levels, and indications for statin therapy are also largely unclear. Sufficiently powered randomized trials are needed to determine whether these observed associations translate into a benefit for statin therapy prescribed perioperatively for the purpose of lowering cardiac event rates surrounding non-cardiac surgery. Utilizing the perioperative period as an opportunity to impact long-term health, consideration should be given to starting statin therapy in patients who meet National Cholesterol Education Program criteria[4,33,34] (**Class I, Level B**).

Eagle et al found that patients undergoing low-risk procedures are unlikely to derive benefit from coronary artery bypass grafting (CABG) before low-risk surgery; however, patients with multivessel disease and severe angina undergoing high-risk surgery might well benefit from revascularization before non-cardiac surgery[35] (**Class II, Level C**).

Successful perioperative evaluation and management of high-risk cardiac patients undergoing non-cardiac surgery requires careful teamwork and communication between surgeon, anesthesiologist, the patient's primary caregiver, and the consultant.[4] For many patients, non-cardiac surgery represents their first opportunity to receive an appropriate assessment of both short- and long-term cardiac risk. Thus, the consultant best serves the patient by making recom-

mendations aimed at lowering the immediate perioperative cardiac risk, as well as assessing the need for subsequent postoperative risk stratification and interventions directed at modifying coronary risk factors.

It is also appropriate to recommend secondary risk reduction in the relatively large number of elective surgery patients in whom cardiovascular abnormalities are detected during preoperative evaluations. Although the occasion of surgery is often taken as a specifically high-risk time, most of the patients who have known or newly detected CAD during their preoperative evaluations will not have any events during elective non-cardiac surgery. A review of a national Medicare population sample identified a cohort of patients (n = 6895) who underwent elective vascular surgery during a 17-month period in 1991 and 1992.[23] The authors noted a relatively high mortality rate (15%) at 1 year of follow-up among patients who did not undergo preoperative stress testing. However, in those patients (19%) undergoing preoperative stress testing with or without subsequent coronary bypass surgery, the mortality rate was lower (less than 6%).[36]

It was postulated that part of this difference may have been due to effective preventive and medical treatment of patients with evident ischemic heart disease. Therefore, it is important to consider which preoperative clinical risk factors and non-invasive testing parameters can be used to help predict long-term cardiac risk.[4]

Randomized controlled trials are still needed to explore the observation that there may be some harm associated with beta-blocker therapy in low-risk patients.

Recent observational studies have shown the benefit of statins during the perioperative period. Future research should be directed at determining the value of routine prophylactic medical therapy versus more extensive diagnostic testing and interventions.

In the approach to the long-term postoperative management of non-cardiac surgery patients, one should first appreciate that the occurrence of an intraoperative non-fatal MI carries a high risk for future cardiac events, including cardiovascular death.[37] Therefore, patients who sustain an acute myocardial injury in the perioperative or postoperative period should receive careful medical evaluation for residual ischemia and overall left ventricular function (**Class I, Level B**).

The ACC/AHA guidelines for post-MI evaluation in these types of patients should be followed as soon as possible after surgical recovery. The use of pharmacologic stress or dynamic exercise for risk stratification should also be a priority in patients to help determine who would benefit from coronary revascularization. In all cases, the appropriate evaluation and management of complications and risk factors such as angina, HF, hypertension, hyperlipidemia, cigarette smoking, diabetes (hyperglycemia), and other cardiac abnormalities should commence before hos-

Table 66.5 Recommendations for use of interventions in patients undergoing non-cardiac surgery

Indication	Class I (indicated)	Class IIa	Class IIb	Class III (not indicated)
Perioperative medical therapy	Beta-blockers required in the recent past to control symptoms of angina or patients with symptomatic arrhythmias or hypertension. Beta-blockers: patients at high cardiac risk owing to the finding of ischemia on preoperative testing who are undergoing vascular surgery.	Beta-blockers: preoperative assessment identifies untreated hypertension, known coronary disease, or major risk factors for coronary disease.	Alpha$_2$-agonists: perioperative control of hypertension, or known CAD or major risk factors for CAD.	Beta-blockers: contraindication to beta-blockade. Alpha$_2$-agonists: contraindication to alpha$_2$-agonists.
Intraoperative nitroglycerin	High-risk patients previously taking nitroglycerin who have active signs of myocardial ischemia without hypotension.	As a prophylactic agent for high-risk patients to prevent myocardial ischemia and cardiac morbidity, particularly in those who have required nitrate therapy to control angina.		Patients with signs of hypovolemia or hypotension.
Intraoperative use of pulmonary artery catheters		Patients at risk for major hemodynamic disturbances that are most easily detected by a pulmonary artery catheter who are undergoing a procedure that is likely to cause these hemodynamic changes (e.g. suprarenal aortic aneurysm repair in a patient with angina) in a setting with experience in interpreting the results.	Either the patient's condition or the surgical procedure (but not both) places the patient at risk for hemodynamic disturbances (e.g., supraceliac aortic aneurysm repair in a patient with a negative stress test).	No risk of hemodynamic disturbances.
Perioperative ST segment monitoring		When available, proper use of computerized ST segment analysis in patients with known CAD or undergoing vascular surgery may provide increased sensitivity to detect myocardial ischemia during the perioperative period and may identify patients who would benefit from further postoperative and long-term interventions.	Patients with single or multiple risk factors for CAD.	Patients at low risk for CAD.

CAD, coronary artery disease. Reproduced with permission from Eagle et al.[2]

pital discharge. It is also important to communicate these new observations and determinations of cardiac status and risk to the physician who will be responsible for arranging subsequent medical care and follow-up (**Class I, Level C**).

References

1. Mangano DT. Perioperative cardiac morbidity. *Anesthesiology* 1990;**72**:153–84.
2. Eagle KA, Berger PB, Calkins H *et al.* ACC/AHA guideline update for perioperative cardiovascular evaluation for non-cardiac surgery. Executive summary: a report of the American College of Cardiology/American Heart Association Task Force on Practice Guidelines (Committee to Update the 1996 Guidelines on Perioperative Cardiovascular Evaluation for Non-cardiac Surgery). *J Am Coll Cardiol* 2002;**39**:542.
3. Fleisher LA, Beckman JA, Brown KA *et al.* ACC/AHA 2006 Guideline Update on Perioperative Cardiovascular Evaluation for Non-cardiac Surgery: Focused Update on Perioperative Beta-Blocker Therapy 2006. *Circulation* 2006;**113**:2662–74.
4. Fleisher LA, Beckman JA, Brown KA *et al.* ACC/AHA 2007 Revised Guidelines on Perioperative Cardiovascular Evaluation and Care for Non-cardiac Surgery. *Circulation* 2007;**116**:e418–e499.
5. Lee TH, Marcantonio ER, Mangione CM *et al.* Derivation and prospective validation of a simple index for prediction

of cardiac risk of major non-cardiac surgery. *Circulation* 1999;**100**:1043–9.

6. Goldman L, Caldera DL, Nussbaum SR, Southwick FS, Krogstad D, Murray B *et al.* Multifactorial index of cardiac risk in non-cardiac surgical procedures. *N Engl J Med* 1977;**297**:845–50.

7. Eagle KA, Coley CM, Newell JB, Brewster JC, Darling RC, Strauss HW *et al.* Combining clinical and thallium data optimizes preoperative assessment of cardiac risk before major vascular surgery. *Ann Intern Med* 1989;**110**(11):859–66.

8. Vanzetto G. Additive value of thallium single-photon emission computed tomography myocardial imaging for prediction of perioperative events in clinically selected high cardiac risk patients having abdominal aortic surgery. *Am J Cardiol* 1996;**77**(2):143–8.

9. Fleisher LA, Eagle KA. Clinical practice. Lowering cardiac risk in non-cardiac surgery. *N Engl J Med* 2001;**345**:1677.

10. Cohn SL, Goldman L. Preoperative risk evaluation and perioperative management of patients with coronary artery disease. *Med Clin North Am* 2003;**87**:111.

11. Furnary AP, Zerr KJ, Grunkemeier GL, Starr A. Continuous intravenous insulin infusion reduces the incidence of deep sternal wound infection in diabetic patients after cardiac surgical procedures. *Ann Thorac Surg* 1999;**67**:352–60.

12. Pomposelli JJ, Baxter JK III, Babineau TJ *et al.* Early postoperative glucose control predicts nosocomial infection rate in diabetic patients. *J Parenter Enteral Nutr* 1998;**22**:77–81.

13. Nelson AH, Fleisher LA, Rosenbaum SH. Relationship between postoperative anemia and cardiac morbidity in high-risk vascular patients in the intensive care unit. *Crit Care Med* 1993;**21**:860–6.

14. Hogue CW Jr, Goodnough LT, Monk TG. Perioperative myocardial ischemic episodes are related to hematocrit level in patients undergoing radical prostatectomy. *Transfusion* 1998;**38**:924–31.

15. Hahn RG, Nilsson A, Farahmand BY, Persson PG. Blood haemoglobin and the long-term incidence of acute myocardial infarction after transurethral resection of the prostate. *Eur Urol* 1997;**31**:199–203.

16. Backer CL, Tinker JH, Robertson DM, Vlietstra RE. Myocardial reinfarction following local anesthesia for ophthalmic surgery. *Anesth Analg* 1980;**59**:257–62.

17. Devereaux PJ, Goldman L, Cook DJ, Gilbert K, Leslie K, Guyatt GH. Perioperative cardiac events in patients undergoing non-cardiac surgery: a review of the magnitude of the problem, the pathophysiology of the events and methods to estimate and communicate risk. *CMAJ* 2005;**173**:627–34.

18. The POISE Trial Investigators, Devereaux PJ *et al.* Rationale, design, and organization of the PeriOperative ISchemic Evaluation (POISE) Trial: a randomized controlled trial of metoprolol versus placebo in patients undergoing non-cardiac surgery. *Am Heart J* 2006;**152**(2):223–30.

19. Grundy SM, Cleeman JI, Merz CN *et al.* Implications of recent clinical trials for the National Cholesterol Education Program Adult Treatment Panel III guidelines. *Circulation* 2004;**110**:227–39.

20. Torsher LC, Shub C, Rettke SR *et al.* Risk of patients with severe aortic stenosis undergoing non-cardiac surgery. *Am J Cardiol* 1998;**81**:448.

21. Mantha S, Roizen MF, Madduri J. Usefulness of routine preoperative testing: a prospective single-observer study. *J Clin Anesth* 2005;**17**(1):51–7.

22. Shaw LJ, Eagle KA, Gersh BJ *et al.* Meta-analysis of intravenous dipyridamole-thallium-201 imaging (1985 to 1994) and dobuta-mine echocardiography (1991 to 1994) for risk stratification before vascular surgery. *J Am Coll Cardiol* 1996;**27**:787.

23. Licker M, Khatchatourian G, Schweizer A *et al.* The impact of a cardioprotective protocol on the incidence of cardiac complications after aortic abdominal surgery. *Anesth Analg* 2002;**95**:1525.

24. Froehlich JB, Karavite D, Russman PL *et al.* American College of Cardiology/American Heart Association preoperative assessment guidelines reduce resource utilization before aortic surgery. *J Vasc Surg* 2002;**36**:758.

25. Lindenauer PK, Pekow P, Wang K, Mamidi DK, Gutierrez B, Benjamin EM. Perioperative beta-blocker therapy and mortality after major non-cardiac surgery. *N Engl J Med* 2005;**353**:349–61.

26. Redelmeier D, Scales D, Kopp A. Beta-blockers for elective surgery in elderly patients: population based retrospective cohort study. *BMJ* 2005;**331**:932.

27. Juul AB, Wetterslev J, Gluud C *et al.* Effect of perioperative beta-blockade in patients with diabetes undergoing major non-cardiac surgery: randomised placebo controlled, blinded multicentre trial. *BMJ* 2006;**332**:1482.

28. Poldermans D, Boersma E, Bax JJ *et al.* The effect of bisoprolol on perioperative mortality and myocardial infarction in high-risk patients undergoing vascular surgery. Dutch Echocardiographic Cardiac Risk Evaluation Applying Stress Echocardiography Study Group. *N Engl J Med* 1999;**341**:1789–94.

29. Mangano DT, Layug EL, Wallace A, Tateo I. Effect of atenolol on mortality and cardiovascular morbidity after non-cardiac surgery. *N Engl J Med* 1996;**335**:1713–20.

30. POISE Study Group; Devereaux PJ *et al.* Effects of extended-release metoprolol succinate in patients undergoing non-cardiac surgery (POISE trial): a randomised controlled trial. *Lancet* 2008;**371**:1839–47.

31. Bangalore S, Wetterslev J, Messerli FH *et al.* Perioperative β blockers in patients having non-cardiac surgery: a meta-analysis. *Lancet* 2008;**372**:1962–76.

32. Durazzo AE, Machado FS, Ikeoka DT, De Bernoche C, Monachini MC, Puech-Leao P, Caramelli B. Reduction in cardiovascular events after vascular surgery with atorvastatin: a randomized trial. *J Vasc Surg* 2004;**39**(5):967–75.

33. Kapoor AS, Kanji H, Buckingham J, Devereaux PJ, McAlister FA. Strength of evidence for perioperative use of statins to reduce cardiovascular risk: systematic review of controlled studies. *BMJ* 2006;**333**(7579):1149.

34. Executive Summary of the Third Report of the National Cholesterol Education Program (NCEP) Expert Panel on Detection, Evaluation, and Treatment of High Blood Cholesterol in Adults (Adult Treatment Panel III). *JAMA* 2001;**285**:2486–97.

35. Eagle KA, Rihal CS, Mickel MC, Holmes DR, Foster ED, Gersh BJ. Cardiac risk of non-cardiac surgery: influence of coronary disease and type of surgery in 3368 operations. CASS Investigators and University of Michigan Heart Care Program. Coronary Artery Surgery Study. *Circulation* 1997;**96**:1882–7.

36. McFalls EO, Ward HB, Santilli S, Scheftel M, Chesler E, Doliszny KM. The influence of perioperative myocardial infarction on long-term prognosis following elective vascular surgery. *Chest* 1998;**113**:681–6.

37. Mangano DT, Browner WS, Hollenberg M, Li J, Tateo IM. Long-term cardiac prognosis following non-cardiac surgery: the Study of Perioperative Ischemia Research Group. *JAMA* 1992;**268**:233–9.

67

Clinical management of diseases of the aorta

Thoralf M Sundt III
Mayo Clinic, Rochester, MN, USA

Introduction

The complexity of the diagnostic and clinical management aspects of thoracic aortic aneurysmal disease is reflected in Sir William Osler's famous aphorism "there is no disease more conducive to clinical humility than aneurysm of the aorta."[1] Shennan drew attention to a particularly lethal aortic pathology – aortic dissection – in his 1934 monograph published by the Medical Research Council.[2] It was, however, only with the advent of successful surgical therapies introduced by DeBakey and Cooley in the 1950s[3,4] that medical attention in these conditions moved from curiosity to cure.

Joyce noted in his seminal observational series of aortic aneurysmal disease in Olmsted County in 1960 that the advent of a realistic surgical option rendered an understanding of the natural history of the disease critical to assessment of the relative risks and benefits of intervention.[5] In this series of patients seen at the Mayo Clinic between 1945 and 1956 with thoracic aortic aneurysmal disease, 50% were dead within 5 years of diagnosis. Even then, he and his co-authors identified aortic diameter as a powerful predictor of rupture, the parameter which has dominated our understanding since. Indeed, it is remarkable that they focused on 6 cm as a particularly critical dimension, with less than 40% of patients presenting with aneurysms greater than 6 cm in diameter alive at 5 years. Follow-up studies from Olmsted County portrayed an even worse prognosis, with only 13% of 72 patients individuals presenting with thoracic aneurysms between 1951 and 1980 alive at 5 years.[6] This may not be surprising as over half of the patients in the latter series presented with rupture as their first indication of the disease, given the limited diagnostic modalities of the day. Perhaps as a reflection of improved radiologic techniques, the apparent natural history would appear to have improved, with more recent studies from the same institution reporting a 20% risk of rupture at 5 years for thoracic aneurysms.[7] At the same time, there was an apparent threefold increase in the incidence of thoracic aortic aneurysms. Incidentally, given our dependence on imaging modalities for detection of aortic disease, this phenomenon of interplay between diagnostic technology and apparent clinical behavior continues to impact our understanding of conditions of the aorta today.

Just as diagnostic modalities have improved over the last several decades, so have therapeutic options. Beginning with DeBakey's introduction of Dacron prosthetic grafts for aortic replacement,[8] landmark improvements have included Bentall's introduction of the technique for root replacement[9] as well as Griepp's introduction of profound hypothermia and circulatory arrest for the management of aneurysmal disease of the aortic arch.[10] Today aortic root replacement can be accomplished with a mortality rate less than 5% in experienced hands[11] and arch replacement with similar risk under elective circumstances.[12,13] Using appropriate adjuncts, the risks have also dropped dramatically in recent years for elective repair of descending thoracic[14] and thoracoabdominal aortic aneurysms[15,16] in centers of excellence. Most recently, endovascular technologies have been introduced for repair of descending thoracic aortic aneurysms, again challenging us to find the balance between risks of the intervention and the natural history of the disease. Equally the advent of valve-sparing aortic root repair has altered the risk/benefit analysis and threshold for recommending prophylactic aortic surgery.[17]

Nomenclature and definitions

By far the majority of aortic conditions presenting in adults requiring surgical intervention are aneurysmal in nature. While coarctation and even interrupted aortic arch may present in adults, these are uncommon and are perhaps most fruitfully discussed in the context of adult congenital heart disease. The majority of aneurysms are "degenerative" in nature, in contrast to traumatic pseudoaneurysms

Evidence-Based Cardiology, 3rd edition. Edited by S. Yusuf, J.A. Cairns, A.J. Camm, E.L. Fallen, and B.J. Gersh. © 2010 Blackwell Publishing, ISBN: 978-1-4051-5925-8.

and chronic dissections. By definition, the wall of a pseudoaneurysm lacks all three layers of the normal aortic wall – intima, media and adventitia – and accordingly chronic dissections fall into this classification as well, although they are seldom referred to as such. Postsurgical anastomotic pseudoaneurysms may also occur, although they are remarkably uncommon.[18]

The term "degenerative" is applied to aneurysms associated with a wide variety of conditions ranging from mundane to exotic. Chronic hypertension, particularly when combined with tobacco abuse, accounts for the majority of aneurysms of the ascending aorta, with connective tissue diseases of defined or undefined type accounting for a smaller but significant fraction.[19] Giant cell arteritis is increasingly recognized as a cause of aneurysmal disease, particularly among women.[20] Finally, ascending aortic aneurysms associated with bicuspid aortic valve disease are also generally considered "degenerative" and account for a considerable fraction of ascending aneurysms coming to surgery today.

The distinction between aortic ectasia and true aneurysmal dilation is subject to some degree of interpretation. Nomograms depicting normal aortic dimensions versus body surface area may be useful,[21] particularly in pediatric populations; however, there is no bright line between enlargement and aneurysm. Furthermore, changes in body mass, which may occur with age, can certainly influence these assessments in the adult. Perhaps a more practical definition of aneurysm as suggested by Crawford is enlargement to greater than twice the diameter of the adjacent normal aorta.[22]

Full characterization of aortic disease must also include a description of the location and extent of the aneurysm itself. This should ideally include distinction between dilation of the ascending aorta and of the root. Either or both may be enlarged. Accordingly, in our institution, we have adopted a classification scheme as depicted in Figure 67.1. Unfortunately this distinction is not always made in the literature. Accordingly there is sometimes confusion over what best to do with a patient having enlargement of the sinuses but not the ascending aorta (Fig. 67.2) when guidelines refer to the ascending aorta specifically. Safi has proposed a classification scheme for aneurysms of the descending thoracic aorta as well (Fig. 67.3), and has demonstrated its correlation with operative risk.[15] Thoracoabdominal aneurysms in turn are conventionally classified according to Crawford's schema as shown in Figure 67.4.[23]

The location and extent of aortic dissection are critical in clinical decision making as well. Acute aortic dissection represents a mechanical failure of the aortic wall with the propagation of a plane of dissection within a weakened media creating a "double-barrel" aorta with a channel of flow into a true and false lumen. Uncommonly, the latter may thrombose completely; more often the false lumen remains at least partially patent and is actually larger than the true lumen. In some instances the false channel may

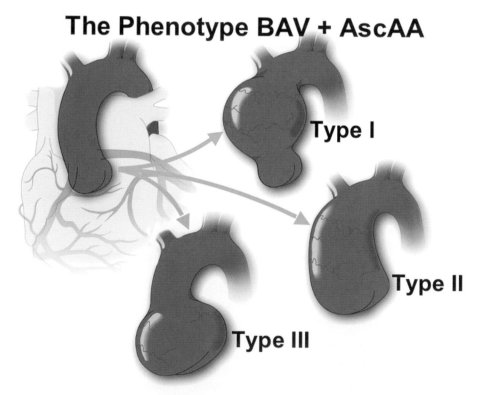

The Phenotype BAV + AscAA

Type I

Type II

Type III

Figure 67.1 Although it is widely recognized that bicuspid aortic valve is associated with ascending aortic aneurysm, in point of fact, there are at least three phenotypes which should be distinguished. The most common is a supracoronary aneurysm confined to the ascending aorta. We refer to this as a Type I aneurysm. The Type II aneurysm demonstrates effacement of the sinotubular junction with generalized enlargement of the ascending aorta and root. This pathology more commonly demands complete root replacement surgically. Type I in contrast can be managed with a separate valve and graft. The least common is Type III with aneurysmal dilatation of the root reminiscent of Marfan syndrome. The ascending aorta can, in fact, be of entirely normal diameter with quite significant enlargement of the sinuses.

compress the true lumen, causing a pseudo-coarctation, or in the extreme may cut off blood flow to end-organs, causing a malperfusion syndrome. Originally classified

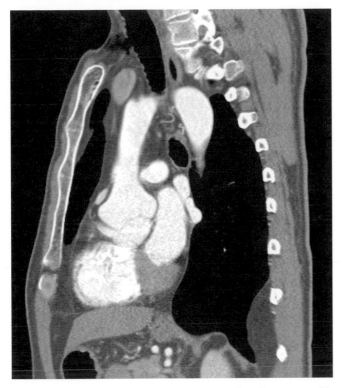

Figure 67.2 This sagittal CT scan demonstrates a Type III aneurysm with significant enlargement of the sinuses of Valsalva but a relatively normal ascending aorta.

by DeBakey into three types (Fig. 67.6),[4] a simpler if somewhat less informative system proposed by Shumway's group (Fig. 67.6)[24] has become more popular, particularly among non-surgeons. In the latter system, those dissections involving the ascending aorta, including both DeBakey type I and II, are classified as "Stanford type A" which is easily remembered ("A" for "ascending") and is of practical value as the immediate clinical management is the same. Those not involving the ascending aorta (DeBakey type III) are by elimination "Stanford type B."

Aortic dissections are also the principal causes of "acute aortic syndromes," a term coined by Vilacosta and Roman in reference to clinical presentation of a variety of aortic pathologies intended to draw attention to these entities in contrast with the much more common causes of chest pain – "acute coronary syndromes."[25] Unfortunately, the former continues frequently to be mistaken for the latter even in today's age of advanced imaging modalities.[26] Given the opposing aims of therapies for each – anticoagulation versus surgical intervention – this misdiagnosis can have tragic consequences.

Other causes of acute aortic syndrome include symptomatic thoracic aortic aneurysm (a relatively uncommon condition) and the so-called "variant forms" of acute dissection – intramural hematoma (IMH) and penetrating atherosclerotic ulcer (PAU). By definition, the term intramural hematoma refers to the presence of hematoma within the wall of the aorta without apparent intimal disruption as described in 1920 by Krukenberg.[27] This definition was created at a time when the diagnosis of intramural hematoma was made at autopsy or, somewhat more recently, at

Figure 67.3 Safi has defined three types of descending thoracic aortic aneurysms with, from right to left, Type A aneurysms involving the upper descending thoracic aorta alone, Type B aneurysms involving the lower descending thoracic aorta and, Type C aneurysms involving the entire descending thoracic aorta. The risks associated with surgical intervention are correspondingly associated with the extent of the disease.

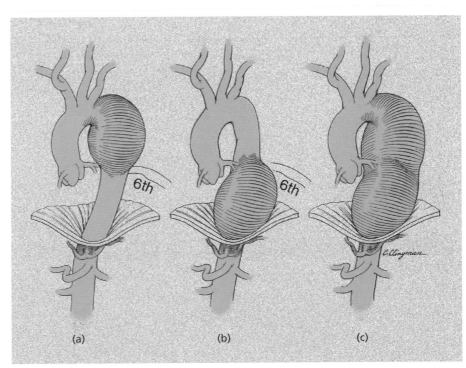

(a) (b) (c)

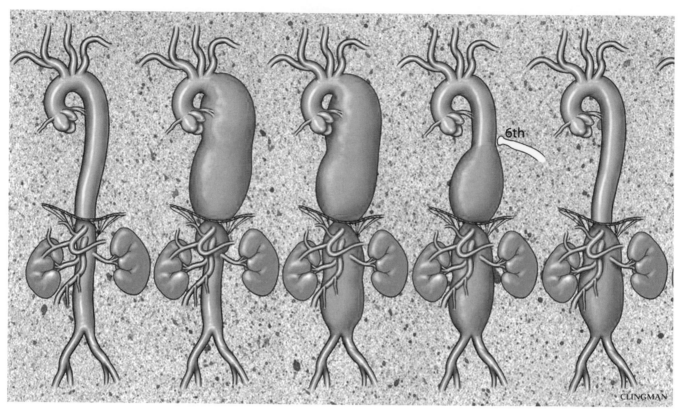

CLINGMAN

Figure 67.4 The Crawford classification of thoracoabdominal aneurysmal disease includes Type I aneurysm with involvement of the entire descending thoracic aorta and upper abdominal aorta including the origins of the visceral vessels, a Type II aneurysm involving the descending thoracic aorta and entire abdominal aorta, Type III – an aneurysm involving the lower descending thoracic aorta and abdominal component and Type IV – perivisceral abdominal aortic aneurysm involving the origins of the visceral vessels but sparing the majority of the descending thoracic aorta.

open surgical intervention. In the current era, the diagnosis of these conditions is most often made radiologically and accordingly a distinction between IMH and so-called "non-communicating dissection" with complete thrombosis of the false lumen can be difficult. Indeed, one could argue that such a distinction is impossible, as it relies upon the demonstration of absence of a disruption. Lack of active flow communication is more straightforward, of course, and from a practical standpoint may be more important as IMH and non-communicating aortic dissection with thrombosis of the false lumen likely behave very much alike.

Penetrating atherosclerotic ulcer as a distinct entity was most clearly defined by Stanson and colleagues in 1986.[28] Penetrating atherosclerotic ulcers represent intimal disruptions with extension into the medial layer. They most often occur in the heavily atherosclerotic descending thoracic aorta with a propensity to arise in the distal descending thoracic aorta. Typically they are surrounded by at least some element of IMH (although if one is adherent to Krukenberg's definition above one would question the use of this term). Penetrating atherosclerotic ulcers are most often discussed in the context of acute aortic syndromes, although a significant percentage are identified as incidental findings during radiologic studies for other reasons.[29] The principal radiologic challenge is differentiating this entity from heavy intraluminal thrombus with surface irregularities.

A variety of congenital conditions can also cause aneurysms of the aorta. Among these the most common is dilation of the origin of an aberrant subclavian artery (Fig. 67.7). Most often this is an aberrant right subclavian artery in the presence of a left aortic arch although the converse may occur as well. The origins of such vessels are often somewhat dilated and again as noted above, the distinction between a diverticulum of Kommeral and true aneurysm is somewhat subjective. The indication for intervention is as often dysphagia lusoria from compression of the esophagus as it is the actual dimensions of the structure.

Incidence

As noted above, both the estimated incidence and apparent natural history of thoracic aortic aneurysmal disease depend to an extraordinary degree on imaging technology, in terms of both technical resolution and clinical application, since most aneurysmal disease is asymptomatic until disaster strikes. Still, in most modern studies the incidence of thoracic aortic aneurysms is estimated at

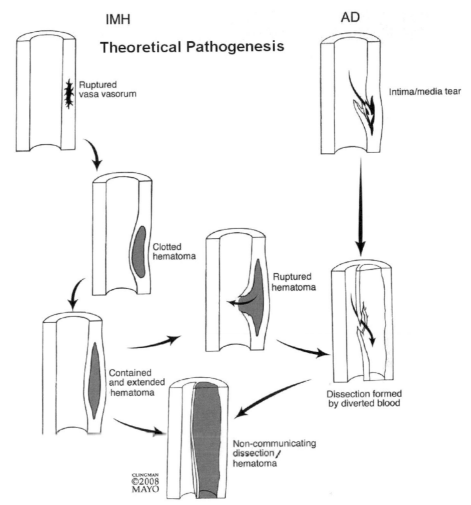

Figure 67.5 The pathogenesis of aortic dissection is thought to originate with an intimal tear which allows blood entry into the media with propagation of the dissection distally. In some instances, the false channel will thrombose resulting in a "noncommunicating dissection." It is currently held that intramural hematoma begins with rupture of the vasorum progressing to a clotted hematoma. In some instances, that hematoma may rupture into the lumen allowing dissection to form.

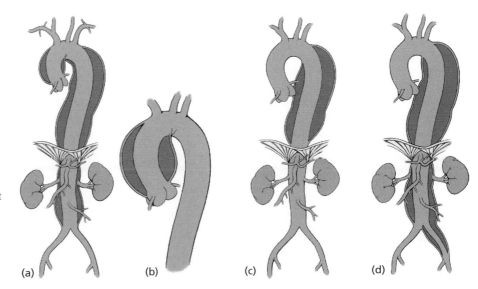

Figure 67.6 The classification of aortic dissection may be either the DeBakey or Stanford classification. From left to right, the most common is the DeBakey Type I or Stanford Type A dissection involving the entire aorta. DeBakey Type II dissection involves the ascending aorta alone. Because it involves the ascending aorta, it is also classified as a Stanford Type A. The DeBakey Type III dissection involves the descending thoracic (III-A) or thoracoabdominal (III-B) aorta and may also be termed a Stanford Type B dissection.

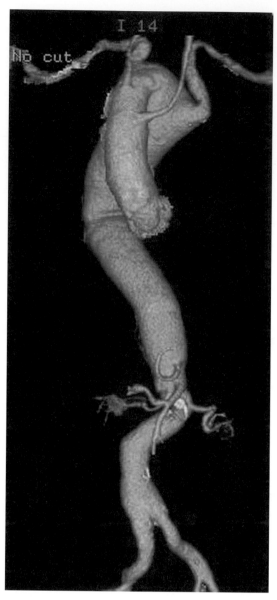

Figure 67.7 Aberrant origin of the left subclavian artery from a right aortic arch with a diverticulum of Kommeral.

between 8 and 12 per 100,000 person-years. In the Olmsted County study mentioned above, Clouse and colleagues estimated the incidence of thoracic aneurysms in that population to be 10.4/100,000 person-years.[7] Perhaps the most comprehensive study of thoracic aortic aneurysmal disease to date was reported by Olsson in 2006, with unique tracking of the population of Sweden over a 16-year period.[30] This study encompasses a population of 8.7 million. Thoracic aortic aneurysms greater than 5 cm in diameter, true dissections and intramural hematomas were tracked. The incidence appeared to gradually rise over the time of the study with approximately 16.3 males/100,000 person-years and 9.1 females/100,000 person-years diagnosed in 2002. As the apparent incidence rose, prognosis

improved with an increasing frequency of surgical procedures performed and a declining operative mortality.

With regard to acute aortic syndromes and aortic dissection, in another Olmsted County study, Clouse and colleagues estimated the incidence of aortic dissection at 2.9 per 100,000 persons per year.[31] Meszaros has estimated the incidence in a Western European study to be 3.5 per 100,000 persons per year.[32] Two-thirds of these dissections involve the ascending aorta.[33] Intramural hematomas are generally thought to represent approximately 5–10% of acute aortic syndromes[34] whereas PAU are far less common. The latter two conditions tend to occur in patients of somewhat more advanced age.

Natural history and prognosis

The natural history of thoracic aortic aneurysmal disease is progressive. The most commonly cited predictor of behavior as identified by Joyce in all subsequent studies is aortic diameter, with risk rising particularly beyond 6 cm.[5,35] In the study by Clouse et al, the rupture risk for aneurysms less than 4 cm in diameter was negligible, while that for aneurysms between 4 and 5.9 cm was 16% and that for aneurysms 6 cm or larger was 31%.[7] Other factors enter play as well, although less well recognized perhaps. Clouse identified female gender and advanced age as risk factors for rupture.[7] Juvonen and Griepp performed a sophisticated analysis of risk factors for rupture of thoracoabdominal aneurysms,[36] confirming these risk factors as well as chronic obstructive pulmonary disease. Not surprisingly, hypertension has been identified as a risk factor as well.[37]

The most comprehensive analysis of the impact of diameter on rupture risk has been performed at Yale University through the efforts of Elefteriades and Rizzo using their thoracic aortic aneurysm database. A number of important publications have derived from this work. Coady identified a hinge point for rupture of the ascending aorta at 6 cm while that for descending thoracic aorta was 7.2 cm.[38] As intervention at this dimension would be at the expense of a significant number of ruptures, most surgeons have adopted 5.5 cm for the ascending aorta and 6.5 cm for the descending thoracic aorta as criteria for intervention (**Class I, Level C**). Subsequent work has demonstrated that the annual risk of aortic catastrophe, taking rupture, dissection or death as the composite endpoint, rises to 15.6% for aneurysms greater than 6 cm in diameter as shown in Figure 67.8.[37] The correlation is even stronger when the diameter is indexed as body surface area: an indexed dimension of 2.75 cm/m^2 is associated with a risk of 4% per year while that greater than 4.25 cm/m^2 is associated with a risk of approximately 20% per year.[39] Unfortunately, the weakness of these data is that they are derived from a surgical database, and therefore may be somewhat biased toward malignant behavior as in any such database the cases entered

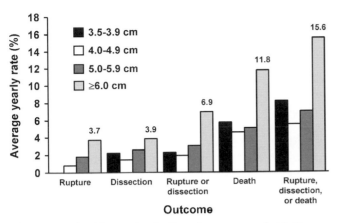

Figure 67.8 The risks associated with aortic aneurysms of various diameter as determined by Davies *et al.* from the Yale University Thoracic Aortic Database.

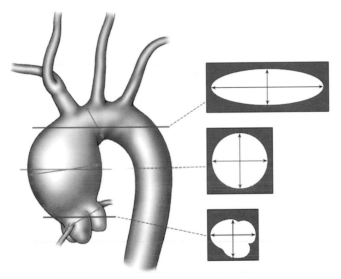

Figure 67.9 The true diameter of the aorta at any given level as derived by 2-D axial imaging will be the smallest diameter as measured on the image at that level. Oblique images will yield an oval, of which the smallest diameter is most accurate assuming a cylindrical structure. Three-D reconstructions permit more accurate assessments measuring the diameter normal to the axis of blood flow.

represent those referred for consideration, in contrast to population-based studies.

Implicit in these guidelines is the accurate measurement of aortic dimensions. Whether by echocardiography or computed tomography, the dimensions measured depend upon the selection of the optimal image with maximal dimensions while appropriately placing the measurement cursor normal to the long axis of the vessel. As shown in Figure 67.9, oblique images will provide deceptively large measures if one is not cautious. Surgeons therefore speak of using the smallest measured diameter on the image with the largest dimensions. On the other hand, asymmetric or saccular aneurysms should be measured in the longer dimension. In our view, the advent of three-dimensional

reconstructions of aortic images has proven very beneficial. It should also be noted that the sinuses of Valsalva are always somewhat larger than the ascending aorta and the majority of studies reporting ascending aortic dimensions do not distinguish whether they were evaluating the ascending aorta or root. In all likelihood, the majority are referable to the ascending aorta. Still, we apply these dimensions even when the dilation is largely in the root. In particular in the setting of Marfan syndrome and some familial thoracic aortic aneurysms, the ascending aorta itself may be remarkably normal in dimension with almost all the dilation in the sinuses themselves. Therefore, one may be just as readily lulled into a false sense of security with a falsely low aortic dimension if only those dimensions in the ascending aorta are considered.

It is likely that the risk of rupture can be reduced through the administration of antihypertensive medications (**Class IIa, Level B**). Among patients with Marfan syndrome, studies by Schor and colleagues[40] and Rossi-Foulkes and co-workers[41] have demonstrated the protective effect of beta-blockers or calcium antagonists respectively on aortic dilation and, in the former case, aortic complications. Yetman and associates have also utilized the angiotensin-converting enzyme enalapril in patients with Marfan syndrome demonstrating improved aortic distensibility, reduced aortic stiffness, and a smaller increase in aortic diameter.[42] Exciting data from the Dietz laboratory at Johns Hopkins have also suggested that use of the angiotensin receptor blocker losartan may have a favorable impact on aortic remodeling as well.[43]

Although the details of the pathophysiologic basis of aortic aneurysmal disease are largely beyond the scope of this chapter, they may have an impact on clinical behavior. This is most obvious in the case of Marfan syndrome in which it is widely accepted that the risks of dissection and rupture are, size for size, greater than for aneurysms of other etiology.[44] The association between mutations in the fibrillin gene and Marfan syndrome has been known for many years now.[45] The pathogenesis was assumed to relate to the critical role of fibrillin in the extracellular matrix as the main component of the 10–20nm microfibrils which associate with elastin in the media. Such mutations have been shown to increase susceptibility to proteolysis and, as a consequence, microfibril and elastin fragmentation. In the last several years, however, intriguing results from the Dietz laboratory have suggested a role for dysregulation of transforming growth factor beta (TGF-β) signaling in Marfan syndrome.[46] Amino acid sequence homology identified in silico between fibrillin-1 and latent TGB-β proteins (LTBPs) suggested that alterations in fibrillin might impact TGB-β levels in the tissues due to decreased binding. Indeed, laboratory studies have shown that alterations in TGB-β signaling may lead to alterations in extracellular matrix homeostasis in the lung as well as the aorta. Subsequent studies have demonstrated an important role for TGB-β in other related aortopathies including mutations in the TGB-β receptor type I and II genes in the "Marfan syndrome II" phenotype and other familial thoracic aortic aneurysm syndromes.[47–49] A particularly malignant form of such a familial syndrome is the recently defined Loeys–Dietz syndrome which may be secondary to mutations in TGF BRI or TGF BRII.[50] Individuals so affected are particularly susceptible to widespread aneurysmal dilation early in life. The clinical significance of such findings is the potential for genetic testing, permitting prophylactic operative repair of the susceptible aortas of family members who may well be susceptible to dissection at lower aortic diameters.

The association between bicuspid aortic valve and ascending aortic dilation has long been recognized.[51] There is mounting evidence that the aortopathy is primary, and not secondary to altered flow dynamics, as it may be present even with a functionally normal valve.[52] Structural abnormalities including gross degenerative histologic abnormalities commonly referred to as "cystic medial necrosis,"[53] thinning of elastic lamellae,[54] smooth muscle cell apoptosis[55] and increased matrix metalloproteinases[56] have been observed in the associated aneurysmal aorta. While there is agreement that the risk of dissection is higher among patients with a bicuspid valve,[57] the relationship between dissection and aortic diameter is less so, with no studies thus far documenting a higher risk of aortic complications at a given dimension than other aortic dilations. Accordingly, while the presence of documented Marfan syndrome or another familial syndrome can be cogently argued as a rationale for predicting a worse outcome and therefore more aggressive approach to management, the same cannot as clearly be said for bicuspid disease. Having said this, a small study by Svensson and colleagues substantiates the notion that patients with bicuspid disease may dissect at dimensions less than 5 cm.[58] Recent data from the IRAD database demonstrate that this may be true even in patients with trileaflet valves,[59] although such studies look only at the numerator and accordingly cannot address actual risk for the population as a whole. Since a very large number of patients have an aortic diameter less than 5.0 or 5.5 cm, the occurrence of dissections among these individuals may take place at a very low incidence – potentially far less than the risk of aortic replacement surgery. The argument for treating patients with bicuspid disease differently with a specifically lower threshold for replacement is therefore weakened. Nonetheless, it is well documented that the ascending aorta may continue to dilate even after aortic valve replacement in the setting of bicuspid disease.[60,61] Accordingly, a number of investigators have advocated prophylactic replacement of the ascending aorta at the time of bicuspid valve repair or replacement should it exceed 4.5–5 cm (**Class IIb, Level C**). These criteria are generally accepted.

Diagnosis

The diagnostic modalities employed in evaluation of aortic disease are similar regardless of the etiology of the condition. By far the most commonly employed technology is computed tomography. This is in part due to its widespread availability. Image acquisition is also less operator dependent although interpretation still requires special expertise. Indeed, the majority of thoracic aortic aneurysms are asymptomatic and are identified at the time of CT scanning for other reasons. CT scanning is also the most common first modality employed in the diagnosis of thoracic aortic dissection.[33] Frequently such a study is performed for the purpose of ruling out pulmonary embolism in the patient with acute-onset chest pain without ECG changes or enzymatic evidence of myocardial infarction. It should be noted that since aortic aneurysmal disease is commonly multifocal,[22,62] complete imaging of the entire thoracic and abdominal aorta should be performed in all patients with a diagnosis of thoracic aortic aneurysm.

Echocardiography is also commonly employed in the evaluation of patients with thoracic aortic disease. Indeed, many ascending aortic aneurysms are discovered incidentally during echocardiography for suspected valvular conditions. This highlights the importance of imaging of the ascending aorta, arch to the extent possible, and descending thoracic aorta as a standard part of routine transthoracic and transesophageal echocardiography. Transesophageal echocardiography is the second most common modality used in the diagnosis of acute dissection and is particularly helpful in that context for evaluating the function of the aortic valve in that setting.[33]

Magnetic resonance imaging is less commonly performed as the initial diagnosis test.[63] It has a greater role perhaps in serial follow-up of patients with aneurysmal disease as it does not subject the patient to radiation. In the case of a young individual, the amount of radiation delivered by annual or biannual CT scanning for follow-up of thoracic aortic aneurysm can be quite considerable. In many cases, MRI is selected as the technique of choice for serial exams. Most surgeons find these images cumbersome, however, and prefer CT scanning.

Management

Management of thoracic aortic aneurysmal disease is dependent upon the location within the aorta, the etiology of the aneurysm and the acuity of its presentation. The thoracic aorta is itself a more complex structure than might be presumed. Far from being a simple tube, it has significant elastin content that serves a "Windkessel function" of storing energy in systole and returning it in diastole.[64] This improves coronary artery blood flow proximally, and likely helps to distribute forces within the vascular tree more effectively. Elastin content varies along the length of the aorta, with the highest content proximally. Given very different forces[65] and mechanical properties,[66] it should come as no surprise that the behavior of pathologic entities such as classic aneurysm, IMH or acute dissection varies according to location. The etiologic basis of the aneurysmal condition may also play a role in determining the optimal management. This is particularly true for individuals with genetic causes of aneurysmal disease including Marfan syndrome, familial thoracic aortic aneurysm, and bicuspid aortic valve in whom the mechanical properties of the aorta itself appear altered.[67] While our understanding of these conditions is still in its adolescence, if not infancy, in general a more aggressive posture is adopted towards those aneurysms and dissections associated with an underlying genetic cause.[68] Finally, the acuity of presentation is an important determinant of the management strategy and will be reflected below by our separation of the management strategies according to this parameter.

Acute aortic syndrome

As noted above, the term acute aortic syndrome was coined in reference to conditions presenting acutely with chest pain secondary to the abnormalities of the thoracic aorta.[25] Accordingly, it includes aortic dissection and its related conditions, IMH and PAU. Broadly speaking, it may also include post-traumatic pseudoaneurysms to the extent that these are acute aortic events. Finally, it may be argued that an acutely symptomatic thoracic aortic aneurysm without dissection should be considered under this heading.

Essentially all causes of acute aortic syndromes are treated acutely with anti-impulse therapy while the diagnosis is made in the interest of reducing hydrodynamic stress.[69] This is accomplished first with beta-blockade to reduce dP/dt.[70] Other vasodilating agents are then added as needed to reduce systolic blood pressure (**Class I, Level C**).

The root, ascending aorta and arch

Acute aortic syndromes involving the ascending aorta are managed surgically in almost all instances. (**Class I, Level C**). The case is most clearly and unequivocally made for acute dissection, an entity for which the non-operative management carries a mortality rate of 50% or more,[33,71] even in the current era. The mortality rate associated with surgical repair varies among series roughly from 10% to 25%,[72–74] depending upon the age and hemodynamic state of the patients preoperatively[75,76] and, likely, the experience of the surgical team.

Early reports of IMH involving the ascending aorta indicated a high mortality rate with non-operative management, leading to recommendations that all such lesions be treated surgically.[77,78] This view was supported by the majority of subsequent studies,[79,80] including a multicenter European study[81] and recent meta-analysis.[82] In recent years, there has been an alternative view of the management of intramural hematoma of the ascending aorta expressed by some Asian authors. Several institutions have reported satisfactory results with an expectant approach to type A IMH.[83–87] Importantly, however, this approach as practiced by these authors involved hospitalization of patients for up to 1 week in the intensive care unit and 1 month in hospital with assiduous blood pressure control, frequent imaging, and a willingness to convert emergently to surgical therapy if the IMH progressed. Among those reported by Kaji's group, for example, 43% had surgery during their hospitalization and 60% eventually progressed,[87] as did 50% of those treated in Moizumi's series.[88] A significant number of late IMH-related deaths occurred in the latter series as well. There may be a cost in terms of operative risk as well, with this approach of necessity bringing patients to surgery under urgent or emergent circumstances rather than semi-electively. In Song's series the operative mortality rate was fully 20%,[89] much higher than that reported by others in the 5% range.[84,90]

Predictors of successful non-operative management include younger age, diameter less than 50 mm and thickness less than 11–12 mm.[87,88,91] The presence of a PAU is seen by most as a predictor of bad outcome, and there seems to be no disagreement that "type A" PAU should be treated operatively.[80]

The principal surgical approach for management of an acutely symptomatic aneurysm or dissection involving the ascending aorta is graft replacement of the affected segment. This is most often accomplished with a Dacron graft, essentially the same as that introduced by DeBakey almost a half-century ago.[8] Aortoplasty procedures for degenerative aneurysms in which a portion of the wall is excised and repaired primarily[92–95] have largely fallen by the wayside due to the risk of recurrent dilation.

Repair of aneurysms of the proximal aorta may be accomplished with or without root replacement/repair (Fig. 67.10). If only the ascending aorta is involved and the valve and sinuses are spared, tube graft replacement of the ascending aorta may be performed. If the valve is dysfunctional but the sinuses of Valsalva are spared, a separate valve replacement and supracoronary graft may be appropriate. Alternatively, if the sinuses of Valsalva are diseased, as may be the case in the setting of acute dissection or in cases of aneurysmal disease secondary to underlying genetic abnormalities such as Marfan syndrome, complete root replacement is appropriate. This may be accomplished with a mechanical valved conduit which is purchased directly from the manufacturer with the valve prosthesis, with the Dacron graft integral to the mechanical prosthesis. For older patients in whom one would likely

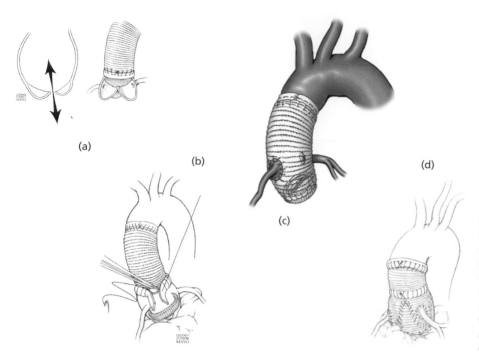

(a)

(b)

(c)

(d)

Figure 67.10 Surgical options for the ascending aorta and root in the presence of valvular disease include: (a) tube-graft replacement of the ascending aorta with correction of the sinotubular junction to correct aortic regurgitation secondary to displacement of he commissures, (b) separate valve-and-graft repair of the supra-coronary aorta, (c) Composite root replacement, and (d) valve-sparing root repair.

select a biologic prosthesis under elective conditions, a biologic root replacement can be accomplished either by using a free-standing biologic root prosthesis such as a human allograft or stentless Porcine xenograft, or simply by fashioning a "home-made" biologic composite by sewing a Dacron graft to a stented tissue valve. The operative risk associated with root replacement has been reported to be less than 5% in experienced hands, although data from the Society of Thoracic Surgeons database suggest that in the practice of cardiac surgery at large, adding root replacement to aortic valve replacement increases operative risk almost threefold.[96]

Finally, for individuals whose valve leaflets are relatively normal and in whom the disease is confined to the aortic wall itself, several valve-sparing root repair procedures have been developed. By far the most popular today is the valve reimplantation technique of David.[17] In this procedure, the aortic wall including aortic sinuses are debrided, leaving the valve itself intact. The Dacron graft is lowered over the root and the valve leaflets resuspended within the Dacron graft itself such that the sinuses have been replaced in their entirety. Coronary arteries are reimplanted into this Dacron graft as they are in the composite and root grafts noted above. There is some uncertainty regarding the longterm durability of this final option as it has been employed for only slightly over a decade. Early results are promising, however, and it is being embraced with increasing enthusiasm by the surgical community.

The extent of distal replacement is dependent upon the extent of disease. In the case of a symptomatic aneurysm confined to the ascending aorta or a DeBakey type II dis-

section or intramural hematoma, replacement of the ascending aorta alone may be all that is required. Very commonly, these procedures are performed under profound hypothermia with circulatory arrest to permit extirpation of the entire ascending aorta right to the orifice of the brachiocephalic trunk. Although data demonstrating an impact of using circulatory arrest for conduct of an "open distal anastomosis" on late outcomes are mixed,[97–99] it has been widely adopted (**Class IIa, Level C**). In the setting of acute dissection, particularly DeBakey type I dissections which extend through the arch, there is greater debate over the extent of repair required. It is commonly stated that the resection must "encompass the distal tear." Unfortunately, from a practical standpoint, there are often multiple tears throughout the arch. Many authors will simply primarily repair the tear and perform hemiarch replacement (Fig. 67.11) in order to avoid total arch replacement.[100]

Total arch replacement is a major technical undertaking, as it demands a thoughtful approach to neurologic protection while the brachiocephalic vessels are being reconstructed. In the setting of acute dissection, authors from Japan have reported outstanding results with mortality rates less than 10%.[101,102] Western authors have been reluctant to advocate the same in the setting of acute dissection despite improving results for arch replacement in elective procedures.[12] This may in part be due to studies published thus far which fail to demonstrate an impact of the more aggressive distal repair on reoperation rate.[103,104] Accordingly, surgeons in the United States have tended to be rather conservative, performing the hemiarch replacement predominantly.

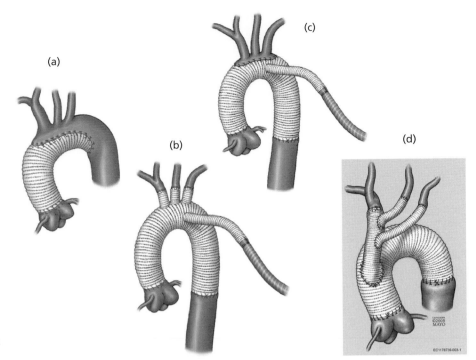

Figure 67.11 Surgical options for the aortic arch include: (a) hemi-arch replacement, (b) total arch replacement with branch-graft reconstruction of the brachiocephalic vessels, (c) total arch replacement with reimplantation of the brachiocephalic vessels as an island, (d) total arch replacement with double-Y graft reconstruction of the brachiocephalic vessels.

Descending thoracic and thoracoabdominal aorta

Those acute aortic syndromes due to pathology involving the descending thoracic aorta are, in general, treated non-operatively (**Class IIa, Level C**). In the classic study by Glower and Miller comparing surgical and medical management of acute (and chronic) type B dissection, early and late survival were equivalent regardless of treatment strategy.[105] As the trend shifted toward medical management unless complications such as continued pain or expansion, rupture or malperfusion due to branch vessel occlusion occurred, more recent studies have demonstrated a higher mortality rate among surgically treated patients. In the large multicenter IRAD database, the in-hospital mortality rate for acute type B dissection was approximately 10% as compared with approximately 30% for the surgical patients.[33,106] While a 10% mortality rate is not low, this number includes both complicated and uncomplicated dissections. If one considers only uncomplicated type B dissections, the mortality rate is in the low single digits.[107] These data of course beg the question of the place of endovascular stent grafting for uncomplicated dissection.

The variant forms IMH and PAU are generally treated non-operatively as well (**Class IIa, Level C**). Malperfusion is uncommon with these entities,[108] drawing an equivalency with uncomplicated dissection in the view of many. A number of studies have documented better behavior of IMH as compared with acute dissection.[34,79,81,87,109] It must be noted, however, that some authors have argued that the plane of dissection in IMH is closer to the adventitia than that for dissection, and they therefore argue for a more aggressive approach.[90,110] Still, the majority view is that type B IMH may be treated pharmacologiacally, a view supported by a comprehensive meta-analysis performed by Maraj and colleagues.[82] Although acute behavior in general is superior with intramural hematoma, this is not to trivialize the risk as IMH may progress rapidly to acute dissection or rupture.[109] Elefteriades has emphasized the importance of careful follow-up.[79]

In the setting of malperfusion manifest as stroke or paraplegia, gastrointestinal ischemia, renal impairment or limb ischemia, intervention is indicated (**Class IIa, Level C**). Unilateral limb ischemia may be addressed by an extra-anatomic bypass such as a femoral–femoral bypass. More complex malperfusion syndromes are better addressed with fenestration, either open[111] or percutaneous,[112,113] or with endovascular stent grafting.[114] Insertion of a covered stent graft proximally with or without distal implantation of uncovered stents has been shown to restore flow in the true lumen, redirecting blood flow and restoring visceral perfusion. While no stent grafts are currently FDA approved in the United States for this application, this is likely the most common indication for stent grafting in the setting of acute dissection in the United States and the world today.

Traumatic transsection

Finally, a special word should be said about the current management of acute aortic transsections with pseudoaneurysm as a cause of acute aortic syndrome. Traumatic transsections occur as a consequence of acute deceleration injury and are typically located adjacent to the ligamentum arteriosum. A variety of mechanisms have been proposed but it is clear that this region of the aorta is subjected to particular stress as it transitions from a relatively fixed mediastinal arch to a more mobile intrathoracic descending thoracic aorta. The aorta is also tethered at this location by the ligamentum arteriosum and this may in turn exert particular traction forces at this location, accounting for the typical location of these pseudoaneurysms on the underside of the arch.

Traditional teaching has been to treat all aortic transsections surgically at the time of diagnosis (**Class IIa, Level C**). This is often complicated by concomitant injuries which have been suffered by these multi-trauma patients. A school of thought has therefore arisen concerning delayed treatment of such pseudoaneurysms with aggressive anti-impulse therapy in the interim.[115] The results of this approach have been reported by only a few groups but seem to be satisfactory. Indeed, if one looks at the original studies of aortic transsection upon which the philosophy of immediate surgical repair is based, the landmark study by Parmely and associates was an autopsy study performed at the Armed Forces Institute of Pathology.[116] Not surprisingly, the majority of these patients died. In point of fact, what this study demonstrates more than anything is the time course of death among patients with transsection who do in fact succumb. It does not address in any way the patients who experience partial transsection who survive. A more recent multicenter study reported by Fabian and associates reinforces this view with significant mortality and morbidity associated with transsection.[117] The majority of patients succumbing, however, do so in the first 36 hours, suggesting that individuals who come to medical attention with this condition beyond this point have "survived the trial of life" and perhaps might be treated non-operatively. The advent of stent grafting provides yet another approach.[114,118–120] The principal limitation here relates to the dimensions of the aorta as many of the individuals suffering traumatic transsection are young and have relatively small aortas for which currently available stent grafts are too large. Nonetheless, this is an appealing application of stent graft technology and likely an area that will grow in importance over time.

Subacute disease

Because of the highly lethal nature of acute aortic syndromes, those presenting subacutely are most often treated similarly to the acute conditions. An exception may be the subacute type A intramural hematoma as noted above. On the basis of the results reported from the Far East, it is likely that patients presenting subacutely who have the aortic characteristics associated with successful non-operative management may be treated with anti-impulse therapy alone (**Class IIb, Level C**). Specifically, those with maximum aortic dimension less than 50 mm and intramural hematoma measuring less than 1 cm in thickness without evidence of intimal disruption to suggest penetrating ulcer or non-communicating dissection may be candidates for aggressive antihypertensive therapy.

Chronic disease

Regarding thoracic aortic aneurysmal disease in the chronic setting, both those due to degenerative disease and those secondary to chronic dissection are discussed together.

Aneurysms of the root, ascending aorta and arch

Aneurysmal dilation of the ascending aorta and arch commonly co-exist and accordingly present a similar challenge from a management standpoint. In general, their appropriate treatment algorithm is dictated primarily by the dimensions of the aorta itself. The majority of natural history studies have demonstrated a profound impact of aortic dimension on risk of rupture, dissection or death as discussed above. The risk of complications secondary to thoracic aortic aneurysm is dictated predominantly by the Law of LaPlace. While tension is related both to the aortic diameter and to internal pressure, the critical dimension for the ascending aorta in numerous series centers about 6 cm. This is as true in the 1963 study by Joyce[5] as it has been in subsequent studies by Perko and colleagues[35] as well as those by Elefteriades, Rizzo and associates at the Yale University Thoracic Aortic Aneurysm Database.[37,38] Recent biomechanical data also from Yale University demonstrate a dramatic increase in wall stress and drop in aortic extensibility as the thoracic aorta reaches 6 cm.[121] This finding is consonant with an observed 27-fold increase in aortic complications when the diameter exceeds 6 cm as reported by these same investigators from their clinical database.

These findings have lead to a general consensus among surgeons that intervention on the ascending aorta is indicated at 5.5 cm in maximum diameter[37](**Class IIa, Level C**). The threshold may be lower for young patients in whom the risk of surgical repair is less and at the same time the risk of lifetime complications related to the aneurysm is greater. In addition, patients with Marfan syndrome or familial thoracic aortic aneurysmal disease, particularly those with a history of dissection, may be treated at even earlier dimensions[68] (**Class IIb, Level C**). There is a current trend to intervene in the setting of Marfan syndrome, even at 4.5 cm. The advent of valve-sparing root operations as described above has promoted this more aggressive approach as the complications associated with implantation of an artificial valve are not imposed upon subjects with such a repair. This is despite thin evidence regarding the long-term durability of this option.[17] Some have argued for indexed criteria, with the predicted risk of rupture being low at less than $2.75\,cm/m^2$ (approximately 4% per year), intermediate at $2.75–4.24\,cm/m^2$ (approximately 8% per year), and high above $4.25\,cm/m^2$ (approximately 20% per year).[39]

Proximal aneurysms due to dissection may be found incidentally after an undiagnosed acute event or after initial successful replacement of the ascending segment with enlargement of the retained root or arch. In the latter setting, similar criteria for intervention are generally applied as for degenerative aneurysms, although there are some data to support the notion that the risk of rupture in the setting of chronic dissection is greater dimension for dimension.[122] Given that such aneurysms are, in fact, pseudoaneurysms, this is perhaps intuitive. When an otherwise unrecognized and untreated type A dissection is identified, however, it is widely accepted that semi-elective repair should be undertaken (**Class IIa, Level C**).

From a technical standpoint, the operative interventions employed for repair of degenerative aneurysms or chronic dissections of the ascending aorta and root are similar to those noted above in an acute setting. These include tube-graft replacement of the ascending aorta, root replacement, and separate valve and graft. In particular, it should be noted that patients with Marfan syndrome or other known connective tissue disorders should undergo a more radical procedure with complete root replacement preferred over leaving the sinuses of Valsalva behind (**Class I, Level C**). This is generally accepted practice for Marfan syndrome and some would argue should be applied for young patients presenting with dissection in whom a suspicion for a familial thoracic aortic aneurysmal disease may be high.

Approaches to the arch in the setting of chronic disease are also dictated by aortic dimensions. If the aortic arch is a normal dimension, the decision is relatively straightforward. Of note, studies of patients with Marfan syndrome have demonstrated a relatively low risk of arch complications and it is the standard of care to replace only the ascending aorta and root at the time of elective root surgery in Marfan syndrome.[123,124] There is no apparent benefit to prophylactic arch replacement in this setting. More commonly, one is faced with moderate aortic arch enlargement in the patient with bicuspid aortic valve disease. The enlargement of the ascending aorta may extend into the proximal aorta with no discrete neck to the aneurysm or transition to a normal dimension (see Fig. 67.11). In this setting, there are no hard and fast rules. There are no data to substantiate a particularly aggressive approach in this setting. Arch dissection and type B dissection are relatively uncommon in patients with bicuspid aortic valve. It is therefore our practice to only perform hemiarch replacement in the setting of bicuspid disease in the presence of arch enlargement exceeding 5 cm.

The contemporary results of elective aortic arch replacement are far superior to those reported only a decade ago.

Technical improvements have included the introduction of adjuncts for neuron protection such as retrograde cerebral perfusion[125,126] whereby the upper body venous system is perfused with cold blood with the intent of providing oxygenated blood to the tissues akin to retrograde cardioplegia. While some surgical groups use this method regularly and report gratifying results,[100,127] others have questioned the real value of this approach[128,129] and have abandoned it in favor of selective antegrade brachiocephalic perfusion.[12,13,130] There has also been a trend in favor of axillary artery cannnulation for arterial inflow,[131,132] a method that provides for flow away from the cerebral vasculature, potentially protecting patients from embolic phenomena. In combination, these techniques, along with branched-graft reconstruction of the brachiocephalic vessels, may be applied with mortality rates for arch replacement below 5% and similar if not lower stroke rates.[13]

When the distal extent of disease includes the descending thoracic or thoracoabdominal aorta, as it may in the setting of chronic dissection or generalized arteriomegaly, arch replacement may be performed using the "elephant-trunk" technique (Fig. 67.12) via median sternotomy, leaving a segment of graft dangling in the descending thoracic aorta for use in subsequent distal repairs.[133–135] This technique obviates the technical difficulties of obtaining proximal control of the aorta in a previously operated field as the surgeon need only open the aneurysmal distal aorta and clamp the dangling graft. In cases in which both the ascending aorta and descending thoracic aorta must be approached at the same procedure, the transverse thoracosternotomy incision which was popular at the inception of cardiac surgery has been reintroduced, providing access to the entire thoracic aorta.[136] Via this incision, the root, ascending aorta, arch and entire descending thoracic aorta may be replaced in a single procedure.

Descending thoracic and thoracoabdominal aorta

Perhaps as a result of lower hemodynamic stresses, the critical diameter at which rupture risk rises for aneurysms of the descending thoracic aorta is estimated to be somewhat higher. The data from the Yale University database indicate an inflection point for a descending thoracic aortic aneurysmal disease at 7.2 cm.[110] Accordingly, there is general agreement that intervention on the descending thoracic aorta should be undertaken at 6.5 cm (**Class I, Level C**). A lower threshold may be appropriate in patients with chronic dissection in whom the risk of rupture or redissection may be higher, as noted above.[122] Additionally, enlargement at a rate exceeding 0.5 cm over 6 months is commonly held as an indication of an actively remodeling aorta, and one for which surgical intervention is indicated. The risks of rupture also increase with advanced age, the presence of chronic obstructive pulmonary disease, and continued

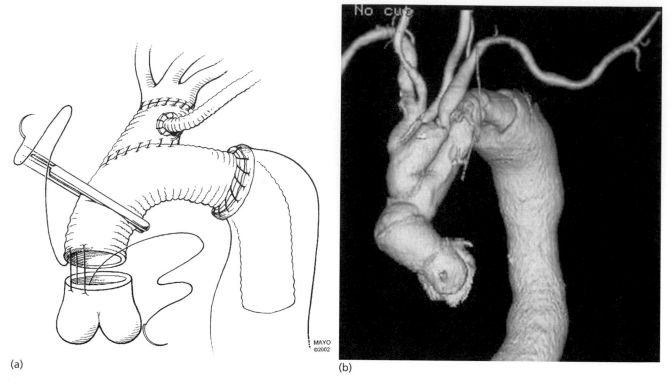

(a)

(b)

MAYO
©2002

Figure 67.12 An "elephant trunk" repair leaves a segment or "trunk" of graft dangling in the descending thoracic aorta to facilitate subsequent repair of the descending thoracic aorta by providing an easily accessible site for proximal anastomosis of the second graft. (a) schematic drawing, (b) postoperative CT scan.

tobacco abuse.[36] Unfortunately, these characteristics also increase the operative risk of open repair.

Non-operative management of patients with descending thoracic and thoracoabdominal aortic aneurysms, like those with ascending aortic aneurysms, should include beta-blockade (**Class I, Level B**). This has been demonstrated to be of value particularly in the setting of intramural hematoma of the descending thoracic aorta in preventing progressive dilation.[81]

In the case of IMH, in the chronic phase, aortic remodeling may progress over time to aneurysm in as many as 30–40%.[77,78,81] Conversely complete resolution of the hematoma has been observed in as many as half of patients within 6 months.[86,137] Predictors of progression include presence of a penetrating ulcer[138] while predictors of resolution include younger age,[137,138] diameter less than 4–4.5 cm[34,137,139] and hematoma thickness less than 1 cm.[34,139] It is important to note that Sueyoshi and colleagues suggested a biphasic modality in the behavior of patients with intramural hematoma including shrinkage in the first year but slow growth thereafter.[139] This emphasizes the importance of long-term monitoring. As compared with type B dissection, survival is superior for IMH at 1 year (100% v 83%), 2 years, (97% v 79%), and 5 years (97% v 79%).[138]

The traditional operative approach is Dacron graft replacement of the involved aortic segment (Fig. 67.13).

With open surgical repair, there is no question that the risks of mortality, as well as morbidity, increase with the extent of resection. The most common morbidity after thoracoabdominal aortic repair is pulmonary failure, followed by renal dysfunction.[140] By far the most dreaded, however, is paraplegia. The blood supply to the anterior spinal cord is highly segmental, with only a single anterior spinal artery in contrast to the paired posterior supply. Further complicating matters, the anterior spinal artery is of highly variable diameter and in some cases may be discontinuous. It is commonly held that the supply to the lower cord is critically dependent upon the arterius radicularis magnus or artery of Adamkiewicz which arises typically between the eighth thoracic and second lumbar vertebra.

As a consequence, repair of aneurysms isolated to the descending thoracic aorta are associated with lower risks of paraplegia than those of thoracoabdominal extent. Safi has classified descending thoracic aneurysms into three type as shown in Figure 67.3. In his series, the incidence of neurologic deficit was 2.3%, with all occurring among patients undergoing replacement of the entire thoracic segment.[14] Similarly, it is well documented that the operative risk as well as risk of neurologic deficit for repair of thoracoabdominal aortic aneurysms correlates with the extent of repair.[16] The risk of repair of thoracoabdominal

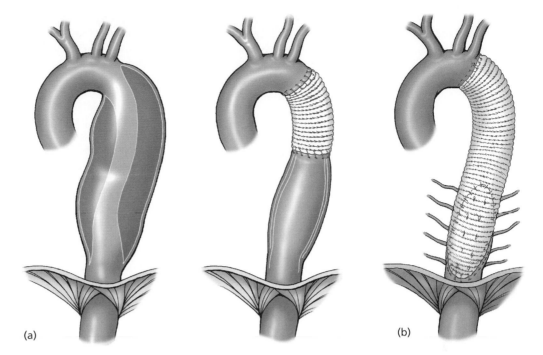

Figure 67.13 Repair of the descending thoracic aorta for chronic dissection may be accomplished with a short segment graft or long-segment with beveled distal anastomosis to preserve intercostal vessels and blood supply to the spinal cord.

(a)

(b)

aortic aneurysm has also been correlated with the experience of the operative surgeon, as well as that of the operative team (hospital).[141] Indeed, the operative risk is half that when a surgeon performs seven such procedures per year as compared with those performing only one per year. Similarly, the risk for procedures performed in hospitals with an annual volume of 12 cases is half that for hospitals performing only one such case per year.[142]

The unsettling incidence of neurologic deficit has stimulated the development of several approaches to intraoperative neurologic protection. The most popular is the provision of distal perfusion during the aortic cross-clamp episode by partial left heart bypass associated with moderate hypothermia.[143] The alternative approach is the use of full cardiopulmonary bypass with profound hypothermia and circulatory arrest.[144] Both methods are imperfect, and the morbidity of the surgical incision itself is significant.

Because of the above risks, the option of endovascular stent grafting has been embraced by physicians and patients alike. For descending thoracic aneurysms, the risks associated with stent grafting appear to be quite low, with mortality rates less than 5% and paraplegia rates of similar magnitude.[142] Of note, the risk of stroke is approximately 5% as well, likely due to atheroembolic material liberated by manipulation of wires in the highly atherosclerotic aortic arch. Stent graft technology as applied to thoracoabdominal aneurysms is complicated by the visceral as well as intercostal vessels. Fenestrated and branched grafts are currently being explored, although none is currently FDA approved for use in the United States.[145,146] Experience is

growing with debranching procedures as well as with extra-anatomic bypass grafts to the visceral vessels. Morbidity associated with these procedures, however, appears to be quite significant.

Conclusion

Thoracic aortic aneurysmal disease is a highly lethal condition if left untreated, and yet it is eminently correctable with appropriate surgical intervention. The results of the latter have improved dramatically in recent years, making early diagnosis and prophylactic treatment even more important. As the maximum diameter of the ascending aorta approaches 6 cm, the risk of rupture or dissection rises dramatically. Accordingly, intervention on the proximal aorta (root or ascending aorta) is indicated at 5.5 cm. In some cases in which the risk of rupture may be judged to be particularly high (Marfan syndrome, family history of dissection) or in which the risk of surgery is particularly low (younger patients), this threshold may be lowered somewhat. The recent advent of aortic valve-sparing procedures has lowered this threshold for Marfan syndrome patients in particular, and in this case some would advocate surgery at 4.5 cm. Likely because of differences in hemodynamic stresses, the risk of rupture of the descending thoracic aorta is lower, with the critical value being closer to 7.0 cm and recommended criteria for intervention at 6.5 cm. Acute aortic syndromes are often misdiagnosed as acute coronary syndromes, with the most important safety measure being a high index of suspicion. When acute dissection, intramural hematoma or penetrating aortic ulcer affects the ascending aorta ("type A"), immediate surgical intervention is indicated. When the descending aorta is involved, however, non-operative management is generally accepted unless complications occur such as malperfusion, rapid aortic expansion or continued pain. Medical therapy is beta-blockade and assiduous control of blood pressure. In complicated dissection, however, surgical repair may be required.

More recently, experience is growing in the endovascular treatment of these conditions, with either percutaneous fenestration for treatment of malperfusion or, more recently, endovascular stent graft placement for malperfusion or rupture. By far the best treatment, however, is prophylactic repair.

References

1. Bean RB. Sir William Osler: aphorisms from his bedside teachings and writings. Vol. **138**. Springfield, IL: Charles C. Thomas, 1961.

2. Shennan T. Dissecting aneurysms. Medical Research Council, Special Report Series, 1934;193.

3. Cooley DA, DeBakey ME. Resection of the thoracic aorta with replacement by homograft for aneurysms and constrictive lesions. *J Thorac Surg* 1955;**29**(1):66–100;discussion 100–4.

4. DeBakey ME, Henly WS, Cooley DA *et al.* Surgical management of dissecting aneurysms of the aorta. *J Thorac Cardiovasc Surg* 1965;**49**:130–49.

5. Joyce JW, Fairbairn JF 2nd, Kincaid OW, Juergen JL. Aneurysms of the thoracic aorta. A clinical study with special reference to prognosis. *Circulation* 1964;**29**:176–81.

6. Bickerstaff LK, Pairolero PC, Hollier LH *et al.* Thoracic aortic aneurysms: a population-based study. *Surgery (St. Louis)* 1982;**92**:1103–9.

7. Clouse WD, Hallett JW Jr, Schaff HV *et al.* Improved prognosis of thoracic aortic aneurysms: a population-based study. *Jama* 1998;**280**(22):1926–9.

8. Debakey ME, Jordan GL Jr, Abbott JP *et al.* The fate of Dacron vascular grafts. *Arch Surg* 1964;**89**:757–82.

9. Bentall H, De Bono A. A technique for complete replacement of the ascending aorta. *Thorax* 1968;**23**(4):338–9.

10. Griepp RB, Stinson EB, Hollingsworth JF, Buehler D. Prosthetic replacement of the aortic arch. *J Thorac Cardiovasc Surg* 1975;**70**(6):1051–63.

11. Zehr KJ, Orszulak TA, Mullany CJ *et al.* Surgery for aneurysms of the aortic root: a 30-year experience. *Circulation* 2004;**110**(11):1364–71.

12. Spielvogel D, Etz CD, Silovitz D *et al.* Aortic arch replacement with a trifurcated graft. *Ann Thorac Surg* 2007;**83**(2):S791–5;discussion S824–31.

13. Sasaki H, Ogino H, Matsuda H *et al.* Integrated total arch replacement using selective cerebral perfusion: a 6-year experience. *Ann Thorac Surg* 2007;**83**(2):S805–10;discussion S824–31.

14. Estrera AL, Miller CC 3rd, Chen EP *et al.* Descending thoracic aortic aneurysm repair: 12-year experience using distal aortic perfusion and cerebrospinal fluid drainage. *Ann Thorac Surg* 2005;**80**(4):1290–6;discussion 1296.

15. Safi HJ, Miller CC 3rd, Huynh TT *et al.* Distal aortic perfusion and cerebrospinal fluid drainage for thoracoabdominal and descending thoracic aortic repair: ten years of organ protection. *Ann Surg* 2003;**238**(3):372–80;discussion 380–1.

16. LeMaire SA, Miller CC 3rd, Conklin LD *et al.* Estimating group mortality and paraplegia rates after thoracoabdominal aortic aneurysm repair. *Ann Thorac Surg* 2003;**75**(2):508–13.

17. David TE, Feindel CM, Webb GD *et al.* Long-term results of aortic valve-sparing operations for aortic root aneurysm. *J Thorac Cardiovasc Surg* 2006;**132**(2):347–54.

18. Strauch JT, Spielvogel D, Lansman SL *et al.* Long-term integrity of teflon felt-supported suture lines in aortic surgery. *Ann Thorac Surg* 2005;**79**(3):796–800.

19. Homme JL, Aubry MC, Edwards WD *et al.* Surgical pathology of the ascending aorta: a clinicopathologic study of 513 cases. *Am J Surg Pathol* 2006;**30**(9):1159–68.

20. Zehr KJ, Mathur A, Orszulak TA *et al.* Surgical treatment of ascending aortic aneurysms in patients with giant cell aortitis. *Ann Thorac Surg* 2005;**79**(5):1512–17.

21. Roman MJ, Devereux RB, Kramer-Fox R, O'Loughlin J. Two-dimensional echocardiographic aortic root dimensions in normal children and adults. *Am J Cardiol* 1989;**64**(8):507–12.

22. Crawford ES, Cohen ES. Aortic aneurysm: a multifocal disease. Presidential address. *Arch Surg* 1982;**117**(11):1393–400.

23. Svensson LG, Crawford ES. Cardiovascular and Vascular Diseases of the Aorta. Philadelphia: Saunders, 1997.

24. Daily PO, Trueblood HW, Stinson EB *et al.* Management of acute aortic dissections. *Ann Thorac Surg* 1970;**10**(3):237–47.

25. Vilacosta I, Roman JA. Acute aortic syndrome. *Heart* 2001;**85**(4):365–8.

26. Hansen MS, Nogareda GJ, Hutchison SJ. Frequency of and inappropriate treatment of misdiagnosis of acute aortic dissection. *Am J Cardiol* 2007;**99**(6):852–6.

27. Krukenberg E. Beitrage zur Frage des Aneurysma dissecans. *Beitr Pathol Anat Allg Pathol* 1920;**67**:329–51.

28. Stanson AW, Kazmier FJ, Hollier LH *et al.* Penetrating atherosclerotic ulcers of the thoracic aorta: natural history and clinicopathologic correlations. *Ann Vasc Surg* 1986;**1**(1):15–23.

29. Cho KR, Stanson AW, Potter DD *et al.* Penetrating atherosclerotic ulcer of the descending thoracic aorta and arch. *J Thorac Cardiovasc Surg* 2004;**127**(5):1393–9;discussion 1399–401.

30. Olsson C, Thelin S, Stahle E *et al.* Thoracic aortic aneurysm and dissection: increasing prevalence and improved outcomes reported in a nationwide population-based study of more than 14,000 cases from 1987 to 2002. *Circulation* 2006;**114**(24):2611–18.

31. Clouse WD, Hallett JW Jr, Schaff HV *et al.* Acute aortic dissection: population-based incidence compared with degenerative aortic aneurysm rupture. *Mayo Clin Proc* 2004;**79**(2):176–80.

32. Meszaros I, Morocz J, Szlavi J *et al.* Epidemiology and clinicopathology of aortic dissection. *Chest* 2000;**117**(5):1271–8.

33. Hagan PG, Nienaber CA, Isselbacher EM *et al.* The International Registry of Acute Aortic Dissection (IRAD): new insights into an old disease. *JAMA* 2000;**283**(7):897–903.

34. Evangelista A, Mukherjee D, Mehta RH *et al.* Acute intramural hematoma of the aorta. A mystery in evolution. *Circulation* 2005;**111**:1063–70.

35. Perko MJ, Norgaard M, Herzog TM *et al.* Unoperated aortic aneurysm: a survey of 170 patients. *Ann Thorac Surg* 1995;**59**(5):1204–9.

36. Juvonen T, Ergin MA, Galla JD *et al.* Prospective study of the natural history of thoracic aortic aneurysms. *Ann Thorac Surg* 1997;**63**(6):1533–45.

37. Davies RR, Goldstein LJ, Coady MA *et al.* Yearly rupture or dissection rates for thoracic aortic aneurysms: simple prediction based on size. *Ann Thorac Surg* 2002;**73**(1):17–27;discussion 27–8.

38. Coady MA, Rizzo JA, Hammond GL *et al.* What is the appropriate size criterion for resection of thoracic aortic aneurysms? *J Thorac Cardiovasc Surg* 1997;**113**(3):476–91;discussion 489–91.

39. Davies RR, Gallo A, Coady MA *et al.* Novel measurement of relative aortic size predicts rupture of thoracic aortic aneurysms. *Ann Thorac Surg* 2006;**81**(1):169–77.

40. Schor JS, Yerlioglu ME, Galla JD *et al.* Selective management of acute type B aortic dissection: long-term follow-up. *Ann Thorac Surg* 1996;**61**(5):1339–41.

41. Rossi-Foulkes R, Roman MJ, Rosen SE *et al.* Phenotypic features and impact of beta blocker or calcium antagonist therapy on aortic lumen size in the Marfan syndrome. *Am J Cardiol* 1999;**83**(9):1364–8.

42. Yetman AT, Bornemeier RA, McCrindle BW. Usefulness of enalapril versus propranolol or atenolol for prevention of aortic dilation in patients with the Marfan syndrome. *Am J Cardiol* 2005;**95**(9):1125–7.

43. Habashi JP, Judge DP, Holm TM *et al.* Losartan, an AT1 antagonist, prevents aortic aneurysm in a mouse model of Marfan syndrome. *Science* 2006;**312**(5770):117–21.

44. Kim SY, Martin N, Hsia EC *et al.* Management of aortic disease in Marfan syndrome: a decision analysis. *Arch Intern Med* 2005;**165**(7):749–55.

45. Dietz HC, Cutting GR, Pyeritz RE *et al.* Marfan syndrome caused by a recurrent de novo missense mutation in the fibrillin gene. *Nature* 1991;**352**(6333):337–9.

46. Neptune ER, Frischmeyer PA, Arking DE *et al.* Dysregulation of TGF-beta activation contributes to pathogenesis in Marfan syndrome. *Nat Genet* 2003;**33**(3):407–11.

47. Hasham SN, Willing MC, Guo DC *et al.* Mapping a locus for familial thoracic aortic aneurysms and dissections (TAAD2) to 3p24–25. *Circulation* 2003;**107**(25):3184–90.

48. Pannu H, Fadulu VT, Chang J *et al.* Mutations in transforming growth factor-beta receptor type II cause familial thoracic aortic aneurysms and dissections. *Circulation* 2005;**112**(4):513–20.

49. Loeys BL, Schwarze U, Holm T *et al.* Aneurysm syndromes caused by mutations in the TGF-beta receptor. *N Engl J Med* 2006;**355**(8):788–98.

50. Loeys BL, Chen J, Neptune ER *et al.* A syndrome of altered cardiovascular, craniofacial, neurocognitive and skeletal development caused by mutations in TGFBR1 or TGFBR2. *Nat Genet* 2005;**37**(3):275–81.

51. McKusick VA. Association of congenital bicuspid aortic valve and erdheim's cystic medial necrosis. *Lancet* 1972;**1**(7758):1026–7.

52. Hahn RT, Roman MJ, Mogtader AH, Devereux RB. Association of aortic dilation with regurgitant, stenotic and functionally normal bicuspid aortic valves. *J Am Coll Cardiol* 1992;**19**(2):283–8.

53. de Sa M, Moshkovitz Y, Butany J, David TE. Histologic abnormalities of the ascending aorta and pulmonary trunk in patients with bicuspid aortic valve disease: clinical relevance to the ross procedure. *J Thorac Cardiovasc Surg* 1999;**118**(4):588–94.

54. Bauer M, Pasic M, Meyer R *et al.* Morphometric analysis of aortic media in patients with bicuspid and tricuspid aortic valve. *Ann Thorac Surg* 2002;**74**(1):58–62.

55. Nataatmadja M, West M, West J *et al.* Abnormal extracellular matrix protein transport associated with increased apoptosis of vascular smooth muscle cells in marfan syndrome and bicuspid aortic valve thoracic aortic aneurysm. *Circulation* 2003;**108**(suppl 1):II329–34.

56. Koullias GJ, Korkolis DP, Ravichandran P *et al.* Tissue microarray detection of matrix metalloproteinases, in diseased tricuspid and bicuspid aortic valves with or without pathology of the ascending aorta. *Eur J Cardiothorac Surg* 2004;**26**(6):1098–103.

57. Edwards WD, Leaf DS, Edwards JE. Dissecting aortic aneurysm associated with congenital bicuspid aortic valve. *Circulation* 1978;**57**:1022–5.

58. Svensson LG, Kim KH, Lytle BW, Cosgrove DM. Relationship of aortic cross-sectional area to height ratio and the risk of aortic dissection in patients with bicuspid aortic valves. *J Thorac Cardiovasc Surg* 2003;**126**(3):892–3.

59. Pape LA, Tsai TT, Isselbacher EM *et al.* Aortic diameter > or = 5.5 cm is not a good predictor of type A aortic dissection: observations from the International Registry of Acute Aortic Dissection (IRAD). *Circulation* 2007;**116**(10):1120–7.

60. Yasuda H, Nakatani S, Stugaard M *et al.* Failure to prevent progressive dilation of ascending aorta by aortic valve replacement in patients with bicuspid aortic valve: comparison with tricuspid aortic valve. *Circulation* 2003;**108**(suppl 1):II291–4.

61. Borger MA, Preston M, Ivanov J *et al.* Should the ascending aorta be replaced more frequently in patients with bicuspid aortic valve disease? *J Thorac Cardiovasc Surg* 2004;**128**(5):677–83.

62. Albornoz G, Coady MA, Roberts M *et al.* Familial thoracic aortic aneurysms and dissections – incidence, modes of inheritance, and phenotypic patterns. *Ann Thorac Surg* 2006;**82**(4):1400–5.

63. Macura KJ, Szarf G, Fishman EK, Bluemke DA. Role of computed tomography and magnetic resonance imaging in assessment of acute aortic syndromes. *Semin Ultrasound CT MR* 2003;**24**(4):232–54.

64. Belz GG. Elastic properties and Windkessel function of the human aorta. *Cardiovasc Drugs Ther* 1995;**9**(1):73–83.

65. Beller CJ, Labrosse MR, Thubrikar MJ, Robicsek F. Finite element modeling of the thoracic aorta: including aortic root motion to evaluate the risk of aortic dissection. *J Med Eng Technol* 2008;**32**(2):167–70.

66. Sokolis DP. Passive mechanical properties and structure of the aorta: segmental analysis. *Acta Physiol (Oxf)* 2007;**190**(4):277–89.

67. Okamoto RJ, Xu H, Kouchoukos NT *et al.* The influence of mechanical properties on wall stress and distensibility of the dilated ascending aorta. *J Thorac Cardiovasc Surg* 2003;**126**(3):842–50.

68. Milewicz DM, Dietz HC, Miller DC. Treatment of aortic disease in patients with Marfan syndrome. *Circulation* 2005;**111**(11):e150–7.

69. Prokop EK, Palmer RF, Wheat MW Jr. Hydrodynamic forces in dissecting aneurysms. In-vitro studies in a Tygon model and in dog aortas. *Circ Res* 1970;**27**(1):121–7.

70. McFarland J, Willerson JT, Dinsmore RE *et al.* The medical treatment of dissecting aortic aneurysms. *N Engl J Med* 1972;**286**(3):115–19.

71. Masuda Y, Yamada Z, Morooka N *et al.* Prognosis of patients with medically treated aortic dissections. *Circulation* 1991;**84**(suppl 5):III7–III13.

72. Ehrlich MP, Ergin MA, McCullough JN *et al.* Results of immediate surgical treatment of all acute type A dissections. *Circulation* 2000;**102**(19 suppl 3):III248–52.

73. Hata M, Shiono M, Inoue T *et al.* Preoperative cardiopulmonary resuscitation is the only predictor for operative mortality of type A acute aortic dissection: a recent 8-year experience. *Ann Thorac Cardiovasc Surg* 2004;**10**(2):101–5.

74. Trimarchi S, Nienaber CA, Rampoldi V *et al.* Contemporary results of surgery in acute type A aortic dissection: the International Registry of Acute Aortic Dissection experience. *J Thorac Cardiovasc Surg* 2005;**129**(1):112–22.

75. Rampoldi V, Trimarchi S, Eagle KA *et al.* Simple risk models to predict surgical mortality in acute type A aortic dissection: the International Registry of Acute Aortic Dissection score. *Ann Thorac Surg* 2007;**83**(1):55–61.

76. Long SM, Tribble CG, Raymond DP *et al.* Preoperative shock determines outcome for acute type A aortic dissection. *Ann Thorac Surg* 2003;**75**(2):520–4.

77. Robbins RC, McManus RP, Mitchell RS *et al.* Management of patients with intramural hematoma of the thoracic aorta. *Circulation.* 1993;**88**(suppl II):II1–II10.

78. Nienaber CA, von Kodolitsch Y, Petersen B *et al.* Intramural hemorrhage of the thoracic aorta. Diagnostic and therapeutic implications. *Circulation* 1995;**92**(6):1465–72.

79. Tittle SL, Lynch RJ, Cole PE *et al.* Midterm follow-up of penetrating ulcer and intramural hematoma of the aorta. *J Thorac Cardiovasc Surg* 2002;**123**(6):1051–9.

80. Ganaha F, Miller DC, Sugimoto K *et al.* Prognosis of aortic intramural hematoma with and without penetrating atherosclerotic ulcer: a clinical and radiological analysis. *Circulation* 2002;**106**(3):342–8.

81. von Kodolitsch Y, Csosz SK, Koschyk DH *et al.* Intramural hematoma of the aorta: predictors of progression to dissection and rupture. *Circulation* 2003;**107**(8):1158–63.

82. Maraj R, Rerkpattanapipat P, Jacobs LE *et al.* Meta-analysis of 143 reported cases of aortic intramural hematoma. *Am J Cardiol* 2000;**86**(6):664–8.

83. Sueyoshi E, Matsuoka Y, Sakamoto I *et al.* Fate of intramural hematoma of the aorta: CT evaluation. *J Comput Assist Tomogr* 1997;**21**(6):931–8.

84. Moriyama Y, Yotsumoto G, Kuriwaki K *et al.* Intramural hematoma of the thoracic aorta. *Eur J Cardiothorac Surg* 1998;**13**(3):230–9.

85. Shimizu H, Yoshino H, Udagawa H *et al.* Prognosis of aortic intramural hemorrhage compared with classic aortic dissection. *Am J Cardiol* 2000;**85**(6):792–5.

86. Song JK, Kim HS, Song JM *et al.* Outcomes of medically treated patients with aortic intramural hematoma. *Am J Med* 2002;**113**(3):181–7.

87. Kaji S, Akasaka T, Horibata Y *et al.* Long-term prognosis of patients with type a aortic intramural hematoma. *Circulation* 2002;**106**(12 suppl 1):I248–52.

88. Moizumi Y, Komatsu T, Motoyoshi N, Tabayashi K. Management of patients with intramural hematoma involving the ascending aorta. *J Thorac Cardiovasc Surg* 2002;**124**(5):918–24.

89. Song JK, Kang SJ, Song JM *et al.* Factors associated with in-hospital mortality in patients with acute aortic syndrome involving the ascending aorta. *Int J Cardiol* 2007;**115**(1):14–18.

90. Uchida K, Imoto K, Takahashi M *et al.* Pathologic characteristics and surgical indications of superacute type A intramural hematoma. *Ann Thorac Surg* 2005;**79**(5):1518–21.

91. Song JM, Kim HS, Song JK *et al.* Usefulness of the initial noninvasive imaging study to predict the adverse outcomes in the medical treatment of acute type A aortic intramural hematoma. *Circulation* 2003;**108**(suppl 1):II324–8.

92. Robicsek F, Cook JW, Reames MK Sr, Skipper ER. Size reduction ascending aortoplasty: is it dead or alive? *J Thorac Cardiovasc Surg* 2004;**128**(4):562–70.

93. Sievers HH. Reflections on reduction ascending aortoplasty's liveliness. *J Thorac Cardiovasc Surg* 2004;**128**(4):499–501.

94. Kuralay E, Demirkilic U, Ozal E *et al.* Surgical approach to ascending aorta in bicuspid aortic valve. *J Card Surg* 2003;**18**(2):173–80.

95. Bauer M, Pasic M, Schaffarzyk R *et al.* Reduction aortoplasty for dilatation of the ascending aorta in patients with bicuspid aortic valve. *Ann Thorac Surg* 2002;**73**(3):720–3;discussion 724.

96. Rankin JS, Hammill BG, Ferguson TB Jr *et al.* Determinants of operative mortality in valvular heart surgery. *J Thorac Cardiovasc Surg* 2006;**131**(3):547–57.

97. Zierer A, Moon MR, Melby SJ *et al.* Impact of perfusion strategy on neurologic recovery in acute type A aortic dissection. *Ann Thorac Surg* 2007;**83**(6):2122–8;discussion 2128–9.

98. Lai DT, Robbins RC, Mitchell RS *et al.* Does profound hypothermic circulatory arrest improve survival in patients with acute type a aortic dissection? *Circulation* 2002;**106**(12 suppl 1):I218–28.

99. Sabik JF, Lytle BW, Blackstone EH *et al.* Long-term effectiveness of operations for ascending aortic dissections. *J Thorac Cardiovasc Surg* 2000;**119**(5):946–62.

100. Bavaria JE, Brinster DR, Gorman RC *et al.* Advances in the treatment of acute type A dissection: an integrated approach. *Ann Thorac Surg* 2002;**74**(5):S1848–52;discussion S1857–63.

101. Watanuki H, Ogino H, Minatoya K *et al.* Is emergency total arch replacement with a modified elephant trunk technique justified for acute type A aortic dissection? *Ann Thorac Surg* 2007;**84**(5):1585–91.

102. Kazui T, Yamashita K, Washiyama N *et al.* Aortic arch replacement using selective cerebral perfusion. *Ann Thorac Surg* 2007;**83**(2):S796–8;discussion S824–31.

103. Moon MR, Sundt TM 3rd, Pasque MK *et al.* Does the extent of proximal or distal resection influence outcome for type A dissections? *Ann Thorac Surg* 2001;**71**(4):1244–9;discussion 1249–50.

104. Geirsson A, Bavaria JE, Swarr D *et al.* Fate of the residual distal and proximal aorta after acute type a dissection repair using a contemporary surgical reconstruction algorithm. *Ann Thorac Surg* 2007;**84**(6):1955–64;discussion 1955–64.

105. Glower DD, Fann JI, Speier RH et al. Comparison of medical and surgical therapy for uncomplicated descending aortic dissection. *Circulation* 1990;**82**(5 suppl):IV39–46.

106. Suzuki T, Mehta RH, Ince H et al. Clinical profiles and outcomes of acute type B aortic dissection in the current era: lessons from the International Registry of Aortic Dissection (IRAD). *Circulation* 2003;**108**(1):9.

107. Estrera AL, Miller CC, Goodrick J et al. Update on outcomes of acute type B aortic dissection. *Ann Thorac Surg* 2007;**83**(2):S842–5;discussion S846–50.

108. Coady MA, Rizzo JA, Elefteriades JA. Pathologic variants of thoracic aortic dissections. Penetrating atherosclerotic ulcers and intramural hematomas. *Cardiol Clin* 1999;**17**(4):637–57.

109. Kaji S, Nishigami K, Akasaka T et al. Prediction of progression or regression of type A aortic intramural hematoma by computed tomography. *Circulation.* 1999;**100**(19 suppl):II281–6.

110. Coady MA, Rizzo JA, Hammond GL et al. Surgical intervention criteria for thoracic aortic aneurysms: a study of growth rates and complications. *Ann Thorac Surg* 1999;**67**(6):1922–6;discussion 1953–8.

111. Elefteriades JA, Hammond GL, Gusberg RJ et al. Fenestration revisited. A safe and effective procedure for descending aortic dissection. *Arch Surg* 1990;**125**(6):786–90.

112. Vedantham S, Picus D, Sanchez LA et al. Percutaneous management of ischemic complications in patients with type-B aortic dissection. *J Vasc Interv Radiol* 2003;**14**(2 Pt 1):181–94.

113. Williams DM, Lee DY, Hamilton BH et al. The dissected aorta: percutaneous treatment of ischemic complications – principles and results. *J Vasc Interv Radiol* 1997;**8**(4):605–25.

114. Kaya A, Heijmen RH, Overtoom TT et al. Thoracic stent grafting for acute aortic pathology. *Ann Thorac Surg* 2006;**82**(2):560–5.

115. Pate JW, Fabian TC, Walker W. Traumatic rupture of the aortic isthmus: an emergency? *World J Surg* 1995;**19**(1):119–25;discussion 125–6.

116. Parmley LF, Mattingly TW, Manion WC, Jahnke EJ Jr. Nonpenetrating traumatic injury of the aorta. *Circulation* 1958;**17**(6):1086–101.

117. Fabian TC, Richardson JD, Croce MA et al. Prospective study of blunt aortic injury: Multicenter Trial of the American Association for the Surgery of Trauma. *J Trauma* 1997;**42**(3):374–80;discussion 380–3.

118. Attia C, Villard J, Boussel L et al. Endovascular repair of localized pathological lesions of the descending thoracic aorta: midterm results. *Cardiovasc Intervent Radiol* 2007;**30**(4):628–37.

119. Stone DH, Brewster DC, Kwolek CJ et al. Stent-graft versus open-surgical repair of the thoracic aorta: mid-term results. *J Vasc Surg* 2006;**44**(6):1188–97.

120. Grabenwoger M, Fleck T, Czerny M et al. Endovascular stent graft placement in patients with acute thoracic aortic syndromes. *Eur J Cardiothorac Surg* 2003;**23**(5):788–93;discussion 793.

121. Koullias G, Modak R, Tranquilli M et al. Mechanical deterioration underlies malignant behavior of aneurysmal human ascending aorta. *J Thorac Cardiovasc Surg* 2005;**130**(3):677–83.

122. Juvonen T, Ergin MA, Galla JD et al. Risk factors for rupture of chronic type B dissections. *J Thorac Cardiovasc Surg* 1999;**117**(4):776–86.

123. Bachet J, Larrazet F, Goudot B et al. When should the aortic arch be replaced in Marfan patients? *Ann Thorac Surg* 2007;**83**(2):S774–9;discussion S785–90.

124. Tagusari O, Ogino H, Kobayashi J et al. Should the transverse aortic arch be replaced simultaneously with aortic root replacement for annuloaortic ectasia in Marfan syndrome? *J Thorac Cardiovasc Surg* 2004;**127**(5):1373–80.

125. Bachet J, Guilmet D, Goudot B et al. Cold cerebroplegia. A new technique of cerebral protection during operations on the transverse aortic arch. *J Thorac Cardiovasc Surg* 1991;**102**(1):85–93;discussion 93–4.

126. Ueda Y, Miki S, Kusuhara K et al. Deep hypothermic systemic circulatory arrest and continuous retrograde cerebral perfusion for surgery of aortic arch aneurysm. *Eur J Cardiothorac Surg* 1992;**6**(1):36–41;discussion 42.

127. Estrera AL, Garami Z, Miller CC 3rd et al. Determination of cerebral blood flow dynamics during retrograde cerebral perfusion using power M-mode transcranial Doppler. *Ann Thorac Surg* 2003;**76**(3):704–9;discussion 709–10.

128. Moon MR, Sundt TM 3rd. Influence of retrograde cerebral perfusion during aortic arch procedures. *Ann Thorac Surg* 2002;**74**(2):426–31;discussion 431.

129. Ehrlich MP, Hagl C, McCullough JN et al. Retrograde cerebral perfusion provides negligible flow through brain capillaries in the pig. *J Thorac Cardiovasc Surg* 2001;**122**(2):331–8.

130. Kazui T, Washiyama N, Muhammad BA et al. Improved results of atherosclerotic arch aneurysm operations with a refined technique. *J Thorac Cardiovasc Surg* 2001;**121**(3):491–9.

131. Svensson LG, Blackstone EH, Rajeswaran J et al. Does the arterial cannulation site for circulatory arrest influence stroke risk? *Ann Thorac Surg* 2004;**78**(4):1274–84;discussion 1274–84.

132. Sabik JF, Nemeh H, Lytle BW et al. Cannulation of the axillary artery with a side graft reduces morbidity. *Ann Thorac Surg* 2004;**77**(4):1315–20.

133. Svensson LG, Kim KH, Blackstone EH et al. Elephant trunk procedure: newer indications and uses. *Ann Thorac Surg* 2004;**78**(1):109–16;discussion 109–16.

134. Heinemann MK, Buehner B, Jurmann MJ, Borst HG. Use of the "elephant trunk technique" in aortic surgery. *Ann Thorac Surg* 1995;**60**(1):2–6;discussion 7.

135. Svensson LG. Rationale and technique for replacement of the ascending aorta, arch, and distal aorta using a modified elephant trunk procedure. *J Card Surg* 1992;**7**(4):301–12.

136. Kouchoukos NT, Mauney MC, Masetti P, Castner CF. Optimization of aortic arch replacement with a one-stage approach. *Ann Thorac Surg* 2007;**83**(2):S811–14;discussion S824–31.

137. Nishigami K, Tsuchiya T, Shono H et al. Disappearance of aortic intramural hematoma and its significance to the prognosis. *Circulation* 2000;**102**(19 suppl 3):III243–7.

138. Kaji S, Akasaka T, Katayama M et al. Long-term prognosis of patients with type B aortic intramural hematoma. *Circulation* 2003;**108**(1):9.

139. Sueyoshi E, Imada T, Sakamoto I et al. Analysis of predictive factors for progression of type B aortic intramural hematoma with computed tomography. *J Vasc Surg* 2002;**35**(6):1179–83.

140. LeMaire SA, Miller CC 3rd, Conklin LD et al. A new predictive model for adverse outcomes after elective thoracoabdominal aortic aneurysm repair. *Ann Thorac Surg* 2001;**71**(4):1233–8.

141. Cowan JA Jr, Dimick JB, Henke PK *et al.* Surgical treatment of intact thoracoabdominal aortic aneurysms in the United States: hospital and surgeon volume-related outcomes. *J Vasc Surg* 2003;**37**(6):1169–74.

142. Makaroun MS, Dillavou ED, Kee ST *et al.* Endovascular treatment of thoracic aortic aneurysms: results of the phase II multicenter trial of the GORE TAG thoracic endoprosthesis. *J Vasc Surg* 2005;**41**(1):1–9.

143. Safi HJ, Hess KR, Randel M *et al.* Cerebrospinal fluid drainage and distal aortic perfusion: reducing neurologic complications in repair of thoracoabdominal aortic aneurysm types I and II. *J Vasc Surg* 1996;**23**(2):223–8;discussion 229.

144. Kouchoukos NT, Masetti P, Rokkas CK, Murphy SF. Hypothermic cardiopulmonary bypass and circulatory arrest for operations on the descending thoracic and thoracoabdominal aorta. *Ann Thorac Surg* 2002;**74**(5):S1885–7;discussion S1892–8.

145. Roselli EE, Greenberg RK, Pfaff K *et al.* Endovascular treatment of thoracoabdominal aortic aneurysms. *J Thorac Cardiovasc Surg* 2007;**133**(6):1474–82.

146. Chuter TA, Rapp JH, Hiramoto JS *et al.* Endovascular treatment of thoracoabdominal aortic aneurysms. *J Vasc Surg* 2008;**47**(1):6–16.

68

Cardiac transplantation: indications and postoperative management

Barry Boilson and Sudhir Kushwaha

William Von Liebig Transplant Center, Mayo Clinic, Rochester, MN, USA

Historical perspective

The original concept of cardiac transplantation dates to the 1890s, with the work of Alexis Carrel and subsequently Mann and colleagues at the Mayo Clinic in the 1930s.[1] The modern era of human cardiac transplantation started with pioneering work by Vladimir Demikhov in Russia in the 1940s[2] and Norman E. Shumway's group at Stanford University throughout the 1950s, the latter associated with the development of cardiopulmonary bypass[3] and perfection of the surgical technique. By the mid 1960s, it was concluded by Shumway that the major barrier to successful mammalian cardiac allotransplantation was rejection.

The first human cardiac transplant was performed by Dr Christiaan Barnard at Cape Town, South Africa, in 1967. Local irradiation, azathioprine, prednisone and actinomycin C were used as immunosuppression. The patient survived 18 days but ultimately succumbed to *Pseudomonas* pneumonia.[4]

Worldwide, further attempts at human cardiac transplantation met with poor outcomes. Most groups discontinued their efforts, but the Stanford group implemented criteria and protocols for detection of acute rejection early post transplant. Initially, this involved ECG, echocardiographic and clinical parameters, but in 1973 histologic criteria on endomyocardial biopsy were developed and remain the mainstay of rejection surveillance. The discovery of ciclosporin A by Professor Jean-François Borel in 1976 and its subsequent introduction into clinical practice after successful animal studies[5] was the breakthrough in the prevention of rejection which allowed successful cardiac transplantation. Despite these advances, the number of transplants performed worldwide has plateaued, primarily due to lack of donor organ supply.[6] This has instigated research and development of new therapeutic avenues such as mechanical device therapy.

Outcomes

The International Society for Heart and Lung Transplantation (ISHLT) has reported outcome data on transplant recipients on an annual basis for the past 24 years. The most recent data are summarized below.[7]

Demographics

The primary indication for cardiac transplantation has remained unchanged in recent years, almost evenly divided between ischemic (41%) and non-ischemic cardiomyopathy (45%). The remaining indications represent a minority of patients with valvular and congenital heart disease and those retransplanted (all 3%). An increasing number of patients are now on inotropic (40%) or mechanical support (including left ventricular assist devices [LVADs], 27%) at the time of cardiac transplantation.

The age of both donors and recipients has increased in the past 20 years. Almost 25% of cardiac transplant recipients in the past year were over the age of 60 years, with a relative fall in numbers of recipients aged 40–49 years. Donors over the age of 50 years now comprise >12% of donors worldwide. Twenty percent of European donors are over 50 years old, whereas in the US that figure is closer to 10%.

Evidence-Based Cardiology, 3rd edition. Edited by S. Yusuf, J.A. Cairns, A.J. Camm, E.L. Fallen, and B.J. Gersh. © 2010 Blackwell Publishing, ISBN: 978-1-4051-5925-8.

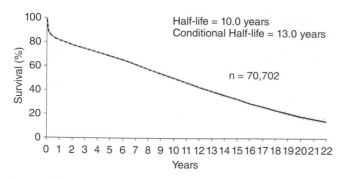

Figure 68.1 Overall survival post cardiac transplantation (ISHLT data 2007).

Outcomes

Since the ISHLT started reporting outcomes in 1982, early survival (up to one year) post transplantation has improved steadily.[8] However, long-term mortality has not changed and the current transplant half-life is 10 years worldwide for adult and pediatric cardiac transplant recipients combined, representing a steady improvement over the past 20 plus years due to the improvements in early survival (Fig. 68.1). In particular, survival for patients retransplanted has improved and is currently similar to those transplanted for the first time (approximately 85% one-year survival in those surviving the first year).

The risk factors for death within one year and, in those surviving the first year, for death within five years are shown in Table 68.1. In the current era, the most significant risk factors for death post cardiac transplantation in the first year remain requirement for short-term extracorporeal mechanical support post transplantation, congenital heart disease as an indication for transplantation and presence of insulin-requiring diabetes mellitus pretransplant. After the first year, the highest risk factors for death within the first five years are need for retransplantation, the development of cardiac allograft vasculopathy and insulin-requiring diabetes mellitus prior to transplantation.

The commonest causes of death up to 30 days, in the first year and up to five years, are shown in Table 68.2. Graft failure remains the commonest cause of death within 30 days, and includes ischemic/reperfusion injury, right heart failure and acute rejection. Beyond 30 days, infection becomes prominent as the commonest cause of death up to the first year (33% of deaths). After this timepoint, cardiac allograft vasculopathy is the most frequent cause of death, representing 30% of all deaths within five years post cardiac transplantation, closely followed by malignancy (22% of deaths).

Recipient selection

The current AHA/ACC recommendations on selection of adult patients for cardiac transplantation are set out in their

Table 68.1 Risk factors for mortality in first year post cardiac transplantation

	95% confidence interval
Risk factors for death within 1 year*	
Need for short-term extracorporeal mechanical support	2.11, 5.42
Adult congenital heart disease	1.47, 3.10
Insulin-requiring diabetes mellitus	1.02, 3.41
Mechanical ventilation at time of transplant	1.36, 2.46
Prior pregnancy	1.05, 1.57
Previous history of CVA	1.00, 1.67
Recent infection (within 2 weeks) requiring IV antibiotics	1.04, 1.55
LVAD *in situ*‡	1.05, 1.55
Prior sternotomy	1.05, 1.42
Risk factors for death within 5 years§	
Retransplantation	1.55, 9.57
Early-onset coronary artery vasculopathy (within first year)	1.55, 2.70
Diabetes mellitus pretransplant	1.25, 1.86
Treated infection during initial transplant hospitalization	1.12, 1.66
Treated rejection episode in first year	1.06, 1.50
Ischemic vs non-ischemic cardiomyopathy pretransplant	0.99, 1.45

Reproduced with permission from reference [6], courtesy of the ISHLT, 2007.
* Data based on transplants performed January 2002 through June 2005, n = 7024.
‡ Data based on a predominance of pulsatile devices having been implanted at the time of audit.
§ Data based on transplants performed January 1999 through June 2001, n = 4079.

Table 68.2 Leading causes of death post cardiac transplantation

	Proportion of all deaths
Up to 30 days (~10% mortality)	
Graft failure	40%
Multiorgan failure	14%
Infection*	13%
Up to 1 year (~15% mortality)	
Infection*	33%
Graft failure	18%
Acute rejection	12%
5 years (~30% mortality)	
Cardiac allograft vasculopathy	30%
Malignancy	22%
Infection*	10%

*Excluding CMV infection

practice guidelines for the management of chronic heart failure in the adult.[9] The primary focus is on patients with severe functional impairment and/or dependence on inotropic support. Rarely, recurrent malignant arrhythmias refractory to medical therapy and debilitating refractory angina pectoris secondary to severe non-revascularizable ischemic heart disease may be indications. Contraindications to cardiac transplantation are all relative and dependent on how modifiable they are before surgery. They include pulmonary disease, pulmonary hypertension, diabetes with complications, systemic disease (including malignancy) and peripheral vascular disease. Age is also included, but this is an area of controversy as data regarding outcomes in older recipients have been conflicting.[10,11] The indications for and contraindications to cardiac transplantation are summarized in Box 68.1.

Donor selection

Selection of a donor requires a number of criteria to be met. First, national (and/or regional criteria where these vary, as in the US) for brain death must be met. The ECG and the echocardiogram should be normal. If a donor older than 45 years is being considered, coronary angiography is performed to exclude significant coronary artery disease. Otherwise, the risk factor profile for coronary artery disease should be low and there should be no evidence of untreated acute infection or systemic malignancy. The HIV and hepatitis screens should be checked and confirmed negative. Potential donors with cardiac trauma are usually excluded.

The matching of a suitable donor to a recipient is dependent on a limited number of key issues.

Blood type

ABO matching is mandatory. Matching of rhesus status is not required.

Body size

Generally, the donor should be at least 80% of the body weight of the recipient.

Pulmonary vascular resistance

Where this is high (generally in excess of 4–5 Wood units) in the recipient, a larger donor heart is usually selected to ensure adequate right ventricular functional reserve. In addition to pulmonary vascular resistance, the pulmonary artery pressure is also considered, and in particular the assessment of reversibility of high pulmonary pressures seen in some patients with chronic heart failure.

BOX 68.1 Cardiac transplantation – indications and contraindications

Absolute indications
- Hemodynamic compromise secondary to heart failure
- Refractory cardiogenic shock
- Dependence on IV inotropic support for adequate organ perfusion
- Peak VO_2 <10 mL/kg/min
- Severely limiting non-revascularizable ischemic heart disease affecting daily living
- Recurrent symptomatic VT refractory to therapy

Relative indications
- Peak VO_2 11–14 mL/kg/min with significant limitation of functional capacity
- Recurrent unstable angina refractory to current therapy
- Recurrently labile fluid balance/renal function in chronic heart failure despite full patient compliance with therapy

Insufficient indications
- Presence of the following without other indications for transplantation:
  - Impaired LV systolic function
  - Previous history of class III–IV heart failure
  - Peak VO_2 >15 mL/kg/min

Contraindications (all relative)
- Pulmonary hypertension (must have evidence of significant reversibility at right heart catheterization)
- Age (controversial – see text)
- Parenchymal lung disease with significant pulmonary function abnormalities (<50% predicted)
- Co-existent systemic illness (e.g. malignancy, infiltrative disorders, infection)
- Acute pulmonary embolus
- Severe peripheral vascular disease
- Irreversible renal and hepatic dysfunction
- Diabetes with severe end-organ damage
- Severe obesity
- Severe osteoporosis
- Psychosocial issues
- Drug addiction, including nicotine

Recipient stability

Where the recipient is unstable (status 1 vs status 2), the urgency of finding a suitable donor heart occasionally requires some compromise on an "ideal" match as outlined above.

Geographic location of donor

This always needs to be considered to ensure the lowest possible cold-ischemic time of the heart after it has been explanted from the donor. Once this rises beyond four hours, outcomes may be compromised. This is accentuated if there is significant hypertrophy of the donor organ.

Anti-HLA antibody titer

Due to the short time window of permitted cold-ischemic time in the setting of heart transplantation, unlike renal transplants, HLA cross-matching is only performed if titer of preformed antibodies in the recipient (PRA level) is significant. The PRA level is part of the routine pretransplant assessment of the recipient. This titer of recipient anti-HLA antibodies reflects the degree of sensitization of the patient to foreign antigens of HLA A, B and DR subtype. This is performed by incubating recipient serum in different wells with a random panel of donor lymphocytes. The result is represented as a percentage of total wells on a panel which show evidence of a positive reaction, hence the term PRA.[12] Numerous variations in methodology exist, and most recently have included flow cytometric virtual cross-match.[13] However, there is also variation in the interpretation of results – most programs consider a titer greater than 10% to be significant. Some institutions have considered any elevation or only titers greater than 20–25% to be of significance.[14]

The importance of the pretransplant PRA level has been known for some time and elevated PRA titers have been associated with increased risk of hyperacute rejection, antibody and cell-mediated rejection, and also cardiac allograft vasculopathy.[15,16] Therefore, patients with significantly elevated pretransplant PRA levels (>10% according to the American Society of Histocompatibility and Immunogenetics and UNOS) require HLA cross-matching to a donor organ.[17]

Operative details

The original operative technique described by Shumway involved removal of the native heart and anastomosis of the recipient heart at mid-atrial level bilaterally (Fig. 68.2).[18] This so-called "biatrial anastomosis" technique was shown to increase the incidence of atrial arrhythmia, right atrial thrombus and tricuspid valve dysfunction.[19,20] The "bicaval technique" involves preservation of the recipient pulmonary veins and anastomosis of a small cuff of recipient left atrial tissue to the donor left atrium, but retaining the anastomosis of the venae cavae and thus sparing integrity of the donor right atrium.[21] Recent evidence has shown short-term clinical benefits of the bicaval technique when compared to the biatrial technique, with enhanced preservation of atrial contractility, sinus node function and tricuspid valve competence, but there is insufficient evidence to date on long-term outcomes.[22]

Postoperative course

Immunosuppression

There are initial induction strategies and long-term chronic immunosuppression regimens. Induction therapy use has increased from 42% in 1995 to 52% in 2005, with use of antithymocyte globulin stable at 20–22% but the more traditional anti-T cell receptor monoclonal antibody OKT3 used in less then 3% of cardiac transplants in 2005.[6] The rationale for induction therapy is to reduce the risk of early acute rejection through enhanced immunosuppression and, in addition, the risk of postoperative renal dysfunc-

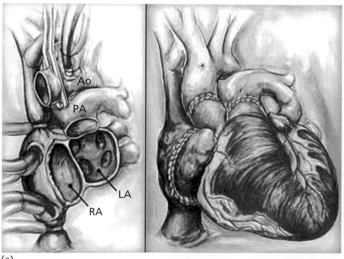
(a)

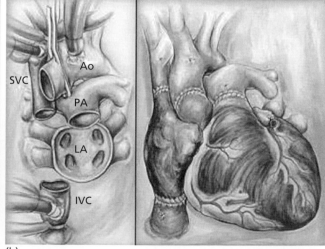
(b)

Figure 68.2 Standard Shumway anastomosis (a) and bicaval anastomosis (b).

tion through a delay in commencement of calcineurin inhibitor therapy.[23] However, induction therapy is not without risk and substantive evidence has linked it to an elevated risk of development of post-transplant lymphoproliferative disorder.[24] Therefore, the use of induction therapy varies, with many centers avoiding its use completely. The newer interleukin-2 antagonists are currently under evaluation.[26]

Maintenance immunosuppression varies among centers. The traditional model of a calcineurin inhibitor (ciclosporin or tacrolimus), an antiproliferative agent (azathioprine or mycophenolate) and a steroid is usual, but use of tacrolimus in preference to ciclosporin has increased in recent years.[6] Two randomized clinical trials have studied tacrolimus in direct comparison with ciclosporin. A European-based multicenter study on over 300 patients showed a significantly lower incidence of severe rejection in the tacrolimus-treated patients at six months but no difference in patient or graft survival at 18 months.[27] A smaller study from the US in which patients did not receive induction therapy showed no difference in survival or incidence of severe rejection between groups but a significantly lower incidence of renal dysfunction and hypertriglyceridemia in the tacrolimus-treated patients.[28] In addition, a non-significant trend was observed towards a lower requirement for antihypertensive therapy in the tacrolimus group.

Mycophenolate is currently used in over 70% of transplanted patients at one year. The advantages of mycophenolate over azathioprine post cardiac transplantation include a reduced incidence of acute rejection and mortality, and possibly even of the incidence of cardiac allograft vasculopathy.[29] The underlying mechanisms for this benefit may include preferential anti-B cell activity compared to azathioprine, and reduced production of anti-HLA antibodies post transplantation.[30,31]

A recent study which compared the ciclosporin/mycophenolate/prednisone, tacrolimus/mycophenolate/prednisone and tacrolimus/sirolimus/prednisone combinations showed a significantly lower incidence of grade >3A or hemodynamically significant rejection at one year in the two tacrolimus-based therapy groups compared to ciclosporin-based therapy.[32] The tacrolimus/mycophenolate/prednisone combination resulted in the most optimal preservation of renal function and the lowest triglyceride levels.

Newer agents such as the mTOR inhibitor rapamycin (sirolimus) are increasingly used due to potent immunosuppressive capacity with minimal nephrotoxicity and possible beneficial effects on the incidence of post-transplant cardiac allograft vasculopathy (CAV). Many centers are now switching patients from calcineurin inhibitors routinely as a renal-sparing maneuver.[33,34] An important side effect of sirolimus is impaired wound healing,[35] and therefore this agent cannot be used early post transplant.

Complications

Early complications

Early complications after cardiac transplantation include primary graft failure, acute and hyperacute rejection, arrhythmia, bleeding and infection.

Primary graft failure includes ischemic/reperfusion injury and right heart failure secondary to pulmonary hypertension. It still accounts for up to 40% of deaths within the first 30 days post cardiac transplantation.[6] Extended cold-ischemic time of the donor heart and elevated pulmonary vascular resistance in the recipient pretransplantation are significant risk factors. Treatment usually requires inotropic support, use of vasodilators to reduce pulmonary and systemic afterload and occasionally mechanical support. In rare circumstances emergency retransplantation is required.

Hyperacute rejection is a rare form of early rejection which is seen as soon as the donor heart is initially perfused with blood from the recipient. This is due to a high titer of preformed donor-specific antibodies in the recipient resulting in severe microvascular injury and thrombosis, with loss of the graft.

Acute rejection is common and usually T-cell mediated (cellular), but sometimes is due to recipient antibodies to donor antigens (humoral). Interestingly, the most recent ISHLT analysis has shown that current practices with induction therapy impact little on this problem. In fact, patients treated with OKT3 induction therapy had more acute rejection episodes in the first year post transplant than patients treated with other forms of induction therapy (i.e. antithymocyte globulin or anti-IL2 antibodies) or no induction therapy at all.[6] Tacrolimus may be superior to ciclosporin early post transplant with fewer rejection episodes in the first year, especially in combination with mycophenolate.[27]

Acute rejection is usually asymptomatic unless fulminant and severe, but its detection is important as frequency of episodes correlates with reduced graft survival (and possibly with the incidence of cardiac allograft vasculopathy).[36] Therefore screening is required with frequent endomyocardial biopsy especially within the first three months post transplant. Alternative approaches are under investigation to reduce the number of endomyocardial biopsies which are associated with an increased risk of tricuspid valve injury. These include the use of microarrays for identification of key (candidate) genes upregulated and downregulated in early rejection.[37] Studies are ongoing to evaluate the utility of this approach for longitudinal analysis of patients in terms of rejection profile.[38]

The ISHLT grading system for acute cellular rejection was changed in 2004. Currently the following system is used (see Plate 68.1):

- Grade 0: no rejection (Plate 68.1a)
- Grade 1 R, mild: interstitial and/or perivascular infiltrate with up to one focus of myocyte damage (Plate 68.1b)
- Grade 2 R, moderate: two or more foci of infiltrate with associated myocyte damage (Plate 68.1c)
- Grade 3 R, severe: diffuse infiltrate with multifocal myocyte damage, with or without edema, hemorrhage or vasculitis (Plate 68.1d).

Humoral or antibody-mediated rejection (AMR) is less well recognized but is associated with an increased incidence of cardiac allograft vasculopathy and mortality.[36,39] Histologically, it is characterized by endothelial swelling and the presence of macrophages and neutrophils in the capillaries with fibrin deposition.[40] Currently, the ISHLT guidelines recommend staining for complement C3d and C4d deposition in interstitial capillaries and for CD68 to highlight macrophages within capillaries.[41] In general, only intense and diffuse (2–3+) staining is considered significant evidence of AMR (Plate 68.2). Analysis of patient serum for the presence of anti-HLA I and II antibodies is also recommended.[42] One recent series has shown that AMR is seen most commonly early post cardiac transplantation and often associated with elevated anti-donor HLA antibodies.[43] However, this is less common in patients developing AMR later in their post-transplant course, where, instead, it is associated with malignancy or recent infection, suggesting activation of antibody-mediated immunity by a new antigen present on an invading pathogen or expressed on tumor cells.[44]

Arrhythmia is common. Frequently, patients are tachycardic due to denervation of the donor heart. Atrial fibrillation can also occur. Bradycardia and junctional rhythms are not unusual, particularly when the cold-ischemic time of the donor heart is prolonged, resulting in sinus and atrioventricular nodal ischemia.[19] Occasionally (4–12% of cases), permanent pacemaker implantation is required before discharging the patient from hospital, and the DDDR mode may be preferable.[45]

Late complications

Coronary allograft vasculopathy (CAV) is the single complication of greatest impact on long-term outcome (see Table 69.2).[42] Allograft vasculopathy occurs in all transplanted solid organs with time.[46] In the transplanted heart, over 50% of adult recipients will have angiographic evidence of CAV at 10 years.[6] However, a high proportion of transplanted patients develop CAV only in the intramyocardial branches of coronary arterioles but with sparing of the smaller arterioles sampled on biopsy, thus making the diagnosis on angiography or endomyocardial biopsy difficult.[47]

Although there is evidence of some reinnervation of cardiac allografts, most transplant recipients do not experience anginal pain with myocardial ischemia or infarction. Therefore, CAV may present as sudden death due to silent myocardial infarction, congestive cardiac failure or arrhythmia.[48]

Risk factors for CAV include hypertension, younger age, male gender and pre-existing coronary artery disease in the donor. The protective effect of older donor age may reflect increased angiographic screening of older donors.[6] Additional risk factors include early and recurrent rejection[49] and metabolic risk factors including diabetes and hyperlipidemia.[37] The role of cytomegalovirus (CMV) infection is controversial – evidence dates back almost 20 years showing an association with CAV.[50,51] However, recent evidence has cast some doubt on the directness of this association.[52]

The diagnosis of CAV has traditionally employed coronary angiography often with intravascular ultrasound (IVUS).[53] However both modalities are limited, the first because CAV involves the entire coronary artery tree longitudinally, and therefore may be missed on angiography; the latter because IVUS only images the larger epicardial arteries and not the smaller vessels and branches. Modalities of additional value for detection of CAV include dobutamine stress echocardiography[54,55] and nuclear scintigraphy[55,56]; cardiac CT and contrast echocardiography may also prove useful in the future as techniques are refined.[57,58]

There is evidence for the role of statins in the prevention of CAV in animal models[59] and in humans.[60] Additional benefits of statins may include prevention of progression of post-transplant renal dysfunction.[61]

There is recent evidence that the use of mTOR inhibitors such as sirolimus (rapamycin) and everolimus, a synthetic derivative, may attenuate the progression of CAV.[34,62,63]

Malignancy is a common complication of long-term immunosuppression.[64] According to current ISHLT figures, by 10 years post cardiac transplantation, the prevalence of malignancy is 32%. Much of this is due to facilitation of chronic opportunistic infection by oncogenic viruses such as Epstein–Barr virus (EBV) in the case of post-transplant lymphoproliferative disorder, HHV8 in Kaposi's sarcoma and human papilloma virus in skin cancers.[65] All immunosuppressive agents have been implicated to some degree, with the possible exception of sirolimus, for which evidence is mounting that the risk of malignancy may be significantly lower.[66] Most of these cancers are skin related (61%), the remainder being solid tumors including prostate, lung, bladder, breast, cervical and renal (total 18%) and lymphoproliferative, including post-transplant lymphoproliferative disorder (PTLD) (6%).[6]

Skin cancer is a common cause of morbidity and rarely mortality post transplant and in the transplant recipient is often recurrent and more aggressive.[67–69] The risk of skin malignancy may vary with different immunosuppressive regimens; recent evidence has suggested that ciclosporin may have a specific carcinogenic effect independent of its immunosuppressive effect[71] and the use of sirolimus as an alternative agent may be protective and may even induce remission of skin cancers in transplant recipients.[71,72]

PTLD has been strongly associated with EBV infection.[73] However, the risk of developing this condition is multifactorial, and also related to immunosuppression and impaired T cell immunity in the setting of foreign antigenicity from the transplanted organ.[74] Other risk factors that have been identified are younger recipient and donor age (<18 years)[75,76] and more than five acute rejection episodes post transplantation.[76] CMV infection may also be a risk factor.[77]

The largest series available on PTLD comes from the Israel Penn International Transplant Tumor Registry based at the University of Cincinatti, Ohio.[78] From their data on 274 cardiac transplant patients with PTLD, the authors reported a 50% mortality within one year. The commonest sites involved were the lung and lymph nodes (34% and 32%), followed by the gastrointestinal tract (24%), the liver (23%), central nervous system (13%), the spleen (11%) and the cardiac allograft itself (10%).

There have been no randomized controlled clinical trials of any treatments currently in use for PTLD. The first strategy employed is minimization of immunosuppressive therapy. The next step is usually anti-B cell monoclonal antibody therapy, most frequently given as rituximab, an anti-CD20 monoclonal antibody, which has had efficacy shown in small studies.[79] Another modality that has been used with success in a small number of patients is anti-IL6 antibody therapy.[80] Failing treatment described above requires salvage chemotherapy, and use of this strategy has recently been described in a small study.[81] A new but promising strategy, adoptive immunotherapy for PTLD, involves the administration of banked HLA-matched or autologous cloned EBV-specific cytotoxic T cells.[82] The results of the first Phase II multicenter clinical trial have been encouraging.[83]

Infection with both the usual community-acquired and opportunistic pathogens is increased in patients on chronic immunosuppression. Common infections include community-acquired pathogens such as common respiratory viruses (e.g. influenza, parainfluenza, respiratory syncytiovirus and adenovirus), and common bacteria such as streptococci, *Mycoplasma*, *Legionella*, *Listeria* and *Salmonella*. Vaccinations for influenza and pneumococcus are recommended but may have reduced efficacy. Endemic organisms such as histoplasma and coccidioides may also be seen in the US.

A specific aspect particular to the transplant population is the issue of reactivation of latent infection and, also, the possibility of acquired latent infection from the donor.

This extends mainly to reactivations of CMV, varicella zoster and herpes simplex virus. However, reactivations of tuberculosis, toxoplasmosis and, in endemic areas, histoplasmosis and blastomycosis may occasionally present.[84–86]

Postoperatively, prophylaxis against cytomegalovirus infection is routine, usually for a period of three months. The benefits of CMV prophylaxis include reduced incidence of acute and chronic rejection, and possibly of CAV and PTLD post transplant.[87] Ganciclovir is the antiviral agent with efficacy against CMV which has been most extensively studied.[88] The major side effect of ganciclovir is myelosuppression.[89] Valganciclovir is a valine ester of ganciclovir which has enhanced oral bioavailability and has proven efficacy as CMV pre-emptive therapy in cardiac transplant recipients.[90] It is rapidly hydrolyzed to ganciclovir, the active metabolite, through enzymes in the gut mucosa and hepatic cells. CMV resistance to ganciclovir (and valganciclovir) has been reported, however.[91] In these cases, foscarnet is the usual agent for CMV therapy but a major dose-limiting side effect of this agent is renal impairment.[89,92] Aciclovir has some efficacy against CMV proven in a meta-analysis of 12 randomized trials.[93] Like ganciclovir, its oral bioavailability is limited but enhanced when delivered as its valyl ester, valaciclovir.[89] Valaciclovir is approved in some European countries for CMV prophylaxis.[89]

The transmission of *Toxoplasma gondii* is a concern in cardiac transplant recipients who are *Toxoplasma* antibody seronegative who receive an organ from a seropositive donor. Therefore, it has been routine to administer anti-*Toxoplasma* prophylactic therapy to this group for at least three months, with pyrimethamine, sulfadiazine or folinic acid. This strategy has been challenged recently, however, as it has been shown that the rates of *Toxoplasma* reactivation in centers which do not employ anti-*Toxoplasma* prophylaxis in at-risk groups is negligible.[94] Efficacy for c-otrimoxazole (trimethoprim-sulfamethoxazole/TMP-SMX) against *Toxoplasma* has also been shown and many groups believe that use of this agent is adequate prophylaxis against both *Pneumocystis jiroveci* and *Toxoplasma*.[95] For cardiac transplant patients (as distinct from heart-lung recipients), antifungal prophylaxis is not routine and not supported by data from clinical trials to date.[96]

Renal insufficiency is seen commonly in cardiac and other solid organ transplant recipients and is multifactorial.[97] However, chronic calcineurin inhibitor therapy is often a major contributor.[98] Analysis of data from 1994 to 2006 has shown that the incidence of renal insufficiency in cardiac transplant recipients has been increasing: at 10 years post cardiac transplant 98% of patients have hypertension, and 14% of patients have renal insufficiency (8% severe with creatinine >2.5 mg/dL and 5% on hemodialysis).[6] There is mounting evidence that replacement of calcineurin inhibitor therapy with sirolimus permits recovery from calcineurin inhibitor-induced renal insufficiency and is associated with stable renal function at least in the medium term.[99,100] The risk of severe renal insufficiency post cardiac transplantation (i.e. creatinine >2.5 mg/dL or requiring renal replacement therapy) correlates with the presence of renal dysfunction, diabetes mellitus and patient age at the time of cardiac transplant.[6] Additional risk factors are a history of pretransplant hypertension, previous history of high PRA levels, inotropic therapy at the time of transplantation, infection requiring intravenous antibiotic therapy within two weeks of transplantation, and recipient weight.[6]

LVADs as long-term cardiac replacement therapy

At the present time, the gold standard of long-term cardiac replacement therapy remains cardiac transplantation, but the number of cardiac transplants performed is limited by donor organ availability.[101] Therefore, there has been great interest in the development of left ventricular assist devices as destination therapy for end-stage chronic heart failure.

Left ventricular assist devices (LVADs) have been in use as a bridge to cardiac transplantation for over 20 years, and the Heartmate XVE ® device (Thoratec Corporation, California, US) was approved by the US Food and Drug Administration (FDA) for this purpose in 1994. Since that time, the Heartmate II ® axial flow device has been FDA approved for use as bridge to transplant in late 2007, and many other LVAD types are currently under evaluation for this indication.

The REMATCH study evaluated the long-term benefit of Heartmate XVE placement compared to optimal medical therapy in end-stage heart failure patients.[102] A 48% reduction in death from all causes was attributable to LVAD therapy compared to best medical therapy in this trial, and on this basis the Heartmate XVE was approved for use as destination therapy in 2002. However, two year survival in the LVAD group was only 23%, with a high incidence of device failure. Furthermore, early mortality was high in both groups of patients, and in this respect Lietz et al. showed that using a novel operative risk score encompassing severity of heart failure, nutritional status, renal function and RV function, the patients with the lowest risk had the best early survival.[103] This underlines the importance of patient selection. Up to the present time, the Heartmate XVE is the only LVAD approved for destination therapy in the US, but the Heartmate II continuous axial flow device, which expected superior durability, is under evaluation for this indication.

The newest generation of centrifugal pumps with a magnetically and/or hydrostatically suspended internal spinning rotor have elimited the need for internal bearings and promise the greatest durability. These pumps such as the Ventrassist ® (Ventracor, Sydney, Australia), Duraheart ® (Terumo Heart, Michigan, US) and HVAD ® (Heartware, Sydney, Australia) devices, are currently under evaluation in clinical trials.

Conclusion

Cardiac replacement therapy in end-stage heart failure is at a crossroads. The art and science of cardiac transplant medicine have been perfected since the first transplant in 1967 and outcomes continue to improve. However, the number of transplants being performed worldwide is far outnumbered by the number of potential candidates, as donor hearts are a very limited resource. Advances in destination device therapy may provide a viable long-term solution for many patients, with either support of the native heart by LVAD therapy or even possibly complete replacement of the heart by a prosthetic device. Completely implantable devices that offer the patient as normal a life as possible with a minimal risk of infection are likely to have the greatest impact in this field. The potential of cell therapy is also under evaluation and the field is still in its infancy but evolving. New insights in this field could potentially open a whole new era in therapy for this devastating condition.

References

1. DiBardino DJ. The history and development of cardiac transplantation. *Tex Heart Inst J* 1999;**26**(3):198–205.
2. Shumacker HB, Jr. A surgeon to remember: notes about Vladimir Demikhov. *Ann Thorac Surg* 1994;**58**(4):1196–1198.
3. Willman VL, Cooper T, Cian LG, Hanlon CR. Autotransplantation of the canine heart. *Surg Gynecol Obstet* 1962;**115**:299–302.
4. Barnard CN. The operation. A human cardiac transplant: an interim report of a successful operation performed at Groote Schuur Hospital, Cape Town. *S Afr Med J* 1967;**41**(48):1271–1274.
5. Christiansen S, Klocke A, Autschbach R. Past, present, and future of long-term mechanical support in adults. *J Card Surg* 2008;**23**(6):664–76.
6. Taylor DO, Edwards LB, Boucek MM *et al.* Registry of the International Society for Heart and Lung Transplantation: twenty-fourth official adult heart transplant report–2007. *J Heart Lung Transplant* 2007;**26**(8):769–781.
7. Taylor DO, Edwards LB, Aurora P *et al.* Registry of the International Society for Heart and Lung Transplantation: twenty-fifth official adult heart transplant report–2008. *J Heart Lung Transplant* 2008;**27**(9):943–56.
8. Lietz K, Miller LW. Improved survival of patients with end-stage heart failure listed for heart transplantation: analysis of

organ procurement and transplantation network/U.S. United Network of Organ Sharing data, 1990 to 2005. *J Am Coll Cardiol* 2007;**50**(13):1282–1290.

9. Hunt SA, Abraham WT, Chin MH *et al*. ACC/AHA 2005 Guideline Update for the Diagnosis and Management of Chronic Heart Failure in the Adult: a report of the American College of Cardiology/American Heart Association Task Force on Practice Guidelines (Writing Committee to Update the 2001 Guidelines for the Evaluation and Management of Heart Failure): developed in collaboration with the American College of Chest Physicians and the International Society for Heart and Lung Transplantation: endorsed by the Heart Rhythm Society. *Circulation* 2005;**112**(12):e154–235.

10. Borkon AM, Muehlebach GF, Jones PG *et al*. An analysis of the effect of age on survival after heart transplant. *J Heart Lung Transplant* 1999;**18**(7):668–74.

11. Morgan JA, John R, Weinberg AD *et al*. Long-term results of cardiac transplantation in patients 65 years of age and older: a comparative analysis. *Ann Thorac Surg* 2003;**76**(6): 1982–7.

12. Nwakanma LU, Williams JA, Weiss ES *et al*. Influence of pre-transplant panel-reactive antibody on outcomes in 8,160 heart transplant recipients in recent era. *Ann Thorac Surg* 2007;**84**(5): 1556–62; discussion 1562–53.

13. Zangwill S, Ellis T, Stendahl G *et al*. Practical application of the virtual crossmatch. *Pediatr Transplant* 2007;**11**(6):650–4.

14. Betkowski AS, Graff R, Chen JJ, Hauptman PJ. Panel-reactive antibody screening practices prior to heart transplantation. *J Heart Lung Transplant* 2002;**21**(6):644–50.

15. Loh E, Bergin JD, Couper GS, Mudge GH, Jr. Role of panel reactive antibody cross reactivity in predicting survival after orthotopic heart transplantation. *J Heart Lung Transplant* 1994;**13**(2):194–201.

16. Leech SH, Lopez-Cepero M, LeFor WM *et al*. Management of the sensitized cardiac recipient: the use of plasmapheresis and intravenous immunoglobulin. *Clin Transplant* 2006;**20**(4): 476–84.

17. UNOS. The United Network for Organ Sharing, Standards for histocompatibility testing. 1998.

18. Shumway NE, Lower RR, Stofer RC. Transplantation of the heart. *Adv Surg* 1966;**2**:265–284.

19. Jacquet L, Ziady G, Stein K *et al*. Cardiac rhythm disturbances early after orthotopic heart transplantation: prevalence and clinical importance of the observed abnormalities. *J Am Coll Cardiol* 1990;**16**(4):832–7.

20. Angermann CE, Spes CH, Tammen A *et al*. Anatomic characteristics and valvular function of the transplanted heart: transthoracic versus transesophageal echocardiographic findings. *J Heart Transplant* 1990;**9**(4):331–8.

21. Sievers HH, Weyand M, Kraatz EG, Bernhard A. An alternative technique for orthotopic cardiac transplantation, with preservation of the normal anatomy of the right atrium. *Thorac Cardiovasc Surg* 1991;**39**:70–2.

22. Schnoor M, Schafer T, Luhmann D, Sievers HH. Bicaval versus standard technique in orthotopic heart transplantation: a systematic review and meta-analysis. *J Thorac Cardiovasc Surg* 2007;**134**(5):1322–31.

23. Uber PA, Mehra MR. Induction therapy in heart transplantation: is there a role? *J Heart Lung Transplant* 2007;**26**(3):205–9.

24. Swinnen LJ, Costanzo-Nordin MR, Fisher SG *et al*. Increased incidence of lymphoproliferative disorder after immunosuppression with the monoclonal antibody OKT3 in cardiac-transplant recipients. *N Engl J Med* 1990;**323**(25):1723–28.

25. Opelz G, Schwarz V, Henderson R *et al*. Non-Hodgkin's lymphoma after kidney or heart transplantation: frequency of occurrence during the first posttransplant year. *Transpl Int* 1994;**7**(Suppl 1):S353–6.

26. Segovia J, Rodriguez-Lambert JL, Crespo-Leiro MG *et al*. A randomized multicenter comparison of basiliximab and muromonab (OKT3) in heart transplantation: SIMCOR study. *Transplantation* 2006;**81**(11):1542–8.

27. Grimm M, Rinaldi M, Yonan NA *et al*. Superior prevention of acute rejection by tacrolimus vs. cyclosporine in heart transplant recipients–a large European trial. *Am J Transplant* 2006;**6**(6):1387–97.

28. Kobashigawa JA, Patel J, Furukawa H *et al*. Five-year results of a randomized, single-center study of tacrolimus vs microemulsion cyclosporine in heart transplant patients. *J Heart Lung Transplant* 2006;**25**(4):434–9.

29. Kobashigawa JA, Meiser BM. Review of major clinical trials with mycophenolate mofetil in cardiac transplantation. *Transplantation* 2005;**80**(2 Suppl):S235–43.

30. Lietz K, John R, Schuster M *et al*. Mycophenolate mofetil reduces anti-HLA antibody production and cellular rejection in heart transplant recipients. *Transplant Proc* 2002;**34**(5): 1828–9.

31. Weigel G, Griesmacher A, Karimi A *et al*. Effect of mycophenolate mofetil therapy on lymphocyte activation in heart transplant recipients. *J Heart Lung Transplant* 2002;**21**(10). 1074–9.

32. Kobashigawa JA, Miller LW, Russell SD *et al*. Tacrolimus with mycophenolate mofetil (MMF) or sirolimus vs. cyclosporine with MMF in cardiac transplant patients: 1-year report. *Am J Transplant* 2006;**6**(6):1377–86.

33. Kushwaha SS, Khalpey Z, Frantz RP *et al*. Sirolimus in cardiac transplantation: use as a primary immunosuppressant in calcineurin inhibitor-induced nephrotoxicity. *J Heart Lung Transplant* 2005;**24**(12):2129–36.

34. Raichlin E, Bae JH, Khalpey Z *et al*. Conversion to Sirolimus as Primary Immunosuppression Attenuates the Progression of Allograft Vasculopathy After Cardiac Transplantation. *Circulation* 2007.

35. Kuppahally S, Al-Khaldi A, Weisshaar D *et al*. Wound healing complications with de novo sirolimus versus mycophenolate mofetil-based regimen in cardiac transplant recipients. *Am J Transplant* 2006;**6**(5 Pt 1):986–92.

36. Michaels PJ, Espejo ML, Kobashigawa J *et al*. Humoral rejection in cardiac transplantation: risk factors, hemodynamic consequences and relationship to transplant coronary artery disease. *J Heart Lung Transplant* 2003;**22**(1):58–69.

37. Deng MC, Eisen HJ, Mehra MR *et al*. Noninvasive discrimination of rejection in cardiac allograft recipients using gene expression profiling. *Am J Transplant* 2006;**6**(1):150–60.

38. Pham MX, Deng MC, Kfoury AG *et al*. Molecular testing for long-term rejection surveillance in heart transplant recipients: design of the Invasive Monitoring Attenuation Through Gene Expression (IMAGE) trial. *J Heart Lung Transplant* 2007;**26**(8): 808–14.

39. Taylor DO, Yowell RL, Kfoury AG et al. Allograft coronary artery disease: clinical correlations with circulating anti-HLA antibodies and the immunohistopathologic pattern of vascular rejection. *J Heart Lung Transplant* 2000;**19**(6):518–21.

40. Uber WE, Self SE, Van Bakel AB, Pereira NL. Acute antibody-mediated rejection following heart transplantation. *Am J Transplant* 2007;**7**(9):2064–74.

41. Stewart S, Winters GL, Fishbein MC et al. Revision of the 1990 working formulation for the standardization of nomenclature in the diagnosis of heart rejection. *J Heart Lung Transplant* 2005;**24**(11):1710–20.

42. Tan CD, Baldwin WM, 3rd, Rodriguez ER. Update on cardiac transplantation pathology. *Arch Pathol Lab Med* 2007;**131**(8):1169–91.

43. Smith RN, Brousaides N, Grazette L et al. C4d deposition in cardiac allografts correlates with alloantibody. *J Heart Lung Transplant* 2005;**24**(9):1202–10.

44. Almuti K, Haythe J, Dwyer E et al. The changing pattern of humoral rejection in cardiac transplant recipients. *Transplantation* 2007;**84**(4):498–503.

45. Roelke M, McNamara D, Osswald S et al. A comparison of VVIR and DDDR pacing following cardiac transplantation. *Pacing Clin Electrophysiol* 1994;**17**(11 Pt 2):2047–51.

46. Radio S, Wood S, Wilson J et al. Allograft vascular disease: comparison of heart and other grafted organs. *Transplant Proc* 1996;**28**(1):496–9.

47. Winters GL, Schoen FJ. Graft arteriosclerosis-induced myocardial pathology in heart transplant recipients: predictive value of endomyocardial biopsy. *J Heart Lung Transplant* 1997;**16**(10):985–93.

48. Bolad IA, Robinson DR, Webb C et al. Impaired left ventricular systolic function early after heart transplantation is associated with cardiac allograft vasculopathy. *Am J Transplant* 2006;**6**(1):161–8.

49. Stoica SC, Cafferty F, Pauriah M et al. The cumulative effect of acute rejection on development of cardiac allograft vasculopathy. *J Heart Lung Transplant* 2006;**25**(4):420–5.

50. Koskinen PK, Nieminen MS, Krogerus LA et al. Cytomegalovirus infection accelerates cardiac allograft vasculopathy: correlation between angiographic and endomyocardial biopsy findings in heart transplant patients. *Transpl Int* 1993;**6**(6):341–7.

51. Hussain T, Burch M, Fenton MJ et al. Positive pretransplantation cytomegalovirus serology is a risk factor for cardiac allograft vasculopathy in children. *Circulation* 2007;**115**(13):1798–1805.

52. Zakliczynski M, Krynicka-Mazurek A, Pyka L et al. The Influence of Cytomegalovirus Infection, Confirmed by pp65 Antigen Presence, on the Development of Cardiac Allograft Vasculopathy. *Transplant Proc* 2007;**39**(9):2866–9.

53. Ramzy D, Rao V, Brahm J et al. Cardiac allograft vasculopathy: a review. *Can J Surg* 2005;**48**(4):319–27.

54. Bacal F, Moreira L, Souza G et al. Dobutamine stress echocardiography predicts cardiac events or death in asymptomatic patients long-term after heart transplantation: 4-year prospective evaluation. *J Heart Lung Transplant* 2004;**23**(11):1238–44.

55. Elhendy A, van Domburg RT, Vantrimpont P et al. Prediction of mortality in heart transplant recipients by stress technetium-99m tetrofosmin myocardial perfusion imaging. *Am J Cardiol* 2002;**89**(8):964–8.

56. Ciliberto GR, Ruffini L, Mangiavacchi M et al. Resting echocardiography and quantitative dipyridamole technetium-99m sestamibi tomography in the identification of cardiac allograft vasculopathy and the prediction of long-term prognosis after heart transplantation. *Eur Heart J* 2001;**22**(11):964–71.

57. Bogot NR, Durst R, Shaham D, Admon D. Cardiac CT of the transplanted heart: indications, technique, appearance, and complications. *Radiographics* 2007;**27**(5):1297–309.

58. Hacker M, Hoyer HX, Uebleis C et al. Quantitative assessment of cardiac allograft vasculopathy by real-time myocardial contrast echocardiography: A comparison with conventional echocardiographic analyses and [Tc99m]-sestamibi SPECT. *Eur J Echocardiogr* 2007.

59. Shirakawa I, Sata M, Saiura A et al. Atorvastatin attenuates transplant-associated coronary arteriosclerosis in a murine model of cardiac transplantation. *Biomed Pharmacother* 2007;**61**(2–3):154–9.

60. Raichlin ER, McConnell JP, Lerman A et al. Systemic inflammation and metabolic syndrome in cardiac allograft vasculopathy. *J Heart Lung Transplant* 2007;**26**(8):826–33.

61. Lubitz SA, Pinney S, Wisnivesky JP et al. Statin therapy associated with a reduced risk of chronic renal failure after cardiac transplantation. *J Heart Lung Transplant* 2007;**26**(3):264–72.

62. Keogh A, Richardson M, Ruygrok P et al. Sirolimus in de novo heart transplant recipients reduces acute rejection and prevents coronary artery disease at 2 years: a randomized clinical trial. *Circulation* 2004;**110**(17):2694–700.

63. Eisen HJ, Tuzcu EM, Dorent R et al. Everolimus for the prevention of allograft rejection and vasculopathy in cardiac-transplant recipients. *N Engl J Med* 2003;**349**(9):847–58.

64. Penn I. Cancers complicating organ transplantation. *N Engl J Med* 1990;**323**(25):1767–69.

65. Dantal J, Soulillou JP. Immunosuppressive drugs and the risk of cancer after organ transplantation. *N Engl J Med* 2005;**352**(13):1371–3.

66. Campistol JM, Eris J, Oberbauer R et al. Sirolimus therapy after early cyclosporine withdrawal reduces the risk for cancer in adult renal transplantation. *J Am Soc Nephrol* 2006;**17**(2):581–9.

67. Penn I. Malignant melanoma in organ allograft recipients. *Transplantation* 1996;**61**(2):274–8.

68. Veness MJ, Quinn DI, Ong CS et al. Aggressive cutaneous malignancies following cardiothoracic transplantation: the Australian experience. *Cancer* 1999;**85**(8):1758–64.

69. Lindelof B, Sigurgeirsson B, Gabel H, Stern RS. Incidence of skin cancer in 5356 patients following organ transplantation. *Br J Dermatol* 2000;**143**(3):513–9.

70. Tiu J, Li H, Rassekh C et al. Molecular basis of posttransplant squamous cell carcinoma: the potential role of cyclosporine a in carcinogenesis. *Laryngoscope* 2006;**116**(5):762–9.

71. Kauffman HM, Cherikh WS, Cheng Y et al. Maintenance immunosuppression with target-of-rapamycin inhibitors is associated with a reduced incidence of de novo malignancies. *Transplantation* 2005;**80**(7):883–9.

72. Mathew T, Kreis H, Friend P. Two-year incidence of malignancy in sirolimus-treated renal transplant recipients: results from five multicenter studies. *Clin Transplant* 2004;**18**(4):446–9.

73. Nalesnik MA, Jaffe R, Starzl TE et al. The pathology of post-transplant lymphoproliferative disorders occurring in the

setting of cyclosporine A-prednisone immunosuppression. *Am J Pathol* 1988;**133**(1):173–92.

74. Birkeland SA, Hamilton-Dutoit S. Is posttransplant lymphoproliferative disorder (PTLD) caused by any specific immunosuppressive drug or by the transplantation per se? *Transplantation* 2003;**76**(6):984–8.

75. Smith JM, Corey L, Healey PJ *et al.* Adolescents are more likely to develop posttransplant lymphoproliferative disorder after primary Epstein-Barr virus infection than younger renal transplant recipients. *Transplantation* 2007;**83**(11):1423–8.

76. Gao SZ, Chaparro SV, Perlroth M *et al.* Post-transplantation lymphoproliferative disease in heart and heart-lung transplant recipients: 30-year experience at Stanford University. *J Heart Lung Transplant* 2003;**22**(5):505–14.

77. Cockfield SM. Identifying the patient at risk for post-transplant lymphoproliferative disorder. *Transpl Infect Dis* 2001;**3**(2):70–8.

78. Aull MJ, Buell JF, Trofe J *et al.* Experience with 274 cardiac transplant recipients with posttransplant lymphoproliferative disorder: a report from the Israel Penn International Transplant Tumor Registry. *Transplantation* 2004;**78**(11):1676–82.

79. Oertel SH, Verschuuren E, Reinke P *et al.* Effect of anti-CD 20 antibody rituximab in patients with post-transplant lymphoproliferative disorder (PTLD). *Am J Transplant* 2005;**5**(12):2901–6.

80. Haddad E, Paczesny S, Leblond V *et al.* Treatment of B-lymphoproliferative disorder with a monoclonal anti-interleukin-6 antibody in 12 patients: a multicenter phase 1–2 clinical trial. *Blood* 2001;**97**(6):1590–7.

81. Trappe R, Riess H, Babel N *et al.* Salvage chemotherapy for refractory and relapsed posttransplant lymphoproliferative disorders (PTLD) after treatment with single-agent rituximab. *Transplantation* 2007;**83**(7):912–8.

82. Preiksaitis JK. New developments in the diagnosis and management of posttransplantation lymphoproliferative disorders in solid organ transplant recipients. *Clin Infect Dis* 2004;**39**(7):1016–23.

83. Haque T, Wilkie GM, Jones MM *et al.* Allogeneic cytotoxic T-cell therapy for EBV-positive posttransplantation lymphoproliferative disease: results of a phase 2 multicenter clinical trial. *Blood* 2007;**110**(4):1123–31.

84. Walker K, Skelton H, Smith K. Cutaneous lesions showing giant yeast forms of Blastomyces dermatitidis. *J Cutan Pathol* 2002;**29**(10):616–8.

85. Masri K, Mahon N, Rosario A *et al.* Reactive hemophagocytic syndrome associated with disseminated histoplasmosis in a heart transplant recipient. *J Heart Lung Transplant* 2003;**22**(4):487–91.

86. Jastrzebski D, Zakliczynski M, Siola M *et al.* Lower respiratory tract infections in patients during hospital stay after heart transplantation. *Ann Transplant* 2003;**8**(1):37–9.

87. Potena L, Holweg CT, Chin C *et al.* Acute rejection and cardiac allograft vascular disease is reduced by suppression of subclinical cytomegalovirus infection. *Transplantation* 2006;**82**(3):398–405.

88. Couchoud C, Cucherat M, Haugh M, Pouteil-Noble C. Cytomegalovirus prophylaxis with antiviral agents in solid organ transplantation: a meta-analysis. *Transplantation* 1998;**65**(5):641–7.

89. Biron KK. Antiviral drugs for cytomegalovirus diseases. *Antiviral Res* 2006;**71**(2–3):154–63.

90. Devyatko E, Zuckermann A, Ruzicka M *et al.* Pre-emptive treatment with oral valganciclovir in management of CMV infection after cardiac transplantation. *J Heart Lung Transplant* 2004;**23**(11):1277–82.

91. Drew WL, Paya CV, Emery V. Cytomegalovirus (CMV) resistance to antivirals. *Am J Transplant* 2001;**1**(4):307–12.

92. Razonable RR, Emery VC. Management of CMV infection and disease in transplant patients. 27–29 February 2004. *Herpes* 2004;**11**(3):77–86.

93. Fiddian P, Sabin CA, Griffiths PD. Valacyclovir provides optimum acyclovir exposure for prevention of cytomegalovirus and related outcomes after organ transplantation. *J Infect Dis* 2002;**186**(Suppl 1):S110–115.

94. Baran DA, Alwarshetty MM, Alvi S *et al.* Is toxoplasmosis prophylaxis necessary in cardiac transplantation? Long-term follow-up at two transplant centers. *J Heart Lung Transplant* 2006;**25**(11):1380–2.

95. Fishman JA. Prevention of infection caused by Pneumocystis carinii in transplant recipients. *Clin Infect Dis* 2001;**33**(8):1397–405.

96. Playford EG, Webster AC, Sorell TC, Craig JC. Antifungal agents for preventing fungal infections in solid organ transplant recipients. *Cochrane Database Syst Rev* 2004;**(3)**:CD004291.

97. Ojo AO, Held PJ, Port FK *et al.* Chronic renal failure after transplantation of a nonrenal organ. *N Engl J Med* 2003;**349**(10):931–40.

98. Olyaei AJ, de Mattos AM, Bennett WM. Immunosuppressant-induced nephropathy: pathophysiology, incidence and management. *Drug Saf* 1999;**21**(6):471–88.

99. Raichlin E, Khalpey Z, Kremers W *et al.* Replacement of calcineurin-inhibitors with sirolimus as primary immunosuppression in stable cardiac transplant recipients. *Transplantation* 2007;**84**(4):467–74.

100. Gustafsson F, Ross HJ, Delgado MS *et al.* Sirolimus-based immunosuppression after cardiac transplantation: predictors of recovery from calcineurin inhibitor-induced renal dysfunction. *J Heart Lung Transplant* 2007;**26**(10):998–1003.

101. Birks EJ, Yacoub MH, Banner NR, Khaghani A. The role of bridge to transplantation: should LVAD patients be transplanted? *Curr Opin Cardiol* 2004;**19**(2):148–53.

102. Rose EA, Gelijns AC, Moskowitz AJ *et al.* Long-term mechanical left ventricular assistance for end-stage heart failure. *N Engl J Med* 2001;**345**(20):1435–43.

103. Lietz K, Long JW, Kfoury AG *et al.* Outcomes of left ventricular assist device implantation as destination therapy in the post-REMATCH era: implications for patient selection. *Circulation* 2007;**116**(5):497–505.

69

Renal dysfunction

Johannes F E Mann[1] *and Ernesto L Schiffrin*[2]

[1] Munich General Hospital, Munich, Germany
[2] Sir Mortimer B Davis-Jewish General Hospital, Montreal, Quebec, Canada

Chronic kidney disease (CKD) affects many people with cardiovascular disease (CVD) but is often undetected. If present in people with CVD, CKD predicts worse cardiovascular outcomes independent of other cardiovascular risk factors. This chapter reviews the evidence regarding proper detection of CKD, gauging the cardiovascular risk associated with CKD, and treating people presenting with both CVD and CKD. As this book is primarily directed at "cardiovascular" readers, we will not discuss underlying diseases causing CKD and the specific therapy of those renal diseases. Rather, we suggest that all people with CKD (and anyone with proteinuria) should be assessed at least once by a nephrologist (and a diabetologist if diabetes is also present) who can identify the underlying reasons of CKD and suggest strategies to halt or inhibit its progression to end-stage renal disease.

Definition of chronic kidney disease

In 2002, efforts of the National Kidney Foundation (USA) and the international KDIGO group (Kidney Disease Initiative to improve Global Outcomes) led to clinical practice guidelines for the evaluation, classification and risk stratification of CKD.[1] CKD was defined as any renal disease lasting for more than three months with histologic or other signs of renal damage. As depicted in Table 69.1, glomerular filtration rate (GFR) may be decreased or normal in affected people.

Kidney damage can be detected in several ways including urinary dipstick and sediment, measurement of urine protein, kidney histology, imaging studies or measurement of markers of GFR such as serum creatinine or cystatin C.

In the vast majority of cases in adults not presenting with kidney-related symptoms, a reduced GFR or an elevated urinary protein excretion will identify CKD.

Glomerular filtration rate

Normal GFR in young men and women averages about 130 and 120 mL/min/1.73 m^2 respectively.[2] After age 40, people tend to lose GFR by approximately 1 mL/min/year; this mean value, however, shows a wide variability, substantially depending on the presence or absence of atherosclerotic vascular disease.[3,4] GFR changes little in elderly people without renal and atherosclerotic vascular disease and is regulated in health and disease by various factors. For example, sodium and protein intake increase GFR and sympathetic drive decreases it.

Exact measurement of GFR by inulin or iothalamate clearance is cumbersome and costly and therefore not practical in routine clinical practice. Serum creatinine is the usual clinical indicator of GFR. However, this indicator (an amino acid derivative of 0.11 KD) is imperfect. First, creatinine is excreted by both glomerular filtration and tubular secretion; second, serum creatinine concentration depends substantially on muscle mass such that individuals with very low muscle mass may exhibit terminal renal failure at serum creatinine concentrations barely above 2 mg/dL (175 μmol/L). Third, dietary intake of creatinine with meat may also affect serum levels. Indeed, GFR may decrease by up to 30% without a corresponding increase in serum creatinine above the normal range.

Despite those obvious shortcomings of serum creatinine as a marker of GFR, it is possible to estimate GFR (eGFR) from the serum creatinine using various formulas that include age, sex, race or weight (Box 69.1).[2] The Cockcroft–Gault (CG) formula was developed to calculate creatinine clearance from regression computation of data in 249 people with GFR of about 30–130 mL/min, comparing serum creatinine and creatinine clearance. The CG formula

Evidence-Based Cardiology, 3rd edition. Edited by S. Yusuf, J.A. Cairns, A.J. Camm, E.L. Fallen, and B.J. Gersh. © 2010 Blackwell Publishing, ISBN: 978-1-4051-5925-8.

Table 69.1 Stages of chronic kidney disease (CKD), its approximate prevalence in Western societies and associated cardiovascular risk

Stage	GFR (mL/min/1.73 m²)	Approx. prevalence (% of population)	CV risk* (odds ratio)
1	>90	3	Depends on degree of proteinuria
2	60–90	3	1.5
3	30–59	4	2–4
4	15–29	0.2	4–10
5	<15	0.1	10–1000

In population studies, GFR was calculated from serum creatinine or cystatin C. The prevalence data are approximated from surveys in North America. The odds of the cardiovascular risk vary substantially with age. For example, the cardiovascular risk of a 20-year-old dialysis patient is about 1000-fold higher than the risk of his age group; at the age of 70 years, it is about 20-fold.

BOX 69.1 Formulas to estimate glomerular filtration rate

Modification of Diet in Renal Disease (MDRD) formula:

$$\text{GFR (mL/min/1.73 m}^2) = 186 \times \text{Screa}^{-1.154} \times \text{age}^{-0.203} \times 0.742 \text{ if female} \times 1.21 \text{ if black}$$

Cockcroft and Gault formula:

$$\text{Ccrea (mL/min)} = \frac{(140 - \text{age}) \times \text{weight} \times 0.85 \text{ if female}}{72 \times \text{Screa}}$$

Formulas derived from serum cystatin C:

$$\text{GFR (mL/min)} = 74:8 \times (\text{Cystatin C})(\text{mg/L})^{-1.333} \text{ (Dade-Behring kit)}$$

$$\text{GFR (mL/min)} = 89:12 \times (\text{Cystatin C})(\text{mg/L})^{-1.675} \text{ (Dako kit)}$$

Screa, serum creatinine; age in years, weight in kg; Ccrea, creatinine clearance; GFR, glomerular filtration rate. There are several formulas developed from the MDRD data set. Above we give the most often used abbreviated formula. Slightly more exact is the following MDRD formula: GFR (mL/min/1.73 m²) = 170 × Screa $^{-0.999}$ × age $^{-0.176}$ × Surea $^{-0.1760}$ × Salbumin $^{+0.318}$ × 0.762 if female × 1.180 if black.

tends to overestimate GFR, especially at low GFR. The MDRD (Modification of Diet in Renal Disease study) formula was based on the relationship between serum creatinine and GFR measured by iothalamate clearance in 1628 people with an elevated serum creatinine. This formula appears to be more accurate than the CG formula, at least in ambulatory people with GFR <60 mL/min, and has been used in people with several renal diseases and different ethnicity. Of note, the calculation of eGFR improves if assays for serum creatinine are calibrated against a standard; a national program for such calibration is in place in the USA. The MDRD tends to underestimate GFR at levels >60 mL/min and may vary from "true" GFR based on inulin clearance by up to 30%. Indeed, above an eGFR of 60 mL/min, the variance of eGFR is so large that many laboratories do not report exact values and just note that the value is >60. The latter approach appears to be reasonable; otherwise eGFR calculations would inflate the number of people with the label "CKD". Thus, people with an eGFR >60 mL/min should only be classified as having CKD if there is other evidence of CKD such as increased urinary protein excretion or kidney damage detected with imaging or histologic studies.

Cystatin C in serum is an alternative to creatinine; it is a 13 KD protein, freely filtered by the glomerulus with extensive tubular reabsorption and catabolism. Its generation as a nuclear degradation product appears to be more stable than the generation of creatinine. Recent data suggest that serum concentration of cystatin C may be a better marker of GFR than creatinine-based eGFR at GFR >60 mL/min. Cystatin C measurements are much more expensive than creatinine (6–10-fold difference) and further research is necessary to establish the role of cystatin C in clinical medicine.

Urine protein

If the kidney leaks proteins, this may reflect underlying renal disease or, in the case of small amounts of albumin, generalized endothelial dysfunction. Common renal diseases are glomerulonephritis, inherited diseases such as polycystic kidney disease, diabetic nephropathy and nephrosclerosis due to smoking or hypertension. Laboratories typically measure either all proteins in the urine or albumin alone; dipsticks detect only albumin. A variety of assays are available and day-to-day variation of urinary protein excretion is substantial, depending on factors such as posture and physical activity. Therefore, urinary protein excretion should be measured more than once to detect kidney damage. Moreover, when urinary protein excretion is measured, it should either be expressed as a ratio to urine creatinine (to account for urine concentration) or as a timed specimen (e.g. per 12 or 24 hours).[1]

Urinary protein excretion is a very strong predictor of cardiovascular risk. This association is progressive; that is, the risk of incident cardiovascular outcomes increases with urinary protein excretion, even within the "normal" range.[5] The term microalbuminuria stems from studies in diabetes and indicates a threshold at which the risk for overt diabetic nephropathy (macroalbuminuria and/or renal insufficiency) suddenly increases severalfold. Such a threshold does not exist in the relationship between urinary albumin excretion and cardiovascular risk. As the term microalbuminuria is well established in clinical medicine, we use it here to describe renal damage and its association with cardiovascular risk.

Low GFR and high urinary protein excretion often coincide. In many studies, however, only one of these standard markers of renal damage is reported, usually serum creatinine. The few studies that documented both parameters suggest that both of these renal-related cardiovascular risk factors are additive and independent of each other.[6,7]

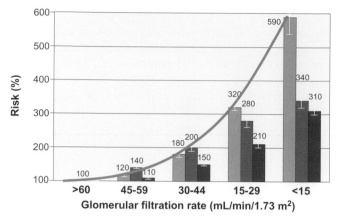

Figure 69.1 Relationship between estimated glomerular filtration rate (eGFR) and cardiovascular outcomes in a general population of >1 million people of a health maintenance organization in California, followed for 2.5 years. Abscissa: GFR estimated from serum creatinine at baseline. Ordinate: relative risk % for death (light gray), for a major cardiovascular event (black) and for hospitalization (gray). Risk of people with a baseline GFR >60 mL/min/1.73 m² was set at 100%. (Modified after Go et al[8], with permission.)

When to measure eGFR and urinary protein excretion?

There is no general consensus regarding when to measure kidney-related cardiovascular risk factors. In general, serum creatinine is measured whenever blood chemistry is ordered. Guidelines support the measurement of serum creatinine whenever a cardiovascular risk profile is evaluated in a person. Urinary protein excretion is usually ordered in the evaluation of kidney disease or at regular intervals in people with diabetes. In a cardiovascular setting, both eGFR and urine protein may be ordered if one is unsure whether to start therapies to prevent cardiovascular disease in a given patient. The presence of increased urinary protein excretion or a low eGFR may then justify such therapy. However, data regarding the additional value of proteinuria and eGFR on top of classic cardiovascular risk are lacking, and some analyses suggest that these measurements are of limited value after accounting for classic cardiovascular disease risk factors.

Population-wide impact of cardiovascular risk associated with renal dysfunction

GFR

A recent systematic review of 39 studies comprising approximately 1.4 million people followed for a median of 4.5 years reported that cardiovascular mortality was increased with reduced eGFR in all but three studies. The univariate risk increase was twofold (range 1–5-fold); this risk was somewhat attenuated after multivariate adjust-

ments.[8] A low eGFR is not consistently associated with cardiovascular risk in the general population[8] due to the low number of cardiovascular outcomes and concomitant low power. However, one study of >1 million participants of the general population in California reported a continuous increase in cardiovascular risk (adjusted hazard ratio) for eGFRs between 45 and 59 mL/min to <15 mL/min from 1.4- to 3.4-fold[9] compared to an eGFR of >60 mL/min (Fig. 69.1); the risk increase for mortality and hospitalization was steeper. Of note, the prevalence of an eGFR <60 mL/min in the general population, especially above age 50, is in the range of 5–10%.[10] Conversely, in people with known cardiovascular disease, the prevalence of an eGFR <60 mL/min is higher than in the general population, in the 15–20% range.[7,10]

Proteinuria

The association of micro- and macroalbuminuria with cardiovascular risk was reported in about 20 longitudinal studies.[7] The overwhelming majority of studies found that both micro- and macroalbuminuria were independent predictors of cardiovascular risk with hazard ratios of 1.5–3.[5,11–13] The association is found in the general population and in high-risk populations. However, the prevalence of increased levels of urinary protein excretion is only 4–7% in the general population and higher (10–30%) in people at high cardiovascular risk, especially in the presence of diabetes.[5,7,12] The largest study in the general population with over 40 000 participants reported that a doubling of urinary protein excretion is associated with a 29% increase of the relative risk for cardiovascular outcomes (Fig. 69.2).[12] In a study of about 10 000 people with known cardiovascular disease or at high risk, any increase in urine albumin excretion by 0.4 mg/mmol creatinine (approx. 3.6 mg/g) was associated with a 6–7% increase in cardiovascular events, myocardial infarction, stroke and cardiovascular death.[5]

The predictive power of classic cardiovascular risk factors and of eGFR or proteinuria was compared by multivariate techniques. Kidney-related factors exhibit hazard or odds ratios that are not different, in absolute terms, from classic risk factors. Moreover, as noted above, when assessing cardiovascular risk in an individual, the renal-related factors add modestly to the classic risk factors.

> Moderately elevated serum creatinine and urine albumin are associated with a doubling in the risk for major cardiovascular events. These two renal-related risk factors are additive, are independent from classic risk factors but add only modestly to classic risk factors for risk calculation.

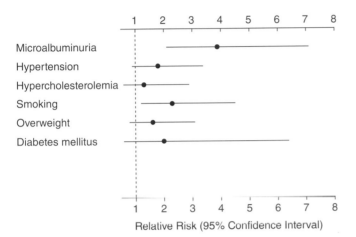

Figure 69.2 Relative risk for death in a general population from a Dutch town, followed for seven years. (From Hillege *et al.*[32].)

Why are low GFR and proteinuria risk factors for vascular disease?

The association of CKD and cardiovascular risk may reflect the (unjustified) fact that people with renal damage receive less therapy to prevent or treat cardiovascular disease than people with no renal damage (Fig. 69.3).[14] Renal damage may also be a marker of the severity of underlying vascular disease.[10,15] In other words, the associated hypertension or peripheral vascular disease may be more severe in people with renal damage. Such differences are not accounted for in adjusted analyses and can be considered as residual confounding. Furthermore, the mechanisms underlying renal and cardiovascular damage are similar. Finally, a reduced GFR accelerates atherosclerosis and vascular calcification.

One of the primary pathophysiologic mechanisms involved in accelerated vascular damage in CKD may be endothelial dysfunction.[16] A number of factors that adversely affect endothelial function are altered in CKD, including activation of the renin-angiotensin system,

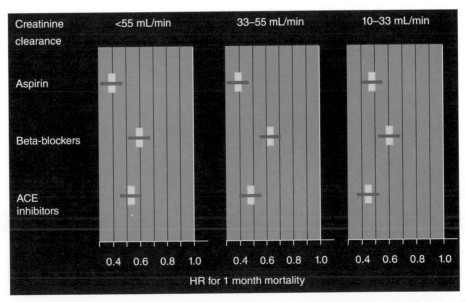

Figure 69.3 Thirty-day mortality in 130 000 people admitted to hospital for acute coronary syndrome. Data are stratified according to creatinine clearance, calculated from serum cratinine at admission according to Cockcroft and Gault. HR, hazard ratio comparing people treated/not treated with the respective drug. (Modified after Shlipak *et al*, *Ann Intern Med* 2002.)

increased oxidative stress, signs of low-grade inflammation with increased circulating cytokines, dyslipidemia and elevated asymmetric dimethylarginin (ADMA), an inhibitor of NO formation.[17–21] Many of those factors occur early in the course of CKD and precede the appearance of vascular and valvular calcifications found in late CKD.[21]

Implications for therapy

The use of cardiovascular drugs in people with kidney disease, specifically with renal insufficiency and a GFR <60 mL/min, may be associated with potential adverse events and potential benefits. We will discuss both aspects and make some general remarks.

Inhibitors of the renin-angiotensin system (RAS), including ACE inhibitors and angiotensin receptor blockers, are given to many people with cardiovascular disease. Acute renal failure and hyperkalemia are among the most feared adverse events of those drugs. Based on the results of the HOPE, ONTARGET and TRANSCEND studies, it appears reasonable to measure serum creatinine and serum potassium in the first few weeks after initiating therapy with an inhibitor of the RAS. In the run-in phase of these three large trials, therapy with an inhibitor of the RAS had to be stopped within the first 2–4 weeks because of increasing serum creatinine in about 0.2% and because of hyperkalemia in about 0.8%.[22,23] During long-term therapy with inhibitors of the RAS, acute renal failure, specifically dialysis dependent, and hyperkalemia were rare (<0.2% during 4–5 years) and not different between inhibitors of the RAS and placebo. As a rule, acute renal failure was related to conditions of potential fluid deprivation.[24] In people with chronic heart failure, the risks of acute renal failure and of hyperkalemia appear to be higher than indicated above, about 1.5% and 0.8% respectively over two years of follow-up and even higher in people with acute heart failure.[25] In people with chronic heart failure, the combined use of ACE inhibitors and angiotensin receptor blockers is sometimes considered. That combination approximately doubles the risk of acute renal failure compared to monotherapy with either ACE inhibitors or angiotensin receptor blockers (ARB).[24,25] Based on pathophysiology, the risk of acute renal failure likely depends on RAS activation. Under conditions of reduced renal perfusion, high renin levels contribute to maintain GFR. Such conditions are typically observed with advanced heart failure, with intravascular, specifically intra-arterial fluid deprivation and with the use of high doses of diuretics. Case reports suggest that the combination of NSAIDs with ACE inhibitors or ARB further increases renal risks when there is fluid deprivation or low cardiac output, especially in people with vascular

disease and potentially reduced capacity for renal autoregulation.

Recommendations: Grade C

- Serum creatinine and potassium should be checked in the first weeks after initiating therapy with inhibitors of the renin-angiotensin system, and during ongoing therapy if there are new signs of intravascular fluid deficiency.
- The concomitant chronic therapy with inhibitors of the renin system and of NSAID is discouraged.

What are the recommendations for the use of inhibitors of the RAS in people with CV disease? It may be wise to inform people treated with inhibitors of the RAS to stop treatment when there is diarrhea, other instances of volume depletion or high-grade fever and to avoid NSAID use apart from low-dose aspirin. When initiating therapy with inhibitors of the RAS or when increasing doses of diuretics, serum creatinine and potassium should be checked.

In chronic heart failure, the potassium-sparing diuretics spironolactone or eplerenone are successfully used. Those aldosterone receptor blockers increase the risk of hyperkalemia with an associated mortality, specifically when used in people with renal insufficiency and at doses higher than used in randomized trials. A cautious recommendation is to avoid such diuretics in people with renal insufficiency. That may not be helpful if people with heart and renal failure exhibit hypokalemia and related arrhythmia. No data are available on how to manage these people. Small trials suggest that hypokalemia is more effectively treated by spironolactone and other potassium-sparing diuretics than by oral potassium supplements. At 25–50 mg/d of spironolactone, serum potassium will increase by approximately 1 mmol/L.

Diuretics should be given at higher doses in people with renal insufficiency, preferentially loop diuretics. With decreasing GFR, less sodium is filtered, so less sodium can be prevented from tubular reabsorption by diuretics. Thus daily negative sodium balance of diuretics in renal insufficiency is reduced and it will take longer to remove excessive sodium and fluid. Sodium output can be easily monitored by collecting urine output. If sodium removal is too slow, hemofiltration may be considered but this procedure is invasive and very expensive. When initiating high-dose diuretic therapy or when large fluid shifts are observed in patients according to a weight change, close monitoring of electrolytes and serum creatinine is mandatory. Negative sodium and volume balance may massively stimulate vasopressin secretion and thirst. Those changes and the reduced free water clearance in renal insufficiency herald a substantial risk of hyponatremia.

Recommendations: Grade B

- Advanced heart failure may be associated with stimulation of thirst and vasopressin secretion. This stimulation may intensify when diuretic therapy is boosted. Hyponatremia in this situation can be prevented by fluid restriction and possibly by vasopressin antagonists.

Anticoagulants and platelet inhibitors can be used in people with renal insufficiency. Low GFR is associated with disordered coagulation and more bleeding. Some anticoagulant drugs, including heparins, act longer with lower GFR. In one study with clopidogrel, the cardiovascular benefits of clopidogrel in the acute coronary syndrome were preserved in those with renal insufficiency but the relative risk for bleeding associated with clopidogrel was actually less than in participants with normal renal function.[26] There are no further data on the balance of benefits and adverse events of anticoagulants in people with CV diseases and concomitant renal insufficiency, so no evidence-based recommendations can be given.

To our knowledge, beta-blockers have not been analyzed for their cardiovascular benefits in subgroups with renal insufficiency. Some of those agents have a prolonged action with decreasing GFR. This prolonged half-life is usually not a clinical problem since the action of beta-blockers can be easily monitored by heart rate.

Statins have similar benefits and adverse effects in people with and without renal insufficiency, according to a thorough meta-analysis.[27] In people with diabetes and treated by chronic dialysis, however, a large trial showed no significant CV benefit of statins. Some statins are partially eliminated via the kidney. Due to a wide safety margin, only minor dose adjustments are suggested with severe renal insufficiency.

From the above it appears reasonable to administer standard CV therapy in people with renal disease but data from registers found that such people receive standard cardiovascular care less frequently than those without renal disease.[10,14] People with renal diseases derive at least as much benefit from standard cardiovascular care as do people without renal damage.[14,24,27,28]

Invasive therapy for acute coronary syndromes clearly saves lives. Such beneficial therapy is often withheld in the presence of renal damage. There is no evidence that benefit or harm of invasive therapy is different in people with and without renal damage. One study found no difference in the relative risks of percutaneous coronary intervention (PCI) in acute coronary syndrome in people with normal and low GFR.[28] Clearly, measures to prevent contrast nephropathy should be instituted. However, the incidence of clinically significant contrast nephropathy is rare except in people with diabetes *and* both a low GFR *and* macroalbuminuria. In these individuals the risk of dialysis dependency after contrast injection is substantial.[29]

Recommendations: Grade B

- Standard cardiovascular therapy is as effective in people with moderate-to-severe renal insufficiency as in people with normal renal function, according to subgroup analyses of major outcome trials.

On the basis of observational data, it has been proposed to target lower blood pressure values in persons with CKD than in the general population, namely below 130/80 mm Hg and even below 125/75 mm Hg if urine protein is above 1 g/d or above 1 g/g creatinine.[10] There is only epidemiologic evidence to support those recommendations.

Many nephrologists assume that proteinuria reflects kidney damage and contributes to progressive renal damage by itself,[1] due to the increasing demand on the resorptive capacity for protein of renal tubular cells. Such tubular cells will then produce cytokines that initiate interstitial renal inflammation, attracting macrophages which will eventually transform into fibroblasts.[30] This hypothesis assumes that any reduction in proteinuria will halt progressive renal damage. Whereas this is consistent with data in both humans and experimental animals, effects of different proteinuria targets have never been tested in a clinical trial.

All the above considerations do not apply to people with end-stage renal disease. In this specific subgroup, mechanisms of vascular disease and of cardiovascular death are different, as are their risk factors.

References

1. Levey AS, Rocco MV. NKF; K/DOQI clinical practice guidelines for chronic kidney disease: evaluation, classification and stratification. *Am J Kidney Dis* 2002;**39**(suppl 1):s1–s266.
2. Stevens LA, Coresh J, Greene T, Levey AS. Assessing kidney function – measured and estimated glomerular filtration rate. *N Engl J Med* 2006;**354**:2473–83.

3. Kasiske BL. Relationship between vascular disease and age-associated changes in human kidney. *Kidney Int* 1987;**31**:1153–9

4. Fliser D, Franek E, Joest M, Block S, Mutschler E, Ritz E. Renal funtion in the elderly: impact of hypertension and cardiac function. *Kidney Int* 1997;**51**:1196–204.

5. Gerstein HC, Mann JFE, Qilong Y *et al.* Albuminuria and cardiovascular events, death and heart failure in diabetic and non-diabetic individuals. *JAMA* 2001;**286**:421–6.

6. Mann JFE, Gerstein HC, Pogue J, Bosch J, Yusuf S. Renal insufficiency as a predictor of cardiovascular outcomes and the impact of ramipril: the HOPE randomized trial. *Ann Intern Med* 2001;**134**:629–36.

7. Mann JFE, Yi QL, Gerstein HC. Albuminuria as a predictor of cardiovascular and renal outcomes in people with known atherosclerotic cardiovascular disease. *Kidney Int* 2004;**66**: S59–S62.

8. Tonelli M, Wiebe N, Culleton B *et al.* Chronic kidney disease and mortality risk: a systematic review. *J Am Soc Nephrol* 2006;**17**:2034–47.

9. Go AS, Chertow GM, Fan D, McCullock CE, Hsu CY. Chronic kidney disease and the risks of death, cardiovascular events, and hospitalization. *N Engl J Med* 2004;**351**:1296–305.

10. Sarnak MJ, Levey AS, Schoolwerth AC *et al.* Kidney disease as a risk factor for development of cardiovascular disease: a statement from the American Heart Association Councils on kidney in cardiovascular disease, high blood pressure research, clinical cardiology, and epidemiology and prevention. *Hypertension* 2003;**42**:1050–65.

11. Dinneen SF, Gerstein HC. The association of microalbuminuria and mortality in non-insulin dependent diabetes mellitus: A systematic overview of the literature. *Arch Int Med* 1997;**157**:1413–8.

12. Hillege HL, Fidler V, Diercks GF *et al.* for the PREVEND Study Group. Urinary albumin excretion predicts cardiovascular and non-cardiovascular mortality in general population. *Circulation* 2002;**106**(14):1777–82.

13. De Zeeuw D, Remuzzi G, Parving HH *et al.* Albuminuria, a therapeutic target for cardiovascular protection in type 2 diabetic patients with nephropathy. *Circulation.* 2004;**110**:921–7.

14. Shlipak MG, Heidenreich PA, Noguchi H *et al.* Association of Renal Insufficiency with Treatment and Outcomes after Myocardial Infarction in Elderly Patients. *Ann Intern Med.* 2002;**137**:555–62.

15. Levin A, Singer J, Thompson CR, Ross H, Lewis M. Prevalent LVH in the predialysis population: Identifying opportunities for intervention. *Am J Kidney Dis.* 1996;**27**:347–54.

16. Endemann DH, Schiffrin EL. Endothelial dysfunction. *J Am Soc Nephrol.* 2004;**15**:1983–92.

17. Schiffrin EL, Lipmann ML, Mann JFE. Chronic kidney disease: effects on the cardiovascular system. *Circulation* 2007;**116**: 85–97.

18. Zoccali C, Bode-Boger SM, Mallamaci F *et al.* Plasma concentration of asymmetrical dimethylarginine and mortality in patients with end-stage renal disease: a prospective study. *The Lancet* 2001;**358**:2113–7.

19. Xu J, Li G, Wang P *et al.* Renalase is a novel, soluble monoamine oxidase that regulates cardiac function and blood pressure. *J Clin Invest* 2005;**115**:1275–80.

20. Meinitzer A, Seelhorst U, Wellnitz B *et al.* Asymmetrical dimethylarginine independently predicts total and cardiovascular mortality in individuals with angiographic coronary artery disease (The Ludwigshafen Risk and Cardiovascular Health Study). *Clin Chem* 2007;**53**:273–83.

21. Russo D, Palmiero G, De Blasio AP, Balletta MM, Andreucci VE. Coronary artery calcification in patients with CRF not undergoing dialysis. *Am J Kidney Dis* 2004;**44**:1024–30.

22. The HOPE investigators. Effects of an angiotensin-converting enzyme inhibitor, ramipril, on death from cardiovascular causes, myocardial infarction, and stroke in high-risk patients. *New Engl J Med* 2000;**342**:145–53.

23. Mann JFE, Schmieder RE, McQueen M *et al.* for the ONTARGET investigators. Renal outcomes with telmisartan, ramipril, or both, in people at high vascular risk (the ONTARGET study): a multicentre, randomized, double-blind, controlled trial. *Lancet* 2008;**372**:547–53.

24. Mann JF, Schmieder RE, McQueen M *et al.* Renal outcomes with telmisartan, ramipril, or both in people at high vascular risk: results from a multicenter, randomised, double-blind, controlled trial. *Lancet* 2008; in press.

25. Phillips CO, Kashani A, Ko DK, Francis G, Krumholz HM. Adverse effects of combination angiotensin II receptor blockers plus angiotensin-converting enzyme inhibitors for left ventricular dysfunction: a quantitative review of data from randomized clinical trials. *Arch Intern Med* 2007;**167**:1930–6.

26. Keltai M, Tonelli M, Mann JFE *et al.* Renal function and outcomes in acute coronary syndrome: impact of clopidogrel. *Eur J Cardiovasc Prevent Rehab* 2007;**14**:312–18.

27. Sandhu S, Wiebe N, Fried LF, Tonelli M. Statins for improving renal outcomes: a meta-analysis. *J Am Soc Nephrol* 2006;**17**: 2006–16.

28. Pinkau T, Mann JFE, Ndrepepa G *et al.* Coronary stenting in people with mild to moderate renal insufficiency: restenosis rate and cardiovascular outcomes. *Am J Kidney Dis* 2004;**44**: 627–35.

29. Parfrey PS, Foley RN. The clinical epidemiology of cardiac disease in chronic uremia. *J Am Soc Nephrol* 1999;**10**: 1053–8.

30. Abbate M, Zoja C, Remuzzi G. How does proeinuria cause progressive renal damage? *J AmSoc Nephrol* 2006;**17**: 2974–84.

31. Giles PD, Fitzmaurice DA. Formula estimation of glomerular filtration rate: have we gone wrong? *BMJ* 2007;**334**:1198–2001.

32. Hillege HL, Girbes AR, De Kam PJ, Boomsma F, De Zeeuw D, Charlesworth A. Renal function, neurohormonal activation and survival in patients with chronic heart failure. *Circulation* 2000;**102**:203–10.

33. Ibsen H, Olsen MH, Wachtell K *et al.* Reduction in albuminuria translates to reduction in cardiovascular events in hypertensive patients – Losartan intervention for endpoint reduction in hypertension study. *J Hypertens* 2005;**45**:198–202.

34. Ruilope LM, Salvetti A, Jamerson K *et al.* Renal function and intensive lowering of blood pressure in hypertensive participants of the Hypertension Optimal Treatment (HOT) Study. *J Am Soc Nephrol* 2001;**12**:218–25.

35. Poggio ED, Wang X, Greene T, van Lente F, Hall PM. Performance of the modification of diet in renal disease and Cockcoft-

Gault equations in the estimation of GFR in health and in chronic kidney disease. *J Am Soc Nephrol* 2005;**16**:459–66.

36. Shulman NB, Ford CE, Hall WD *et al.* prognostic value of serum creatinine and the effect of treatment of hypertension on renal function. Results from the hypertension detection and follow-up program. The Hypertension Detection and Follow-up Program Cooperative Group. *Hypertension* 1989;**13**(suppl):I80–I93.

37. Wang TJ, Gona P, Larson MG *et al.* Multiple biomarkers for the prediction of first major cardiovascular events and death. *N Engl J Med* 2006;**355**:2631–9.

70 Pulmonary hypertension

Brendan P Madden

St George's Hospital, London, UK

Introduction

Pulmonary hypertension is defined as a mean pulmonary artery pressure of greater than 25 mm Hg at rest or 30 mm Hg with exercise. The term pulmonary arterial hypertension (PAH) denotes a series of apparently unrelated disorders many of which share the histopathologic entity of plexogenic pulmonary arteriopathy (PPA). Typically in PAH the mean pulmonary capillary wedge pressure is less than 15 mm Hg.

Examples of PAH include idiopathic PAH, familial PAH and pulmonary hypertension associated with scleroderma, hepatic cirrhosis, HIV infection and Eisenmenger's syndrome. It has also been described in association with ingestion of slimming agents, e.g dexfenfluramine, and with other unusual conditions including pulmonary veno-occlusive disease and glycogen storage disorders (Box 70.1).

Pulmonary hypertension can also occur in association with cardiac and respiratory diseases. Examples of the former include left ventricular failure, chronic left atrial hypertension and mitral valve disease and of the latter chronic obstructive pulmonary disease (COPD), interstitial lung disease, disorders of pulmonary development and sleep apnea syndrome. Chronic thromboembolic pulmonary hypertension (CTEPH) affecting proximal or distal pulmonary arteries may occur for unknown cause or may be associated with thrombophilia abnormalities such as protein S and C deficiency or abnormalities in factor V. Prothrombotic states can also accompany connective tissue disorders or malignancy. In addition, pulmonary hypertension can result from other unusual conditions, e.g. lymphangioleiomyomatosis (see Box 70.1).

Idiopathic PAH was initially described by Romberg as "sclerosis of the pulmonary arteries" over 100 years ago.[1] Dresdale and colleagues termed the condition primary pulmonary hypertension some 50 years later.[2] Wood observed a reduction in pulmonary arterial pressure in response to intravenous administration of acetylcholine and suggested that a "vasoconstrictive factor" was responsible for its pathogenesis.[3] Subsequently clinical experience with vasodilator therapy was disappointing and this was consistent with reports from Wagenvoort and Wagenvoort[4] (4) and Caslin and colleagues which suggested that more extensive vascular injury and remodeling occurred in this process (Fig. 70.1).[5-7] Over the years that followed the term PAH was defined as an umbrella term to link a number of apparently different disease processes which shared similar histopathologic appearances and were associated with severe elevation in pulmonary vascular resistance (PVR). Authors described pulmonary hypertension occurring in association with ingestion of aminorex fumarate (an appetite suppressant) in Western Europe,[8] in association with connective tissue disease,[9] hepatic cirrhosis and portal hypertension[10] and with HIV infection.[11] Traditionally idiopathic PAH was described in young females although with increasing awareness, the condition is now diagnosed in patients beyond the fourth and fifth decades of life. The incidence and prevalence of idiopathic PAH are estimated to be four per million and ten per million of the population respectively. Overall, the prevalence of PAH is estimated to be in the region of 100 per million of the population. The incidence and prevalence of pulmonary hypertension in patients with cardiac and respiratory disorders are not precisely known although they are believed to be considerably higher than for PAH. PAH is associated with a poor survival and a poor quality of life. There is no cure, limited treatment options and incomplete understanding of the disease.[12,13]

Evidence-Based Cardiology, 3rd edition. Edited by S. Yusuf, J.A. Cairns, A.J. Camm, E.L. Fallen, and B.J. Gersh. © 2010 Blackwell Publishing, ISBN: 978-1-4051-5925-8.

Pulmonary arterial hypertension (PAH)
- Idiopathic PAH
- Familial PAH
- Related to:
  - Connective tissue diseases
  - HIV
  - Portal hypertension
  - Anorexigens
  - Congenital heart diseases
- Pulmonary capillary hemangiosis
- Pulmonary veno-occlusive disease
- Others (e.g. glycogen storage disease, splenectomy)

Associated with left heart disease
- Atrial or ventricular dysfunction
- Valvular disease

Associated with lung disease/hypoxemia
- COPD
- Interstitial lung diseases
- Sleep-disordered breathing
- Developmental abnormalities
- Chronic exposure to high altitude

Associated with chronic thrombotic and/or embolic disease
- Obstruction of proximal pulmonary artery
- Obstruction of distal pulmonary artery
- Non-thrombotic pulmonary emboli (e.g. tumor)

Miscellaneous
- Histiocytosis
- Lymphangioleiomyomatosis
- Sarcoidosis
- Compression of pulmonary vessels (adenopathy, tumor, mediastinal fibrosis)

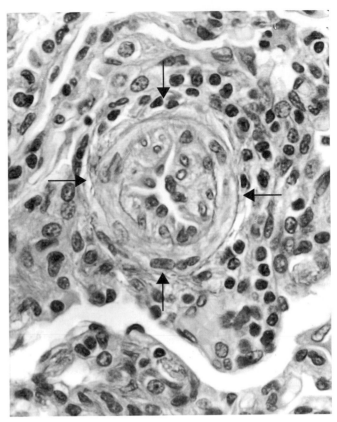

Figure 70.1 Pulmonary arteriole from a patient with PAH showing extensive reduction in vessel lumen as a consequence of smooth muscle cell migration from the inner half of the media. Once in the lumen, the cells become myofibroblasts and proliferate. Note also a surrounding inflammatory infiltrate (H&E, medium power).

Pathology

PPA occurs in a select group of disorders. It is unclear why this histopathologic entity occurs although it is possible that the lung has only a finite number of responses to injury which feed into final common pathway mechanisms. This may explain why similarities occur in patients with conditions such as obliterative bronchiolitis following lung transplantation and those with obliterative bronchiolitis associated with rheumatoid lung disease or respiratory syncytial virus infection in childhood. Similarly many conditions have been implicated as causative in the acute respiratory distress syndrome yet the pathology is similar regardless of etiology.

In PPA the pathophysiologic triggers are not clear. Following initial vasoconstriction smooth muscle migration occurs from the inner half of the media of muscular pulmonary arterioles into the vessel lumen where these cells become myofibroblasts capable of laying down either smooth muscle or fibrous tissue. Once in the lumen, the cells proliferate in a concentric fashion and ultimately obliterate the lumen (see Fig. 70.1). As this process develops the radius of the vessel lessens and in accordance with Poiseuille's law, the resistance to flow increases. When sectioned, these vessels have the appearance under the microscope of a cut onion and the process has been described as "onion skin proliferation". Interestingly, in COPD smooth muscle cells migrate into the vessel lumen but migrate in a longitudinal fashion and although reduced, there is less compromise to the radius than with PPA. At proximal points of weakness in the vessel (often at areas of branching), the vessel distends and ruptures. Hemorrhage follows and primitive blood vessels grow into this area in a haphazard or plexiform arrangement. The combination of concentric laminar intimal ("onion skin") proliferation and plexiform lesions is referred to as PPA. Some authors believe that plexiform lesions represent a type of collateral circulation.

It is not clear why these particular changes occur in diseases with such diverse etiology and clinical presentation. Immunoreactive cells in the lung for gastrin-releasing peptide and calcitonin may be important factors in the smooth muscle cell migration process.[14] Endothelial injury as a consequence of damage by toxins or genetic factors may also be important and indeed, overexpression of endothelin-1 and reduced levels of prostacyclin synthase have been noted in plexiform lesions.[15–20] There is ongoing extensive research into endothelial dysfunction in patients with PAH.

Survival

The natural history of idiopathic PAH has been described and the National Institute of Health Registry followed up 194 patients with this condition enrolled at 32 medical centers between 1981 and 1985. The median survival was 2.8 years with one-, three- and five-year survival rates of 68%, 48% and 34% respectively.[21] Indeed, actuarial five-year survival for untreated patients with PAH who are in class IV New York Heart Association (NYHA) status is significant lower than that for patients with lung, breast, prostate, colon and gastric carcinoma. The following factors are useful in predicting mortality in PAH:

- etiology
- unctional capacity (NYHA or PAH class)
- xercise capacity (unencouraged six-minute walk test)
- hemodynamics (severity of right ventricular dysfunction)
- echocardiographic parameters.

It appears that survival for patients with PAH associated with scleroderma is worse than for patients with idiopathic PAH[22] while survival for patients with PAH associated with HIV infections is similar to those patients with idiopathic PAH.[23] Interestingly, in a number of studies most deaths in patients with HIV infection and PAH were related to PAH. Patients with congenital heart disease may have a better prognosis than those with idiopathic PAH although further experience is necessary to validate this.[24]

As in adults, the prognosis in children with PAH is linked to the underlying etiology.

The incidence and prevalence of pulmonary hypertension in patients with cardiac and respiratory disorders are not precisely known but are believed to be considerably higher than for the causes of PAH. In these conditions expert medical treatment focusing on the underlying cardiac, pulmonary or hematologic abnormalities is key to the management of the co-existing pulmonary hypertension, at least in the first instance.

Higher NYHA functional class (III or IV) is associated with increased mortality in both treated and untreated patients with idiopathic PAH.[21,22,25] Failure to improve NYHA functional class or deterioration in NYHA functional class while on therapy may of itself be predictive of a poor outcome. The unencouraged six-minute walk test is an easy-to-perform and reproducible modality of assessing exercise capacity in patients with PAH and may be an independent predictor of survival for these patients. One study suggested that a six-minute walk test of less than 332 meters was associated with a significantly lower survival rate than for patients whose six-minute walk test exceeded this distance.[26]

In patients with suspected pulmonary hypertension right heart catheterization is performed to confirm the presence and severity of pulmonary hypertension and to help establish the underlying diagnosis. Furthermore, right heart catheterization is required to guide therapeutic intervention. The PVR (mm Hg/L/min) is calculated as follows:

$$\frac{\text{Mean pulmonary} \_ \text{mean pulmonary capillary}}{\text{Cardiac output}}$$
$$\frac{\text{artery pressure} \quad \text{wedge pressure}}{}$$

Echocardiography is an integral part of the evaluation of a patient with pulmonary hypertension. Common findings in patients with PAH include right atrial and right ventricular enlargement, reduced right ventricular function, paradoxic movement of the intraventricular septum and tricuspid regurgitation (Fig. 70.2). The presence of a pericardial effusion seems to be associated with a poorer prognosis.[27] Another indicator of an adverse outcome is an elevated Doppler echocardiography right ventricular index.[28]

Correlation between estimated pulmonary artery systolic pressure on echocardiography and at right heart catheterization is not always close. Echocardiographic measurements are usually dependent on assessment of the tricuspid regurgitant velocity and errors with this measurement and with subsequent formulae employed often contribute to inaccuracy.

Quality of life

Patients with PAH have similar quality of life scores when compared with those for patients with COPD and with end-stage renal failure.

Natural history

Early on in the course of their illness, patients with PAH may be asymptomatic or experience dyspnea with exertion. In the early stages of the disease the non-specific nature of the symptoms may lead to either failure of diagnosis or incorrect diagnosis. Many patients have had their symptoms attributed to depression. As the condition

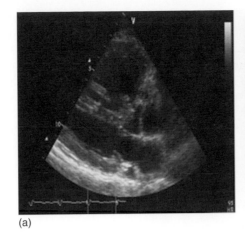
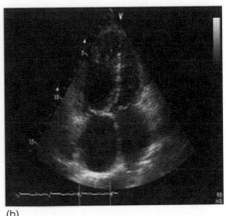

(a) (b)

Figure 70.2 Two-dimensional echocardiography from a patient with PAH showing right ventricular enlargement and paradoxic encroachment of the intraventricular septum from the right ventricle into the left ventricle. (a) parasternal long axis view. (b) Apical four-chamber view.

progresses, the PVR rises and the cardiac output falls. At this stage patients may change from having relatively few symptoms to experiencing dyspnea, palpitations, chest pain (right ventricular angina), presyncope or syncope. Initially these symptoms may occur with exertion and subsequently at rest. As the condition progresses further peripheral edema, ascites, plethora and more profound fatigue develop as right ventricular dysfunction and tricuspid regurgitation evolve. Ultimately right heart failure and death occur.[12]

Disease progression and response to therapy can be functionally assessed using the World Health Organization classification of functional capacity which is an adaptation of the NYHA system (Table 70.1).

Diagnosis

Since PAH can occur in association with other conditions, symptomatic evidence of a related illness should be considered. For example, orthopnea and paroxysmal nocturnal dyspnea suggest elevated pulmonary venous pressure and pulmonary congestion due to left-sided heart disease or pulmonary veno-occlusive disease. Features such as Raynaud's phenomenon or arthralgias or rash may suggest the possibility of an underlying connective tissue disease. Other lung diseases such as lung fibrosis, COPD and obstructive sleep apnea can be associated with pulmonary hypertension and will need to be assessed and potentially treated in addition to the primary lung disease. One should also exclude pulmonary thromboembolic disease by performing either a ventilation/perfusion (V/Q) or computed tomographic pulmonary angiography (CTPA) scan (Fig. 70.3) or pulmonary angiography. For many patients with pulmonary hypertension associated with other conditions, treatment of the primary condition will significantly improve their pulmonary hypertension.

Table 70.1 WHO classification of functional status of patients with pulmonary hypertension (PH)*

Class	Description
I	Patients with PH in whom there is no limitation of usual physical activity; ordinary physical activity does not cause increased dyspnea, fatigue, chest pain or presyncope
II	Patients with PH who have mild limitation of physical activity. There is no discomfort at rest, but normal physical activity causes increased dyspnea, fatigue, chest pain or presyncope
III	Patients with PH who have a marked limitation of physical activity. There is no discomfort at rest, but less than ordinary activity causes increased dyspnea, fatigue, chest pain or presyncope
IV	Patients with PH who are unable to perform any physical activity and who have signs of right ventricular failure. Dyspnea and/or fatigue may be present at rest, and symptoms are increased by almost any physical activity

* Rich S. *Primary Pulmonary Hypertension: Executive Summary*. Evian, France: World Health Organisation, 1998.

Physical examination

The clinical features of pulmonary hypertension can be subtle and may be missed on physical examination. Important features to identify are a loud pulmonary component to the secondary heart sound which reflects increased force of pulmonary valve closure secondary to elevated pulmonary artery pressure. Other auscultatory abnormalities include an early systolic ejection click due to sudden inter-

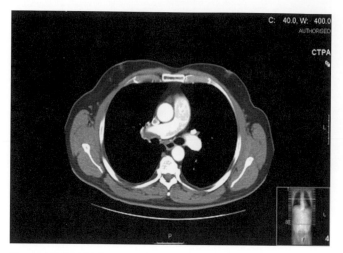

Figure 70.3 CTPA from a patient with pulmonary hypertension associated with pulmonary thromboembolic disease.

ruption of pulmonary valve opening, a midsystolic ejection murmur caused by turbulent transvalvular pulmonary flow and a right ventricular fourth heart sound. Additional features include a palpable left parasternal lift as a consequence of right ventricular hypertrophy and a prominent jugular "a" wave which suggests high right ventricular filling pressures. As the condition develops further a diastolic murmur of pulmonary regurgitation may be noted together with a pansystolic murmur of tricuspid regurgitation. Tricuspid regurgitation may also be detected by inspection of the neck demonstrating an elevated jugular venous pressure with accentuated V waves, a hepatojugular reflux and a pulsatile liver. Right ventricular failure is associated with a right ventricular third heart sound, distension of the jugular veins, pulsatile hepatomegaly, ascites and peripheral edema. As the disease progresses hypotension and poor peripheral perfusion indicate significant reduction of cardiac output with elevated peripheral vascular resistance. Cyanosis is noted in 20% of patients with idiopathic PAH; clubbing is rare.[12] Other cardiac and respiratory abnormalities may give further clues to other diagnoses and in particular, one must exclude CTEPH and potential underlying causes of this condition.

Routine investigations

In addition to routine hematologic and biochemical indices (full blood count, urea, creatinine and electrolytes, liver function test), one should screen for autoimmune diseases and clotting abnormalities and check arterial blood gas analysis on room air. Genetic screening is also important. A chest X-ray may show enlarged main and hilar pulmonary arteries, peripheral pruning of pulmonary vessels and cardiomegaly of right ventricular configuration. ECG may

be normal, may identify right axis deviation and right ventricular strain or show evidence of right atrial or right ventricular hypertrophy or arrhythmias. Two-dimensional echocardiography can provide useful information of right and left heart function and valvular abnormalities and can provide an estimate of the pulmonary artery systolic pressure. Ventilation perfusion and CTPA scanning can help exclude CTEPH and right heart catheterization can help confirm the presence of pulmonary hypertension and provide important information as to its origin. Full lung function tests may be normal or show abnormalities consistent with other diagnoses, e.g. low transfer factor for patients with lung fibrosis, left heart failure or CTEPH.

Evidence for diagnostic tests in patients with suspected pulmonary arterial hypertension

As PAH is a relatively rare condition, the literature is lacking in large series of appropriately conducted clinical trials which help establish firm guidelines for diagnosis and treatment. Furthermore, there is no effective cure and many treatments available will at best reduce the rate of deterioration of the illness and improve quality of life. Additionally, there is an important cost implication, particularly for long-term use of prostanoids and endothelin receptor antagonists. Therapies such as lung transplantation are limited by donor organ availability. Finally PAH represents a series of diverse conditions which interface at the level of the pulmonary circulation. Efforts to rationalize diagnostic modalities and treatment options are clearly difficult.

As a consequence, a number of expert consensus group meetings were organized to obtain broad agreement as to how patients with PAH should be diagnosed and treated.[13] What is reported in this chapter represents a distillation of current international opinion. Often such expert opinion is based on clinical experience in conjunction with results obtained from clinical trials. Many of these trials provide encouraging results but may be criticized because of design, duration and relatively small numbers of patients. In the light of early results further prospective trials are under way. It should also be stressed that there are currently no firm data based on properly constructed clinical trials to advocate specific management strategies for patients whose pulmonary hypertension is associated with primary cardiac and pulmonary diseases.

Consensus of opinion recommends that for patients with suspected PAH routine hematologic and biochemical investigations be performed and that autoimmune profile and HIV status is assessed (**Class I**). Chest X-ray is considered routine as is 12-lead ECG. Doppler echocardiography is a good screening tool to detect PAH (**Class I**) and is useful at assessing morphology and abnormalities and in estimating right ventricular and pulmonary arterial systolic pressures (**Class IIa**), to assess left ventricular function (**Class I**) and (with contrast) intracardiac shunting (**Class IIa**).

V/Q scan or CT pulmonary angiography is recommended to exclude chronic pulmonary thromboembolic disease (**Class IIa**) and pulmonary angiography is advocated prior to considering pulmonary thromboendarterectomy (**Class I**). Lung function tests and arterial blood gas analysis are routinely performed (**Class IIa**). Estimate of gas transfer is useful in patients with PAH and scleroderma (**Class IIa**) and chronic pulmonary thromboembolism (**Class IIa**). Lung biopsy is not routinely advocated (**Class I**). Right heart catheter (Box 70.2) is required to confirm the presence of pulmonary hypertension, establish the specific diagnosis and determine its severity (**Class I**) and also to help guide treatment (**Class IIa**). Genetic testing and counseling should be offered to patients with familial PAH (**Class I**) and patients with idiopathic PAH should be

advised of the availability of genetic counseling and testing for their relatives (**Class I**).[13]

Genetic aspects

Disease-causing mutations in bone morphogenetic protein receptor II (BMPR2) may underlie familial PAH.[29,30] Mutations have been detected in 55%[29] of families and show autosomal dominance with incomplete penetrance. Thus far up to 26% of sporadic cases (idiopathic PAH) have BMPR2 mutations.[30] Bone morphogenetic proteins are a family of secreted growth factors. BMPR2 regulates cell proliferation in response to ligand binding. Mutations in either BMPR2 or downstream ligand binding or activation lead to a loss of the inhibitory action of bone morphogenetic protein on vascular smooth muscle cell growth. As a consequence of this lack of inhibition, inappropriate cellular proliferation can occur and this may be important in the vascular remodeling that develops in PAH.

Current theories on the pathophysiology of pulmonary arterial hypertension

Patients may have a genetic predisposition (e.g. BMPR2 mutation) or have a risk factor such as autoimmune disease or HIV which can facilitate vascular injury. When vascular injury occurs endothelial cell dysfunction follows, giving rise to loss of regulation of local vasomotor tone, inflammation, smooth muscle migration and *in situ* thrombosis. As a consequence, vascular remodeling ensues, disease progression occurs, the PVR rises and cardiac output falls (Fig. 70.4). It should be stressed that the precise

---

BOX 70.2 Right heart catheter from a patient with idiopathic PAH

RA mean	14 mm Hg
RV	80 mm Hg
EDP	15 mm Hg
PA	80/14 mm Hg, mean 36 mm Hg
PCWP mean	12 mm Hg
Cardiac output mean	3 L/min
PVR	12 Wood units

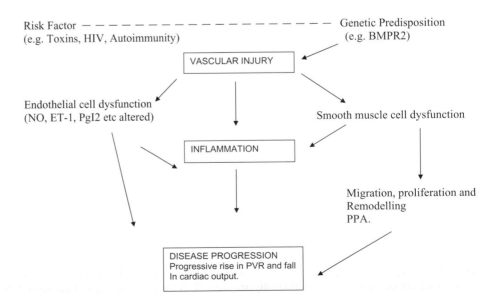

Figure 70.4 Factors involved in the pathogenesis of PAH.

mechanisms underpinning the pathogenesis of PAH are not fully understood.

Therapeutic targets

Abnormalities in endothelial function with respect to vasoreactivity, intimal proliferation and thrombus formation are believed to be important in the pathogenesis of PAH. Increasing attention has been given to endothelin-1 which is a potent vasoconstrictor and smooth muscle mitogen that may contribute to the vascular remodeling and increased PVR seen in PAH.[15–18] Elevated endothelin-1 production expression and concentration in plasma and in plexiform lesions are demonstrated in patients with PAH.[15–19] There are two distinct endothelin receptor isoforms, namely ET_A and ET_B.[31] When the ET_A receptor is activated vasoconstriction and vascular smooth muscle cell proliferation are facilitated. ET_B receptors are believed to be involved in endothelin clearance, particularly in the pulmonary and renal vascular beds, and they may also be involved in causing vasodilation and nitric oxide release.[31] At present it is unclear whether it is preferable to block both ET_A and ET_B receptors (with agents such as bosentan) or to primarily target the ET_A receptor alone (e.g. with agents such as sitaxsentan). Both bosentan and sitaxsentan have undergone randomied and controlled clinical trials in patients with PAH.[32–36]

Prostacyclin is a metabolite of arachidonic acid produced primarily in vascular endothelium. It is a potent vasodilator of both the pulmonary and systemic circulation and also has important antiplatelet aggregatory effects. There is evidence suggesting that a relative deficiency of prostacyclin may contribute to the pathogenesis of PAH. As a consequence there would be reduced local vasodilation and a tendency to platelet aggregation and it is known that PAH is associated with the presence of *in situ* thromboses. Prostacyclin acts by increasing cyclic adenosine monophosphate (cAMP) and in addition to potentiating vasodilation, it may be antiproliferative. Clinical studies have suggested benefit from long-term treatment with exogenous prostacyclin analogs by intravenous,[37] nebulised[38,39] or subcutaneous[40] administration.

Nitric oxide (NO) acts via cyclic guanosine 3′ 5′ monophosphate (cGMP) to promote vasodilation and it too may be antiproliferative. It is an important local regulator of vascular function and structure.[41,42] NO is generated by three isoforms of nitric oxide synthase (NOS) which are present in multiple and differing cell types. They are continuously active (constitutive types I and III) in endothelium or inducible (type II) in other cells such as macrophages, bronchial epithelium and vascular smooth muscle. L-arginine is the sole substrate for NOS and the regulation of NOS is multifactorial and is influenced by growth factors,

hormones, oxygen tension and hemodynamics, among others. In the endothelium arginine reaches the interior of the cell by active transport[43] and in the endothelium this transporter is tightly co-localized with NOS.[44] If this linkage were to be disrupted by endothelial injury normal extracellular levels might become insufficient for NO generation and as a consequence, NO deficiency may occur. Indeed, arginine deficiency has been shown to accompany persistent pulmonary hypertension of the newborn[45] and acute L-arginine infusion in infants with this condition has been shown to favorably improve PaO_2 levels.[46] When it became clear that NO production from L-arginine is the endothelium-derived relaxation factor,[47] inhaled NO was found to have a role in the management of a number of different types of conditions associated with pulmonary hypertension.[48]

The vasodilator effects of NO are dependent on its ability to augment and sustain cGMP content in vascular smooth muscle. Once produced, NO directly activates soluble guanylate cyclase. This leads to an increase in cGMP production which activates cGMP kinase which in turn opens potassium channels and promotes vasorelaxation. The effects of intracellular cGMP are transient as it is rapidly degraded by phosphodiesterases.[49,50] These latter enzymes hydrolyze cAMP and cGMP and limit their intracellular signaling properties by generating the inactive products 5′cAMP and 5′GMP. There are at least five classes of phosphodiesterase enzymes in the human body and the highest concentration of phosphodiesterase type V is in the lung and urologic tract. As a consequence, agents which selectively inhibit phosphodiesterase type V pathways should augment pulmonary vasodilation by potentiating the effects of endogenous or inhaled NO.[51] Sildenafil, which is a potent and highly specific phosphodiesterase type V inhibitor, may be useful for selected patients with pulmonary hypertension.[52–57]

A summary of the mechanism of action of prostaglandins, nitric oxide, phosphodiesterase V inhibitors and endothelin receptor antagonists is outlined in Figure 70.5.

Therapeutic options

Current drugs available have improved quality of life and prolonged survival for some patients with PAH. Therapies can be classified into medical and surgical. Examples of medical therapies include:
- supplemental oxygen
- diuretics
- digoxin
- inotropes
- anticoagulants
- calcium channel blockers

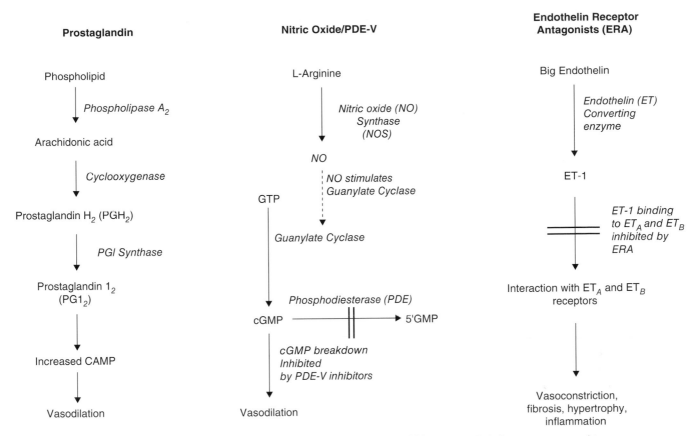

Figure 70.5 Mechanism of action of prostaglandins, nitric oxide, phosphodiesterase V inhibitors and endothelin receptor antagonists.

- angiotensin-converting enzyme inhibitors or receptor blockers
- prostanoids
- L-arginine
- endothelin receptor antagonists
- phosphodiesterase inhibitors
- nitric oxide.

Surgical therapies include:

- atrial septostomy
- bilateral lung or heart and lung transplantation
- pulmonary thromboendarterectomy.

What defines acute vasoreactivity is controversial. An agent such as NO is administered at the time of right heart catheterization. Initially a positive response was defined as a 30% reduction in PVR with a corresponding increase in cardiac output. More recently, it has been defined as a reduction in mean pulmonary artery pressure close to or indeed to normal values with a documented increase in or an unchanged cardiac output. The European Society of Cardiology defined a positive vasodilator response as a fall of mean pulmonary artery pressure of at least 10 mm Hg to less than or equivalent to 40 mm Hg with an increased or unchanged cardiac output. Patients with idiopathic PAH who demonstrate an acute vasodilator response have an

---

BOX 70.3 Current approach to management of patients with pulmonary hypertension (**Class I**)

Step 1. Fully evaluate the patient; assess whether he or she has PAH or pulmonary hypertension associated with other conditions.

Step 2. Refer patients with an underlying cause to an appropriate specialist, e.g. cardiologist and cardiothoracic surgeon for patients who have pulmonary hypertension associated with mitral valve disease.

Step 3. If the patient has PAH and is in functional classes II, III or IV consider general measures such as anticoagulants (**Class IIa**), diuretics (**Class IIa**), oxygen (as necessary to maintain saturations over 90%) (**Class I**) and digoxin (**Class IIa**). These patients should be managed in centers specializing in diagnosing and treating patients with PAH (**Class I**).

Step 4. If the patient has PAH perform right heart catheter and assess for acute vasoreactivity (**Class I**). The usefulness of acute vasoreactivity in patients with scleroderma or congenital heart disease is less clear (**Class IIb**).

improved survival with long-term use of a calcium channel blocker (**Class IIa**). In practice, however, only a minority of patients with PAH (less than 10%) will respond to oral calcium channel-blocking agents. These patients will require long-term follow-up to assess whether their response is sustained. If not, further treatments may be required. Calcium channel blockers should not be used to treat patients with PAH unless acute vasoreactivity has been demonstrated (**Class I**).

Those patients who are in functional class III who have failed or who are not candidates for calcium channel blockers should be treated with endothelin receptor antagonists (**Class I, Level C1**) or chronic IV epoprostenol (**Class I, Level C1**) or prostonoid analogs (subcutaneous treprostinil, inhaled iloprost or oral beraprost (**Class IIa**) or phosphodiesterase V inhibitors (e.g. sildenafil (**Class I**)). Combination of agents may be necessary. Patients who are in functional class IV are also treated with these agents. In addition, patients in functional class III or IV should be referred to a transplant center for work-up (**Class I**). Atrial septostomy has been used (**Class IIb, Level C2**) to palliate patients with advanced PAH due to its potential to decompress the failing right ventricle and to improve cardiac index.[58] Some patients who have CTEPH may be candidates for pulmonary thromboendarterectomy (**Class I, Level C1**)[59] and others may be suitable for lung transplantation. However, shortage of donor organs and the late complication of obliterative bronchiolitis are limiting factors (**Class I, Level C1**).[60]

The management of PAH is complex and requires multidisciplinary input from physicians, surgeons, nurse specialists, physiotherapists, dieticians and pharmacists in a specialized environment. Additionally, the management of pulmonary hypertension associated with cardiac and pulmonary disease and thrombotic conditions requires management by a multidisciplinary team of many specialists interfacing at the level of the pulmonary circulation. There are no specific guidelines to manage patients with pulmonary hypertension secondary to cardiac and lung diseases. Information is available from non-randomized, non-controlled studies on small numbers of patients.

A number of emerging therapies are being considered in the management of PAH but evidence is at present inconclusive and many studies are currently at an early stage of development and recruitment. In the rat hypoxic model sustained vasoconstriction and increased vasoreactivity are influenced by rho-kinase mediated calcium sensitization.[61] When such animals are treated with the rho-kinase inhibitor fasudil a reduction in pulmonary artery pressure is observed.[62] In a small clinical trial intravenous fasudil was associated with a slight reduction in mean pulmonary artery pressure together with an increase in cardiac index in nine patients with severe PAH although the results did not attain statistical significance. There was, however, a significant decrease in PVR.[63] It is possible that the benefit of phosphodiesterase type V inhibitors could in part be mediated by rho-kinase inhibition.[64,65]

Platelet-derived growth factor (PDGF) may be important in endothelial cell dysfunction and vascular remodeling in patients with PAH. Interestingly, chronic myeloproliferative disorders such as myelofibrosis are associated with a high incidence of PAH,[66] suggesting an association between PAH and marrow fibrosis.[67] Imatinib is a PDGF receptor antagonist which has obtained approval to treat patients with chronic myeloid leukemia and recently this agent has been used for selected patients with PAH. There are some case reports suggesting that imatinib may be efficient in managing patients with severe PAH[68] although cardiac toxicity is an important long-term concern which may limit its use.[69]

Simvastatin may improve BMPR type II signaling in pulmonary artery smooth muscle and microvascular endothelial cells.[70] In theory, therefore, simvastatin may enhance endothelial function. It may also be effective in inducing apoptosis in plexiform lesions and areas of vascular remodeling.[71] A study demonstrated an improvement in six-minute walk in 16 patients receiving between 20 mg and 80 mg of simvastatin daily.[72] Other potential treatments include ghrelin, an endogenous vasodilator peptide which can also stimulate growth hormone release,[73] and bradykinin which may modulate endothelial function and also potentially induce apoptosis via local nitric oxide and prostacyclin synthesis.[74] Other compounds being explored include vasoactive intestinal peptide (which can promote bronchodilation and systemic and pulmonary vasodilation[75]) which has produced some benefit in patients with PAH when administered as an aerosol.[76] Interestingly, vasoactive intestinal peptide may be reduced in the lung parenchyma and serum of patients with PAH.[76] There is increased lung expression of the 5-hydroxy tryptamine transporter in patients with PAH. This transporter may be involved in the development of PAH by facilitating smooth muscle migration.[77] Fluoxetine is a selective 5-hydroxy tryptamine transporter inhibitor and this agent has been shown to have a beneficial effect on PAH in the monocrotaline animal model.[78] This transporter promotes smooth muscle cell proliferation and demonstrates increased pulmonary expression in patients with PAH. There is also interest in clarifying the role of voltage-gated potassium channels in the pathogenesis of PAH.[79]

Special circumstances

Children

Treatment for children with severe PAH is similar to that for adults with idiopathic PAH (**Class IIa**). Indeed, although there are limited data, children with severe PAH treated with long-term epoprostenol infusions appear to have at least as good a response as seen with adults with idiopathic PAH.[80] Diagnostic evaluation for pediatric patients is similar to that for adults and in addition acute vasoreactivity is assessed during cardiac catheterization to determine whether some patients may respond to long-term oral calcium channel-blocking agents (**Class I**).

Although treatment regimes are similar for adult and pediatric patients, the doses per kilogram for many of the medications used (e.g. epoprostenol and calcium channel blockers) are often significantly greater for children. Anticoagulants such as warfarin are typically prescribed for children with right heart failure or for those who have a hypercoagulable state (**Class IIa**). Line-related complications appear to be more frequently encountered in younger children than adults. The pharmacokinetics, safety and response to bosentan in the pediatric population have been reported[81] but specific information with regard to pediatric response to prostanoids is lacking in the medical literature.

Neonatal patients with severe PAH are much more responsive than adults to inhaled nitric oxide and multicenter randomized controlled trials have demonstrated benefit with low-dose inhaled NO in the treatment of term newborns with persistent pulmonary hypertension (**Class I, Level A**).[82] Experience with type V phosphodiesterase inhibitors such as dipyridamole or sildenafil is limited in children to small series and anecdotes (**Class IIb, Level C2**).[83]

Pregnancy

Many patients with idiopathic PAH are women of childbearing age. During pregnancy significant physiologic change occurs with increasing blood volume of between 30% and 50% and a corresponding increase in cardiac output, heart rate (10–20 beats/min), stroke volume and a reduction in systemic blood pressure and vascular resistance. These changes commence during the first trimester and are maximal between 20 and 24 weeks of gestation. Further increases in cardiac output occur during labor and blood pressure increases with uterine contractions. Immediately following delivery cardiac filling pressures increase markedly as a consequence of decompression of the vena cava and return of uterine blood into the systemic circulation. It takes approximately six weeks after delivery for the hemodynamic changes associated with pregnancy to normalize.

Not surprisingly, such circulatory changes present a significant risk and mortality rates between 30% and 50% have been described for pregnant women with idiopathic PAH.[84,85] As a consequence many doctors recommend effective contraception and some advocate early fetal termination.[86]

Aside from hemodynamic issues, hormonal influences may be important adverse factors. There are some reports of mothers who successfully delivered a term infant whose pulmonary hypertension progressed during pregnancy and deteriorated further after delivery. There is also some evidence suggesting an increased incidence of children born with congenital anomalies and born small for gestational age to mothers with idiopathic PAH.

Treatment of PAH in pregnancy is anecdotal. Some encouraging reports have been described using long-term IV epoprostenol,[87] inhaled NO[88] and oral calcium channel blockers.[89] It is believed, however, that such reports are insufficient at present to establish recommendations for the management of PAH during pregnancy. Normally women with PAH are admitted to hospital for monitoring, supportive therapy with appropriate fluid regimes, oxygen, diuretics and perhaps inotropic support if required. It is usually advocated to deploy a pulmonary artery catheter during labor or in cases of deterioration during gestation. This helps not only to provide a fuller picture of the hemodynamic situation but also to guide appropriate therapy.

The optimum mode of delivery for women with PAH is controversial. Normal delivery as opposed to caesarean section may be preferred.[90]

Current guidelines from the American Heart Association and the American College of Cardiology advocate that pregnancy be avoided or terminated in women with cyanotic congenital heart disease, pulmonary hypertension and Eisenmenger's syndrome (**Class I, Level C2**). Maternal mortality may be as high as 36% in Eisenmenger's syndrome, 30% in idiopathic PAH and 56% in pulmonary hypertension secondary to other conditions.[85]

Endothelin receptor antagonists are not recommended during pregnancy (**Class I**).

Portopulmonary hypertension

Patients with chronic late-stage liver disease have an increased prevalence of pulmonary hypertension when compared to the normal population.[91,92] The reason behind this is not clear. Two forms of pulmonary vascular disease have been described in patients with chronic liver disease: the hepatopulmonary syndrome and portopulmonary hypertension. Usually these present independently although occasionally features suggestive of both conditions have been described in a single patient. Both conditions can increase the risks attendant on liver transplantation.

Typical features of the hepatopulmonary syndrome are hypoxia (with low oxygen saturation on room air and failure to appropriately increase oxygen saturation with supplemental oxygen) and intrapulmonary shunting. Other features include orthodeoxia (lower oxygen saturation in the standing position as opposed to lying supine). Treatment is supportive with supplemental oxygen and in some patients improvement has been noted following successful liver transplantation. Although the histologic appearance of PPA has been described in patients with portopulmonary hypertension, the mechanisms for this are unclear. Some theories suggest that an inability of the liver to detoxify potentially toxic metabolites is causative.

Some differences have been described between portopulmonary hypertension and the clinical presentation of idiopathic PAH. In the former condition, the pulmonary arterial diastolic and mean pressures and systemic and pulmonary vascular resistances seem to be lower and cardiac output higher.[93] As the disease progresses the hemodynamic features approximate to those of idiopathic PAH. Full work-up is of course mandatory for any of these patients to ensure that other disease processes are not contributory (**Class I**).

Data on the treatment of portopulmonary hypertension are limited. This condition can significantly increase the risks attendant on liver transplantation. Current treatment advocates supplemental oxygen and diuretic therapy (**Class IIa**). Anticoagulants should normally be avoided, particularly if patients have significant clotting disturbances and gastroesophageal varices (**Class I**). Acute vasoreactivity testing should be determined as some patients may respond to calcium channel blockers (**Class I**). The dose of calcium channel blockers should be kept as low as possible as higher doses may precipitate liver failure. As with idiopathic PAH, failure to respond acutely to IV epoprostenol does not necessarily predict a failure to respond to this agent when it is administered by long-term IV infusion. Some patients may demonstrate an improvement in pulmonary hemodynamics following liver transplantation[94] although for other patients worsening of pulmonary hypertension after hepatic transplantation has been described. It is therefore very important not to wean patients off pulmonary vasodilator therapy until careful evaluation of their pulmonary hemodynamics has been made.

As endothelin receptor antagonists can cause hepatic toxicity, their use is generally avoided in patients with pulmonary hypertension associated with liver disease (**Class I**).

HIV disease

There is an increased incidence of PAH in patients with HIV although the precise relationship between these two conditions is not clear.[95] The clinical hemodynamic and histologic findings of pulmonary hypertension accompanying HIV infection are similar to that found in patients with idiopathic PAH. Virus and viral DNA is absent in pulmonary endothelial cells[96] and perhaps an indirect action of the virus through second messengers including cytokines and growth factors[97] or endothelin[98] is important. Since the condition only affects a minority of HIV-infected patients genetic factors may also be important.

Currently, uncontrolled studies suggest that patients with severe PAH associated with HIV infection should be considered for long-term infusion of epoprostenol together with combination antiretroviral therapy (**Class IIa, Level C2**). Further experience with other agents used in the management of patients with PAH is awaited before recommendations can be made on the application of these therapies to patients with HIV infection and pulmonary hypertension. Lung transplantation is usually contraindicated for this patient group (**Class I**).

Conclusion

PAH is a progressive and lethal disease whose initial symptoms can be non-specific. A comprehensive diagnostic approach is essential to identify associated medical conditions and to characterize hemodynamics and functional profiles. Although at present there is no cure for PAH, many of the agents currently employed are associated with an improvement in survival and quality of life. It is hoped that by increasing awareness and understanding of disease mechanisms, the development of more effective treatment modalities will be facilitated.

Interestingly, many of the lessons learned from PAH are being applied to patients with other forms of pulmonary hypertension. This not only helps to facilitate diagnostic awareness and physician training but has led to the successful application of a variety of drugs currently employed in the management of PAH to patients with pulmonary hypertension associated with cardiac, respiratory and thromboembolic disease.

References

1. Romberg E. Ueber sklerose der lungen arterie. *Dsch Arc Klin Med* 1891;**48**:197–206.
2. Dresdale DT, Schultz M, Michtom RJ. Primary pulmonary hypertension: 1. Clinical and hemodynamic study. *Am J Med* 1951;**11**:686–705.
3. Wood P. Pulmonary hypertension with special reference to the vasoconstrictive factor. *Br Heart J* 1958;**21**:557–70.
4. Wagenvoort CA, Wagenvoort H. Primary pulmonary hypertension: a pathologic study of the lung vessels in 156 classically diagnosed cases. *Circulation* 1970;**42**:1163–84.
5. Caslin AW, Heath D, Madden B, Yacoub M, Gosney JR, Smith P. The histopathology of 36 cases of plexogenic pulmonary arteriopathy. *Histopathology* 1990;**16**:9–19.
6. Smith P, Heath D, Yacoub M, Madden B, Caslin A, Gosney J. The ultra structure of plexogenic pulmonary arteriopathy. *J Pathol* 1990;**160**:111–21.
7. Madden B, Gosney J, Coghlan J *et al*. Pre-transplant clinicopathological correlation in end-stage primary pulmonary hypertension. *Eur Respir J* 1994;**7**:672–8.

8. Gurtner HP. Pulmonary hypertension, "plexogenic pulmonary arteriopathy" and the appetite depressant drug aminorex: post or propter? *Bull Eur Pathophysiol Resp* 1979;**15**:897–923.

9. Battle RW, Davitt MA, Cooper SM *et al.* Prevalence of pulmonary hypertension in limited and diffuse scleroderma. *Chest* 1996;**110**:1515–19.

10. Hadengue A, Benhayoun MK, Lebrec D *et al.* Pulmonary hypertension complicating portal hypertension: prevalence and relation to splanchnic haemodynamics. *Gastroenterology* 1991;**100**:520–8.

11. Petitpretz P, Brenot F, Azarian R *et al.* Pulmonary hypertension in patients with human immunodeficiency virus infection: comparison with primary pulmonary hypertension. *Circulation* 1994;**89**:2722–7.

12. Rich S, Dantzker DR, Ayres SM *et al.* Primary pulmonary hypertension: a national prospective study. *Ann Intern Med* 1987;**107**:216–23.

13. Rubin LJ, Abman S, Ahearn G *et al.* Diagnosis and management of pulmonary arterial hypertension: ACCP evidence based clinical practice guidelines. *Chest* 2004;**126**(1):S1–S92.

14. Heath D, Yacoub M, Gosney J, Madden B, Caslin A, Smith P. Pulmonary endocrine cells in hypertensive pulmonary vascular disease. *Histopathology* 1990;**16**:21–8.

15. MacLean MR. Endothelin-1: a mediator of pulmonary hypertension? *Pulm Pharmacol Ther* 1998;**11**:125–32.

16. Kim H, Yung GL, Marsh JJ *et al.* Endothelin mediates pulmonary vascular remodelling in a canine model of chronic embolic pulmonary hypertension. *Eur Respir J* 2000;**15**:640–8.

17. Yamane K. Endothelin and collagen vascular disease: a review with special reference to Raynaud's phenomenon and systemic sclerosis. *Intern Med* 1994;**33**:579–82.

18. Giaid A, Yanagisawa M, Langleben D *et al.* Expression of endothelin-1 in the lungs of patients with pulmonary hypertension. *N Engl J Med* 1993;**328**:1732–9.

19. Christman BW, McPherson CD, Newman JH *et al.* An imbalance between the excretion of thromboxane and prostacyclin metabolites in pulmonary hypertension. *N Engl J Med* 1992;**327**:70–5.

20. Tuder RM, Cool CD, Geraci MW *et al.* Prostacyclin synthase expression is decreased in lungs from patients with severe pulmonary hypertension. *Am J Respir Crit Care Med* 1999;**159**:1925–32.

21. D'Alonzo GE, Barst RJ, Ayres SM *et al.* Survival in patients with primary pulmonary hypertension: results from a national prospective registry. *Ann Intern Med* 1991;**115**:343–9.

22. Kuhn KP, Byrne DW, Arbogast PG *et al.* Outcome in 91 consecutive patients with pulmonary arterial hypertension receiving epoprostenol. *Am J Respir Crit Care Med* 2003;**167**:580–6.

23. Opravil M, Pechere M, Speich R *et al.* HIV-associated primary pulmonary hypertension: a case control study; Swiss HIV Cohort Study. *Am J Respir Crit Care Med* 1997;**155**:990–5.

24. Hopkins WE, Ochoa LL, Richardson GW *et al.* Comparison of the haemodynamics and survival of adults with severe primary pulmonary hypertension or Eisenmenger syndrome. *J Heart Lung Transplant* 1996;**15**:100–5.

25. Higenbottam T, Butt AY, McMahon A *et al.* Long term intravenous prostaglandin (epoprostenol or iloprost) for treatment of severe pulmonary hypertension. *Heart* 1998;**80**:151–5.

26. Miyamoto S, Nagaya N, Satoh T *et al.* Clinical correlates and prognostic significance of six-minute walk test in patients with primary pulmonary hypertension: comparison with cardiopulmonary exercise testing. *Am J Respir Crit Care Med* 2000;**161**:487–92.

27. Hinderliter AL, Willis PW 4th, Long W *et al.* Frequency and prognostic significance of pericardial effusion in primary pulmonary hypertension. PPH Study Group. *Am J Cardiol* 1999;**84**:481–484, A10.

28. Yeo TC, Dujardin KS, Tei C *et al.* Value of a doppler derived index combining systolic and diastolic time intervals in predicting outcome in primary pulmonary hypertension. *Am J Cardiol* 1998;**81**:1157–61.

29. Machado RD, Pauciulo MW, Thomson JR *et al.* BMPR2 haploinsufficiency as the inherited molecular mechanism for primary pulmonary hypertension. *Am J Hum Genet* 2001;**68**:92–102.

30. Thompson JR, Machado RD, Pauciulo MW *et al.* Sporadic primary pulmonary hypertension is associated with germline mutations of the gene encoding BMPR-II, a receptor member of the TGF-β family. *J Med Genet* 2000;**37**:741–5.

31. Benigni A, Remuzzi G. Endothelin antagonists. *Lancet* 1999;**353**:133–8.

32. Channick RN, Simonneau G, Sitbon O *et al.* Effects of the dual endothelin-receptor antagonist Bosentan in patients with pulmonary hypertension: a randomised placebo-controlled study. *Lancet* 2001;**358**:1119–23.

33. Rubin LJ, Badesch DB, Barst RJ, Galie N *et al.* Bosentan therapy for pulmonary arterial hypertension. *N Engl J Med* 2002;**346**:896–903.

34. Galie N, Rubin LJ, Hoeper M *et al.* Treatment of patients with mildly symptomatic pulmonary arterial hypertension with bosentan (EARLY study): a double blind, randomised controlled trial. *Lancet* 2008;**371**:2093–100.

35. Barst RJ, Langleben D, Frost A *et al.* Sitaxsentan therapy for pulmonary arterial hypertension. *Am J Respir Crit Care Med* 2004;**169**:441–7.

36. Barst RJ, Langleben D, Badesch D *et al.* Treatment of pulmonary arterial hypertension with the selective endothelin-A receptor antagonist sitaxsentan. *J Am Coll Cardiol* 2006;**47**:2049–56.

37. Barst RJ, Rubin LJ, Long WA *et al.* A comparison of continuous intravenous epoprostenol (prostacyclin) with conventional therapy for primary pulmonary hypertension. The Primary Pulmonary Hypertension Study Group. *N Engl J Med* 1996;**334**:296–302.

38. Olschewski H, Ghofrani HA, Schmehl T *et al.* Inhaled Iloprost to treat severe pulmonary hypertension: an uncontrolled trial. German PPH Study Group. *Ann Intern Med* 2000;**132**:435–43.

39. Olschewski H, Simonneau G, Galie N *et al* for the AIR Study Group. Inhaled iloprost in severe pulmonary hypertension. *N Engl J Med* 2002;**347**:322–9.

40. Simonneau G, Barst RJ, Galie N *et al.* Continuous subcutaneous infusion of Treprostinil, a prostacyclin analogue, in patients with pulmonary arterial hypertension: a double blind, randomized, placebo-controlled trial. *Am J Respir Crit Care Med* 2002;**165**:800–4.

41. Moncada S, Palmer RM, Higgs EA. Nitric oxide: physiology, pathophysiology and pharmacology. *Pharmacol Rev* 1991;**43**:109–42.

42. Stamler JS, Loh E, Roddy MA *et al.* Nitric oxide regulates basal systemic and pulmonary vascular resistance in healthy humans. *Circulation* 1994;**89**:2035–40.

43. Vasta V, Meacci E, Farnararo M *et al.* Identification of a specific transport system for L-arginine in human platelets. *Biochem Biophys Res Commun* 1995;**206**:878–84.

44. McDonald KK, Zharikov S, Block ER *et al.* A caveolar complex between the cationic amino acid transporter 1 and endothelial nitric-oxide synthase may explain the "arginine paradox". *J Biol Chem* 1997;**272**:31213–16.

45. Vostka RJ, Kashyap S, Trifiletti RR. Arginine deficiency accompanies persistent pulmonary hypertension of the new-born. *Biol Neonate* 1994;**66**:65–70.

46. McCaffrey MJ, Bose CL, Reiter PD *et al.* Effect of L-arginine infusion on infants with persistent pulmonary hypertension of the new-born. *Biol Neonate* 1995;**67**:240–3.

47. Palmer RM, Ferrige AG, Moncada S, Nitric oxide release accounts for the biological activity of endothelium-derived relaxing factor. *Nature* 1987;**327**:524–6.

48. Zapol WM, Falke KJ, Hurford WE *et al.* Inhaling nitric oxide: a selective pulmonary vasodilator and bronchodilator. *Chest* 1994;**105**:87S–91S.

49. Beavo JA, Reifsnyder DH. Primary sequence of cyclic nucleotide phosphodiesterase isozymes and the design of selective inhibitors. *Trends Pharmacol Sci* 1990;**11**:150–5.

50. Ahn H, Foster M, Cable M *et al.* Ca/CaM-stimulated and cGMP-specific phosphodiesterases in vascular and non vascular tissues. *Adv Exp Med Biol* 1991;**308**:191–7.

51. Braner DA, Fineman JR, Chang R *et al.* M&B 22948, a cGMP phosphodiesterase inhibitor, is a pulmonary vasodilator in lambs. *Am J Physiol* 1993;**264**:H252–H258.

52. Michelakis E, Tymchak W, Lien D *et al.* Oral sildenafil is an effective and specific pulmonary vasodilator in patients with pulmonary arterial hypertension: comparison with inhaled nitric oxide. *Circulation* 2002;**105**:2398–403.

53. Sheth A, Park JS, Ong YE, Ho T, Madden BP. Early haemodynamic benefit of sildenafil in patients with co-existing chronic thromboembolic pulmonary hypertension and left ventricular dysfunction. *Vasc Pharmacol* 2005;**42**:41–5.

54. Madden BP, Allenby M, Loke TK, Sheth A. A potential role for sildenafil in the management of pulmonary hypertension associated with parenchymal lung disease. *Vasc Pharmacol* 2006;**44**(5):372–6.

55. Madden BP, Sheth A, Wilde M, Ong YE. Does sildenafil produce a sustained benefit in patients with pulmonary hypertension associated with parenchymal lung and cardiac disease? *Vasc Pharmacol* 2007;**47**:184–8.

56. Madden BP, Sheth A, Ho T, Kanagasabay R. A potential role for sildenafil in the management of perioperative pulmonary hypertension and right ventricular dysfunction following cardiac surgery. *Br J Anaesthesia* 2004;**93**(1):155–6.

57. Galie N, Ghofrani HA, Torbicki A *et al.* The Sildenafil Use in Pulmonary Arterial Hypertension (SUPER) Study Group. Sildenafil citrate therapy for pulmonary arterial hypertension. *N Engl J Med* 2005;**353**:2148–57.

58. Nihill MR, O'Laughlin MP, Mullins CE. Effects of atrial septostomy in patients with terminal cor pulmonale due to pulmonary vascular disease. *Cathet Cardiovasc Diagn* 1991;**24**:166–72.

59. Moser KM, Spragg RG, Utley J *et al.* Chronic thrombotic obstruction of major pulmonary arteries: result of thromboendarterectomy in 15 patients. *Ann Intern Med* 1983;**99**:299–305.

60. Madden B, Hodson M, Tsang V, Radley-Smith R, Khaghani A, Yacob M. Intermediate term results of heart-lung transplantation for cystic fibrosis. *Lancet* 1992;**339**:1583–7.

61. Nagaoka T, Gebb SA, Karoor V *et al.* Involvement of RhoA/Rho kinase signalling in pulmonary hypertension of the fawn-hooded rat. *J Appl Physiol* 2006;**100**:996–1002.

62. Abe K, Shimokawa H, Morikawa K *et al.* Long-term treatment with a Rho-kinase inhibitor improves monocrotaline-induced fatal pulmonary hypertension in rats. *Circ Res* 2004;**94**:385–93.

63. Ishikura K, Yamada N, Ito M *et al.* Beneficial acute effects of rho-kinase inhibitor in patients with pulmonary arterial hypertension. *Circ J* 2006;**70**:174–8.

64. Guilluy C, Sauzeau V, Rolli-Derkinderen M *et al.* Inhibition of RhoA/Rho kinase pathway is involved in the beneficial effect of sildenafil on pulmonary hypertension. *Br J Pharmacol* 2005;**146**:1010–18.

65. Barst RJ. PDGF Signalling in pulmonary arterial hypertension. *J Clin Invest* 2005;**115**:2691–4.

66. Dingli D, Utz JP, Krowka MJ *et al.* Unexplained pulmonary hypertension in chronic myeloproliferative disorders. *Chest* 2001;**120**:801–8.

67. Hoffman R, Xu M. Is bone marrow fibrosis the real problem? *Blood* 2006;**107**:3421–2.

68. Patterson KC, Weissmann A, Ahmadi T *et al.* Imatinib mesylate in the treatment of refractory idiopathic pulmonary arterial hypertension. *Ann Intern Med* 2006;**145**:152–3.

69. Kerkela R, Grazette L, Yacobi R *et al.* Cardiotoxicity of the cancer therapeutic agent Imatinib mesylate. *Nat Med* 2006;**12**:908–16.

70. Hu H, Sung A, Zhao G *et al.* Simvastatin enhances bone morphogenetic protein receptor type II expression. *Biochem Biophys Res Commun* 2006;**339**:59–64.

71. Taraseviciene-Stewart L, Scerbavicius R, Choe KH *et al.* Simvastatin causes endothelial cell apoptosis and attenuates severe pulmonary hypertension. *Am J Physiol Lung Cell Mol Physiol* 2006;**291**:L668–L676.

72. Kao PN. Simvastatin treatment of pulmonary hypertension: an observational case series. *Chest* 2005;**127**:1446–52.

73. Henriques-Coelho T, Roncon-Albuquerque Junior R, Lourenco AP *et al.* Ghrelin reverses molecular, structural and haemodynamic alterations of the right ventricle in pulmonary hypertension. *Rev Port Cardiol* 2006;**25**:55–63.

74. Taraseviciene-Stewart L, Scerbavicius R, Stewart JM *et al.* Treatment of severe pulmonary hypertension: a bradykinin receptor 2 agonist B9972 causes reduction of pulmonary artery pressure and right ventricular hypertrophy. *Peptides* 2005;**26**:1292–300.

75. Petkov V, Gentscheva T, Schamberger C *et al.* The vasoactive intestinal peptide receptor turnover in pulmonary arteries indicates an important role for VIP in the rat lung circulation. *Ann NY Acad Sci* 2006;**1070**:481–3.

76. Petkov V, Mosgoeller W, Ziesche R *et al.* Vasoactive intestinal peptide as a new drug for treatment of primary pulmonary hypertension. *J Clin Invest* 2003;**111**:1339–46.

77. Marcos E, Fadel E, Sanchez O *et al.* Serotonin-induced smooth muscle hyperplasia in various forms of human pulmonary hypertension. *Circ Res* 2004;**94**:1263–70.

78. Guignabert C, Raffenstin B, Benferhat R *et al.* Serotonin transporter inhibition prevents and reverses monocrotaline-induced pulmonary hypertension in rats. *Circulation* 2005;**111**:2812–19.

79. Michelakis ED, McMurtry MS, Sonnerberg B *et al.* The NO-K+ channel axis in pulmonary arterial hypertension. Activation by experimental oral therapies. *Adv Exp Med Biol* 2003;**543**:293–322.

80. Barst RJ, Maislin Fishman AP. Vasodilator therapy for primary pulmonary hypertension in children. *Circulation* 1999;**99**: 1197–208.

81. Barst RJ, Ivy D, Dingemanse J *et al.* Pharmacokinetics, safety and efficacy of Bosentan in pediatric patients with pulmonary arterial hypertension. *Clin Pharmacol Ther* 2003;**73**:372–82.

82. Neonatal Inhaled Nitric Oxide Society Group.Inhaled nitric oxide in full-term and nearly full-term infants with hypoxic respiratory failure. *N Engl J Med* 1997;**336**:597–604.

83. Ivy DD, Ziegler JW, Kinsella JP *et al.* Hemodynamic effects of dipyridamole and inhaled nitric oxide in pediatric patients with pulmonary hypertension [abstract]. *Chest* 1998;**114**:17S.

84. McCaffrey RN, Dunn LH. Primary pulmonary hypertension in pregnancy. *Obstet Gynecol Surv* 1964;**19**:567–91.

85. Weiss BM, Zemp L, Seifert B *et al.* Outcome of pulmonary vascular disease in pregnancy: a systemic overview from 1978 through 1996. *J Am Coll Cardiol* 1998;**31**:1650–7.

86. Elkayam U, Dave R, Bokhari SWH. Primary pulmonary hypertension in pregnancy. In: Elkayam U, Gleicher N (eds) Cardiac Problems in Pregnancy. New York: Wiley-Liss, 1998:183–90.

87. Badalian SS, Silverman RK, Aubry RH *et al.* Twin pregnancy in a woman on long-term epoprostenol therapy for primary pulmonary hypertension: a case report. *J Reprod Med* 2000;**45**:149–52.

88. Lam GK, Stafford RE, Thorp J *et al.* Inhaled nitric oxide for primary pulmonary hypertension in pregnancy. *Obstet Gynecol* 2001;**98**:895–8.

89. Kiss H, Egarter C, Asseryanis E *et al.* Primary pulmonary hypertension in pregnancy: a case report. *Am J Obstet Gynecol* 1995;**172**:1052–4.

90. Smedstad KG, Cramb R, Morison DH. Pulmonary hypertension and pregnancy: a series of eight cases. *Can J Anaesth* 1994;**41**:502–12.

91. Niemann C, Mandell S. Pulmonary hypertension and liver transplantation. *Pulm Perspect* 2003;**20**:4–6.

92. Schraufnagel DE, Kay JM. Structural and pathologic changes in the lung vasculature in chronic liver disease. *Clin Chest Med* 1996;**17**:1–15.

93. Groves B, Brundage B, Elliott C *et al.* Pulmonary hypertension associated with hepatic cirrhosis. In: Fishman AP (ed) The Pulmonary Circulation: Normal and Abnormal. Philadelphia, PA: University of Pennsylvania, 1990:359–69.

94. Schott R, Chaouat A, Launoy A *et al.* Improvement of pulmonary hypertension after liver transplantation. *Chest* 1999;**115**:1748–9.

95. Mehta NJ, Khan IA, Mehta RN *et al.* HIV-related pulmonary hypertension: analytic review of 131 cases. *Chest* 2000;**118**: 1133–41.

96. Mette SA, Palevsky HI, Pietra GG *et al.* Primary pulmonary hypertension in association with human immunodeficiency virus infection: a possible viral etiology for some forms of hypertensive pulmonary arteriopathy. *Am Rev Respir Dis* 1992;**145**: 1196–200.

97. Humbert M, Monti G, Fartoukh M *et al.* Platelet-derived growth factor expression in primary pulmonary hypertension: comparison of HIV seropositive and HIV seronegative patients. *Eur Respir J* 1998;**11**:554–9.

98. Ehrenreich H, Rieckmann P, Sinowatz F *et al.* Potent stimulation of monocytic endothelin-1 production by HIV-1 glycoprotein 120. *J Immunol* 1993;**150**:4601–9.

IV Clinical applications

Ernest L. Fallen, Editor

71 Clinical applications of external evidence

Ernest L Fallen and Salim Yusuf

McMaster University, Faculty of Health Sciences, Hamilton, Ontario, Canada

External evidence derived from randomized clinical trials (RCTs) provides the practicing physician with a sound, rigorous and secure basis for making management decisions on individual patients. However, even vociferous advocates of evidence-based medicine will caution against the use of external evidence as the sole criterion for treating all patients. It is well to bear in mind that evidence obtained from clinical trials is derived from large population databases. More often than not, the entry criteria tend to define the boundaries of specified interest (for example, acute myocardial infarction), whereas exclusion criteria, such as age, sex, co-morbid disease states, etc., may well have denied entry to the individual patient now awaiting treatment. These exclusions may be based on concerns related to patient safety, lack of applicability, historic considerations or confounders (for example, significant non-cardiac illness) that can affect the evaluation of treatment. Nevertheless, the practicing physician is left inquiring, "Where can I find my patient within the trial's data set?". Here is where interpretation and the application of external evidence require a logical integration of overall trial results with a knowledge of biologic mechanisms, patient risk and clinical circumstances.

Evidence-based versus patient-centered medicine? Not an either/or choice

Few would deny an approach to therapeutic decision making based on proven external evidence combined with clinical experience, knowledge of pathophysiology and sensitivity to individual patient needs. To marry the two effectively is to recognize, and hence to avoid, their respective limitations if either were to be applied alone.

Evidence-Based Cardiology, 3rd edition. Edited by S. Yusuf, J.A. Cairns, A.J. Camm, E.L. Fallen, and B.J. Gersh. © 2010 Blackwell Publishing, ISBN: 978-1-4051-5925-8.

Recognizing the limitations of external evidence

For most RCTs, proving therapeutic efficacy necessitates certain constraints in patient selection. It is not uncommon that many patients in a physician's practice would not have fulfilled the restrictive entrance criteria of most moderate-sized RCTs. For example, some RCTs have an age cut-off that actually excludes more than half of all patients with the disorder. This by no means implies that the reputed benefit of the test drug is not applicable (effective) to the patients excluded, but it does beg the question. Entry criteria alone should never be the sole basis for denying a patient the benefit of proven therapy. Interpatient variability is inevitable in all RCTs and contributes much to the "random errors" seen in small and moderate-sized trials. However, the larger the trial, the smaller the random error, and the more likely that benefit can be reliably extrapolated to some patients who do not necessarily qualify for entry.[1,2] For example, one may observe that the benefits are consistent across different subgroups, suggesting that the results may be applicable beyond the boundaries of patient selection. On the other hand there may emerge reliable evidence for a lack of benefit in certain subgroups.

Evidence-based medicine that depends solely on external evidence is disease oriented rather than patient oriented. In other words, the verifiability of RCT data is often dependent on having a given diagnosis, as opposed to a clinical spectrum of risk associated with the diagnosis. This is the so-called "labeling" dilemma. For example, patients labeled as having "acute coronary syndrome" simply because they present with chest pain associated with non-ST segment elevation are often treated alike in an RCT, whereas the clinical expression of this entity may encompass a wide range from very low- to very high-risk patients. Translating external evidence based solely on a unified diagnosis into practice guidelines or clinical pathways has the unfortunate consequence of making management decisions dependent on a label rather than the presenting clinical circumstances and risk of the underlying disorder.

Another nagging problem with the "bottom line" of clinical trials is the emphasis on primary endpoints that are measurable. Statistical dependency on hard data such as mortality rates, prespecified clinical outcome events, rehospitalizations, etc., fails to acknowledge the significance of clinically relevant "soft" data, such as impact on symptoms, quality of life, psychosocial well-being, attitudes, economic realities and patient preferences.

Finally, clinical trials all have finite time limits and, not uncommonly, the duration may be inadequate to assess long-term benefits and risks, especially for any new drug. In such cases the information from RCTs may have to be supplemented by other sources of non-randomized evidence.

Recognizing the limitations of patient-centered medicine

Who would have guessed that aspirin could reduce the relative risk of death and adverse coronary events in post-myocardial infarction patients by 25%? Or that beta-blockers would be so effective in class II/III chronic heart failure? Or that inotropic agents, despite improving hemodynamics and clinical well-being in patients with advanced heart failure, do so at the expense of shortened survival? Or that some antiarrhythmic agents, although they achieve cosmetic cleansing of so-called malignant ventricular ectopy from the electrocardiogram, are potentially hazardous?

Previously held concepts of disease mechanisms as the basis for initiating new therapies or persisting with old therapies have been challenged by clinical trials results. And so, what is apparent as a "logical" management approach to a given clinical problem may commit even the most experienced physician to inappropriate prescribing practices. Patient-centered medicine is not a concept that is firmly rooted in empiric medicine.[3] It does not guarantee that a physician, feeling secure in his or her realm of expertise, will be kept abreast of therapeutic advances based on clinical trial results. Unfortunately, this can lead to a tendency to persist in outmoded approaches.

Surely a cogent argument can be made to blend the positive features of patient-centered and evidence-based approaches through a constant awareness of their respective limitations.

Some principles of application

Knowing the person who has the disease is as important as knowing the disease that the patient has.[4] Clinical

decision making ought to incorporate the following three ingredients:
- intelligent use of external evidence based on well-established clinical trial results and epidemiologic data whenever available
- clinical expertise, knowledge of fundamental mechanisms of disease, and willingness to listen to the testimony of one's patients
- sensitivity to patients' preferences, values, needs and beliefs.

It is well to bear in mind that for any given diagnosis (label), patients at the greatest risk of a disease will usually derive the greatest benefit from an established treatment, as the absolute benefit usually increases with risk whereas harm due to the treatment remains comparatively fixed across the risk spectrum.[5] Therefore, to avoid the hazard of labeling, it is critical to risk stratify the patient. It is only after one has listened carefully to the testimony of the patient, performed a proper examination and conducted the relevant tests that one can formulate a degree of attributable risk. Remember, it is just as important to identify the patient at very low risk, thereby sparing him or her unnecessary aggressive investigation and/or therapy, as it is to identify the high-risk patient for whom aggressive treatment can be life saving.

The absence of external evidence should not lead to therapeutic nihilism. Not all consensus recommendations are supported by Grade A evidence. In fact, many consensus panel recommendations and clinical practice pathways are based on evidence that ranges from the use of clinical judgment, albeit under a cloud of uncertainty, to Grade B through Grade A evidence.[6,7] When external evidence is lacking, one's own clinical experience, knowledge of pathophysiology, reasoned judgment and awareness of the patient's needs are indispensable substitutes.

One should avoid using the trial entry criteria to determine whether a particular patient would benefit from the active treatment.[2,5] Failure to qualify for entry is determined by many factors, few of which necessarily compromise the potential for therapeutic benefit. For example, if a trial's age cut-off was 65 years then a reasonable risk/benefit assessment can be done for those older by assessing whether, within the trial, age modified the treatment effect.

One should always try to use the best available external evidence science has to offer, but never at the expense of ignoring the patient's psychosocial conditions, beliefs, values and preferences. As medical decisions become more codified, one should not fail to recognize and honor the importance of patient preferences.[8] A patient's medical decision based on his or her particular needs, preferences and beliefs should always be respected, as the patient is given the opportunity to hear the nature of the external evidence. Consensus recommendations are guidelines only. They represent an active process subject to continual review as new and as yet untested information emerges. When following any recommendation based on external evidence, the physician should always exercise clinical judgment based on a close working interaction with the patient.

knowledge of cardiovascular pathophysiology and sensitivity to the patient's needs and preferences.

Section preview

In the day-to-day practice of clinical medicine, it is not sufficient to know *what* the available external evidence is but also *how* and *when* to apply it to the individual patient. This section is made up of individual case reports that attempt to put a clinical face to a statistical bottom line by illustrating practical solutions to both common and uncommon problems in clinical cardiology. These case studies, encompassing 10 disease categories, are real-life presentations drawn from the files of distinguished consultant cardiologists. Here one finds therapeutic decisions made on the basis of both external evidence and clinical reasoning skills. For each case scenario, the story is presented. A question is posed at each decision point and a commentary follows. The commentary demonstrates how best external evidence is used in the management of the patient while recognizing the importance of sound judgment, a careful examination,

References

1. Yusuf S, Held P, Teo KK. Selection of patients for randomized controlled trials: implications of wide or narrow eligibility criteria. *Stat Med* 1990;**9**:73–86.
2. Yusuf S, Wittes HJ, Probstfield J, Tyroler HA. Analysis and interpretation of treatment effects in subgroups of patients in randomized clinical trials. *JAMA* 1991;**266**:93–8.
3. Bensing J. Bridging the gap. The separate worlds of evidence-based and patient-centered medicine. *Patient Educ Counseling* 2000;**39**:17–25.
4. McCormick J. Death of the personal doctor. *Lancet* 1996;**348**:667–8.
5. Glasziou PP, Irwig LM. An evidence based approach to individualising treatment. *BMJ* 1995;**311**:1356–9.
6. Fallen EL, Cairns J, Dafoe W *et al.* Management of the postmyocardial infarction patient: a consensus report. *Can J Cardiol* 1995;**11**:477–86.
7. Hayward RS, Wilson MC, Tunis SR *et al.* User's guide to the medical literature. VIII. How to use clinical practice guidelines. A. Are the recommendations valid? *JAMA* 1995;**274**:570–4.
8. Kassirer JP. Incorporating patients' preferences in medical decisions. *N Engl J Med* 1994;**330**:1895–6.

72

Stable angina: choice of PCI versus CABG versus medical therapy

William S Weintraub

Christiana Care Health System, Newark, DE, USA

Case history

A 58-year-old salesman presents to his primary care physician with a chief complaint of chest pain for 3 months. On further questioning, the chest pain is found to happen several times per week, occurring with exertion such as carrying packages up several flights of stairs. The pain is relieved by rest and has never occurred at rest. There have been several episodes, however, occurring with emotional stress. The patient does note that he has been under financial pressure at work and has had some family difficulties at home. The pain does impose some physical limitation on his activity, but it is felt to be mild. The pain does interfere with his quality of life, and the patient notes that he is fearful and worried about the pain. The pain has not been getting worse. The patient has never had a myocardial infarction and has never been hospitalized for his heart.

The patient has known risk factors for coronary artery disease. He has mild, controlled hypertension, taking only a diuretic. In addition, he has a 40-pack/year smoking history. He has no history of diabetes. He does have a history of hyperlipidemia and takes a statin. The patient has had a history of depression, but states that while he is anxious, he is not depressed at present. His lifestyle is entirely sedentary.

On physical exam he is a mildly anxious, slightly obese white male appearing his stated age. His waist circumference is 39 inches and his BMI 29.4. His pulse is 74, blood pressure 136/84. His peripheral pulses are full without bruits. His lung fields are clear. His cardiac exam reveals a barely perceptible apical impulse in the fifth intercostal space, in the mid-clavicular line. His heart sounds reveal an S1 and physiologically split S2, with no murmurs, gallops or rubs.

There is no peripheral edema and the exam is otherwise unremarkable. An electrocardiogram reveals normal sinus rhythm, QRS axis of 60°, normal intervals, somewhat high-voltage QRS complexes, and some T-wave flattening. Laboratory work reveals normal CBC and electrolytes. His fasting blood sugar is 103, HDL 38 and LDL 98 and triglycerides 168. Other than his statin and diuretic, the patient takes no medications.

- What is the diagnosis?
- What tests should be performed?
- What are the best therapeutic choices?

Comment

The patient gives a classic story for angina pectoris.[1] The probability of this being angina pectoris secondary to atherosclerotic cardiovascular disease is very high, probably in excess of 90%. At this level of probability, there is little need for non-invasive testing to establish the diagnosis. Non-invasive testing is most useful in the mid-range of probabilities, when the diagnosis is uncertain.[2] However, the patient also has risk factors which are not well controlled. The patient's blood pressure is controlled but not below the optimal level, below 120/80.[3]. His LDL choles-terol is below 100. Recent changes to the NCEP ATP guidelines would suggest that this is adequate control, but they recommend an LDL below 70 for high-risk patients.[4,5] That control of LDL cholesterol will reduce cardiovascular events has been shown in multiple trials, and there is evidence that with lower LDL, the event rate will be even lower.[5,6] The patient's blood sugar is also of concern. Recent guidelines from the American Diabetic Association diagnose impaired fasting glucose to be above 100.[7] His lifestyle is a concern. He is sedentary and overweight. In fact, the patient has the metabolic syndrome, being overweight with a history of hypertension, elevated fasting blood glucose, low HDL cholesterol and elevated triglycerides.[8] He actually has all five components of the metabolic syndrome, but the diagnosis could actually be made with just three of these components. He is also not taking aspirin.

Evidence-Based Cardiology, 3rd edition. Edited by S. Yusuf, J.A. Cairns, A.J. Camm, E.L. Fallen, and B.J. Gersh. © 2010 Blackwell Publishing, ISBN: 978-1-4051-5925-8.

Antiplatelet therapy with aspirin has been shown to reduce events in patients with vascular disease in multiple clinical trials, with greater benefit in higher risk patients.[9,10] He also continues to smoke, a major risk factor for cardiovascular events. Smoking cessation advice is highly cost-effective and should be routinely given.[11] The patient also had a history of depression. Patients with depression are at higher risk of cardiovascular disease and should be treated for their depression.[12] However, it is not clear that such treatment can prevent cardiovascular events.

Case history *continued*

His primary care physician recognizes that this may be angina pectoris secondary to coronary artery disease. She also recognizes that he has the metabolic syndrome. She starts him on aspirin, 81 mg, a day as well as sublingual nitrates for episodes of chest pain. She assesses his history of depression carefully, noting that he is not currently depressed. She counsels him strongly on the need to stop smoking. She continues his other medications and refers him to a cardiologist for further evaluation.

The consulting cardiologist confirms the history, physical examination and laboratory values. He also agrees with the diagnosis of almost certain angina pectoris due to atherosclerotic cardiovascular disease. He notes that the pattern of angina has been stable for several months, with no rest pain. He therefore makes a presumptive diagnosis of chronic coronary artery disease. He reiterates the need for the patient to stop smoking.

The diagnosis has been made and initial therapy started. What are the next diagnostic and therapeutic steps?

Comment

The diagnosis of chronic coronary disease was straightforward for the cardiologist, but the next steps are less clear. It would be acceptable at this point to begin to treat the patient medically, deferring diagnostic testing. Smoking cessation advice and aspirin have already been started. The blood pressure control could be strengthened. ACE inhibition has been shown in two clinical trials to reduce the incidence of cardiovascular events in moderately high-risk patients, although this was not confirmed in a third trial.[13–15] Increased physical activity and diet have been shown to be effective in reducing fasting blood sugar and preventing diabetes.[16] The patient's LDL is controlled, although not to the most aggressive level. HDL is also low at 38 and triglycerides mildly elevated. Patients with increased physical activity are also at lower risk of events, although physical activity has not been shown to decrease events in clinical trials.

The major issues concern additional testing, possible cardiac catheterization with coronary arteriography and possible revascularization. Patients can be further risk stratified by stress testing with myocardial perfusion imaging.[17] Patients with reversible ischemia on myocardial perfusion imaging are at increased risk.[18] However, it is not clear that reversal of the ischemia with revascularization reduces risk. Patients who can exercise on a treadmill are also at lower risk than those who cannot.[19,20] There are patients with chronic coronary disease in whom coronary artery bypass grafting (CABG) reduces risk.[21–23]

Case history *continued*

The cardiologist counsels the patient on diet and recommends seeing a nutritionist. The patient declines to see the nutritionist, saying he knows what to do about diet but has trouble doing it. The cardiologist advises the patient to begin a walking program, pointing out that walking is the exercise of choice for adults, and that a more strenuous exercise program is not necessary. He hopes that the exercise program will result in amelioration of multiple components of the metabolic syndrome, lessening the need for additional therapy for serum lipids and driving the fasting blood sugar below 100. He begins a beta-blocker to treat the angina and also to further lower the blood pressure. He is also worried about the electrocardiogram, which suggests left ventricular hypertrophy. Left ventricular hypertrophy can also increase risk, and tight blood pressure control may help reduce it.[26] In order to risk stratify, he orders a stress test with myocardial perfusion imaging. The patient walks on the Bruce protocol for 5 minutes and 40 seconds, without ST changes on his electrocardiogram, but he does have some chest pain at peak exercise. His myocardial perfusion imaging reveals mild reversible ischemia and also shows that his left ventricular function is normal. The cardiologist is now comfortable that while the patient has chronic coronary artery disease, he is not at high risk. He elects to continue medical therapy, deferring catheterization and possible revascularization.

The patient returns 3 months later. He has begun a walking program and is feeling better, with decreased chest pain. He says that the walking program has also improved his overall sense of well-being. He has stopped smoking but has not lost weight. He fasting blood sugar has fallen to 98 and HDL has risen to 41. His LDL is essentially unchanged. His blood pressure is 132/81. His physical exam remains normal and electrocardiogram unchanged. As his blood pressure is not optimal and considering the results of the HOPE and EUROPA trials, the cardiologist begins the patient on an ACE inhibitor and continues his other medications.[13,14] He is now on aspirin, ACE inhibitor, beta-blocker and a statin. He returns 3 months later with blood pressure of 124/76, but now complains that he continues to have chest pain. Given the recurring angina, the physician elects to perform cardiac catheterization, with coronary arteriography and left ventriculography. The catheterization shows an 80% blockage in the left anterior descending coronary artery and a 70% blockage in the right coronary artery. There was mild diffuse disease and normal left ventricular function.

How should this patient be treated now?

In particular, these are patients with left main disease and three-vessel disease with abnormal left ventricular function. These patient groups were defined in the three major clinical trials of CABG from the late 1970s to early 1980s. However, these trials are somewhat historic and do not reflect contemporary medical therapy. There is no group of patients with chronic coronary artery disease in whom percutaneous coronary intervention (PCI) has been shown to decrease the incidence of cardiovascular events. Inability of PCI to prevent events has been shown in multiple clinical trials and recently confirmed in the COURAGE trial.[24,25]

Comment

The COURAGE trial has shown that an initial management strategy of optimal medical therapy will offer the same event rate over 7 years as initial medical strategy of PCI plus optimal medical therapy.[25] However, about one-third of patients in COURAGE crossed over from medical therapy to have revascularization at a median time of 10 months. COURAGE did show that there is better control of angina with PCI. Most of these crossovers were for failure to adequately control angina. There have also been multiple trials comparing balloon angioplasty to CABG and, more recently, coronary stenting to CABG. These trials generally show better control of angina with CABG, but little difference in event rates, except in diabetics, where several studies have favored CABG. As this patient has two-vessel disease and continuing angina on optimal medical therapy, he is a candidate for revascularization with either PCI or CABG.[27-29] PCI can be performed with either drug-eluting or bare metal stents, with little difference in death or myocardial infarction during follow-up, but less restenosis with drug-eluting stents.[30]

Case history *continued*

The patient undergoes stenting of the left anterior descending and right coronary arteries with drug-eluting stents. The procedure is uncomplicated. He has amelioration but not complete resolution of his angina. He is much more functional. His only additional medication is a thienopyridine to prevent stent thrombosis.[31] This is continued for 1 year. He continues his walking program, takes his five medications and does not smoke. He is not rehospitalized for heart-related problems. While the patient does not lose weight, he otherwise continues to do well.

Conclusion

This is a classic story of angina pectoris and chronic stable coronary artery disease. Optimal medical therapy, both pharmaceutic and lifestyle, has been shown in multiple

clinical trials to be associated with a good outcome, and has played a significant role in the reduction in cardiovascular disease mortality in recent decades. Except in special groups, revascularization is largely a treatment for angina. Where angina is disabling, revascularization can have a dramatic effect on quality of life. By beginning with optimal medical therapy, clinical trial data have shown that revascularization can be safely deferred in many patients. When angina pectoris does not improve over time in the medically treated patient, then revascularization with PCI or CABG is indicated.[25]

References

1. Blackwelder WC, Kagan A, Gordon T, Rhoads GG. Comparison of methods for diagnosing angina pectoris: the Honolulu heart study. *Int J Epidemiol* 1981;**10**(3):211–15.
2. Diamond GA, Forrester JS. Analysis of probability as an aid in the clinical diagnosis of coronary-artery disease. *N Engl J Med* 1979;**300**(24):1350–8.
3. Chobanian AV, Bakris GL, Black HR *et al.* The Seventh Report of the Joint National Committee on Prevention, Detection, Evaluation, and Treatment of High Blood Pressure: the JNC 7 report. *JAMA* 2003;**289**(19):2560–72.
4. Update on Cholesterol Guidelines: More Intensive Treatment Options for Higher Risk Patients. 2004. (Accessed 12/17/07, 2007, at http://www.nhlbi.nih.gov/new/press/04-07-12.htm.)
5. Collins R, Armitage J, Parish S. MRC/BHF Heart Protection Study of antioxidant vitamin supplementation in 20,536 high-risk individuals: a randomized placebo-controlled trial. *Lancet* 2002;**360**:23–33.
6. No authors listed. Randomised trial of cholesterol lowering in 4444 patients with coronary heart disease: the Scandinavian Simvastatin Survival Study (4S). *Lancet* 1994;**344**(8934): 1383–9.
7. Nathan DM, Davidson MB, DeFronzo RA *et al.* Impaired fasting glucose and impaired glucose tolerance: implications for care. *Diabetes Care* 2007;**30**(3):753–9.
8. Grundy SM, Brewer HB Jr, Cleeman JI, Smith SC Jr, Lenfant C. Definition of metabolic syndrome: report of the National Heart, Lung, and Blood Institute/American Heart Association conference on scientific issues related to definition. *Arterioscler Thromb Vasc Biol* 2004;**24**(2):e13–18.
9. Hayden M, Pignone M, Phillips C, Mulrow C. Aspirin for the primary prevention of cardiovascular events: a summary of the evidence for the U.S. Preventive Services Task Force. *Ann Intern Med* 2002;**136**(2):161–72.
10. Collins R, Peto R, Baigent C, Sleight P. Aspirin, heparin, and fibrinolytic therapy in suspected acute myocardial infarction. *N Engl J Med* 1997;**336**(12):847–60.
11. Krumholz HM, Cohen BJ, Tsevat J, Pasternak RC, Weinstein MC. Cost-effectiveness of a smoking cessation program after myocardial infarction. *J Am Coll Cardiol* 1993;**22**(6):1697–702.
12. Rumsfeld JS, Magid DJ, Plomondon ME *et al.* History of depression, angina, and quality of life after acute coronary syndromes. *Am Heart J* 2003;**145**(3):493–9.

13. Yusuf S, Sleight P, Pogue J, Bosch J, Davies R, Dagenais G. Effects of an angiotensin-converting-enzyme inhibitor, ramipril, on cardiovascular events in high-risk patients. The Heart Outcomes Prevention Evaluation Study Investigators. *N Engl J Med* 2000;**342**(3):145–53.

14. Fox KM. Efficacy of perindopril in reduction of cardiovascular events among patients with stable coronary artery disease: randomised, double-blind, placebo-controlled, multicentre trial (the EUROPA study). *Lancet* 2003;**362**(9386):782–8.

15. Solomon SD, Rice MM, Jablonski AK *et al.* Renal function and effectiveness of angiotensin-converting enzyme inhibitor therapy in patients with chronic stable coronary disease in the Prevention of Events with ACE inhibition (PEACE) trial. *Circulation* 2006;**114**(1):26–31.

16. Knowler WC, Barrett-Connor E, Fowler SE *et al.* Reduction in the incidence of type 2 diabetes with lifestyle intervention or metformin. *N Engl J Med* 2002;**346**(6):393–403.

17. Hachamovitch R, Berman DS, Kiat H, Cohen I, Friedman JD, Shaw LJ. Value of stress myocardial perfusion single photon emission computed tomography in patients with normal resting electrocardiograms: an evaluation of incremental prognostic value and cost-effectiveness. *Circulation* 2002;**105**(7):823–9.

18. Klocke FJ, Baird MG, Lorell BH *et al.* ACC/AHA/ASNC guidelines for the clinical use of cardiac radionuclide imaging – executive summary: a report of the American College of Cardiology/American Heart Association Task Force on Practice Guidelines (ACC/AHA/ASNC Committee to Revise the 1995 Guidelines for the Clinical Use of Cardiac Radionuclide Imaging). *Circulation* 2003;**108**(11):1404–18.

19. Gibbons RJ, Balady GJ, Beasley JW *et al.* ACC/AHA Guidelines for Exercise Testing. A report of the American College of Cardiology/American Heart Association Task Force on Practice Guidelines (Committee on Exercise Testing). *J Am Coll Cardiol* 1997;**30**(1):260–311.

20. Marwick TH, Shaw L, Case C, Vasey C, Thomas JD. Clinical and economic impact of exercise electrocardiography and exercise echocardiography in clinical practice. *Eur Heart J* 2003;**24**(12):1153–63.

21. Veterans Administration Coronary Artery Bypass Surgery Cooperative Study Group. Eleven-year survival in the Veterans Administration randomized trial of coronary bypass surgery for stable angina. *N Engl J Med* 1984;**311**(21):1333–9.

22. Passamani E, Davis KB, Gillespie MJ, Killip T. A randomized trial of coronary artery bypass surgery. Survival of patients with a low ejection fraction. *N Engl J Med* 1985;**312**(26):1665–71.

23. European Coronary Surgery Study Group. Long-term results of prospective randomised study of coronary artery bypass surgery in stable angina pectoris. *Lancet* 1982;**2**(8309):1173–80.

24. Katritsis DG, Ioannidis JP. Percutaneous coronary intervention versus conservative therapy in nonacute coronary artery disease: a meta-analysis. *Circulation* 2005;**111**(22):2906–12.

25. Boden WE, O'Rourke RA, Teo KK *et al.* Optimal medical therapy with or without PCI for stable coronary disease. *N Engl J Med* 2007;**356**(15):1503–16.

26. Levy D, Garrison RJ, Savage DD, Kannel WB, Castelli WP. Prognostic implications of echocardiographically determined left ventricular mass in the Framingham Heart Study. *N Engl J Med* 1990;**322**(22):1561–6.

27. King SB 3rd, Lembo NJ, Weintraub WS *et al.* A randomized trial comparing coronary angioplasty with coronary bypass surgery. Emory Angioplasty versus Surgery Trial (EAST). *N Engl J Med* 1994;**331**(16):1044–50.

28. Bypass Angioplasty Revascularization Investigation (BARI) Investigators. Comparison of coronary bypass surgery with angioplasty in patients with multivessel disease. *N Engl J Med* 1996;**335**(4):217–25.

29. SoS Investigator. Coronary artery bypass surgery versus percutaneous coronary intervention with stent implantation in patients with multivessel coronary artery disease (the Stent or Surgery trial): a randomised controlled trial. *Lancet* 2002;**360**(9338):965–70.

30. Moses JW, Leon MB, Popma JJ *et al.* Sirolimus-eluting stents versus standard stents in patients with stenosis in a native coronary artery. *N Engl J Med* 2003;**349**(14):1315–23.

31. Grines CL, Bonow RO, Casey DE Jr *et al.* Prevention of premature discontinuation of dual antiplatelet therapy in patients with coronary artery stents: a science advisory from the American Heart Association, American College of Cardiology, Society for Cardiovascular Angiography and Interventions, American College of Surgeons, and American Dental Association, with representation from the American College of Physicians. *J Am Coll Cardiol* 2007;**49**(6):734–9.

73 Non-ST segment elevation acute coronary syndrome

David Fitchett
St Michael's Hospital, Toronto, Ontario, Canada

Case history

A 78-year-old woman with a past history of hypertension and type 2 diabetes awoke with dyspnea and burning chest discomfort. Despite taking antacids the symptoms persisted for 45 minutes. She arrived in the emergency department about one hour later. At the time of arrival she had no symptoms.

Her medications included metformin, hydrochlorothiazide, and amlodipine. She was a lifelong non-smoker. Her parents died in a car crash at a young age and she had no siblings.

The vital signs were normal (heart rate 84 bpm, BP 140/85, O_2 saturation 97%), The venous pressure was not elevated, but there were scattered crepitations in both lung bases. The heart sounds were normal.

The ECG showed 1 mm T-wave inversion in V1–4.

The biochemical profile showed normal electrolytes, creatinine 112 µmol/L (eGFR 35 mL/min/1.73 m^2), blood glucose 10.7 mmol/L. The cardiac troponin I taken within 10 minutes of arrival was 0.05 ng/L (99 percentile 0.06 ng/L).

Question

What is your management of this patient?

Comment

This older patient with diabetes and hypertension presents with symptoms that may be attributable to an acute coronary syndrome (ACS). Older patients and those with diabetes not infrequently have atypical symptoms, with dyspnea predominating over chest pain. The level of sus-

picion for ACS is high, yet there are no objective or high-risk features at the time of presentation, such as specific ECG abnormalities indicative of myocardial ischemia or elevation of the biomarker (troponin) of cardiac injury.

As an initial management step, it is necessary to recognize that both ECG and troponin abnormalities may take several hours to become abnormal. Hence it is important that this patient, with a high suspicion for ACS, is observed and both the ECG and troponin are repeated 6–9 hours after the initial presentation. Studies of patients with possible ACS indicate it will take up to 12–14 hours for all patients to develop a positive troponin. Thus even the currently recommended observation period of six hours may not detect an important number of patients with ACS and elevated troponin.

Risk stratification of the patient with a possible ACS is an essential step in the choice of appropriate management. For ACS with no ST segment elevation there are two specific reasons for risk stratification: only high-risk patients benefit from an early invasive strategy, and antithrombotic and antiplatelet therapy has evidence-based support in patients with objective high-risk features.

Features that are associated with a higher risk of adverse outcomes in patients with ACS are shown in Box 73.1. The risk factors are divided between those that will immediately impact on management decisions and those which although associated with increased risk, are unlikely to change the management strategy on their own. For example, a patient with symptoms compatible with an ACS, yet normal ECG and no troponin elevation is unlikely to benefit from an early invasive strategy just because of older age or the presence of diabetes. Yet a similar patient with increased background risk due to diabetes, impaired renal function or known coronary artery disease probably should receive clopidogrel and a heparin during the observation period.

The patient with any one of the high-risk features described in Box 73.1 is at higher risk of an adverse outcome,

Evidence-Based Cardiology, 3rd edition. Edited by S. Yusuf, J.A. Cairns, A.J. Camm, E.L. Fallen, and B.J. Gersh. © 2010 Blackwell Publishing, ISBN: 978-1-4051-5925-8.

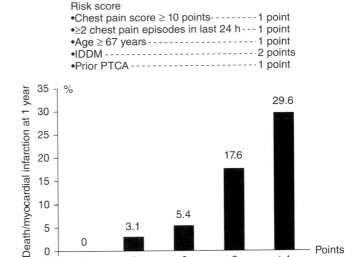

Figure 73.1 Death and non-fatal myocardial infarction rates over one year, in patients with symptoms compatible with an acute coronary syndrome yet no increased troponin and no high-risk ECG findings.[1,2,60] A chest pain score >10 is for chest pain symptoms that are likely to have been due to myocardial ischemia.

and justifies an early invasive management strategy. However, the patient with no high-risk features is not necessarily at low risk, especially over the medium and longer term. A recently developed scoring system[1] to identify high-risk patients who have no troponin elevation nor high-risk ECG features is shown in Figure 73.1. This scoring system shows that patients with a score >3 have outcomes similar to a patient with an elevated troponin[2] and in this patient population, the score was a better predictor of outcomes than the thrombolysis in myocardial infarction (TIMI) risk score.

Our patient has no high-risk features that would by themselves indicate high risk. Yet age and the history of diabetes give her a score of 3 according to the scoring system in Figure 73.1. She received dual antiplatelet therapy with aspirin and clopidogrel. An anticoagulant (a heparin, fondaparinux or bivalirudin) was not given.

Case history *continued*

The blood sample taken at six hours after the patient arrived in the emergency department shows the troponin I has increased to 0.15 ng/L (99 percentile reference level 0.06 ng/L). Would this result change your management?

Comment

The presence of an elevated troponin I level in a patient with symptoms and circumstances compatible with an ACS is objective evidence supportive of the diagnosis of ACS, and indicates:

- a higher risk for recurrent ACS
- benefit from an early invasive strategy of coronary angiography and revascularization when appropriate
- benefit from immediate use of antiplatelet and antithrombotic treatment.

Outcomes related to elevated troponin

The relationship between elevated biomarkers of myocardial necrosis and outcomes has been recognized for many years. The patient with a myocardial infarction and increased biomarkers (transaminases, lactate dehydrogenase (LDH) or creatine kinase (CK)) has substantially increased mortality when compared to the patient presenting with rest pain and no biochemical evidence of infarction, i.e. unstable angina. With the development of troponin as a highly sensitive and specific marker of myocardial injury, approximately 30% of patients with a previously designated diagnosis of unstable angina and normal CK and CKMB have increased troponin. Whereas early mortality relates to both the maximal CKMB and troponin levels, the risk of early myocardial (re-) infarction is more related to low levels of troponin.[3] Small increases in troponin I or T in a patient with a clinical history compatible with an acute coronary syndrome indicate increased risk of recurrent ACS and the need for more aggressive treatment. It should be recognized that many other clinical situations such as pulmonary embolism, septic shock, acute heart failure and renal failure are associated with minor degrees of myocardial injury indicated by elevation of troponin, that are not due to thrombotic coronary occlusion. The troponin elevation should be evaluated in the clinical context.

Early invasive strategy or conservative management?

The strategy of early cardiac catheterization and revascularization (when appropriate) reduces early recurrent acute coronary syndromes and long-term mortality when compared to a conservative strategy of cardiac catheterization only if the patient has recurrent ischemia or high-risk noninvasive testing.

Four meta-analyses[4–7] have showed that an early (during the index hospitalization) invasive strategy is superior to a selectively invasive approach. A meta-analysis of the seven most recent trials, included 9212 patients and showed that death or myocardial infarction was reduced by 18% (odds ratio (OR) 0.82, 95% confidence interval (CI) 0.72–0.93) over a follow-up period of 17 months (range 6–24 months) with routine early coronary angiography and revascularization (when appropriate), compared to a selective approach[5] (Fig. 73.2). An analysis showed improved outcomes, including reduced mortality, were only achieved when coronary stenting and an aggressive antiplatelet strategy were employed.[6] The early benefit from an invasive strategy is mainly from a reduction of myocardial infarction. However, long-term mortality was reduced in the FRISC 2[8] and the RITA 3[9,10] trials with a 26–30% reduction in 1–5-year mortality compared to patients managed conservatively. High-risk patients with elevated troponin or greater TIMI risk scores benefit the most from the early invasive strategy.[11–13]

Early revascularization within 48 hours in high-risk patients with non-ST segment elevation (NSTE) ACS is supported by data from the CRUSADE registry[14] and the TACTICS/TIMI 18 study.[11] Furthermore, the ISAR COOL trial[15] indicated that there was no benefit from a 72-hour period of medical stabilization with an aggressive protocol of heparin, acetylsalicylic acid (ASA), clopidogrel and glycoprotein (GP) IIb/IIIa inhibitors compared to immediate cardiac catheterization within six hours. Ischemic events occurred more frequently prior to percutaneous coronary intervention (PCI) in the medical stabilization group despite the vigorous treatment. Hence the current evidence supports early angiography within the first 48 hours in the majority of patients identified as being at high risk. For patients with frequent episodes of ischemia, heart failure or hypotension, even more urgent coronary angiography allows immediate revascularization in very high-risk individuals.

The 2007 ACC/AHA guidelines[16] for the management of NSTE ACS have recommended that an initially conservative management strategy can be considered for initially stabilized patients even with high-risk features (**Class IIb, Level C**). This recommendation is based on the results of the ICTUS trial.[17] Patients included had rest pain, elevated troponin and either ECG abnormalities or a known coronary artery disease. The study compared an early invasive management strategy, with coronary angiography and revascularization where feasible within 24–48 hours, with a selectively invasive approach that only progressed to an invasive management with recurrent ischemia or a high-risk stress ECG. In the ICTUS study myocardial infarction was defined as any increase in CKMB beyond the normal range, with no higher threshold for patients undergoing PCI or bypass surgery. During the index hospitalization 98% of the early invasive group and 53% of the selectively

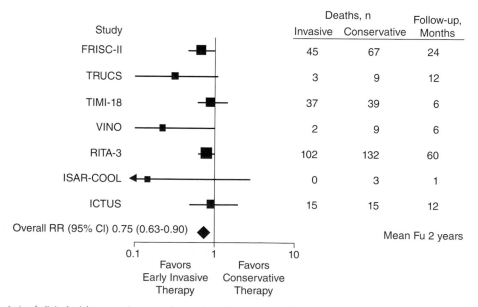

Figure 73.2 Meta-analysis of clinical trials comparing an early invasive with a conservative strategy in the management of patients with NSTE ACS.[61]

invasive group underwent coronary angiography. One year after the index ACS event, 67% of the selectively invasive group had undergone coronary angiography. At one year after the ACS event, there was no difference in the primary outcome of death/recurrent myocardial infarction or unstable angina. The ICTUS patients had a low incidence of cardiovascular events (one-year mortality 2.5%). Almost two-thirds of the conservative group underwent coronary angiography and revascularization by the end of the first year. Thus the management strategies mainly differed by the timing of the invasive strategy and the study compared an early invasive with a delayed invasive strategy. It is unlikely therefore that this study alone will change practice.

Antithrombotic and antiplatelet therapy

The vast majority of acute coronary syndromes result from arterial thrombosis occurring with either atherosclerotic plaque erosion that denudes endothelial cells or plaque rupture exposing thrombogenic collagen and tissue factor to the blood. Propagating thrombus may occlude the vessel. However, the size of the thrombus and the activity of intrinsic fibrinolysis may determine whether the vessel remains occluded or is spontaneously recanalized. A high proportion of patients with NSTE ACS have patent culprit coronary arteries when investigated within the first 24 hours. This is in contrast to ST segment elevation ACS (STE ACS) where 80% of patients have an occluded infarct-related artery. In the patient with NSTE ACS the rationale of therapy is to prevent recurrent ACS due to reocclusion of both the culprit artery and other sites of plaque rupture or vulnerability, by using medications (antiplatelet and antithrombotic agents) and revascularization when feasible and indicated.

Medications to reduce thrombosis are the mainstay of early therapy in patients with acute coronary syndromes. Drugs reducing platelet activation and aggregation such as ASA, clopidogrel and GP IIb/IIIa inhibitors, and agents interfering with blood coagulation such as heparins, fondaparinux and bivalirudin have been shown to reduce recurrent ischemic events when administered in the first few hours after the onset of symptoms. The clinical trials for many agents were performed in an era when cardiac catheterization was performed less frequently and usually much later than has become current practice. Consequently, application of the results to current practice requires interpretation and extrapolation often beyond information provided by the individual trials.

Antiplatelet therapy ASA was studied in patients with unstable angina and shown to reduce recurrent events both early and over many months. The benefit was observed in patients receiving no antithrombotic treatment and before

the days of frequent revascularization. In patients with NSTE ACS the CURE trial[18] demonstrated that the addition of clopidogrel 75 mg daily to ASA reduced the primary endpoint (cardiovascular mortality, myocardial infarction or stroke) by a relative 20% (2% absolute risk reduction) over the nine-month period of treatment. Within hours of administration of the 300 mg loading dose, there was a significant reduction of the combined endpoint of cardiovascular death, myocardial infarction (MI) and recurrent severe ischemia. The majority of patients included in the CURE trial had either ECG abnormalities or positive biochemical markers (usually CKMB). However, for the first 3000 patients enrolled, age greater than 60 and a history of coronary artery disease were entry criteria. Across a wide risk spectrum, there was a constant relative risk reduction with clopidogrel. The benefits were achieved with a 1% absolute increase in major bleeding, mainly determined by a 50 g/L fall in hemoglobin or need for transfusion, yet with no increase in life-threatening bleeding. Approximately one-third of patients underwent revascularization after randomization. Patients undergoing both percutaneous coronary intervention[19] and coronary artery bypass surgery[20] had benefit from pretreatment with clopidogrel before revascularization. However, for the few patients undergoing coronary bypass surgery within five days of receiving clopidogrel, major bleeding was increased 50%.[18]

The intravenously administered GP IIb/IIIa inhibitors abciximab, tirofiban and eptifibatide were studied in patients with NSTE ACS before clopidogrel was used in the early management of these patients. A meta-analysis of clinical trials that included over 31 000 patients suggested a modest benefit with one fewer death or MI at 30 days per 100 patients treated.[21] The greatest benefit was observed in higher risk patients, such as those with troponin elevation,[22,23] and diabetes mellitus.[24]

Currently it is unclear whether the addition of a GP IIb/IIIa inhibitor to dual antiplatelet therapy with ASA and clopidogrel improves outcomes. The ISAR React 2 study evaluated the use of abciximab at the time of PCI in patients with recent NSTE ACS pretreated with clopidogrel. Those receiving both clopidogrel and abciximab and with elevated troponin had a 25% reduction of the combined endpoint of death/non-fatal myocardial infarction or urgent target vessel revascularization.

Antithrombotic treatment Activation of the coagulation pathway by agents such as tissue factor initiates a positive feedback system activating platelets and resulting in rapid growth and propagation of the thrombus. Control of the coagulation pathway is important to prevent recurrent ischemic events in patients with acute coronary syndromes. Available agents and their interaction with the coagulation pathway are shown in Figure 73.3.

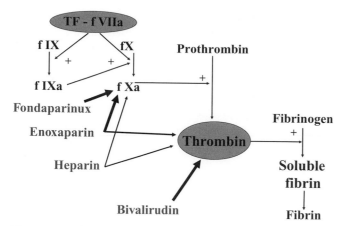

Figure 73.3 The sites of action of the antithrombin agents currently used in the management of patients with NSTE ACS.

Unfractionated heparin (UFH) An analysis of six clinical trials in patients with NSTE ACS that compared UFH with placebo showed a 33% reduction of death and MI over the short term (OR 0.66, 95% CI 0.44–0.99, *P* = 0.045).[25] When UFH is combined with ASA and compared to ASA alone, there is a trend to a benefit with the combined therapy.[26] Studies that compare either UFH or low molecular weight heparin combined with ASA with ASA alone show a 39% reduction of death and MI.

Low molecular weight heparin (LMWH) When compared with placebo in patients with NSTE ACS, there is benefit from LMWH (death/MI OR 0.34, 95% CI 0.20–0.58, *P* < 0.0001).[27] However in this meta-analysis LMWH was not superior to UFH (OR 0.88, 95% CI 0.69–1.12, *P* = 0.34). However, individual LMWH preparations may be superior to UFH. When enoxaparin is compared to UFH a meta-analysis showed no difference in mortality outcomes at 30 days (OR 1.00, 95% CI 0.85–1.17). Yet death/MI was reduced 9% by enoxaparin (OR 0.91, 95% CI 0.83–0.99).[28] In this analysis there was no increase in bleeding as defined by major bleeding or transfusion needs when enoxaparin was used. A more contemporary use of enoxaparin in the SYNERGY trial[29] included 9978 high-risk patients with NSTE ACS destined to undergo very early coronary angiography and revascularization. Patients were randomized to receive either enoxaparin or UFH. Coronary angiography was performed an average 22 hours after randomization. In the context of aggressive, very early invasive management, enoxaparin was not shown to be superior to UFH. There was a trend to increased major bleeding in patients receiving enoxaparin (OR 1.17, 95% CI 0.99–1.39). As a result of the SYNERGY trial, UFH is preferred over enoxaparin if the patient is likely to go to the catheterization laboratory within the first 24 hours after presentation.

Fondaparinux The synthetic anti-factor Xa inhibitor fondaparinux was evaluated in the large outcome study OASIS 5 (Organisation to Assess Strategies for Ischemic Syndromes 5).[18] In this study, 20 078 patients with NSTE ACS were randomized to receive either fondaparinux or enoxaparin for an average of six days. The primary efficacy endpoint (death, MI or refractory ischemia at nine days) of the two treatment groups (fondaparinux 5.8% vs enoxaparin 5.7%) was not statistically different and satisfied predetermined non-inferiority criteria. The composite efficacy and safety endpoint (death, MI, refractory ischemia or major bleeding) was significantly reduced in patients receiving fondaparinux (fondaparinux 7.3% vs enoxaparin 9.0%). Major bleeding was increased in patients receiving enoxaparin compared to fondaparinux, and was an independent predictor of medium- and long-term mortality (six-month mortality: fondaparinux 5.8%, enoxaparin 6.5%, *P* = 0.05). The increased mortality at 30 days and at six months in patients receiving enoxaparin is almost entirely accounted for by the increase in major bleeding. The reduced bleeding associated with fondaparinux compared to enoxaparin treatment was observed in a very wide range of patient baseline observations and management strategies. Older patients, women, and those with renal insufficiency had less major bleeding with fondaparinux. Patients undergoing early cardiac catheterization (even within the first 24 hours) and those receiving either a GP IIb/IIIa inhibitor or heparin at the time of the procedure had less major bleeding when they received fondaparinux compared to the enoxaparin group.[30]

Guide catheter thrombosis at the time of PCI was observed more frequently in fondaparinux-treated patients (0.9% vs 0.4%, *P* < 0.001). Although the additional use of unfractionated heparin with fondaparinux at the time of PCI appears to reduce the incidence of guide catheter thrombosis, the safety of the combined treatment needs further assessment. Fondaparinux has a similar efficacy to enoxaparin for the prevention of recurrent ischemic events but in the protocol used in the OASIS 5 study, the reduction of major bleeding translated into a significantly lower mortality.

Bivalirudin Direct thrombin inhibitors such as bivalirudin were shown in a meta-analysis to be more effective than heparin in reducing death or reinfarction in patients with ACS undergoing early percutaneous coronary intervention.[31] Bivalirudin was evaluated in patients with NSTE ACS in the ACUITY trial.[32] Although there was no difference in the ischemic endpoint between the three strategies of heparin and GP IIb/IIIa inhibitor, bivalirudin and GP IIb/IIIa inhibitor, and bivalirudin alone, patients receiving bivalirudin alone had less major bleeding than those in the other two groups. Bivalirudin is an attractive antithrombin in moderate- to high-risk NSTE ACS patients who will undergo very early cardiac catheterization in the first 12–24 hours.

Case history *continued*

Our patient now has evidence for a high-risk non-ST segment ACS. Evidence shown above supports referral for early coronary angiography and revascularization, and the use of both antithrombotic and antiplatelet agents.

She was already receiving dual antiplatelet therapy with ASA 81 mg and clopidogrel 75 mg daily (after a 300 mg loading dose). The ASA dose was maintained at 81 mg to minimize the incidence of gastrointestinal bleeding. In the CURE trial the incidence of major bleeding in patients receiving combined clopidogrel 75 mg daily and ASA 75–100 mg daily was less than for those receiving only ASA 325 mg.

On the basis of the ESSENCE[33] and TIMI 11b[34] trials, our patient was given enoxaparin 1 mg/kg daily. It was recognized that she had moderate renal insufficiency with an estimated glomerular filtration rate (eGFR) of 35 mL/min. LMWH and fondaparinux are excreted renally. Although it is recommended that the dose of enoxaparin be reduced 50% to 1 mg daily for patients with eGFR < 30 mL/min, there are no safety data to support this recommendation. The patient was admitted to an ECG monitored bed. A referral was sent to the local cardiac center for coronary angiography, and arrangements made for transfer within the next 48 hours.

Over the next 24 hours our patient had a further episode of chest pain and dyspnea with associated ST segment depression in ECG leads V1–V4. The pain resolved within 10 minutes after administration of nitroglycerin 0.4 mg sublingually.

How will you manage this patient now?

Comment

Our patient now has refractory myocardial ischemia with associated ECG abnormalities. Prior to the current era of the use of early cardiac catheterization and multiple antithrombotic agents, refractory ischemia was the factor most predictive of future adverse outcomes.[35] More recently, the GUSTO 2b study[36] showed that mortality was threefold greater in patients receiving ASA and heparin who developed refractory ischemia associated with ECG changes.

The patient requires urgent transfer to a cardiac center for angiography and, if possible, PCI. The question now is whethere there is benefit to starting other medication to reduce recurrent ischemic events. The patient's chest pain did appear to resolve with sublingual nitroglycerin. Thus many physicians would use an infusion of intravenous nitroglycerin at doses of 20–150 μg/h. The use of an intravenous GP IIb/IIIa inhibitor for patients with refractory ischemia has never been evaluated. The clinical trials of GP

IIb/IIIa inhibition in patients with NSTE ACS have either recruited patients at the time of presentation[37–39] or during the waiting period for PCI, when the coronary anatomy was known.[40]

Case history *continued*

Our patient is started on an infusion of nitroglycerin at 60 μg/h. It was decided not to use a GP IIb/IIIa inhibitor in addition to ASA, clopidogrel and enoxaparin, because the patient's gender, age, and impaired renal function would substantially increase the bleeding risk. The cardiac center was called and transfer arranged in the next four hours.

At coronary angiography a severe proximal left anterior descending coronary stenosis was found. There were minor stenoses in the other coronary vessels. Left ventricular function was not assessed at this procedure.

Arrangements were made for immediate PCI. As the patient had received enoxaparin four hours previously, no additional anticoagulant was given. However, eptifibatide was started prior to the procedure. The artery was successfully dilated and a 4.0 mm paclitaxel drug-eluting stent deployed. The final result showed no residual stenosis.

Comment

Successful dilation and stenting of the culprit stenosis is not the end of the story. The patient may have other vulnerable coronary plaques that could cause further acute coronary events unrelated to the original culprit lesion; acute stent thrombosis, although rare, may occur and there is a short- and long-term risk of bleeding resulting from the multiple antithrombotic agents. In addition, there is need for evidence-based vascular protective medication and lifestyle modification to reduce progression and atherothrombotic complications of atherosclerosis.

Case history *continued*

Following the successful PCI, our patient returned to the cardiology ward of the cardiac center. The arterial access sheath had been closed with a vascular closure device. There was no hematoma or evidence of bleeding when the patient returned to the ward. An order had been written to discontinue enoxaparin, but to continue eptifibatide at the standard infusion rate of 2 μg/kg/minute for the next 18 hours. In addition, the ASA dose was increased to 325 mg and clopidogrel 75 mg daily continued.

Six hours after the PCI our patient complained of lower back pain and pain over the front of the thigh. The blood pressure had initially been 140/85, but with the onset of pain fell to 90/50.

Question

What is the current problem, how will you make a diagnosis, what is the management, and will it influence long-term outcomes?

Comment

The onset of back and thigh pain in a patient receiving powerful antiplatelet or anticoagulant therapy should raise a high level of suspicion for a retroperitoneal bleed.

There was no visible or palpable hematoma at the femoral access site. The abdominal examination was unremarkable and bowel sounds were present. With the administration of 1.5 litres of 0.9% saline, the blood pressure was restored to the baseline level. The eptifibatide was discontinued. Our patient was sent for a CT scan of the abdomen that confirmed the presence of a large retroperitoneal hemorrhage, on the contralateral side to the arterial access site. The hemoglobin fell from a baseline 135 g/L to 85 g/L when measured the next day. The patient was transfused 2 units of packed red blood cells.

Question

Was this major bleeding event predictable and preventable?

Comment

With the greater use of both antithrombotic medications and early revascularization, bleeding has become an increasingly important problem for patients admitted to hospital with ACS. In fact, major bleeding and the need for transfusion is the most common adverse event and exceeds the incidence of death, myocardial infarction and heart failure.[41] Not only does bleeding result in an immediate threat, but it is also associated with increased coronary heart disease mortality and reinfarction. The older patient, females, those with anemia, renal dysfunction, high-risk ACS, diabetes, hypertension and those undergoing invasive procedures are at high risk for bleeding. Major bleeding, from whatever cause or site, is associated with a 60% increased risk of in-hospital death and a fivefold increase in one-year mortality and reinfarction.[42,43] In addition, patients receiving blood transfusion had a fourfold increase in mortality.[41] Yet the causal link between bleeding, transfusion and increased coronary heart disease events is unproven.

The current paradigm for the management of ACS is to minimize recurrent ischemic events but also to minimize the risk of bleeding. Such a strategy includes matching the ACS risk to the most appropriate treatment, assessing the bleeding risk, using vascular access techniques to minimize bleeding, selecting the antithrombotic agent that is best for the patient, minimizing the duration of exposure to antithrombotic agents, using the correct dose of medications, and recognizing early signs of bleeding.

Our patient had a number of higher risk features that increased her chance for major bleeding. These included: older age, female gender, hypertension, diabetes, renal insufficiency, and recent femoral arterial vascular access. Furthermore, she had received enoxaparin and eptifibatide at standard doses, despite moderately severe renal insufficiency. Excessive dosing of anticoagulants and antiplatelet agents, due to inaccurate estimates of weight and failure to correct doses for renal impairment, is responsible for bleeding in an important number of cases.[44]

Case history *continued*

Fortunately our patient made a good recovery from the retroperitoneal bleeding and left hospital five days after the PCI procedure. She was given a discharge prescription that included ASA 81 mg daily, clopidogrel 75 mg daily, ramipril 10 mg daily, hydrochlorothiazide 25 mg daily, atorvastatin 80 mg daily, metoprolol 50 mg twice daily, and metformin 500 mg bid.

Comment

Vascular protective measures that reduce recurrent ischemic events have a large impact on long-term outcomes. These measures include lifestyle changes and pharmacologic treatment. All patients admitted to hospital for an ACS should receive lifestyle counseling. This should include smoking cessation advice and referral to a smoking cessation clinic. Weight control, increased physical activity and dietary advice are frequently required. Vascular protective medications for patients who have had an ACS should include ASA, a statin, an ACE inhibitor and a beta-blocker. In addition, glycemic and blood pressure control should be optimized.

Long-term treatment: the discharge prescription

Lifestyle counseling is started in hospital prior to discharge. Efforts to promote smoking cessation after an acute coronary event are likely to be more successful than at any other time. However, it is recognized that for success with lifestyle modification, ongoing support in a cardiac rehabilitation center is most likely to result in long term gains.

Abnormal glucose metabolism is present in two-thirds of patients with acute coronary syndromes[45,46] (30% have known diabetes, 15% have newly diagnosed diabetes, 22% have impaired glucose tolerance (IGT), and 5% have impaired fasting glucose (IFG)). The earlier detection and treatment of diabetes will prevent microvascular disease and may have an impact on preventing recurrent cardiac events.

Statin treatment reduces death, MI and stroke in patients with stable coronary heart disease over a wide range of baseline LDL cholesterol. The MIRACL[47] and PROVE-IT-TIMI 22[48] studies showed that cardiovascular events were reduced within 30 days of initiating treatment by vigorously reducing LDL-C in patients with a recent ACS.[49] Current evidence supports treatment early after an ACS with an intensive statin regimen such as atorvastatin 80 mg daily. Angiotensin-converting enzyme inhibitors or angiotensin receptor blockers (ARB) should be considered in patients with ACS and heart failure or impaired LV ejection fraction (LVEF < 40%) to prevent the development of heart failure and reduce mortality.[50] The VALIANT study demonstrated that the ARB valsartan was not inferior to the ACE inhibitor captopril for the prevention of cardiovascular events in patients with recent myocardial infarction and either heart failure or LVEF < 40%. The SAVE trial[50] also demonstrated that early treatment with captopril reduced recurrent myocardial infarction. A combined analysis[51] of the HOPE,[52] EUROPA[53] and PEACE[54] clinical trials showed that ACE inhibition resulted in a 14% reduction of cardiovascular mortality and 18% reduction of myocardial infarction. The ONTARGET trial[55] showed that the ARB telmisartan was not inferior to ramipril for the prevention of cardiovascular events in high-risk patients. However, none of these four studies with ACE inhibitors or ARB included patients during the first 1–3 months after acute MI. Yet it is likely that ACE inhibitors or ARBs started early after an acute MI will prevent recurrent MI, as suggested by the SAVE results.[50]

Antiplatelet therapy with ASA and clopidogrel, initiated on admission and continued for nine months, was shown in the CURE trial[56] to reduce the combined outcome of death/MI/stroke by 20%. Many patients with NSTE ACS will receive an intracoronary stent as part of an early intervention and revascularization strategy. These patients benefit from combined ASA and clopidogrel continued for one year. Beyond one year, treatment with dual antiplatelet therapy remains controversial. Patients receiving drug-eluting stents, especially with complex anatomy or high-risk locations, may benefit from longer term treatment to prevent late stent thrombosis. The CHARISMA trial[57] in patients with either clinically evident cardiovascular disease or multiple risk factors showed no overall advantage of combined ASA and clopidogrel beyond ASA alone. However, an analysis of patients with established vascular disease showed a significant, albeit modest benefit.[58]

Beta-adrenergic blockers reduce mortality by approximately 25% in patients with MI during treatment for two years or more after the acute event.[59] Patients with non-Q wave infarction were included in these studies.

References

1. Sanchis J, Bodi V, Nunez J et al. New risk score for patients with acute chest pain, non-ST-segment deviation, and normal troponin concentrations. A comparison with the TIMI Risk Score. _J Am Coll Cardiol_ 2006;**46**:443–9.

2. Sanchis J, Bodi V, Nunez J et al. A practical approach with outcome for the prognostic assessment of non-ST-segment elevation chest pain and normal troponin. _Am J Cardiol_ 2007;**99**:797–801.

3. Lindahl B, Diderholm E, Lagerqvist B et al. Mechanisms behind the prognostic value of troponin T in unstable coronary artery disease. _J Am Coll Cardiol_ 2001;**38**:987–90.

4. Choudhry NK, Singh JM, Barolet A, Tomlinson GA, Detsky AS. How should patients with unstable angina and non-ST-segment elevation myocardial infarction be managed? A meta-analysis of randomized trials. _Am J Med_ 2005;**118**:465–74.

5. Mehta SR, Cannon CP, Fox KAA et al. Routine vs selective invasive strategies in patients with acute coronary syndromes. _JAMA_ 2005;**293**:2908–17.

6. Biondi-Zoccai GGL, Abbate A, Agostoni P et al. Long-term benefits of an early invasive management in acute coronary syndromes depend on intracoronary stenting and aggressive antiplatelet treatment: A metaregression. _Am Heart J_ 2005;**149**:504–11.

7. Bavry AA, Kumbhani DJ, Quiroz R, Ramchandani SR, Kenchaiah S, Antman EM. Invasive therapy along with glycoprotein IIb/IIIa inhibitors and intracoronary stents improves survival in non-ST-segment elevation acute coronary syndromes: a meta-analysis and review of the literature. _Am J Cardiol_ 2004;**93**:830–5.

8. FRagmin and Fast Revascularisation during InStability in Coronary artery disease Investigators. Invasive compared with non-invasive treatment in unstable coronary-artery disease: FRISC II prospective randomised multicentre study. _Lancet_ 1999;**354**:708–15.

9. Fox KAA, Poole-Wilson P, Henderson, RA et al. Interventional versus conservative treatment for patients with unstable angina or non-ST segment elevation myocardial infarction: the British Heart Foundation Randomised RITA 3 Trial. _Lancet_ 2002;**360**:743–51.

10. Fox KAA, Poole-Wilson P, Clayton TC et al. Five Year outcome of an interventional strategy in non-ST elevation acute coronary syndromes. The British Heart Foundation RITA-3 randomised trial. _Lancet_ 2005;**366**:914–20.

11. Cannon CP, Weintraub WS, Demopoulos L et al. Comparison of early invasive and conservative strategies in patients with unstable coronary syndromes treated with the glycoprotein IIb/IIIa inhibitor tirofiban. N Eng J Med 2001;**344**:1879–87.

12. Solomon DH, Stone PH, Glynn RJ et al. Use of risk stratification to identify patients with unstable angina likeliest to benefit from an invasive versus conservative management strategy. J Am Coll Cardiol 2001;**38**:969–76.

13. Cantor WJ, Goodman SG, Cannon CP et al. Early cardiac catheterization is associated with lower mortality only among high-risk patients with ST- and non-ST-elevation acute coronary syndromes: observations from the OPUS-TIMI 16 trial. Am Heart J 2005;**149**:275–83.

14. Bhatt DL, Roe MT, Peterson ED et al. Utilization of early invasive management strategies for high-risk patients with non-ST-segment elevation acute coronary syndromes: results from the CRUSADE Quality Improvement Initiative. JAMA 2004;**292**:2096–104.

15. Neumann FJ, Kastrati A, Pogatsa-Murray G et al. Evaluation of prolonged pre-treatment (cooling off strategy) before intervention in patients with unstable coronary syndromes: a randomised controlled trial. JAMA 2003;**290**:1593–9.

16. Anderson JL, Adams CD, Antman EM et al. ACC/AHA 2007 guidelines for the management of patients with unstable angina/non-ST-elevation myocardial infarction – executive summary: a report of the American College of Cardiology/American Heart Association Task Force on Practice Guidelines (Writing Committee to Revise the 2002 Guidelines for the Management of Patients With Unstable Angina/Non-ST-Elevation myocardial Infarction): developed in collaboration with the American College of Emergency Physicians, American College of Physicians, Society for Academic Emergency Medicine, Society for Cardiovascular Angiography and Interventions, and Society of Thoracic Surgeons. J Am Coll Cardiol 2007;**50**:652–726.

17. De Winter RJ, Windhausen F, Cornel JH et al. Early invasive versus selectively invasive management for acute coronary syndromes. N Eng J Med 2005;**353**:1095–104.

18. Clopidogrel in Unstable Angina to Prevent recurrent Events Trial Investigators. Effects of clopidogrel in addition to ASA in patients with acute coronay syndromes without ST segment elevation. N Engl J Med 2001;**345**:494–502.

19. Mehta SR, Yusuf S, Peters RJG et al. Effects of pretreatment with clopidogrel and aspirin followed by long term therapy in patients undergoing percutaneous coronary intervention: the PCI CURE Study. Lancet 2001;**358**:527–33.

20. Fox KA, Mehta SR, Peters R et al. Benefits and risks of the combination of clopidogrel and aspirin in patients undergoing surgical revascularization for non-ST-elevation acute coronary syndrome: the Clopidogrel in Unstable angina to prevent Recurrent ischemic Events (CURE) Trial. Circulation 2004;**110**:1202–8.

21. Boersma E, Harrington RA, Moliterno DJ et al. Platelet glycoprotein IIb/IIIa inhibitors in acute coronary syndromes: a meta-analysis of all major randomised clinical trials. Lancet 2002;**359**:189–98.

22. Heeschen C, Hamm CW, Goldmann B, Deu A, Langenbrink L, White HD. Troponin concentrations for stratification of patients with acute coronary syndromes in relation to therapeutic efficacy of tirofiban. PRISM Study Investigators. Platelet Receptor Inhibition in Ischemic Syndrome Management. Lancet 1999;**354**:1757–62.

23. Newby LK, Ohman EM, Christenson RH et al. Benefit of glycoprotein IIb/IIIa inhibition in patients with acute coronary syndromes and troponin T positive status. Circulation 2001;**103**:2891–6.

24. Roffi M, Chew DP, Mukherjee D et al. Platelet glycoprotein IIb/IIIa inhibitors reduce mortality in diabetic patients with non-ST segment elevation acute coronary syndromes. Circulation 2001;**104**:2767–71.

25. Hirsh J, Raschke R. Heparin and low molecular weight hepain: the Seventh ACCP Conference on Antithrombotic and Thrombolytic Therapy. Chest 2004;**126**:188S–203S.

26. Oler A, Whooley MA, Oler J, Grady D. Adding heparin to aspirin reduces the incidence of myocardial infarction and death in patients with unstable angina. A meta-analysis. JAMA 1996;**276**:811–15.

27. Eikelboom JW, Anand SS, Malmberg K, Weitz JI, Ginsberg JS, Yusuf S. Unfractionated heparin and low-molecular-weight heparin in acute coronary syndrome without ST elevation: a meta-analysis. Lancet 2000;**355**:1936–42.

28. Petersen JL, Mahaffey KW, Hasselblad V et al. Efficacy and bleedin complications among patients randomized to enoxaparin or unfractionated heparin for anti-thrombin therapy in non-ST segment elevation acute coronary syndromes. JAMA 2004;**292**:89–96.

29. SYNERGY Trial Investigators. Enoxaparin vs unfractionated heparin in high-risk patients with non-ST-segment elevation acute coronary syndromes managed with an intended early invasive strategy. Primary results of the SYNERGY randomized trial. JAMA 2004;**292**:45–54.

30. Mehta SR, Granger CB, Eikelboom JW et al. Efficacy and safety of fondaparinux versus enoxaparin in patients with acute coronary syndromes undergoing percutaneous coronary intervention: results from the OASIS-5 trial. J Am Coll Cardiol 2007;**50**:1742–51.

31. Sinnaeve PR, Simes J, Yusuf S et al. Direct thrombin inhibitors in acute coronary syndromes:effect in patients undergoing early percutaneous coronary intervention. Eur Heart J 2005;**26**:2396–403.

32. Stone GW, McLaurin BT, Cox DA et al. Bivalirudin for patients with acute coronary syndromes. N Engl J Med 2006;**355**:2203–16.

33. Cohen M, Demers C, Gurfinkel EP et al. Low-molecular-weight heparins in non-ST-segment elevation ischemia: the ESSENCE trial. Efficacy and Safety of Subcutaneous Enoxaparin versus intravenous unfractionated heparin, in Non-Q-wave Coronary Events. Am J Cardiol 1998;**82**:19L–24L.

34. Antman EM, McCabe CH, Gurfinkel EP et al. Treatment benefit of enoxaparin in unstable angina/non-Q wave myocardial infarction is maintained at one year followup in TIMI 11B. Circulation 1999;**100**: I-497.

35. Murphy JJ, Connell PA, Hampton JR. Predictors of risk in patients with unstable angina admitted to a district general hospital. Br Heart J 1992;**67**:395–401.

36. Armstrong PW, Fu Y, Chang WC et al. Acute coronary syndromes in the GUSTO-IIb trial: prognostic insights and impact of recurrent ischemia. The GUSTO-IIb Investigators. Circulation 1998;**98**:1860–8.

37. Platelet Receptor Inhibition in Ischemic Syndrome Management in Patients Limited by Unstable Signs and Symptoms (PRISM-PLUS) Study Investigators. Inhibition of the platelet glycoprotein IIb/IIIa receptor with tirofiban in unstable angina and non-Q-wave myocardial infarction. [published erratum appears in *N Engl J Med* 1998;**339**(6):415]. *N Engl J Med* 1998;**338**:1488–97.

38. Platelet Receptor Inhibition in Ischemic Syndrome Management (PRISM) Study Investigator. A comparison of aspirin plus tirofiban with aspirin plus heparin for unstable angina. *N Engl J Med* 1998;**338**:1498–505.

39. PURSUIT Trial Investigators. Inhibition of platelet glycoprotein IIb/IIIa with eptifibatide in patients with acute coronary syndromes. Platelet Glycoprotein IIb/IIIa in Unstable Angina: Receptor Suppression Using Integrilin Therapy [see comments]. *N Engl J Med* 1998;**339**:436–43.

40. Hamm CW, Heeschen C, Goldmann B *et al*. Benefit of abciximab in patients with refractory unstable angina in relation to serum troponin T levels. c7E3 Fab Antiplatelet Therapy in Unstable Refractory Angina (CAPTURE) Study Investigators. *N Engl J Med* 1999;**340**:1623–9.

41. Yang X, Alexander KP, Chen AY *et al*. The implications of blood transfusions for patients with non-ST-segment elevation acute coronary syndromes: results from the CRUSADE National Quality Improvement Initiative. *J Am Coll Cardiol* 2005;**46**:1490–5.

42. Moscucci M, Fox KA, Cannon CP *et al*. Predictors of major bleeding in acute coronary syndromes: the Global Registry of Acute Coronary Events (GRACE). *Eur Heart J* 2003;**24**:1815–23.

43. Segev A, Strauss BH, Tan M, Constance C, Langer A, Goodman SG. Predictors and 1-year outcome of major bleeding in patients with non-ST elevation acute coronary syndromes: Insights from the Canadian Acute Coronary Syndrome Registries. *Am Heart J* 2005;**150**:690–4.

44. Alexander KP, Chen AY, Roe MT *et al*. Excess Dosing of antiplatelet and antithrombin agents in the treatment of non-ST-segment elevation acute coronary syndromes. *JAMA* 2005;**294**:3108–116.

45. Bartnick M, Malmberg K, Norhammar A, Tenerz A, Ohrvik J, Ryden L. Newly detected abnormal glucose tolerance: an important predictor of long-term outcome after myocardial infarction. *Eur Heart J* 2004;**25**:1990–7.

46. Bartnik M, Malmberg K, Hamsten A *et al*. Abnormal glucose tolerance – a common risk factor in patients with acute myocardial infarction in comparison with population-based controls. *J Intern Med* 2004;**256**:288–97.

47. Schwartz GG, Olsson AG, Ezekowitz MD *et al*. Effects of atorvastatin on early recurrent ischemic events in acute coronary syndromes: the MIRACL study: a randomized controlled trial. *JAMA* 2001;**285**:1711–18.

48. Cannon CP, Braunwald E, McCabe CH *et al*. Intensive versus moderate lipid lowering with statins after acute coronary syndromes. *N Engl J Med* 2004;**350**:1495–504.

49. Ray KK, Cannon CP, McCabe CH *et al*, for the PROVE-IT-TIMI 22 Investigators. Early and late benfits of high-dose atorvastatin in patients with acute coronary syndromes. Results from the PROVE-IT-TIMI 22 Trial. *J Am Coll Cardiol* 2005;**46**:1405–10.

50. Pfeffer MA, Braunwald E, Moye LA *et al*. Effect of captopril on mortality and morbidity in patients with left ventricular dysfunction after myocardial infarction. Results of the survival and ventricular enlargement trial. The SAVE Investigators. *N Engl J Med* 1992;**327**:669–77.

51. Dagenais GR, Pogue J, Fox K, Simoons ML, Yusuf S. Angiotensin-converting-enzyme inhibitors in stable vascular disease without left ventricular systolic dysfunction or heart failure: a combined analysis of three trials. *Lancet* 2006;**368**:581–8.

52. Yusuf S, Sleight P, Pogue J, Bosch J, Davies R, Dagenais G. Effects of an angiotensin-converting-enzyme inhibitor, ramipril, on cardiovascular events in high-risk patients. The Heart Outcomes Prevention Evaluation Study Investigators. *N Engl J Med* 2000;**342**:145–53.

53. EURopean trial On reduction of cardiac events with Perindopril in stable coronary Artery disease Investigators. Efficacy of perindopril in reduction of cardiovascular events among patients with stable coronary artery disease: randomised, double-blind, placebo-controlled, multicentre trial (the EUROPA study). *Lancet* 2003;**362**:782–8.

54. PEACE Investigators. Angiotensin-converting enzyme inhibition in stable coronary artery disease. *N Engl J Med* 2004;**351**: 2058–68.

55. Yusuf S, Teo KK, Pogue J *et al*. Telmisartan, ramipril, or both in patients at high risk for vascular events. *N Engl J Med* 2008;**358**:1547–59.

56. Yusuf S, Zhao F, Mehta SR, Chrolavicius S, Tognoni G, Fox KK. Effects of clopidogrel in addition to aspirin in patients with acute coronary syndromes without ST-segment elevation. *N Engl J Med* 2001;**345**:494–502.

57. Bhatt DL, Fox KA, Hacke W *et al*. Clopidogrel and aspirin versus aspirin alone for the prevention of atherothrombotic events. *N Engl J Med* 2006;**354**(16):1706–17.

58. Bhatt DL, Flather MD, Hacke W *et al*. Patients with prior myocardial infarction, stroke, or symptomatic peripheral arterial disease in the CHARISMA trial. *J Am Coll Cardiol* 2007;**49**:1982–8.

59. Yusuf S, Peto R, Lewis J, Collins R, Sleight P. Beta blockade during and after myocardial infarction: an overview of the randomized trials. *Prog Cardiovasc Dis* 1985;**27**:335–71.

60. Sanchis J, Bodi V, Nunez J *et al*. New risk score for patients with acute chest pain, non-ST-segment deviation, and normal troponin concentrations: a comparison with the TIMI risk score. *J Am Coll Cardiol* 2005;**46**:443–9.

61. Bavry AA, Kumbhani DJ, Rassi AN, Bhatt DL, Askari AT. Benefit of early invasive therapy in acute coronary syndromes: a meta-analysis of contemporary randomized clinical trials. *J Am Coll Cardiol* 2006;**48**:1319–25.

74

Acute ST segment elevation myocardial infarction

Ernest L Fallen

McMaster University, Faculty of Health Sciences, Hamilton, Ontario, Canada

Case history

A 55-year-old self-employed male truck driver suddenly experiences, for the first time, severe retrosternal chest pain accompanied by weakness, nausea, and shortness of breath. When his distress fails to abate he presents, within 30 minutes, to the emergency room of a hospital without heart catheterization facilities.

Physical exam reveals a pale, anxious, diaphoretic overweight man with a blood pressure of 110/90 and a regular heart rate of 98 beats per minute. There are sibilant rales at both lung bases bilaterally but his neck veins are flat. On auscultation there is a soft apical systolic murmur and an S4 gallop rhythm. His risk factors include a 10-year history of hypertension for which he is on a thiazide diuretic as his only medication. He is a 40 pack/year smoker with a strong family history of a sister with an MI at age 58 and a father who suffered an MI in his 40s. He is not diabetic and his lipid status is unknown.

An ECG is immediately ordered (Fig. 74.1).

Question

What is your clinical assessment and what action should be taken at this juncture?

Comment

The clinical presentation of persistent chest pain, nausea, weakness, dyspnea and diaphoresis coupled with characteristic ECG findings of elevated ST segments in more than two contiguous leads points to the diagnosis of an acute ST segment elevation myocardial infarction (STEMI) of the

Evidence-Based Cardiology, 3rd edition. Edited by S. Yusuf, J.A. Cairns, A.J. Camm, E.L. Fallen, and B.J. Gersh. © 2010 Blackwell Publishing, ISBN: 978-1-4051-5925-8.

anterior wall. The objectives of management at this stage are: (a) relief of symptoms with oxygen, morphine and an intravenous beta-blocker, and (b) rapid restoration of nutrient blood flow through the occluded coronary artery. As to the latter, time is of the essence! There are three therapeutic options:

- fibrinolytic therapy with streptokinase or intravenous tissue plasminogen activator (e.g. reteplase, tenectoplase or alteplase)
- primary percutaneous coronary intervention (PCI)
- facilitated PCI.

Although fibrinolytic therapy is a proven effective strategy for reducing both morbidity and mortality in STEMI,[1] there is now persuasive Level A evidence that primary PCI achieves better short-term (4–6 weeks) and long-term (6–18 months) outcomes when compared to fibrinolytic therapy.[2] The outcomes measured were mortality rates, non-fatal reinfarction, strokes and major bleeds.

Timing and access must be taken into consideration. The earlier the arrival of the patient (less than 30 minutes), the less the advantage of PCI over fibrinolysis becomes apparent, especially if there is an anticipated time delay in transporting the patient across town to another facility.[3] Conversely, many studies have shown the superiority of primary PCI for those patients who require emergency transport to another facility especially if the "time to balloon" can be achieved within 60–90 minutes.[4] The degree of risk has not always been carefully integrated in trial analyses. However, it is safe to assume that those patients at higher risk, as with any of the established interventions, benefit the most. Our patient is an ideal candidate for primary PCI. He is at moderate to high risk (anterior myocardial infarction with evidence of some cardiac decompensation), he appears within the recommended window of 30–60 minutes and has no major contraindications.

Should there be no ready access to an angiographic facility, the preferred treatment would be aspirin 150–

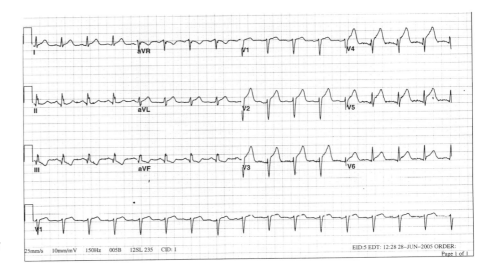

Figure 74.1 12-lead ECG of acute anterior ST elevation myocardial infarction.

350 mg followed immediately by fibrinolysis with, in this particular case, a tissue plaminogen activator. An antithrombin agent is added to help maintain patency of the culprit artery. It should be borne in mind that the combined use of fibrinolytics, antiplatelets and antithrombin agents reduces mortality rates and non-fatal reinfarction at the expense of an increased risk of major and minor bleeding.[5] While low molecular weight heparin offers better outcomes than weight-adjusted unfractionated heparin, the net clinical benefit (i.e. adjusted for major bleeding rates) is less apparent because of the higher rates of bleeding with low molecular weight heparin.[6] The presence of pulmonary rales and an S4 gallop rhythm in this patient with a suspected large anterior wall infarction mitigates against intravenous beta-blocker therapy as long as the chest pain can be ameliorated with oxygen and morphine.[7]

What about opting for a strategy of immediate thrombolysis followed by PCI? This is so-called facilitated PCI. Theoretically, this approach offers quicker patency of the culprit artery on the way to restoration of coronary blood flow with PCI. The 2007 ACC/AHA focused update no longer recommends facilitated PCI for STEMI.[7] Recent analyses have shown a worse outcome with facilitated PCI compared to primary PCI for STEMI.[8]

Case history *continued*

On the basis of the PCI-CURE study, our patient is quickly administered two antiplatelet agents: 150 mg of chewable aspirin and 300 mg clopidogrel loading dose.[9] He is quickly transported to a cardiovascular center situated within one mile of the index hospital. At 90 minutes post symptom onset, a paclitaxel drug-eluting stent (DES) is deployed at the site of an occlusive thrombus in the proximal left anterior descending artery. His angiogram also demonstrates an old distal occlusion of a dominant right coronary artery and a 30% lesion in the obtuse marginal branch of the circumflex artery. He tolerates the procedure without incident. His blood pressure is now 132/70 and he is not in heart failure. He is started on a well-established secondary prevention regimen of an oral beta-blocker (metoprolol 50 mg bid), an angiotensin-converting enzyme (ACE) inhibitor in the form of ramipril starting at 5 mg qam and a HMG Co-A reductase inhibitor (atorvastatin) at 20 mg qhs.[1] Aspirin at 81 mg and clopidogrel 75 mg daily are continued.

The following day he complains of a sharp left parasternal pain exacerbated by movement, coughing and/or taking a deep breath. On his ECG we now see that the ST segment elevation has failed to descend following deployment of the stent and there is new ST elevation in leads II and III (Fig. 74.2). Furthermore, the tachycardia has returned despite the institution of a beta-blocker and clear lung fields. Physical examination confirms the presence of a pericardial friction rub. His blood pressure remains stable at 130/80. His internal jugular veins are not distended.

An echocardiogram shows severe anteroapical hypokinesis of the left ventricle, a pedunculated apical thrombus and an estimated global ejection fraction of 35%. There is no significant pericardial effusion. His troponin I levels increase from 0.8 to 4.5 ng/mL (normal < 0.04). His routine serum electrolytes, urea, creatinine and blood sugars are normal. His white count is only slightly elevated. His hemoglobin on admission was 140 gm/L. It is now 119.

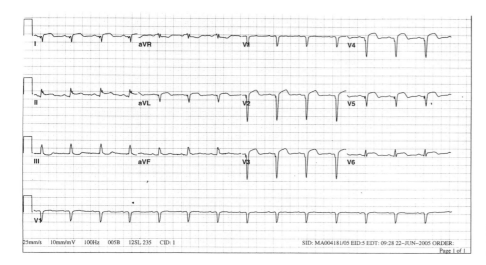

Figure 74.2 Note the new ST elevation in lead II with further ST depression in AVR—all consistent with an acute pericardial reaction.

Question

How would you manage the pericarditis and how aggressive should you be with the LV apical aneurysm and endocardial thrombus?

Comment

In the acute phase of a full-thickness myocardial infarction, pericarditis is not an uncommon complication. It rarely poses a threat and usually runs a benign course. For pain relief a short course of an anti-inflammatory agent, either an increased dose of aspirin (650 mg qid) or a non-steroidal anti-inflammatory agent, suffices. Ibuprofen should probably be avoided as it interferes with the antiplatelet effect of aspirin.[10] It is interesting that in the thrombolytic era, the incidence of pericarditis associated with STEMI has decreased significantly, presumably due to smaller infarct sizes.[11] However, this is also the era of double antiplatelet agents, anticoagulants, antithrombin agents, platelet glycoprotein IIb/IIIa inhibitors and fibrinolytics. Despite these agents the incidence of serious hemorrhagic pericardial effusion in the acute stage of STEMI remains low.

The presence of a pedunculated apical thrombus poses a more sinister threat of systemic embolism. The patient is already on clopidogrel and aspirin. His hemoglobin is falling. What to do? The 2004 ACC/AHA guidelines for treatment of STEMI issue a Level B recommendation for three months of warfarin preventive therapy for patients with a mural thrombus.[1] The decision to add warfarin to this patient's double antiplatelet regimen (already a Level A recommendation) poses a hazard of a major bleed of 0.62%/year[12] versus the risk of a systemic embolus (<0.1%). The mural thrombus is not static and will likely endothelialize within two months. A judgment is made to forego the warfarin.

Case history *continued*

Our patient's condition is now stabilized. He is ambulating well without symptoms. On day four of his hospital course he suddenly develops a severe retrosternal pain not unlike that of his infarct. His ECG (Fig. 74.3) shows evolutionary changes only. However, his troponin I level rebounds from 0.08 to 3.5 ng/mL, clearly indicating new myocardial injury. An urgent coronary angiogram reveals an occlusive thrombus at the site of the drug-eluting stent. An intravenous platelet glycoprotein IIb/IIIa inhibitor (eptifibatide) is quickly administered and the lesion is restented using, once again, a paclitaxel-eluting (Taxus) stent. Shortly following the procedure, our patient develops rigors, fever and an urticarial rash.

Questions

- Do these events alter your management plans?
- What precipitated the allergic reaction?

Comment

Persuasive evidence exists that deployment of drug-eluting stents (DES) such as paclitaxel reduces the incidence of in-stent restenosis compared to bare metal stents.[13] But thrombotic restenosis at the site of a DES is said to occur at a rate of 0.6% at one year.[14] Under these circumstances, the choice of a glycoprotein IIb/IIIa inhibitor such as eptifibatide (Integrilin) appears to offer slightly better protection by improving outcome following stent insertion, according to the ESPRIT study.[15] The propensity for a serious bleed should be borne in mind whenever a third antiplatelet agent is added to aspirin and clopidogrel. This again is a judgment call because the occurrence of an early thrombotic occlusion of his DES does not place our patient neatly into any of the large-scale clinical trials.

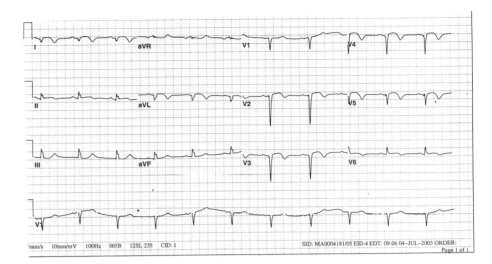

Figure 74.3 Evolutionary changes of an acute anterior myocardial infarction.

Other approaches to prevent restenosis have been proposed. One of these is intracoronary gamma radiation, so-called brachytherapy.[16] This is a highly specialized procedure and so far its superiority in preventing restenosis when compared with DES has not been demonstrated.[17] The evidence for the optimum choice in preventing in-stent restenosis at the site of a compromised DES is sparse and requires further study.

As for the allergic reaction, one can only surmise that it was more related to the contrast agent since the incidence of acute allergy to Integrilin was shown to be identical (0.15%) between the placebo group and the drug group in the PURSUIT study.[18]

The allergic event responds well to intravenous corticosteroid and diphenhydramine, following which our patient goes on to make a gradual but satisfactory recovery. There are no appreciable hemodynamic, ischemic or electrical sequelae. At the time of hospital discharge he is pain free and ambulating well. Despite his trials and tribulations, our patient has a new DES in place with restoration of satisfactory flow through an occluded artery. He is pain free and failure free and he is now recovering without major mishap. He is ready for discharge and it is time for a chat.

The objectives of post-MI management are threefold:

1 to restore patient confidence by outlining an activities program commensurate with the gradual healing process of his injured myocardium

2 to advocate and prescribe secondary prophylactic medications proven to be effective in reducing reinfarction and death. These include enteric-coated aspirin, clopidogrel (at least 12 months), a statin, an ACE inhibitor and, preferably, a beta-blocker[1]

3 to advise on risk factor modification and to promote lifestyle changes. The latter include a regular exercise program (initially supervised), weight reduction, nutri-

tional advice and maintenance of a low lipid profile (see Chapters 12, 15, 23).

All this will certainly be a challenge insofar as our patient, who has just sworn off cigarettes, is a self-employed transport driver with erratic eating habits.

What about alternative strategies such as implantation of an intracardiac defibrillator (ICD) to prevent sudden cardiac death? He doesn't quite fulfill the entry criteria for the MADIT II study.[19] His LV ejection fraction at the time of hospital discharge eight days post STEMI is now 40% and probably rising. Besides, the LV ejection fraction during the first week post STEMI is a questionable determinant of future malignant events. His QRS duration is less than 120 msec. Among the several untoward events that complicated this patient's hospital course, a sinister arrhythmia was not one of them.

Conclusion

Clinical decision making is a fine balancing act between application of external best evidence and what the physician deems best for the patient. Here is a case where on two separate occasions rapid restoration of coronary blood flow was indispensable. In both instances the strategies employed were guided by evidence derived from major clinical trials despite unforeseen complications such as acute pericarditis, depressed LV function, mild heart failure, allergic reactions, the presence of a large apical mural thrombus and the threat of a major bleed.

The case also cautions against blind adherence to every consensus recommendation for the individual patient with unique complications. Here is where the physician's clinical judgment ought to be weighed carefully. For example, in this case the decision to add an anticoagulant (warfarin) because of the mural thrombus had to be weighed against the threat of a major bleed in a patient already on two antiplatelet drugs. The decision not to implant an ICD was a judgment call based on borderline criteria. With deployment of the second stent, the decision to add a platelet glycoprotein IIb/IIIa inhibitor was not based on external evidence pertaining to that particular circumstance but on a supposition that the site of the occluded DES was particularly prone to repeat thrombosis.

References

1. ACC/AHA. Guidelines for the management of patients with ST-elevation myocardial infarction. *J Am Coll Cardiol* 2004; **44**:671–719.
2. Keeley EC, Boura JA, Grimes CL. Primary angioplasty versus intravenous thrombolytic therapy for acute myocardial infarction. A quantitative review of 23 randomized trials. *Lancet* 2003;**361**:13–20.
3. Mauro M, Kim E. Door to balloon time in primary percutaneous coronary intervention. *Circulation* 2006;**113**:1048–50.
4. Dalby M, Bouzamondo A, Lechat P *et al.* Transfer for primary angioplasty vs immediate thrombolysis in acute myocardial infarction. A meta analysis. *Circulation* 2003;**108**:1809–14.
5. Antithrombotic Trialists' Collaboration. Collaborative meta analysis of randomized trials of antiplatelet therapy for prevention of death, myocardial infarction and stroke in high risk patients. *BMJ* 2002;**324**:71–86.
6. Antman EM, Morrow DA, McCabe CH *et al.* Enoxaparin vs unfractionated heparin with fibrinolysis for ST elevation myocardial infarction. *N Engl J Med* 2006;**354**:1477–88.
7. Antman EM, Hand M, Armstrong PW *et al.* 2007 focused update of the ACC/AHA 2004 guidelines for the management of patients with ST elevation myocardial infarction. *J Am Coll Cardiol* 2008;**51**:210.
8. Keeley EC, Boura JA, Grines CL *et al.* Comparison of primary and facilitated percutaneous coronary intervention for ST elevation myocardial infarction: quantitative review of randomized trials. *Lancet* 2006;**367**:579–88.
9. Mehta SR, Yusuf S, Peters RJ *et al.* Effects of pre-treatment with clopidogrel and aspirin followed by long term therapy in patients undergoing percutaneous coronary intervention: the PCI-CURE Study. *Lancet* 2001;**358**:527–33.
10. Catella-Lawson F, Reilly MP, Kapoor SC *et al.* Cyclooxygenase inhibitors and the antiplatelet effect of aspirin. *N Engl J Med* 2001;**345**:1809–17.
11. Correale E, Maggioni AP, Romano S *et al.* Comparison of frequency, diagnostic and prognostic significance of pericardial involvement in acute myocardial infarction treated with and without thrombolytics. GISSI Study. *Am J Cardiol* 1993;**71**:1377–81.
12. Hurlen M, Abdelnoor M, Smith P *et al.* Warfarin, aspirin or both after myocardial infarction. *N Engl J Med* 2002;**347**:969–74.
13. Stone GW, Ellis SG, Cannon L *et al.* Comparison of a polymer based Paclitaxil eluting stent with a bare metal stent in patients with complex coronary artery disease. *JAMA* 2005;**294**:1268–70.
14. Bavry AA, Kumbhani DJ, Helton TJ *et al.* What is the risk of stent thrombosis associated with the use of Paclitaxel eluting stents for percutaneous cotonary intervention? A meta analysis. *Evid Based Cardiovasc Med* 2005;**3**:187–9.
15. O'Shea JC, Hafley GE, Greenberg S *et al.* Platelet glycoprotein IIb/IIIa integren blockade with eptifibatide in coronary stent intervention: the ESPRIT trial. *JAMA* 2001;**285**:2468–73.
16. Ajani AE, Waksman R, Sharma AK *et al.* Three year followup after coronary gamma radiation therapy for in-stent restenosis. Original WRIST trial. *Cardiovasc Rad Med* 2001;**4**:200–4.
17. TAXUS Investigators. Paclitaxel-eluting stents vs vascular brachytherapy for in-stent restenosis within bare metal stents. The Taxus V ISR randomized trial. *JAMA* 2006;**295**:1307–9.
18. PURSUIT Investigators. Inhibition of platelet glycoprotein IIb/IIIa with eptifidamide in patients with acute coronary syndromes. *N Engl J Med* 1998;**339**:436–43.
19. Moss AJ, Zareba W, Hall WJ *et al.* Prophylactic implantation of a defibrillator in patients with myocardial infarction and reduced ejection fraction. *N Engl J Med* 2002;**346**:877–83.

75 Secondary prevention strategies post myocardial infarction

Jacques Genest

McGill University Health Center/Royal Victoria Hospital, Montreal, Canada

Case history

The patient is a 69-year-old man who sustained an acute non-ST-elevation myocardial infarction. He has a family history of premature coronary artery disease (CAD), with a brother who had coronary bypass surgery at age 54 and his father died suddenly at age 60. He is a cigarette smoker (1/2 pack per day). The ECG showed ST segment depression in the anterior leads and plasma levels of troponin I (TnI) reached 3.18 u/L (normal <0.01). A coronary angiogram showed a proximal 90% stenosis of the left anterior decending (LAD) coronary artery and the decision was taken to place a bare metal stent in the proximal LAD lesion. The left ventricular ejection fraction (LVEF) was 55% with mild anterior wall hypokinesis. The patient was discharged the following day.

Six months later, he is referred for evaluation of a low high-density lipoprotein cholesterol (HDL-C). He is presently on atorvastatin 40 mg and ASA 81 mg; clopidogrel was discontinued after 3 months. He stopped beta-blockers on his own because they made him feel "sluggish". He is currently asymptomatic, in Canadian Cardiovascular Society angina class 1, and his exercise stress test showed no ischemia at a workload of 10 METS.

On physical examination, the BP is 130/82, the heart rate 72 and his Body Mass Index (BMI) is 28. The rest of the examination is normal. The lipoprotein profile is as follows: cholesterol 3.72 mmol/L, low-density lipoprotein cholesterol (LDL)-C 2.1 mmol/L, HDL-C 0.8 mmol/L, triglycerides 1.8 mmol/L, Chol/HDL-C ratio 4.65 (Table 75.1). The thyroid-stimulating hormone (TSH) is normally suppressed, Serum levels of creatine kinase (CK) and alanine transaminase (ALT) are normal.

Question

Are further interventions warranted to further reduce cardiovascular risk?

Evidence-Based Cardiology, 3rd edition. Edited by S. Yusuf, J.A. Cairns, A.J. Camm, E.L. Fallen, and B.J. Gersh. © 2010 Blackwell Publishing, ISBN: 978-1-4051-5925-8.

Comment

This case is seen frequently in the secondary prevention setting. The patient is nearly at the LDL-C goal of <2.0 mmol/L. The argument can be made that in the absence of mortality benefit of lowering the LDL-C <2.0 in the TNT and IDEAL trials, the patient is treated according to the current standard of care. The low HDL-C remains problematic. There is presently a paucity of evidence supporting raising HDL-C pharmacologically on a background of statin treatment. This evidence is derived, in part, from *post hoc* analysis of large-scale studies or from pooled analysis of data. The approach to this patient must first involve lifestyle changes (cigarette cessation, quality of diet, weight reduction, exercise, and possibly moderate alcohol intake) which stand on their own merits, irrespective of their effects on HDL-C levels. Indeed, an elevated serum level of HDL-C might be considered a biomarker for cardiovascular health.

While each lifestyle change is expected to raise HDL-C by ~5%, the cumulative effect of these changes may bring the HDL-C into the low-normal range for age and gender. Unfortunately, few patients implement such changes. Smoking cessation should be a priority of treatment in this patient. My own approach would be to further reduce LDL-C by optimizing the dose of statin. (Table 75.1) shows the expected effects of various pharmacologic manipulations including (1) keeping the current treatment, (2) increasing atorvastatin to 80 mg, (3) switching to rosuvastatin 40 mg, (4) adding niacin (extended release) 2 g, (5) adding fenofibrate 200 mg or (6) adding ezetimibe to atorvastatin 40 mg.

While the lipoprotein profile is improved by the five additional options suggested here, the improvement is relatively small and the clinical significance is uncertain. Niacin extended release seems to have the most favorable improvement in both HDL-C and the Chol/HDL-C ratio. Increasing the statin dose is another option and favors

Table 75.1 Expected effects on LDL-C, HDL-C and the Chol/HDL-C ratio if the current treatment is maintained, if niacin 2 g/d is added, if atorvastatin is increased to 80 mg/d, if atorvastatin is substituted for rosuvastatin 40 mg/d and if ezetimibe 10 mg/d is added. Data are based on large-scale clinical trials (see Table 75.2).

Expected → Treatment ↓	%Δ HDL-C %Δ LDL-C	HDL-C LDL-C (mmol/L)	Chol/ HDL-C	Evidence-based?
Current treatment Atorvastatin 40 mg	No Δ No Δ	0.80 2.1	4.65	Yes*
Atorvastatin 80 mg	No Δ −10%	0.80 1.9	4.39	Yes
Rosuvastatin 40 mg	No Δ −10%	0.80 1.9	4.39	Yes*
Niacin 2 g added	+20% −18%	0.96 1.72	3.45	No
Fenofibrate 200 mg added	+6% No Δ	0.9 2.1	4.04	No
Ezetimibe 10 mg added	No Δ −20%	0.80 1.7	4.14	No

* Based on clinical trials of LDL-C reduction to prevent primary or recurrent cardiovascular events in high-risk populations.

monotherapy. It should be pointed out that of the options presented here, only statins (at either the maximal dose or used to decrease LDL-C <2.5 mmol/L) are currently supported by evidence-based literature. The use of fenofibrate is less well supported by clinical trial data, especially in light of the FIELD trial. Other fibrates, especially gemfibrozil, should not be combined with statins because of the risk of rhabdomyolysis. The addition of ezetimibe to statin monotherapy has the advantage of reducing LDL-C to a greater extent than simply doubling the dose of statin and avoiding side effects and adverse events associated with high-dose statins.

General comments on secondary preventive strategies

National guidelines for the secondary prevention of cardiovascular disease emphasize lifestyle changes (smoking cessation, quality of the diet, in terms of reducing saturated fats, weight reduction, physical activity and decrease in psychologic stress[1-3]). In this case, the immediate period following acute myocardial infarction was discussed, with emphasis on treatment and prevention of thrombotic episodes. Here, we will review an aspect of metabolic heart disease that is more controversial and much less supported by evidence-based medicine.

The data supporting lowering LDL-C for the prevention of recurrent events are well established and entrenched in

clinical practice. Pharmacologic therapy is indicated to reach an LDL-C <2.0 mmol/L and a Chol/HDL-C ratio <4.0. Aspirin is indicated in all subjects unless contraindicated. Beta-adrenergic blockers are indicated post myocardial infarction as are ACE inhibitors if the LVEF is decreased. A goal for HDL-C has not been set because of a lack of effective therapies to raise HDL-C and a lack of solid clinical evidence supporting raising HDL-C pharmacologically for cardiovascular disease prevention. While a low HDL-C is considered a categoric cardiovascular risk factor[2-4] and is the most frequent lipoprotein disorder in premature CAD,[5,6] there is still controversy surrounding the causal role of a low HDL-C in atherosclerosis. Experimental evidence shows that the atheroprotective effects of HDL extend far beyond removing cholesterol from lipid-laden macrophages in the atherosclerotic plaque, an effect known as the reverse cholesterol transport. HDL have anti-inflammatory effects, prevent oxidation of LDL, have antithrombotic properties, modulate vasomotor tone and may improve endothelial cell survival (by preventing apoptosis), migration and proliferation.[7,8]

Current approaches to raising HDL-C pharmacologically include statins, fibrates and niacin. Large-scale clinical studies using statins or fibric acid derivatives (fibrates) have shown a modest effect of these two classes of medication on HDL-C levels, usually in the order of 5–10%, much less than reported in smaller studies[9] (Table 75.2). The drug torcetrapib, an inhibitor of cholesteryl ester transfer protein (CETP), led to marked improvement in all lipoprotein classes when used with atorvastatin, but proved toxic in the large-scale clinical trial ILLUMINATE[10] and showed no benefits on surrogate markers of atherosclerosis such as intravascular ultrasound[11] or carotid intima-media thickness.[12,13] Whether other CETP inhibitors will prove cardioprotective will have to be determined in appropriate clinical trials.

Effects of statins

Statins have a modest effect on HDL-C which may be mediated by the decrease in plasma triglycerides and an indirect effect on the transcriptional regulation of apolipoprotein AI (apo AI).[14] There are presently six large-scale secondary or high-risk prevention trials that have examined the effect of statins on major cardiovascular events, coronary heart disease (CHD) mortality and total mortality[15-20]; the SEARCH trial[21] will compare simvastatin 20 mg to atorvastatin 80 mg. These findings are summarized in Table 76.2. Overall, the increase in HDL-C is modest, between 0% and 10%. The reduction in LDL-C is far more impressive and is considered to be a major factor in the reduction in cardiovascular morbidity and mortality. Meta-analysis of cholesterol reduction trials shows unambiguously the benefits of lowering LDL-C for cardiovascular disease prevention, especially in high-risk individuals.[22] The results of these trials have been incorporated in national treatment guidelines for the prevention of CAD.[1,2]

Table 75.2 Major high-risk studies of lipid-modifying therapies in high-risk patients.

Study	Intervention (dose in mg/day)	n	% HDL-C	Endpoints
Statin studies				
4S[15]	Simva 20–40	4444	+8%	Total mortality
CARE[16]	Prava 40	4159	+5%	CHD mortality, non-fatal MI
LIPID[17]	Prava 40	9014	+5%	CHD mortality
HPS[18]	Simva 40	20556	+0.03 mmol/L	Total mortality
"Incremental"s tatin studies				
TNT[19]	Atorva 10–80	10001	No	CHD mortality
IDEAL[20]	Atorva 10–80	8888	+0.03 mmol/L	Neutral*
SEARCH[21]	Simva 20 or 80	12064	NA	Expected 2009
Fibrate studies				
VA-HIT[23]	Gem 1200	2531	+6%	Death, non-fatal MI
BIP[24]	Beza 400	3090	+18%	Neutral*
FIELD[25]	Feno 200	9785	+6%	CHD deaths, MI
Niacin studies				
Coronary Drug Project[27]	Niacin 3 g	3908	+15–35%	Total mortality
Stockholm IHD study[28]	Niacin 3 g+ clofibrate 2 g	555	NA	Total CHD mortality

* Primary endpoint not statistically significant. Combined secondary endpoints significant.[20]

Simva, simvastatin; Prava, pravastatin; Atorva, atorvastatin; Gem, gemfibrozil; Beza, bezafibrate; Feno, fenofibrate.

Effect of fibrates

The use of fibrates for the prevention of cardiovascular diseases had led to more nuanced results. The VA-HIT trial showed a 22% reduction in major cardiovascular events with the drug gemfibrozil in patients with low HDL-C.[23] Conversely, bezafibrate showed no benefits overall in patients post MI in an Israeli study.[24] The FIELD study, in stable diabetic subjects, showed a neutral effect of fenofibrate on cardiovascular endpoints.[25] These studies showed potential benefits of fibrates in subgroup analysis which were, for the most part, not prespecified. Meta-analysis of fibrate trials, based on 17 studies,[26] not including the FIELD trial, suggests that fibrates have a neutral effect on cardiovascular mortality. Generally, fibrates use will increase HDL-C by 5–15%, reduce triglycerides by 20–40% and cause a variable change in LDL-C. In moderate hypertriglyceridemia, fibrates can cause an elevation in LDL-C, because of an increase in lipoprotein lipase activity and increased conversion of VLDL to LDL.

Effects of niacin

Only two relatively large trials, both predating the statin era, have studied the effects of niacin on cardiovascular outcomes. The Coronary Drug Project examined the effects of 3 g/day of nicotinic acid on CHD events.[27] After 6.5 years, there was a reduction in CHD events, but not cardiovascular mortality. A *post hoc* analysis performed 10 years after the end of the study revealed a significant 11% reduction in total mortality, even when most patients were off study drug. The Stockholm Ischemic Heart Disease Study examined the combined effects of clofibrate 2 g/d with niacin 3 g/day in MI survivors. Total mortality was reduced by 26% and cardiovascular mortality by 36%.[28] Niacin has broad and beneficial effects on all lipoprotein subclasses, including lipoprotein Lp(a).[29] An in-depth analysis of all subsequent trials, most of which are angiographic regression studies or surrogate endpoints of atherosclerosis, and underpowered to evaluate cardiovascular morbidity and mortality, suggests that niacin has potent antiatherosclerotic effects.[30] It should be noted that the currently recommended dose of niacin (either in a slow- or extended-release form) is 2 g/d. At this dose, one can expect an increase in HDL-C in the order of 20–25%, a reduction in LDL-C of 15–20% and a reduction in triglycerides of 20–30%, depending on baseline values.

Clinical trial evidence Niacin has been used clinically for the past 50 years, since the observation by Canadian pathologist Aschtul that it can decrease total serum cholesterol.[31] For many years, niacin was one of the few medications available to treat patients with dyslipidemias. The use of bile acid-binding resins and fibrates in the 1970s increased the physician's armamentarium. However, the many side effects of niacin led to a decreased enthusiasm for its continued use in favor of statins which were first used in the mid 1980s. The side effects of niacin include flushing, now known to be caused by the release of prostaglandin G2 by the Langerhans cells in the epidermis. Blocking the PgG2 receptor DP1 markedly decreases episodes of flushing and may make niacin easier to tolerate.[32] A decrease in flushing is also seen in extended-release forms of niacin, by taking the drug with a small amount of food and taking aspirin which may work by decreasing prostaglandin release. Other side effects include gastritis, elevation of hepatic transaminases, worsening of dysglycemia and diabetes control, and an unusual form of acanthosis nigricans affecting the skin. These side effects, especially vasomotor flushing, cause a marked decrease in compliance, with less than half of the patients continuing treatment at one year.

A recent meta-analysis of published trials with niacin, statins or fibrates in combination concluded that the simultaneous reduction of LDL-C and elevation of HDL-C are associated with independent and synergistic effects of these two approaches.[30] This analysis and another review of IVUS studies[33] suggest that HDL-C elevation brings additional benefits to those observed by lowering LDL-C alone.

Novel approaches to raising HDL-C

CETP inhibitors CETP is a serum enzyme that facilitates the equimolar exchange of cholesteryl esters within HDL particles for triglycerides in triglyceride-rich lipoproteins, such as VLDL. Its role is to facilitate the reverse cholesterol transport from HDL to the liver. Rare deficiencies of CETP in man are associated with a marked increase in large HDL particles that appear biologically functional, in terms of promoting cellular cholesterol efflux.[34] Several CETP inhibitors have been or are in the process of being developed. Initial clinical data on torcetrapib and JTT705[35,36] showed that these agents increase HDL-C in a dose-dependent fashion. Unfortunately, clinical trials with torcetrapib have led to the conclusion that despite a marked (and beneficial) improvement in all lipoprotein subclasses, the drug has toxic features unrelated to its HDL-C rising effects.[10] Whether other CETP inhibitors will show similar problems will be determined clinically. In light of the increased mortality in the ILLUMINATE trial with torcetrapib, it is likely that regulatory agencies will scrutinize this class of products very closely.

Endocannabinoid receptor CB1 antagonists The first of its class, the CB1 blocker rimonabant is designed to be used for the reduction of cardiometabolic risk in subjects with obesity and elevated cardiovascular risk. In large clinical trials of weight reduction, HDL-C increased by ~8%, a finding closely related to weight reduction.[37] This is likely to represent an appealing therapeutic option in patients with abdominal obesity and at elevated cardiovascular

risk. Rinomabant is no longer approved because of concerns about depression and suicide.

Oral phospholipid supplements Lipoprotein researchers have known for some time that phospholipids, the major lipid constituent of nascent HDL particles, can increase HDL-C. A novel approach, the use of orally administered phosphatidylinositol, has been associated with a modest rise in HDL-C when taken in large doses (3–5 g/d).[38] This approach is limited because of a high incidence of gastrointestinal side effects (mostly diarrhea) at the highest doses in small-scale clinical trials.

Intravenous injections of apo AI proteoliposomes A proteoliposome is an artificially reconstituted small (nascent) HDL particle. It consists of apo AI mixed with phospholipids (usually phosphatidylcholine – PC) in a specific ratio of approximately two molecules of apo AI to ~200 molecules of PC. This results in the formation of disk-like structures that have many of the proprietes of nascent HDL particles. Apo AI Milano (Apo AI_M) is a naturally occurring mutant of apo AI found in a single kindred living in the northern Italian region of Limone sul Garde. Carriers of Apo AI_M have very low levels of HDL-C but do not develop atherosclerosis and appear to benefit from longevity.[39] In a small clinical trial, apo AI_M proteoliposomes were injected intravenously weekly for five weeks in 47 subjects presenting with an acute coronary syndrome. Intravascular ultrasound of the coronary arteries documented a small but significant 4.2% regression of coronary artery atherosclerotic plaques, suggesting that apo AI_M has rapid antiatherosclerotic effects.[40] A similar trial used wild-type (i.e. normal) apo AI proteoliposomes in patients with acute coronary syndromes. The results of this study showed no evidence of regression of CAD on intravascular ultrasound (IVUS), compared to placebo.[41] Large-scale trials with clinical events are needed to assess the impact of apo AI_M on cardiovascular events. The cost of repeated injections with a protein, the stability and shelf-life of proteoliposomes preparations remain concerns.

The potential benefits of peptide-mimetic substances that share similar properties of the amphipathic α-helical structural domains of apo AI were examined using the synthetic peptide D4F that appears to have anti-inflammatory effects similar to apo AI. The advantage of this compound is that it can be administered orally. In animal studies, D4F has been shown to act synergistically with statins to prevent atherosclerosis in the apo $E^{-/-}$ mouse model.[42] Clinical trials in man have not yet been reported.

Molecular approaches to increasing HDL-C
Drugs that increase the production of apo AI have the potential benefit of raising HDL-C. Statins and fibrates both increase apo AI production.

Patients infected with the human immunodeficiency virus (HIV) who are treated with highly active antiretroviral therapy (HAART) develop, in some instances, a dyslipidemia similar to that observed in partial lipodystrophy and the metabolic syndrome, with a low HDL-C and elevated triglycerides. The non-nucleoside reverse transcriptase inhibitors nevirapine and efavirenz are associated with an increase in apo AI and HDL-C, likely caused by an increased production of apo AI.[43] While the effect on atherosclerotic cardiovascular disease of these compounds has yet to be reported, they represent interesting alternatives in patients on HAART who develop a dyslipidemia. In theory, a compound that increases the transcriptional regulation of apo AI in the liver and intestine could lead to the formation of nascent HDL particles. Several compounds, such as statins and fibrates, may increase apo AI production, albeit weakly.[14] Novel molecules that increase apo AI are currently being explored. Similarly, compounds that increase the ABCA1 transporter may increase the formation of HDL particles. The ABCA1 gene is under the regulatory control of the liver-specific receptor (LxR) family of transcriptional regulators. Several LxR agonists are available for *in vitro* experiments, but these lack specificity for the ABCA1 gene and may cause the upregulation of a multitude of genes, especially in fatty acid metabolism. The search for selective ABCA1 LxR agonists holds theoretic promise.[44]

Conclusion

The prevention of cardiovascular events in high-risk individuals or those at high risk of recurrent events in secondary prevention of CAD requires a multifactorial approach, combining lifestyle changes and intensive medical therapy. The interventions explain more than half the observed reduction in CHD observed between 1980 and 2000.[45] Such therapy has been shown to preclude the necessity of coronary revascularization in patients with chronic, stable angina.[46] The role of LDL-C lowering is well established and current guidelines emphasize this point. The issue of raising HDL-C is presently uncertain.[47] Epidemiologic evidence has consistently shown the inverse relationship between HDL-C and CAD. It has yet to be shown that raising HDL-C pharmacologically prevents atherosclerosis. The current therapies available to clinicians are limited, especially after the failure of torcetrapib to reduce cardiovascular events. The only drug that raises HDL-C reliably is niacin. Statins, fibrates and ezetimibe have a more modest effect on HDL-C. An argument can be made that aggressive lowering of LDL-C is presently the only treatment unequivocally shown to reduce cardiovascular risk. Drug therapy aimed at increasing HDL-C (other than niacin) has been disappointing and the data supporting niacin are weaker than that for statins.

Two large-scale trials are currently under way to assess the effects of HDL-C elevation with niacin on cardiovascular morbidity and mortality. These two trials will examine the effects of adding niacin to the current standard of care in patients at high risk of cardiovascular diseases (information available at http://clinicaltrials.gov/) The AIM-HIGH study will randomize 3300 subjects with atherogenic dyslipidemia to a combination of extended-release niacin and simvastatin or simvastatin alone in the prevention of heart disease. The primary objective will be to examine the composite endpoints of CHD death, non-fatal MI, ischemic stroke or hospitalization for high-risk non-ST segment elevation acute coronary syndrome. The trial is expected to last four years. The HPS THRIVE trial will examine the effects of MK0264a (niacin 2 g/day with the PgG2 DP1 blocker laropiprant 40 mg) or placebo in 20 000 subjects at high cardiovascular risk from the UK, Scandinavia and China over a background treatment with simvastatin 40 mg or simvastatin 40 mg plus ezetimibe 10 mg to reach LDL-C goals. The follow-up will be approximately four years for an expected number of major cardiovascular events of 2300. Results are expected by 2013.

References

1. McPherson R, Frohlich J, Fodor G, Genest J, Canadian Cardiovascular Society. Canadian Cardiovascular Society position statement – recommendations for the diagnosis and treatment of dyslipidemia and prevention of cardiovascular disease. *Can J Cardiol* 2006;**22**:913–27.
2. Grundy SM, Cleeman JI, Merz CN *et al*. National Heart, Lung, and Blood Institute; American College of Cardiology Foundation; American Heart Association. Implications of recent clinical trials for the National Cholesterol Education Program Adult Treatment Panel III guidelines. *Circulation* 2004;**110**(2): 227–39.
3. Yusuf S, Hawken S, Ounpuu S *et al*. Effect of potentially modifiable risk factors associated with myocardial infarction in 52 countries (the INTERHEART Study): case-control study. *Lancet* 2004;**364**(9438):937–52.
4. Assmann G, Schulte H, von Eckardstein A, Huang Y. High-density lipoprotein cholesterol as a predictor of coronary heart disease risk. The PROCAM experience and pathophysiological implications for reverse cholesterol transport. *Atherosclerosis* 1996;**124**:S11–20.
5. Genest J Jr, Martin-Munley SS, McNamara JR *et al*. Familial lipoprotein disorders in patients with premature coronary artery disease. *Circulation* 1992;**85**:2025–33.
6. Despres JP, Lemieux I, Dagenais GR, Cantin B, Lamarche B. HDL-cholesterol as a marker of coronary heart disease risk: the Quebec cardiovascular study. *Atherosclerosis* 2000;**153**(2):263–72.
7. Assmann G, Nofer JR. Atheroprotective effects of high-density lipoproteins. *Annu Rev Med* 2003;**54**:321–41.

8. Barter PJ. Cardioprotective effects of high-density lipoproteins: the evidence strengthens. *Arterioscler Thromb Vasc Biol* 2005; **25**(7):1305–6.

9. Genest J, Pedersen TR. Prevention of cardiovascular ischemic disease: high-risk and secondary prevention. *Circulation* 2003; **107**:2059–65

10. Barter PJ, Caulfield M, Eriksson M *et al*. ILLUMINATE Investigators. Effects of torcetrapib in patients at high risk for coronary events. *N Engl J Med* 2007;**357**(21):2109–22.

11. Nissen SE, Tardif JC, Nicholls SJ *et al*. ILLUSTRATE Investigators. Effect of torcetrapib on the progression of coronary atherosclerosis. *N Engl J Med* 2007;**356**(13):1304–16

12. Kastelein JJ, van Leuven SI, Burgess L *et al*. RADIANCE 1 Investigators. Effect of torcetrapib on carotid atherosclerosis in familial hypercholesterolemia. *N Engl J Med* 2007;**356**:1620–30.

13. Bots ML, Visseren FL, Evans GW *et al*. RADIANCE 2 Investigators. Torcetrapib and carotid intima-media thickness in mixed dyslipidaemia (RADIANCE 2 study): a randomised, double-blind trial. *Lancet* 2007;**370**(9582):153–60.

14. Martin G, Duez H, Blanquart C, Berezowski V, Poulain P, Fruchart JC, Najib-Fruchart J, Glineur C, Staels B. Statin-induced inhibition of the Rho-signaling pathway activates PPARalpha and induces HDL apoA-I. *J Clin Invest* 2001;**107**:1423–3.

15. Pedersen TR, Kjekshus J, Berg K *et al*. Randomised trial of cholesterol lowering in 4444 patients with coronary heart disease: the Scandinavian Simvastatin Survival Study (4S). *Lancet* 1994;**344**:1383–9.

16. Sacks FM, Pfeffer MA, Moye LA *et al*. The effect of pravastatin on coronary events after myocardial infarction in patients with average cholesterol levels. *N Engl J Med* 1996; **335**:1001–9.

17. Long-term Intervention with Pravastatin in Ischemic Disease (LIPID) Study Group. Prevention of cardiovascular events and death with pravastatin in patients with coronary heart disease and a broad range of initial cholesterol levels. *N Engl J Med* 1998;**339**:1349–57.

18. Heart Protection Study Collaborative Group. MRC/BHF Heart Protection Study of cholesterol lowering with simvastatin in 20,536 high-risk individuals: a randomised placebo-controlled trial. *Lancet* 2002;**360**:7–22.

19. Larosa JC, Grundy SM, Waters DD *et al*. Intensive lipid lowering with atorvastatin in patients with stable coronary disease. *N Engl J Med* 2005;**352**(14):1425–35.

20. Pedersen TR, Faergeman O, Kastelein JJP *et al*. High-dose atorvastatin vs usual dose simvastatin for secondary prevention after myocardial infarction – the IDEAL Study: a randomized controlled trial. *JAMA* 2005;**294**(19):2437–4.

21. MacMahon M, Kirkpatrick C, Cummings CE, Clayton A, Robinson PJ, Tomiak RH, Liu M, Kush D, Tobert J. A pilot study with simvastatin and folic acid/vitamin B12 in preparation for the Study of the Effectiveness of Additional Reductions in Cholesterol and Homocysteine (SEARCH). *Nutr Metab Cardiovasc Dis* 2000;**10**:195–203.

22. Cholesterol Treatment Trialists. Efficacy and safety of cholesterol-lowering treatment: prospective meta-analysis of data from 90 056 participants in 14 randomised trials of statins. *Lancet* 2005;**366**:1267–78.

23. Rubins HB, Robins SJ, Collins D *et al*. Gemfibrozil for the secondary prevention of coronary heart disease in men with low levels of high-density lipoprotein cholesterol. Veterans Affairs High-Density Lipoprotein Cholesterol Intervention Trial Study Group. *N Engl J Med* 1999;**341**(6):410–18.

24. BIP Study Group. Secondary prevention by raising HDL cholesterol and reducing triglycerides in patients with coronary artery disease: the Bezafibrate Infarction Prevention (BIP) study. *Circulation* 2000;**102**:21–7.

25. Keech A, Simes RJ, Barter P *et al*. FIELD study investigators. Effects of long-term fenofibrate therapy on cardiovascular events in 9795 people with type 2 diabetes mellitus (the FIELD study): randomised controlled trial. *Lancet* 2005; **366**(9500):1849–61.

26. Studer M, Briel M, Leimenstoll B, Glass TR, Bucher HC. Effect of different antilipidemic agents and diets on mortality: a systematic review. *Arch Intern Med* 2005;**165**:725–30.

27. Canner PL, Berge KG, Wenger NK, Stamler J, Friedman L, Prineas RJ, Friedewald W. Fifteen year mortality in Coronary Drug Project patients: long-term benefit with niacin. *J Am Coll Cardiol* 1986;**8**:1245–55.

28. Carlson LA, Rosenhamer G. Reduction of mortality in the Stockholm Ischaemic Heart Disease Secondary Prevention Study by combined treatment with clofibrate and nicotinic acid. *Acta Med Scand* 1988;**223**:405–18.

29. Carlson LA. Nicotinic acid: the broad-spectrum lipid drug. A 50 anniversary review. *J Intern Med* 2005;**258**:94–114.

30. Brown BG, Stukovsky KH, Zhao XQ. Simultaneous low-density lipoprotein-C lowering and high-density lipoprotein-C elevation for optimum cardiovascular disease prevention with various drug classes, and their combinations: a meta-analysis of 23 randomized lipid trials. *Curr Opin Lipidol* 2006;**17**:631–6.

31. Altschul R, Hoffer A. Influence of nicotinic acid on serum cholesterol in man. *Arch Biochem* 1955;**54**:558–8.

32. Cheng K, Wu TJ, Wu KK, Sturino C, Metters K, Gottesdiener K, Wright SD, Wang Z, O'Neill G, Lai E, Waters MG. Antagonism of the prostaglandin D2 receptor 1 suppresses nicotinic acid-induced vasodilation in mice and humans. *Proc Natl Acad Sci USA* 2006;**103**:6682–7.

33. Nicholls SJ, Tuzcu EM, Sipahi I, Grasso AW, Schoenhagen P, Hu T, Wolski K, Crowe T, Desai MY, Hazen SL, Kapadia SR, Nissen SE. Statins, high-density lipoprotein cholesterol, and regression of coronary atherosclerosis. *JAMA* 2007;**29**:499–508.

34. Matsuura F, Wang N, Chen W, Jiang XC, Tall AR. HDL from CETP-deficient subjects shows enhanced ability to promote cholesterol efflux from macrophages in an apoE- and ABCG1-dependent pathway. *J Clin Invest* 2006;**116**:1435–42.

35. Brousseau ME, Schaefer EJ, Wolfe ML, Bloedon LT, Digenio AG, Clark RW, Mancuso JP, Rader DJ. Effects of an inhibitor of cholesteryl ester transfer protein on HDL cholesterol. *N Engl J Med* 2004;**350**(15):1505–15.

36. Kuivenhoven JA, de Grooth GJ, Kawamura H, Klerkx AH, Wilhelm F, Trip MD, Kastelein JJ. Effectiveness of inhibition of cholesteryl ester transfer protein by JTT-705 in combination with pravastatin in type II dyslipidemia. *Am J Cardiol* 2005;**95**(9):1085–8.

37. Despres JP, Golay A, Sjostrom L; Rimonabant in Obesity-Lipids Study Group. Effects of rimonabant on metabolic risk factors in overweight patients with dyslipidemia. *N Engl J Med* 2005;**353**(20):2121–34.

38. Burgess JW, Neville TA, Rouillard P, Harder Z, Beanlands DS, Sparks DL. Phosphatidylinositol increases HDL-C levels in humans. *J Lipid Res* 2005;**46**(2):350–5.

39. Sirtori CR, Calabresi L, Franceschini G, Baldassarre D, Amato M, Johansson J, Salvetti M, Monteduro C, Zulli R, Muiesan ML, Agabiti-Rosei E. Cardiovascular status of carriers of the apolipoprotein A-I(Milano) mutant: the Limone sul Garda study. *Circulation* 2001;**103**(15):1949–54.

40. Nissen SE, Tsunoda T, Tuzcu EM, Schoenhagen P, Cooper CJ, Yasin M, Eaton GM, Lauer MA, Sheldon WS, Grines CL, Halpern S, Crowe T, Blankenship JC, Kerensky R. Effect of recombinant ApoA-I Milano on coronary atherosclerosis in patients with acute coronary syndromes: a randomized controlled trial. *JAMA* 2003;**290**(17):2292–300.

41. Tardif JC, Gregoire J, L'Allier PL, Ibrahim R, Lesperance J, Heinonen TM, Kouz S, Berry C, Basser R, Lavoie MA, Guertin MC, Rodes-Cabau J; Effect of rHDL on Atherosclerosis-Safety and Efficacy (ERASE) Investigators. Effects of reconstituted high-density lipoprotein infusions on coronary atherosclerosis: a randomized controlled trial. *JAMA* 2007;**297**(15):1675–82.

42. Li X, Chyu KY, Faria Neto JR, Yano J, Nathwani N, Ferreira C, Dimayuga PC, Cercek B, Kaul S, Shah PK. Differential effects of apolipoprotein A-I-mimetic peptide on evolving and established atherosclerosis in apolipoprotein E-null mice. *Circulation* 2004;**110**:1701–5.

43. Young J, Weber R, Rickenbach M, Furrer H, Bernasconi E, Hirschel B, Tarr PE, Vernazza P, Battegay M, Bucher HC. Lipid profiles for antiretroviral-naive patients starting PI- and NNRTI-based therapy in the Swiss HIV cohort study. *Antivir Ther* 2005;**10**(5):585–9.

44. Miao B, Zondlo S, Gibbs S, Cromley D, Hosagrahara VP, Kirchgessner TG, Billheimer J, Mukherjee R. Raising HDL cholesterol without inducing hepatic steatosis and hypertriglyceridemia by a selective LXR modulator. *J Lipid Res* 2004;**45**:1410–17.

45. Ford ES, Ajani UA, Croft JB, Critchley JA, Labarthe DR, Kottke TE, Giles WH, Capewell S. Explaining the decrease in U.S. deaths from coronary disease, 1980–2000. *N Engl J Med* 2007;**356**:2388–98.

46. Boden WE, O'Rourke RA, Teo KK, Hartigan PM, Maron DJ, Kostuk WJ, Knudtson M, Dada M, Casperson P, Harris CL, Chaitman BR, Shaw L, Gosselin G, Nawaz S, Title LM, Gau G, Blaustein AS, Booth DC, Bates ER, Spertus JA, Berman DS, Mancini GB, Weintraub WS; COURAGE Trial Research Group. Optimal medical therapy with or without PCI for stable coronary disease. *N Engl J Med* 2007;**356**:1503–16.

47. Alrasadi K, Awan Z, Alwaili K *et al.* Comparison of treatment of severe high-density lipoprotein cholesterol deficiency in men with daily atorvastatin (20 mg) versus fenobibrate (200 mg) versus extended-release niacin (2 g). *Am J Cardiol* 2008;**102**(10): 1341–7.

Heart failure

Michael M Givertz and Garrick C Stewart
Brigham and Women's Hospital, Harvard Medical School, Boston, MA, USA

Case history

A 60-year-old man with type 2 diabetes mellitus and coronary artery disease presents to your office with progressive dyspnea on exertion and lower extremity edema. He is status post anterior myocardial infarction five years ago. Following cardiac rehabilitation, he returned to work full-time as an electrical engineer and remained asymptomatic without angina or heart failure until one year ago when he started to "slow down". Over the last several months, he has noted increasing shortness of breath with usual daily activities, and more recently the onset of bilateral lower extremity edema. He can no longer play with his grandchildren due to fatigue. He denies chest pain, palpitations or lightheadedness. He sleeps comfortably on two pillows and has had no recent change in his weight or appetite. His current medications include captopril 12. 5 mg tid, furosemide 20 mg qd, rosiglitazone 4 mg qd and aspirin 81 mg qd.

On physical exam, he is a well-nourished older-appearing man who appears comfortable lying supine. Blood pressure is 130/70 mmHg and heart rate is 95 beats per minute and regular. Jugular venous pressure is 10 cm of water. Lungs are clear bilaterally. Cardiac exam reveals a laterally displaced point of maximal impulse, grade 2 over 6 holosystolic murmur at the apex, and soft S_3 gallop. The liver edge is palpable 2 cm below the right costal margin, and there is 1+ pitting edema to the mid-calves bilaterally. His feet are warm with intact distal pulses. Lab tests are notable for serum sodium of 136 mmol/L, creatinine of 1. 6 mg/dL and hemoglobin A1c of 6.2%. His electrocardiogram reveals normal sinus rhythm with an intraventricular conduction delay (QRS duration 150 msec) and old anterior myocardial infarction. A transthoracic echocardiogram demonstrates moderate left ventricular dilation (end-diastolic dimension 63 mm) with anteroapical akinesis, left ventricular ejection fraction of 25%, mild right ventricular dysfunction, and 2+ mitral regurgitation with a structurally normal valve.

Question

How would you manage this patient?

Comment

This is a middle-aged man with diabetes and an ischemic cardiomyopathy who presents with New York Heart Association (NYHA) functional class III heart failure. There is clinical and laboratory evidence of left ventricular systolic dysfunction, and "bedside" hemodynamic assessment reveals volume overload without evidence of decreased systemic perfusion. In addition, his echocardiogram shows findings consistent with left ventricular remodeling without intracavitary thrombus formation. He has been compliant with his medications and fluid and salt restriction, and does not drink alcohol. His blood sugars have been well controlled, and he has had no recent infection. A complete blood count and thyroid function tests should be checked to rule out anemia and hyperthyroidism, respectively. One possible precipitating factor in this case is his use of a thiazolidinedione for glucose control, a class of medications that has been shown to worsen heart failure symptoms and may increase the risk of cardiovascular events.[1,2] The patient should be switched to an alternative antidiabetic medication, such as a sulfonylurea or insulin. Metformin is relatively contraindicated in patients with heart failure and renal dysfunction due to a small risk of lactic acidosis.

After identifying and addressing a precipitating factor, it is reasonable to consider treatment of the underlying cause of heart failure.[3] The patient is a diabetic status post myocardial infarction several years ago and may have developed recurrent ischemia, either silent or with dyspnea as an anginal equivalent. An exercise study with imaging should be performed to rule out reversible ischemia. If this is negative, an assessment of myocardial viability with low-dose dobutamine stress echocardiography, resting

Evidence-Based Cardiology, 3rd edition. Edited by S. Yusuf, J.A. Cairns, A.J. Camm, E.L. Fallen, and B.J. Gersh. © 2010 Blackwell Publishing, ISBN: 978-1-4051-5925-8.

thallium scintigraphy or positron emission tomography should be considered.[4] Several studies have shown that patients with ischemic cardiomyopathy and viable myocardium have significant improvement in left ventricular function following surgical revascularization. However, in the absence of angina or inducible ischemia, the superiority of surgery over medical therapy in prolonging survival in patients with ischemic cardiomyopathy remains unproven.

Sleep-disordered breathing is a common co-morbidity in heart failure. As many as 30–40% of heart failure patients may have obstructive or central sleep apnea, or both.[5] Frequent apneic episodes lead to sympathetic activation, hypertension and diastolic dysfunction, which may worsen heart failure symptoms. The most extreme form of central sleep apnea, Cheyne–Stokes periodic breathing, is present in more severe forms of heart failure. Routine screening for sleep apnea should be performed in all heart failure patients by asking the patient and spouse about snoring, nocturnal apneic episodes, and daytime somnolence.[6] The cornerstone of sleep apnea therapy is positive airway pressure, often with supplemental oxygen. Positive pressure therapy has been shown to improve ejection fraction and six-minute walk distance, but not survival.[7] Prospective studies are needed to evaluate the impact of sleep apnea on heart failure outcomes, including sudden death.

The overall goals in the management of heart failure are to eliminate symptoms, improve quality of life, and prolong survival. Non-pharmacologic management of heart failure should be reviewed with the patient and family. The importance of salt and fluid restriction and daily weight monitoring should be reinforced, and alcohol moderation or cessation should be advised. Once euvolemia has been achieved, a submaximal aerobic exercise program (e.g. walking, stationary bicycle) should be encouraged. Exercise training may result in improvement in symptoms and functional capacity, enhanced blood flow and skeletal muscle metabolism, and reduced heart failure hospitalizations.[8,9] In a National Institutes of Health-sponsored trial (HF-ACTION), exercise training had no significant effect on survival in heart failure.[10]

Pharmacologic therapy should be optimized according to consensus guidelines.[11–13] The patient is currently taking captopril, an angiotensin-converting enzyme (ACE) inhibitor, at a relatively low dose. Several large prospective randomized controlled trials have demonstrated the beneficial effects of ACE inhibitors on exercise tolerance, salt and water balance, symptoms, neurohormonal activation, quality of life and survival in patients with chronic heart failure.[14] As demonstrated in SAVE, captopril reduces the risk of recurrent myocardial infarction and stroke in patients with post-MI left ventricular dysfunction.[15] In this patient with mild diabetic nephropathy, ACE inhibitor or angiotensin-II receptor blocker (ARB) therapy may also slow the progression of renal dysfunction. The optimal

dosing of ACE inhibitors remains controversial. One prospective study (ATLAS) demonstrated the modest superiority of high-dose versus low-dose ACE inhibitor therapy in patients with chronic heart failure without increased toxicity.[16] Current guidelines recommend increasing the dose of captopril to 50 mg tid as blood pressure and renal function tolerate. For improved medication compliance, a change to once-daily ACE inhibitor dosing may also be considered since these drugs exhibit a class effect. Despite previous concerns that aspirin use may attenuate ACE inhibition, recent studies indicated no adverse effects of combining aspirin and ACE inhibitors.[17,18] Therefore it is reasonable to continue low-dose aspirin for secondary prevention of coronary artery disease.

Treatment of systemic and pulmonary venous congestion warrants more aggressive diuresis. The daily dose of furosemide or other loop diuretic should be increased until the required response is achieved (e.g. absence of jugular venous distension, hepatomegaly and edema). This "dry weight" should be recorded and used as a euvolemic baseline to guide future diuretic therapy, although further weight loss in advanced heart failure may be due to cardiac cachexia.[19] If this strategy is not effective, combination therapy with a thiazide diuretic should be tried. Adequate diuresis will generally result in improved symptoms and may slow the progression of chamber dilation by reducing ventricular filling pressures. However, diuretic therapy may also cause renal dysfunction, electrolyte depletion and neurohormonal activation. It should be emphasized that there have been no randomized controlled trials demonstrating the long-term efficacy and safety of diuretic therapy in patients with heart failure. Furthermore, studies are needed to address the safety and efficacy of diuretic withdrawal in stable heart failure patients.

Case history *continued*

The patient undergoes rest and stress imaging with positron emission tomography, which is negative for ischemia and demonstrates no significant viability of the anterior wall. He diureses eight pounds on an increased dose of oral furosemide, and captopril is titrated to 37.5 mg tid. Jugular venous distension and lower extremity edema resolve, while blood pressure, heart rate, and renal function are unchanged. Despite adjustment of ACE inhibitor and diuretic therapy, there is minimal improvement in his exertional dyspnea and fatigue.

Question

The patient remains moderately symptomatic despite treatment with an ACE inhibitor and diuretic. What is the next step?

Comment

The next step is to initiate beta-adrenergic antagonist therapy. Multiple randomized controlled trials have demonstrated that beta-blockers improve symptoms and cardiac function, and reduce morbidity and mortality in patients with chronic heart failure due to left ventricular systolic dysfunction.[20–23] Consensus guidelines recommend using beta-blockers, in addition to ACE inhibitors and diuretics, in the management of patients with left ventricular systolic dysfunction.[11] Once euvolemia has been achieved, beta-blocker therapy with carvedilol, bisoprolol or sustained-release metoprolol can be initiated safely at a low dose and titrated gradually at regular intervals (e.g. every 1–2 weeks). Despite concerns that beta-blockers may increase insulin resistance, reduce insulin secretion or mask hypoglycemia, they have been shown to be safe and effective in treating symptomatic systolic dysfunction in diabetic patients.[24] In heart failure patients, carvedilol, a non-selective beta-blocker with alpha$_1$-blocking properties, has a lower rate of new-onset diabetes and diabetic events when compared to metoprolol.[25]

Given this patient's multiple exacerbations of chronic heart failure, complicated by diabetes and renal insufficiency, it would be appropriate to refer him to a comprehensive disease management program in heart failure. Either clinic or home-based disease management programs significantly reduce readmission rates and costs, while improving functional status and quality of life for heart failure patients.[26,27] Such programs promote self-care, emphasize behavioral strategies to increase adherence, increase access to providers, and give early attention to signs and symptoms of fluid overload.[28]

Case history *continued*

Carvedilol is initiated at a dose of 3.125 mg bid. One week later, the patient returns to your office with complaints of increased exertional dyspnea and pedal edema. His clinical evaluation is consistent with worsening heart failure, a known adverse effect of beta-blocker therapy initiation. This responds to a doubling of the furosemide dose for two days. The patient is also enrolled in a heart failure disease management program for comprehensive care. Over the next three months, carvedilol is titrated to a target dose of 25 mg bid. During this period, an exacerbation of heart failure symptoms occurs on one additional occasion. Close monitoring of symptoms and weight, and adjustments in diuretic dosing, enable the patient to achieve a target dose of beta-blocker therapy. Repeat echocardiogram reveals a modest decrease in the left ventricular end-diastolic dimension and an increase in the left ventricular ejection fraction to 30%.

Question

What are your next steps in pharmacologic management if the patient continues to have symptomatic heart failure?

Comment

For persistent heart failure symptoms despite optimal dosing of ACE inhibitor, beta-blocker and diuretic, several adjunctive medications may be considered. Given the patient's reduced ejection fraction and relatively preserved renal function, an aldosterone antagonist is a reasonable next step. Aldosterone, an adrenal mineralocorticoid, plays an important role in the pathophysiology of heart failure, contributing to salt and fluid retention, cardiac and vascular remodeling and ventricular arrhythmias.[29] The addition of spironolactone to standard therapy was shown to reduce mortality in patients with NYHA functional class III–IV heart failure in the RALES trial.[30] Although spironolactone is generally well tolerated, it has antiandrogenic and progesterone-like effects and is associated with a small risk of painful gynecomastia, often prompting a switch to the more selective aldosterone antagonist eplerenone. Eplerenone has been shown to reduce mortality if added to standard therapy within two weeks of myocardial infarction complicated by reduced ejection fraction or heart failure.[31] Both spirinolactone and eplerenone can produce hyperkalemia, a particular risk in older patients with compromised renal function on ACE inhibitors, ARBs or potassium supplements.[32] Serum potassium and creatinine levels must be checked frequently during initiation and titration of aldosterone antagonists. Potassium supplementation should be discontinued unless there is evidence of persistent hypokalemia with serum potassium levels <4 mmol/L. The addition of an ARB to ACE inhibitor and beta-blocker therapy may be considered for heart failure patients with reduced ejection fraction and preserved blood pressure.[33] ARBs have also been recommended for use in heart failure patients with systolic dysfunction who are intolerant of ACE inhibitors, or in addition to ACE inhibitors in patients not treated with beta-blockers.[34]

Another class of medications that may provide symptomatic benefit in heart failure patients is the organic nitrates. Nitrates may be used to reduce both systemic and pulmonary venous congestion and prevent ischemia. As with diuretics, nitrates alone have not been shown to reduce morbidity and mortality in patients with chronic heart failure. However, a fixed combination of hydralazine and isosorbide dinitrate has been shown to reduce morbidity and mortality and improve quality of life in self-identified blacks with heart failure already treated with ACE inhibitors and beta-blockers.[35]

Digoxin is an oral positive inotropic agent with antiadrenergic effects that has been shown to be safe and effective in patients with symptomatic heart failure. While the DIG trial showed no difference in survival in heart failure patients treated with digoxin versus placebo, there were fewer heart failure hospitalizations and a trend toward reduced death from progressive heart failure in the digoxin-treated group.[36] For heart failure patients in sinus rhythm, digoxin dosing should be based on lean body mass and renal function, and serum digoxin levels should be maintained less than 0.8–1.0 ng/mL.[37]

Question

Which device-based therapies may be considered for this patient with symptomatic heart failure and reduced ejection fraction?

Comment

In recent years there has been considerable enthusiasm for cardiac resynchronization therapy (CRT) as adjunctive treatment for patients with advanced heart failure. Dyssynchronous contraction, as occurs with left bundle branch block or other intraventricular conduction delays, is mechanically inefficient and over time may lead to a reduction in left ventricular ejection fraction and cardiac output.[38] Simultaneous pacing of the left and right ventricles (biventricular pacing) to resynchronize ventricular contraction has been shown to improve both functional capacity and quality of life as early as one month after device implantation, and is associated with reverse ventricular remodeling as early as six months.[39,40] Two clinical trials, COMPANION and CARE-HF, evaluated the effect of CRT on survival.[41,42] In both trials the risk of all-cause mortality was reduced by CRT as compared to no pacing, although only CARE-HF reached statistical significance. Current indications for CRT include dilated cardiomyopathy of any cause with a left ventricular ejection fraction <35%, intraventricular conduction delay as measured by a QRS interval of at least 120 msec, and NYHA functional class III or stable class IV heart failure despite optimal medical therapy.[43] The REVERSE trial also showed benefits of CRT on hospitalization and ventricular remodeling in patients with mildly symptomatic HF.[44] Of concern, 20–30% of patients will not have significant clinical or echocardiographic improvement with CRT. Establishing criteria to identify CRT responders prior to device implantation is an active area of investigation.

Heart failure patients with reduced ejection fraction are also at increased risk for sudden cardiac death.[45] Implantable cardioverter-defibrillators (ICDs) have been shown to improve survival in patients with left ventricular ejection fraction <30–35% and heart failure due to either ischemic or non-ischemic causes.[46,47] In SCD-HeFT, ICD implantation was superior to both antiarrhythmic therapy with amiodarone and placebo on primary prevention of sudden cardiac death in symptomatic heart failure patients with low ejection fraction.[48] As with CRT, ICDs are not recommended for end-stage, refractory heart failure patients with little prospect of clinical improvement or survival beyond one year.[49] Primary prevention therapy with an ICD may be considered if there is a persistently reduced ejection fraction despite 3–6 months of optimal medical therapy, including an ACE inhibitor and beta-blocker. Most candidates for CRT are also candidates for ICD placement. An ongoing trial (MADIT-CRT) will evaluate the role of ICDs with or without CRT in a large cohort of minimally symptomatic patients with NYHA class I or II heart failure.

Case history *continued*

The patient is started on spironolactone 12. 5 mg once daily and eventually titrated to 25 mg, with close monitoring of his renal function and serum potassium level. Despite these maneuvers, he still has recurrent symptomatic heart failure and elects to undergo implantation of a CRTD (CRT plus ICD) device. The patient responds clinically to CRT and experiences an improvement in his exercise capacity and quality of life. Two months after implantation he is playing with his grandchildren again with minimal dyspnea. A repeat echocardiogram obtained six months later shows reduced LV dimensions and an increase in ejection fraction to 35%.

References

1. Lago RM, Singh PP, Nesto RW. Congestive heart failure and cardiovascular death in patients with prediabetes and type 2 diabetes given thiazolidinediones: a meta-analysis of randomised clinical trials. *Lancet* 2007;**370**(9593):1129–36.
2. Lipscombe LL, Gomes T, Levesque LE, Hux JE, Juurlink DN, Alter DA. Thiazolidinediones and cardiovascular outcomes in older patients with diabetes. *JAMA* 2007;**298**(22):2634–43.
3. Givertz MM, Colucci WS, Braunwald E. Clinical aspects of heart failure; pulmonary edema, high-output heart failure. In: Zipes DP, Libby P, Bonow RO, Braunwald E (eds) *Heart Disease: A Textbook of Cardiovascular Medicine*. Philadelphia: WB Saunders, 2005: 539–68.
4. Bourque JM, Hasselblad V, Velazquez EJ, Borges-Neto S, O'Connor CM. Revascularization in patients with coronary artery disease, left ventricular dysfunction, and viability: a meta-analysis. *Am Heart J* 2003;**146**(4):621–7.
5. Shamsuzzaman AS, Gersh BJ, Somers VK. Obstructive sleep apnea: implications for cardiac and vascular disease. *JAMA* 2003;**290**(14):1906–14.
6. Pepin JL, Chouri-Pontarollo N, Tamisier R, Levy P. Cheyne–Stokes respiration with central sleep apnoea in chronic heart failure: proposals for a diagnostic and therapeutic strategy. *Sleep Med Rev* 2006;**10**(1):33–47.
7. Bradley TD, Logan AG, Kimoff RJ *et al.* Continuous positive airway pressure for central sleep apnea and heart failure. *N Engl J Med* 2005;**353**(19):2025–33.
8. Coats AJ, Adamopoulos S, Radaelli A *et al.* Controlled trial of physical training in chronic heart failure. Exercise performance,

hemodynamics, ventilation, and autonomic function. *Circulation* 1992;**85**(6):2119–31.

9. McKelvie RS, Teo KK, McCartney N, Humen D, Montague T, Yusuf S. Effects of exercise training in patients with congestive heart failure: a critical review. *J Am Coll Cardiol* 1995;**25**(3):789–96.

10. O'Connor CM, Whellan DJ, Lee KL *et al*. HF-ACTION Investigators. Efficacy and safety of exercise training in patients with chronic heart failure: HF-ACTION randomized controlled trial. *JAMA* 2009;**301**(14):1439–50.

11. Hunt SA, Abraham WT, Chin MH *et al*. 2009 focused update incorporated into the ACC/AHA 2005 Guidelines for the Diagnosis and Management of Heart Failure in Adults: a report of the American College of Cardiology Foundation/American Heart Association task Force on Practice Guidelines: developed in collaboration with the International Society for Heart and Lung Transplantation. *Circulation* 2009;**119**(14):e391–479. Epub 2009 Mar 26.

12. Heart Failure Society of America Executive Summary. HFSA 2006 Comprehensive Heart Failure Practice Guideline. *J Cardiac Fail* 2006;**12**(1):10–38.

13. Swedberg K, Cleland J, Dargie H *et al*. Guidelines for the diagnosis and treatment of chronic heart failure: executive summary (update 2005): The Task Force for the Diagnosis and Treatment of Chronic Heart Failure of the European Society of Cardiology. *Eur Heart J* 2005;**26**(11):1115–40.

14. Garg R, Yusuf S. Overview of randomized trials of angiotensin-converting enzyme inhibitors on mortality and morbidity in patients with heart failure. Collaborative Group on ACE Inhibitor Trials. *JAMA* 1995;**273**(18):1450–6.

15. Loh E, Sutton MS, Wun CC *et al*. Ventricular dysfunction and the risk of stroke after myocardial infarction. *N Engl J Med* 1997;**336**(4):251–7.

16. Packer M, Poole-Wilson PA, Armstrong PW *et al*. Comparative effects of low and high doses of the angiotensin-converting enzyme inhibitor, lisinopril, on morbidity and mortality in chronic heart failure. ATLAS Study Group. *Circulation* 1999;**100**(23):2312–18.

17. Teo KK, Yusuf S, Pfeffer M *et al*. Effects of long-term treatment with angiotensin-converting-enzyme inhibitors in the presence or absence of aspirin: a systematic review. *Lancet* 2002; **360**(9339):1037–43.

18. McAlister FA, Ghali WA, Gong Y, Fang J, Armstrong PW, Tu JV. Aspirin use and outcomes in a community-based cohort of 7352 patients discharged after first hospitalization for heart failure. *Circulation* 2006;**113**(22):2572–78.

19. Anker SD, Steinborn W, Strassburg S. Cardiac cachexia. *Ann Med* 2004;**36**(7):518–29.

20. Packer M, Bristow MR, Cohn JN *et al*. The effect of carvedilol on morbidity and mortality in patients with chronic heart failure. U.S. Carvedilol Heart Failure Study Group. *N Engl J Med* 1996;**334**(21):1349–55.

21. CIBIS-II Investigators and Committees. Cardiac Insufficiency Bisoprolol Study II (CIBIS-II): a randomised trial. *Lancet* 1999;**353**(9146):9–13.

22. MERIT-HF Study Group. Effect of metoprolol CR/XL in chronic heart failure: Metoprolol CR/XL Randomised Intervention Trial in Congestive Heart Failure (MERIT-HF). *Lancet* 1999;**353**(9169): 2001–7.

23. Packer M, Coats AJ, Fowler MB *et al*. Effect of carvedilol on survival in severe chronic heart failure. *N Engl J Med* 2001; **344**(22):1651–8.

24. Haas SJ, Vos T, Gilbert RE, Krum H. Are beta-blockers as efficacious in patients with diabetes mellitus as in patients without diabetes mellitus who have chronic heart failure? A meta-analysis of large-scale clinical trials. *Am Heart J* 2003; **146**(5):848–53.

25. Torp-Pedersen C, Metra M, Charlesworth A *et al*. Effects of metoprolol and carvedilol on pre-existing and new onset diabetes in patients with chronic heart failure: data from the Carvedilol Or Metoprolol European Trial (COMET). *Heart (British Cardiac Society)* 2007;**93**(8):968–73.

26. Stewart S, Marley JE, Horowitz JD. Effects of a multidisciplinary, home-based intervention on unplanned readmissions and survival among patients with chronic congestive heart failure: a randomised controlled study. *Lancet* 1999; **354**(9184):1077–83.

27. Fonarow GC, Stevenson LW, Walden JA *et al*. Impact of a comprehensive heart failure management program on hospital readmission and functional status of patients with advanced heart failure. *J Am Coll Cardiol* 1997;**30**(3):725–32.

28. Stromberg A, Martensson J, Fridlund B, Levin LA, Karlsson JE, Dahlstrom U. Nurse-led heart failure clinics improve survival and self-care behaviour in patients with heart failure: results from a prospective, randomised trial. *Eur Heart J* 2003; **24**(11):1014–23.

29. Weber KT. Aldosterone in congestive heart failure. *N Engl J Med* 2001;**345**(23):1689–97.

30. Pitt B, Zannad F, Remme WJ *et al*. The effect of spironolactone on morbidity and mortality in patients with severe heart failure. Randomized Aldactone Evaluation Study Investigators. *N Engl J Med* 1999;**341**(10):709–17.

31. Pitt B, Remme W, Zannad F *et al*. Eplerenone, a selective aldosterone blocker, in patients with left ventricular dysfunction after myocardial infarction. *N Engl J Med* 2003; **348**(14):1309–21.

32. Juurlink DN, Mamdani MM, Lee DS *et al*. Rates of hyperkalemia after publication of the Randomized Aldactone Evaluation Study. *N Engl J Med* 2004;**351**(6):543–51.

33. Cohn JN, Tognoni G. A randomized trial of the angiotensin-receptor blocker valsartan in chronic heart failure. *N Engl J Med* 2001;**345**(23):1667–75.

34. McMurray JJ, Ostergren J, Swedberg K *et al*. Effects of candesartan in patients with chronic heart failure and reduced left-ventricular systolic function taking angiotensin-converting-enzyme inhibitors: the CHARM-Added trial. *Lancet* 2003;**362**(9386):767–71.

35. Taylor AL, Ziesche S, Yancy C *et al*. Combination of isosorbide dinitrate and hydralazine in blacks with heart failure. *N Engl J Med* 2004;**351**(20):2049–57.

36. Digitalis Investigation Group. The effect of digoxin on mortality and morbidity in patients with heart failure. *N Engl J Med* 1997;**336**(8):525–33.

37. Rathore SS, Curtis JP, Wang Y, Bristow MR, Krumholz HM. Association of serum digoxin concentration and outcomes in patients with heart failure. *JAMA* 2003;**289**(7):871–8.

38. Abraham WT, Hayes DL. Cardiac resynchronization therapy for heart failure. *Circulation* 2003;**108**(21):2596–603.

39. Abraham WT, Fisher WG, Smith AL *et al*. Cardiac resynchronization in chronic heart failure. *N Engl J Med* 2002; **346**(24):1845–53.

40. Sutton MG, Plappert T, Hilpisch KE, Abraham WT, Hayes DL, Chinchoy E. Sustained reverse left ventricular structural remodeling with cardiac resynchronization at one year is a function of etiology: quantitative Doppler echocardiographic evidence from the Multicenter InSync Randomized Clinical Evaluation (MIRACLE). *Circulation* 2006;**113**(2):266–72.

41. Bristow MR, Saxon LA, Boehmer J *et al*. Cardiac-resynchronization therapy with or without an implantable defibrillator in advanced chronic heart failure. *N Engl J Med* 2004; **350**(21):2140–50.

42. Cleland JG, Daubert JC, Erdmann E *et al*. The effect of cardiac resynchronization on morbidity and mortality in heart failure. *N Engl J Med* 2005;**352**(15):1539–49.

43. Jarcho JA. Biventricular pacing. *N Engl J Med* 2006; **355**(3):288–94.

44. Linde C, Abraham WT, Gold MR, St John Sutton M, Ghio S, Daubert C, REVERSE (REsynchronization reVErses Remodeling in Systolic left vEntricular dysfunction) Study Group. Randomized trial of cardiac resynchronization in mildly symptomatic heart failure patients and in asymptomatic patients with left ventricular dysfunction and previous heart failure symptoms. *J Am Coll Cardiol* 2008;**52**(23):1834–43. Epub 2008 Nov 7.

45. Josephson M, Wellens HJ. Implantable defibrillators and sudden cardiac death. *Circulation* 2004;**109**(22):2685–91.

46. Moss AJ, Zareba W, Hall WJ *et al*. Prophylactic implantation of a defibrillator in patients with myocardial infarction and reduced ejection fraction. *N Engl J Med* 2002;**346**(12):877–83.

47. Desai AS, Fang JC, Maisel WH, Baughman KL. Implantable defibrillators for the prevention of mortality in patients with nonischemic cardiomyopathy: a meta-analysis of randomized controlled trials. *JAMA* 2004;**292**(23):2874–9.

48. Bardy GH, Lee KL, Mark DB *et al*. Amiodarone or an implantable cardioverter-defibrillator for congestive heart failure. *N Engl J Med* 2005;**352**(3):225–37.

49. Stevenson LW, Desai AS. Selecting patients for discussion of the ICD as primary prevention for sudden death in heart failure. *J Cardiac Fail* 2006;**12**(6):407–12.

77 Atrial fibrillation

Michael Klein
Boston University Medical Center, Boston, MA, USA

Case history

A 40-year-old male was evaluated for intermittent chest tightness without shortness of breath or palpitations. Symptoms occurred with nervousness but not exertion. Family history was notable for the death of his mother at 57 with chronic heart failure and a brother at age 16 of sudden cardiac death while jogging. His father was 75 and previously had both aortic valve replacement and abdominal aortic aneurysm surgery. Personal habits included no smoking, two cups of caffeinated coffee daily, modest alcohol, on weekends mostly. He was physically active including bike riding and water skiing.

Physical exam revealed a robust male with normal peripheral pulses and no bruits or edema. The BP was 136/90 mmHg sitting and 130/86 mmHg right arm after 30 seconds standing. Pulse was 80 and regular. Fundoscopy was normal. The chest was muscular with left precordial hypertrophy. S1 was normal, S2 normally split with $A_2 > P_2$; apical fourth and third heart sounds were audible together with a Grade 2/6 midsystolic murmur. Occasional extrasystoles were noted. ECG (Fig. 77.1) showed normal sinus rhythm with normal PR, QRS, QT intervals, a QRS axis of 9 degrees, narrow Q-waves in aVF. Increased voltage of left ventricular hypertrophy (LVH) with strain effect and left atrial enlargement were present.

A tentative diagnosis of cardiomyopathy with possible outflow tract obstruction was made.[1] Because of the worrisome pattern of LVH with strain which has been associated with non-fatal and fatal cardiovascular events,[2] the family history, and the angina-like symptoms, cardiac catheterization was undertaken.

Coronary angiography revealed a 60–70% left anterior descending artery stenosis. Minimal atherosclerosis was evident elsewhere. Pressures were 107/18 mmHg in the LV, 24/13 mmHg in the PA, and 29/7 mmHg in the RV without evidence for either left- or right-sided outflow tract obstruction at rest. By echocardiogram, the LV was normal in size and had concentric hypertrophy with an interventricular septal thickness of 16 mm. The LVEF was 40%. Left atrial volume was modestly increased at 36 mL/m² with an

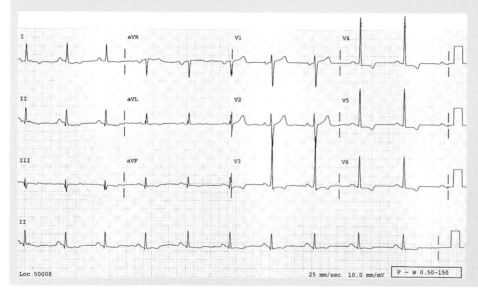

Figure 77.1 Initial encounter ECG showing sinus rhythm, left atrial enlargement, left ventricular strain.

emptying time of 190 msec. Mitral inflow velocity profile showed a E/A ratio of 1.2. The low septal early diastolic mitral annular velocity e' was 8 cm/sec with increased E/e' ratio. Grade II diastolic dysfunction was calculated.[3]

Based upon these findings, drug therapy was begun with beta-blocker, aspirin, statin and low-dose angiotensin-converting enzyme (ACE) inhibition. Goals included:

- slowing the resting heart rate to 50–60 to maximize diastolic flow-time into the hypertrophied LV
- affording some protection against atrial or ventricular ectopy
- lowering LDL cholesterol to below 130 mg/dL.[4,5]

Four years later the patient developed palpitations and exertional dyspnea. ECG revealed atrial flutter-fibrillation (Fig. 77.2). Transesophageal echocardiography excluded left atrial thrombus or smoke.

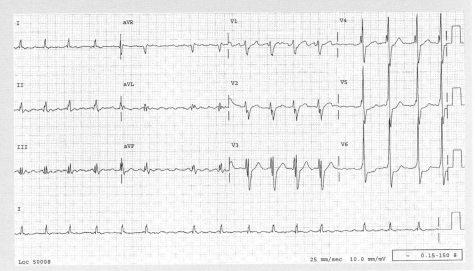

Figure 77.2 Four years later. ECG shows atrial flutter fibrillation.

Question

What action would you take at this juncture?

Comment

Sinus rhythm was re-established by cardioversion. Restoration of rhythm control, as opposed to rate control, was believed likely to alleviate symptoms of exertional dyspnea and palpitations, thereby improving lifestyle,[6] even if it did not confer an additional benefit of stroke risk protection.[7] Sequential atrioventricular contraction would maximize diastolic filling of the hypertrophied left ventricle while lowering left atrial pressure and normalizing exertional heart rate increments, enhancing exercise capacity.[8]

Anticoaulation with warfarin to INR 2.0–3.0 was initiated to reduce the risk of atrial fibrillation-induced thromboembolic (TE) stroke.[9] Even though the patient's CHADS$_2$ score was only one, implying an intermediate risk for such TE stroke origin, both this metric and other risk stratification schemes used to predict stroke risk in atrial fibrillation exhibit poor discriminatory ability with c-statistic of 0.56–0.62, distant from the ideal of 1.0.[10] The advanced left ventricular hypertrophy and diastolic dysfunction associated with the patient's cardiomyopathy was likely to result in recurrent atrial fibrillation with sluggish left atrial appendage inflow and outflow velocities posing an appendicular thrombus risk.

Case history *continued*

Within six months, however, palpitations recurred and the ECG documented atrial flutter. An electrophysiology study confirmed the presence of atrial flutter with a 230 msec cycle length and typical cavotricuspid isthmus (CTI) and counterclockwise rotation.

Question

How should you proceed with this information?

Comment

The atrial flutter was thought to present an even greater problem with heart rate control with the potential for quantum jumps in ventricular rate with exertion. Radiofrequency catheter ablation was performed and terminated the flutter with bidirectional conal block documented at the ablation site.[11] The atrial flutter was thought to be related to previous fibrillation-flutter functionally, wherein a line of block (LoB) in the right atrium in the CTI formed.[12] Medical therapy with low-dose aspirin and warfarin was continued. Beta-blocker, angiotensin-converting enzyme inhibitor and statin therapy were also maintained to slow the process of electrical ventricular remodeling associated with hypertrophic cardiomyopathy[13] and retard the processes of mechanical and electrical atrial remodeling predisposing to atrial fibrillation.[14–16]

Case history *continued*

During office visits over the next several years, the patient reported episodes of palpitations and recrudescent atrial fibrillation documented by ECG. INR control was managed via an anticoagulation clinic with documented INRs between 2.0 and 3.0 for more than 85% of measurements. Cardioversion to sinus rhythm was successfully accomplished on two separate occasions nine months apart. Amiodarone, 200 mg/day, was added to the medical regimen in an effort to electrically stabilize the atria and preserve sinus rhythm.[17] However, though remaining physically very active, the patient continued to have palpitations, sporadic chest pressure or dyspnea and a new fatigue and occasional light-headedness. Repeat ECG showed sinus bradycardia of 46–50/min, infrequent single late cycle ventricular premature beats, and an unchanged left ventricular hypertrophy with strain. Blood tests showed a thyroid-stimulating hormone (TSH) of 3.5, HCt 42%, Cr of 0.8 mg/dL, BUN 12 mg/dL, glucose 88, NA 144 mEq/L, K 4.5 mEq/L, cholesterol 188 mg/dL, HDL 45 mg/dL, triglyceride 160 mg/dL, with calculated LDL of 111 mg/dL. A stress echo was performed to clarify the symptoms of exertional chest pressure and shortness of breath. With the BRUCE protocol the patient exercised for 8.2 minutes, stopping with fatigue and chest pressure at a peak heart rate of 114 per minute. The ECG was obscured by LVH with strain. Occasional ventricular and atrial premature beats were observed. Echo recordings indicated preserved LV systolic function, Grade II diastolic dysfunction, and recruitment (thickening) on all regions of the left ventricle except the septum. Based upon these findings, repeat coronary angiography was done which indicated persistent 60–70% left anterior descending artery stenosis and minimal atherosclerosis elsewhere. Symptoms of exertional dyspnea and chest pressure were ascribed to diastolic dysfunction and, possibly, abnormal coronary vasodilator reserve capacity.[18] Amiodarone was discontinued because of fatigue and sinus bradycardia.

On return evaluation six months later, atrial fibrillation was again documented by ECG. The ventricular response rate was 48 per minute. Fatigue and light-headedness symptoms were more prominent and interfering with the patient's active lifestyle and work.

Question

What, if any, intervention should be considered now?

Comment

An electrophysiologic radiofrequency ablation procedure was proposed to the patient because:
- beta-blockers to constrain the atrial fibrillation might have contributed to unacceptable bradycardia
- electrical and mechanical remodeling of the atria might have progressed to a degree where drug therapy alone could no longer suppress the atrial fibrillation

- restoration of co-ordinated atrioventricular contraction would be expected to lower left heart filling pressures and mitigate exertional dyspnea and chest discomfort.[19]

A wide area of substrate radiofrequency ablation was accomplished with the catheter procedure lasting 5.5 hours.[20–22] Sinus rhythm was restored without ensuing complications (Fig. 77.3). Effort dyspnea and fatigue were alleviated. Follow-up Holter monitoring one year later revealed persistent sinus rhythm with occasional isolated ventricular premature beats (VPB) and rare VPB couplets. Repeat echocardiography indicated moderate left atrial volume enlargement of 39 ml/m² but recurrent atrial fibrillation was not observed.[23,24] Medical therapy with

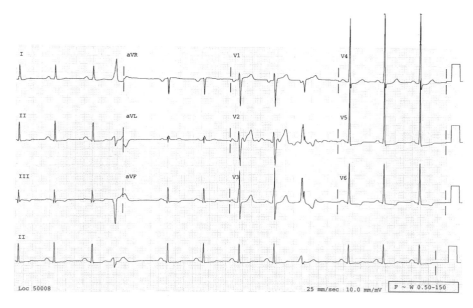

Figure 77.3 Restoration of sinus rhythm following successful cardioversion. Left ventricular hypertrophy with strain is seen again. Ventricular premature beats are present.

beta-blocker, ACE inhibitor, statin, low-dose aspirin, and warfarin was continued. During a repeat treadmill exercise test, to 6.5 metabolic equivalents, sinus rhythm was maintained. VPB and VPB couplets were observed but no ventricular tachycardia (VT). Blood pressure rose from 110/70 to 140/70 mmHg with exertion. Recall the patient's family history that included his brother's sudden cardiac death in adolescence and his mother's mid-life demise with chronic heart failure. Although his ventricular wall thickness of less than 20 mm placed him in a low-risk cohort for sudden death,[25] his combination of coronary and myopathic heart disease and family history presented an unusual hazard for sudden death. He was offered an implantable defibrillator, but declined.

References

1. Maron BJ. Hypertrophic cardiomyopathy. *Lancet* 1997; **350**:127–33.

2. Levy B, Salomon M, D'Agostino RB, Belanger AJ, Kannel WB. Prognostic implications of baseline electrocardiographic features and their serial changes in subjects with left ventricular hypertrophy. *Circulation* 1994; **90**:1786–93.

3. Lester SJ, Tajik J, Nishimura RA, Oh JK, Khandheria BK, Sevard JB. Unlocking the mysteries of diastolic function: deciphering the Rosetta Stone ten years later. *J Am Coll Cardiol* 2008; **51**:679–89.

4. Reiter MJ, Mann DE, Reiffel JE, Hahn E, Hartz V. Significance and incidence of concordance of drug efficacy predictions by Holter monitoring and electrophysiologic study in the ESVEM Trial. *Circulation* 1995; **91**:1988–95.

5. Downs JR, Clearfield M, Weis S *et al*. Primary prevention of acute coronary events with Lovastatin in men and women with average cholesterol levels. Results of the AFCAPS/TexCaps. *JAMA* 1998; **279**:1615–22.

6. Thrall G, Lane, D, Carroll D, Lip GY. Quality of life in patients with atrial fibrillation: a systematic review. *Am J Med* 2006;**119**: 448.

7. AFFIRM Investigators. A comparison of rate control and rhythm control in patients with atrial fibrillation. *N Engl J Med* 2002; **347**:1834–40.

8. Singh SN, Tang XC, Singh BN *et al*, for the SAFE-T Investigators. Quality of life and exercise performance in patients in sinus rhythm versus persistent atrial fibrillation. A Veterans Affairs Cooperative Studies Program substudy. *J Am Coll Cardiol* 2006; **48**:721–30.

9. Hylek EM, Skates SJ, Sheehan MA, Singer DE. An analysis of the lowest effective intensity of prophylactic anticoagulation for patients with non-rheumatic atrial fibrillation. *N Engl J Med* 1996; **335**:540–6.

10. Fang MC, Go AS, Chang Y, Borowsky L, Pomernacki NK, Singer DE, for the ATRIA Study Group. Comparison of risk stratification schemes to predict thromboembolism in people with non-valvular atrial fibrillation. *J Am Coll Cardiol* 2008; **51**:810–15.

11. Kirkorian G, Moncada E, Chevalier P *et al*. Radiofrequency ablation of atrial flutter. Efficacy of an anatomically guided approach. *Circulation* 1994; **90**:2804–14.

12. Waldo AL, Feld GK. Inter-relationships of atrial fibrillation and atrial flutter. *J Am Coll Cardiol* 2008; **51**:779–86.

13. Jeyarah B, Wilson LB, Zhong J *et al*. Mechanoelectrical feedback as a novel mechanism of cardiac electrical remodeling. *Circulation* 2007; **115**:3145–55.

14. Madrid AH, Peng J, Zamora J *et al*. The role of angiotensin receptor blockers and/or angiotensin converting enzyme inhibitors and atrial fibrillation in patients with cardiovascular diseases: meta-analysis of randomized controlled clinical trials. *PACE* 2004; **27**:1405–10.

15. Cardin S, Vanshi L, Thorin-Trescases N, Tack-Ki L, Thorin E, Nattel S. Evolution of the atrial fibrillation substrate in experimental congestive heart failure: angiotensin-dependent and independent pathways. *Cardiovasc Res* 2003; **60**:315–25.

16. Olshansky B. Can lipid lowering medication reduce the prevalence of atrial fibrillation in patients with left ventricular dysfunction? *Nat Clin Pract* 2007; **4**:16–17.

17. Singh BN, Singh SN, Reda DJ *et al*. Sotalol, Amiodarone, Atrial Fibrillation Efficacy Trial (SAFE-T) Investigators. Amiodarone versus sotalol for atrial fibrillation. *N Engl J Med* 2005; **352**:1861–72.

18. Christensen CW, Rosen LB, Gal RA, Haseeb M, Lassar TA, Port SC. Coronary vasodilator reserve. Comparison of the effects of papaverine and adenosine on coronary flow, ventricular function, and myocardial metabolism. *Circulation* 1991; **83**: 294–303.

19. Braunwald E, Frahm CJ. Studies on Starling's Law of the Heart: IV. Observations on the hemodynamic functions of the left atrium in man. *Circulation* 1961; **24**:633–42.

20. Khan R. Identifying and understanding the role of pulmonary vein activity in atrial fibrillation. *Cardiovasc Res* 2004; **64**:387–94.

21. Calkins H, Brugada J, Packer DL *et al*. HRS/EHRA/ECAS expert consensus statement on catheter and surgical ablation of atrial fibrillation: recommendations for personnel, policy, procedures and follow-up. *Heart Rhythm* 2007; **4**(6):1–46.

22. Pappone C, Augello G, Sala S *et al*. A randomized trial of circumferential pulmonary vein ablation versus anti-arrhythmic drug therapy in paroxysmal atrial fibrillation. The APAF Study. *J Am Coll Cardiol* 2006; **48**:2340–7.

23. Tsang TS, Barnes ME, Bailey KR *et al*. Left atrial volume: important risk marker of incident atrial fibrillation in 1,665 older men and women. *Mayo Clin Proc* 2001; **76**:467–75.

24. Tani T, Tenabe K, Ono M *et al*. Left atrial volume in the risk of paroxysmal atrial fibrillation in patients with hypertrophic cardiomyopathy. *J Am Soc Echocardiogr* 2004; **17**:644–8.

25. Spirito P, Bellone P, Harris KM, Benabo P, Bruzzi P, Maron BJ. Magnitude of left ventricular hypertrophy and risk of sudden death in hypertrophic cardiomyopathy. *N Engl J Med* 2000; **342**:1778–85.

78

The case for and against implantable cardioverter defibrillators in patients with coronary artery disease

Jeffrey S Healey
Hamilton Health Science, Hamilton, Ontario, Canada

Case history

A 50-year-old steelworker experiences severe retrosternal chest pain. He is brought to a tertiary care hospital by one of his co-workers, approximately two hours after the onset of chest pain. On examination, the patient's pulse is regular at 95 beats per minute and his blood pressure is 145/90. The lungs are clear bilaterally and there is an S4, but no murmurs. The patient's father died of a myocardial infarction at age 52. He has no significant prior medical history and does not have regular health maintenance visits with a physician or nurse. He does not smoke, but is overweight (Body Mass Index is 29) and eats a "fast food" diet. He is physically active at work, but does not engage in additional regular exercise.

An ECG is done in the emergency department which shows evidence of an acute, lateral wall myocardial infarction. He is given 160 mg of aspirin and a total of three doses (0.4 mg) of sublingual nitroglycerin. Approximately 15 minutes later, while a subsequent ECG is being done (Fig. 78.1), the patient loses consciousness. His nurse recognizes that the patient has developed ventricular fibrillation and promptly defibrillates him with a 200 J biphasic shock. The patient is returned to sinus rhythm and regains consciousness. He is given a total of 15 mg of intravenous metoprolol and 300 mg of clopidogrel and is taken promptly to the catheterization laboratory. There he is found to have single-vessel disease, with an occluded proximal circumflex artery. Percutaneous coronary intervention (PCI) is successfully performed and a bare metal stent inserted. With the re-establishment of TIMI-3 flow, it is

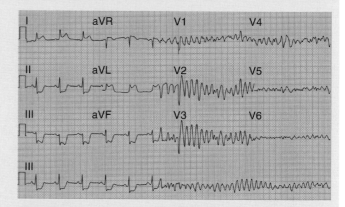

Figure 78.1 Patient's ECG in the emergency department.

apparent that the non-dominant circumflex supplies three large marginal branches. A left ventricular angiogram is performed which shows hypokinesia of the entire lateral wall, with an estimated ejection fraction of 35%.

Three days following his myocardial infarction, the patient is doing well. He has had no heart failure, no recurrent angina and no evidence of heart block or ventricular arrhythmias. He is receiving aspirin 81 mg daily, clopidogrel 75 mg daily, metoprolol 50 mg bid, ramipril 5 mg daily and pravastatin 40 mg daily.

Question

What else can be done to reduce the chance of this patient dying suddenly?

Comment

This patient has suffered an acute ST elevation myocardial infarction that was complicated (<48 hours) by the

development of ventricular fibrillation. In this context, the arrhythmia is often referred to as "primary ventricular fibrillation"[1] although this term is often a source of confusion, as the arrhythmia is actually *secondary* to the acute myocardial infarction. Given the potential for confusion with "idiopathic ventricular fibrillation", this term should probably be abandoned.

It is traditionally felt that ventricular fibrillation (VF) occurring within 48 hours of a myocardial infarction does not confer an increased risk of arrhythmic death and thus does not warrant specific therapy, such as an implantable defibrillator (ICD) or antiarrhythmic drugs.[2] This is based

Evidence-Based Cardiology, 3rd edition. Edited by S. Yusuf, J.A. Cairns, A.J. Camm, E.L. Fallen, and B.J. Gersh. © 2010 Blackwell Publishing, ISBN: 978-1-4051-5925-8.

on data from the GISSI-1 trial, which suggests that patients with this type of arrhythmia in the acute phase of an acute (AMI) have a similar prognosis to patients with comparable myocardial infarctions without VF.[3] Accordingly, current guidelines suggest that an implantable defibrillator is *not* indicated in this setting (**Class III**).[2]

However, this decision is contingent on two key facts. First, the arrhythmia in question must be polymorphic ventricular tachycardia or ventricular fibrillation, as the occurrence of monomorphic ventricular tachycardia generally implies the existence of an arrhythmogenic substrate[4] and an unfavorable prognosis,[5] warranting specific therapy. Secondly, it should be clear that the arrhythmia in question occurred in the context of a definite myocardial infarction. As sustained ventricular arrhythmias may increase serum troponin (even in the absence of coronary artery disease), clinicians should have other corroborating evidence of myocardial infarction (history of chest pain, ECG changes, wall motion abnormality, occluded artery) before attributing a potentially lethal ventricular arrhythmia to an acute myocardial infarction.[6] In practice, it can sometimes be difficult to make this distinction, and if there is any doubt, it is generally advisable to pursue specific treatment of the ventricular arrhythmia.

More recently, several reports have called into question the "benign" nature of ventricular fibrillation occurring within 48 hours of acute myocardial infarction.[7,8] It is possible that in the modern therapeutic era for myocardial infarction, the prognostic significance of early ventricular arrhythmias has changed. However, there have been no randomized trials demonstrating a benefit with implantable defibrillators in this group of patients and current guidelines have not been changed.[2,9] Left ventricular ejection fraction remains the strongest predictor of all-cause and arrhythmic mortality following myocardial infarction[10] and arrhythmic mortality remains an important cause of death during the first year following myocardial infarction, in patients with a low ejection fraction.[10]

With the emergence of the ICD as the treatment of choice for cardiac arrest survivors, the DINAMIT study was conducted to determine if the routine use of ICD, 6–40 days following myocardial infarction, in patients with an ejection fraction of ≤35% and with low heart rate variability, reduced mortality.[9] Surprisingly, it did not.[9] Although the implantation of an ICD significantly reduced arrhythmic death, ICD-treated patients experienced a significant *increase* in heart failure death, such that all-cause mortality was unchanged.[9] The increase in heart failure was not due to right ventricular pacing[11] as patients in DINAMIT were only paced in VVI-40 mode.[9] Furthermore, patients dying of heart failure typically had received appropriate ICD shocks before death.[9] In essence, the use of the ICD in these high-risk patients merely converted sudden death to heart failure death.

Given the negative results of DINAMIT, the prophylactic implantation of an ICD early after myocardial infarction is not indicated (**Class III, Level B**).[2] However, if a patient similar to the one described were to develop atrioventricular block requiring permanent pacing, it would be reasonable to implant an ICD instead, given the potential for benefit and the minimal incremental risk to the patient.

Case history *continued*

The patient was discharged home on the fourth day following myocardial infarction. In addition to the usual secondary prophylactic agents, he was also instructed to take 1 g/day of omega-3 fatty acid supplements (EPA/DHA), as this intervention has been shown in the GISSI-Prevenzione trial to lower the risk of arrhythmic death.[12] An ICD was not implanted; however, a follow-up radionuclide angiogram was scheduled in three months' time, to re-evaluate the patient's left ventricular ejection fraction.

Guidelines typically suggest waiting at least 40 days following myocardial infarction and 90 days following revascularization, to allow time for ventricular remodeling (positive or negative) and to ensure that the patient survives the early postmyocardial infarction period.[2,13]

Three months later, the patient was asymptomatic and still taking his medications. The follow-up ejection fraction was 38%. A Holter monitor was also completed and did not show any evidence of ventricular arrhythmias. The patient was seen in consultation by an electrophysiologist who discussed the potential role of an ICD (and its potential complications). A determination was made that an ICD was not indicated at the present time.

Comment

The current ACC/AHA/ESC guidelines suggest that a prophylactic ICD should be considered in patients with coronary artery disease, who are at least 40 days following myocardial infarction and who have a left ventricular ejection fraction of ≤30–40% (**Class I, Level A**).[2] However, not a single randomized trial has demonstrated a benefit for the ICD in patients with an ejection fraction of 36 – 40%. The only ICD trial to include a small number of such patients was the MUSTT trial; however, this was not a randomized trial of the ICD, but rather a strategy of EP testing in patients with coronary artery disease, left ventricular dysfunction and non-sustained ventricular tachycardia.[14] Appreciating that there is a measurement error associated with assessment of left ventricular ejection fraction (even when using radionuclide angiography), many clinicians continue to recommend an ICD to individual patients with a left ventricular ejection fraction of between 35% and 40%. However, there is insufficient evidence to warrant a Class I, Level A recommendation for this group as a whole.

Case history *continued*

The patient was lost to follow-up for two years, but then returned to his primary care physician, having stopped his ramipril and beta-blocker due to side effects. His clopidogrel had already been stopped one year following his myocardial infarction. He remained asymptomatic with no shortness of breath on exertion, angina, syncope or palpitation. His blood pressure was now 175/100 and his ECG showed sinus rhythm at 80 beats per minute and an incomplete left bundle branch block (QRS width of 130 msec) and left axis deviation.

He was eventually restarted on a different beta-blocker and full doses of an angiotensin receptor-blocking agent. A follow-up radionuclide angiogram was done three months later and revealed a left ventricular ejection fraction of 29%. A repeat coronary angiogram showed a patent circumflex stent and no new coronary lesions. An echocardiogram showed a large posterolateral wall motion abnormality, an estimated left ventricular ejection fraction of 30–35%, moderate left ventricular hypertrophy and moderate mitral regurgitation. The primary care physician was reluctant to consider an ICD because the patient "was doing well" (i.e. no clinical symptoms). However, the patient had been doing some reading on the internet and wished to see his electrophysiologist to discuss his options.

Comment

It appears that the patient's left ventricle has suffered late, negative remodeling, perhaps as a result of uncontrolled hypertension. In the short term, it is important to re-initiate evidence-based therapy for left ventricular dysfunction and to gain control of his blood pressure. Time should be given for this therapy to impact ventricular function before re-evaluating the ejection fraction.

It is a common misconception that if patients are doing well and are many years following myocardial infarction, they do not warrant consideration for an ICD. Although some trials (SCD-HeFT, COMPANION) did require symptomatic heart failure as an inclusion criterion,[15,16] others (MADIT-II) did not.[17] In fact, cost-effectiveness analyses suggest that it is among minimally symptomatic patients that the ICD is the most cost-effective.[18]

Despite the patient's low ejection fraction and prolonged QRS duration, there is currently no indication to implant a cardiac resynchronization device. All major, published studies of this therapy have been in patients with NYHA class III or IV heart failure. Two studies are ongoing (RAFT, MADIT-CRT) that will help determine if this therapy can reduce the incidence of death and heart failure in patients with NYHA class I or II heart failure. Given the increased cost and complexity of cardiac resynchronization devices, pending the results of these two trials, the use of cardiac resynchronization in these patients is not recommended.

Case history *continued*

The patient undergoes an uneventful placement of a single-chamber implantable defibrillator. Two years later, he has been compliant with medications and has not received any therapy from the ICD, nor suffered any adverse consequence.

Conclusion

The decision to implant an ICD in this patient was based on robust scientific evidence and good clinical judgment.[17] However, unlike most other prophylactic interventions (i.e. vaccines, aspirin), physicians can determine if a specific patient actually derived benefit from their ICD given the ICD's capacity to capture and store records of arrhythmia. Over 21 months mean follow-up, only 23% of similar ICD recipients would be expected to receive an appropriate therapy from the ICD.[19] The fact that this patient has not received therapy from his device should not cause physicians to reconsider the appropriateness of the ICD for this patient, as the application of these guidelines to a population of similar patients is expected to produce a net benefit, with a very respectable number needed-to-treat of only 8 patients, for three years to prevent one death.[20] However, efforts are ongoing to more precisely define patients at risk of ventricular arrhythmias.[21]

References

1. Gheeraert PJ, DeBuyzere ML, Taeymans YM *et al.* Risk factors for primary ventricular fibrillation during acute myocardial infarction: a systematic review and meta-analysis. *Eur Heart J* 2006;**27**:2499–510.

2. Zipes DP, Camm AJ, Borggrefe M *et al.* ACC/AHA/ESC 2006 guidelines for the management of patients with ventricular arrhythmias and the prevention of sudden cardiac death: a report of the American College of Cardiology/American Heart Association Task Force and the European Society of Cardiology Committee for the Management of Patients with Ventricular Arrhythmias and Prevention of Sudden Cardiac Death. *Circulation* 2006;**114**:e385–e484.

3. Volpi A, Cavailli A, Santoro L, Negri E. Incidence and prognosis of early ventricular fibrillation in acute myocardial infarction – results of the Gruppo Italiano per lo Studio della Spravvivenza nell'Infarto Miocardico (GISSI-2) database. *Am J Cardiol* 1998;**82**:265–71.

4. Stevenson WG, Khan H, Sager P *et al.* Identification of reentry circuit sites during catheter mapping and radiofrequency ablation of ventricular tachycardia late after myocardial infarction. *Circulation* 1993;**88**:1647–70.

5. Hatzinikolaou E, Tziakas D, Hotidis A *et al.* Could sustained monomorphic ventricular tachycardia in the early phase of a prime acute myocardial infarction affect patient outcome? *J Electrocardiol* 2007;**40**(1):72–7.

6. Machoado MN, Suzuki FA, Mouco OC, Hernandes ME, Lemos MA, Maia LN. Positive troponin T in a chagasic patient with sustained ventricular tachycardia and no obstructive lesions on cine coronary angiography. *Arq Bras Cardiol* 2005;**84**(2):182–4.

7. Wyse DG, Friedman P, Brodsky MA *et al.* Life-threatening ventricular arrhythmias due to transient or correctable causes: high risk for death in follow-up. *J Am Coll Cardiol* 2001;**38**(6):1725–7.

8. Al-Khatib SM, Stebbins AL, Califf RM *et al.* Sustained ventricular arrhythmias and mortality among patients with acute myocardial infarction: results from the GUSTO-III trial. *Am Heart J* 2003;**145**(3):515–21.

9. Hohnloser SH, Kuck KH, Dorian P *et al.* Prophylactic use of an implantable cardioverter-defibrillator after acute myocardial infarction. *N Engl J Med* 2004;**351**(24):2481–8.

10. Solomon SD, Zelenkofske S, McMurray JJ *et al.* Sudden death in patients with myocardial infarction and left ventricular dysfunction, heart failure, or both. *N Engl J Med* 2005;**352**(25):2581–8.

11. DAVID Trial Investigators. Dual-chamber pacing or ventricular backup pacing in patients with an implantable defibrillator (DAVID) trial. *JAMA* 2002;**288**(24):3115–23.

12. GISSI-Prevenzione Investigators. Dietary supplementation with n3-polyunsaturated fatty acids and vitamin E after myocardial infarction: results of the GISSI-Prevenzione trial. *Lancet* 1999;**354**:447–55.

13. Tang AS, Ross H, Simpson CS *et al.* Canadian Cardiovascular Society/Canadian Heart Rhythm Society position paper on implantable cardioverter defibrillator use in Canada. *Can J Cardiol* 2005;**21**(suppl A):11A–8A.

14. Buxton AE, Lee KL, Fisher JD *et al.* A randomized study of the prevention of sudden death in patients with coronary artery disease. *N Engl J Med* 1999;**341**:1882–90.

15. Bristow MR, Saxon LA, Boehmer J *et al.* Cardiac-resynchronization therapy with or without an implantable defibrillator in advanced heart failure. *N Engl J Med* 2004;**347**:2140–50.

16. Bardy GH, Lee KL, Mark DB *et al.* Amiodarone or an implantable cardioverter-defibrillator for congestive heart failure. *N Engl J Med* 2005;**352**:225–37.

17. Moss AJ, Zareba W, Hall WJ *et al.* Prophylactic implantation of a defibrillator in patients with myocardial infarction and reduced ejection fraction. *N Engl J Med* 2002;**346**(12):877–83.

18. Sanders GD, Hlatky MA, Owens DK. Cost-effectiveness of implantable cardioverter-defibrillators. *N Engl J Med* 2005;**353**:1471–80.

19. Moss AJ, Greenberg H, Case RB *et al.* Long-term clinical course of patients after termination of ventricular tachyarrhythmia by an implanted defibrillator. *Circulation* 2004;**110**:3760–5.

20. Zwanziger J, Hall WJ, Dick AW *et al.* The cost effectiveness of implantable cardioverter-defibrillators: results from the Multicenter Automatic Defibrillator Implantation Trial (MADIT)-II. *J Am Coll Cardiol* 2006;**47**(11):2310–18.

21. Al-Khatib SM, Sanders GD, Bigger JT *et al.* Preventing tomorrow's sudden cardiac death today: part I: Current data on risk stratification for sudden cardiac death. *Am Heart J* 2007;**153**(6):941–50.

79 Bradyarrhythmias – choice of pacemakers

Pablo B Nery[1] and Carlos A Morillo[2]
[1]University of Ottawa Heart Institute, Ottawa, Ontario, Canada
[2]Hamilton Health Sciences, McMaster University, Hamilton, Ontario, Canada

Case history 1

A 58-year-old woman presents to your office with a three-month history of recurrent presyncope and progressive fatigue on exertion. There is no history of chest pain or dyspnea. She has had two syncopal episodes over the last 10 months, both without prodromes. During the last episode she suffered a Colles' fracture.

Physical examination reveals a patient in no acute distress with a blood pressure of 120/68 and a regular heart rate of 42 beats per minute. Chest exam shows good bilateral air entry and lungs are clear. Neck veins are flat. Heart sounds show a normal S1 and S2. No added sounds or murmurs on auscultation. She was diagnosed with hypertension five years ago for which she is on a thiazide diuretic as her only medication. She is not a smoker and she has no history of diabetes, coronary artery disease, dyslipidemia or syncope until last year. Her family history is non-contributory. Anemia and thyroid disease were ruled out by her family doctor. Her two-dimensional echocardiogram revealed normal left ventricular size and function.

Baseline 12-lead ECG (Fig. 79.1) and 24-hour Holter monitor were ordered. Of note, she had a presyncopal episode during Holter recording (Fig. 79.2).

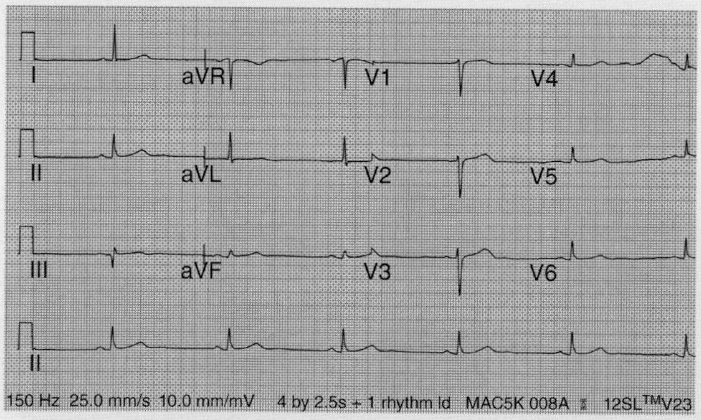

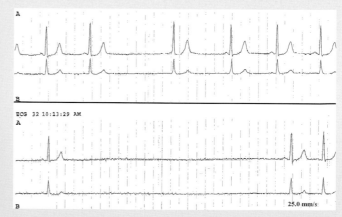

Figure 79.2 Holter monitor recording from Case 1 showing significant bradycardia and a sinus pause lasting 5.8 seconds. This pause was associated with severe presyncope.

Figure 79.1 Twelve-lead ECG from Case 1 showing severe sinus bradycardia at a rate of 37 bpm.

Evidence-Based Cardiology, 3rd edition. Edited by S. Yusuf, J.A. Cairns, A.J. Camm, E.L. Fallen, and B.J. Gersh. © 2010 Blackwell Publishing, ISBN: 978-1-4051-5925-8.

Case history 2

A 72-year-old man is brought to the emergency department by his daughter after a syncopal episode. He was sitting on a chair when he suddenly lost consciousness for approximately 40 seconds. He recovered with no residual symptoms. When asked, he denied any prodromes but his daughter noticed transient cyanosis during the episode. Past medical history is significant for hypertension which was controlled after weight loss and low-salt diet.

Physical examination reveals no acute distress with a blood pressure of 112/62 and a regular heart rate of 48 beats per minute. Chest exam shows good bilateral air entry and lungs are clear. Neck veins are 3 cm above the sternal angle. Normal S1 and S2. No added sounds or murmurs on auscultation. He is not a smoker and he has no history of stroke, coronary artery disease or diabetes. There is no previous history of syncope. A recent two-dimensional echocardiogram (three months ago) measured his left ventricular ejection fraction at 60%. A 12-lead ECG was obtained (Fig. 79.3).

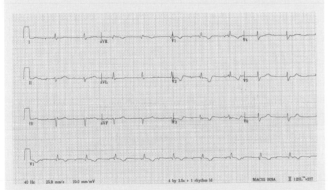

Figure 79.3 Twelve-lead ECG from Case 2 showing complete third-degree heart block with right bundle branch block.

Question

What is your diagnosis and what therapy is indicated for each patient?

Comment

In Case 1 the clinical presentation of syncope, presyncope and fatigue, temporarily related to sinus pauses on both the 12-lead ECG and Holter monitor, point to a diagnosis of sinus node dysfunction (SND). Before confirming the diagnosis, it is of key importance to exclude secondary causes of sinus bradycardia such as hypothyroidism or pharmacologically induced bradycardia.

SND constitutes a spectrum of cardiac arrhythmias including sinus bradycardia, sinus arrest, sinoatrial block, and paroxysmal supraventricular tachycardia alternating with periods of bradycardia or asystole. Patients with the latter condition may be symptomatic from paroxysmal tachycardia, bradycardia or both. Correlation of symptoms with the above-mentioned arrhythmias by use of 12-lead ECG, Holter monitoring or event recorder is essential.

Sinus node dysfunction may present as chronotropic incompetence in which there is an inadequate response to exercise or stress. Chronotropic incompetence is defined as failure to achieve 85% of the predicted maximal heart rate during a treadmill stress test. Other more common causes of syncope such as vasovagal syncope should always be ruled out. However, this diagnosis is unlikely given the clinical presentation of syncope, presyncope and progressive fatigue induced by exercise in addition to symptom correlation of presyncope and a sinus pause >3 seconds (see Fig. 79.2).

Simple historic criteria have recently been described and a point score to rule out vasovagal syncope, known as the Calgary Syncope Score, that includes age of onset of syncope before age 35, classic prodrome, evidence of ECG alterations, and other clinical characteristics, has been validated.[1] A point score <–2 had a high sensitivity and specificity for the diagnosis of vasovagal syncope. In both cases the Calgary Syncope Score was –7, which rules out vasovagal syncope. Case 1 has typical clinical and ECG features of SND and has a **Class I, Level C** indication for a permanent pacemaker.[2,3] Sinus bradycardia is a physiologic finding in trained athletes, who frequently have resting heart rates between 40 and 50 bpm at rest. Moreover, rhythm changes during sleep such as sinus pauses >2 seconds, sinus bradycardia (<40 bpm), first-degree atrioventricular (AV) block and type I second-degree AV block are observed in up to 24% of healthy subjects.[4] The patient presented in Case 1 has a **Class I, Level C** indication for a permanent pacemaker. Current **Class I, Level C** indications for sinus bradycardia syndromes are as follows; permanent pacemaker implantation is indicated for:

• SND with documented symptomatic bradycardia, including frequent sinus pauses that produce symptoms
• symptomatic chronotropic incompetence
• symptomatic sinus bradycardia that results from required drug therapy for medical conditions.

The patient presented in Case 2 has a clear presentation of abrupt syncope with no prodrome and ECG documentation of third-degree AV block associated with right bundle branch block (see Fig. 79.3). Patients diagnosed with high-degree AV block – third-degree or second-degree type 2 – are clearly at risk for adverse cardiovascular events if not treated with permanent pacemaker implantation.[5,6] Therefore, this patient unquestionably benefits from a permanent pacemaker and also has a **Class I, Level C** indication.

Both cases may benefit from a single-chamber pacemaker. In Case 1 an atrial-based single-chamber pacemaker is appropriate and in Case 2 a single-chamber ventricular pacemaker may also be adequate. The need for a temporary transvenous wire is advocated by current ACLS guidelines[7] for patients with second-degree AV block type 2 or third-degree AV block associated with signs or symptoms of poor perfusion secondary to bradycardia. Transvenous pacing may increase the risk of postoperative infection[8] and cardiac perforation[9] and should be reserved for carefully selected patients although these issues have not been addressed by randomized controlled studies.

Question

Which is the most beneficial pacing mode for each patient?

Comment

The use of dual-chamber pacing offers theoretic advantages over ventricular pacing, such as maintenance of AV synchrony and preservation of normal ventricular activation through the His–Purkinje system (only in SND and depending upon a programmed long AV delay). Given the higher cost, greater complexity and increased complications of dual-chamber permanent pacemaker (PPM), several clinical studies assessed their potential benefit. In patients with SND, retrospective studies involving approximately 1400 patients suggest a significant survival benefit of dual-chamber PPM.[10–16] However, this is observational information and randomized clinical trials are needed to establish the benefit of dual-chamber pacing.

The first prospective, randomized controlled trial was published in 1994 by Andersen and colleagues.[17] This study assigned 225 patients with SND to receive a single-chamber atrial or ventricular PPM. A second analysis was published when the mean follow-up in these patients was 5.5 years[18] showing a significant lower risk of atrial fibrillation in the atrial pacing group, with a relative risk reduction of 0.54 ($P = 0.012$). There was also a reduced incidence of thromboembolic events and cardiovascular death. These results should be interpreted with caution since this study was small. The second analysis was *post hoc*. Thus no conclusive information could be derived but the exercise was useful as hypothesis generating.

The Danish group provided important data on the safety of atrial pacing in carefully selected patients with SND.[17,18] They excluded patients with bifascicular bundle branch block, atrial fibrillation with R-R interval longer than 3 seconds, PQ interval >220 ms (or >260 ms if age >70 years), and those who could not support 1:1 AV conduction with atrial pacing at 100 bpm. The population studied was shown to be at low risk for AV block, with an incidence of 0.6% per year.[18] The final word on atrial-based pacing for SND will be provided by the DANPACE study, a randomized multicenter study comparing single-chamber atrial pacemaker (AAI) versus dual-chamber pacemaker (DDD) pacing in patients with sick sinus syndrome which will complete enrollment in 2008.

The Mode Selection Trial (MOST) in SND followed 2010 patients for a median of 33.1 months. No advantage for dual-chamber pacing over single-chamber ventricular pacing in terms of the trial's primary endpoint – death from any cause or non-fatal stroke – was observed.[19] However, there was a significant reduction in the incidence of atrial fibrillation, with a relative risk reduction of 0.21 ($P = 0.008$). The effect of dual-chamber pacing was probably underestimated in this study since more than 30% of patients randomized to ventricular pacing were crossed over to dual-chamber mode. Moreover, the potential benefit of dual-chamber pacing may have been counteracted by the hazardous effects of unnecessary right ventricular pacing associated with short AV delay programmed in patients with SND and dual-chamber devices.[20,21]

The Canadian Trial of Physiological Pacing (CTOPP) compared clinical outcomes in 2568 patients who were randomized to atrial-based or ventricular pacing for a mean follow-up period of 3.5 years. Among the study population, SND was the indication for pacing in 42% and AV block in 58%. The study found no difference between the two groups in the combined incidence of stroke or death or in the likelihood of hospitalization for heart failure. Nevertheless, after two years of follow-up, physiologic pacing was associated with 18% relative risk reduction in the development of chronic atrial fibrillation (AF). The subgroup of patients paced for SND showed no benefit from physiologic pacing in terms of mortality or stroke.

The United Kingdom Pacing and Cardiovascular Events (UKPACE) was the most recently published of the major trials. It randomized 2023 patients greater than 70 years of age with high-grade AV block to dual- or single-chamber devices, showing no significant difference in overall survival after a mean follow-up period of 4.6 years. The incidence of stroke, atrial fibrillation or heart failure hospitalizations did not differ between groups. The UKPACE was the largest appraisal of pacing mode in patients with AV block and hence provides the best estimate of treatment effect in this population.

The Pacemaker Selection in the Elderly (PASE) trial – the only randomized trial specially designed to address quality of life (QoL) – enrolled 407 patients with indication for pacing, half of them with AV block. No significant difference in total mortality was shown between treatment groups (rate-responsive, single-chamber ventricular pacemaker [VVIR] vs. rate-responsive, dual-chamber pacemaker [DDDR]). Nevertheless, QoL improved after 30 months, corroborating with data from MOST and CTOPP substudies.[22] Of note, QoL improvement in PASE and MOST was mainly through a reduction in pacemaker syndrome, a "questionable" endpoint showing distinct incidence among series.[23]

A recently published meta-analysis confirmed that the bulk of data available to date is inconclusive for pacing mode selection and survival. Nevertheless, this meticulous review showed that atrial-based pacing reduces the incidence of atrial fibrillation.[24] This careful analysis suggests that the benefit was mainly observed in patients with SND. It also verified the higher complication rate associated with atrial-based PPM, generally secondary to lead dislodgment. Of note, atrial-based pacing translates to dual-chamber pacing in all studies but the first published by Andersen and colleagues.[17] Also, dual-chamber devices cost more, do not last as long and have a higher incidence of minor complications.[24] A few retrospective studies[25–27] as well as current guidelines[2,3] support the use of single-lead capable of dual sensing and ventricular pacing devices – so-called

VVD pacemakers – in patients with atrioventricular block and preserved sinus node function. Table 79.1 summarizes the current recommendations on mode selection in patients requiring permanent pacemaker implantation.

Conclusion

What about our patients? Case 1 has SND and is at low risk for complete heart block given her normal PR interval and QRS width less than 120 msec. The first choice for a PPM in her case would be a single-chamber atrial device.[2] Implanting a dual-chamber device capable of minimizing ventricular pacing would be an acceptable option as well in patients considered at higher risk for AV block (**Class IIa**) and indeed, the recommended mode when AV block was previously documented (**Class I, Level C**). Both strategies intend to avoid or reduce unnecessary ventricular pacing and may decrease the burden of atrial fibrillation in patients with SND.[18,28] Case 1 underwent an AAI pacemaker implantation after documenting 1:1 AV conduction when atrial paced at 110 pulses per minute, a simple test performed during the procedure.

It is well recognized in patients with AV block (as is also true for SND) that mortality is mainly a reflection of the severity of underlying disease, and less dependent on the conduction system status or pacing mode. Thus, it is not surprising that no significant difference in mortality between single- or dual-chamber PPM has been encountered to date. In view of the above, Case 2 underwent a single-chamber ventricular (VVIR) PPM implantation.

Table 79.1 Pacemaker mode in selected indications for pacing[2]

Pacemaker Generator	Sinus Node Dysfunction	Atrioventricular Block
Single-chamber atrial pacemaker	No suspected abnormality of atrioventricular conduction and not at increased risk for future atrioventricular block Maintenance of atrioventricular synchrony during pacing desired	Not appropriate
Single-chamber ventricular pacemaker	Maintenance of atrioventricular synchrony during pacing not necessary Rate response available if desired	Chronic atrial fibrillation or other atrial tachyarrhythmia or maintenance of atrioventricular synchrony during pacing not necessary Rate response available if desired
Dual-chamber pacemaker	Atrioventricular synchrony during pacing desired Suspected abnormality of atrioventricular conduction or increased risk for future atrioventricular block Rate response available if desired	Rate response available if desired Atrioventricular synchrony during pacing desired Atrial pacing desired Rate response available if desired
Single-lead, atrial-sensing ventricular pacemaker	Not appropriate	Desire to limit the number of pacemaker leads

References

1. Sheldon R, Rose S, Connolly S, Ritchie D, Koshman ML, Frenneaux M. Diagnostic criteria for vasovagal syncope based on a quantitative history. *Eur Heart J* 2006;**27**(3):344–50.
2. Epstein AE, DiMarco JP, Ellenbogen KA *et al.* ACC/AHA/HRS/2008 guidelines for device-based therapy of cardiac rhythm abnormalities: a report of the American College of Cardiology/American Heart Association Task Force on Practice Guidelines. *Circulation* 2008;**117**(21):e350–408.
3. Vardas PE, Auricchio A, Blanc JJ *et al.* Guidelines for cardiac pacing and cardiac resynchronization therapy: the Task Force for Cardiac Pacing and Cardiac Resynchronization Therapy of the European Society of Cardiology. Developed in Collaboration with the European Heart Rhythm Association. *Eur Heart J* 2007;**28**(18):2256–95.
4. Gula LJ, Krahn AD, Skanes AC, Yee R, Klein GJ. Clinical relevance of arrhythmias during sleep: guidance for clinicians. *Heart* 2004;**90**(3):347–52.
5. Edhag O, Swahn A. Prognosis of patients with complete heart block or arrhythmic syncope who were not treated with artificial pacemakers: a long-term follow-up study of 101 patients. *Acta Med Scand* 1976;**200**:457–63.

6. Johansson BW. Complete heart block: a clinical, hemodynamic and pharmacological study in patients with and without an artificial pacemaker. *Acta Med Scand* 1966;**180**(suppl 451):1–127.

7. ECC Committee, Subcommittees and Task Forces of the American Heart Association. American Heart Association guidelines for cardiopulmonary resuscitation and emergency cardiovascular care. *Circulation* 2005 13;**112**(24 suppl):IV1–203.

8. Sohail MR, Uslan DZ, Khan AH *et al.* Risk factor analysis of permanent pacemaker infection. *Clin Infect Dis* 2007;**45**(2):166–73.

9. Mahapatra S, Bybee KA, Bunch TJ *et al.* Incidence and predictors of cardiac perforation after permanent pacemaker placement. *Heart Rhythm* 2005;**2**(9):907–11.

10. Rosenqvist M, Brandt J, Schuller H. Long-term pacing in sinus node disease: effects of stimulation mode on cardiovascular morbidity and mortality. *Am Heart J* 1988;**116**(1 Pt 1):16–22.

11. Sasaki Y, Shimotori M, Akahane K *et al.* Long-term follow-up of patients with sick sinus syndrome: a comparison of clinical aspects among unpaced, ventricular inhibited paced, and physiologically paced groups. *Pacing Clin Electrophysiol* 1988;**11**(11 Pt 1):1575–83.

12. Bianconi L, Boccademo R, Di Fiorio A *et al.* Atrial versus ventricular stimulation in sick sinus syndrome: effects on morbidity and mortality. *Pacing Clin Electrophysiol* 1989;**12**:1236A.

13. Santini M, Alexidou G, Ansalone G, Cacciatore G, Cini R, Turitto G. Relation of prognosis in sick sinus syndrome to age, conduction defects and modes of permanent cardiac pacing. *Am J Cardiol* 1990;**65**(11):729–35.

14. Nurnberg M, Frohner K, Podczeck A *et al.* Is VVI pacing more dangerous than AV-sequential pacing in patients with sick sinus syndrome? *Pacing Clin Electrophysiol* 1991;**14**:674A.

15. Hesselson AB, Parsonnet V, Bernstein AD, Bonavita GJ. Deleterious effects of long-term single-chamber ventricular pacing in patients with sick sinus syndrome: the hidden benefits of dual-chamber pacing. *J Am Coll Cardiol* 1992;**19**(7):1542–9.

16. Sgarbossa EB, Pinski SL, Maloney JD. The role of pacing modality in determining long-term survival in the sick sinus syndrome. *Ann Intern Med* 1993;**119**(5):359–65.

17. Andersen HR, Thuesen L, Bagger JP, Vesterlund T, Thomsen PE. Prospective randomised trial of atrial versus ventricular pacing in sick-sinus syndrome. *Lancet* 1994;**344**(8936):1523–8.

18. Andersen HR, Nielsen JC, Thomsen PE *et al.* Atrioventricular conduction during long-term follow-up of patients with sick sinus syndrome. *Circulation* 1998;**98**(13):1315–21.

19. Lamas GA, Lee KL, Sweeney MO *et al.* Ventricular pacing or dual-chamber pacing for sinus-node dysfunction. *N Engl J Med* 2002;**346**(24):1854–62.

20. Sweeney MO, Hellkamp AS, Ellenbogen KA *et al.* Adverse effect of ventricular pacing on heart failure and atrial fibrillation among patients with normal baseline QRS duration in a clinical trial of pacemaker therapy for sinus node dysfunction. *Circulation* 2003;**107**(23):2932–7.

21. Nielsen JC, Kristensen L, Andersen HR, Mortensen PT, Pedersen OL, Pedersen AK. A randomized comparison of atrial and dual-chamber pacing in 177 consecutive patients with sick sinus syndrome: echocardiographic and clinical outcome. *J Am Coll Cardiol* 2003;**42**(4):614–23.

22. Newman D, Lau C, Tang AS *et al.* Effect of pacing mode on health-related quality of life in the Canadian Trial of Physiologic Pacing. *Am Heart J* 2003;**145**(3):430–7.

23. Link MS, Hellkamp AS, Estes NA3rd *et al.* High incidence of pacemaker syndrome in patients with sinus node dysfunction treated with ventricular-based pacing in the Mode Selection Trial (MOST). *J Am Coll Cardiol* 2004;**43**(11):2066–71.

24. Healey JS, Toff WD, Lamas GA *et al.* Cardiovascular outcomes with atrial-based pacing compared with ventricular pacing: meta-analysis of randomized trials, using individual patient data. *Circulation* 2006 ;**114**(1):11–17.

25. Huang M, Krahn AD, Yee R, Klein GJ, Skanes AC. Optimal pacing for symptomatic AV block: a comparison of VDD and DDD pacing. *Pacing Clin Electrophysiol* 2004;**27**(1):19–23.

26. Wiegand UK, Bode F, Bonnemeier H, Eberhard F, Schlei M, Peters W. Long-term complication rates in ventricular, single lead VDD, and dual chamber pacing. *Pacing Clin Electrophysiol* 2003;**26**(10):1961–9.

27. Wiegand UK, Potratz J, Bode F *et al.* Cost-effectiveness of dual-chamber pacemaker therapy: does single lead VDD pacing reduce treatment costs of atrioventricular block? *Eur Heart J* 2001;**22**(2):174–80.

28. Sweeney MO, Bank AJ, Nsah E *et al.* Minimizing ventricular pacing to reduce atrial fibrillation in sinus-node disease. *N Engl J Med* 2007;**357**(10):1000–8.

80   Peripheral arterial disease with suspect coronary artery disease

Victor Aboyans[1] and Michael H Criqui[2]
[1]Department of Thoracic and Cardiovascular Surgery and Angiology, Dupytren University Hospital, Limoges, France
[2]Department of Medicine, University of California, San Diego, CA, USA

Case history 1

A 63-year-old man presents with progressive right leg discomfort, with his walking distance gradually decreasing to less than one block over the last 2 months. Standing still provides complete relief within 5 minutes. His claudication is now very disabling. He has smoked 20 cigarettes daily for 40 years. He is treated with ramipril for hypertension and takes 325 mg of aspirin daily since a transient ischemic attack (TIA) 3 years ago.

On examination, his blood pressure is 140/90 mmHg in the right arm and 130/85 mmHg in the left arm. His resting pulse is regular at 85 bpm. He does not report any chest pain or shortness of breath. Chest and neck auscultation are normal. There is a right femoral bruit, with reduced femoral and popliteal pulses and absent pulses distally. On the left side, a reduced femoral pulse is present, and none of the other pulses are palpable. The remainder of the physical examination is normal.

A resting ECG reveals normal sinus rhythm with no abnormality. The chest radiograph is normal. Routine hematology and chemistry values are normal except for an abnormal fasting blood lipid profile: triglycerides, 280 mg/dL; total cholesterol, 305 mg/dL; HDL cholesterol, 42 mg/dL; LDL cholesterol, 195 mg/dL.

The Ankle Brachial Indexes (ABI) are 0.70 on the right, 0.45 on the left. After walking 99 yards (90 m) on a treadmill (10% incline, 1.5 mph) and the occurrence of bilateral (left > right) hip and thigh claudication, his post-exercise ABIs are 0.25 on the right and 0.20 on the left, consistent with severe peripheral arterial occlusive disease. Duplex ultrasound reveals a 2.5 inch (6 cm) long severe stenosis (90%) at the level of the right common and external iliac arteries, and an occlusion of the left external iliac artery, with femoral reperfusion by collaterals. An MRA confirms these observations. The arteries below these lesions are free of any significant stenosis.

You decide to refer the patient to a vascular surgeon who eventually schedules an aortic–bifemoral bypass.

Evidence-Based Cardiology, 3rd edition. Edited by S. Yusuf, J.A. Cairns, A.J. Camm, E.L. Fallen, and B.J. Gersh. © 2010 Blackwell Publishing, ISBN: 978-1-4051-5925-8.

Question

In this patient, what is your strategy to avoid any cardiac ischemic events during the perioperative period?

Comment

We are confronted here with a middle-aged patient with severe proximal peripheral arterial disease (PAD), without any clinical evidence of coronary artery disease (CAD). In the classic study of Hertzer *et al*,[1] performing systematic coronary angiography in 1000 patients undergoing peripheral vascular surgery, the prevalence of >70% coronary stenosis was 60%. More recently, using rest and stress echocardiography in a similar population, Feringa *et al*[2] reported a prevalence of 23% and 28% of unrecognized myocardial infarction and silent ischemia, respectively.

Several risk scores are used to assess the risk of perioperative cardiovascular events in non-cardiac surgery. According to the 2007 ACC/AHA guidelines,[3] the clinical risk factors are: ischemic heart disease, compensated or prior heart failure, diabetes mellitus, renal failure and cerebrovascular disease. This leads us to classify our patient at intermediate risk level with one risk factor (prior TIA suggestive of cerebrovascular disease). According to these guidelines,[3] preoperative heart rate control with beta-blockers is recommended. Of note, it still remains unclear whether lowering heart rate alone or the use of beta-blockers *per se* is beneficial. No substantial data regarding the potential interest of other treatments reducing heart rate (i.e. calcium channel blockers) are currently available. In addition, even the interest in beta-blockers according to these guidelines might be tempered by more recent data. In the POISE trial,[4] the benefit of metoprolol versus placebo to prevent myocardial infarction during non-cardiac surgery was counterbalanced by an excess risk of death and disabling stroke, although the high dosage of metoprolol and the lack of titration in this study have been criticized. Besides, in a retrospective analysis of a large database in the United States, Lindenauer et al[5] found a neutral effect of preoperative use of beta-blockers. However, beta-blockers appeared harmful in patients at low risk of perioperative events, but beneficial for those at a high level of perioperative risk.

According to the ACC/AHA guidelines,[3] non-invasive testing might only be considered if it could change management. The randomized Coronary Artery Revascularization Prophylaxis (CARP) trial[6] failed to demonstrate any additional prognostic benefit of preoperative coronary revascularization in such cases, but led to extended vascular surgery delays.

Beyond the perioperative period, the Clinical Outcomes Utilizing Revascularization and Aggressive Drug Evaluation (COURAGE) trial[7] also failed to demonstrate any prognostic improvement of patients with stable coronary artery disease when undergoing coronary revascularization, compared to those with optimal medical management. In the DECREASE-II study,[8] patients at intermediate risk prior to vascular surgery were randomized into two strategies comparing tight heart rate control (60–65 bpm) using beta-blockers with the use of non-invasive testing followed by coronary angiography and revascularization when appropriate. At 3 years, the cardiac event rates were similar between both groups.

Thus, we propose for our patient an optimal medical management. Smoking cessation is essential to improve the long-term vital prognosis[9] and reduce the progression of PAD.[10] Additionally, smoking cessation within the weeks prior to surgery is associated with a significant reduction of perioperative complications.[11] Beta-blockers could be proposed to decrease his resting heart rate to within the 60–65 bpm range, being careful to avoid a large drop in systolic blood pressure. In a longitudinal study,[12] patients who had their beta-blocker therapy prolonged beyond the perioperative period presented a better prognosis than those who had their treatment discontinued. Finally, the use of statins (and possibly combined lipid-lowering therapy) is highly recommended for the long-term management of this patient, with the aim to lower LDL cholesterol below 100 mg/dL.[13] The use of statins can also be beneficial in the first months following revascularization: in a randomized study comparing atorvastatin 10 mg with placebo in patients undergoing vascular surgery,[14] an 18% event risk reduction was noted in the statin group.

Case history 2

A 72-year-old woman presents with progressive leg pain atypical for claudication in the right calf and ankle over the past year. Standing still provides complete relief but her walking distance has gradually shortened to two blocks. She also sometimes experiences this pain at rest when sitting on a chair or during the night. She notes similar but less severe discomfort in the left ankle, occurring only when walking. When asking for other cardiovascular symptoms, she also reports occasional epigastric pain when climbing a flight of stairs, and sometimes even at rest. The pain does not radiate elsewhere and usually disappears after a couple of minutes.

She has taken metformin for type 2 diabetes for 12 years. She stopped smoking 5 years ago (overall amount is 35 pack-years). She is hypertensive, treated by hydrochlorothiazide 25 mg daily.

On examination her blood pressure is 150/90 mmHg (both arms), resting pulse is regular at 90 bpm. Chest and neck auscultation are normal. The popliteal, posterior tibial and dorsalis pedis pulses are absent on the right. On the left, the popliteal and posterior tibial pulses are moderately reduced. The dorsalis pedis pulse is absent.

Resting ECG (Fig. 80.1) shows normal sinus rhythm with Q-waves located at leads II, III and aVF, associated with abnormal repolarization in the same leads as well at V3–V6 and D1 and aVL, suggesting past inferior myocardial infarction as well as apical and lateral silent ischemia. Routine hematology and chemistry values are normal but glycosylated hemoglobin is elevated at 9%. Blood lipids profile is as follows: total cholesterol, 180 mg/dL; HDL-C,

52 mg/dL; LDL-C, 118 mg/dL. Resting ABI is 0.8 on the right but cannot be measured on the left due to incompressible arteries. Duplex ultrasound reveals an occlusion of the right popliteal artery and a very attenuated flow through a calcified fibular artery. Left distal arteries (posterior tibial, fibular and anterior tibial) present multiple stenoses and diffuse calcifications.

You decide to assess her coronary state prior to referring her to a diabetes care center. She undergoes dobutamine stress echocardiography (DSE). At rest, the prior myocardial infarction is confirmed by the presence of akinesis at the inferior wall (basal, mid and apical segments). The ejection fraction is estimated at 52%. After dobutamine infusion, an extended hypokinesia of the anterior and lateral walls occurs at the level of 68% of the maximal theoretical heart rate. She denies any chest pain.

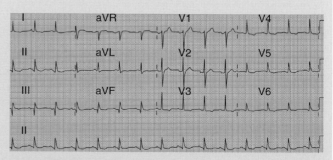

Figure 80.1 Case 2 – ECG at rest.

Question

How would you proceed at this point?

Comment

This case deals with the management of multifocal atherosclerotic disease in an elderly diabetic patient. Clinical symptoms may be atypical and may occur at a more advanced stage of the disease, possibly due to the associated diabetic neuropathy with impaired sensory feedback.[15] In addition, walking impairment related to PAD may reduce the patient's physical efforts and limit the occurrence of angina. In this case, the modest limb symptoms, the absence of critical ischemia and the poor distal arterial state preclude peripheral revascularization at this point. However, the coronary artery disease revealed by interrogation and ECG is a matter for concern.

Dobutamine stress echocardiography is a valuable tool to detect CAD in PAD patients with limited ability to perform a satisfactory exercise test.[16] The DSE data in this patient are highly suspect for severe CAD, possibly affecting several arteries, which is frequent in diabetic patients.[17] In this situation, revascularization can improve prognosis.[18] Thus, we referred the patient for coronary angiography. This exam revealed triple-vessel disease, including a 80% stenosis of the left main coronary artery. Of note, in the COURAGE trial[19] comparing percutaneous coronary revascularization to optimal medical treatment alone, patients with these types of severe lesions were excluded from the study.

The patient was referred for coronary artery bypass grafting, which was ultimately successful despite a prolonged intensive care unit stay for poorly tolerated atrial fibrillation. Overall, the long-term management of CAD in PAD is similar to any other patient.[20] It should, however, be emphasized that in cases of concomitant PAD, the short- and long-term prognosis of patients with CAD is more severe, even with revascularization.[21,22] Beyond coronary revascularization, our patient should benefit from statins with the aim of lowering LDL below 70 mg/dL. Beta-blockers are also indicated because of the history of myocardial infarction.[23] Finally, according to the results of the HOPE[24] and EUROPA[25] trials, she should benefit from an ACE inhibitor. Blood pressure should be controlled under 130/80 mmHg in this diabetic patient.

References

1. Hertzer NR, Beven EG, Young JR et al. Coronary artery disease in peripheral vascular patients. Classification of 1000 coronary angiograms and results of surgical management. *Ann Surg* 1984;**199**:223–33.

2. Feringa HHH, Karagiannis SE, Vidakovic R et al. The prevalence and prognosis of unrecognized myocardial infarction and silent myocardial ischemia in patients undergoing major vascular surgery. *Coron Art Dis* 2007;**18**:571–6.

3. Fleisher LA, Beckman JA, Brown KA et al. ACC/AHA 2007 guidelines on perioperative cardiovascular evaluation and care for noncardiac surgery: a report of the American College of Cardiology/American Heart Association Task Force on Practice Guidelines. *Circulation* 2007;**116**:e418–e499.

4. POISE Study Group, Devereaux PJ, Yang H et al. Effects of extended-release metoprolol succinate in patients undergoing non-cardiac surgery (POISE trial): a randomised controlled trial. *Lancet* 2008;**371**:1839–47.

5. Lindenauer PK, Pekow P, Wang K, Mamidi DK, Gutierrez B, Benjamin EM. Perioperative beta-blocker therapy and mortality after major noncardiac surgery. *N Engl J Med* 2005;**353**:349–61.

6. McFalls EO, Ward HB, Moritz TE et al. Coronary-artery revascularization before elective major vascular surgery. *N Engl J Med* 2004;**351**:2795–804.

7. Boden WE, O'Rourke RA, Teo KK et al. COURAGE Trial Research Group. Optimal medical therapy with or without PCI for stable coronary disease. *N Engl J Med* 2007;**356**:1503–16.

8. Poldermans D, Bax JJ, Schouten O et al. Should major vascular surgery be delayed because of preoperative cardiac testing in intermediate-risk patients receiving beta-blocker therapy with tight heart rate control? *J Am Coll Cardiol* 2006;**48**:964–9.

9. Khan S, Cleanthis M, Smout J, Flather M, Stansby G. Life-style modification in peripheral arterial disease. *Eur J Vasc Endovasc Surg* 2005;**29**:2–9.

10. Aboyans V, Criqui MH, Denenberg JO, Knoke JD, Ridker PM, Fronek A. Risk factors for progression of peripheral arterial disease in large and small vessels. *Circulation* 2006;**113**:2623–9.

11. Møller AM, Villebro N, Pedersen T, Tønnesen H. Effect of preoperative smoking intervention on postoperative complications: a randomised clinical trial. *Lancet* 2002;**359**:114–17.

12. Hoeks SE, Scholte Op Reimer WJ, van Urk H et al. Increase of 1-year mortality after perioperative beta-blocker withdrawal in endovascular and vascular surgery patients. *Eur J Vasc Endovasc Surg* 2007;**33**:13–19.

13. Norgren L, Hiatt WR, Dormandy JA, Nehler MR, Harris KA, Fowkes FGR, on behalf of the TASC II Working Group. Inter-society consensus for the management of peripheral arterial disease (TASC II). *Eur J Vasc Endovasc Surg* 2007;**33**:S1–S75.

14. Durazzo AES, Machado FS, Ikeoka DT et al. Reduction in cardiovascular events after vascular surgery with atorvastatin: a randomized trial. *J Vasc Surg* 2004;**39**:967–76.

15. American Diabetes Association. Peripheral arterial disease in people with diabetes. *Diabetes Care* 2003;**26**:3333–41.

16. Feringa HH, Elhendy A, Karagiannis SE et al. Improving risk assessment with cardiac testing in peripheral arterial disease. *Am J Med* 2007;**120**:531–8.

17. Bax JJ, Young LH, Frye RL, Bonow RO, Steinberg HO, Barrett EJ. Screening for coronary artery disease in patients with diabetes. *Diabetes Care* 2007;**30**:2729–36.

18. Eagle KA, Guyton RA, Davidoff R et al. American College of Cardiology/American Heart Association 2004 guideline update for coronary artery bypass graft surgery: a report of the American College of Cardiology/American Heart Association Task Force on Practice Guidelines. *Circulation* 2004;**110**(14):e340–437.

19. Boden WE, O'Rourke RA, Teo KK *et al.* COURAGE Trial Research Group. Optimal medical therapy with or without PCI for stable coronary disease. *N Engl J Med* 2007;**356**:1503–16.

20. Grundy SM, Cleeman JI, Merz CN *et al.* Implications of recent clinical trials for the National Cholesterol Education Program Adult Treatment Panel III guidelines. *Circulation* 2004;**110**:227–39.

21. Saw J, Bhatt DL, Moliterno DJ *et al.* The influence of peripheral arterial disease on outcomes: a pooled analysis of mortality in eight large randomized percutaneous coronary intervention trials. *J Am Coll Cardiol* 2006;**48**:1567–72.

22. Aboyans V, Lacroix P, Postil A *et al.* Subclinical peripheral arterial disease and incompressible ankle arteries are both long-term prognostic factors in patients undergoing coronary artery bypass grafting. *J Am Coll Cardiol* 2005;**46**:815–20.

23. Yusuf S, Peto R, Lewis J, Collins R, Sleight P. Beta blockade during and after myocardial infarction: an overview of the randomized trials. *Prog Cardiovasc Dis* 1985;**27**:335–71.

24. HOPE Investigators. Effects of ramipril on cardiovascular and microvascular outcomes in people with diabetes mellitus: results of the HOPE study and MICRO-HOPE substudy. Heart Outcomes Prevention Evaluation Study Investigators. *Lancet* 2000;**355**:253–9.

25. Fox KM. EURopean trial On reduction of cardiac events with Perindopril in stable coronary Artery disease Investigators. Efficacy of perindopril in reduction of cardiovascular events among patients with stable coronary artery disease: randomised, double-blind, placebo-controlled, multicentre trial (the EUROPA study). *Lancet* 2003;**362**:782–8.

81 Valvular heart disease: timing of surgery

Jon-David R Schwalm and Victor Chu
McMaster University/Hamilton Health Sciences, Hamilton, Ontario, Canada

Case history 1

A 63-year-old male carpenter is referred to a cardiologist for consultation regarding a newly diagnosed systolic ejection murmur noted by his family physician during his annual physical examination. His medical history is significant for a remote 20 pack-year smoking history and type 2 diabetes mellitus for which he is on an oral hypoglycemic agent. Upon close questioning, he does not report any cardiovascular limitations despite an active lifestyle. Specifically, he denies any symptoms of shortness of breath, angina, exertional presyncope or syncope.

Physical examination by the consulting cardiologist reveals a grade IV–VI, late-peaking, systolic murmur at the right upper sternal border with radiation to both carotid arteries. S2 is diminished and an apical-carotid delay is noted. The heart rate is 72 beats per minute and the blood pressure 110/88 mmHg.

His baseline electrocardiogram is within normal limits, demonstrating no evidence of left ventricular hypertrophy. Transthoracic echocardiogram confirms a calcific bicuspid aortic valve with an area of $0.9\,cm^2$, and a mean transvalvular gradient of 46 mmHg. There is mild aortic insufficiency and the aortic root dimension is within normal limits. There is preserved left ventricular function with no wall motion abnormalities and no evidence of left ventricular hypertrophy.

Question

What is the appropriate initial management and follow-up for this patient? Is aortic valve replacement indicated at this time?

Comment

This case is meant to highlight the appropriate investigations, follow-up, and management of patients found to have an asymptomatic murmur of severe aortic stenosis on routine physical exam. Aortic stenosis is the most common

Evidence-Based Cardiology, 3rd edition. Edited by S. Yusuf, J.A. Cairns, A.J. Camm, E.L. Fallen, and B.J. Gersh. © 2010 Blackwell Publishing, ISBN: 978-1-4051-5925-8.

valvular condition across Europe and North America, affecting 2–7% of individuals over the age of 65 years.[1] The most common cause of aortic stenosis is calcification of either a congenitally bicuspid valve (more common if under 70 years of age) or a tricuspid valve (more common over 70 years of age).[2]

Aortic stenosis is a progressive condition with significant interpatient variability. A prospective study has shown an average increase in mean aortic gradients of 7 mmHg per year and a decrease in valve area of $0.1\,cm^2$ per year.[3]

While severe aortic stenosis carries an increased risk of sudden cardiac death, this rarely occurs (<1%/year) without the development of any of the classic symptoms including angina, heart failure, and syncope.[3] Symptoms tend to develop when the aortic valve area is less than $1\,cm^2$ or the mean transvalvular gradient is more than 40 mmHg. Thus, severe aortic stenosis is defined as a valve area less than $1\,cm^2$, mean gradient greater than 40 mmHg or jet velocity greater than 4.0 m per second.[4] Following the onset of symptom development in patients with severe aortic stenosis, the mean survival is 2–3 years without surgical intervention.[5] Conversely, aortic valve replacement is not indicated in asymptomatic patients despite having severe aortic stenosis and preserved left ventricular function.

Given the strong association of increased mortality with symptom development, close clinical follow-up is recommended. The frequency of clinical follow-up depends on multiple factors including the degree of stenosis, left ventricular function, functional capacity, and patient compliance. Patient education regarding the natural history of aortic stenosis and how to properly interpret their symptoms is essential to clinical follow-up. Often, patients will not report one or more of the classic triad of symptoms. A slight change in exercise capacity or exertional dyspnea may be their only tell-tale sign of progressing disease. Due to the gradual onset of symptoms related to aortic stenosis, it is not uncommon for patients to fully appreciate the severity of their symptoms after their aortic valve has been replaced. The ACC/AHA 2006 practice guidelines recommend (**Class I**) that patients with severe aortic stenosis undergo yearly echocardiograms to evaluate the severity of aortic stenosis, left ventricular hypertrophy, and function.[4]

Until recently, aortic stenosis was a **Class I** indication for the use of antibiotics in preventing bacterial endocarditis.[6] However, more recent guidelines have removed acquired and congenital valvular disease as an indication for the use of prophylactic antibiotics in the prevention of bacterial endocarditis. Antibiotics continue to be recommended with dental procedures in patients with a prosthetic valve.[7]

Case history 1 *continued*

The patient returns for his one-year follow-up visit. He remains asymptomatic with no significant change noted on either physical examination or echocardiogram. He states that he has joined a cycling club and plans to undertake some long-distance trips. Given this planned increase in exercise, an exercise stress test is arranged.

He exercises on the bicycle ergometer for 8 minutes and 57 seconds, reaching a peak heart rate of 127 beats. His blood pressure rises appropriately with exercise and he has no anginal symptoms. The reason for terminating the test is leg fatigue and significant ST segment depression of 3 mm. After review of the exercise stress test results, his consulting cardiologist is concerned regarding possible silent ischemia and the patient is advanced for cardiac catheterization. Catheterization reveals no flow-limiting coronary artery disease with a mean gradient across the aortic valve of 45 mmHg.

Question

Can this patient with severe but asymptomatic aortic stenosis undergo activities requiring significant exertion? What is the role of exercise stress testing in aortic stenosis? Was the cardiac catheterization indicated at this time?

Comment

This patient, with a history of severe but asymptomatic aortic stenosis, wants to undertake a new level of exercise. The ACC/AHA practice guidelines recommend against competitive sports with high dynamic or static muscular demands.[4] However, can we risk stratify the average patient who wants to undertake an increase in exercise?

Currently, the evidence suggests that routine exercise stress testing of patients with aortic stenosis is not warranted.[8] With confounding variables such as left ventricular hypertrophy and reduced coronary flow reserve, ST segment depression during exercise stress testing of patients with aortic stenosis adds little prognostic value. Electrocardiographic ST segment depression during exercise occurs in 80% of patients with asymptomatic aortic stenosis. However, exercise stress testing in patients with asymptomatic severe aortic stenosis may add other prognostic information including exercise-induced symptoms and abnormal blood pressure response (fall of >10 mmHg or a blunted blood pressure rise of <20 mmHg).[4,8] Stress

testing may also help provide the patient with an exercise prescription.[9] Exercise testing should not be performed in symptomatic patients with severe aortic stenosis.

Cardiac catheterization is recommended for patients before planned aortic valve replacement who are at risk of coronary artery disease or to help clarify the severity of aortic stenosis in symptomatic patients when non-invasive imaging was inconclusive.[4] Given that ST segment depression is common with aortic stenosis during exercise stress testing and the patient was asymptomatic with a normal blood pressure response, cardiac catheterization could be postponed at this time.

In summary, this patient remains asymptomatic with respect to his severe aortic stenosis. Despite close clinical and echocardiographic follow-up, he has not demonstrated progression of his disease. Given these findings, he should not be advanced for aortic valve replacement. As per the ACC/AHA 2006 guidelines, patients should not undergo aortic valve replacement until they become symptomatic, develop left ventricular dysfunction (ejection fraction less than 50%) or are scheduled to undergo another cardiac surgical procedure (e.g. coronary bypass surgery).[4]

Despite these fairly simple and clear-cut guidelines, timing of valve replacement surgery for patients with "asymptomatic" severe aortic stenosis remains one of the more common dilemmas in clinical practice. Many factors, such as patient age, surgical risk profiles, choice of prosthesis types, and the need for long-term anticoagulation, can play a significant role in the decision process. It is important for the treating physician to carefully balance the risks and the potential pitfalls of continued medical therapy against the risks of an elective operative procedure before making a recommendation to the patient.

Case history 2

An 86-year-old retired office manager is referred to a cardiologist for review of progressive symptoms of exertional syncope and Canadian Cardiovascular Society class III angina. She has multiple co-morbidities including poorly controlled diabetes mellitus, hypertension, obesity, current cigarette smoking with a 50 pack-year history, chronic obstructive lung disease, and atrial fibrillation. Despite these co-morbidities, she has a reasonable quality of life but is significantly limited by her cardiovascular symptoms. Her medications include insulin, metformin, salbutamol inhalers, ramipril, simvastatin, diltiazem, and warfarin.

Her electrocardiogram demonstrates controlled atrial fibrillation averaging 78 beats per minute and left ventricular hypertrophy with strain pattern. Transthoracic echocardiogram reveals severe aortic stenosis with a valve area of $0.7 \, cm^2$ and a mean gradient of 50 mmHg. She has mild left ventricular dysfunction with an ejection fraction of 45%. Left ventricular hypertrophy with a mass index of $140 \, g/m^2$ is noted. Cardiac catheterization reveals a peak-to-peak gradient of 45 mmHg but no flow-limiting coronary artery disease is seen.

Question

Is this patient considered to be too high a risk for traditional aortic valve replacement? Are there other management options available for the treatment of aortic stenosis?

Comment

This case is meant to highlight the risk stratification of patients being considered for traditional aortic valve replacement surgery and to address possible alternative interventions for high-risk elderly patients with multiple co-morbidities.

Aortic valve replacement surgery is a well-established procedure which has been perfected since the early 1960s. The average perioperative mortality is 3% for isolated aortic valve replacement and 6% when combined with coronary bypass surgery.[10] However, the 30-day mortality rate for the octogenarian population is approximately 17%, with 40% mortality after one year.[11] These rates are highly center dependent.

For our patient, the perioperative morbidity and mortality are considered to be prohibitively high with traditional aortic valve replacement as estimated using the EuroSCORE.[12] Considering the yearly rate of sudden death with severe aortic stenosis is 1% (the patient is 86 years old), the upfront risk of the surgery far outweighs the expected reduction in mortality with aortic valve replacement. However, the patient may accept an increased perioperative mortality risk considering she is significantly limited by her symptoms. Often, octogenarians undergo aortic valve replacement to improve their quality of life, rather than for an improvement in overall prognosis. Unfortunately medical therapy does not offer a significant reduction in morbidity or mortality. Aortic stenosis is a mechanical problem, requiring a mechanical solution. While percutaneous balloon aortic valvotomy is indicated in treating the pediatric population and young adults, its only indication for treating aortic stenosis in the adult population is for palliation in inoperable patients or as a bridge to surgery.[4]

Another novel and still experimental option is that of percutaneous aortic valve replacement. This procedure was first reported in a human subject in 2002 using a Cribier–Edwards valve (Edwards Lifesciences Inc, Irvine, CA), constructed from a tubular slotted stainless steel stent with an attached equine pericardial trileaflet valve.[13] This procedure is done without the need for cardiopulmonary bypass and two approaches are currently being studied. The first method is via a femoral transarterial approach with retrograde access to the aortic valve.[14] More recently, a transapical approach has been developed, which is particularly effective in patients with significant peripheral vascular disease, thus limiting a peripheral approach.[15] For all methods of percutaneous aortic valve implantation, rapid pacing of the ventricle is required at the time of valve deployment to reduce both transaortic flow and cardiac motion.

Percutaneous aortic valve implantation is a reasonable option for patients deemed to be too high a risk for traditional aortic valve replacement. However, this procedure is still under development with immediate hemodynamic and early clinical improvement only reported in a small number of patients.

This 86-year-old patient was deemed to be too high a risk for traditional aortic valve replacement surgery. She is currently being evaluated for percutaneous aortic valve replacement.

References

1. Stewart BF, Siscovick D, Lind BK *et al*. Clinical factors associated with calcific aortic stenosis. *J Am Coll Cardiol* 1997;**29**:630–4.
2. Roberts WC, Ko JM. Frequency by decades of unicuspid, bicuspid, and tricuspid aortic valves in adults having isolated aortic valve replacement for aortic stenosis, with or without associated aortic regurgitation. *Circulation* 2005;**111**(7):920–5.
3. Otto CM, Burwash IG, Legget ME *et al*. A prospective study of asymptomatic valvular aortic stenosis: clinical, echocardiographic and exercise predictors of outcome. *Circulation* 1997;**95**:2262–70.
4. Bonow, RO, Carabello, BA, Chatterjee, K *et al*. ACC/AHA 2006 practice guidelines for the management of patients with valvular heart disease. *J Am Coll Cardiol* 2006;**48**:e1.
5. Schwartz F, Baumann P, Manthey J *et al*. The effect of aortic valve replacement of survival. *Circulation* 1982;**66**:1105–10.
6. Dajani AS, Taubert KA, Wilson W *et al*. Prevention of bacterial endocarditis. Recommendations by the American Heart Association. *Circulation* 1997;**96**:358–66.
7. Nishimura RA, Carabello BA, Faxon DP *et al*. ACC/AHA 2008 Guideline Update on Valvular Heart Disease: focused update on infective endocarditis. *J Am Coll Cardiol* 2008;**52**:676–85.
8. Otto CM. Valvular aortic stenosis: disease severity and timing of intervention. *J Am Coll Cardiol* 2006;**47**(11):2141–51.
9. Chung EH, Gaasch WH. Exercise testing in aortic stenosis. *Curr Cardiol Rep* 2005;**7**(2):105–7.
10. Edwards FH, Peterson ED, Coombs LP *et al*. Prediction of operative mortality after valve replacement surgery. *J Am Coll Cardiol* 2001;**37**:885–92.
11. Edwards MB, Taylor KM. Outcomes in nonagenarians after heart valve replacement operation. *Ann Thorac Surg* 2003;**75**:830–4.
12. Nashed SA, Roques F, Michel P *et al*. European system for cardiac operative risk evaluation (EuroSCORE). *Eur J Cardiothorac Surg* 1999;**16**:9.
13. Cribier A, Eltchaninoff H, Bash A *et al*. Percutaneous transcatheter implantation of an aortic valve prosthesis for calcific aortic stenosis. *Circulation* 2002;**106**:3006–8.
14. Webb JG, Chandavimol M, Thompson C *et al*. Percutaneous aortic valve implantation retrograde from the femoral artery. *Circulation* 2006;**113**:842–50.
15. Lichtenstein SV, Cheung A, Ye J *et al*. Transapical transcatheter aortic valve implantation in humans: initial clinical experience. *Circulation* 2006;**114**(6):591–6.

Index

Note: page numbers in *italics* refer to figures; those in **bold** to tables or boxes.

A list of abbreviations used in subheadings can be found on page xvii.

Index

Index